Alters & Schiff

Essential Concepts for Healthy Living

SEVENTH EDITION

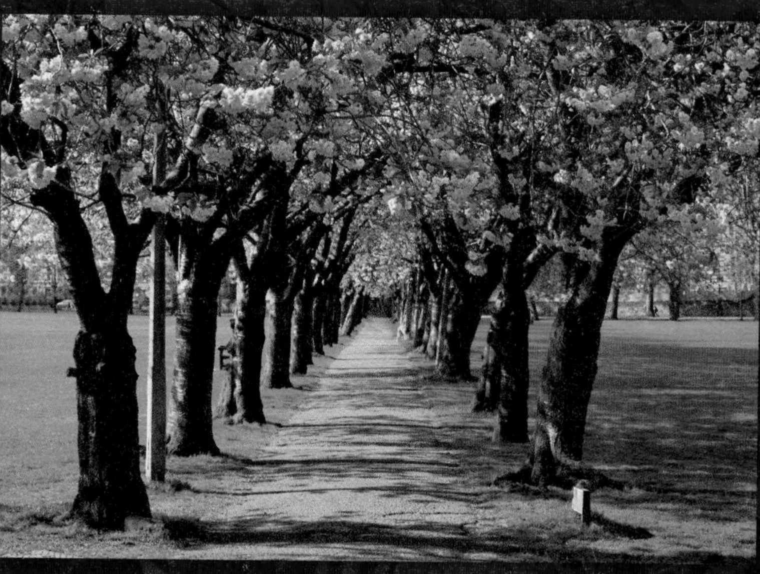

Jeff Housman, PhD, MCHES
Department of Health and Human Performance
Texas State University
Mary Odum, PhD, CHES
Department of Health and Human Performance
Texas State University

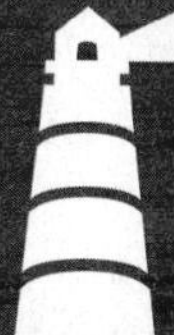

JONES & BARTLETT
LEARNING

World Headquarters
Jones & Bartlett Learning
5 Wall Street
Burlington, MA 01803
978-443-5000
info@jblearning.com
www.jblearning.com

Jones & Bartlett Learning books and products are available through most bookstores and online booksellers. To contact Jones & Bartlett Learning directly, call 800-832-0034, fax 978-443-8000, or visit our website, www.jblearning.com.

Substantial discounts on bulk quantities of Jones & Bartlett Learning publications are available to corporations, professional associations, and other qualified organizations. For details and specific discount information, contact the special sales department at Jones & Bartlett Learning via the above contact information or send an email to specialsales@jblearning.com.

07573-1

Production Credits
Chief Executive Officer: Ty Field
President: James Homer
Chief Product Officer: Eduardo Moura
VP, Executive Publisher: David D. Cella
Publisher: Cathy L. Esperti
Associate Acquisitions Editor: Kayla Dos Santos
Editorial Assistant: Sara J. Peterson
Production Editor: Leah Corrigan
Senior Marketing Manager: Andrea DeFronzo
VP, Manufacturing and Inventory Control: Therese Connell
Composition: Cenveo Publisher® Services
Cover Design: Kristin E. Parker
Rights and Media Coordinator: Amy Rathburn
Media Development Assistant: Shannon Sheehan
Cover Image: © SergeBertasiusPhotography/ShutterStock
Printing and Binding: Courier Companies
Cover Printing: Courier Companies

Library of Congress Cataloging-in-Publication Data

Library of Congress Cataloging-in-Publication Data unavailable at time of printing.

ISBN: 978-1-284-04997-8

6048

Printed in the United States of America
19 18 17 16 15 10 9 8 7 6 5 4 3 2 1

Brief Contents

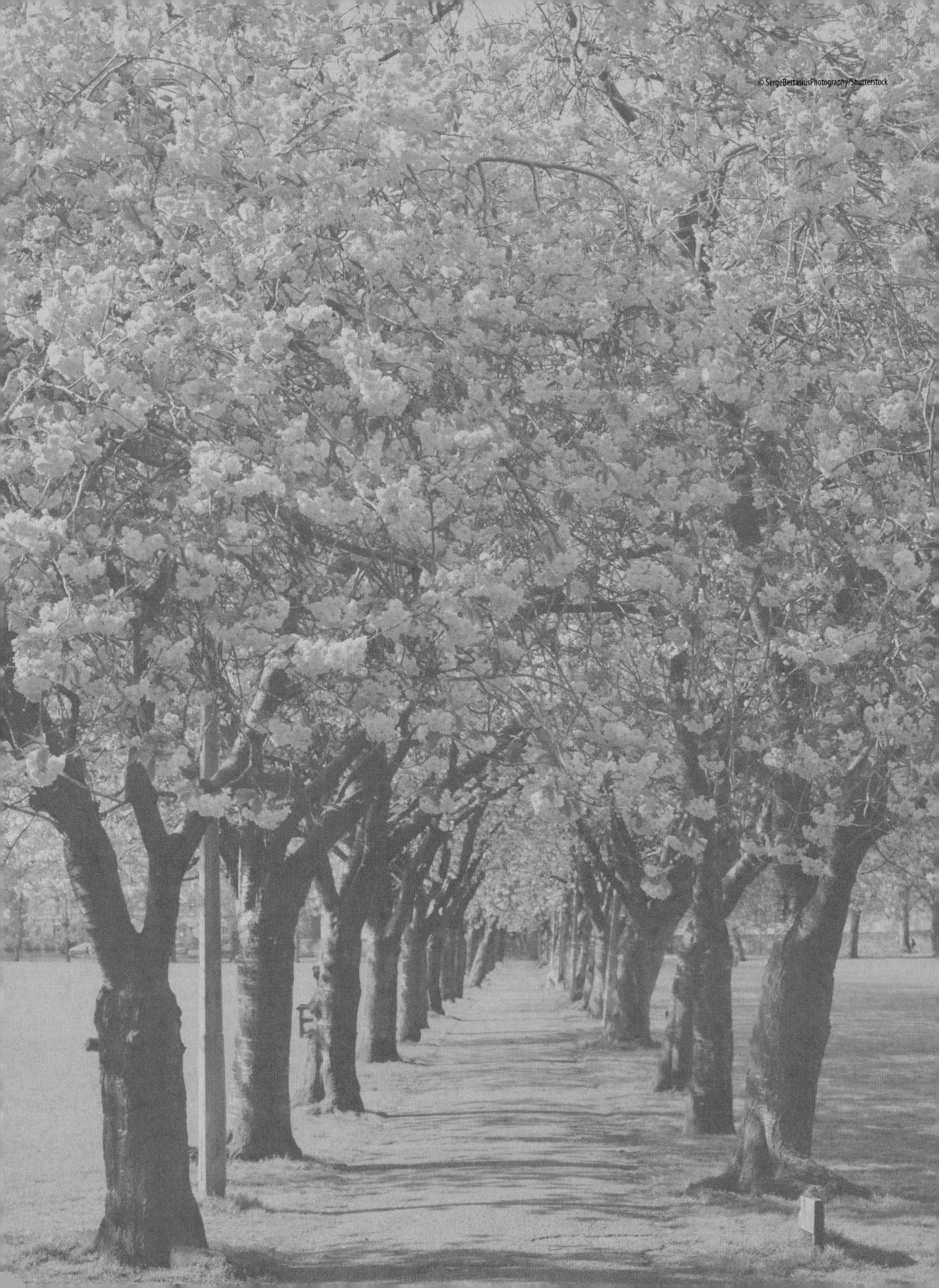

Contents

© SergeBertasiusPhotography/ShutterStock

Features

© SergeBertasiusPhotography/ShutterStock

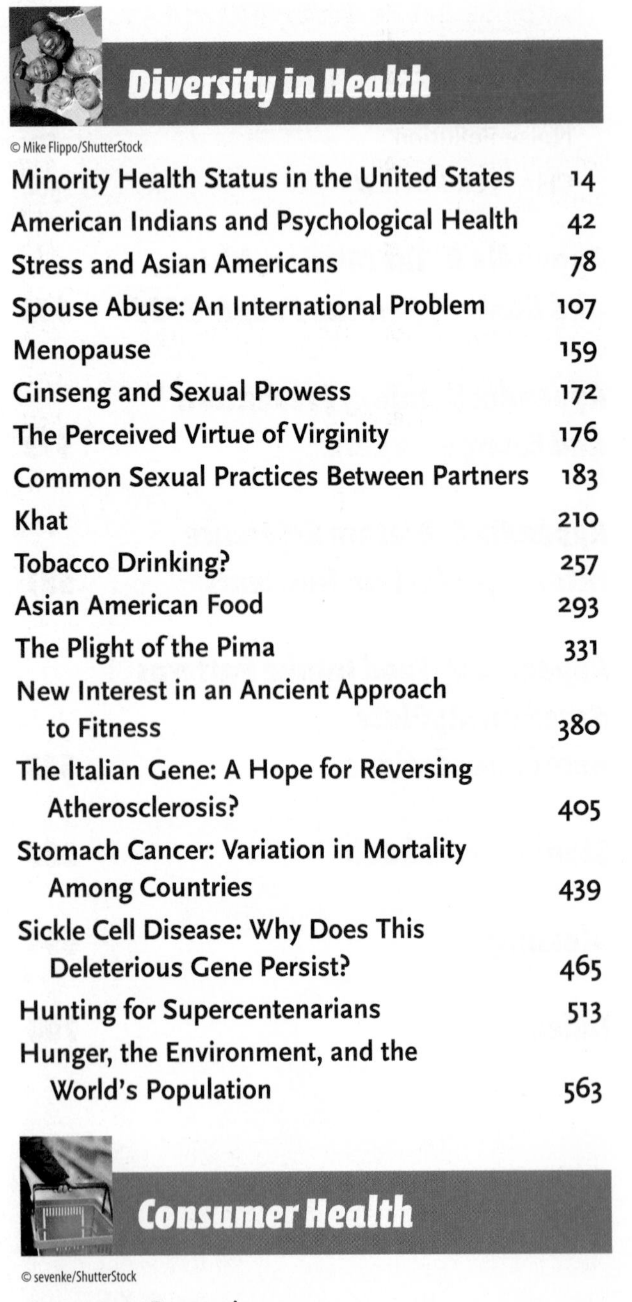

Diversity in Health

© Mike Flippo/ShutterStock

Consumer Health

© sevenke/ShutterStock

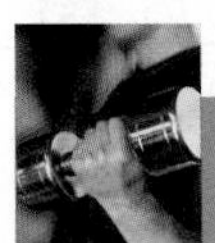

Managing Your Health

© Kzenon/ShutterStock

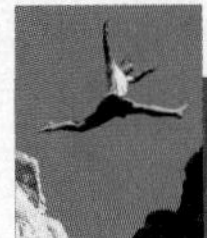

Across the Life Span

Focus on Critical Thinking

As the title suggests, *Alters & Schiff Essential Concepts for Healthy Living* was written to provide students with current information on how to live and age well. Our textbook combines evidence-based information with critical thinking activities to guide students towards healthy living through analysis of their own health behavior. We challenge students to think seriously about health-related information by using critical-thinking strategies.

What Is Critical Thinking? What Does a Critical-Thinking Textbook Do?

Critical thinking encompasses a variety of cognitive skills such as

- Synthesizing
- Analyzing
- Applying
- Evaluating

Throughout the textbook, a critical-thinking icon identifies features that focus specifically on these skills.

In the health sciences, critical-thinking skills are necessary to understand and evaluate health information as well as apply it to daily life. This book teaches critical-thinking skills that help students develop expertise in important cognitive functions:

- Differentiating between verifiable facts and value statements
- Distinguishing relevant information from irrelevant information
- Determining the factual accuracy of health claims
- Making responsible health-related decisions

To think critically, students need a solid foundation of personal health information. *Alters & Schiff Essential Concepts for Healthy Living* has been developed from the latest scientific and medical research, relying heavily on primary sources, which are cited in the text. Because understanding health involves understanding science, this text includes basic scientific information that relates to health and presents it in an easy-to-understand manner.

What Is New and Improved in This Edition?

The *Seventh Edition* is updated to provide the most current statistical data on a comprehensive array of health and wellness topics and issues, including the latest information on:

- Healthcare costs
- American adults and teenagers affected by stress
- Mental illness
- Violent crime statistics, including aggravated assault, forcible rape, abuse, homicide, domestic partner violence, intimate partner violence, stalking, and female on male violence
- Legalization of same-sex marriages worldwide
- Physical activity and health
- Eating disorders and disordered eating
- Drug use and abuse
- Legalization of marijuana

As with each new edition, this revision continues to discuss major health topics such as:

- Chapter 1
  - Genomics
  - *Healthy People 2020*
  - Extended discussion of individual, social and environmental factors that influence health behavior, and how understanding these factors can assists us in changing health behaviors
  - Updated recommendations for routine health care
- Chapter 2
  - Updated discussion of mental health and mental health disorders, incorporating changes from the DSM-5
  - Extended discussion of suicide and suicide prevention
- Chapter 3
  - Updated discussion regarding stress management strategies

- Chapter 4
  - Expanded discussion regarding sexual assaults on college campuses
  - Extended discussion of workplace violence to include military violence
- Chapter 5
  - Updated information about the Plan B One-Step® emergency contraception
  - Expanded instructions for male condom usage
  - Updated recommendations for menopause hormone replacement therapy
- Chapter 6
  - Extended explanation of the difference between *gender* and *sex*
  - Expanded discussion of sexual orientation, gender identity, and gender roles
- Chapter 7
  - Updated and extended discussion regarding student use of stimulants for academic performance
  - Updated discussion of bath salts
- Chapter 8
  - Updates on proposed graphic warning labels on cigarette packages
  - Extended discussion on e-cigarette use and regulation
- Chapter 9
  - Updated discussion regarding functional foods, including the current definition and marketer claims
  - Updated and extended discussion of *omega-3* and *omega-6* fatty acids, including suggested consumption and impact on health
  - Discussion of "healthy option" menus at restaurants and how to eat healthily when eating out
- Chapter 10
  - Updated information on popular diet plans for weight loss
  - Updated discussion regarding FDA-approved prescription drugs for weight loss
- Chapter 11
  - Discussion of measures of physical activity, including calories, METS, and PAL
  - Inclusion of ACSM guidelines for physical activity
  - Extended discussion of flexibility, including dynamic and PNF stretching
  - Inclusion of the FITT principle for development of an exercise program
- Chapter 12
  - Extended discussion of AEDs, including suggested use and public AED locations
  - Updated information on performing CPR using the American Heart Associations *Two Steps for Stayin' Alive*
  - Extended discussion of cholesterol, including LDL, HDL cholesterol, and their functions in the body
  - Updated discussion of C-reactive protein and high-sensitivity C-reactive protein test
- Chapter 13
  - Updated information on Surgeon General's statement on skin cancer and mandate for warnings on tanning beds
- Chapter 14
  - Updated discussion and graphic of the chain of infection, describing all six links in the chain
- Chapter 15
  - Inclusion of physical activity recommendations for older adults
  - Discussion of the impact of social and psychological health on well-being in older adults
  - Discussion of the impact of brain training, or mind games, on mental health in older adults
- Chapter 16
  - Updated references
  - New objectives

How to Use This Book

Analyzing health-related information activities included throughout the text provide students with examples of common advertisement techniques and other forms of media, and asks them to determine whether the information presented is valid. Because health information is readily available through many forms of media, we believe it is important for students to be able to distinguish evidence-based information from unreliable health information.

We believe that students will find these activities and tools easy to use and, if students read each chapter carefully and complete each activity thoroughly, they will gain a good understanding of major concepts of healthy living that can be applied to their personal lives, as well as future health-related careers.

Key Features

Alters & Schiff Essential Concepts for Healthy Living focuses on teaching behavior change, personal decision-making, and up-to-date personal health concepts. The critical-thinking approach encourages students to consider their own behaviors in light of the knowledge they are gaining. The pedagogical aids that appear in the chapters are described in the following pages.

The organization of ideas is an integral part of learning comprehension. The chapters are structured with a consistent format throughout the text. Each chapter begins and ends with a section that points out the key concepts and ties the information together.

Chapter-Opening Pedagogy

Each chapter-opening spread shows students the organization of the chapter using a chapter overview and a list of the special boxed features. It also lists activities in the companion Student Workbook (included at the back of this text).

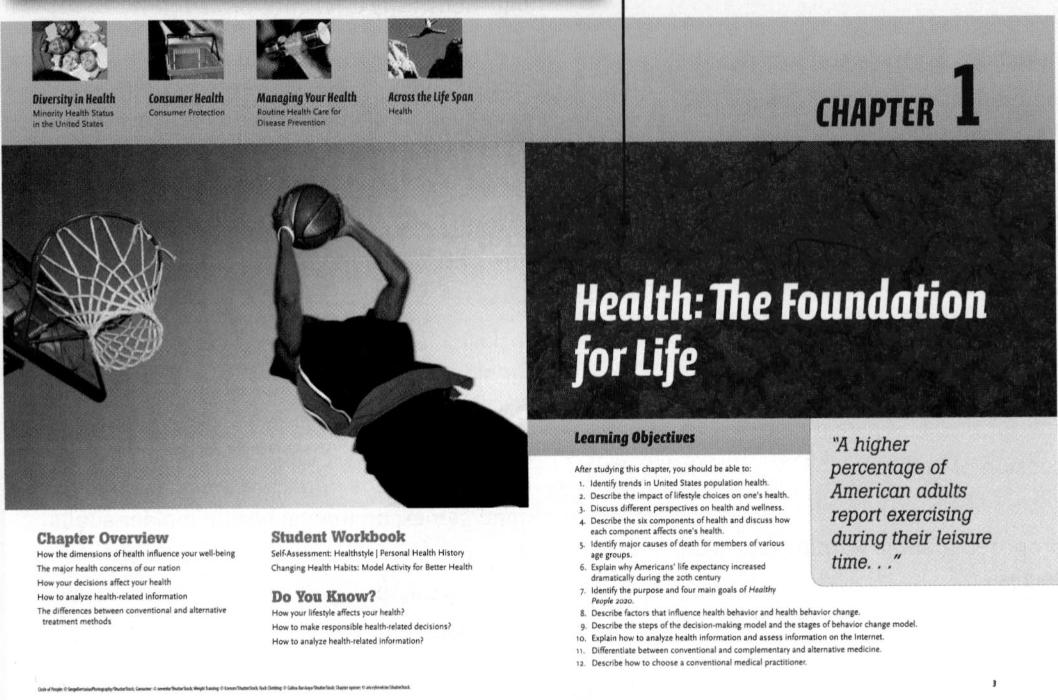

Diversity in Health
Minority Health Status in the United States

Consumer Health
Consumer Protection

Managing Your Health
Routine Health Care for Disease Prevention

Across the Life Span
Health

CHAPTER 1

Health: The Foundation for Life

Learning Objectives

After studying this chapter, you should be able to:

1. Identify trends in United States population health.
2. Describe the impact of lifestyle choices on one's health.
3. Discuss different perspectives on health and wellness.
4. Describe the six components of health and discuss how each component affects one's health.
5. Identify major causes of death for members of various age groups.
6. Explain why Americans' life expectancy increased dramatically during the 20th century
7. Identify the purpose and four main goals of *Healthy People 2020*.
8. Describe factors that influence health behavior and health behavior change.
9. Describe the steps of the decision-making model and the stages of behavior change model.
10. Explain how to analyze health information and assess information on the Internet.
11. Differentiate between conventional and complementary and alternative medicine.
12. Describe how to choose a conventional medical practitioner.

"A higher percentage of American adults report exercising during their leisure time. . ."

Chapter Overview

How the dimensions of health influence your well-being
The major health concerns of our nation
How your decisions affect your health
How to analyze health-related information
The differences between conventional and alternative treatment methods

Student Workbook

Self-Assessment: Healthstyle | Personal Health History
Changing Health Habits: Model Activity for Better Health

Do You Know?

How your lifestyle affects your health?
How to make responsible health-related decisions?
How to analyze health-related information?

3

Chapter Summaries

Research says that students learn how to identify the key ideas of stories in elementary school, but that they often have difficulty identifying key ideas in textbooks in their later schooling. Chapter summaries help students with this task. The chapter summaries follow the organization of the chapter.

CHAPTER REVIEW

Summary

Lifestyle includes behaviors that promote or deter good health and well-being. Optimal wellness is an optimal degree of health. The holistic approach to health integrates physical, psychological, social, intellectual, spiritual, and environmental dimensions. Contemporary definitions of *health* reflect not only how an individual functions but also what that person can achieve, given his or her circumstances.

Heart disease and cancer are the major killers of Americans. Lifestyle choices contribute to the development of these and many other life-threatening diseases. The distribution of health problems differs among the various ethnic and racial groups in the United States. Poverty and cultural differences are often barriers to good health care.

Experiences, knowledge, needs, and values affect one's motivation to change health-related behaviors. People are motivated to take action if they feel that a sufficient threat to their health exists and that the results of changing their behavior will be worthwhile.

Although no one can guarantee good health, many factors contribute to one's chances of enjoying a long and productive lifetime of good health. Several of these factors are the result of lifestyle choices that people can make, while they are still young, to prevent or delay disease. Responsible health-related lifestyle choices involve a systematic approach to decision making.

People can become more careful consumers of health-related information, products, and services by learning to recognize misinformation. To obtain reliable health-related information, check with experts in federal, state, and local agencies and organizations.

Conventional medicine relies on modern scientific principles, modern technologies, and scientifically proven methods to prevent, diagnose, and treat health conditions. Complementary and alternative medicine (CAM) is an unconventional and diverse system of preventing, diagnosing, and treating diseases that emphasizes spirituality, self-healing, and harmonious interaction with the environment. Conventional medical practitioners are likely to be skeptical of CAM techniques that have not been shown scientifically to be safe and effective. Until supportive data are available, consumers should be wary of CAM practices.

Throughout the life span, health concerns vary. The most common causes of infant deaths are birth defects, low birth weights, and prematurity. Preventable injuries are the major causes of death for children and youth. Additional serious public health concerns for adolescents are suicide, homicide, drug abuse, obesity, pregnancy, and sexually transmitted infections (including HIV).

Applying What You Have Learned

1. Develop a plan to improve your health by selecting a health behavior you'd like to change. **Application**
2. Select a health-related advertisement from the Internet and evaluate the validity of its information. Use the information provided in the "Analyzing Health Information" section to help you answer the following questions. **Analysis**
3. Identify several sources of health information that you have used in the past year. Using the criteria from the "Analyzing Health Information" section, explain why you think each source is reliable or unreliable. **Synthesis**
4. Think of a health-related decision that you made recently. For example, did you decide to turn down an offer to use a mind-altering drug, wear a helmet while riding a motorcycle, lose a few pounds, or use an herbal product to treat a condition? When you made this decision, did you use the decision-making process described in this chapter or did you act impulsively? Explain why you would or would not make the same decision today. **Evaluation**

34 Chapter 1 Health: The Foundation for Life

How to Use This Book to Adopt Healthier Lifestyles

Alters & Schiff Essential Concepts for Healthy Living, Seventh Edition encourages students to adopt healthier lifestyles, and the boxed features throughout the text recommend practical ways to do so.

Healthy Living Practices

Unique to this text, these short lists of bulleted statements throughout the chapters summarize key points and concisely state concrete yet simple actions students can take to improve their own health.

Managing Your Health

This feature contains short essays or lists of tips that focus on ways to live a healthier life.

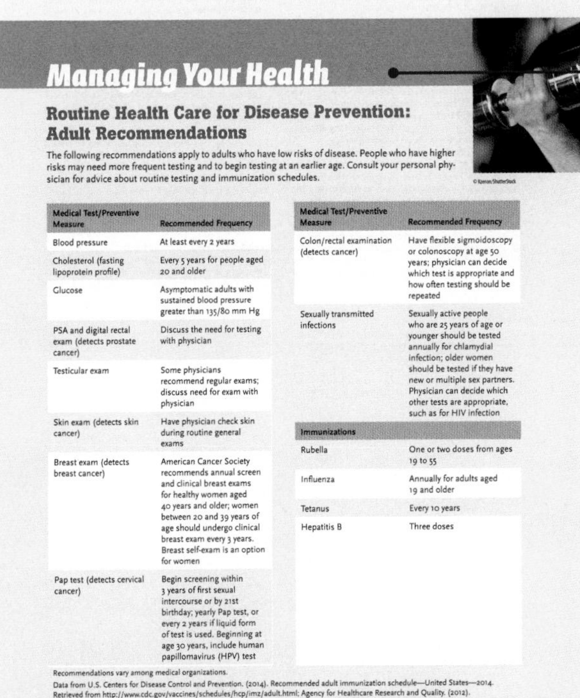

Managing Your Health

Routine Health Care for Disease Prevention: Adult Recommendations

The following recommendations apply to adults who have low risks of disease. People who have higher risks may need more frequent testing and to begin testing at an earlier age. Consult your personal physician for advice about routine testing and immunization schedules.

© Kzenon/ShutterStock

Medical Test/Preventive Measure	Recommended Frequency
Blood pressure	At least every 2 years
Cholesterol (fasting lipoprotein profile)	Every 5 years for people aged 20 and older
Glucose	Asymptomatic adults with sustained blood pressure greater than 135/80 mm Hg
PSA and digital rectal exam (detects prostate cancer)	Discuss the need for testing with physician
Testicular exam	Some physicians recommend regular exams; discuss need for exam with physician
Skin exam (detects skin cancer)	Have physician check skin during routine general exams
Breast exam (detects breast cancer)	American Cancer Society recommends annual screen and clinical breast exams for healthy women aged 40 years and older; women between 20 and 39 years of age should undergo clinical breast exam every 3 years. Breast self-exam is an option for women
Pap test (detects cervical cancer)	Begin screening within 3 years of first sexual intercourse or by 21st birthday; yearly Pap test, or every 2 years if liquid form of test is used. Beginning at age 30 years, include human papillomavirus (HPV) test
Colon/rectal examination (detects cancer)	Have flexible sigmoidoscopy or colonoscopy at age 50 years; physician can decide which test is appropriate and how often testing should be repeated
Sexually transmitted infections	Sexually active people who are 25 years of age or younger should be tested annually for chlamydial infection; older women should be tested if they have new or multiple sex partners. Physician can decide which other tests are appropriate, such as for HIV infection
Immunizations	
Rubella	One or two doses from ages 19 to 55
Influenza	Annually for adults aged 19 and older
Tetanus	Every 10 years
Hepatitis B	Three doses

Recommendations vary among medical organizations.

Data from U.S. Centers for Disease Control and Prevention. (2014). Recommended adult immunization schedule—United States—2014. Retrieved from http://www.cdc.gov/vaccines/schedules/hcp/imz/adult.html; Agency for Healthcare Research and Quality. (2012). Guide to Clinical and Preventive Services, 2012. Retrieved from http://www.ahrq.gov/professionals/clinicians-providers/guidelines-recommendations/guide/section1.html#ref12; Centers for Disease Control and Prevention. (n.d.) National HIV and STD testing resources. Retrieved from http://hivtest.cdc.gov/faq.aspx#stdtest; American Cancer Society. (2013). American Cancer Society guidelines for early detection of cancer. Retrieved from http://www.cancer.org/healthy/findcancerearly/cancerscreeningguidelines/american-cancer-society-guidelines-for-the-early-detection-of-cancer

The Goal of Prevention 19

anecdotes Personal reports of individual experiences.

testimonials Individual claims about the value of a product.

Analyzing Health Information

"Take antioxidants to live longer." "Drink red wine to prevent heart attacks." "Improve your memory with ginkgo." Every day Americans are barraged with a confusing array of health-related information in newspapers, magazines, television and radio shows, commercials, and infomercials. Family members, friends, medical professionals, and the Internet also supply information about health and health-related products. Are these sources reliable? Not necessarily. No laws prevent anyone from making statements or writing books about health, even if their information is false. The First Amendment to the U.S. Constitution protects freedom of speech and freedom of the press. This protection extends to talk show hosts and guests, authors, and salespeople in health food stores who might provide health misinformation.

Companies and individuals can make considerable amounts of money by selling untested remedies, worthless cures, unnecessary herbal supplements, and books filled with misinformation. Health frauds include the promotion or sale of substances or devices that are touted as being effective to diagnose, prevent, cure, or treat health problems, but the scientific evidence to support their safety and effectiveness is lacking.

Despite the regulatory activities of the Food and Drug Administration (FDA) and Federal Trade Commission (FTC), the sale of fraudulent products and services and the circulation of false or misleading health information continue to be concerns of medical experts. For information about the roles of the FDA and FTC in regulating health-related information, see the Consumer Health feature that follows.

Becoming a Wary Consumer of Health Information

Maybe you have read an article or an ad about the health benefits of an herbal supplement or a weight loss device that you might buy. Perhaps you watched a physician promote his "antiaging, high-energy" diet on a TV show. How do you know if health-related information and claims that are in the media and from other sources are true? Will the supplement, device, product, or diet do what its promoters claim? Or will you merely be wasting your money?

20 Chapter 1 Health: The Foundation for Life

As shown in Figure 1-6, information is a crucial element of decision making. Although health information from some sources is based on scientific evidence and can be extremely useful, that from other sources may be unreliable. Relying on flawed information can waste time and money and can even be dangerous. To be a wary consumer of health information, you need to learn how to analyze it.

Analysis Model Analyzing something simply means breaking it down into its component parts for study. Analyzing information is easier to do if you follow a particular model of analysis. The following model is a series of questions that will help you evaluate health information and determine if it is reliable, regardless of its source.

© djgis/ShutterStock

Healthy Living Practices

- To change your health-related behaviors, you must determine that you need to change and that you value the change.
- Use a decision-making plan as a tool to help you make responsible decisions.
- Take charge of your health by having regular physical examinations and monitoring your health.

1. **Which statements are verifiable facts, and which are unverified statements or value claims?** In the context of this model, *verifiable facts* are conclusions drawn from scientific research. *Unverified statements* are conclusions that have no such support. *Value claims* are statements suggesting that something is useful, or effective, or has other worthwhile characteristics. Look for unverified statements and value claims; such information may or may not be true. Also, be wary of claims that "sound too good to be true."

Look for *red-flag* terms, expressions that indicate the possibility of irrelevant information or misinformation, such as "patented formula," "all-natural," "no risk," "chemical-free," "clinically tested," "scientifically proven," or "everyone is using." Claims that the product or service provides "quick," "painless," "effortless," or "guaranteed" cure or other desirable results are also red flags.

Ignore *anecdotes* and *testimonials*. **Anecdotes** are personal reports of individual experiences, such as "I take vitamin C and zinc pills, and I never get colds." **Testimonials** are claims individuals make concerning the value of a product. Advertisers often rely on paid celebrities to provide testimonials. Anecdotes may be interesting and testimonials may be persuasive, but these sources of information reflect the experiences of individuals and may not be true for most people. More compelling evidence, on the other hand, involves results of studies of hundreds or thousands of people. Such findings are more likely to be generalized to a wide population.

Look for *disclaimers* on product labels or in advertisements, such as "This statement has not been evaluated by the FDA," "This product is not intended to diagnose, treat, cure, or prevent disease," or "Results are not typical." In televised or written ads, disclaimers usually appear in small print near the end of the ad. Disclaimers may provide important information to consider.

2. **What are the credentials of the person who makes health-related claims? Does this person have the appropriate background and education in the topic area? What can you do to check the person's credentials?** Often it is difficult to tell if a health "expert" is qualified to make claims. Articles and books usually include the name and credentials of the author, but the credentials may be fraudulent. Anyone can call himself or herself a "nutritionist," "doctor," or "health expert." Therefore, a PhD or the title "Certified . . ." after someone's name is no guarantee that this person has had extensive training in a health or science field from an accredited educational institution. Individuals can buy certain doctorate degrees through the mail or Internet from unaccredited colleges called "diploma mills." To determine if a college or university is accredited, visit the U.S. Department of Education's website (www.ed.gov).

One way to investigate an author's medical or scientific expertise is to see if his or her work has been published in reputable journals. To conduct

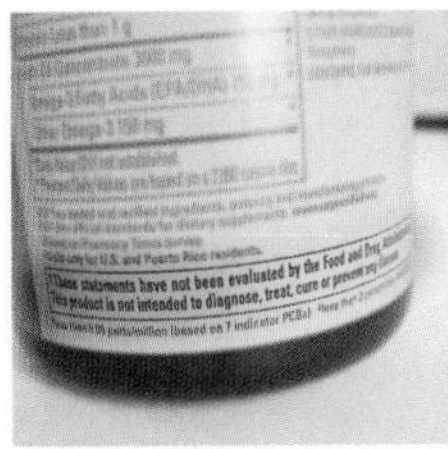

Disclaimer on a dietary supplement label.
Courtesy of Wendy Schiff

Analyzing Health Information 21

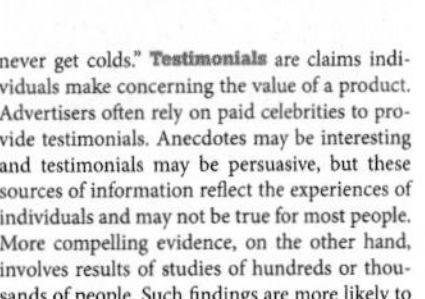

Consumer Health

Consumer Protection

The U.S. government has laws and agencies to protect consumers against health fraud.

The federal agencies that enforce consumer protection laws include the Food and Drug Administration (FDA) and the Federal Trade Commission (FTC). The FDA protects consumers by regulating the information that manufacturers can place on food or drug product labels. In addition, FDA personnel alert consumers about fraudulent health practices and can seize untested or unsafe medical devices and drugs. The manufacturers of such products can be punished (usually fined) for their illegal practices. The FTC regulates claims made in advertisements for products and services. Both agencies regulate only products and services involved in interstate commerce. The FDA's website is www.fda.gov, and the FTC's website is www.ftc.gov.

To avoid being victims of health frauds, people must take the initiative and be very critical when judging the reliability of health-related information. If you suspect fraudulent activity, you can file a complaint with the local office of the FDA or your state's attorney general. You can also file a lawsuit if you have been injured as a result of following the advice or using the services or products of unscrupulous practitioners and manufacturers.

Consumer Health

These commentaries and tips provide practical information and suggestions to help students become more careful consumers of health-related goods and services. In addition to being highlighted in this feature, consumer topics are integrated throughout the book and are the subject of scrutiny in the Analyzing Health-Related Information activities.

How to Use This Book to Enforce Critical Thinking

The focus of education today is not simply to give students information, but to teach them how to acquire and evaluate information. Unlike other personal health textbooks, the critical-thinking features in this text teach students higher-order thinking skills and give them ways to practice these skills in every chapter.

Diversity in Health

This feature cultivates an interest in and an appreciation for the health status and practices of various ethnic, cultural, and racial groups in the United States, as well as people around the world. Although the diversity essays focus specifically on multiculturalism, additional multicultural information is woven throughout the book.

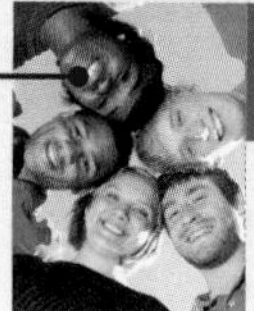

© Mike Flippo/ShutterStock

Diversity in Health

Minority Health Status in the United States

Did you know that African Americans are more likely to die of cancer than are Whites? Did you know that Hispanics are more likely to die in accidents than as the result of strokes? The differences in death and illness rates for various population subgroups reflect numerous factors, such as socioeconomic status and access to health insurance and medical care. By investigating reasons for these differences, medical researchers have learned a great deal about the health of American minorities. A major goal of the U.S. Department of Health and Human Services is improving the health of all Americans through research, education, and better access to health care.

Hispanic or Latino People

Hispanic, or Latino, people have immigrated to the United States or have ancestors from countries in which Spanish is the primary language, especially Mexico, Puerto Rico, Central and South America, and Cuba. Hispanics are the largest minority group in the United States, making up 16.7% of the population in 2011.[25]

In 2011, the leading causes of death for Hispanics were cancer, heart disease, accidental injuries, stroke, and diabetes.[20] Some Hispanic/Latino population groups have a high prevalence of asthma, obesity, chronic lung diseases, HIV infection, tuberculosis (TB), and diabetes.

Poverty, lack of health insurance, and poor education are barriers to good health for many Hispanics. About 26.6% of this minority lives in poverty.[25] Health disorders associated with poverty, such as tuberculosis and obesity, are more common in certain Spanish-speaking subgroups. In 2010, almost 31% of Hispanic Americans did not have health insurance.[22] Hispanic persons, especially those of Mexican ancestry, are more likely to be uninsured than non-Hispanic Whites. Regardless of one's ethnic/racial background, not having health insurance is a major obstacle to obtaining good health care in the United States.

African or Black Americans

In the United States, African Americans comprised 14.2% of the population in 2012; they are the second largest minority group.[24] Despite recent improvements, the health status of Black Americans is generally poorer than that of other minorities. The life expectancies of Whites and Blacks reflect their health status. In 2011, the life expectancy of African American females was 78.7 years; the life expectancy of White American females was 81.3 years. At the same time, the life expectancy of African American males was 72.1 years and that of White males was 76.6 years.[24]

The major causes of death of Black Americans are similar to those of non-Hispanic Whites. Although Black Americans are less likely to die from chronic lung diseases, Alzheimer's disease, and suicide, members of this minority are more likely to die of homicide, cancer, stroke, diabetes, HIV infection, and heart disease than are White Americans.[26] Black women are more likely to die of breast, cervical, colon, and stomach cancers than White women are, and Black men are more likely to die of lung, prostate, colon, and stomach cancers than White men are.[26]

Childbearing is riskier for an African American woman; in 2008, she was almost three times more likely to die during pregnancy or childbirth than a White woman was.29 In addition, Black infants are more likely to die during the first month of life than other babies are. In 2008, the infant death rate among Black infants was more than twice that of White babies.[26]

In 2007–2010, African Americans were more likely to have hypertension than non-Hispanic White Americans or Mexican Americans.[26] The reason for this high prevalence is unclear, but scientists think diet, genetics, stress, and smoking play roles. Overweight also increases the risk of hypertension. Black women are more likely to have excess body fat than are other Americans. In the period from 2007 to 2010, 53% of non-Hispanic Black women were obese.[26]

Asian and Pacific Islanders

As one of the fastest-growing minority groups, Asian Americans and Pacific Islanders (APIs) are a diverse group of people who immigrated to the United States

14 Chapter 1 Health: The Foundation for Life

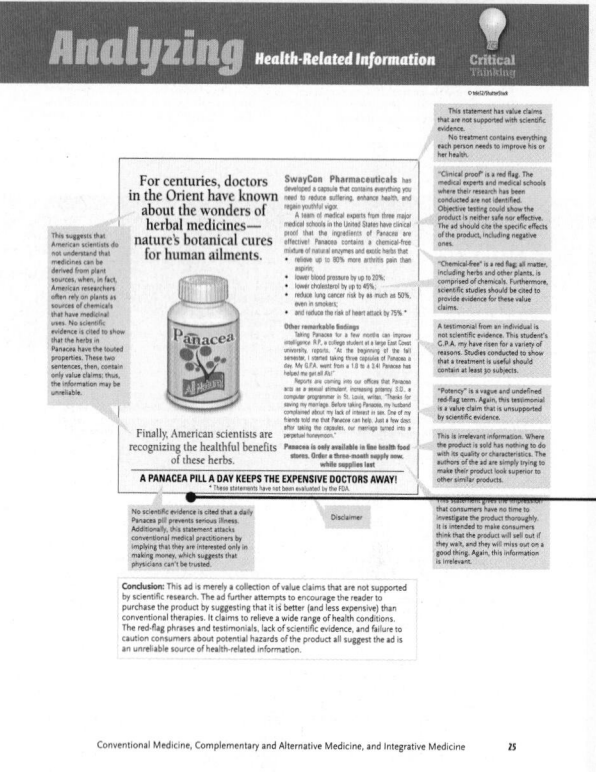

Analyzing Health-Related Information — Critical Thinking

© tele52/ShutterStock

For centuries, doctors in the Orient have known about the wonders of herbal medicines—nature's botanical cures for human ailments.

SwayCon Pharmaceuticals has developed a capsule that contains everything you need to reduce suffering, enhance health, and regain youthful vigor.

A team of medical experts from three major medical schools in the United States have clinical proof that the ingredients of Panacea are effective! Panacea contains a chemical-free mixture of natural enzymes and exotic herbs that

- relieve up to 80% more arthritis pain than aspirin;
- lower blood pressure by up to 20%;
- lower cholesterol by up to 45%;
- reduce lung cancer risk by as much as 50%, even in smokers;
- and reduce the risk of heart attack by 75%.*

Other remarkable findings

Taking Panacea for a few months can improve intelligence. R.P., a college student at a large East Coast university, reports, "At the beginning of the fall semester, I started taking three capsules of Panacea a day. My G.P.A. went from a 1.8 to a 3.4! Panacea has helped me get all A's!"

Reports are coming into our offices that Panacea acts as a sexual stimulant, increasing potency. S.D., a computer programmer in St. Louis, writes, "Thanks for saving my marriage. Before taking Panacea, my husband complained about my lack of interest in sex. One of my friends told me that Panacea can help. Just a few days after taking the capsules, our marriage turned into a perpetual honeymoon."

Finally, American scientists are recognizing the healthful benefits of these herbs.

Panacea is only available in fine health food stores. Order a three-month supply now, while supplies last

A PANACEA PILL A DAY KEEPS THE EXPENSIVE DOCTORS AWAY!

* These statements have not been evaluated by the FDA.

This suggests that American scientists do not understand that medicines can be derived from plant sources, when, in fact, American researchers often rely on plants as sources of chemicals that have medicinal uses. No scientific evidence is cited to show that the herbs in Panacea have the touted properties. These two sentences, then, contain only value claims; thus, the information may be unreliable.

This statement has value claims that are not supported with scientific evidence.

No treatment contains everything each person needs to improve his or her health.

"Clinical proof" is a red flag. The medical experts and medical schools where their research has been conducted are not identified. Objective testing could show the product is neither safe nor effective. The ad should cite the specific effects of the product, including negative ones.

"Chemical-free" is a red flag; all matter, including herbs and other plants, is comprised of chemicals. Furthermore, scientific studies should be cited to provide evidence for these value claims.

A testimonial from an individual is not scientific evidence. This student's G.P.A. my have risen for a variety of reasons. Studies conducted to show that a treatment is useful should contain at least 30 subjects.

"Potency" is a vague and undefined red-flag term. Again, this testimonial is a value claim that is unsupported by scientific evidence.

This is irrelevant information. Where the product is sold has nothing to do with its quality or characteristics. The authors of the ad are simply trying to make their product look superior to other similar products.

This statement gives the impression that consumers have no time to investigate the product thoroughly. It is intended to make consumers think that the product will sell out if they wait, and they will miss out on a good thing. Again, this information is irrelevant.

No scientific evidence is cited that a daily Panacea pill prevents serious illness. Additionally, this statement attacks conventional medical practitioners by implying that they are interested only in making money, which suggests that physicians can't be trusted.

Disclaimer

Conclusion: This ad is merely a collection of value claims that are not supported by scientific research. The ad further attempts to encourage the reader to purchase the product by suggesting that it is better (and less expensive) than conventional therapies. It claims to relieve a wide range of health conditions. The red-flag phrases and testimonials, lack of scientific evidence, and failure to caution consumers about potential hazards of the product all suggest the ad is an unreliable source of health-related information.

Conventional Medicine, Complementary and Alternative Medicine, and Integrative Medicine 25

Analyzing Health-Related Information

This innovative feature teaches students the critical-thinking skill of analysis. Students use this skill and the model provided to determine the reliability of health-related information in articles, advertisements, websites, and other sources. Learning such a skill and practicing it helps students become knowledgeable consumers of health-related information and products.

Reflecting on Your Health

This end-of-chapter journal-writing activity stimulates students to consider what they have learned and to understand how their thoughts and feelings about health might have changed as a result of their new knowledge. Compiling these activities and reviewing them from time to time, especially at the end of the semester, can offer tangible evidence of changes and psychological and intellectual growth.

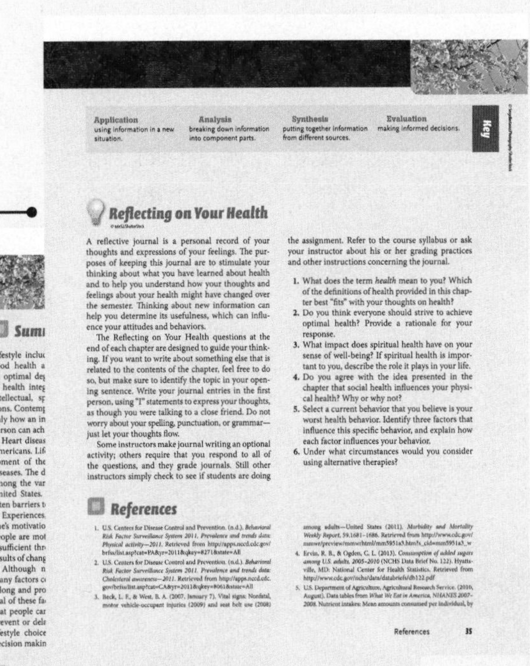
Key

Application using information in a new situation.
Analysis breaking down information into component parts.
Synthesis putting together information from different sources.
Evaluation making informed decisions.

Reflecting on Your Health

A reflective journal is a personal record of your thoughts and expressions of your feelings. The purposes of keeping this journal are to stimulate your thinking about what you have learned about health and to help you understand how your thoughts and feelings about your health might have changed over the semester. Thinking about new information can help you determine its usefulness, which can influence your attitudes and behaviors.

The Reflecting on Your Health questions at the end of each chapter are designed to guide your thinking. If you want to write about something else that is related to the contents of the chapter, feel free to do so, but make sure to identify the topic in your opening sentence. Write your journal entries in the first person, using "I" statements to express your thoughts, as though you were talking to a close friend. Do not worry about your spelling, punctuation, or grammar—just let your thoughts flow.

Some instructors make journal writing an optional activity; others require that you respond to all of the questions, and they grade journals. Still other instructors simply check to see if students are doing the assignment. Refer to the course syllabus or ask your instructor about his or her grading practices and other instructions concerning the journal.

1. What does the term *health* mean to you? Which of the definitions of health provided in this chapter best "fits" with your thoughts on health?
2. Do you think everyone should strive to achieve optimal health? Provide a rationale for your response.
3. What impact does spiritual health have on your sense of well-being? If spiritual health is important to you, describe the role it plays in your life.
4. Do you agree with the idea presented in the chapter that social health influences your physical health? Why or why not?
5. Select a current behavior that you believe is your worst health behavior. Identify three factors that influence this specific behavior, and explain how each factor influences your behavior.
6. Under what circumstances would you consider using alternative therapies?

References

1. U.S. Centers for Disease Control and Prevention. (n.d.). *Behavioral Risk Factor Surveillance System 2011. Prevalence and trends data: Physical activity—2011.* Retrieved from http://apps.nccd.cdc.gov/brfss/list.asp?cat=PA&yr=2011&qkey=8271&state=All
2. U.S. Centers for Disease Control and Prevention. (n.d.). *Behavioral Risk Factor Surveillance System 2011. Prevalence and trends data: Cholesterol awareness—2011.* Retrieved from http://apps.nccd.cdc.gov/brfss/list.asp?cat=CA&yr=2011&qkey=8061&state=All
3. Beck, L. F., & West, B. A. (2007, January 7). Vital signs: Nonfatal, motor vehicle-occupant injuries (2009) and seat belt use (2008) among adults—United States (2011). *Morbidity and Mortality Weekly Report,* 59.1681–1686. Retrieved from http://www.cdc.gov/mmwr/preview/mmwrhtml/mm5951a3.htm?s_cid=mm5951a3_w
4. Ervin, R. B., & Ogden, C. L. (2013). *Consumption of added sugars among U.S. adults, 2005–2010* (NCHS Data Brief No. 122). Hyattsville, MD: National Center for Health Statistics. Retrieved from http://www.cdc.gov/nchs/data/databriefs/db122.pdf
5. U.S. Department of Agriculture, Agricultural Research Service. (2010, August). Data tables from *What We Eat in America,* NHANES 2007–2008. Nutrient intakes: Mean amounts consumed per individual, by

References 35

Applying What You Have Learned

This unique end-of-chapter feature is a series of questions and activities that require critical thinking—application, analysis, synthesis, and evaluation. Each question is labeled with what type of critical thinking is required, and a key provides a brief explanation of the process students need to follow to complete the question or activity.

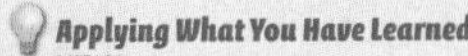

Applying What You Have Learned

1. Develop a plan to improve your health by selecting a health behavior you'd like to change. **Application**
2. Select a health-related advertisement from the Internet and evaluate the validity of its information. Use the information provided in the "Analyzing Health Information" section to help you answer the following questions. **Analysis**
3. Identify several sources of health information that you have used in the past year. Using the criteria from the "Analyzing Health Information" section, explain why you think each source is reliable or unreliable. **Synthesis**
4. Think of a health-related decision that you made recently. For example, did you decide to turn down an offer to use a mind-altering drug, wear a helmet while riding a motorcycle, lose a few pounds, or use an herbal product to treat a condition? When you made this decision, did you use the decision-making process described in this chapter or did you act impulsively? Explain why you would or would not make the same decision today. **Evaluation**

34 Chapter 1 Health: The Foundation for Life

The Integrated Teaching and Learning Package

Integrating the text and ancillaries is crucial to deriving their full benefit. Based on feedback from instructors and students, the following supplements are offered with *Alters & Schiff Essential Concepts for Healthy Living, Seventh Edition*.

Instructor Resources

- Robust Test Bank
- Slides in Power Point Format
- Image Bank
- Instructor Manuals
- Transition Guide
- Sample Syllabus

Student Workbook

In addition, the *Seventh Edition* contains a built-in critical-thinking workbook that allows students to assess and improve their health-related behaviors and attitudes. (See the Student Workbook at the end of this text for more information.)

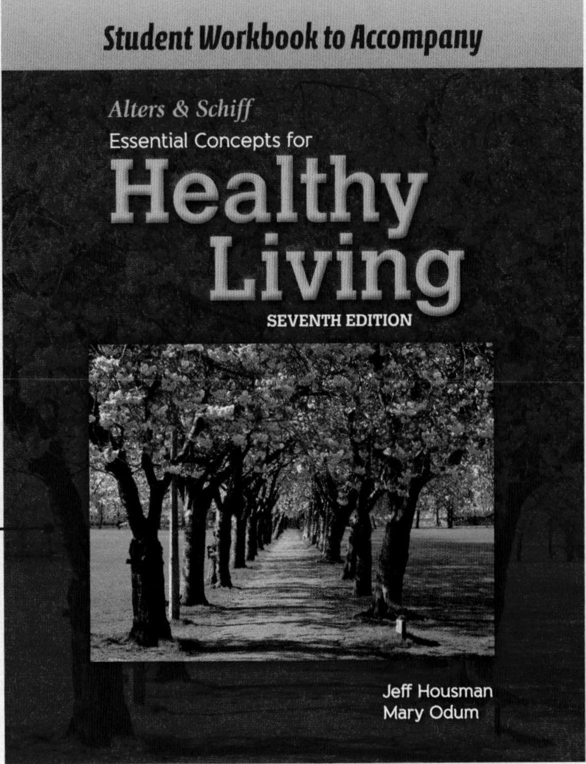

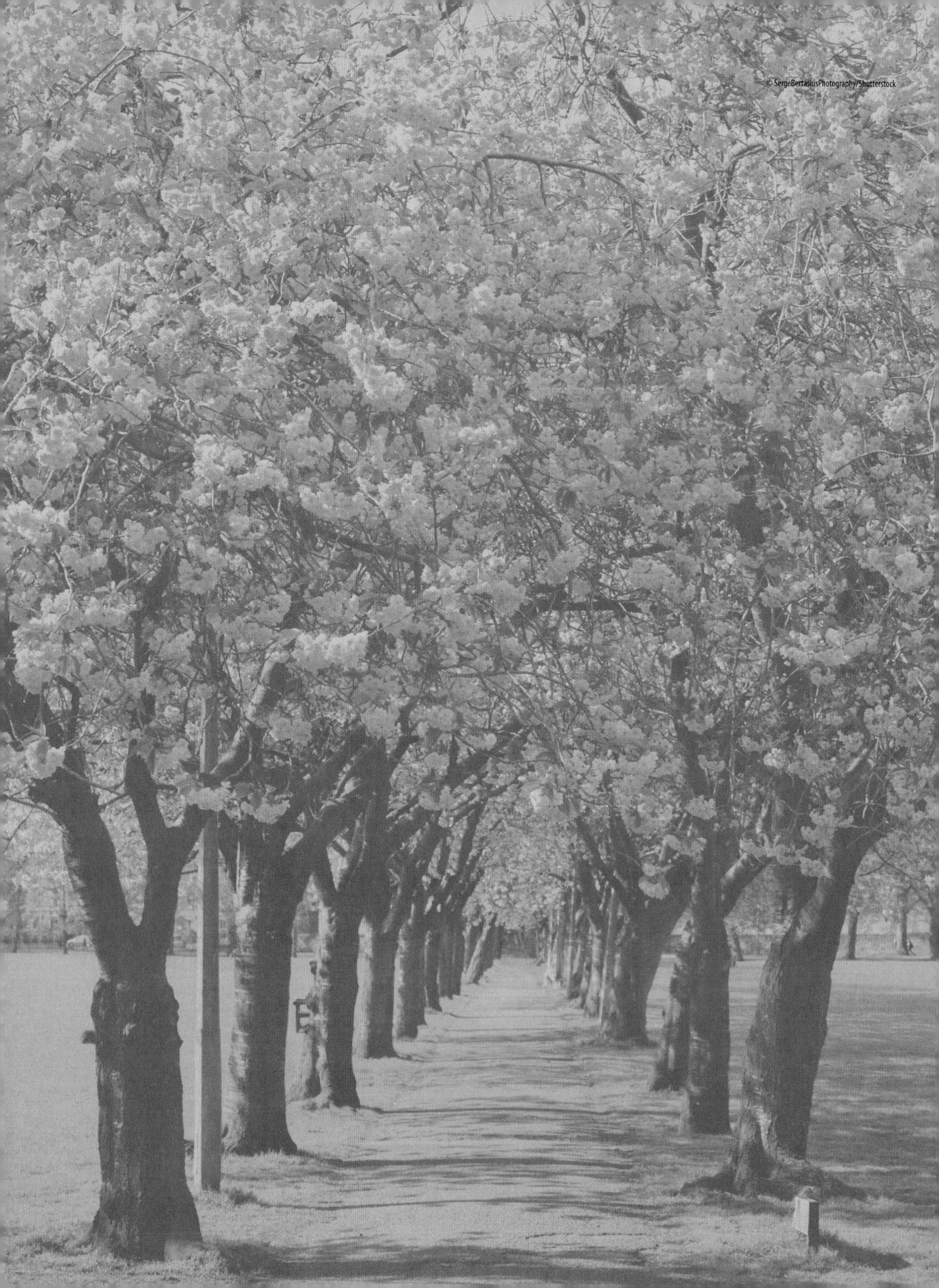

Dedication for Sandy Alters

SergeBertasiusPhotography/ShutterStock

My life has been extraordinary, but it wouldn't have been so if I hadn't been touched by an extraordinary person: ***Sandy Alters***. For over 20 years, my relationship with Sandy spanned several levels. Initially, she was my professor. Then she became my mentor, then my colleague, my coauthor, and finally, my best friend and confidant. She had enormous talent as a science writer and was an exemplary college educator. Sandy was one of those rare individuals who was secure enough in her own abilities to help others develop their own.

I mourn the loss of my best friend. There are no more emails, phone chats, and hilarious birthday cards to look forward to receiving. She died too young. It makes me feel better to know that I told Sandy, on several occasions, how much she meant to me and that I attributed my success as a college textbook author to her. Thus, I dedicate the seventh edition of *Alters & Schiff Essential Concepts for Healthy Living* to Sandra Alters.

Most sincerely,
Wendy Schiff

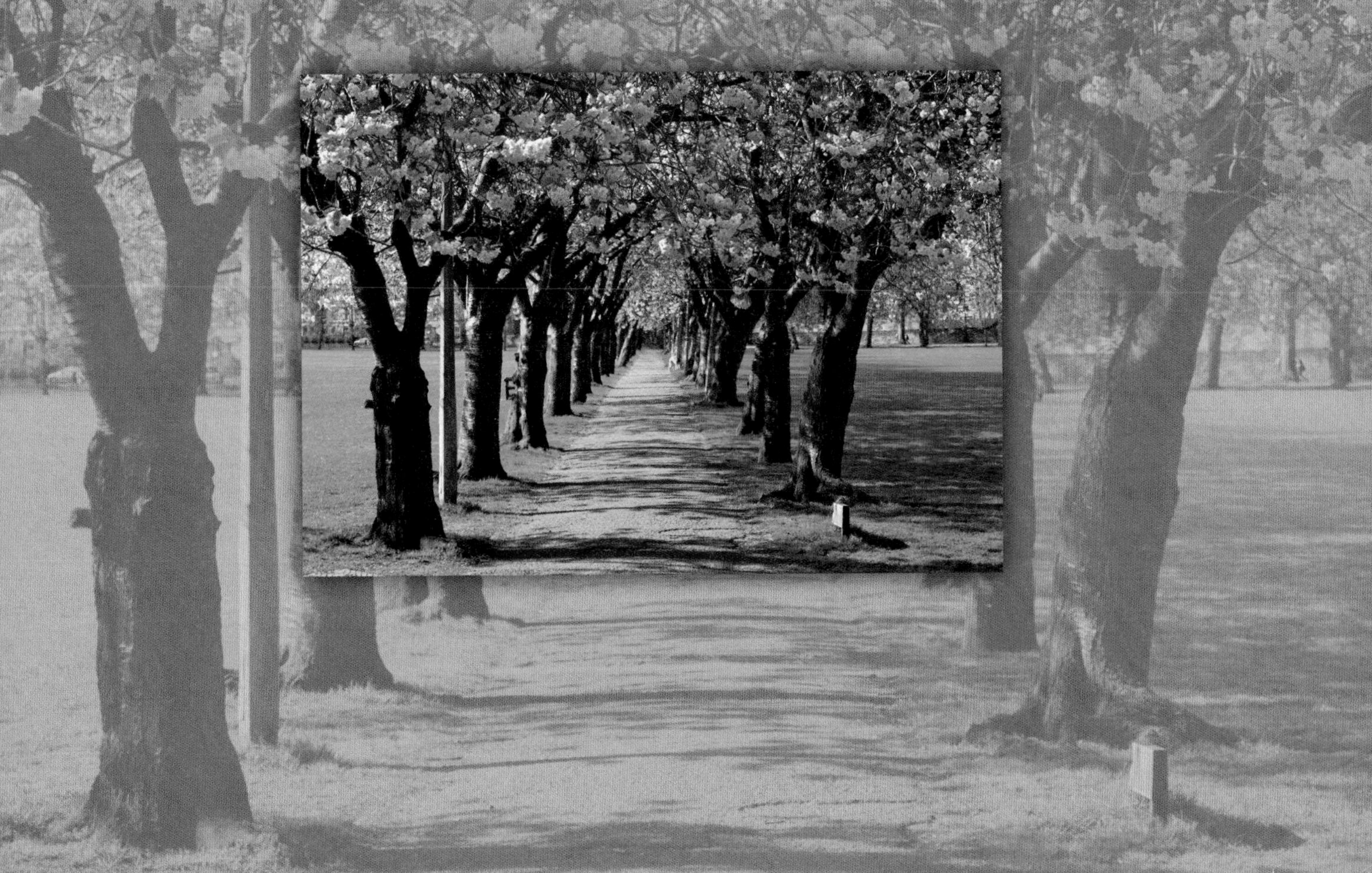

Reviewers

© SergeBertasiusPhotography/Shutterstock

Many health teachers and researchers have made significant contributions to the development of this book. Our gratitude goes to the following reviewers whose expertise gave invaluable direction to the development of the seventh edition of *Alters & Schiff Essential Concepts for Healthy Living*:

Brandy Hancock Adelsberger
Fontbonne University
St. Louis, Montana

Liza Allen
Mesa Community College
Mesa, Arizona

Leigh Poirier Ball
Orange Coast College
Costa Mesa, California

Amanda L. Divin
Western Illinois University
Macomb, Illinois

Chris Eisenbarth
Weber State University
Ogden, Utah

Jacqueline M. Franz
Mercer County Community College
West Windsor Township, New Jersey

Linda J. Hoffman
Community College of Allegheny County
Pittsburgh, Pennsylvania

Walter Hook
Eastern University
St. Davids, Pennsylvania

Donna McGill-Cameron
Woodland Community College
Woodland, California

J. Dirk Nelson
West Texas A&M University
Canyon, Texas

David J. Pearson
Baptist University
Riverside, California

Grace Pokorny
Long Beach City College
Long Beach, California

Mikel Stone
Shawnee University
Portsmouth, Ohio

Nanette Tummers
Eastern Connecticut State University
Willimantic, Connecticut

Julia VanderMolen
Davenport University
Grand Rapids, Michigan

About the Authors

© SergeBertasiusPhotography/Shutterstock

Alters & Schiff Essential Concepts for Healthy Living, Seventh Edition was written by an author team with extensive credentials and backgrounds in health, exercise science, human sexuality, nutrition, health behavior, and education.

Jeff Housman

Jeff Housman holds a doctorate degree in health education and a master's degree in kinesiology and is a tenured associate professor in health and human performance at Texas State University, where he teaches courses in health education, community health, school health, behavior theory, and research and statistics. Understanding the importance of research, as well as remaining current with the industry, Dr. Housman's research interests include health behavior, substance use, and program evaluation. He has authored multiple peer-reviewed articles and several textbook chapters, in addition to *Alters & Schiff Essential Concepts for Healthy Living*. He has also contributed to several professional publications, including *A Competency-Based Framework for Health Education Specialists*, for the National Commision for Health Education Credentialing, Inc., and he serves as a consulting editor for the *Journal of American College Health*. Dr. Housman is a member of multiple professional organizations, including the *Eta Sigma Gamma* Health Education Honorary, the American College Health Association, the American School Health Association, and the Society for Public Health Education. As the new lead author on *Alters & Schiff Essential Concepts for Healthy Living, Seventh Edition*, Dr. Housman brings his education expertise, background in health, exercise science, and health behavior, as well as his extensive writing experience, to this best-selling product and author team.

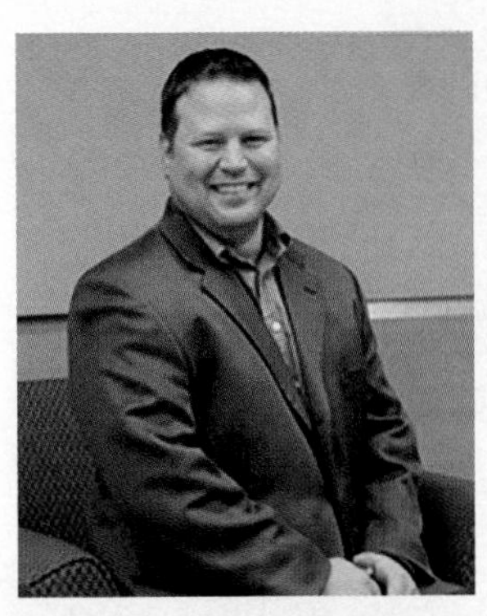

Mary Odum

Mary Odum holds a doctorate degree in health education, a master's degree in health, exercise and sport sciences, and a bachelor's degree in psychology. She holds a full-time faculty appointment at Texas State University and an adjunct position at Texas A&M University, where she teaches courses in health education, program planning and evaluation, women's health, human sexuality, and worksite health. Dr. Odum's research interests include child health and maternal health, and she serves as a review editor for *Frontiers in Public Health: Public Health Education and Promotion*. Dr. Odum is a member of multiple professional organizations, including the *Eta Sigma Gamma* Health Education Honorary, the American Public Health Association, and the Text and Academic Authors Association.

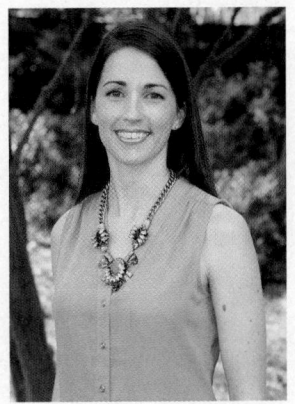

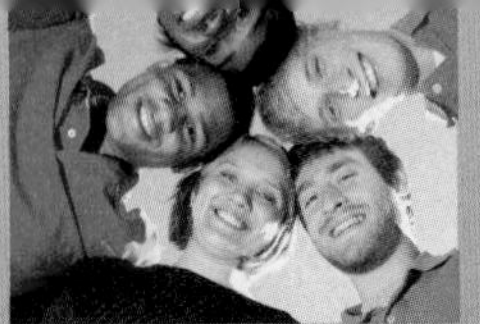

Diversity in Health
Minority Health Status in the United States

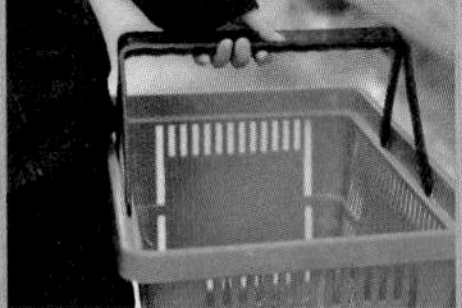

Consumer Health
Consumer Protection

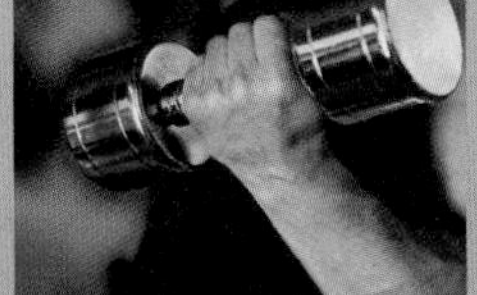

Managing Your Health
Routine Health Care for Disease Prevention

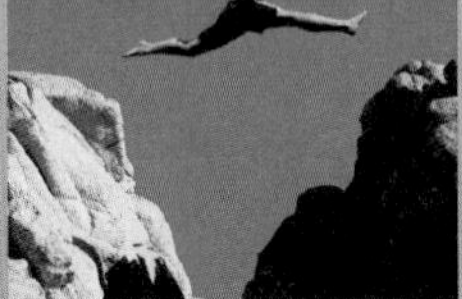

Across the Life Span
Health

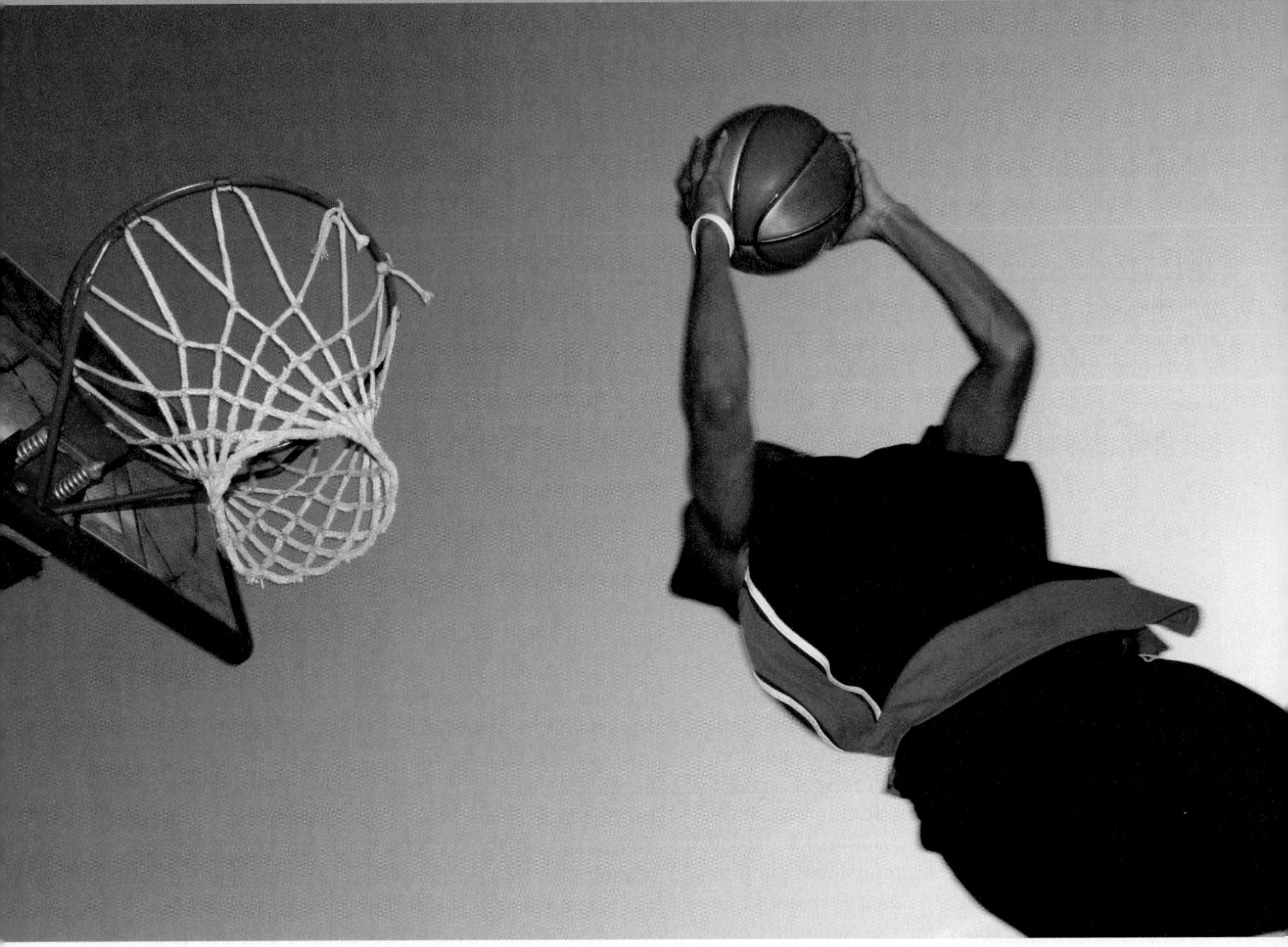

Chapter Overview

How the dimensions of health influence your well-being

The major health concerns of our nation

How your decisions affect your health

How to analyze health-related information

The differences between conventional and alternative treatment methods

Student Workbook

Self-Assessment: Healthstyle | Personal Health History

Changing Health Habits: Model Activity for Better Health

Do You Know?

How your lifestyle affects your health?

How to make responsible health-related decisions?

How to analyze health-related information?

CHAPTER 1

Health: The Foundation for Life

Learning Objectives

After studying this chapter, you should be able to:

1. Identify trends in United States population health.
2. Describe the impact of lifestyle choices on one's health.
3. Discuss different perspectives on health and wellness.
4. Describe the six components of health and discuss how each component affects one's health.
5. Identify major causes of death for members of various age groups.
6. Explain why Americans' life expectancy increased dramatically during the 20th century
7. Identify the purpose and four main goals of *Healthy People 2020*.
8. Describe factors that influence health behavior and health behavior change.
9. Describe the steps of the decision-making model and the stages of behavior change model.
10. Explain how to analyze health information and assess information on the Internet.
11. Differentiate between conventional and complementary and alternative medicine.
12. Describe how to choose a conventional medical practitioner.

"A higher percentage of American adults report exercising during their leisure time. . ."

life expectancy The average number of years that an individual of a particular age can expect to live.

lifestyle A way of living, including behaviors that promote or impair good health and longevity.

risk factor A characteristic that increases an individual's chances of developing a health problem.

In the United States, there are some encouraging signs that more people are concerned about improving and protecting their health than in the past. A higher percentage of American adults met physical activity guidelines for aerobic physical activity (i.e., at least 150 minutes or more a week) in 2011 than in previous years.[1] In 1995, 71% of adults reported that their blood cholesterol level had been checked. By 2013, that percentage had increased to 79.2% of adults.[2] Between 1988 and 2008, the percentage of Americans wearing seat belts while riding in motor vehicles increased dramatically.[3] In some respects, Americans have also improved their eating habits. Between 2005 and 2010, on average adolescents consumed more than 16% of their total calories from added sugar, slightly above the recommended 15%. Most adults aged 20 or older, however, met recommended sugar consumption guidelines. In addition, Americans are consuming more calcium and more dietary fiber.[4,5] In 2009, fewer Americans died of cancer than in 1999.[6] Finally, Americans are living longer than in the 1980s. **Life expectancy** is the average number of years that an individual of a particular age can expect to live. In 1990, the life expectancy of an infant in the United States was 75.4 years.[7] By 2010, Americans' life expectancy at birth had increased to 76 years for males and 81 years for females.[7]

Other findings about Americans' current health status and health-related behaviors, however, are less encouraging. Although the overall rate of cigarette smoking has decreased slightly, consumption of cigars and loose-leaf tobacco (e.g., pipe tobacco) increased from 2000 to 2011. The greatest increase in loose-leaf tobacco consumption occurred after the federal tobacco excise tax increased in 2009, making cigarettes more expensive than loose-leaf tobacco.[8] Additionally, alcohol abuse is a widespread behavior, particularly among young people. Tobacco use remains the leading cause of preventable illness and death in the United States. In 2009, adults smoked fewer cigarettes than in 1985, but about 18% of Americans who were 18 years of age and older smoked cigarettes.[8] U.S. public health officials are also concerned about Americans who use alcohol irresponsibly. In 2011, excessive alcohol consumption was the third leading cause of preventable deaths in the United States, including traffic-related fatalities.[9] Approximately 17% of adult Americans reported binge drinking in 2011[10] and 25% of high school students reported that they engaged in *binge drinking* in 2011.[11] Binge drinking is defined as consuming five or more alcoholic drinks per occasion (males) and four or more drinks per occasion (females). Americans who are 18 to 24 years of age are more likely to binge drink than other members of the population. According to results of one study, about one in four college students indicated that their drinking behaviors contributed to serious academic problems, including missing classes, performing poorly on exams, and lowering their grade point averages.[12] The typical American does not meet the federal government's recommendations concerning healthy food choices. The majority of the U.S. population does not eat enough vegetables, whole grains, fruits, milk, and oils ("healthy" fats).[13] An important sign of Americans' poor nutritional practices is the high prevalence of *obesity* in the United States. Between 1988 and 1994, 10% of children[14] and almost 23% of adults[14] were obese. By 2010, 17% of American children and more than 36% of American adults were obese.[15] Between 1994 and 2008, the prevalence of obesity increased dramatically among all groups of Americans regardless of their age, sex, race, ethnicity, socioeconomic status, region of the country, and educational level. Excess body fat is associated with the development of many serious diseases, including high blood pressure, heart disease, certain cancers, and *type 2 diabetes*, a serious disorder characterized by the body's inability to regulate blood sugar normally.

Although Americans are living longer than in the past, living longer is not always a sign that people are living *better*. Many older adults suffer from conditions that reduce their ability to enjoy life and perform important daily activities such as bathing and dressing. Heart disease, stroke, cancer, Alzheimer's disease, impaired vision, hearing loss, osteoporosis, and depression create much misery not only for millions of older adults but also for the family members who struggle to care for their disabled relatives.

The results of many studies show that exercising regularly, eating a more nutritious diet, and avoiding smoking and excess alcohol consumption promote good health. Incorporating these and other healthy habits into your *lifestyle*, while you are still young, can improve your health and well-being and increase your chances of living a longer and healthier life than your parents and grandparents.

Lifestyle is a way of living. As a college student, your lifestyle includes a variety of behaviors that promote or impair good health and longevity. Although you may be unable to prevent severe birth defects or inherited disorders from affecting your health, you can modify many health *risk factors*, reducing the likelihood that you will develop serious medical problems. A **risk factor** is a characteristic that increases an individual's chances of developing a health problem. For example, physical inactivity, tobacco use, emotional stress, and obesity are risk factors for heart disease, *hypertension* (persistent high blood pressure), and certain types of cancers. You can dramatically lower your chances of developing these conditions by incorporating exercise into your daily schedule, choosing not to use tobacco products, practicing relaxation techniques, and eating a more nutritious diet.

Are you concerned about your health? What are you doing to protect it? What steps can you take to enhance your state of health so that you can enjoy life more fully? Where can you find reliable information concerning health? This text presents findings from current scientific research for you to use in making choices that will improve your health.

The Dimensions of Health

What Is Health?

Most people can describe how it feels to be healthy or ill, but trying to define *health* is not an easy task. In 1948, the World Health Organization (WHO) constitution defined health as "a state of complete physical, mental, and social well-being and not merely the absence of disease or infirmity."[16] Some, however, consider this definition too limited and suggest health cannot be a state because our health is ever changing. Consider the people in **Figure 1.1**. Although they are in wheelchairs, they are able to compete as athletes. If you judged their state of health using WHO's 1948 definition, you might conclude that they are unhealthy. Many physically disabled people are able to function adequately in society and do not consider themselves ill or infirm.

The Ottawa Charter for Health Promotion defines *health* as "a resource for everyday life . . . a positive concept emphasizing social and personal resources, as well as physical capabilities."[17] According to this charter, health requires "peace, shelter, education, food, income, a stable ecosystem, sustainable resources, social justice and equity." In addition to these conditions, most healthy adults want to

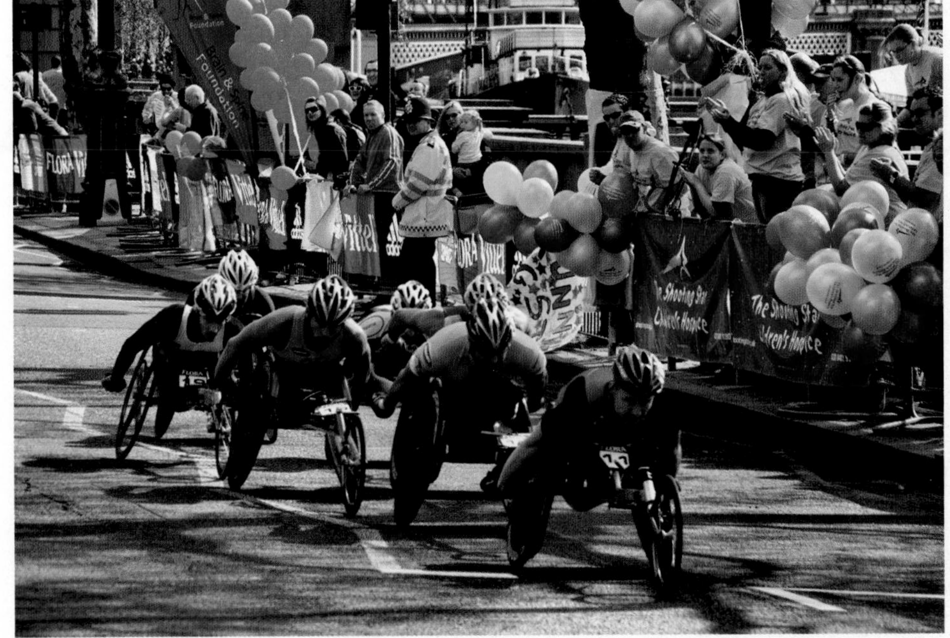

Figure 1.1

Wheelchair Athletes. Many physically disabled people do not consider themselves ill or infirm because they can function well in society. According to Hochbaum's definition of health, individuals with physical disabilities can be healthy and enjoy life.

good health The ability to function adequately and independently in a constantly changing environment.

optimal wellness A sense that one is functioning at his or her best level.

holistic (hole-IS-tic) A characteristic involving all aspects of the person.

signs Observable and measurable features of an illness.

symptoms Subjective complaints of illness.

acute A condition or illness that tends to develop quickly and resolve within a few days or weeks.

chronic A condition or disease that often takes months or years to develop, progresses in severity, and can affect a person over a long period.

function independently; enjoy eating, sexual, and physical activities; feel good about themselves; and enjoy being with family and friends.

Behavioral scientist Godfrey Hochbaum proposed a simple definition for health: "Health is what helps me be what I want to be . . . do what I want to do . . . [and] live the way I would like to live."[18] Using Hochbaum's definition, you might conclude that the wheelchair-bound athletes in **Figure 1.1** are as healthy as people who are capable of running. In this text, we use concepts from all of these perspectives and define *health* as "a dynamic state or condition of the human organism that is multidimensional (i.e., physical, emotional, social, intellectual, spiritual, and occupational) in nature, a resource for living, and results from a person's interactions with an adaptations to his or her environment".[19]

Health and Wellness

Health and wellness are related concepts. **Good health** enables one to function adequately and independently in a constantly changing environment; **optimal wellness** is a sense that one is functioning at one's best level. **Figure 1.2** illustrates the concept of health as a continuum; there are degrees of health. The absence of functioning (premature death) is at one end of this continuum, and the highest level of functioning (optimal well-being) is at the other end. Many people accept responsibility for the quality of their health and well-being. These people are willing to take various steps to improve their health, achieving a higher degree of wellness in the process.

Most health educators agree that health and wellness are **holistic**; that is, they involve all aspects of the individual. Thus, the holistic concept of health encompasses not only the physical, psychological, and social aspects but also the intellectual, spiritual, and environmental dimensions of a person. Each dimension is an integral part of a person's health, and any change in the quality of one component of health affects the others. For example, individuals who exercise with others to increase their level of physical health often report a sense of improved psychological and social health.

The Components of Health

Physical Health *Physical health* refers to the overall condition of the organ systems, such as the cardiovascular system (heart and blood vessels), respiratory system (lungs), reproductive system, and nervous system. A healthy person's systems function properly; the individual feels well and is free of disease. When organs do not function adequately, a person has various signs and symptoms of illness. **Signs** are the observable and measurable features of an illness, such as fever, rash, and abnormal behavior. **Symptoms** are the subjective complaints of an illness, such as reports of fatigue, headaches, and numbness. An **acute** condition or illness, such as the common cold or a food-borne infection, tends to develop quickly and resolve within a few days or weeks. A **chronic** condition or disease often takes months or years to

Figure 1.2

A Health Continuum. Some people view health as a continuum; that is, there are degrees of health. Premature death is at one end of this continuum, and optimal well-being is at the other end.

Modified from Ebersole, P., & Hess, P. (1994). *Toward Healthy Aging* (4th ed.). St. Louis: Mosby. Copyright © 1994 with permission from Elsevier.

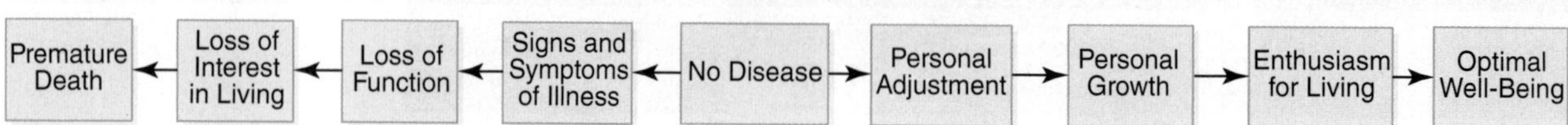

develop, progresses in severity, and can affect a person over a longer period, in some cases, throughout his or her lifetime.

Psychological Health Psychological (mental) health involves the ability to deal effectively with the psychological challenges of life. Psychologically healthy people accept responsibility for their behavior, feel good about themselves and others, are comfortable with their emotions (feelings), and have positive, realistic outlooks on life. Although experiences such as losing a job or a family member cause stress or grief, psychologically healthy people are able to limit the extent to which crises affect their lives.

Social Health Social health is the sense of well-being that an individual achieves by forming emotionally supportive and intellectually stimulating relationships with family members, friends, and associates. Living in communities rather than in isolation, identifying with social groups, and belonging to organizations strengthen the social dimension of health. When social networks break down, health declines.

Intellectual Health Intellectual health is the ability to use problem solving and other higher-order thinking skills to deal effectively with life's challenges. Healthy people analyze situations, determine alternative courses of action, and make decisions. After making decisions, intellectually healthy individuals are able to judge the effectiveness of their choices and learn from their experiences. Effective intellectual skills enable people to feel in control of their lives.

Spiritual Health Spiritual health is the belief that one is a part of a larger scheme of life and that one's life has purpose. Identifying with a religion and having religious beliefs influence the spiritual health of many people. However, spirituality is not confined to those who belong to organized religious groups or have religious beliefs. People can develop spirituality without practicing a particular religion or believing in the power of a supreme being. Whatever the nature of their spirituality, many individuals achieve a sense of inner peace and harmony as well as emotional fulfillment by believing that their lives have a purpose. As in the other wellness dimensions, a breakdown in spiritual health can have a negative impact on one's well-being.

Environmental Health Nothing affects the quality of wellness components as much as the state of the environment—the conditions in which people live, work, and play. Environmental concerns that influence wellness include the provision of clean water and air, the management of wastes, and the control of distressing social problems such as crime and family violence. Humans cannot achieve a high degree of wellness if their environment is polluted or unsafe (**Figure 1.3**).

Figure 1.4 is a model that illustrates how these six components of health are related and integrated into a holistic approach to understanding wellness. This model has the physical and psychological health components at the core of the larger environmental component. The social, intellectual, and

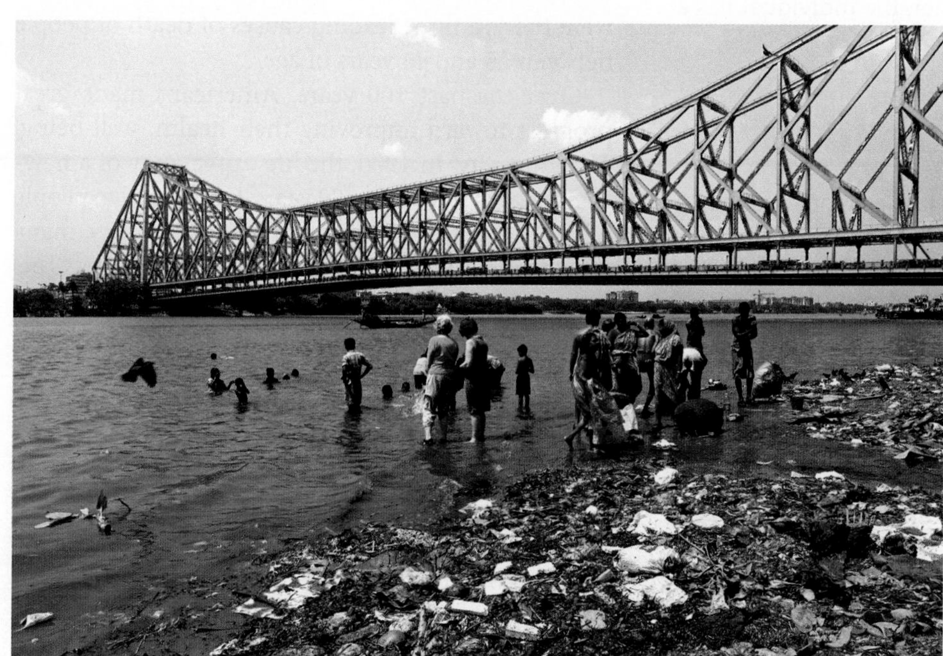

Figure 1.3

Environmental Health. The state of the environment in which people live, work, and play affects the quality of their health. People cannot achieve a high degree of wellness if their environment is polluted or unsafe.

Figure 1.4

The Components of Health. The components of health are interrelated. According to this model, the social, intellectual, and spiritual components of health are in the larger spheres of physical and psychological health, which are in the largest sphere of environmental health.

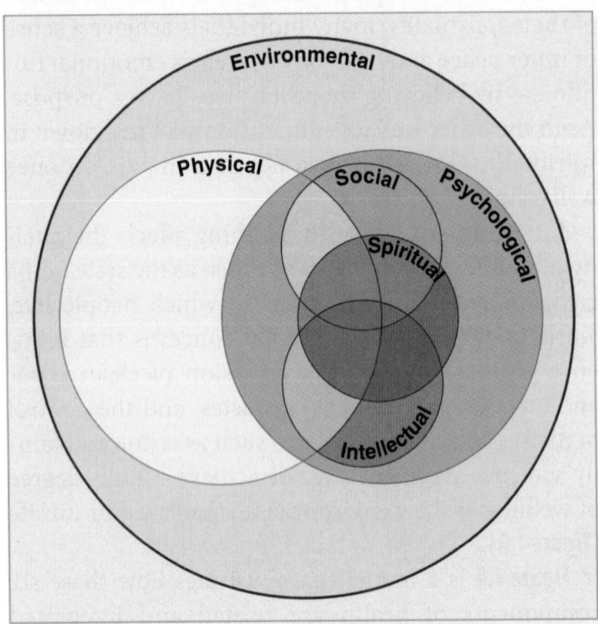

spiritual components involve thought processes; therefore, they are found in the psychological health dimension. Note how the physical and psychological spheres overlap to illustrate how the body and mind are closely integrated. When the components of health function well together, the individual has a sense of well-being.

The Nation's Health

Health involves more than just personal health—health is a national concern, too. Many of the crucial social, political, and economic issues facing this country are health related, such as domestic violence, terrorism, care of the aged, and access to health care and insurance.

Lack of health insurance and the high cost of health care are major barriers to obtaining routine preventive medical care and proper treatment. The United States spends more on health-related care per person than any other country.[7] According to the U.S. Department of Health and Human Services, total healthcare costs reached $2.7 *trillion* in 2011 and were projected to reach $5 trillion in 2022.[20] Americans generally rely on themselves and their employers, as well as private and public health insurance programs, to pay for some of their health care. Millions of Americans, however, do not have health insurance or they have inadequate insurance coverage. In 2013, an estimated 16.9% of Americans younger than 65 years of age were not covered by health insurance.[20] A major illness, serious accident, or hospitalization can quickly exhaust a person's financial resources and create enormous personal debt; therefore, it is important to have adequate health insurance to cover such expenses. The Affordable Care Act is projected to reduce the number of uninsured Americans by 30 million by 2022.[20]

Tracking the Nation's Health

The U.S. government, particularly the Public Health Service of the Department of Health and Human Services, monitors the nation's health in a variety of ways. One way is by recording cases of certain diseases and causes of death. **Table 1.1** shows preliminary data for the 10 leading causes of death for all Americans in 2010. In the United States, heart disease was the leading cause of death, followed by cancer, chronic lower respiratory disease, and stroke.[21]

The major causes of death differ for members of various age groups. **Table 1.2** shows preliminary data concerning the leading causes of death in two age categories: 15 to 24 years and 25 to 44 years. In 2009, unintentional injuries (accidents), homicide, and suicide were the top three leading causes of death of people between 15 and 24 years of age. Note that unintentional injuries, cancer, and heart disease were the top three leading causes of death of people between 25 and 44 years of age.

Over the past 100 years, Americans made great progress toward improving their health, well-being, and longevity. In 1900, the life expectancy of a newborn baby was less than 50 years. Compared to people who lived in the first half of the 20th century, many Americans can now expect to live longer lives. This progress occurred largely because various government agencies provided greater access to health care, promoted preventive healthcare efforts, funded health education and research programs, and regulated the safety of the environment. For example, childhood vaccination programs have removed the threat of polio and controlled other infectious diseases such as measles, diphtheria, rubella, and tetanus. Food fortification programs have nearly eliminated nutritional deficiency diseases such as goiter, rickets, and pellagra. Efforts to educate the public concerning the

Table 1.1

The 10 Major Causes of Death in the United States (2010)

Rank	Cause	Approx. Percentage of Deaths
1	Heart disease	24.2
2	Cancer	23.3
3	Chronic lower respiratory diseases	5.6
4	Stroke	5.2
5	Accidents/unintentional injuries	4.9
6	Alzheimer's disease	3.4
7	Diabetes mellitus	2.8
8	Pneumonia/influenza	2.0
9	Kidney disease	2.0
10	Suicide	1.6
—	Other causes	25

Modified from Heron, M. (2013). Deaths: Leading causes for 2010. *National Vital Statistics Reports*, 62(6), 1–96.

Table 1.2

Causes of Death: All Races, Selected Age Groups of American (Preliminary Data, 2010)

Ages 10-24	
Rank	**Cause**
1	Unintentional injuries
2	Suicide
3	Homicide
4	Cancer
5	Heart disease
Ages 25-44	
Rank	**Cause**
1	Unintentional injuries
2	Cancer
3	Heart disease
4	Suicide
5	Homicide

Data from Heron, M. (2013). Deaths: Leading causes for 2010. *National Vital Statistics Reports*, 62(6), 1–96.

importance of early and routine *prenatal care* (medical care for pregnant women) have helped reduce the infant death rate.

Although the life expectancy of Americans has increased, many people still die prematurely, that is, before they reach 75 years of age. According to health experts at the Centers for Disease Control and Prevention in Atlanta, actual causes of death are the underlying reasons that are not reported on death certificates. In 2000, for example, about 18% of all deaths were the result of tobacco use, including secondhand exposure to tobacco smoke; poor diet and lack of physical activity accounted for about 15% of deaths.[21] Leading causes of death tables such as **Table 1.1**, however, integrate those deaths within the number of deaths resulting primarily from heart disease, cancer, chronic lower respiratory diseases, and stroke. Health experts predict that the combination of poor diet and physical inactivity will soon replace tobacco use as the leading actual cause of death in the United States. In many instances, actual causes of death are associated with lifestyle choices, such as tobacco use or physical inactivity. By changing these and other health-related behaviors, people may avoid dying prematurely.

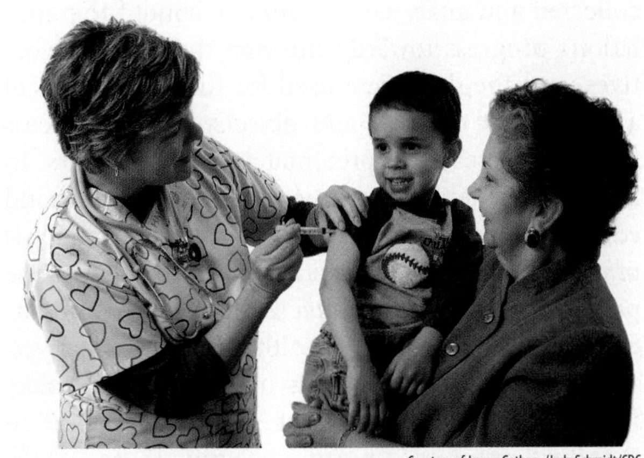

Courtesy of James Gathany/Judy Schmidt/CDC.

Health Promotion: Development of *Healthy People 2020*

Health promotion is the practice of helping people become healthier by encouraging them to take more control over their health and change their lifestyles. Health promotional efforts strive to *prevent* rather than treat disease and injury. Federal, state, and local governments can help the population develop healthy lifestyles by funding and providing educational programs and preventive medical care services. When planning effective health promotional programs, public health experts and government officials need to identify which aspects of the population's health should receive the most attention. How does the federal government identify serious health concerns and monitor the health of its citizens? What is being done to improve the nation's health?

In the late 1980s, a team of concerned health experts, health educators, and U.S. government officials analyzed the results of reports, recommendations, and studies that provided data concerning the health status of Americans. In 1991, these experts published their findings in a report called *Healthy People 2000*.[23]

Healthy People 2000 had three general goals: increase the healthy life span of Americans, improve the health status of American minorities, and extend the accessibility of preventive health services to all Americans. *Healthy People 2000* also established numerous health-related objectives that related to each goal, such as increasing the percentage of children who engaged in 20 minutes or more of vigorous physical activity at least 3 days a week. The overall aim was for Americans to achieve the health objectives by the year 2000; as more *Healthy People 2000* objectives were met, the overall health status of Americans would improve. By 2000, public health experts had collected and analyzed information about the population's progress toward achieving the health objectives, and the data were used for the publication of a revised set of goals and objectives. This process would be repeated approximately every 10 years. In 2000, the federal government released the second edition of the plan, *Healthy People 2010*. The analysis of data obtained from *Healthy People 2010* led to the publication of *Healthy People 2020*, the third and latest edition of the national health goals and objectives.

Table 1.3 indicates the four main goals of *Healthy People 2020* and factors that will be measured to monitor progress toward meeting those goals.

Table 1.3

***Healthy People 2020*: Foundation Health Measures**

Main Goals of *Healthy People 2020*	Measures of Progress
General Health Status Attain high quality, longer lives free of preventable disease, disability, injury, and premature death	Life expectancy; healthy life expectancy Years of potential life lost Physically and mentally unhealthy days Self-assessed health status Limitation of activity Chronic disease prevalence
Disparities and Inequity Achieve health equity, eliminate disparities, and improve the health of all groups	Race/ethnicity Socioeconomic status Sex; sexual orientation Disability status Geography
Social Determinants of Health Create social and physical environments that promote good health for all	Social and economic factors Natural and built environments Policies and programs
Health-Related Quality of Life and Well-Being Promote quality of life, healthy development, and healthy behaviors	Self-reports of well-being and satisfaction Quality of life Participation in common activities

Adapted from U.S. Department of Health and Human Services, Office of Disease Prevention and Health Promotion. (2010). *Healthy People 2020*. Retrieved from http://www.healthypeople.gov/2020/about/Foundation-Health-Measures

Healthy People 2020 identifies 42 "objective topic areas," including "physical activity" and "injury and violence prevention" as well as nearly 600 health objectives. An *objective* identifies target populations and a specific health concern. One of the physical activity objectives, for example, is "Increase the proportion of adults who meet current federal physical activity guidelines for aerobic physical activity and for muscle strengthening activity."

Staff of various federal, state, and local agencies are responsible for developing and implementing health education efforts, such as community and school-based programs to reduce the prevalence of childhood obesity, that support *Healthy People 2020* objectives. In addition, staff will monitor Americans' progress in meeting these health objectives. You can learn more about *Healthy People 2020* by visiting the government's website www.healthypeople.gov/2020/default.aspx.

Minority Health Status

For hundreds of years, immigrants from around the world have been changing the face of the United States as they settle in this country. Each new group of immigrants brings different cultural traditions and various ethnic identities with them (**Figure 1.5**). *Culture* consists of the unique social characteristics of a population, such as its customs, rituals, and health beliefs and practices, which are passed down from generation to generation. An ethnic group is one in which members share a common national, religious, racial, or ancestral identity. According to the U.S. Department of Health and Human Services, the major American racial/ethnic subpopulations are Caucasians (Whites), African Americans (Blacks), Latinos (Hispanics), American Indian/Alaska Natives, and Asian/Pacific Islanders. The same terms, however, are not used by all agencies. Throughout this text, terms such as *Caucasian* may be used in one context and *Whites* in another; when reporting statistics or results of research studies, the text reflects the language of the agency or researcher.

Figure 1.5

An American Family. Culture consists of the unique social characteristics of a population, such as its customs, rituals, and health practices. Immigrants who settle in the United States contribute much to the racial, ethnic, and cultural diversity of the population.

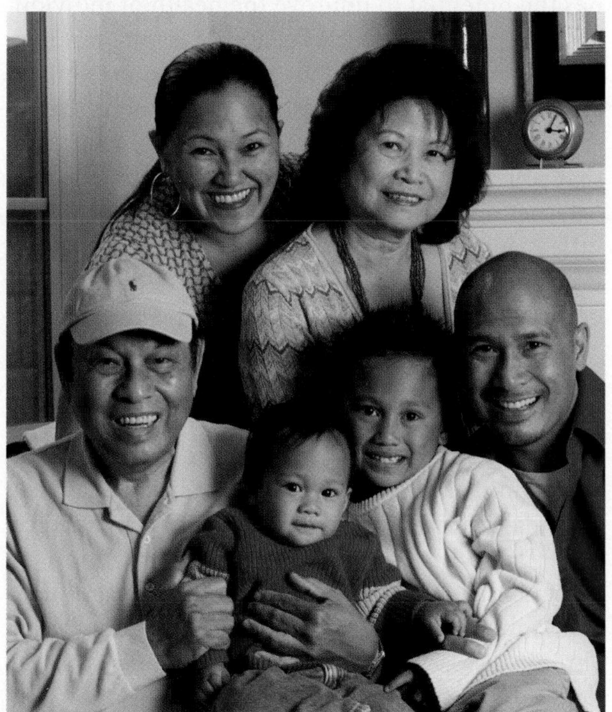

In the United States, the majority of Americans have European ancestry, particularly northern European. The National Center for Health Statistics refers to this population as "white, non-Hispanic." In 2008–2012, 74.2% of the U.S. population identified itself as "White."[24]

Differences in death and illness rates between the nation's men and women, as well as among its diverse ethnic and racial groups, are major public health concerns. For example, American men generally do not live as long as American women and are more likely to die from each of the 10 leading causes of death. More African Americans die of cancers and diseases of the heart and blood vessels than members of other ethnic and racial groups. The reasons for these differences are unclear, but socioeconomic status, environmental conditions, and lifestyle choices are major contributing factors. The term minority, however, is not strictly limited to race or ethnicity. In the U.S., minorities groups also include religious minorities (e.g., Mormons, Muslims), sexual minorities (e.g., lesbian, gay, bisexual, and transgender), age minorities (e.g., the very young or very old) and people with disabilities (e.g., those with autism).

The Diversity in Health essay addresses topics that concern a variety of populations in the United States as well as around the world. The Diversity in Health essay in this chapter, "Minority Health Status in the United States," discusses differences in the overall health of major minority groups in the United States.

Genetics and Genomics

Your lifestyle and environment influence your health status, but your *genes* also play a role in determining your health. With the exception of red blood cells, all cells in your body contain genes. **Genes** are segments of *DNA*, a complex chemical compound that codes

genes Segments of DNA that code for specific proteins.

genomics (Jee-nom-iks) The scientific study of an organism's entire set of genes.

for the production of proteins. Cells use proteins for a variety of functions, including building, maintaining, and repairing structures, such as bones and other tissues. Mistakes in the genetic code can result in the production of faulty proteins that can cause disease and even death. Genes are *inherited*, that is, their coded instructions for protein synthesis are passed on to subsequent generations.

Genetics is the scientific study of genes and the way they pass certain traits, such as the risk of breast cancer, or medical conditions, such as birth defects, from one generation to another. Thus, genetics can help people understand how certain life-threatening medical conditions, including sickle cell anemia and cystic fibrosis, tend to "run in families." Scientists have developed tests to identify the gene or genes for hundreds of diseases, most of which are rare genetic disorders such as Duchenne muscular dystrophy and certain breast and ovarian cancers.

Most of the 10 leading causes of death in the United States, particularly heart disease, cancer, stroke, diabetes, and Alzheimer's disease, have a genetic component. Unlike cases of rare genetic conditions, these common chronic diseases generally develop partly as a result of *multiple* genes interacting with behavioral and environmental risk factors, such as poor food choices, lack of physical activity, and exposure to tobacco smoke.

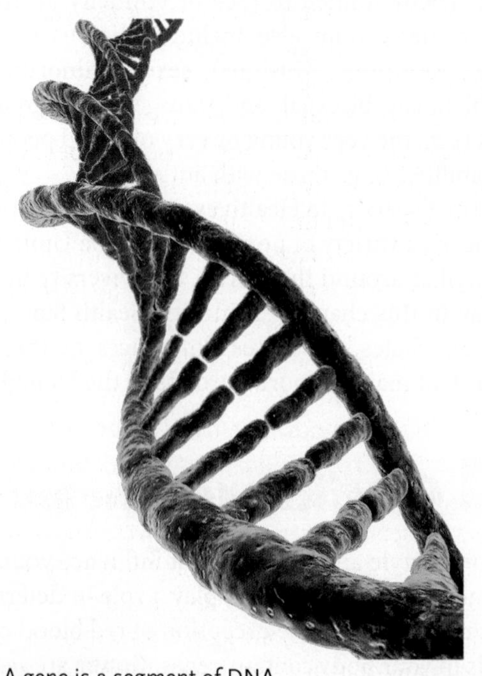

A gene is a segment of DNA.
© Hemera/Thinkstock

Genomics is the study of all of a person's genes (*genome*), including the complex ways the genes interact with each other and the environment to influence the individual's health. A person's genome can provide medical researchers with important biological clues about the individual's health status, disease risk, and responses to treatments. Scientific analysis of individual genomes may help explain why people who share similar environments or health-related behaviors do not always develop the same health conditions.

Genes play roles in a person's ability to achieve and maintain good health. Medical researchers use genetics to learn more about diseases that are caused by genes. Researchers use genomics to understand how multiple genes contribute to the development of complex diseases and how these particular genes interact with other factors, such as lifestyle and environment. As a result of such analyses, medical researchers can develop better ways to prevent, diagnose, and treat diseases.

Genomics is a relatively new science, and genomic testing, which involves combinations of biochemical and molecular methods to analyze a cell's genes, has the potential to improve the health of individuals. However, the value of genomic testing for diagnosing, predicting, and treating common chronic diseases has not been established. Public health experts are concerned about *personal genomic tests* that are directly marketed to consumers through Internet and other media outlets. At present, very little scientific evidence supports the validity and usefulness of the results of such *direct-to-consumer* genomic tests.

More research is needed to establish the usefulness of adding information obtained by genomic testing to the standard medical history that healthcare practitioners routinely collect from their patients. Maintaining a record of your health history can help you make a positive contribution to your medical care. How? When you share this information with your physicians, the medical practitioners can consider inherited factors to predict your risk of certain chronic diseases and develop ways (*interventions*) to help you prevent or forestall those diseases.

motivation The force or drive that leads people to take action.

self-efficacy (EF-fih-ka-see) Regarding health education, the belief that one is capable of changing his or her behavior.

Understanding Health Behavior

Regardless of their cultural and ethnic background, not all Americans share the same level of concern for their health. How many times have you heard a smoker say, "I can stop smoking whenever I want to; now is just not a good time" or "You've got to die of something; it might as well be lung cancer." You may know people who eat too many fatty foods, do not exercise regularly, drink too much alcohol, and smoke cigarettes. You may know other people who follow a nutritious diet, walk at a brisk pace for 45 minutes nearly every day, and avoid drugs such as alcohol and tobacco. Why do some people adopt more positive health-related behaviors than others do?

Changing Health Behavior

"I wish I had the willpower to stop smoking." "I just can't seem to find the motivation to exercise more often." Do these statements sound familiar? Is having a lot of willpower the key to becoming healthier? Is willpower alone enough to change health behavior and overcome barriers?

Health educators often use the term **motivation** to describe what is commonly referred to as willpower. Motivation, sometimes called attitude, is one of the forces or drives that lead people to take action. Past experiences, perceived needs and barriers, and personal beliefs and values influence one's motivation. For example, a person who has tried unsuccessfully to stop smoking several times and claims to enjoy smoking may have little motivation to make another attempt to quit.

Self-efficacy, individuals' belief in their ability to perform a behavior that will lead to the desired outcome, is also an important factor in changing health behavior. For example, someone who believes he or she has the ability to attend smoking cessation counseling sessions is more likely to attempt to quit smoking than someone who doesn't believe he or she has time to attend. Various barriers, such as poor education or lack of support from family members, can interfere with self-efficacy development and reduce someone's motivation to change behaviors.

Knowledge about risky behaviors and the seriousness of a health condition is another important for behavior change. Someone who smokes cigarettes, and does not know smoking causes lung cancer, will not usually be motivated to quit. On the other hand, someone who smokes and understands health risks associated with smoking, may have a different attitude toward smoking and may be motivated to quit. As we've seen, however, many other factors also influence our health behavior. For example, many people know that seat belts reduce the possibility of a serious injury in an automobile accident and that most states require them to wear seat belts in a car. Nevertheless, some people cite discomfort, restricted movement, and individual choice as reasons for not wearing seat belts regularly. Many students enrolled in personal health classes can correctly identify behaviors that promote optimal health, yet they do not regularly practice these behaviors. Acquiring knowledge about health is important, but motivation to adopt a healthier lifestyle is essential for making long-term changes that benefit our health.

Taking an active role in achieving and maintaining good health depends on certain personal factors: degree of perceived vulnerability, motivation (attitude), sense of control, and perceived value of the behavior. Health behavior research indicates people are motivated to take action if they feel that a sufficient threat to their health exists and that the consequences of changing the behavior are worthwhile. Furthermore, people are more likely to attempt a behavior if they value the behavior (i.e., the behavior is important to them), they believe the behavior (e.g., regular exercise) will lead to desired outcomes (e.g., weight loss), and they believe they have control over the behavior (i.e., I can exercise regularly if I want to).

Assume, for example, that diabetes affects several members of your family. You have heard that diabetes may be inherited; therefore, you are aware that you have a good chance of developing this condition (*vulnerability*). You know that family members who have diabetes suffer from kidney damage, blindness, and premature heart disease. Because you want to avoid these consequences, you are motivated to change certain behaviors (*motivation*). Moreover, you believe that your actions influence the quality of your health (*sense of control*). Concerned, you decide to learn more about diabetes and determine what actions can reduce your risk of developing the disease. You now

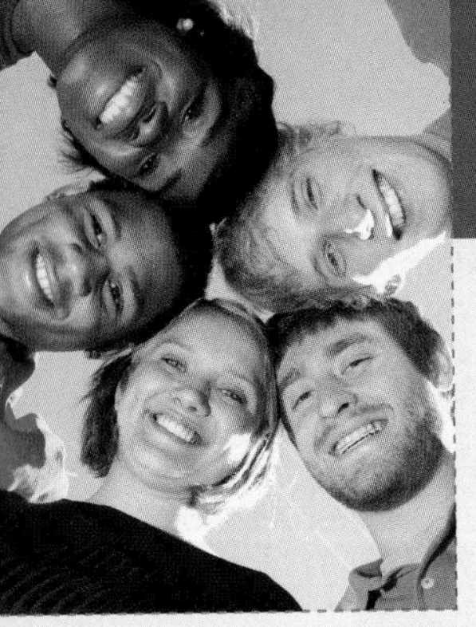
© Mike Flippo/ShutterStock

Diversity in Health

Minority Health Status in the United States

Did you know that African Americans are more likely to die of cancer than are Whites? Did you know that Hispanics are more likely to die in accidents than as the result of strokes? The differences in death and illness rates for various population subgroups reflect numerous factors, such as socioeconomic status and access to health insurance and medical care. By investigating reasons for these differences, medical researchers have learned a great deal about the health of American minorities. A major goal of the U.S. Department of Health and Human Services is improving the health of all Americans through research, education, and better access to health care.

Hispanic or Latino People

Hispanic, or Latino, people have immigrated to the United States or have ancestors from countries in which Spanish is the primary language, especially Mexico, Puerto Rico, Central and South America, and Cuba. Hispanics are the largest minority group in the United States, making up 16.7% of the population in 2011.[25]

In 2011, the leading causes of death for Hispanics were cancer, heart disease, accidental injuries, stroke, and diabetes.[20] Some Hispanic/Latino population groups have a high prevalence of asthma, obesity, chronic lung diseases, HIV infection, tuberculosis (TB), and diabetes.

Poverty, lack of health insurance, and poor education are barriers to good health for many Hispanics. About 26.6% of this minority lives in poverty.[25] Health disorders associated with poverty, such as tuberculosis and obesity, are more common in certain Spanish-speaking subgroups. In 2010, almost 31% of Hispanic Americans did not have health insurance.[22] Hispanic persons, especially those of Mexican ancestry, are more likely to be uninsured than non-Hispanic Whites. Regardless of one's ethnic/racial background, not having health insurance is a major obstacle to obtaining good health care in the United States.

African or Black Americans

In the United States, African Americans comprised 14.2% of the population in 2012; they are the second largest minority group.[24] Despite recent improvements, the health status of Black Americans is generally poorer than that of other minorities. The life expectancies of Whites and Blacks reflect their health status. In 2011, the life expectancy of African American females was 78.7 years; the life expectancy of White American females was 81.3 years. At the same time, the life expectancy of African American males was 72.1 years and that of White males was 76.6 years.[24]

The major causes of death of Black Americans are similar to those of non-Hispanic Whites. Although Black Americans are less likely to die from chronic lung diseases, Alzheimer's disease, and suicide, members of this minority are more likely to die of homicide, cancer, stroke, diabetes, HIV infection, and heart disease than are White Americans.[26] Black women are more likely to die of breast, cervical, colon, and stomach cancers than White women are, and Black men are more likely to die of lung, prostate, colon, and stomach cancers than White men are.[26]

Childbearing is riskier for an African American woman; in 2008, she was almost three times more likely to die during pregnancy or childbirth than a White woman was.29 In addition, Black infants are more likely to die during the first month of life than other babies are. In 2008, the infant death rate among Black infants was more than twice that of White babies.[26]

In 2007–2010, African Americans were more likely to have hypertension than non-Hispanic White Americans or Mexican Americans.[26] The reason for this high prevalence is unclear, but scientists think diet, genetics, stress, and smoking play roles. Overweight also increases the risk of hypertension. Black women are more likely to have excess body fat than are other Americans. In the period from 2007 to 2010, 53% of non-Hispanic Black women were obese.[26]

Asian and Pacific Islanders

As one of the fastest-growing minority groups, Asian Americans and Pacific Islanders (APIs) are a diverse group of people who immigrated to the United States from China, Japan, Vietnam, Korea, India, the Philippines, and other Pacific Islands. In 2010, Asian Americans made up about 5% of the U.S. population.[27] Asian Americans generally have lower *age-adjusted* death rates for the 10 major causes of death than do Whites and members of other minority groups.[7] This means that an average 30-year-old Asian American is less likely to die of any major cause of death, including heart disease and cancer, than is an average 30-year-old American who is a White person or a member of another minority population. Compared with other minority groups of Americans, Asian American women have the highest life expectancy.[28] Asian American women, however, are more likely to die from stomach cancer than other American women are.[27] People who immigrated recently from Asia and the Pacific Islands are more likely to suffer from hepatitis, a serious liver disease, and tuberculosis than are people who have lived in the United States for longer periods of time. Factors that contribute to the poor health status of some Asian Americans include language and cultural barriers; social disgrace (*stigma*) associated with certain conditions, especially mental illness; and lack of health insurance.[29]

American Indians and Alaska Natives

American Indian and Alaska Natives (AI/ANs) are a diverse group of people comprising only about 2% of the American population in 2011.[24] About 22% this minority population live in designated areas such as reservations or reservation trust areas, whereas 60% live in metropolitan areas. AI/ANs generally have more health problems than do Whites. Geographic isolation, poverty, inadequate sewage disposal, and cultural barriers are some of the reasons why health among AI/ANs is poorer than it is among other groups of Americans.[30]

American Indian/Alaska Native infants and children are more likely to die than other American infants and children.[28] AI/ANs are more likely to be smokers than members of other racial/ethnic groups, and binge drinking is a serious health concern of AI/ANs. Diabetes poses a health threat for many members of this minority. The rate of diabetes among AI/ANs is twice as high as the rate among Whites.[31] In addition to diabetes, mental health problems and alcohol-related deaths such as accidents, homicides, and suicides are major health concerns for AI/ANs.

The Impact of Social Conditions on Health Status

Although genetic factors may be the primary cause of many health problems, income level, health insurance coverage, educational attainment, and years living in the United States play major roles in determining a particular group's state of health. Many chronic diseases, such as tuberculosis and malnutrition, are associated with poor standards of living. Other health threats often associated with poverty include substance abuse, homicide, and lead poisoning. Poverty, however, is not limited to any single population group in the United States. Regardless of their racial or ethnic background, individuals who achieve a higher level of education usually have higher incomes and better health than those with less education.

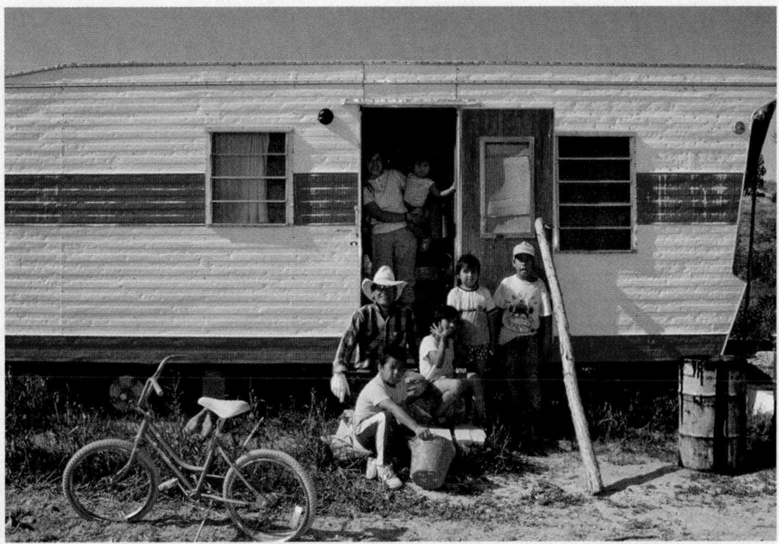

In the United States, many chronic diseases are associated with poor standards of living.

have a reason to take action because you believe it is important (*value*) to prevent this disease, even if it means making lifestyle changes now while you are still healthy.

Making Positive Health-Related Decisions

How I Quit Smoking

About a month ago I was a smoker—about 10 cigarettes a day during the week and up to a pack a day on weekends. After thinking about quitting for about a year, it happened. Without even giving it any consideration, I was able to not buy a pack for 2 days. On day 3, I realized my success and told myself I would never buy a pack again. I miss it, especially after a drink or a meal, but I'm glad I've gone this far. There have been times when I've really wanted one, but that's when you realize how powerful of a drug it is. At least that's how I talk myself out of having one. Before, I never thought of myself as being addicted—too harsh of a word—but I was just like all of the other smokers out there. It's a filthy habit—I'm glad I stopped.

Although this college student smoked less than a pack of cigarettes a day, he took about a year to quit smoking. He made the final decision to stop smoking while listening to other students' habit-breaking experiences in his health class. Some people take less time to make health-related decisions than others do, and some people have less difficulty making lifestyle changes than others do. **Figure 1.6** illustrates the complex process of decision making.

Stages of Behavior Change According to many health education experts, the process of changing behaviors involves the five stages shown in **Figure 1.7**.[35] We use the example of smoking to illustrate this process. The first stage is *precontemplation*. In this stage, smokers show no interest in quitting tobacco use, do not see a need to quit, and may avoid discussing their smoking behavior with others. Smokers move into the *contemplation* stage when they realize or admit tobacco use is unhealthy, and they intend to quit smoking in the next 6 months. In the *preparation* stage of change, smokers may have made unsuccessful attempts to quit smoking, yet they express the desire to stop within the next month. Smokers in the *action* stage of change take steps to quit smoking, such as "going cold turkey" or using a nicotine patch. They succeed in quitting for up to 6 months. Finally, smokers in the *maintenance* stage develop practices to avoid relapsing into using tobacco. Former smokers, for example, might socialize with nonsmokers or use exercise as a substitute for smoking. According to health education researchers, 40% of people who engage in risky behaviors such as smoking or being physically inactive are in the precontemplation stage,

Figure 1.6

Decision-Making Model. Decision making can be a complex process. Information, personal attitudes, and personal experiences influence your decision-making process. To change health-related behaviors, you must recognize the need to change, that the change has personal value, and that it is consistent with your beliefs.

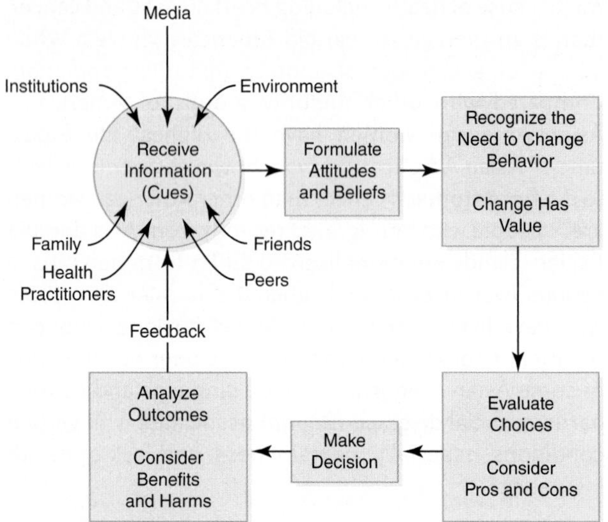

Figure 1.7

Stages of Behavior Change. According to many health education experts, the process of changing behaviors involves these five stages.

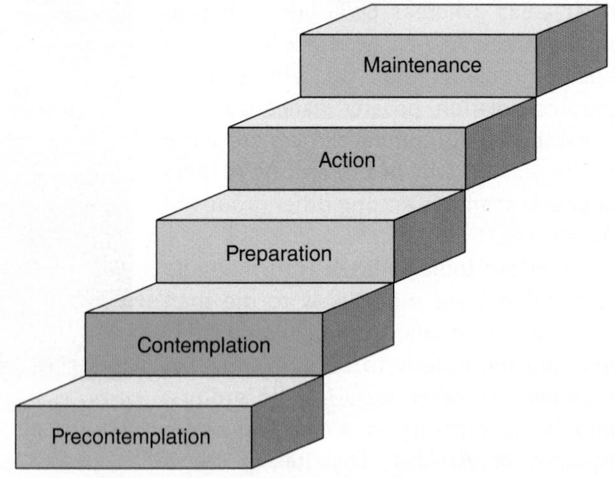

40% are in the contemplation stage, and the remaining 20% are preparing to change the unhealthy behaviors.[32]

When people *relapse*, they return to an earlier stage of change and usually feel like failures as a result of their inability to maintain the new behaviors. In the case of smokers, they may even return to the precontemplation stage in which they stop thinking about quitting. However, the majority of people who relapse eventually decide to stop smoking again, and they tend to try a different method of quitting. People who seriously want to quit smoking, for example, typically make three to four efforts to stop before they actually succeed.[33]

When changing a behavior, people use various strategies to increase their chances of success, including stimulus control, counterconditioning, rewards, and social support. *Stimulus control* involves altering cues to modify responses (behaviors). Cues can be sensory triggers, such as seeing a billboard advertisement for cigarettes or smelling someone else's cigarette smoke. Cues can also be emotional states or thoughts. For example, a person may smoke to relieve stress or because he or she associates smoking with celebrities or sophisticated people. As a result, this person is likely to light up a cigarette when tense or in certain social situations.

If you are a smoker who wants to quit, you may need to identify and eliminate the various cues that signal this unhealthy behavior. You may realize, for example, that seeing ashtrays and lighters are your smoking cues. Throwing out or giving away your ashtrays and lighters are ways of avoiding these cues. If feeling tense triggers your desire to smoke, then learning and practicing relaxation techniques whenever you feel stressed out may help you resist the urge to buy a pack of cigarettes.

Counterconditioning involves replacing unhealthy behaviors with less destructive or healthier ones. When you desire a cigarette, you may be able to eliminate the craving by exercising, taking a warm bath, or calling someone who supports your efforts to quit. Chewing sugarless gum, eating raw vegetables or fruit, or drinking a glass of water whenever you feel the urge to smoke may also reduce the craving.

Rewards are incentives for positive behaviors. Some former smokers keep a jar in which they save the money that would have been used to buy cigarettes. At the end of a week or two, they spend that money on something fun such as a movie, DVD, or another type of reward to help maintain the new behavior. Other former tobacco users are rewarded by the return of their sense of taste or the praise they receive from nonsmokers for adopting a smoke-free lifestyle.

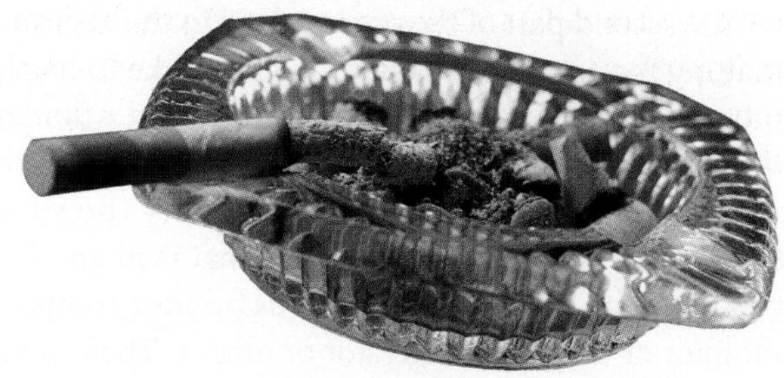

Cues are sensory triggers for behaviors, such as seeing cigarette butts as a cue for smoking.
© AbleStock

Obtaining social support by enlisting the help of others is very important for changing a negative behavior and maintaining a positive one. If you are a smoker in the contemplation stage of change and most of your friends are smokers in the precontemplation stage, they are not likely to support your efforts to quit. Therefore, you may have to associate with nonsmokers or people in later stages of change to provide the help, encouragement, and positive reinforcement you need to quit tobacco use.

A systematic model for the decision-making process can help you improve your health and well-being. A model is a plan or pattern that can be used as a guide.

The first part of the decision-making process involves identifying a problem behavior that you want to change, a goal that you would like to reach, or a question that you would like to answer. For example, you might want to quit smoking, lose 20 pounds, or determine whether you are ready to end an abusive relationship. Because the process of altering a behavior can have its unpleasant aspects, particularly if you have to overcome side effects or cravings, it is important to determine your level of commitment. To determine if you are ready to change a behavior or situation, it is helpful to make a list of the benefits, or pros, as well as the harms, or cons, of changing. After you make the list, think about each pro and con's value or importance to you. Assign a point value from 1 to 5 to each pro and con; a rating of 5 points would be the highest value. Then, find the sums of each list. If the sum of the cons list is greater than that of the pros list, you are probably in the precontemplation stage and not ready to make the change. On the other hand, if the sum of your pros is higher, you are likely in the contemplation stage and ready to make the change.

The second part of the process used in the decision-making model describes steps you can take to implement the change and evaluate your progress. After you decide to make a change, set a target date to begin the new behavior, reach the goal, or modify the situation. Mark that date on a calendar that is in an obvious place for you to notice, such as by your computer monitor or on your refrigerator or mirror. Then, make a list of factors that will increase the chances that you will be successful in making the change, such as enlisting the help of friends or obtaining advice from a medical expert. Because there are often barriers to making changes, make another list of factors that will hinder your chances for success, such as having little time to practice new behaviors or friends who will not support your decision to change.

The third major step in the process involves preparing an action plan that provides specific steps you will take to change your behavior or situation. You should be able to identify more than one way to reach your goal. To quit smoking, for example, you might quit "cold turkey," gradually reduce the number of cigarettes smoked over a 4-week period, or use a medically approved nicotine-containing product. At this point, you need to learn about the pros and cons of each method and consider the factors that can help or hinder your effort to change. How are you going to handle cravings or social situations that promote the behavior you are trying to change? Now you are ready to make the change by implementing your action plan. Keep a daily record of your progress, including strategies that are helpful and your feelings about the process. When you reach the goal date, analyze your success in attaining the goal. How well did your plan work? What can you learn from the experience?

To enjoy a long, healthy, and productive life, it is important for you to make numerous health-related decisions every day. If you act impulsively and base these decisions simply on cues, attitudes, and emotions, you may make poor choices. However, you are likely to make responsible choices if you follow a systematic method of decision making such as the one we describe. Changing habits often requires learning new information and practicing new skills.

The Goal of Prevention

A primary focus of health promotion is preventing diseases, infections, injuries, birth defects, and other serious health conditions. Preventing a health problem is a far better and less costly option than trying to treat it. In addition to adopting healthy lifestyle practices, serious health problems can also be prevented by having routine physical examinations. The Managing Your Health box that follows provides recommendations for the frequency of routine screening procedures such as blood pressure, cholesterol, mammograms, prostate exams, and Pap smears (cervical cancer detection). Some examinations, such as testicular and breast self-exams, can be done in the privacy of your home. Some college students do not believe routine physical evaluations are important; however, having regular medical checkups enables you and your physician to monitor your physical and psychological health status. Furthermore, your physician may be able to identify a problem before it results in serious damage to your health and well-being.

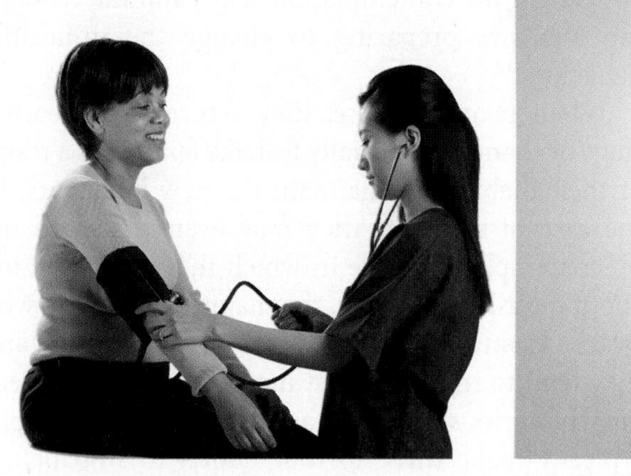

Can Good Health Be Prescribed?

No one has a crystal ball that predicts future health, and neither can anyone guarantee good health. Numerous factors contribute to an individual's chances of enjoying a long and productive lifetime of good health. Several of these factors are the result of lifestyle choices that people can make, while they are still young, to prevent or delay disease. You may know someone or have heard about individuals who avoided exercise, smoked a pack of cigarettes, and consumed a six-pack of beer each day, yet lived to a ripe old age. Such behavior defies nearly every reasonable prescription for good health. Perhaps these people inherited genes that foster the hardiness to withstand the effects of their risky lifestyles. You might wonder if these people enjoyed good health throughout their lives, or if they spent their last years in poor health. Would their lives have been even longer and healthier if they had followed more health-conscious behaviors?

Managing Your Health

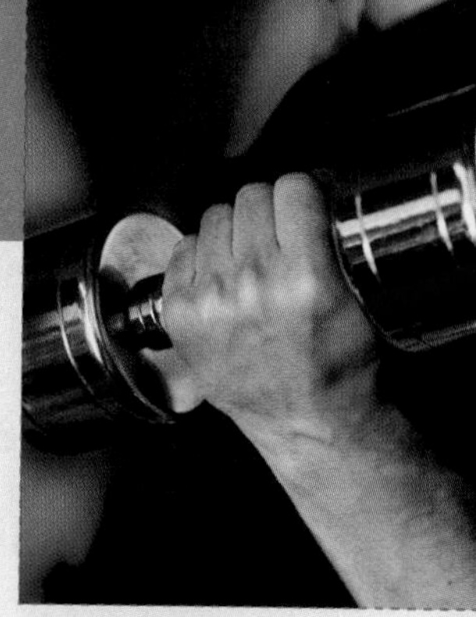

© Kzenon/ShutterStock

Routine Health Care for Disease Prevention: Adult Recommendations

The following recommendations apply to adults who have low risks of disease. People who have higher risks may need more frequent testing and to begin testing at an earlier age. Consult your personal physician for advice about routine testing and immunization schedules.

Medical Test/Preventive Measure	Recommended Frequency
Blood pressure	At least every 2 years
Cholesterol (fasting lipoprotein profile)	Every 5 years for people aged 20 and older
Glucose	Asymptomatic adults with sustained blood pressure greater than 135/80 mm Hg
PSA and digital rectal exam (detects prostate cancer)	Discuss the need for testing with physician
Testicular exam	Some physicians recommend regular exams; discuss need for exam with physician
Skin exam (detects skin cancer)	Have physician check skin during routine general exams
Breast exam (detects breast cancer)	American Cancer Society recommends annual screen and clinical breast exams for healthy women aged 40 years and older; women between 20 and 39 years of age should undergo clinical breast exam every 3 years. Breast self-exam is an option for women
Pap test (detects cervical cancer)	Begin screening within 3 years of first sexual intercourse or by 21st birthday; yearly Pap test, or every 2 years if liquid form of test is used. Beginning at age 30 years, include human papillomavirus (HPV) test
Colon/rectal examination (detects cancer)	Have flexible sigmoidoscopy or colonoscopy at age 50 years; physician can decide which test is appropriate and how often testing should be repeated
Sexually transmitted infections	Sexually active people who are 25 years of age or younger should be tested annually for chlamydial infection; older women should be tested if they have new or multiple sex partners. Physician can decide which other tests are appropriate, such as for HIV infection
Immunizations	
Rubella	One or two doses from ages 19 to 55
Influenza	Annually for adults aged 19 and older
Tetanus	Every 10 years
Hepatitis B	Three doses

Recommendations vary among medical organizations.

Data from U.S. Centers for Disease Control and Prevention. (2014). Recommended adult immunization schedule—United States—2014. Retrieved from http://www.cdc.gov/vaccines/schedules/hcp/imz/adult.html; Agency for Healthcare Research and Quality. (2012). Guide to Clinical and Preventive Services, 2012. Retrieved from http://www.ahrq.gov/professionals/clinicians-providers/guidelines-recommendations/guide/section1.html#ref12; Centers for Disease Control and Prevention. (n.d.) National HIV and STD testing resources. Retrieved from http://hivtest.cdc.gov/faq.aspx#stdtest; American Cancer Society. (2013). American Cancer Society guidelines for early detection of cancer. Retrieved from http://www.cancer.org/healthy/findcancerearly/cancerscreeningguidelines/american-cancer-society-guidelines-for-the-early-detection-of-cancer

anecdotes Personal reports of individual experiences.

testimonials Individual claims about the value of a product.

Analyzing Health Information

"Take antioxidants to live longer." "Drink red wine to prevent heart attacks." "Improve your memory with ginkgo." Every day Americans are barraged with a confusing array of health-related information in newspapers, magazines, television and radio shows, commercials, and infomercials. Family members, friends, medical professionals, and the Internet also supply information about health and health-related products. Are these sources reliable? Not necessarily. No laws prevent anyone from making statements or writing books about health, even if their information is false. The First Amendment to the U.S. Constitution protects freedom of speech and freedom of the press. This protection extends to talk show hosts and guests, authors, and salespeople in health food stores who might provide health misinformation.

Companies and individuals can make considerable amounts of money by selling untested remedies, worthless cures, unnecessary herbal supplements, and books filled with misinformation. Health frauds include the promotion or sale of substances or devices that are touted as being effective to diagnose, prevent, cure, or treat health problems, but the scientific evidence to support their safety and effectiveness is lacking.

Despite the regulatory activities of the Food and Drug Administration (FDA) and Federal Trade Commission (FTC), the sale of fraudulent products and services and the circulation of false or misleading health information continue to be concerns of medical experts. For information about the roles of the FDA and FTC in regulating health-related information, see the Consumer Health feature that follows.

Becoming a Wary Consumer of Health Information

Maybe you have read an article or an ad about the health benefits of an herbal supplement or a weight loss device that you might buy. Perhaps you watched a physician promote his "antiaging, high-energy" diet on a TV show. How do you know if health-related information and claims that are in the media and from other sources are true? Will the supplement, device, product, or diet do what its promoters claim? Or will you merely be wasting your money?

As shown in Figure 1-6, information is a crucial element of decision making. Although health information from some sources is based on scientific evidence and can be extremely useful, that from other sources may be unreliable. Relying on flawed information can waste time and money and can even be dangerous. To be a wary consumer of health information, you need to learn how to analyze it.

Analysis Model Analyzing something simply means breaking it down into its component parts for study. Analyzing information is easier to do if you follow a particular model of analysis. The following model is a series of questions that will help you evaluate health information and determine if it is reliable, regardless of its source.

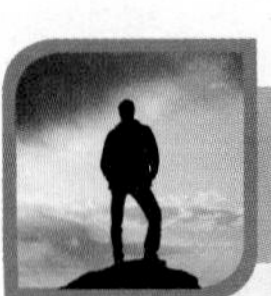

© djgis/ShutterStock

Healthy Living Practices

- To change your health-related behaviors, you must determine that you need to change and that you value the change.
- Use a decision-making plan as a tool to help you make responsible decisions.
- Take charge of your health by having regular physical examinations and monitoring your health.

1. **Which statements are verifiable facts, and which are unverified statements or value claims?** In the context of this model, *verifiable facts* are conclusions drawn from scientific research. *Unverified statements* are conclusions that have no such support. *Value claims* are statements suggesting that something is useful, or effective, or has other worthwhile characteristics. Look for unverified statements and value claims; such information may or may not be true. Also, be wary of claims that "sound too good to be true."

   Look for *red-flag* terms, expressions that indicate the possibility of irrelevant information or misinformation, such as "patented formula," "all-natural," "no risk," "chemical-free," "clinically tested," "scientifically proven," or "everyone is using." Claims that the product or service provides "quick," "painless," "effortless," or "guaranteed" cure or other desirable results are also red flags.

   Ignore *anecdotes* and *testimonials*. **Anecdotes** are personal reports of individual experiences, such as "I take vitamin C and zinc pills, and I

Consumer Health

Consumer Protection

The U.S. government has laws and agencies to protect consumers against health fraud.

The federal agencies that enforce consumer protection laws include the Food and Drug Administration (FDA) and the Federal Trade Commission (FTC). The FDA protects consumers by regulating the information that manufacturers can place on food or drug product labels. In addition, FDA personnel alert consumers about fraudulent health practices and can seize untested or unsafe medical devices and drugs. The manufacturers of such products can be punished (usually fined) for their illegal practices. The FTC regulates claims made in advertisements for products and services. Both agencies regulate only products and services involved in interstate commerce. The FDA's website is www.fda.gov, and the FTC's website is www.ftc.gov.

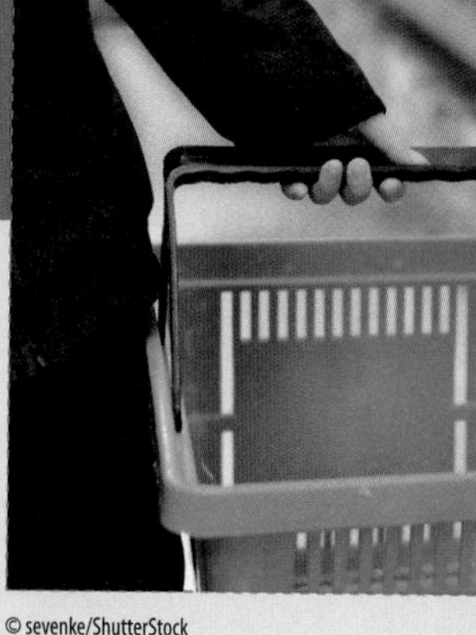
© sevenke/ShutterStock

To avoid being victims of health frauds, people must take the initiative and be very critical when judging the reliability of health-related information. If you suspect fraudulent activity, you can file a complaint with the local office of the FDA or your state's attorney general. You can also file a lawsuit if you have been injured as a result of following the advice or using the services or products of unscrupulous practitioners and manufacturers.

never get colds." **Testimonials** are claims individuals make concerning the value of a product. Advertisers often rely on paid celebrities to provide testimonials. Anecdotes may be interesting and testimonials may be persuasive, but these sources of information reflect the experiences of individuals and may not be true for most people. More compelling evidence, on the other hand, involves results of studies of hundreds or thousands of people. Such findings are more likely to be generalized to a wide population.

Look for *disclaimers* on product labels or in advertisements, such as "This statement has not been evaluated by the FDA," "This product is not intended to diagnose, treat, cure, or prevent disease," or "Results are not typical." In televised or written ads, disclaimers usually appear in small print near the end of the ad. Disclaimers may provide important information to consider.

2. **What are the credentials of the person who makes health-related claims? Does this person have the appropriate background and education in the topic area? What can you do to check the person's credentials?** Often it is difficult to tell if a health "expert" is qualified to make claims. Articles and books usually include the name and credentials of the author, but the credentials may be fraudulent. Anyone can call himself or herself a "nutritionist," "doctor," or "health expert." Therefore, a PhD or the title "Certified . . ." after someone's name is no guarantee that this person has had extensive training in a health or science field from an accredited educational institution. Individuals can buy certain doctorate degrees through the mail or Internet from unaccredited colleges called "diploma mills." To determine if a college or university is accredited, visit the U.S. Department of Education's website (www.ed.gov).

One way to investigate an author's medical or scientific expertise is to see if his or her work has been published in reputable journals. To conduct

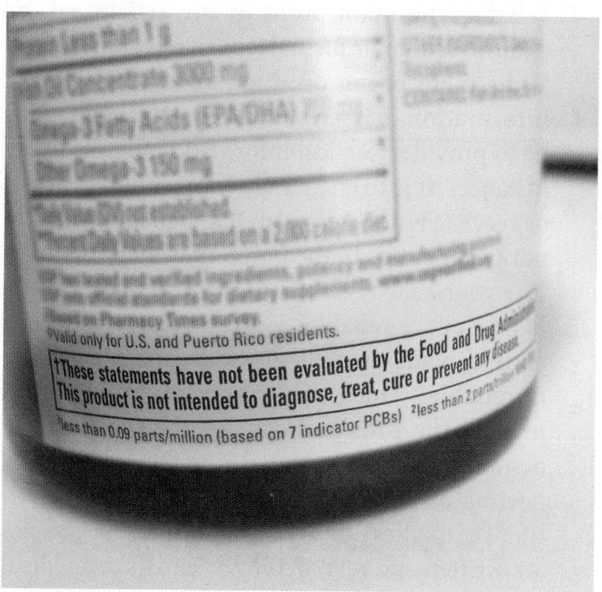

Disclaimer on a dietary supplement label.
Courtesy of Wendy Schiff.

quackery The practice of medicine without having the proper training and credentials.

a literature search, use a site such as PubMed, which is sponsored by the National Library of Medicine (www.ncbi.nlm.nih.gov/pubmed/).

Quackery is the practice of medicine without having the proper training and credentials. *Quackwatch* is a website operated by retired psychiatrist Stephen Barrett, vice president of the Institute for Science and Medicine and a fellow of the Committee for Skeptical Inquiry. Quackwatch (www.quackwatch.com/) provides information about health-related frauds as well as people, popular books, and organizations that are sources of questionable health information.

3. **What might be the motives and biases of the person making the claims?** *Motive* is the incentive, purpose, or reason for which someone promotes health misinformation. People profit from the sales of books as well as bogus treatments and products. Thus, ads are always written to motivate the consumer to buy the treatment, product, or service. A *bias* is the tendency to have a particular point of view. The author of a book or article, for example, may present information that supports his or her bias and ignores opposing views or research findings that do not support the bias. When analyzing health-related information, it is important to take into account the motives and biases of the people providing the information as you draw conclusions from it.
4. **What is the main point of the article, ad, or claim? Which information is relevant to the issue, main point, product, or service? Which information is irrelevant?** The main point may be to provide practical information, but in many instances, it is to encourage you to buy a product or service. Ignore terms and information that are not pertinent or to the point; they will only confuse your analysis.
5. **Is the source reliable? What evidence supports your conclusion that the source is reliable or unreliable? Does the source of information present the pros and cons of the topic or the benefits and risks of the product?** Look for supporting or more in-depth information in scientific or medical journals because their articles are written and reviewed by scientists or medical experts. Articles in reputable scientific journals have been *peer reviewed*, meaning their content was critiqued by experts in that field before it was accepted for publication. If peer reviewers think a study was poorly designed or provides questionable conclusions, the article describing the study is likely to be rejected by the journal's editor.

   Be wary of sources, such as magazines, books, and journals that look like bona fide providers of health information, but may not be. In many instances, they are actually designed to sell products or services. Such publications have articles about the benefits of healthcare products and include advertisements and instructions for ordering these products, often in the article or next to it.

   Be skeptical of promoters, articles, or ads that do not present the risks along with the benefits of using a health product or service. For example, a reliable article about taking bee pollen supplements should present scientific evidence from peer-reviewed journals to support as well as refute health claims. Moreover, reliable sources of information often caution people about the hazards of using treatments, and they may include recommendations to seek the advice of more than one medical expert.
6. **Does the source of information attack the credibility of conventional scientists or medical authorities?** In some instances, people making health claims try to confuse readers by implying that evidence-based medicine is unreliable. For example, an ad for a treatment to relieve back pain may include claims that the technique is "unknown to Western medicine" or "used for centuries in China." Such claims suggest that conventional medical practitioners, including physicians, dietitians, and nurse practitioners, lag behind ancient systems of health care in finding cures or treatments. Statements that attack the reliability of conventional (scientific) medical practitioners are usually indications that the information is unreliable.

Finding reliable sources of health-related information can be challenging. You can usually obtain reliable answers to your questions from experts at state and local health departments, universities and colleges, local hospitals, and federal health agencies.

Assessing Information on the Internet

The Internet can be a valuable source of health-related information. The U.S. government maintains

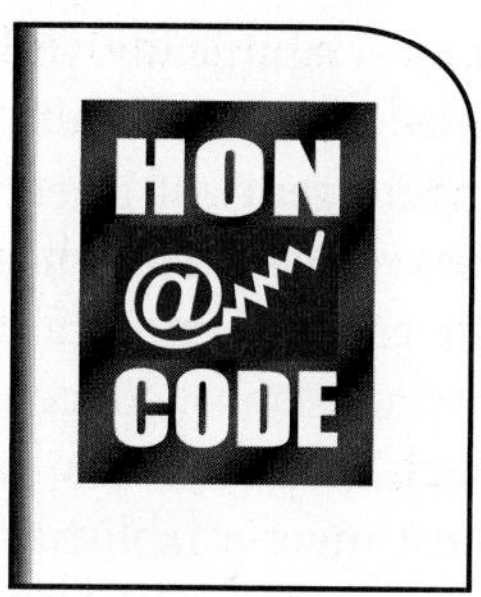

© Health On the Net Foundation

websites for health-related information, including the sites of the Centers for Disease Control and Prevention (www.cdc.gov), Food and Drug Administration (www.fda.gov), and National Institutes of Health (www.nih.gov). Additionally, the Department of Health and Human Services sponsors www.healthfinder.gov, a general health information site that provides links to reliable sources, including government agencies, universities, and nonprofit health organizations.

Websites that are accredited by the Health on the Net (HON) Foundation (www.healthonnet.org/pat.html) are reliable sources of health-related or medical information. This nonprofit organization is headquartered in Switzerland and provides a widely recognized and accepted code of ethics. Websites can become certified by adhering to the HONcode. The HON site also provides a search engine to research trustworthy sources of health information (www.healthonnet.org/HONsearch/Patients/index.html).

Although HON monitors the websites it certifies, no organization regulates the quality and truthfulness of all the health information on the Internet. Many websites are sources of inaccurate and potentially harmful information. Therefore, you need to analyze the reliability of health information from websites as critically and carefully as you analyze health information from other sources. In addition, when researching a health topic, seek information from more than one Internet source and consult a medical professional before following advice from the Web.

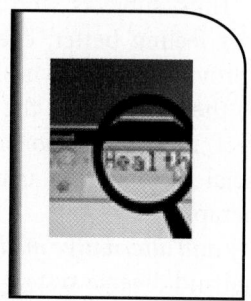

© Health On the Net Foundation

When using a website as a source of health-related information, determine answers to the following questions to help you establish credibility of the site.

- **What is the source of the information?** Websites sponsored by individuals may give questionable advice that is based on personal experiences, biases, or opinions rather than medical expertise and scientific evidence, unless the individuals are credentialed experts. Commercial sites (.com) may or may not contain misinformation, but keep in mind that their purpose is generally commercial not educational. As with any commercial endeavor, the focus is usually selling products, so what is stated is meant to entice the buyer. Websites sponsored by organizations (.org) may or may not provide credible information as well. However, there are many good .com and .org sources of health-related information. Asking yourself the next questions will help you determine which of those sites likely provides reliable health-related information.
- **Is the site sponsored by a nationally known health or medical organization or affiliated with a well-known medical research institution or major university? If not, is the site staffed by well-respected and credentialed experts in the field?** Such sites usually provide accurate and timely health information. Some have independent review boards to ensure that the site maintains accuracy and timeliness. Websites providing credible health-related information usually include documentation of the expertise of the staff and the background of the institution or organization.
- **Does the site include up-to-date references from well-known, respected medical or scientific journals or links to reputable websites, such as nationally recognized medical organizations?** Such information generally helps support the claims or information on the site and provides ways to research the claims in-depth. Providing such references also shows that the information is based on published research.
- **Is the information at the website current?** Health information is constantly changing; the site should indicate when the information was posted and updated.

conventional medicine The form of medicine that relies on modern scientific principles, modern technologies, and scientifically proven methods to prevent, diagnose, and treat health conditions.

placebo A sham treatment that has no known physical effects; an inactive substance.

Applying What You Have Learned

The Analyzing Health-Related Information feature in this text provides examples of ads, articles, and websites to help you determine the value of health-related information. To sharpen your critical thinking skills, analyze the information in these features using the six points of the analysis model. When you analyze a website, use the questions posed in the previous section. If you determine that the website is highly credible, your analysis is completed. If, however, you are unsure of the credibility of the site after answering the Web analysis questions, then continue with the six Analyzing Health-Related Information questions. Additionally, the Consumer Health features provide tips to help you become a better consumer of health information.

To obtain reliable answers for your health-related questions, consult experts at clinics or hospitals, state and local health departments, universities and colleges, federal health agencies, and nationally recognized health associations and foundations.

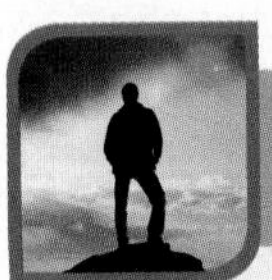

© djgis/ShutterStock

Healthy Living Practices

- Use the model for analyzing health-related information and the questions for analyzing websites to evaluate information from the media and other sources.

Conventional Medicine, Complementary and Alternative Medicine, and Integrative Medicine

Conventional medicine (scientific medicine) relies on modern scientific principles, modern technologies, and scientifically proven methods to prevent, diagnose, and treat health conditions. The notion that certain agents of infection such as bacteria and viruses cause many health disorders is accepted by conventional medical practitioners. To practice in their professions, conventional healthcare practitioners, such as physicians, nurses, dietitians, and dentists, must meet established national and/or state standards concerning their education and pass licensing examinations. To maintain their professional certification or licensing, many types of conventional healthcare practitioners must update their medical backgrounds regularly by participating in continuing education programs. Most Americans use the services of conventional medical practitioners.

Before adopting a method of treatment, conventional medical practitioners want to know if it is safe and effective. To determine the safety and effectiveness of a treatment, medical researchers usually conduct studies on animals before testing humans in *clinical studies*. A clinical study should contain at least 30 subjects, preferably hundreds or thousands, if possible. The greater the number of participants in the study, the more likely the findings did not occur by chance and are the result of the treatment.

In designing clinical studies, researchers take a group of volunteers with similar characteristics and randomly divide them into two groups: a treatment group and a control group. Subjects in the treatment group receive the experimental treatment; members of the control group are given a placebo. A **placebo**, often referred to as a "sugar pill," is a sham treatment that has no known physical effects. Because a person's positive expectations can result in positive findings, placebos help rule out the effects of such wishful thinking.

Researchers give subjects placebos to compare their responses to responses of subjects who receive the actual treatment. In *double-blind studies*, subjects and researchers are unaware of the identity of those taking placebos. Placebos can temporarily relieve subjective complaints, such as pain, lack of energy, and poor mood. Thus, subjects who are given placebos often report feeling better, even though the placebo did not provide any known physical effects. Scientists refer to these reports as the *placebo effect*. The placebo effect may be responsible for many claims of beneficial results from using unconventional medical therapies.

Complementary and alternative medicine (*CAM*) is an unconventional and diverse system of preventing, diagnosing, and treating diseases that emphasizes

Analyzing Health-Related Information

For centuries, doctors in the Orient have known about the wonders of herbal medicines—nature's botanical cures for human ailments.

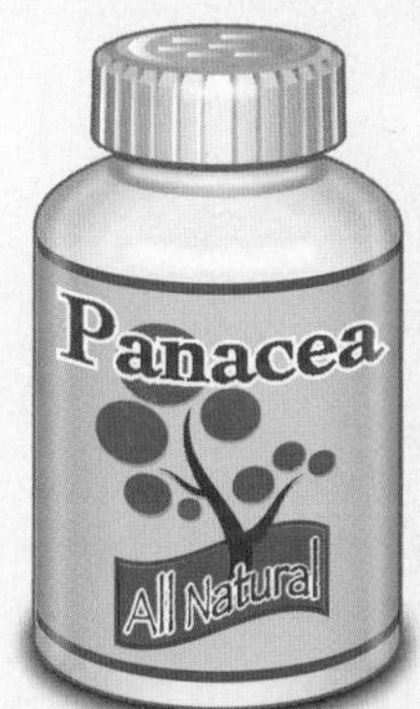

Finally, American scientists are recognizing the healthful benefits of these herbs.

SwayCon Pharmaceuticals has developed a capsule that contains everything you need to reduce suffering, enhance health, and regain youthful vigor.

A team of medical experts from three major medical schools in the United States have clinical proof that the ingredients of Panacea are effective! Panacea contains a chemical-free mixture of natural enzymes and exotic herbs that

- relieve up to 80% more arthritis pain than aspirin;
- lower blood pressure by up to 20%;
- lower cholesterol by up to 45%;
- reduce lung cancer risk by as much as 50%, even in smokers;
- and reduce the risk of heart attack by 75%.*

Other remarkable findings

Taking Panacea for a few months can improve intelligence. R.P., a college student at a large East Coast university, reports, "At the beginning of the fall semester, I started taking three capsules of Panacea a day. My G.P.A. went from a 1.8 to a 3.4! Panacea has helped me get all A's!"

Reports are coming into our offices that Panacea acts as a sexual stimulant, increasing potency. S.D., a computer programmer in St. Louis, writes, "Thanks for saving my marriage. Before taking Panacea, my husband complained about my lack of interest in sex. One of my friends told me that Panacea can help. Just a few days after taking the capsules, our marriage turned into a perpetual honeymoon."

Panacea is only available in fine health food stores. Order a three-month supply now, while supplies last

A PANACEA PILL A DAY KEEPS THE EXPENSIVE DOCTORS AWAY!

* These statements have not been evaluated by the FDA.

This suggests that American scientists do not understand that medicines can be derived from plant sources, when, in fact, American researchers often rely on plants as sources of chemicals that have medicinal uses. No scientific evidence is cited to show that the herbs in Panacea have the touted properties. These two sentences, then, contain only value claims; thus, the information may be unreliable.

This statement has value claims that are not supported with scientific evidence.

No treatment contains everything each person needs to improve his or her health.

"Clinical proof" is a red flag. The medical experts and medical schools where their research has been conducted are not identified. Objective testing could show the product is neither safe nor effective. The ad should cite the specific effects of the product, including negative ones.

"Chemical-free" is a red flag; all matter, including herbs and other plants, is comprised of chemicals. Furthermore, scientific studies should be cited to provide evidence for these value claims.

A testimonial from an individual is not scientific evidence. This student's G.P.A. my have risen for a variety of reasons. Studies conducted to show that a treatment is useful should contain at least 30 subjects.

"Potency" is a vague and undefined red-flag term. Again, this testimonial is a value claim that is unsupported by scientific evidence.

This is irrelevant information. Where the product is sold has nothing to do with its quality or characteristics. The authors of the ad are simply trying to make their product look superior to other similar products.

This statement gives the impression that consumers have no time to investigate the product thoroughly. It is intended to make consumers think that the product will sell out if they wait, and they will miss out on a good thing. Again, this information is irrelevant.

No scientific evidence is cited that a daily Panacea pill prevents serious illness. Additionally, this statement attacks conventional medical practitioners by implying that they are interested only in making money, which suggests that physicians can't be trusted.

Disclaimer

Conclusion: This ad is merely a collection of value claims that are not supported by scientific research. The ad further attempts to encourage the reader to purchase the product by suggesting that it is better (and less expensive) than conventional therapies. It claims to relieve a wide range of health conditions. The red-flag phrases and testimonials, lack of scientific evidence, and failure to caution consumers about potential hazards of the product all suggest the ad is an unreliable source of health-related information.

integrative medicine System of medical care that emphasizes personalized health care and disease prevention.

dietary supplement A product that is consumed to add nutrients, herbs, or other plant materials to a person's diet.

spirituality, self-healing, and harmonious interaction with the environment.[34] A treatment is *complementary* when it is used along with scientific medical care. A young man with liver cancer, for example, may use yoga and meditation to accompany the conventional medical treatments prescribed by his physician. An *alternative* therapy replaces conventional medical therapy. If the patient with liver cancer stops his prescribed treatments and substitutes fasting and coffee enemas in hopes of a cure, he is relying on alternative forms of medical care.

CAM can be classified as follows:

- *Alternative medical systems*, such as Ayurveda, traditional Chinese medicine, homeopathy, and naturopathy
- *Manipulative therapies*, such as spinal manipulation (chiropractic), osteopathy, reflexology, rolfing, and therapeutic massage
- *Mind–body interventions*, such as meditation, biofeedback, prayer, and creative arts healing (music therapy, for example)
- *Biologically based treatments*, such as aromatherapy, special foods (probiotic yogurt, for example), herbal teas, and large doses of vitamins
- *Energy therapies*, such as acupuncture, acupressure, and use of magnets

Figure 1.8

Acupuncture. Some physicians combine acupuncture with conventional forms of medical care. Acupuncture may stimulate the body to release natural pain-relieving compounds, but its effectiveness is difficult to test scientifically.

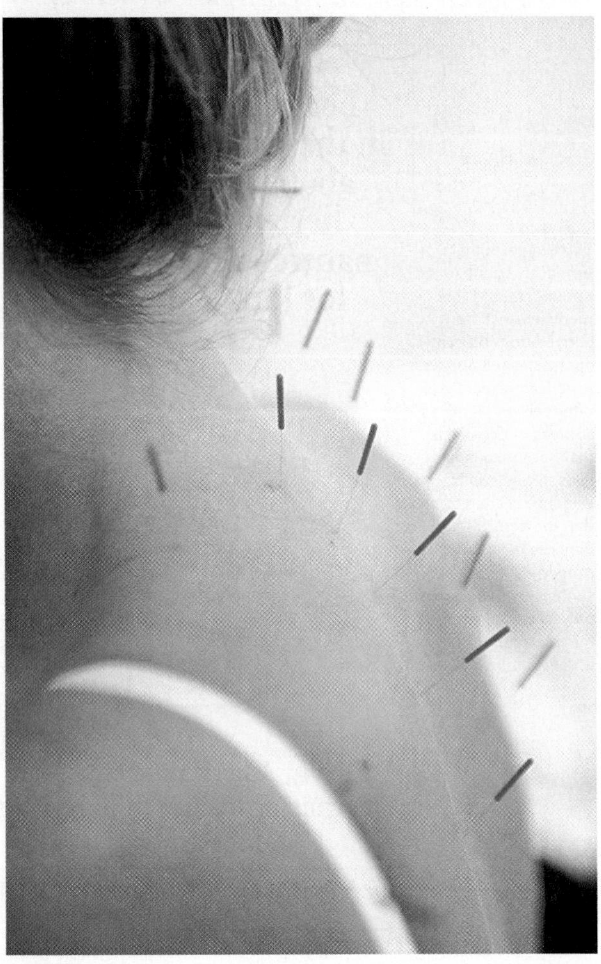

Certain CAM therapies have positive effects on the body and mind. For example, acupuncture (**Figure 1.8**) can relieve the nausea and vomiting that often occur after surgery or that are associated with early pregnancy and lower back pain.[35] Although difficult to test scientifically, aromatherapy and therapeutic massage can be soothing and relaxing. **Table 1.4** provides information about popular CAM practices, including homeopathy and reflexology.

Promoters of certain CAM practices claim diseases can be prevented or cured by "cleansing" tissues, "eliminating toxins" from the body, and "balancing chi." To support claims of their method's effectiveness, promoters often use anecdotal reports and testimonials. Nevertheless, the effectiveness of most CAM therapies is not supported by results of well-designed clinical studies.

Conventional medicine focuses on the "disease-oriented" approach, which seeks to diagnose and treat illnesses. Many physicians practice **integrative medicine**, which emphasizes personalized health care and disease prevention. Integrative medical practitioners focus on ways to encourage people to take greater responsibility for achieving and maintaining good health and well-being. Such practitioners also recognize the potential value of incorporating forms of alternative medicine that have scientific support into their preventive healthcare practices.

Table 1.4

Common Alternative Medical Practices

Type	Claims and Principles of Practice	Results of Scientific Research
Acupuncture	Used to treat a variety of common ailments. Based on an ancient Chinese medical practice in which thin needles are inserted into the skin or underlying muscles at specific places and stimulated to regulate the flow of "chi," the life force.	Testing acupuncture scientifically is difficult. It may relieve nausea and vomiting associated with "morning sickness," recovery from surgery, and cancer chemotherapy. Acupuncture may stimulate the body to release natural pain-relieving compounds.
Ayurvedic medicine	According to ancient Hindu religious beliefs, one achieves good health by meditating; eating grains, ghee (a form of butter), milk, fruits, and vegetables; and using herbs. Lack of balance between "energies" causes health problems. Fasting and enemas are used to treat severe ailments.	Meditation relieves stress; fruits, vegetables, and dairy products are nutritious foods; and some herbs have medicinal value. Ghee, however, can be fattening, and fasting can be dangerous for unhealthy people. Enemas are unnecessary for good health and should be used only under a physician's instructions.
Chiropractic medicine	According to some chiropractors, misaligned spinal bones cause disease. Spinal manipulation prevents or cures disease by correcting the spine. Other practitioners use spinal manipulation, but accept the germ theory of disease.	Can be effective in treating certain types of back pain, but some spinal conditions require medications and surgery that only a physician can provide. There is no scientific evidence that any disease can be treated by spinal adjustment.*
Homeopathy	Use of extremely dilute solutions of natural substances to treat specific illness symptoms.	Studies do not indicate that homeopathy is effective.
Naturopathy or natural medicine	Practice based on natural healing. Practitioners believe diseases occur as the body rids itself of wastes and toxins. Treatments include fasting, enemas, acupuncture, and "natural" drugs.	Lack of standardized medical training for practitioners called "naturopaths."
Therapeutic massage, reflexology, or zone therapy	Specific areas of the body correspond to certain organs. To alleviate pain or treat certain diseases, practitioners massage or press on the area that is related to the affected tissues.	The practice may stimulate the body to release pain-relieving compounds, but testing "touch" therapies scientifically is difficult. In general, scientific evidence does not indicate that pressing on body parts is an effective method of diagnosing or treating ailments.

*Data from: Ernst, E. (2008). Chiropractic: A critical evaluation. *Journal of Pain and Symptom Management, 35*(5), 544–562. Ernst, E., & Posaszki, P. (2011). An independent review of NCCAM-funded studies of chiropractic. *Clinical Rheumatology, 30*(5), 593–600.

Herbs as Medicines

Many Americans ingest pills or teas made from herbs and other plants because they think these products are natural and harmless ways to cure various disorders or achieve optimal health and well-being. The U.S. government classifies herbal products as *dietary supplements.* A **dietary supplement** is a product that is consumed to add nutrients, herbs, or other plant materials to a person's diet. Dietary supplements are not regulated by the FDA like medications are. As a result, the FDA does not require dietary supplement manufacturers to register their products and submit clinical evidence indicating that the products have been tested for safety and effectiveness prior to being marketed. In 2007, the FDA established a new rule that required manufacturers of dietary supplements to test the purity, strength, and composition of their products before marketing them to consumers. As a result, dietary supplements sold in the United States should be accurately labeled, contain the ingredients listed on the label, and provide standard amounts of the substances.

When the FDA determines that an ingredient contained in dietary supplements is dangerous, the agency can ban its use. Furthermore, the FDA can remove a dietary supplement from the market if its label states claims about the product's health benefits that are not supported by scientific evidence. The FDA permits herbal supplement manufacturers to include certain structure/function claims on the product's label. For example, the claims "maintains a healthy circulatory system" and "improves urine flow" describe how supplements can affect body functions. Unless given prior approval by the FDA, herbal supplement manufacturers cannot indicate on the label that a supplement can prevent, diagnose, treat, improve, or cure diseases. Results of clinical studies indicate that specific herbs can provide measurable health benefits. St. John's wort, for example, can relieve symptoms of mild to moderate depression and appears to be relatively safe when not combined with prescription medications.[36] Ginseng is a top-selling dietary supplement in the United States. People use the herb for a variety of purposes, including as a sedative, antidepressant, and aphrodisiac. There is scientific evidence that taking *American ginseng* before meals may improve blood sugar values of people with type 2 diabetes.[37] Ingesting an extract made from the herb regularly may reduce the risk of respiratory tract infections, such as the common cold. Although evidence that ginseng provides other healthful benefits is lacking, scientists continue to investigate the herb's potential uses.

Not every herbal product has measurable beneficial effects on health. Ginkgo is a popular dietary supplement, but scientific evidence to support claims that extracts made from ginkgo leaves improve memory is weak or inconsistent.[38] Many people take echinacea to prevent or treat the common cold, but the usefulness of this practice does not have widespread scientific support.[38,39,40] More research is needed to determine whether taking ginkgo, echinacea, and many other dietary supplements has measureable health benefits.

A "natural" therapy is not necessarily a safe one. Many plants, including comfrey, chaparral, pennyroyal, kava, birthwort, snakeroot, and germander, contain chemicals that can be harmful and even deadly when consumed. Ingesting *kava*, an herb that is promoted for relieving anxiety, can result in serious liver damage.[41] In 2004, the FDA banned the sale of most dietary supplements that contained *ephedra*, a naturally occurring stimulant drug that is often called ma huang. Traditional Chinese remedies and herbal teas that contain ephedra were exempt from the ban. Consuming ephedra can result in stroke, heart attack, and death.[42] In 2003, a weight-loss supplement that contained the toxic herb contributed to the sudden death of Steve Bechler, a 23-year-old professional pitcher for the Baltimore Orioles baseball team.

Consumers need to be aware that medicinal herbs may interact with prescription medications or other herbs, producing serious side effects. These products may also be contaminated with pesticides or highly toxic metals. Many dietary supplements are expensive and useless in promoting good health. **Table 1.5** includes information about the safety and effectiveness of some popular herbal supplements. For reliable information about herbs and other dietary supplements, check the following government websites: http://nccam.nih.gov/health/atoz.htm and www.ods.od.nih.gov.

Some herbal supplement manufacturers claim their products have been clinically tested and shown to provide health benefits. The reliability of these claims may be questionable, however, because they are often based on results obtained from animal research or few, poorly designed human studies. Given the lack of scientific evidence that most medicinal herbs are safe and effective, the amount of money

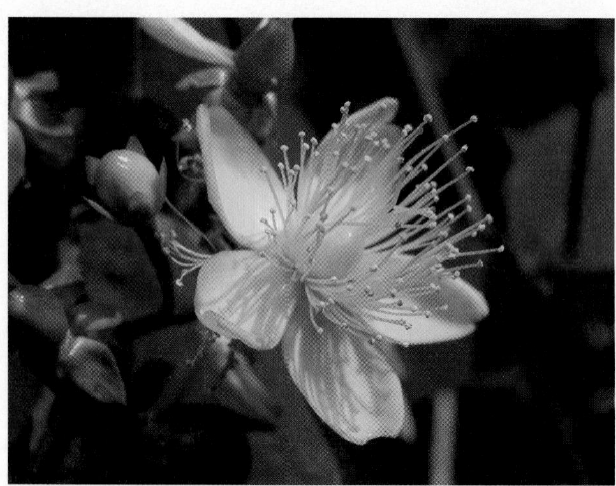

St. John's wort.

Table 1.5

Popular Herbal Supplements

Supplement	Common Claims	Research Findings: Uses	Research Findings: Risks
St. John's wort	Relieves depression	May reduce mild to moderate depression symptoms; no value for major depression	Can interfere with birth control pills and other prescribed medicines, increase sensitivity to sunlight, and cause stomach upset
Saw palmetto	Improves urine flow	May reduce symptoms of prostate enlargement that are not caused by cancer	May interfere with prostate-specific antigen (PSA) test to detect prostate cancer
Feverfew	Relieves headaches, fever, arthritis pain	Contains a chemical that may prevent migraines or reduce their severity	May cause dangerous interactions with aspirin or Coumadin (warfarin; a prescribed drug)
Echinacea	Prevents colds and influenza	Does not prevent colds or reduce their severity	May cause allergic response and be a liver toxin
Ginkgo biloba	Enhances memory and sense of well-being; prevents dementia	Weak or inconsistent scientific evidence to support claims	May interfere with normal blood clotting, cause intestinal upset, and increase blood pressure
Ginseng	Enhances sexual, mental, and exercise performance; increases energy; relieves stress and depression	Has no mood-enhancing effects. May reduce risk of respiratory infections and improve blood sugar values of people with diabetes	Can cause "jitters," insomnia, hypertension, and diarrhea and can be addictive; can be contaminated with pesticides and the toxic mineral lead
Yohimbe	Enhances muscle development and sexual performance	Dilates blood vessels but has no beneficial effects on muscle growth or sex drive of humans	Can produce abnormal behavior, high blood pressure, and heart attacks
Guarana	Boosts energy and enhances weight loss	Acts as a stimulant drug	May cause nausea, anxiety, and irregular heartbeat
Kava	Relieves anxiety and induces sleep	Acts as a depressant drug	May cause serious liver damage; do not use when driving

consumers pay for these products is astonishing. In 2012, for example, Americans spent more than $5.6 billion on herbal supplements.[43]

CAM Therapies in Perspective

National surveys provide estimates of the extent to which Americans use unconventional medical therapies. According to the National Health Interview Survey, 38% of adults used forms of CAM in 2007.[48] Other commonly used CAM treatments were natural products, deep breathing exercises, meditation, and chiropractic care. In most cases, CAM was used to treat back, neck, and joint problems; colds; anxiety; and depression.

The natural or exotic nature of many alternative therapies such as herbal pills and teas, coffee enemas, shark cartilage, and reflexology may appeal to people who distrust modern technology or have lost faith in conventional medical care. Others use alternative therapies to prevent or treat ailments because they want to take more control over their health. Conventional medical practitioners are concerned when persons with serious conditions forgo or delay conventional treatments and rely instead on questionable alternative therapies. These could be life-threatening decisions. Many forms of cancer, for example, respond well to conventional treatments, particularly if the disease is in an early stage.

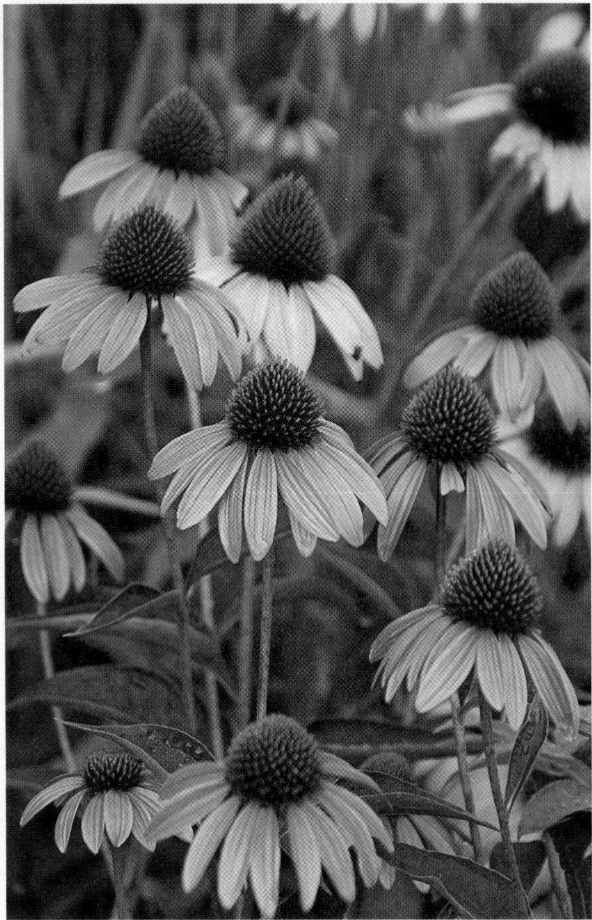

Echinacea.
© Zina Seletskaya/ShutterStock

Many adults who use alternative medical therapies choose them to complement rather than replace conventional treatments.[44]

Regardless of treatment, people suffering from acute conditions such as low back pain, common colds, and gastrointestinal disturbances generally recover with time. Individuals with chronic health problems such as osteoarthritis and multiple sclerosis often report *remissions*, times when their conditions improve. If people use alternative therapies when they are recovering or their illnesses are in remission, they are likely to think the nonconventional treatment cured or helped them. Additionally, people who combine alternative therapies with conventional medical care may attribute any improvement in their health only to the alternative treatments.

Conventional medical practitioners are likely to be skeptical of CAM techniques if they have not been shown scientifically in large-scale clinical studies to be safe or more helpful than placebos. The National Center for Complementary and Alternative Medicine within the National Institutes of Health funds research to determine the safety and effectiveness of alternative medical practices. Until supportive data are available from well-designed studies, consumers should be wary of CAM practices.

Before using alternative therapies, discuss your options with your physician and consider taking the following steps to protect yourself:

- Contact a variety of reliable sources of information to determine the risks and benefits of the treatment. For example, ask people who have used the treatment to describe its effectiveness and side effects. Conduct a review of medical literature, and recognize that popular sources of information such as health magazines and the Internet may be unreliable. Look for articles in medical journals or news magazines that have information concerning the usefulness of conventional as well as alternative medical approaches to care.
- Ask people who administer the treatment to provide proof of their medical training. Investigate the validity of their educational credentials. People who promote certain alternative medical practices often have little or no medical and scientific training.
- Determine the cost of treatment and whether your health insurance covers the particular alternative therapy. If it does not, find out why. You may find that your health insurer considers the treatment risky or ineffective.
- Ask your primary care physician for his or her opinion of the treatment. If you still have questions about the treatment, seek a second opinion from one or more other physicians.
- If you decide to use an alternative therapy, do not use it along with conventional therapy or abandon conventional treatment for any medical problem without consulting your physician.
- Investigate the possibility that the alternative medicine or herbal supplement can interact with conventional medications that you take and produce serious side effects. Investigate the possibility that taking combinations of herbal supplements can be harmful.
- If you are pregnant or breastfeeding, do not use herbal supplements or alternative therapies without consulting your physician.
- Do not give herbal supplements or alternative therapies to children.

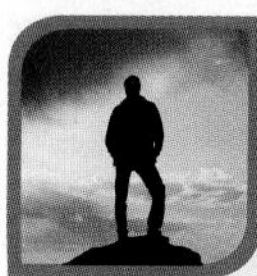
© djgis/ShutterStock

Healthy Living Practices

- Before using an herbal supplement or alternative therapy, obtain reliable information concerning the pros and cons of the treatment and discuss your options with your physician.

Choosing Conventional Medical Practitioners

Scientific research, technological advancements, and a systematic approach to medical education make the conventional healthcare system in the United States among the best in the world. Conventional medicine, however, has its limitations; not every condition can be prevented, managed, or cured.

Americans generally consider conventional medical care practitioners, such as physicians, dentists, nurses, and dietitians, to be experts in their fields. How do you choose the best medical professionals? A good way is to ask family and friends for their recommendations. If you are enrolled in certain health insurance plans, you generally must select from approved lists of providers. After you obtain some names of physicians or other conventional practitioners, check your health insurance plan's list of healthcare providers to determine whether the recommended individuals are listed.

To help ensure high-quality conventional health care, consumers should choose physicians who have certain personal and professional characteristics, including appropriate training and excellent medical credentials (**Table 1.6**). For example, a physician who is *board certified* or *board eligible* in a specialty, such as internal medicine, is well trained in that particular field of practice. In addition to considering a prospective physician's qualifications, you should evaluate his or her personality and office conditions. Make an appointment to meet with the physician and prepare a list of questions to ask him or her. For example, which health insurance plans are accepted? Where did the practitioner receive his or her medical training? With which hospitals does the physician have affiliations? When you are in the practitioner's waiting room, observe its cleanliness and the staff's attitude and friendliness. When you interview the physician, observe his or her body language and judge the person's verbal responses to your questions. After the interview, evaluate the physician's level of comfort with you, his or her answers to your questions, and office conditions. Was the physician friendly and interested in you and your health history? Did he or she provide satisfactory answers to your questions? Was the office clean and staff courteous? If you answered "yes" to these questions, you are likely to enjoy a good relationship with this physician and receive good medical care.

Ideally, people should be able to form a trusting relationship with their conventional medical practitioners, including physicians. To develop these relationships, patients need to acknowledge that they are largely responsible for their health status. For

Table 1.6

Characteristics of Good Personal Physicians

A good personal physician:

- Is intelligent and well qualified in his or her field of practice
- Spends adequate time with patients and listens to patients' concerns
- Is willing to modify treatment to meet patients' concerns and values
- Is caring and sympathetic
- Enlists patients' active participation in health-related decisions
- Is willing to admit when his or her medical knowledge is lacking
- Recognizes the limitations of his or her expertise and is willing to refer patients to other medical professionals when necessary
- Provides thorough physical examinations and orders appropriate testing, such as blood tests or x-rays
- Is available for telephone consultations when necessary
- Is available to handle emergencies or has a competent backup physician to take care of such situations
- Does not delay in seeing patients with urgent care needs
- Is on staff at one or more nearby accredited hospitals
- Keeps up to date by attending professional educational meetings or reading medical journals
- Has a well-managed, well-equipped office with friendly, courteous staff

Table 1.7

Life Stages

Stage	Approximate Age
Infants and toddlers	0–3 years
Children	4–11 years
Adolescents and teens	12–19
Adults	20–64
Older adults	65 or older

example, patients should adopt healthy lifestyles, obtain regular checkups, and seek medical attention for ailments that do not improve within a few days or have serious signs or symptoms. Moreover, patients should follow their healthcare practitioners' advice and communicate with them should concerns about their medical care arise.

Healthcare practitioners can foster positive relationships with patients by spending adequate time with them, listening to their concerns carefully, and showing an interest in knowing more about them, not just their physical signs and symptoms. In addition, it is important for practitioners to be caring, sensitive, and understanding; to modify treatment to meet the patient's concerns and values; and to enlist the patient's active participation in health-related decisions.

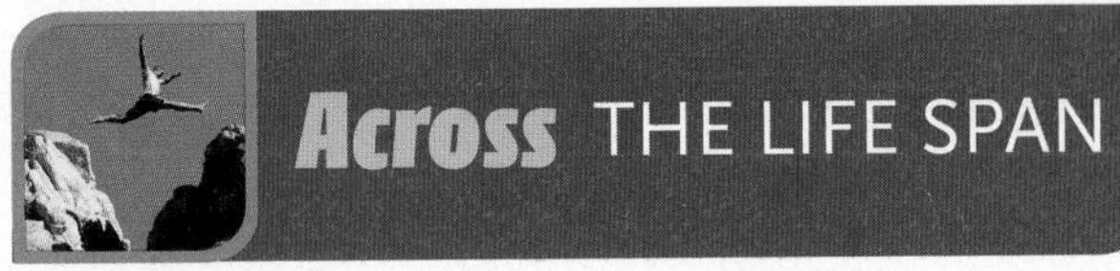

HEALTH

Although the focus of this text is adult health, the Across the Life Span feature briefly describes health concerns that are specific to other stages of life, such as infancy, childhood, adolescence, and the older adult years. **Table 1.7** indicates the approximate age groupings for these life stages.

Why should college students learn about health conditions that can affect very young or very old members of the population? This information is relevant because many college students have younger siblings, some students have children, and those who are not parents may have children in the future. Many college students are middle aged or have elderly parents and grandparents. The following information highlights some major life cycle health concerns of Americans.

In the United States in 2010, about 6 babies in 1,000 died during the first year after birth.[7] Most of these deaths were due to birth defects, low birth weights, and breathing difficulties that arose from *prematurity*—being born too early (**Figure 1.9**). Public health efforts aimed at educating and providing medical care for pregnant women can reduce the number of infant deaths.

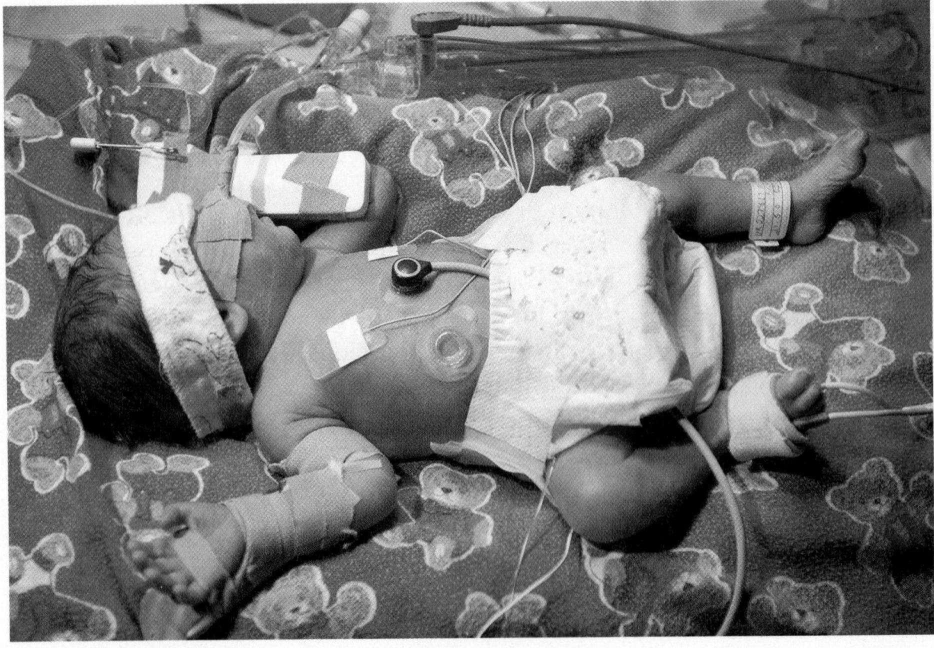

Figure 1.9

Premature Newborns. Infants born prematurely have a greater risk of serious health problems than do healthy full-term infants.

Unintentional injuries are the major health threat to children between 1 and 14 years of age. Most deaths from unintentional injuries, such as deaths due to motor vehicle crashes, drownings, and house fires, are preventable.

Adolescence is a time when youngsters establish behaviors that may last a lifetime and when experimentation with risky behaviors usually begins. In 2011, about 8% of high school students reported driving a car or other vehicle after consuming alcohol, and 16.6% had carried a weapon on at least one day during the 30 days preceding the survey.[45] About 9% reported that they had been physically abused intentionally by a boyfriend or girlfriend and 30% of these students reported being overweight or obese. Unintentional injuries (accidents), homicide, and suicide are major causes of death for people aged 15 to 24. In 2010, motor vehicle accidents accounted for almost two-thirds of deaths resulting from unintentional injuries for Americans in this age group.[7]

In 2011, the teenage birth rate declined to its lowest level in nearly 70 years of recordkeeping in the United States.[46] However, sexually transmitted infections (STIs) continue to be major health problems for adolescents. People between 15 and 24 years of age contract about 50% of all new cases of sexually transmitted infections.[17] AIDS is primarily a sexually transmitted infection; sexually active adolescents are at risk of becoming infected with HIV, the virus that causes AIDS.

In 2012, people 65 years of age and older made up nearly 14% of the U.S. population. The percentage of older adults in the population is expected to increase rapidly over the next 40 years.[47]

CHAPTER REVIEW

© SergeBertasiusPhotography/ShutterStock

Summary

Lifestyle includes behaviors that promote or deter good health and well-being. Optimal wellness is an optimal degree of health. The holistic approach to health integrates physical, psychological, social, intellectual, spiritual, and environmental dimensions. Contemporary definitions of *health* reflect not only how an individual functions but also what that person can achieve, given his or her circumstances.

Heart disease and cancer are the major killers of Americans. Lifestyle choices contribute to the development of these and many other life-threatening diseases. The distribution of health problems differs among the various ethnic and racial groups in the United States. Poverty and cultural differences are often barriers to good health care.

Experiences, knowledge, needs, and values affect one's motivation to change health-related behaviors. People are motivated to take action if they feel that a sufficient threat to their health exists and that the results of changing their behavior will be worthwhile.

Although no one can guarantee good health, many factors contribute to one's chances of enjoying a long and productive lifetime of good health. Several of these factors are the result of lifestyle choices that people can make, while they are still young, to prevent or delay disease. Responsible health-related lifestyle choices involve a systematic approach to decision making.

People can become more careful consumers of health-related information, products, and services by learning to recognize misinformation. To obtain reliable health-related information, check with experts in federal, state, and local agencies and organizations.

Conventional medicine relies on modern scientific principles, modern technologies, and scientifically proven methods to prevent, diagnose, and treat health conditions. Complementary and alternative medicine (CAM) is an unconventional and diverse system of preventing, diagnosing, and treating diseases that emphasizes spirituality, self-healing, and harmonious interaction with the environment. Conventional medical practitioners are likely to be skeptical of CAM techniques that have not been shown scientifically to be safe and effective. Until supportive data are available, consumers should be wary of CAM practices.

Throughout the life span, health concerns vary. The most common causes of infant deaths are birth defects, low birth weights, and prematurity. Preventable injuries are the major causes of death for children and youth. Additional serious public health concerns for adolescents are suicide, homicide, drug abuse, obesity, pregnancy, and sexually transmitted infections (including HIV).

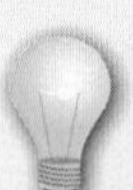

Applying What You Have Learned

© tele52/ShutterStock

1. Develop a plan to improve your health by selecting a health behavior you'd like to change. **Application**
2. Select a health-related advertisement from the Internet and evaluate the validity of its information. Use the information provided in the "Analyzing Health Information" section to help you answer the following questions. **Analysis**
3. Identify several sources of health information that you have used in the past year. Using the criteria from the "Analyzing Health Information" section, explain why you think each source is reliable or unreliable. **Synthesis**
4. Think of a health-related decision that you made recently. For example, did you decide to turn down an offer to use a mind-altering drug, wear a helmet while riding a motorcycle, lose a few pounds, or use an herbal product to treat a condition? When you made this decision, did you use the decision-making process described in this chapter or did you act impulsively? Explain why you would or would not make the same decision today. **Evaluation**

Application	Analysis	Synthesis	Evaluation	Key
using information in a new situation.	breaking down information into component parts.	putting together information from different sources.	making informed decisions.	

© SergeBertasiusPhotography/ShutterStock

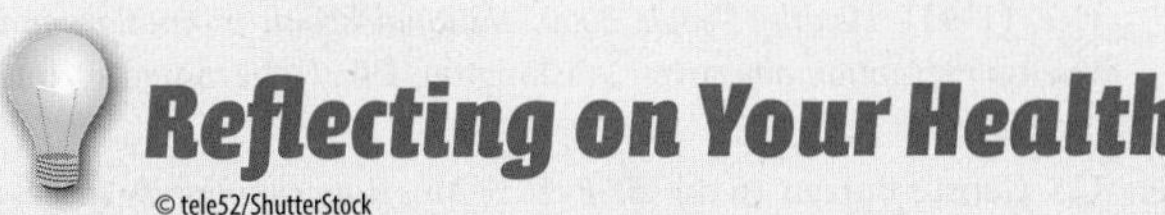

© tele52/ShutterStock

A reflective journal is a personal record of your thoughts and expressions of your feelings. The purposes of keeping this journal are to stimulate your thinking about what you have learned about health and to help you understand how your thoughts and feelings about your health might have changed over the semester. Thinking about new information can help you determine its usefulness, which can influence your attitudes and behaviors.

The Reflecting on Your Health questions at the end of each chapter are designed to guide your thinking. If you want to write about something else that is related to the contents of the chapter, feel free to do so, but make sure to identify the topic in your opening sentence. Write your journal entries in the first person, using "I" statements to express your thoughts, as though you were talking to a close friend. Do not worry about your spelling, punctuation, or grammar—just let your thoughts flow.

Some instructors make journal writing an optional activity; others require that you respond to all of the questions, and they grade journals. Still other instructors simply check to see if students are doing the assignment. Refer to the course syllabus or ask your instructor about his or her grading practices and other instructions concerning the journal.

1. What does the term *health* mean to you? Which of the definitions of health provided in this chapter best "fits" with your thoughts on health?
2. Do you think everyone should strive to achieve optimal health? Provide a rationale for your response.
3. What impact does spiritual health have on your sense of well-being? If spiritual health is important to you, describe the role it plays in your life.
4. Do you agree with the idea presented in the chapter that social health influences your physical health? Why or why not?
5. Select a current behavior that you believe is your worst health behavior. Identify three factors that influence this specific behavior, and explain how each factor influences your behavior.
6. Under what circumstances would you consider using alternative therapies?

References

1. U.S. Centers for Disease Control and Prevention. (n.d.). *Behavioral Risk Factor Surveillance System 2011. Prevalence and trends data: Physical activity—2011.* Retrieved from http://apps.nccd.cdc.gov/brfss/list.asp?cat=PA&yr=2011&qkey=8271&state=All
2. U.S. Centers for Disease Control and Prevention. (n.d.). *Behavioral Risk Factor Surveillance System 2011. Prevalence and trends data: Cholesterol awareness—2011.* Retrieved from http://apps.nccd.cdc.gov/brfss/list.asp?cat=CA&yr=2011&qkey=8061&state=All
3. Beck, L. F., & West, B. A. (2007, January 7). Vital signs: Nonfatal, motor vehicle-occupant injuries (2009) and seat belt use (2008) among adults—United States (2011). *Morbidity and Mortality Weekly Report,* 59,1681–1686. Retrieved from http://www.cdc.gov/mmwr/preview/mmwrhtml/mm5951a3.htm?s_cid=mm5951a3_w
4. Ervin, R. B., & Ogden, C. L. (2013). *Consumption of added sugars among U.S. adults, 2005–2010* (NCHS Data Brief No. 122). Hyattsville, MD: National Center for Health Statistics. Retrieved from http://www.cdc.gov/nchs/data/databriefs/db122.pdf
5. U.S. Department of Agriculture, Agricultural Research Service. (2010, August). Data tables from *What We Eat in America, NHANES 2007–2008.* Nutrient intakes: Mean amounts consumed per individual, by

CHAPTER REVIEW

gender and age, in the United States, 2007–2008. Retrieved from http://www.ars.usda.gov/SP2UserFiles/Place/12355000/pdf/ 0708/Table_1_NIN_GEN_07.pdf

6. U.S. Centers for Disease Control and Prevention. (n.d.). *U.S. cancer statistics: An interactive atlas.* Retrieved from http://apps.nccd.cdc.gov/DCPC_INCA/DCPC_INCA.aspx
7. U.S. Centers for Disease Control and Prevention, National Center for Health Statistics. (2013). *Health, United States, 2012.* Retrieved from http://www.cdc.gov/nchs/data/hus/hus12.pdf
8. U.S. Centers for Disease Control and Prevention. (2012). Consumption of cigarettes and combustible tobacco—United States, 2000–2011. *Morbidity and Mortality Weekly Report,* 61(30): 565–569. Retrieved from http://www.cdc.gov/mmwr/preview/mmwrhtml/mm6130a1.htm
9. U.S. Census Bureau. (n.d.). *Statistical abstract of the United States: 2011.* Table 1112. Alcohol involvement for drivers in fatal crashes: 1998 and 2008. Retrieved from http://www.census.gov/compendia/statab/2011/tables/11s1112.pdf
10. U.S. Centers for Disease Control and Prevention. (n.d.). Behavioral Risk Factor Surveillance System 2011. Prevalence and trends data: Alcohol consumption—2012. Retrieved from http://apps.nccd.cdc.gov/brfss/list.asp?cat=AC&yr=2012&qkey=8371&state=All
11. U.S. Centers for Disease Control and Prevention. (2013). Binge drinking—United States, 2011. *Morbidity and Mortality Weekly Report,* 62(03), 77–80. Retrieved from http://www.cdc.gov/mmwr/preview/mmwrhtml/su6203a13.htm
12. National Institute on Alcohol Abuse and Alcoholism. (2013). *A snapshot of annual high-risk college drinking consequences.* Retrieved from http://www.collegedrinkingprevention.gov/StatsSummaries/snapshot.aspx
13. Krebs-Smith, S. (2010). Americans do not meet federal dietary recommendations. *Journal of Nutrition,* 140(10),1832–1838.
14. Ogden, C., Carroll, M., Kit, B., & Flegal, K. (2012). *Prevalence of obesity in the United States, 2009–2010* (NCHS Data Brief No. 82). Retrieved from http://www.cdc.gov/nchs/data/databriefs/db82.pdf
15. Fryar, C., Carroll, M. D., & Ogden, C. (2012). *Health E-Stat: Prevalence of overweight, obesity, and extreme obesity among adults: United States, trends 1960–1962 through 2009–2010.* Retrieved from http://www.cdc.gov/nchs/data/hestat/obesity_adult_09_10/obesity_adult_09_10.pdf
16. World Health Organization. (1948). *Official records of the World Health Organization, no. 2. Proceedings and final acts of the international health conference held in New York from 19 June to 22 July 1946.* New York, NY: United Nations WHO Interim Commission.
17. World Health Organization. (1986). *Ottawa charter for health promotion.* Copenhagen, Denmark: Author.
18. Hochbaum, G. M. (1979). An alternative approach to health education. *Health Values,* 3, 197–201.
19. McKenzie, J. F., Pinger, R. R., & Kotecki, J. E. (2012). *An introduction to community Health* (7th ed.). Burlington, MA: Jones & Bartlett Learning.
20. U.S. Department of Health and Human Services, Centers for Medicare and Medicaid Services. (2012). *National health expenditure projections 2012–2022, forecast summary.* Retrieved from http://www.cms.gov/Research-Statistics-Data-and-Systems/Statistics-Trends-and-Reports/NationalHealthExpendData/Downloads/Proj2012.pdf
21. Heron, M. (2013). Deaths: Leading causes for 2010. *National Vital Statistics Reports,* 62(6). Hyattsville, MD: National Center for Health Statistics. Retrieved from http://www.cdc.gov/nchs/data/nvsr/nvsr62/nvsr62_06.pdf
22. Mokdad, A. H., et al. (2004). Actual causes of death in the United States, 2000. *Journal of the American Medical Association,* 291(10),1238–1245. [Published correction appears in *Journal of the American Medical Association, 293*(3), 293–294.]
23. U.S. Department of Health and Human Services, Public Health Service. (1991). *Healthy People 2000: National health promotion and disease prevention objectives.* Washington, DC: Government Printing Office.
24. U.S. Census Bureau. (n.d.). *2008–2012 American community survey.* Retrieved from http://factfinder2.census.gov/faces/tableservices/jsf/pages/productview.xhtml?pid=ACS_12_5YR_DP05
25. U.S. Centers for Disease Control and Prevention, Minority Health. (2013). *Hispanic or Latino populations.* Retrieved from http://www.cdc.gov/minorityhealth/populations/REMP/hispanic.html#10
26. U.S. Centers for Disease Control and Prevention, Minority Health. (2013). *Black or African American populations.* Retrieved from http://www.cdc.gov/minorityhealth/populations/REMP/black.html
27. National Cancer Institute. (2013). *SEER Cancer Statistics Review 1975–2010.* Retrieved from http://seer.cancer.gov/csr/1975_2010/
28. Meyer, P. A., Yoon, P. W., & Kaufmann, R. B. (2013). Health disparities and inequalities report—United States, 2013. *Morbidity and Mortality Weekly Report,* 62(03), 77–80. Retrieved from http://www.cdc.gov/mmwr/pdf/other/su6203.pdf
29. U.S. Centers for Disease Control and Prevention, Office of Minority Health and Health Disparities. (2013). *Asian American populations.* Retrieved from http://www.cdc.gov/minorityhealth/populations/REMP/asian.html
30. U.S. Centers for Disease Control and Prevention, Office of Minority Health and Health Disparities. (2013). *American Indian/Alaskan Native profile.* Retrieved from http://www.cdc.gov/minorityhealth/populations/REMP/aian.html
31. U.S. National Institute of Diabetes and Kidney and Digestive Diseases, National Diabetes Information Clearinghouse (NDIC). (2014). *National diabetes statistics, 2014.* Retrieved from http://www.cdc.gov/diabetes/pubs/statsreport14/national-diabetes-report-web.pdf http://diabetes.niddk.nih.gov/dm/pubs/statistics/#fast
32. Norcross, J. C., & Prochaska, J. O. (2002). Using the stages of change. *Harvard Mental Health Letter,* 18(11),5–7.
33. Prochaska, J. O., & Velicer, W. F. (1997). The transtheoretical model of health behavior change. *American Journal of Health Promotion,* 12(1), 38–48.
34. Eskinazi, D. P. (1998). Factors that shape alternative medicine. *Journal of the American Medical Association,* 280(18), 1621–1623.
35. Vanderploeg, K., & Yi, X. (2009). Acupuncture in modern society. *Journal of Acupuncture and Meridian Studies,* 2(1), 26–33.
36. U.S. National Institutes of Health, National Center for Complementary and Alternative Medicine. (2013). *St. John's wort.* Retrieved from http://nccam.nih.gov/health/stjohnswort
37. U.S. National Institutes of Health, National Library of Medicine, MedlinePlus. (2013). *Ginseng, American.* Retrieved from http://www.nlm.nih.gov/medlineplus/druginfo/natural/967.html

38. Fransen, H. P., Pelgrom, S. M., Stewart-Knox, B., de Kaste, D., & Verhagen, H. (2010). Assessment of health claims, content, and safety of herbal supplements containing *Ginkgo biloba*. *Food & Nutrition Research*, 54, 5221. doi:10.3402/fnr.v54i0.5221
39. Barrett, B., et al. (2010). Echinacea for treating the common cold. A randomized trial. *Annals of Internal Medicine*, 153(12), 769–777.
40. Karsch-Volk, M., et al. (2014). Echinacea for preventing and treating the common cold. *The Cochrane Database of Systematic Reviews*, 20(2), 1–90.
41. U.S. National Institutes of Health, National Center for Complementary and Alternative Medicine. (2012). *Kava*. Retrieved from http://nccam.nih.gov/health/kava/
42. U.S. National Institutes of Health, National Center for Complementary and Alternative Medicine. (2013). *Ephedra*. Retrieved from http://nccam.nih.gov/health/ephedra/
43. American Botanical Council. (2013). *Herbal dietary supplement retail sales up 5.5% in 2012*. Retrieved from http://cms.herbalgram.org/press/2013/2012_Market_Report.html
44. Barnes, P. M., et al. (2008). Complementary and alternative medicine use among adults and children: United States, 2007. *National Health Statistics Reports*, No. 12. Hyattsville, MD: National Center for Health Statistics.
45. U.S. Centers for Disease Control and Prevention. *YRBSS: Youth Risk Behavior Surveillance System, 2009 results*. Trends in prevalence of behaviors that contributed to violence, National YRBS: 1991–2011. Retrieved from http://www.cdc.gov/healthyyouth/yrbs/pdf/us_violence_trend_yrbs.pdf
46. Martin, J., et al. (2013). Births: Final data for 2012. *National Vital Statistics Reports*, 62(9), 1–87. Retrieved from http://www.cdc.gov/nchs/data/nvsr/nvsr62/nvsr62_09.pdf#table02
47. U.S. Census Bureau. Fact Sheet. (n.d.). *2008–2012 American Community Survey 5-year estimates United States*. Retrieved from http://factfinder2.census.gov/faces/tableservices/jsf/pages/productview.xhtml?pid=ACS_12_5YR_DP05&prodType=table

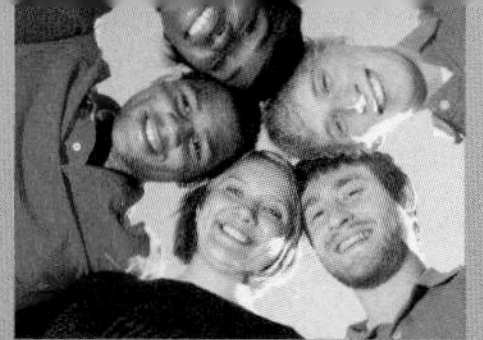

Diversity in Health
American Indians and Psychological Health

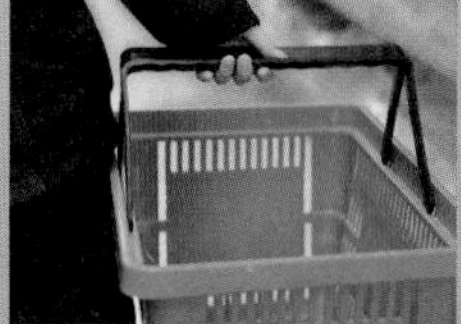

Consumer Health
Locating and Selecting Mental Health Therapists

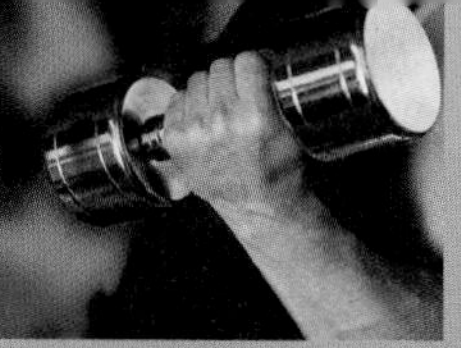

Managing Your Health
Resolving Interpersonal Conflicts Constructively

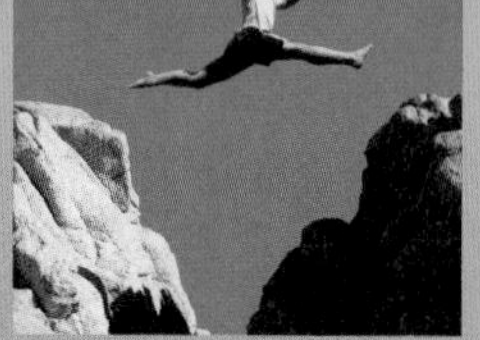

Across the Life Span
Psychological Health

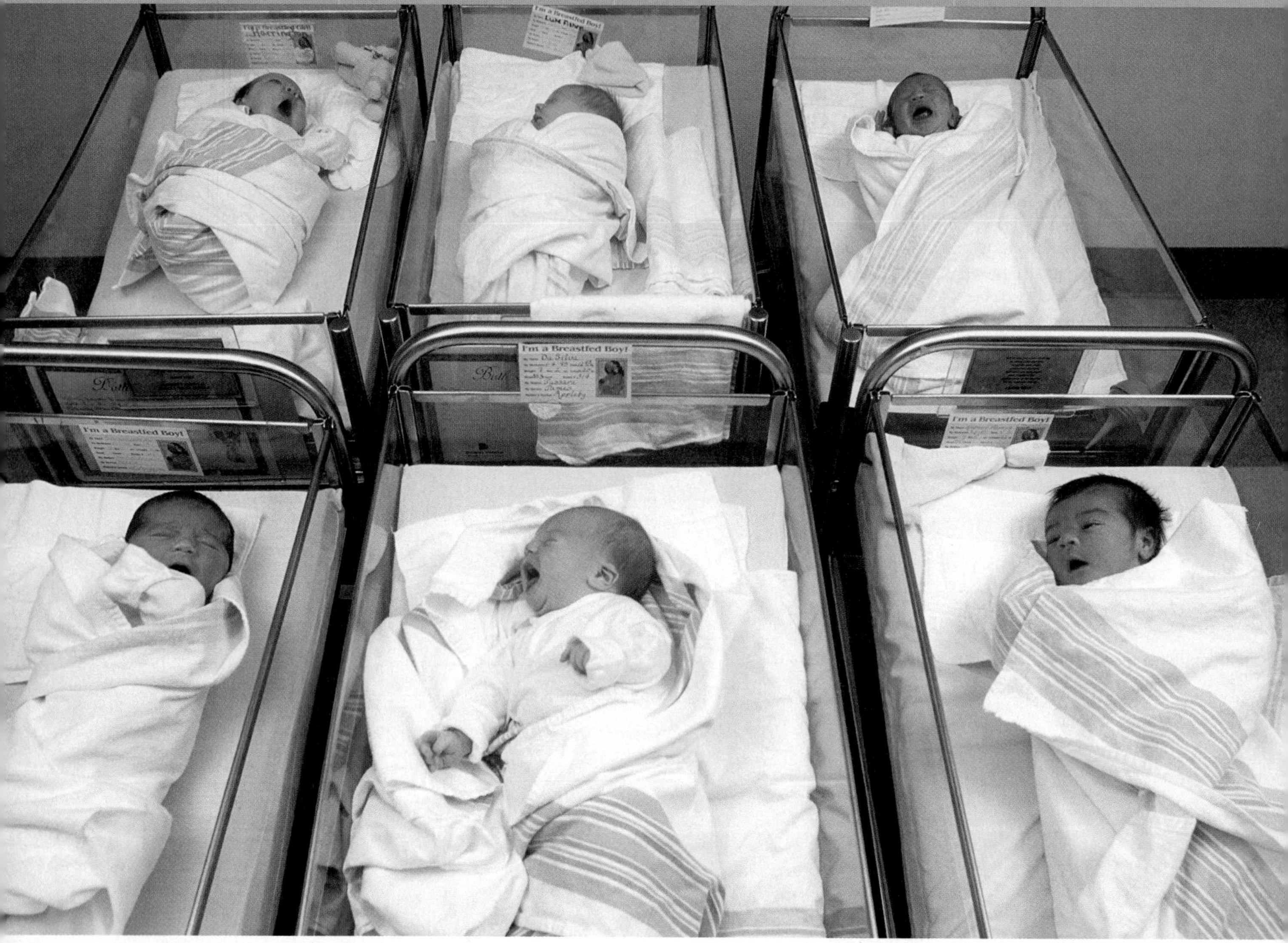

Chapter Overview

How your nervous system affects your psychological health

How biological, social, and cultural forces interact to mold personality

How psychological adjustment leads to psychological growth

How to identify common psychological disorders

How to recognize suicidal behavior and prevent suicide

Student Workbook

Self-Assessment: Self-Esteem Inventory

Changing Health Habits: Are You Ready to Improve Your Psychological Health?

Do You Know?

If you are psychologically healthy?

Why emotions are useful?

How to resolve conflicts in a healthy manner?

Circle of People: © SergeBertasiusPhotography/Shutterstock; Consumer: © sevenke/ShutterStock; Weight Training: © Kzenon/ShutterStock; Rock Climbing: © Galina Barskaya/ShutterStock; Chapter opener: © Blaine Harrington III/Alamy Images

CHAPTER 2

Psychological Health

Learning Objectives

"Each newborn is a unique person."

After studying this chapter, you should be able to:

1. Explain the basics of psychological health and list characteristics of psychologically healthy people.
2. Compare and contrast theories of personality development.
3. List common defense mechanisms and provide an example of each.
4. Identify levels of Maslow's hierarchy of needs and characteristics of a self-actualized person.
5. Define psychological adjustment and growth.
6. Describe the relationships between psychological health, self-esteem, and autonomy.
7. Differentiate between healthy and unhealthy emotional responses.
8. Identify common psychological health disorders and describe the major symptoms of each.
9. List and describe common methods for treating psychological disorders.
10. Identify warning signs of suicide and describe methods of suicide prevention.

psychology The study of the mental processes that influence human behavior.

physiology The study of bodily functions.

central nervous system (CNS) Of the two primary divisions of the nervous system, the one that consists of brain and spinal cord.

peripheral nervous system (PNS) Of the two primary divisions of the nervous system, the one that consists of nerves, which relay information to and from the CNS.

neurotransmitters Chemicals produced and released by nerves that convey information between most nerve cells.

Observing newborn infants in a hospital nursery is a fascinating experience. Some of the babies sleep peacefully; others are awake, calmly gazing around at their surroundings while gently sucking their pacifiers. A few of the newborns are restless. Although tightly wrapped in swaddling, one infant tries to stretch her hand into the air as though she were reaching for something hanging above the bassinet. Another fussy baby frowns and closes his eyes tightly before spitting out his pacifier, kicking his feet, and howling in pain. Moments later, several other babies begin to grow fussy. Soon a chorus of crying babies shatters the calmness of the nursery. The infants' caregivers scurry to each bassinet, trying to determine which babies are truly in need of their attention and the reasons why. Why do some newborns respond differently when all of them are in the same situation?

Each newborn is a unique person. All infants, however, have basic physical needs that must be met if they are to survive. These needs include nutritious food and a safe environment. Additionally, children have psychological needs for belonging, love, social acceptance, and respect that must be met if they are to mature into healthy adults. What if there was a crystal ball in the nursery that would enable you to predict each baby's future? Which of these infants will be psychologically healthy, achieving personal fulfillment and being satisfied with themselves and their lives? Which ones will be emotionally distressed and lead troubled lives?

Psychology is the study of the thinking or mental (cognitive) processes that influence human behavior. Psychological (mental) health involves the ability to deal effectively with the psychological challenges of life. Psychological health is dynamic, becoming more positive or negative as a person responds to a constantly changing environment. Many individuals, however, manage to maintain high degrees of positive psychological functioning throughout their lives. People with positive mental health are able to deal effectively with the psychological challenges of life. Such people accept themselves, have realistic and optimistic outlooks on life, function independently, form satisfying interpersonal relationships, and cope effectively with change (**Table 2.1**). In addition to these traits, psychologically healthy individuals resolve their problems without resorting to substance abuse or violence, and they assert themselves in social situations.

Table 2.1

Characteristics of Psychologically Healthy People

Psychologically healthy people:

- Accept themselves and others
- Display creative abilities
- Respond to changing situations with spontaneity
- Show appropriate emotional responses
- Desire privacy
- Are aware of reality
- Function independently
- Are concerned about the needs of others
- Enjoy interpersonal relationships
- Have goals in life

Adapted from Maslow, A. H. (1970). *Motivation and Personality* (2nd ed.). New York, NY: Harper & Row.

The quality of one's psychological health often affects the other components of health, such as social, spiritual, and physical health. This chapter discusses factors that influence positive psychological health as well as those that contribute to the development of psychological disorders.

The Basics of Psychological Health

Understanding psychological health involves learning about **physiology**, the study of body functions, and psychology. Cognitive processes such as thinking, decision making, and remembering rely on the functioning of the nervous system. The nervous

personality A set of distinct thoughts and behaviors that characterizes a person's response to situations.

heredity The transmission of biological information, coded within genes, from parents to offspring.

Figure 2.1

The Nervous System. The nervous system consists of the brain, the spinal cord, and peripheral nerves.

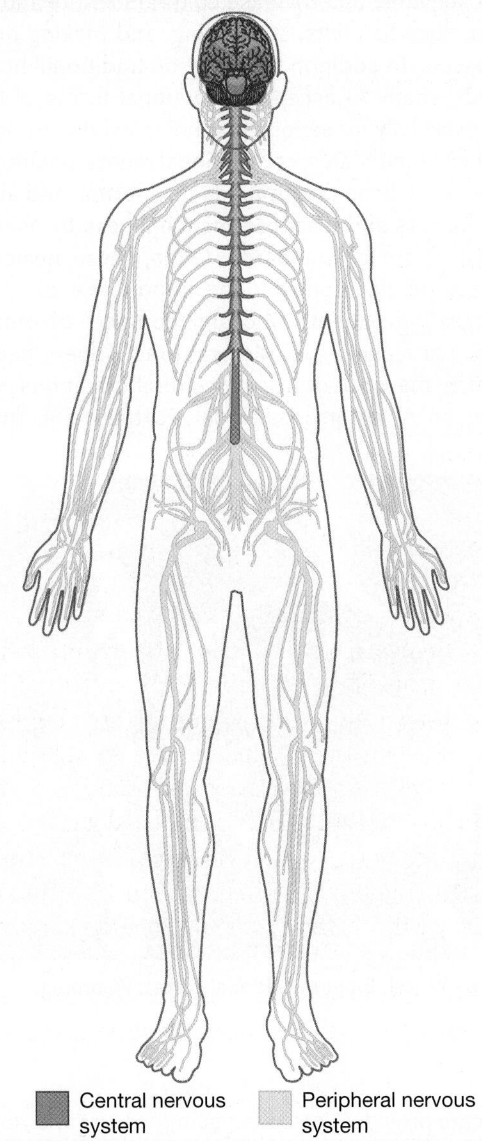

system is an elaborate biological communications network that contains billions of nerve cells, or neurons, which are designed to receive, send, and interpret messages in your body by means of electrical and chemical signals. As you can see in **Figure 2.1**, this network consists of two interrelated parts: the **central nervous system (CNS)**, the brain and spinal cord; and the **peripheral nervous system (PNS)**, nerves that relay information to and from the CNS.

Most nerves produce and release **neurotransmitters**, chemicals such as acetylcholine, dopamine, and serotonin that convey information between nerve cells. By altering the levels of various neurotransmitters, the nervous system transmits information and produces physical responses, thoughts, and emotions.

Emotions are a way of communicating our moods to others. Emotions are associated with typical behavioral and physical responses, including changes in speech patterns as well as facial expressions and other forms of body language. Happiness, sadness, anger, and fear are among the basic emotions that we often call *feelings*. A psychologically healthy person is able to express his or her emotions appropriately. Much of the disability that is associated with psychological illness results from abnormal or extreme emotional responses to situations.

Parts of the brain, collectively referred to as *the mind*, process various types of information received from the rest of the body and the environment. As a result, the mind thinks about what takes place, finds meaning in events, considers actions, makes decisions, directs responses, evaluates and remembers consequences, and plans for the future. These activities involve neurotransmitters in the brain. Certain conditions can negatively affect the mind by altering neurotransmitter levels and disrupting normal brain chemistry and functioning. As a result, inappropriate moods, unrealistic thoughts, and *maladaptive* behaviors occur. Maladaptive behaviors interfere with one's ability to be productive, interact well socially, and adjust to the demands of everyday living. In many instances, treating these conditions involves taking medication that corrects abnormal neurotransmitter levels as well as learning how to change distorted ways of thinking.

Personality Development

Personality is a set of distinct thoughts and behaviors, including emotional responses, that characterizes the way a person responds to situations. Many factors, including biological, cultural, social, and psychological forces, interact to mold personality.

Biological Influences **Heredity** is the transmission of biological information, coded within genes, from parents to offspring. This information determines, in part, an individual's physical, emotional,

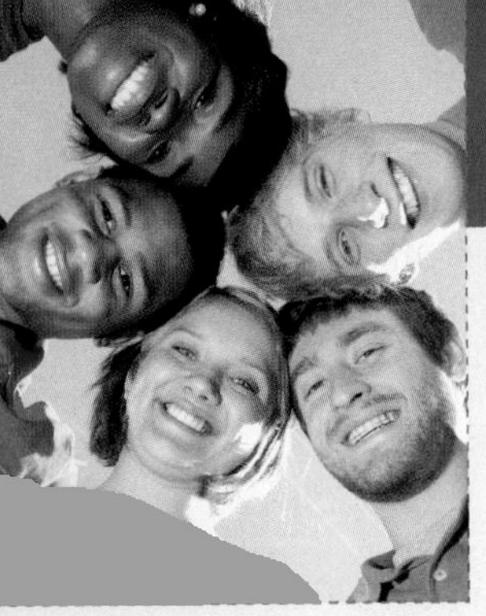

© Mike Flippo/ShutterStock

Diversity in Health

American Indians and Psychological Health

Major health concerns affecting American Indians (AIs) include problems associated with poor psychological health such as alcoholism, suicide, and accidents. According to the results of a major survey conducted from 2009–2010, AI adults were more likely to have experienced serious psychological distress—feeling sad, restless, hopeless, nervous, or worthless—during the past 30 days than adults of other racial or ethnic groups. Rates of suicide deaths and attempts for AI teens in 2009 was significantly higher than teens in other racial categories, and AI teens were significantly more likely to think about committing suicide. A study of more than 3,000 Northern Plains and Southwest tribal members indicated that alcoholism and major depression were common among subjects. Factors that may contribute to AIs' generally poor mental health status include poverty, low educational level, exposure to violence, and discrimination. AIs can obtain professional help for mental health problems through the Indian Health Service (IHS); however, AI adults are less likely to seek or receive psychological counselling or use prescription medications for mental health treatment. Many AIs have more confidence in traditional healing practices than in therapies provided by conventional medical practitioners.

The traditional AI concept of health involves the *medicine wheel*, a circle divided into four equal parts representing the major aspects of health: context (natural environment and social setting), mind, body, and spirit. When the four components of the medicine wheel are balanced with each other, people enjoy wellness or "harmony." When people are not in harmony with nature, their community, or themselves, they suffer from physical and psychological illnesses. According to some traditional AI beliefs, an emotionally disturbed individual is in a state of disharmony with the rest of nature or in a hopeless state of health. In other AI traditions, the symptoms of mental illnesses result from supernatural forces exerting control over the person.

Traditionally, AIs view alcohol abuse and other mental health problems as imbalances in the spiritual component of the medicine wheel. Because spiritual health is linked closely with psychological health, treatments are spiritual in nature and may involve prayer, sweat lodges, or purification ceremonies led by natural healers. Efforts to restore spiritual balance may also include participation in activities that increase cultural identity and self-esteem, such as crafts, storytelling, and making drums and baskets. In addition to relying on traditional healing methods, many AI accept conventional forms of treatment, especially for serious psychological disturbances.

In the United States, conventional mental health practitioners have been taught to identify normal and abnormal behaviors and diagnose mental illness by using an established set of standards. Often, these healthcare providers do not consider the importance of culture when treating patients who are members of minority groups, particularly AIs. Medical practitioners need to recognize the importance of cultural traditions when treating an AI or any individual. Furthermore, mental healthcare providers can often gain the trust and respect of clients from various cultural backgrounds by learning about traditional healing methods. As a result, patients are more likely to accept the healthcare provider's advice and suggestions for conventional treatment.

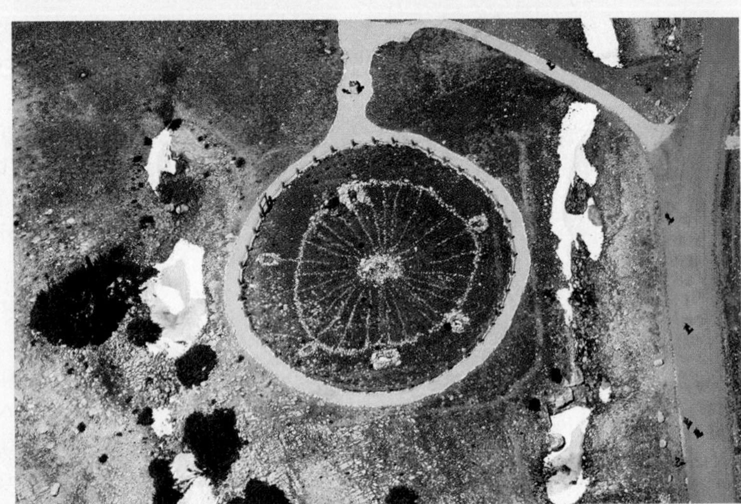

Aerial view of Medicine Wheel, Bighorn National Forest, Wyoming.

© Jim Wark/Lonely Planet Images/Alamy Images

Data from U.S. Centers for Disease Control and Prevention, Office of Minority Health and Health Disparities. (2012). *Mental health and American Indians/Alaskan Natives.* Retrieved from http://minorityhealth.hhs.gov/templates/content.aspx?lvl=3&lvlID=9&ID=6475; Beals, J., et al. (2005). Prevalence of DSM-IV disorders and attendant help-seeking in 2 American Indian reservation populations. *Archives of General Psychiatry*, 62(1), 99–108; Walls, M. L., et al. (2006). Mental health and substance abuse services preferences among American Indian people of the Northern Midwest. *Community Mental Health Journal*, 42(6), 521–535.

temperament The predictable way an individual responds to situations and others, such as being pleasant, outgoing, or shy.

and intellectual characteristics. Much of a person's **temperament**, the predictable way an individual responds to the environment, is inherited. Soon after birth, parents can usually describe their children's temperamental styles, such as irritable, fearful, or pleasant. As children mature, social and cultural influences modify their temperaments.

Social and Cultural Influences From the moment of birth, the social environment, such as interactions with parents and other family members, influences the psychological development of an individual. Most people learn how to respond to situations in socially and culturally acceptable ways when they are children. The circumstances surrounding a situation influence the kind and extent of an emotional display. Consider, for example, emotions that are appropriate to express while attending the funeral of a child.

A person's cultural and ethnic background can influence his or her responses to situations and perceptions of mental health disturbances. Although psychological problems affect people from every culture, symptoms of these problems may differ among cultures. The Diversity in Health essay "American Indians and Psychological Health" discusses a traditional American Indian concept of health, the *medicine wheel*, and healing methods.

Theories of Personality Development

Freud's Framework of Personality More than 100 years ago, physician Sigmund Freud pioneered modern approaches to the diagnosis and treatment of psychological disturbances. Freud observed that people have an element of the mind that lacks awareness of certain thoughts, feelings, and impulses. He proposed that this "unconscious" component of the mind influences much of an individual's behavior. The unconscious mind, for example, engages various defense mechanisms such as repression and avoidance to cope with anxiety and guilt.

Defense mechanisms are ways of thinking and behaving that reduce or eliminate anxiety and guilt feelings by altering the individual's perception of reality. Nearly everyone uses defense mechanisms to protect their minds against psychological conflicts and threats. A basic defense mechanism is *repression*, the unconscious forgetting of anxiety-producing feelings, thoughts, or impulses. For example, adults who were sexually or physically abused as children may repress the memories of the abuse. Students who blame teachers for their lack of academic success, instead of themselves for skipping classes or not studying, may be using *rationalization* as a defense mechanism. **Table 2.2** lists repression, projection, and some other common defense mechanisms and describes instances in which the unconscious mind employs them. Although these strategies may protect the mind and reduce anxiety in the short run, defense mechanisms usually do not provide long-term solutions to problems.

Freud believed that unconscious desires or drives, particularly the *libido*, or sex drive, control human behavior by creating psychological tension. Relieving this tension produces pleasurable sensations. However, members of society establish *moral values*, rules for good and bad behavior that often prevent individuals from satisfying all of their desires. If a person who accepts the moral values of society acts or thinks in ways that conflict with these rules, he or she usually feels anxious and guilty. Many people use moral values as guidelines to judge their behavior, themselves, and others.

Erikson's Psychosocial Stages of Development Psychoanalyst Erik Erikson modified Freud's ideas by proposing that social influences play a greater role in shaping personalities than do sexual drives.[1] According to Erikson, individuals progress through eight psychosocial stages during their lifetimes (**Table 2.3**). Each stage has major social crises or conflicts that people must manage or resolve to achieve a sense of emotional well-being.

Infants require a considerable amount of care and nurturing from adults to survive and to develop normally. Erikson thought that babies learn to *trust* other individuals if their parents or other caregivers meet their basic physical and emotional needs. Establishing trusting relationships with caring and loving adults enables infants to begin the process of developing high degrees of psychological well-being later in life.

Erikson viewed adolescence as a critical period in which youth develop a sense of *identity*. During this stage, adolescents become increasingly responsible for making their own decisions. They begin to function separately from their families and define who they are as well as what their future roles will be. According to Erikson, the three major areas of concern that adolescents must clarify relate to their sexuality, future occupation, and social conduct.

Table 2.2

Defense Mechanisms

Defense Mechanism	Behavior	Example
Repression	Blocking unpleasant thoughts or feelings	A woman suppresses the memory of being sexually abused as a child.
Rationalization	Making up false or self-serving excuses for unpleasant behavior or situations	A man makes excuses for not being hired for a job.
Denial	Refusing to acknowledge unpleasant situations or feelings	A young man does not accept the fact he has been diagnosed with a terminal illness.
Projection	Attributing unacceptable thoughts, feelings, or urges to someone else	A woman accuses her boyfriend of being unfaithful while repressing her desire to have an affair.
Displacement	Redirecting a feeling or response toward a target that usually is less of a threat	An abused wife does not fight back but mistreats her child instead.
Avoidance	Taking action to prevent situations that produce powerful feelings	A woman will not date because she is afraid of falling in love.
Regression	Reducing anxiety by acting immature to feel more secure	A 6-year-old child begins to suck his thumb after the birth of his baby brother.

Adolescents begin to establish their identities when they begin to clarify their feelings and positions about their roles in life. Identity confusion results when they are unable to develop sound self-concepts and function independently of their families.

Table 2.3

Erikson's Psychosocial Stages of Personality Development

Conflicts	Approximate Age Ranges
Trust vs. mistrust	Birth to 1 year
Autonomy vs. doubt and shame	1 to 3 years
Initiative vs. guilt	3 to 6 years
Industry vs. inferiority	6 to 12 years
Identity vs. identity confusion	12 to 18 years
Intimacy vs. isolation	Young adulthood
Generativity vs. stagnation	Middle age
Integrity vs. despair	Old age

As adolescents mature into young adulthood, they face the challenge of *intimacy*, forming close and loving relationships with others. Adults who did not develop a sense of trust earlier in their lives or have not clarified their identities may be unable to establish intimate relationships and thus feel isolated. During middle age, individuals who have mastered previous developmental tasks often focus on meeting the needs of others through activities such as raising families and performing community service. Erikson coined the term *generativity* to refer to these psychosocial tasks. In the final stage of life, people seek *integrity*, a feeling that their lives have been fulfilling and complete.

Maslow's Hierarchy of Needs According to psychologist Abraham Maslow, individuals behave in response to their values rather than to their unconscious drives.[2] Maslow thought that healthy people value the freedom to achieve personal fulfillment by developing their talents and competencies. This freedom becomes a psychological need that drives personality development. Maslow created a hierarchy of five human needs, from the most basic biological requirements that contribute to human survival to the one that is most essential for psychological fulfillment, self-actualization (**Figure 2.2**). To achieve *self-actualization*, each level of needs from

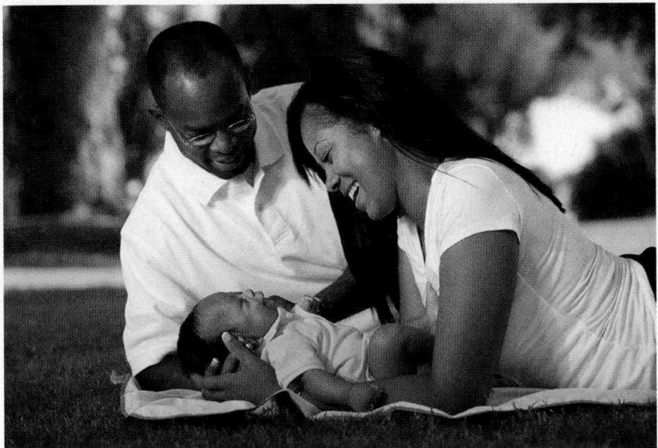

Establishing trusting relationships with loving adults enables infants to begin developing psychological well-being.

psychological adjustment Changing one's thoughts, attitudes, and behaviors to cope effectively with the demands of the environment.

psychological growth The process of learning from one's experiences.

the base to the top of the hierarchy must be met, in order.

Self-actualized persons are psychologically healthy and mature. They feel free to pursue their creative and intellectual capabilities. The possibility of self-actualization exists in all people, but unless the prerequisite needs are met, individuals can never fully realize their potential. According to Maslow and others, only about 1 person in 100 will reach the top of the human needs hierarchy. Nevertheless, Maslow admitted that many people are satisfied with their lives even if they have not achieved self-actualization.

Figure 2.2

Maslow's Hierarchy of Human Needs. Maslow created a hierarchy of five human needs, from the basic biological survival requirements to psychological fulfillment (self-actualization). Before achieving self-actualization, a person must satisfy all of the preceding needs.

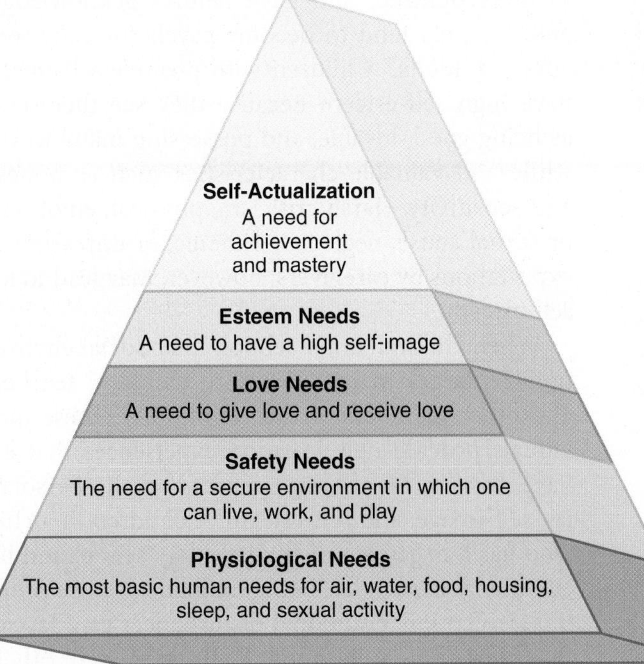
Self-Actualization
A need for achievement and mastery
Esteem Needs
A need to have a high self-image
Love Needs
A need to give love and receive love
Safety Needs
The need for a secure environment in which one can live, work, and play
Physiological Needs
The most basic human needs for air, water, food, housing, sleep, and sexual activity

Adjustment and Growth

Each day, individuals respond to the demands of other people, their physical environment, and themselves. Throughout life, these demands are changing constantly. Being in college is especially demanding, but consider how your life will change after you graduate. What do you think your life will be like 10, 20, or 30 years after graduation? What kinds of adaptations do you expect to make over your lifetime?

Adapting to change, which is called *adjustment*, involves the responses people make to cope with the demands of life. **Psychological adjustment** occurs when an individual learns that certain responses meet these demands more effectively than others do. For example, one way a new student might psychologically adjust to college life is by scheduling time each week for various tasks, such as studying, attending classes, and going to work. Maintaining the new schedule may be challenging, particularly if the student followed a less structured lifestyle in the past.

Psychological growth occurs when a person discovers that certain adjustment strategies, such as studying more or planning for the future, enhance one's sense of freedom and control over oneself and the environment. To adjust in beneficial ways and to experience psychological growth, an individual needs to obtain reliable information, set realistic goals, plan effective ways to achieve those goals, take actions that are based on reasonable judgments and decisions, and evaluate the consequences of his or her choices.

If not managed effectively, interpersonal conflicts can hinder psychological adjustment and growth. Such conflicts often arise

autonomy Sense of independence.

self-esteem The extent to which a person feels worthy and useful.

self-compassion Treating yourself with the same empathy you show others.

when people do not share opinions, values, needs, or beliefs. In these situations, many individuals respond by expressing anger or aggression. *Aggressive* reactions often injure other people physically or psychologically; therefore, these responses do not facilitate social interactions.

Assertiveness is a way of reacting to social situations by maintaining one's rights without interfering with the rights of other people and without harming them. Consider how students respond to an instructor who failed to consider certain possible answers to an essay question. An aggressive student might take class time to argue a point, verbally lashing out at the teacher. An assertive student might arrange to meet with the instructor after class, using the time to discuss his or her case in a more thoughtful and rational manner.

Another way healthy people constructively resolve interpersonal conflicts is by using compromise. An individual who disagrees with a friend over an issue, for example, may decide that preserving the friendship is more valuable in the long run than "winning" the argument. This person is willing to compromise by modifying his or her attitudes. The Managing Your Health feature provides additional suggestions for resolving conflicts constructively.

Psychological growth fosters the development of **autonomy**. People with a high degree of autonomy tend to function independently and display positive **self-esteem**, the extent to which a person feels worthy and useful.

Self-Esteem

Self-esteem is a key component of personality that influences an individual's thoughts, actions, and feelings. Positive self-esteem is a characteristic of psychologically healthy people. Individuals who have positive or high self-esteem tend to:

- Have a high degree of autonomy
- Display self-confidence and self-respect
- Be satisfied with themselves
- Accept challenges and work well with others
- Develop supportive and loving relationships
- Adjust more easily to change
- Accept responsibility for actions when they make mistakes

People with low self-esteem tend to:

- Have more difficulty making decisions
- Resist changing their behavior
- Resent any form of criticism, even if it is constructive
- Put down others to make themselves look or feel better
- Experience more stress and anxiety
- Have difficulty developing friendships or romantic relationships
- Be more vulnerable to drug and alcohol abuse

The "Self-Esteem Inventory" in the Student Workbook at the end of this text can help you assess your self-esteem.

People begin developing self-esteem early in childhood. Parents and other caregivers play a crucial role in determining their children's level of self-esteem. By interacting with parents and other family members, for example, young children learn that certain behaviors are good or bad. Children use this information to begin forming their *self-image*, the way they view themselves. Caregivers play an essential role in the development of children's self-esteem. Children who are listened to, spoken to with respect, given appropriate attention and affection, have accomplishment recognized, and have failures acknowledged and accepted tend to become psychologically well-adjusted adults.[3] Children with positive self-images have high self-esteem because they see themselves as being good, lovable, and possessing many worthwhile and valuable characteristics such as honesty and sensitivity. Harsh criticism, physical, emotional, or sexual abuse, neglect or ridicule, or unreasonable expectations by caregivers, however, may lead to low self-esteem.

When children enter school, their social environment enlarges to include more children, teachers, and other members of the community. These individuals provide new learning experiences that can have positive or negative impacts on the personality, self-image, and self-esteem of children. If a child who has a negative self-image enters school and has experiences, such as being bullied, that reinforce this perception, emotional disturbances can develop that persist into adulthood. With the help of others,

Managing Your Health

Resolving Interpersonal Conflicts Constructively

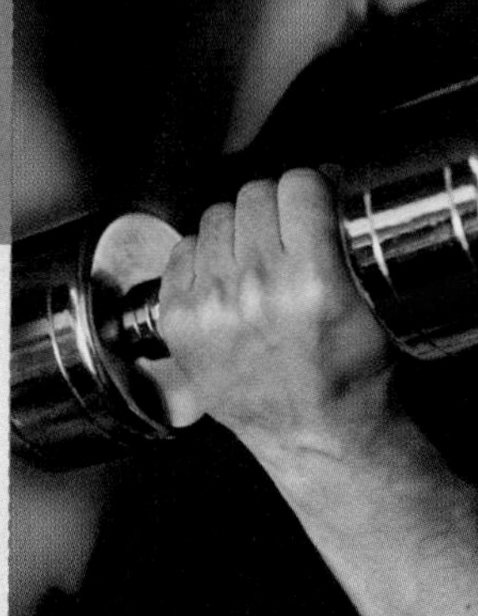

© Kzenon/ShutterStock

In addition to compromise, consider using the following tips to resolve conflicts constructively:

1. Focus on one issue; state your perception of the problem as clearly as possible.
2. Consider the feelings of others; avoid criticizing, name-calling, threats, or sarcasm.
3. Use "I feel" statements. "You" statements make others defensive. For example, say, "I feel angry when you . . ." instead of "You make me angry."
4. Do not assume how other people feel, what they believe, or how they will react.
5. Discuss the current concern; avoid dredging up past arguments.
6. Think before you speak; choose your words carefully to avoid confusion.
7. Listen carefully to others; avoid interrupting them while they talk.
8. Accept responsibility for your actions. Apologize for making mistakes.
9. Offer reasonable solutions.
10. Give others time to consider, accept, or reject your ideas.
11. Be patient; keep the door open for future communication.

children can develop positive self-concepts that establish the foundation for a lifetime of wellness. Parents and other adults help children feel good about themselves by spending time with them, listening to their concerns, and treating them with respect.

During adulthood, experiences at school, work, and home and a variety of social factors, including relationships, influence self-esteem. Relationships and experiences that are rewarding, enriching, and satisfying support positive self-esteem. In addition to having self-respect, people with a high degree of self-esteem gain the respect and approval of colleagues and others.

Self-esteem is a deep-rooted aspect of an individual. Although self-esteem may rise or fall over the course of a day, its basic nature remains fairly stable over longer periods. Individuals with persistent low self-esteem can improve their negative thoughts and feelings about themselves. By analyzing their situations, these people can determine factors that contribute to their poor self-concepts. For example, working in a dull job or remaining in an abusive relationship can affect self-esteem negatively. In these instances, people may improve their situations and feelings of self-worth by finding new jobs or ending the self-destructive relationships.

Self-esteem can be improved by identifying and learning to appreciate positive traits and abilities, while accepting our weaknesses (we all have them). Practicing **self-compassion**, or treating yourself with the empathy you show others, can also help facilitate self-esteem improvement. Accepting *constructive criticism* can support personal growth; therefore, is it also important to recognize that not all criticism is destructive or insensitive.[4] Making a few lifestyle changes, such as developing new interests, changing some bad habits, exercising regularly, or taking an assertiveness training class, can improve a person's psychological outlook. To overcome low self-esteem, psychological counseling may be necessary to help individuals develop the ability to evaluate themselves realistically and form accurate self-perceptions.

Improving Your Psychological Health

What can you do to improve your psychological health? You can enhance the quality of your mental health primarily by improving the other dimensions of your health. Exercising regularly may boost your mood.[3,5] Getting enough sleep, eating a nutritious diet, and maintaining a healthy weight for your height may also enhance psychological health by improving physical health. In addition to taking good care of your physical needs, fostering positive social contacts, whether with family, friends,

affect Observable expressions of mood.

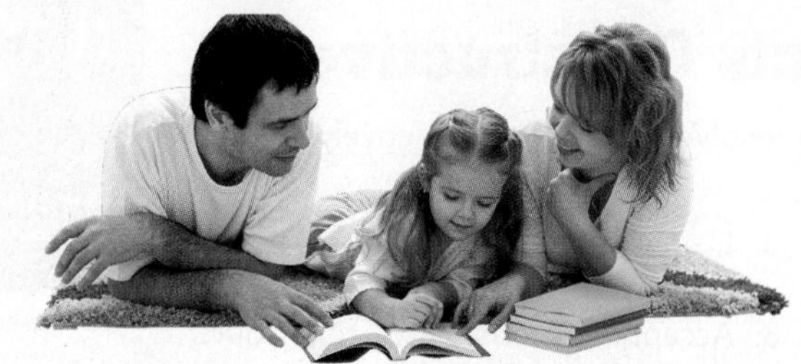

Caregivers play a crucial role in determining children's level of self-esteem.

© Ilike/ShutterStock

or colleagues, is very important. Everyone needs to communicate with other people on a regular basis. For example, one goal to improve your psychological health could be to make and maintain at least one new social contact each year. You can improve your intellectual health by reading challenging books, playing mind-stimulating games such as crossword puzzles or chess, or serving as a tutor. Some people find that keeping a journal or diary in which they record their most private feelings helps them cope with the challenges of daily life. Attending to your spiritual needs can provide personal fulfillment also. For example, you can volunteer to serve as a mentor for troubled children or become involved in your religious organization. Finally, taking an active role in ensuring and protecting the quality of your environment will support all dimensions of your health.

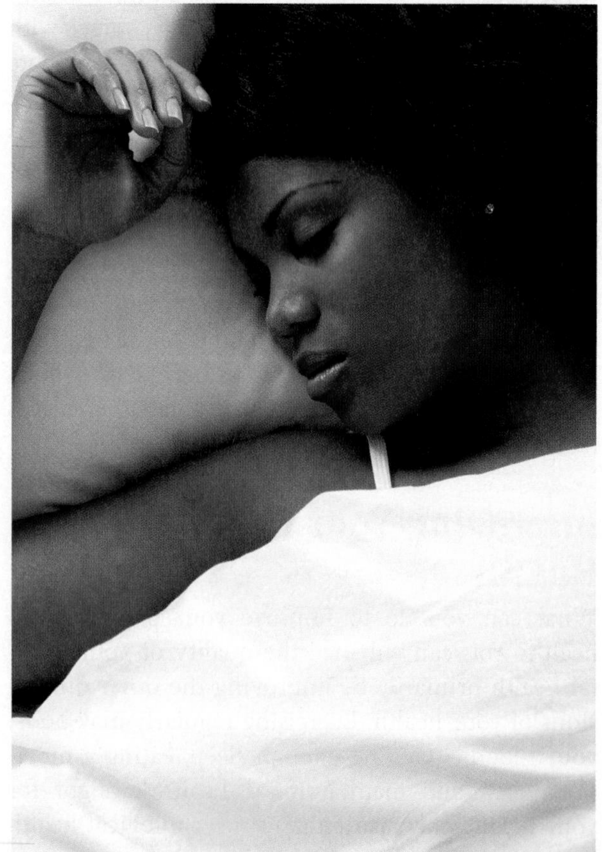

Adequate sleep can enhance psychological health by improving physical health.

© auremar/ShutterStock

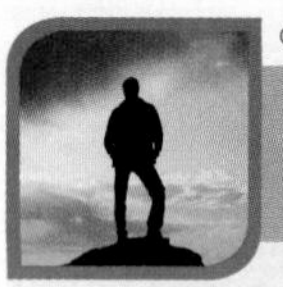

© djgis/ShutterStock

Healthy Living Practices

- To experience psychological adjustment and growth, set realistic goals, plan effective ways to achieve those goals, take actions that are based on reasonable judgments and decisions, and evaluate the consequences of your choices.
- To facilitate your psychological adjustment, learn ways to manage interpersonal conflicts constructively, without being aggressive. When such conflicts arise, decide when it is best to compromise or assert your position.
- To improve your self-esteem, avoid making negative statements about yourself. Identify and be realistic about your strengths and weaknesses; focus on your accomplishments and positive characteristics.
- To improve your psychological health, take steps to improve the quality of the other dimensions of your health.

Understanding Psychological (Mental) Illness

Having "the blues," feeling "scared to death," or being "worried sick"—perhaps you can recall situations in which you experienced these strong emotions or uncomfortable sensations. Occasionally, healthy people have disturbing thoughts, experience unpleasant feelings, or display inappropriate behaviors. In most instances, these are normal responses and adaptive reactions to unpleasant or threatening situations. For example, it is normal to be sad after learning about the death of a friend or to be afraid when a snake crosses your path. Given a reasonable amount of time, however, the strong emotional responses or unpleasant thoughts and feelings resolve, and you regain your sense of well-being.

The observable physical and behavioral changes that signal emotional state are referred to as **affect**

delusions Inaccurate and unreasonable beliefs that often result in decision-making errors.

hallucinations False sensory perceptions that have no apparent external cause.

or mood. Expressing emotions appropriately is a characteristic of a psychologically healthy individual; extreme or improper emotional responses can indicate a serious psychological disturbance. The key features that distinguish a normal emotional response from an abnormal one are the intensity and duration of the feelings. Mentally ill individuals experience abnormal feelings, thoughts, and behaviors that persist, interfere with daily life, and hinder psychological adjustment and growth.

A *psychosis* is a severe type of mental illness characterized by disorganized thoughts and unreal perceptions that result in strange behavior, isolation, delusions, and hallucinations. **Delusions** are inaccurate and unreasonable beliefs that often result in decision-making errors. For example, a person suffering from a delusion might think that he or she can fly, so this individual jumps off a tall building. **Hallucinations** are false sensory perceptions that have no apparent external cause, but they are real to the psychotic individual. Examples of hallucinations include hearing instructions from pictures, seeing ghostly images, or feeling insects crawling underneath skin. Psychotic conditions (psychoses) can be acute or chronic, and they can result from brain damage, chemical imbalances in the brain, or substance abuse.

Situations and cultures provide the context in which behaviors are judged as normal or abnormal. If a person who is living in a country torn apart by civil war bombs a crowded marketplace, people may view this individual as a terrorist or a hero but not necessarily mentally ill. However, if this bombing occurs in an American shopping mall, and the bomber says that a dog gave the order to perform the deed, you might suspect that this person is psychotic.

The Impact of Psychological Illness

Why is it important to learn about psychological illness? Most Americans have one or more family members who suffer from a psychological illness. Between 2006 and 2010, about 1 in 10 adult Americans reported experiencing "frequent mental distress" for 14 or more days during the previous 30 days.[6] According to data from the National Comorbidity Survey Replication, depression and alcohol dependence are the most common psychological disturbances that affect Americans (**Table 2.4**).[7] In 2012, 21% of adults aged 26 to 49 had a mental illness, whereas 19.6% of those aged 18 to 25 and 15.8% of those aged 50 or older had some form of mental illness, respectively.[8] Women and American Indians had the highest rates of mental illness in 2012.

The emotional and economic costs of mental illness are high not only for affected individuals and their families but also for society. People may drop out of college or abuse alcohol and other drugs because of unresolved emotional problems or underlying psychological disorders. Mental illness frequently has a negative impact on the quality of life and the productivity of workers.

Table 2.4

Lifetime Prevalence of Mental Health Disorders

Disorder	Percentage of Americans Affected*
Any mental health disorder	46.4
Any anxiety disorder	28.8
Panic disorder	4.7
Specific phobia	12.5
Social phobia	12.1
Generalized anxiety disorder	5.1
Obsessive-compulsive disorder	1.6
Impulse control disorders	24.8
Attention-deficit hyperactivity disorder	8.1
Any substance abuse/dependence	14.6
Alcohol abuse	13.2
Alcoholism	5.4
Drug dependence other than alcoholism	3.0
Any mood disorder	20.8
Major depressive episode	16.6
Bipolar disorders	3.9

*The sum of these percentages is more than 100 because many individuals suffer from more than one disorder.

Data from Kessler, R. C., et al. (2005). Lifetime prevalence and age-of-onset distributions of DSM-IV disorders in the National Comorbidity Survey Replication. *Archives of General Psychiatry, 62*(6), 593–602.

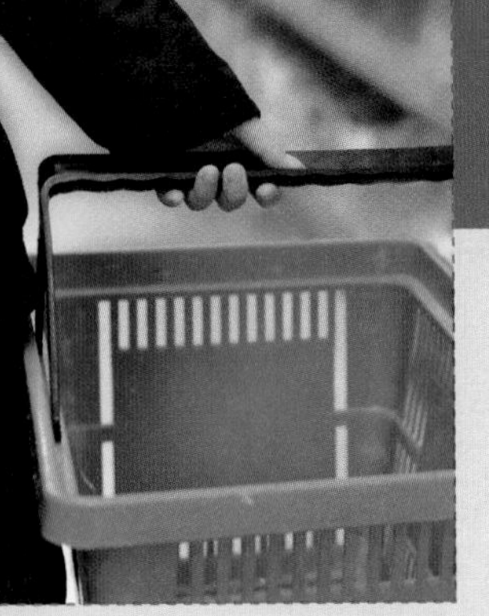
© sevenke/ShutterStock

Consumer Health

Locating and Selecting Mental Health Therapists

The following tips can help you find and select qualified mental health specialists:

- Discuss psychological health concerns with your personal physician or with medical staff at your student health center. These individuals can assess your health and refer you to qualified mental health specialists if necessary.
- Contact local mental health associations or agencies for information about psychological health. Members of these associations can give you information about local support groups and mental health services.
- Contact your state's social welfare department or the social services department of a local hospital to identify qualified therapists.
- Interview therapists before making any agreements for services.
- Ask therapists about treatment philosophies, methods, insurance coverage, and payment expectations before agreeing to use their services.

In the past, psychologically disturbed individuals were often misunderstood and mistreated. Having a mental illness was considered disgraceful by people who associated the condition with bizarre behaviors, violent acts, and long stays in mental healthcare facilities. Today, being diagnosed with a psychological disorder is no longer a hopeless situation, because scientists understand more about the various biological, environmental, and social factors that influence behaviors than in the past. Nevertheless, these disorders do not receive the kind of interest and concern from public health officials that conditions such as heart disease, cancer, and stroke generate. Why? Mental illnesses may not get much attention because of the stigma associated with them and the lack of major risk factors that can be modified to prevent them.

Although mental health disorders are common and can be quite disabling, mental illnesses are often not treated adequately worldwide.[9] In 2011, fewer than 50% of Americans who have these conditions sought treatment.[8] Approximately 50% of respondents to the *2012 National Survey on Drug Use and Health* indicated the most significant barrier to treatment was cost. Believing they could handle the problem themselves or that treatment wouldn't work, not knowing where to go for mental health services, and negative attitudes toward mental illness were identified as major reasons for not seeking beneficial therapy. To many medical and health professionals, however, seeking professional help for psychological problems is a sign of personal strength, not weakness.

What Causes Psychological Disorders?

There are numerous psychological disorders, and in each case, it may be impossible to determine a single cause. Alterations in the normal chemical and physical environment of the brain often produce mental illness. In many instances, these alterations are the result of genetic defects that adversely affect neurotransmitter levels. People whose brains have been physically damaged by injuries, tumors, or infections often display abnormal behavior. When introduced into the body, drugs such as cocaine can interfere with the brain's ability to produce, use, or eliminate neurotransmitters. Furthermore, pollutants such as pesticides and toxic minerals, including lead, mercury, and arsenic, can damage the brain.

Scientists note that certain mental illnesses such as schizophrenia and most major mood disorders tend to occur within the same family. These observations support the role of inheritance in their development. Genetic factors alone, however, do not explain the development of every psychological disorder. Several members of a family could develop similar forms of mental illness because they are more likely to experience the same physical, economic, and social environments than unrelated individuals.

Environmental conditions influence the expression of many inborn traits, including psychological responses. Children, for example, often learn ways of reacting to situations by observing their parents. Think about how you respond when angered or frustrated. Are your responses like those of your mother or father?

Personal experiences can trigger the onset and influence the severity of some psychological disturbances. Some experts think that a child's brain can be altered by exposure to extremely stressful situations, increasing the youngster's risk of developing depression later in life. However, researchers have yet to understand completely the extent to which biological, social, and environmental factors interact to influence psychological health.

Treating Psychological Disorders

Many people with psychological disorders respond well to treatment. Treating these conditions involves the cooperation of the affected individuals and their families and, in many instances, the assistance of mental health therapists who have specialized training. **Table 2.5** lists the major types of mental health therapists and some information concerning their qualifications.

Many people learn to cope with various psychological problems, such as drug addictions or the loss of loved ones, by joining *support groups*. The support group is an informal approach to treatment. Support group participants have regular meetings in which they can discuss personal adjustment problems. Group members usually conduct these meetings rather than mental health therapists. In addition to attending regular meetings, some group members may need to obtain professional counseling.

Mental health therapists can offer a variety of effective psychotherapies (treatments) that enable many individuals with psychological disorders to lead normal, productive lives. Psychotherapy uses many methods to provide counseling, including *cognitive behavioral therapy*, group therapy, and medications. Cognitive behavioral therapy can help people who are anxious, angry, or depressed identify and change negative or inaccurate ways in which they think about themselves and their situations. As mentioned

Table 2.5

Major Types of Mental Health Therapists

Therapist	Training and Degrees
Counseling and clinical psychologists	M.A., Ph.D., or Psy.D. in psychology; 5 or more years in psychotherapy methods, research, and assessment
Psychiatrists	Medical (M.D. or O.D.) degree and at least 3 years of specialized training in psychiatry
Psychoanalysts	Have undergone personal psychoanalysis and completed 7 to 10 years of part-time psychoanalytic training (most are psychiatrists)
Psychiatric social workers	M.S.W.; most states require certification by the Academy of Certified Social Workers
Clinical mental health counselors	Master's degree (or equivalent) and 2 years of counseling experience; certified by National Academy of Certified Clinical Mental Health Counselors
Psychiatric nurse practitioners	Registered nurses with additional education and experience working in psychiatric settings
Marital and family therapists	Master's degree. Licensed or certified in about one-half of the states; member of the American Association for Marriage and Family Therapy
Sexual therapists	Minimum of a master's degree, a license in related field, specialized sex education and sex-therapist training, extensive supervised individual and group therapy experience; the American Association of Sex Educators, Counselors and Therapists provides certification
Abuse counselors	Substance abuse training; often counselors are recovering substance abusers
Clergy	Religious training; may have spiritual and family counseling training

Data from Cornacchia, H. J., & Barrett, S. (1993). *Consumer health*. St. Louis, MO: Mosby.

earlier, medication can correct neurotransmitter imbalances in the brain.

More than one form of treatment may be necessary to alleviate or control the disorder. In severe cases, people suffering from major psychological conditions may require hospitalization for treatment and to prevent self-injury or harm to others. If you or someone you know needs mental health care, the Consumer Health box titled "Locating and Selecting Mental Health Therapists" provides some suggestions for finding and choosing qualified help.

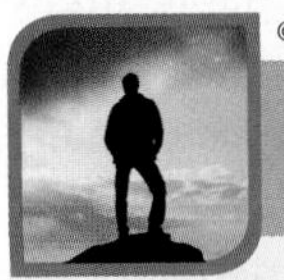

Healthy Living Practices

- Many psychological problems respond well to treatment. If you think you may have a mental health disorder, ask your personal physician or the medical staff at your campus health center for help.

Common Psychological Disorders

Anxiety Disorders

Do you feel uneasy when you ride in an elevator, enter a classroom to take a test, or give a speech? Nearly everyone experiences anxiety, the uncomfortable feeling of apprehension or uneasiness that results while expecting a vague threat. The physical changes associated with anxiety states include increased heart rate, rapid breathing, and elevated blood pressure. Anxious people may report feeling tense, distressed, or worried; and they may be emotionally upset, sweating, and trembling.[9] Anxiety disorders are common; according to the results of the National Comorbidity Survey Replication, nearly 30% of Americans suffer from these conditions at some time in their lives.[10]

Generalized Anxiety Disorder When you perceive a threat, it is normal to feel mildly anxious as your body physically prepares to deal with the danger. However, if the anxiety interferes with your ability to perform daily activities, the condition is abnormal. During their lifetimes, about 5% of the population suffers from **generalized anxiety disorder**, a condition characterized by uncontrollable chronic worrying, anxiousness, and nervousness. People with this disorder have unrealistic and excessive concerns about their jobs, children, health, or minor situations such as making home repairs. They are tense, irritable, and restless, and they often experience sleeping problems. Treatment usually includes antianxiety and antidepressant medications as well as cognitive behavioral therapy.

Phobias A **phobia** is an intense and irrational fear of a situation or object. *Agoraphobia* is the fear of open places or public areas. *Social phobias* are fears of performing in situations that involve people, such as giving speeches or taking tests. *Specific phobias* (formerly called simple phobias) are fears of certain objects or situations, such as snakes or flying. According to the results of the National Comorbidity Survey Replication, phobias are among the most common psychological disturbances in the United States.[10] About 12% of Americans report having social phobias, and about 12.5% of Americans report experiencing specific phobias. It is not uncommon for a person to be affected by more than one phobia. Although people who suffer from phobias know that their behavior is irrational, they still become anxious in the situations that arouse their fears (**Figure 2.3**).

Most cases of phobia are mild; affected individuals often learn to live with this condition by avoiding situations that arouse the anxiety. Severe phobias can interfere with normal social functioning. For example, people with agoraphobia may refuse to leave their homes. Individuals who are severely affected by phobias can seek professional treatment that includes behavioral therapy and medications to control irrational feelings and reduce anxiety.

Figure 2.3

Phobias. Phobias are intense and irrational fears of certain situations or objects that can interfere with functioning. Many people have a fear of flying.

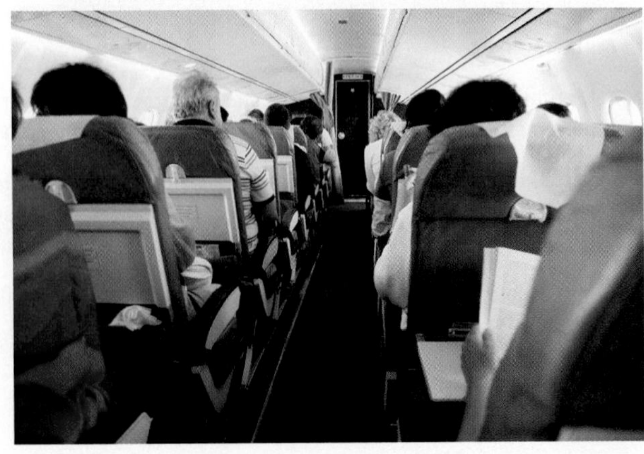

generalized anxiety disorder A condition characterized by uncontrollable chronic worrying and nervousness.

phobia An intense and irrational fear of an object or a situation.

panic disorder Psychological condition that features panic attacks, unpredictable episodes of extreme anxiety, and loss of emotional control.

Panic Disorder An estimated 3 million Americans suffer from *panic disorders* that feature *panic attacks*, unpredictable episodes of extreme anxiety and loss of emotional control. During a panic attack, people usually experience shortness of breath, shakiness, faintness, nausea, and a rapid, pounding heartbeat. Affected individuals often feel terrified because they think they are becoming insane or having a heart attack. Severe phobias, certain drugs, or frightening experiences may trigger panic attacks, but they can occur spontaneously.

Therapists often combine cognitive behavioral therapy and medications to treat panic disorders. People who have frequent panic attacks should seek medical help because studies indicate that they are at risk of committing suicide.

Trauma- and Stressor-Related Disorders

Psychological disorders in this category differ from anxiety disorders because exposure to a traumatic or stressful event is explicitly listed as a criterion for diagnosis.[10] For example, someone can experience *Post-Traumatic Stress Disorder (PTSD)* when they survive extraordinary life events such as a sexual assault, military combat, or a natural disaster may develop post-traumatic stress disorder (**Figure 2.4**). The diagnostic criteria for PTSD include (1) reexperiencing the traumatic event (e.g., recurrent dreams), (2) heightened arousal (e.g., aggressiveness, sleep disturbances, hypervigilance), (3) avoidance (e.g., blocking reminders of the traumatic event), and (4) negative thoughts, moods, or feelings (e.g., distorted sense of self-blame, estrangement from others).

Figure 2.4

Surviving a Disaster. Rescuers pull a boy from beneath a collapsed wall at Plaza Towers Elementary School after an EF-5 tornado destroyed it and thousands of homes in Moore, Oklahoma on May 20, 2013.

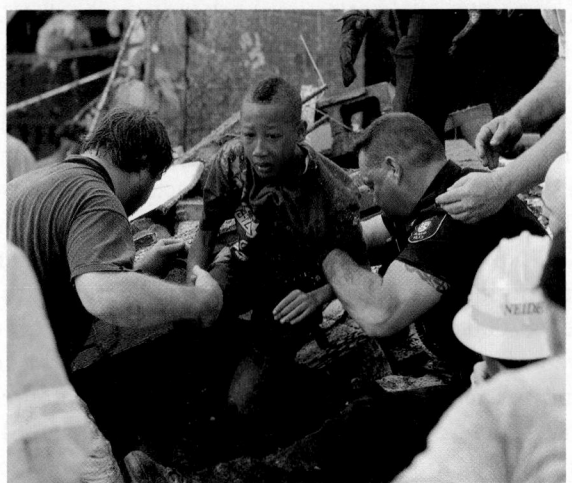

Symptoms of PTSD may take months to develop fully and include having disturbing recollections or nightmares of the event, and in severe cases, feeling emotionally "numb." Affected people often avoid thinking about or discussing the traumatic experiences, and they may smoke heavily, overeat, or abuse drugs as a way of coping. Treatment of PTSD includes antianxiety medication and trauma-focused cognitive behavioral therapy that encourages survivors to talk about the traumatic events with others.[11]

Acute Stress Disorder Characterized by severe anxiety, disassociation, and other symptoms, *acute stress disorder* occurs within 1 month of exposure to a traumatic stressor.[9] People suffering from acute stress disorder display decreased emotional responsiveness, including feelings of guilt about pursuing usual life tasks and may find it difficult to experience pleasure in previously enjoyable activities. In many cases, people experiencing acute stress disorder have difficulty concentrating or recalling specific details of the traumatic event, and report feeling detached from their bodies. For acute stress disorder to be diagnosed, someone must experience distress or impairment in social, occupational, or other important areas of function and inhibit the individual's ability to pursue necessary tasks. Furthermore, symptoms must persist for a minimum of 2 days and a maximum of 4 weeks and must not be associated with substance use or abuse.

Adjustment Disorders An *adjustment disorder* is a stress-related disorder often consisting of a group of symptoms, including feeling sad or physical symptoms (e.g., twitching, skipping heartbeats, or nervousness) that occur after a stressful life event. Symptoms occur when someone has a difficult time coping with events such as death of a loved one, worries about money, sexuality issues, or major illness. Adjustment disorder is often diagnosed when a person's reaction to a stressful event if stronger or greater than expected. In many cases, symptoms of adjustment disorder mirror acute stress disorder but do not meet clinical criteria for diagnosis.

Obsessive-Compulsive and Related Disorders

Obsessive-Compulsive Disorder In the new *Diagnostic and Statistical Manual of Mental Disorders*, DSM-5, *obsessive-compulsive disorder (OCD)* was placed in the new obsessive compulsive and related disorders category. An *obsession* is a persistent, inappropriate, and repetitive thought or impulse that produces anxious feelings. Obsessions are often related to self-doubt or fears. A *compulsion* is the behavior that usually follows the obsessive thoughts or impulses. Compulsive behaviors reduce the obsessed individual's anxiety. A young person, for example, might have recurring thoughts of injuring a family member. This individual may wash his or her hands hundreds of times a day and take numerous long showers to reduce anxious feelings. Other typical compulsive behaviors include hoarding cats and dogs or useless items like plastic containers or making repetitive actions such as checking the oven frequently to see if it is turned off. Affected individuals often think that their obsessions and compulsions are repulsive or troublesome, but efforts to stop create more anxiety. Treatment includes medication and psychological counseling. In most cases, the longer the obsessive-compulsive behavior pattern has been in place, the more difficult the disorder is to treat.

Other disorders, including hoarding disorder, trichotillomania, and excoriation disorder are considered related disorders, as they also indicated obsessive tendencies. *Hoarding disorder* reflects persistent difficulty discarding or parting with possessions due to a perceived need to save the items and distress associated with discarding them. *Tricholtillomania* (hair-pulling disorder) is a compulsive urge to pull out, and in some cases eat, one's own hair, and *excoriation disorder* (skin picking) is characterized by compulsively picking at one's skin for no apparent reason. Treatment for compulsive disorders begins with proper diagnosis by a mental health professional.

Neurodevelopmental Disorders

Neurodevelopmental disorders refer to deficits in social communication and social interaction. Those with a neurodevelopmental disorder may display repetitive or restrictive behaviors, may have difficulty coping with change, and may experience great distress when required to change focus or action. *Attention-deficit hyperactivity disorder (ADHD)* and *autism spectrum disorder* are common neurodevelopmental disorders.

Attention-Deficit Hyperactivity Disorder ADHD is characterized by short attention span and/or hyperactivity-impulsivity that results in serious social impairment. An estimated 4.4% of American adults have ADHD; men are more likely to be diagnosed with ADHD than are women.[12] The causes of ADHD are unclear, but genetics plays a role in the development of the condition.

People with ADHD have difficulty focusing and maintaining their attention on tasks, such as performing work-related responsibilities, studying, or completing assignments. Unemployment, sleep disturbances, accident proneness, and cigarette smoking are associated with adult ADHD.[12]

There is no generally accepted test for diagnosing adult ADHD, and the condition is often more difficult to recognize in adults than in children because the signs are less obvious.[12] Adults with ADHD frequently suffer from anxiety, mood, and drug abuse disorders. Treatment may include stimulants such as methylphenidate (Ritalin) and psychological counseling. According to the results of one survey, only about 10% of adults with ADHD reported receiving treatment for the condition during the past 12 months.[12] More consumer and physician awareness programs are needed to alert the public about adult ADHD and its treatments. If you would like more information about ADHD, visit the Centers for Disease Control and Prevention's website at www.cdc.gov/ncbddd/adhd/.

Autism Spectrum Disorder (ASD) encompasses autistic disorder, Asperger's disorder, childhood disintegrative disorder, and pervasive developmental disorder—not otherwise classified (or atypical autism). People with ASD tend to have difficulty communicating, may respond inappropriately in conversation, misread nonverbal interactions, and have difficulty building and maintaining relationships. Additionally, people with ASD are highly dependent on routine and sensitive to change.[10] Between the years 2000 and 2008, approximately 1 in 88 children were diagnosed with ASD[13]. There is currently no known cause for ASD, although most scientists agree that genetics play a large role. The beliefs that ASD is linked to poor parenting or routine vaccination, however, are not supported by evidence.[14] Diagnosis of ASD can be difficult and requires trained medical professionals. For more information about ASD, visit the Centers for Disease Control and Prevention's website at www.cdc.gov/ncbddd/autism/index.html.

Substance-Related and Addictive Disorders

Substance Use Disorder Excess use of ten classes of drugs, including alcohol, caffeine, cannabis, inhalants, opioids, sedatives, hypnotics, and stimulants, is classified as substance-related disorder.[10] Drugs taken in excess activate the brain's reward system and create a feeling of pleasure, often referred to as a "high." By doing so, drug abuse behavior is reinforced. For some people, activation of the reward system is so intense, normal activities may be neglected. People with lower levels of self-control, which may reflect impairments of the brain inhibitory mechanism, may be predisposed to substance use disorders. Generational pattern, in which people are exposed to drug use in their family, social, or community environments, are also major contributors to increased risk for addiction.

Problem Gambling Nearly every state permits some form of gambling, such as lotteries, track racing, or casinos. For most people who place bets, the activity is entertaining, occasional, and controllable. However, about 1% of adult Americans are problem gamblers who gamble compulsively, excessively, and at the expense of their families, jobs, and relationships.[15] Men are more likely to be compulsive gamblers than women are. Psychological disorders, including depression and anxiety disorders, and risky behaviors such as binge drinking and illegal drug use often accompany problem gambling behavior. **Table 2.6** lists typical features of problem gamblers.

Gamblers Anonymous is a self-help group that can enable problem gamblers to control their troublesome behavior (www.gamblersanonymous.org). Many problem gamblers, however, do not remain in treatment. Some counselors have certification to treat compulsive gambling, but health insurance providers may not cover their services. More research is needed to determine effective ways to prevent as well as treat this condition.

Table 2.6

Typical Features of Problem Gambling

The problem gambler:

- Seems to think only about gambling or how to get money to gamble
- Loses friends, family members, and jobs because of his or her behavior
- Gambles more often over time
- Has no control over the impulse to gamble
- Becomes restless, angry, or agitated when he or she tries to gamble less often (withdrawal)
- Gambles to escape problems or cope with depression, guilt, or anxiety
- Gambles again, trying to recover losses
- Lies to cover up the behavior
- Has others financially bail him or her out
- Resorts to illegal acts, such as forging checks and stealing money, to obtain money for gambling
- Abuses mind-altering drugs

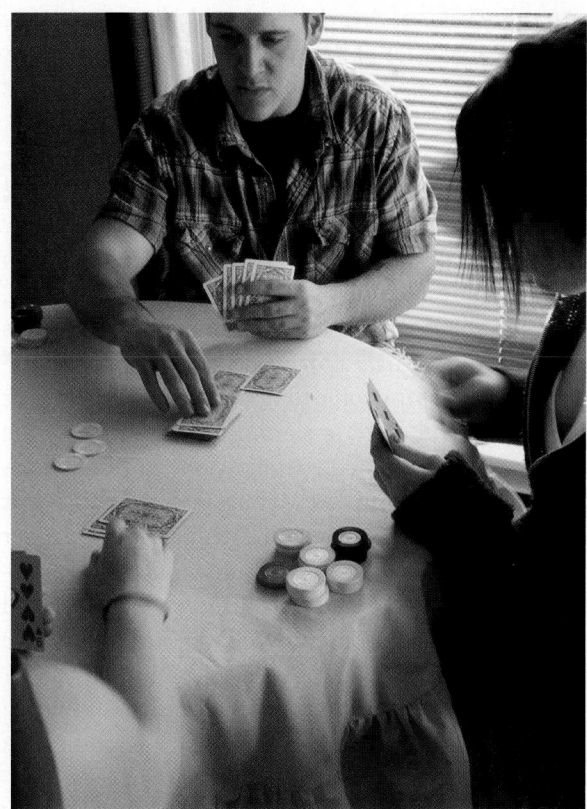

Do you know someone who is a problem gambler?

© neal and molly jansen/Alamy Images

Mood Disorders

Until a few years ago, the two words that best described my life were fear and loneliness. *As a child, I experienced physical, emotional, and verbal abuse from my parents. There were some instances when the beatings*

major depressive disorder A mood disorder characterized by persistent and profound sadness, hopelessness, helplessness, and feelings of worthlessness; lack of energy; loss of interest in usual activities; loss of the ability to concentrate; suicidal thoughts; and appetite and sleep disturbances.

were so severe, I just forgot about them. I married a man who also physically abused me. Having no savings or college degree, I lacked the self-confidence to walk out of the marriage. I felt trapped. Deep depression set in; I cried a lot of the time and felt guilty because I was unable to carry out the normal daily responsibilities of cooking and cleaning the house. I began to think suicidal thoughts.

Finally, I entered a hospital that had a stress unit. Between the group sessions and private therapy, I learned a lot about those who abuse others and how to handle stress. However, spending 3 weeks in the hospital did not cure my depression. I realized that the only thing that would do that would be to remove myself from its cause. I separated from my husband and started college.

It has been a struggle financially, but I am determined to make it. I am preparing to graduate this semester with a Bachelor of Arts degree, and I plan to continue on to get a Master of Arts degree. The best change is my new self-confidence gained from overcoming the obstacles and becoming independent.

This middle-aged college student's case illustrates not only the harsh origins of her depression but also how an emotionally resilient person can recover from depression, resolve problems, and regain self-esteem. How can you distinguish a normal period of sadness from one that signals a major depressive disorder?

It is normal for people to feel "down" after a loss or disappointment. After a significant loss, such as the death of a close friend or relative, one normally feels grief, an intense sadness that may persist up to a year after the loss. Most grieving individuals soon recover their emotional balance and resume their usual activities. Grieving people are probably severely depressed if they become so profoundly sad that they withdraw and isolate themselves for several months and harbor feelings of guilt, low self-worth, and suicide. Enduring other stressful experiences, such as a difficult relationship or experiencing severe physical or emotional trauma, can trigger the first episode of depression in susceptible persons.

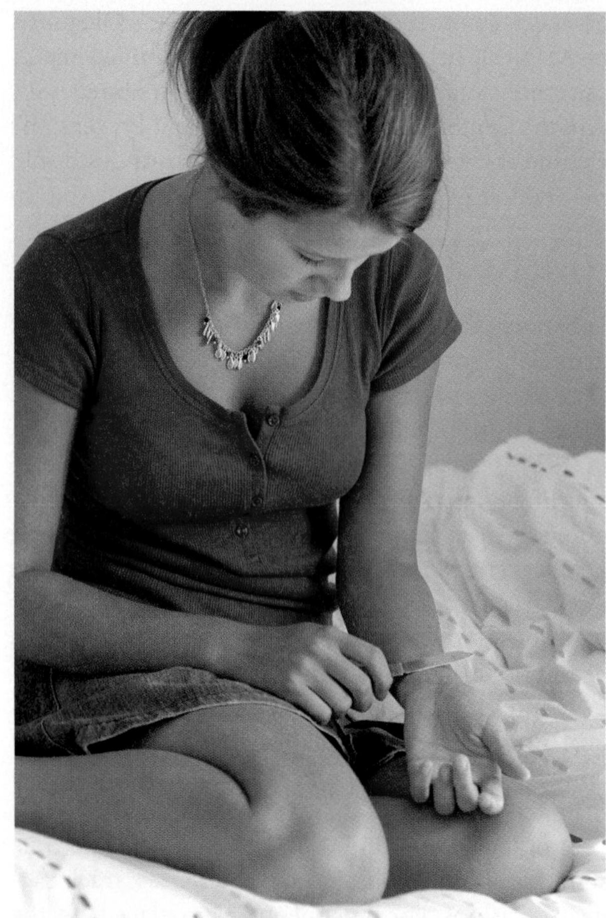

"Cutting" can be a sign of depression.

People suffering from **major depressive disorder** generally experience the following:

- Persistent sad, "empty," or hopeless feelings
- Feelings of guilt, worthlessness, or helplessness
- Loss of interest or pleasure in activities that used to be enjoyed
- Unexplainable fatigue
- Difficulty concentrating, remembering, or making decisions
- Frequent insomnia, early-morning wakening, or oversleeping
- Changes in appetite resulting in weight loss or gain
- Restlessness
- Physical complaints that do not respond to treatment, such as chronic headaches, intestinal tract disturbances, and pain
- Thoughts about death, suicide, or attempting suicide

These symptoms last for 2 weeks or more and interfere with relationships and responsibilities related to school, work, and home. Depressed people may be anxious and irritable, and they often use alcohol or illegal drugs to alter their emotional state. Self-mutilation (for example, "cutting") can also be a sign of depression. Depression can be devastating for individuals and their families. About 7% of men with a history of depression commit suicide, whereas only 1% of women with a history of depression will take their own lives.[16]

According to results of a survey conducted in 2006–2008, almost 10% of U.S. adults were depressed at the time of the study, and about one-third of those persons were suffering from *major* depression.[17] The people who were most likely to have major depression were:

- Between 45 and 64 years of age
- Women
- Blacks and Hispanics
- People who had dropped out of high school
- Divorced persons
- People who were unable to work or find work
- People without health insurance coverage

What Causes Depression? Depressive illnesses are disorders of the brain that have no single cause. The condition probably results from a complex combination of genetic, biochemical, and environmental factors as well as learned behavioral responses to situations. Some types of depression tend to run in families; however, depression also occurs in people who do not have family histories of the disorder.[18] Researchers have detected abnormal neurotransmitter levels in depressed people's brains.[18] As a result, the parts of the brain that regulate mood, thoughts, sleep, appetite, and behavior function abnormally.

For reasons that are unclear but that may be related to hormonal fluctuations, women are more likely to become depressed than are men. Men, however, tend to experience depression differently from how women experience it. Men are more likely to be irritable, report lack of interest in formerly pleasurable activities, be unusually fatigued, and have sleep disturbances; women are more likely to report feeling sad, worthless, and guilty.[18]

Like diabetes and high blood pressure, depression is a chronic but treatable disease. Many people who are severely and chronically depressed can obtain dramatic relief from their disabling symptoms by receiving therapies that include prescribed antidepressant medications and psychotherapy, which teaches patients to focus on positive rather than negative thoughts. However, physicians who are not psychiatrists often fail to diagnose the condition in their patients. As a result, many people with depression are not treated or are improperly treated.[19,20] Younger people with depression, typically those 18 to 25 years of age, are less likely than older adults to receive mental health treatment.[21]

Alternative remedies for depression are becoming popular in the United States. The herb St. John's wort may be helpful as a treatment for mild to moderate depression.[22] St. John's wort has been reported to interact with certain prescription drugs and cause side effects, so individuals should not take this substance without consulting a physician.

People who are depressed often feel better when engaging in regular physical activity. According to the Surgeon General's report *Physical Activity and Health*,[23] a moderate amount of physical activity each day may reduce symptoms of anxiety and depression and improve mood and a sense of well-being.

Managing Mild Depression If you experience mild depression, you can help yourself by:

- Setting priorities at work, home, or school
- Avoiding excess responsibilities
- Maintaining social contacts and confiding in someone you can trust
- Participating in a few enjoyable activities, especially if they are social and improve your mood
- Exercising regularly
- Relaxing
- Focusing on positive rather than negative thoughts
- Volunteering to help others in need

By taking these actions, your mood should gradually improve. If you still feel depressed after a couple of weeks, or your mood worsens, seek professional help. For more information about depression, visit the National Institute of Mental Health's website: http://www.nimh.nih.gov/health/topics/depression/index.shtml?utm_source=BrainLine.org&utm_medium=Twitter.

Bipolar Disorder *Bipolar disorder*, formerly called manic depression, is characterized by unusual shifts in mood, energy and physical activity levels, and

eating disorders Persistent, abnormal eating patterns that can threaten a person's health and well-being.

ability to carry out daily tasks. A person with bipolar disorder typically experiences distinct episodes of intense positive and negative emotional states. The extremely happy and excited emotional state is called *mania*. Individuals with mania typically brag about themselves and their accomplishments, engage in excessive physical activity and rapid talking, and sleep very little. Another characteristic of mania is excessive participation in pleasurable and risky activities that can lead to unwelcome consequences, such as careless sexual encounters or costly shopping sprees. After the manic episode subsides, the person's behavior and mood become more "normal." In time, however, his or her emotional state swings to the negative mood (severe depression) state, and this person feels extremely sad and hopeless.

During each phase of bipolar disorder, the mood of the affected person gradually reaches an extreme level, and the affected person may not be able to function normally. When this occurs, the person with bipolar disorder may become suicidal and require hospitalization.

In addition to the extremes of mania and severe depression, bipolar disorder can cause a range of moods. People with bipolar disorder may develop *hypomania*, an emotional state that is characterized by increased energy and activity levels, which are not as excessive as in the manic state. A person with hypomania tends to feel very well and be highly productive. Although close associates of this individual may recognize that he or she is not behaving and functioning normally, the affected person may feel fine. Unless people with hypomania receive proper treatment, they may develop severe mania or depression. **Table 2.7** lists typical symptoms of manic and depressive states, and **Figure 2.5** shows the cyclic pattern of bipolar disorder.

Bipolar disorder tends to develop during the late teens or young adult years—before 25 years of age. People with the bipolar disorder tend to have a family history of the illness, so medical researchers suspect the condition may be inherited.[24]

The cyclic mood shifts that characterize the bipolar disorder may recur several times during an individual's life. In many cases, however, the symptoms are not easy to recognize or distinguish from normal emotional responses. As a result, the illness may not be diagnosed or treated properly. There is no cure for bipolar disorder, but in many cases, the condition can be managed with medications.

Table 2.7

Typical Symptoms of Bipolar Disorder

Mania Symptoms	Depressive Symptoms
Experiences an unusually long period of acting "high" or being extremely happy or outgoing	Experiences an unusually long period of feeling worried or empty
Is extremely irritable; appears jumpy or "wired"	Loses interest in activities that he or she had enjoyed
Talks very fast, jumps from one idea to another, has "racing" thoughts	Feels tired or in "slow motion"
Is easily distracted	Has difficulty concentrating, remembering, and making decisions
Takes on several new projects but does not complete them or performs poorly	Is restless and irritable
Is restless and sleeps very little	Experiences changes in usual eating, sleeping, and other habits
Has unrealistic beliefs about his or her abilities	Thinks about death or suicide, or attempting suicide
Behaves impulsively and engages in risky behaviors	

Seasonal Affective Disorder Besides bipolar disorder, other mood disorders occur in cycles. People with *seasonal affective disorder (SAD)* become depressed around mid- to late fall, and their depression ends in late winter or early spring. Besides feeling depressed and tired, people with SAD also report craving sweets and gaining weight. Because these symptoms resolve when the daylight period

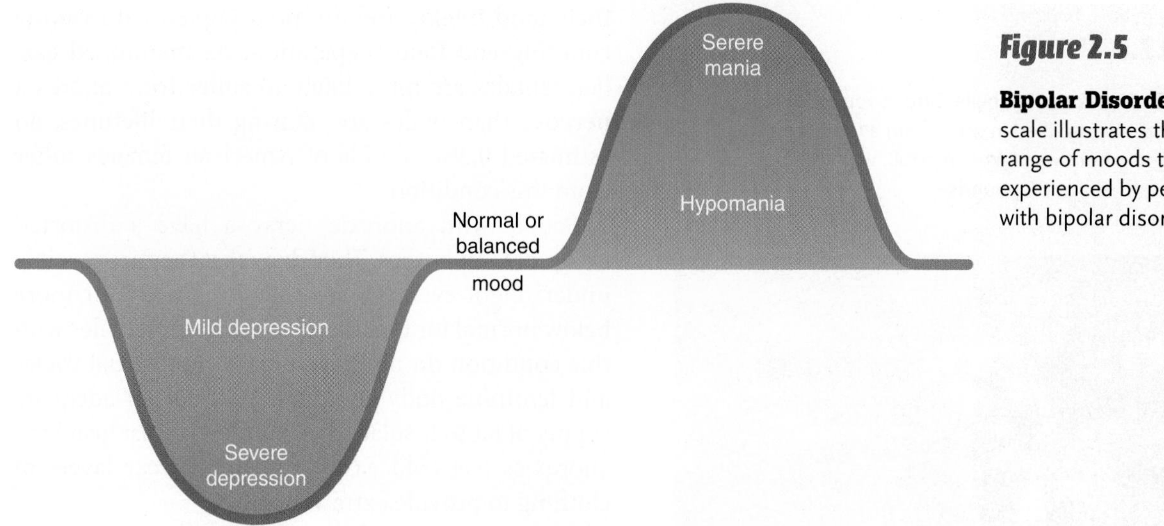

Figure 2.5

Bipolar Disorder. This scale illustrates the range of moods typically experienced by people with bipolar disorder.

lengthens or when people with the condition spend time in sunnier climates, medical experts think SAD may be related to a lack of exposure to bright light. Light therapy is an effective form of treatment for this disorder.[25]

Feeding and Eating Disorders

A female college athlete habitually skips breakfast. For lunch, she typically drinks an 8-ounce canned milkshake that is marketed as a weight loss supplement. By the time dinner is served in her dormitory, she describes herself as "starving." A male college student whose height is 5′ 9″ and weight only 125 pounds also skips breakfast. Nearly every day, he eats cheeseburgers and french fries from a fast-food restaurant that is within walking distance of his campus. He rarely eats fruits or green vegetables. A young man who describes himself as a vegetarian eats only brown rice, fruit, and tea. Are these behaviors examples of eating disorders?

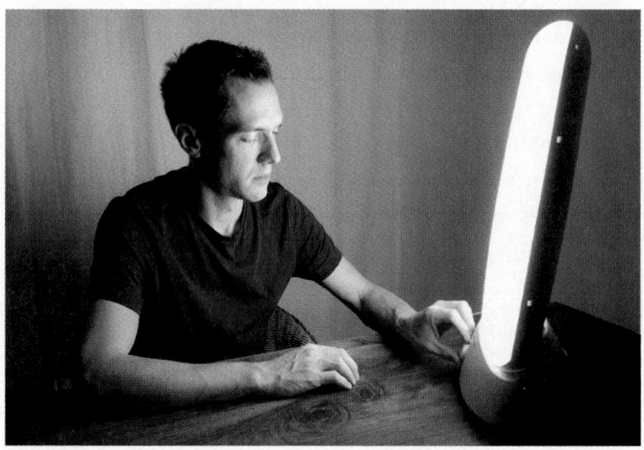

Light therapy is an effective treatment for SAD.

Occasionally, most people engage in unusual eating practices, such as skipping meals, fasting, or avoiding sweets in an effort to lose a few pounds. *Disordered eating* practices are mild and often temporary changes in an individual's otherwise normal food-related behaviors. In many instances, a person uses these behaviors to improve health or appearance. Disordered eating practices, however, can become eating disorders. **Eating disorders** are persistent, abnormal eating patterns that can threaten a person's health and well-being. Each year, millions of American lives are disrupted by the three major eating disorders—bulimia nervosa, anorexia nervosa, and binge eating disorder. These conditions often develop in adolescence or young adulthood, and they are more likely to affect females than males. An estimated 85% to 95% of the people with anorexia nervosa and 65% of those suffering from bulimia nervosa are female.

Hormonal, genetic, psychological, and sociocultural factors influence the development of eating disorders. Risk factors include family history, childhood abuse, depression and anxiety, low self-esteem, and family conflict.[26,27] Additionally, homosexual males may have a higher risk of eating disorders than heterosexual males.[26,27]

Although it is true that excess body fat is not healthy, a society that emphasizes thinness as a sign of physical attractiveness makes many young people overly concerned about and dissatisfied with their body size and shape, even when it is normal. As a result of societal influences, many American females admire the bodies of actresses, fashion models, and

Figure 2.6

Anorexia Nervosa. Isabelle Caro, a young Italian model and actress, died in 2010 from a long-term illness. This photo was taken in 2008, when Caro weighed only about 66 pounds.

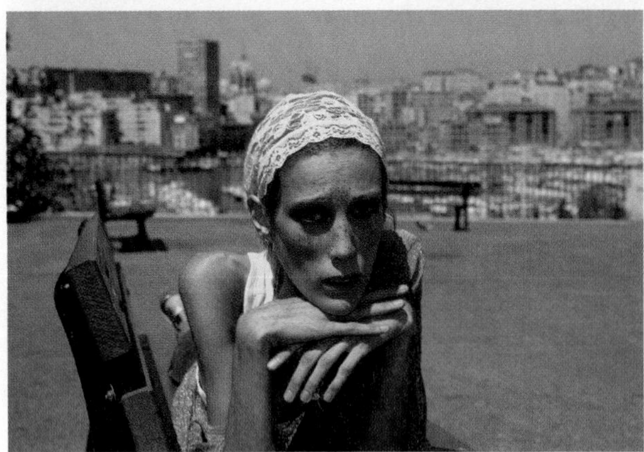

ballet dancers who look as though they are starving (**Figure 2.6**). Young males, on the other hand, may equate optimal health and attractiveness with the massive, well-defined muscles of action heroes that are typically portrayed in comic books and movies. Such efforts to achieve an ideal body shape can evolve into a disastrous and obsessive preoccupation with body weight and composition, food intake, and physical activity level. It is interesting to note that eating disorders are uncommon in regions of the world where the food supply is limited and starvation is an everyday occurrence.

Although usually considered nutritional problems, eating disorders are often associated with psychological disturbances, including obsessive-compulsive and mood disorders as well as substance abuse. Goals of counseling include encouraging patients to cooperate in their recovery and change their unhealthy attitudes toward food and their bodies. Treating underlying psychological and family-related problems may help resolve the eating disorder or reduce the frequency of the abnormal eating behavior.

Anorexia Nervosa Occasionally, nearly everyone has *anorexia*, appetite loss that can occur under various circumstances, such as excitement or fever. **Anorexia nervosa**, however, is a severe psychological disturbance in which an individual refuses to eat enough food to maintain a healthy body weight. People with anorexia nervosa have an irrational fear of becoming fat, usually maintain strict control over their food intake, and are preoccupied with calorie counting and food preparation. As mentioned earlier, females are more likely to suffer from anorexia nervosa than males are. During their lifetimes, an estimated 0.3% to 3.7% of American females suffer from this condition.[27]

People with anorexia nervosa have a distorted image of their bodies. They deny that they are severely underweight even though they weigh 15% or more below normal for their height. Typically, females with this condition do not have normal menstrual cycles and feminine body contours. Without an adequate supply of fat to insulate their bodies against heat loss, anorexics feel cold easily and often wear layers of clothing to provide extra warmth.

Some people suffering from anorexia nervosa occasionally lose control over their food intake and eat excessive amounts of food (*bingeing*). To avoid gaining weight, these individuals induce vomiting, give themselves frequent enemas, or abuse laxatives (*purging*). People with anorexia nervosa often exercise excessively to "burn up" calories. **Table 2.8** lists these and other typical signs of anorexia nervosa.

Table 2.8
Typical Signs of Anorexia Nervosa

In addition to refusing to gain weight despite weighing 15% or more below that which is healthy, a person who has anorexia nervosa typically:

- Has an intense drive to achieve a thin body
- Seems unaware that body size has changed
- Denies malnourished appearance
- Derives little satisfaction from his or her body shape
- Fears losing control over appetite
- Becomes full after eating small amounts of food
- Is a "picky" eater; avoids foods that contain fat, starch, or sugar
- Exercises excessively
- Lacks menstrual periods (females)
- Is depressed
- Has low self-esteem
- Has perfectionist tendencies

Data from Garfinkel, P. (1992). Classification and diagnosis. In K. A. Halmi (Ed.), *Psychobiology and treatment of anorexia nervosa and bulimia nervosa*. Washington, DC: American Psychiatric Press.

Treatment for anorexia nervosa includes individual and family counseling; patients must reach about 85% of their normal body weight before antidepressant therapy is useful. In severe cases, people with anorexia nervosa can die unless they are given special feedings and monitored closely in hospitals. Earlier estimates of the percentage of deaths that resulted from anorexia nervosa may have been too high. According to several recent studies in which the long-term outcomes of patients with anorexia nervosa were analyzed, about 5% of the patients died, in most instances from suicide, and less than 50% recovered completely.[28,29] The remaining individuals with anorexia nervosa were improved or remained chronically ill with the disorder.

Bulimia Nervosa Whereas people with anorexia nervosa are so thin they are easy to identify, those with bulimia nervosa may be more difficult to recognize because their weights are often normal. **Bulimia nervosa** is a craving for food that is difficult to satisfy; bulimic people typically eat excessive amounts of food at one time because they are depressed or anxious rather than hungry (**Table 2.9**). Some bulimic persons are able to maintain normal body weights because after bingeing, they purge by fasting, practicing self-induced vomiting, taking laxatives and diuretics, or exercising excessively. Vomiting prevents the body from absorbing and using the nutrients in food and beverages. Laxatives speed up the movement of the intestinal tract and can lead to watery diarrhea; diuretics increase urine production and elimination. Vomiting and abusing laxatives and diuretics can seriously disrupt the body's normal fluid and chemical balance, which can be life threatening.

anorexia nervosa A severe psychological disturbance in which an individual refuses to eat enough food to maintain a healthy weight.

bulimia nervosa An eating disorder characterized by a craving for food that is difficult to satisfy.

binge eating disorder A pattern of eating excessive amounts of food in response to distress such as anxiety or depression.

Table 2.9

Typical Signs of Bulimia Nervosa

- Evidence of consuming excessive amounts of food in short periods, such as empty food containers, without gaining weight
- Evidence of efforts to avoid digesting large amounts of food
- Spending time in the bathroom during meals or immediately after eating
- Odor of vomit in bathroom
- Presence of empty laxative or diuretic packages
- Sores or scars on knuckles that result from self-induced vomiting
- Dental decay from frequent contact with acidic stomach contents
- Preoccupation with obtaining food and exercising
- Social withdrawal

Occasional episodes of bulimic behavior are common among young women who are trying to control their weight. It is estimated that about 1% to 4% of females suffer from bulimia nervosa during their lifetimes.[27] Men may also have bulimia nervosa if they regularly consume too much food along with excessive amounts of alcohol and then vomit afterward. Furthermore, some young men who participate in sports that require maintaining a particular weight, such as wrestling and gymnastics, practice the behaviors associated with bulimia nervosa to remain competitive.

Many people who binge and follow up with purging are disgusted with their disordered eating behavior, and they hide it from roommates, friends, and family members. Some people practice bingeing and purging twice a week; in severe cases, affected individuals engage in these behaviors several times a day. Severely bulimic people can become so preoccupied with eating that they shoplift food to supply their binges and experience legal problems as a consequence. College students with bulimia nervosa frequently encounter academic problems after they neglect to attend their classes.

Typically, bulimic individuals are more socially outgoing than people with anorexia nervosa, yet they experience low self-esteem, anxiety, and depression. Eating temporarily relieves the bulimic person's anxiety. Although antidepressant medications and psychotherapy are useful treatments, people with bulimia nervosa often do not seek help for their behavior. Affected women tend to improve over time, but 10 years following diagnosis, about 30% still suffer from the condition.[27]

Binge Eating Disorder About one-third of overweight people engage in regular episodes of binge eating that are rarely followed up with purging or heavy exercise.[28] This behavior is called **binge eating disorder**. Some binge eaters report *blackouts*,

schizophrenia A form of psychosis.

periods of time that they cannot recall when they had overeating episodes, but empty food containers provide them with evidence of the incidents. Like persons with bulimia nervosa, binge eaters have poor self-esteem, and they often feel disgusted, depressed, and guilty about their eating behavior and physical appearance. These feelings may trigger additional episodes of overeating. *Night eating syndrome*, which is more common among obese than normal-weight persons, may be a variation of binge eating disorder. People with night eating syndrome are not hungry during the day, but have difficulty staying asleep at night; they awake often and frequently get out of bed to eat large amounts of food.

If you or someone you know suffers from an eating disorder such as bulimia nervosa or binge eating, ask the staff at your campus health center or your personal physician to recommend conventional mental health practitioners, such as psychiatrists, who specialize in treating these conditions. Additionally, check hospitals in your area because many have self-help groups for people with eating disorders.

Other Disordered Eating Conditions Athletes involved in sports that tend to emphasize leanness, such as gymnastics, wrestling, light-weight rowing, horse racing, figure skating, body building, and distance running, have an increased risk of developing eating disorders. As many as 62% of female athletes and 33% of male athletes suffer from eating disorders.[30] A relatively small number of female athletes develop the *female athlete triad*, a condition characterized by low energy intake, menstrual cycle abnormalities, and bone mineral irregularities, such as *osteopenia* (low bone density). Osteopenia is generally associated with postmenopausal women, not healthy young women.

Although most females with the female athlete triad do not show every sign of illness associated with anorexia nervosa or bulimia nervosa, their food-related practices, such as bingeing and self-induced vomiting, are similar. To prevent this condition, it is important to teach young athletes about healthy eating practices and body weights. Furthermore, parents need to be aware of factors that contribute to the triad, such as having low self-esteem and few friends, identifying thin physiques with ideal body shapes, being preoccupied with weigh-ins, and having overly demanding coaches who criticize the young athlete for being "fat" and insist on weight loss.

In the United States, many men experience social pressure to attain larger, more muscular body builds. *Muscle dysmorphia* ("bigorexia") is a psychological condition that affects weightlifters, particularly bodybuilders.[31] Despite their very muscular body builds, people suffering from this condition are not satisfied with the size of their bodies, and as a result, they spend hours working out each day, particularly lifting weights. Moreover, they are ashamed of their bodies and reluctant to expose themselves in public places such as beaches. Individuals with muscle dysmorphia are obsessed with the need to gain muscle without adding body fat; they have a high risk of eating disorders and abuse of *anabolic steroids*, drugs that can increase muscle size. At this point, little is known about the prevalence of muscle dysmorphia or effective ways to treat the condition.

We've discussed several major eating disorders in this section; however, people with disordered eating habits do not always display clear or consistent eating patterns easily diagnosable as an eating disorder. Emotional eating, overeating, and similar unhealthy eating patterns can also indicate an eating disorder. For more information about eating disorders and disordered eating, visit www.nationaleatingdisorders.org.

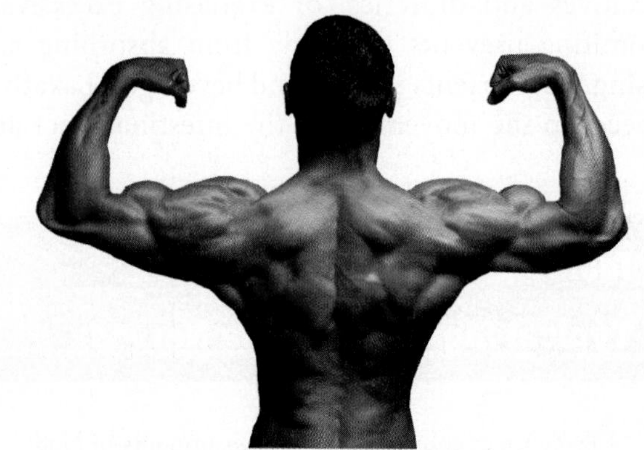

Could this be a case of muscle dysmorphia?

Schizophrenia

An estimated 1% of Americans suffer from **schizophrenia**, a type of psychosis.[32] Laypeople often believe schizophrenia means "split" or "multiple personalities;" actually, people with schizophrenia experience extremely disorganized thought processes, including hallucinations and delusions. People with *paranoid* delusions may think someone is trying to harm them. Individuals with schizophrenia often display strange behavior and inappropriate emotions. Communicating with some affected

Table 2.10

Common Symptoms of Schizophrenia

- Hallucinations, particularly hearing "voices" (auditory hallucinations)
- Delusions, including bizarre beliefs or paranoid beliefs
- Difficulty organizing thoughts; illogical thoughts
- Garbled speech and use of meaningless words
- Agitated body movements
- Dull, monotonous voice
- Little or no speaking
- Neglect of personal hygiene
- Inability to focus attention
- Difficulty using recently learned information

individuals is difficult because their speech often consists of words strung together into meaningless sentences. **Table 2.10** lists common symptoms of schizophrenia.

The brains of people with schizophrenia tend to have biochemical or structural defects that many medical experts think are inherited. A person who has a parent with schizophrenia has a 10% likelihood of developing the condition.[32] If a person has an identical twin with schizophrenia, he or she has a 45% to 65% chance of developing the illness.

Schizophrenia usually develops early in adulthood. Some affected people have one schizophrenic episode and recover, but others experience recurrent episodes and require long-term treatment. By taking special medications, many people with schizophrenia experience relief from their symptoms and live as productive members of society. Individuals with severe forms of schizophrenia must live in mental healthcare facilities because their behavior is unmanageable or dangerous to themselves or others.

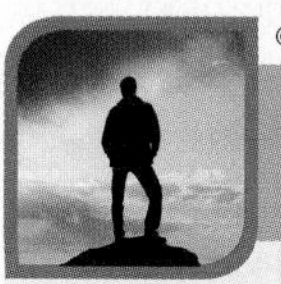

Healthy Living Practices

- If you or someone you know has an eating or other psychological disorder, seek help from the medical staff at the campus health center or from your personal physician.

Suicide

Suicide, the deliberate ending of one's own life, is not a mental illness. However, such extreme violence against oneself is often the behavioral consequence of a severe psychological disorder. Most people who choose to end their lives feel overwhelmed by the demands of life; they are unable to solve their problems or adapt to their situations.

Overall, suicide accounts for only a small percentage of deaths in the United States. In 2011 about 1.6% of deaths were attributed to suicide.[33] Suicide was the third leading cause of death for Americans between 18 and 24 years of age. Males are almost four times more likely to kill themselves than are females.[34]

Despite what many people believe, the Christmas holiday season is not the time that suicide rates peak; intentional deaths are generally low in winter, and high in late spring and early summer.[35] Although women are more likely to attempt suicide, men are more likely to complete the act of killing themselves. Most people use a firearm to end their lives; however, taking drug overdoses and crashing motor vehicles are also frequent suicide methods. Thus, it is difficult to determine the actual number of suicides that occurs each year.

Preventing Suicide

Psychological disturbance, particularly a mood disorder that may have included substance abuse, is strongly associated with suicide.[34] Other characteristics associated with a high risk of committing suicide are previous suicide attempts, family history of suicide, being abused as a child, loss (relational, work, or financial), illness, and feeling socially isolated.[35] Some individuals with severe or terminal health problems seek the help of others, particularly family members or physicians, to commit suicide. People who know or treat individuals with these characteristics or conditions should be aware of their suicide risk and initiate intervention methods to prevent them from ending their lives.

Suicidal persons usually demonstrate *suicide ideation*, or thinking about, considering, or planning for suicide. In many cases, suicidal people will communicate their intentions to friends or family members. These individuals might say "everyone would be better off if I were dead" or "I am going to kill myself," discuss the pros and cons of various suicide methods, talk about being a burden to others, increase drug or alcohol use, act anxious or agitated, or isolate themselves. After deciding to kill themselves, suicidal individuals often seem cheerful and relaxed. Friends, family members, or acquaintances often recall the positive emotional state of someone who committed suicide and may report that they showed no signs of distress prior to dying.

Occasionally people express suicidal thoughts to family or friends. It is always important to take suicidal conversations or gestures seriously and react in a supportive manner. Most people are surprised by suicidal conversation and may try to reduce tension by saying things like "it's not that bad" or try to point out the positives in the person's life. Although this reaction is natural, it can also deny the person's feelings and cause them to stop speaking. Psychologists recommend speaking directly by asking the person why they want to kill themself.[36] Then, listen carefully with nonjudgmental empathy and concern, while firmly and patiently obtaining professional help immediately. It is common for suicidal people to resist help and say they were only joking; however, it is important for the friend or family member to be firm and, if necessary, make an appointment with a professional. For more information about common presuicide behavior and suicide prevention, visit www.suicide.org.

Mental health centers with trained counselors who provide 24-hour crisis intervention services are available in most communities. On college campuses, student health centers offer mental health services and can refer students to mental health professionals when necessary. You may also find local suicide prevention resources using Internet search engines and websites (e.g., yellowpages.com) by searching for "suicide" or "suicide prevention centers." For more information, or if you or someone you know is thinking of committing suicide, call the National Suicide Prevention Lifeline at 1-800-273-TALK (8255), or visit their website (www.suicidepreventionlifeline.org/) for help.

Suicide prevention begins long before suicidal thoughts occur. Protective factors, factors that reduce suicide risk, exist on multiple levels; therefore, suicide prevention requires individual, community, and legislative cooperation. Factors that protect against suicide include strong family and community connections, development of problem-solving and conflict resolution skills, and cultural and religious beliefs that support self-preservation. Furthermore, easy access to effective clinical care for mental, physical, and substance abuse disorders and ongoing, supportive medical and mental health care relationships reduce suicide risk.[37,38] As demonstrated by this list, suicide prevention is not an individual behavior. Instead, prevention of suicide requires families to support psychological health and skill development, communities to develop and maintain healthy connections, and citizens and politicians advocate for and develop policy making treatment more available.

Table 2.11 lists these and other behavioral warning signs of suicidal persons.

© djgis/ShutterStock

Healthy Living Practices

- If you are or someone you know is suicidal, immediately contact a suicide prevention center to obtain specific instructions concerning ways to prevent yourself or another from committing this act.

Table 2.11

Behavioral Warning Signs of Suicide

- Discussing, joking, or writing about suicide or death
- Giving away prized possessions
- Making final arrangements: planning a will or making funeral plans
- Displaying severe depressive symptoms
- Reporting feelings of hopelessness and helplessness
- Performing risky behaviors: playing with guns, driving while drunk, or performing daredevil stunts
- Injuring oneself by cutting, burning, or hitting
- Behaving in a manner that is different from usual: showing no interest in usual activities, becoming socially withdrawn
- Planning the suicide: buying a gun or hoarding a supply of barbiturates
- Expressing anxiety over an impending action: worrying about a divorce, dropping out of school, or losing a job
- Showing physical signs of a previous suicide attempt: cut or scarred wrists, neck bruises

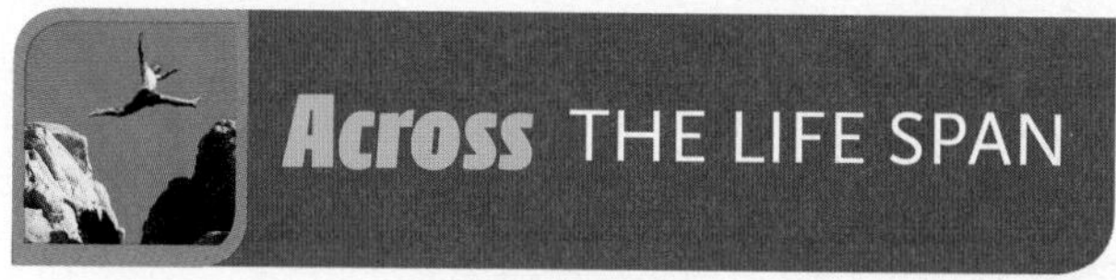

Across THE LIFE SPAN

© Galina Barskaya/ShutterStock

PSYCHOLOGICAL HEALTH

Children and adolescents establish the foundation for a lifetime of good mental health by developing positive self-concepts. Parents can help their children feel good about themselves by spending time with them, listening to their concerns, and helping them learn to adjust to a changing world (**Figure 2.7**).

School-age children who live in dysfunctional families are vulnerable to developing emotional disorders such as depression and school anxiety. However, childhood depression can occur in any child who experiences a traumatic event, such as the loss of a parent through death or divorce. Children who are anxious about going to school often complain of morning headaches and stomach upsets before leaving for school, and they return home in a distressed state. Parents and teachers need to recognize the symptoms of childhood depression and anxiety. By receiving individual and family counseling, many distressed children and their families can learn positive ways of handling crisis situations.

Attention-deficit hyperactivity disorder (ADHD) is a common childhood behavioral disorder. In 2011, nearly 11% of American school-age children, mostly boys, were reported to have ADHD.[39] This condition is characterized by an inability to focus and maintain attention on tasks, such as doing homework or following simple instructions. Children with ADHD also display excessive levels of physical activity and restlessness. They cannot sit still; they rush through meals, dash away from their caregivers, and resist efforts to relax or fall asleep. Their attention spans are so short they are often unable to follow instructions or complete tasks. Children with this condition demonstrate impulsive behaviors such as interrupting conversations, talking when it is inappropriate, and acting before thinking. Some children with ADHD are aggressive, argumentative, and defiant. Not surprisingly, children with ADHD frequently have low self-esteem and conflicts with their family members, peers, and teachers.

In addition to prescribing medications, many physicians recommend behavioral and family counseling to treat the disorder. Recently, some people expressed concerns that ADHD is overdiagnosed and that too many children are being treated with stimulant medications, such as Ritalin, in the United States. In addition, questions were raised about the negative effects of stimulants on children's growth and the potential for substance abuse among children treated with these medications. Although some studies indicate stimulants can mildly suppress the growth rates of children with ADHD, more long-term research is needed.

During the maturation process, an adolescent undergoes numerous hormonal, physical, social, and other changes necessary to become an independent adult. Many youth make this transition smoothly with a minimum of serious problems, but for some, the teenage years are filled with emotional turmoil and family conflict. Certain forms of mental illness, including major depression and eating disorders, are likely to develop during this period. As mentioned earlier, suicide is a major cause of death for adolescents.

Figure 2.7

Establishing Good Mental Health. Parents can help their children feel good about themselves by spending time with them.

© Photodisc

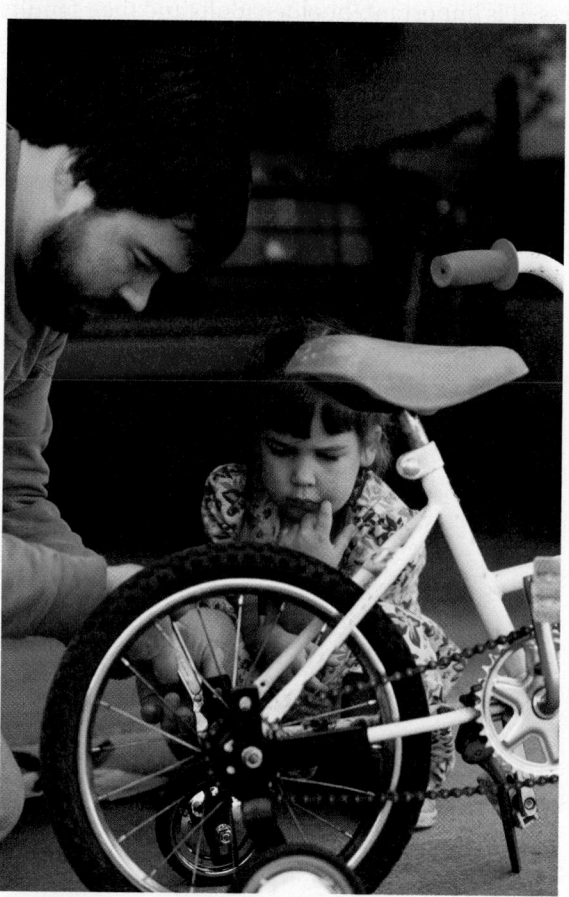

Older adults who approach the end of their lives with a sense of satisfaction about their accomplishments are likely to feel emotionally fulfilled.

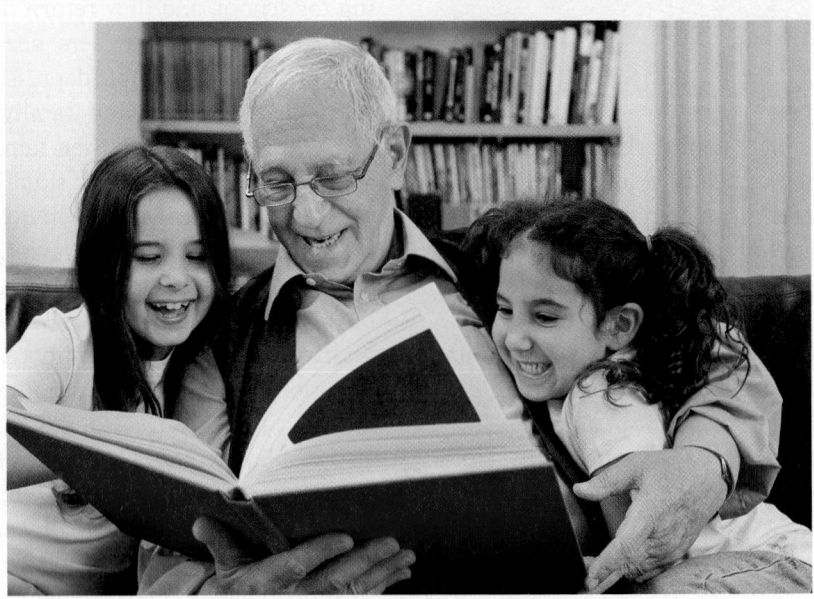

By the time people reach late adulthood, they may have raised a family, retired from working outside of the home, and maintained a network of friends and family. Older adults who approach the end of their lives with a sense of satisfaction with their accomplishments are likely to feel emotionally fulfilled. Many elderly people, however, suffer from sleep disturbances and depression after the death of a spouse and friends, family separation or disintegration, financial instability, or a disabling physical illness. It is important for older adults and their families to recognize the symptoms of depression and obtain professional help.

Analyzing Health-Related Information

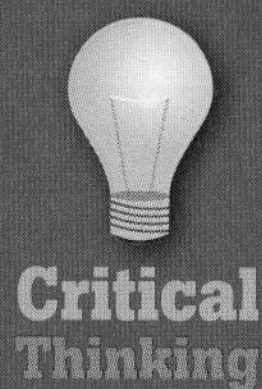

© tele52/ShutterStock

The following ad promotes a series of compact discs designed to improve mood and reduce anxiety. Read the advertisement and evaluate it using the model for analyzing health-related information. The main points of the model are noted here.

1. Which statements in the ad are verifiable facts, and which are unverified statements or value claims?
2. What might be the motives and biases of the person making the claims?
3. What is the main point of the ad? Which information is relevant to the product? Which information is irrelevant?
4. Is the source of information reliable? What evidence supports your conclusion that the source is reliable or unreliable? Does the source of information present the benefits and risks of the product? Does the ad include a disclaimer?
5. Does the source of information attack the credibility of conventional scientists or medical authorities?

Based on your analysis, do you think that this ad is a reliable source of health-related information? Explain why you would or would not buy the CDs. Summarize your reasons for coming to this conclusion.

ADVERTISEMENT ADVERTISEMENT ADVERTISEMENT ADVERTISEMENT

Feeling sad? Hopeless? Anxious?
Have you lost interest in usual activities? If you answered "yes" to one or more of these questions. You are depressed.

Fortunately, you can learn how to cure depression and prevent anxiety from ruining your life. Now you can benefit from the latest discovery in subliminal microtechnology that produces phenomenal advances in brain functioning. Scientists from around the world are predicting that this incredible breakthrough will be the greatest medical discovery of the 21st century!

"How can I ever thank you? I've tried three other neurotechnology products, but BRAINFIT was the only one that worked." B. J., London, England

"Please send another copy of the miraculous BRAINFIT CD—my sister took mine and won't return it!" S. A., New Delhi, India

Our amazing new **BRAINFIT** CD can improve your mood without the need for potentially harmful drugs. Listening to the CD has been scientifically proven to decrease anxiety by up to 35%, enhance positive feelings by up to 28%, and boost enthusiasm for living by up to 55%.* Millions of people in 60 countries report that BRAINFIT really works!

For the first time, BRAINFIT is available in the United States. Order your copy now. We guarantee that

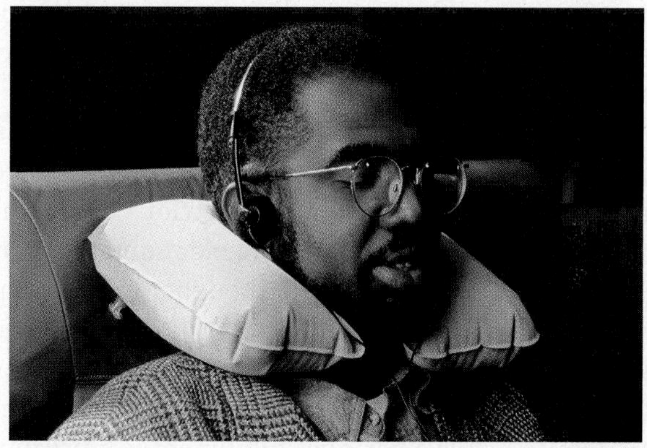

© Jack Hollingsworth/Photodisc

BRAINFIT will improve your mental health, and we'll add our clinically tested antianxiety pillow to your order—free! BRAINFIT is easy to use at home, work, or even as you drive your car!

For your personalized copy of BRAINFIT, send a money order for $69.95 to: BRAINFIT

*This statement has not been evaluated by the Food and Drug Administration.

CHAPTER REVIEW

Summary

A person's psychological health affects and is affected by other wellness components such as physical and social health. Psychological health is dynamic, improving or declining as an individual responds to a constantly changing environment. Psychologically healthy people accept themselves, are assertive, have realistic and optimistic outlooks on life, function independently, form satisfying interpersonal relationships, cope with change, and find effective solutions to their problems.

Understanding mental health involves the study of physiology and psychology. Biochemical changes in the brain elicit myriad human responses, including thoughts, emotions, and behaviors. Conditions that alter normal brain chemistry can disrupt the mind, producing negative moods or abnormal behaviors.

Personality is a set of distinct thoughts and behaviors, including emotional responses that characterize the way an individual responds to situations. Biological, cultural, social, and psychological forces interact to mold a person's personality.

Over the past 100 years, numerous psychologists, including Freud, Erikson, and Maslow, provided valuable insights into human behavior, laying the foundation for our present understanding of personality development. Freud thought unconscious drives control human behavior. Erikson identified eight stages of the life span in which different social forces influence personality. Maslow believed that the freedom to achieve personal fulfillment is a psychological need that motivates human behavior.

Psychological adjustment and growth occur when one adapts effectively to the demands of life by altering one's thoughts, attitudes, and responses. Self-esteem, a feeling of self-worth, is a key component of personality. Positive self-esteem is a characteristic of psychologically healthy people.

Intensity and duration are the key features that distinguish a normal emotional response from an abnormal one. Mentally ill individuals experience abnormal feelings, thoughts, and behaviors that persist, interfere with daily life, and hinder psychological adjustment and growth.

There are numerous psychological disorders; each may have multiple causes. Alterations in the normal chemical and physical environment of the brain often produce mental illness. These alterations may be the result of genetic defects, injuries, tumors, infections, or exposure to certain drugs or pollutants. Social interactions, including those with one's family, also contribute to the quality of an individual's psychological health.

In many cases, medications and/or behavioral therapies are effective treatments for mental health problems. People can learn to cope with various problems by seeking the help of conventional mental health therapists or by joining self-help groups.

It is common for individuals to experience phobias, anxiety, panic attacks, or mood disorders at some time in their lives. In many cases, these disorders are mild and do not interfere with the affected person's ability to function in society. In other instances, psychological illnesses such as schizophrenia, generalized anxiety, or major depression impair functioning to the extent that affected individuals require professional treatment.

Eating disorders are often symptoms of underlying mental illnesses, particularly depression and obsessive-compulsive disorders. Self-imposed starvation and denial of thinness characterize anorexia nervosa. Bulimic individuals and some people with anorexia nervosa engage in food bingeing and purging practices. Binge eaters overeat but rarely follow up with purging.

Suicide is not a mental illness, but in many instances suicide is the behavioral consequence of a major depressive illness that includes substance abuse. Individuals who are contemplating suicide often discuss their feelings and intentions with others. Thus, people should take someone's suicidal conversations or gestures seriously and assist the individual by obtaining immediate intervention.

Parents can help their children feel good about themselves by spending time with them, listening to their concerns, and helping them learn to adjust to a changing world. Some children develop psychological disturbances, particularly anxiety and depression. Attention-deficit hyperactivity disorder is a common childhood behavioral disorder. Most adolescents experience relatively few emotional problems as they mature into adults, but for some, the teenage years are filled with turmoil. Certain forms of mental illness, including major depression and eating disorders, are likely to develop during this period of life. Older adults who approach the end of their lives with a sense of satisfaction with their accomplishments are likely to feel emotionally fulfilled.

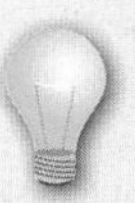

Applying What You Have Learned

1. Investigate several factors that facilitate self-esteem development. Create three recommendations for parents to foster children's self-esteem development. **Application**
2. Determine your current position on Maslow's human needs hierarchy. Explain, in detail, how you arrived at your conclusion, including discussion of psychological adjustment and growth, and autonomy. **Analysis**
3. In the United States, cultural perceptions of mental illness often lead to social stigma. Explain how the media may contribute to these perceptions. **Synthesis**
4. Consider your current state of psychological health. Rate your psychological health as excellent, good, fair, or poor. Explain how you determined this rating, and explain what steps you might take to improve your psychological health, if necessary. **Evaluation**

Key

Application	**Analysis**	**Synthesis**	**Evaluation**
using information in a new situation.	breaking down information into component parts.	putting together information from different sources.	making informed decisions.

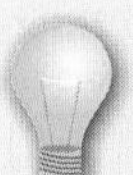

Reflecting on Your Health

1. As described in this chapter, self-esteem develops during childhood. When you were a child, how did your interactions with family members, peers, and teachers influence the development of your self-esteem?
2. Using Table 2-1, Characteristics of Psychologically Healthy People, identify the characteristics that describe you best. Why did you choose those traits?
3. What have you done to boost your psychological health by improving your physical, social, intellectual, spiritual, and environmental health? How did your actions help?
4. As mentioned in this chapter, people often have negative feelings toward psychologically disturbed persons. How would you feel if you, a close friend, or a family member were diagnosed with a psychological disorder? If you, a close friend, or a family member has a serious psychological disorder, how does it affect you?
5. People older than 65 years of age have a high risk of depression. What could you do or have you done to enhance the psychological health of an elderly person whom you know, such as a grandparent?

CHAPTER REVIEW

© SergeBertasiusPhotography/ShutterStock

References

1. Erikson, E. H. (1982). *The life cycle completed.* New York, NY: Morton. (Original work published 1964)
2. Maslow, A. H. (1968). *Toward a psychology of being* (2nd ed.). New York, NY: Van Nostrand Reinhold.
3. Stanton, R., & Peter, R. (2014). Exercise and the treatment of depression: A review of the exercise program variables. *Journal of Science & Medicine in Sport*, 17(2), 177–182.
4. UT Counseling and Mental Health Center. (2013). *Self-esteem.* Retrieved from http://cmhc.utexas.edu/selfesteem.html
5. Rimer, J., et al. (2012) Exercise for depression. *Cochrane Database Systematic Review*, 7.
6. U.S. Centers for Disease Control and Prevention, National Center for Chronic Disease Prevention and Health Promotion. (2012). *Health-related quality of life, BRFSS trend data, annual trend data.* Retrieved from http://apps.nccd.cdc.gov/HRQOL/
7. Kessler, R. C., et al. (2005). Lifetime prevalence and age-of-onset distributions of *DSM-IV* disorders in the National Comorbidity Survey Replication. *Archives of General Psychiatry*, 62(6), 593–602.
8. Substance Abuse and Mental Health Services Administration. (2013). *Results from the 2012 National Survey on Drug Use and Health: Mental Health Findings*, NSDUH Series H-47, HHS Publication No. (SMA) 13-4805. Rockville, MD. Retrieved from http://www.samhsa.gov/data/NSDUH/2k12MH_FindingsandDetTables/2K12MHF/NSDUHmhfr2012.htm
9. Demyttenaere, K., et al. (2004). Prevalence, severity, and unmet need for treatment of mental disorders in the World Health Organization world mental health surveys. *Journal of the American Medical Association*, 291(21), 2581–2590.
10. American Psychiatric Association. (2013). *Diagnostic and statistical manual of mental disorders* (5th ed.). Arlington, VA: American Psychiatric Publishing.
11. U.S. Department of Veterans Affairs, National Center for PTSD. (2014). *Treatment of PTSD.* Retrieved from http://www.ptsd.va.gov/public/pages/treatment-ptsd.asp
12. Kessler, R. C., et al. (2006). The prevalence and correlates of adult ADHD in the United States: Results from the National Comorbidity Survey Replication. *American Journal of Psychiatry*, 163(4), 716–723.
13. U.S. Centers for Disease Control and Prevention. (2014). *Autism Spectrum Disorder: Data and statistics.* Retrieved from http://www.cdc.gov/ncbddd/autism/data.html
14. U.S. Centers for Disease Control and Prevention. (2014). *Autism Spectrum Disorder: Facts about ASD.* Retrieved from http://www.cdc.gov/ncbddd/autism/facts.html
15. Kessler, R. C., et al. (2008). The prevalence and correlates of *DSM-IV* pathological gambling in the National Comorbidity Survey Replication. *Psychological Medicine*, 38(9), 1351–1360.
16. U.S. Department of Health and Human Services. (n.d.). Does depression increase the risk of suicide? Retrieved from http://answers.hhs.gov/questions/3200
17. Gonzalez, O., et al. (2012). Current depression among adults—United States, 2006–2008. *Morbidity and Mortality Weekly Report*, 59(38), 1229–1235.
18. National Institute of Mental Health. (2011). *Depression.* Retrieved from http://www.nimh.nih.gov/health/publications/depression/complete-index.shtml#pub5
19. Kocsis, J. H., et al. (2008). Chronic forms of major depression are still undertreated in the 21st century: Systematic assessment of 801 patients presenting for treatment. *Journal of Affective Disorders*, 111(1–2), 55–61.
20. U.S. Department of Health and Human Services, Substance Abuse & Mental Health Services Administration, Office of Applied Studies. (2009, July). *The NSDUH report—serious psychological distress and receipt of mental health services.* Retrieved from http://www.oas.samhsa.gov/2k9/SPDtx/SPDtx.cfm
21. Sharpley, C. F., & Bitsika, V. (2010, December 11). Joining the dots: Neurobiological links in a functional analysis of depression. *Behavioral and Brain Functions*, 6, 73. doi:10.1186/1744-9081-6-73
22. National Center for Complementary and Alternative Medicine. (2012). *Herbs at a glance. St. John's wort.* Retrieved from http://nccam.nih.gov/health/stjohnswort/ataglance.htm
23. U.S. Centers for Disease Control and Prevention. (1996). *Physical activity and health: A report of the Surgeon General.* Atlanta, GA: Author. Retrieved from http://www.cdc.gov/nccdphp/sgr/summary.htm
24. National Institute of Mental Health. (2014). *Bipolar disorder.* Retrieved from http://www.nimh.nih.gov/health/topics/bipolar-disorder/index.shtml
25. Howland, R. H. (2009). Somatic therapies for seasonal affective disorder. *Journal of Psychosocial Nursing and Mental Health Services*, 47(1), 17–20.
26. American Psychiatric Association Work Group on Eating Disorders. (2006). *Treatment of patients with eating disorders* (3rd ed.). Washington, DC: American Psychiatric Association.
27. National Institute of Mental Health. (2011). *What are eating disorders?* Retrieved from http://www.nimh.nih.gov/health/publications/eating-disorders/complete-index.shtml
28. Grucza, R. A., et al. (2007). Prevalence and correlates of binge eating disorder in a community sample. *Comprehensive Psychiatry*, 48(2), 124–131.
29. Crow, S. J., et al. (2009). Increased mortality in bulimia nervosa and other eating disorders. *American Journal of Psychiatry*, 166(12), 1342–1346.
30. Bonci, C. M., et al. (2008). National Athletic Trainers' Association position statement: Preventing, detecting, and managing disordered eating in athletes. *Journal of Athletic Training*, 43(1), 80–108.
31. Knoesen, N., et al. (2009). To be superman: The male looks obsession. *Australian Family Physician*, 38(3), 131–133.
32. National Institute of Mental Health. (2009). *What is schizophrenia?* Retrieved from http://www.nimh.nih.gov/health/publications/schizophrenia/complete-index.shtml

33. Murphy, S. L., Xu, J., & Kochanek, K. D. (2013). Deaths: Final data for 2010. *National Vital Statistics Reports*, 61(4). Retrieved from http://www.cdc.gov/nchs/data/nvsr/nvsr61/nvsr61_04.pdf

34. National Institute of Mental Health. (2010, September). *Suicide in the U.S.: Statistics and prevention*. Retrieved from http://www.nimh.nih.gov/health/publications/suicide-in-the-us-statistics-and-prevention/index.shtml

35. Voracek, M., et al. (2007). Facts and myths about seasonal variation in suicide. *Psychological Reports*, 100(3 Pt 1), 810–814.

36. Edlin, G., & Golanty, E. (2014). *Health & wellness* (11th ed.). Burlington, MA: Jones & Bartlett Learning.

37. U.S. Centers for Disease Control and Prevention. (2008). *Suicide prevention, scientific information: Risk and protective factors, risk factors for suicide*. Retrieved from http://www.cdc.gov/ViolencePrevention/suicide/

38. Suicide Prevention Resource Center. (2012). *About suicide prevention*. Retrieved from http://www.sprc.org/basics/about-suicide-prevention

39. U.S. Centers for Disease Control and Prevention. (2013). *Attention-deficit/hyperactivity disorder: Data and statistics*. Retrieved from http://www.cdc.gov/ncbddd/adhd/data.html

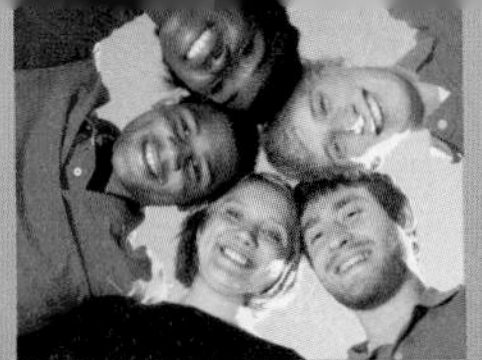

Diversity in Health
Stress and Asian Americans

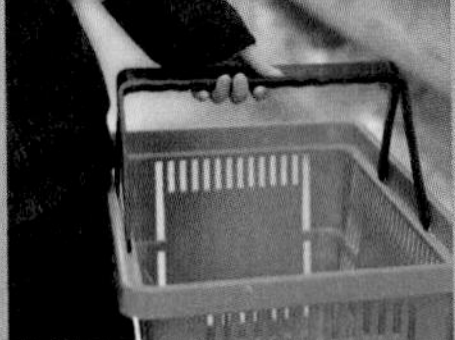

Consumer Health
Herbal Remedies for Stress Symptoms

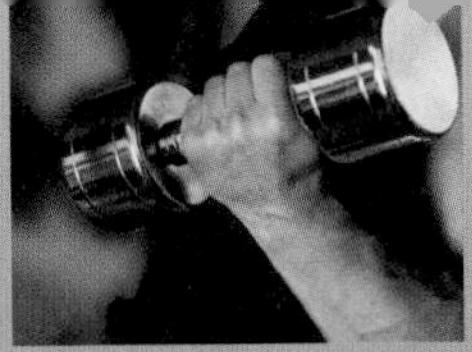

Managing Your Health
A Technique for Progressive Muscular Relaxation

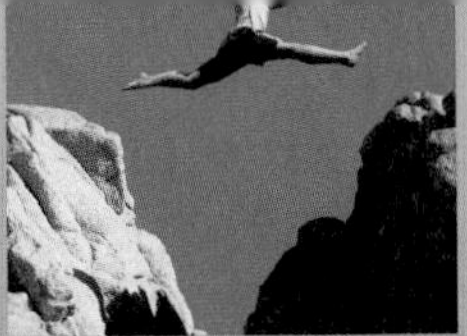

Across the Life Span
Stress

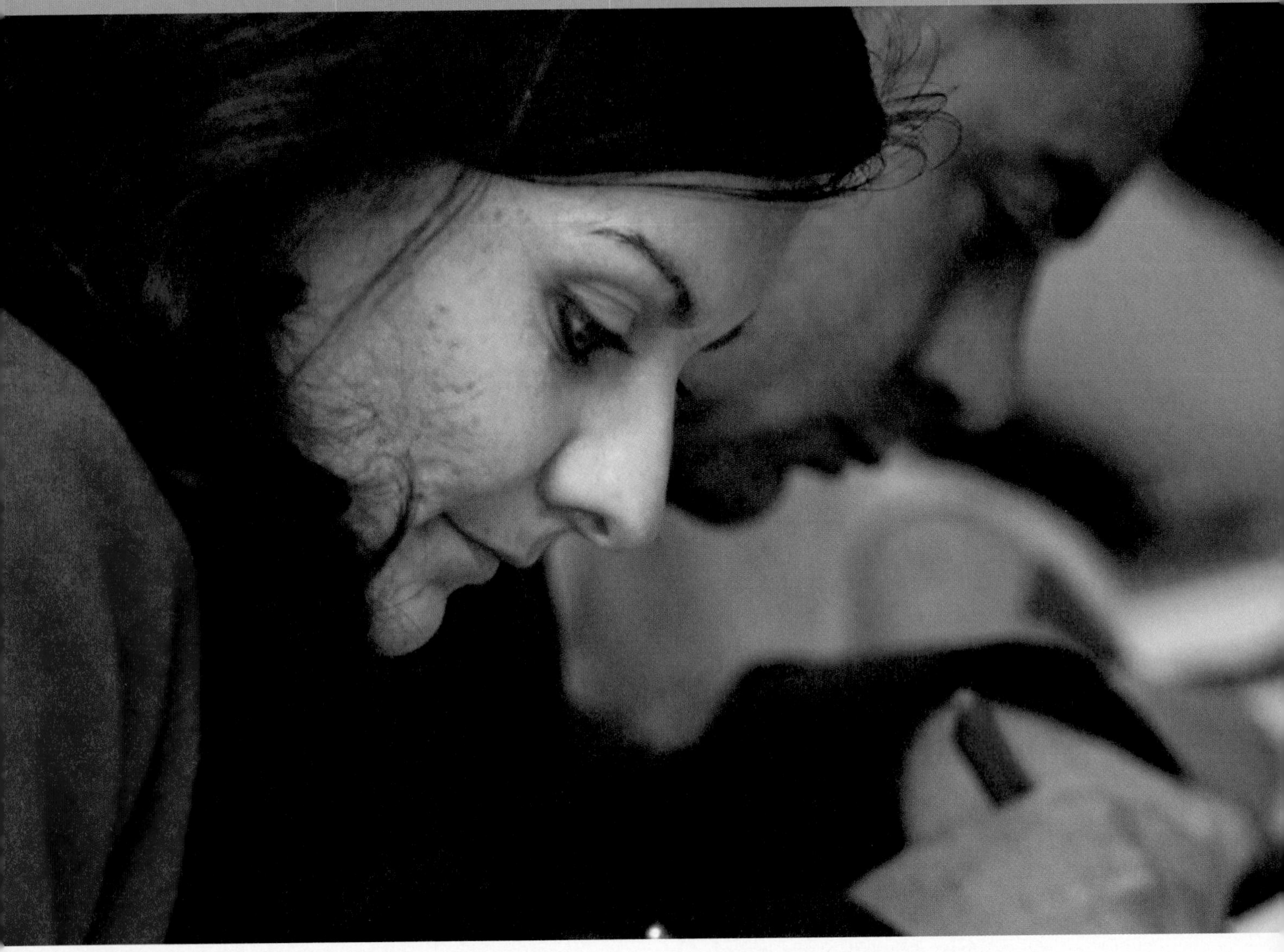

Chapter Overview

The different meanings of stress

The ways your body responds to stress

How stressful life events can affect your health

Strategies for coping with stress

Skills that can help you manage stress

Student Workbook

Self-Assessment: How Much Stress Have You Had Lately?

K6 Serious Psychological Distress Assessment

Changing Health Habits: Taking Steps to Reduce Your Stress

Do You Know?

An easy way to manage your time more effectively?

If having a pet can reduce stress?

How to relax within just a few minutes?

If stress can be good for you?

CHAPTER 3

Stress and Its Management

Learning Objectives

After studying this chapter, you should be able to:

1. Define stress and stressors.
2. Differentiate between distress and eustress.
3. Differentiate between physical and psychological responses to stressors.
4. Describe the three stages of the general adaptation syndrome.
5. Describe how health is affected by stress and how personality distinguishes responses to stress.
6. Explain how stress affects chronic health problems.
7. Describe various positive and negative ways of coping with stress.
8. Highlight the difference between problem- and emotion-focused strategies of coping with stress.
9. Identify three stress reduction techniques.

"Going to college places considerable demands on your time and mind. . ."

stress A complex series of psychological and physical reactions that occur as one responds to a situation.

stressors Events that produce physical or psychological demands on an individual.

If you ask students to identify what makes college life stressful, you will receive a long list of situations, including taking exams, preparing term papers and lab reports, applying for loans, and juggling hours to fit part-time jobs into their class schedules. College students probably cannot imagine any other period in their lives that will demand so much of their time, energy, and finances.

How would you respond to the question, "What was the most stressful situation that you've experienced in the past year?" Three college students enrolled in a health course wrote the following answers to this question.

The most stressful situation I've encountered in the past 12 months must be the discovery that my wife was pregnant and our financial security was at risk because the only source of income for us is her wages. I'm wondering if I will be able to continue pursuing my degree after the baby is born—this adds to my stress day by day.

I went away to a university last year and was the victim of a rape. The whole ordeal of talking to the police, confronting the man who did it, and telling my boyfriend was horrible, but the most stressful part was having to tell my parents.

The most stressful situation was the death of both of my grandparents within 6 months of each other. I watched them suffer as they passed away. It was very difficult. Also, my choice of a major was a mistake; I've had to change it.

Each of these students had to cope with a stressful situation. You may have had to cope with similar distressing events. Although going to college places considerable demands on your time and mind, you can expect stressful situations to arise during every phase of your life, so learning how to identify and manage stressful situationsis a life skill that will serve you well for the rest of your life.

What is stress? What effects can it have on your health and well-being? Can stress be good for you? What factors make a situation stressful? Is it possible to reduce the negative effects that stress can have on your health? This chapter examines the nature of stress, how it can affect you physically and mentally, and how you can manage your stress.

 What Is Stress?

Stress can refer to the situations that threaten or place demands on your mind and body. Stressful situations can be physical, such as being confronted by an angry dog, or psychological, such as worrying over your future employment possibilities. Stress can also describe your responses to a threatening situation; in other words, how you *feel* stress. Imagine that you have three exams in 1 day; how do you feel?

Stress is commonly defined as a complex series of psychological and physical reactions that occur as one responds to a demanding or threatening situation. Given the uniqueness of each person's views on what is demanding or threatening, how one appraises a situation to determine whether it will have positive, negative, or neutral consequences varies widely. In addition, a person determines his or her ability to manage the situation according to his or her previous experiences and personality characteristics. For example, how would you respond if a friend were to ask you to go skydiving with her? Would you be excited to join your friend? Would you be "stressed out" at the idea of skydiving and decline the invitation? If you have never gone skydiving, look forward to trying new and potentially dangerous activities,and have no major concern about the safety surroundingskydiving, you might accept your friend's invitation. However, if jumping out of a plane with only a parachute to keep you from free falling is not something you would look forward to doing, you probably would be very "stressed out" in anticipation of the activity and would turn down your friend's request. On the other hand, if you have gone skydiving before and found the activity thrilling and enjoyable, you would likely be excited to accompany your friend. Thus, it is possible for different individuals to form different appraisals of the same event; as a result, stress responses are as unique and different as people.

Stressors

Stressors are situations that create stress. *Physiologic (physical) stressors* include engaging in exercise; experiencing illness, pain, or injury; and being exposed to dangerous pollutants or extreme temperature changes. *Psychological stressors* include managing extreme emotions, handling difficult social situations, and dealing with troublesome thoughts and relationships. Certain psychologically demanding situations can add just enough stress to make life more challenging and interesting, but enduring too much stress, physical or psychological, can have negative effects on health and well-being. This chapter focuses on the impacts of psychological stressors.

The nature of psychological stressors has a major role in determining its impact on health. When people think of stress, they usually think of **distress**, that is, events that are difficult to control and that have unwanted or negative outcomes. Distressing experiences include having problems with one's education, job, family, and relationships. Other situations create positive stress, or **eustress**. Becoming a new parent, competing in an athletic event, and accepting a desired job are examples of events that can have positive outcomes by making people feel happy, challenged, or successful.

Experiencing stressors with positive psychological consequences may reduce the unhealthy effects of negative stressors. Eustress, however, still has negative effects on the body and mind because any event that creates stress requires specific physical and psychological adjustments. These changes can damage the body and disturb the mind. In this chapter, the terms stress and distress are used interchangeably when referring to negative psychological stressors.

According to the results of the American Psychological Association's Stress in America™ 2013 nationwide survey, 71% of American adults reported concern over their financial situations as a major stressor.[1] The following section describes the stress response and its effects on health.

distress Events or conditions that produce unwanted or negative outcomes.

eustress (YOU-stress) Events or conditions that create positive effects, such as making one feel happy, challenged, or successful.

hormones Chemical messengers that convey information from a gland to other cells in the body.

endocrine system A group of glands that produce hormones.

Stress Responses

Physical Responses

The environment constantly exposes people to stressful situations; to survive, they must deal physically with these stressors. The body has a variety of ways to manage stressors, including the release of certain hormones. **Hormones** are chemical messengers that convey information from a gland to other cells in the body. The glands of the **endocrine system** produce several different hormones and secrete them directly into the bloodstream (**Figure 3.1**). Some endocrine

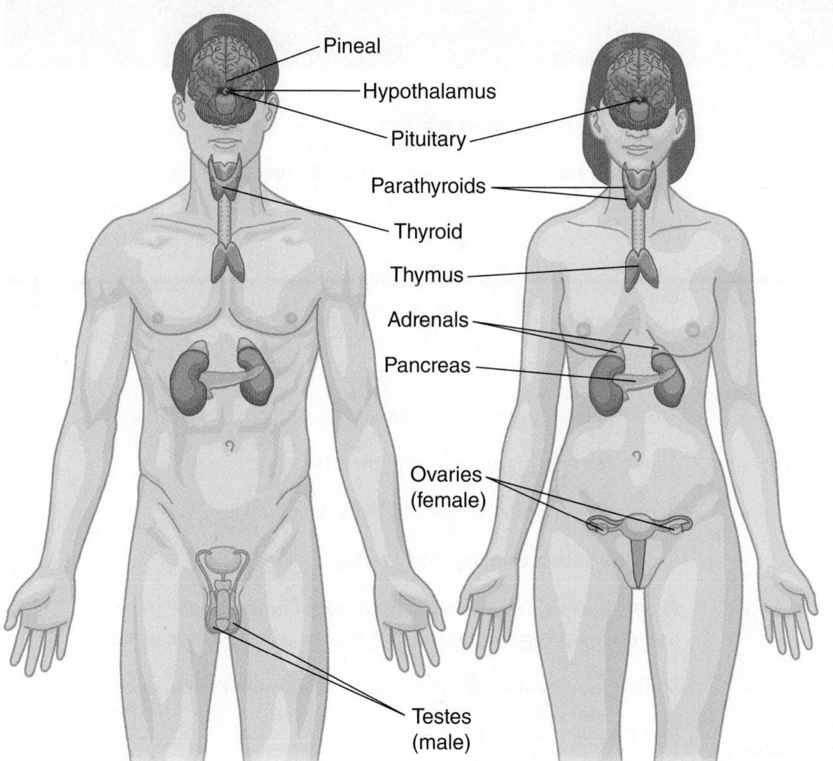

Figure 3.1

The Endocrine System. The glands of the endocrine system produce chemical messengers called *hormones*, which enter the bloodstream via small ducts.

fight-or-flight response The physical responses to stressful situations that enable the body to confront or leave dangerous situations.

general adaptation syndrome (GAS) The three-stage manner in which the human body responds to stress: alarm, resistance, and exhaustion.

hormones regulate growth and development. Other hormones regulate body processes, including those necessary to function during stress.

In emergencies, a person's nervous system instantly activates the adrenal glands that are on top of the kidneys to release cortisol, epinephrine (adrenaline), and norepinephrine (noradrenaline). These hormones are often referred to as the "stress hormones" because they can prepare the body to respond rapidly when danger threatens. As a result, the person's body is able to confront or leave the dangerous situation quickly (**fight-or-flight response**).

Stress hormones increase heart rate, blood pressure, central nervous system (CNS) activity, and blood flow to the heart and skeletal muscles. These hormones also increase the metabolic rate, the rate at which cells use energy. At the same time, the stress hormones reduce blood flow to the skin, kidneys, and intestinal organs. Under the influence of cortisol, certain cells release fat and glucose (blood sugar) into the bloodstream, which transports these energy nutrients to active muscle or nerve cells.

The nervous system also participates directly in the body's response to stressors. When the body is exercising or under emotional stress, the CNS produces and releases a group of chemical messengers that have pain-killing properties, including endorphins. Temporary reduction in pain sensation may be a valuable adaptation during stressful situations, especially if an injured person has to react quickly when threatened. **Table 3.1** lists major immediate or short-term physical adaptations to stress and their possible survival value.

Selye's General Adaptation Syndrome The classic research of Hans Selye paved the way for our understanding of the relationship between the mind and body.[2] Selye first used the term *stress* to describe the responses that allow a person to adapt physically or psychologically to any demand. As a result of his classic observations, Selye developed a three-stage description of the physical responses to stressors, the **general adaptation syndrome (GAS)**. Selye identified the

Table 3.1

Acute Physical Adaptations to Stress

Physical Change	Immediate or Short-Term Effect
Central nervous system activity increases	Increases mental alertness and reduces reaction times
Pupils enlarge	Improves vision
Energy nutrients released from storage	Supplies fuels for muscular activity
Heart rate increases	Pumps more blood and faster
Blood pressure increases	Provides more pressure to circulate blood
Blood clots more easily	Prevents bleeding
Skeletal muscles become tense and can work longer	Allows for fighting or escaping threats
Sweating increases	Removes extra heat created by muscular activity
Saliva flow decreases	Avoids wasting valuable body water
Respiratory tract (the smaller airways) dilates	Allows more air to move into and out of lungs, supplying more oxygen for energy and removing more carbon dioxide waste
Gastrointestinal tract movements decrease	Shifts blood to skeletal muscles for their more critical needs
Endorphin levels increase	Reduces sensations of pain

three GAS stages as alarm, resistance, and exhaustion; he described the physical status of the body in each stage.

When you think about or see a stressor, your brain sends an alarm through your nerves to your adrenal glands. Almost immediately, these glands release stress hormones to prepare your body to deal with the stressful event (*alarm stage*). In the alarm stage, your entire body undergoes the dramatic physical changes listed in Table 3.1. Consider, for example, how quickly you respond to an unexpected loud noise that sounds like a gunshot.

If you manage to survive the initial encounter but the stressor persists, your body enters the *resistance phase* of the response. During this stage, your body maintains its protective physical reactions to the stressor. As the threatening situation eases, your body recovers its normal physical state. Generally, by resting and avoiding additional exposure to stressors, your body can repair any damage that has occurred.

If the stressful situation persists, your body will not be able to maintain its resistance, and it will enter the *exhaustion stage*. In this stage, physical stress defenses are weakened, and you become more susceptible to infections. Prolonged exposure to stress may lead to death, if the body depletes its response mechanisms.

The stress response evolved to enable humans to react immediately to physical threats. Indeed, when people are in life-threatening situations, these dramatic physical changes may be essential for their survival. The same dramatic adaptations, however, take place when people deal with everyday hassles and concerns. Although these situations may be worrisome, they usually do not represent direct or serious threats to people's physical well-being. Nevertheless, such stressors elicit the unnecessary release of stress hormones into the bloodstream.

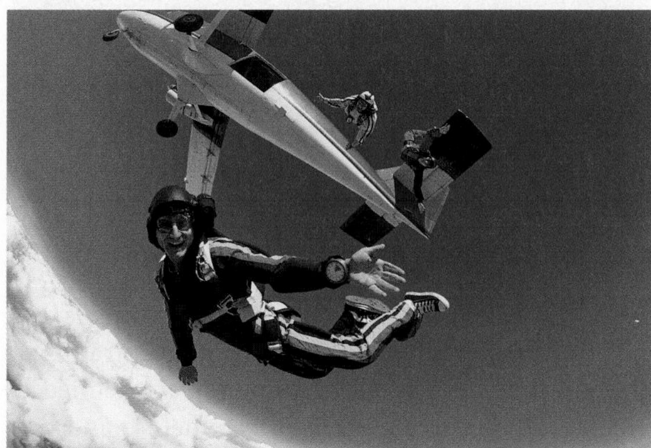

Would you find skydiving distressing or thrilling?

People with higher than normal levels of stress hormones, fat, and glucose in their blood are likely to develop chronic high blood pressure and other diseases of the heart and blood vessels. Enhanced blood clotting is a beneficial adaptation to an immediate, life-threatening situation. Blood clots, however, pose a serious danger when they form too easily and block blood flow in arteries and veins. Stress hormones also increase appetite; elevated cortisol levels are associated with increased body fat and weight gain.[3] The Diversity in Health feature in this chapter discusses the effects of severe stress on the psychological health of Asian immigrants, particularly Asian women, in the United States.

Psychological Responses Stressful situations affect the mind as well as the body, but the psychological impacts are not easy to test, observe, or measure. Several mental health conditions, including post-traumatic stress disorder and depression, have direct links to stressful life events.

Distressed individuals are more likely to report psychological symptoms such as frustration, anxiety, and anger. They may be irritable most of the time, eat too much (or too little) food, or abuse drugs. "Stressed-out" people often have difficulty focusing their attention, making decisions, and sleeping.

Burnout can be a consequence of experiencing too much psychological stress. People who are burned out feel as though they have exhausted their physical and psychological abilities to cope with stressors.[8] Typical signs and symptoms of burnout are loss of enthusiasm for job, school, or others; increased feelings of dissatisfaction, irritation, frustration, and pessimism; loss of concern for others; and anxiety and depression. Burnout often results from unrealistic beliefs or expectations concerning one's occupation and workplace situation, but caregivers and college students can also experience the condition. The stress management skills presented in this chapter, especially coping mechanisms based on social support, can help reduce the effects of burnout.

To some extent, stress can have positive effects on the mind. Low levels of psychological stress can enhance performance by increasing one's effort and attention to the task. As the degree of stress increases, however, the individual may respond by worrying too much about performance, which creates even more psychological stress. This response can reduce the ability of actors, athletes, and

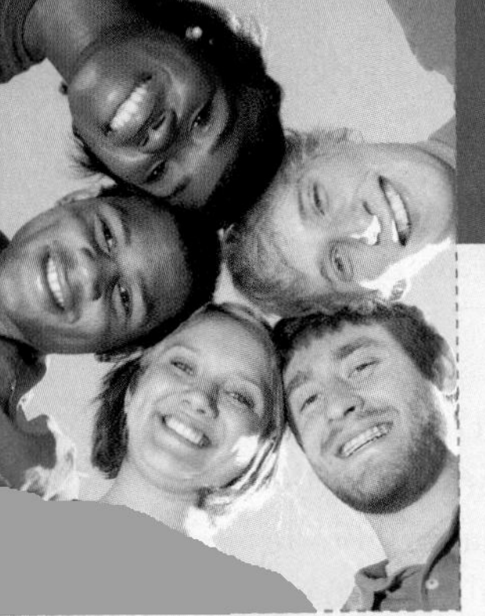
© Mike Flippo/ShutterStock

Diversity in Health

Stress and Asian Americans

In the United States, the majority of recent Asian American immigrants are from China, the Philippines, India, Korea, and Vietnam. The new immigrants to this country often face a variety of unfamiliar situations, as well as new and conflicting demands. Many of the immigrants must cope with being separated from friends and family members who remain in their homeland, learning an unfamiliar language, and adjusting to a very different culture.

The cultural "shock" that often results after settling in the United States creates numerous psychological conflicts for immigrants. Many members of this population experience homesickness, discrimination, unemployment, racial stereotyping, language barriers, and social isolation. The stress of immigrating and adjusting to a new culture may lead to depression.[4]

Asian Americans who espouse traditional beliefs think that fate determines much of what occurs in their lives, and they often deny or hide feelings of sadness, disappointment, and anxiety. As a result, Asian Americans may avoid expressing negative feelings.

Recent immigrants from Asia tend to follow traditional gender-specific roles. Men are accustomed to having a dominant role over women, especially in making decisions, and they expect their wives to maintain households and take care of children. Although wives may work outside the home, their incomes often are not crucial for supporting their families. In the United States, people who are descendants of immigrants who came to this country several decades ago tend to accept more equitable roles at work and home for men and women. Therefore, many women who recently immigrated to this country from Asia perceive their status in society as very low, and they experience much psychological stress as a result.[5]

Instead of seeking treatment for anxiety or depression, distressed Asian American women often visit conventional medical practitioners, such as their personal physicians, for treatment of various physical symptoms such as appetite loss, headaches, and fatigue.[6] The effects of unrecognized and untreated stress can be devastating. Suicide is the second leading cause of death for Asian American women who are between 15 and 24 years of age, and the third leading cause of death the 10–14 and 25–34 age ranges.[7]

Regardless of one's ethnic/racial background, the unwillingness to reveal conflicting feelings can produce stress. The serious effects of stress on the health and well-being of Asian American immigrants underscore the need for conventional medical practitioners to be culturally sensitive and recognize symptoms of emotional distress in members of this minority group.

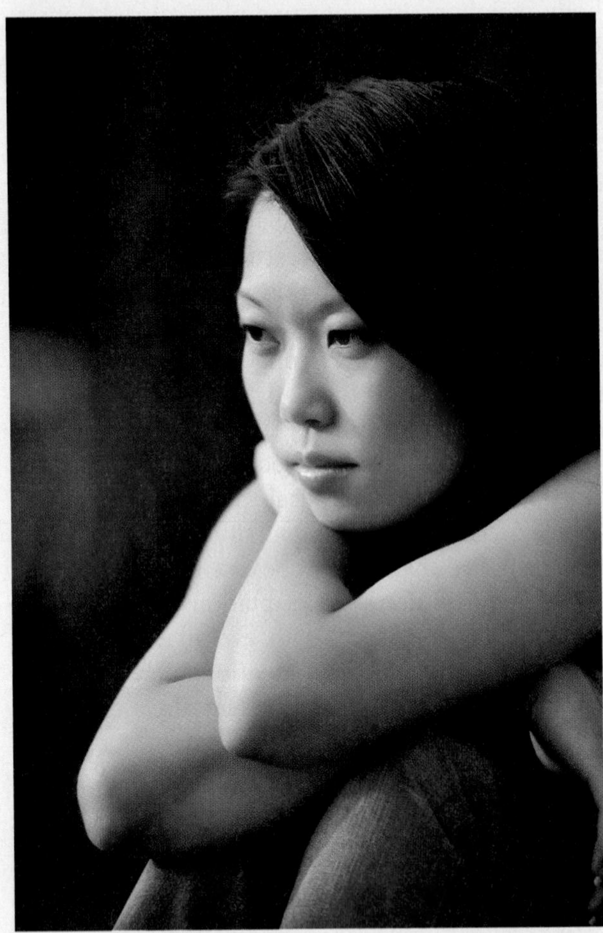
© Serget Skleznev/ShutterStock

college students to concentrate on and perform tasks. Stage fright affects the best veteran actors, and many superb athletes "choke" under competitive pressure.

Taking tests is stressful for many college students, but students with test anxiety overreact emotionally to the testing situation. As a result, such students have difficulty recalling information and concentrating on test questions. To avoid becoming overwhelmed by anxiety, students can learn to relax before and during exams by using the stress management skills presented later in this chapter.

The Impact of Stress on Health

Stressful Life Events

In 1967, Thomas Holmes and Richard Rahe introduced the Social Readjustment Rating Scale (SRRS), maintaining that people who experience numerous major life events within a short time span are likely to develop illnesses.[9] Holmes and Rahe developed this scale by asking nearly 400 people to rate life events according to the average amount of social change the individuals thought would be needed to deal with the situation. Death of a spouse, for example, received the maximum score of 100 points (see **Table 3.2**). In studies using the SRRS, Rahe found that subjects who

Table 3.2

Social Readjustment Rating Scale

Rank	Life Event	Value	Rank	Life Event	Value
1	Death of spouse	100	23	Son or daughter leaving home	29
2	Divorce	73	24	Trouble with in-laws	29
3	Marital separation	65	25	Outstanding personal achievement	28
4	Jail term	63	26	Wife begins or stops work	26
5	Death of close family member	63	27	Begin or end school	26
6	Personal injury or illness	53	28	Change in living conditions	25
7	Marriage	50	29	Revision of personal habits	24
8	Fired at work	47	30	Trouble with boss	23
9	Marital reconciliation	45	31	Change in work hours or conditions	20
10	Retirement	45	32	Change in residence	20
11	Change in health of family member	44	33	Change in schools	20
12	Pregnancy	40	34	Change in recreation	19
13	Sexual difficulties	39	35	Change in religious activities	19
14	Gain a new family member	39	36	Change in social activities	18
15	Business readjustment	39	37	Mortgage or loan less than $10,000	17
16	Change in financial state	38	38	Change in sleeping habits	16
17	Death of close friend	37	39	Change in number of family get-togethers	15
18	Change to different line of work	36	40	Change in eating habits	15
19	Change in the number of arguments with spouse	35	41	Vacation	13
20	Mortgage over $10,000	31	42	Christmas	12
21	Foreclosure of mortgage or loan	30	43	Minor violations of the law	11
22	Change in responsibilities at work	29			

Reproduced from Holmes, T. H., & Rahe, R. H. (1967). The social readjustment rating scale. *Journal of Psychosomatic Research*, 11, 213–218. Reprinted with permission from Elsevier Science.

psychoneuroimmunology (SIGH-ko-NEW-ro-im-mu-NOL-lo-gee) The study of the relationships between the nervous and immune systems.

immune system The specific defenses of the body that include combating infectious agents.

accumulated higher scores, because they had experienced more major life events in a year, were more likely to become ill at some time in the following year.

Although a few items on the original SRRS are outdated, such as "mortgage over $10,000," this scale has been a popular measurement of stress levels. Many stress experts, however, question the scale's ability to predict the onset of illness. Also, the SRRS might not capture the top stressors faced by many college students. Using the SRRS as a model, Martin Marx and his colleagues developed the College Schedule of Recent Experience to assess the level of stress experienced by college freshmen.[10] First-year college students often have difficulty coping with the unfamiliarity and demands of college life. Not surprisingly, these individuals have a high dropout rate. Concerned with the negative impact of change on first-year students, college administrators often establish academic, social, and counseling programs to ease the stress new students feel during their first year in school. What resources does your school provide for students?

Medical experts generally agree with the idea that stressful life events are related to illness. However, observing an association between stressful events and the onset of illnesses does not mean that stress *causes* health problems. An indirect link between stress and illness is widely accepted. For example, distressed people may follow unhealthy lifestyles: They may not exercise regularly, eat nutritious foods, or get enough sleep. Such behaviors are likely to result in poorer health. The following section explores the connections between psychological stress and physical health.

Figure 3.2

The Immune System. The immune system defends the body against disease-causing agents. The organs of the immune system include the thymus gland, spleen, and lymph nodes.

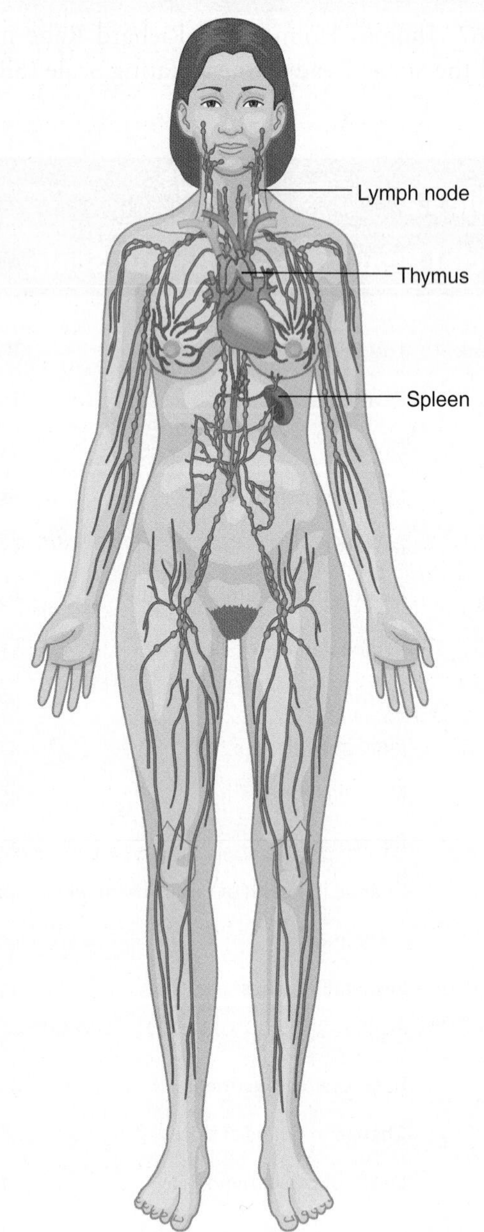

The Mind–Body Relationship

Psychoneuroimmunology, the study of the relationships among the nervous, endocrine, and immune systems, is the field of medical research that explores the connection between mind and body. The **immune system**, which includes the red bone marrow, spleen, lymph nodes, white blood cells, and thymus gland, defends the body against disease-causing agents (**Figure 3.2**). The white blood cells are the key soldiers of the immune system, serving as the body's internal scouts and commandos. These special cells find, identify, and destroy many agents that can endanger one's health. *Inflammation* is a normal result of the immune system's response to infection or injury and can assist in the recovery process.

The immune system functions in harmony with the nervous and endocrine body systems. By using nerves and neurotransmitters, the brain relays information about the person's emotional state to the places where white blood cells are made and located in the body. These specialized cells produce their own chemical messengers that enable them to communicate information about the state of the body back to the brain and the endocrine system.

Scientists have discovered links between the nervous and immune systems that explain how some emotional responses affect physical health. Stress alters the normal functioning of the brain, which in turn, affects immune system functioning. Stress depresses some aspects of the immune system, resulting in delayed wound healing and increased susceptibility to infection. Stress may also stimulate other components of the body's immune response, resulting in inflammation. Immune system cells produce *cytokines*, a group of compounds that regulate the immune response and communicate with the nervous system. Stress increases the production of cytokines that promote inflammation. Under these circumstances, the inflammatory processes are not necessary and cause harmful effects on the body. Chronic mild inflammation is thought to be associated with the development of many serious diseases, including heart and other blood vessel diseases, obesity, diabetes, smoking, rheumatoid arthritis, inflammatory bowel disorders, certain cancers, and Alzheimer's disease.[11–13]

Autoimmune diseases occur when the immune system malfunctions and the system's defense mechanisms become aimed at the body's own healthy cells. Rheumatoid arthritis, lupus, celiac disease, psoriasis, type 1 diabetes, and multiple sclerosis are autoimmune diseases. Although these chronic health problems have a genetic component, stress may contribute to their development.

Psychological stress can cause existing conditions to flare or worsen (**Table 3.3**). For example, people with chronic health problems such as asthma, rheumatoid arthritis, migraines, and genital herpes report that the signs and symptoms of their illness tend to recur or worsen during stressful periods.[14] Therefore, stress management techniques may indirectly improve health by decreasing one's response to stressful events.

Psychological, environmental, and biological forces influence health in complex ways. Many people reap health benefits by modifying the way they respond to stress. For example, a group of women with heart disease who participated in a group-based stress management program lived longer than participants who did not receive the stress reduction training.[15] Stress reduction techniques are presented in a later section of this chapter.

Table 3.3

Common Disorders Linked to Psychological State

Eating disorders	Itchy skin
Tension headaches	Rapid or irregular heart rate
Migraines	Intestinal ulcers
Muscle spasms	Nausea and vomiting
Chest pains	Frequent urination
Excessive menstrual cramps	Irritable bowel syndrome
Acne	Rheumatoid arthritis flare-ups
Recurring herpes simplex	Asthma attacks
Chronic fatigue syndrome	Premenstrual syndrome (PMS)
Fibromyalgia syndrome	

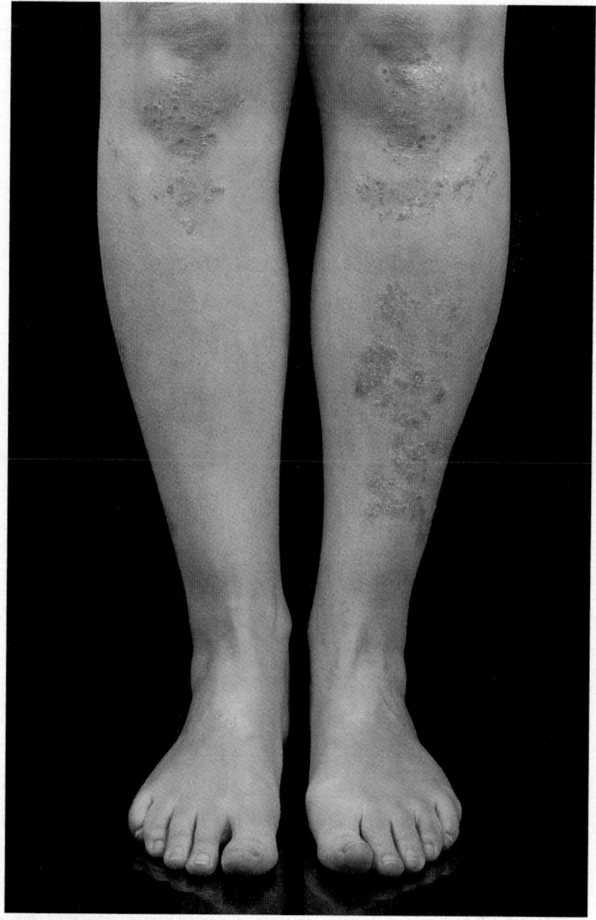

Psoriasis.

peptic ulcer A sore in the lining of the esophagus, stomach, or duodenum.

Personality and Stress

Although exposure to any stress can increase an individual's susceptibility to illnesses, the same stressful situation can have a different impact on different individuals. Why do people often respond differently to a stressor? Each person's unique combination of personality traits and background experiences contributes to his or her stress response.

People who see only the negative aspects of a stressor may view a difficult situation as impossible to overcome and be more vulnerable to stress than those who make positive appraisals of the situation. As a result of this vulnerability, people may be more likely to become anxious, angry, and depressed and to make poor decisions, thus adding to their stress. Distressed individuals may engage in behaviors that undermine their health, such as eating too much or too little, sleeping too little, smoking cigarettes, or abusing drugs. Although such behaviors may be seen as a "quick fix," they actually exacerbate the problem.

Stress and Chronic Health Problems

As mentioned previously, some common chronic health problems are associated with stress. You or someone you know may have irritable bowel syndrome, fibromyalgia, intestinal ulcers, or severe headaches, including migraines. Unwanted weight gain is also associated with stress. The following sections take a closer look at these conditions.

Irritable Bowel Syndrome (IBS) Anxiety and stress worsen the signs and symptoms of irritable bowel syndrome (IBS). People with IBS have recurrent bouts of intestinal cramps, constipation, diarrhea, and mucus in bowel movements. Medical testing and physical examination, however, fail to find a physical cause for the condition. Studies estimates that 10–15% of the U.S. adult population experiences IBS, that twice as many women as men are affected, and that it occurs most often among people younger than age 45.[16]

Irritable bowel syndrome often occurs with *fibromyalgia syndrome* (*FMS*), a condition characterized by extreme fatigue, muscle and joint pain, headaches, and sleep disturbances for which no physical cause can be found. In some instances, a stressful event seems to trigger FMS.[17] People suffering from FMS tend to be depressed and anxious; however, these negative psychological states may be the result of the symptoms of the disorder, rather than the cause.

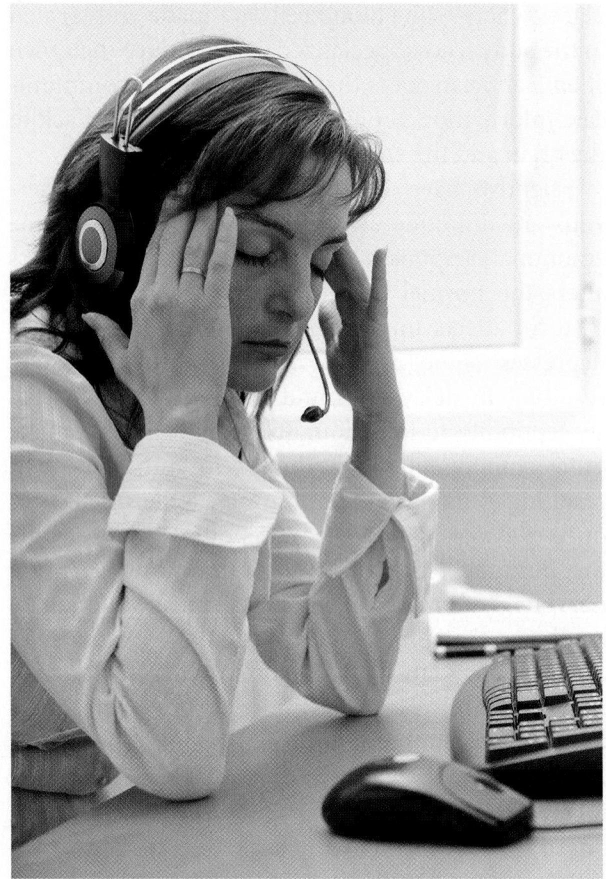

The most common type of headache is the "tension" headache.

Peptic Ulcers Each year, about a half million Americans develop **peptic ulcers**.[18] Such ulcers are sores in the lining of the esophagus (the "food tube"), stomach, or *duodenum*, which is the first part of the small intestine that leads from the stomach. Ulcers form in the stomach ("peptic" or "gastric" ulcers) when its protective lining and overlying mucous layers do not resist the normal amount of hydrochloric acid that is secreted by the stomach. Ulcers of the esophagus develop when the acidic contents of the stomach chronically enter the structure and damage it. This action, *acid reflux*, often occurs when the ring muscle that serves as the "doorway" to the stomach from the esophagus relaxes. Cigarette smoking, alcohol, chocolate, fats, and peppermints can relax this muscle. In addition, lying down immediately after eating or overeating promotes acid reflux. People with intestinal ulcers usually experience burning or aching sensations in the middle of their abdomens from 30 minutes to 2 hours after eating. They may also feel bloated and nauseated after meals.

In many cases, the protective lining of the stomach may be chronically infected with the bacterium *Helicobacter pylori* (*H. pylori*). This microscopic organism is thought to weaken the stomach lining and make the person more susceptible to ulcers. However, not all individuals who are infected with *H. pylori* develop ulcers. Aspirin and ibuprofen (NSAIDs) are other common causes of peptic ulcers.[18]

Unavoidable risk factors associated with ulcers are age and family history. As you age, your risk for ulcers increases; most ulcers are diagnosed in persons older than 40 years of age. Infection with *H. pylori* is an additional risk factor, although most people do not know if they are infected. The avoidable risk factors are cigarette smoking, chronic alcohol use, and regular use of anti-inflammatory drugs such as aspirin and ibuprofen.

Many people think that the "typical" individual who develops an ulcer has a hard-driving personality and endures a great deal of stress. Although stress does not cause peptic ulcers, it seems to worsen ulcer symptoms.[18] Furthermore, distressed people may smoke, drink too much alcohol, and not get enough sleep. Such unhealthy behaviors can negatively affect the immune system, reducing the body's ability to control *H. pylori* infection and making ulcers more likely.

Ulcers can be serious, especially if they bleed. Signs and symptoms of a bleeding intestinal ulcer include dark, tarry stools; a bloated sensation; and weakness. If you think you have a bleeding ulcer, seek medical attention immediately.

Headaches Nearly everyone has had a headache at one time or another. People who drink caffeinated beverages regularly may get headaches when they do not consume them, and physical ailments such as sinus infections often cause headaches. The most common type of headache is the *tension-type* ("tension") *headache*. People suffering from tension headaches report that the pain feels like a tight band has been placed around their forehead. The mechanisms that result in tension headaches are unknown, but stress can trigger tension headaches.[19] The typical tension headache is *not* accompanied by visual problems, stiff neck, nausea, vomiting, or fever.

Over-the-counter painkillers are usually effective for relieving tension-type headaches. For some people, simply applying hot packs to the head or neck and relaxing by having a massage are helpful. It is important to note that "rebound headaches" can occur when remedies that contain caffeine are used regularly to treat headaches.

Migraines are another type of recurring headache. About 12% of Americans suffer from migraine headaches, which are characterized by throbbing, intense pain that often affects one side of the head.[19] The cause of migraine headaches is unclear but thought to be related to genetic factors that affect potassium ion channels.[20] Sometimes a migraine attack is preceded by *aura*, a nerve-related symptom that usually lasts for less than an hour. In most cases, the aura includes visual disturbances such as flashing lights or zigzag lines, but "pins and needles" sensations, numbness, and speech problems may occur as well (**Figure 3.3**). In addition to being disabled by the headache, people with migraines often experience nausea and vomiting. Because their headaches are aggravated by light, sound, and routine physical activity,

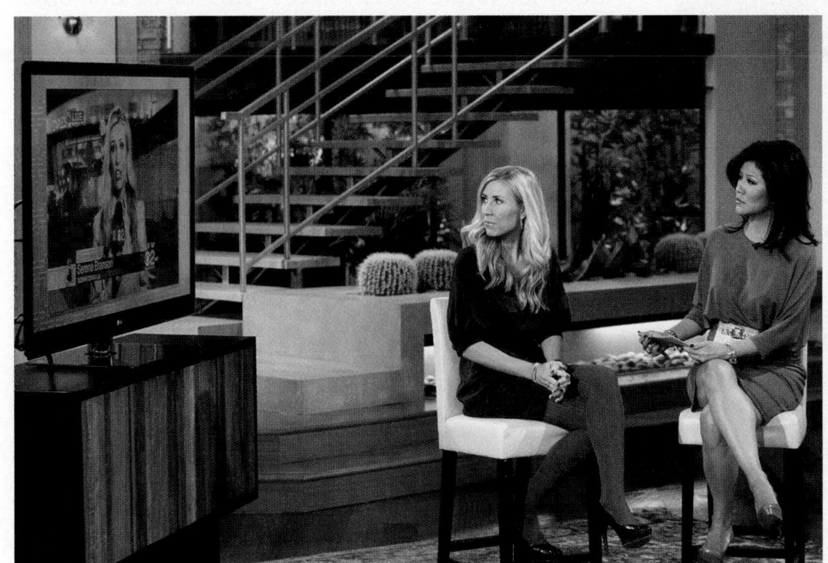

Figure 3.3

Migraines. In 2011, Los Angeles TV news reporter Serene Branson was broadcasting "live," when she began to garble her words. Although she appeared to have had a stroke, doctors later determined she had a severe migraine headache. Difficulty speaking is a sign of severe migraines as well as strokes.

people with a migraine headache usually retreat to a darkened, quiet room to rest and recover. Migraine headaches often persist for several hours and are quite debilitating.

The first line of defense against migraines is identifying and avoiding their triggers. Some people develop migraines when they are anxious or under a lot of emotional stress. Others report having migraines when they do not get enough sleep or they have disrupted sleep patterns. In these cases, maintaining a regular, sufficient sleep schedule is crucial to avoiding attacks. Other persons have migraines that are triggered by consuming certain foods, including chocolate, aged cheeses, and red wines, and foods containing aspartame and monosodium glutamate (MSG). Keeping a food diary can be important to determine which foods bring on headaches and then avoiding those triggers. In addition to managing or avoiding triggers, many people who have recurrent migraine headaches can take prescription medications to prevent the attacks. Natural treatments are sometimes used, including magnesium, coenzyme Q10, butterbur, and vitamin B2.[21]

The Consumer Health feature in this chapter discusses the usefulness of the herb feverfew as a natural means to prevent migraines.

If you suffer from frequent tension or migraine headaches, seek help from your physician. Headaches rarely signal life-threatening conditions. **Table 3.4** describes circumstances under which you should seek *immediate* medical attention for a headache.

Table 3.4

Serious Headache Signs and Symptoms

Consult a physician if a headache:

- Is accompanied by stiff neck, confusion, weakness, double vision, unconsciousness, or convulsions
- Occurs after a blow to the head
- Is persistent in someone who has been free of headaches previously
- Worsens over days or weeks
- Is accompanied by fever, shortness of breath, nausea, or vomiting
- Is recurrent, especially in children

Modified from National Institutes of Health, National Institute of Neurological Disorders and Stroke. *Headache: Hope through research*. Retrieved from http://www.ninds.nih.gov/disorders/headache/detail_headache.htm

Overweight and Obesity Do you lose your appetite or look for something sweet and creamy to eat when you are experiencing a lot of stress? About 80% of people alter their eating habits when they feel stressed out.[24] About half of the people who change their eating practices consume less food; the other half eats more food than usual and is referred to as *emotional eaters*. When under stress, emotional eaters usually choose tasty foods. Such "comfort foods" tend to be high in sugar and/or fat, such as cookies, cake, and ice cream.[24]

As mentioned earlier in this chapter, stress increases the level of the stress hormone cortisol in the bloodstream. In response to increased blood cortisol levels, the pancreas releases the hormone insulin. The combined effect of cortisol and insulin is an increased desire to consume pleasurable, energy-rich foods—fatty and/or sweet foods. These hormonal adaptations are beneficial because the body needs a source of energy to fuel an immediate fight-or-flight response to threatening situations. In today's world, however, threats to well-being are usually chronic and not life threatening, such as stressors generated by going to school, working, and dealing with family relationships and responsibilities. Furthermore, stressed-out Americans usually do not have to spend a lot of time hunting or searching for something tasty to eat, as their ancestors did hundreds of years ago. Adults can simply stop at a convenience store to buy a large sugar-sweetened drink, donuts, and candy bars as they drive to work, school, or home. When the extra energy is not needed to cope physically with a stressful situation, it is stored as fat in the body for future energy needs. This adaptation often results in undesirable weight gain.

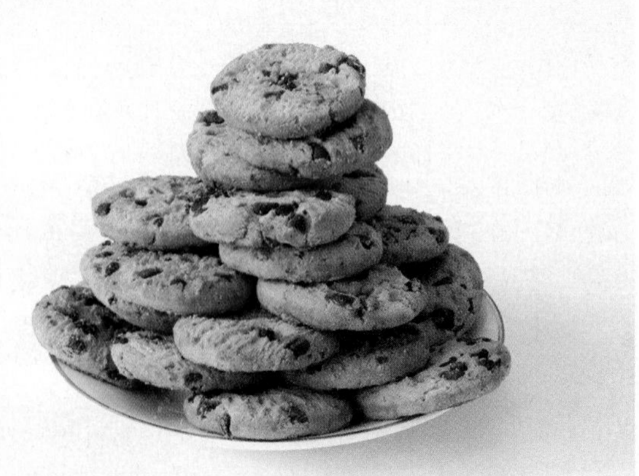

Are you an emotional eater?

Consumer Health

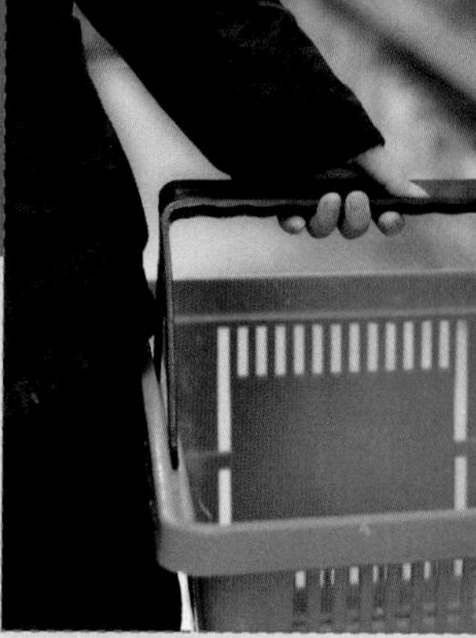

© sevenke/ShutterStock

Herbal Remedies for Stress Symptoms

Since ancient times, people have treated their stress symptoms with herbs and other plants. Many plants contain chemicals that have medicinal properties. Recently, many Americans have tried kava, valerian, and feverfew to relax or treat their stress-related symptoms. Does kava induce relaxation? Is valerian effective for treating insomnia? Can feverfew prevent migraines? Are these alternative therapies safe?

For hundreds of years, a ceremonial beverage made from the roots of the kava plant (*Piper methysticum*) has been used by South Pacific Islanders to reduce anxiety, relax muscles, and induce sleep. Although kava may relieve anxiety, the U.S. Food and Drug Administration issued a warning that kava can cause serious liver damage, including liver failure, which can be deadly.[21] Furthermore, kava may interact with other drugs and intensify the effects of depressant drugs, including alcohol. Therefore, check with your physician before consuming products made from this herb.

Ancient Romans were aware of the medicinal value of the heliotrope plant, commonly known as valerian (*Valeriana officinalis*). Hippocrates, the father of modern medicine, described the medicinal uses of valerian and the Greek physician Galen of Pergamon prescribed it for insomnia.[22] Roots of the plant are dried and then brewed into a tea that is used to induce sleep. Valerian is available in pills or mixed with alcohol to make a tincture. Valerian may have usefulness as a sleep inducer, but more studies need to be conducted to assess if it works for anxiety or depression.[22] When taken for short periods of time (4–6 weeks), valerian has been found generally safe to use; it can cause side effects such as headaches, dizziness, upset stomach, and tiredness the morning following its use.[22] The safety of taking valerian for longer than 6-week periods is unknown.[22] It is a good idea to consult your physician before taking valerian.

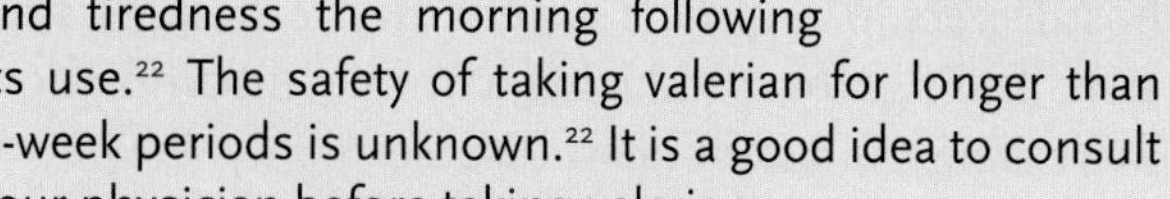

Feverfew (*Tanacetum parthenium* or *Chrysanthemum parthenium*) has been used for centuries to treat headaches, menstrual problems, stomachaches, toothaches, insect bites and fever. Before supplements were available, people would chew the leaves of the plant, but this practice caused sores in the mouth and loss of taste. Feverfew may reduce the risk of migraines, but more research is needed to confirm this finding. There is not enough scientific evidence to support the use of feverfew for other health problems.[23]

Feverfew does not seem to be toxic when consumed in recommended amounts.[24] Pregnant women, however, should not take the herb because it may cause the uterus to contract, increasing the risk of miscarriage or premature delivery. People who are allergic to ragweed and chrysanthemums are likely to be allergic to feverfew as well, so they should be careful when using the herb. Stop taking feverfew (or any herbal product) if you have adverse reactions. As in the case of all herbal treatments, check with your physician before trying feverfew.

Heart Disease and Cancer Chronic stress increases the risk of cardiovascular disease.[25] Some people's minds overreact to stressors, and their bodies respond by releasing excessive amounts of stress hormones into the bloodstream. This response may lead to inflammatory processes that cause high blood pressure and other physical changes that damage the inside walls of certain blood vessels. In addition, scientists have found that platelets, cell fragments that participate in the blood clotting process, become stickier when a person is distressed.[25] When a blood vessel is damaged and bleeding occurs, platelets clump together and form a plug that may stop blood loss. If a person is injured during a fight for survival, the ease with which the platelets form blood clots can be lifesaving. Many stressful experiences, however, do not include the risk of bleeding, yet the enhanced ability for blood clotting still occurs. In these instances, blood clots can be life threatening, particularly when a clot forms and blocks the blood flow to the heart muscle or the brain. A heart attack results when blood flow to the heart is blocked; a stroke can occur when blood cannot circulate through the brain.

Are there specific personality types that increase a person's risk of heart disease? For years, the popular belief is that people who have a *type A personality* (ambitious, restless, competitive, impatient, and hostile) are more likely to develop heart disease than people who do not have these characteristics. During the 1980s, medical researchers recognized that many people with type A personalities did not

coping strategies Behavioral responses and thought processes that people use to deal with stressors.

develop heart disease. More recently, scientists have associated a specific personality trait, *hostility*, with the development of heart and blood vessel diseases (cardiovascular disease). Hostile people harbor negative feelings, such as anger, hostility, and mistrust. A hostile person's immune system may respond to negative feelings by producing chronic inflammation, increasing the risk of heart disease.[26]

The stress response can reduce the effectiveness of the immune system, possibly interfering with its ability to detect and destroy cells that become cancerous. Most scientific studies, however, do not show an association between stress and cancer onset.[27] However, the effects of stress on the immune, nervous, and endocrine systems may lead to biochemical changes in the body that aid the growth of cancerous tumors. More research is needed to determine whether stress has tumor-promoting effects.

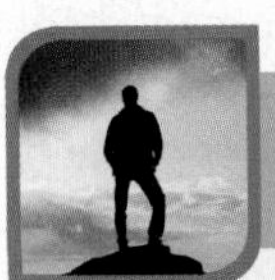

© djgis/ShutterStock

Healthy Living Practices

- To reduce the risk of peptic ulcers, avoid cigarette smoking and chronic alcohol use, lying down after eating, overeating, and chronic use of anti-inflammatory drugs.
- If you experience a burning or aching sensation in the middle of your abdomen after eating, or feel bloated and nauseated after meals, you may have a peptic ulcer. See your personal physician for diagnosis and treatment.
- To reduce the risk of tension headaches, learn relaxation techniques. Consult a physician if you have severe headaches.

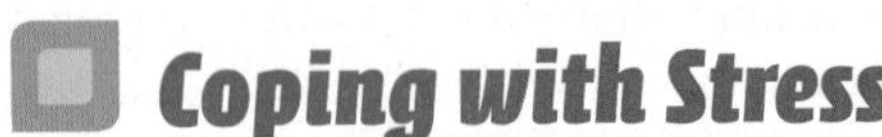

Coping with Stress

Stress is a consequence of living. In today's world, many people cannot fight or escape some of their stressors because the sources of stressors are difficult to pinpoint and control. In other instances, distressed individuals can identify their stressors, but they lack the resources to improve their situations. By learning ways to lessen the overall impact of everyday stressors on their health, many people can minimize the unhealthy impact of stress. Some healthy coping strategies include lifestyle behaviors such as getting enough rest, exercising regularly, and becoming involved with spiritually uplifting activities.

Coping strategies are behavioral responses and thought processes that individuals use to deal actively with sources of stress. Coping strategies can be problem-focused, emotion-focused, or social support methods of managing stressful situations. Although many coping strategies are useful, some can be harmful to health.

According to the results of the American Psychological Association's Stress in America™ 2013 survey, American adults most commonly reported coping with stress by listening to music (48%), exercising or walking (43%), going online (42%), watching TV or movies (40%), and reading (39%).[1] Participants were also asked to gauge the effectiveness of their stress management activities and reported exercise/walking as the most effective (62%), followed by listening to music (65%) and reading (49%).

Problem-Focused Strategies

Problem-focused strategies, such as planning, confronting, and problem-solving activities, are behaviors that can directly reduce or eliminate the negative effects of stressors. For example, setting priorities, managing money and time, planning for retirement, and retraining for a career change are strategies that can make people feel more in control of stressful situations. When individuals identify the sources of their stress and think that they have some control over their stressors, they feel less distress and experience fewer health problems.

Managing Your Time One of the most useful stress-reduction skills that you can learn is effective time management. Begin by making a list of all work, school, family, and leisure activities that you perform in a day. Then, analyze the list so that you can rank the activities according to level of priority. High-priority activities are those that must be accomplished if you are to meet your most important goals. Are some activities, such as watching television, chatting online, texting, or talking on the phone, relatively unimportant or "time wasters"? If so, these activities have low priority. To allocate and use time well, you may decide to eliminate some low-priority activities from your daily schedule.

After analyzing and ranking the high-priority activities, determine the amount of time that is

Analyzing Health-Related Information

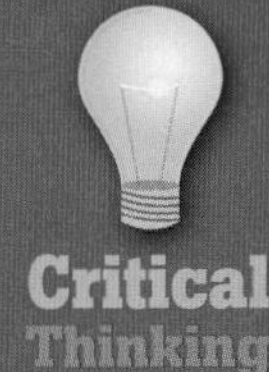

Critical Thinking

© tele52/ShutterStock

The following article about sleep appeared in *FDA Consumer*. Read the article and explain why you think it is a reliable or an unreliable source of information. Use the model for analyzing health information to guide your thinking; the main points of the model are noted here.

1. Which statements are verifiable facts, and which are unverified statements or value claims?
2. What are the credentials of the person who wrote the article? Does this person have the appropriate background and education in the topic area? What can you do to check the person's credentials?
3. What might be the motives and biases of the person who wrote the article?
4. What is the main point of the article? Which information is relevant to the main point? Which information is irrelevant?
5. Is the source reliable? What evidence supports your conclusion that the source is reliable or unreliable?
6. Does the author attack the credibility of conventional scientists or medical authorities?

Based on your analysis, do you think that this article is a reliable source of health-related information? Summarize your reasons for coming to this conclusion.

Sleepless Society

Tamar Nordenberg, staff writer for *FDA Consumer*

Millions of Americans undersleep by choice, burning the candle at both ends because of hectic work and family schedules. Americans sleep 7 hours each night on average, down from 9 hours in 1910 when people generally went to sleep as darkness fell.

"People don't respect sleep enough," says Daniel O'Hearn, a sleep disorders specialist at Johns Hopkins University. "They feel they can do more—have more time for work and family—by allowing themselves less time for sleep. But they do sleep; they sleep at work, or driving to work."

Like drunk driving, drowsy driving can kill. The National Highway Traffic Safety Administration estimates that more than 200,000 crashes each year involve drivers falling asleep at the wheel, and that thousands of Americans die in such accidents annually.

"Besides being an unpleasant sensation, when we're tired, we're less alert and less able to respond," says FDA drug reviewer Bob Rappaport, M.D. Lack of sleep can cause memory and mood problems, too, Rappaport says, and may affect immune function, which could lead to an increased incidence of infection and other illnesses. In studies performed on rats, prolonged sleep deprivation resulted in death.

©lightpoet/ShutterStock

Beyond the observable consequences of sleep deprivation, why humans—or any animal, for that matter—need sleep remains largely a mystery. "What we do know is that sleep is an important biological need, like food and drink, and that the brain is very active while we're sleeping," says James Kiley, director of the National Center for Sleep Disorders Research of the National Institutes of Health.

So just how much sleep does a person need? That can change throughout one's life based on age and other factors. For most people, though, 7.5 to 8.5 hours of sleep each night fulfills the basic physical need, but this is "very individual" and can range from as few as 4 or 5 hours to as many as 9 or 10. The Mayo Clinic of Rochester, Minnesota, defines an adequate amount of sleep as whatever produces daytime alertness and a feeling of well-being. People should not need an alarm clock to wake them, if they are getting enough sleep.

Data from Nordenberg, T. (1998). Sleepless society. *FDA Consumer*, 32(4), 11.

needed to carry them out. Allow more time to complete the highest priority tasks than for those of lesser importance. Perform the high-priority tasks first. Putting off an important task (*procrastination*) often results from fear—fear of failure or doing a less-than-perfect job. If the task appears overwhelming, break it into smaller jobs that can be checked off as they are completed. Also consider when your "best time" of the day is; plan to do the most challenging tasks during that period. To be successful in college, for example, you should allow time to attend all classes and prepare for each class, which includes setting some time aside daily for out-of-class tasks (e.g., reading, taking/reviewing notes, homework).

To manage time, using a calendar or personal computer to record appointments and important due dates for papers and exams are given can be helpful. Many people also make daily lists of "things to do," especially on very busy days. Allow some time for unexpected situations; it is not necessary to lock yourself into a rigid work schedule.

Of course, you also need time to relax, eat, exercise, socialize, and sleep. Arrange your schedule so that you can obtain 7 to 8 hours of sleep each night. Many college students are sleep deprived, and to stay alert, they often drink caffeinated beverages. Because excessive caffeine can interfere with relaxation, you may need to reduce your consumption of these drinks.

If you work or have family responsibilities while you are in school, planning your time carefully is even more crucial. Individuals who balance the time that they spend performing task-centered responsibilities with that spent engaging in pleasurable activities are often able to improve their performance and feel a sense of accomplishment.

Journal Writing

In the past, I have seen a psychiatrist. There were times when I didn't want to go, either because I didn't have anything to say or I was in a good mood. But, I learned that no matter how I felt, it made me feel better just to talk about my life. Journaling acts somewhat like a psychiatrist or even a friend. It allows you to "get it off your chest" . . . by writing down your feelings, you receive feedback from yourself.

Coping with daily stressors may be easier if you keep a written record of personal events, thoughts, and feelings. Entering your thoughts in a journal regularly can help you focus on your emotional responses to situations. There are no rules to writing effective therapeutic journals. You do not have to write the passages in prose; some people express their feelings in poetry or as letters that are not to be mailed. Identify distressing problems or situations, and then write your thoughts concerning them, including ways to resolve these problems or manage the troublesome situations (see the Reflecting on Your Health activity at the end of this chapter).

Emotion-Focused Strategies

Instead of directly dealing with stressors, many individuals use *emotion-focused strategies* to alter their appraisal of stressful situations. These strategies involve reducing a person's negative emotional response associated with a stressful event. Such alterations can improve mood and reduce anxiety by making the events seem less threatening. For example, many successful athletes cope with the stress of competition by appraising each competitive event as an opportunity to challenge themselves and achieve excellence in their sport. By viewing the competition as a challenge rather than a threat, athletes are less likely to experience the emotionally and physically destructive effects of stress on their performance.

Another emotion-focused coping strategy that encourages more positive thinking is humor. Humor can serve as a "stress buffer," lessening the negative health effects of both daily hassles and major life events.[28] For example, the homeowners who posted a "For Sale" sign in front of their hurricane-damaged house were using humor to relieve some of their distress. Forming constructive rather than destructive appraisals of stressful situations is another useful emotion-focused strategy.

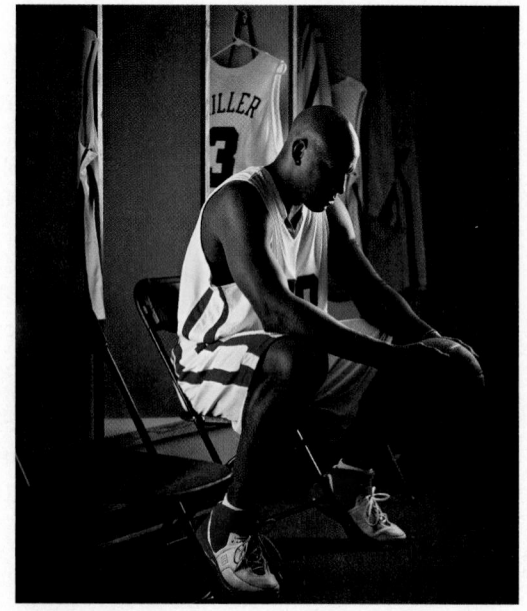

© Thomas Barwick/Getty Images

However, emotion-focused strategies can have harmful impacts when used as a means to avoid or deny the existence of stressors. Defense mechanisms, such as denial and projection, serve as emotion-focused coping strategies to defend one's mind against threats. Some people overeat or abuse alcohol to feel better during stressful periods. These unhealthy lifestyles generally relieve stress for the short term, but the consequences of overeating and drinking often create even more stress in the long term.

Social Support Strategies

Many individuals use *social support strategies* to cope with stressful situations. Social support strategies include seeking the advice, assistance, or consolation of close friends and relatives; participating in support groups; and obtaining spiritual help from members of the clergy or religious congregations.

When a major disaster occurs in a community, relief organizations such as the Red Cross provide valuable social and financial support services that reduce the impact of the catastrophe on people's lives. The knowledge that other people, even strangers, are willing to provide assistance is comforting and reassuring for many distressed individuals. Humans are not the sole providers of social support; lonely people who love animals often find comfort in the companionship of their pets (**Figure 3.4**).

Figure 3.4

Pets as Friends. People who love animals often find comfort in the companionship of their pets.

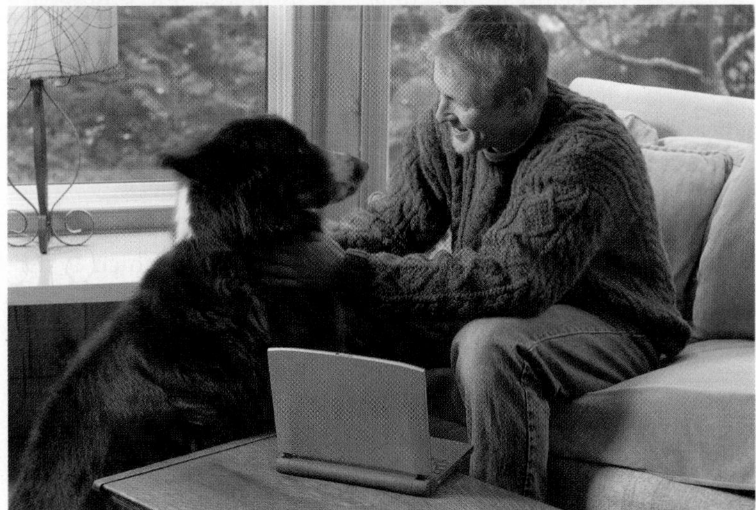

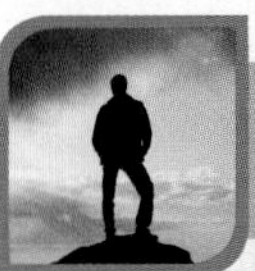

Healthy Living Practices

- Accepting stress as a part of life can reduce the negative or harmful impact of stress on your health.
- Planning for the future, setting priorities, and managing time can help you feel more in control of your life.
- Recording your thoughts and feelings in a journal can help you manage stress.
- Viewing challenging situations as opportunities to experience psychological growth can help you manage your stress.
- Seeking the companionship and social support of others can reduce your stress.

Relaxation Techniques

Although no one can eliminate stress, you can use a variety of relaxation techniques to reduce its impact on your health. Furthermore, relaxation techniques help redirect your attention away from stressors and toward more pleasant thoughts and relieve physical tension.

As you relax, your intestinal functioning becomes normal, your breathing and heart rate slow, and your blood pressure declines. Practicing relaxation techniques when you feel stressed can help restore many body processes to normal, which reduces the potentially damaging effects that stress can have on your body. Relaxation activities often involve learning how to identify and relax your tense skeletal muscles while remaining mentally alert.

Most relaxation methods are relatively easy to learn, but to be effective, one needs a high degree of motivation, self-control, and willingness to practice the skills for about 10 to 20 minutes daily. Learn each technique to determine which ones are effective for you. At first, learning to relax may be difficult, but by practicing at least one of these techniques every day, you should be able to master the activity within a couple of weeks.

temporomandibular (TEM-pe-row-man-DIB-you-ler) joint The place where the lower jaw bone (mandible) attaches to the temporal bone of the skull.

meditation An activity in which one relaxes by mentally focusing on a single word, object, or thought.

Deep Breathing

While having panic attacks, people often *hyperventilate* (pant for air) and feel as though they are suffocating. Hyperventilation alters the chemistry of the blood, which increases the heart rate and causes dizziness. By deliberately breathing more slowly and deeply, distressed people can feel more relaxed as their blood chemistry values return to normal. Concentrating on breathing more deeply allows people to shift their attention away from stressors and toward the breathing activity.

Under normal conditions, you breathe an average of 12 to 18 times per minute, but to relax, you need to breathe only 8 to 10 times per minute. The key is to take several deep breaths, using your abdominal muscles, and recognize how deep breathing feels different from your usual breathing pattern. Results from studies show that deep breathing is a quick and simple method to reduce the impact of stress on your health. You can use this breathing technique whenever you begin to feel excited or stressed; so, before your next exam, speech, or job interview, relax by simply breathing deeply.

Of all the relaxation techniques we learned this semester, the deep breathing method was the most helpful. I can remember many situations when I've had to use it. While driving home from school, somebody pulled out in front of me and I had to make a ridiculous move to avoid hitting him head on. I didn't turn my car around and try to find him, which I would have done 6 months ago; I simply took some deep breaths and was thankful that no one, including myself, was injured.

Progressive Muscular Relaxation

Although some degree of skeletal muscular tension is necessary to maintain a comfortable body posture, excess tension in forehead, scalp, jaw, and neck muscles may contribute to the development of tension headaches. Distressed individuals often look tense because of their tightened facial muscles or clenched fists. Even when they are resting, stressed people still report feeling excess muscle tension. Teeth grinding is a common sign of stress that often occurs during sleep and may lead to headaches and pain in the **temporomandibular joint**, the joint where the lower jaw attaches to the skull in front of the ear (**Figure 3.5**).

Figure 3.5

The Temporomandibular Joint. The temporomandibular joint is the point at which the lower jaw attaches to the skull in front of the ear. Pain in the temporomandibular joint may result from grinding teeth during sleep, a common sign of stress.

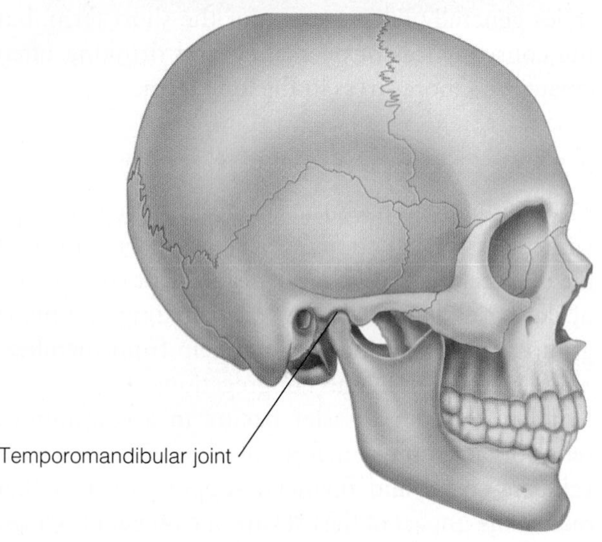

The *progressive muscular relaxation technique* teaches people how to recognize the differences between a tensed muscle and a relaxed one. Individuals learn how to release muscle tension voluntarily, becoming aware of the relaxed sensations. When a person's skeletal muscles are completely relaxed, the individual is limp and feels calm. People often use the technique to fall asleep. The Managing Your Health feature titled "A Technique for Progressive Muscular Relaxation" highlights the steps of this particular stress reduction method.

Meditation and the Relaxation Response

For some people, praying or meditating reduces stress. **Meditation** is an activity in which a person relaxes by mentally focusing on a single word, object, or thought. *Mindfulness meditation* involves a variety of relaxation methods that focus your attention completely and in a nonjudgmental way on what you are doing or experiencing at the moment. Instead of repeating one word or thinking about a single thing or object, you allow your thoughts to

Managing Your Health

A Technique for Progressive Muscular Relaxation

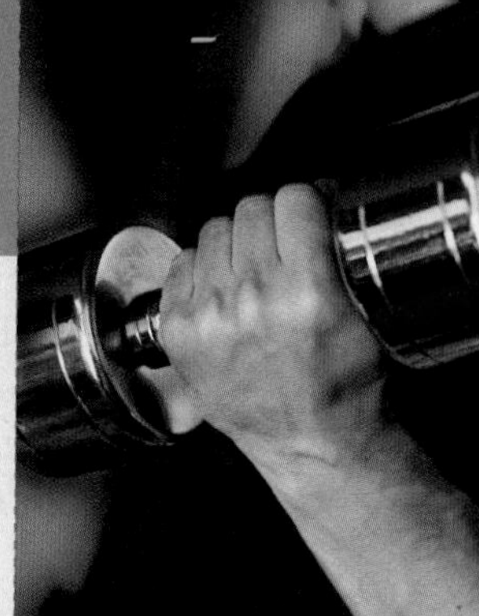
© Kzenon/ShutterStock

1. Choose a quiet location and sit in a comfortable position, hands down at your sides, and both feet flat on the floor.
2. Close your eyes and take a few deep breaths; concentrate on becoming as relaxed as possible.
3. With your arms at your sides, make a fist with one of your hands. Hold your clenched fist for about 5 seconds, release your hand from this position, and concentrate on the feeling as the muscular tension "drains" out of your hand.

This basic exercise is repeated as you tense muscles, hold the tensed position for 5 seconds, and then relax the major muscle groups in your body. It is important to focus on recognizing the difference between muscular tension and relaxation sensations. Continue breathing normally as the activity progresses. Begin with your head.

1. Tense your forehead and scalp muscles; feel the tight muscular sensations as you hold this position for 5 seconds; relax these muscles.
2. Tense your facial muscles; hold this position for 5 seconds; relax.
3. Tense the muscles of your neck and jaw; hold this position; relax.
4. Tense your back muscles—but not too tight; hold this position; relax.
5. Tense your right arm; hold; relax.
6. Tense your left arm; hold; relax.
7. Tense your chest muscles; hold; relax.
8. Tense your stomach muscles; hold; relax.
9. Tense your buttocks; hold; relax.
10. Tense your right leg—but not too tight; hold; relax.
11. Tense your left leg—but not too tight; hold; relax.

Now, imagine traveling back through your body searching for muscles that are not relaxed. As you find tense muscles, relax them. Maintain this position for several minutes, concentrating on your breathing. In this relaxed state, you may practice tranquil imagery and positive self-talk. To regain your normal physical activity, open your eyes, stand, and stretch your muscles.

flow and experience as much as you can about what you are sensing and thinking. According to results of scientific studies, people who practice mindfulness meditation are better able to regulate their emotional responses, and they report lower levels of emotional stress, anxiety, depression, and anger than people who do not use meditation to relax.[28]

You can engage in mindfulness-based stress reduction while performing ordinary activities such as eating or walking, or by studying an interesting photograph, painting, or object such as a seashell. By practicing this relaxation technique regularly, you can learn to regulate your attention and reduce your negative reactions to stress.

Herbert Benson incorporated features of meditation into his relaxation response, claiming that this method is effective for reducing blood pressure and drug abuse.[29] To practice Benson's method, find a quiet place where you can sit comfortably for 10 to 20 minutes. Close your eyes, breathe normally, and concentrate on repeating a simple word or maintaining a pleasant thought. Progressively relax groups of muscles, starting at your feet and moving up your body to your face. After relaxing your muscles, maintain this pose for at least 10 minutes. When you are ready to regain your usual degree of alertness, open your eyes, stand up, and stretch.

Imagery

Imagery is a mental activity that is often combined with progressive muscular relaxation exercises to enhance physical relaxation. The technique is simple. After relaxing his or her muscles, the person thinks of a peaceful, pleasurable scene, using imagination or past experiences as a guide. While relaxed, the person "sees" the scene in his or her mind and imagines other sensations as well. For example, someone who enjoys outdoor activities might recall floating down a small stream in a canoe. This individual would imagine the peaceful feeling of floating gently on the water as well as the sound of birds singing and water flowing. Imagery, or visualization, can be a creative and enjoyable way to relax as it disengages the mind from thinking about problems. Relaxation tapes or CDs often incorporate nature sounds with slow tempo music to facilitate imagery.

Athletes, actors, and other performers often use imagery to reduce their stress and enhance their performance. Before an event, for example, a pole vaulter often visualizes the entire sequence of events that takes place when approaching and vaulting over the pole. Although imagery is not a substitute for actually practicing the required skills, the technique is a useful training activity for many competitive athletes.

You do not have to be an athlete or an actor to use imagery to reduce your stress levels. Before facing a stressful situation, such as giving a speech or interviewing for a job, imagine the setting. Also imagine the other people's responses and your own behavior. Mentally rehearsing the situation can reduce your anxiety by making you feel better prepared. Then, immediately before the stressful event, breathe deeply to relax.

Self-Talk

At times, people may have irrational or negative thoughts concerning their abilities to deal effectively with their stressors. Individuals can reduce their stress levels by identifying these self-defeating thoughts and replacing them with positive self-talk statements. Positive self-talk reflects a person's attributes and boosts self-confidence. However, thinking about oneself in a positive manner may be difficult for individuals who have low self-esteem. People with poor self-esteem often have self-degrading or self-critical thoughts, and they are unaccustomed to acknowledging their positive characteristics.

To practice positive self-talk, think of at least three affirmative statements to say about yourself, including your feelings, accomplishments, skills, and characteristics. Self-talk can be personal compliments ("I look great today"), statements of encouragement ("I can handle this problem"), or statements that reflect personal strengths ("I know I can ace that test"). Write these positive statements on a small card and place the card where you will see it daily. Repeat these statements to yourself every day and when you are feeling "stressed out." You can begin your daily relaxation sessions with progressive muscular relaxation followed by imagery, and then complete the stress management activity by repeating your positive self-statements.

Physical Exercise

Whether it is gardening or ballroom dancing, physical activity can reduce stress by shifting one's attention away from stressors and toward the enjoyable aspects of the activity. Besides this psychological benefit, physical activity can metabolize the extra energy released during the stress response, lessening the impact of stress on the body. Engaging in physical activity with others can also enhance social and spiritual well-being. Nearly everyone can think of at least one physical activity that they can enjoy on a regular basis.

Regular exercise improves mood and self-image while reducing anxiety and stress.[30] Exercising regularly enhances the functioning of the immune system and may reduce symptoms of depression and anxiety.[31] Too much physical activity, however, can cause exhaustion or muscle damage, creating emotional stress. Athletes who engage in endurance activities and extensive physical training may have less effective immune systems while they are in active training.

During strenuous physical activity, such as running, the nervous system releases endorphins that may be responsible for creating the "runner's high," the heightened sense of well-being that long-distance runners often experience. As mentioned earlier in this chapter, endorphins can relieve pain, but they also can reduce the activity of certain components of the immune system. However most people can gain far more health benefits than harmful effects from regular, moderate exercise.

Tai Chi and Yoga *Tai chi*, a form of martial art that originated in China, emphasizes relaxation of the mind while the body is in motion. As people perform the gentle, gliding movements of tai chi, they

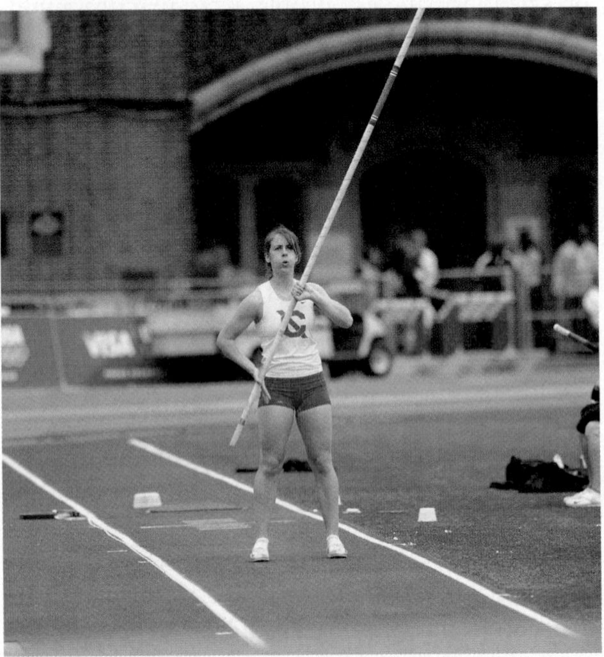

Imagery can help reduce stress and enhance performance.

focus their attention on this physical activity and disregard all other thoughts. In addition to tai chi, the other martial arts can be effective in reducing stress, increasing the body's flexibility, and boosting self-confidence. Tai chi, however, may be preferred by less physically active older adults because the exercises are less strenuous.

Yoga, a philosophy of living that originated in India thousands of years ago, includes specific physical exercises, breathing techniques, meditation activities, and dietary restrictions to promote a healthier body and manage stress (**Figure 3.6**). As individuals practice the yoga exercises, they slowly move their bodies into positions that stretch their skeletal muscles. After maintaining these positions, trained individuals usually report feeling relaxed and refreshed. Although some of yoga's teachings concerning nutrition and the health benefits of stretching organs are not based on modern medical concepts, these exercises can enhance the body's muscular flexibility and reduce stress.[32]

Interest in tai chi and yoga is increasing in the United States. If you would like to learn the activities, check with the physical education department on your campus or the local fitness club to determine if they offer tai chi and yoga classes. Before beginning any new physical activity program, especially the martial arts and yoga, it is advisable to receive approval from your personal physician.

Figure 3.6

Managing Stress with Yoga. Yoga includes specific physical exercises, breathing techniques, meditation activities, and dietary restrictions to promote a healthier body. After practicing yoga, trained individuals usually report feeling relaxed and refreshed.

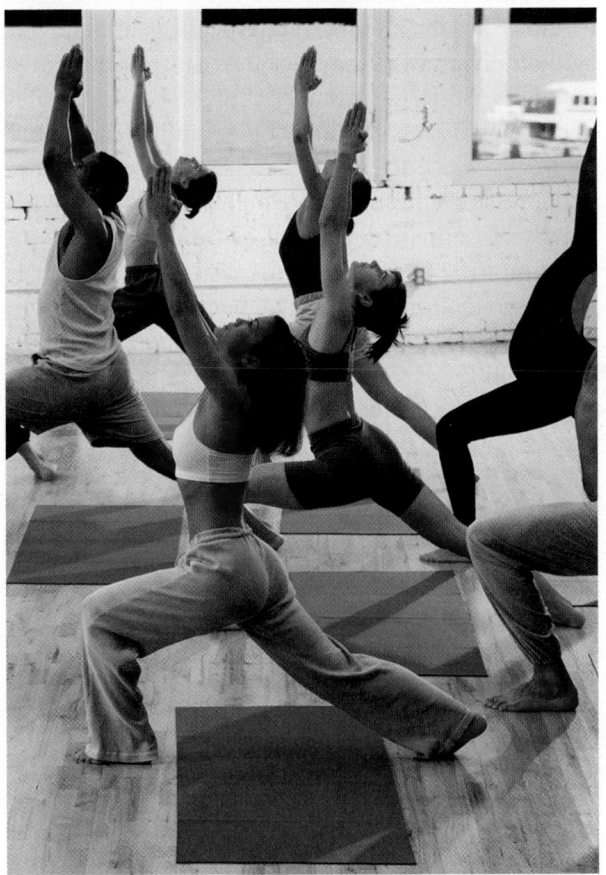

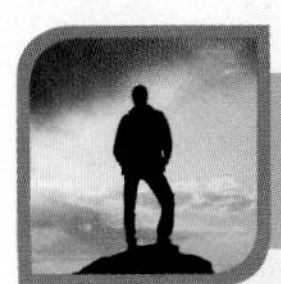

Healthy Living Practices

- If dwelling on negative self-thoughts creates stress for you, think about your strengths and develop a list of affirmative self-statements to repeat regularly.
- Consider setting aside some time to relax every day, perhaps by using the techniques discussed in this chapter.
- Try breathing slowly and deeply before or during a stressful situation as a simple but effective way to relax.
- Engaging in tai chi, yoga, and moderate exercise and physical activity on a regular basis can reduce your stress.

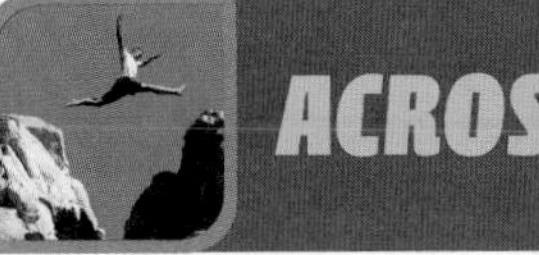

ACROSS THE LIFE SPAN

STRESS

Distressed adults may recall images of a carefree childhood, but children also experience stress. Common stressors for children include separation from a parent through divorce or death, moving to a new neighborhood and changing schools, and illness of a close family member.

When children are distressed, they often exhibit regressive behaviors, like clinging to and acting more dependent on their parents. In addition to acting immature, distressed youngsters may become

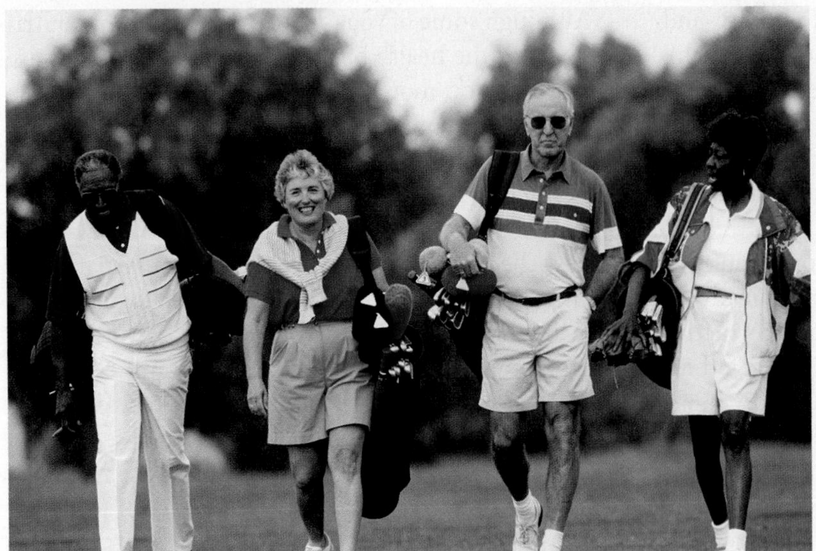

Figure 3.7

Social Interaction Among Older Adults. Many communities offer social and physical programs for older adults that can combat the stress of isolation.

depressed and withdrawn; suffer sleep disturbances, headaches, and stomachaches; or experience problems at school. Parents can help their children learn healthy ways to cope with stressful situations by teaching them problem-solving skills and relaxation exercises.

The adolescent years are stressful because individuals undergo numerous physical and social changes during this time. The most recent Stress in America™ survey found that teens, like their adult counterparts, report having stress levels far higher than what they deem healthy and that stress is negatively impacting their lives.[1] Distressed youth who do not have effective and healthy coping mechanisms are likely to suffer from depression, abuse drugs, have serious traffic accidents, and experience problems with parents and school authorities. If an adolescent's stress response persists or is severe, professional counseling is necessary.

For many people, the older adult years can be very stressful. Aging individuals often feel bored or useless, especially if they have retired from the responsibilities of a job or raising a family. On the other hand, many older adults are distressed because they must work to supply an income, or they must raise their grandchildren. Older adults frequently experience distress when they must care for spouses with debilitating mental or physical illnesses.

Coping with loneliness and the deaths of friends or close family members is especially difficult for aging individuals as they face the reality of their own mortality. Suffering from disabling illnesses creates additional distress for many older adults. The inability to cope with stress can have serious results; rates of depression and suicide are high among the isolated elderly. To enhance the well-being of older adults, communities often have programs that encourage social interaction among aged members of the population (**Figure 3.7**). Elderly residents of most long-term care facilities can participate in social and physical activities that combat the stress of isolation.

CHAPTER REVIEW

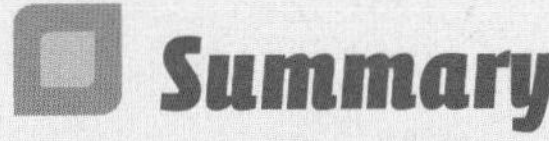

Summary

Stress can refer to a threatening or demanding situation, a person's responses to a situation, or the interactions that take place between a person and a situation. Various situations or conditions, referred to as stressors, create stress. Individuals, however, can appraise the same situation differently. Situations with unwanted or negative outcomes produce distress, those with positive outcomes produce eustress. Stress can make life more challenging and interesting, but too much can make life miserable.

In a combined response, the nervous, endocrine, and immune systems prepare the body to confront or leave dangerous situations. Hans Selye proposed the general adaptation syndrome to describe the three stages of the body's adaptive physical responses to stressors. The stress response produces physical changes that include altering the activity and effectiveness of the immune system. As a result, enduring too many stressful life events can increase one's susceptibility to disease.

People often use problem-focused, emotion-focused, or social support coping strategies to deal with stressful situations. Although these strategies can be effective methods of helping people take control over their stressors, some coping methods can be harmful to health. For example, emotional eating and avoiding and denying stressors are coping mechanisms that usually do not eliminate the sources of stress. Adopting healthy lifestyles can help one manage stress effectively.

Many stress management activities involve learning skills that enable one to relax. Relaxation can reverse many of the normal but damaging physical responses to stress. Relaxation techniques include deep breathing exercises, progressive muscular relaxation, meditation, and mental imagery. Journal writing, effective time management, positive self-talk, and moderate physical activity can also reduce stress.

Common childhood stressors include separation from a parent through divorce or death, moving to a new neighborhood and changing schools, and the illness of a close family member. Older distressed youths are often depressed, abuse drugs, and experience problems with parents and school authorities. Aging people often find that coping with loneliness, disability, and the deaths of friends or close family members is especially stressful.

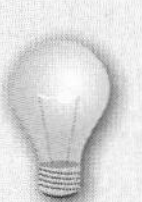

Applying What You Have Learned

1. Using the techniques described in this chapter, develop a personal stress-reduction program that you can incorporate into your daily schedule. **Application**
2. You have two final exams scheduled for the same day. Describe how you could use a negative coping strategy to reduce your stress. Describe how you could use a positive coping method to deal with the same situation. **Application**
3. Plan a program that uses social support as a coping strategy to help distressed older adults who live in your community. **Synthesis**
4. Evaluate your present situation. Identify and list the sources of distress in your life. **Evaluation**

Key

Application
using information in a new situation.

Synthesis
putting together information from different sources.

Evaluation
making informed decisions.

CHAPTER REVIEW

© SergeBertasiusPhotography/ShutterStock

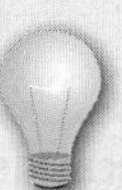
© tele52/ShutterStock

Reflecting on Your Health

1. Review the physical adaptations to stress listed in Table 3.1. The last time you were faced with a stressful situation, did you experience these changes? How did you feel?
2. Recall that stress can have positive outcomes. Reflect on a stressful experience that made you feel happy, challenged, or successful. Why did the experience make you feel this way?
3. Each person can appraise a situation differently; what is distressing to one can be thrilling to another. Choose a situation that distresses you. Why do you think it affects you in this manner? Do you think other people would find this situation distressing? Why or why not?
4. Chronic stress can have negative effects on health. What was the most stressful situation that you had to endure in the past year? How did this experience affect your health and well-being?
5. How do you usually react when faced with stressful situations? Are your responses positive or negative? How do you think you could reduce the impact of stress on your health?

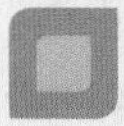

References

1. American Psychological Association. (2014, March). *Stress in America™ 2013 highlights: Are teens adopting adults' stress habits?* Retrieved from http://www.apa.org/news/press/releases/2014/02/teen-stress.aspx
2. Selye, H. (1976). *The stress of life* (2nd ed.). New York, NY: McGraw-Hill.
3. Black, P. H. (2006). The inflammatory consequences of psychologic stress: Relationship to insulin resistance, obesity, atherosclerosis, and diabetes mellitus, type II. *Medical Hypotheses*, 67(4), 879–891.
4. Ayers, J. W., et al. (2009). Sorting out the competing effects of acculturation, immigrant stress, and social support on depression: A report on Korean women in California. *Journal of Nervous and Mental Disease*, 197(10), 742–747.
5. Ibrahim, F. A., & Ohnishi, H. (2001). Posttraumatic stress disorder and the minority experience. In D. B. Pope-Davis & H. L. K. Coleman (Eds.), *The intersection of race, class, and gender in multicultural counseling* (pp. 89–126). Thousand Oaks, CA: Sage Publications.
6. Ro, M. (2002). Moving forward: Addressing the health of Asian American and Pacific Islander women. *American Journal of Public Health*, 92, 516–519.
7. Heron, M. (2013). Deaths: Leading cause for 2010. *National Vital Statistics Reports*, 68(6), 1–97.
8. Blonna, R. (2005). *Coping with stress in a changing world* (3rd ed.). Boston, MA: McGraw-Hill.
9. Holmes, T. H., & Rahe, R. H. (1967). The social readjustment rating scale. *Journal of Psychosomatic Research*, 11, 213–218.
10. Marx, M. B., Garrity, T. F., & Bowers, F. R. (1975). The influence of recent life experiences on the health of college students. *Journal of Psychosomatic Research*, 19, 87–98.
11. Holmes, C., et al. (2009). Systemic inflammation and disease progression in Alzheimer disease. *Neurology*, 73(10),768–774.
12. Kiecolt-Glaser, J. K., et al. (2003). Chronic stress and age-related increases in the proinflammatory cytokine IL-6. *Proceedings of the National Academy of Sciences*, 100(15), 9090–9095.
13. Wong, C. M. (2002). Post-traumatic stress disorder: Advances in psychoneuroimmunology. *Psychiatric Clinics of North America*, 25(2), 369–383.
14. Levenson, J. L. (2003). Psychological factors affecting medical conditions. In R. E. Hales, et al. (Eds.), *Textbook of psychiatry* (3rd ed., pp. 635–661). Washington, DC: American Psychiatric Press.
15. Orth-Gomér, K., et al. (2009). Stress reduction prolongs life in women with coronary artery disease: The Stockholm Women's Intervention Trial for Coronary Heart Disease. *Circulation, Cardiovascular Quality and Outcomes*, 2, 25–32.
16. National Institutes of Health, National Institute of Diabetes and Digestive and Kidney Diseases. (2014, March). *Irritable bowel syndrome*. Retrieved from http://digestive.niddk.nih.gov/ddiseases/pubs/ibs/
17. National Institutes of Health, National Institute of Arthritis and Neuromuscular and Skin Diseases. (2014, March). *Fibromyalgia*. Retrieved from http://www.niams.nih.gov/Health_Info/Fibromyalgia/default.asp
18. National Institutes of Health, National Institute of Diabetes and Digestive and Kidney Diseases. (2014, March). H. pylori *and peptic ulcers*. Retrieved from http://digestive.niddk.nih.gov/ddiseases/pubs/hpylori/index.aspx
19. National Institutes of Health, National Institute of Neurological Disorders and Stroke. (2014, March). *Headache: Hope through research*. Retrieved from http://www.ninds.nih.gov/disorders/headache/detail_headache.htm
20. National Institutes of Health, National Institute of Neurological Disorders and Stroke. (2014, March). *NINDS migraine information page*. Retrieved from http://www.ninds.nih.gov/disorders/migraine/migraine.htm

21. National Institutes of Health, National Center for Complementary and Alternative Medicine. (2014, March)). *Herbs at a glance. Kava.* Retrieved from http://nccam.nih.gov/health/kava/
22. National Institutes of Health, National Center for Complementary and Alternative Medicine. (2014, March). *Herbs at a glance. Valerian.* Retrieved from http://nccam.nih.gov/health/valerian/
23. National Institutes of Health, National Center for Complementary and Alternative Medicine. (2014, March). *Herbs at a glance. Feverfew.* Retrieved from http://nccam.nih.gov/health/feverfew
24. Dallman, M. R. (2010). Stress-induced obesity and the emotional nervous system. *Trends in Endocrinology & Metabolism*, 21(3), 159–165.
25. Ho, R. C. M., et al. (2010). Research on psychoneuroimmunology: Does stress influence immunity and cause coronary artery disease? *Annals of the Academy of Medicine of Singapore*, 39(3), 191–196.
26. Brydon, L., et al. (2010). Hostility and physiological responses to laboratory stress in acute coronary syndrome patients. *Journal of Psychosomatic Research*, 68(2), 109–116.
27. Ross, K. (2008). Mapping pathways from stress to cancer progression. *Journal of the National Cancer Institute*, 100(13), 914–915, 917.
28. Greeson, J. M. (2009). Mindfulness research update: 2008. *Complementary Health Practice Review*, 14(1), 10–18.
29. Benson, H. (1975). *The relaxation response*. New York, NY: William Morrow.
30. Kruk, J. (2009). Physical activity and health. *Asian Pacific Journal of Cancer Prevention*, 10(5), 721–728.
31. Tsatsoulis, A., & Fountoulakis, S. (2006). The protective role of exercise on stress, stress system dysregulation, and comorbidities. *Annals of the New York Academy of Science*, 1083, 196–213.
32. Kiecolt-Glaser, J. K., et al. (2010). Stress, inflammation, and yoga practice. *Psychosomatic Medicine*, 72(2), 113. doi:10.1097/PSY.0b013e3181cb9377

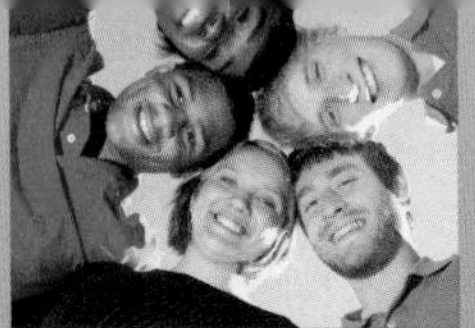

Diversity in Health
Spouse Abuse: An International Problem

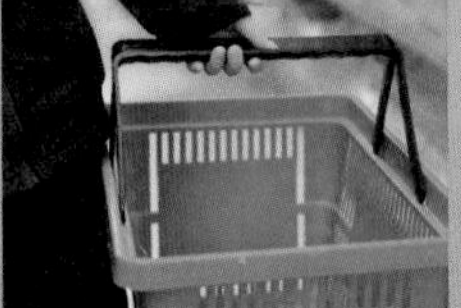

Consumer Health
Natural Defense: Pepper Spray

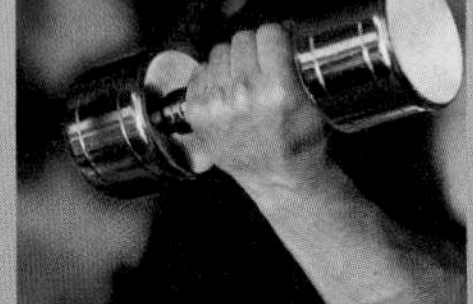

Managing Your Health
Sexual Assault: Reducing Your Risk

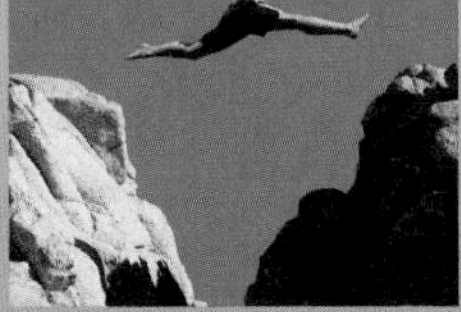

Across the Life Span
Violence and Abuse

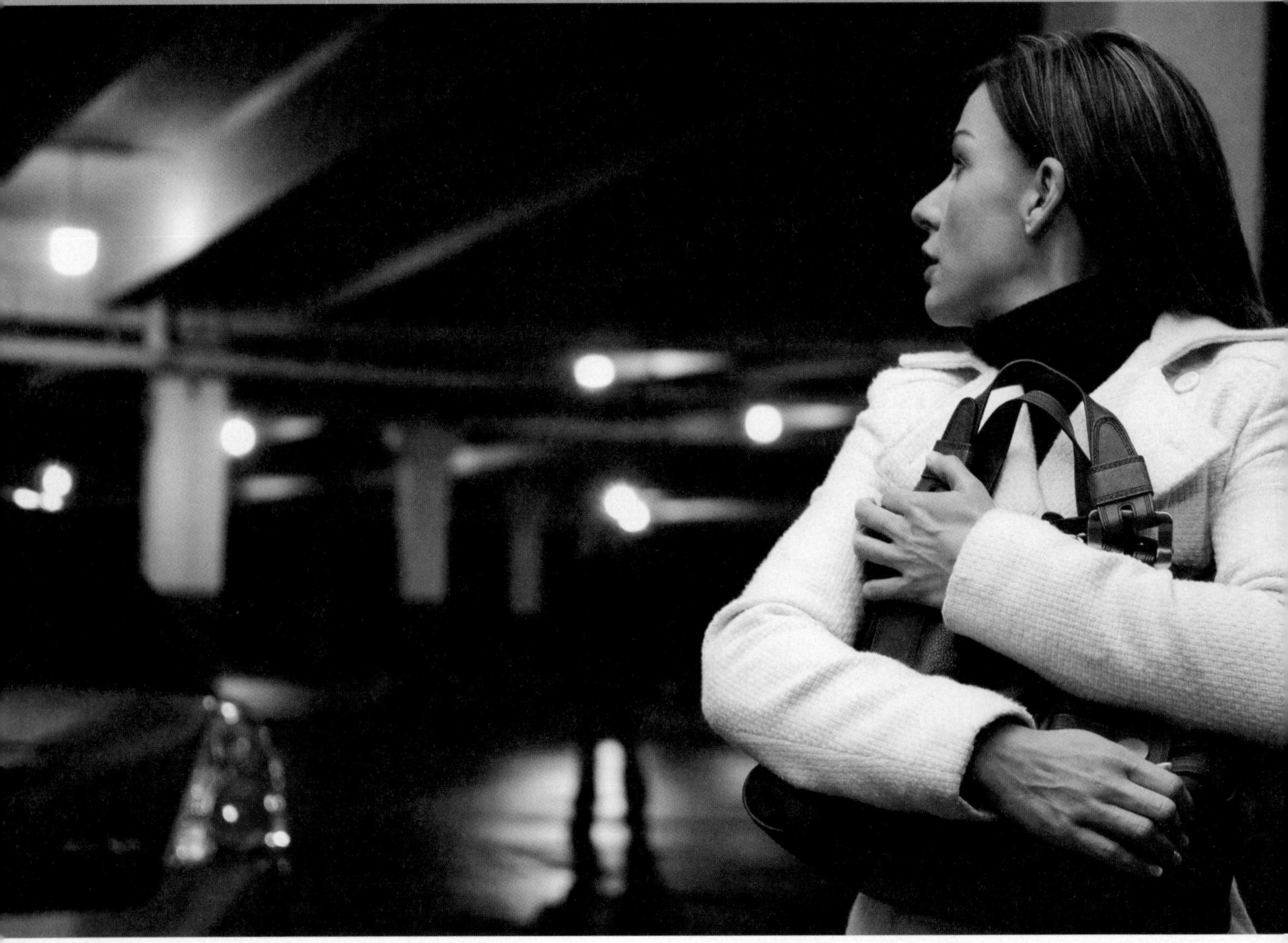

Chapter Overview

How violence affects your health

Factors that contribute to violence

Major types of violence and abuse

How to assess your risk of becoming a victim of violence

What you can do to prevent and avoid violence

Student Workbook

Self-Assessment: Am I in an Abusive Intimate Relationship?

Changing Health Habits: Can You Reduce Your Risk of Violence?

Do You Know?

Whether watching violent television shows can encourage violent behavior?

How to tell if your partner is likely to become physically abusive?

What to do if you are sexually harassed?

CHAPTER 4

Violence and Abuse

Learning Objectives

After studying this chapter, you should be able to:

1. Describe the effects of violence on society and personal health.
2. Classify various forms of violence.
3. Identify factors that contribute to violent behavior.
4. Identify actions that you can take to reduce your risk of violence.
5. Explain why cases of violence are often unreported to the police.
6. Define sexual harassment and steps you can take to report such abuse.
7. Define terms such as "pedophile," "child molester," and "elder abuse."

". . .one aggravated assault occurred about every 42 seconds. . ."

violence Interpersonal uses of force that are not socially sanctioned.

assault The intentional use of force to injure another person physically.

abuse Taking advantage of a relationship to mistreat a person.

Most of the campus security notices seemed to be for women, and I had a high school letter in wrestling, so I wasn't worried. Late one night, I was walking across campus, hardly watching where I was going, when a guy with a gun jumped out of some bushes and demanded my money. I gave him my watch and wallet, but he still hit me in the face with the gun barrel. I needed several stitches to close the wound.

According to the Federal Bureau of Investigation (FBI), in 2011 one violent crime happened about every 26.2 seconds in the United States.[1] Of these crimes, one aggravated assault occurred about every 42 seconds, one forcible rape took place almost every 6.3 minutes, and one murder happened nearly every 36 minutes.

In 2012, an estimated 686,000 children were abused or neglected in the United States, and an estimated 1,640 children died as a result.[2] Partner-against-partner violence is common in the United States. During their lifetimes, 1 in every 4 American women and 1 in every 14 American men suffer sexual and/or physical abuse at the hands of their intimate partners.[3] For many Americans, violence is a way of life.

Every society tolerates certain controlled uses of force, for example, spanking a misbehaving child or playing contact sports. In this chapter, **violence** refers to interpersonal uses of force that are not socially sanctioned. Such violence occurs when at least one person intentionally applies or threatens physical force against one or more people. These incidents are usually onesided—for example, a perpetrator attacking a victim—but they are sometimes mutual, such as in a barroom brawl, a schoolyard scuffle, or a fight between a husband and wife.

No one is exempt from violence; it may be directed against infants, children, adolescents, and older adults. Certain groups of people, such as African Americans, homosexuals, and Jews, are often targets of violence (*hate crimes*). Over the past 20 years, American citizens have become victims of violence as domestic and foreign terrorists waged deadly attacks in the United States.

Most physical violence in the United States could be regarded as nonsexual crimes against persons, primarily assault, robbery, and homicide. **Assault** is the intentional use of force to injure someone physically. **Abuse** occurs when one takes advantage of a relationship to mistreat a person, often by using frequent threats of force. Examples of abuse include spouse abuse, child abuse, elder abuse, and sexual harassment.

At some time in your life, you may have been a victim of abuse or violence, or you may have been indirectly involved in violent incidents. As a child, you may have been verbally abused by a parent or punched or kicked by a playground bully. As a teenager, you may have been slapped, shoved, or forced to have sex by someone you dated. As an adult, you may have been threatened or assaulted by a person with a weapon, as was the male college student in the chapter opener. How likely are you to become a victim of abuse or violence in the days to come?

Many Americans feel that their lives are more dangerous than in the past, but national rates of violent crime have declined dramatically since 2002: the homicide rate declined by 49% between 2002 and 2011, which is the lowest level in 50 years.[4] In 2009, the estimated number of murders, rapes, and aggravated assaults decreased by about 7.5% from the 2000 estimate.[5] Nevertheless, males, Blacks, American Indians, teens, and young adults experienced higher rates of violent crime than did others.[6] This chapter explores the causes of violence and describes its effects on health. It provides practical steps you can take to reduce your risk of being a victim.

How Violence Affects Health

Many patients who seek treatment in hospital emergency rooms are victims of violence. Although some victims just need medical attention for minor cuts or bruises, others have more serious injuries such as lost teeth, broken bones, and firearm or knife wounds thatmay require hospitalization (**Figure 4.1**). Victims of rape or attempted rape may also need immediate treatment to reduce the risk of sexually transmitted infections (STIs) and unintentional pregnancies.

In some cases, victims of violence suffer serious permanent physical disabilities such as blindness, brain damage, and loss of body movement (*paralysis*). Additionally, the stress of fighting or living in an abusive situation alters the functioning

Figure 4.1

The Aftermath of Violence. Injuries resulting from violence often require medical treatment.

© Jonathan Nourok/PhotoEdit

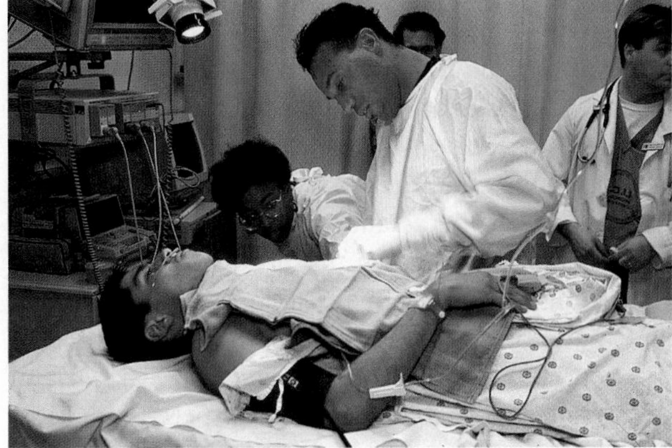

of the immune system, which can lower one's resistance against infectious illnesses. Death is, of course, the most serious consequence of violence. In 2010, homicide was the second and third leading causes of death for Americans 15 to 19 and 20 to 34 years of age, respectively; was the second leading cause of death among American males 15 to 24 years old; and was the number one cause of death among African Americans aged 15 to 34.[7]

Experiencing violence also causes psychological damage—including anxiety and depression, which can heighten one's risk of abusing drugs, developing eating disorders, and having suicidal thoughts. Violence caused by persons outside the home can create serious problems for the victims' family life. Family relationships may become strained, suspended, or even ended as a consequence. Violence that occurs within a family setting is very harmful. Cases of marital separation or divorce often involve violence against a spouse or child. To recover from the psychological effects of violence, one should seek help from qualified mental health professionals.

A possible social effect is the *intergenerational* transmission of violence, in which child victims of abuse mature and become abusive as parents, perpetuating family violence.[8] This particular effect, however, occurs only among some abused children; others have personality factors that buffer them from the long-term effects of child abuse. Overall, the financial costs of violence on physical, psychological, and social health are staggering; the cost in human misery is immeasurable.

What Causes Violent Behavior?

Violence is complex; there is no single cause of violent behavior. Indeed, several factors contribute to violence including "frustration, exposure to violent media, violence in the home or neighborhood and a tendency to see other people's actions as hostile even when they're not. Certain situations also increase the risk of aggression, such as drinking, insults and other provocations and environmental factors like heat and overcrowding."[9,para.1] In many instances, violence is learned behavior: children who are exposed to violence in their homes are more likely to be abusive or violent as adults than children who do not witness violence.

Does exposure to violent screen media, particularly movies, video games, and television programs, contribute to violent behavior? The average American 3rd to 12th grader spends more than 6 hours per day using various forms of screen media.[10] In general, children who watch acts of violence in screen media are more likely to exhibit aggressive and violent behavior than children who do not view violence in such media.[10] How do television shows and other forms of screen media contribute to violence in the United States?

Screen media, such as violent computer games and movies, offer opportunities for young people to learn violent behavior. Watching violent movies, for example, provides indirect ways to participate in the violence, experience emotional states associated with being violent, and observe the outcomes of violence. Television programs and movies often glamorize violent and abusive people, and the perpetrators may avoid punishment. If violence is portrayed as an effective way of getting what one wants, an impressionable

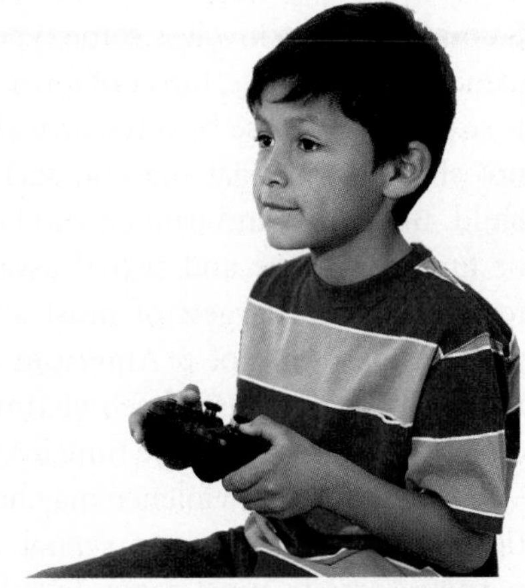

Violent video games offer opportunities for children to learn violent behavior.

© Digital Media Pro/ShutterStock

sexual violence Gaining sexual activity through force or threat of force.

rape Sexual intercourse by force or with a person who is incapable of legal consent.

young observer may resort to violence when he or she is in similar situations. Another concern is that young people who often use violent forms of screen media for entertainment may become "desensitized" to real cases of violence and tolerate such behavior as a result.

Televisions are equipped with "V-chips" that enable adults to block certain programs from being viewed by children, but only 20% of parents use this control.[8] The screen media industry provides various rating systems to help parents select software and programs with acceptable content for children. Many parents find the ratings confusing, and some children misuse the ratings to find violent programs. Thus, parents still must exercise good judgment concerning which media are appropriate for their children and monitor their offsprings' use of screen media as a form of entertainment.

Major Types of Violence and Abuse

Sexual Violence

My first sexual experience was very unpleasant. It happened on San Padre Island over Spring Break when I was a freshman. I was 18, and he was 25 years old. He took me to an area where no one could see him or hear me. I was naive and thought I could stop him, but I couldn't. I had wanted to wait until I was married, or at least in love with the person.

Sexual violence involves some type of sexual activity gained through force, threat of force, or coercion. **Rape** is sexual intercourse by force or with a person who is not able to give legal consent, such as a 12-year-old child. Both men and women can be the perpetrators or targets of rape and sexual assault. Nevertheless, females are the targets of most attempted or completed rapes. One of 6 American women and 1 of 33 American men have been victims of an attempted or completed rape at some time in their lives.[11]

Although sexual violence may happen in any relationship, most victims of sexual assault know the perpetrator.[12] In most cases, female victims of rape know the attacker—often a current or former husband, current or ex-boyfriend, a date, classmate, or live-in (*cohabiting*) partner. Although men are not as likely to be raped as women, male victims are usually raped by male strangers and acquaintances.[11] *Marital rape* generally refers to the use or threat of violence against one's spouse to force sexual activity. *Acquaintance rape* is forced sexual activity that occurs between unmarried adults who know each other. If the couple is involved in a dating relationship, forced sexual activity is called *date rape*.

Sexual assaults on college campuses have a similar gender pattern: college women are more likely than college men to be assaulted and are more likely to be assaulted by a known person than by a stranger. According to one major research report, about 1 in 36 female college students are victims of a completed or attempted rape during an academic year; 90% of these college women knew the perpetrator.[13] Most of the completed rapes occur in campus residential housing; the remainder of these assaults took place in fraternity houses. The Campus Sexual Assault Study, funded by the U.S. Department of Justice, found freshman and sophomores to be at higher risk for sexual assault than upperclassmen, and the majority of sexual assaults occurred when the victims were incapacitated due to substances, namely alcohol.[14] The use of alcohol or other drugs may weaken a person's inhibitions and alter his or her usual behavior. For example, while intoxicated, a person may act more sexually aggressive toward her/his date or partner, or be less able to prevent forced sex. The deliberate use of Rohypnol and other so-called date-rape drugs to sexually assault unsuspecting persons (primarily women) is a growing problem in the United States. Rohypnol causes not only loss of consciousness but also loss of memory concerning events that occurred when the drug was taken.

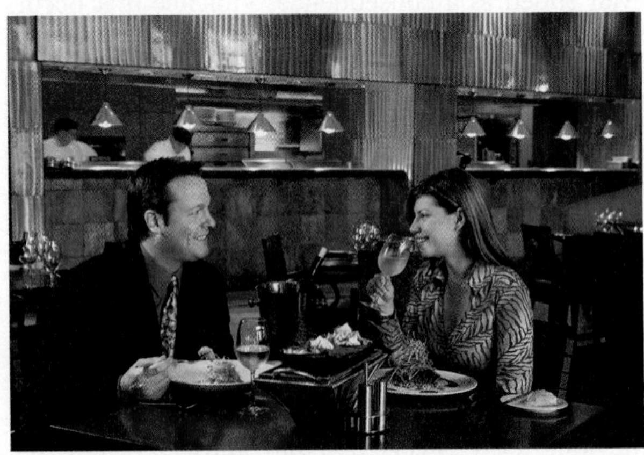

When intoxicated, a person may act more sexually aggressive toward his or her date or partner, or be less able to prevent forced sex.

Managing Your Health

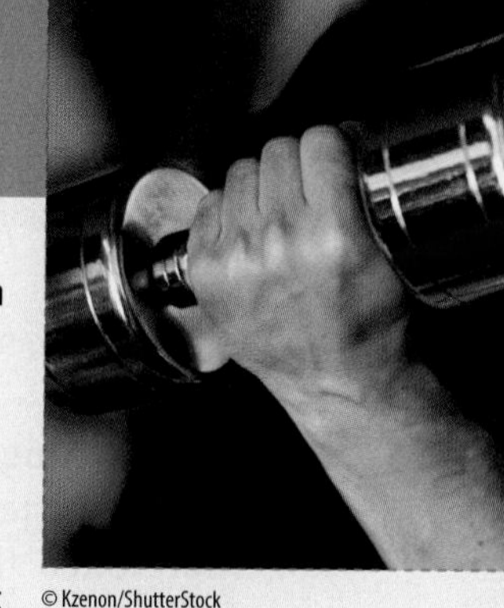
© Kzenon/ShutterStock

Sexual Assault: Reducing Your Risk

Sexual assault is a crime of motive and opportunity; there is no guaranteed way to completely protect yourself from being attacked. However, there are some actions you can take to help reduce your risk of being assaulted.

Avoiding Dangerous Situations:

- **Be aware** of your surroundings. Knowing where you are and who is around you may help you to find a way to get out of a bad situation.
- Try to **avoid isolated areas**. It is more difficult to get help if no one is around.
- **Walk with purpose**. Even if you don't know where you are going, act like you do.
- **Trust your instincts**. If a situation or location feels unsafe or uncomfortable, it probably isn't the best place to be.
- **Try not to load yourself down** with packages or bags because this can make you appear more vulnerable.
- **Make sure your cell phone is with you** and charged and that you have cab money.
- **Don't allow yourself to be isolated** with someone you don't trust or someone you don't know.
- **Avoid putting music headphones in both ears** so that you can be more aware of your surroundings, especially if you are walking alone.

In a Social Situation:

- **When you go to a social gathering, go with a group of friends**. Arrive together, check in with each other throughout the evening, and leave together. Knowing where you are and who is around you may help you to find a way out of a bad situation.
- **Trust your instincts**. If you feel unsafe in any situation, go with your gut. If you see something suspicious, contact law enforcement immediately (local authorities can be reached by calling 911 in most areas of the United States).
- **Don't leave your drink unattended** while talking, dancing, using the restroom, or making a phone call. If you've left your drink alone, just get a new one.
- **Don't accept drinks from people you don't know or trust**. If you choose to accept a drink, go with the person to the bar to order it, watch it being poured, and carry it yourself. At parties, don't drink from punch bowls or other large, common open containers.
- **Watch out for your friends and vice versa**. If a friend seems out of it, is way too intoxicated for the amount of alcohol they've had, or is acting out of character, get him or her to a safe place immediately.
- **If you suspect you or a friend has been drugged, contact law enforcement immediately (local authorities can be reached by calling 911 in most areas of the United States)**. Be explicit with doctors so they can give you the correct tests (you will need a urine test and possibly others).

If Someone is Pressuring You:

- **Remember that being in this situation is not your fault**. You did not do anything wrong; it is the person who is making you uncomfortable that is to blame.
- **Be true to yourself**. Don't feel obligated to do anything you don't want to do. "I don't want to" is always a good enough reason. Do what feels right to you and what you are comfortable with.
- **Have a code word with your friends or family** so that if you don't feel comfortable you can call them and communicate your discomfort without the person you are with knowing. Your friends or family can then come to get you or make up an excuse for you to leave.
- **Lie**. If you don't want to hurt the person's feelings it is better to lie and make up a reason to leave than to stay and be uncomfortable, scared, or worse. Some excuses you could use are needing to take care of a friend or family member, not feeling well, having somewhere else that you need to be, etc.
- **Try to think of an escape route**. How would you try to get out of the room? Where are the doors? Windows? Are there people around who might be able to help you? Is there an emergency phone nearby?
- **If you and/or the other person have been drinking**, you can say that you would rather wait until you both have your full judgment before doing anything you may regret later.

Computer Safety:

- Find a safe computer.
- Edit privacy settings on social media (see https://www.rainn.org/get-information/computer-safety for how to manage personal information on Facebook and Twitter).
- Clear history/cache on Internet browsers (Firefox, Internet Explorer, Safari, etc.) on mobile devices and computers (see https://www.rainn.org/get-information/computer-safety for how to clear this information).

Adapted from RAINN. (2014). Ways to reduce your risk of sexual assault. Retrieved from https://www.rainn.org/get-information/sexual-assault-prevention

family (domestic) violence Violence or abuse between family members, people who are involved in intimate relationships, or unrelated individuals who live together.

Reporting Sexual Assault Data from crime surveys consistently suggest that sexual crimes occur more often than reported. Rape victims frequently feel ashamed and embarrassed and are often reluctant to report their experiences to the authorities. Moreover, they may fear further victimization by the assailant or negative reactions from family, friends, and coworkers. Some victims, however, fail to report the assault because they do not want to become involved in the criminal justice system. Many victims of acquaintance rape are often unwilling to report the incidents because they feel partially to blame. For example, a female college student may feel that if she had consumed less alcohol or smoked less marijuana at a party, she would have been able to resist the sexual advances of others. These examples highlight the social stigma associated with sexual assaults, in which victim-blaming may occur, a trend that does not hold true in other crimes (e.g., victims of muggings are generally not blamed for being attacked).

Many organizations are actively combating the social stigma of sexual assault by providing education to the public and support to those affected by sexual assault. For example, RAINN (Rape, Abuse & Incest National Network)—the largest antisexual violence organization in the United States—provides a variety of free, confidential services, including a National Sexual Assault Web-based hotline (www.rainn.org) and a 24/7 phone hotline (800-656-HOPE) for sexual assault victims, friends, and family members.[15] In addition, the *DoD Safe Helpline* (877-995-5247), which is contracted out to RAINN as an independent, anonymous service, offers sexual assault support for member of the DoD (Department of Defense) community.[16] Such services may alter the current social perceptions of sexual violence, which, in turn, may lower the perceived barriers of reporting sexual assault crimes.

Sexual assault victims may obtain immediate medical attention for their injuries and to preserve any physical evidence in case they choose to prosecute the perpetrator. The preservation of physical evidence—such as semen and pubic hair—is vital to assist law enforcement with identifying the attacker; therefore, victims should not wash any part of their bodies or change clothes before receiving medical attention. Hospital emergency rooms often have staff who are trained to respond to sexual assault victims with sensitivity, and local sexual assault crisis centers may have volunteers on standby to offer assistance. In addition to receiving treatment for physical injuries, many rape victims need testing for sexually transmitted infections, medication to prevent pregnancy, and counseling to cope with the situation.

Family Violence

Family (domestic) violence is a pattern of behavior characterized by physical assaults, including sexual violence; psychological/emotional abuse; and threats to cause harm that occur among family members, couples in intimate relationships, or unrelated individuals who live together. Such violence includes assaults and murders of spouses, children, and older family members. Between 2003 and 2012, domestic violence accounted for 21% of all violent victimizations, was predominantly committed against women (76%), was most often committed by current or former boy/girlfriends, and persons ages 18–24 had the highest rate of victimization.[17] In 2009, family members were responsible for almost one-fourth of all murders.[18] Child and elder abuse are often classified as forms of family violence; the Across the Life Span feature of this chapter provides information concerning these forms of family violence.

Intimate Partner Violence *Intimate partner violene (IPV)* involves actual or threatened physical or sexual violence, as well as emotional abuse, by a spouse, ex-spouse, lover, former lover, or date. Although the rates of IPV have mostly declined over the past few decades, the rate for women is over three times larger than the rate for men, as of 2011 (4.7 and 1.5 per 1,000 persons, respectively.[18]

In many instances, perpetrators of IPV emotionally abuse their partners for a period before they become overtly violent toward them.[19] Violent acts may range from slapping, shoving, and punching to beating and murder. Typically, verbal and/or emotional abuse accompany the physical violence. *Dating violence*, the threat or use of force against one's partner during courtship, is quite common. About 10% of high school students reported that they had been hit, slapped, or physically hurt (on purpose) by their boyfriend or girlfriend in 2009.[20] Furthermore, 10% of the female students and about 5% of the male high school students reported that they had been forced to have sex at some point in their lives.

Compared to women, men are more likely to seriously injure or murder their female intimate partners (**Figure 4.2**).[19] In 2014, Baltimore Ravens running back Ray Rice assaulted his then-fiance, knocking her

Figure 4.2

A Case of Domestic Violence. A woman is far more likely than a man to be seriously injured as the result of domestic violence.

© Tatiana Belova/ShutterStock

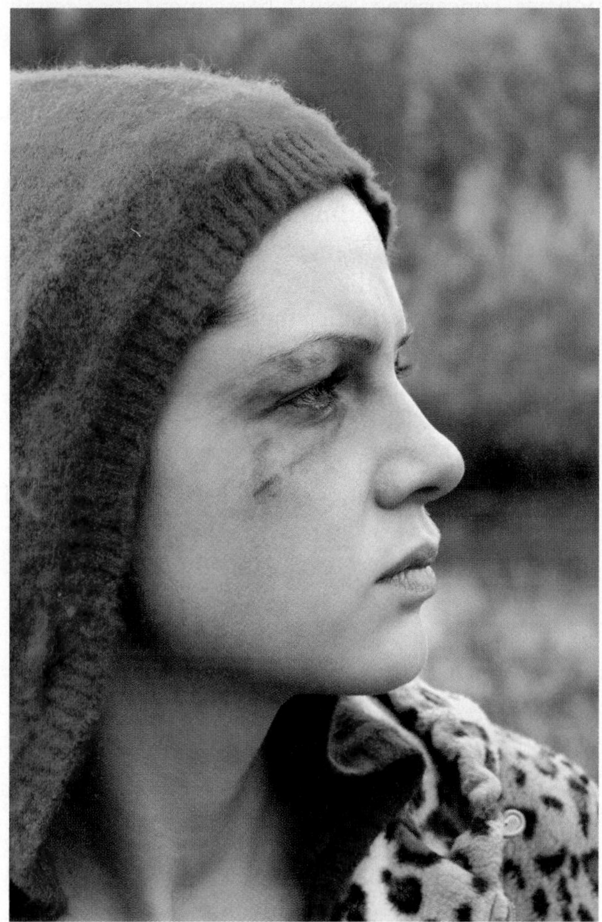

unconscious; the publicity ensuing after a video of the assault was posted online caused a national outcry and prompted the National Football League to revisit its policies regarding domestic violence cases. In 2010, of the female murder victims for whom their relationships to the offenders were known, about 51% were murdered by their intimate partner, compared to approximately 6% for male homicide victims.[18] Although both sexes commit violent acts against their dates or partners, women usually engage in violence against their male partners as acts of self-defense.

What factors contribute to violence between intimate partners? Such violence exists within every racial, ethnic, socioeconomic, and religious group. The rates of intimate partner violence, however, are higher among those who have a lower socioeconomic status, are unemployed, or are employed in low-status occupations. Children who are exposed to violence between their parents have a greater risk of abusing their intimate partners later in life.[21] As a result of witnessing violence between their parents, children may grow up thinking such abuse is a "normal" aspect of intimate relationships.

Another major factor that contributes to intimate partner violence is drug use. Often, one or both partners have consumed alcohol or used other mind-altering drugs when the violence between them erupts. Both perpetrators and victims tend to have low self-esteem and be highly dependent on their partners. Some men and women have difficulty asserting themselves without becoming angry and resort to aggressive behavior to control and intimidate their partners. The activity "Am I in an Abusive Relationship?" in the Student Workbook at the end of the book can help you determine if your partner is abusive. Furthermore, **Table 4.1** lists certain behaviors

Table 4.1

Signs of Danger in a Relationship

A partner who is likely to become physically abusive:

- Insists that you do things that you do not want to do and prevents you from doing things that you would like to do
- Argues with you over any issue
- Does not accept responsibility for his or her mistakes and blames you or other persons for his or her problems
- Prevents you from associating with your family and friends and threatens to end the relationship if you do not stop interacting with others
- Displays excessive jealousy or is too possessive
- Attempts to control your behavior, for example, tells you how to dress or wear your hair
- Is verbally abusive, for example, criticizes you or says degrading things to you either in private or in public
- Expects you to do everything perfectly and according to his or her wishes, and expects you to know what they are, even without being told
- Pushes, slaps, or shoves you during disagreements
- Reacts violently ("loses control" over his or her behavior) toward you or others when things go wrong or not according to his or her wishes
- Exhibits cruelty to other persons or animals, usually without remorse

Data from Mariani, C. (1996). *Domestic Violence Survival Guide.* Flushing, NY: Looseleaf Law Publications.

sexual harassment Intentional use of unwelcome sexually related comments or behaviors to intimidate or coerce people into unwanted sexual activity.

and attitudes that often characterize individuals who are physically abusive. Because dating violence is often a precursor of marital violence, identifying abuse in a dating relationship can help you determine whether you wish to remain in the relationship. It is important to recognize that abuse usually does not lessen when the relationship moves from dating to marital status and can even worsen.

Why do men and women stay in abusive relationships? Women often remain in these situations because of their emotional attachment to and economic dependency on the abuser. They often feel trapped and isolated.[22] Furthermore, an abusive partner may be apologetic and loving after episodes of violence, raising the victim's hopes that the violence has ended. Spousal abuse is a worldwide concern: the Diversity in Health feature "Spouse Abuse: An International Problem" discusses the nature of this behavior in non-Western societies.

Sexual Harassment

Sexual harassment is the intentional use of unwelcome and offensive sexually related comments or behaviors to intimidate people or coerce them into unwanted sexual activity. Such abusive behavior can include unwelcome requests for dates, sexually offensive jokes, lewd comments, or touching and fondling. It is difficult to determine the scope of the problem because surveys often use different definitions of *sexual harassment*. Furthermore, sexual harassment is not always easy to recognize. For example, if someone tells a sexually offensive joke, under what circumstances would you consider this sexual harassment?

Sexual harassment can happen anywhere. College instructors, for example, engage in sexual harassment if they provide special treatment, such as awarding a passing grade, to students who submit to their sexual advances. In addition to schools, sexual harassment frequently occurs in the workplace, where it creates stress and reduces employees' job satisfaction, performance, and loyalty. It is especially devastating for individuals who feel that their grade, job, or career depends on enduring the harassment or submitting to the intimidating person.

How can one handle a person who engages in sexual harassment? Some people simply avoid or ignore harassing persons; others choose to confront their tormentors by telling them, verbally or in writing, to stop the annoying and unprofessional comments or behaviors. If the harassment persists, victims can pursue more aggressive steps, including reporting the behavior to management or taking legal action. Many educational institutions and businesses have policies concerning sexual harassment that follow guidelines established by the federal government's *Equal Employment Opportunity Commission* (*EEOC*). These policies usually identify steps that people can take to file harassment-related complaints. Before initiating such action, a person should document episodes of sexual intimidation, recording the date and nature of the unwanted comments or behaviors. In many instances, the abusive person has harassed other workers or students; therefore, a victim may be able to strengthen his or her case against this person by asking other victims to serve as witnesses.

Stalking

Sensational stories about celebrities who are pursued relentlessly by overly aggressive, obsessive fans have led to interest and research into *stalking* behavior. Anyone, however, can be the victim of a stalking. Stalking is defined by the U.S. Department of Justice as "a pattern of repeated and unwanted attention, harassment, contact, or any other course of conduct directed at a specific person that would cause a reasonable person to feel fear" The term "stalker" generally refers to a person who willfully and repeatedly harasses or threatens another person. Stalking behavior typically includes following the targeted individual, hanging around this person's home, making harassing or threatening phone calls, leaving threatening voicemail or electronic messages, or vandalizing his or her property. Other examples of harassment include sending unwanted text messages or gifts and making unwelcome visits to the targeted person's workplace (see **Table 4.2**).

An estimated 6.6 million people are stalked annually in the United States; 1 in 4 women and 1 in 13 men report being the stalked at some point in their lives.[25] In only about 10% of the cases, the stalker was a stranger to his or her victim; according to victims, most of the stalkers were a former intimate partner or a friend, roommate, or neighbor.[25] Women are disproportionally affected by stalking: Sixty-six percent of female victims are stalked by a current or former intimate partner (compared to 41% of male victims); more than three-quarters of intimate partner femicide victims were stalked by intimate partners; and, more than half of femicide victims reported their

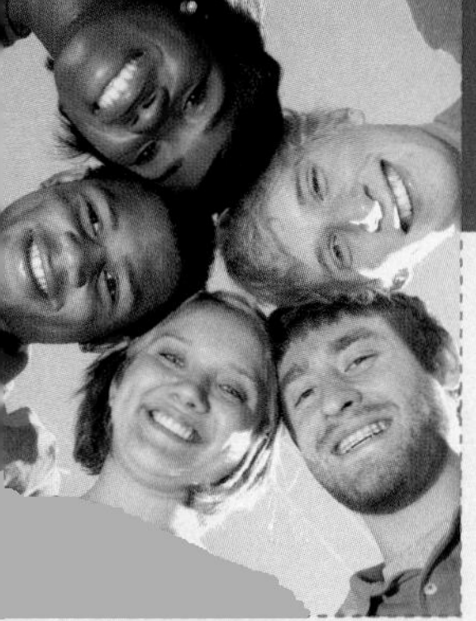
© Mike Flippo/ShutterStock

Diversity in Health

Spouse Abuse: An International Problem

Throughout the world, women of all cultural, religious, ethnic, and socioeconomic groups are abused by their intimate partners. Throughout the world, at least one-third of all women have experienced violence or abuse on one or more occasions during their lifetimes.[23] According to results of a study conducted by the World Health Organization, rates of IPV ranged from 15% in Japan to about 70% in Peru and Ethiopia.[24] In many societies, husbands are not punished for acting out violently against their wives, and female victims often accept blame for their mistreatment.

Why does spouse abuse persist? Certain non-Western cultures ascribe low status to women. Many men living in these societies do not consider wife battering and other forms of mistreatment of their spouses as violence or abuse. In addition, certain practices in such cultures increase the financial dependence of women on their spouses, which makes it difficult for them to leave their abusive husbands. For example, women living in some countries lose their inheritance or the opportunity to earn an income outside of the home when they marry. The economic power in these countries is unequally distributed in favor of men, and as a result, husbands feel entitled to control their wives and families. Male domination continues at community and state levels as women are often denied access to education and government positions. Thus, they lack the knowledge and political power necessary to change public policy. To eliminate violence against women, people from around the world must work to change the attitudes, behaviors, and laws that negatively affect the status of women.

Table 4.2

Typical Stalking Behaviors

- Follow you and show up wherever you are
- Send unwanted gifts, letters, cards, or e-mails
- Damage your home, car, or other property
- Monitor your phone calls or computer use
- Use technology, like hidden cameras or global positioning systems (GPS), to track where you go
- Drive by or hang out at your home, school, or work
- Threaten to hurt you, your family, friends, or pets
- Find out about you by using public records or online search services, hiring investigators, going through your garbage, or contacting friends, family, neighbors, or coworkers
- Posting information or spreading rumors about you on the Internet, in a public place, or by word of mouth
- Taking other actions that control, track, or frighten you

Data from Stalking Resource Center, The National Center for Victims of Crime. (2012). *Stalking Fact Sheet.* Retrieved from http://www.victimsofcrime.org/docs/src/stalking-fact-sheet_english.pdf?sfvrsn=4

stalkers' behavior to law enforcement before being killed by their stalkers.[25]

The majority of stalkers are males; the largest group of stalkers is composed of lonely men who are emotionally unstable and have been rejected by their partners.[26] Despite his expartner's efforts to avoid him, the stalker often hopes he can convince her to rekindle the relationship. When she ignores or rebuffs his efforts, he becomes angry with her and wants to harm her emotionally or physically.

Stalking can lead to violence, including homicide. Stalkers physically attack an estimated one-fourth to about one-third of their victims.[27] Warning signs of a violent stalker include the use of verbal threats and prior involvement in an intimate relationship with the victim. Even if the victim is not physically threatened or harmed, he or she usually experiences extreme emotional distress and often seeks legal means to make the stalker stop the harassing behavior. Victims often continue to suffer severe emotional effects long after the stalking ends, and they may need treatment for depression and post-traumatic stress disorder.

If you are being stalked, what can you do to discourage the stalker and end his or her terrifying behavior? If the stalker is a former intimate partner,

community violence Violence between strangers or acquaintances that occurs in public settings.

experts advise that either you or a family member confront the stalker to tell him or her that the relationship is over and you have no interest in renewing it. After that, avoid all communication with the person but keep records of his or her harassing behavior. If the stalker persistently telephones you, have an answering machine record calls on that line and get a separate, unlisted phone number for other callers. If the stalker uses e-mail messages or text messages to annoy you (*cyberstalking*), contact your Internet service (ISP) or cell phone service provider for help. Additionally, seek support and help from family, friends, neighbors, and coworkers by telling them about the stalking incidents. Finally, make sure your home is secure, and if you feel threatened by the stalker, notify the police.

Community Violence

Community violence refers to violence that happens in public settings such as street corners, bars, and public places. Among youths, community violence often occurs as *gang violence*. Typical members of a gang are males between 8 and 24 years of age who share similar racial or ethnic backgrounds. Such gangs are prevalent in certain neighborhoods of U.S. cities and are becoming more common in many suburbs. Between 2002 and 2011, the number of gangs increased by almost 36%.[28] According to one government estimate, approximately 1.4 million gang members were involved in criminal activity throughout the United States during 2011.[29] Gang-related criminal activities include armed robberies, drug trafficking, car theft, identity theft, and murder.[23]

Violence is a characteristic of gang activities—gang members often resort to violence to defend their territory. Violent gang activities are more likely to occur on city streets during weekend evenings. The late-night drive-by shooting, for example, has come to be associated with gang violence.

Why are some youths attracted to gangs, placing themselves at high risk for serious injury and even death? Adolescents may join gangs for social reasons, especially if their communities offer few opportunities for safe social activities. Gang membership provides an opportunity for some youths to belong to a group and find self-identity, that is, to "be someone." Involvement with gangs, however, dramatically increases one's risk of being murdered. In 2010, homicide was the number one cause of death for African American and Hispanic males between 15 and 34 years of age.[7]

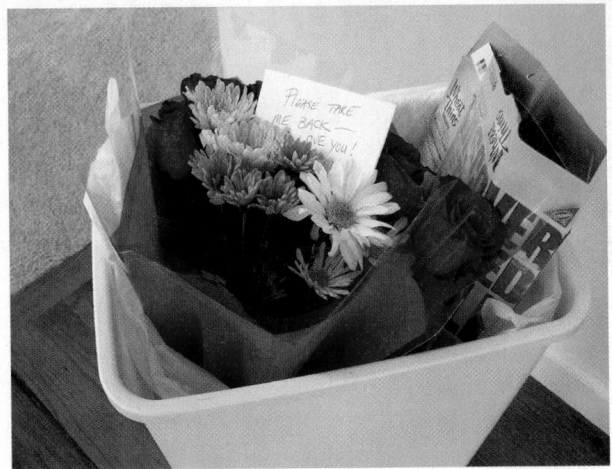

Men who stalk women may send unwanted gifts, such as bouquets of flowers, to their victims.
Courtesy of Wendy Schiff.

Institutional Violence

School Violence Most acts of **institutional violence** occur in schools, where students attack their peers or even their teachers and school administrators. Earlier generations of students may have shoved and punched to settle arguments; today's students may use guns and knives.

In the past few years, several incidents in which students used guns to kill their classmates and teachers made headline news. Such terrible events, however, are rare. Less than 1% of murders involving youth take place on school property. In 2009, American youth were much less likely to carry weapons to school and engage in fighting than in 1993.[20]

What can be done to reduce the risk of violence at school? Many urban schools now resort to using metal detectors and hiring uniformed police in an attempt to curb school violence. Other steps to manage the problem include training elementary school teachers and administrators to identify potential troublemakers in their classrooms. Children who are prone to become violent often model the aggressive behaviors of their parents. Such high-risk children have difficulty controlling their anger; tend to poke, shove, or annoy other people; act impulsively; bully other children; and defy authorities, including parents and teachers. In many communities, schools now offer conflict resolution classes for children that emphasize socially acceptable ways of settling disputes.

Violence on College Campuses On April 16, 2007, Cho Seung-Hui, a 23-year-old psychologically

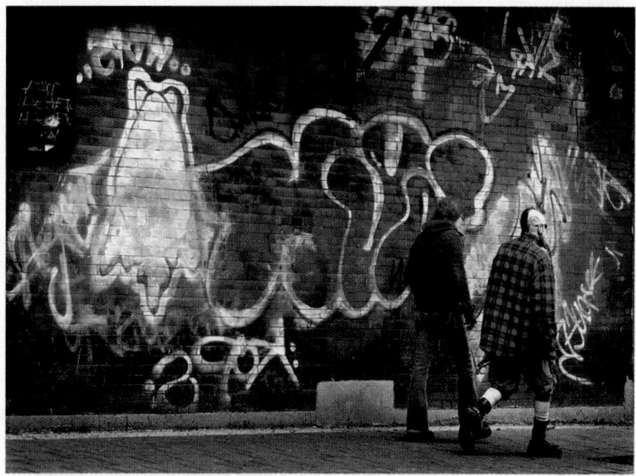
© Galina Barskaya/ShutterStock

institutional violence Violence that occurs mainly in institutional settings such as college campuses or workplaces.

disturbed college student, shot 32 students and faculty to death on the Virginia Polytechnic Institute (Virginia Tech) campus before taking his own life (**Figure 4.3**). The violent incident raised serious questions about the safety of American university students and sparked efforts to improve campus security and identify troubled college students before they react violently. Prior to the Virginia Tech shootings, the results of nationwide surveys conducted between 1995 and 2002 indicate college students were less likely to be victims of violent crime than nonstudents of the same age.[30] According to these surveys, the majority of violent crimes against college students occurred off campus and during the evening or at night (6 P.M. to 6 A.M.). Only about one-third of the violent crimes committed against college students were reported to the police.

The *Student Right to Know and Campus Security Act* requires administrators of colleges and universities that receive federal funds to report information concerning the number of murders, assaults, rapes, and other specific crimes that take place on their campuses. The administrators must also develop programs that are designed to educate students about personal safety and campus security. To reduce the violence on their campuses, many college administrators have adopted security measures such as restricting access to campus buildings, setting up emergency call boxes on campus, improving lighting near walkways and parking lots, limiting visitation hours in residence halls, and initiating escort services for female students. For information about the types and extent of crime at your college or university, visit the Department of Education's Office of Postsecondary Education website http://ope.ed.gov/security/GetOneInstitutionData.aspx for an interactive tool that provides data concerning numbers of reported crimes on college campuses. You can also contact staff at the campus police department.

Workplace Violence

Workplace violence is any act of violence or abuse directed toward an individual who is performing his

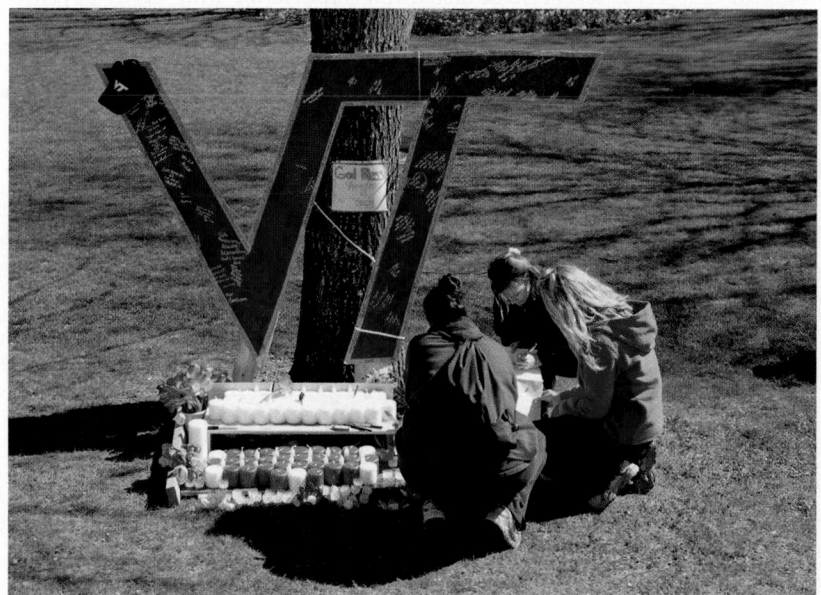

Figure 4.3

College Violence. On April 16, 2007, a psychologically disturbed college student shot 32 students and faculty to death on the Virginia Polytechnic Institute campus before taking his own life.
© Kevin Lamarque/Reuters/Landov

or her job. Although most people will never experience the most dangerous types of workplaces, such as psychiatric hospitals and prisons, any workplace can be a setting for violence. In 2012, homicide was the cause of 1 in 10 fatal occupational injuries for U.S. workers.[31] The stereotype of workplace violence as vengeful acts committed by disgruntled former workers is misleading. Work-related homicides are most likely to occur during armed robberies of retail businesses such as grocery stores, restaurants, bars, and gas stations. Employees with the highest risk of being murdered while working are cab drivers, convenience store attendants, police, and security guards.

Certain workers have a high risk of becoming violent, particularly when they are laid off, fired, or not promoted. Persons most likely to resort to workplace violence are men between the ages of 25 and 40 who are loners, have marital and other family problems, appear angry and paranoid, abuse alcohol and/or other drugs, and blame others for their problems. Women are less likely to commit violent acts in workplaces, but they are more likely to be victims.

One military base receiving much media attention is Fort Hood, Texas, the site of two tragic shootings within a 5-year period. In each case, the shooters were soldiers who were involved in verbal altercations before the shootings that resulted in multiple fatalities.[32,33] During the November 5, 2009 shooting, 13 people were killed and 32 wounded.[32] In the April 2, 2014 shooting 3 soldiers died and 16 others were wounded.[33]

Terrorism

Terrorism is intentional violent acts against civilians to produce extreme fear, severe property damage, and numerous deaths. Terrorists may attack specific cultural or political symbols, such as places of worship or government buildings; or more random targets, such as restaurants, subway stations, and airplanes (**Figure 4.4**). Regardless of whether terrorists are citizens of the country they attack or foreigners, a major purpose of terrorism is to frighten the general population and make them feel vulnerable and helpless.

The use of conventional bombs by terrorists is not new, but recently, terrorists have adopted more sinister methods of killing civilians and destroying property. The arsenal of terrorist weapons now includes poisonous chemicals, life-threatening infectious agents such as the bacterium that causes anthrax, and explosives strapped to suicidal individuals who intentionally blow themselves up in crowded places.

Figure 4.4

New York City, September 11, 2001. On this day, foreign terrorists used commercial jets to attack the World Trade Center and the Pentagon.

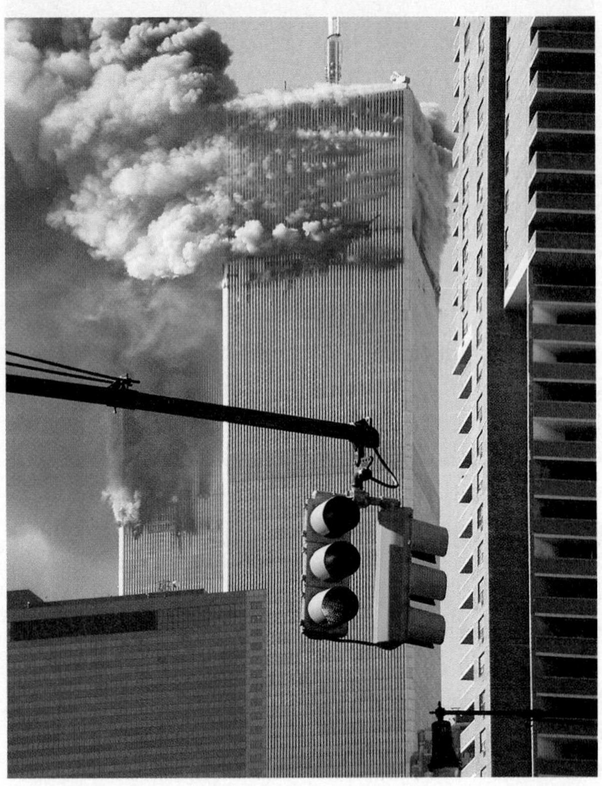

In addition to physical injuries, survivors of a terrorist attack often experience long-term psychological consequences such as post-traumatic stress disorder (PTSD) and depression. Extensive media reporting of the disastrous event, however, indirectly affects the psychological health of those outside the zone of destruction. National surveys conducted after the September 11, 2001, attacks on the World Trade Centers and Pentagon indicate many Americans who were not directly affected by the attacks suffered from extreme psychological stress symptoms as a result of the terrorism.[34,35] After September 11, 2001, U.S. government officials took steps to reduce the risk of terrorism by, for example, erecting video surveillance cameras in public places and increasing airport security. Nevertheless, many Americans think additional terrorist attacks in the United States are likely. Living with such fear increases the risk of stress-related health problems.

Assessing Your Risk of Violence

What are the chances that you, or some of the people you care about deeply, are at risk for violence? The risk is difficult to determine because many violent incidents, especially rapes and spouse battering, are never reported to the police. Nevertheless, some people are more likely to suffer serious or fatal injury than others. The likelihood of a particular person experiencing such harm depends on specific risk factors, including his or her family situation, living conditions, personality, and activities.

Family disruption is a major risk factor for family and community violence. Parental conflict that leads to separation, divorce, or desertion contributes to family disruption, as does the presence of a parent with a criminal or drug-use history. Neighborhood conditions, such as high rates of unemployment, can lead to high rates of family disruption. Other risk factors for family violence are social isolation, the presence of children with special needs, and a large number of children in the family. Factors that increase a youth's risk for engaging in school violence include a history of violence, poor grades, drug use (including alcohol and tobacco), community poverty, and poor family functioning.[36]

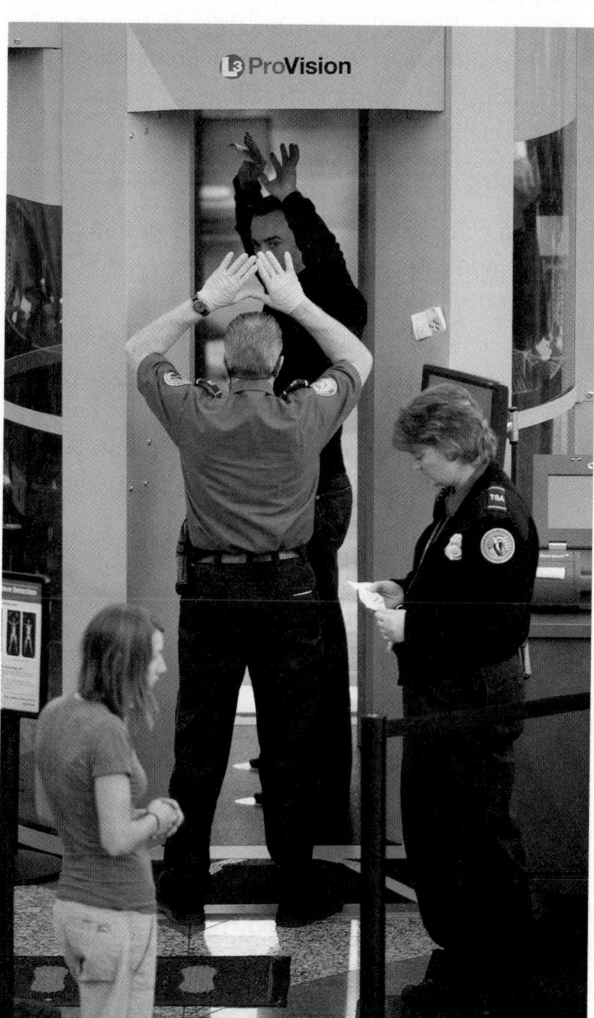

Increased airport security measures were an outcome of the September 11, 2001 terrorist attacks.

© GARY C. CASKEY/UPI/Landov

As mentioned earlier in this chapter, the availability of alcohol, other drugs, and guns dramatically escalates the likelihood of serious injury or death in violent situations. A significant percentage of people who commit violent crimes test positive for alcohol, marijuana, cocaine, or combinations of mind-altering drugs at the time of their arrest. In 2012, firearms were used in about 69% of the nation's murders, 41% of robberies, and 22% of aggravated assaults.[37]

Certain individuals are more likely than others to find themselves in places and situations in which violence is likely to occur. Age is a major risk factor. Americans younger than 25 years old are more likely to become involved in violence than persons over 25. In both 2011 and 2012, the 12–24 age group experienced higher rates of violent victimization than those aged 35 and older.[38] Americans between 18 and 24 years of age experienced the highest rate of homicide and the greatest decline (about 22%) from 2002 to 2011.[38]

Another key risk factor is sex. The average homicide rate for males was 3.6 times greater than the rate for females between 2002 and 2011.[38] In 2012, males experienced higher rates of both violent victimization and serious violent victimization than their female counterparts.[40] While in their homes, women are as likely as men to use force, but in community settings they are far less likely to do so. Men are more likely than women to be arrested for perpetrating crimes of violence, and they are more likely to be the victims of such crimes. Women, however, have a greater risk of being killed by their spouses than men do.

Race and ethnicity are two other characteristics strongly associated with involvement in violent incidents. In 2009, African Americans were more likely than Whites to be victims of sexual assault and aggravated assault.[39] In that year, however, almost half of the murder victims were White and half of the victims were African Americans. In 2012, the rate of violent victimization for African Americans was nearly 36% higher than for Whites and nearly 40% higher than for Hispanics.[40] In 2011, the average homicide rate was 6.3 times higher for African Americans than for Whites.[38]

An objective of *Healthy People 2020* is to reduce the homicide rate from 6.1 per 100,000 (the rate in 2007) to 5.5 per 100,000 Americans by 2020. This is one national health indicator in which progress has been made; the homicide rate decreased to 5.3 murders per 100,000 Americans in 2010. Another *Healthy People 2020* objective is to reduce firearm-related deaths from 10.3 per 100,000 (the 2007 rate) to 9.3. Although the rate has dropped some (10.1 in 2010), the firearm-related death rate has remained relatively stable between 1999 and 2010, with rates ranging from 10.0–10.4.[41]

Preventing and Avoiding Violence

To reduce violent crime, communities are turning increasingly to environmental measures such as improved street lighting, neighborhood watch organizations, and surveillance by closed-circuit cameras. Many large companies have taken specific steps to reduce workplace violence, such as hiring security staff, controlling access to offices, requiring employees to wear identification badges, and offering employee assistance programs that provide referrals for counseling services.

You can take numerous practical steps to reduce your personal risk of victimization. Many avoidance measures are simple, inexpensive, and effective. To be effective, however, these measures must become part of your routine. The most effective action is staying away from high-risk situations and people. For example, a college student might decide not to attend a party where binge drinking and drug usage are likely to occur. Simply put, people should avoid high-risk places and dangerous persons when realistically possible.

Another preventive measure is to avoid using destructive responses such as angry verbal exchanges, including insults and name calling, to manage interpersonal conflicts. Arguments are the most frequently cited circumstances that result in murder. In 2012, for example, arguments were involved in about 4 of 10 murders in which the circumstances were known.[42] If you become involved in a heated dispute or threatening situation, keeping calm may prevent the situation from escalating into a violent one. For example, breathe deeply, count to 10, "bite your tongue," or make some excuse and quickly leave the scene. Relaxation techniques can help you maintain your composure in such situations. If you have a "short fuse" and get angry easily, counseling can help you learn conflict management strategies such as impulse control, anger management, and negotiation techniques.

Home Security Measures

Improving your home's security can discourage and possibly prevent criminals from victimizing you. In many break-ins, the intruder simply came through an unlocked door or window. Before you leave your residence, check to see if it is secure. The most important safety measure is to have and always use good deadbolt locks on doors. If your entry door does not have windows, consider having a peephole installed in the door. When someone knocks at your door, do not open it until you have peered through the peephole and are certain that you can safely welcome the visitor into your home. Also, keep windows securely locked, especially when you are not home. Contact your police department or the campus security center to see if they will perform a free safety inspection of your residence. If you can keep a pet at your residence, consider getting a large dog for a companion and "bodyguard."

Following are other helpful safety measures:

- When you go out of your home, leave some lights and a radio on to give the impression that someone is there.
- When you return to your home, do not enter if you see signs of a break-in or suspicious persons in the area. Go instead to a neighbor's or public place and call the police. If surprised, burglars often become assailants and attack the robbery victims.
- Lock the door immediately after entering your home or dorm room.

Community Security Measures

If you live in a dangerous neighborhood, consider moving to a safer one if you can. This is the most effective measure you can take to avoid violence. If you cannot leave the neighborhood, look for a place to live that is farther away from the most dangerous streets. If the new area looks safer, ask a few residents, and even local police, if they would prefer to live elsewhere. The police may have local crime statistics, so you can compare crime rates of various neighborhoods.

Daily life is filled with people and situations that cannot be avoided, but you can use certain tactics to reduce your chances of victimization. If your usual routine requires traveling through dangerous neighborhoods, remove yourself from these high-risk areas by taking safer routes, when possible, even if they are out of your way. Avoid isolated places, especially when you are alone. Jogging trails in parks, deserted buildings, infrequently used sections of libraries, and nearly empty parking lots and garages are places where violent incidents are more likely to occur.

A considerable percentage of violent crimes, especially sexual assaults, happen between 6 P.M. and midnight. Thus, if you must go out at night, do not go alone. Stay in places where you can see other people. Being in the presence of others greatly reduces your risk of violence. If you are alone at night and on campus, use the college's escort service or usethe "buddy system" when walking to and from buildings.

Following are other community safety measures:

- Do not walk, jog, or bike alone, especially at night.
- Wear a whistle to signal an alarm or carry a can of pepper spray to use if threatened (see the Consumer Health feature).
- Look alert.
- Park in a well-lit, busy area. Check inside and underneath the car before entering. If you need to use public transportation, choose well-populated stops.
- If violence erupts anywhere near you, run away if you can.

Reducing the Risk of Violence While in a Car

Regardless of the time of day, as soon as you enter your car, lock the doors. Keep your car doors locked, and take the keys with you, even when you leave the car for a minute. Do not give rides to strangers or stop to help others. If you spend a lot of time in your car, keep a charged cell phone with you to call for assistance in any emergency. If you are involved in a minor accident, stay in your car; call the police, and keep the doors locked and the windows rolled up until they arrive.

If someone demands that you surrender your car, do not argue with or resist the person: Get out of the car and quickly move away from the area. Then, contact the police. If you are driving and someone in a nearby vehicle drives aggressively and irresponsibly, avoid getting angry with the person. If a driver tailgates your car, flashes high beams at you, or makes angry gestures, do not stop to discuss the matter. Avoid making eye contact with this individual. In this situation, *do not* drive to your home because he or she is likely to follow you and confront you when you get out of your car. You can discourage this person from continuing to follow you by driving to a busy highway or other high-traffic area. If you still feel threatened, drive to a well-lit public place: police and fire stations are the best choices.

Workplace Safety Measures

In the workplace, learn your company's security measures, for example, the locations of fire alarms, so that you can activate one in case of any trouble. Keep your cell phone with you at all times. Perhaps most important, strive to get along with coworkers and the public. Help create a positive working environment and relationships by displaying a friendly attitude, good manners, tact, and diplomacy. The "Changing Health Habits" activity in the Student Workbook at the end of the book can help you identify and change habits that may increase your risk of becoming a victim of violence.

Self-Protection

When faced with the threat of force, your actions can influence the outcome of the situation; however, it is important to remember that victims of violence are not responsible for their victimization. For example, you may obtain help from others by calling the police, pressing an alarm button, blowing a whistle, or screaming "Fire" to attract attention. When cornered and facing a threatening person alone, you can try to defuse the situation verbally by reasoning with your assailant. If you become overwhelmed by fear or conclude that you cannot escape, your response may be to offer no resistance. However, the gut responses to danger are fight-or-flight reactions. Sometimes flight—simply running away—is the best means of escaping threatening situations. The opposite response is to defend yourself by fighting. Many Americans carry with them, or keep handy in their homes, a weapon for self-defense such as a gun, knife, or chemical defense spray. When danger threatens, other people may rely on improvised weapons such as car keys, scissors, or a flashlight. Some people seek training in personal defense or in firearm use to enhance their ability to defend themselves (**Figure 4.5**).

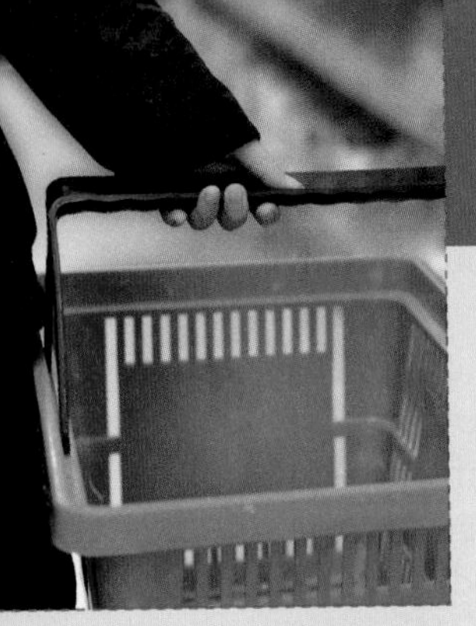

© sevenke/ShutterStock

Consumer Health

Natural Defense: Pepper Spray

One way to protect yourself against an aggressor is to use pepper spray. Pepper spray contains capsaicin, a compound that is found in hot chili peppers. When sprayed in an assailant's eyes, pepper spray produces a painful burning sensation. Almost immediately, the person's eyelids swell shut and tears begin to flow. The spray also causes the attacker to experience difficulty breathing and lose control over body movements. These effects last about 20 to 30 minutes, which gives you time to escape the situation and call police. Pepper spray is an effective and safe way to subdue an attacker, but it may take a few seconds to work on enraged or drugged individuals.

Hardware or variety stores often sell pepper spray in small canisters that can be carried on a key chain or in a coat pocket or purse. Some states may impose age or other restrictions concerning the use of pepper spray. Therefore, before buying the product, check with local law enforcement agencies to determine if it is legal to use pepper spray. Always follow the package directions when using it as a defense and keep the canister out of the reach of children and irresponsible persons.

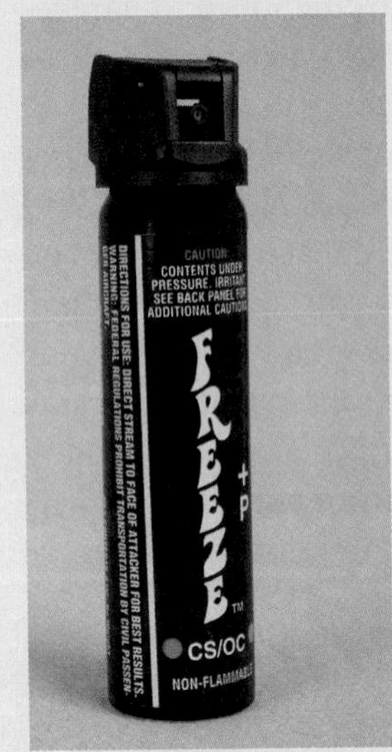

Should victims always resist their attackers? No uniform answer can be given. Each potential victim must assess each situation quickly to decide how to respond underthe circumstances. In situations involving intimate partner abuse or stalking, civil protection orders that separateand prohibit contact between the abuser or stalker and the victim can be effective in preventing further abuse.

Figure 4.5

In Self-Defense. Fighting back is one way of responding to violent situations.

© Hemera Technologies/AbleStock.com/Thinkstock

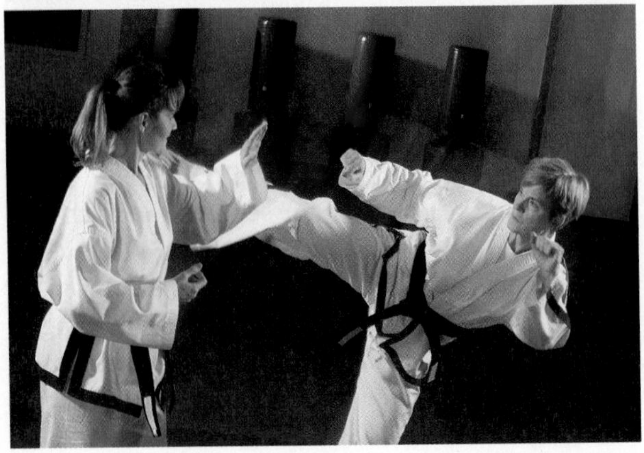

Reporting Violence

If you are attacked, you must decide whether to report the incident. You should report any attempted or completed crime of violence by strangers or acquaintances to the police. Most large police departments include specially trained family violence and sexual assault units that provide sympathetic and appropriate responses. A 911 call usually gains access to the appropriate emergency services.

In certain instances, you may feel reluctant to inform police about what happened to you. Consider reporting the incident to an agency, such as a rape crisis center or a women's self-help service that can assist you in dealing with legal authorities and medical establishments. Nationwide, a 24-hour, toll-free family violence hotline can be reached at 800-799-7233.

Seeking help is beneficial to the victim's recovery from violence. Managing the short- and long-term effects of the violent incident on the victim's family

child physical abuse Physical violence against a child who is under 18 years of age.

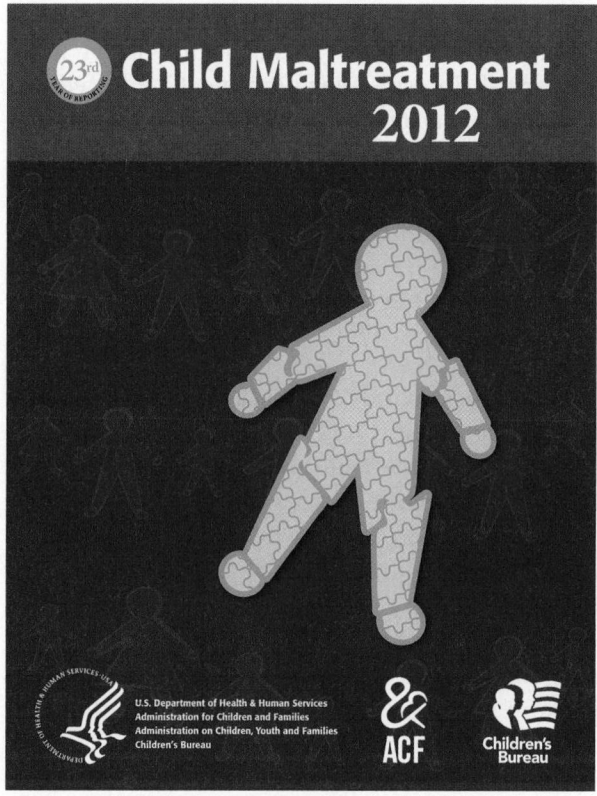

Reproduced from U.S. Department of Health and Human Services, Administration on Children, Youth, and Families. (2013). *Child Maltreatment 2012*. Retrieved from http://www.acf.hhs.gov/programs/cb/resource/child-maltreatment-2012.

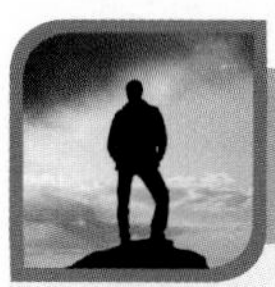

© djgis/ShutterStock

Healthy Living Practices

- To reduce your risk of violence, avoid high-risk places and dangerous people. Take steps to make your environment safe.
- If a dispute turns into a heated argument, try to keep calm to prevent the threatening situation from escalating into a violent one.
- Conflict-management skills can help defuse tense, angry situations. Some college campuses offer courses in conflict management; consider taking a class to learn these techniques.
- There is no single way to react whenever someone threatens your safety; therefore, assess each situation to decide how to respond under the circumstances.
- If you are a victim of violence, report the attack to police. In addition, obtain prompt treatment of your physical injuries and emotional distress.

and friends also is important. Useful services include marital counseling, couple therapy, financial and legal aid, and family therapy. Access to such services and information concerning local self-help groups can usually be arranged through your campus student health center or through social service agencies in your community.

Studies show that abused children behave more aggressively at every stage of the life span. As adults, they are more likely to be violent against dates, spouses, their children, and, later, their elderly parents.

Why do some parents abuse their children? Parents who are physically abusive to each other have a high risk of abusing their own children. Abusive parents generally lack effective parenting skills and frequently have faulty or unrealistic expectations about their children's behavior. For example, a parent may shake a 3-month-old infant to make him or her stop crying or kick a 2-year-old child for not using the toilet. Abusive parents tend to be under tremendous psychological stress and often are isolated from people who could provide helpful advice and social support. Regardless of the parents' situation, suspected or observed cases of child neglect or abuse

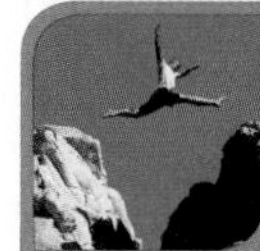

Across THE LIFE SPAN

© Galina Barskaya/ShutterStock

VIOLENCE AND ABUSE

Child physical abuse includes beating, squeezing, burning, cutting, suffocating, binding, and poisoning a child who is younger than 18 years of age. Although child physical abuse takes place in institutional settings, such as day care centers and schools, homes are by far the most common setting. Most physical violence against children is not committed by strangers or casual acquaintances but by parents and other adults known to the victims, such as neighbors, babysitters, and family friends. Abused children younger than 2 years of age are at greatest risk of fatalities, primarily from head injuries. Many children, however, receive less severe injuries on a regular basis. Such violence is not confined to impoverished families or to any particular racial or ethnic group.

child sexual abuse Sexual activity involving a child that takes place as a result of force or threat.

pedophile (PE-doe-file) An individual who is sexually attracted to children.

incest Sexual relations between family members who are not spouses.

elder abuse Use of physical or sexual violence against an elderly person.

can be reported anonymously by calling the *Childhelp National Child Abuse* hotline (800-422-4453). In some states, a person must report suspected cases of child abuse or neglect to authorities.

Data from various studies indicate that many adults were victims of sexual abuse during childhood. **Child sexual abuse** refers to sexual activity with a child that takes place as a result of force or threat or by taking advantage of an age difference or a caretaking relationship. A **pedophile** is an individual who is sexually attracted to children and fantasizes about having physical contact with them. A *child molester* acts on his or her urges by having sexual activity with vulnerable children. Most molesters are heterosexual males who generally target girls between 8 and 10 years old. The abuse usually involves fondling a child's body, but it may include completed or attempted vaginal, anal, or oral sex. According to a survey of more than 17,300 adult Americans, 16% of men and about 25% of women experienced sexual abuse as children.[43] Such abuse often causes long-term serious psychological problems.[44]

Many people think that child molesters are strangers who are mentally ill, looking for children to kidnap, rape, and murder. In fact, most cases involve adults whom the children know and trust, such as babysitters, family friends, relatives, teachers, camp counselors, coaches, and clergy. Only 3% of murdered children younger than 5 years of age were killed by strangers.[45] However, children who have unsupervised access to personal computers provide a way for sophisticated child abusers to communicate with and befriend vulnerable children through Internet chat rooms, social networking sites, or electronic bulletin boards. Adult caregivers can teach their children safety tips to lessen their risk of being targeted electronicallyby potential perpetrators.

Incest refers to sexual experiences between family members who are not married to each other. In many instances, incest involves an adult and his or her young children, stepchildren, or grandchildren. Victims may be boys, although girls are at much greater risk. Incest is often nonviolent but forced, and it typically escalates over time. Ignorance or fear may keep the child from disclosing the abuse to others. Because of its psychological and physical impact on the youthful victim, incest is a serious form of sexual abuse. The risk factors for incest are similar to those of nonsexual abuse: childhood sexual victimization of the perpetrator and high levels of stress within the family.

To reduce child sexual abuse risk, parents should teach their young children how to recognize and report sexual abuse, regardless of their relationships with perpetrators. Because most cases involve perpetrators known to the child victim, telling children "Don't talk to strangers" is insufficient. Very young children need to learn which parts of their bodies are private. Additionally, children need to learn that if anyone touches them in ways that make them feel uncomfortable, they should report the incidents to parents, teachers, or other responsible adults.

Elder abuse is the use of physical or sexual violence against an older adult; some researchers include verbal threats and neglect in their definitions. Physical and psychological abuse of older persons takes place not only in institutional settings such as hospitals and nursing homes, but especially in family settings. Such abuse occurs in all racial and ethnic groups and at all socioeconomic levels. An estimated 3% of older Americans experience abuse.[46] As the average age of the American population increases, many experts expect that the prevalence of elder abuse will increase as well.

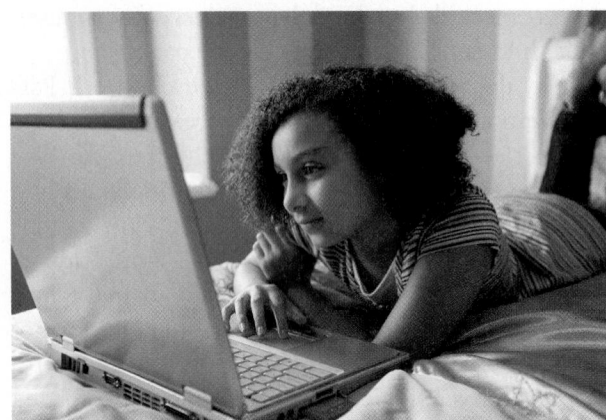

Some child abusers target and befriend vulnerable children who have unsupervised access to personal computers.

The causes of elder abuse are complex. Older adults with chronic health conditions are most likely to be victimized by their spouses or adult children who must care for them. Caring for frail, aged relatives can be frustrating and stressful. Furthermore, the caregiver may depend on the older adult relative for his or her housing and income. In such situations, resentful caregivers may resort to abusive behavior. In severe cases, violence against older adults is associated with certain mental illnesses and drug (usually alcohol) abuse. If you observe an older adult being abused or neglected, report the situation to a local adult protective services agency.

Analyzing Health-Related Information

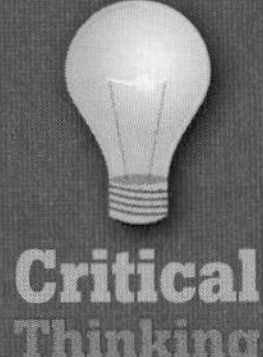

Critical Thinking

© tele52/ShutterStock

The following article promotes an herbal tea formulated to reduce a person's level of anger. Read the article and evaluate it using the model for analyzing health-related information. The main points of the model are noted here.

1. Which statements are verifiable facts, and which are unverified statements or value claims?
2. What are the credentials of the person who wrote the article? Does this person have the appropriate background and education in the topic area? What can you do to check the person's credentials?
3. What might be the motives and biases of the person making the claims?
4. What is the main point of the article? Which information is relevant to the main point of the article? Which information is irrelevant?
5. Is the source reliable? What evidence supports your conclusion that the source is reliable or unreliable? Does the source of information present the pros and cons of the topic or the benefits and risks of the tea?
6. Does the source of information attack the credibility of conventional scientists or medical authorities?

Based on your analysis, do you think that this article is a reliable source of health-related information? Summarize your reasons for coming to this conclusion.

Aunt Annie's Tranquility Tea

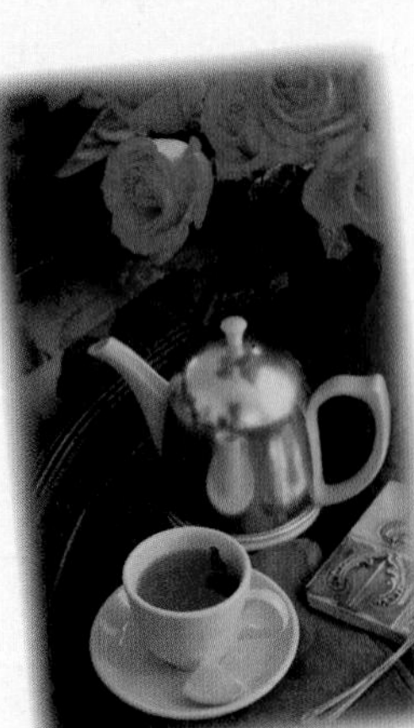

© Janis Christie/Photodisc

As you know, I've been using herbs all my life to treat everything from acne to zinc deficiency. Most of my knowledge about herbs didn't come from books or the Internet; it was passed down to me in my Great Aunt Annie's diary. Annie had a fabulous herb garden in the back of her house. One afternoon in 1914 she made the most amazing discovery, which she later recorded in her diary. She had dug up some comfrey root and picked a bunch of pennyroyal and lobelia leaves from the garden. Since coltsfoot was blooming, she thought it might be a nice change to add some of its leaves to her usual tea recipe. She brewed a pot of tea from the mixture and drank about 2 cups of it. The tea was delicious. Very soothing.

Less than an hour later, Great Uncle Jeb came in from the barn, tracking dirt all over Aunt Annie's new carpet. Now I need to tell you that Annie had a terrible temper—she was only 4' 8" tall, but she used to push big old Jeb around a lot. Needless to say, Uncle Jeb was expecting the worst from his wife. But this time, instead of flying off the handle and kicking Jeb, as she was prone to do, Aunt Annie laughed and hugged him. Happy as a kitten rolling in catnip, Annie cleaned up the mess. Uncle Jeb suspected Annie had added something different to her usual tea recipe, so he had her sit down and recall the herb mixture. Using her recipe, Jeb made a pot of that tea for Annie to drink every day for the rest of her life. When Uncle Jeb began making whiskey in the barn and staying out late with his friends, Annie never raised a fuss. She just sat in the bent oak rocking chair, sipping her tea.

If you want to try Aunt Annie's Tranquillity Tea on someone you know who's got a bad temper, I'll send the recipe to you. I'm the editor of this magazine, so just send $10 for shipping and handling to my address, which is on the inside of the front cover. I'd love to hear about your experiences with the tea; be sure and let me know how it worked for you.

Your friend,

Herb

Herb Z.Gardenia

CHAPTER REVIEW

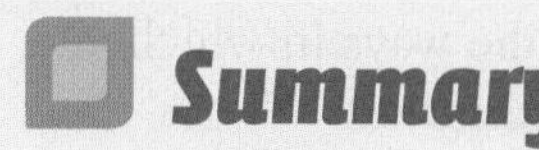

Summary

Violence refers to interpersonal uses of force that are not socially sanctioned. A violent social incident occurs when at least one person intentionally applies or threatens physical force on others. Violence is a major public health problem because it produces staggering physical, psychological, and social consequences. For many Americans, violence is a way of life; no one is exempt from violence.

Assault is the intentional use of force to injure someone physically; abuse occurs when one takes advantage of a relationship to mistreat a person. Examples of abuse include spouse abuse, child abuse, and sexual harassment.

Regardless of whether physical harm occurs, violent victimization damages psychological health. Psychological effects of violence include anxiety, depression, and suicidal thinking, which can lead to drug abuse or other unhealthy "coping" strategies. Family relationships may become strained or end as a result of violence. Furthermore, intergenerational transmission of violence occurs when abused children mature and abuse their own children. To recover from the psychological effects of violence, one should seek help from mental healthcare professionals.

Violence is complex; there is no single cause of violence, and neither is violent behavior limited to a particular group of persons. Factors that contribute to violence include poverty, substance abuse, certain psychological disorders, and poor self-esteem. In many instances, violence is learned behavior. Watching violent media, for example, may contribute to violent behavior.

Sexual violence involves areas of the body that are sensitive to sexual arousal. Such violence involves sexual activity gained through force, threat of force, or coercion. The majority of sexual assaults are committed not by strangers but by acquaintances, friends, family members, and spouses. Family (domestic) violence encompasses both friends and family members and usually takes place in homes. Community violence includes acts that occur between strangers or acquaintances, usually in public places. Institutional violence occurs mainly within institutional environments such as schools, workplaces, or prisons. Terrorism involves violent acts against civilians to produce extreme fear, severe property damage, and numerous deaths.

To reduce the likelihood of becoming a victim of violence, individuals should limit their exposure to risky situations and take steps to make their residences secure. When faced with a violent situation, a person can obtain help from others by attracting attention, defuse the situation by reasoning with an assailant, or simply run away. In some instances, the threatened individual may need to defend himself or herself physically.

Most physical violence against children is committed by adults known to the victims, such as relatives, neighbors, or babysitters. Most violence against children occurs in their homes. Girls, especially those between the ages of 8 and 10 years, are more likely to be targets of sexual abuse than are boys. Parents and caregivers should teach their young children how to recognize and report sexual abuse. Children who experience violence often suffer emotional and social injuries that remain long after physical injuries have healed.

Elder abuse occurs in all racial and ethnic groups and at all socioeconomic levels. Family members are responsible for the vast majority of abuse directed toward older adults. As the average age of the American population increases, many experts predict that the incidence of elder abuse will also increase.

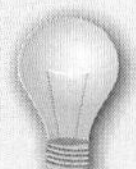

Applying What You Have Learned

1. If your friend reports being sexually harassed by a college professor, what advice could you give to him or her? **Application**
2. You have to attend classes or work at a job in the evenings. Determine at least two steps you can take to reduce your risk of violence on campus or at work. **Analysis**
3. Plan a program to increase security in your dorm or on your campus. Consider forwarding it to an official at the university who might be interested

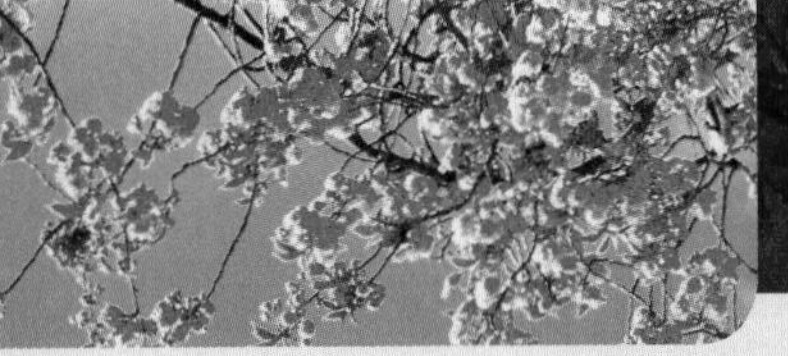

CHAPTER REVIEW

in your plan, such as the Dean of Student Affairs. **Synthesis**

4. Evaluate your present security situation. Determine situations in your life that provide some risk of violence and describe ways in which you can reduce these risks. **Evaluation**

Key

Application	Analysis	Synthesis	Evaluation
using information in a new situation.	breaking down information into component parts.	putting together information from different sources.	making informed decisions.

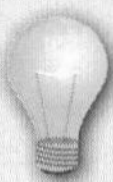

Reflecting on Your Health

1. As mentioned in this chapter, visual media can influence a person's attitudes toward violence. Choose a violent movie or television show that you watched recently. What impact, if any, did it have on your feelings about violence?
2. Do you like to play violent computer games? If so, how does this activity affect your attitudes toward violence?
3. What could you do to avoid getting into an abusive relationship with an intimate partner? If you are already in an abusive relationship, what are your feelings about your partner? What would make you change your current situation?
4. How safe do you feel at home or in the dorm? What worries you most about the safety of your environment? What steps could you take to make your residence more secure?
5. If you were out walking alone at night and realized someone was following you, describe what you would do to reduce your risk of being attacked. Do you think that it is safe for you to walk alone at night? Why or why not?

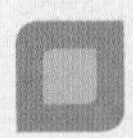

References

1. U.S. Department of Justice, Federal Bureau of Investigation. (2011). *2011 crime clock statistics*. Retrieved April 14, 2014 from http://www.fbi.gov/about-us/cjis/ucr/crime-in-the-u.s/2011/crime-in-the-u.s.-2011/offenses-known-to-law-enforcement/crime-clock
2. U.S. Department of Health and Human Services, Administration on Children, Youth, and Families. (2012). *Child maltreatment 2012*. Retrieved April 14, 2014 from http://www.acf.hhs.gov/sites/default/files/cb/cm2012.pdf
3. Tjaden, P., & Thoennes, N. (2000). *Extent, nature, and consequences of intimate partner violence: Findings from the National Violence Against Women Survey* (Publication NCJ 181867). Washington, DC: U.S. Department of Justice, Office of Justice Programs.
4. Cooper, A., & Smith, E. L. (2013 December 30). *Homicide in the U.S. known to law enforcement, 2011*. Retrieved April 14, 2014 from http://www.bjs.gov/index.cfm?ty=pbdetail&iid=4863
5. U.S. Department of Justice, Federal Bureau of Investigation. (2010). *Crime in the United States, 2009*. Retrieved March 23, 2011, from http://www2.fbi.gov/ucr/cius2009/index.html
6. U.S. Department of Justice, Bureau of Justice Statistics. (2010, March 1). *Key facts: Violent crime*. Retrieved March 30, 2011, from http://bjs.gov/index.cfm?ty=kftp&tid=31
7. Heron, M. (2010). Deaths: Leading causes for 2010. *National Vital Statistics Report*, 62(6), 17–54. Retrieved April 11, 2014 from http://www.cdc.gov/nchs/data/nvsr/nvsr62/nvsr62_06.pdf
8. Tremblay, R. E., et al. (2005). Physical aggression during early childhood: Trajectories and predictors. *Canadian Child and Adolescent Psychiatry Review*, 14(1), 3–9.
9. American Psychological Association. (2014). *Violence*. Retrieved May 13, 2014, from http://www.apa.org/topics/violence/
10. American Academy of Pediatrics. (2009). Policy statement—media violence. *Pediatrics*, 124(5), 1495–1503.
11. Tjaden, P., & Thoennes, N. (2006). *Extent, nature, and consequences of rape victimization: Findings from the National Violence Against Women Survey*. Atlanta, GA: National Institute of Justice and the Centers for Disease Control and Prevention.
12. Office of Justice Programs, National Institute of Justice. (2010, October 26). *Victims and perpetrators*. Retrieved April 15, 2014 from http://www.nij.gov/topics/crime/rape-sexual-violence/Pages/victims-perpetrators.aspx#note1
13. Fisher, B. S., et al. (2000). *The sexual victimization of college women* (Publication NCJ 182369). Washington, DC: National Institute of Justice, Bureau of Justice Statistics, U.S. Department of Justice.

14. Krebs, C. P., et al. (2007). *The campus sexual assault (CSA) study.* (Publication NCJ 221153). Washington, DC: National Institute of Justice, U.S. Department of Justice. Retrieved April 15, 2014 from https://www.ncjrs.gov/pdffiles1/nij/grants/221153.pdf
15. RAINN. (2014). *National sexual assault online hotline.* Retrieved April 15, 2014 from https://ohl.rainn.org/online/
16. DoD Safe Helpline. (2014). *About Department of Defense (DoD) Safe Helpline.* Retrieved April 15, 2014 from https://www.safehelpline.org/about-dod-safe-helpline
17. Morgan, R. E., & Truman, J. L. (2014). *Nonfatal domestic violence, 2003–2012.* (Publication NCJ 244697). Retrieved May 13, 2014, from http://www.bjs.gov/index.cfm?ty=pbdetail&iid=4985
18. Cantalano, S. (2013). *Intimate partner violence: Attributes of victimization, 1993–2011.* (Publication NCJ 243300). Retrieved May 13, 2014, from http://www.bjs.gov/content/pub/pdf/ipvav9311.pdf
19. U.S. Centers for Disease Control and Prevention, National Center for Injury Prevention and Control, Division of Violence Prevention. (2011). *Understanding intimate partner violence.* Retrieved March 25, 2011, from http://www.cdc.gov/violenceprevention/pdf/IPV_factsheet-a.pdf
20. Eaton, D. K., et al. (2010). Youth risk behavior surveillance—United States, 2009. *Morbidity and Mortality Weekly Report, Surveillance Summaries,* 59(SS5), 1–148.
21. McKinney, C. M., et al. (2009). Childhood family violence and perpetration and victimization of intimate partner violence: Findings from a national population-based study of couples. *Annals of Epidemiology,* 19(1), 25–32.
22. Frank, J. B., & Rodowski, M. F. (1999). Review of psychological issues in victims of domestic violence seen in emergency settings. *Emergency Medical Clinics of North America,* 17(3), 657–677.
23. World Health Organization. (2010). *International day for elimination of violence against women.* Retrieved March 25, 2011, from http://www.who.int/violence_injury_prevention/media/news/2010/25_11/en/index.html
24. World Health Organization/London School of Hygiene and Tropical Medicine. (2010). *Preventing intimate partner and sexual violence against women: Taking action and generating evidence.* Geneva, Switzerland: Author.
25. Stalking Resource Center, The National Center for Victims of Crime. (2012). *Stalking fact sheet.* Retrieved May 17, 2014 from http://www.victimsofcrime.org/docs/src/stalking-fact-sheet_english.pdf?sfvrsn=4.
26. Lamberg, L. (2001). Stalking disrupts lives, leaves emotional scars. *Journal of the American Medical Association,* 286(5), 519, 522–523.
27. U.S. Centers for Disease Control and Prevention. (2008). Notice to readers: National Stalking Awareness Month—January 2008. *Morbidity and Mortality Monthly Report,* 57(3), 72.
28. Egley, A., Jr., & Howell, H. C. (2013, September). Highlights of the 2011 National Youth Gang Survey. *OJDP Fact Sheet.* Retrieved May 17, 2014, from http://www.ojjdp.gov/pubs/242884.pdf
29. The Federal Bureau of Investigation. (2011). *2011 National Gang Threat Assessment: Emerging Trends* (Document ID: 2009-M0335-001). Retrieved May 17, 2014, from http://www.fbi.gov/stats-services/publications/2011-national-gang-threat-assessment/2011-national-gang-threat-assessment-emerging-trends
30. Baum, K., & Klaus, P. (2005). *Violent victimization of college students, 1995–2002* (Publication NCJ 206836). Washington, DC: U.S. Department of Justice, Bureau of Justice Statistics, Office of Justice Programs. Retrieved March 26, 2011, from http://www.bjs.gov/index.cfm?ty=pbdetail&iid=593
31. U.S. Department of Labor, Bureau of Labor Statistics. (2014). *Census of fatal occupational injuries charts, 1992-2012 (revised data).* Retrieved May 17, 2014, from http://www.bls.gov/iif/oshwc/cfoi/cfch0011.pdf
32. U.S. Department of Defense. (2009). *Special report: Tragedy at Fort Hood.* Retrieved May 18, 2014 from http://www.defense.gov/home/features/2009/1109_ft_hood/
33. U.S. Department of Defense. (2014). *Fort Hood Shooting: April 2, 2014.* Retrieved May 18, 2014 from http://www.defense.gov/home/features/2014/0414_forthood/
34. Holman, E. A., et al. (2008). Terrorism, acute stress, and cardiovascular health: A three-year national study following the September 11th attacks. *Archives of General Psychiatry,* 65(1), 73–80.
35. Galea, S., et al. (2005). Posttraumatic stress disorder in the general population after mass terrorist incidents: Considerations about the nature of exposure. *CNS Spectrums,* 10(2), 107–115.
36. Centers for Disease Control and Prevention. (2013). *Understanding school violence.* Retrieved May 17, 2014 from http://www.cdc.gov/violenceprevention/pdf/school_violence_fact_sheet-a.pdf
37. U.S. Department of Justice, Federal Bureau of Investigation. (2013). *Crime in the United States, 2012.* Retrieved May 17, 2014, from http://www.fbi.gov/about-us/cjis/ucr/crime-in-the-u.s/2012/crime-in-the-u.s.-2012/violent-crime/violent-crime
38. Smith. E. L., & Cooper, A. (2013 December). *Homicide in the U.S. known to law enforcement, 2011.* Retrieved May 18, 2014, from http://www.bjs.gov/content/pub/pdf/hus11.pdf36.
39. U.S. Department of Justice, Bureau of Justice Statistics. (2011, March 30). Victim characteristics. *National Crime Victimization Survey.* Retrieved March 30, 2011, from http://www.bjs.gov/-index.cfm?ty=tp&tid=92
40. Langton, L., Planty, M., & Truman, J. (2013, October). *Criminal victimization, 2012.* Retrieved May 18, 2014 from http://www.bjs.gov/index.cfm?ty=pbdetail&iid=4781
41. U.S. Department of Health and Human Services, Public Health Service, Healthy People 2020. (2013, August). 2020 topics and objectives, injury and violence prevention. Retrieved May 18, 2014, from http://www.healthypeople.gov/2020/TopicsObjectives2020/ObjectivesList.aspx?topicid=24#45
42. U.S. Department of Justice, Federal Bureau of Investigation. (2012). Expanded homicide data table 10: Murder circumstances by relationship, 2012. *Crime in the United States, 2012.* Retrieved May 18, 2014, from http://www.fbi.gov/about-us/cjis/ucr/crime-in-the-u.s/2012/crime-in-the-u.s.-2012/offenses-known-to-law-enforcement/expanded-homicide/expanded_homicide_data_table_10_murder_circumstances_by_relationship_2012.xls
43. Middlebrooks, J. S., & Audage, N. C. (2008). *Effects of childhood stress on health across the lifespan.* Atlanta, GA: Centers for Disease Control and Prevention, National Center for Injury Prevention and Control.
44. Huyer, D. (2005). Childhood sexual abuse and family physicians. *Canadian Family Physician,* 51, 1317–1319.
45. U.S. Department of Justice, Bureau of Justice Statistics. (2011, March 30). *Homicide trends in the United States: Infanticide.* Retrieved March 30, 2011, from http://www.bjs.gov/content/-homicide/-children.cfm
46. Gibbs, L. M., & Mosqueda, L. (2007). The importance of reporting mistreatment of the elderly. *American Family Physician,* 75(5), 628.

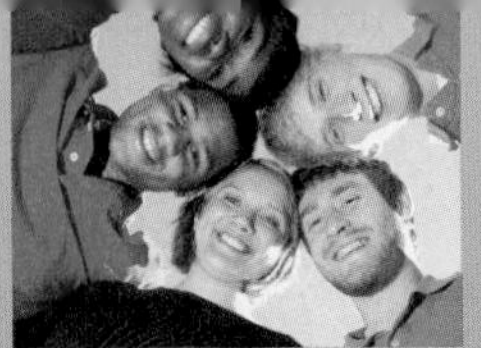

Diversity in Health
Menopause

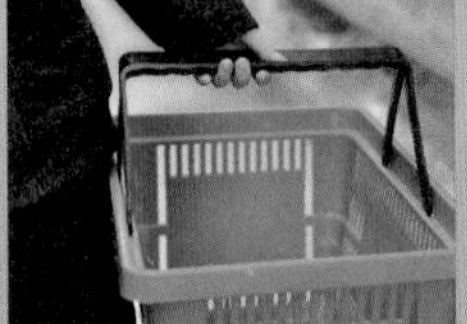

Consumer Health
Home Pregnancy Tests

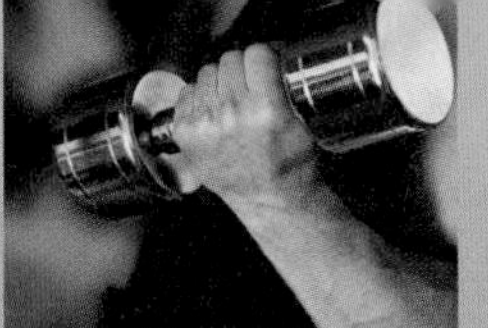

Managing Your Health
Genetic Counseling and Prenatal Diagnosis
Enlargement of the Prostate

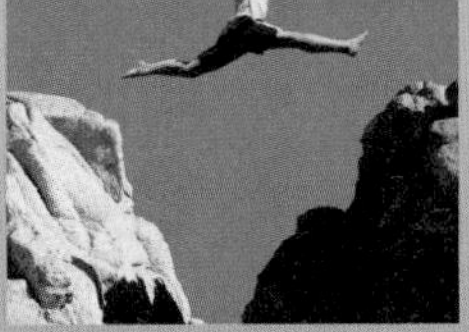

Across the Life Span
Sexual Development

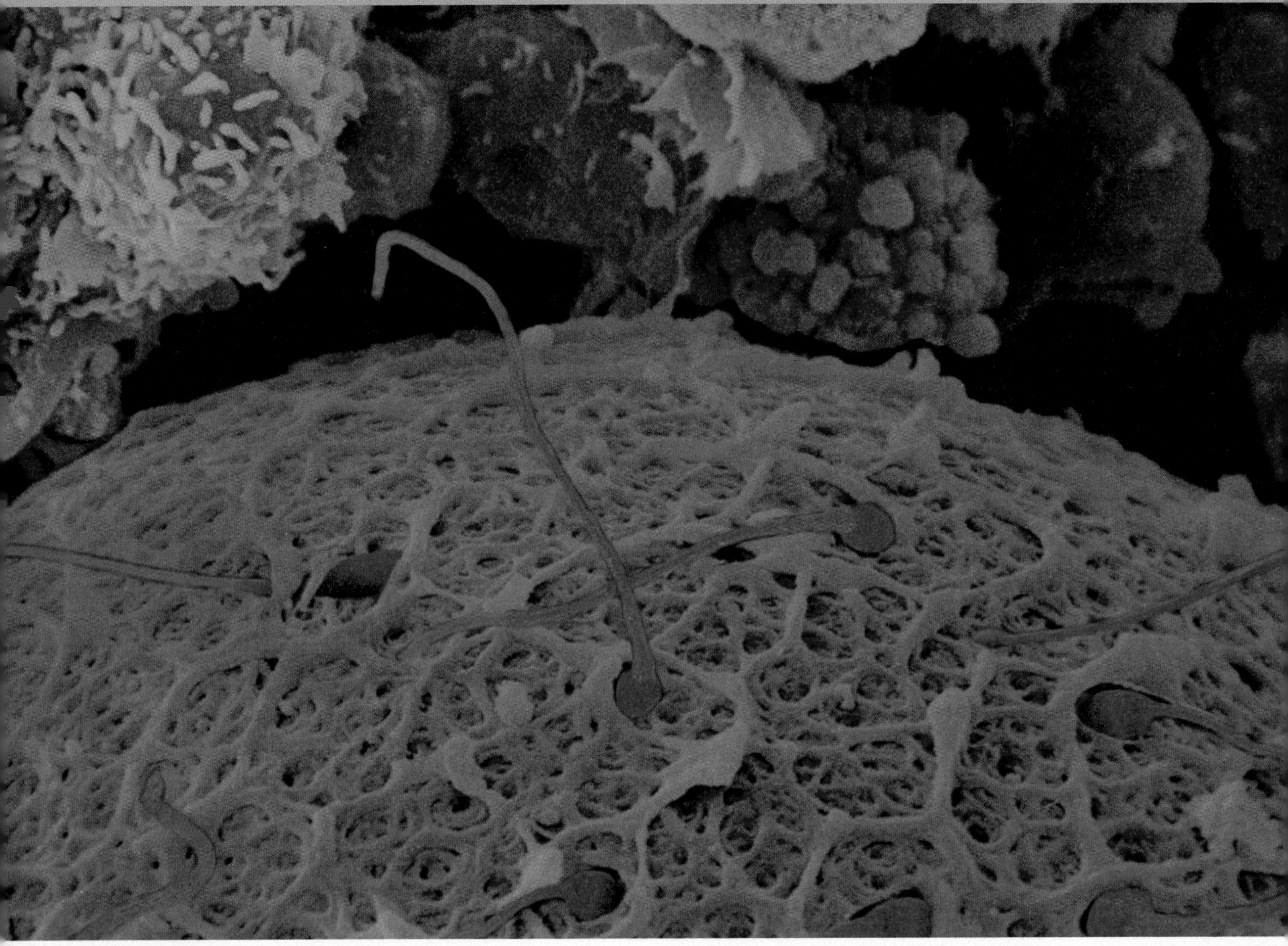

Chapter Overview

The functions and structures of the male and female reproductive systems

What happens throughout the menstrual cycle

How a woman can prepare her body for pregnancy

How a fetus develops

The changes in a pregnant woman from conception through the postpartum period

The causes of and treatments for infertility

The benefits and drawbacks of contraceptive methods

Student Workbook

Self-Assessment: Contraceptive Comfort and Confidence Scale | Attitudes Toward Timing of Parenthood Scale

Changing Health Habits: Do You Want to Improve Your Reproductive Health?

Do You Know?

How well your contraceptive method works compared to others?

What causes birth defects?

When a woman is most likely to get pregnant?

CHAPTER 5

Reproductive Health

Learning Objectives

After studying this chapter, you should be able to:

1. Identify parts of the male and female reproductive systems and describe the function and location of each part.
2. Identify actions that women can take to increase their chances of having healthy pregnancies and healthy babies.
3. Describe events that occur during each stage of the birth process.
4. Identify the various types of contraception, discuss how couples use each method correctly and rate the effectiveness of each method.
5. List the pros and cons of using each method of contraception and the effectiveness of each.
6. Identify three clinical abortion methods and describe when a particular method is used.
7. Describe how puberty affects the reproductive system and how aging affects reproductive health.

"The striking chapter opening photograph depicts the essence of sexual reproduction: the fertilization of an egg (ovum) by a sperm. . ."

sexual reproduction The fertilization of an egg (*ovum*; plural, *ova*) by a sperm.

testes (TES-tease) The male reproductive organs that produce sperm (the male sex cells) and testosterone (a male sex hormone).

scrotum (SKRO-tum) The sac of skin in which the testes are enclosed and hang outside the body.

epididymis (EP-ih-DID-ih-mis) A coiled tube that lies on the back of each testis and in which sperm mature.

The striking chapter opening photograph depicts the essence of **sexual reproduction**: the fertilization of an egg (ovum) by a sperm, a process also called conception. The photograph is color enhanced; the outside of the egg is shown as orange and the sperm as blue. A layer of cells that extend from the egg covers its surface. During the maturation of the egg, these outer cells secrete a thick gel-like material that covers the egg beneath. Together, the gel and the outer cells form a protective covering, which sperm must penetrate by means of digestive enzymes in their heads. Although it is difficult to see in this photograph, the head of only one sperm is making its way through these outer layers to ultimately fertilize this egg.

When the sperm enters the egg, it triggers the egg's final maturation. Following this process, the hereditary material from the sperm and the mature egg unite, forming a new cell—the zygote. This single cell has the potential to develop into a new person.

Fertility is the ability to conceive a child, whereas infertility is the inability of a couple to conceive a child after 1 year of unprotected sex. Couples may have reduced fertility for a variety of reasons; it is not necessarily because of "a problem" with one partner or the other. Factors that slightly impair the fertility of both sexual partners may interact to render a couple infertile. These factors include a low sperm count, a high percentage of abnormally shaped sperm, scarring in the female genital tract, structural defects of the uterus, and hormonal imbalances. Treatments for infertility are specific to the causes and include surgical procedures, hormone therapy, medication, and lifestyle changes. In addition to these therapies, physicians can harvest eggs and sperm to assist fertilization and implantation.

Whether physician-assisted or accomplished with no intervention at all, fertilization is preceded by a variety of physiologic processes that make it all possible, and that is where we begin this chapter.

The Male Reproductive System

The male reproductive system is structured for the development and maturation of sperm and for delivering sperm to the vagina. **Figure 5.1** is a diagram of a posterior view (a) and a lengthwise section of the male reproductive tract (b).

The Internal Organs of Sexual Reproduction

Sperm Development Sperm are produced in the **testes** (singular, *testis*), which hang outside the body (in the angle formed between the legs) encased in a sac of skin called the **scrotum**. The testes have two major functions: production of the sex hormone testosterone and production of sperm cells. The testes are packed with hundreds of feet of tubes (called *seminiferous tubules*) in which sperm are made. Each day, the testes of an adult male produce hundreds of millions of sperm. Various conditions are necessary for proper sperm production.

In a review of environmental and lifestyle effects on the development of sperm, Richard Sharpe notes that factors that result in a rise in scrotal temperature have a negative effect on sperm development. The testes must be cooler than body temperature to produce normal sperm; the position of the scrotum keeps the temperature of the testes below that of the rest of the body. However, behaviors that result in the scrotum not being able to dissipate heat can result in increased temperature of the testes. Such behaviors include taking long, hot baths and staying seated for long periods, especially when wearing tight pants. Obesity in men has also been shown to adversely affect sperm development.[1]

Semen Formation After sperm are manufactured in the seminiferous tubules, they are gently moved along by the fluid in which they are suspended. The sperm move through a network of ducts to the **epididymis** (plural, *epididymides*). The epididymis is a coiled tube that lies on the back of each testis. Here is where the sperm mature, developing the ability to swim and to fertilize an egg.

Rhythmic contractions of the muscular walls of the epididymis slowly move the sperm to the **vas deferens** when maturation is complete. The vas deferens is a tube that links the epididymis and the urethra, the passageway through which sperm exit the body. Sperm are stored in the vas deferens until they are released from the body during **ejaculation**, their emission from the penis during **orgasm**, the peak of sexual excitement. Sperm can be stored for a few days in these ducts. If not ejaculated within that time, the sperm die and are ingested by the body's white blood cells and newly synthesized sperm take their place. For this reason, men who have had vasectomies should not be concerned that sperm are accumulating in their bodies.

The sperm are suspended in relatively little fluid while stored in the vas deferens. A variety of organs referred to as accessory sex glands add fluid to the sperm as they exit the body during ejaculation. This fluid contains nutrients to fuel the sperm as they journey up the female reproductive tract, alkaline substances to neutralize the acidity of the vagina, and other chemicals to aid sperm movement. The secretions of the accessory sex glands (called seminal fluid) and the sperm make up the **semen**, or *ejaculate*.

During ejaculation, sperm are swiftly propelled through the vas deferens by the rhythmic contractions of its muscular walls. Just prior to the merging of the two vasa deferentia where they meet the

vas deferens (VAS DEF-er-enz) A tube that links the epididymis and the urethra, the passageway through which sperm exit the body.

ejaculation The emission of semen from the penis during orgasm.

orgasm The peak of sexual excitement.

semen The ejaculate; the secretions of the accessory sex glands (called seminal fluid) and sperm.

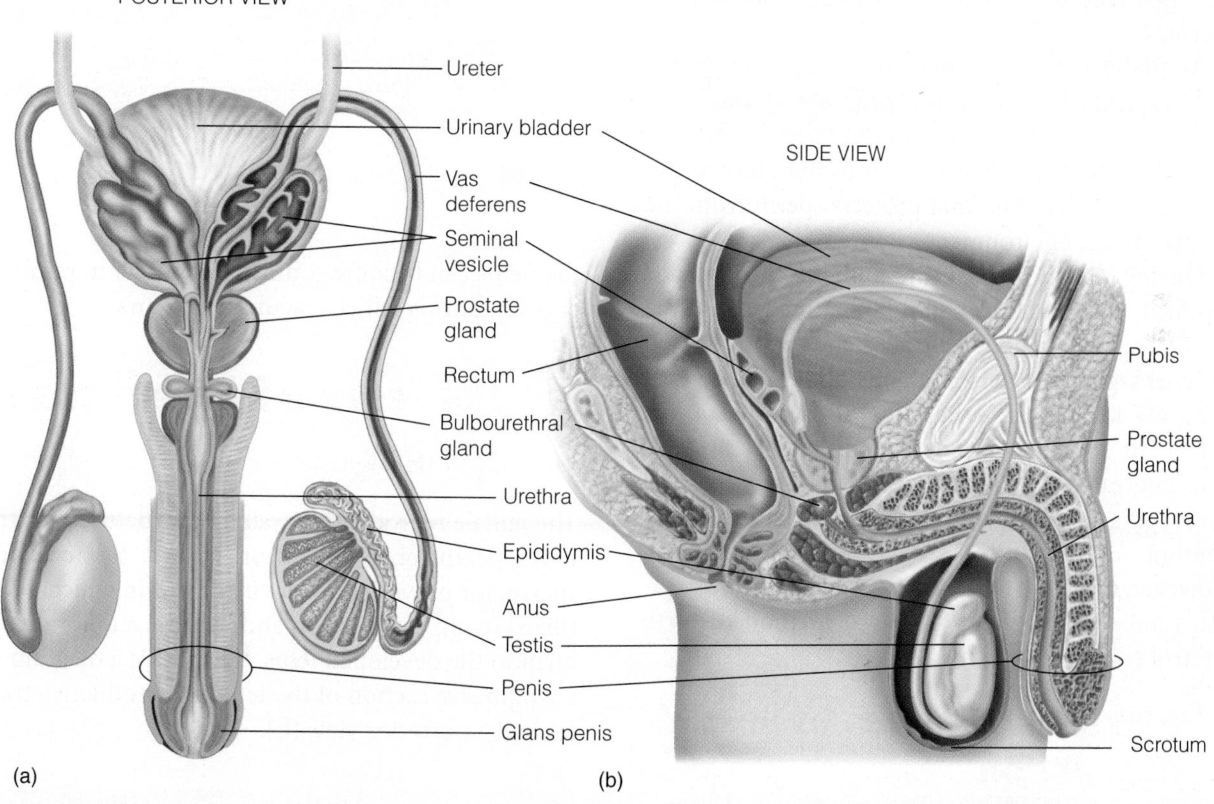

Figure 5.1

The Male Reproductive System. (a) Posterior view of the internal organs, and (b) lengthwise section (side view) of the internal organs.

seminal vesicles (SEM-ih-nal VES-ih-klz) Paired male sex organs located near the junction of the two vasa deferentia, which produce thick fructose-containing secretions that are added to the ejaculate.

prostate gland A single, walnut-sized gland that lies just below the bladder, surrounding the urethra. The prostate produces a milky alkaline fluid that is added to the ejaculate.

penis A cylindrical external organ of sexual reproduction in males, which hangs in front of the scrotum.

ovaries Internal organs of female sexual reproduction within which eggs (ova) develop.

follicles Masses of cells in the ovaries that contain immature ova (eggs) in various stages of development. Each follicle contains one ovum.

urethra, the secretions of the paired seminal vesicles flow into the ejaculate. The thick secretions of the **seminal vesicles** add much of the volume to the ejaculate (approximately 60%) and contain the sugar fructose, which provides nutrition for the sperm.

As the ejaculate continues traveling through the male reproductive tract, the **prostate gland** adds its secretion. This single, walnut-sized gland lies just below the bladder. It surrounds the urethra and produces a milky fluid that protects sperm from the vagina's acidic environment.

During sexual arousal, the bulbourethral glands produce a mucus-like fluid that precedes the ejaculate. The bulbourethral glands (also called Cowper's glands), paired glands about the size of peas, are located on either side of the urethra just below the prostate. The secretions of these glands help neutralize the acidity of the male urethra and the vagina. These glands also contribute a small amount of lubrication for sexual intercourse. However, this fluid may contain sperm: For this reason (and others), the withdrawal method of birth control is not reliable.

The External Organs of Sexual Reproduction

The scrotum and the **penis** are the external organs of sexual reproduction (external genitals) in males (see Figure 5.1). Three columns of spongy tissue in the inner structure of the penis (**Figure 5.2**) become filled with blood during sexual arousal, which causes the penis to enlarge and become firm so that it can be inserted into the vagina. During sexual intercourse, the penis can become stimulated enough to result in orgasm, during which ejaculation occurs.

Figure 5.2

The Erect and Flaccid Penis. (a) During an erection, blood fills the spongy erectile tissue of the penis. (b) When the blood drains from this tissue, as it does after orgasm, the penis becomes flaccid.

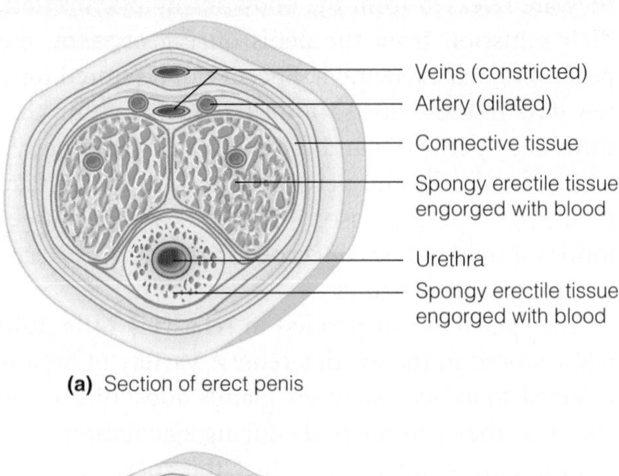

(a) Section of erect penis

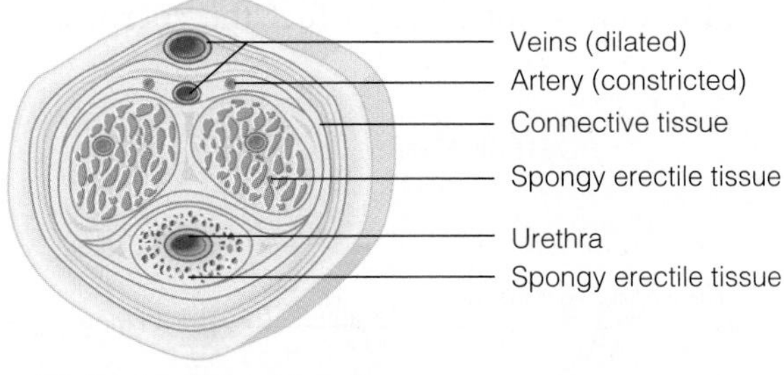

(b) Section of flaccid penis

The Female Reproductive System

The female reproductive system is structured for the development and maturation of ova, for receiving sperm, for providing an environment in which a fertilized ovum can develop and mature, and for giving birth to the developed fetus. **Figure 5.3** is a diagram of a lengthwise section of the female reproductive tract (a) and a posterior view (b).

The Internal Organs of Sexual Reproduction

Egg Development Ova are produced in the **ovaries**, which are two oval organs suspended by ligaments (a type of connective tissue) in the pelvic cavity. The almond-sized ovaries contain **follicles**, which are

Figure 5.3

The Female Reproductive System. (a) Side view (lengthwise section) of the internal organs, and (b) posterior view of the internal organs.

(a)

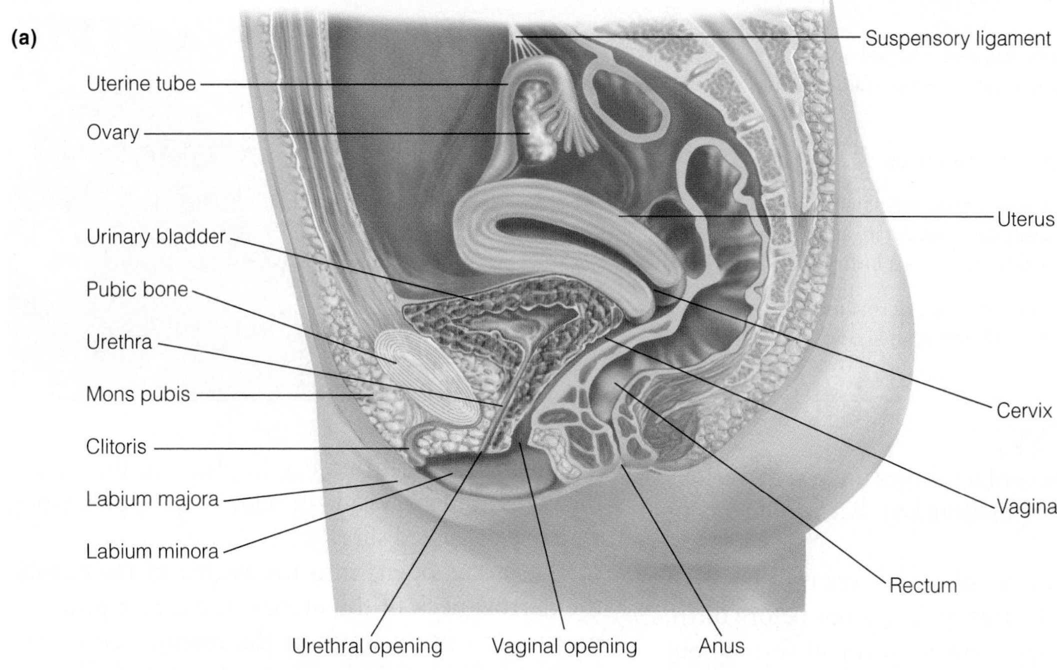

(b)

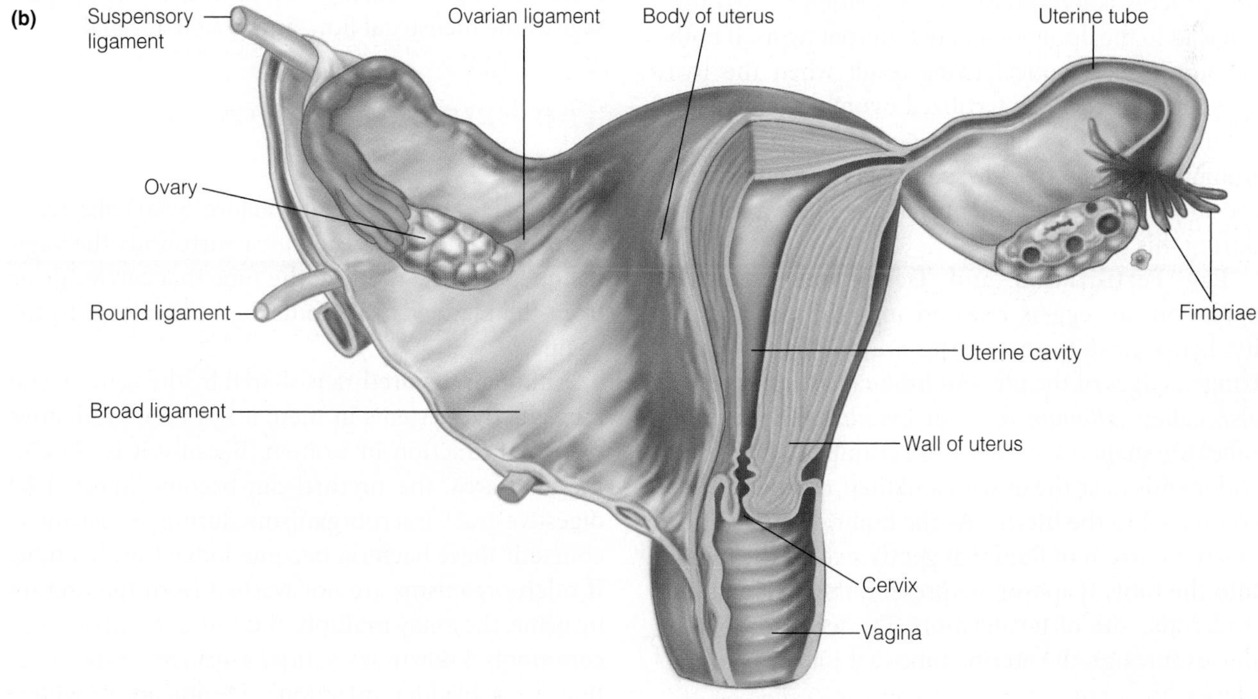

puberty (PEW-ber-tea) A stage of sexual development during which the endocrine (hormone) and reproductive systems mature.

ovulation The maturation and release of an egg from an ovary, usually each month from puberty to menopause.

uterine tubes Passageways that extend from each ovary to the uterus.

uterus A hollow, muscular, pear-shaped organ that protects and nourishes the embryo/fetus during development.

cervix The narrow neck of the uterus.

vagina A tube about 10 cm (approximately 4 in.) long that receives the penis during intercourse, allows the passage of the menstrual flow, and is a birth canal.

vulva The collective term for the external female genitals. The vulva surrounds the vaginal opening.

Figure 5.4

The Developing Ovum. A highly magnified, colorized photograph of a developing ovarian follicle with developing egg (ovum).

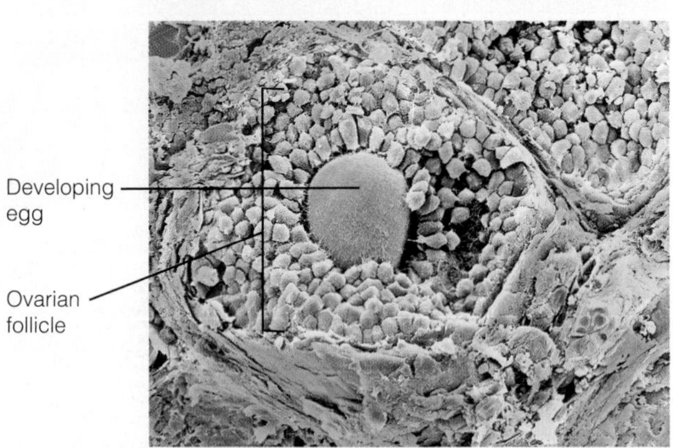

masses of cells that contain immature ova in various stages of development (**Figure 5.4**). Each follicle contains one ovum.

Unlike male sex cells, *all* female sex cells begin to develop before birth. This process stops before birth, and the potential eggs remain dormant throughout childhood. Each month after the onset of sexual maturity, or **puberty**, but prior to menopause, a few ova continue their development. Most of the time one ovum matures and bursts from an ovary each month; this process is **ovulation**. The ovulation of two ova can lead to the development of fraternal twins, if both are fertilized. Identical twins result when the two cells formed from the fertilized ovum's first division continue development as independent organisms. A woman's reproductive life span lasts from puberty to age 50 years (on average); only about 400 ova mature during this period.

Egg Fertilization and Development During ovulation, an egg is released into the pelvic cavity. Lying close to the ovaries are the fimbriae, the fringed edges of the **uterine tubes** (see Figure 5.3), also called *fallopian tubes* or *oviducts*. The uterine tubes are shaped somewhat like trumpets, with their wider ends near the ovaries and their narrower ends connected to the uterus. As the fimbriae move, they create a current of fluid that gently sweeps the ovum into the tube. If sperm are present, the uterine tube is also the site of fertilization. The fertilized ovum moves through the uterine tube as it journeys to the uterus.

The **uterus** is a hollow, muscular, pear-shaped organ that protects and nourishes the developing organism. The fertilized egg implants in the wall of the uterus and grows and develops during pregnancy, which is discussed shortly.

The uterus opens into the vagina at the **cervix**, the narrow neck of the uterus. The cervix produces mucus. At certain times of the month, the consistency of the cervical mucus changes, facilitating sperm movement into the uterus around the time of ovulation and hindering it at other times. The **vagina** is a tube about 10 cm (approximately 4 in.) long. It receives the penis during intercourse, allows the passage of the menstrual flow, and is a birth canal.

The External Organs of Sexual Reproduction

The female external genitals (Figure 5.3a) collectively are called the **vulva**. The vulva surrounds the vaginal opening. The urethra, the tube that carries urine from the bladder to the outside, lies anterior to the vagina.

Although the urethra is shared by the urinary and reproductive systems in men, it has no reproductive or sexual function in women. Because it is close to the anal area, the urethra can become infected by digestive tract microorganisms during sexual intercourse if these bacteria become lodged in this tube. If microorganisms are not washed from the urethra by urine, they may multiply and cause urethritis (also commonly known as cystitis, a urinary tract infection, or a bladder infection). Healthcare providers recommend that women who often develop such infections urinate after sexual intercourse and drink plenty of fluids to keep the urethra washed free of bacteria.

Located under a protective hood of tissue, the **clitoris** lies anterior to the urethra. This tiny structure has spongy tissue like that of the penis and becomes engorged with blood during sexual arousal. Like the penis, it has numerous nerve endings that send messages to the brain, which are interpreted as sensations of sexual pleasure when this organ is stimulated indirectly during sexual activity. Stimulating the clitoris directly may result in discomfort for some women.

Extending from over the clitoris to an area behind the vagina, two thin, hairless folds of skin called the **labia minora** (meaning "small lips") cover and protect the vaginal opening and urethra. Within the area bounded by the labia minora, lying near the vaginal and urethral openings and the clitoris, are various glands that secrete lubricating substances during sexual activity. Next to these skin folds are the hairy, more rounded, and thicker **labia majora** ("large lips"). The labia majora extend forward to unite in a mound of fatty tissue called the **mons pubis**. The mons pubis provides a cushion over the pubic bone, a portion of the pelvic bones that is in front of the genitals.

The breasts are also external organs of sex and reproduction in women. Breasts primarily consist of fat and glandular tissue (**Figure 5.5**). Exercise will not increase breast size; it can develop only the underlying pectoral muscles. Although their major purpose is the production of milk to sustain an infant after birth, the breasts are also sensitive to sexual stimulation. The nipples contain nerve endings that are sensitive to touch; smooth muscles in the nipples contract during sexual arousal, causing the nipples to become erect.

clitoris (KLIT-oh-ris) A female organ of sexual arousal. Located under a protective hood of tissue, the clitoris lies in front of the urethra.

labia minora (LAY-bee-ah my NOR-ah) Two thin, hairless folds of skin that extend from over the clitoris to an area behind the vagina. The labia minora cover and protect the vaginal opening and urethra.

labia majora (LAY-bee-ah mah-JOR-ah) Hairy, rounded, and thick folds of skin that lie adjacent to the labia minora and extend forward to unite at the mons pubis.

mons pubis A mound of fatty tissue that lies over the pubic bone, cushioning it.

menstrual (MEN-strool-al) cycle The monthly changes in the levels of the female sex hormones that orchestrate physiological changes in the ovaries and uterus.

menses (MEN-seez) The menstrual period; the sloughing of the endometrium.

endometrium (EN-doe-ME-tree-um) The inner lining of the uterus.

estrogen (ES-tro-jen) A hormone secreted by ovarian follicles, the groups of cells within which ova mature. With progesterone, estrogen stimulates the continued development and thickening of the uterine lining.

progesterone (pro-JES-te-rone) A hormone secreted by the corpus luteum. With estrogen, progesterone stimulates the continued development and thickening of the uterine lining.

corpus luteum (KOR-pus LOO-tea-um) The ruptured follicle left behind after ovulation.

The Menstrual Cycle

Women, unlike men, experience a cyclic waxing and waning of their sex hormones each month. These hormonal changes orchestrate physiologic changes in the ovaries and uterus. These changes are collectively called the **menstrual cycle**, which literally means "monthly cycle." The average length of a cycle is 28 days, but menstrual cycles generally vary from 21 to 45 days in teens and 21 to 35 days in adults.[2]

The menstrual cycle is usually described as beginning on the first day of the **menses** (menstrual period; **Figure 5.6**). The menses are the sloughing of the inner lining of the uterus, which is the **endometrium**. This lining develops gradually during the cycle, preparing for the implantation of a fertilized egg. If fertilization and implantation do not occur, the ovum dissolves and hormonal changes result in the lining being cast from the body. Each cycle a new lining develops.

What happens to the uterine lining is controlled by the hormones estrogen and progesterone. **Estrogen** is a hormone secreted by ovarian follicles, the groups of cells within which ova mature (Figure 5.4); **progesterone** is secreted by the **corpus luteum**, the remnant of a follicle that has released its ovum (Figure 5.6).

Each cycle (roughly each month) during her childbearing years, a woman's body prepares for a pregnancy. Usually only one ovarian follicle reaches the final stage of development in any particular cycle. About midcycle, hormonal changes trigger ovulation, the release of the egg from the ovary. The corpus luteum (meaning "yellow body") secretes high

placenta (plah-SEN-tah) A structure that develops after implantation of a fertilized ovum in the uterine wall and consists of maternal and fetal tissues that secrete hormones that help maintain the pregnancy.

amounts of progesterone and lesser amounts of estrogen, which cause the uterine lining to grow, thicken, and develop a rich blood supply in preparation for the implantation of a fertilized ovum. If fertilization does not occur, the corpus luteum degenerates and stops producing hormones. Without hormonal stimulation, the uterine lining degenerates and is passed out of the body through the vagina during the menses.

If fertilization occurs, the corpus luteum does not degenerate. It produces estrogen and progesterone throughout pregnancy, maintaining the lining of the uterus. As the pregnancy develops, so does the **placenta**, a structure consisting of maternal and fetal tissues that also secretes hormones that help maintain the pregnancy. In addition, oxygen, nutrients, and wastes move between mother and fetus across the placenta, which is connected to the fetus by the umbilical cord.

Premenstrual Syndrome

Approximately 70% to 90% of American women in their reproductive years report mild to moderate discomfort during the week prior to menstruation as their hormonal levels drop. More than 20% report that premenstrual symptoms such as anxiety/tension, mood swings, decreased interest in activities, appetite changes/food cravings, aches, and cramps interfere with their relationships and their daily activities.[3] This condition, originally termed *premenstrual tension syndrome* because most women experiencing it reported tension and anxiety among their symptoms, is now simply referred to as

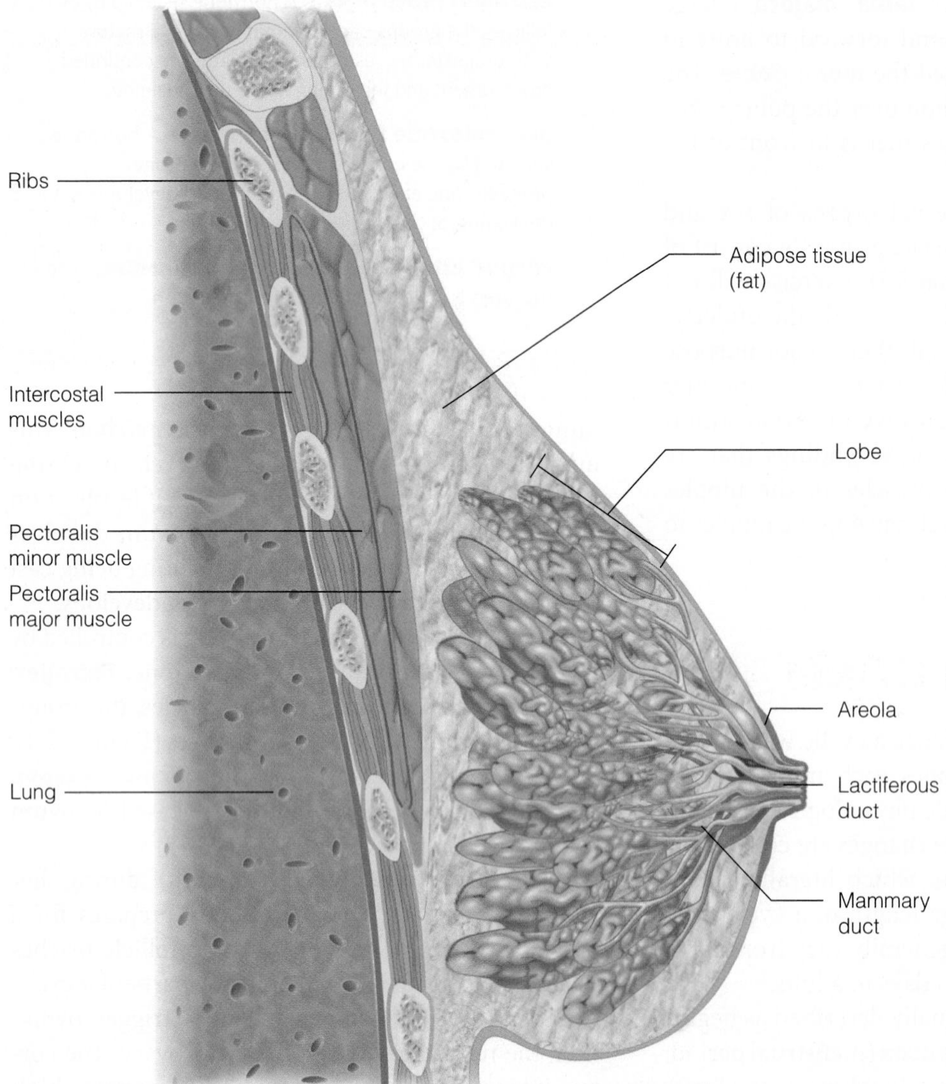

Figure 5.5

Mammary Gland Anatomy. The breasts, external organs of sex and reproduction in women, consist primarily of fat and glandular tissue.

premenstrual syndrome (PMS) Symptoms such as anxiety, mood swings, aches, and cramps that occur prior to the menses and that significantly interfere with daily life.

premenstrual syndrome, or **PMS**. A range of 5% to 8% of women report severe impairment of their daily activities because of PMS symptoms.[3] This debilitating condition is called *premenstrual dysphoric disorder* (PMDD). Research results provide some evidence that both PMS and PMDD may be partly the result of interactions between sex hormone levels and certain brain neurotransmitters.[4]

Most women with mild to moderate PMS are helped by one or more of the following treatments: counseling, lifestyle modification such as including exercise in their daily regimen, or medications prescribed for specific symptoms. Fluoxetine (Prozac) has shown usefulness in the treatment of PMS, acting to reduce symptoms of depression and anxiety that are linked to problems with the proper regulation of serotonin, a brain neurotransmitter. Many women are helped by using low-dose, combined oral contraceptives. Nutritional treatments include a diet low in salt, alcohol, caffeine, and sugar. Taking calcium supplements may reduce the severity of symptoms of PMS. Women with more severe symptoms of PMS and with PMDD may benefit from medications prescribed for their specific situation and symptoms.[4]

Toxic Shock Syndrome

A disease called *toxic shock syndrome (TSS)* is associated with the menses. This disease became well known in the 1980s, when hundreds of women who used certain high-absorbency tampons during their menstrual periods were stricken. In TSS, staphylococcal (STAFF-ih-low-KAH-kul) bacteria grow in the blood-soaked tampon and in vaginal tissues, producing toxins that can enter the woman's bloodstream. TSS is associated with a wide variety of surgical conditions unrelated to the menses (such as skin, bone, and soft-tissue infections); fewer than 50% of TSS cases are associated with tampon use during menstruation.[5] TSS can also occur from use

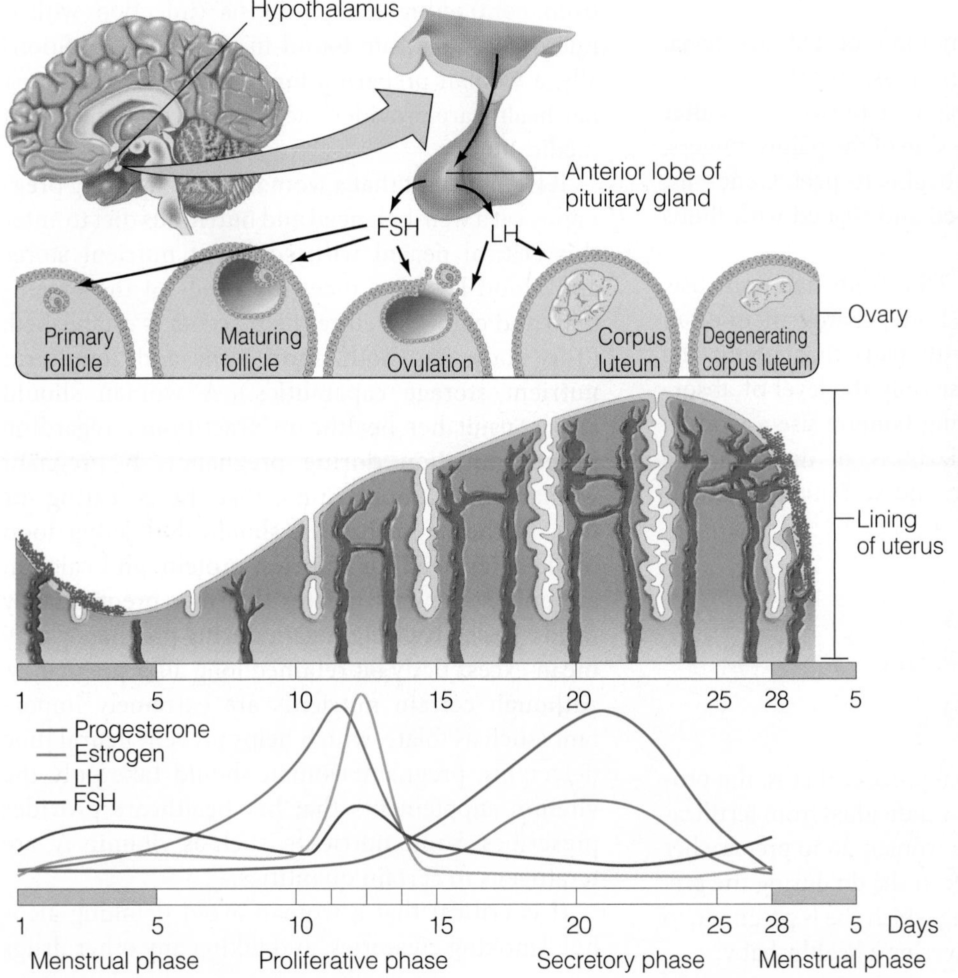

Figure 5.6

The Menstrual Cycle. The cycle begins on the first day of the menses. Hormones from the hypothalamus control the release of the hormones follicle-stimulating hormone (FSH) and luteinizing hormone (LH) from the anterior pituitary. Estrogen is secreted by the ovarian follicles, and progesterone is secreted by the corpus luteum. The rise and fall of hormone levels are related to ovulation and to the building up and sloughing off of the uterine lining.

pregnancy The gestational process; the process of development of a new individual from fertilization until birth.

teratogens Various environmental influences such as drugs, alcohol, viruses, and dietary deficiencies that can damage the embryo or fetus early in pregnancy.

amniocentesis A prenatal test performed generally between the 15th and 18th weeks of gestation, in which some of the amniotic fluid that surrounds the fetus is removed and studied to determine whether the fetus has a genetic abnormality.

chorionic villus sampling (CVS) A prenatal test performed generally between the 10th and 12th weeks of gestation, in which some of the fetal extraembryonic tissue is removed and analyzed to determine whether the fetus has a genetic abnormality.

human chorionic gonadotropin (hCG) In a pregnant woman, a hormone produced by embryonic tissues destined to become the placenta. Pregnancy tests rely on the detection of this hormone in the blood.

of contraceptive diaphragms and sponges, but such occurrences are rare. Although TSS is an uncommon disease, women from 15 to 34 years old are at the highest risk.

The most common symptoms of TSS are fever, muscle pain, headache, dizziness, diarrhea, vomiting, and a sunburn-like rash. One to two weeks after the onset of the disease, the skin of the palms, fingers, toes, and soles of the feet begins to peel. Generally, TSS patients are hospitalized and treated with fluids and antibiotics.

To avoid contracting TSS from tampon use, women who use tampons should change them often and alternate their use with pads throughout the menses. Women should use only the level of absorbency they require. If during tampon use a woman experiences fever, rash, dizziness, or diarrhea, she should remove the tampon and seek medical attention immediately.

Pregnancy and Human Development

Pregnancy is the gestational process, that is, the process of development of a new individual from fertilization until birth. What can a woman do to prepare her body for pregnancy? What can she do during the *prenatal* period, the time during which she is pregnant, to increase her chances of delivering a healthy baby?

Prepregnancy and Prenatal Care

Various **teratogens**, environmental influences such as drugs, alcohol, viruses, cigarette smoking, and dietary deficiencies, can damage the embryo or fetus. The most highly sensitive periods of the developing structures of the embryo and fetus to teratogens occur primarily during the first 8 weeks after conception, possibly before a woman knows that she's pregnant. Therefore, if you are trying to become pregnant, to avoid birth defects you should take care of your body as if you were pregnant. The Analyzing Health-Related Information feature found later in this chapter discusses folic acid (folate), a B vitamin critical to proper neural tube development of the embryo. **Table 5.1** lists various teratogens and their detrimental effects on the embryo/fetus.

A woman preparing for pregnancy should have a medical checkup to determine if her level of antibodies against rubella (German measles) is sufficient. She should also be screened for sexually transmitted infections (STIs), especially HIV, and should avoid changing the cat's litter box to protect herself from contracting toxoplasmosis (infection with a microscopic parasite found in cat feces). Additionally, a woman preparing for pregnancy should seek her healthcare provider's advice regarding the use of medications.

It is important that a woman contemplating pregnancy eat a well-balanced and nutritious diet to enter this critical period with sufficient nutrient stores and blood levels to meet the needs of the preembryo and embryo before the placenta is established. (The body has both short-term and long-term nutrient storage capabilities.) A woman should also consult her healthcare practitioner regarding proper nutrition during pregnancy. A pregnant woman should not assume that she is "eating for two" in the sense that she should double her food intake. Her need for calories, protein, and calcium are only somewhat greater than her prepregnancy needs. Excessive weight gain during pregnancy may mean excess body fat retained long after pregnancy. Although certain nutrients are extremely important (such as folate, which helps prevent neural tube defects), a pregnant woman should take only the vitamin supplements that her healthcare provider prescribes. Some nutrients, such as vitamin A, are teratogens in certain quantities.

It is critical that a woman avoid drinking alcohol, smoking cigarettes, and taking any other drugs

Table 5.1

Selected Teratogens Known to Cause Birth Defects

Teratogen	Explanation
Maternal Infectious or Noninfectious Disease	
Cytomegalovirus	A herpes-type virus that can cross the placenta and infect the embryo. Found in about 1% of newborns. Most defects affect the nervous system. Risk of brain damage is 50% after infection early in pregnancy. One in 10 affected fetuses die.
Diabetes mellitus	Risk of major malformations is about 18%. Heart malformations and neural tube defects are most frequent. Risk is greatest in uncontrolled or poorly controlled diabetes.
Phenylketonuria (PKU), untreated	Excess phenylalanine, not the defective gene, causes birth defects such as intellectual disability and malformations of the heart.
Rubella	The German measles virus can cross the placenta and infect the embryo. Infection during the first 3 months of pregnancy is likely to result in abnormalities such as deafness, heart defects, and intellectual disability.
Drugs, Other Chemicals, and Radiation	
Alcohol	Main characteristics of the birth defects caused by maternal alcohol consumption are growth deficiency, hyperactivity, distractibility, small head, under-development of the brain, and intellectual disability. No safe level of alcohol consumption during pregnancy is known.
Anticonvulsant medication	Probability of birth defects varies with medications, dosage, and stage of pregnancy.
Chemotherapeutic agents	Drugs used to treat cancer can also harm the embryo or fetus.
Cocaine	Some possible birth defects from cocaine use during pregnancy are bleeding in the brain, death of part of the brain tissue, underdeveloped head and brain, prematurity, and seizures.
Diethylstilbestrol (DES)	A drug formerly prescribed for women who were in danger of having a miscarriage. This drug affected some of their female offspring, causing unusual vaginal, cervical, and uterine changes beginning in adolescence. Increased risk for developing a certain type of vaginal and cervical cancer.
Ionizing radiation	Extremely high exposure to x-rays or exposure to radiation used in cancer therapy can affect the embryo or fetus and result in an underdeveloped head and brain.
Accutane	This synthetic form of vitamin A is used to treat certain types of acne. Birth defects that may result from use during pregnancy (when taken by mouth) include malformations of the ear, brain, and heart. Healthcare providers also suggest avoiding megadoses (more than 10,000 I.U.) of vitamin A during pregnancy.
Thalidomide	A drug taken for morning sickness in the 1960s. Taking this drug between 20 days and 36 days after conception resulted in major anatomic deformities of the limbs and heart.

(unless they have been prescribed) when preparing for pregnancy and during pregnancy. Alcohol consumption can cause a fetal alcohol spectrum disorder, which can result in a variety of birth defects, including intellectual disability, growth deficiency, and hyperactivity. Smoking a pack or more of cigarettes per day can result in a low-birth-weight baby who is weak, has a reduced brain size, and is vulnerable to illness. If a pregnant woman is addicted to a drug, her baby will be born addicted as well. In addition, she is more likely to experience complications during pregnancy and have a baby with severe birth defects. Taking drugs—including alcohol—occasionally can also damage the embryo or fetus. No safe level of these teratogens has been determined.

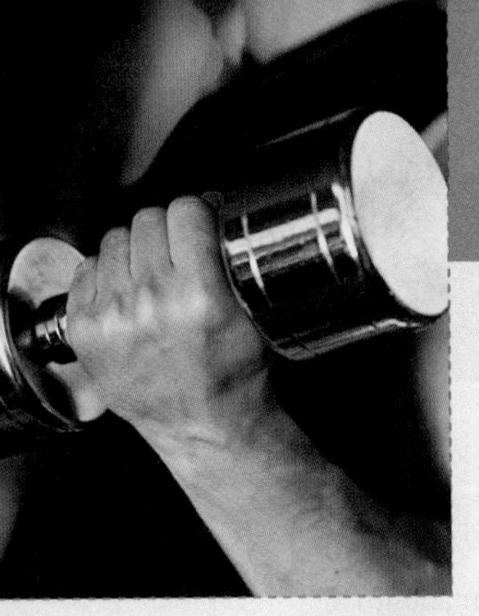

© sevenke/ShutterStock

Managing Your Health

Genetic Counseling and Prenatal Diagnosis

You and your partner have decided it's time to have a baby. You are both worried that a genetic disease may run in one of your families. (A genetic disease is caused by problems with the hereditary, or genetic, material.) Also, you're worried about the risk of birth defects because "mom" will be far past age 35 when she gives birth, and the likelihood of genetic diseases is higher then than at younger ages. What can you both do to ensure the genetic health of your baby?

Your first step might be to discuss your concerns with an obstetrician/gynecologist. Your healthcare practitioner may send both of you to a genetic counselor to explore the incidence of genetic disease in your families and to determine the probability of you and your partner having a child with a genetic disorder.

There are many reasons to seek genetic counseling. Parents with a child who has a genetic disease often choose genetic counseling to determine the probability that future children will be affected. In populations at high risk for certain genetic diseases, such as African Americans and sickle cell anemia, or Ashkenazi Jews and Tay-Sachs disease, families or prospective parents may visit genetics centers to undergo screening tests. Once screening has been done and the carriers and non-carriers of the disease have been identified, the genetic counselor can advise them of their probability of passing on problem genes to children.

After the baby is conceived and prior to birth, various techniques are available to tell for sure if the baby is affected with any of a wide variety of disorders. Tests performed on the fetus (or related tissues) to determine its health are called prenatal diagnoses. Methods that are frequently used are ultrasound, **amniocentesis**, and chorionic villus sampling (CVS). These methods can detect many, but not all, fetal abnormalities.

Ultrasound scanning, or sonography, is a common, painless, safe, and relatively inexpensive procedure for prenatal diagnosis that has been used since the 1960s. Ultrasound uses high-frequency sound waves to visualize the fetus, which can be seen as early as 7 weeks of development. The ultrasound probe is moved over the woman's abdomen. Sound waves enter the uterus and bounce off fetal structures in ways that reflect their density and makeup. The reflected waves are projected on a monitor screen (**Figure 5.A**), and their patterns are interpreted by a healthcare provider. Using this technique, a healthcare provider can detect many structural abnormalities, estimate the age of the fetus, confirm if multiple fetuses are present, and confirm fetal position. In addition, ultrasound is often used to help guide needle placement in amniocentesis, fetal blood sampling, and chorionic villus sampling.

Another common type of prenatal diagnosis is amniocentesis, which was developed in the 1960s and was widely used by the 1970s. Amniocentesis involves the removal of some of the amniotic fluid that surrounds the fetus. This watery fluid protects the baby from jarring movements and contains waste products and some cells from the fetus. Geneticists observe these cells to determine whether the fetus will be born with a genetic abnormality. In addition, medical technicians can perform tests on the fluid to determine the presence of substances that are indicators of various conditions, such as certain neural tube defects and Rh disease (a blood incompatibility problem between mother and fetus).

To extract some amniotic fluid and cells from around the fetus, the physician inserts a thin, long needle through theabdominal and uterine walls of the mother until the needle pierces the amniotic sac (**Figure 5.B**). (The physician guides the needle using ultrasound so that it will not injure the fetus and anesthetizes the

Figure 5.A

Ultrasound in Pregnancy. The ultrasound probe produces sound waves that bounce off fetal tissues. As the probe is moved across a pregnant woman's abdomen, images that provide information about the position, size, and physical condition of the fetus are visualized on a screen.

© Chris Ryan/OJO Images/Getty Images

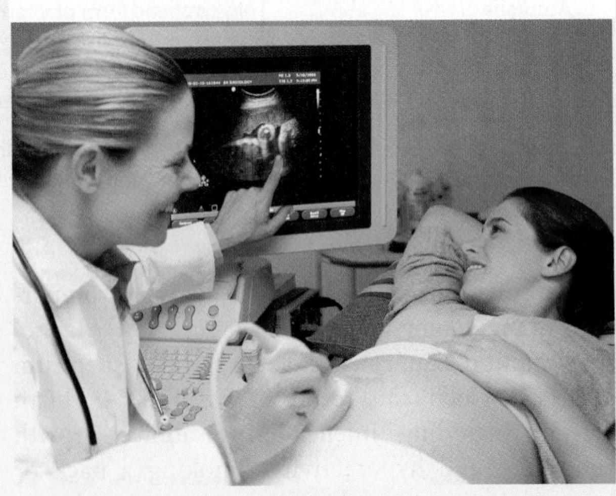

Figure 5.B

Amniocentesis. In the amniocentesis procedure, a long, thin needle is used to pierce the mother's abdominal wall and uterus and withdraw amniotic fluid. Free fetal cells are found in this fluid and can be analyzed for the fetus's gender, age, and indications of chromosomal abnormalities.

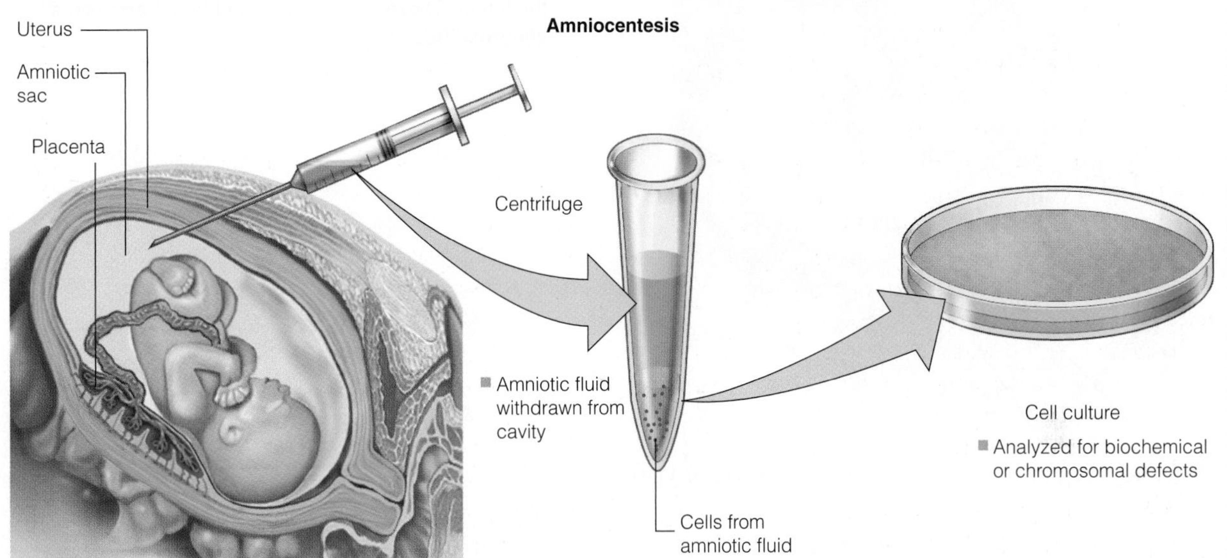

abdominal wall with a local anesthetic.) After the fluid is withdrawn, the cells must be grown, or cultured, which takes approximately 4 weeks. This technique is now performed as early as 11 weeks of gestation but is routinely performed between 15 and 18 weeks, so diagnosis is generally completed by the 19th to 22nd week. This procedure is considered safe; the risk of miscarriage resulting from amniocentesis is 0.2% to 0.3% (1 in 300 to 500).

Fetal blood sampling was developed in the 1970s. Extracting blood from the fetus is risky; however, blood can be withdrawn safely from the umbilical vein. With this technique, physicians can screen infants for various blood disorders such as sickle cell anemia and hemophilia and check for fetal oxygen levels or infection. The risk of miscarriage with this technique is up to 2% (2 in 100). This technique is least risky when performed between weeks 18 and 21 of pregnancy but can be done as early as week 17.

Chorionic villus sampling (CVS) was also developed around 1970 but came into wide use in the 1980s. The chorion is the outermost of the fetal membranes (**Figure 5.C**) that facilitate the exchange of nutrients, gases, and other materials such as waste products between the fetus and the mother. The umbilical cord extends from the fetus to the chorion. Finger-like projections called villi (singular, *villus*) extend from the chorion into maternal tissues at the placenta, the part of the chorion that joins mother and fetus. In this way, the blood of the fetus, circulating through blood vessels in the chorion and its villi, comes into close contact (but does not mix) with maternal blood vessels. To perform CVS, a physician inserts a thin tube or a needle into the vagina and up into the uterus or can enter the uterus by puncturing the abdomen. The instrument vacuums up a tiny sample of villi. Although this technique has the advantages of early testing (weeks 10 to 12) and quick analysis of cells (no culturing is needed), the risk of miscarriage is approximately 1% (1 in 100). CVS was previously thought to cause birth defects of the limbs in some pregnancies, but it has been determined that such defects occur at the same rate as in pregnancies without CVS.

Today, using ultrasound to guide them, physicians are able to sample fetal skin and certain other tissues. In addition, some conditions can be treated before birth with a blood transfusion or one of the forms of fetal surgery currently available. The choices that remain are terminating the pregnancy or carrying the fetus to term. If the second choice is made, prenatal diagnosis is extremely helpful to ensure that the baby receives the best possible medical care for its condition, beginning from his/her first breath.

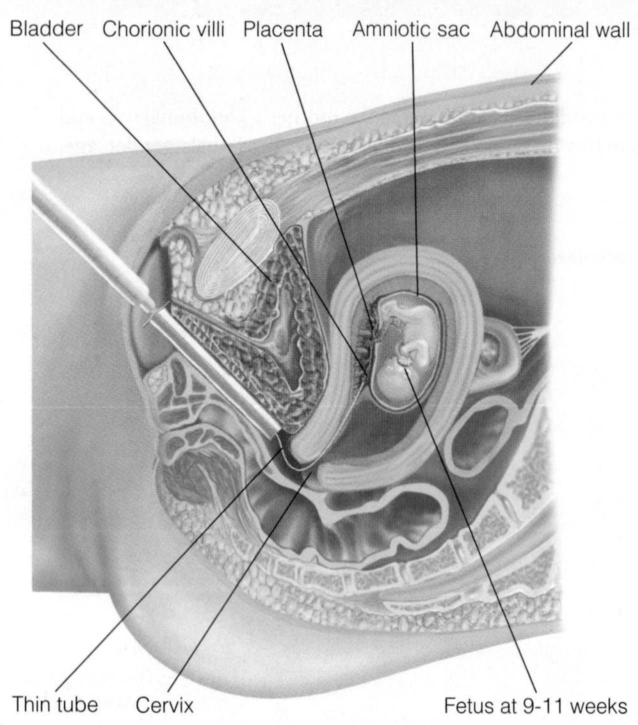

Figure 5.C

Chorionic Villus Sampling. One way to perform CVS is to insert a tube, or catheter, into the vagina, up through the cervix, and into the uterus. This tube is used to collect pieces of chorionic villi, which are part of the outer fetal tissue called the chorion (not part of the fetus). These cells are analyzed for chromosomal abnormalities.

Women older than 35 years of age have a higher risk of having babies with Down syndrome (a genetic abnormality resulting in intellectual disability) than younger women. Older women may choose to have diagnostic tests such as amniocentesis and chorionic villus sampling during pregnancy to detect possible genetic disease or other abnormalities in the fetus. In addition, couples often seek genetic counseling before becoming pregnant. If anyone in a couple's family has a genetic disease, seeking genetic counseling may be prudent. (The Managing Your Health essay "Genetic Counseling and Prenatal Diagnosis" discusses prenatal tests and counseling.)

Many women want to know if exercising during pregnancy will hurt the fetus. Generally, if a woman was exercising before she became pregnant, she can continue exercising while she is pregnant. However, a healthcare provider may suggest modifications in a pregnant woman's workout regimen. Also, some healthcare providers recommend that their previously sedentary patients start a mild exercise program to help them become stronger and develop stamina for the birth process.

Determining If You Are or Your Partner Is Pregnant

How do you know if you or your partner is pregnant? By noticing certain physical signs, you may become aware of this condition. A pregnant woman will not menstruate, so a missed menstrual period may be the first sign. However, a pregnant woman may experience *implantation bleeding* about a week before the expected time of the menstrual period. This small amount of blood flow from the uterus occurs when the fertilized ovum nestles into the uterine wall. The breasts may feel sore, she may feel nauseated at certain times during the day or all day, and she may feel tired, moody, or both. These signs are bodily reactions to changes in hormone levels during pregnancy.

If a woman suspects that she is pregnant, she may choose to conduct a home pregnancy test or visit her gynecologist/obstetrician for such a test. The Consumer Health feature "Home Pregnancy Tests" discusses how pregnancy tests work and provides guidelines for conducting such a test.

If a woman has missed more than one menstrual period and is certain that she is not pregnant, she

Consumer Health

Home Pregnancy Tests

Most pregnancy tests rely on the detection of the hormone **human chorionic gonadotropin (hCG)**. This hormone is produced by embryonic tissues destined to become the placenta, the organ that allows the exchange of nutrients, gases, and wastes between the fetus and a pregnant woman. Pregnancy tests to detect hCG can be conducted on either blood or urine. Urine tests are most frequently used to detect hCG because urine is easier to collect than blood. This is the type of test in home test kits.

The way pregnancy tests work is that hCG binds with specific antibodies in the test kit. If a woman is not pregnant, hCG will not be present in her urine, binding will not occur, and the test will be negative. If a woman is pregnant, hCG will be present in her urine, binding will occur, and the test will be positive.

Home pregnancy tests are easy to use. These tests contain either a plastic stick with an absorbent part that is placed in the urine flow or immersed in a container of collected urine, or a plastic device with an opening containing absorbent material into which drops of urine are placed. While a woman waits, the urine moves through the absorbent material inside either type of device, and the hCG (if present) attaches to an antibody that has a color label such as blue or red. The hCG-antibody complex then moves to another window where it binds to a second antibody attached to the absorbent material in either a line, symbol, color, or the word *pregnant*. If hCG is not present in a woman's urine, the line, symbol, color, or the word *pregnant* will not appear.

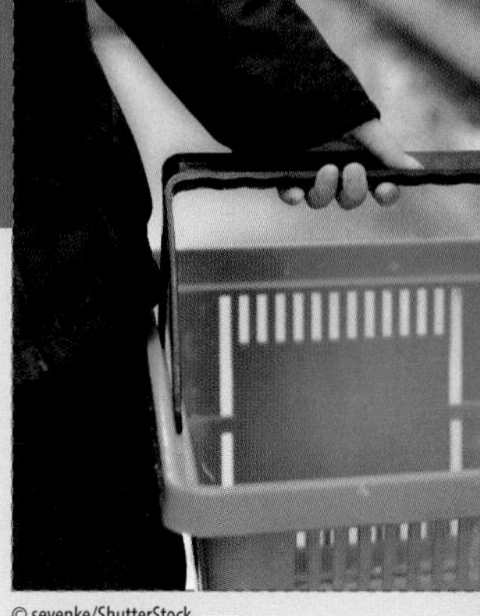

It is important to follow the directions of a home test carefully and wait the prescribed length of time to "read" the result. Testing the first urine of the day is best because hCG is most concentrated in the first urine. The manufacturers of home pregnancy tests claim that a woman can test her urine on the first day of her missed period or before and that she will obtain results that are 99% accurate. However, hCG levels are usually quite low this early in pregnancy. It may be advisable to obtain a blood test from a healthcare practitioner for a reliable early result or to wait at least a week after one's missed period to use a home pregnancy test, using the first urine of the day. It is advisable to check the expiration date on the package and use only tests that have not expired. One may also decide to repeat the test after a few days no matter the result of the initial test.

If you are unsure which test to choose, ask a pharmacist for help. A woman who has a positive test should see her healthcare provider immediately for a confirmatory test and appropriate prenatal care.

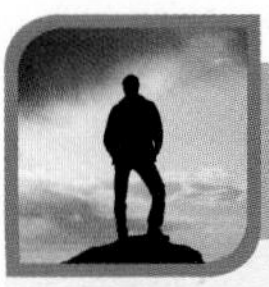

Healthy Living Practices

- Women preparing for pregnancy should have a medical checkup, eat a well-balanced and nutritious diet, and avoid drinking alcohol, smoking cigarettes, or using other drugs.
- Women and men concerned about the possibility of passing a genetic condition on to their offspring can seek genetic counseling when considering pregnancy.

should see her healthcare provider. *Amenorrhea* (ah-MEN-oh-REE-ah), or abnormal stoppage of the menses, is most often caused by stress, weight loss, or strenuous exercise regimens. However, it can have more serious causes, such as hormonal imbalances or tumorous growths.

Pregnancy and Fetal Development

Pregnancy usually lasts 38 weeks, or approximately 9 months. The delivery date is calculated to be 40 weeks from a woman's last menstrual period because *conception* (fertilization) usually occurs in the middle of the cycle. Typically pregnancy is described in terms of trimesters, or 3-month periods, during which certain developmental events take place. (Because months are more than 4 weeks, the month-to-week correlations given here are approximate.)

The first trimester is a crucial time of development when all the organ systems of the body are forming and becoming functional. Cells in the embryo migrate to key developmental positions, shaping the individual as it takes on a human form. In contrast, the second and third trimesters are periods of growth and refinement of the organ systems. **Figure 5.7**

labor (parturition) (PAR-too-RISH-un) The process of childbirth.

through **Figure 5.11** depict the development of the *preembryo* (the first 2 weeks of development), the *embryo* (weeks 3 through 8), and the fetus (weeks 9 through 38). Figure 5.7 also describes ectopic pregnancy, implantation of the embryo outside of the uterus.

While the fetus is developing, changing, and growing over 9 months, changes also take place in the mother's body. **Figure 5.12** summarizes these changes. In addition, the pregnant woman may experience nausea, vomiting, frequent urination, leg cramps, vaginal discharge, fatigue, and constipation during the first trimester. Nausea, vomiting, and leg cramps (if present) usually subside by the second trimester. At that time, additional changes may take place. In her last two trimesters, a pregnant woman may experience swelling of the legs and feet, varicose veins, backache, heartburn, and shortness of breath, in addition to continuing vaginal discharge, frequent urination, fatigue, and constipation. **Table 5.2** lists various problematic conditions that may occur during pregnancy. As women of childbearing age get older, their risks for pregnancy complications and adverse outcomes increase.[6]

The Birth Process

No one is certain what events signal the beginning of **labor**, the process of childbirth. Labor, also called **parturition**, takes place in three stages: cervical dilation, fetal delivery, and placental delivery. The birth process normally takes about 13 hours for the woman

Figure 5.7

Fertilization and Implantation. The first event in human development is fertilization, which takes place in the uterine (fallopian) tube. The fertilized ovum begins to divide as it moves along the tube to the uterus and is now referred to as a pre-embryo. At 4 days after fertilization, the developing ball of cells begins to fill with fluid, a stage of pre-embryonic development termed the blastocyst. Approximately 6 days after fertilization, the blastocyst implants in the back wall of the uterus. During implantation, the embryo attaches firmly to the inner lining of the uterus. This illustration shows the journey of the fertilized ovum from the fallopian tube to the uterus. Occasionally, implantation takes place outside of the uterus, a condition known as ectopic pregnancy. Pre-embryos may implant on an ovary, on the intestine, or in a fallopian tube. All ectopic pregnancies endanger the mother's life.

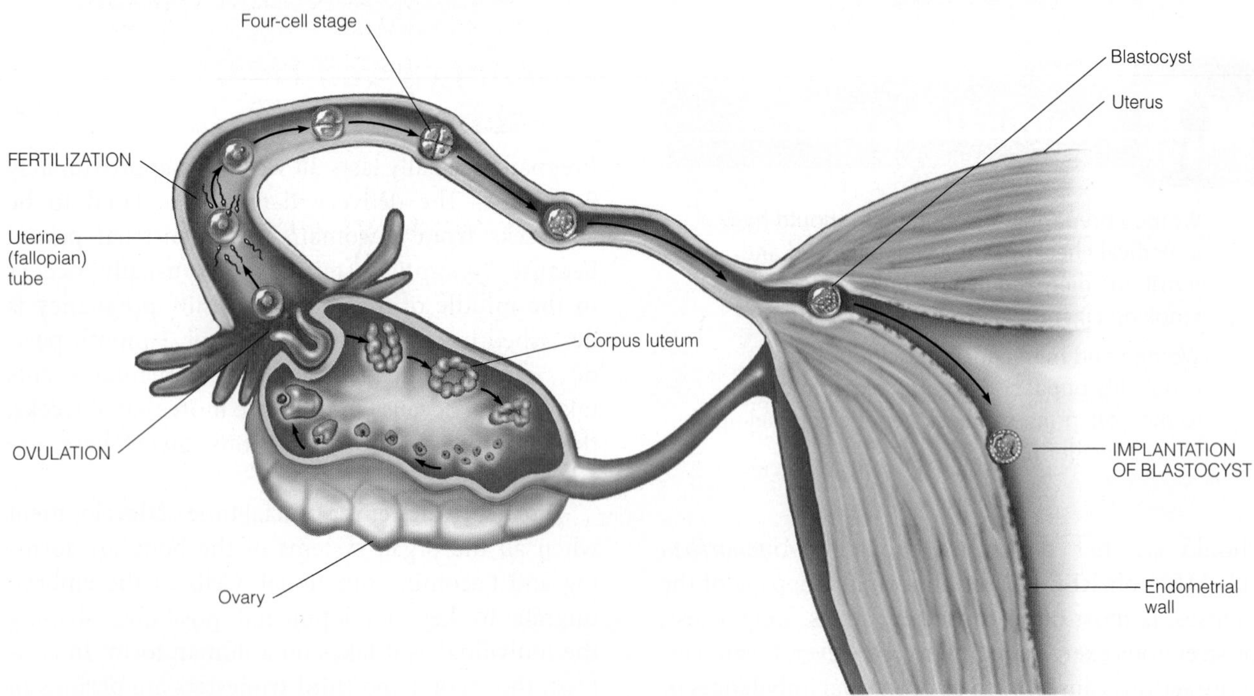

Figure 5.8

Human Embryo Between 4 and 5 Weeks of Development. As the pregnancy moves into the 3rd week, the pre-embryo is only 0.10 in. long. The flattened pre-embryo develops into a cylindrical embryo. Some of the organs, such as the heart, begin to develop. This 4.5-week-old embryo has established the beginnings of most of the major organ systems of the body. Its C-shaped body has a featureless head, a middle with the heart and liver bulging from the body, and a tail. During the 5th week, the embryo doubles in length from 4 mm (0.18 in.) to 8 mm (0.38 in.). The brain grows rapidly. Wrists, fingers, and ears begin to form during the 6th week of development. Although development has been rapid, growth has not. By the end of the 6th week, the embryo is a mere half-inch long.

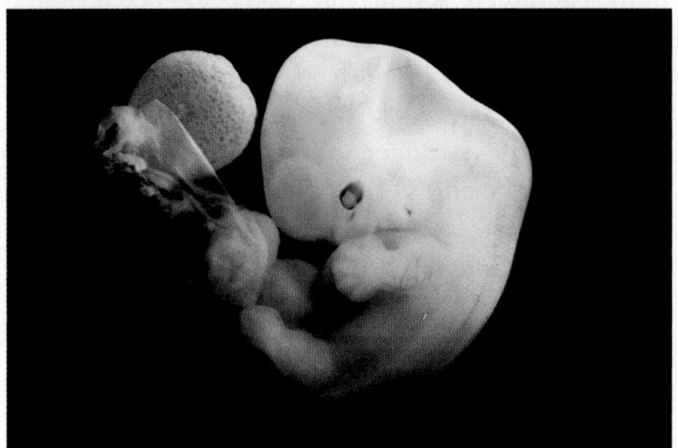

Figure 5.9

Human Fetus About 11 to 12 Weeks of Development. During the 7th week, eyelids begin to cover the eyes, and the face begins to look somewhat human. By the 8th week, the last week in the embryonic period, the embryo grows to about an inch. Most of the body systems are functional by this time. The fetal period begins at week 9, lasts throughout the rest of the pregnancy, and is characterized by growth and functional maturation of the organs. During weeks 9 through 13 (the 3rd month), facial features become more well developed, with eyelids completely covering the eyes and then fusing shut. (The eyes can be seen through the thin eyelids.) The genitals begin to develop, and the heart is now a four-chambered structure.

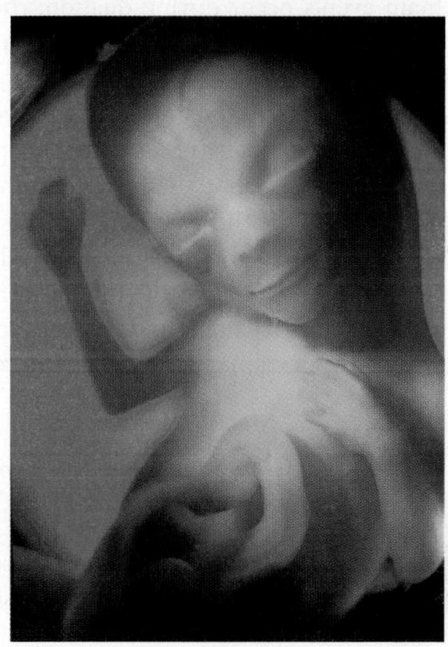

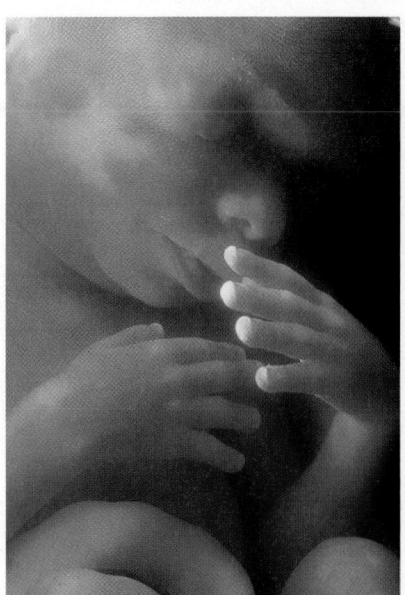

Figure 5.10

Human Fetus About 5 Months (20 Weeks) of Development. The second trimester comprises the 4th, 5th, and 6th months of development, or weeks 14 through 26. The organs that developed during the first trimester mature and grow during this trimester. As the 4th month passes, the genitals become fully formed. The sensory organs nearly finish their development and refinements of body structures occur. The mother becomes aware of fetal movements around the 5th month of pregnancy, the stage of development of the fetus in the photo. By the end of the 5th month, as fat deposits are laid down, the fetus begins to look more like a baby. Only 12 inches long and weighing 1 pound, it probably could not survive on its own. However, if born by the end of the 6th month, the fetus has a chance of surviving with special medical care.

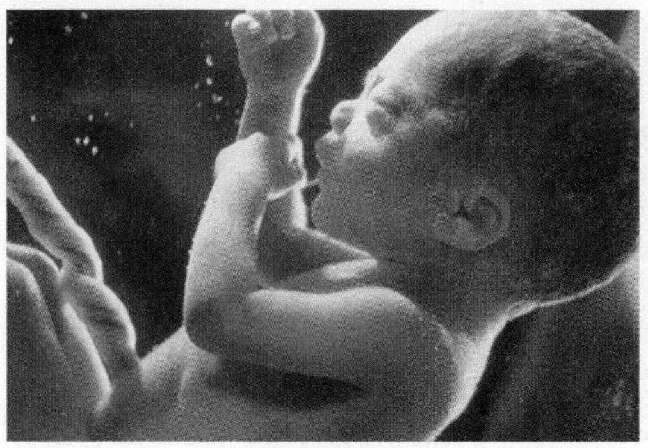

Figure 5.11

Human Fetus Nearly Full Term—8 to 9 Months. During the third trimester, months 7 through 9 or weeks 27 through 38, the fetus primarily gains weight. Its lungs develop more fully, eyelids open, and the nervous system undergoes further development. However, the nervous system is not fully developed and its maturation continues after birth. At the end of the third trimester, the average fetus weighs about 7.5 pounds and is 20 inches long.

who is giving birth for the first time. In women who have previously given birth, the time shortens considerably and is about 8 hours.

Two main events occur during dilation: rhythmic contractions of the uterine muscles cause the cervix (the opening of the uterus) to dilate (widen) and to efface (thin out). In the nonpregnant state, the cervix is hard and tubelike with an extremely narrow opening. During the first stage of labor, the cervix becomes soft. The opening widens and the tissue stretches so that by the end of the first stage of labor the cervical opening is 3.5 in. to 4 in. wide and the tubular cervix no longer exists as such—it flattens and becomes continuous with the lower portion of the uterus (**Figure 5.13**). During this time—or prior to labor in some cases—the amniotic sac ruptures (the water breaks), releasing the amniotic fluid. This fluid cushions the fetus during development. The baby must be born within 24 hours of the rupture, or serious infection could occur.

In the beginning of her labor, a woman's uterine contractions may last for 30 seconds and be 15 to 20 minutes apart. As labor progresses, the contractions become stronger, longer, and more closely spaced. By the end of the first stage of labor, during a period called transition, contractions occur every 1 to 2 minutes and last up to a minute each.

Some women experience preparatory contractions that are not a part of labor, which are called

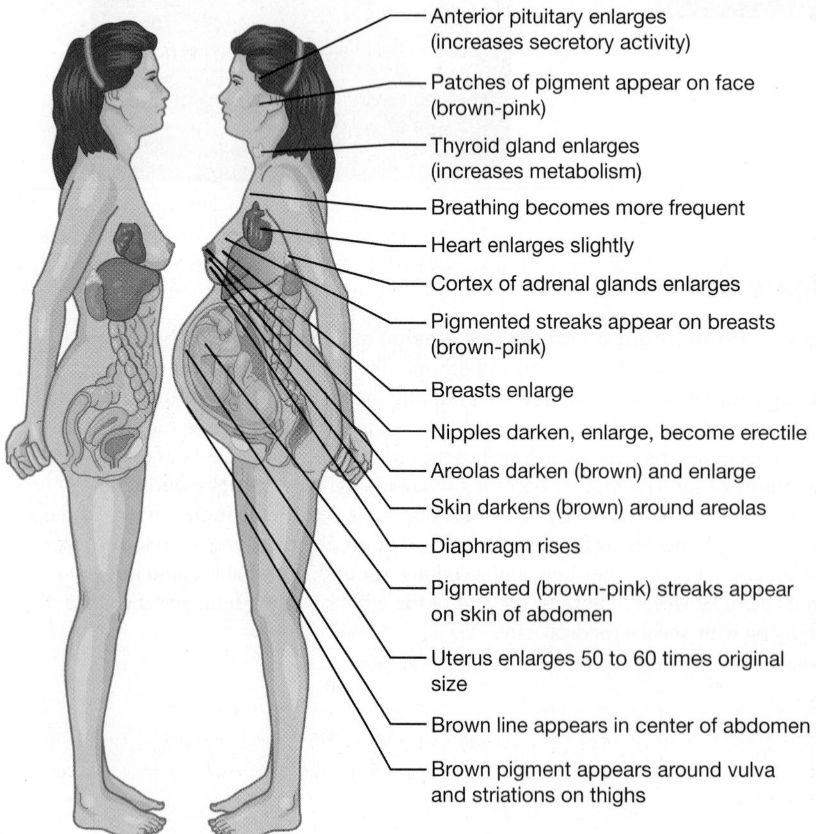
Anterior pituitary enlarges (increases secretory activity)
Patches of pigment appear on face (brown-pink)
Thyroid gland enlarges (increases metabolism)
Breathing becomes more frequent
Heart enlarges slightly
Cortex of adrenal glands enlarges
Pigmented streaks appear on breasts (brown-pink)
Breasts enlarge
Nipples darken, enlarge, become erectile
Areolas darken (brown) and enlarge
Skin darkens (brown) around areolas
Diaphragm rises
Pigmented (brown-pink) streaks appear on skin of abdomen
Uterus enlarges 50 to 60 times original size
Brown line appears in center of abdomen
Brown pigment appears around vulva and striations on thighs

Figure 5.12

A Summary of the Physical Changes That Take Place During Pregnancy. (Left) The unpregnant female body; (Right) Changes that appear by 30 weeks of fetal development.

Braxton-Hicks contractions False labor; preparatory contractions that are not a part of labor.

Braxton-Hicks contractions, or false labor. False labor contractions can be distinguished from the contractions of true labor in that they occur irregularly, the intervals between contractions do not shorten, and the contractions do not increase in strength. A woman experiencing these contractions should consult her physician to confirm that she is not in labor.

Table 5.2

Pregnancy Problems and Symptoms

Name of Condition (Alternative or former names)	Definition	Cause	Symptoms	Treatment
Ectopic pregnancy	Fertilized egg implants outside the uterus. Majority occur in the uterine tube.	Problems with anatomy of uterine tubes, possibly resulting from pelvic inflammatory disease, uterine surgery, or use of IUD	Loss of menses, pelvic or abdominal pain, abnormal vaginal bleeding.	Surgery to remove embryo. Nonsurgical treatments may be used in certain situations.
Pregnancy-induced hypertension [PIH] (Preeclampsia) (Toxemia of pregnancy)	A group of metabolic disturbances.	Unknown.	High blood pressure, water retention, and an excess of protein in the urine, occurring in the third trimester. Primarily a disease of first pregnancy. Occurs with higher frequency in adolescent women and those older than 35 years.	Bed rest. Medication to reduce blood pressure and prevent seizures. Delivery usually cures the condition.
Eclampsia	An extension of PIH to the point of seizure, coma, or both.	Unknown.	Increase in blood pressure from that in PIH, abdominal pain, blurry vision, headache, shakiness. May occur in third trimester or postpartum.	Convulsions and high blood pressure are treated with medication. Delivery takes place as soon as patient is stabilized.
Diabetes mellitus associated with pregnancy (Gestational diabetes mellitus [GDM])	A metabolic disorder that leads to high glucose levels in the blood (see Chapter 9). In pregnancy, poor control of blood glucose levels can lead to fetal abnormalities.	Hormonal changes of pregnancy often result in a display of diabetes in women with risk factors for the disease.	See Table 9.5. Women with risk factors for diabetes (obesity and family history) should be screened prior to and during pregnancy for this disease.	Control of blood glucose level with diet and/or insulin injections.

Data from Rivlin, M. E., & Martin, R. W. (Eds.). (2000). *Manual of Clinical Problems in Obstetrics and Gynecology* (5th ed.). Philadelphia: Lippincott, Williams & Wilkins; and Zuspan, F. P., & Quilligan, E. J. (1998). *Handbook of Obstetrics, Gynecology, and Primary Care*. St. Louis, MO: Mosby.

breech birth A delivery in which the baby presents feet or buttocks first instead of the usual head-first position.

episiotomy (uh-pee-zee-OT-uh-me) A cut in the tissue surrounding the vaginal opening to widen it during a vaginal delivery so that the surrounding skin and tissues will be less likely to tear.

During the second stage of labor, the baby is born. The average time for this stage is 30 to 60 minutes. Uterine contractions continue and move the baby into the birth canal (vagina). The woman pushes and bears down, aiding this process. The head usually appears first, but some babies are born in the breech position, feet or buttocks first. A **breech birth** is a more complicated delivery than a head-first delivery and may require surgical removal of the baby through the abdominal wall—a cesarean section. During a vaginal delivery, the physician may perform an **episiotomy**, making a cut in the tissue surrounding the vaginal opening to widen the opening. This cut is usually made in the direction of the anus. Without this procedure, the skin and surrounding tissues may sustain more damage and heal with more difficulty than surgically cut tissue does.

After the baby is born, her/his nose and mouth are cleared of mucus by suctioning. The umbilical cord is clamped in two places and cut between the clamps to prevent bleeding. Healthcare practitioners assess the baby's ability to adjust to life outside the uterus at 1 minute and then 5 minutes after birth.

Within 15 to 30 minutes after delivery of the baby, the uterus continues to contract, separating the fetal placental tissues from maternal tissues. During this

Figure 5.13

The Stages of Labor. (a) The position of the fetus at the beginning of labor. (b) Dilation, the cervix (the opening to the uterus) widens and thins. (c) Expulsion, the baby is born. (d) Placental delivery.

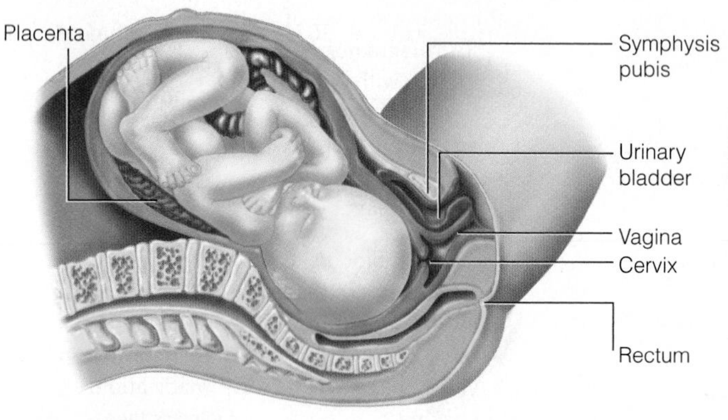

(a) Early first-stage labor

Ruptured amniotic sac

(b) Later first-stage labor: the transition

Placenta

(c) Early second-stage labor

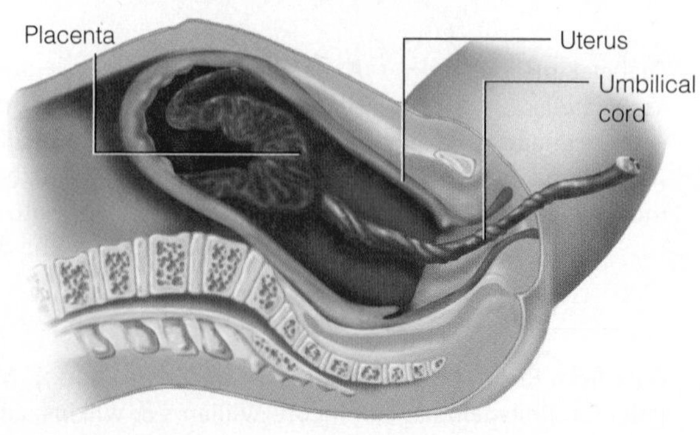

(d) Third-stage labor: delivery of placenta

third stage of labor, the placenta is expelled from the uterus. Figure 5.13 visually summarizes the birth process, showing the three stages of labor.

Circumcision

Although few data are available, the CDC's National Hospital Discharge Survey show that approximately 56% of male newborns are circumcised in the United States.[7] In some groups, such as followers of the Jewish and Islamic faiths, circumcision rates approximate 100% because the procedure is practiced for religious and cultural reasons. *Circumcision* is a surgical procedure to remove the foreskin of the penis, which is a fold of skin covering the end of the penis. The photos in **Figure 5.14** show both an uncircumcised and a circumcised penis.

Existing scientific evidence demonstrates potential medical benefits of newborn male circumcision, such as lowered risk of urinary tract infections, especially in infants younger than 1 year of age, lowered risk of penile cancer, and lowered risk of STIs, especially herpes (HSV-2) and HIV infection. Circumcision also reduces the prevalence and transmission of human papillomavirus, which is linked to the development of cervical cancer.[8] However, the policy statement of the American Academy of Pediatrics (AAP),[9] which was reaffirmed in 2005[10] and again in 2012,[11] notes that, in general, the differences in risk are small and the data are not sufficient to recommend routine circumcision of male newborns at this time. In addition, circumcision has some risks as does any surgical procedure, though complications are rare and usually minor. Therefore, the AAP suggests that parents, in conjunction with their pediatricians, decide what is in the best interest of the child. If the decision is made for circumcision, the academy strongly recommends giving the infant pain relief medication.

The Postpartum Period

The *postpartum period* is the 6 weeks after childbirth during which a mother's body returns to its prepregnant state. One of the areas of the body affected greatly, of course, is the reproductive system. The uterus returns nearly to its original size. Within 2 weeks, the cervical opening closes to a slit, and tissue damage that occurred to it during the birth process heals. The vagina, bruised and swollen from the newborn traveling through it, returns to normal after about 3 weeks. The episiotomy and any torn tissues surrounding the vaginal opening heal within 1 week.

A variety of other organ systems and tissues in the mother's body change during pregnancy and return to their prepregnant state during the postpartum period and beyond. For example, muscles in the pelvic region gradually regain their original tone, but

Figure 5.14

Circumcision. (a) Uncircumcised penis. (b) Circumcised penis.

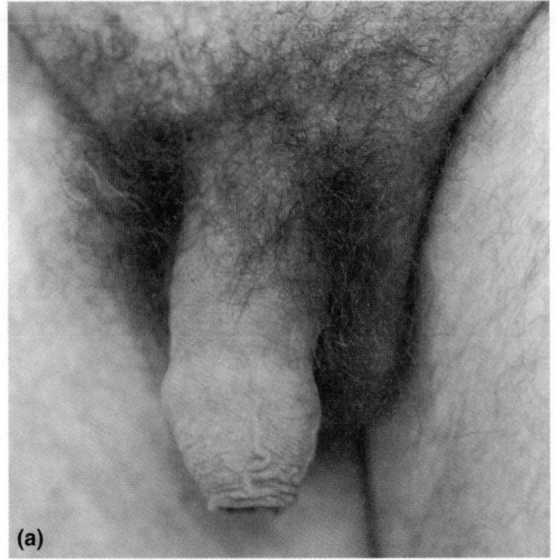

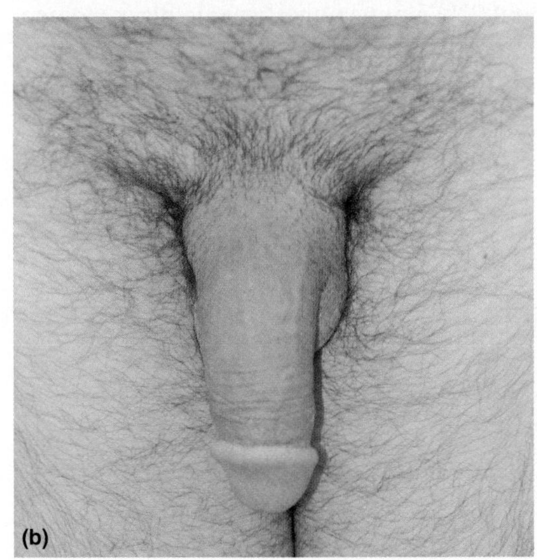

infertility Inability to conceive a child after 1 year of unprotected sex.

this process may take up to 6 months. During the first few days after delivery, a woman may have trouble urinating due to bruising of the bladder, the effects of anesthetics, and swelling of the ureters (tubes that lead from the kidneys to the bladder). The ureters may remain swollen for up to 3 months, although problems with urination usually last only a few days. During the birth process and the expulsion of the placenta, a woman loses blood. Her blood plasma and red blood cell volumes usually return to the normal nonpregnant state by the end of the postpartum period but may take a few additional weeks. Hormonal changes are comparatively rapid after delivery; some return to normal levels by the end of the first postpartum day, but others take 1 to 2 weeks to normalize.

Many women experience *postpartum depression*, especially in the week after delivery. Approximately 40% to 85% of women experience mild depression, often referred to as "the baby blues." This mild form of depression, often accompanied by mood swings, is thought to be a result of the physical and mental stresses of childbirth, as well as the variety of physical (including hormonal) changes that take place during that time. Symptoms include periods of crying, sleep disturbances, loss of appetite, and confusion. Whereas the baby blues do not require medical attention, more serious postpartum depression does. This disorder can occur up to 1 year after giving birth and affects 10% to 15% of mothers.[12] The prevalence of postpartum depression varied by age (ranging from about 23% of women aged 19 or younger to 10% women in their thirties), race/ethnicity (ranging from about 22% among non-Hispanic Black women, 17% among Hispanic women, and 12% among non-Hispanic White women), and geographic location (ranging from about 21% in Tennessee to just under 10% in Minnesota).[13]

At the beginning of the postpartum period, many women also start breastfeeding their infants.

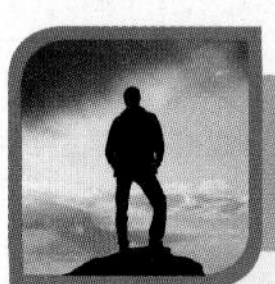

Healthy Living Practices

- If you are female and in your reproductive years, have missed a period, are nauseated at times, feel tired often, and are experiencing moodiness, check with a healthcare practitioner; you may be pregnant.
- Manufacturers claim that home pregnancy tests can be used prior to or on the day of a missed period or thereafter to determine pregnancy. However, early results may be unreliable. A healthcare practitioner can provide laboratory testing to confirm pregnancy.

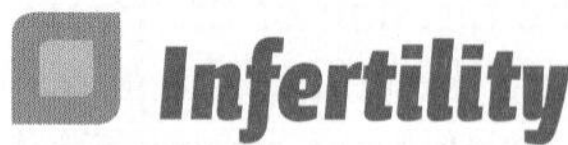

Infertility

Infertility is the inability of a couple to conceive a child after 1 year of unprotected sex and affects 10.9% of women aged 15 to 44 in the United States.[14] Some infertility experts suggest that couples wait for 2 years before seeking help for infertility. Infertility is not necessarily the result of "a problem" with one partner or the other. Factors that slightly impair the fertility of both sexual partners may interact to render a couple infertile.

Factors That Affect Fertility

One reason for male infertility is faulty sperm production. In normal sperm production, the semen contains approximately 80 million to 120 million sperm per milliliter (mL). Because the ejaculate volume ranges from 2 to 8 mL (slightly less than a teaspoon to nearly 2 teaspoons), the total sperm ejaculated ranges from about 200 million to 800 million. A sperm count lower than 20 million sperm per mL (40 million to 160 million total) in the ejaculate may impair fertility.

In addition to a low sperm count, a high percentage (usually more than 40%) of abnormally shaped sperm can affect male fertility. Abnormally shaped sperm such as those with two heads or abnormally shaped heads or tails (**Figure 5.15**) may not be able to swim well. These defects may reduce their chances of reaching the egg.

Male infertility is often related to a variety of environmental factors or diseases. Cigarette smoking, chronic alcoholism, various medications, and prolonged illnesses with accompanying fever all affect sperm production. Infection with the mumps virus can render a man sterile.

A man can also have a problem with sperm transport, which can cause infertility even if the sperm count is adequate for conception. Infections caused by certain STIs can block the vas deferens and injure

Figure 5.15

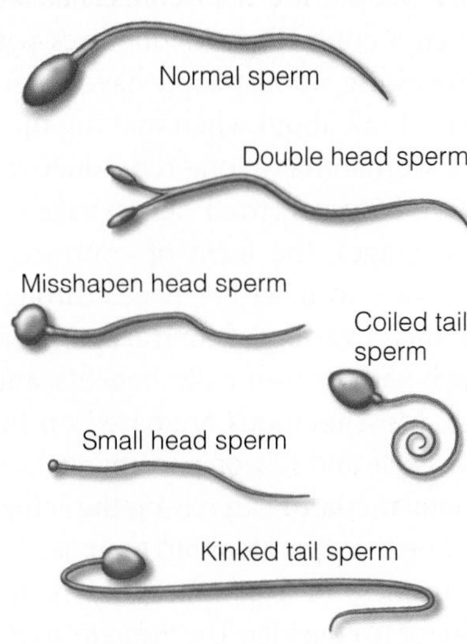

Abnormal Sperm. Abnormal sperm exhibit various types of malformations. A normal sperm is shown at the top.

these tubes. Erectile dysfunction is also a common cause of infertility if a man is unable to ejaculate.

There is a variety of causes of infertility in women. In some instances, the vagina cannot be penetrated because of an intact hymen (a membrane that partially covers the vagina and that is usually ruptured at the first intercourse) or due to vaginismus (involuntary, painful contractions of the vagina). Some abnormalities in the structure of the vagina, which may be present at birth or caused by scarring from STIs or trauma, allow only partial penetration. Unknowingly complicating the problem, couples having trouble with penetration often use lubricants that kill sperm. For example, one type of the popular K-Y Jelly has spermicidal properties.

Once sperm travel up the vagina, they must pass through the cervix to reach the uterus and the fallopian tubes. Secretion of mucus by the cervix is important for sperm motility. Infection can damage the glands that secrete mucus or result in the presence of white blood cells. The properties of this mucus also change if a woman has an estrogen deficiency. Such changes in the quality and quantity of mucus can impair the sperm's ability to reach an egg.

Structural defects of the uterus do not usually cause infertility; usually such problems result in repeated miscarriage. However, the uterine (fallopian) tubes can be another fertility trouble spot. Infection with *Neisseria gonorrhoeae* or *Chlamydia trachomatis* can result in severe tissue destruction, completely blocking the tubes and causing sterility. Infections of other origins, such as from appendicitis or intrauterine device (IUD) complications, may result in less severe blockage. Pregnancy may occur, but the risk is increased for ectopic pregnancy. Endometriosis, the growth of abnormal tissue in the abdomen, is another cause of sterility, ectopic pregnancy, or both.

The ovaries can be the source of impaired fertility. Hormonal imbalances can interfere with ovulation, and a mumps infection, radiation, and chemotherapy can damage the ovaries. Function of the ovaries declines as a woman ages, reducing her ability to conceive. Occasionally, because of an unknown cause, a young woman can experience a decline in the function of the ovaries known as primary ovarian insufficiency, in which she prematurely "runs out" of cells destined to become eggs.[15] Dietary deficiencies, frequent strenuous exercise, smoking, and obesity have also been shown to negatively affect ovary function and the ability to conceive.[16–18]

Treating Infertility

To treat infertility, a physician skilled in this practice begins with extensive histories of the couple's health. This may be followed by a series of relatively simple tests such as a sperm count to rule out common causes of infertility. Other, more extensive, physical examinations may be necessary to determine the cause. In some instances, the cause cannot be determined. Treatments are specific to the known causes of the infertility and include surgical procedures, hormone therapy, medication, and lifestyle changes. In addition, nutritional treatment is currently being investigated. Research results reveal that either sperm quality or pregnancy rate rose in men after treatment with oral antioxidants, such as vitamins C and E, zinc, and folate.[19]

In addition to these therapies, physicians can harvest ova and obtain semen to assist fertilization and implantation. For example, if a couple has problems with sperm reaching the cervix, cervical conditions that are hostile to sperm, or the health of the sperm themselves, a physician may suggest artificial insemination, which has been practiced in the United States for more than 50 years. During this procedure, semen is placed in the cervical opening during the time of ovulation. With intrauterine insemination, concentrated sperm are placed in the uterus.

birth control (contraception) Methods to prevent pregnancy.

abstinence A method of birth control that involves refraining from vaginal intercourse.

Women who have no uterine tubes or blocked tubes that do not respond to surgery often choose in vitro fertilization (IVF) to conceive. *In vitro* means "in a test tube" or "in the laboratory." In vitro fertilization involves fertilization of ova with sperm in laboratory glassware, with subsequent implantation of zygotes (fertilized eggs) in the woman's uterus. The birth of the first baby conceived through in vitro fertilization took place in 1978.

In 1992, a new IVF technique called intracytoplasmic sperm injection, or ICSI, was developed to fertilize eggs directly. Early IVF techniques involved putting eggs and sperm together and allowing sperm to swim to and fertilize the eggs. In the late 1980s, a technique was developed in which a few sperm were injected into the space between the egg and its barrier, increasing the chance of fertilization. The ICSI technique involves injecting a single sperm directly into the egg. It is used when men have a very low sperm count, nonmotile sperm, or sperm unable to penetrate the chemical barrier that protects the egg.

Any treatment of infertility in which the sperm and eggs are both handled outside of the body is called assisted reproductive technology. Although assisted reproductive technology has been helpful, studies urge some caution. The use of assisted reproductive technology increases the risk of multiple births and infants born with low birth weights (under 5.5 pounds) for both multiple births and single births. These risks increase the chances of long-term neurological problems such as cerebral palsy.[20]

Contraception

Most of the time, people engage in sexual intercourse for nonreproductive reasons. The timing may not be right for a pregnancy, or their family may be complete. Therefore, couples usually use some form of **birth control (contraception)**, which are methods to avoid pregnancy. You can assess your attitude toward the timing of parenthood by using the self-assessment scale in the Student Workbook pages at the end of the book.

Couples and individuals have many factors to consider when choosing a birth control method. They might consider its cost, effectiveness, reversibility, side effects, ease of use, convenience, and effectiveness against STIs. They must also consider their age and whether they need contraception on a regular basis or if they have only infrequent contraceptive needs. Many people are also concerned about the ways in which a contraceptive interferes with or fits in with their sex life. Some people have religious considerations to think about when making this choice.

Because a woman has a long reproductive life lasting some 30 to 35 years (from her teenage years until age 50, on average), the form of contraception she chooses may vary to meet her needs throughout the stages of her life. A variety of contraceptive methods is available, each with its own risks, benefits, and level of effectiveness. Most methods are based on the female reproductive cycle and rely on a woman taking action. However, many methods can rely on the action of both partners and be incorporated into their sex life.

The effectiveness of a contraceptive method is an important factor to consider. The *theoretical effectiveness* of a contraceptive refers to the number of women who will *not* become pregnant out of 100 couples using a method consistently and properly as their only means of birth control for 1 year. For example, if a method is 80% effective, 80 of 100 women using this method will not become pregnant over a year; 20 women will become pregnant. *Actual effectiveness* refers to the number of women who will *not* become pregnant of 100 couples using a method under usual conditions. Many people forget to use the method or use it improperly, lowering its effectiveness. (Unprotected sex has an effectiveness rate of 15%; 85 out of 100 women will become pregnant over a year.) **Table 5.3** lists the effectiveness of the various forms of birth control.

The "Contraceptive Comfort and Confidence Scale" in the Student Workbook pages at the end of the book can help you assess whether the method of contraception that you are using or considering is, or will be, effective for you.

Abstinence and Natural Methods

With respect to contraception, **abstinence** means refraining from vaginal intercourse. Without this act, a woman cannot get pregnant (unless sperm are introduced artificially into her reproductive tract by a physician or possibly if sperm are deposited at the opening to the vagina and are able to travel into the vagina and then into the uterus). Abstinence is 100% effective and is an excellent alternative for young men and women who feel they are not ready to have sex.

natural family planning (fertility awareness) Formerly called the rhythm method; a group of birth control techniques in which a couple abstains from sexual intercourse during the time of the month when a woman is most likely to conceive.

Table 5.3

Effectiveness of Various Birth Control Methods

Method	Actual Effectiveness (%)	Theoretical Effectiveness (%)
Abstinence	—	100
Fertility awareness	70	91–99
Coitus interruptus (withdrawal)	78	96
Spermicides	72	82
Diaphragm	88	94
Contraceptive sponge (women who have not given birth)	88	91
Contraceptive sponge (women who have given birth)	76	80
Male condom	82	98
Female condom	79	95
Combined oral contraceptives (the pill)	91	99.7
Progestin-only pill (the mini-pill)	91	99.5
Contraceptive patch (Ortho Evra)	91	99.7
Contraceptive vaginal ring (NuvaRing)	91	99.7
Contraceptive implant (Implanon)	99.95	99.95
Depo-Provera	94	99.7
IUDs (across types)	99.2–99.8	99.4–99.9
Female sterilization	99	99.5
Male sterilization	99	99.9

Data from Centers for Disease control and Prevention. (2014). Contraception. Retrieved July 12, 2014, from http://www.cdc.gov/reproductivehealth/UnintendedPregnancy/Contraception.htm

Also, people choose to abstain from sex during various periods of their lives for varied reasons.

Natural family planning, or **fertility awareness** (formerly called the *rhythm method*), is a group of birth control techniques in which a couple abstains from sexual intercourse during the time of the month when a woman is most likely to conceive. Although the theoretical effectiveness of natural family planning/fertility awareness is high—91% to 99% depending on the method—the actual effectiveness of these methods is about 75% because it is often difficult to determine when ovulation has occurred and fertilization can take place. However, when couples consistently use two indicators of fertility, mucus inspection and temperature (the mucothermal method), and strictly adhere to the guidelines of using these methods together, the methods have been shown to be more than 98% effective.[21]

Ovulation usually (but not always) takes place about 14 days before the woman's next menstrual period. If she has sex up to 72 hours before ovulation, she can become pregnant because sperm live approximately this long. The egg survives for approximately 24 hours, so fertilization can occur for 1 day after ovulation also. In summary, fertilization can take place up to 3 days before and 1 day after ovulation.

The time of ovulation varies with the length of a woman's cycle and may vary within cycles of a consistent length. In fact, a woman can ovulate anytime during her cycle and can even become pregnant during her menstrual period. The following are four ways to determine (but without 100% certainty) when ovulation takes place: the temperature method, the calendar method, mucus inspection, and the mucothermal method. All but the calendar method are based on changes that take place in a woman's body around the time of ovulation.

To use the *temperature method*, a woman takes her temperature with a special basal thermometer before she gets out of bed every day for a few months. Because the body temperature usually dips just before and rises just after ovulation (**Figure 5.16**), charting body temperature for a few months can help a woman determine when she ovulates and if ovulation is regular.

coitus interruptus (withdrawal) (KO-ih-tus in-ter-RUP-tus) A form of birth control in which the man removes his penis from his partner's vagina and genital area, interrupting intercourse before ejaculation.

spermicides Chemicals that kill sperm.

To use *mucus inspection*, a woman notes when her cervical mucus changes consistency. Four days before ovulation, cervical mucus (which flows to the vagina) becomes clearer and thinner. She should avoid intercourse from this time until the mucus changes back to its cloudier, thicker appearance. The *mucothermal method* combines this method with the temperature method described in the previous paragraph.

To use the *calendar method*, the woman records the length of her menstrual cycles for a year, beginning on day 1 of menstrual bleeding. After determining the length of her shortest and longest cycles, she uses a chart or formula provided by her healthcare practitioner to determine which days of the month she could become pregnant. This method works best when a woman has cycles that are consistently the same length. If a woman's cycle varies greatly, "safe" times within her cycle will be shorter than if her cycles are more regular.

Figure 5.16

Basal Body Temperature Variations During the Menstrual Cycle. In this graph, basal body temperature is shown to vary during this "model" menstrual cycle. The time of ovulation is determined by noting the fall in temperature just before ovulation and the rise over 3 days just after. Remember, most menstrual cycles are not as regular as this model cycle. Safe days vary widely among women and may vary widely among an individual woman's cycles. The days prior to ovulation are considered "unsafe" because a woman does not yet know whether ovulation has occurred.

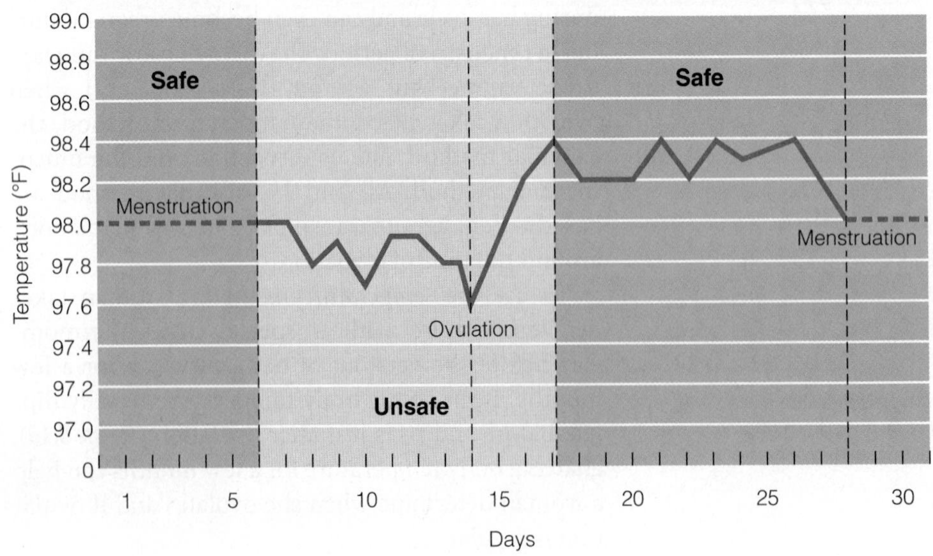

Coitus interruptus, or **withdrawal**, is another natural form of birth control. To use this method, the man senses when he is close to ejaculation, and then removes his penis from his partner's vagina and genital area, interrupting intercourse. There are many problems with this method. A man must exercise a great deal of self-control, removing his penis from the vagina at a time when his desire may be to thrust more deeply. Also, he must be able to sense when he has enough time to remove himself before ejaculation. Additionally, sperm from a recent ejaculation may be present in the urethra and may be carried to the tip of the penis with drops of preejaculatory fluid and result in pregnancy. To reduce the possibility of sperm in the preejaculate, a man should urinate after ejaculation and carefully clean all semen from the penis. With perfect use, coitus interruptus is 96% effective. However, during actual use this form of contraception is only 78% effective. None of the natural methods of birth control protects against the transmission of STIs.

Chemical Methods

Spermicides are chemicals that kill sperm. The most common active ingredient in spermicides marketed in the United States is nonoxynol-9. The inactive ingredients make up the carrier, or base, of the spermicides, which are sold as foams, creams, jellies, films, suppositories, and tablets. (Spermicides are also added to many brands of condoms.) The carrier distributes the spermicide in the vaginal canal. Shortly before vaginal sex, foams, creams, and jellies are placed high in the vagina near the cervix using an applicator, as shown in **Figure 5.17** (a and b). Spermicidal films are placed near the cervix. Suppositories and tablets are placed in the vagina and given time to dissolve. Correct placement of the spermicide and timing of insertion are critical to the spermicide's effectiveness, which is 82% if these products are used correctly and consistently (i.e., theoretical effectiveness), and the actual effectiveness is 72%.

Advantages to using spermicides are that the side effects (such as allergy and vaginal irritation or infection) are minimal, they are used only when birth control is needed, and they are easy products to obtain over the counter. Disadvantages are a low rate of effectiveness and an increase in the frequency of genital irritation and lesions caused by nonoxynol-9. The presence of genital lesions and irritated membranes increase the risk of contracting a sexually transmitted infection such as HIV during intercourse with an infected partner.[22]

douching (DOOSH-ing) The use of specially prepared solutions to cleanse the vagina; not an effective birth control method.

Some women use **douching** as a contraceptive method. Douching is the use of specially prepared solutions to cleanse the vagina. Douching is *not* effective for contraception. By the time a woman can

Figure 5.17

Contraceptive Foam and Jelly, Diaphragm, FemCap, and Lea's Shield. (a) Contraceptive foam or jelly is placed high up in the vagina, covering the cervix, using a plunger-type applicator. (b) Contraceptive jelly and applicator. (c) The diaphragm is ringed with contraceptive spermicide prior to insertion. The diaphragm is pinched to narrow it and is then placed high in the vagina, covering the cervix. (d) Diaphragm.

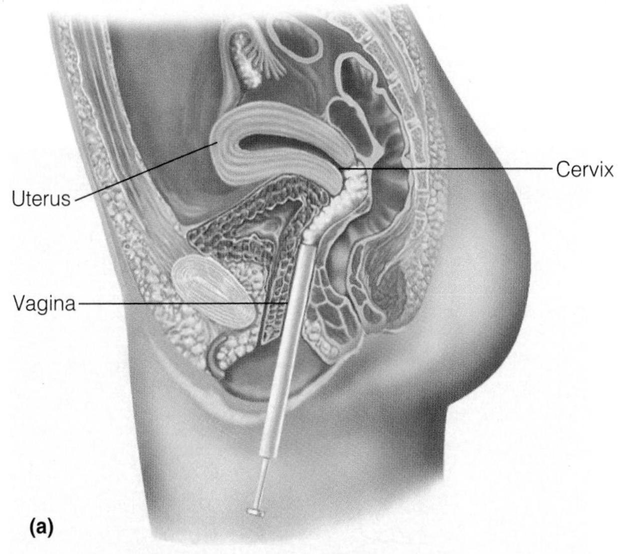

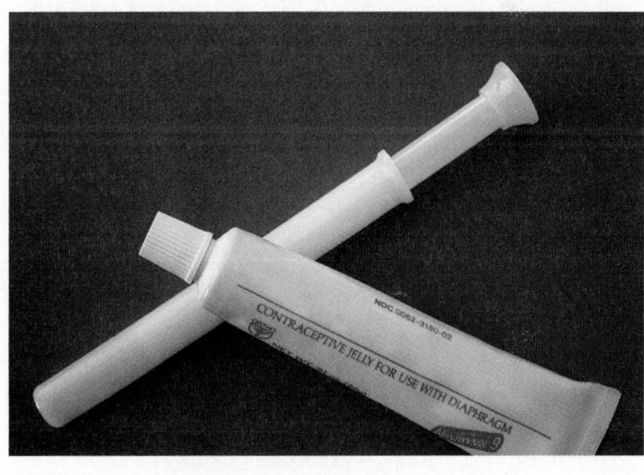

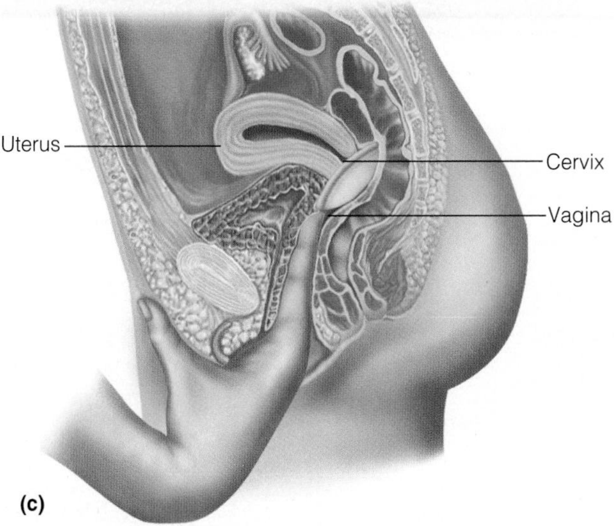

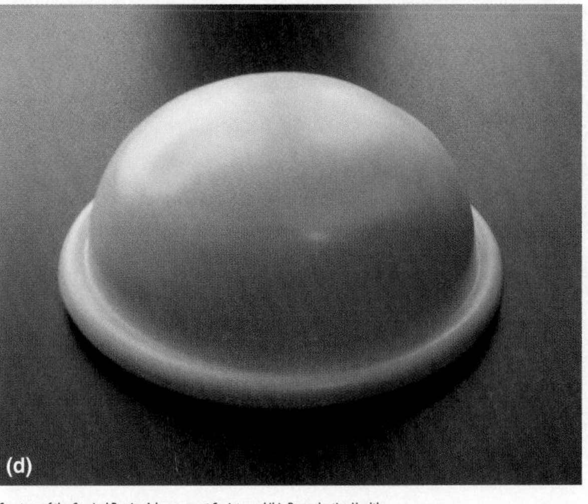

Courtesy of the Cervical Barrier Advancement Society and Ibis Reproductive Health.

barrier methods Types of birth control that block the path that sperm must take to reach the ovum; these forms of contraception include male condoms, female condoms, diaphragms, and cervical caps.

douche after sexual intercourse, sperm have already reached the cervix and uterus and cannot be washed away. In addition, if a woman has used a contraceptive product containing spermicide or has used spermicide alone as a contraceptive, douching may wash away the chemical and render it inactive.

Barrier Methods

Barrier methods of contraception block the path that sperm must take to reach the ovum. These forms of contraception include diaphragms, cervical caps, male condoms, and female condoms.

Diaphragms and Diaphragm-like Products The diaphragm has been in use in the United States for over 60 years. Shown in Figure 5.17c and Figure 5.17d, a *diaphragm* is a dome-shaped rubber cup bordered by a flexible spring that is designed to cover the cervix and surrounding area. This

Figure 5.17 (Continued)

(e) A small amount of spermicide is spread on the rim and brim of the side of the FemCap that will face outward, away from the cervix. A larger amount of spermicide is spread in the groove on the side of the FemCap that will face inward, toward the cervix. The FemCap is pinched to narrow it and is then placed high in the vagina with the bowl facing upward and the long brim entering first. The FemCap is placed to cover the cervix completely. (f) FemCap. (g) Lea's Shield. This contraceptive device is also pinched for insertion and pushed up into the vagina as far as it can go. It is used in conjunction with spermicide.

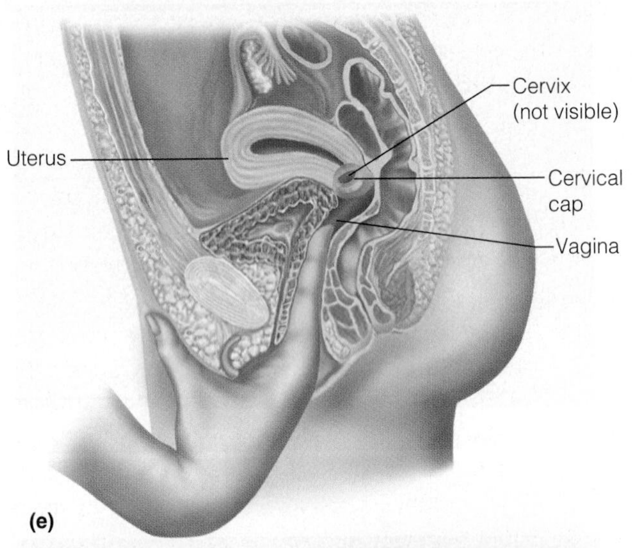

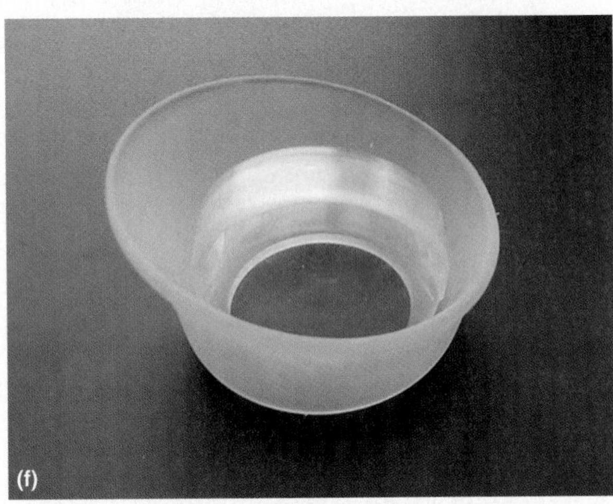

Courtesy of the Cervical Barrier Advancement Society and Ibis Reproductive Health.

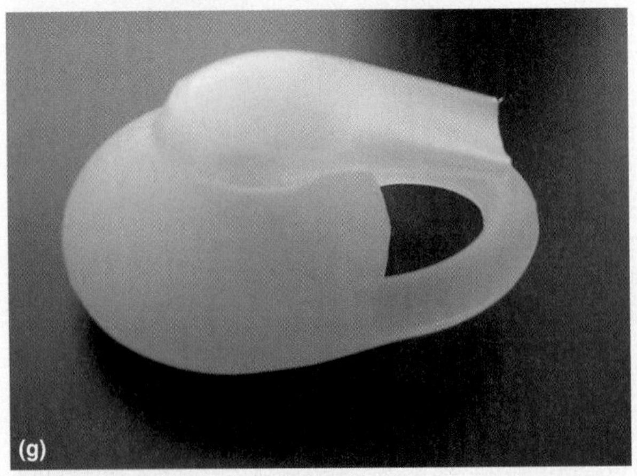

Courtesy of the Cervical Barrier Advancement Society and Ibis Reproductive Health.

prescription item must be fitted by a healthcare practitioner.

Before inserting a diaphragm, place spermicide on both its sides and around its rim. Compress the spring, collapsing the diaphragm so that it can be inserted into the vagina. When the diaphragm reaches the cervical area, its spring pops open, causing the diaphragm to assume its dome shape and to be held firmly in place over the cervix.

After insertion, a diaphragm is effective for 6 hours, so a woman could insert the diaphragm well before sexual intercourse. However, spermicide must be added before each additional act of intercourse. After the last intercourse, the diaphragm must be left in place for at least 6 hours but must not be worn for more than 24 hours because of risk of infection. Used properly and consistently, the diaphragm is 94% effective.

The Today Vaginal Contraceptive Sponge, an over-the-counter single-use, disposable *sponge* that contains spermicide and is used like a diaphragm, was taken off the market in the United States in 1995. The Food and Drug Administration (FDA) discovered that the water system used in the manufacture of the product was contaminated with bacteria that cause diarrhea, although the sponges were never shown to be contaminated with this pathogen. A New Jersey pharmaceutical company purchased the Today sponge from its original manufacturer in 1999. The FDA approved U.S. sales of the Today sponge in April 2005.

In 2002, the FDA approved *Lea's Shield*, a diaphragm-like vaginal barrier contraceptive. The shield, shown in Figure 5.17g, is composed of three parts: a bowl, a one-way valve, and a loop. After coating the inside of the bowl around the hole, the front of the rim, and the outer part of the valve with spermicide, pinch the rim of the shield and slide the device high up in the vagina. The bowl of the shield covers the cervix. The valve vents air during insertion, which creates a suction that helps hold the shield in place.

The loop is used to remove the device and to prevent its rotation during use. Lea's Shield can be inserted up to 24 hours prior to intercourse and should remain in place for 8 hours afterward but for no longer than 48 hours total. The actual effectiveness of the shield is 85%.

The *cervical cap* works much the same way as the diaphragm, but it is smaller and covers only the cervix. In 2003, the FDA approved the FemCap (Figure 5.17f). Like Lea's Shield, the FemCap can be inserted up to 24 hours prior to intercourse and should remain in place for 8 hours afterward but for no longer than 48 hours total. Before inserting, put a small amount of spermicide in the dome of the FemCap, spread a thin layer on the brim, and put a small amount in the folded area between the brim and the dome. The FemCap is inserted with the long brim entering first and the dome-side down. The actual effectiveness of the FemCap is 86%.

Condoms A **condom** is a sheath, usually made of thin latex or polyurethane, that covers the erect penis (male condom) or lines the vagina and covers the labia (female condom) to provide a barrier against fertilization or sexually transmitted infections.

Male condoms, the only form of birth control presently available for men other than vasectomy, are one of the most popular forms of birth control in the United States. Used for the prevention of pregnancy, condoms are 82% effective with actual use and 98% effective with consistent and proper use.

Figure 5.18 illustrates the correct procedure for putting on a male condom. Always read and follow the instructions provided by the manufacturer. Before opening a condom, verify that it has not expired and that there is an air bubble inside the wrapper by holding the condom between—and gently pressing with—your thumb and index finger. Do not used expired condoms or condoms that come from packaging that is torn or looks brittle or worn. Carefully open the wrapper, being sure not to tear or rip the condom. Visually inspect the condom to make sure it does not have any defects. Hold the tip of the condom away from the penis to determine which way it rolls. If you place the condom on the tip of the penis and it will not roll down, do not flip it over; discard the condom and select a new condom. Put the condom on after the penis has become erect but before there is genital contact with a partner. Hold the top half-inch of the condom, squeezing the air out. This space will form a reservoir for semen. If air is not removed from this space, the semen cannot collect at the condom tip, and the condom is more likely to break during intercourse. Place the rolled-up condom over the head of the penis (Figure 5.18a). While still holding the tip, unroll the condom to cover the penis to its base (Figure 5.18b and c). Gently smooth out any air that may have been trapped between the condom and the penis. After ejaculation, hold the condom firmly at its base to prevent slippage while you withdraw the still-erect penis from your partner's body. Remove the condom from the penis (Figure 5.18d), being careful not to spill semen on your partner and not to touch the exterior of the condom to your genital area, because the outside of the condom may have become

combined oral contraceptives "The pill" suppresses ovulation through the combined actions of estrogen and progestin.

contaminated from an infected partner. Check the used condom carefully to ensure it was not ruptured during intercourse; if any ruptures are found, other methods of contraception and STI prevention can be used. Discard the used condom.

Approved by the FDA in 1993, the Reality female condom, a polyurethane sheath with a ring at each end, lines the vagina. Female condoms, used consistently and properly as a form of birth control, are approximately 95% effective. Their actual effectiveness, however, is 79%.

Figure 5.19 shows a female condom and the correct procedure for inserting one: Holding the closed end of the condom, squeeze the ring inside the condom so that it flattens and can be inserted into the vagina (Figure 5.19a). Insert the flattened ring and condom into the vagina (Figure 5.19b), gently pushing it up to the cervix as shown in Figure 5.19c. You should be able to feel the ring positioned past the pubic bone. Straighten out the part of the condom lining the vagina if it is twisted. The outside ring should cover the labia, as shown in Figure 5.19d. After intercourse, first twist the condom to close it at the vaginal opening, which will prevent sperm and pathogens from touching your genital area. Remove the condom with gentle pulling and discard. Female and male condoms are intended for one-time use.

Hormonal Methods

There are two basic types of hormonal contraception: combined estrogen and progestin contraceptives, and progestin-only contraceptives. With the exception of progesterone-only mini-pills, hormonal methods of birth control prevent pregnancy by suppressing ovulation.

Combined Estrogen and Progestin Contraceptives **Combined oral contraceptives** (COCs; "the pill") suppress ovulation through the combined actions of estrogen and progestin (a synthetic form

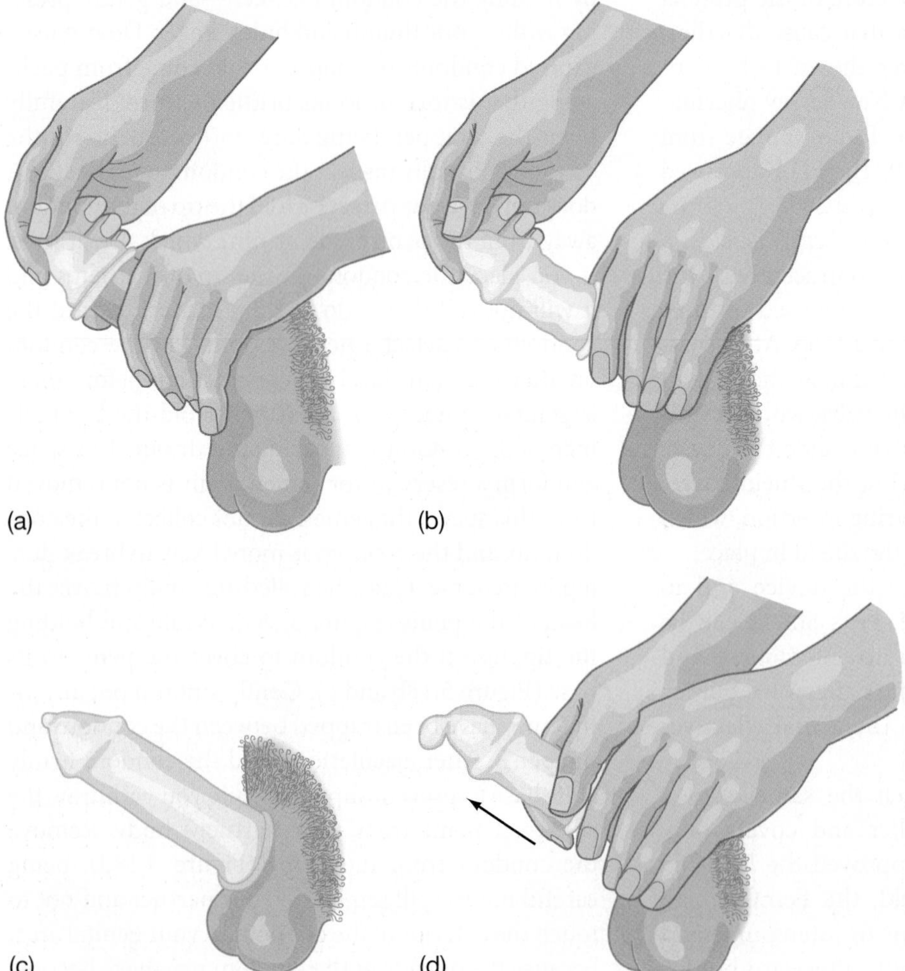

Figure 5.18

How to Put on a Male Condom. The text explains each step.

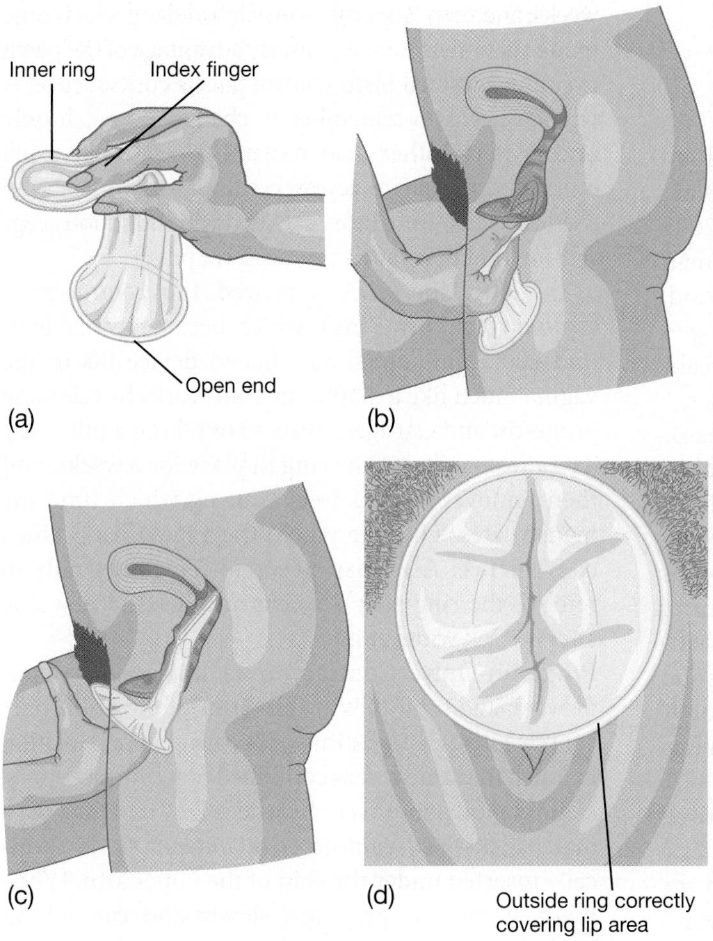

Figure 5.19

How to Insert a Female Condom. The text explains each step.

of progesterone). With the exception of extended-cycle oral contraceptives (Seasonale and Seasonique) and Lybrel, which are described later in this section, menstruation occurs monthly.

The Guttmacher Institute notes that the pill is the most common method of birth control reported by women who use birth control methods (64%).[23] The pill has numerous advantages. It is highly effective, decreases menstrual cramps, decreases the length of the menses and the amount of blood lost, has a protective effect against pelvic inflammatory disease, reduces the risk for ovarian and endometrial cancer (cancer of the uterine lining), reduces the risk for benign (noncancerous) breast disease, and helps prevent osteoporosis (thinning of the bones). The pill is a readily reversible form of contraception.

COCs have been available since 1960 and are some of the best-studied prescription medications. The amount of estrogen and progestin in pills has decreased over the years, so today's pills are much safer than pills of the past. Cardiovascular disease is the most serious complication of the pill. Women at high risk for developing this complication of COC use are those who are older than 50 years of age or who are older than 35 years of age and smoke cigarettes. Women who are sedentary, overweight, and have high blood pressure, diabetes mellitus, or an elevated serum cholesterol level are also at high risk. **Table 5.4** lists symptoms that may warn of a potential health complication when using the pill. The mnemonic (memory aid) ACHES can help you remember these symptoms.

A review of studies on the risk of cervical cancer in women taking COCs reveals that risk increases with increasing duration of use.[24] The studies included women on combined oral contraceptives and some on progestin-only preparations, which are discussed shortly. Risk was shown to decline after use stopped. After 10 years, the risk was the same as that for women who never used oral contraceptives.

Extended-cycle oral contraceptives contain lower doses of hormones than conventional birth control pills and are taken for 84 days instead of the usual 21 before menstruation occurs. With this pill, a woman has only four menstrual periods per year, one each season, instead of the usual 13. In addition

intrauterine device (IUD) A small contraceptive device that either is covered with copper or contains a reservoir of progestin and is inserted into the uterus.

to suppressing ovulation, this pill prevents buildup of the lining of the uterus. Therefore, the menses are light. Seasonale was approved by the FDA in 2003 and Seasonique in 2006. With Seasonale, a woman takes an inactive pill during the days of her period, and with Seasonique, she takes a low-dose estrogen pill. The low-dose estrogen appears to reduce breakthrough bleeding during the time between menses.

Lybrel was approved by the FDA in 2007. Like Seasonale and Seasonique it is a low-dose pill, but it is taken 365 days per year. Over time menstruation stops, but a woman may experience some breakthrough bleeding and spotting, especially during the first few months of use. Thus, a woman choosing to use this form of COC should weigh the convenience of not menstruating with the uncertainty of breakthrough bleeding and spotting. The health benefits, health risks, and theoretical effectiveness of Lybrel, Seasonale, and Seasonique are comparable to other COCs.

The *contraceptive patch* (Ortho Evra) was approved by the FDA in 2001 and became available in late April 2002. The patch delivers hormones through the skin for 1 week. A woman uses three patches over 3 weeks, and then "goes off" the patch, during which time menstruation occurs. A primary advantage of the patch over conventional birth control pills is convenience: A woman needs to remember to change the patch only once a week rather than remembering to take a pill every day. Results of research show that women who used the patch were more satisfied with this contraceptive method than with contraceptive pills.[25]

In 2001, the FDA approved the *contraceptive vaginal ring* (NuvaRing), which became available in mid-2002. This doughnut-shaped device fits in the vagina much like a diaphragm but works by releasing progestin and estrogen. Instead of taking a pill every day, a woman keeps the ring in place for 3 weeks, and then removes it for 1 week, during which time she menstruates. Like the patch, the vaginal ring offers convenience: A woman needs to remember only to remove the ring after 3 weeks and insert a new one after a week without it.

Progestin-Only Contraceptives Implanon, Depo-Provera, and mini-pills are all forms of progestin-only contraceptives. Progestin works to suppress ovulation in much the same way as combined oral contraceptives.

Implanon, approved by the FDA in 2006, is a matchstick-sized *contraceptive implant*. It is surgically inserted under the skin of the upper arm. While there, it releases progestin slowly and can inhibit ovulation for 3 years.

Depo-Provera, which has been used in the United States since 1992, is an injection of progestin that inhibits ovulation for 3 months. *Mini-pills* are progestin-only pills that are taken continually, which were introduced in 1970.

Although highly effective, progestin-only contraceptives have a few serious disadvantages. These contraceptives change a woman's menstrual cycle. In addition to amenorrhea (no periods), these changes can include opposite effects: an increased number of days of menstruation with light bleeding or an increased number of days with heavy bleeding. Women find some of these changes unacceptable. Another disadvantage is that long-term use of progestin-only contraceptives may cause thinning of the bones because of low estrogen.

Table 5.4

Warning Signs and Symptoms of a Potential Health Complication When Using "The Pill" or an IUD

Pill	IUD
A Abdominal pain (severe)	**P** Period is late; abnormal spotting or bleeding
C Chest pain (severe), shortness of breath	**A** Abdominal pain or pain with intercourse
H Headache (severe), may include dizziness, weakness, numbness	**I** Infection (sexually transmitted) exposure, abnormal discharge
E Eye problems: vision loss, blurring, double vision, flashing lights	**N** Not feeling well, fever, chills
S Sudden, severe leg or arm pain; leg or arm numbness	**S** String is missing or is shorter or longer

Intrauterine Devices

An **intrauterine device (IUD)** is a small apparatus that a healthcare practitioner inserts into the uterus (**Figure 5.20**). A string hangs from the base of the IUD and extends into the vagina; the presence of the string is an indication that the IUD is still in place. The active ingredient of the IUD is either copper, which covers the IUD, or progestin, which is contained in a reservoir within the IUD.

IUDs are among the safest, most effective, and least expensive reversible contraceptives available. Although their modes of action aren't precisely understood, IUDs seem to work primarily by inhibiting the ability of sperm to reach and fertilize the egg. IUDs also appear to thin the uterine lining and sometimes may prevent ovulation. Table 5.4 lists signs and symptoms that may warn of a potential health complication when using an IUD. The mnemonic PAINS can help you remember these symptoms.

Emergency Contraception

Emergency contraception (EC) helps prevent pregnancy *after* sexual intercourse, rather than before or during sex. Therefore, some types of EC are called "the morning-after pill." Despite the nickname, EC does not have to be used right away but can be used up to 3 to 5 days after sex, depending on the method. Women often choose EC if they did not use another form of contraception or if they think their method did not work (e.g., a condom was used, but it ruptured). EC can also be used in cases of rape.

Emergency contraception methods are not 100% effective, but they reduce the likelihood that a woman will become pregnant by about 75% after unprotected sex or after sex with a method that has failed. Because of the lower level of effectiveness of EC compared to other birth control methods, it is not a wise choice for use as a woman's primary method. Like most forms of birth control, EC does not protect against sexually transmitted infections.

Three types of emergency contraception are currently available in the United States: a progestin-only pill (Plan B One-Step®), various brands of combined oral contraceptives, and insertion of the copper IUD. Both types of emergency contraceptive pills do one of three things, depending when in the cycle they are taken and whether fertilization has already taken place: They temporarily stop the release of an egg from the ovary, they prevent fertilization, or they prevent a fertilized egg from implanting in the uterine wall. Emergency contraception will not abort an embryo already implanted. Insertion of the copper IUD works in the latter two ways as emergency contraception. The Plan B One-Step® emergency contraceptive was first approved for use without a

> **emergency contraception (EC)** Birth control methods that help prevent pregnancy after sexual intercourse, rather than before or during sex.

Figure 5.20

The Intrauterine Device. An IUD is a small apparatus that is inserted into the uterus. The active ingredient of an IUD is either copper or progestin. The far right photo shows two typical IUDs.

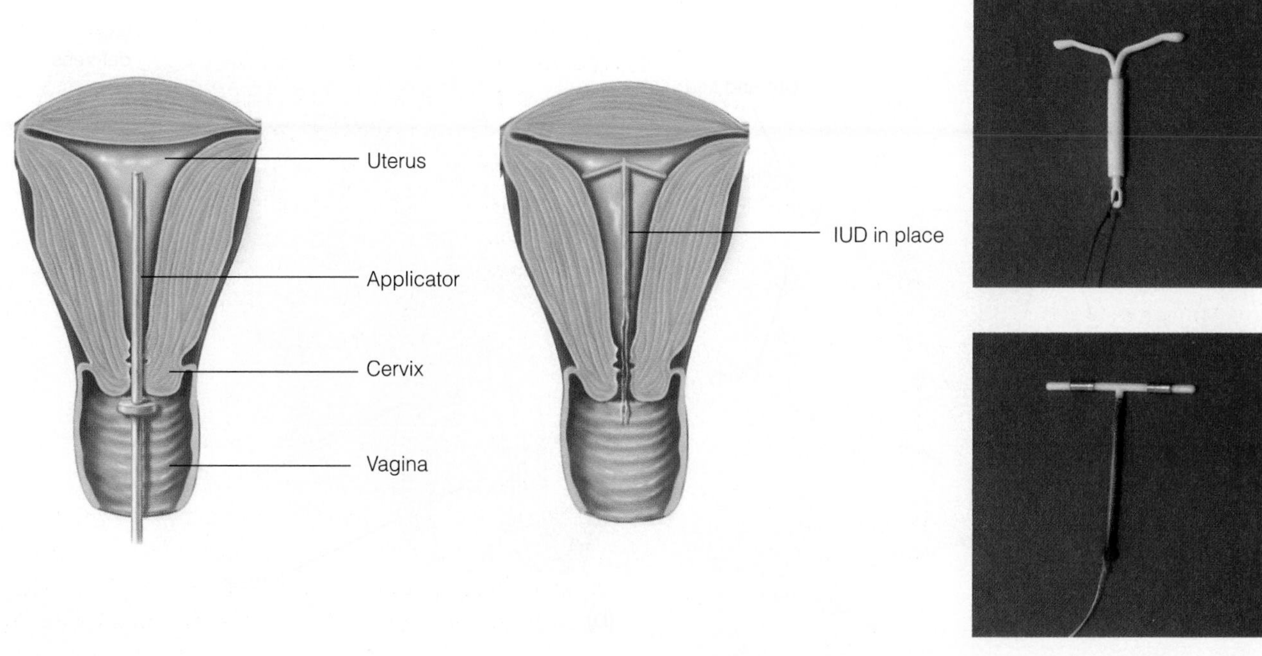

sterilization A permanent form of birth control that requires a surgical procedure.

tubal ligation Female sterilization that is performed by cutting and tying off the uterine tubes so that the sperm and egg cannot unite.

vasectomy Male sterilization that is performed by cutting and tying off the vas deferens to prevent sperm from becoming part of the ejaculate.

prescription in 2009 but was limited to women age 17 and older; in 2013, the FDA approvedits use as an over-the-counter product for all women of child-bearing age, which removed the age restriction, thus making it available to all women of all ages.[26] IUDs still require a prescription, and insertion by a trained medical practitioner.

Sterilization

Sterilization is a permanent form of birth control. In the past, sterilization was available only as a surgical procedure, but in 2002 the FDA approved a nonsurgical, irreversible method of female sterilization called Essure. Using a local anesthetic, a physician inserts a tiny spring into each fallopian tube by passing it through the vagina and then the uterus. Over 3 months, the spring irritates the tube, causing it to produce scar tissue that blocks the tube. After the 3-month period, a physician injects dye into the uterus and up into the tubes. An x-ray of the dye-injected area shows whether the tubes are fully blocked.

The surgical form of female sterilization is a **tubal ligation**, which involves cutting and tying off the uterine tubes by means of clips, rings, or burning so that the sperm and egg cannot unite. Male sterilization is a **vasectomy**, which involves cutting and tying off the vas deferens to prevent sperm from becoming part of the ejaculate. Tubal ligation is a medically more complicated and more costly procedure than vasectomy, but both are highly effective. Failure is most often the result of surgical error or the spontaneous rejoining of the tubes. **Figure 5.21** illustrates tubal ligation and vasectomy.

The surgical forms of sterilization can be reversed, but subsequent pregnancy rates vary depending on factors such as the type of procedure that was performed, the health of the tubes being rejoined, and the health and age of the patient. Microsurgical techniques provide excellent success rates.

Abortion

Sometimes contraceptive methods fail and an unplanned pregnancy occurs that a woman or a couple chooses to terminate. Sometimes pregnancy

Figure 5.21

Sterilization Methods. Female sterilization (a), or tubal ligation, involves cutting and tying off the fallopian tubes. Male sterilization (b), or vasectomy, involves cutting and tying off the vas deferens.

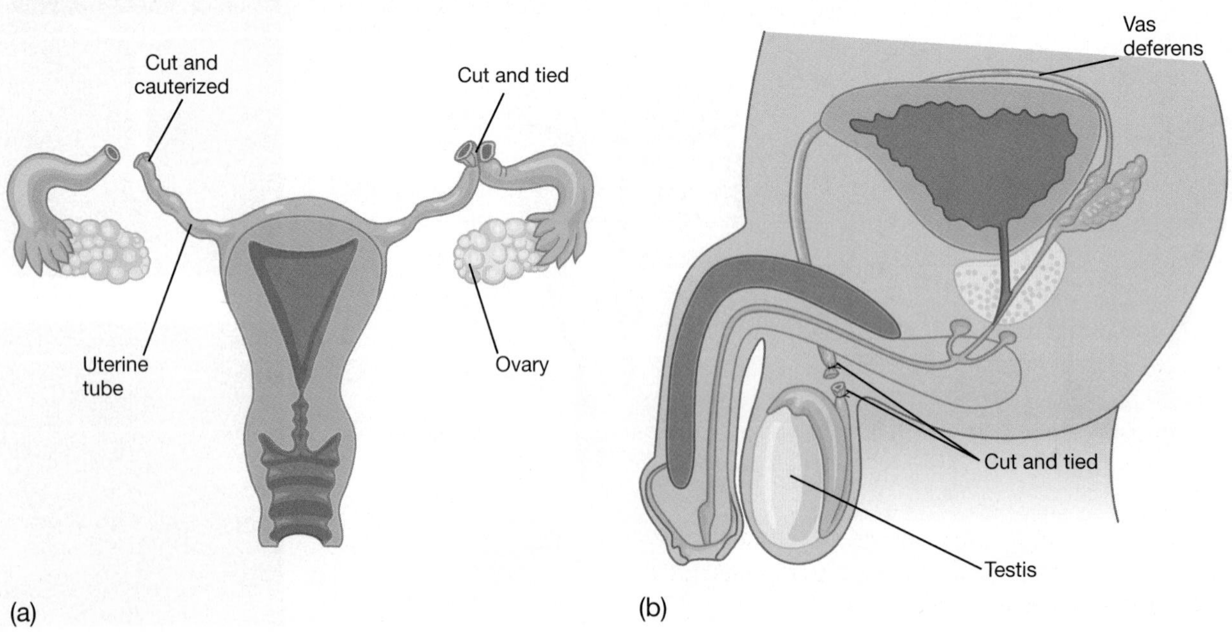

seriously jeopardizes a woman's health and ending the pregnancy is the only means of saving her life. There are numerous other reasons why women and couples choose to terminate a pregnancy.

A controversial 1973 United States Supreme Court decision (*Roe v. Wade*) ruled that induced abortion is a legal medical procedure. States may regulate abortions in the second trimester to protect the health of the pregnant woman, but the decision to end a pregnancy during the first trimester is the private concern of a woman and her healthcare practitioner.

An **abortion** is the removal of the embryo or fetus from the uterus before it is able to survive on its own. During a *spontaneous abortion*, the body expels the embryo, usually because of serious genetic defects, although there may be other causes. Spontaneous abortions (miscarriages) generally occur during the first trimester. Ten percent to 20% of pregnancies end in spontaneous abortion.

An *induced abortion* is one that does not happen on its own. It is caused by taking certain drugs (a medical abortion) or by having certain physical procedures performed (a surgical abortion). During the first trimester, both types of abortions can be performed.

A **medical abortion** can be performed within 9 weeks of the first day of the last period and uses a combination of the drugs mifepristone and misoprostol. Mifepristone causes changes in the pregnant woman's body so that it cannot sustain the pregnancy and the embryo/fetus detaches from the uterine wall. Misoprostol causes the uterus to contract and expel its contents. According to the Centers for Disease Control and Prevention (CDC), about 13% of abortions are performed this way.[24]

In a **surgical abortion**, a physician physically removes the contents of the uterus. *Vacuum (suction) aspiration* is used from 3 to 12 weeks of gestation. It can be performed in the physician's office in approximately 10 to 20 minutes with the use of a local anesthetic. To perform a vacuum aspiration, the physician dilates (widens) the cervix slightly and inserts a slender, hollow plastic tube through the vagina and cervix into the uterus. The tube is connected to a suction aspirator, which draws the tissue out of the uterus and into a container (**Figure 5.22**).

Vacuum aspiration is used for 78% of abortions;[27] the embryo is less than an inch long at this time. Thus, 91–92% of abortions are performed either medically (using drugs) or with vacuum aspiration early in pregnancy. According to CDC data, most abortions—almost two-thirds—are performed at 8 weeks or less of gestation.[27]

abortion Removal of the embryo or fetus from the uterus before it is able to survive on its own.

medical abortion A method of drug-induced abortion performed within 9 weeks of the first day of the last period.

surgical abortion Includes various methods of induced abortion in which the contents of the uterus are physically removed.

If the abortion is performed between 12 and 15 weeks of gestation, the uterus is often scraped with a tool called a curette after the vacuum aspiration is completed. This procedure is commonly called a *D&C*, which means dilation and curettage.

Abortions that are performed during 15 to 21 weeks of development are performed somewhat like a D&C, but forceps are also used to remove larger pieces of tissue. Therefore, the cervix must be dilated to a greater extent to allow the entry of the forceps. This procedure is called a dilation and evacuation, or *D&E*. General anesthesia is often used for this procedure. According to the CDC, only about 7% of abortions are performed between 14 and 20 weeks of gestation.[27]

Figure 5.22

Vacuum (Suction) Aspiration. During this procedure, a thin, hollow tube is inserted through the vagina and cervix to the uterus. A suction aspirator (vacuum pump) draws tissue out of the uterus and into a container.

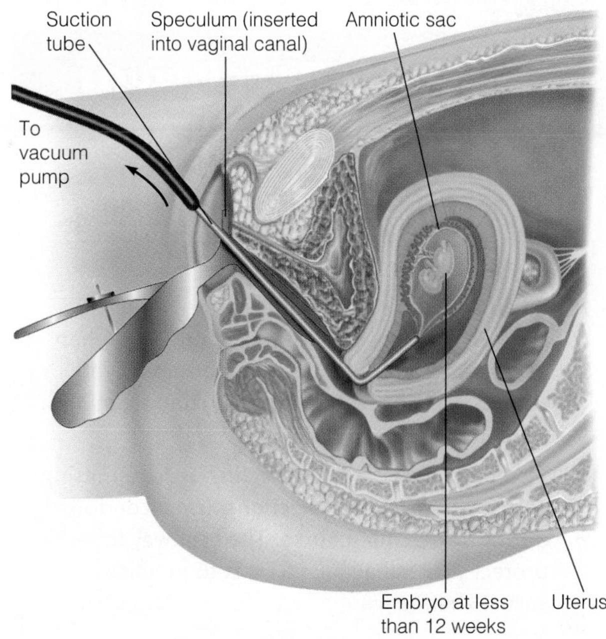

menarche (meh-NAR-key) The first menstruation.

There are two basic methods of abortion for the 1% that is performed at 21 weeks of gestation or more: induction, and intact dilation and extraction. *Induction* is a form of abortion in which labor is artificially induced (started). Saline abortions are one method of induction: A physician inserts a long needle through the abdominal wall and into the amniotic sac. A salt solution is injected into the sac, which causes the quick death of the fetus. The uterus begins contractions within 12 to 24 hours, and the woman delivers a dead fetus. This procedure is performed using a local anesthetic. Other types of solutions and prostaglandins (hormone-like substances that cause the uterus to contract) are also used for induction.

A special type of D&E procedure called an *intact dilation and extraction* (IDX or intact D&X) is the so-called partial birth abortion procedure. President George W. Bush signed the Partial-Birth Abortion Ban Act in November 2003, which criminalizes the procedure. Physicians from many states challenged the constitutionality of the law. Three federal judges from California, New York, and Nebraska ruled that the legislation had many constitutional defects and rejected the ban. The question of the constitutionality of the law went to the Supreme Court, and on April 18, 2007, the high court ruled in a 5–4 decision that the federal Partial-Birth Abortion Ban Act of 2003 was constitutional.

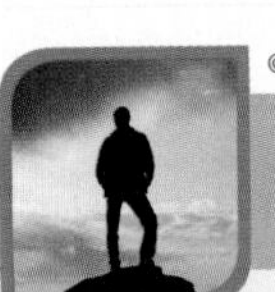

© djgis/ShutterStock

Healthy Living Practices

- The most effective means to prevent an unwanted pregnancy are sexual abstinence, the use of an IUD, and sterilization, followed closely by hormonal methods.
- If you are using a hormonal method of birth control, consult your healthcare provider when you are taking antibiotics to determine if you should use a backup method of contraception while taking this medication.
- To reduce the risk of contracting or transmitting sexually transmitted infections, use a condom during sexual intercourse. The best way to protect yourself against STIs is to practice sexual abstinence.

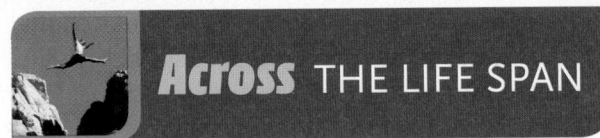

Across THE LIFE SPAN

© Galina Barskaya/ShutterStock

SEXUAL DEVELOPMENT

The gender of an individual is set at the time of fertilization and is determined by the type of sex chromosomes (genes) it receives from its parents. Females have two X chromosomes; males have an X and a Y.

During the 7th week of development, the embryo with a Y chromosome begins to develop testes. The developing testes secrete male hormones collectively called androgens. These hormones direct the development of a male reproductive system. Embryos and fetuses without a Y chromosome begin to develop ovaries during the 9th week. The absence of androgens results in the development of a female reproductive system.

After birth, the secretion of the androgen testosterone in male babies nearly ceases and does not resume until puberty, the time of sexual maturation. The female reproductive system does not become active until that time as well.

Puberty is a stage of development during which the endocrine (hormone) and reproductive systems mature. Puberty begins at approximately 10 to 11 years of age and concludes about 5 or 6 years later. Girls usually enter puberty about 2 years earlier than boys do. Scientists do not know what triggers this developmental process.

During childhood, the production of a hormone that stimulates the release of male and female sex hormones is suppressed. At the onset of puberty, the suppression ceases and the brain begins releasing the hormone that regulates the production of testosterone in males and estrogen in females. As puberty proceeds, the brain secretes greater and greater amounts of this hormone; thus more and more testosterone or estrogen is secreted. These hormones stimulate the physical changes of puberty. These changes include growth spurts resulting from the growth of the skeleton (especially the long bones), the development of pubic and underarm hair, and the growth and maturation of the reproductive tract.

In males, building levels of testosterone result in an enlarging of the testes and penis, deepening of the voice as a result of an enlargement of the voice box, development of facial hair, broadening of the shoulders, and enlargement of the arm, chest, and leg muscles. Under the direction of testosterone, the seminiferous tubules

Diversity in Health

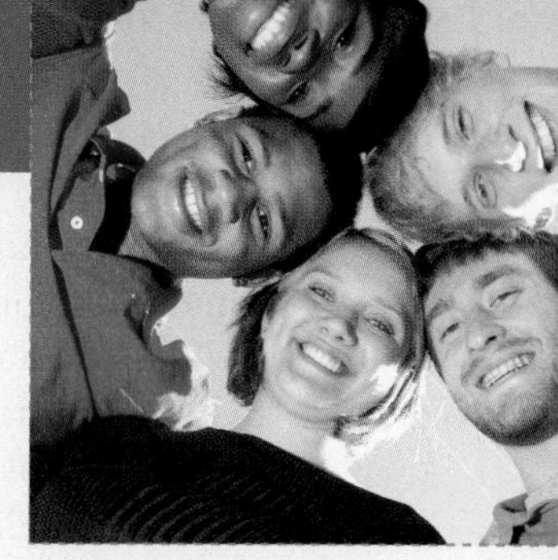
© Mike Flippo/ShutterStock

Menopause

Menopause is a time of transition for every woman who reaches her 50s, but transition is about the only thing women universally experience during this time. The symptoms of menopause and attitudes regarding this process vary extensively among women across cultures. Why do these differences exist?

One hypothesis is that if a society regards menopause as a positive time, the symptoms of menopause reported by its women will decrease in number and severity. Certain evidence seems to support this hypothesis. For example, during their childbearing years, the Rajput women of Northern India are socially constrained and cannot move about freely in their villages. Those who no longer menstruate are freed of this constraint. Interestingly, these women report no symptoms of menopause. Similarly, Mayan women look upon menopause as a lifting of the burden of childbearing. They, too, report no symptoms of hot flashes or cold sweats such as are typically reported by North American women. Yanomamo women (forest-dwellers who live near the border between Brazil and Venezuela) eagerly await menopause, which is considered the time of "older age," for this time of life bringsincreased status and decision-making power in their society.

In a multiethnic study of U.S. women, Green and Santoro found that most menopausal symptoms varied by ethnicity and culture as well. Night sweats and hot flashes were reported more often by African American and Hispanic women, whereas vaginal dryness was reported most often by Hispanic women. And even though other menopausal symptoms varied among Hispanic women, the symptoms correlated with their country of origin.

Nevertheless, the diversity of the symptoms and experiences of women of various cultures regarding menopause cannot be attributed solely to differences in culture. Ayers, Forshaw, and Hunter took a broader look at the correlation between menopausal symptoms and attitudes toward menopause, conducting a review of cross-cultural studies on the subject. The researchers determined that women with more negative attitudes toward menopause reported more symptoms of menopause when experiencing this life transition, and those with less negative attitudes experienced fewer symptoms.

Menopausal symptoms and experiences must also be evaluated in the context of risk factors for death and disease. But just as it affects attitudes, culture affects lifestyle, and lifestyle affects health. Thus, culturally influenced lifestyles affect susceptibility to disease, the aging process, and the quality of life and, in turn, may account for some of the differences in the perception of menopausal symptoms among women. Cultural differences in the experience of menopause exist but appear to be so intertwined with the various facets of a woman's life that the effect of culture alone may be difficult to assess.

Data from Ayers, B., et al. (2010). The impact of attitudes towards the menopause on women's symptom experience: A systematic review. *Maturitas, 65*(1), 28–36; Green, R., & Santoro, N. (2009). Menopausal symptoms and ethnicity: The study of women's health across the nation. *Women's Health, 5*(2), 127–133; and Melby, M. K., et al. (2005). Culture and symptom reporting at menopause. *Human Reproduction Update, 11*, 495–512.

begin manufacturing sperm. A significant developmental event in pubertal boys is semen emission during sleep, called nocturnal emissions or wet dreams. Initially, sperm are not present in the semen.

In females, estrogen results in the development of the breasts and the rounding of the hips. Females experience **menarche**, the first menstruation, at around 12 years of age. The normal range for menarche is 8 to 15 years of age. A delay of the menarche may occur in girls with chronic diseases, such as diabetes mellitus; those with disorders that affect their nutritional status, such as anorexia nervosa; and those undergoing strenuous training, such as Olympic hopefuls.

When a woman reaches 45 to 55 years of age, most of her ovarian follicles (eggs) have matured, and the remaining follicles are aged. During some months, these aging follicles do not reach maturity and ovulation does not take place. Without mature egg follicles, the normal cyclic secretion of estrogen and progesterone does not occur, and the menses become irregular. Eventually, all follicles stop maturing, estrogen and progesterone are no longer secreted, and the menses cease. The cessation of the menses is called menopause. This term means the final menstrual period, but it is widely used to refer to the few years of transition when a woman passes from her reproductive years to her nonreproductive years. The Diversity in Health essay discusses menopausal symptoms and attitudes across cultures.

As the hormonal changes of menopause take place, women usually experience symptoms such as hot flashes and physiologic changes such as thinning of the vaginal walls and vaginal dryness. In addition, the loss of estrogen results in an increased risk of osteoporosis and heart disease.

In a 2013 report, the International Menopause Society (IMS) updated recommendations on menopausal hormone therapy (MHT), clarifying the sometimes confusing and conflicting information.[28] In 2002, data from the Women's Health Initiative (WHI) trial showed that MHT did not protect postmenopausal women against heart attacks as previously thought.[29] Since the initial 2002 report more information has become available, and more importance has been placed on the fact that the study population for the WHI trial was women with a mean age of recruitment of 63 years.

The IMS recommends that "consideration of MHT should be part of an overall strategy including lifestyle recommendations regarding diet, exercise, smoking cessation and safe levels of alcohol consumption for maintaining the health of peri- and postmenopausal women." The IMS notes that, if used, MHT and its dosage should be tailored to each patient by her physician and that menopausal women should become knowledgeable of the risks and benefits of the therapy. The IMS concludes that "MHT is the most effective treatment for moderate to severe menopausal symptoms and is most beneficial before the age of 60 years or within 10 years after menopause," is effective "for the prevention of fracture in at-risk women before age 60 years or within 10 years after menopause," and "reduces the risk of diabetes and, through improving insulin action in women with insulin resistance, it has positive effects on other related risk factors for cardiovascular disease such as thelipid profile and metabolic syndrome." Regarding potential serious adverse effects of MHT, the IMS concludes that the possible risk of breast cancer is less than 0.1% per year and that "the risk of venous thromboembolic events and ischemic stroke increases with oral MHT but the absolute risk is rare below age 60 years."[28]

Men also undergo changes in their reproductive systems during middle age. Men are fertile throughout their lives, although the number of healthy, active sperm they produce decreases as they grow older. Middle-aged men experience a decline in testosterone, ejaculate with less force and less volume, and take longer to regain an erection after orgasm. In addition, the prostate gland usually enlarges. See the Managing Your Health essay "Enlargement of the Prostate."

Although both men and women undergo changes in their reproductive systems beginning at middle age, these changes do not have to impair their ability to have a healthy, enjoyable sex life extending into their elderly years.

Managing Your Health

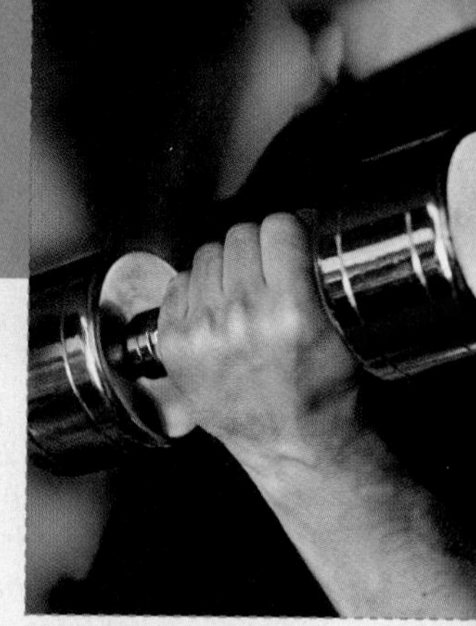

© Kzenon/ShutterStock

Enlargement of the Prostate

If you are male and older than 45 years, your prostate may be enlarging slowly; if you are not yet 45 years old, prostate enlargement may be in your future. This process of enlargement is common for middle-aged and older men; it is part of the aging process and may never be a cause for concern. However, about 50% of men in their 60s and about 90% of men in their 70s and 80s complain of problems caused by an enlarged prostate gland, also known as prostatic hyperplasia, or benign prostatic hypertrophy (BPH).

How can an enlarged prostate affect your health? Notice in Figure 5-1 that the prostate gland surrounds the urethra beneath the urinary bladder. As the prostate enlarges, it may squeeze the urethra, hampering the flow of urine through this tube. Therefore, the symptoms that may appear first as a result of BPH are difficulty in beginning to urinate, a decrease in the force of the urine stream, a dribbling of urine after urinating, a sensation of a full bladder after urinating, and a need to urinate 5 or 10 minutes after urinating.

As the prostate squeezes the urethra more and more, the muscles of the bladder wall respond by thickening as they forcefully push urine through the constricted urethra. This thickened bladder is irritated easily, however, and contracts more readily. Therefore, the following symptoms develop: an urgency to urinate and/or leaking of urine; more frequent urination, especially at night; and painful urination. Eventually, urine flow can be blocked to the point that emergency treatment is necessary.

There are several treatments for BPH. Surgery is usually undertaken when symptoms are severe. During the surgery, the portion of the prostate squeezing the urethra is removed. Laser therapy, radio frequency therapy, or microwave therapy can be used to destroy the enlarged prostate tissue as well. These procedures are less invasive than traditional surgical techniques are and usually have fewer long-term side effects and complications.

Another treatment is balloon dilatation. During this procedure, an inflatable device is inserted into the urethra through the opening at the tip of the penis. The device is inflated at the area of constriction and is then removed. This procedure widens the urethra to alleviate symptoms. Various medications also ease the symptoms of BPH.

Enlargement of the prostate may also be caused by prostate cancer. This cancer is the second most common cause of cancer deaths in men (lung cancer being the first). However, it usually does not appear in men younger than 55 years, and it is generally a slow-growing form of cancer. Its symptoms overlap with those of BPH and include difficult, frequent, and painful urination and blood in the urine.

The symptoms of BPH and prostate cancer are more than just a nuisance. The restriction or blockage of urine flow can damage the kidneys; prostate cancer can spread, resulting in death. To avoid the discomforts and possible serious consequences of these conditions, therefore, the prostate should be examined regularly. The American Cancer Society recommends that men older than 50 years have a digital rectal examination every year. During this examination, the physician inserts a gloved, lubricated finger into the rectum. Because the prostate lies next to the rectum (*Figure 5.D*), the physician can palpate (feel by pressing lightly) the size of the prostate.

Newer diagnostic techniques include transrectal ultrasound, in which the physician inserts an ultrasound probe into the rectum that results in an image of the prostate on a monitor.

A blood test has been developed to help detect prostate cancer. This test is known as prostate-specific antigen (PSA) and helps find many prostate cancers years before they would otherwise be detected.

Figure 5.D

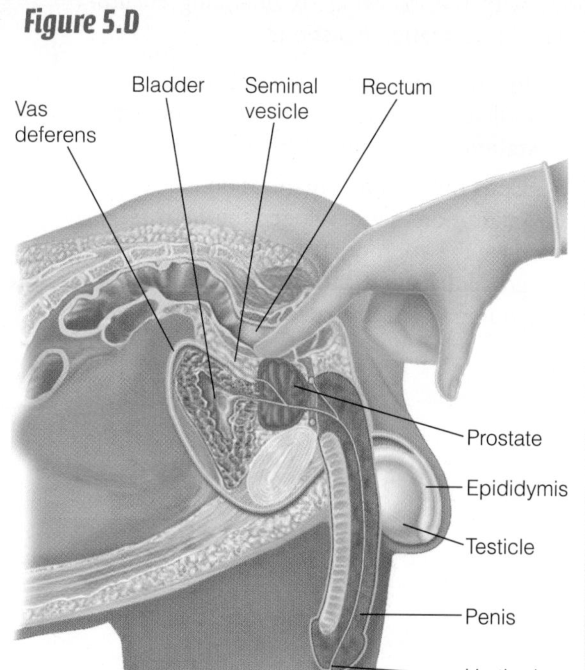

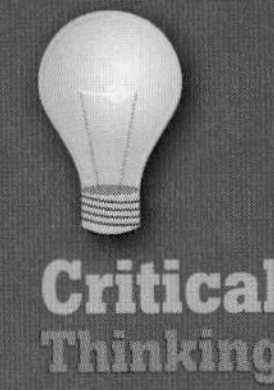

Explain why you think this web page about folic acid is a reliable or an unreliable source of information. Use the "Assessing Information on the Internet" portion of the model for analyzing health-related information to guide your thinking; the main points of the model are noted here. If you wish to visit this site, the web address is www.cdc.gov/ncbddd/folicacid.

- What is the source of the information?
- Is the site sponsored by a nationally known health or medical organization or affiliated with a well-known medical research institution or major university? If not, is the site staffed by well-respected and credentialed experts in the field?
- Does the site include up-to-date references from a well-known, respected medical or scientific journal or links to reputable websites, such as nationally recognized medical organizations?
- Is the information at the website current?

Based on your analysis, do you think that this web page is a reliable source of health-related information? Summarize your reasons for coming to this conclusion.

If you are unsure of the credibility of the site after answering the preceding questions, continue with the following six Analyzing Health-Related Information questions.

1. Which statements on the website are verifiable facts, and which are unverified statements or value claims?
2. Does the person, organization, or institution that developed the website have the appropriate background and credentials in the topic area? What can you do to check credentials?
3. What might be the motives and biases inherent to the website?
4. What is the main point of the article, ad, or claim made on the site? Which information is relevant to the issue, main point, product, or service? Which information is irrelevant?
5. Does the source of information present the pros and cons of the topic or the benefits and risks of the product?
6. Does the source of information attack the credibility of conventional scientists or medical authorities?

Based on your additional analysis, do you think that this web page is a reliable source of health-related information? Summarize your reasons for coming to this conclusion.

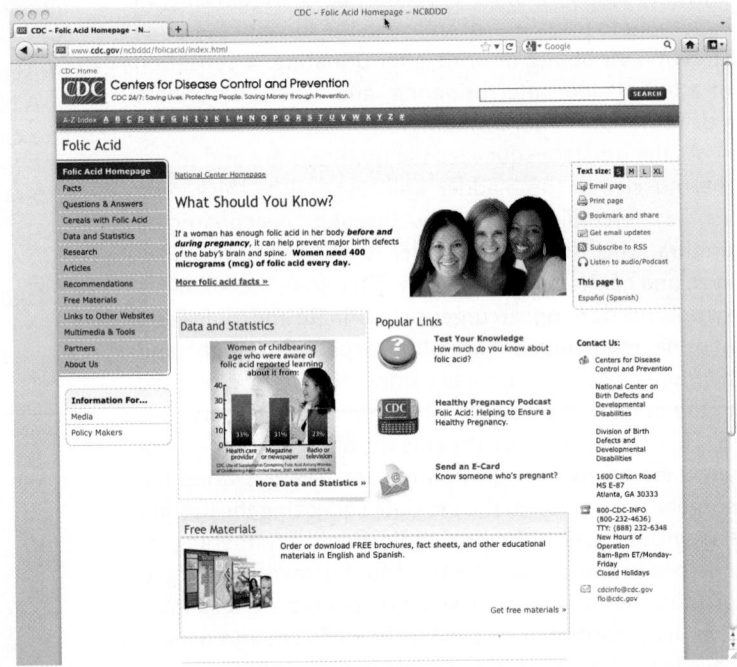

Courtesy of CDC.

CHAPTER REVIEW

Summary

Sexual reproduction involves the fertilization of an egg by a sperm, forming the first cell of a new individual. The male reproductive system produces sperm (male sex cells) and delivers them to the vagina of the female. Sperm are produced in the testes and are moved along the male reproductive tract with the seminal fluid secreted by accessory sex glands during ejaculation.

Eggs (ova; female sex cells) develop and mature in the female reproductive system, which also receives sperm and provides an environment in which a fertilized ovum can develop. Eggs mature in the ovaries, are fertilized in the uterine tubes, and develop in the uterus during pregnancy.

Women experience cyclic monthly hormonal changes that orchestrate physiologic changes that take place in the ovaries and uterus. The changes are collectively called the menstrual cycle. During the menstrual cycle, an ovum matures and is released from the ovary while the lining of the uterus thickens in preparation for the implantation of a fertilized ovum. If pregnancy does not occur, the uterine lining sloughs off during the menses.

If fertilization takes place, the embryo/fetus develops in the uterus of the female. This developmental process is termed pregnancy, or gestation. Various environmental influences (teratogens) such as drugs, alcohol, viruses, and dietary deficiencies can damage the embryo or fetus early in pregnancy. A woman preparing for pregnancy should have a medical checkup; eat a well-balanced and nutritious diet; avoid drinking alcohol, smoking cigarettes, and taking drugs; and possibly seek genetic counseling.

Women who become pregnant may notice physical signs of this condition such as a missed period, nausea, fatigue, and moodiness. A woman can conduct a home pregnancy test or have a laboratory test performed to determine if she is pregnant.

Pregnancy lasts about 38 weeks and is typically described in terms of trimesters, or 3-month periods. During the first trimester, all the organ systems of the body form and become functional. The second and third trimesters are periods of growth and refinement of the organ systems.

The process of childbirth (labor) takes place in three stages: dilation, expulsion, and placental delivery. During dilation, the uterine muscles contract, causing the cervix to widen (dilate) and thin out (efface). During the second stage of labor the baby is born. Within 15 to 30 minutes after delivery of the baby, the placenta is expelled from the uterus.

Couples often want to avoid pregnancy for various reasons, so they choose some form of birth control, or contraception. Contraceptive methods are varied and can be grouped into seven categories: abstinence and natural methods, chemical methods, barrier methods, hormonal methods, intrauterine devices, sterilization, and emergency contraception. Each method has different advantages, disadvantages, and levels of effectiveness. Abstinence, sterilization, IUDs, and hormonal methods are the most effective means of contraception. Using condoms and practicing abstinence are the best ways to prevent the transmission of sexually transmitted infections while at the same time preventing pregnancy.

Sometimes contraceptive methods fail and an unplanned pregnancy occurs that a woman or a couple chooses to terminate. Women and couples choose to terminate a pregnancy for other reasons, including health concerns of the mother. Terminating a pregnancy involves the removal of the embryo or fetus from the uterus before it is able to survive on its own. This process is called an induced abortion. In the United States today, there is great controversy over a woman's right to choose induced abortion. More than 90% of abortions are performed either medically (using drugs) or with vacuum aspiration early in pregnancy; almost two-thirds are performed at 8 weeks or less of gestation.

The sex of an individual is set at the time of fertilization and is determined by the type of sex chromosomes (genes) that the embryo receives from its parents. The male and female reproductive tracts develop during gestation. Further maturation does not continue until puberty, the time of sexual maturation, which begins at approximately 10 to 11 years of age and concludes about 5 or 6 years later. Men and women both undergo changes to their reproductive

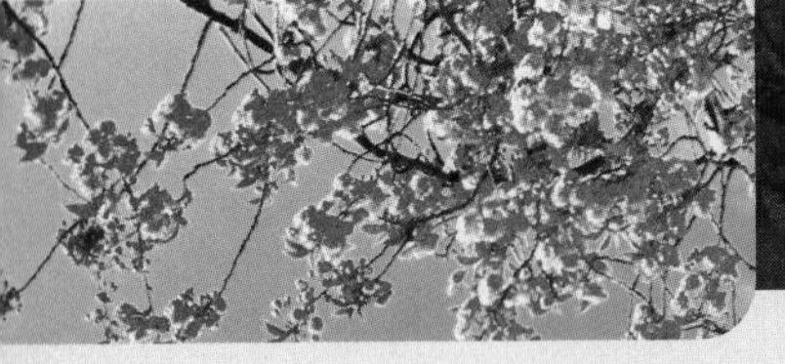

CHAPTER REVIEW

function during middle age. Women have a cessation of the menses (menopause) as a result of physiologic and hormonal changes and can no longer reproduce. Men can reproduce throughout their lives but at middle age experience a decline in testosterone and sexual functioning.

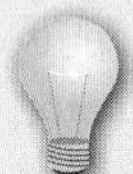

Applying What You Have Learned

1. A woman is 42 years old, unmarried, and has sex regularly with a single sexual partner. She has been using an intrauterine device but has developed an infection with the insertion of her most recent IUD. She must change to another method of birth control. If you were this woman, which method would you choose? Provide evidence that your choice is prudent. **Application**
2. In this chapter, much attention is given to the theoretical and actual effectiveness of various types of birth control. When you look at Table 5.3, which column should carry more weight in your decision making—the theoretical or the actual effectiveness? Give reasons for your answer. **Analysis**
3. You have been asked to lead a discussion in your health class about maximizing maternal and fetal health during pregnancy. You may discuss any information in this chapter relevant to this issue. (You may add topics not mentioned in this chapter as well.) List the topics you will discuss and briefly describe the importance of each. **Synthesis**
4. Devise an assessment that will help people evaluate their attitudes toward abortion. Explain why you think that your assessment tool will accurately evaluate these attitudes. **Evaluation**

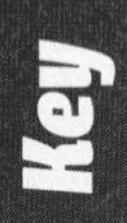

Key

Application	**Analysis**	**Synthesis**	**Evaluation**
using information in a new situation.	breaking down information into component parts.	putting together information from different sources.	making informed decisions.

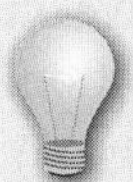

Reflecting on Your Health

1. Contracting sexually transmitted infections can endanger your health and your ability to have children. What is the relationship between responsible sexual behavior and reproductive health in your life?
2. If you are a man, what did you learn in this chapter about female reproductive health that was new to you? If you are a woman, what did you learn in this chapter about male reproductive health that was new to you? How will this new knowledge affect your behavior toward the opposite sex? How might it affect your attitudes?
3. Most contraceptive methods focus on the female reproductive system. Because of this focus, should women have the primary responsibility for contraception? Why or why not?
4. In the United States, a woman's right to choose to have an abortion (other than a "partial-birth" abortion) is protected by law. Do you think that the law should be changed to criminalize abortion in general? If so, why? Should abortion be legal only in certain circumstances? If so, when?
5. Table 5.1 lists selected teratogens. If a woman knowingly exposes her embryo or fetus to teratogenic drugs such as alcohol, should she be prosecuted in the criminal justice system? Why or why not?

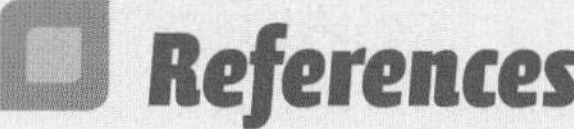

References

1. Sharpe, R. M. (2010). Environmental/lifestyle effects on spermatogenesis. *Philosophical Transactions of The Royal Society B*, 365, 1697–1712.
2. U.S. Department of Health and Human Services, Office on Women's Health. (2014). *Menstruation and the menstrual cycle*. Retrieved July 10, 2014, from http://www.womenshealth.gov/publications/our-publications/fact-sheet/menstruation.pdf
3. Freeman, E. W., et al. (2011). Core symptoms that discriminate premenstrual syndrome. *Journal of Women's Health*, 20(1), 29–35.
4. Shulman, L. P. (2010). Gynecological management of premenstrual symptoms. *Current Pain and Headache Reports*, 14(5), 367–375.
5. Medline Plus, U.S. National Library of Medicine, National Institutes of Health. (2012, August 15). *Toxic shock syndrome*. Retrieved July 10, 2014, from http://www.nlm.nih.gov/medlineplus/ency/article/000653.htm
6. Luke, B., & Brown, M. B. (2007). Elevated risks of pregnancy complication and adverse outcomes with increasing maternal age. *Human Reproduction*, 22, 1264–1272.
7. Centers for Disease Control and Prevention. (2008). *Estimated number of male newborn infants, and percent circumcised during birth hospitalization, by geographic region: United States, 1979–2008*. Retrieved July 11, 2014 from http://www.cdc.gov/nchs/nhds/nhds_tables.htm#male
8. Tobian, A. A. R., et al. (2009). Male circumcision for the prevention of HSV-2 and HPV infections and syphilis. *New England Journal of Medicine*, 360, 1298–1309.
9. American Academy of Pediatrics. (1999). Circumcision policy statement. *Pediatrics*, 103(3), 686–693.
10. American Academy of Pediatrics. (2005). AAP publications retired and reaffirmed. *Pediatrics*, 116(3), 796.
11. American Academy of Pediatrics. (2012). Circumcision policy statement. *Pediatrics*, 130(3), 585–586.
12. Brett, K., & Barfield, W. (2008). Prevalence of self-reported postpartum depressive dymptoms—17 states, 2004–2005. *Morbidity and Mortality Weekly Report*, 57, 361–366.
13. Reeves, W. C., et al. (2011). Mental illness surveillance among adults in the United States. *Morbidity and Mortality Weekly Report*, 60(03), 1–32.
14. Centers for Disease Control and Prevention. (2014). *Infertility*. Retrieved July 11, 2014, from http://www.cdc.gov/nchs/fastats/infertility.htm
15. De Vos, M., et al. (2010). Primary ovarian insufficiency. *Lancet*, 376(9744), 911–921.
16. Olive, D. L. (2010). Exercise and fertility: An update. *Current Opinions in Obstetrics and Gynecology*, 22(4), 259–263.
17. Brewer, C. J., & Balen, A. H. (2010). The adverse effects of obesity on conception and implantation. *Reproduction*, 140(3), 347–364.
18. Anderson, K., et al. (2010). Lifestyle factors in people seeking infertility treatment—A review. *Australian and New Zealand Journal of Obstetrics and Gynaecology*, 50(1), 8–20.
19. Ross, C., et al. (2010). A systematic review of the effect of oral antioxidants on male infertility. *Reproductive Biomedicine Online*, 20(6), 711–723.
20. Basatemur, E., & Sutcliffe, A. (2008). Follow-up of children born after ART. *Placenta*, 29, S135–S140.
21. Frank-Herrmann, P., et al. (2007). The effectiveness of a fertility awareness based method to avoid pregnancy in relation to a couple's sexual behavior during the fertile time: A prospective longitudinal study. *Human Reproduction*, 22, 1310–1319.
22. Herold, B. C., et al. (2011). Female genital tract secretions and semen impact the development of microbicides for the prevention of HIV and other sexually transmitted infections. *American Journal of Reproductive Immunology*, 65, 325–333.
23. Guttmacher Institute. (June 2014). *Contraceptive use in the United States*. Retrieved July 11, 2014, from http://www.guttmacher.org/pubs/fb_contr_use.html
24. International Collaboration of Epidemiological Studies of Cervical Cancer, Appleby, P., et al. (2007). Cervical cancer and hormonal contraceptives: collaborative reanalysis of individual data for 16,573 women with cervical cancer and 35,509 women without cervical cancer from 24 epidemiological studies. *Lancet*, 370, 1609–1621.
25. Wan, G. J., et al. (2007). Treatment satisfaction with a transdermal contraceptive patch or oral contraceptives. *Contraception*, 75, 281–284.
26. U.S. Food and Drug Administration. (2013). FDA approves Plan B One-Step emergency contraceptive for use without a prescription for all women of child-bearing potential. Retrieved July 12, 2014, from http://www.fda.gov/newsevents/newsroom/pressannouncements/ucm358082.htm
27. Pazol, K., et al. (2011). Abortion surveillance—United States, 2007. *Morbidity and Mortality Weekly Update*, 60(1), 1–39. Retrieved February 25, 2011, from http://www.cdc.gov/mmwr/pdf/ss/ss6001.pdf
28. Villiers, T. J., et al. on behalf of the Board of the International Menopause Society. (2013). Updated 2013 International Menopause Society recommendations on menopausal hormone therapy and preventive strategies for midlife health. *Climacteric*, 16, 316–337.
29. Women's Health Initiative Memory Study Investigators. (2004). Conjugated equine estrogens and global cognitive function in postmenopausal women: Women's health initiative memory study. *Journal of the American Medical Association*, 291(24), 2959–2968.

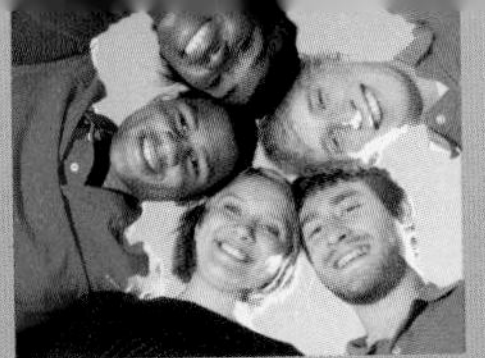

Diversity in Health
The Virtue of Virginity

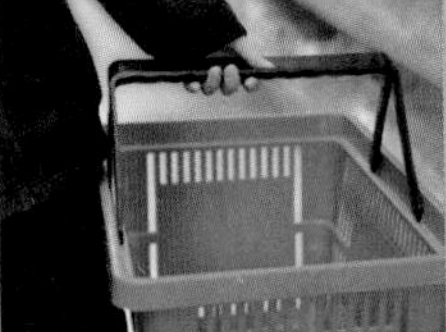

Consumer Health
Ginseng and Sexual Prowess

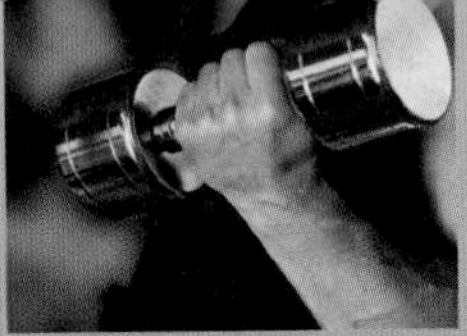

Managing Your Health
Minding Your Sexual Manners

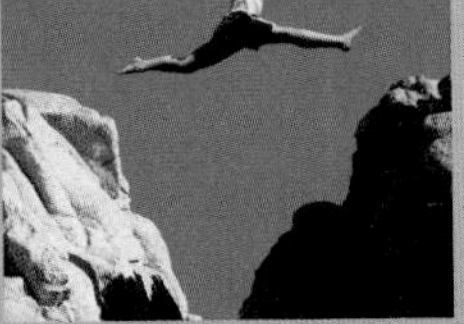

Across the Life Span
Sexuality

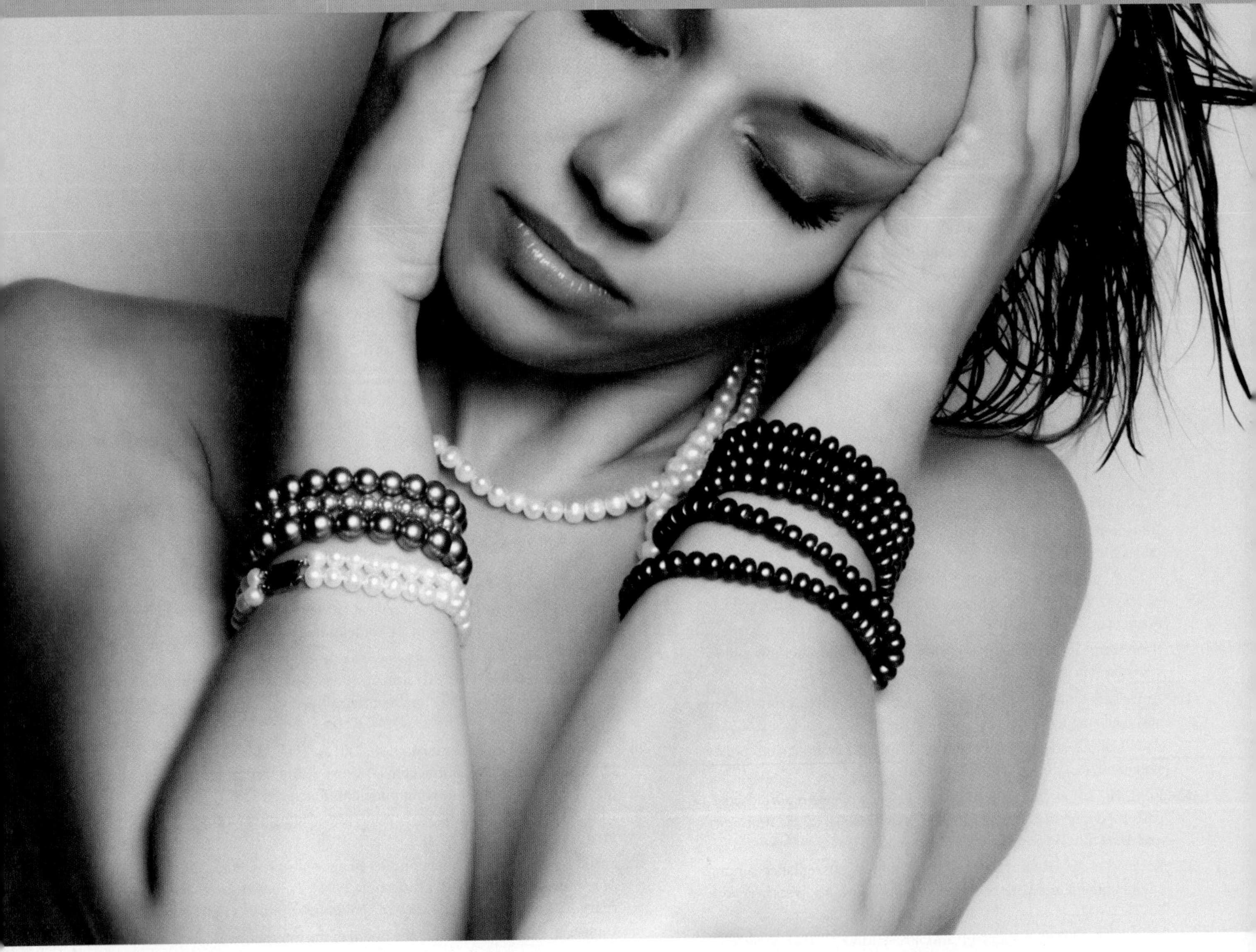

Chapter Overview

How biological and psychological factors influence sexual behavior

The phases of sexual response cycles

Symptoms of and treatments for sexual dysfunctions

How culture affects sexuality

Nature versus nurture and sexual orientation

The diversity of sexual behavior

Definitions and theories of love and commitment

Student Workbook

Self-Assessment: Male Sexual Quotient Self-Assessment Questionnaire | The Love Attitudes Scale

Changing Health Habits: Would a Behavior Change Improve Your Relationship?

Do You Know?

What are common sexual practices?

How living together affects future marriage?

How to communicate effectively?

Circle of People: © SergeBertasiusPhotography/ShutterStock; Consumer: © sevenke/ShutterStock; Weight Training: © Kzenon/ShutterStock; Rock Climbing: © Galina Barskaya/ShutterStock; Chapter opener: © dpaint/ShutterStock.

CHAPTER 6

Romantic Relationships and Sexuality

© Sara Bertasi/Photography/Alamy Stock

Learning Objectives

"... promoters and advertisers know that 'sex sells.'"

After studying this chapter, you should be able to:

1. Define sexuality.
2. Describe factors that influence a person's desire to form intimate relationships.
3. List the characteristics of loving relationships.
4. Identify factors that contribute to compatibility.
5. Define homosexuality, heterosexuality, and bisexuality.
6. Explain how culture and society influence sexual behavior.
7. Differentiate between passionate and companionate love.
8. Describe factors that are associated with long-term loving relationships.
9. Discuss the biological origins and social ramifications of gender roles.
10. Identify the phases of the human sexual response and the physiological changes that occur in males and females during each phase.
11. Describe common sexual dysfunctions and their causes and treatments.
12. Describe the impact of aging on sexuality.

sex The biological or physiological differences that distinguish one as female or male.

gender Socially constructed differences (or psychological identity) that distinguish one as female or male.

sexuality The aspect of personality that encompasses a person's sexual thoughts, feelings, attitudes, and actions.

Sex is everywhere in our society. You can find sexually explicit images and information in movies, books, TV shows, advertisements, social media, online, and in song lyrics. If you browse through magazines or online you are likely to see pictures of attractive young men and women in advertisements for clothes, perfumes, and cars. Whether their product is a movie, jewelry, or pair of jeans, promoters and advertisers know that "sex sells." What does sex mean to you?

The term **sex** refers to the physiological differences between men and women. In other words, sex is a term that identifies whether one is biologically female or biologically male (e.g., men have testes; women have ovaries). This biological sex is changeable only via a surgical operation. Sex can also refer to behavior (e.g., sexual intercourse, oral sex). **Gender** is a related, yet distinct, term: it refers to the socially constructed distinctions between men and women. Gendered distinctions accepted by society are socially constructed norms—the accepted and expected behavior—that identify what is expected of one based on her (or his) biological sex. For example, in the United States, it is generally acceptable and sometimes expected that girls wear dresses: however, it is not generally acceptable and is rarely expected that boys wear dresses. Gender also refers to one's psychological identity (more on gender identity later in the chapter). Gender, and gendered norms, evolve as society evolves, whereas biological sex remains constant. Thus, both *sex* and *gender* refer to differences between men and women: *sex* refers to the biological, physiological differences, and *gender* refers to the social differences. **Sexuality**, however, is more than gender or reproductive organs. Sexuality is the aspect of personality that encompasses an individual's sexual thoughts, feelings, attitudes, and actions. Each person has a unique collection of private and public sexual experiences that shapes his or her sexuality.

Numerous biological, psychological, social, and cultural forces interact to influence a person's sexual development, sexual health, and interpersonal relationships (**Figure 6.1**). Sexuality is woven into every aspect of human life; sex affects a person's identity, self-esteem, emotions, personality, relationships, lifestyle, and overall health.

Figure 6.1

Sexuality Model. Numerous biological, psychological, social, and cultural forces interact to influence sexual development, sexual health, and interpersonal relationships.

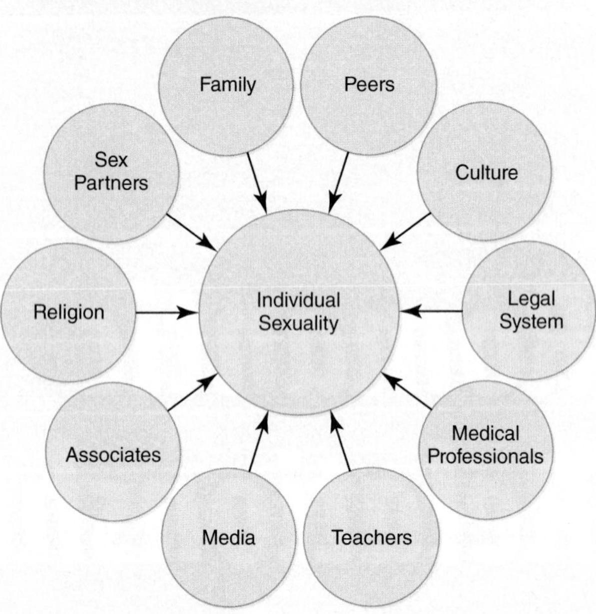

Being knowledgeable about sexuality is important for maintaining good health and optimal well-being. Misinformation can lead to serious consequences, such as unintentional pregnancies or sexually transmitted infections. Additionally, people who are well informed about sexuality can communicate effectively with their medical practitioners and sexual partners regarding reproductive or sexual concerns.

Throughout life, you make various sexually related decisions, such as deciding with whom to have an intimate sexual relationship. Such decisions can have serious effects on your health and well-being, as well as those of others. By considering how your actions may affect yourself and your sexual partners, you can become a more sexually responsible person.

Human Sexual Behavior

The reproductive activity of most complex animals includes behaviors commonly referred to as courtship and mating. Unlike other animals, humans exhibit a variety of complex sexual behaviors that do not necessarily result in reproduction. People often engage in sexual activity for pleasure and relaxation or to help maintain the emotional bonds of their intimate relationships. Some individuals, however, use their sexuality to dominate, exploit, or harm others. What factors influence human sexual behavior?

The Biology of Sexual Behavior

The motivation to pursue sexual activity—the sex drive, or *libido*—is an instinctual behavior moderated by the sex hormones. The ovaries and the testes, glands that make up part of the hormonal (endocrine) system, secrete these chemical messengers. The endocrine system is so named because of the endocrine glands, such as the ovaries and the testes, which secrete the hormones. Glands are individual cells or groups of cells that secrete substances. They are called *endocrine* because they release substances within (*endo-*) the body, rather than secreting substances that exit the body, such as sweat.

The endocrine system plays an important role in sexual functioning. The pituitary, located in the brain, and the ovaries and testes produce hormones that affect sexual functioning (**Figure 6.2**). The hypothalamus, located above the pituitary, produces hormones that trigger the secretion of pituitary hormones. During puberty in males, pituitary hormones activate the maturation of the male reproductive structures and the release of increased levels of the male sex hormone, testosterone. Testosterone plays a role in the maturation of the male reproductive structures, stimulates the development of sperm, and triggers and maintains the development of the secondary sexual characteristics such as the growth of a beard and the deepening of the voice. During puberty in females, pituitary hormones cause maturation of the ovaries, which then begin secreting the female sex hormones estrogen and progesterone. Estrogen stimulates maturation of the uterus and vagina, development of the female secondary sexual characteristics such as the development of breasts, and a change in the distribution of body fat.

During middle age, the production of sex hormones declines. After 40 years of age, men produce less testosterone and fewer sperm, although accelerated declines appear to be slowed by practicing healthy behaviors, such as avoiding overweight and obesity.[1] Despite these reductions, elderly men can still father children. When women reach menopause, usually between 45 and 55 years of age, their

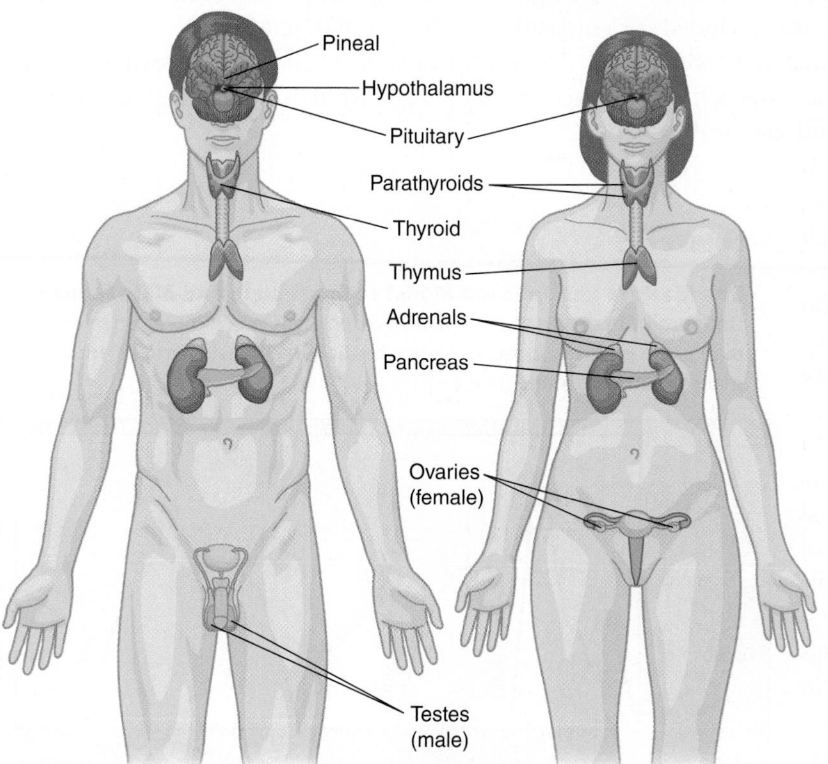

Figure 6.2

Endocrine Glands. The pituitary, ovaries, and testes produce hormones that affect sexual functioning. The hypothalamus produces hormones that trigger the secretion of pituitary hormones.

sexologists Scientists who study human sexuality.

testosterone A male sex hormone (androgen) that plays a role in the development of functionally mature sperm and is responsible for the development and maintenance of male secondary sexual characteristics such as the deepening of the voice and the growth of facial hair.

vasocongestion A condition in which the spongy tissue of the penis and clitoris expands with blood during sexual arousal.

myotonia An increase in muscle tension throughout the body during sexual arousal.

estrogen and progesterone levels decrease dramatically. As a result, menopausal women are no longer fertile. However, most healthy elderly men and women continue to have an interest in sex, and they engage in sexual activity. Research conducted for the 2010 AARP Survey of Midlife and Older Adults reveals that among those older than 70 years of age, 80% of men and 39% of women believed that a satisfying sexual relationship was important to the overall quality of life. In addition, 15% of men and 5% of women older than 70 years reported engaging in sexual intercourse at least once a week.[2]

The Psychology of Sexual Behavior

Certain thoughts, sensations, and emotions modulate sexual behavior, as do the sex hormones. Included in this psychological mix are factors that can influence sexual behavior positively, such as satisfaction with one's body, good physical and emotional health, absence of beliefs that can hinder sexual responsiveness or enjoyment, previous positive sexual experiences, and high self-esteem.

Many **sexologists**, scientists who study human sexuality, report that people who have high self-esteem are more likely to have positive attitudes concerning their sexuality than persons with poor self-concepts. However, people frequently judge their bodies and sexual prowess against unrealistic standards of physical attractiveness and sexual ability that are presented in the media. As a result, some individuals develop feelings of sexual inadequacy and low self-esteem because they feel sexually unattractive or inept. People who have these feelings may be unable to enjoy their sexuality and may be unable to form fulfilling intimate relationships.

If you are male, you may want to assess your level of sexual function and satisfaction by taking the "Male Sexual Quotient Self-Assessment Questionnaire" in the Student Workbook pages at the end of this book.

The Sexual Response

The sexual response in both males and females is governed primarily by the nervous system rather than by hormones. Hormones are chemicals secreted in one part of the body that have an effect in another. **Testosterone**, the "male" hormone (women also secrete testosterone), helps maintain the sex drive, or libido.

The two major physical changes that occur during sexual arousal are vasocongestion and myotonia. **Vasocongestion** occurs as blood flow away from the sexual organs is reduced. The spongy tissue of the penis and clitoris expands with blood and these structures become erect. **Myotonia**, an increase in muscle tension, occurs throughout the body.

The Masters and Johnson Model Both sexes have broader responses than just these events. This pattern of responses is termed the *sexual response cycle*. First defined by Masters and Johnson, the cycle is usually thought of as having four phases: excitement, plateau, orgasm, and resolution (**Figure 6.3**).

During the *excitement phase* of the sexual response cycle, both men and women have a heightened sexual

Figure 6.3

The Masters and Johnson Model of the Female and Male Human Orgasmic Responses. The female response is much more variable than is the male response, as shown by the three female patterns and one male pattern illustrated here.

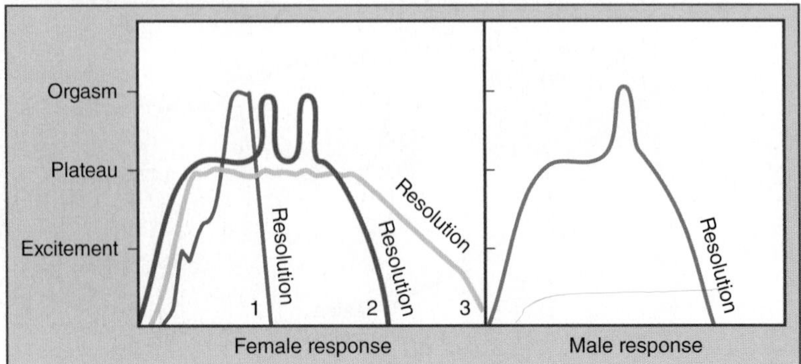

awareness. Certain thoughts, sights, touches, and even sounds or odors lead to a rush of blood to the clitoris and vaginal opening in women and to the penis in men.

In men, the penis expands as blood fills spaces in its columns of spongy tissue. As a result, the penis becomes erect, and the expansion of the tissue compresses the veins that take blood away from this organ. Consequently, as blood flow into the penis increases, blood flow out of the penis decreases. This decrease in outward blood flow maintains the erection.

In women, glands in the vulvar area secrete mucus-like fluid. The congestion of blood in the vulvar area and in the vagina swells the labia and pushes fluid through the vaginal wall. These fluids are lubricants for sexual intercourse. Blood also rushes to the breasts. In response, the breasts swell. The nipples become erect as smooth muscles contract. Many women also exhibit a sex flush at this time, a reddening of the skin as blood flow through it increases.

As sexual excitement continues, the *plateau phase* begins. The heart rate, blood pressure, respiration rate, and level of muscle tension all increase. During the plateau phase, the erection of the male intensifies as the penis is massaged rhythmically by intercourse (anal or vaginal), manual stimulation, or oral stimulation. Sensory impulses from tactile sensations in both sexes reinforce their sexual sensations. In women, the lower third of the vagina constricts around the penis. The upper two-thirds of the vagina widens as the uterus and cervix lift up, creating a space for the semen. Continued stimulation of the clitoris and penis leads to the next phase of the sexual response—the orgasmic phase.

In men, ejaculation occurs during the *orgasmic phase*. This involuntary response (over which men can exert some voluntary control) results when the nervous system sends messages to muscles in the walls of the vas deferens and urethra to contract. At the same time, the seminal vesicles and prostate receive messages to release their secretions. The pelvic muscles also rhythmically contract. Orgasm in women is characterized by rhythmic contractions of the pelvic muscles and vaginal walls. Both sexes experience a peak of sexual pleasure at orgasm. Erection and ejaculation are the two primary components of the male sex act. The clitoris of the female becomes erect during sexual activity and she achieves orgasm, but women do not ejaculate like men.

During the *resolution phase* the body returns to its prearousal state. The heart rate, blood pressure, and respiration slow; the muscles relax. In males, the erection subsides (the penis becomes flaccid) and sometimes fatigue sets in. Depending on the man and his age, he will not be able to develop another erection for a few minutes to a few hours. This time is the *refractory period*. Unlike men, women have the capacity to reach the orgasmic phase again (have multiple orgasms) in sequence or rather quickly after dropping to the plateau phase.

The Masters and Johnson model is considered a biological and linear model of sexual response. It is considered biological because it encompasses only physiologic aspects of the sexual response and not emotional or psychological aspects. It is considered linear because it has a beginning, middle, and end, starting at one place and ending at another. Although this model may reflect the male sexual response well, it may not be as reflective of the female sexual response.

Other Sexual Response Models Whipple and Brash-McGreer developed a circular model of female sexual response based on a previous linear four-stage model developed by Reed. The circular model shows that a woman's reflection on a sexual encounter affects her desire for the next sexual encounter. Satisfying sexual experiences reinforce her desire for another, whereas negative sexual experiences detract from her desire. This circular model recognizes that the pleasure and emotional satisfaction derived from one sexual experience can lead to desire for the next sexual experience.[3]

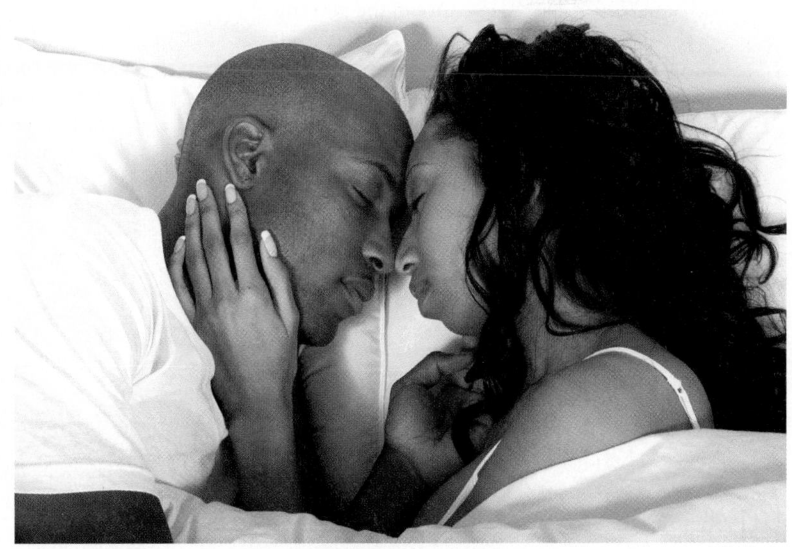

Consumer Health

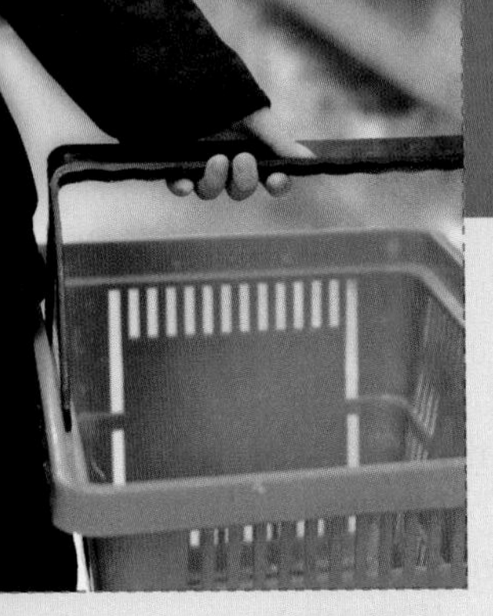

© sevenke/ShutterStock.

Ginseng and Sexual Prowess

You've probably seen ads for ginseng in magazines, on television, or on the Web. The ads often make claims such as "Ginseng will boost your energy and sexual stamina," or "Ginseng has been used for centuries in maintaining overall health and vitality," or "Ginseng will reduce stress and the effects of aging." "Can it do that?" you might wonder.

Ginseng is an herb that grows wild or is cultivated in eastern Asia and North America. For hundreds of years, the root of the plant has been used in Asia for medicinal purposes and as an aphrodisiac because it often looks like a human body (**Figure 6.A**). But what do we know about ginseng? Will it make you more sexually "potent"? Can it harm you or, alternatively, enhance your health?

On the positive side, sperm motility and ability to fertilize an egg (capacitation) are enhanced after sperm are incubated with extracts of ginseng. Are sperm motility and capacitation enhanced in men who take ginseng? There is still no answer to that question. Does ginseng affect sexual arousal or performance? Ginseng has been shown to significantly enhance libido and copulatory behavior in male rats and mice. This herb appears to have a direct effect on penile tissue, which could be responsible for its copulatory performance-enhancing actions and has been used to treat erectile dysfunction.

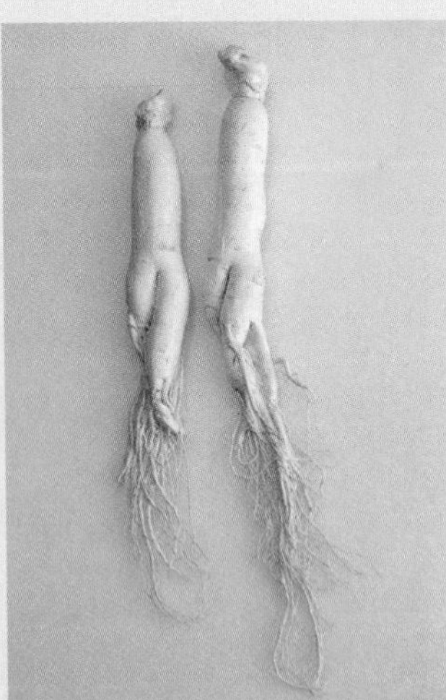

Figure 6.A

Ginseng root. The use of the ginseng root as an aphrodesiac presumably began because it looks like a human body.

© Blue Jean Images/Digital Vision/Thinkstock

On the negative side, medical researchers know that drug interactions occur with many herbals. Ginseng, in particular, may alter bleeding (or clotting) time, the time it takes for blood to stop flowing from a tiny wound. Ginseng also interacts with anticoagulant drugs, which "thin" the blood; that is, they decrease the ability of the blood to clot. Therefore, anticoagulants and ginseng should not be taken together. Ginseng also may interfere with the heart medication digoxin (digitalis), which affects the force and rate at which the heart beats.

In addition to its interaction with anticoagulants and digoxin, ginseng should not be used if a person is taking estrogens or corticosteroid drugs such as cortisone because of possible additive effects. Ginseng may also affect blood glucose levels, so it should not be taken by persons with diabetes mellitus. For those on the antidepressant drug phenelzine sulfate (Nardil), ginseng could provoke a manic episode (an extreme excited state). Its general side effects may include headache and involuntary muscular contractions.

Should you take ginseng to boost your sexual prowess? This herb is commonly used in Asia to treat sexual dysfunction in humans. In addition, animal studies provide evidence that ginseng may be useful in such treatment, and it may enhance libido and copulatory behavior in males. Results of one small-scale study show that Korean red ginseng improved sexual arousal in menopausal women. However, a review published in the *Journal of Sexual Medicine* in 2010 states that "although there's a positive trend towards recommending ginseng as an effective aphrodisiac, however, more in depth studies involving [a] large number of subjects and its mechanism of action are needed before definite conclusions could be reached." With all this evidence in mind, you might not want to rely on ginseng for better bedroom calisthenics just yet.

Data from De Andrade, E., et al. (2007). Study of the efficacy of Korean red ginseng in the treatment of erectile dysfunction. *Asian Journal of Andrology*, 9, 241–244.; Zhang, H., et al. (2007). Ginsenoside Re promotes human sperm capacitation through nitric oxide-dependent pathway. *Molecular Reproduction and Development*, *74*, 497–501.

Basson also developed a cyclical model of the female sexual response, which is shown in **Figure 6.4**.[4] This model heavily incorporates emotional and psychosocial aspects. Sexual stimuli act on the sex drive as biologic and psychological factors come into play, such as satisfaction with her sex partner, her self-image, and previous sexual experiences. A positive psychological state can lead to sexual arousal and then sexual desire. The resulting emotional and physical satisfaction she experiences from sexual activity leads to emotional intimacy with her partner and reinforces her being receptive to the next sexual encounter.

erectile dysfunction (ED) A sexual dysfunction in which a man is unable to develop and/or sustain an erection firm enough for penetration of the vagina. Also called impotence.

Sexual Dysfunctions

A *dysfunction* is an impaired bodily process or a behavior that hinders the development or maintenance of healthy relationships. *Sexual dysfunctions* relate to the psychological and physical conditions that interfere with the sexual response.

Erectile Dysfunction (Impotence)

A common problem with the sexual response that occurs in men, particularly middle-aged and older men, is *impotence*. More properly called **erectile dysfunction (ED)**, impotence is the inability of a man to develop and/or sustain an erection firm enough for penetration. The incidence of ED rises as men age: 5% in men aged 20 to 39 years, 15% in men aged 40 to 59 years, 44% in men aged 60 to 69 years, and 70% in men 70 years or older.[5] Some men with various degrees of erectile dysfunction are able, with proper stimulation, to reach orgasm and ejaculate.

Until recently, impotence was thought to be primarily a psychological problem, a conclusion based on research studies conducted by well-known sex therapists Masters and Johnson. However, medical researchers have discovered that approximately 70% to 80% of cases of impotence are caused by physical problems. The most common cause of physically based impotence is blood vessel disease. Lifestyle factors that affect ED are smoking, alcohol consumption, and physical activity. Smoking increases the risk of ED and is associated with its progression. Physical activity decreases the risk of ED, while moderate alcohol consumption (two drinks per day for men) decreases the risk of ED compared to no alcohol consumption or heavier consumption.[6]

To develop and maintain an erection, blood must fill the spongy tissue of the penis and compress the veins that bring blood away from the penis. If a man has fatty deposits clogging his penile arteries, blood flow to the penis may be insufficient to develop and maintain an erection. The drugs Viagra (sildenafil), Levitra (vardenafil), and Cialis (tadalafil) work by widening blood vessels in the penis, thus increasing blood flow.

Figure 6.4

Basson's Blended Intimacy-Based and Sexual Drive-Based Circular Model of the Female Sexual Response. Women seek sexual intimacy for reasons beyond the physiologic sex drive, such as a desire to increase emotional closeness. This model shows that both the sex drive and the desire for emotional intimacy may motivate a woman to be responsive to sexual stimuli. In addition, biological and psychological factors combine to determine whether she becomes sexually aroused. For example, past sexual abuse may interfere with arousal even if she desires intimacy with her partner. Positive past experiences, however, will promote arousal. Her emotional and physical satisfaction from the sexual experience will then increase her desire for emotional intimacy, continuing the cycle of response.

Reproduced from Basson, R. (2001). Female sexual response: The role of drugs in the management of sexual dysfunction. *Obstetrics and Gynecology*, 98(2),350–353.

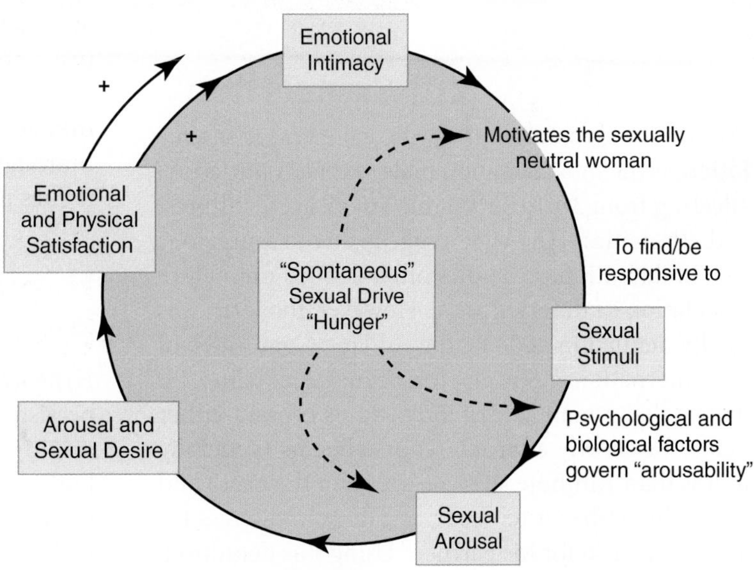

premature (rapid) ejaculation A common male sexual dysfunction in which a man consistently attains orgasm either before or shortly after intercourse begins and before he wishes it to occur.

Erectile dysfunction can also be caused by a variety of other conditions, such as diabetes mellitus;[5] damage to the spinal nerves or other nerves involved in erection; damage to the arteries that bring blood to the penis; certain medications used to control high blood pressure, anxiety, or depression; illness or injury that damages the penis; and hormonal imbalances. Research results show that use of a testosterone patch improves sexual function in men aged 50 to 70 years who exhibit symptoms of hormonal imbalance.[7]

Alcohol and illegal drugs such as marijuana, heroin, and cocaine have also been shown to affect penile function negatively. In addition, stress can be a cause of erectile difficulties. Epinephrine (adrenaline), a chemical released by the body during the stress reaction, impedes a man's ability to have an erection.

Physicians warn that minor physical problems can cause erectile difficulties that can worry a man and lead to psychological problems with erection. A significant finding to help distinguish between a physical and psychological cause for impotence is whether the man has a normal pattern of erections while asleep but not while engaged in sex with his partner. Men are encouraged to seek medical help for impotence immediately so that underlying, and possibly serious, physical problems can be diagnosed and treated promptly. If physical problems are not the cause, the psychological health of the patient as well as the health of his relationships should be explored.

Premature (Rapid) Ejaculation

Premature ejaculation (PE), also called **rapid ejaculation**, is the most common male sexual dysfunction, affecting from 3% to 30% of men of all ages, cultures, and ethnicities.[8] The wide range is due to a previous lack of definition, so studies often defined premature ejaculation in differing ways. However, the term was finally defined in 2008 by the Ad Hoc Committee of the International Society for Sexual Medicine. PE means that a man consistently attains orgasm either before or shortly after intercourse begins (generally in less than 1 minute all or nearly all of the time) and before he wishes it to occur, resulting in distress for a man and also for his partner.[7] Using this definition, the International Society for Sexual Medicine expects that the proportion of men affected by PE may be less than 3%.[8]

The cause of PE is a controversial topic among medical researchers and psychologists who study sex-related disorders. One hypothesis suggests that PE is related to anxiety. Another hypothesis is that men who exhibit premature ejaculation may be physically more sensitive to sexual stimulation. In the past decade, however, the focus has shifted from psychological factors to biological factors that may underlie PE, such as genetically based differences in ejaculation or neurotransmitter problems. (Neurotransmitters are chemical messengers that allow nerve cells to communicate with one another.) Consequently, treatment focus is shifting from behavioral techniques to drugs.[9] Nonetheless, specialists in sexual dysfunction advise that a variety of therapies may be useful in helping men with PE and suggest that a man or couple with this problem see a sex therapist as well as a physician.

Dapoxetine is a drug that is currently being considered for approval by the FDA for the treatment of PE, although the drug was rejected initially by the FDA in 2005. Dapoxetine is a short-acting antidepressant that allows the neurotransmitter serotonin to be used more effectively by the brain. (Serotonin is a brain chemical that affects emotions, behavior, and thought.) If approved, dapoxetine would be the first drug approved to treat PE. Although the drug appears to be effective and generally well tolerated by patients, it has serious side effects with long-term use, which include psychiatric problems, weight gain, skin reactions, lowered sex drive, nausea, and headache. These side effects have been one stumbling block in the FDA approval process. Another similar drug called Escitalopram, which has received tentative—not final—FDA approval, is also in development. Topical anesthetic creams are available, but they are messy, must be applied prior to sex and then thoroughly washed off, and may numb the partner's tissues if not removed completely.[9]

Hypoactive Sexual Desire Disorder

Hypoactive sexual desire disorder (HSDD) refers to a persistent low interest in sex with personal distress resulting from this low desire.[10] This disorder affects both men and women, although HSDD occurs more often in women. Interest in sex declines with age in both men and women as hormone levels drop.

Thus, older women and men may not be as distressed as younger persons by a lowered sex drive and may consider it part of the normal aging process. Consequently, HSDD may have a lower frequency in older persons than in younger persons.

A study of a large national sample of U.S. women using the Women's International Study of Health and Sexuality (WISHeS) questionnaire supports this hypothesis.[11] Results of the study reveal that 24% to 36% of women between the ages of 20 and 70 years had low sexual desire. Nonetheless, not all of these women had HSDD because not all of them experienced personal distress as a result of their low desire. In premenopausal women aged 20 to 49 years, 24% had low sexual desire. In naturally postmenopausal women aged 50 to 70 years (those who had not had menopause induced surgically by removal of the ovaries), 29% had low sexual desire. However, a much larger proportion of the younger women were distressed by their low desire: 59% of the younger age group who experienced low sexual desire versus 33% of the older age group. Thus, in calculating HSDD in these two groups of women, the researchers determined that the younger women had a higher rate of HSDD (14%) than the older women did (9%).

Hypoactive sexual desire disorder has a variety of psychological and physical causes, such as restrictive views regarding sex, a history of sexual abuse, relationship problems, certain chronic diseases such as rheumatoid arthritis, fatigue, stress, illness, and abnormal hormone levels. Stahl suggests that HSDD may be the result of a dysfunction of certain "reward pathway" neurotransmitters in the brain.[10]

Treatment of HSDD includes the identification and elimination of the cause. Problems within the relationship or conflicting personal feelings and beliefs regarding sexuality are best identified and resolved via counseling and therapy. Other treatments include relaxation techniques, hormone treatments, and changes in medications that a patient may be taking. Drugs that act on the dysfunctional "reward" pathways in the brain may hold promise for the future treatment of HSDD as well.[12]

Female Sexual Arousal Disorder

When a woman becomes sexually excited, the blood vessels in the pelvic area widen, tissues expand, and fluid seeps through the walls of the blood vessels in the vaginal area, providing lubrication for sexual intercourse. *Female sexual arousal disorder* (FSAD) is a condition in which a woman is continually unable, over an extended period of time, to attain or maintain adequate lubrication along with the swelling response during sexual activity. The causes of FSAD include depression, stress, relationship problems, past sexual or emotional abuse, and self-image problems. If the absence of this response is the result of a physiologic cause, such as the changes of menopause, injuries to the genital area, damage to nerves, the side effect of medications, or illness, the condition is considered a sexual dysfunction resulting from a medical condition, and it is not considered FSAD.

Treatments for the absence of adequate lubrication during sexual activity vary depending on the cause. Treatments for sexual dysfunction caused by a medical condition include hormone replacement therapy, prescription intravaginal hormone creams, and nonprescription lubricants. The EROS clinical therapy device, which is a small vacuum pump designed to increase blood flow to the area, helps some women. In addition, research results show sildenafil citrate (Viagra) to be a moderately useful treatment.[13] Treatments for FSAD include sex therapy and psychological therapy.

vaginismus A sexual dysfunction of women in which the lower portion of the vagina contracts involuntarily at the anticipation of penetration, preventing it.

Vaginismus

Vaginismus is a sexual dysfunction of women in which the muscles of the lower third of the vaginal canal contract involuntarily (and often painfully) at the anticipation of sexual intercourse, the insertion of tampons, or a pelvic examination, causing distress. The muscular contractions are strong enough to prevent penetration. Women with vaginismus do not usually have other sexual dysfunctions and can achieve orgasm by stimulating the clitoris.

Vaginismus appears to have both physical and psychological causes. A variety of physical conditions can cause pain during intercourse (*dyspareunia*; dis-pah-ROO-nee-ah) and result in vaginismus. Causes of dyspareunia include a poorly healed episiotomy (an incision made to widen the vaginal opening during the birth process); infections, sores, or lesions of the vagina or vulva; estrogen deficiency; sexually transmitted infections (STIs); or inadequate lubrication during intercourse. If a woman experiences pain during intercourse because of one or more of these

Diversity in Health

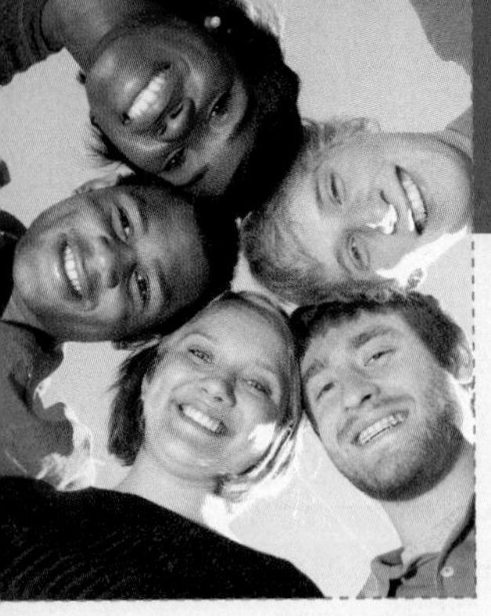

© Mike Flippo/ShutterStock

The Perceived Virtue of Virginity

In many cultures and to many people, virginity is a virtue that is presented on the wedding night to one's spouse. Since ancient times, people from various cultures have used the condition of a bride's hymen to determine if this virtue is intact. Although the hymen has no known biological function, this thin membranous tissue usually covers part of the outer entrance to the vagina. Most hymens have at least one opening that is wide enough to permit the discharge of menstrual blood. In many instances, this opening is too narrow for a penis to penetrate without tearing the surrounding tissue, but the hymen can also be torn while engaging in nonsexual activities, such as riding a bicycle, exercising, or using tampons.

According to the Old Testament of the Bible, a man who thought that his bride was not a virgin on their wedding night was entitled to have his townspeople stone her to death. In some ancient societies, a newly wed woman who could not prove her virginity might be banished from her hometown, tortured, or killed. Her lover, if known, often received the same treatment. Today, virginity is still an important criterion for selecting a mate in some places, especially in India, Indonesia, China, Taiwan, Iran, Turkey, and Arab nations. In most of these places, however, a new bride with sexual experience usually receives less harsh treatment than in the past. She may be rejected by her husband and returned to her family as "used goods." Facing embarrassment and ridicule from neighbors, the woman's family may disown her.

According to Islamic tradition, a woman's virginity is the basis for her honor and that of her family, her future groom, and his family. Muslims, followers of Islam, would arrange early marriages for their female children to ensure that these girls entered puberty as virgin brides. Fatima Mernissi, a sociologist in the African country of Morocco, thinks that Muslim men maintain their respect and pride by controlling the sexuality of their wives, daughters, and sisters. In many Muslim communities, young women are required to be heavily veiled in the presence of strange men and in public (**Figure 6.B**). If they do not wear veils, young women may be punished severely.

Marriage and social customs in rural parts of Africa, Asia, and the Mediterranean often include some ritual that "proves" the bride has lost her virginity on her wedding night. In parts of Greece, the groom's friends gather outside the window of the newly married couple on the morning after the wedding to receive the news that the bride is no longer a virgin. After the groom makes the expected announcement, the gathering of friends celebrates by firing guns into the air. In many Middle Eastern villages it is customary for the groom to display bloodstained sheets as evidence of wedding night virginity loss. In some societies with such traditions, new brides keep a small amount of chicken blood handy to drip on sheets during the wedding night, or they make a small cut near the vaginal opening that will bleed during sexual intercourse. The social value of virginity is so powerful that cosmetic surgeons in Japan and Italy routinely reconstruct hymens so that

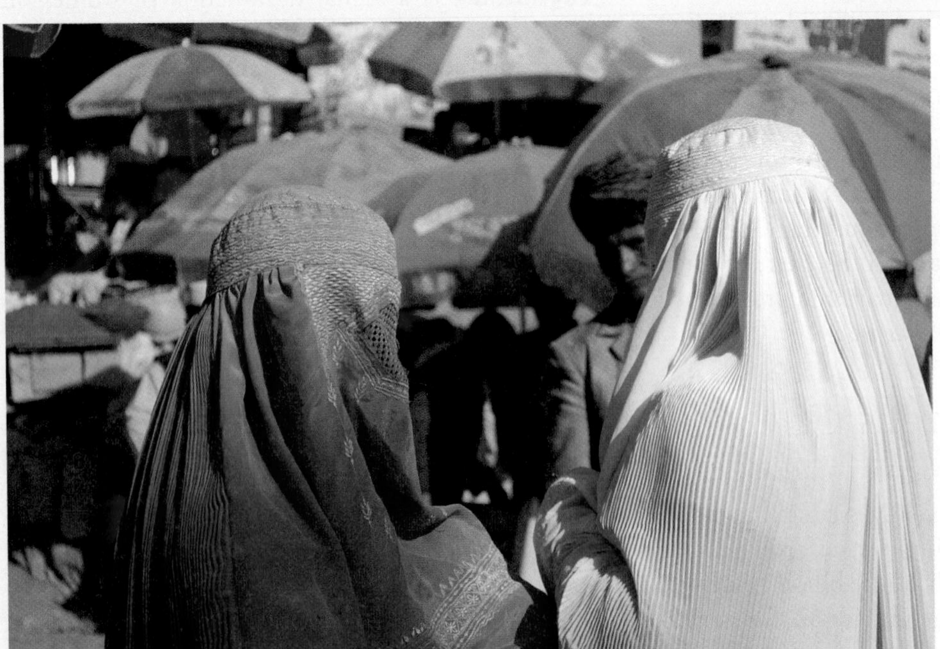

Figure 6.B

Culturally Appropriate Clothing. In some Islamic traditions women wear the body-covering burka in public. A mesh screen covers the eyes. These women are at a bazaar in Afghanistan.

© Lizette Potgieter/ShutterStock

their unmarried female patients who have been sexually active or have torn hymens for reasons unrelated to sex can present themselves with the needed tissues intact.

Economic factors also play a major role in perpetuating the value of premarital virginity. In many cultures, property is handed down from fathers to sons. Therefore, families strive to protect their financial interests and lines of inheritance by seeking virgin brides for male relatives. An unmarried woman who is not a virgin could be pregnant with a male child whose father is from another family. Without DNA testing to confirm a child's paternity, rural people in underdeveloped regions rely on an intact hymen as a sign of virginity. Along with this view of women as property, cultural norms of sexual chastity, female virginity, pure bloodlines, and family honor may also serve to control women's behavior.

In some societies, virginity tests, which usually involve inspection of the hymen, are used to document premarital virginity. For example, virginity testing existed in Turkey until 2002 when laws were changed that had previously allowed school administrators to require virginity testing for female students. In 2010, the Indonesian government was urged by Amnesty International to block attempts to institute virginity and pregnancy testing for high school girls, which it did.

Virginity testing has also been reported as retaliation for women political protesters. In 2011, women protesters in Egypt were forced to undergo virginity testing while under military detention; 1 year later, the military doctor was acquitted of any wrongdoing for performing the tests. Women protesters in Sudan also reported being subjected to virginity testing while under military detention.

In some areas of South Africa, virginity "tests" that are born of ancient tribal customs and that have no relationship to whether a young woman is really a virgin are still practiced alongside public genital inspection for an intact hymen (**Figure 6.C**). South Africans who support virginity testing explain that this tradition is important not only to retain long-held customs but also to promote sexual abstinence in a country with a high rate of HIV/AIDS.

Is disease prevention the "new" virtue of virginity? It may be, but promoting virginity by means of virginity testing is viewed by its opponents as nothing more than degrading abuse. Virginity testing is placing ancient cultures and human rights on a collision course and makes virginity look less like a virtue and more like a condition to endure.

How do you view virginity? As something that is good, bad, or neither good nor bad? Do you agree or disagree with the statement, "virginity testing is a violation of human rights;" why?

Data from Amnesty International. (2010, November 11). Indonesia urged to block discriminatory pregnancy tests for school girls. Retrieved March 7, 2011, from http://www.amnesty.org/en/news-and-updates/indonesia-urged-block-discriminatory-pregnancy-tests-schoolgirls-2010-11-11; Amnesty International. (2013, February 6). Egypt: Impunity fuels sexual violence. Retrieved July 18, 2014 from http://www.amnesty.org/en/for-media/press-releases/egypt-impunity-fuels-sexual-violence-2013-02-06; Brulliard, K. (2008, September 26). Zulus eagerly defy ban on virginity test: S. Africa's progressive constitution collides with tribal customs. *Washington Post*. Retrieved March 7, 2011, from http://www.washingtonpost.com/wp-dyn/content/article/2008/09/25/AR2008092504625.html; Mernissi, F. (2003). *Beyond the veil: Male–female dynamics in Muslim society*. London, England: Saqi Books; Mthethwa, B. (2009, December 12). Virginity testing keeps boys pure. Retrieved on March 7, 2011, from http://www.timeslive.co.za/sundaytimes/article231102.ece

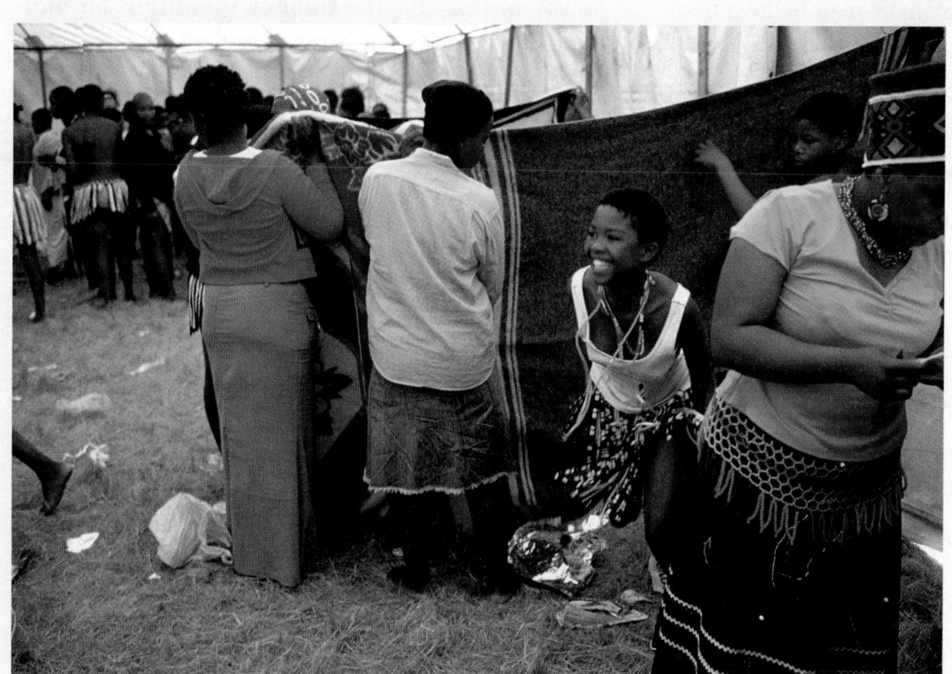

Figure 6.C

This smiling girl has just completed her virginity testing in rural Natal, South Africa.

value The belief that an idea, object, or action has worth.

gender identity An individual's perception of himself or herself as male or female.

gender role Patterns of behavior, attitudes, and personality attributes that are traditionally considered in a particular culture to be feminine or masculine.

sexual (gender) stereotype The widespread association of certain perceptions with one gender.

conditions, involuntary vaginal contractions may occur as the body attempts to protect itself from penetration and subsequent pain. If the cause of the pain eventually subsides, the contractions may still occur as a conditioned response. Recent research suggests that vaginismus and dispareunia should be considered as one "genito-pelvic penetration/pain disorder" because the two conditions generally occur together, and reliable diagnosis of vaginal spasm is difficult.[14]

Psychogenic vaginismus usually begins without a physical cause. The results of studies show that this type of vaginismus occurs as a protective response to perceived pain or violation of the body, with common causes being child sexual abuse, early traumatic sexual experiences, early traumatic gynecological examinations, inadequate sex information, and cultural and religious taboos.

Treatments for vaginismus are usually tailored to the individual and are multidimensional. Education helps correct misconceptions a woman may have about the genitals in general and the vagina in particular. (For example, a woman may believe that the vagina is particularly narrow and delicate and therefore easily harmed by penetration.) Psychiatric or psychological therapy may be useful for a woman alone or for her and her partner. Physical treatment generally includes using vaginal inserts of graded sizes to slowly help a woman overcome her fear of penetration, but this step can be taken only when a woman feels ready.

Culture and Sexuality

Society strongly influences the sexual attitudes and behaviors of a population by identifying acceptable sexual activities and placing restrictions on others. For example, some cultures value sexual abstinence before marriage; others value sexual experimentation during childhood. A **value** is a belief that an idea, object, or action has worth. The Diversity in Health essay "The Virtue of Virginity" provides a cross-cultural perspective concerning the value of sexual abstinence before marriage.

An individual usually formulates a personal value system before adulthood. A *value system* is a collection of beliefs that helps a person identify and classify things as being good or bad, or neither good nor bad. This value system guides the reasoning and behavior of the individual, especially in sexual decision making.

Many Americans derive their sexual values from Judeo-Christian religious teachings. However, people in the culturally diverse U.S. population adhere to a variety of sexual values, some of which conflict with traditional Judeo-Christian teachings. No universally accepted set of sexual values applies to Americans.

Widely accepted values can help people determine behavioral norms, but these norms often change over time and across cultures. Before World War I, for example, it was socially unacceptable for "proper" American men or women to expose much of their bodies in public. Today, most Americans think that it is acceptable for people to wear clothing that exposes much of their bodies, especially in warm weather. However, in some cultures, persons are punished severely if they appear in public dressed in revealing outfits; the only acceptable style of clothing is that which has been worn for centuries (**Figure 6.B**).

Gender Identity and Roles

Gender is the socially constructed differences that distinguish one as female or male, as defined previously in this chapter. **Gender identity** is an individual's perception of himself or herself as male or female. Most people have a gender identity that is congruent with their biological sex. Various biological, social, and environmental forces mold a child's gender identity.

Before birth, genetic and hormonal factors influence the sexual development of the embryonic brain. After birth, social factors have a major impact on gender identity. As children interact with people, they observe and learn gender roles and sexual stereotypes. A **gender role** refers to patterns of behavior, attitudes, and personality attributes that are traditionally considered in a particular culture to be feminine or masculine. For example, women have traditionally borne more responsibility for child-rearing and household management and men have traditionally been viewed as the protectors and providers for their families. A **sexual (gender) stereotype** is the widespread association of certain perceptions with one gender. Examples of sexual stereotypes are associating household chores or child-care activities with women (e.g., cleaning the house and staying home to care for children is "women's work") or associating the responsibility for earning the family income with men (e.g., it is a man's responsibility to provide for his family).

Throughout the world, obvious biological differences between the sexes form the basis for many traditional gender roles. Women being responsible for routine child-rearing and household management likely developed for a variety of reasons, such as a woman's biological role in giving birth and nursing infants. It is also likely that because men, in general, are physically stronger than women are, their customary roles have been protecting and providing for their families, especially in hunter-gatherer or agrarian societies.

In addition to biological factors, culture and religion heavily influence sexual attitudes and behaviors. In many cultures, men learn to be sexually aggressive and women learn to be sexually passive. According to these sexual stereotypes, men are always eager for sex, and they are expected to demonstrate their interest and aggressiveness by initiating sexual encounters. Women are expected to be less interested in sex than men are but to accept the sexual advances of men (such as their partners) willingly.

In the United States, parents, friends, teachers, and the media influence children's perceptions of gender roles. Academic engagement, peers, and women's studies courses appear to be relevant in shaping college students' perceptions of gender roles.[15]

Some Americans reject traditional gender stereotypes because these attitudes and practices can create and foster sexism. **Sexism**, discrimination and bias against one sex, is common in many societies. For many women in the United States and other countries, sexist practices affect their status and health at work, school, and home. Sexual harassment and violence against women are forms of sexism. Men can experience sexism as well; males sometimes feel the object of sexist practices in the workplace when hiring guidelines favor females.

Over the past 2 decades, societal norms in the United States have moved to a more liberal interpretation of appropriate role behaviors for women. Women are now more comfortable initiating dates. Men and women may feel free to initiate or refuse sexual activity. Additionally, a growing number of Americans feel free to choose nontraditional careers and adopt flexible gender roles. For example, many mothers work outside of the home; also, some fathers stay at home to care for their children and manage household tasks.

sexism Discrimination and bias against one sex.

transgender An umbrella term for various groups of people who do not conform to traditional gender roles.

Transgender

Transgender is an umbrella term that is commonly used—but not universally accepted—for various groups of people who do not conform to traditional gender roles for appearance (gender expression) or whose gender identity differs from the societal norm.[16] The transgender category can include transsexuals, crossdressers, intersex persons, drag performers, and androgynes. According to data released in 2011 from the Williams Institute at the University of California, Los Angeles (UCLA), 0.3% of the U.S. adult population is transgender.[17]

Transsexuals are persons whose gender identity conflicts with his or her biological sex, a condition known as *gender dysphoria*. In many cases, an individual feels trapped in the body of the opposite sex. Persons with gender dysphoria often seek psychotherapy and/or hormonal treatments in an effort to cope with their gender identity conflicts; some choose to have sex reassignment surgery to align their physical body with their gender identity. Physicians who perform sex reassignment surgeries usually remove certain reproductive organs and reconstruct the genitals of the patient to make them resemble those of the opposite sex. After gender reassignment surgery, however, the newly fashioned reproductive organs do not function like the organs of people who were born with them. **Figure 6.5** is a before and after photo of Chaz Bono—actor, writer, musician, transgender activist, and son of Sonny Bono and Cher—who underwent a female to male gender reassignment surgery.

Unlike transsexuals, *crossdressers* are comfortable with their gender, but they occasionally dress and act like the opposite sex. Most crossdressers are heterosexual men. *Drag performers* dress like the opposite sex as well, but they do it as a job or as play; it is not an identity for them.

Intersex persons have disorders of sex development (DSD) resulting in some combination of male and female internal and external sexual organs. These characteristics are the result of the action of genes and are present at birth. In 2010, a gene that influences

sexual orientation The direction of a person's romantic thoughts, feelings, and attractions toward people of the same or different sex.

heterosexual A person who is sexually attracted to members of the opposite sex.

homosexual A person who is sexually attracted to members of his or her own sex.

bisexual A person who is sexually attracted to members of both sexes.

Figure 6.5

Chastity Bono to Chaz Bono. Born the daughter of Sonny Bono and Cher, Bono's transition from female to male began in 2008, was physically completed in 2009 with gender reassignment surgery, and was legally completed in 2010 when a California court agreed to change Bono's gender and name. (a) Chastity Bono in 1998. (b) Chaz Bono in 2011.

(a) © Susan Sterner/AP Images; (b) © Helga Esteb/ShutterStock

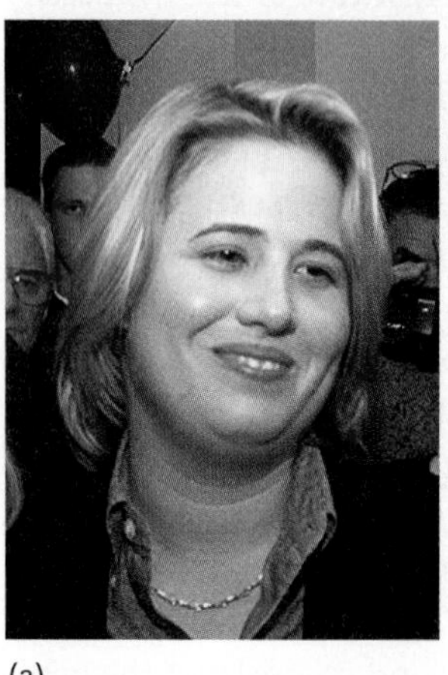

(a)

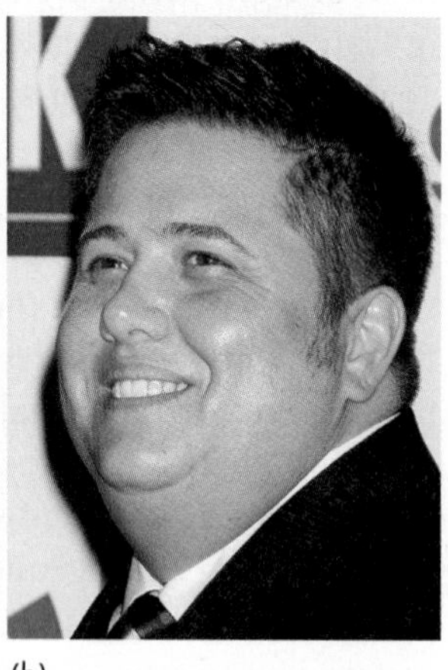

(b)

the activity of other genes involved in human sex determination was discovered.[18] With 1 in 1,000 individuals affected by DSD, research is ongoing to better understand the genes involved in the development of a person's sex and how they work.

Androgynous persons, or *androgynes*, have traits with no gender value—they do not fit easily into male or female categories—or they have traits attributed to the opposite sex. These characteristics may be physical or behavioral.

Sexual Orientation

One of the most emotionally charged aspects of human sexuality is **sexual orientation**, that is, the direction of a person's romantic thoughts, feelings, and attractions. Results of one study reveal that of a nationally representative sample of 9,400 U.S. college and university students, 93.9% identified themselves as **heterosexual** (sexually attracted to members of the opposite sex).[19] Of the remainder, 2.4% identified themselves as **homosexual**, and 3.7% as **bisexual**. One who is homosexual is sexually attracted to members of her or his own sex; one who is bisexual is sexually attracted to both sexes.

Men and women who identify as homosexual are commonly referred to as *gay*; homosexual women are also called *lesbians*. Sexologist Alfred Kinsey proposed that sexual orientation is a continuum with exclusively heterosexual and homosexual designations at opposite ends and degrees of bisexuality within this continuum (**Figure 6.6**).[20] Sexual orientation percentages hold fairly consistent across sociodemographic groups.[21]

For the first time in its 57-year history, the 2013 National Health Interview Study—conducted by the Centers for Disease Control and Prevention (CDC)—included questions regarding sexual orientation. According to the results, published in July 2014, of the 34,557 respondents 18 years and older, 96.6% identified as straight (heterosexual), 1.6% identified as gay or lesbian, 0.7% identified as bisexual, 0.2% identified as "something else." Although this study did not find any significant differences in the percentages of men and women identifying as gay, lesbian, or straight, the percentage of women identifying as bisexual was more than twice as high as their male counterparts (0.9% and 0.4%, respectively). Age differences were reported among those identifying as gay or lesbian: The percentages of those aged 18–44 and 45–64 who identified as gay or lesbian were more than 2.5 times higher than the percentage of those 65 and older. Age differences were also reported for those identifying as bisexual: The percentage of those aged 18–44 who identified as bisexual was 2.75 times higher than the percentage of those aged 45–64 and 5.5 times higher than for those aged 65 and older.[22]

Results from the National Survey of Family Growth (NSFG), also conducted by researchers at the CDC, and most recently published in 2011, show that 6% of men and 12% of women aged 25 to 44 years engaged in sex with a same-sex partner at least once over their lifetime (**Figure 6.7**). Of the homosexual population in the study, 55% were males and 45% were females. Of the bisexual population in the study, 29% were males and 71% were females. These percentages of sexual orientation are similar to the results of many other studies.[21]

Figure 6.6

Kinsey's Continuum of Sexual Orientation. Sexuality researcher Alfred Kinsey thought that sexual orientation is a continuum with exclusively heterosexual and homosexual designations on the ends and degrees of bisexuality between them.

100% Heterosexual	A few homosexual fantasies or experiences	More heterosexual than homosexual	Bisexual	More homosexual than heterosexual	A few heterosexual fantasies or experiences	100% Homosexual

Nature or Nurture?

Do people choose their sexual orientation? Formerly, there was widespread belief that homosexuality was learned behavior and that children became homosexual by having early social and sexual experiences with gay individuals. At present, researchers cannot find a common childhood characteristic that predicts adult sexual orientation. Children may have same-sex experiences with other children, but most develop heterosexual orientations as they mature. Some gays and lesbians report that they knew they were different at an early age, but they did not recognize their homosexuality until they were in their teens or early 20s.

Today, researchers and mental health experts generally agree that people do not decide their sexual orientation and cannot alter their sexual preferences, whether they are at either end of the sexual orientation continuum or somewhere in-between. Researchers have been studying the biological basis of homosexuality, and results of studies of the early 1990s show physical differences in small groups of cells in the hypothalamus of the brains of heterosexual and homosexual men.[23] In 1993, molecular geneticist Dean Hamer and his colleagues announced that a particular region of the X chromosome in homosexual males was involved in male sexual orientation in some, but not all, gay men.[24] Males inherit this sex chromosome (condensed piece of hereditary material) from their mothers. The particular region of the X chromosome was dubbed the "gay gene." However, the results of more recent research suggest that homosexuality is under the control of more than a single gene. Scientists are now studying how genes

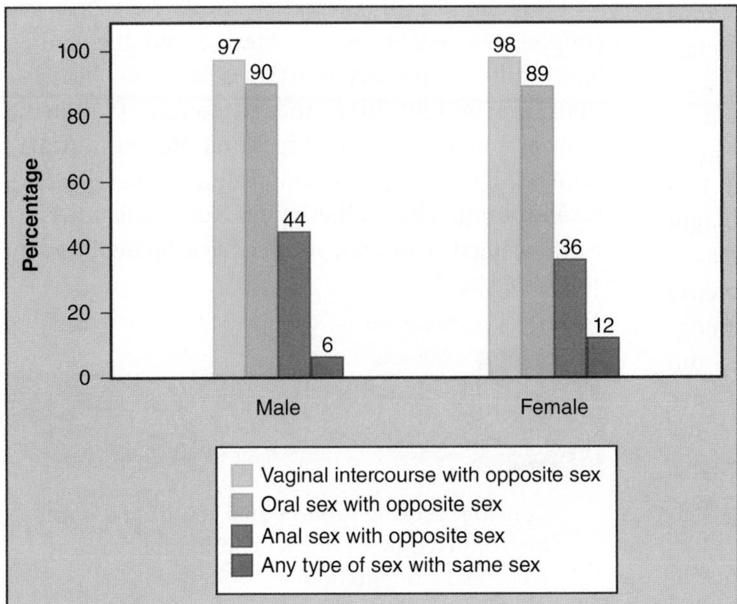

Figure 6.7

Sexual Behavior. Sexual behavior in lifetime among males and females 25–44 years of age: United States.

Reproduced from Chandra, A., et al (2011, March 3). Sexual behavior, sexual attraction, and sexual identity in the United States: Data from the 2006–2008 National Survey of Family Growth. *National Health Statistics Reports*, no. 36. Retrieved July 20, 2014, from http://www.cdc.gov/nchs/data/nhsr/nhsr036.pdf

homophobia An intense fear of or hostility toward homosexuals.

sexual intercourse Penetration of the vagina by a penis.

coitus (KO-ih-tus) The act of a penis penetrating a vagina, often referred to as vaginal intercourse.

cunnilingus Use of the mouth and tongue to stimulate a woman's genitals.

fellatio Use of the mouth and tongue to stimulate a male's genitals.

that control homosexuality are maintained in the population.[25]

Sexual Orientation and Society

Since ancient times, homosexuality has existed in most societies. Homosexuals are members of every racial, ethnic, socioeconomic, religious, and occupational group. Although many homosexuals choose to conceal their sexual orientation, others have decided to express their sexual preferences openly.

Homophobia is an intense fear of or hostility toward homosexuals. However, not every person who objects to homosexuality is afraid of gay people or is hostile toward them. Therefore, *antihomosexual* may be a more descriptive term than *homophobic* to describe people who harbor such fears and hostilities.

Many heterosexuals do not accept homosexuality because they think gay sexual behavior is unnatural or it contradicts their religious beliefs. Other people are afraid of contact with gays because they associate acquired immune deficiency syndrome (AIDS) with homosexuality. Results of a May 2014 Gallup poll on tolerance for gay rights revealed that 66% of respondents thought that gay and lesbian relations should be legal, up from 44% in 1996, whereas 30% thought it should not be legal, down from 47% in 1996.[26]

U.S. President Bill Clinton signed the Defense of Marriage Act in 1996, which does not recognize marriages between same-sex individuals and allows states to ignore same-sex marriages that have been performed in other states. Gay couples, however, often cohabit and form lifetime commitments, commonly called domestic partnerships. Because domestic partners often contribute to the economic survival of their households, share property, and raise children, they want the same legal rights and protections that opposite-sex married couples have, such as the right to claim insurance benefits when their partners die.

In 2012 U.S. President Barak Obama became the first sitting president to announce support for same-sex marriage. Also in 2012, three states (Maine, Maryland, and Washington) became the first to legalize same-sex marriage through popular vote. In 2013, the Supreme Court struck down part of the Defense of Marriage Act, thus requiring the federal government to recognize same-sex marriages from the states in which they are legal. In 2014, federal courts struck down same-sex marriage bans in nine states: Utah, Oklahoma, Virginia, Texas, Michigan, Idaho, Wisconsin, Indiana, and Kentucky.[27] When asked in 2014 whether marriages between same-sex couples should or should not be recognized by the law as valid, with the same rights as traditional marriages, 55% of Gallup poll respondents said they should be valid, up from 27% in 1996, whereas 42% said they should not be valid, down from 68% in 1996.[26]

As of June 2014, 19 states—California, Connecticut, Delaware, Hawaii, Illinois, Iowa, Maine, Maryland, Massachusetts, Minnesota, New Hampshire, New Jersey, New Mexico, New York, Oregon, Pennsylvania, Rhode Island, Vermont, and Washington—and the District of Columbia have legalized gay marriage. Colorado, Nevada, and Wisconsin have civil unions or domestic partnership provisions for gay couples, but most states in the United States still ban same-sex marriage or refer to marriage as being between a man and a woman.[27] Domestic partnerships grant nearly all or some state-level spousal rights to unmarried couples.

There are very few places in the world where gay couples can legally marry. Mexico and the United States allow same-sex marriages in some jurisdictions. As of July 2014, the 18 countries allowing same-sex marriage were Argentina, Belgium, Brazil, Canada, Denmark, England/Wales, France, Iceland, Luxembourg, The Netherlands, New Zealand, Norway, Portugal, Scotland, South Africa, Spain, Sweden, and Uruguay.[28]

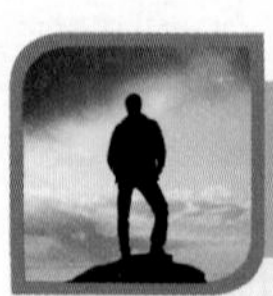

© djgis/ShutterStock

Healthy Living Practices

- Consider seeking professional counseling if you are confused by, or not yet comfortable with, your sexual orientation.

Diversity in Health

Common Sexual Practices Between Partners

Most heterosexuals are familiar with the notion of "having sex" or **sexual intercourse** as vaginal sex, the insertion of a penis into a vagina. Vaginal sex, or **coitus**, is the most common and popular form of intimate sexual activity between partners. According to findings from the National Survey of Sexual Health and Behavior (NSSHB) conducted by researchers from the Center for Sexual Health Promotion at Indiana University, about three-fourths of men and women aged 25 to 39 years and more than half aged 20–24 and 40–49 years engaged in vaginal intercourse in the month prior to taking the survey.[29] Results from the NSFG show that 97% of men and 98% of women aged 25–44 years had vaginal intercourse at least once over their lifetime (see Figure 6.7).

The report *American Sexual Behavior: Trends, Sociodemographic Differences, and Risk Behavior* from the University of Chicago's National Opinion Research Center states that, on average, adult Americans say that they engage in vaginal intercourse about once a week. Married individuals report having vaginal sex more frequently than never-married, divorced, or widowed persons. The results of various surveys indicate that the longer a couple has been married, the less frequently they engage in coitus.[21]

Men engaging in *anal intercourse*—whether with other men or with women—was reported much less frequently than vaginal intercourse. The highest incidence of past-month homosexual/heterosexual "insertive" anal intercourse (inserted penis into anus) was among men aged 25–29 years at 10.3%.[29] Lifetime heterosexual anal sex for men aged 25–44 years was reported as 44% on the NSFG (see Figure 6-7). The highest incidence of homosexual past-month "receptive" anal intercourse (received penis in anus) was among men aged 50–59 years at 2.9%.[29]

For women, the incidence of anal intercourse is low. The highest incidence of past-month anal intercourse reported on the NSSHB was among those aged 18–24 years at about 7% to 8%.[29] Lifetime anal sex for females aged 25–44 years was reported as 36% on the NSFG (see Figure 6-7).

Many women and men find receptive anal intercourse unappealing because the practice can be painful, it increases the risk of contracting sexually transmitted infections, especially HIV, and it increases the risk of developing urinary tract infections. The lining of the rectum tears easily—much more easily than the vagina—elevating the risk of bacteria and viruses entering the bloodstream. Lubricants that are often used with anal sex may irritate the tissues, increasing the risk further. Using latex condoms during anal sex reduces but does not eliminate this risk. For women, if anal intercourse is followed by vaginal intercourse, bacteria can be spread from the rectum into the vagina or the *urethra*, the tube that carries urine from the bladder. After anal sex, one should wash the fingers and penis thoroughly before engaging in additional sexual activity, and a fresh condom should be used. Women should urinate after vaginal sex to help remove some of the bacteria that have entered the urethra, reducing the risk of a bladder infection.

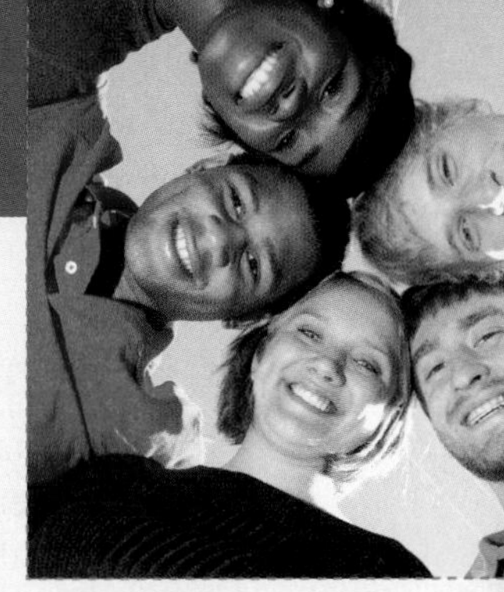

© Mike Flippo/ShutterStock

People often engage in *petting*, more recently called *mutual masturbation*, as a pleasurable substitute for or a prelude to intercourse. During these activities, two or more people stimulate themselves or another sexually, often with the hands, without vaginal or anal intercourse. Mutual masturbation activities include a variety of sex acts that range from kissing and fondling breasts to performing oral sex. Additionally, people may rub their genital areas together, without penetration. For people who want to reduce their risk of pregnancy or sexually transmitted infections, mutual masturbation can be a safer alternative to vaginal or anal sex.

Although not as popular as vaginal intercourse, oral sex is a common sexual activity. **Cunnilingus** is the use of the mouth and tongue to stimulate a woman's genitals; **fellatio** refers to oral stimulation of a male's genitals. In the early part of the 20th century, heterosexuals, even those who were married, rarely practiced oral sex. By the 1970s, sex manuals and sexuality textbooks had begun to suggest that couples incorporate oral sex into their sexual routines. Women who are unable to have orgasms during coitus are often able to have them while receiving oral sex.

In a study of more than 2,000 college students using an anonymous online survey, researcher Wendy Chambers of the University of Georgia found that 39.1% of virgins had given oral sex to someone in their lifetime and that 95.5% of nonvirgins had. Of the respondents, 53.5% considered oral sex to be an intimate act, compared to 91% who considered sexual intercourse to be an intimate act.[30]

Results of the NSSHB show that the percentage of males who gave oral sex to a female within the month before the survey peaks at ages 25–29 years at 40%, and the percentage of males who gave oral sex to a male within the month is highest at ages 20–24 years at 5.2% and at 50–59 years at 6.4%. The percentage at other ages is much lower for male-on-male oral sex within the month. Results of the NSSHB also show that the percentage of females who gave oral sex to a male within the month before the survey peaks at ages 25–29 years at 49.9%, and the percentage of females who gave oral sex to a female within the month peaks at ages 16–17 years at 4.2%. The percentage at other ages is much lower for female-on-female oral sex within the month.[30] On the NSFG, lifetime percentages for oral sex with the opposite sex were 90% for men aged 25–44 years and 89% for women of the same age group (see Figure 6-7).

celibacy (sexual abstinence) Refrainment from sexual intercourse, usually by choice.

Solitary Sexual Behavior

In 1994, statements on masturbation by the U.S. Surgeon General M. Joycelyn Elders resulted in her being forced to resign her post. Her comments were in response to a question at a United Nations conference on AIDS and suggested that masturbation might be taught as a means to limit the spread of HIV/AIDS. Although masturbation was a taboo subject to speak about publicly at that time, Elders recognized in 2010 that "we have finally included masturbation in our national conversation" as she discussed the reports from the National Survey of Sexual Health and Behavior (NSSHB).[31]

Data from the NSSHB show that solo masturbation is a common sexual practice in the United States. From 28% to 69% of men report that they masturbated alone within the month prior to the survey and from 12% to 52% of women did as well. Percentages varied by age group, with the lowest percentages reported by the oldest age group (70+ years old) and the highest percentages reported by those aged 25 to 29 years. This was true for both men and women.[29] The NSSHB research team also reported data on solo masturbation within the past year by gender and age; although these data held a similar gender and age pattern, they were slightly higher than the past month percentages. From 46% to 84% of men reported that they masturbated alone within the last year and from 33% to 72% of women did, as well. As with past month data, the lowest percentages were reported by the oldest age group (70+ years old), and the highest percentages reported by those aged 25–29 years, for both men and women.[32] A British survey released in 2008 had similar findings: 73% of men and nearly 37% of women aged 16 to 44 years reported masturbating within the month prior to the survey.[33]

Celibacy

Celibacy, or **sexual abstinence**, is refrainment from sexual intercourse, usually by choice. Celibacy can be a way of life; the clergy of some religions practice sexual abstinence. Some celibate individuals engage in alternative sexual practices such as masturbation. Temporary sexual abstinence during the woman's peak period of fertility is a feature of natural family planning methods. Late in pregnancy, couples may decide to avoid vaginal intercourse, especially if the activity is too awkward and uncomfortable.

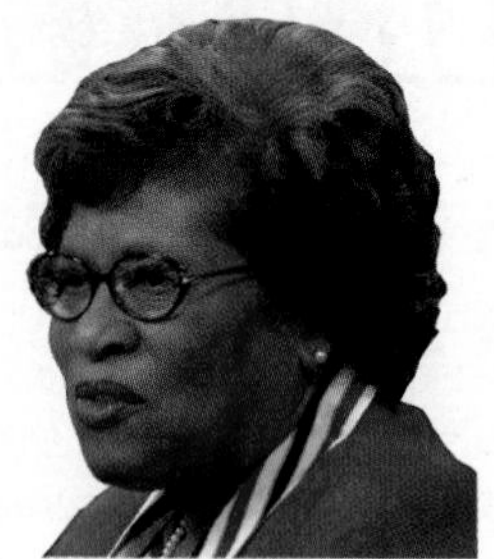

Former U.S. Surgeon General M. Jocelyn Elders.
© Mike Wintroath/AP Images

Celibacy is not known to be harmful; indeed, it is the most effective measure for preventing pregnancies and sexually transmitted infections.

© djgis/ShutterStock

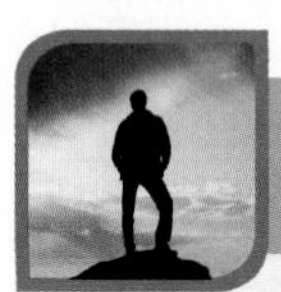

Healthy Living Practices

- Wash after touching the anal area so as not to spread bacteria that live in the rectum to other parts of the body.
- To reduce the risk of transmitting the virus that causes AIDS, use latex condoms during vaginal or anal intercourse.
- Practicing sexual abstinence is the most reliable way to avoid pregnancy and sexually transmitted infections.

Romantic Relationships

Defining Love

Giving and receiving love are so important to a person's well-being that social scientists have speculated about love and studied its origins, characteristics, and stages. What is love? Why do people fall in love?

Love is difficult to define because the term has different meanings for different people. One definition is that love is a collection of behaviors, thoughts, and emotions that are associated with a psychological attraction toward other individuals. There are numerous kinds or degrees of love and a variety of feelings associated with love. Liking, fondness, affection, attraction, infatuation, and lust are feelings related to love. Also, the love of two friends can be quite different from the feelings between parent and child or husband and wife. According to sexologists William H. Masters and Virginia E. Johnson, all forms of love involve the element of **caring**, the expression of concern for someone's well-being.

Zick Rubin, one of the first psychologists to develop a questionnaire to measure the meanings of love, attempted to differentiate between loving and liking. He found that loving had characteristics of intimacy, attachment, caring, and commitment whereas liking had characteristics of affection and respect.[34] **Intimacy** is the disclosure of one's most personal thoughts and emotions to a trusted individual. **Attachment** is the desire to spend time with someone to give and receive emotional support. **Commitment** is the determination to maintain the relationship even when times are difficult. **Affection** is a feeling of fondness toward another. **Respect** is the feeling that another has value and deserves attention.

Most humans seek loving relationships with other individuals to meet their emotional needs. Love that is fulfilling is reciprocal; that is, when one loves another, he or she is loved in return. Individuals who are in love feel free to achieve self-actualization because their relationship fosters mutual independence as well as emotional, social, and spiritual growth.

caring The expression of concern for someone's well-being.

intimacy Disclosure of one's most personal thoughts and emotions to a trusted individual.

attachment The desire to spend time with someone to give and receive emotional support.

commitment The determination to maintain a relationship even when times are difficult.

affection Fondness.

respect The feeling that another has value and deserves attention.

Psychologists' Theories About Love

Beginning with Sigmund Freud in 1922, psychologists have tried to explain the phenomenon of love. Early "love theorists" such as Freud were clinical psychologists, professionals who diagnose, treat, and study mental or emotional problems and disabilities. Most of their theories relied on ideas that people loved others as a remedy for their own problems or deficiencies, rather than loving others for themselves.

In recent decades, social psychologists have formulated theories on love. These professionals explore questions by examining the individual in a social context while taking into account personality, which is the distinctive pattern of behavior, thoughts, motives, and emotions that characterizes an individual.

In 1956, Eric Fromm presented his ideas about love in *The Art of Loving*.[35] A basic idea in Fromm's book, as noted in its title, is that loving is an art and, as such, must be learned and practiced. Fromm also distinguishes between types of love, such as motherly love and erotic love.

In 1973, John Alan Lee theorized that six styles of loving exist.[36] His ideas have since been upheld by results of studies of other researchers. **Table 6.1** lists these styles with their names (derived from the Greek), meanings, and characteristics. To see with which of Lee's style you most closely align, take "The Love Attitudes Scale" provided in the Student Workbook section at the end of this book.

In 1986, Robert Sternberg developed a triangular theory of love that incorporates three components—intimacy, commitment, and passion—as symbolized by the points of a triangle, shown in **Figure 6.8**.[37] His intimacy component includes behaviors that foster a feeling of warmth, whereas the commitment component refers to the decision to love as well as to make

Table 6.1

Lee's Six Styles of Loving

Name	Meaning	Characteristics
Ludus	Game-playing love	Enjoying "chasing" love interests but not "catching" them
Eros	Romantic, passionate love	Believing in "true" love and "instant" chemistry
Storge	Affectionate, friendly love	Believing that love grows out of friendship
Mania	Possessive, dependent love	Believing that your lover's attention is all that matters
Pragma	Logical, practical love	Thinking that the best lover for you will fit a predetermined set of criteria
Agape	Selfless love	Wanting to bear your lover's burdens so that he or she does not suffer

Figure 6.8

Sternberg's Love Triangle. Psychologist Robert Sternberg created a model that incorporates three components of love—intimacy, commitment, and passion—at the points of a triangle. Couples with identical "love triangles" (a) are more likely to be satisfied with their relationships because they share more sexual feelings and attitudes than couples with similar (b) or highly mismatched triangles (c).

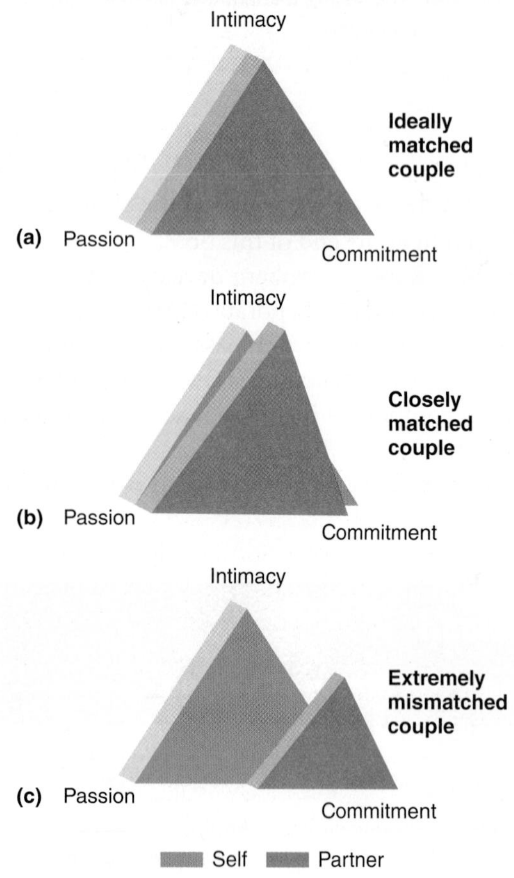

a relationship last. Passion, in the love triangle, refers not only to sexual passion but also to the fulfillment of needs that elicit a passionate response. The balance of these three components affects the shape of the triangle. Amount of love affects the area of the triangle.

People in a love relationship often have feelings of intimacy, commitment, and passion that differ from those of their partners. Although two people may be in love with each other, their "love triangles" will not match if one loves the other more than is reciprocated and if one differs from the other in the balances of the three kinds of love. According to Sternberg, couples with similar love triangles are more likely to be satisfied with their relationships because they share more love-related feelings and attitudes, as Figure 6-8b shows, there are couples with mismatched triangles, as in Figure 6-8c. Sternberg has developed a questionnaire to measure love according to his love triangles theory.[38,39]

Finally, Sternberg asserts that although there are only three components of love, these three components combine in various ways to produce seven kinds of love.[39] For example, an absence of all three components (intimacy, commitment, and passion) results in nonlove. The presence of all three components results in consummate love. **Figure 6.9** lists Sternberg's kinds of love and their components.

Love Attachments

The early bonds, or attachments, that develop between parents and their offspring may influence the ability of the children to form close, secure relationships when they are adults. *Attachment* is a biological drive in which a child seeks nearness to or contact with a specific person, such as a parent, when he or she is frightened, tired, hungry, or ill. A child will exhibit attachment behavior, such as eye contact, smiling, crying, and clinging, to obtain or maintain desired proximity to this person. How the person responds to the child largely determines the type of attachment the child will form: secure, ambivalent, or avoidant.

For example, when an infant is hungry, he or she will exhibit attachment behavior, such as crying, which usually evokes a nurturing response from the attachment figure (e.g., mom or dad). A nurturing response to this need usually includes touching, eye contact, smiling, and providing milk. When the infant receives this nurturing response consistently, trust is built. When the infant does not receive this response consistently, the child may develop mistrust and may stop his or her attachment behavior. Over time, symptoms may emerge such as lack of eye contact, destructive behavior, and poor peer relationships. Some children who have poor attachments to their parents may avoid becoming emotionally close to people in adulthood.

Experts think that children who have emotionally distant and neglectful parents may mature into anxious lovers. *Anxious lovers* often have considerable doubts about the quality of their sexual relationships, are unable to trust their partners, and may be unable to form long-term commitments. However, if parents meet the emotional needs of their children and frequently display affection toward them, the children are likely to mature into secure lovers. Secure lovers are more likely to form trusting and committed relationships with other adults than are anxious lovers.

Some people experience *infatuation*, a passionate but unrealistic attraction to someone. Infatuated

Figure 6.9

Sternberg's Seven Kinds of Love

Modified from *Cupid's Arrow: The Course of Love Through Time* by Dr. Robert J. Sternberg, Cambridge University Press, 1998.

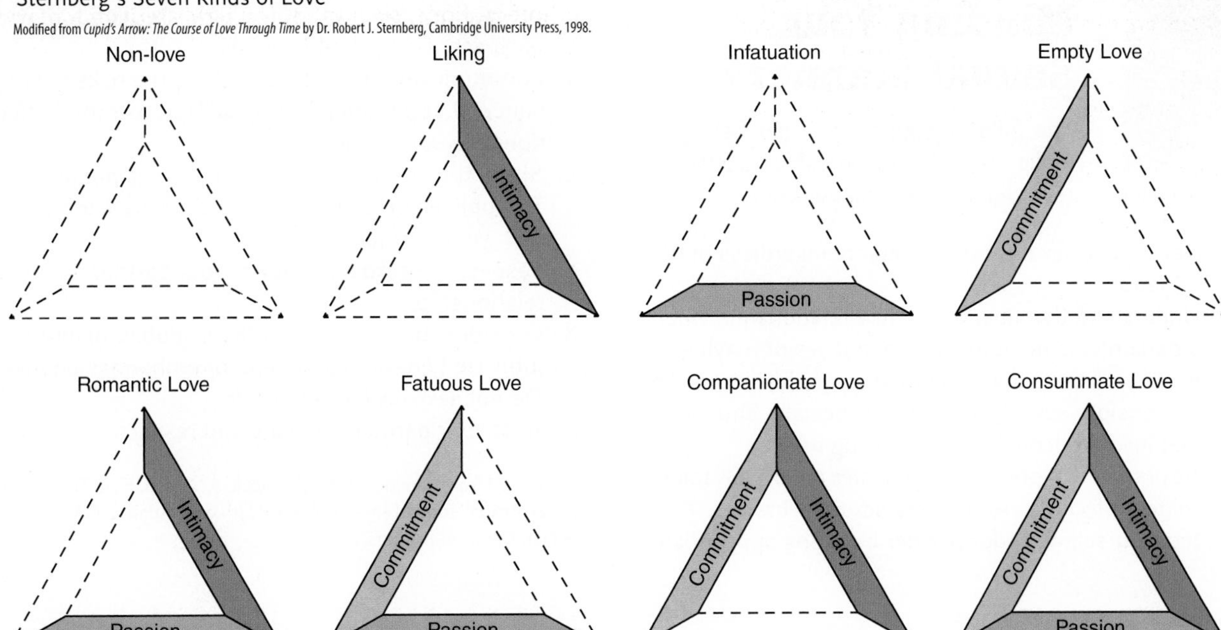

individuals often exaggerate the positive characteristics of their partners while ignoring their faults. A relationship that is based on infatuation may not survive, especially when one or both lovers become aware of their partners' weaknesses and find these faults unacceptable.

Eventually, the intense sexual attraction that characterizes the initial stage of a romantic relationship subsides. The couple, if sexually active, usually engages in sex less frequently than in the earlier phase of their relationship. They enjoy being together, but they can endure separations. Other aspects of their relationship, such as companionship, often deepen. Although couples in this stage of love have conflicts, committed partners usually try to resolve their problems.

Not every couple experiences the stages of love in this order. Sometimes passionate love affairs evolve from companionate relationships, such as when friends become lovers. Whatever the course of a romantic relationship, however, it will have phases of growth and change.

The following Managing Your Health feature "Minding Your Sexual Manners" provides suggestions for socially responsible sexually related behaviors.

Establishing Romantic Commitments

Have you ever been in love? Why did you fall in love with that person? Studies have shown that physical attraction is the most important factor that determines whether two individuals become romantically interested in one another. People often use other criteria as well, such as social status, occupation, and wealth, to select their sexual partners. Not surprisingly, Americans spend millions of dollars annually to enhance their "sex appeal" by purchasing makeup, jewelry, clothing, and expensive cars.

Initially, two people who are physically attracted to each other usually make and hold eye contact.

Love Changes over Time

Early in a relationship, when physical attraction is greatest and partners know very little about one another, their passion is high. Preoccupied with their sexual desire for each other, passionate lovers think about their partners and want to be with them constantly.

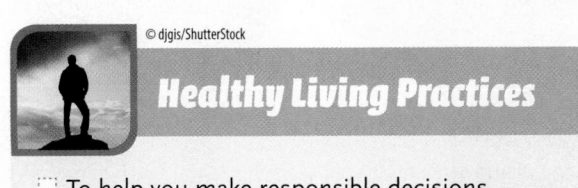

© djgis/ShutterStock

Healthy Living Practices

- To help you make responsible decisions concerning your sexuality, consider how your sexual behavior affects yourself and others.

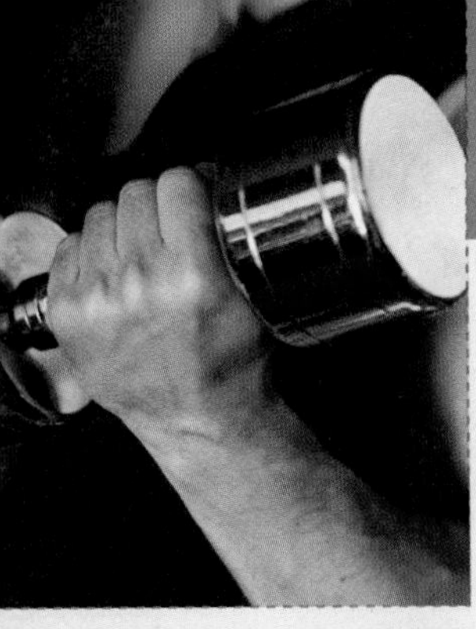

© Kzenon/ShutterStock

Managing Your Health

Minding Your Sexual Manners

The following guidelines can help you make socially responsible decisions regarding your sexual behavior.

1. Never force sex on another person, regardless of the situation.
2. Understand that at any time in a relationship, when a person says no, it means no, not yes or maybe.
3. Avoid situations that can impair your ability to make responsible sexual decisions, especially situations that involve alcohol and other drug use.
4. Be prepared to prevent pregnancies or sexually transmitted infections. Avoid risky sexual behaviors. Protect yourself and your partner by taking appropriate precautions, such as using a new latex condom with each act of sexual intercourse.
5. Communicate your concerns about the risks of pregnancy (if applicable) and sexually transmitted infections to your partner.
6. Share the responsibility of preventing pregnancies (if applicable) and sexually transmitted infections with your partner.
7. Respect the sexual privacy of your partner and your relationship.
8. Consider the feelings of others. Public displays of intimate behavior can offend or embarrass people.
9. Do not sexually harass others.
10. Treat your partner with care and respect.

Reproduced from Hatcher, R. A., Colestock, S., Pluhar, E., & Thrasher, C. (2002). Sexual etiquette 101 and more (4th ed.). Atlanta, GA: Bridging the Gap Communications.

Couples may describe this behavior as "falling in love at first sight." After two people find each other physically appealing, they need to determine if they are **compatible**; that is, if they are capable of existing together in harmony.

Which characteristics are important for establishing long-term satisfying and compatible relationships? Individuals in such relationships are usually close in age, and they usually share similar racial, ethnic, religious, and educational backgrounds (**Figure 6.10**). Members of couples who have extremely different backgrounds or many dissimilar characteristics can certainly form satisfying and lasting relationships, but these situations are less common than those described previously.

Sexual satisfaction is another characteristic related to the establishment of long-term satisfying and compatible relationships. Several studies show an association between sexual satisfaction and overall relationship satisfaction.[40] One study focused on the association between sexual satisfaction and relationship quality in premarital heterosexual couples.[41]

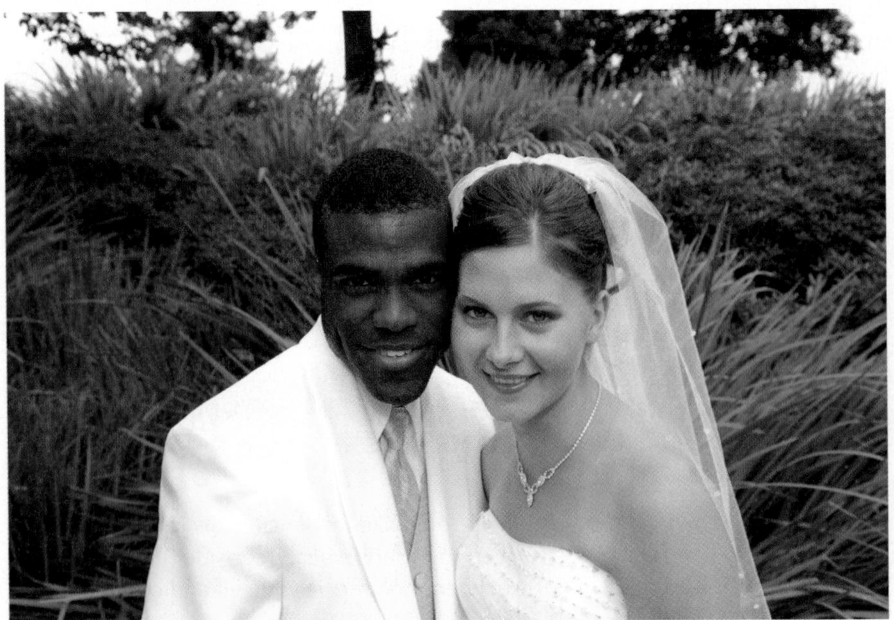

Figure 6.10

Many Personal Characteristics Contribute to Compatibility. Although this man and woman do not share the same racial background, they are similar in age and may have other similarities that foster their compatibility as a couple.

© Bassittart/ShutterStock

compatible Capable of existing together in harmony.

cohabitation Unmarried persons living together.

Research results showed that over time, sexual satisfaction was positively associated with relationship satisfaction, love, and commitment for both men and women. When change occurred in sexual satisfaction over time, change also occurred in relationship satisfaction, love, and commitment. Overall, sexual satisfaction had stronger links with relationship quality for men than for women.

Types of Romantic Commitments

Cohabitation In the second half of the 20th century, a growing number of unmarried people decided to live with their heterosexual partners. Between 1960 and 2011, the number of adult heterosexual couples living together rose more than 17-fold.[42] The practice of unmarried couples living together is called **cohabitation**.

Why do people live together rather than get married? One reason is that marriage is not a legal option for everyone. For example, same-sex couples or those in plural (polygamous) relationships are unable to legally marry. In some states, domestic partnerships and civil unions are options for those who cannot legally marry. Other reasons include convenience, economics, and recent changes in societal norms. Cohabitation is emerging as a significant experience for young adults and is replacing marriage as the first living-together union. Researchers estimate that approximately 25% of unmarried women in the United States between the ages of 25 and 39 are currently living with a heterosexual partner. An additional 25% are estimated to have cohabited at one time.[42]

Research presents conflicting results regarding cohabitation outcomes. Some research reports that people who cohabit before marriage (with the exception of those who are engaged and have set a wedding date) are *not* more likely to enjoy longer and happier marriages than individuals who do not live together before marrying. Studies conducted in the United States, Sweden, and Canada document higher divorce rates among couples who cohabited before marriage than among those who did not. Research results suggest that this increased risk of divorce may be due to the result of self-selection; that is, persons who are less able to sustain long-term relationships may choose to cohabit prior to marriage, rather than to marry without first living with their partners.[42] Additionally, research data show that multiple cohabiting experiences do not help people learn to have better relationships. In fact, persons with multiple cohabiting experiences are more likely to have failed future relationships than persons who do not cohabit.[43]

Other—more recent—research presents differing perspectives. One study found more similarities between cohabitation and marriage than differences.[44] This study found no statistical difference between cohabitating and married partners' depression or relationship with family and friends. However, differences were reported: married partners fared better in health whereas cohabiters were happier and had higher self-esteem.

Although much research links marriage and cohabitation, Guzzo points out that many cohabitors enter into cohabitation without plans of marriage, in part, because cohabitation is gaining societal acceptance and today's young adults may receive less pressure to marry than earlier cohorts. Therefore, cohabitation may simply be viewed as a convenient arrangement rather than part of a marriage precursor.[45]

Marriage In the United States and in most other countries, marriage is a legally binding commitment between an adult man and an adult woman. Same-sex marriages and plural marriages (between more than two people) are legal only in select places. Most Americans desire marriage as a lifelong and loving partnership, and expect sexual faithfulness, emotional support, mutual trust, and lasting commitment. However, research results show a moderate decline in marital quality since the 1970s (**Figure 6.11**).

Along with being less satisfied with their marriages, Americans are also marrying a bit later in life today than in recent decades. In 1960, the median age at first marriage was 20.3 years for women and 22.8 years for men. (The median is the point below which 50% of the scores fall.) By 2011, the median age of first marriage had increased to 26.5 years for women and 28.7 years for men. Americans have also become less likely to marry; from 1970 to 2010 the annual number of new marriages per 1,000 unmarried women aged 15 years and older declined more than 50%.[42]

What factors help make a marriage successful? Partners in successful marriages often demonstrate positive problem-solving and communication skills. When conflicts arise, couples with these skills can openly discuss their feelings, and they are willing to negotiate and compromise to find solutions. In addition, partners in successful marriages share basic values, have mutual concerns, and exhibit high degrees of physical intimacy.

Extrarelational Sex Some people have sexual relationships with individuals who are not their spouses or primary sex partners. Although most Americans

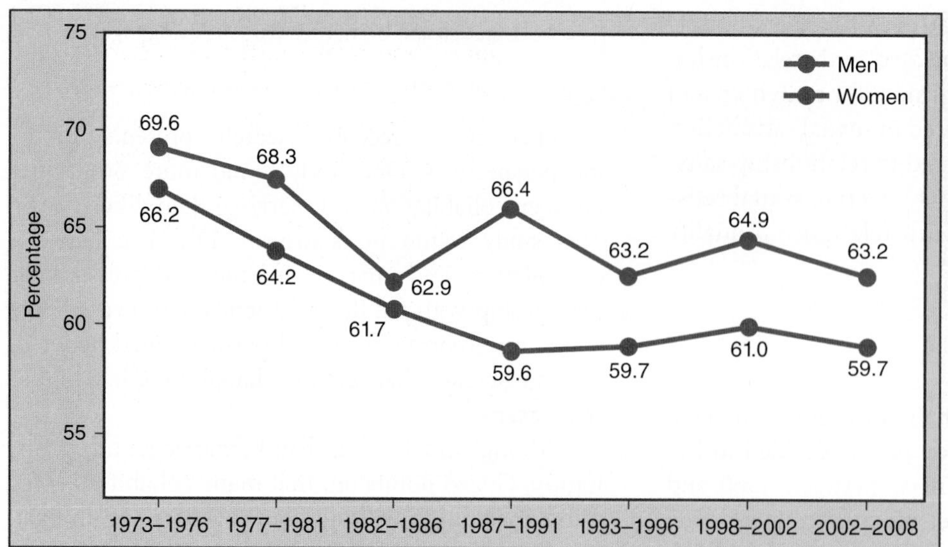

Figure 6.11

Percentage of Married Persons Age 18 Years and Older Who Said Their Marriages Were "Very Happy," by Period, United States.

Reproduced from General Social Survey, conducted by the National Opinion Research Center of the University of Chicago. Sprecher, S. (2002). Sexual satisfaction in premarital relationships: Associations with satisfaction, love, commitment, and stability. *Journal of Sex Research*, 39(3), 190–196, with permission from Taylor & Francis Ltd.

disapprove of such extrarelational sex, particularly when married couples are involved, results from the General Social Survey on American Sexual Behavior show that 21.7% of men and 12.6% of women had sexual relations with a person other than their spouse while married.[19] Rates are highest among persons who are "not too happy" with their marriage (30%), those who rarely attend church (22%), and those who are separated (39.4%). Having sex with someone other than one's spouse is commonly referred to as *extramarital sex* or *adultery*. The majority of married Americans report that they are faithful to their spouses.

Separation and Divorce Despite having high hopes for happiness and success during their wedding celebrations, many couples see their marriages end in separation or divorce. Nearly half of recent first marriages may end in divorce; the divorce rate for younger persons has risen in recent years. Accurate data concerning the number of married persons who separate permanently are unavailable. Teenage marriages are especially vulnerable to dissolution. Women who marry when they are younger than 20 years of age are much more likely to be in a failed marriage than women who marry when they are at least 20 years of age. In addition, divorce rates are higher for high school dropouts than for college graduates, and for marriages in which there is conflict over money matters, an extramarital affair has taken place, or an alcohol/drug problem exists.[42]

Early in the 20th century, divorce was uncommon: In 1940, the U.S. divorce rate was 2 divorces per 1,000 persons. The divorce rate rose during World War II and peaked at more than 4 divorces per 1,000 at the war's end. The rate fell during the 1950s to nearly prewar rates, and rose again in the 1960s and 1970s. From 1979 through 1981, the U.S. divorce rate was at its highest level of the 20th century, slightly more than 5 divorces per 1,000. The decline in the divorce rate has been relatively steady since that time, and in 2011 (the most recent data available mid-2014) was at 3.6 for every 1,000 persons (**Figure 6.12**).

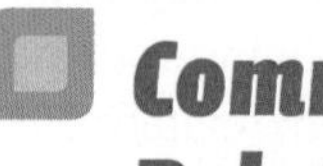

Communication in Relationships

Effective communication is a cornerstone of interpersonal and sexual relationships. To communicate effectively, people must express themselves as accurately and as clearly as possible but also must listen with attentiveness, openness, and patience. To express yourself accurately and clearly, first say exactly what you mean. If you avoid being straightforward so that you will not hurt someone's feelings, for example, the person with whom you're communicating may not understand your message. Second, your statements must be specific, not vague. For example, telling your partner that you would like him to be more spontaneous will probably make him question what you really mean. Do you always want him to act in a spontaneous manner? Has he never been spontaneous? Or do you really mean that you had wanted him to accept yesterday's last-minute party invitation, and wished that he could have just dropped what he was doing, changed his clothes, and dashed out the door with you? Third, avoid sending mixed messages. For example, don't tell your partner that everything is fine when she can tell from your behavior and expression that you are really feeling "down."

Figure 6.12

U.S. Divorce Rates: 1940 to 2011. Since 1981, the divorce rate has declined in the United States.

Data from U.S. Bureau of the Census, National Center for Health Statistics.

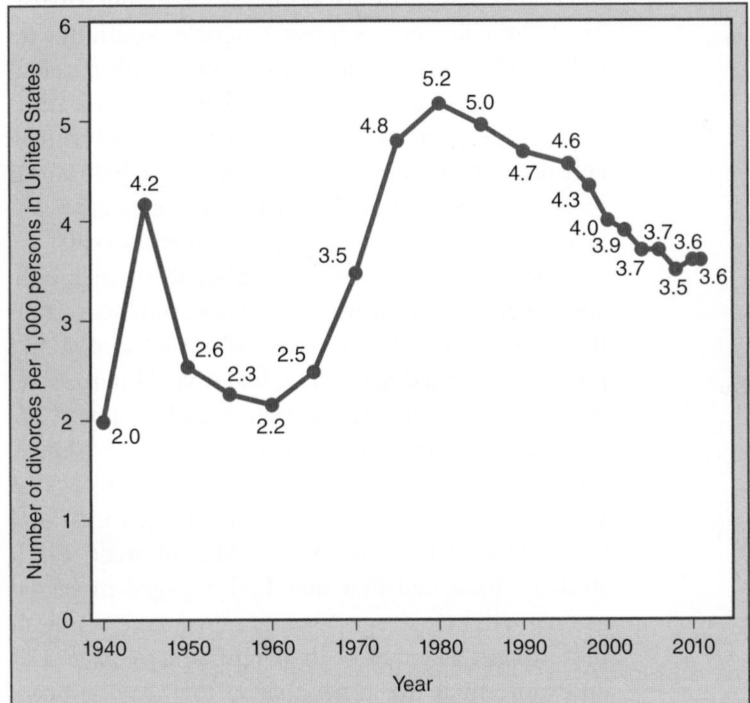

Another mechanism to foster effective communication is to express your feelings using "I" statements when discussing issues with a partner. Then, go on to say what you need to try to maintain (or change) the feeling. Statements that begin with "You" can hinder open communication between partners, particularly if the speaker is criticizing the listener's behavior or blaming this person for something. For example, instead of saying "You always spend too much time with your friends," you could say, "I feel lonely and miss you terribly when you are out with your friends." (Express the feeling.) "Could I join you on those occasions so that we could spend more time together?" (State the remedy.) Try not to fall into the trap of "false" I statements: "I feel like you spend too much time with your friends" is really a "you" statement.

Besides being able to express oneself clearly, an effective communicator has good listening skills. Failure to hear information accurately or completely can create misunderstandings that result in conflicts. In discussions, good listeners restate or paraphrase what they have heard their partners say. This practice allows speakers, if necessary, to correct or clarify what they have said. For example, if your partner says, "When we get together with your friends or your family, you always ignore me," you could respond by saying, "I didn't realize that you feel neglected in those situations. What can I do to make you feel more included?"

In addition to words, people use nonverbal forms of communication, such as body positioning (body language) and facial gestures, to express their thoughts (**Figure 6.13**). Touching is a form of nonverbal communication that can convey important information about intimate sexual feelings. Many people report that being held, kissed, massaged, or fondled by their partners is as sexually gratifying as sexual intercourse. Sensual touching does not have to involve the genitals; gently massaging your partner's back, for example, can convey your feelings of love to this individual.

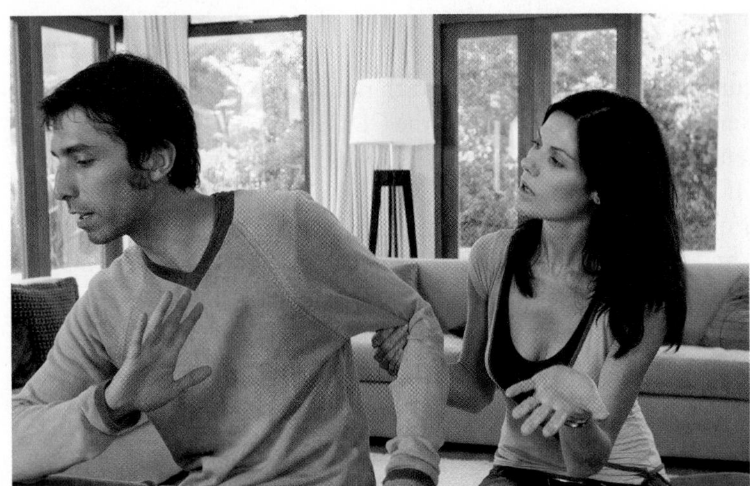

Figure 6.13

Nonverbal Communication. Nonverbal forms of communication, such as body postures and facial gestures, can convey thoughts. What do this couple's nonverbal signals communicate?

© Pixland/Thinkstock

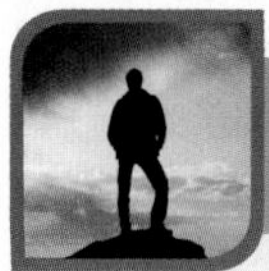

© djgis/ShutterStock

Healthy Living Practices

- To increase your child's chances of being able to form secure and trusting relationships as an adult, consider ways to be more attentive to his or her emotional needs; display your affection frequently.
- To increase your likelihood of having a happy and long-term romantic relationship, communicate as effectively as possible with your partner.
- To encourage discussions between you and your partner about issues that concern the relationship, use "I" statements to express your feelings and avoid using "You" statements. "You" statements can anger or belittle your partner.
- Listen carefully to your partner during your discussions. Repeat what your partner says to avoid misunderstandings. If your partner gives unclear responses to your questions, ask for additional information.

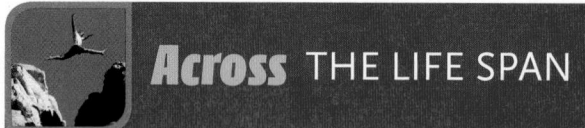

© Galina Barskaya/ShutterStock

SEXUALITY

Most preschoolers masturbate. Parents who think masturbation is a healthy and normal aspect of sexuality usually let their children know that the behavior is inappropriate in public but do not attempt to stop this behavior in private. Preschool children typically play games in which they act out adult gender roles. By this age, children have learned that there are differences between the sexes. Children are curious about sexuality; they may "play doctor" by examining each other's genitals. Young children often ask questions such as "Where did I come from?" If parents are uncertain how to answer this or other questions about sexual matters, they can usually find a collection of age-appropriate sexuality books at their libraries that they can read with their children after reading them themselves.

It is not unusual for elementary school-age children to engage in mutual sex play, activities that may include rehearsing adult sexual behaviors. Sex experts consider such sex play normal behavior when it is playful, occurs infrequently, and does not involve coercion.

The ability to reproduce begins during puberty. Many teens avoid sexual activity because they fear becoming pregnant, contracting sexually transmitted infections, and losing self-esteem or parental trust. The media, however, expose American youth to sexually explicit images that may conflict with parental values and encourage sexual experimentation. Additionally, peers or older persons can exert considerable pressure on teens to engage in sex. To help youth maintain their abstinence, parents and educators can teach teens how to use sexual assertiveness skills.

Despite efforts to promote teenage abstinence, only about half of American high school students refrain from having sex. By grade 10, about 42% of young girls in the United States have had sexual intercourse. By grade 12, about 63% have engaged in coitus.[46]

Results of the Youth Risk Behavior Surveillance, 2013, conducted by the CDC revealed that by age 13 years, more boys reported having engaged in sexual intercourse than girls. About 24% of male Black students indicated that they had engaged in sexual intercourse before age 13; this percentage was well more than twice that of their Hispanic peers (9.2%) and more than five times that of their White peers (4.4%). Overall, 14% of Black students, 6.4% of Hispanic students, and 3.3% of White students initiated sexual intercourse before 13 years of age. In comparing behavior trends from 1991 to 2013, initiation of sexual intercourse before 13 years of age decreased substantially (from 10.2% to 5.6%).[46]

In comparing behavior trends in youth from 1991 through 2013, the CDC has found that the percentage of high school students who have ever had sexual intercourse has decreased from about 54% in 1991 to about 47% in 2013. More students are using condoms; in 1991 about 46% of sexually active students used a condom during their last sexual intercourse, whereas in 2013, 59.1% reported having done so.[46]

The teenage birth rate in 2010 was the lowest it has ever been since the CDC began keeping track of birth rates for teenagers in 1960 (**Figure 6.14**). The preliminary 2010 birth rates (the most recent data available mid-2014) for teenagers 18 to 19 years old was 58.3 births per 1,000 females of that age group. This rate was about 65% lower than in 1960 (166.7 per 1,000) and 38% lower than in 1991 (94.0 births per 1,000). For those in the 15- to 17-year-old age group, birth rates fell to 17.3 per 1,000 young women, which is 55% lower than in 1991 (38.6 births per 1,000) and 60% lower than in 1960 (43.9 births per 1,000).[47]

Figure 6.14

Birth Rates for Teenagers by Age: United States, 1960–2010.

Reproduced from Hamilton, B. E., & Ventura, S. J. (2012). Birth Rates for U.S. teenagers reach historic lows for all age and ethnic groups. NCHS Data Brief, no. 89. Retrieved July 21, 2014 from http://www.cdc.gov/nchs/data/databriefs/db89.pdf

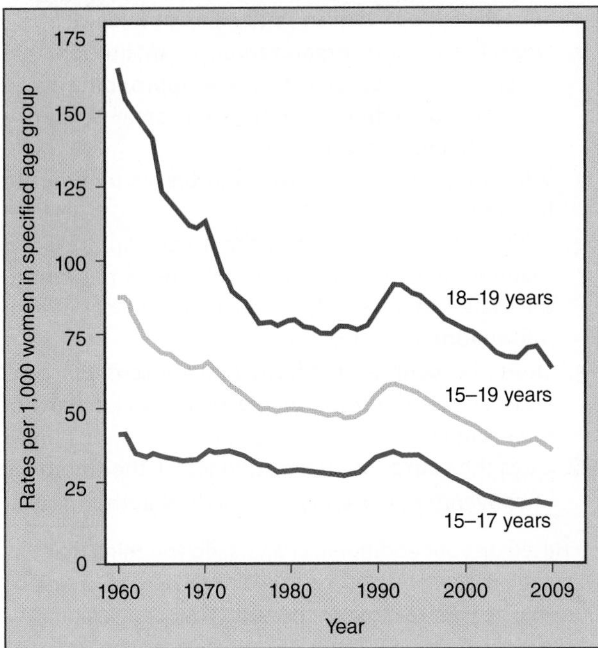

Compared to women in their 20s, pregnant teenagers have a greater risk of experiencing serious complications during pregnancy and delivery as well as of giving birth to premature, underweight babies. Premature infants are born before the 37th week of pregnancy. The risk of giving birth to a premature, low-birth-weight infant is especially high for pregnant adolescents between 10 and 14 years of age. Underweight premature newborns have a greater risk of serious health and developmental problems than do normal-weight newborns who are born at term, that is, between the 37th and 41st weeks of pregnancy.

Most unmarried teenage girls who give birth to live infants keep their babies rather than give them up for adoption. Adolescent mothers are more likely to be unmarried, poor, and have less education than mothers who give birth when they are older. Many teenage mothers have difficulty improving their educational and socioeconomic levels when they become adults.

Teenaged fathers do not usually marry the teenaged mothers of their children, even though the relationship between the teens may have been ongoing for 6 months or longer. If the father is 20 years or older, he is more likely than his teenaged counterpart to marry the mother. As the child becomes older, the teenaged father typically becomes less and less involved with the child. When asked why they did not live with or marry their children's mothers, teenaged fathers cite financial concerns as one major issue.[48]

With respect to older adults, sex has enduring importance. Sexuality does not end because a person is older. According to findings from the National Survey of Sexual Health and Behavior, 20% of Americans who are 70 to 79 years of age engage in sexual intercourse a few times per year, 20% a few times per month, and 5% two or three times per week. Those aged 80 years and older enjoy sexual intercourse as well; almost 19% in this age group had sexual intercourse a few times per month. Twenty-one percent of those in their 70s received oral sex and 25% gave oral sex within the past year. Fifteen percent of those aged 80 years and older received oral sex and 22% gave oral sex within the past year.[49] Sexual inactivity in the later years of life is more often the result of medical disabilities or lack of a sexual partner rather than lack of desire.

Older adults experience a gradual decline in sexual functioning. Therefore, elderly individuals should recognize that their sexual responses are likely to be different from when they were young adults. For example, it usually takes longer for the older adult to become adequately sexually stimulated before sex, and orgasms are less intense. Chronic diseases such as diabetes and heart disease can further limit an aged person's sexual responses or interest in sex. Certain antihypertensive and antidepressant medications can produce side effects that impair sexual functioning; affected individuals should discuss their sexual problems with their physicians. Frequently, changing medications can be helpful. In some cases, medical treatments are available that can improve sexual functioning. Elderly individuals who have sexual impairments that do not respond to treatment can rely on noncoital forms of sexual expression such as kissing, caressing, cuddling, and oral sex to obtain pleasure and fulfillment. For some, affectionate behavior is more crucial to happiness than sex is.

Besides physical factors, significant social changes such as the loss of a spouse or moving into a nursing home can have negative impacts on the sexuality of aged individuals. Widows and widowers may have difficulty meeting sexual partners. Elderly nursing home residents may not feel free to express their sexuality because they lack privacy. As the number of elderly Americans rises, addressing sexual needs in this age group will become an increasingly important issue.

Analyzing Health-Related Information

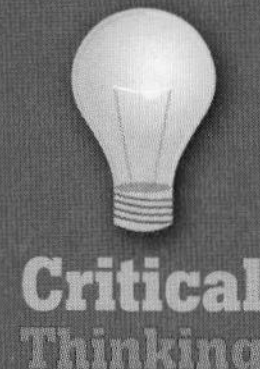

© tele52/ShutterStock

Search the word *impotence* using Google or another search engine. Choose a website that sells an impotence product. Explain why you think the website you chose is a reliable or an unreliable source of information. Use the "Assessing Information on the Internet" portion of the model for analyzing health-related information to guide your thinking; the main points of the model are noted here.

- What is the source of the information?
- Is the site sponsored by a nationally known health or medical organization or affiliated with a well-known medical research institution or major university? If not, is the site staffed by well-respected and credentialed experts in the field?
- Does the site include up-to-date references from a well-known, respected medical or scientific journal or links to reputable websites, such as nationally recognized medical organizations?
- Is the information at the website current?

Based on your analysis, do you think that this web page is a reliable source of health-related information? Summarize your reasons for drawing your conclusion.

If you are unsure of the credibility of the site after answering the preceding questions, continue with the following six Analyzing Health-Related Information questions:

1. Which statements on the website are verifiable facts, and which are unverified statements or value claims?
2. Does the person, organization, or institution that developed the website have the appropriate background and credentials in the topic area? What can you do to check credentials?
3. What might be the motives and biases inherent to the website?
4. What is the main point of the article, ad, or claim made on the site? Which information is relevant to the issue, main point, product, or service? Which information is irrelevant?
5. Does the source of information present the pros and cons of the topic or the benefits and risks of the product?
6. Does the source of information attack the credibility of conventional scientists or medical authorities?

Based on your additional analysis, do you think that this web page is a reliable source of health-related information? Summarize your reasons for drawing your conclusion.

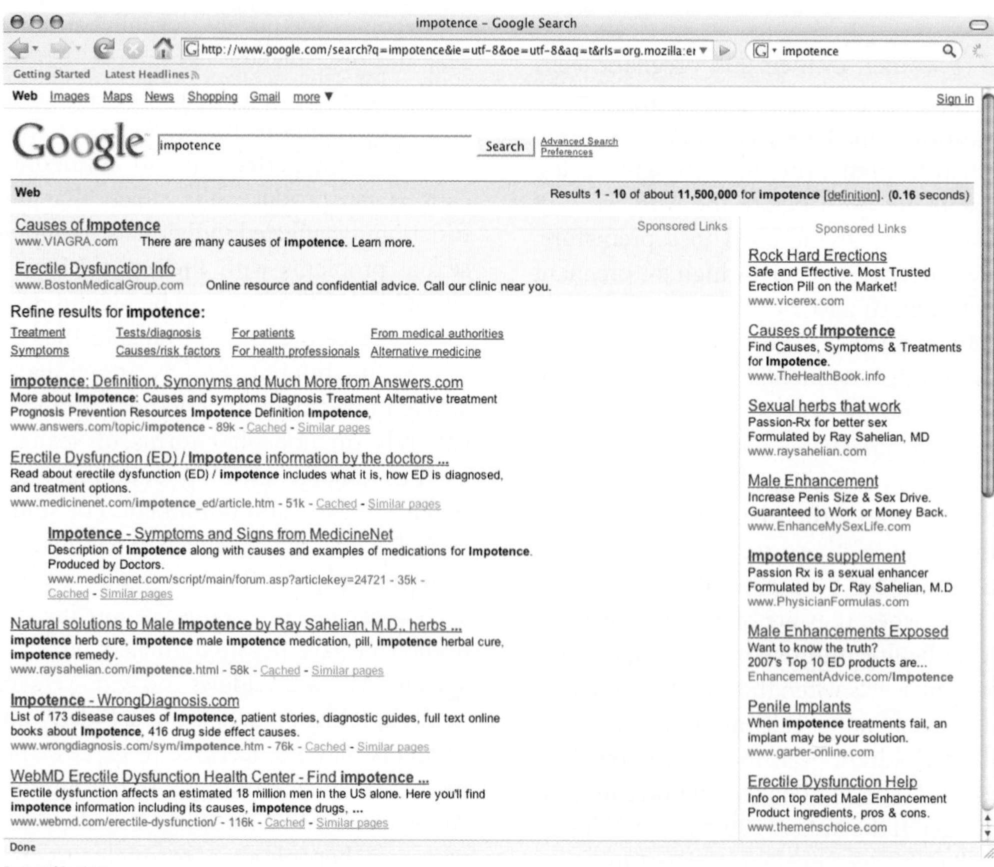

Courtesy of Google, Inc.

CHAPTER REVIEW

Summary

Human sexuality is a complex set of thoughts, feelings, attitudes, and behaviors that are related to reproduction as well as to being male or female. Numerous biological, psychological, social, and cultural forces interact to influence sexuality. Sexuality influences all aspects of an individual's life, including identity, self-esteem, emotions, personality, relationships, lifestyle, and health. Being knowledgeable about sexuality is important for maintaining good health and optimal well-being.

The sexual response of individuals engaging in sexual activity is usually described in phases. During the excitement phase, both men and women have a heightened sexual awareness. During the plateau phase, the heart rate, blood pressure, respiration rate, and level of muscle tension all increase and the erection of the male intensifies. During the orgasmic phase, men ejaculate, and women's vaginal walls contract rhythmically. During the resolution phase, the body returns to its prearousal state. Other models of the sexual response include emotional or psychological aspects as well as these physiologic aspects.

Some people have sexual dysfunctions that interfere with their sexual response. Common sexual dysfunctions include erectile dysfunction, the inability of a man to develop and/or sustain an erection firm enough for penetration; premature ejaculation, consistently attaining orgasm either before or shortly after intercourse begins and before he wishes it to occur; hypoactive sexual desire, a low interest in sex that causes distress, which occurs in both sexes but is more prevalent in women; and vaginismus, a sexual dysfunction of women in which the muscles of the lower third of the vaginal canal contract involuntarily at the anticipation of vaginal penetration.

Instincts, sensations, and hormones drive reproductive behavior, but social, cultural, and religious factors heavily influence a person's sexual attitudes, values, and behaviors. Sexually responsible people consider how their sexual behavior affects themselves and others.

Gender is the classification of the sex of a person based on many criteria, among them anatomic and chromosomal characteristics. Gender identity is an individual's perception of himself or herself as male or female. Various biological, social, and environmental forces mold a child's gender identity. A *gender role* refers to patterns of behavior, attitudes, and personality attributes that, in a particular culture, are traditionally considered feminine or masculine. In the United States today, gender roles are undergoing dramatic changes and are becoming more flexible than in the past.

Sexual orientation, the direction of one's romantic thoughts, feelings, and attractions, can be toward the same sex, the opposite sex, or both sexes. Today, researchers and mental health experts generally agree that people do not decide their sexual orientation and cannot alter their sexual preferences, whether they are at either end of the sexual orientation continuum or somewhere in between.

Sexual partners may engage in a variety of intimate activities, including mutual masturbation as well as vaginal, oral, and anal sex. However, sex does not require a partner for it to be a pleasurable experience—most people solo masturbate at some point during their lives. Some people choose to refrain from sexual activity for a variety of reasons, such as health concerns or religious beliefs. Abstaining from sexual activity is not known to be harmful, and it is an effective measure for preventing pregnancies and sexually transmitted infections.

People need to establish and maintain satisfying attachments to others for optimal health and well-being. People who have high self-esteem, are satisfied with their bodies, are in good health, and have positive feelings about their sexuality are likely to form fulfilling intimate relationships. Although love is difficult to define, people in loving relationships share feelings of caring, respect, attachment, commitment, and intimacy.

CHAPTER REVIEW

Various psychologists have developed theories about love. However, experts generally agree that love changes over time. Early in a relationship, when physical attraction is greatest and partners know very little about one another, their passion is high. Eventually, the intense sexual attraction that characterizes a romantic relationship in its initial stages subsides. Other aspects of the relationship, such as companionship, often deepen. Compatibility, the ability to exist in harmony, is crucial in the development of a healthy emotional attraction between partners. Usually important for establishing a compatible relationship is the sharing of similar interests, attitudes, and values.

More couples are choosing to cohabit before marriage, but this practice results in a higher risk of divorce than not living together prior to marriage. Those who are married are less satisfied with their marriages and are marrying later in life than in recent decades. Effective communication is an essential ingredient for maintaining satisfying and successful marriages and intimate relationships.

Children are curious about sex; they frequently play sex games with other children and ask their parents questions about sex. Children's sex play is normal behavior when it is playful, occurs infrequently, and does not involve coercion.

The teenage birth rate has declined dramatically since the 1960s. Compared with women in their 20s, pregnant teenagers have a greater risk of serious complications during pregnancy and delivery, as well as of giving birth to premature and underweight newborns. Additionally, adolescent mothers are more likely to be unmarried, poor, and have less education than mothers who give birth when they are older. Many teenage mothers have difficulty improving their educational and socioeconomic levels when they become adults.

Sexuality does not end at a particular age. Most healthy elderly men and women continue to be interested and participate in sexual activity. However, sexual functioning declines with aging; sexual responses in older persons are different from when they were young adults. As the number of elderly Americans rises, addressing sexuality needs in this age group will become an increasingly important issue.

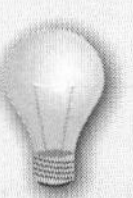

Applying What You Have Learned

1. Develop a plan to improve the way you convey your feelings in relationships. **Application**
2. Analyze your present intimate relationship or a past one. Explain why you think it will be (or was) a short-term or long-term relationship. **Analysis**
3. Propose a checklist of characteristics that you could use to select a suitable partner. Explain why these characteristics are important. **Synthesis**
4. Develop a position concerning the promotion of masturbation as a safe sex alternative. How would you defend your position? **Evaluation**

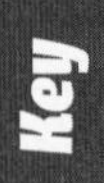

Key

Application using information in a new situation.

Analysis breaking down information into component parts.

Synthesis putting together information from different sources.

Evaluation making informed decisions.

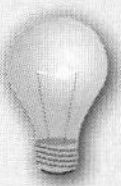

Reflecting on Your Health

1. What is the source of your sexual values (e.g., your parents, your religious upbringing)? Do you feel comfortable with those values? Why or why not? Do you feel as though your peers share some or all of your values, or do you feel intimidated or pressured to change your values?
2. Do you think that "traditional" gender roles are appropriate in American society today? If you think that some are appropriate and some are not, pick one example from each category and explain your feelings about their appropriateness or inappropriateness.
3. Do you agree with former Surgeon General Jocelyn Elders's opinion that sex education in U.S. schools could include instruction about masturbation particularly for the purpose of reducing the spread of sexually transmitted infections, especially HIV/AIDS? Why or why not?
4. Think about a current or former intimate relationship you had. Do you think that your love relationship fits one of Lee's six styles of loving or one of Sternberg's kinds of love? How does it fit or not fit?
5. Think about the nature of your verbal interactions with someone important to you—a parent or spouse, for example. How could you communicate more effectively with that person using suggestions in this chapter?

References

1. Travison, T. G., et al. (2007). The relative contributions of aging, health, and lifestyle factors to serum testosterone decline in men. *Journal of Clinical Endocrinology and Metabolism*, 92, 549–555.
2. Fisher, L. L., et al. (2010). *Sex, romance, and relationships: AARP survey of midlife and older adults.* Retrieved March 3, 2011, from http://assets.aarp.org/rgcenter/general/srr_09.pdf
3. Whipple, B. (2002). Women's sexual pleasure and satisfaction. A new view of female sexual function. *The Female Patient*, 27, 39–44.
4. Basson, R. (2001). Female sexual response: The role of drugs in the management of sexual dysfunction. *Obstetrics and Gynecology*, 98, 350–353.
5. Selvin, E., et al. (2007). Prevalence and risk factors for erectile dysfunction in the US. *American Journal of Medicine*, 120, 151–157.
6. Kupelian, V., et al. (2010). Relative contributions of modifiable risk factors to erectile dysfunction: Results from the Boston Area Community Health (BACH) Survey. *Preventive Medicine*, 50(1–2), 19–25.
7. Kazi, M., et al. (2007). Considerations for the diagnosis and treatment of testosterone deficiency in elderly men. *The American Journal of Medicine*, 120, 835–840.
8. International Society for Sexual Medicine. (2010). *Premature ejaculation: Advice for men from the International Society for Sexual Medicine* [Patient information sheet]. Retrieved March 6, 2011, from http://www.issm.info/v4/data/education/patient/patient.asp
9. Hellstrom, W. J. (2011). Update on treatments for premature ejaculation. *International Journal of Clinical Practice*, 65(1), 16–26.

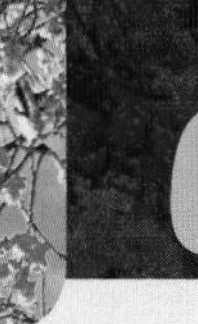

CHAPTER REVIEW

10. Stahl, S. M. (2010). Circuits of sexual desire in hypoactive sexual desire disorder. *Journal of Clinical Psychiatry*, 71(5), 518–519.
11. Leiblum, S. R., et al. (2006). Hypoactive sexual desire disorder in postmenopausal women: US results from the Women's International Study of Health and Sexuality (WISHeS). *Menopause*, 13, 46–56.
12. Stahl, S. M. (2010). Targeting circuits of sexual desire as a treatment strategy for hypoactive sexual desire disorder. *Journal of Clinical Psychiatry*, 71(7), 821–822.
13. Schoen, C., & Bachmann, G. (2009). Sildenafil citrate for female sexual arousal disorder: A future possibility? *Nature Reviews Urology*, 6(4), 216–222.
14. Binik, Y. M. (2010). The *DSM* diagnostic criteria for vaginismus. *Archives of Sexual Behavior*, 39, 278–291.
15. Bryant, A. N. (2003). Changes in attitudes toward women's roles: Predicting gender-role traditionalism among college students. *Sex Roles*, 48(3/4), 131–142.
16. Eliason, M. J. (2014). An exploration of terminology related to sexuality and gender: Arguments for standardizing the language. *Social Work in Public Health*, 29(2), 162–175.
17. Gates, G. J. (2011, April). *How many people are lesbian, gay, bisexual, and transgender?* The Williams Institute, School of Law, University of California Los Angeles. Retrieved September 1, 2014, from http://williamsinstitute.law.ucla.edu/wp-content/uploads/Gates-How-Many-People-LGBT-Apr-2011.pdf
18. Pearlman, A., et al. (2010). Mutations in MAP3K1 cause 46,XY disorders of sex development and implicate a common signal transduction pathway in human testis determination. *The American Journal of Human Genetics*, 87, 898–904.
19. Ford, J. A., & Jasinski, J. L. (2005). Sexual orientation and substance use among college students. *Addictive Behaviors*, 31, 404–413.
20. Kinsey, A. C., et al. (1953). *Sexual behavior in the human female*. Philadelphia, PA: W.B. Saunders.
21. Smith, T. W. (2006). *American sexual behavior: Trends, socio-demographic differences, and risk behavior* (GSS Topical Report No. 25). Chicago, IL: University of Chicago, National Opinion Research Center.
22. Ward, B.W., Dalhamer, J. M., Galinky, A. M., Joestl, S. S. for the CDC's National Health Statistics Reports. (2014, July 15). *Sexual orientation and health among U.S. adults: National Health Interview Survey*, 2013 (No. 77). Retrieved July 20, 2014 from http://www.cdc.gov/nchs/nhis.htm
23. LeVay, S. (1991). A difference in hypothalamic structure between heterosexual and homosexual men. *Science*, 253, 1034–1037.
24. Hamer, D. H., et al. (1993). A linkage between DNA markers on the X chromosome and male sexual orientation. *Science*, 26, 321–327.
25. Iemmola, F., & Camperio Ciani, A. (2009). New evidence of genetic factors influencing sexual orientation in men: Female fecundity increase in the maternal line. *Archives of Sexual Behavior*, 38, 393–399.
26. Gallup Poll. (2014). *Gay and lesbian rights*. Retrieved July 20, 2014, from http://www.gallup.com/poll/1651/Gay-Lesbian-Rights.aspx
27. Pew Research Center. (2014, June 25). *Same-sex marriage state-by-state*. Retrieved July 21, 2014 from http://www.pewforum.org/2014/06/25/same-sex-marriage-state-by-state/
28. Pew Research Center. (2014, June 19). *Gay marriage around the world*. Retrieved July 21, 2014 from http://www.pewforum.org/2013/12/19/gay-marriage-around-the-world-2013/#some
29. Herbenick, D., et al. (2010). Sexual behavior in the United States: Results from a national probability sample of men and women ages 14–94. *The Journal of Sexual Medicine*, 7(Suppl 5), 255–265.
30. Chambers, W. C. (2007). Oral sex: Varied behaviors and perceptions in a college population. *Journal of Sex Research*, 44, 28–42.
31. Elders, M. J. (2010). Sex for health and pleasure throughout a lifetime. *The Journal of Sexual Medicine*, 7(Suppl 5), 248–249.
32. Reece, M., et al. (2014). *The National Survey of Sexual Health and Behavior (NSSHB)*. Retrieved July 21, 2014 from http://www.nationalsexstudy.indiana.edu/graph.html
33. Gerressu, M., et al. (2008). Prevalence of masturbation and associated factors in a British national probability survey. *Archives of Sexual Behavior*, 37, 266–278.
34. Rubin, Z. (1973). *Liking and loving*. New York, NY: Holt, Rinehart, & Winston.
35. Fromm, E. (1956). *The art of loving*. New York, NY: Harper.
36. Lee, J. A. (1973). *The colours of love*. Ontario, Canada: New Press.
37. Sternberg, R. J. (1986). A triangular theory of love. *Psychological Review*, 93, 119–135.
38. Sternberg, R. J. (1997). Construct validation of a triangular love scale. *European Journal of Social Psychology*, 27, 313–335.
39. Sternberg, R. J. (1998). *Cupid's arrow: The course of love through time*. Cambridge, England: Cambridge University Press.
40. Rosen, R. C., & Bachmann, G. A. (2008). Sexual well-being, happiness, and satisfaction, in women: The case for a new conceptual paradigm. *Journal of Sex & Marital Therapy*, 34, 291–297.
41. Sprecher, S. (2002). Sexual satisfaction in premarital relationships: Associations with satisfaction, love, commitment, and stability. *Journal of Sex Research*, 39(3), 190–196.
42. Marquardt, E., et al. (2012). *The state of our unions: Marriage in America 2012*. Charlottesville, VA: National Marriage Project and Institute for American Values.
43. Popenoe, D. (2008). *Cohabitation, marriage and child wellbeing*. Piscataway, NJ: Rutgers University and The National Marriage Project. Retrieved October 22, 2014, from http://www.jdsupra.com/legalnews/national-marriage-project-cohabitation-34400/
44. Musick, K., & Bumpass, L. (2012). Reexamining the case for marriage: Union formation and changes in well-being. *Journal of Marriage and Family*, 72, 1–18.
45. Guzzo, K. B. (2014). Trends in cohabitation outcomes: Compositional changes and engagement among never-married young adults. *Journal of Marriage and Family*, 76, 826–842.

46. Centers for Disease Control and Prevention. (2014, June 13). Youth Risk Behavior Surveillance—United States, 2013. *Morbidity and Mortality Weekly Report*, 63(4). Retrieved July 21, 2014, from http://www.cdc.gov/mmwr/pdf/ss/ss6304.pdf
47. Hamilton, B. E., & Ventura, S. J. (2012). Birth rates for U.S. teenagers reach historic lows for all age and ethnic groups. *NCHS Data Brief*, no. 89. Retrieved July 21, 2014 from http://www.cdc.gov/nchs/data/databriefs/db89.pdf
48. Elfenbein, D. S., & Felice, M. E. (2003). Adolescent pregnancy. *Pediatric Clinics of North America*, 50, 781–800.
49. Schick, V., et al. (2010). Sexual behaviors, condom use, and sexual health of Americans over 50: Implications for sexual health promotion for older adults. *The Journal of Sexual Medicine*, 7(Suppl 5), 315–329.

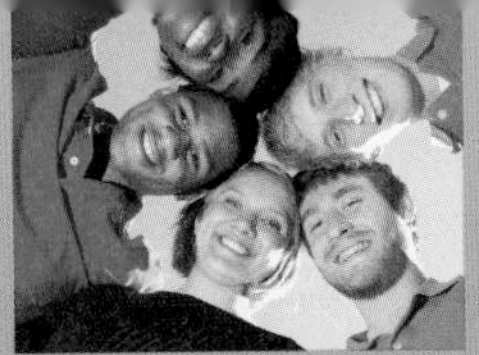

Diversity in Health
Khat

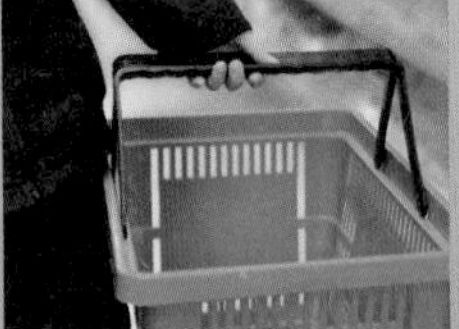

Consumer Health
Over-the-Counter Medicines: Safety and the FDA

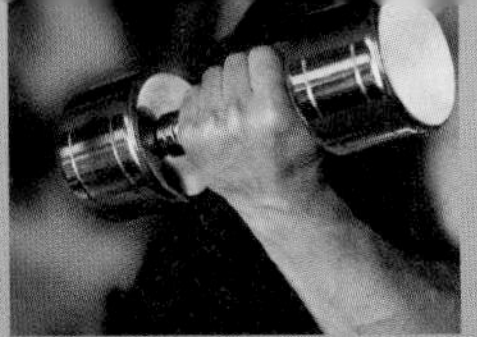

Managing Your Health
Falling Asleep Without Prescriptions

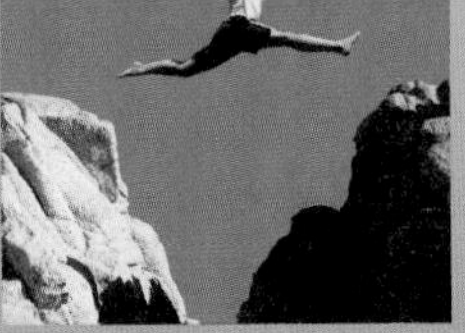

Across the Life Span
Drug Use and Abuse

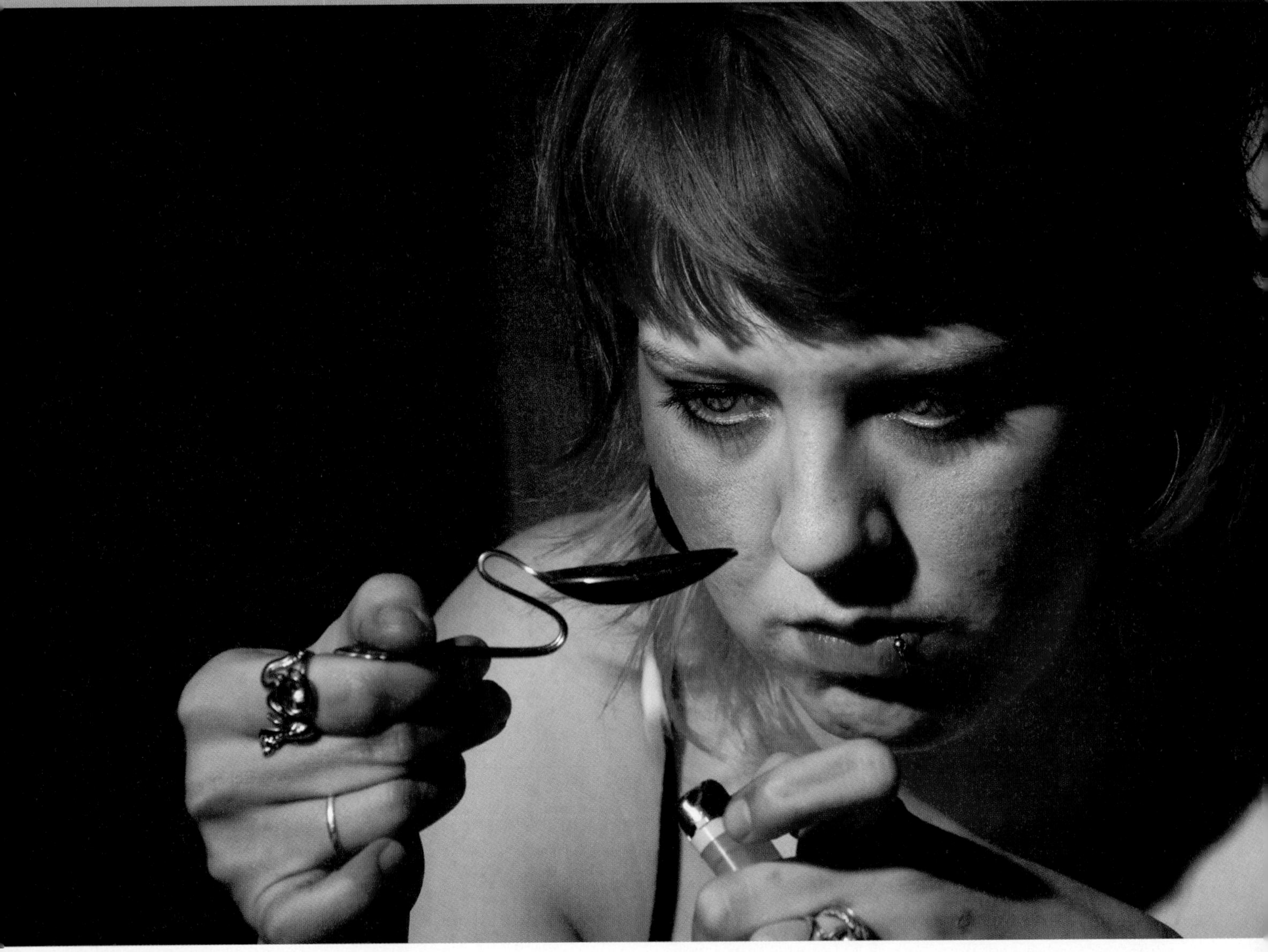

Chapter Overview

Differences between drug use, misuse, and abuse

The effects of psychoactive drugs on the mind and body

Why people use psychoactive drugs

Patterns of drug use in the United States

How physiologic and psychological drug dependence develop

The risk factors for drug dependence

The long-term effects of drug abuse

How the FDA regulates over-the-counter drugs

Goals and strategies for drug treatment and prevention

Student Workbook

Self-Assessment: Are You Dependent on Drugs?

Changing Health Habits: Are You Using Drugs Inappropriately?

Do You Know?

How drugs can affect the brain?

If smoking marijuana is safer than smoking cigarettes?

Which dietary supplements contain drugs that may be dangerous?

CHAPTER 7

Drug Use and Abuse

Learning Objectives

After studying this chapter, you should be able to:

1. Define drug-related terms.
2. Describe the psychological and physical effects of psychoactive drugs.
3. Differentiate between drug use, misuse, and abuse.
4. Explain why drugs are classified into five drug schedules and describe each schedule.
5. Define drug addiction or dependence, and differentiate between psychological and physical dependence.
6. Discuss risk factors for drug use, abuse, and dependency.
7. Describe current trends related to licit and illicit drug use in the United States.
8. Describe ways in which over-the-counter drugs may be abused.
9. Describe common elements of drug treatment and prevention and drug programs.
10. Identify protective factors for drug abuse among young people.

"Drugs . . . can have serious negative effects on the health and well-being of individuals when used improperly."

drugs Nonfood chemicals that alter the way a person thinks, feels, functions, or behaves.

psychoactive Having mind-altering or mood-altering effects.

drug misuse The temporary and improper use of a legal drug.

Drugs. For many people, this word produces thoughts of shadowy characters secretively injecting illegal and dangerous compounds into their veins. This word may also evoke images of boarded-up crack houses, young people cooking heroin to liquefy it for injection, and women being assaulted while under the influence of date-rape drugs. To others, the word *drugs* brings positive thoughts, such as physicians prescribing medicines to relieve the signs and symptoms of illness. Other images might include your sitting comfortably in the dentist's chair while drugs block the pain of the drill or a person with cancer being treated with powerful chemical therapies to eliminate deadly abnormal cells. What are drugs? Why do drugs elicit both negative and positive images?

Drugs are nonfood chemicals that alter the way a person thinks, feels, functions, or behaves. For thousands of years, people have taken naturally occurring drugs that produce medicinal benefits or **psychoactive** (mood-altering or mind-altering) effects. Nearly everyone uses drugs, for a variety of reasons. Most people have taken aspirin or other pain relievers to treat headaches, sipped cups of coffee or caffeinated soft drinks to stay awake, or drunk alcoholic beverages to celebrate special occasions or to complement meals. Each of these familiar products contains drugs that have beneficial uses, but they can have serious negative effects on the health and well-being of individuals when used improperly. Additionally, inappropriate drug use contributes to numerous social problems that plague our society, such as crime, unemployment, and family violence and dissolution.

This chapter examines the effects of certain drugs on the functioning of the brain, the general nature of drug use and abuse, and the various problems associated with the use of these chemicals. Summary Table 7.7 at the end of this chapter lists the major types of drugs that affect brain functioning and provides examples of each. Many Americans use alcoholic beverages and tobacco. Some people take steroid hormones to improve their appearance.

Drug Use, Misuse, and Abuse

The typical American household has a supply of pain relievers, cold remedies, cough syrups, and other medications. Medications are drugs that have beneficial uses such as treating diseases or correcting physiologic abnormalities. Medicinal drugs are frequently misused. **Drug misuse** is the temporary and improper use of a legal drug. **Table 7.1** lists some typical misuses of drugs.

A prescription is necessary to legitimately purchase the most powerful and potentially hazardous medications. Most of the active compounds in prescription drugs have been tested scientifically for safety and effectiveness.

Nonetheless, mixing prescription drugs with other prescription or nonprescription drugs can be fatal. On January 22, 2008, actor Heath Ledger died from an accidental overdose of prescription drugs (**Figure 7.1**). The Academy Award nominee took a

Table 7.1

Typical Drug Misuse Behaviors

Behavior	Example
Discontinuing the use of prescribed medications prematurely even though you have been instructed to take it for a longer period	Taking an antibiotic only until symptoms disappear
Mixing drugs	Taking barbiturates and drinking alcohol at a party (combining these depressant drugs can be fatal)
Taking more than the recommended dosage	Consuming ten multiple vitamin and mineral supplements instead of one daily
Saving and using medications past their expiration date	Taking a pain reliever that was prescribed 5 years ago
Sharing medicines	Giving your prescribed allergy medicine to a friend

drug abuse The intentional improper or nonmedical use of any drug.

Figure 7.1

Mixing Prescription Drugs. Academy Award nominee Heath Ledger died accidentally at the age of 28 from the abuse of prescription medications. The drugs Ledger took that resulted in his death included painkillers, tranquilizers, and antihistamines. Six prescription medications were found in Ledger's body.

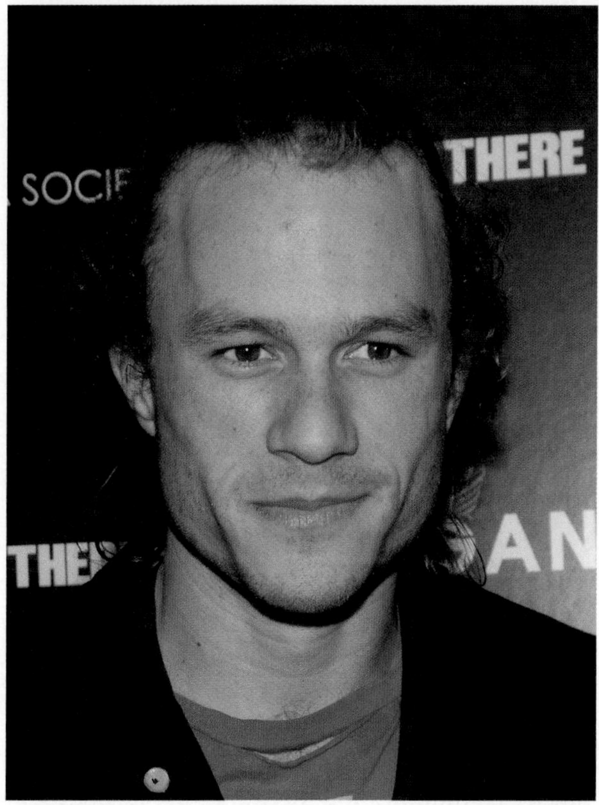

combination of painkillers, antianxiety drugs, and sleeping pills, and their combined effects led to his death. Together, these drugs can cause the brain and brainstem to stop sending messages to the heart and respiratory system. As happened with Ledger, the heartbeat and breathing stopped.

People can buy thousands of medicines without prescriptions, commonly called over-the-counter, or OTC, drugs. Many over-the-counter remedies contain chemicals that have not been evaluated scientifically. Although people often think that OTC drugs are completely safe, any substance that has druglike effects can be dangerous if used improperly. Aspirin and antihistamines, for example, are toxic (poisonous) when ingested in high doses. A later section of this chapter examines problems associated with the use of certain OTC drugs.

Foods are not considered drugs, but many foods contain substances such as caffeine that affect the body. Furthermore, when some vitamins and minerals are consumed in large doses, they have druglike activity in the body. For example, physicians occasionally prescribe large doses of niacin (a B vitamin) to lower the blood cholesterol levels of certain patients. Many people, however, take massive doses of vitamins and minerals without consulting physicians because they think these nutrients are always safe to ingest. However, many vitamins and minerals are toxic when taken in such high doses.

In some instances, drug use becomes **drug abuse**, the intentional improper or nonmedical use of any drug. Drug abuse occurs whenever the use of a substance negatively affects the health and well-being of the user, his or her family, or society. People are more likely to abuse psychoactive drugs than other drugs because of their effects on the mind.

The government controls the use of most psychoactive drugs because of their potential for abuse. Title II of the Comprehensive Drug Abuse Prevention and Control Act of 1970, usually referred to as the Controlled Substances Act, is the legal foundation of narcotics enforcement in the United States. It classifies psychoactive substances into five drug schedules according to their potential for abuse, medical usefulness, and safety (**Table 7.2**). Schedule I drugs have the most stringent control status. They are commonly abused, have little medicinal value (although the medicinal value of marijuana is hotly debated), and lack accepted safety for use. In the United States, it is illegal to use, possess, or sell Schedule I drugs. Schedule V drugs have the least stringent control status. They are infrequently abused, have important medicinal uses, and are considered safe when taken as directed. Schedule II, III, IV, and V drugs are available by prescription.

Officials with the Drug Enforcement Administration (DEA) evaluate medical and scientific information from the U.S. Department of Health and Human Services (HHS) before classifying a drug as a controlled substance. Although classified together, drugs in each schedule do not necessarily have the same potential for producing harmful effects. Heroin and marijuana are Schedule I drugs, for example, but the effects of abusing heroin are more serious than those

Table 7.2

Drug Schedules

Schedule	Examples of Drugs	Description
I	Heroin, LSD, mescaline, peyote, psilocybin, marijuana, GHB, China white	No current accepted medical use; high potential for abuse
II	Ritalin, PCP, Dilaudid, cocaine, methadone, Demerol, morphine, OxyContin, codeine, opium	Current accepted medical use; high potential for abuse
III	Paregoric, anabolic steroids, Tylenol with codeine, Vicodin, Marinol	Current accepted medical use; medium potential for abuse
IV	Rohypnol* ("roofies" or the "date-rape drug"), MDMA, Valium, Librium, Serax, Halcion, Darvon, Placidyl, phenobarbital, Xanax, khat	Current accepted medical use; low potential for abuse
V	Robitussin A–C, Lomotil, Motofen, Parepectolin	Current accepted medical use; lowest potential for abuse

*Penalties for the possession, trafficking, or distribution of Rohypnol are the same as for Schedule I drugs.

Data from U.S. Department of Justice, Drug Enforcement Administration.

of abusing marijuana. In addition, drugs classified in a more stringently controlled schedule do not necessarily have a greater potential for producing harmful effects as drugs in a less stringently controlled schedule or drugs that are not scheduled. For instance, alcohol and nicotine are not scheduled drugs, yet the widespread abuse of these addictive substances is responsible for disabling and killing more people each year than the combined use of all controlled drugs.

People abuse illegal drugs such as cocaine, legally available psychoactive substances such as alcohol, some prescription drugs, and OTC remedies. Many individuals abuse a combination of legal and illegal drugs. Regardless of its legal status, no drug is completely safe. The risk that a drug will cause serious side effects largely depends on the type of drug, the amount taken over time, and the health of the person using the drug.

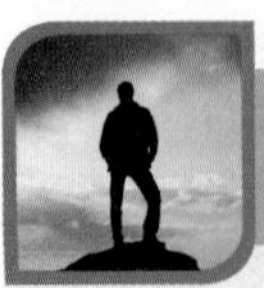

Healthy Living Practices

- Because no drug is completely safe, consider the effects a drug can have on your health and well-being before using it.

Psychoactive Drugs: Effects on the Mind and Body

How Psychoactive Drugs Affect the Brain

Psychoactive drugs affect the nervous system—the "quick" communication network of the body—by changing the way the brain perceives and processes information received from the environment. The nervous system includes the brain and spinal cord (central nervous system, or CNS) and the sensory and motor nerves that transmit messages to and from the central nervous system.

Psychoactive drugs interact with nerve cells in the brain, altering the activity of chemical transmitters that carry messages from one nerve to another. As a result, these drugs influence perceptions, thought processes, feelings, and behaviors. Many commonly abused drugs affect specific regions of the brain, referred to as reward centers because they have a positive influence on mood and alertness. As a result, when used initially, these drugs often produce **euphoria**, an intense feeling of well-being commonly called a "high." Although altering the normal internal chemical environment of the brain affects a person's mood and behavior, external conditions can modify these responses.

What Happens to Drugs in the Body?

After being taken, psychoactive drugs enter the bloodstream and eventually reach the brain, where they produce their characteristic effects. As drugs circulate, the body may eliminate small amounts of these substances in urine, feces, or exhaled breath. In most cases, the remaining drugs undergo **detoxification**, the process of converting harmful substances into less dangerous compounds that can be excreted. Detoxification usually occurs in the liver. The body stores some drugs, primarily in fat, for days and possibly weeks after exposure, particularly when detoxification occurs slowly. Until the body completely eliminates a drug, small amounts of the substance may be detectable in blood or urine.

A state of **intoxication** occurs when the amount of a substance reaches poisonous levels in the body. This level varies among individuals, but genetic factors, body size, physical health, and prior drug exposure influence a person's ability to metabolize, or process, a drug. The signs and symptoms of intoxication include slurred speech, poor muscular coordination, and mental confusion.

An *overdose* occurs when an excessive amount of a drug circulates in the bloodstream and overwhelms the ability of the body to detoxify or eliminate the substance rapidly. Overdoses of OTC, prescription, and illegal drugs can damage or destroy tissues. In some instances, drug overdoses can be fatal. Table 7.7 (at the end of this chapter) describes some signs and symptoms of overdoses of various psychoactive drugs.

Polyabuse, abusing more than one drug at a time, is a common practice. For example, individuals often drink alcoholic beverages while they use heroin, barbiturates, cocaine, or other drugs. When people take different drugs that have similar actions, the effects of each drug may be greatly multiplied. This phenomenon, called **synergism**, can be deadly. Alcohol and barbiturates, for example, are depressant drugs that slow the functioning of the central nervous system. If a person drinks a few alcoholic beverages while taking barbiturates, the combined effects of these substances can depress respiration severely, producing coma or death. Polyabuse can cause drug interactions in addition to synergism that can have serious and even fatal outcomes. Many people are not aware that drinking alcohol while taking acetaminophen, a compound contained in popular over-the-counter pain relievers, can cause liver failure and death.

euphoria (you-FOR-ee-a) An intense feeling of well-being commonly called a "high."

detoxification The process of converting harmful substances into less dangerous compounds.

intoxication The state of being poisoned by a drug or other toxic substance.

polyabuse Abusing more than one drug at a time.

synergism (SIH-ner-jism) The multiplied effects produced by taking combinations of certain drugs.

Illicit Drug Use in the United States

The Prevalence of Illicit Drug Use

Illegal drugs, such as heroin, lysergic acid diethylamide (LSD) and marijuana, are those having no currently accepted medical use in the United States, although some states allow medical marijuana use (**Figure 7.2**). Except for research purposes, it is illegal to buy, sell, possess, and use these drugs. They are listed as Schedule I drugs (see Table 7.2). Only registered, qualified researchers can obtain illegal drugs in the United States.

Legal drugs are those for which sale, possession, and use as intended are not forbidden by law; however, use may be restricted. Restricted drugs, such as narcotics, depressants, and stimulants, are called *controlled substances* and are available with a prescription.

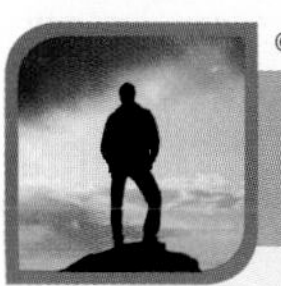

© djgis/ShutterStock

Healthy Living Practices

- Do not combine drugs, including alcohol and OTC medicines, without consulting a physician or registered pharmacist. *Mixing drugs can kill you!*

Illicit drugs are defined by the Substance Abuse and Mental Health Services Administration as illegal drugs and controlled substances held without a legal prescription.

Periodic (e.g., annual) surveys and interviews are used to estimate the prevalence of illicit drug use in the United States. Tens of thousands of Americans

Figure 7.2

Medical Marijuana. As of late 2013, 20 states and the District of Columbia allowed the use of marijuana for medical purposes, and 4 states had legislation pending. In these states, registered outlets, such as the one in Denver, Colorado shown in this 2011 photo, sold marijuana to people with a license. A variety of medical marijuana strains are shown on the dispensary shelves.

© Rick Wilking/Reuters/Landov

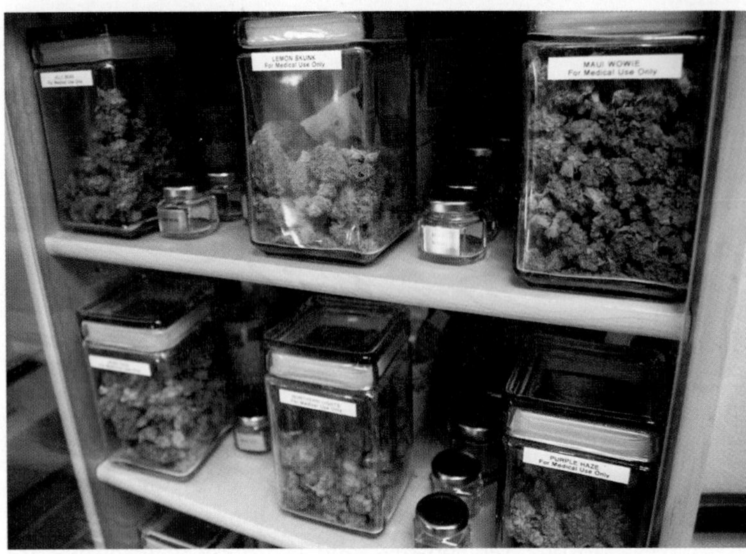

12 years of age or older complete the National Survey on Drug Use and Health (NSDUH), annually. NSDUH data from 2012 indicated an estimated 23.9 million Americans, or 9.2%, of Americans aged 12 years and older were current illicit drug users, meaning respondents used an illicit drug in the month prior to the interview (see Figure 7.9). The 2012 figure represents an increase in illicit drug users from 2008 (8%).[1] These data indicate fewer Americans used illicit substances in 2012 than in the late 1970s, a time in which approximately 25 million Americans used illicit drugs.

NSHUH 2012 data also suggest slightly more men than women currently use illicit drugs, 7.5% and 7.0%, respectively. Furthermore, certain segments of the American population use illicit drugs more than do other groups; for example, 18.1% of unemployed adults were current users of illicit drugs in 2012, whereas only 8% of full-time employed adults used illegal substances. Among people aged 18 years and older in 2012, those who lacked high school diplomas had the highest rate of current illicit drug use (11.1%), and college graduates had the lowest rate of current use (6.6%).[1]

Rates of illicit drug use are especially high among teenagers and young adults. **Figure 7.3** shows that drug use peaks at ages 18 to 20 years, with more than one out of five persons in this age group reporting past-month illicit drug use in both 2011 and 2012. Current illicit drug use was reported by more than 10% of young people aged 16 to 29 years in 2012, with a slight decrease through the early to mid 30s.

Since 1975, researchers at the University of Michigan's Institute for Social Research have conducted Monitoring the Future (MTF), an annual survey of American high school and college students, to ascertain their use of drugs. Data from the 2012 survey indicate that 37.3% of full-time college students aged 19 to 22 years took at least one illicit drugs during 2012, up from 30.6% in 1992. In 2012, 36.4% of college students used marijuana at least once during the year, up from 27.7% in 1992. Additionally, the use of LSD ("acid") rose in the mid-1990s from 1989, and has since begun to fall. Furthermore, 1.9% of college students reported taking LSD during the previous 12 months in 2012. In 1994, this figure was about 5%; in 1989, it was 3.4%.[2]

Why Do People Use Psychoactive Drugs?

Drug users often provide numerous reasons to explain why they began taking psychoactive substances. Most people begin taking mood-altering drugs for nonmedical purposes. Some individuals use alcohol or other drugs simply as a pleasurable experience. Others use drugs to cope with their psychological problems, reduce stress, or escape from unpleasant aspects of their lives. Curiosity often motivates many teenagers and young adults to experiment with drugs. Movies and advertisements may stimulate this curiosity by showing, for example, sophisticated and attractive people smoking cigarettes or cigars or drinking alcoholic beverages while engaging in enjoyable activities (**Figure 7.4**). Additionally, teenagers may use drugs to experience new behaviors, relieve peer pressure, or enhance social interactions.

Patterns of Psychoactive Drug Use

Drug experimentation and illicit use often occurs during the teen years and peaks between the ages

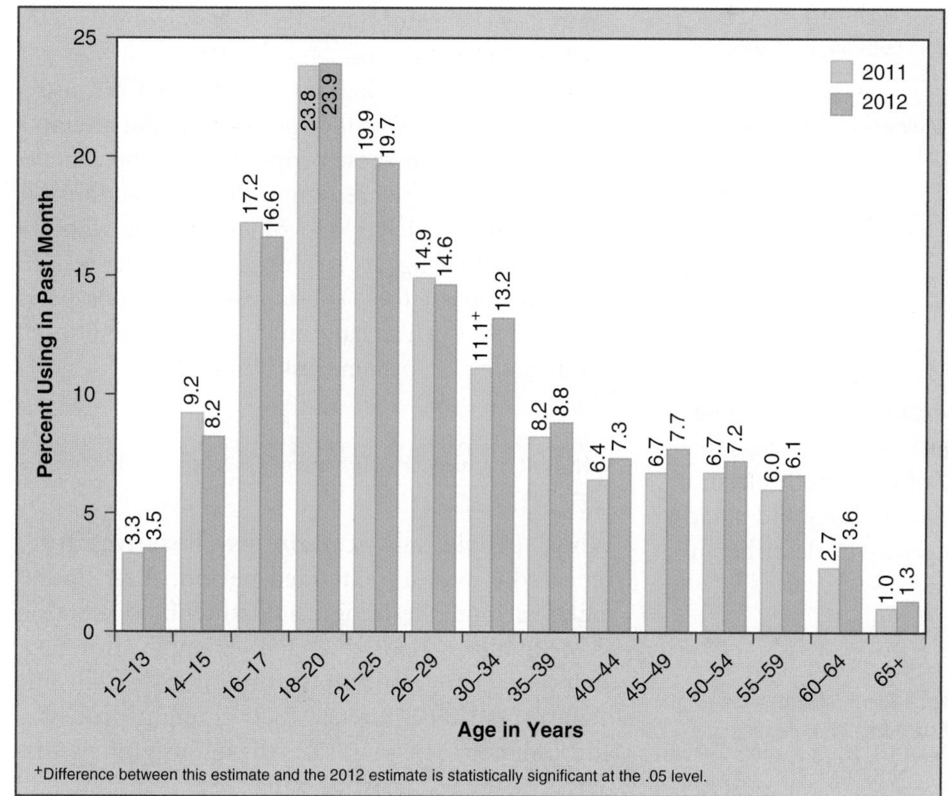

Figure 7.3

Past-Month Illicit Drug Use Among Persons Aged 12 Years and Older, by Age: 2011 and 2012.

Reproduced from Substance Abuse and Mental Health Services Administration. (2013). Results from the 2012 National Survey on Drug Use and Health: Summary of National Findings (HHS Publication No. SMA 13-4795). Retrieved from http://www.samhsa.gov/data/NSDUH/2012SummNatFindDetTables/NationalFindings/NSDUHresults2012.pdf

of 18 and 20 years (see Figure 7.3). Most drug abusers in this age group begin by smoking cigarettes, and then they consume alcoholic beverages such as beer or wine. Some youth inhale chemicals such as those in aerosols and plastic cements to obtain their mind-altering effects. Alcohol, nicotine, marijuana, and inhalants are often referred to as "gateway" drugs because adolescents use these substances before moving on to other psychoactive drugs.[3]

Many adolescents stop experimenting with new drugs after using alcohol or nicotine; however, those who continue to experiment with drugs often, try marijuana next. The rate of marijuana use among 8th and 10th graders in the United States remained relatively consistent between 2011 and 2011. Approximately 11% of 8th graders and, 28% of 10th graders survey in the MTF reported trying marijuana in 2012. On the other hand, a slight increase in marijuana use, from 33% up 2011 to 36% in 2012, was seen among 12th graders.[2]

Any combination of stimulants, depressants, or hallucinogens may follow marijuana use. After trying these drugs, some young people move on to use opiates; however, not every youthful drug user follows this stepping-stone pattern of drug experimentation. For example, many teenagers who experiment with alcohol or marijuana do not try other psychoactive drugs.

The recreational use of illegal drugs generally declines with increasing age beyond age 20 years as traditional adult roles, including marriage, parenthood, and careers, are adopted. As they age, many individuals recognize that abusing illicit drugs can be self-destructive. Nevertheless, elderly persons who feel socially isolated and depressed, and those with a history of substance abuse, are at greater risk of abusing prescription drugs than are adolescents and young adults.[4]

Drug Dependence

Most people who use psychoactive drugs such as alcohol or marijuana take them for pleasure, to relax, or to feel comfortable in social settings, which is termed *recreational drug use.* To assess your use of drugs, complete the questionnaire in the exercise entitled "Are You Dependent on Drugs?" in the Student Workbook pages at the end of this book.

drug dependence (addiction) Occurs when users develop a habitual pattern of taking drugs that produces a compulsive need, which is both physical and psychological.

tolerance An adaptation to drugs in which the usual dose no longer produces the anticipated degree of physical or psychological effects.

withdrawal A temporary physical and psychological state that occurs when certain drugs are discontinued.

Drug dependence or **addiction** occurs when users develop a habitual pattern of taking drugs that produces a compulsive need, which is both physical and psychological. The terms *dependency* and *addiction* are often used interchangeably to describe any compulsive behavior that interferes with one's health, work, and relationships.

Dependent individuals are unable to avoid using drugs; most have a history of unsuccessful attempts to stop. Over time, these people escalate their intake of drugs even as they recognize that their actions are harmful to themselves and others. People who are dependent on drugs are so preoccupied with the need to obtain and use these substances that other aspects of their lives, such as handling the responsibilities of family and work, become less important.

Figure 7.4

Grammy-winning British singer Amy Winehouse at Balans café bar in Soho, London. The media frequently portray sophisticated and attractive people smoking or binge drinking while engaging in enjoyable activities. As a result, some young people copy these unhealthy behaviors. Winehouse evidenced many other unhealthy behaviors. She died on July 23, 2011 at the age of 27, from accidental alcohol poisoning, drinking heavily after weeks of abstinence.

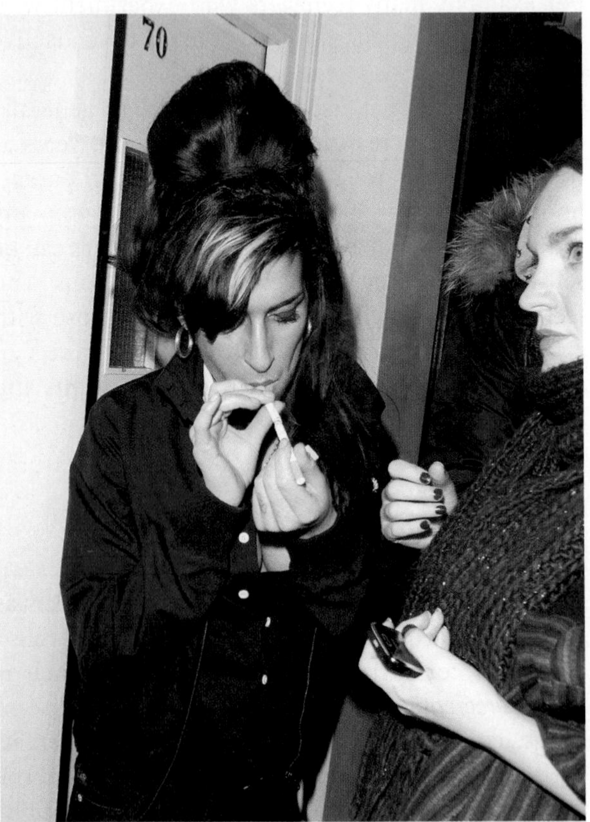

Physiologic and Psychological Dependence

When people take certain psychoactive drugs repeatedly over an extended period, their bodies make various physiologic adjustments to function as normally as possible. For example, dramatic chemical changes occur in the brains of chronic drug users that influence their thought processes and behaviors. As a result, these individuals display the characteristic signs and symptoms of *physical dependence* or *physical addiction*: drug tolerance and withdrawal.

After chronic exposure to certain drugs, the body develops **tolerance**, the ability to endure larger amounts of these substances while the adverse effects decrease. When this occurs, users discover that their usual dose of drugs no longer produces the desired degree of physical or psychological effects. To get the desired effects, people must take larger quantities, which results in increased tolerance. This upward spiral is more difficult to break at each successive level, increasing the risk of overdose.

Withdrawal is a temporary physical and psychological state that occurs when certain drugs are discontinued. The signs and symptoms of withdrawal include trembling, anxiety, and pain. In cases of barbiturate addiction, withdrawal symptoms are so severe they can cause death. Table 7.7 at the end of this chapter indicates psychoactive drugs' potentials for producing tolerance, withdrawal, and addiction.

Psychological dependence is a person's need to use certain psychoactive drugs regularly to obtain their pleasurable effects and to relieve boredom, anxiety, or stress. Psychologically dependent people experience powerful cravings for these substances, which motivates drug-seeking behavior. However, it may be difficult to distinguish psychological dependence from physical dependence. As mentioned earlier, psychoactive drugs produce physiologic changes in the brain that influence behavior. Thus, these changes may affect a person's emotional responses, including feelings about the need to take psychoactive substances.

Not everyone who habitually uses or abuses psychoactive substances becomes dependent on their use. For example, individuals who drive after becoming drunk at bars or parties are abusing alcohol, but they are not necessarily alcoholics. It is difficult to determine when the habitual use of a psychoactive substance becomes a dependency. Scientists are interested in determining why some people seem to be more susceptible to drug dependency and addiction than others are.

Risk Factors for Drug Dependency

Like many other health problems, there is no single risk factor for drug dependency. Substance addiction results from complex interactions among biological, personal, social, and environmental factors. Results of research conducted by the National Institute on Drug Abuse (NIDA) and reported in its most recent edition of *Preventing Drug Use Among Children and Adolescents: A Research-Based Guide* suggest that certain conditions in the home are probably the most crucial risk factors for children becoming drug abusers.[5] Such factors include home environments in which parents abuse drugs or suffer from mental illness; ineffective parenting, particularly with children who have difficult temperaments or conduct disorders; and a lack of mutual child–parent attachments and parental nurturing. Risk factors for drug abuse that relate to a child's behavior outside of the home include inappropriately shy or aggressive behavior in the classroom; poor school performance; poor social skills; friendships with peers who use drugs; and a belief that parents, the school, peers, and the community approve of drug use. Conversely, *protective factors*, those associated with reduced potential for drug abuse, include strong family and school ties; parental monitoring of behavior with clear rules of conduct; involvement of parents in the lives of children; academic success in school; and the belief that parents, the school, peers, and the community do not approve of drug use.

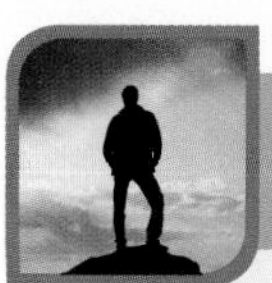

© djgis/ShutterStock

Healthy Living Practices

- To avoid the destructive effects of a drug dependency or addiction, do not use psychoactive substances unless you are under a physician's care.

Stimulants

Throughout the world, people have used various stimulant drugs for thousands of years to relieve fatigue, suppress appetite, and improve mood. (See the Diversity in Health essay "Khat.") Stimulants enhance chemical activity in parts of the brain that influence emotions, sleep, attention, and learning. Within minutes after taking stimulants, users are more alert, excitable, and restless. These drugs also increase blood pressure levels and heart rates.

Amphetamines and Methamphetamines

Synthetic stimulants are amphetamines, methamphetamines, and nonamphetamines (see Table 7.7). Amphetamines such as Dexedrine (dextroamphetamine) increase energy and alertness, lessen the need to sleep, produce euphoria, and suppress appetite. In the early 1980s, 21% to 22% of college students reported using amphetamines within the past year. Their use dropped significantly each year from 1983 to 1992, when only 3.6% of college students reported using this drug. From 1993 to 2001, amphetamine use rose again, ranging from 4.2% in 1993 to 7.2% in 2001. By 2012, 11.1% of full-time college students reported using amphetamines, but only 1.8% reported using methamphetamines. Methamphetamine use in U.S. college students has steadily declined from its height of 3.3% in 1999 to 0.2% in 2011.[2]

Methamphetamines ("speed") are powerful forms of amphetamines that have few medically approved uses. Methamphetamine is taken orally (usually as a pill), or the powder is snorted. It can also be injected or smoked. In small doses, methamphetamines produce euphoria, appetite loss, excessive perspiration, and pounding heartbeats. The effects of taking larger doses can be frightening: chest pains, irregular heartbeat, fever, hallucinations, and convulsions. People who drive while on methamphetamines exhibit erratic driving patterns and are often involved in high-speed collisions.

Methamphetamine use is associated with weakening of the heart muscle in young people (those aged 45 years or younger).[6] Overdoses of methamphetamines

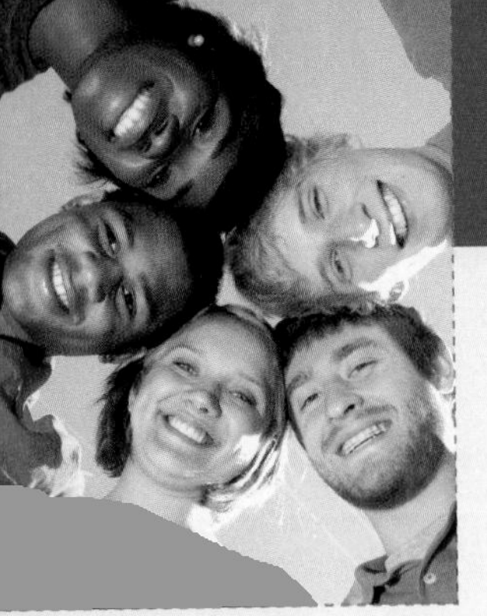

© Mike Flippo/ShutterStock

Diversity in Health

Khat

Which psychoactive drug is associated with weddings and weekends? If your answer is alcohol, you may be wrong with respect to certain cultures. In the East African countries of Somalia and Ethiopia, and on the nearby Arabian peninsula in Yemen, people chew khat, the leaf buds and leaves of the native bush *Catha edulis*, to celebrate weddings and other special events (**Figure 7.A**). For centuries, people from these cultures have chewed or smoked khat or drunk tea brewed from its leaves as a socially acceptable and enjoyable pastime. Many homes in Somalia have a special room in which family members and their friends (primarily men) gather to munch khat and chat. Like alcohol and other psychoactive substances that are more familiar to Americans, khat contains chemicals that are known to produce both pleasurable and harmful side effects.

Khat contains cathionine, more potent and found in fresh leaves, and cathine, less potent and found in older leaves. These compounds are chemically similar to amphetamines and produce psychological and physiologic responses that resemble those produced by amphetamines and other stimulants. After using khat, people report feeling euphoric and alert; they have little desire to eat, sleep, or engage in sex. Khat users experience elevated blood pressures and heart rates. After the stimulating and mood-elevating effects of the drug subside, khat users feel anxious and irritable.

Khat impairs thought processes such as mental concentration and judgment; therefore, driving while under its influence can be hazardous. Men who use khat regularly may develop permanent impotence; women who use khat during pregnancy are at risk of giving birth to underweight newborns. Overdosing on khat can produce aggressive, paranoid, and psychotic behavior. Khat has also been found to be a significant risk factor for acute coronary syndrome, a range of life-threatening heart-related disorders.

In the early 1990s, thousands of Somalis and Ethiopians fled the civil unrest raging in their homelands and sought refuge in Western countries, including England and the United States. After settling in the West, many of these immigrants maintained their habit of using khat. To satisfy their demand, the immigrants purchase khat leaves that have been flown into North America or the United Kingdom from East Africa.

Concerned about the drug's effects on the central nervous system, officials at the U.S. Drug Enforcement Administration added cathine to its list of controlled substances in 1988 as a Schedule IV drug. In 1993, the Food and Drug Administration issued an import alert that recommended detention of khat by customs officials to prevent its entry into the United States. Currently, khat use does not pose a major drug enforcement problem.

Sources: Valente, M. J., et al. (2014). Khat and synthetic cathinones: A review. *Archives of Toxicology, 88*(1), 15–45.; Al-Hebshi, N. N., & Skaug, N. (2005). Khat (*Catha edulis*)— an updated review. *Addiction Biology, 10*, 299–307.; El-Wajeh, Y. A., & Thornhill, M. H. (2009). Qat and its health effects. *British Dental Journal, 206*, 17–21.; and Mwenda, J. M., et al. (2003). Effects of khat (*Catha edulis*) consumption on reproductive functions: A review. *East African Medical Journal, 80*, 318–323.

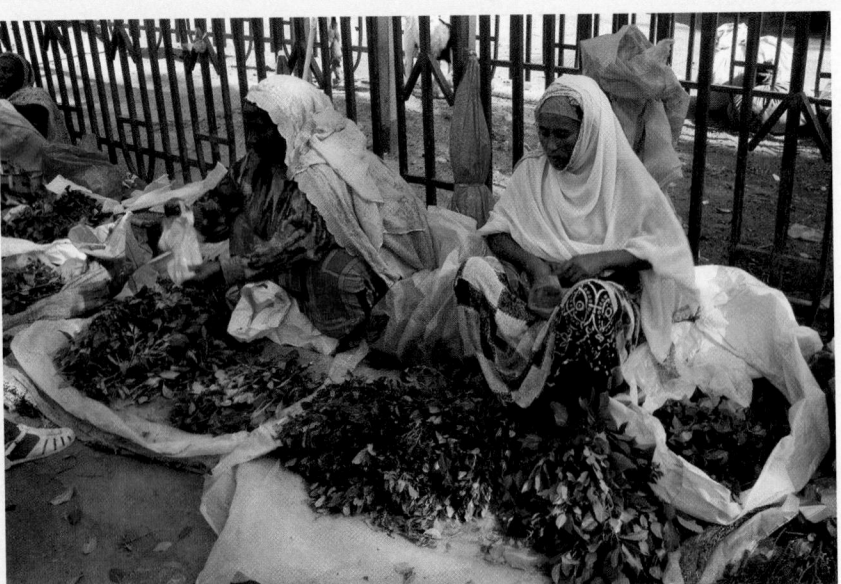

Figure 7.A

Women selling khat in Ethiopia.

© Peter Smolka/dpa/Landov

Figure 7.5

Brain Decay Caused by Methamphetamine Use. This magnetic resonance imaging (MRI) image of one hemisphere of the brain shows areas of brain-volume loss in a methamphetamine user.

Courtesy of Paul Thompson, Kiralee Hayashi, Arthur Toga, Edythe London/UCLA.

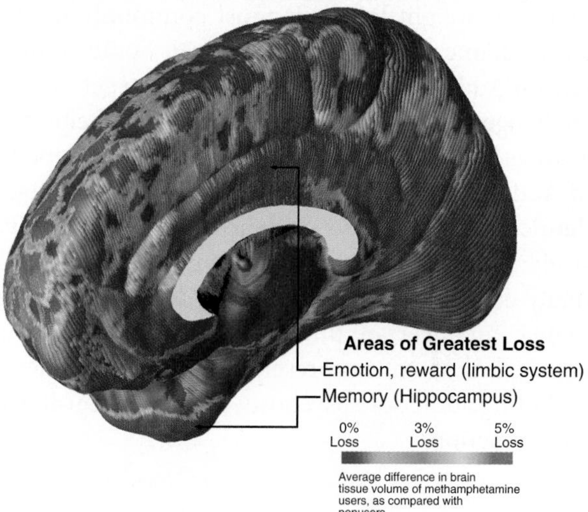

Figure 7.6

Before and After Using Crystal Meth. The mug shot on the left is of a woman who committed a felony prior to using crystal meth. The mug shot on the right is of the same woman after 2.5 years of using this drug.

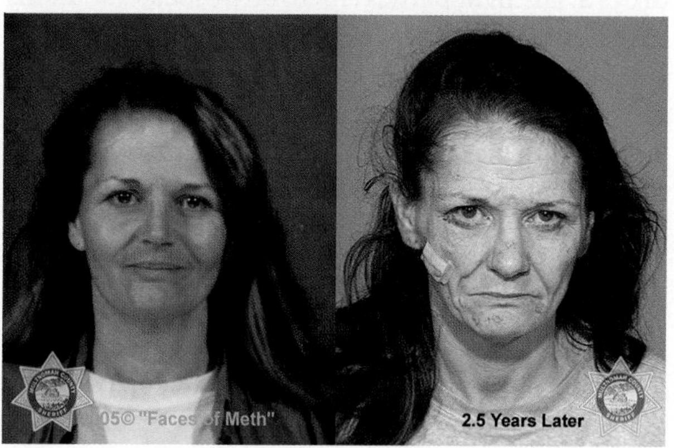

can be deadly by resulting in cardiovascular collapse or strokes. When taken by pregnant women, the drug can stunt fetal growth and negatively affect the development of the fetal brain.[7,8]

Brain damage is a hallmark of chronic methamphetamine abuse. **Figure 7.5** shows this damage in a user: The red areas are those with the greatest tissue loss. The limbic region, which is involved in drug craving, reward, mood, and emotion, lost 11% of its tissue in this user's brain. The hippocampus, which is involved in memory making, lost 8% of its tissue. The persons examined in the study were in their 30s and had used methamphetamine for 10 years, primarily by smoking it approximately every other day, using 4 g per week.[9] Withdrawal from methamphetamines often results in anxiety, fatigue, sleeplessness, paranoia, delusions, and severe depression.

In the 1980s, drug suppliers from Korea, Taiwan, and the Philippines introduced an illegal crystalline form of methamphetamine called *crystal meth* (also referred to as *meth*, *crank*, *ice*, and *glass*). An extremely potent and addictive drug, crystal meth can produce violent behavior and damage the liver, kidneys, and lungs as well as the physical appearance (**Figure 7.6**).

Both methamphetamine and crystal meth are synthetic drugs; that is, they are not made directly from plant material as are opium or cocaine but are made in laboratories from other chemicals, called precursor chemicals. Drug suppliers manufacture the drug using temporary homemade labs that they move from place to place to evade law enforcement.

The ingredients for making meth are lithium from batteries, acetone from paint thinner, lye, and ephedrine/pseudoephedrine, which are found in cold remedies and sinus medications. However, the Domestic Chemical Diversion Control Act of 1993 made it illegal to sell ephedrine over the counter (although it could still be sold in pills containing other active ingredients), and the Comprehensive Methamphetamine Control Act of 1996 placed additional controls on products containing ephedrine and pseudoephedrine. More recently, the Combat Methamphetamine Epidemic Act enacted in 2006 placed restrictions on the amount of medications containing ephedrine and pseudoephedrine that could be sold in one day and over a 30-day period to an individual. To circumvent the law, methamphetamine "manufacturers" often use the drug ephedra (ma huang) as a substitute or have many individuals purchase the drugs up to the daily and monthly limit, a practice called "smurfing."

Party Drugs Amphetamines and methamphetamines are two drugs in a group called *party drugs* (*club drugs*). Party drugs also include alcohol, GHB, GBL, and Rohypnol (depressants); LSD (acid) and ketamine (special K) (both are hallucinogens); and MDMA (ecstasy, a drug with mixed effects).

anesthetic Substance that interferes with normal sensations.

Adolescents, teenagers, and young adults use these drugs at all-night parties and in other social situations to reduce anxiety, induce euphoria, or build energy to keep on dancing or partying. However, these drugs are not harmless "fun" drugs because they can have long-lasting negative effects on the brain. (We discuss these drugs in this chapter.)

Ritalin, Adderall, and Other Medically Useful Stimulants Amphetamines and chemically related stimulants have a few medical uses, such as treatment of the sleep disorder narcolepsy, short-term weight loss, and attention control. One medicinally useful stimulant is Ritalin (methylphenidate), prescribed for people with attention disorders. Ritalin is abused, however, by persons who do not need the drug for its prescribed use but use it for its stimulant effect.

The annual prevalence of nonprescription Ritalin use for high school seniors from 1976 to 1993 was very low and ranged from 0.1% to 0.7%. In 1994, Ritalin use by high school seniors rose to 1% from 0.4% in 1993 and reached a peak of 3.9% in 2004. Since then, prevalence of use has fallen and was 1.3% in 2009.[10] In 2001, MTF researchers changed the way they asked the question about nonprescription Ritalin use, and the results yielded higher prevalence rates, from 5.1% in 2001, decreasing to 2.1% in 2009, and have remained steady at 2.6 to 2.7% from 2010 to 2012.[2] The results from asking both questions suggest an ongoing, gradual decline in Ritalin use in recent years.

The stimulant Adderall (amphetamine and dextroamphetamine) is more recently used for the treatment of attention-deficit hyperactivity disorder (ADHD), and the MTF researchers began asking questions of seniors regarding its use in 2007. In that year, 2.8% of high school seniors reported using the drug, and that figure rose to 3.3% by 2009.[10] Using a revised question as with Ritalin, the prevalence of Adderall use by seniors in 2012 was 7.6%.[2] MTF researchers suggest that the decrease in Ritalin use may be occurring because it is being replaced by Adderall use.

Among college students, the annual prevalence of Ritalin use is about the same as with high school seniors. MTF began asking the question of college students in 2002, using the revised format. Nonprescription prevalence of use for college students was 5.7% in 2002 but fell through 2012 to a rate of 1.8%. The annual prevalence of use for young adults aged 19 to 28 years not enrolled in college was lower than for college students from 2002 to 2008 but was the same in 2012 at 1.7%. Use of Adderall was high in college students in 2012 at 9.0% and was 7.4% for young adults not enrolled in college.[2]

Although Adderall is used by some college students for weight lost, it is most commonly used as an academic performance enhancer. Some students rely on Adderall for mental endurance to get through challenges of school and believe it will help them achieve better grades. Despite student perceptions of Adderall's ability to help them perform better academically, there is no evidence Adderall improves student grades or learning outcomes. Unfortunately, many college student who use Adderall as a performance enhancer are unware of negative health outcomes linked to nonprescription use of Adderall, including addiction, psychosis, and severe cardiovascular reaction.

Cocaine

Cocaine is a white powdery substance extracted from the leaves of the coca bush, which is not the same plant as the cacao tree from which cocoa and chocolate are derived. Crack is a rock crystal form of cocaine that can be heated and its vapors smoked (inhaled); its name comes from the cracking sound that is heard during the heating process. The powdered form of cocaine can be snorted (inhaled through the nose) or dissolved in water and injected. Most people snort, rather than inject, cocaine.

This potent stimulant has some medical uses, particularly as an **anesthetic**, a substance that interferes with normal sensations. However, cocaine was the most widely used illegal stimulant in the United States during the late 1970s and early 1980s, a time during which the public was misinformed about the drug and its dangers. Additionally, many health-care practitioners did not understand the dangers of cocaine use or its addictive nature; as a consequence, cocaine was viewed as glamorous and was used by many celebrities as well as millions of other Americans. The popularity of cocaine declined dramatically between 1985 and 1992, most likely from public understanding that accompanied increased knowledge about this drug and its dangerous effects.[3] The level of cocaine use has not changed significantly since 1992, but it has dropped somewhat in recent years. Experts estimate that approximately 1.6 million Americans were current cocaine users in 2012, down from 2.4 million in 2006 (see Figure 7.9).[1]

Cocaine is highly addictive. In laboratory studies of the drug's effects, animals prefer to self-administer cocaine rather than engage in reproductive behavior or obtain food. Many people who are dependent on cocaine demonstrate similar responses. Cocaine abusers often dissociate themselves from their families, friends, and associates.

Chronic cocaine abuse produces serious health problems (see Table 7.7). People who snort cocaine regularly often suffer from chronic irritation of their nasal passages. This irritation causes nosebleeds, and it can destroy the septum, the cartilaginous tissue that divides the area between the two nostrils (**Figure 7.7**). Snorting cocaine and smoking crack damage lung tissue and increase susceptibility to respiratory tract infections.

Long-term use of cocaine may interfere with normal sexual functioning. Men who use cocaine regularly often experience an inability to achieve erections and a reduced sexual drive. Women who are chronic users may experience infertility, menstrual problems, and difficulty achieving orgasms.

Cocaine use can have deadly consequences. People with hepatitis or AIDS can spread these diseases by sharing their used hypodermic needles with uninfected drug users. Additionally, cocaine use increases the risk of dying suddenly from life-threatening disorders of the circulatory system such as irregular and rapid heartbeat, high blood pressure, stroke, and heart attacks. Death is especially likely when people take cocaine with other psychoactive substances such as alcohol and heroin. During the past 2 decades, several well-known individuals have died as a result of using cocaine, such as comedian/actor John Belushi, comic Chris Farley, and bassist John Entwistle of the rock band The Who.

While under the influence of cocaine, some individuals experience severe psychotic reactions, including paranoia, which may result in violent behavior. It is not uncommon for cocaine abusers to report having delusions such as the sensation that bugs are crawling beneath their skin. The psychological symptoms of cocaine intoxication also lead some users to attempt suicide, and a number of them succeed.

Figure 7.7

Perforated Nasal Septum. The nostril is being held open with a nasal speculum, showing the nasal passage and mucosa. The septum divides the inner passageways. The perforation (hole) in the septum, a common result of snorting cocaine, may cause symptoms such as bleeding, crusting, whistling, and difficulty breathing.

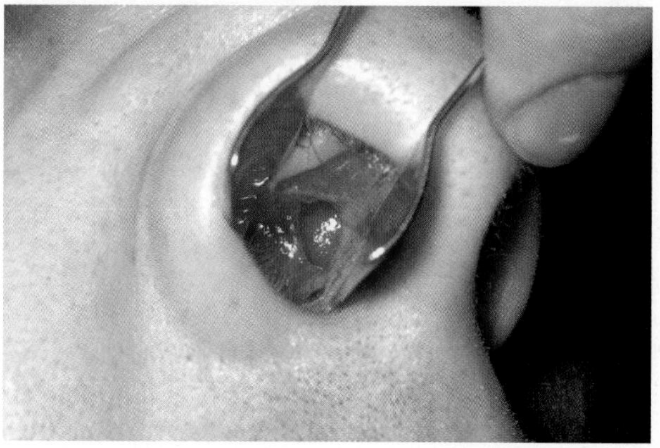

Caffeine

Worldwide, caffeine is the most widely used psychoactive substance. Caffeine and its related chemical compounds occur naturally in several varieties of plants that we use to make foods and beverages, including coffee, tea, and cocoa. People may ingest caffeine when they consume caffeinated soft drinks or they take certain over-the-counter medications. **Table 7.3** lists the amounts of caffeine contained in certain beverages, foods, and over-the-counter products.

Caffeine has been generally recognized as a stimulant that causes limited dependence. The average American consumes about 200 mg of caffeine daily—the equivalent of about two cups of coffee or five cola beverages. Typical patterns of moderate caffeine consumption do not appear to be harmful to healthy persons.

The Center for Science in the Public Interest notes that—on the positive side—people who consume caffeine regularly have a lower risk of developing Parkinson's disease and gallstones. In addition, caffeine intake improves alertness and reaction time, lifts the mood, helps the body burn fat, blunts pain, and helps relieve headache pain. On the negative side, however, caffeine can disturb sleep and provoke migraine headaches in those prone to them. Consuming 200 mg or more per day may increase the risk of miscarriage.[11]

After abstaining from caffeine for about half a day, a person who is accustomed to taking the drug typically experiences withdrawal symptoms that include headache, tiredness, irritability, and depression. Individuals who consume more than 600 mg per day often experience psychological as well as physical problems known as *caffeinism*. The manifestations of caffeinism include nervousness, trembling, irritation of the stomach lining, insomnia, increased urine production, diarrhea, sweating, and rapid heart rate.

sedatives Drugs that produce calming effects.

hypnotics Drugs that produce trancelike effects.

People who do not regularly consume caffeine or who are sensitive to it may develop caffeinism after taking as little as 250 mg of the drug daily.

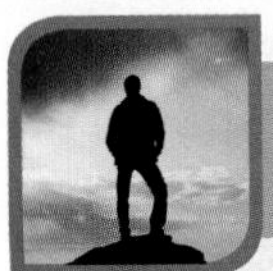

© djgis/ShutterStock

Healthy Living Practices

- If you have ill effects such as anxiety or sleep disturbances from consuming too much caffeine, gradually wean yourself from the drug to avoid its withdrawal symptoms, especially headaches.

Depressants

Depressants produce **sedative** (calming) and **hypnotic** (trancelike) effects as well as drowsiness. These drugs slow the activity of the cerebral cortex, the part of the brain that is responsible for thought processes. Depressant drugs include alcohol, barbiturates such as phenobarbital (Luminal), and minor tranquilizers such as diazepam (Valium).

Dangerous side effects can result when people misuse depressants. All of these drugs slow the heart and respiratory rates, which increases the risk of dying from respiratory failure after taking an overdose. Combining depressants—for example, drinking alcohol while taking Valium—produces synergistic (combined) effects. Such synergism of depressants can be life threatening.

Table 7.3

Caffeine Content of Popular Beverages, Foods, and Products

Beverage, Food, or Product	Typical Amount/ Range (mg)
Coffee	
Cappuccino (2 oz)	100
Espresso (2 oz)	100
Brewed, drip method (5 oz)	60–180
Brewed, percolator (5 oz)	40–170
Instant (5 oz)	30–120
Decaffeinated, brewed (5 oz)	2–5
Decaffeinated, instant (5 oz)	1–5
Tea	
Brewed, U.S. brands (5 oz)	0–90
Brewed, imported brands (5 oz)	25–110
Instant (5 oz)	25–50
Iced (5 oz)	28–32
Cocoa-Containing Products	
Cocoa (5 oz)	2–20
Chocolate milk (5 oz)	1–4

Beverage, Food, or Product	Typical Amount/ Range (mg)
Milk chocolate (1 oz)	1–15
Dark chocolate, semi-sweet (1 oz)	5–35
Chocolate-flavored syrup (1 oz)	4
Soft Drinks (12 oz)	
Dr. Pepper	40
Cola-type beverages	
Regular	30–46
Diet	2–58
Caffeine-free	0
Mountain Dew, Mello Yello	52
Jolt	75–100
Over-the-Counter Medications	
Vivarin (1 pill)	200
Nodoz (1 pill)	100
Anacin, Empirin, or Midol (2 pills)	64

Data from Caffeine: Grounds for concern? (1994). *University of California at Berkeley Wellness Letter*, 10(6), 5.; Goldberg, R. (2005). *Drugs across the spectrum*. Belmont, CA: Brooks/Cole; and Sizer, F., & Whitnet, E. (2005). *Nutrition: Concepts and controversies*. Belmont, CA: Wadsworth Publishing Co.

Managing Your Health

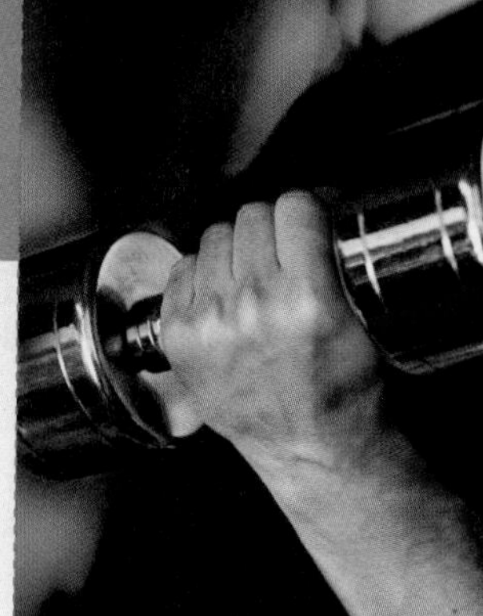

© Kzenon/ShutterStock

Falling Asleep Without Prescriptions

If you experience occasional sleepless nights, the following self-treatment tips for insomnia may be helpful:

1. Try to adhere to a regular sleeping and waking schedule, even on weekends, to foster natural sleep–wake timing.
2. Don't eat big meals or drink large amounts of fluids in the evening. Have a light snack before bedtime if you like, but avoid alcohol, caffeine, and over-the-counter (OTC) pain relievers that contain caffeine.
3. Reserve time for vigorous regular exercise earlier in the day and no closer than 2 hours before bedtime.
4. Practice a prebedtime relaxing routine, such as taking a warm bath or shower.
5. Keep your bedroom dark, cool, and as quiet as possible.
6. Practice progressive muscular relaxation while in bed.
7. Don't stay in bed if you can't fall asleep; get out of bed and read a dull book. Avoid watching TV or any screen; the flickering light stimulates the brain. Return to bed when you begin to feel sleepy.
8. Take an OTC sleep aid only as a last resort. Recognize that most of these medications contain antihistamines that lose their effectiveness if used regularly.

Tolerance and dependency occur with regular use of depressants. Withdrawal from these drugs can cause *delirium* (mental confusion and disorientation) and *seizures* (abnormal brain activity that results in uncontrollable muscular movements). Some addicted people die while undergoing withdrawal from depressants.

Sedatives and Tranquilizers

Physicians frequently prescribe sedatives and minor tranquilizers, especially for people suffering from insomnia or mild anxiety. In many instances, people can treat their mild anxiety or insomnia without powerful depressants. Anxious individuals can try to reduce their feelings of stress by practicing relaxation techniques. The Managing Your Health feature "Falling Asleep Without Prescriptions" provides suggestions that may induce sleep without the use of depressants or other drugs. Prescription medications used to treat anxiety and sleep disorders are often abused. In 2012, 2.1 million people abused tranquilizers and 270,000 abused sedatives.[1]

Rohypnol

Rohypnol (row-HIP-nole), commonly called *roofies* (along with a variety of other street names), is one of a few "date-rape drugs." (See the section titled "GHB and GBL" that follows.) While under the influence of Rohypnol, women are unable to resist rapists, and they cannot recall, for various lengths of time, what happened to them while under the influence. Because of concern about Rohypnol and other similarly abused sedative–hypnotics, Congress passed the Drug-Induced Rape Prevention and Punishment Act of 1996 to increase federal penalties for use of any controlled substance to aid in sexual assault. After 1996, Rohypnol use declined. It was used by only 1.5% of high school seniors in 2012 and less than 0.1% of college students, which appears on MTF tables as 0%.[2]

Although not approved for use in the United States, this drug is widely available in Mexico, Colombia, and Europe, where it is used for the treatment of insomnia. Like other depressants, its effects include sedation, muscle relaxation, and anxiety reduction. It also causes dizziness, loss of motor control, lack of coordination, slurred speech, confusion, and gastrointestinal disturbances, all of which can last 12 hours or more.

GHB and GBL

Gamma hydroxybutyrate, better known as *GHB*, was formerly sold in health food stores as a dietary supplement to induce sleep and build muscle. Its over-the-counter sale was banned by the Food and Drug Administration (FDA) in 1990. The longer periods of sleep it induced were supposed to allow release of human growth hormone, which has been linked

analgesics (an-al-GEEZ-iks) Drugs that alleviate pain.

narcotics Drugs that induce euphoria and sleep as well as alter the perception of pain.

with increased muscle mass. However, GHB users reported unpleasant side effects such as nausea and shaking. More dangerously, this drug has induced seizures and coma in some users and can also cause irregular heartbeat, slowed breathing, hypothermia, and vomiting.[12] With legislation passed in February 2000, GHB became a Schedule I drug.

In January 1999, the FDA warned consumers about a drug related to GHB: gamma butyrolactone, or *GBL*. After ingestion, the body converts GBL to GHB. Some products labeled as dietary supplements contain GBL and claim to build muscles, improve physical performance, enhance sex, reduce stress, and induce sleep. However, GBL-related products have been associated with reports of at least 55 adverse health effects, including seizures, vomiting, slowed breathing, slowed heartbeat rate, and coma. One death had been reported from GBL at the time of the FDA warning. The FDA considers GBL an unapproved drug. After the FDA warning, all but one manufacturer of GBL-related products agreed to recall these drugs and to stop their manufacture and distribution.

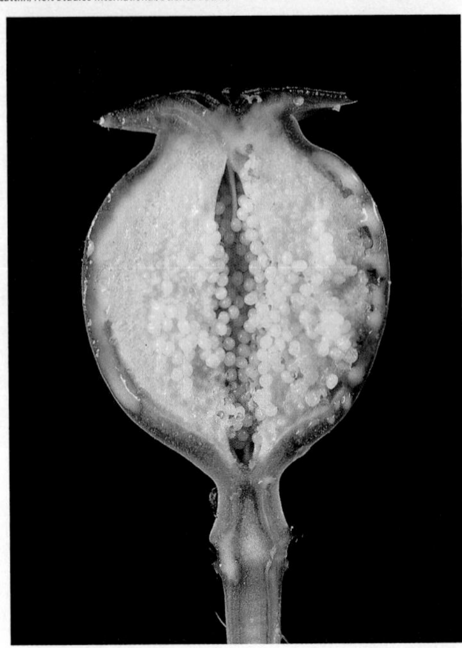

Figure 7.8

Longitudinal Section Through a Seedpod of the Opium Poppy. The dried sap extracted from opium poppy seedpods is used to make the narcotic opium. Some white sap can be seen on the cut edge of this seedpod.

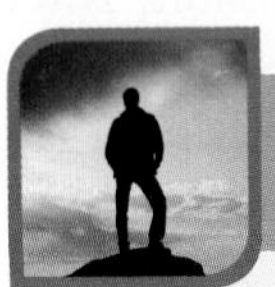

Healthy Living Practices

- Do not accept drinks from casual acquaintances or strangers; they may contain dangerous drugs.
- Do not drive or operate machinery while under the influence of depressant drugs because these substances can impair your thought processes and muscular coordination.
- Do not drink alcohol while taking other depressants. The synergistic effect of combining these compounds can be deadly.

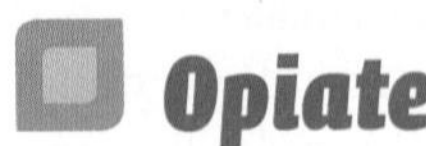

Opiates

Opiates include *opium*, the dried sap extracted from seedpods of opium poppies shown in **Figure 7.8**, and drugs such as codeine, morphine, heroin, and Percodan (aspirin and oxycodone hydrochloride) that are derived from opium. Synthetic opiates include Darvon (propoxyphene) and Demerol (meperidine). These compounds have important medical uses as sedatives, analgesics, and narcotics. **Analgesics** alleviate pain; **narcotics** alter the perception of pain and induce euphoria and sleep. (Many people incorrectly use the term *narcotic* to describe any illegal drug.)

In addition to relieving pain, opiates slow the activity of the intestinal tract, so they are useful in treating severe diarrhea. In addition, physicians frequently prescribe codeine-containing syrups to subdue severe coughing. Despite their medicinal value, opiates are extremely dangerous when taken in an uncontrolled manner. These drugs are highly addictive; people who use opiates daily develop dependence and tolerance within a few weeks.

Using opiates, especially heroin, can cause a variety of serious health problems as well as death. Excessive doses of opiates depress the CNS, slowing respiration and reducing mental functioning. Such overdoses require immediate medical attention. Sharing needles that are used to inject heroin intravenously can cause life-threatening bacterial infections and viral diseases, such as AIDS and hepatitis.

Opium and Heroin

After it enters this country, opium is chemically converted to heroin by drug dealers. They also add various materials, such as quinine or cornstarch, to dilute the drug's concentration. Substances that dilute the concentration of a drug are called *adulterants*. Because heroin abusers lack information concerning the potency of their drug purchases after chemical conversion by drug dealers, they risk taking overdoses or having allergic reactions to the adulterants.

Heroin is one of the most widely abused illegal drugs worldwide;[3] however, survey data indicate that it is not very popular with young people in the United States. Only 0.6% of American high school seniors and 0.1% of college students used heroin in 2012.[2] In the United States overall, only 0.4% of those aged 12 years and older used heroin in 2012 (see **Figure 7.9**).

OxyContin and Vicodin

In 2001, news reports of abuse of the time-released opiate pain reliever OxyContin became common. OxyContin (oxycodone) is a medication prescribed primarily for patients with terminal cancer and other illnesses that cause moderate to severe chronic pain. By 2002, hundreds of people had died from OxyContin abuse, and researchers began collecting data on the use of OxyContin by high school students, college students, and adults. In 2012, the percentages of eighth, tenth, and twelfth graders, college students, and adults aged 19 to 28 years using OxyContin during the year prior to being surveyed (the annual prevalence) were 1.6%, 3.0%, 4.3%, 1.2%, and 2.3%, respectively. The annual prevalence of use of OxyContin increased for all groups through 2009; however, rates steadily declined in all age groups through 2012. The figures show that the highest use among high school seniors since 2010.[2]

OxyContin is a time-release medication with the synthetic opiate oxycodone as its active ingredient.

Persons who abuse this prescription medication chew, crush, or dissolve the pills and then inject, inhale, or take them orally, which delivers the medication all at once rather than slowly over time. The result is a rapid and intense euphoria that does not occur when the drug is taken as prescribed, but such ingestion carries the dangers of opiates mentioned previously. Abusers also take OxyContin with other pills, marijuana, or alcohol, which can result in serious injury or death.

Vicodin (hydrocodone bitartrate and acetaminophen) is also a drug prescribed to reduce pain. Abuse of this drug is more prevalent than abuse of OxyContin. In 2012, the annual prevalence of abuse of Vicodin among eighth, tenth, and twelfth graders, college

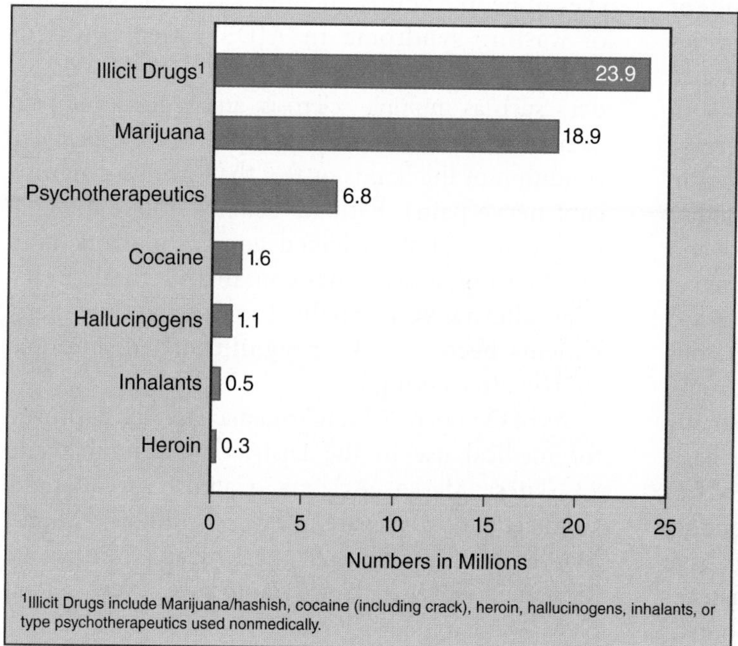

Figure 7.9

Past-Month Illicit Drug Use Among Persons Aged 12 Years and Older: 2012. Marijuana was the most widely used illicit drug in the United States in 2012. Here, the category "psychotherapeutics" includes four prescription-type drug groups: pain relievers, tranquilizers, stimulants, and sedatives.

Reproduced from Substance Abuse and Mental Health Services Administration. (2013). Results from the 2012 National Survey on Drug Use and Health: Summary of National Findings (HHS Publication No. SMA 13-4795). Retrieved from http://www.samhsa.gov/data/NSDUH/2012SummNatFindDetTables/NationalFindings/NSDUHresults2012.pdf

[1]Illicit drugs include marijuana/hashish, cocaine (including crack), heroin, hallucinogens, inhalants, and prescription-type psychotherapeutics used nonmedically.

students, and adults aged 19 to 28 years was 1.3%, 4.4%, 7.5%, 3.8%, and 6.3%, respectively. The annual prevalence of use of Vicodin rose for all groups between 2002 and 2009; however, the prevalence rate for all age groups has steadily declined since 2009. In 2012, the annual prevalence of use was highest for twelfth graders.[2]

Marijuana

Marijuana is the most widely used illicit drug in the United States. An estimated 18.9 million Americans aged 12 years and older were current users of marijuana in 2009 (Figure 7.9).

The marijuana plant (*Cannabis sativa*) contains the psychoactive compound delta-9-tetrahydrocannabinol, or THC. *Hashish* is a dried resin made from marijuana flowers, which contain a higher concentration of THC than the leaves of the plant. Also extracted from marijuana flowers, hashish oil contains a greater percentage of THC than hashish. A few drops of hashish oil added to a cigarette produce psychoactive effects that are the same as smoking a marijuana cigarette, or *joint*.

When people smoke marijuana or hashish, THC enters the brain rapidly. THC alters muscular coordination and normal thought processes such as mental concentration, problem solving, time perception, and short-term memory. Not only are these effects likely to decrease educational achievement, but also they can have serious consequences for drivers. Results of studies on the effects of marijuana on driving abilities reveal that marijuana impairs driving performance in a dose-related manner, just like alcohol does. In addition, recent use of marijuana appears to increase the risk of a driver's being involved in a car crash. Smoking marijuana and drinking alcohol together has significant additive effects on driving ability and sharply increases a driver's risk of a car crash, even at low doses.[13]

Marijuana and hashish smoke contain numerous irritants that can damage the bronchial tubes and lungs. Respiratory symptoms reported consistently by those who smoke these drugs on a regular basis include chronic bronchitis; shortness of breath; frequent coughing, wheezing, and phlegm production; and pneumonia. Long-term marijuana smokers have an increased risk for developing chronic obstructive pulmonary disease (COPD), which is a group of lung diseases that makes it hard to breathe. COPD can range from mild to life threatening. Physical and behavioral dependence occurs in about 7% to 10% of users and is more likely in those who begin using this drug at an early age.[13]

Although many users think that marijuana enhances their sexual responsiveness, results of some studies have found that the drug interferes with reproductive functioning. Men who use marijuana may experience a temporary reduction of their normal testosterone levels. Testosterone is a sex hormone that maintains sex drive and sperm production. This effect decreases the sperm count and increases the proportion of abnormal sperm, qualities that are associated with reduced fertility and an increased probability of fetal abnormalities. Babies born of women who smoked marijuana during their pregnancy face an increased risk of low birthweight and mild developmental abnormalities.[3,13]

Most Americans who smoke marijuana use the drug occasionally, particularly while they are in social settings. Although low-THC cannabis (the form generally available in the United States) rarely produces physical dependence when taken infrequently and in low doses, it can cause psychological dependence. Psychologically addicted persons mentally crave the euphoric effects of THC; experience a heightened sensitivity to and distortion of sight, smell, taste, and sound; have mood changes; and have a slowed reaction time.[3,13]

Among marijuana's medical uses is that it helps control seizures, reduces the fluid pressure in the eyes of people with glaucoma, eases the symptoms of wasting syndrome in AIDS patients, lessens muscle spasms in patients with muscle disorders such as multiple sclerosis, and reduces the pain of migraine headaches and peripheral neuropathy (a condition of the hands or feet that produces significant nerve pain). Patients usually smoke medical marijuana, eat it in baked goods, or drink it in tea. Marinol, a drug that contains synthetic THC, is an alternative to medical marijuana, but many patients become sick or significantly disoriented shortly after taking it.

As of October, 2014, marijuana has been approved for medical use in the District of Columbia and 23 states: Alaska, Arizona, California, Colorado, Connecticut, Delaware, Hawaii, Illinois, Maine, Maryland, Massachusetts, Michigan, Minnesota, Montana, Nevada, New Hampshire, New Jersey, New Mexico, New York, Oregon, Rhode Island, Vermont, and Washington. Laws in these states also remove state-level criminal penalties for cultivation, possession, and use of medical marijuana. Also, as of October, 2014, Florida, Ohio, and Pennsylvania had legislation pending to legalize use of medical marijuana, and Alabama, Iowa, Florida, Kansas, Kentucky, Mississippi, Missouri, North Carolina, Oklahoma, South Dakota, Texas, and West Virginia had legislation pending that was favorable to medical marijuana use but would not legalize it. Furthermore, two states, Washington and Colorado, have legalized nonmedicinal use of marijuana.

In June 2005, the U.S. Supreme Court ruled that federal authorities may prosecute patients whose physicians prescribe marijuana for their medical use, and that state laws do not protect users from the federal ban on the drug. Although against federal law, the sale, purchase, and use of medical marijuana by licensed individuals in accordance with state law was not prosecuted during the Obama administration (see Figure 7.2) until October 2011, when federal prosecutors in California targeted growers and dispensaries they believed were involved in drug trafficking. Many medical societies support legal protection for those using marijuana medically and support research into its usefulness as a medicinal treatment.

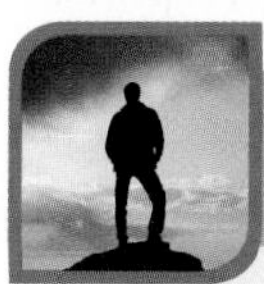

© djgis/ShutterStock

Healthy Living Practices

- Smoking marijuana can impair your thought processes and ability to drive, damage your lungs, reduce your fertility, and lessen your motivation to work. To avoid these serious effects, abstain from using this drug unless prescribed for medical reasons.

Hallucinogens

When taken internally, hallucinogens produce *hallucinations*, abnormal and unreal sensations such as seeing distorted and vividly colored images. Many people report feeling pleasantly detached from their bodies or united with their environment while using hallucinogens. Hallucinogens, however, can produce frightening psychological responses such as anxiety, depression, and the feeling of losing control over your mind. The physical side effects of hallucinogens include elevated blood pressure, dilated pupils, and increased body temperature. Although chronic users of these drugs may develop psychological dependence and tolerance, physical addiction and withdrawal do not occur.

In the United States, the most potent and commonly abused hallucinogens are LSD, mescaline, psilocybin (SIGH-low-SIGH-bin), PCP, and ketamine. These drugs have no approved medical uses, and their recreational use is illegal. Native Americans, however, are permitted to use peyote, a cactus that contains mescaline, in certain religious rites.

LSD

LSD (lysergic acid diethylamide) is a colorless, odorless, flavorless compound that is manufactured in pill, solution, and powder form. It is an extremely potent drug; taking very small amounts produces vivid hallucinations that can last up to 12 hours. While taking LSD, some people have severe psychotic reactions, such as paranoid delusions. Additionally, for weeks or months after taking LSD, some users may have "flashbacks" in which they experience mild hallucinations. Flashbacks usually subside over time and few long-term psychological problems seem to result from hallucinogen use. LSD can stimulate uterine contractions, so pregnant women should avoid it.

During the early 1980s, LSD use by college students declined dramatically, from 6.3% in 1982 to 2.2% in 1985. By 1992, however, LSD use among college students had climbed to 5.7% and peaked in 1995 at 6.9%. Use then steadily declined to 0.7% in 2005, with the exception of a spike in 1999 of 5.4%. After 2005, LSD use among college students began to climb again; in 2012, 1.9% of college students had used LSD in the past year.[2]

Mescaline

A small, round, spineless cactus that grows in Mexico and Texas produces the hallucinogen mescaline, or peyote (**Figure 7.10**). After eating peyote, people have hallucinations that last 1 to 2 hours. These "trips" are milder and easier to control than LSD trips. Because pure mescaline is difficult to produce for illicit sale, most mescaline sold on the streets contains LSD as the psychoactive agent.

Psilocybin

Many mushrooms, including several wild-growing varieties that are found throughout the United States, contain psilocybin. After eating these fungi,

analogs Drugs that are chemically similar but have different effects on the body.

Figure 7.10

Peyote Cactus (*Lophophora williamsii*). This small, round, spineless cactus grows in Mexico and Texas and produces the hallucinogen mescaline, or peyote.

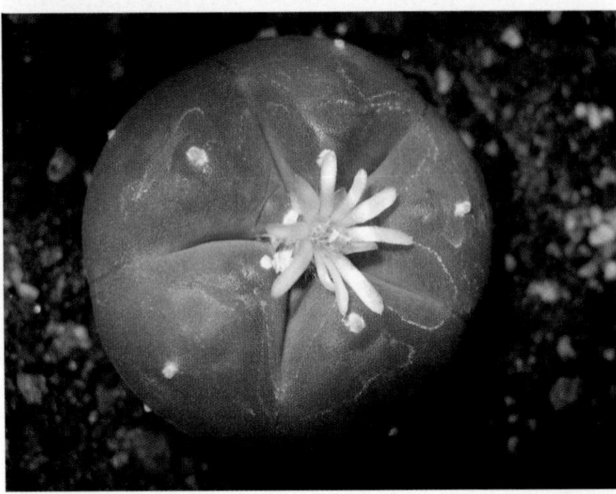

sometimes called *magic mushrooms*, people experience elevated blood pressure, body temperature, and pulse rate. Psilocybin produces euphoria and hallucinations, but these psychoactive effects are not as intense or long lasting as those produced by LSD. Unpleasant responses to psilocybin ingestion include wide mood swings and uncontrollable movements of arms and legs. Although fatal overdoses from psilocybin have not been reported, users may die if they eat other wild mushrooms that are poisonous.

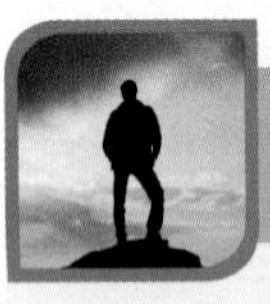

Healthy Living Practices

- Do not eat wild mushrooms. Some are poisonous and can cause death.

PCP

PCP (commonly called *angel dust* or *rocket fuel*) is difficult to classify because the drug produces hallucinogenic, depressant, stimulant, or anesthetic effects depending on the dose in which it is taken. Within a few minutes after taking PCP, users begin to experience its psychoactive effects, which can last up to 6 hours.

Unlike other hallucinogenic drugs, high doses of PCP can cause severe toxic reactions. Taking 1 mg to 5 mg of PCP produces confusion and loss of muscular coordination; users also feel warm, sweaty, relaxed, and euphoric. As the level of intake increases to about 10 mg, users become confused, paranoid, and agitated; they act drunk, have hallucinations, and report numbness in their arms and legs. Taking 10 mg to 25 mg produces the signs and symptoms of PCP toxicity, including trancelike or psychotic behavior. Doses that exceed 25 mg to 50 mg can produce fever, convulsions, coma, elevated blood pressure, and death. People who survive the acute toxic effects of PCP often feel depressed and anxious. In addition, they may show signs of brain damage such as confusion and disorientation that can take weeks to disappear.

Ketamine

In the 1960s, drug researchers developed ketamine, a PCP analog that has fewer troublesome side effects than PCP. An **analog** is chemically similar to another drug and may or may not produce similar responses. Today, legally manufactured PCP analogs such as Ketalar (ketamine hydrochloride) have limited human and veterinary medical use as anesthetics.

Teens and young adults most commonly abuse ketamine by snorting the drug for its dreamlike or hallucinatory effects. In addition, the drug can be swallowed, smoked, drunk, or injected intramuscularly. Ketamine injection is highly risky because multiple injections typically occur during a single "session" in large groups, and the drug is drawn from shared bottles of liquid ketamine. These behaviors put ketamine injectors at risk of infectious diseases such as hepatitis C and HIV. At high doses, ketamine can cause delirium, amnesia, impaired motor function, high blood pressure, and potentially fatal respiratory problems. These effects are magnified when the drug is taken with sedatives or depressants, such as alcohol, which is a common practice.

Inhalants

Inhalants are gases (fumes) that are breathed in and produce euphoria, dizziness, confusion, and drowsiness. Most inhalants are taken to induce mood changes, but nitrites are used as a sexual enhancer

Table 7.4

Types of Toxic Inhalants and Common Examples

Types of Toxic Inhalants	What Are They?	Examples
Volatile solvents	Liquids that form gases at room temperature	Paint thinner, paint remover, dry-cleaning fluid, gasoline, glues, felt-tip marker fluids
Aerosols	Sprays that contain propellants and solvents	Spray paint, spray deodorant, hairspray, fabric protector sprays
Gases	Medical anesthetics and other gases used in everyday products	Examples of toxic gases: ether, chloroform, nitrous oxide (laughing gas) Examples of products containing toxic gases: whipped cream dispensers, butane lighters, propane tanks, refrigerants
Nitrites	Chemicals that dilate blood vessels and relax muscles	Known as "poppers" or "snappers"; sold in small bottles labeled as video head cleaner, room odorizer, leather cleaner, or liquid aroma

Data from the National Institute on Drug Abuse.

because they dilate (widen) blood vessels. **Table 7.4** lists the types of inhalants.

Inhalants are taken into the body in a variety of ways. Fumes can be sniffed from a container, or aerosols can be sprayed directly into the nose or mouth. Alternatively, fumes or sprays can be sniffed directly or inhaled from a bag, a practice called "bagging." Another approach is "huffing," in which a rag is soaked with the inhalant and the rag is pressed to the mouth and nose. Nitrous oxide can be inhaled from balloons filled with the gas or from poppers, small bottles of the gas (see Table 7.4).

Inhalants irritate the mucous membranes lining the eyes, mouth, nose, throat, and lungs. Inhalant abusers often develop watery, reddened eyes and a persistent cough. Some users experience double vision, nausea, vomiting, fainting, and a ringing sensation in their ears. Many teenagers are unaware of the serious health effects of inhalant use: brain damage, irregular heartbeat, anemia, liver damage, kidney failure, coma, or death.

Inhalant use begins at young ages—sometimes in the fifth grade—and its use drops as students grow older. Inhalants are the second most widely used class of illicit drugs for eighth graders (after marijuana). In 2012, the annual prevalence for inhalant use for eighth graders was 7.0%; for tenth graders, 4.5%; and for twelfth graders, 3.2%. Lowest use was by college students and young adults at 0.9% and 0.8%, respectively.[2] Inhalant use has gradually decreased in all age groups since 2008.

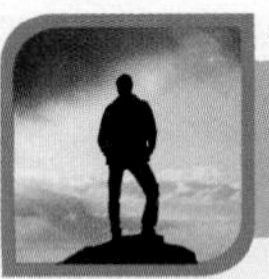

Healthy Living Practices

- Use household products that release toxic fumes, such as paints, glues, and lighter fluids, in well-ventilated areas to avoid inhaling these chemicals.

Designer Drugs: Drugs with Mixed Effects

People who have some knowledge of chemistry can alter the chemical structure of a controlled substance to make a new compound that is not classified as a controlled drug. The new compound, called a *designer drug*, usually produces psychoactive responses similar to the drug from which it was produced. Designer drugs are relatively easy and inexpensive to produce. Thus, people who make these drug analogs can reap considerable profits from selling them.

After officials with the DEA determine that a designer drug has the potential to be abused, they can classify the compound as a controlled substance. However, underground chemists often avoid prosecution by continuing to modify the substance, producing new generations of the drug that the DEA does not control. **Table 7.5** lists some of the best-known designer drugs, their psychoactive effects, and potential health risks.

Designer drugs are often more toxic than the compounds from which they are derived. China white, for example, is 1,000 times more potent than its parent drug, fentanyl, a powerful synthetic opioid often used for general anesthesia or in the treatment of chronic pain. In 2008, the Centers for Disease Control and Prevention (CDC) reported that illicitly manufactured fentanyl and its analogs were

Table 7.5

Popular Designer Drugs

Designer Drug	Original Drugs	Psychoactive Effects	Possible Health Risks
MPPP MPTP	Meperidine (Demerol)	Heroin-like euphoria (depressant)	Parkinsonian syndrome: drooling, uncontrollable skeletal muscle movements, muscle rigidity (permanent)
China white	Fentanyl (Sublimaze)	Euphoria, respiratory depression	Death from respiratory failure
Ecstasy, XTC, Adam, M & M, MDMA	Mescaline–methamphetamine	Euphoria, CNS stimulant, hallucinations	Panic, anxiety, paranoia, increased and irregular heart rate, fever, hypertension, brain damage, seizures, death
Love drug (MDA)	Mescaline–methamphetamine	Euphoria, talkativeness, increased need to make friends	Fever, rapid heart rate, hypertension, seizures, death

responsible for more than 1,000 deaths in the United States from April 2005 to March 2007 alone.[14] This was the most recent report from the CDC on fentanyl deaths as of March 2011.

Ecstasy

The illegal designer drug *ecstasy*, or *MDMA* (3,4-methylenedioxymethamphetamine), became a controlled substance in 1985. Chemically similar to mescaline and methamphetamine, ecstasy produces both hallucinogenic and stimulant effects. Ecstasy users report that the drug improves their self-esteem and increases their desire to have intimate contacts with other people. However, users may experience panic and anxiety, hallucinations, tremors, rapid heart rate, loss of coordination, and psychotic behavior. Some users report more serious side effects such as irregular heartbeat, hypertension, fever, memory loss, and seizures. Since the 1980s, several people have died after taking this drug.

The use of ecstasy by high school students, college students, and young adults rose sharply between 1999 and 2001. Use declined since then in all three groups. In 2012, annual prevalence rates for eighth, tenth, and twelfth graders were 1.1%, 3.0%, and 3.8%, respectively. For college students and for young adults aged 19 to 28 years and not in college, the prevalence rates were 5.8% and 4.1%, respectively.[2] These data indicate a decrease in ecstasy use among high school students since 2009; however, use among college students and young adults has increased gradually since 2007.

K2

K2 is a drug that is made in the laboratory and works in the brain much like the THC of marijuana. It is sprayed on herbal and spice plant products and smoked. First synthesized and used recreationally in the mid-1990s, K2 became popular again in 2006. Although nicknamed "fake weed," this drug is not marijuana and is much more potent and dangerous than marijuana. Some of K2's side effects are severe potentially life-threatening hallucinations, dangerously elevated blood pressure and heart rate, pale skin, vomiting, and seizures.

Bath Salts

Despite its name, this stimulant designer drug has nothing to do with the bath salts you put in your soaking tub. The name is only a disguise for a cocaine-like, life-threatening drug that raises the blood pressure and heart rate, increases the risk of heart attack and stroke, and can cause hallucinations, delusions, and paranoia—possibly long term. Marketed under names like Zoom 2, Vanilla Sky, and Ocean Wave (**Figure 7.11**), reports of this drug began in 2010, and by 2011 legislation was under way to make "bath salts" a controlled substance. Data on bath salt use was first collected in the 2012 version of the Monitoring the Future survey. In 2012, bath salt use rates for eight, tenth, twelth graders, college students, and young adults were 0.8%, 0.6%, 1.3%, 0.2%, and 0.8%, respectively.[2]

Figure 7.11

"Bath Salts" Can Be Deadly. They are not for the bathtub but contain synthetic stimulants that can kill.

Courtesy of DEA.

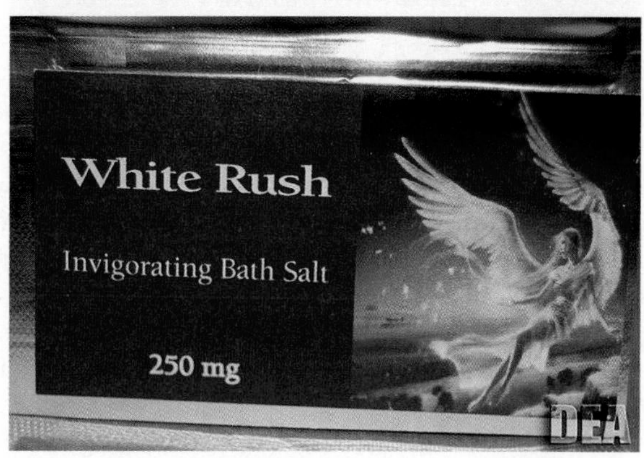

Over-the-Counter Drugs

The FDA regulates the production and marketing of prescription and nonprescription medications in the United States. To be sold in this country, an OTC medicine must be effective and safe when people follow the product information that comes with it (in packages or on labels). Although the FDA does not evaluate the safety or effectiveness of every OTC product that is marketed, the agency requires that active ingredients in products be evaluated for safety and usefulness. *Active* ingredients have an effect on the body; *inert* ingredients do not affect the body. Products that contain unsafe or ineffective ingredients or that have dishonest labeling cannot be sold. Herbal products that are sold as food supplements in health food stores are not regulated by the FDA. Some of these products contain substances that produce druglike effects and are toxic (see the Consumer Health box in this chapter).

Consumer Health

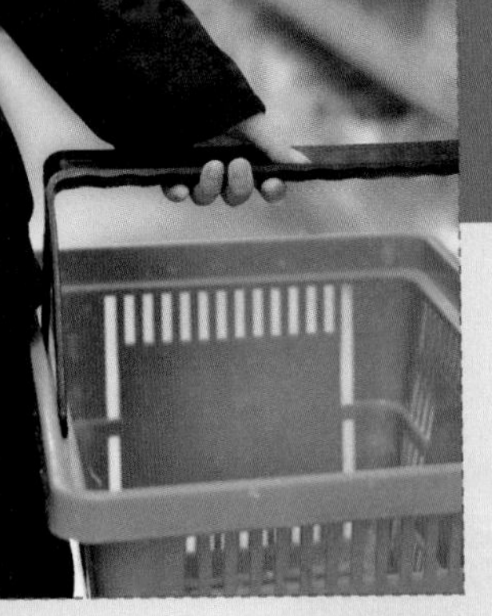

© sevenke/ShutterStock

Over-the-Counter Medicines: Safety and the FDA

To protect consumers, the Food and Drug Administration (FDA) regulates the testing, production, marketing, and labeling of medical devices and medications; the safety of foods and truthfulness of information on their labels; and the safety of cosmetics. A medical device or OTC medicine that is sold in the United States must be effective for its intended use and safe when its instructions are followed.

The FDA also requires that the active ingredients in OTC products be evaluated for safety and usefulness. Active ingredients have an impact on the body; inert ingredients do not affect the body. The FDA allows manufacturers of OTC products to use ingredients that are generally recognized as safe (GRAS), generally recognized as effective (GRAE), and generally recognized as honestly labeled (GRAHL). The FDA employs investigators who review information that appears on the labels of OTC products. Products that contain unsafe or ineffective ingredients, or that have labels displaying dishonest information, cannot be sold.

In 1998, the FDA proposed an easy-to-read and easy-to-understand labeling format for OTC drugs. Figure 7.B shows the information that must appear on the labels of an OTC medicinal product. Note that the label clearly displays warnings concerning the safe use of the product. Always follow instructions on the package or label concerning the use of any OTC medication.

Individuals, physicians, and staff of healthcare facilities can report cases of harm that result from using medicinal and nutritional products. If you have any problem with a medication, medical device, or dietary supplement, report the problem to the FDA's MedWatch hotline by calling 1-800-332-1088 or go to www.fda.gov/MedWatch/report.htm.

Data from Food and Drug Administration.

Figure 7.B

Certain information must appear on the labels of an OTC medicinal product. (a) Front of label, and (b) back of label.

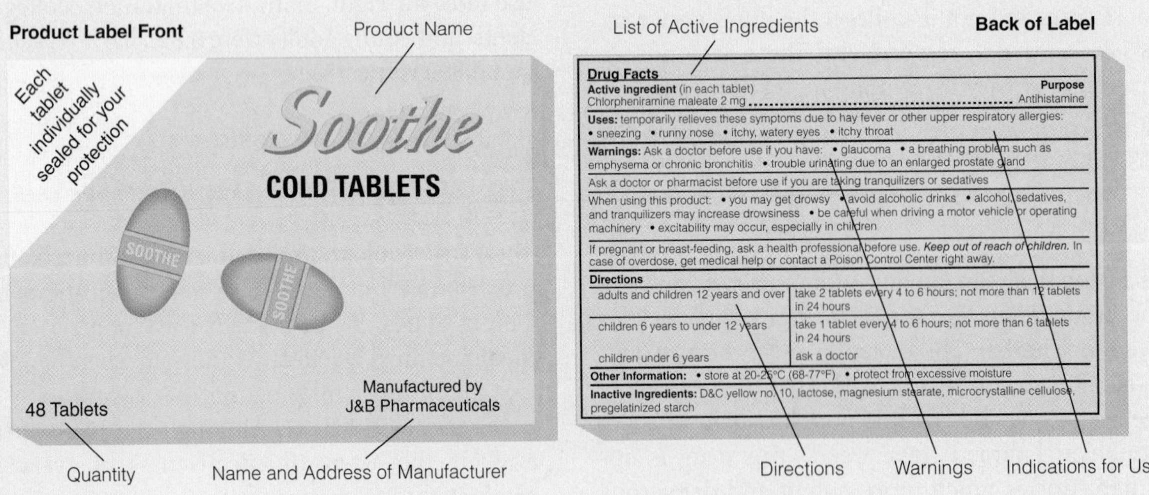

Individuals, physicians, and staff of healthcare facilities can report cases of harm that result from using medicinal and nutritional products. If you have any problem with a medication, medical device, or dietary supplement, report the problem to the FDA's MedWatch hotline by calling 1-800-332-1088 or go to www.fda.gov/MedWatch/report.htm.

Misuse and abuse of OTC medicines are common. As mentioned in the beginning of this chapter, the improper use of these medications can be harmful. Furthermore, some OTC products contain substances that can produce serious psychoactive effects, especially when they are taken in large doses.

An example of the potential dangers of abusing OTC medications is the tragic death of a 17-year-old track star in June 2007 from an overdose of methyl salicylate. This chemical compound is an active ingredient in a popular sports muscle pain cream and other OTC medications. The young woman used the sports cream liberally on her legs between runs while also using two other OTC medications containing methyl salicylate. This drug is an anticlotting agent, and at high doses it can cause internal bleeding, changes in heart rhythm, and liver damage. The death of the young woman emphasizes the need to use even seemingly harmless OTC medications according to directions and in moderation, and to remember that taking more than one medication simultaneously—even OTC preparations—may be risky.

Look-Alike Drugs

The active ingredient in "stay-awake" pills is the stimulant caffeine. Some manufacturers produce caffeine-containing capsules or pills that look like prescription amphetamines or related prescribed stimulants. The production and sale of these look-alike drugs are difficult to regulate because they contain caffeine, an allowed substance. Frequently, people who sell street drugs misrepresent look-alike stimulants as amphetamines to unsuspecting users.

Weight Loss Aids

Nearly anyone who has tried to lose weight knows that it is frustrating and that hunger seems to be constant. Many overweight people have taken various pills, powders, beverages, and foods for years to promote weight loss and prevent hunger.

Ephedrine/Ephedra

Ephedrine and pseudoephedrine are found in various OTC preparations such as weight loss aids and cold remedies, and they act as a stimulant, appetite suppressant, concentration aid, and decongestant. Because ephedrine and pseudoephedrine act as mild stimulants, some individuals misuse medicines that contain these compounds to pep themselves up. However, ephedrine-containing drugs can produce high blood pressure, sleeplessness, irregular and rapid heart rate, and restlessness; taking high doses of either substance may evoke psychotic symptoms.

Ephedra, known in Chinese as ma huang, is a plant extract that is the source of ephedrine and pseudoephedrine. Many laws control the sale of ephedrine-, pseudoephedrine-, and ephedra-containing products. For example, in 2004 FDA officials banned the sale of ephedra-containing dietary supplements because of their dangerous side effects. The ban targeted supplements that had been advertised for weight loss, muscle building, and athletic performance. In 2003, ephedra was implicated in the death of 23-year-old Steve Bechler, a prospective pitcher for the Baltimore Orioles.

In addition to ephedra, numerous other herbs or plant extracts—such as lobelia, comfrey, yohimbine, *Ginkgo biloba*, or sassafras—contain substances that can produce harmful side effects when ingested as supplements or teas (**Figure 7.12**).

Figure 7.12

Hazardous Herbs. Numerous plants can be toxic. For example, when taken internally, comfrey (shown here) can cause hepatic veno-occlusive disease (VOD), in which some of the small veins of the liver are blocked. VOD can lead to liver failure and death.

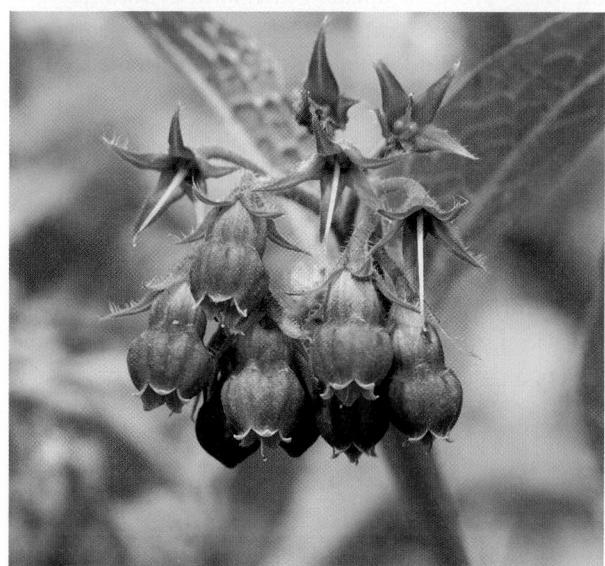

Drug Treatment and Prevention

Treating Drug Dependency

The goal of drug treatment is to stop the drug abuse and reduce the likelihood that abusers will return to their previous drug use behaviors. Currently, three major forms of long-term drug abuse treatment exist:

methadone maintenance, outpatient drug-free programs, and residential therapeutic communities.

Methadone maintenance is used to treat addiction to opiates; methadone reduces the cravings for these drugs. This controversial treatment is often used after other attempts at treatment have failed. Methadone is taken orally, diluted in juice. When taken this way, the drug prevents opiate withdrawal symptoms and reduces cravings, but it does not produce euphoria or cloud the mind. In addition, it blocks the effects of heroin and other opiates, which reduces the desire of addicts to continue taking these drugs. Thus, methadone treatment helps people stop taking opiates while at the same time allowing them to go to work, go to school, and take care of themselves and their family. Some drug rehabilitation programs prescribe methadone during opiate detoxification and then taper off methadone use. However, other programs allow people to stay on methadone as long as they feel it is necessary.

Most abusers prefer *outpatient drug-free programs* that provide medical care and a wide variety of counseling and psychotherapy approaches while patients continue to live with their families and work in their communities. These programs do not include use of methadone.

Self-help groups are a popular and useful adjunct to professional outpatient drug treatment. Individuals recovering from drug dependency attend regular meetings to receive encouragement and social support from other former substance abusers. Alcoholics Anonymous (AA) is one of the oldest, most effective self-help programs. Many other community-based self-help programs that treat drug abuse, such as Narcotics Anonymous, are modeled after AA.

In severe cases, drug abusers may undergo detoxification and then live for several months in controlled environments called *residential therapeutic communities* or *group homes*. Living in these communities reduces the likelihood that patients will be exposed to drugs while they resocialize, or readjust to general society.

While in group homes, patients also receive medical care, social services, and psychological counseling. After they leave residential therapeutic communities, individuals usually attend community- or hospital-based counseling sessions to prevent *relapse*, the return to drug abuse. For people who lack health insurance, the high cost of medical care is a major barrier to obtaining treatment in a therapeutic community.

Most drug treatment programs that last fewer than 3 months have limited long-term effectiveness.[15] According to the Partnership for a Drug-Free America, results of studies show that length of time in drug treatment is the best single predictor of positive posttreatment outcomes. Many drug-dependent people need more than 3 months of outpatient care or living in controlled environments to change their substance-related behaviors and attitudes. Additionally, recovering addicts often need to acquire job skills while they are in therapy to improve their chances of becoming drug-free, productive members of society.

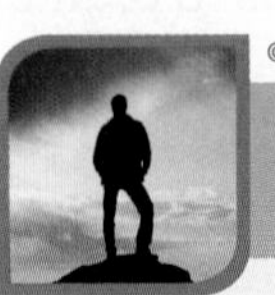

© djgis/ShutterStock

Healthy Living Practices

- Ask your physician about the need to use over-the-counter medications. If it is necessary for you to take these drugs, follow the labels' instructions concerning their safe use. Your pharmacist is also a source of reliable information concerning the safe use of OTC drugs.
- Obtain reliable information concerning the safety and effectiveness of herbal products before you take them.

A considerable number of patients finish treatment but relapse within a few weeks or months of abstinence. Former addicts are more likely to relapse if they have severe mental illness or polyabuse, and if they return to communities where illicit drugs are available and are widely used. Recovering drug addicts are more likely to abstain from using drugs if they are married or in stable relationships, supported by their families, and employed. In 2009, 2.6 million Americans received treatment for their drug use, including alcohol use.[1]

Antidrug Vaccines

Many drug treatment programs use medications to help individuals break their addictions. These medications help by suppressing drug withdrawal symptoms, reducing drug cravings, and helping reestablish proper brain function. One new type of drug that is being developed to help in drug treatment is the antidrug vaccine.

An antidrug vaccine works by stimulating the immune system to develop antibodies against a particular drug, such as an anticocaine vaccine or an antimorphine vaccine. These antibodies attach to the drug in the bloodstream, making the molecules of the drug too large to pass through the membranous blood–brain barrier. If the drug does not reach the brain, the vaccinated person will not feel the effects of the drug because the pleasure centers of the brain would not be stimulated. With no "reward" for taking the drug, the addicted person soon loses the craving sensations that are a part of drug addiction.

One problem is that drug vaccines do not always elicit a robust antibody response in an individual. If the antibody response is weak, only some of the drug would be bound by the vaccine and some would remain free and able to pass to the brain. In this situation, if the drug addict took a high-enough dose of the drug, he or she could likely attain their usual "high." Researchers are working to resolve problems such as this and also note that counseling and behavior therapy in conjunction with vaccines would likely produce the best results.[16]

Preventing Drug Misuse and Abuse

The U.S. government devotes much of its drug prevention efforts to reducing the supply of illicit drugs. These efforts include destroying crops such as marijuana and coca plants; stopping the flow of illegal substances through U.S. borders; and prosecuting individuals who manufacture, sell, and purchase drugs illegally. Such measures, however, are not effectively reducing the demand for illicit drugs in this country. Many people think that social and economic programs to reduce poverty and unemployment would decrease the demand for illicit drugs. Educational programs that promote drug-free lifestyles, especially among children and young adults, may help reduce the prevalence of drug abuse.

The National Institute on Drug Abuse conducted research for 25 years to determine which drug prevention programs have the highest degree of long-term effectiveness. They found that successful prevention programs:

- Enhance protective factors and reverse or reduce known risk factors
- Use interactive methods such as peer discussion groups
- Target all forms of drug use
- Teach skills to resist drugs when offered
- Strengthen personal commitments against drug use
- Increase social skills and assertiveness
- Reinforce attitudes against drug use

Additionally, drug education programs that involve parents, media, and the community are more successful than programs that limit educational activities to classrooms.[17]

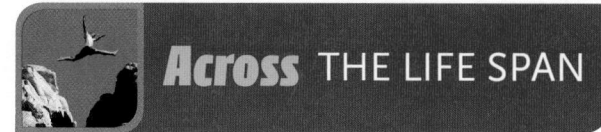

© Galina Barskaya/ShutterStock

DRUG USE AND ABUSE

Pregnant drug users are at risk for miscarriage, *ectopic* ("tubal") pregnancy, and stillbirth (giving birth to a dead infant). Babies born to women who used cocaine, opiates, amphetamines, or marijuana regularly during pregnancy are more likely to be premature (born too soon) and smaller than infants who were not exposed to these drugs before birth. Compared to other infants, premature, underweight, and prenatally drug-exposed newborns are more likely to have serious health problems early in life. Drug-exposed newborns also tend to have smaller than normal head circumferences, a sign that brain growth has been negatively affected. Pregnant women should consult their physicians before taking any drug.

Adolescents who have certain risk factors are more likely to use alcohol and other drugs than adolescents without these characteristics. **Table 7.6** lists risk factors and protective factors in drug use prevention.

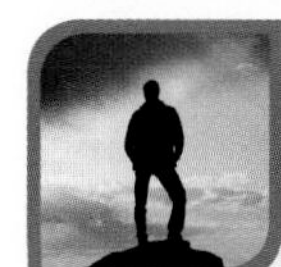

© djgis/ShutterStock

Healthy Living Practices

- [ ] If you or someone you know is abusing drugs, obtain help from local substance abuse programs or from your healthcare practitioner.

Despite living in situations that promote substance use and abuse, many young people abstain from taking psychoactive drugs. Teenagers who stay in high school, attend classes regularly, make good grades, and get along well with their parents generally avoid using drugs. These children have personality traits that are collectively referred to as resilience. Resilient children accept responsibility, adapt to change, manage stress, solve problems, and are achievement and success oriented. Resilient young people have the ability to remain psychologically, socially, and

Table 7.6
Risk and Protective Factors for Drug Abuse Among Youth

Protective Factors
Strong and positive family bonds
Parental monitoring of children's activities and peers
Clear rules of conduct that are consistently enforced within the family
Involvement of parents in the lives of their children
Success in school performance
Strong bonds with institutions, such as school and religious organizations
Adoption of conventional norms about drug use
Risk Factors
Chaotic home environments, particularly in which parents abuse substances or suffer from mental illnesses
Ineffective parenting, especially with children with difficult temperaments or conduct disorders
Lack of parent–child attachments and nurturing
Inappropriately shy or aggressive behavior in the classroom
Failure in school performance
Poor social coping skills
Affiliations with peers displaying deviant behaviors
Perceptions of approval of drug-using behaviors in family, work, school, peer, and community environments

Reproduced from National Institute on Drug Abuse. (2002, February). Risk and protective factors in drug abuse prevention. *NIDA Notes*, 16(6). Retrieved on March 21, 2011, from http://archives.drugabuse.gov/nida_notes/nnvol16n6/Risk.html

spiritually healthy even if their families are dysfunctional or not supportive.

The abuse of illicit drugs is not a widespread problem among older adults in the United States. However, many older adults take a variety of prescribed medications to treat problems such as insomnia, depression, hypertension, and heart disease. These aged individuals have a higher risk of becoming intoxicated from taking medications because their bodies do not detoxify and eliminate the substances as effectively as younger people do. More research is needed to determine medication levels that are safe and effective for elderly individuals.

The risk of serious drug interactions and drug synergism is high among aged people who take more than one prescribed drug. In many instances, elderly persons appear to have suffered a stroke, developed Alzheimer's disease, or become severely depressed when actually their confusion and weakness are the side effects of taking numerous prescribed medicines in bad combinations or the wrong amounts or schedules.

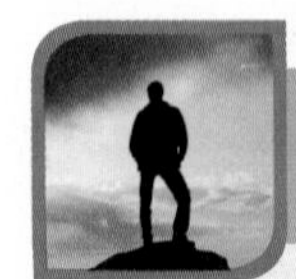
© djgis/ShutterStock

Healthy Living Practices

- Do not use drugs of any kind during pregnancy without the approval of your physician.

Table 7.7

Summary of Psychoactive Drugs: Effects on the Body

Drug Category	Trade or Other Names	Physical Dependence	Psychological Dependence	Tolerance	Possible Side Effects	Overdose Effects	Withdrawal Effects
Stimulants	Caffeine, cocaine (snow, big c), methamphetamine, crystal meth (crystals), Preludin, Ritalin, Dexadrine or "dex," black beauties, black hollies	Possible	High	Yes	Alertness, euphoria, increased pulse rate and blood pressure, sleeplessness, lack of appetite	Fever, hallucinations, convulsions, death	Prolonged sleep, irritability, depression, anxiety, moodiness, headaches
Depressants	Alcohol,* barbiturates (goofballs), Valium, Halcion, Quaalude, GHB, GBL, "roofies" (Rohypnol)	Varies	Varies	Yes	Slurred speech, drunken behavior	Depressed breathing, dilated pupils, coma, death	Depression, anxiety, sleeplessness, convulsions, death
Opiates	Heroin (China white), morphine, codeinecontaining products, methadone, Demerol, Oxy-Contin, Vicodin, Darvon, Percodan	Moderate to high	Moderate to high	Yes	Euphoria, sleepiness, depressed breathing, nausea	Slowed breathing, convulsions, coma, death	Teary eyes, watery nose, yawning, tremors, anxiety, abdominal cramps
Marijuana (cannabis)	Pot, hash, hashish oil, Acapulco gold, blunts, buds, Colombo, weed	Unknown	Moderate	Possible	Euphoria, relaxation, increased appetite, distorted time perception	Anxiety, paranoia	Anxiety, depression
Hallucinogens	LSD blotters, mescaline, STP, psilocybin, high doses of PCP, peyote, psychedelic mushrooms, ketamine	None (LSD and mescaline) Others: unknown	Unknown	Yes	Euphoria, hallucinations, poor time perception	Anxiety, psychotic behavior	None reported
Inhalants	Gasoline, paint thinners and removers, freon, aerosols, butyl nitrate	None	Possible	No	Euphoria, sleepiness, confusion, slurred speech	Brain, kidney, or liver damage; headaches; death	Anxiety
Drugs with mixed effects	Nicotine,* PCP, MDMA (Ecstasy)	Unknown	High (PCP) Unknown (MDMA)	Yes	Hallucinations and altered perceptions (PCP)	Psychosis, possible death (PCP)	Unknown

*See Chapter 8.

Data from *Drugs of abuse*. (2005). Washington, DC: U.S. Department of Justice, Drug Enforcement Administration; Goldberg, R. (2009). *Drugs across the spectrum*. Belmont, CA: Brooks/Cole; and Hanson, G. R., et al. (2011). *Drugs and society*. Burlington, MA: Jones & Bartlett Learning.

Analyzing Health-Related Information

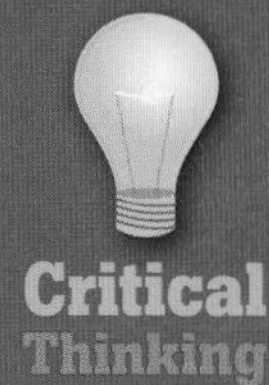

Critical Thinking

© tele52/ShutterStock

The following ad promotes a book that describes how to eliminate addictive urges. Read the advertisement and evaluate it using the model for analyzing health-related information. The main points of the model are noted here.

1. Which statements are verifiable facts, and which are unverified statements or value claims?
2. What are the credentials of the person who makes health-related claims? Does this person have the appropriate background and education in the topic area? What can you do to check the person's credentials?
3. What might be the motives and biases of the person making the claims?
4. What is the main point of the ad? Which information is relevant to the issue, main point, product, or service? Which information is irrelevant?
5. Is the source reliable? What evidence supports your conclusion that the source is reliable or unreliable? Does the source of information present the pros and cons of the topic or the benefits and risks of the product?
6. Does the source of information attack the credibility of conventional scientists or medical authorities?

Based on your analysis, do you think that this ad and the book are reliable sources of health-related information? Explain why you would or would not buy the book. Summarize your reasons for coming to this conclusion.

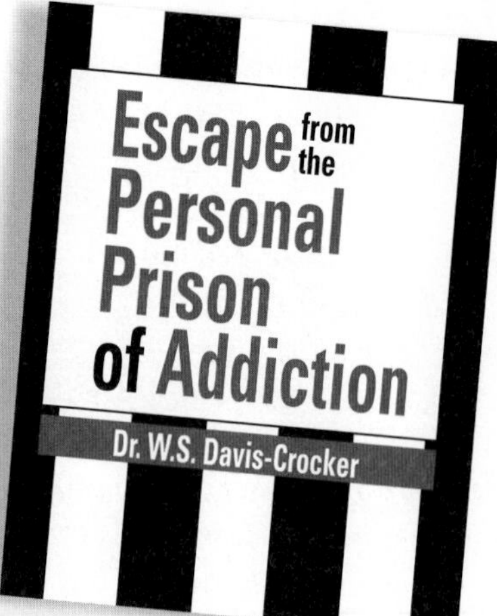

Escape from the Personal Prison of Addiction

Dr. W. S. Davis-Crocker

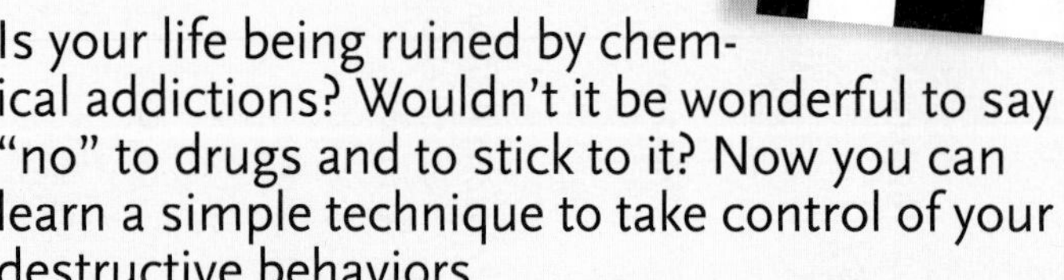

Is your life being ruined by chemical addictions? Wouldn't it be wonderful to say "no" to drugs and to stick to it? Now you can learn a simple technique to take control of your destructive behaviors.

After years of scientific research, Dr. W. S. Davis-Crocker has unlocked the neurobiochemical secrets of addiction. In her newest book, *Escape from the Personal Prison of Addiction*, Dr. Davis-Crocker, world-renowned author and founder of the Davis-Crocker Institute for the Study of Habituation, describes how to rid yourself of addictions painlessly.

Finally, there is hope for addicts. In just three days of practicing the advice in her book, your cravings for alcohol, cigarettes, heroin, and even chocolate will vanish! There is no need for you to use special medications or costly psychotherapy.

To order your copy of *Escape from the Personal Prison of Addiction*, call [illegible]. All major credit cards accepted.

Also register to attend Dr. Davis-Crocker's next seminar in your area. Enrollment is limited, so call the toll-free number now to reserve your seat, and we'll send you our informative pamphlet *Why Me?* at no charge.

CHAPTER REVIEW

© SergeBertasiusPhotography/ShutterStock

Summary

Drugs are nonfood chemicals that alter the way a person thinks, feels, functions, or behaves. Many drugs have beneficial uses as medicines, but these substances can have serious negative effects on the health and well-being of people who use them improperly. People often abuse psychoactive, or mood-altering, drugs. Drug abuse contributes to numerous social problems that plague our society, such as crime, unemployment, and family violence and dissolution.

By interacting with nerve cells in the brain, psychoactive drugs influence perceptions, thought processes, feelings, and behaviors. Additionally, environmental factors can affect how people act and feel while under the influence of psychoactive drugs.

In most instances, the liver converts drugs into less dangerous compounds that can be eliminated in urine, feces, or exhaled breath. When the body is unable to detoxify and eliminate excessive amounts of a drug rapidly, the characteristic signs and symptoms of intoxication occur. Drug overdoses and polyabuse may produce serious, even deadly, effects.

In 2009, an estimated 21.8 million Americans older than 12 years of age were current illicit drug users. Rates of illicit drug use are especially high among teenagers and young adults. Initially, these individuals typically use alcohol, nicotine, or inhalants; they then may move on to marijuana. Some persons experiment with or use other illicit drugs after marijuana. In general, illicit drug use declines after age 20 years.

Dependency and addiction describe any habitual behavior that interferes with a person's health, work, and relationships. Drug dependence or addiction occurs when users develop a pattern of taking drugs that usually produces a compulsive need to use these substances, a tolerance for them, and withdrawal when they are discontinued. The type of substance taken, the social environment of the person, his or her personality, and genetics influence an individual's chances of developing a drug dependency.

Depressants such as alcohol and barbiturates slow the activity of the cerebral cortex, producing sedative and hypnotic effects as well as drowsiness. Thus, people should not drive or operate machinery while under the influence of depressants. Misusing depressants can be deadly.

Stimulants enhance chemical activity in parts of the brain that influence emotions, sleep, attention, and learning. Caffeine is the most commonly consumed legal stimulant in this country. Stimulants such as Ritalin and cocaine have few medical uses. Cocaine is addictive and frequently abused. Methamphetamine use in U.S. college students has declined since 1999, from 3.3% in that year to 0.3% in 2009.

Opiates have important medical uses as sedatives, analgesics, and narcotics. When misused, opiates are highly addictive and extremely dangerous.

Marijuana, which contains THC as its major psychoactive compound, is the most widely used illicit drug in the United States. Although marijuana does not produce physiologic dependence, some people become compulsive users. Marijuana smoke contains numerous irritants that can damage the bronchial tubes and lungs.

Hallucinogens alter the brain's ability to perceive sensory information, producing abnormal and unreal sensations. In the United States, the most potent and commonly abused hallucinogens are mescaline, psilocybin, LSD, ketamine, and PCP. High doses of PCP and ketamine can be deadly.

Many common household products release toxic fumes that can produce psychoactive effects when inhaled. Teenagers may use inhalants before they move on to other psychoactive drugs. Inhalants can depress respiration, resulting in coma or death.

Designer drugs are made by altering the chemical structures of controlled substances. In some cases, these drug analogs are more toxic than the compounds from which they were derived.

The FDA regulates the production and marketing of all medications in the United States. Some health food and OTC products contain substances that are harmful or that produce psychoactive effects, especially when they are misused or abused.

The primary goal of drug treatment is to help abusers become drug-free. Drug treatment usually involves participation in outpatient treatment programs and self-help groups. Drug prevention programs that target school-age children typically provide information about drugs and teach drug resistance and refusal skills.

CHAPTER REVIEW

Drug use during pregnancy increases the risk of miscarriage, ectopic pregnancy, and stillbirth. Women who use cocaine, opiates, amphetamines, and marijuana regularly during pregnancy are more likely to give birth to premature and smaller infants than pregnant women who do not use these drugs. The extent to which prenatal drug exposure influences the long-term mental and physical development of children is unclear.

Adolescents who are more likely to use drugs are those who have parents and friends who abuse drugs, are failing in school, have poor social coping skills, and have a lack of parent–child attachment.

Although drug abuse is rare among older adults, these individuals may experience harmful effects from taking prescribed medicines because they do not detoxify and eliminate drugs as effectively as younger individuals do or because they misuse or become confused by multiple prescriptions.

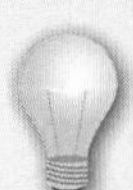

Applying What You Have Learned

1. Why do some people abuse certain drugs, such as cocaine, and not others, such as aspirin? **Application**
2. Think of a time you have misused a drug (i.e. use a drug for a reason other than its intended use). Describe your misuse of the drug and reflect on why you engaged in this behavior. **Analysis**
3. Plan an educational program for fifth-grade students that discourages illicit drug use. Include at least three main ideas you want to convey and at least three activities you will use to deliver the information **Synthesis**
4. One of your friends thinks that marijuana is safe and that its use should be decriminalized. Evaluate this person's position by considering potential health effects on the population, both positive and negative, if marijuana were legalized. **Evaluation**

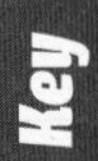

Key

Application	**Analysis**	**Synthesis**	**Evaluation**
using information in a new situation.	breaking down information into component parts.	putting together information from different sources.	making informed decisions.

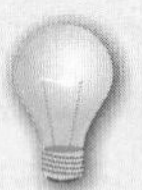

Reflecting on Your Health

1. Do you use drugs responsibly? Explain why you do or do not.
2. Under what circumstances would you intervene to stop a friend from abusing drugs?
3. What are you currently doing or what would you do to encourage your children not to use illegal drugs?
4. What kinds of over-the-counter drugs do you use? Do you think that your use of these drugs is helpful or harmful to your health?
5. If you abuse drugs, do you think that your health or the health of others is adversely affected by your behavior? Why or why not? After reading this chapter and learning about the health effects of illegal drugs, are you motivated to stop your drug abuse? Why or why not?

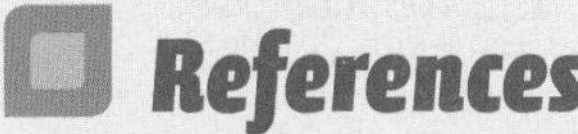

References

1. Johnston, L. D., et al. (2013). *Monitoring the future: National survey results on drug use, 1975–2012: Vol. 2. College students and adults ages 19–50.* Ann Arbor: Institute for Social Research, The University of Michigan. Retrieved from http://monitoringthefuture.org//pubs/monographs/mtf-vol2_2012.pdf
2. Hanson, G., Fleckenstein, A. E., & Venturelli, P. J. (2012). *Drugs and society* (11th ed.). Burlington, MA: Jones & Bartlett Learning.
3. Hanson, G., Fleckenstein, A. E., & Venturelli, P. J. (2012). *Drugs and society* (11th ed.). Burlington, MA: Jones & Bartlett Learning.
4. Culberson, J. W., & Ziska, M. (2008). Prescription drug misuse/abuse in the elderly. *Geriatrics, 63*, 22–31.
5. National Institute on Drug Abuse. (2003). *Preventing drug use among children and adolescents: A research-based guide* (2nd ed.). Washington, DC: U.S. Government Printing Office. Retrieved March 16, 2011, from http://www.nida.nih.gov/pdf/prevention/RedBook.pdf
6. Yeo, K.-K., et al. (2007). The association of methamphetamine use and cardiomyopathy in young patients. *American Journal of Medicine, 120*, 165–171.
7. Nguyen, D., et al. (2010). Intrauterine growth of infants exposed to prenatal methamphetamine: Results from the infant development, environment, and lifestyle study. *Journal of Pediatrics, 157*(2), 337–339.
8. Roussotte, F., et al. (2010). Structural, metabolic, and functional brain abnormalities as a result of prenatal exposure to drugs of abuse: Evidence from neuroimaging. *Neuropsychology Review, 20*(4), 376–397.
9. Thompson, P. M., et al. (2004). Structural abnormalities in the brains of human subjects who use methamphetamine. *Journal of Neuroscience, 24*, 6028–6036.
10. Johnston, L. D., et al. (2010). *Monitoring the future: National survey results on drug use, 1975–2009: Vol. 1. Secondary school students* (NIH Publication No. 10-7584). Bethesda, MD: National Institute on Drug Abuse. Retrieved on March 17, 2011, from http://www.monitoringthefuture.org/pubs/monographs/vol1_2009.pdf
11. Schardt, D. (2008, March). Caffeine: The good, the bad, and the maybe. *Nutrition Action Health Letter,* Center for Science in the Public Interest. Retrieved March 17, 2011, from http://www.cspinet.org/nah/02_08/caffeine.pdf
12. Drasbek, K. R., et al. (2006). Gamma-hydroxy-butyrate—A drug of abuse. *Acta Neurologica Scandinavica, 114*, 145–156.
13. Hall, W., & Degenhardt, L. (2009). Adverse health effects of non-medical cannabis use. *Lancet, 374*(9698), 1383–1391.
14. Centers for Disease Control and Prevention. (2008, July 25). Non-pharmaceutical fentanyl-related deaths—Multiple states, April 2005 to March 2007. *Morbidity and Mortality Weekly Report, 57*, 793–796.
15. National Institute on Drug Abuse. (2009). *Principles of drug addiction treatment: A research-based guide* (NIH Publication No. 09-4180). Washington, DC: National Institutes of Health, National Institute on Drug Abuse. Retrieved March 21, 2011, from http://www.nida.nih.gov/PDF/PODAT/PODAT.pdf
16. Kinsey, B. M., et al. (2009). Anti-drug vaccines to treat substance abuse. *Immunology and Cell Biology, 87*(4), 309–314.
17. National Institute on Drug Abuse. (2004). Lessons from prevention research. *NIDA InfoFacts.* Retrieved from http://www.drugabuse.gov/sites/default/files/prevention_0.pdf

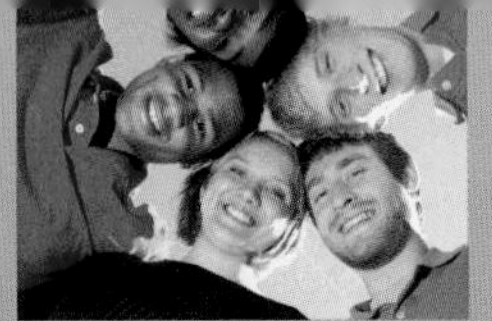

Diversity in Health

Tobacco Drinking?

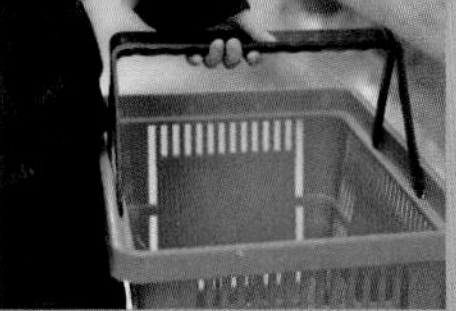

Consumer Health

Kretecks and Bidis: Unwrapping the Facts

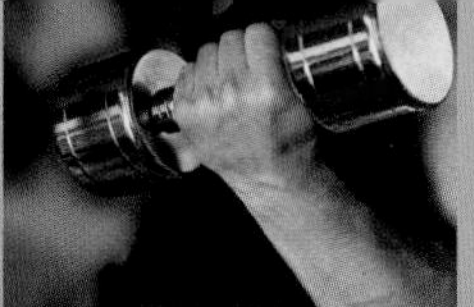

Managing Your Health

Drinking and Date-Rape Drugs: Safety Tips for Women | Guidelines for Safer Drinking | How to Say No to Secondhand Smoke | Tips for Quitters

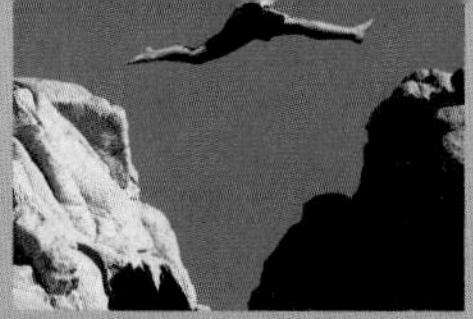

Across the Life Span

The Effects of Alcohol and Tobacco Use

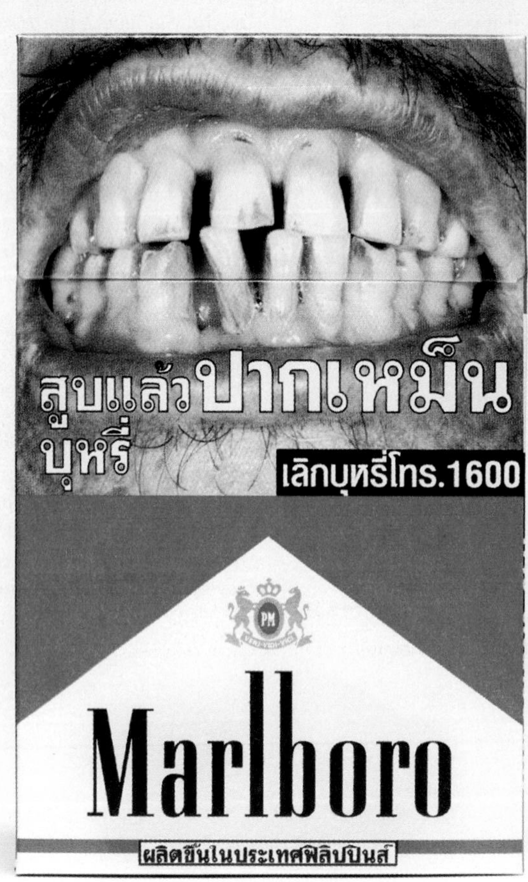

Chapter Overview

Factors related to and consequences of alcohol abuse and dependence

Alcohol's effects on college students

How to control your alcohol consumption

How alcoholism is diagnosed and treated

Who uses tobacco products and why

The short- and long-term health effects of tobacco use

The benefits and process of quitting

Student Workbook

Self Assessment: Why Do You Smoke?

Changing Health Habits: Do You Want to Change a Smoking or Drinking Habit?

Do You Know?

Whether clove cigarettes are safer than regular cigarettes?

The major reasons why college students drink?

How smoking can affect your sex life?

Circle of People: © SergeBertasiusPhotography/ShutterStock; Consumer: © sevenke/ShutterStock; Weight Training: © Kzenon/ShutterStock; Rock Climbing: © Galina Barskaya/ShutterStock; Chapter opener: © ShutterWorx/iStockphoto.com

CHAPTER 8

Alcohol and Tobacco

Learning Objectives

After studying this chapter, should will be able to:

1. Describe the effects of alcohol on health.
2. Identify factors that influence alcohol consumption.
3. Distinguish between alcohol use, abuse, and dependence.
4. Identify signs of alcohol abuse and dependence.
5. Describe programs for prevention and treatment of alcohol abuse and dependence.
6. Identify short- and long-term effects of tobacco use on health.
7. Discuss the impact of environmental tobacco smoke on non-smokers.
8. Describe programs for quitting cigarettes or tobacco use.
9. Identify benefits of quitting cigarette or tobacco use.
10. Describe the impact of alcohol and tobacco use during pregnancy.

For 28 years—from 1984 to 2014—the health warnings on cigarette packs in the United States have been small and text only.

The graphic and sobering warnings shown on the facing page are among those that appear on cigarette packs and advertisements in Canada, Brazil, and Malaysia. For 30 years—from 1984 to 2014—the health warning on cigarette packs in the United States have been small and text only. A major change occurred with the passage of the Tobacco Control Act, which was signed into law on June 22, 2009. With this law, the U.S. Food and Drug Administration (FDA) became empowered to regulate the manufacture, marketing, and distribution of tobacco products. The law also stipulates that the FDA develop color graphics—photos or drawings—to accompany nine new health warnings written to educate the American public about the dangers of smoking, similar to those in other countries. The goal of the educational warnings was to reduce the rate of smoking in the United States to 12% by 2020. The new warnings were mandated to cover at least half of the front and back of each cigarette pack and at least one-fifth of the area of an advertisement.

However, five tobacco companies filed a lawsuit against the federal government in August 2011. The companies contended that these huge graphics and accompanying statements advocate that people not buy cigarettes, rather than simply warning them of the risks of smoking. In 2012, two separate courts ruled the newly proposed graphic warning labels go beyond simple factual warnings and are a form of advocacy imposed by the government and, therefore, violate the First Amendment. As of March 2014, the U.S. Food and Drug Administration was undertaking new research to address issues identified by the court and has postponed implementation of the graphic warning labels.

Other countries, however, continue to require graphic images and strong health warnings on their cigarette packages, including Australia, Brazil, Canada, Malaysia, Singapore, and Thailand. Do these warning labels work to deter people from smoking?

To find out, researchers from the Centers for Disease Control and Prevention (CDC) asked smokers and nonsmokers aged 18 to 24 years to explain their reactions to large graphic and text cigarette warnings on packs of Canadian cigarettes compared to the much smaller text-only U.S. warnings.[1] The results from this investigation and other studies cited by the CDC revealed that the large graphic images along with specific information, such as those on the Canadian cigarette packs, were more likely to be noticed, read, and believed than the smaller, text-only, less-specific messages on U.S. cigarette packs. Percentages, facts, and corresponding graphic images had more effect on the thinking of young adults than did vague text-only messages such as "Quitting smoking now greatly reduces serious risks to your health." The CDC concluded that "stronger warnings on U.S. cigarette packages that include graphic images and factual messages may help consumers make more informed decisions about using tobacco products."

Smoking cigarettes and drinking alcohol are behaviors that usually begin in the preteen and teen years. Although many factors influence young people's decision to use tobacco or alcohol, tobacco and alcohol industry ads and products often target young people and can persuade young people to engage in alcohol or tobacco use.[2] Although tobacco companies are not allowed to advertise, market, and promote their products to those younger than 18 years as part of the 1998 Master Settlement Agreement (MSA) between the states and the tobacco industry, they still do. Results of a study conducted by researchers at the Cancer Prevention and Control Program at the University of California San Diego Cancer Center indicated that "recent RJ Reynolds advertising may be effectively targeting adolescent girls."[2] The researchers were referring to the Camel No. 9 advertising campaign, which associated the thin cigarettes with romance, glamour, and Chanel perfumes. One of the Camel No. 9 advertisements is shown in **Figure 8.1**.

Hanewinkel et al. studied cigarette ads versus noncigarette ads and the effect of each on smoking initiation among adolescents and teens. The data revealed an association between cigarette ads and smoking initiation in youth aged 10 to 17 years but revealed no association between exposure to ads in general and smoking initiation in this age group. The researchers explain that cigarette ads are powerful mechanisms that draw young persons to smoking because they contain images to which this age group aspires—images of "masculinity (for boys), thinness (for girls), independence, extroversion, and sex appeal." The researchers note:

Cigarette marketers have created brands with multiple aspirational images, each designed to fit the needs common among adolescents. Adolescents are in the process of identity formation, when they face emotional instability and social self-consciousness. Aspirational imagery used in cigarette advertising is especially appealing, because it associates the

Figure 8.1

Camel No. 9 Cigarette Advertisement. The magazine ads attracted adolescent and teen girls with flowery images and vintage fashion. The cigarette packs were a high-style glossy black with hot pink and teal blue borders Promotional giveaways were hot pink as well and included cell phone jewelry and tiny purses.

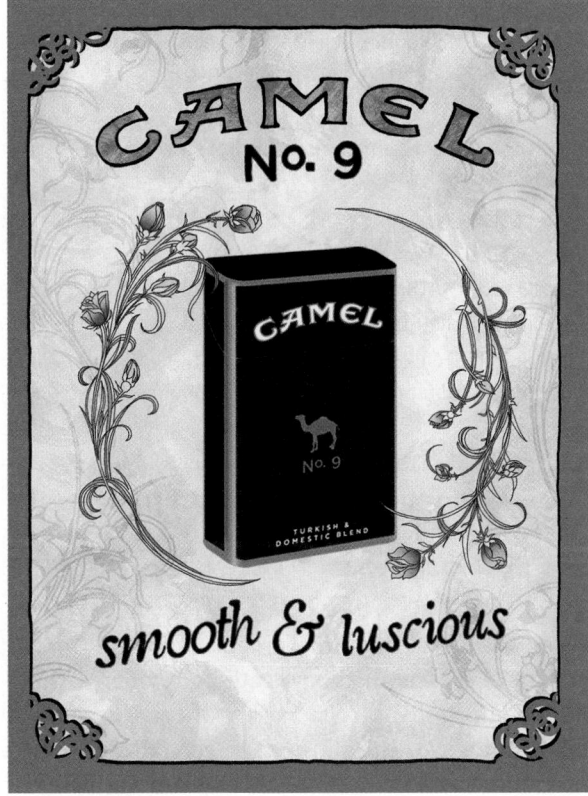

behavior, smoking, with characteristics adolescents are trying to assimilate.[3]

Many medical researchers and healthcare professionals think that advertising alcohol and other drug-related products such as cigarettes encourages the use of drugs, in general. The practice of promoting alcohol and tobacco use is particularly dangerous because they are two primary "gateway" drugs; that is, most people who abuse drugs have followed a progression in drug use from alcohol and/or tobacco to marijuana and "hard" drugs.

Both tobacco and alcohol can have negative effects on health, with some consequences being severe. The National Cancer Institute's quiz "Why Do You Smoke?" will help you understand the roots of your smoking behavior. If you do not smoke cigarettes or drink alcoholic beverages, you probably know family members, coworkers, or friends who may benefit from these self-assessments. Taking these tests could be their first steps to healthier lifestyles.

harmful use Drinking alcoholic beverages while knowingly damaging one's physical and/or psychological health.

alcohol abuse Includes the symptoms of harmful use, but when drinking the abuser exhibits long-term social interaction problems and uses alcohol in physically dangerous situations.

Alcohol

Alcohol Use, Abuse, and Dependence

Alcohol use is quite common in the United States. According to the 2012 National Survey on Drug Use and Health, 52.1% of Americans older than 12 years are current alcohol users, which means that they had at least one drink in the month before they took the survey.[4] This group includes binge alcohol users and heavy alcohol users. For the purposes of the survey, binge alcohol users had five or more drinks on the same occasion at least once in the month prior to the survey. Heavy alcohol users had five or more drinks on the same occasion on at least five days in the month prior to the survey. (All heavy alcohol users are also binge alcohol users.) **Table 8.1** lists the number of drinks consumed by light to heavier drinkers as measured in standard drinks.

Alcohol use becomes **harmful use** when a person drinks alcoholic beverages while knowingly damaging his or her health. For example, a person who drinks heavily on a regular basis (see Table 8.1), gets injured often while drinking, or becomes depressed from drinking is engaging in harmful use.

Alcohol abuse includes the symptoms of harmful use but adds a social dimension. When drinking, the alcohol abuser has problems interacting with people in his or her family, in social settings, or at work. Typically, the abuser uses alcohol in physically dangerous situations, such as when driving a car. However, he or she does not develop tolerance to the drug, exhibit withdrawal symptoms when not drinking, or compulsively use alcohol. Both harmful use and alcohol abuse are patterns of behavior, not just one-time occurrences. Both are usually considered to be present if the behavior has occurred for at least 1 month or has occurred repeatedly over a longer period of time.

alcohol dependence (alcoholism) A syndrome characterized by at least three of the following symptoms: a compulsion to drink, difficulty in controlling the amount of alcohol consumed, withdrawal symptoms when alcohol is not consumed, evidence of tolerance, progressive neglect of other interests because of drinking, and continuing to use alcohol despite its physical and psychological effects on the user.

Alcohol abuse becomes **alcohol dependence**, or **alcoholism**, when certain other symptoms occur that are part of the *alcohol dependence syndrome.* **Table 8.2** lists the symptoms of this syndrome. A diagnosis of dependence is usually made if a person exhibits three or more of these symptoms over a year's time. According to the CDC, excessive alcohol use is the third leading cause of preventable death in the United States, accounting for approximately 79,000 deaths per year.[5]

Factors Related to Alcohol Abuse and Dependence

About 100 years ago, alcoholics were thought simply to have a "weak character" or to suffer from "moral weakness." Since that time, especially within the past 50 years or so, scientists have gathered evidence showing that alcoholism has a variety of origins, many of them biological. In addition, research results show the importance of the interactions among heredity, brain effects, and psychological, social, and developmental factors in the development of alcoholism. Researchers are increasingly studying the roles of the interaction between genes and the environment in alcohol use and dependence.[6] A cause of alcoholism is unknown.

Table 8.1

Drinking Levels as Shown in Standard Drinks*

Drinking Level	Amount
Abstainer	Fewer than 12 drinks in lifetime or no drinks in the past year
Light	Three or fewer drinks/week
Moderate	More than 3 drinks/week but no more than 7 drinks/week for women and no more than 14 drinks/week for men
Heavy or highrisk	Women: More than 3 drinks on any day or more than 7 drinks/week. Men: More than 4 drinks on any day or more than 14 drinks/week.

*One standard drink is 0.5 oz absolute alcohol, 12 oz beer, 5 oz wine, or 1.5 oz 80-proof liquor. (Amounts for beer and wine vary depending on their alcohol content.)
Data from U.S. Department of Agriculture and U.S. Department of Health and Human Services. (2010). Dietary guidelines for Americans, 2010 (7th ed.). Washington, DC: U.S. Government Printing Office; and National Institute on Alcohol Abuse and Alcoholism.

Table 8.2

Alcohol Dependence Syndrome

Having three or more of the following symptoms over a year usually indicates alcohol dependence syndrome:

- A strong desire or compulsion to drink
- Difficulty in controlling the amount of alcohol consumed and when it is consumed
- Withdrawal symptoms when alcohol is not consumed, or consuming alcohol to avoid withdrawal symptoms
- Evidence of tolerance, that is, increased amounts of alcohol are needed to achieve the effects originally produced by lower amounts
- Progressive neglect of other interests because of drinking, while spending an increased amount of time obtaining and drinking alcohol, and recovering from its effects
- Continued use of alcohol despite clear evidence of its physical and/or psychological effects on the user

Heredity For centuries, people have observed that alcoholism runs in families. Researchers have explored environmental and hereditary (genetic) factors of alcoholics to determine which are significant in the development of alcoholism.

By studying the family history of alcoholics, scientists determined that people who have a first-degree relative (parent, brother, or sister) with alcoholism have a higher risk of developing alcoholism than do people in the general population. Scientists estimate this risk to be from four to seven times higher. Sons of alcoholic fathers are at greatest risk. Additionally, data from adoption, twin, and animal studies indicate that there is a genetic component to alcoholism.

intoxication Impairment of the functioning of the central nervous system as a result of ingesting toxic substances such as alcohol.

Scientists also study the reactions of people at risk for developing alcoholism (those who have a first-degree alcoholic relative) compared to those not at risk for alcoholism. In general, those at risk do not react to the consumption of alcohol with the same intensity as those not at risk. Some scientists think that persons at risk for alcoholism may not perceive that they are becoming intoxicated until they have had far more to drink than those not at risk for alcoholism.

Two other genetically linked factors are thought to influence the development of alcoholism: behavior and temperament. *Behavior* is the way people act—what they do. *Temperament* means disposition—the characteristic way in which people emotionally respond to the things and people around them. Behavior and temperament are thought to be inherited traits that are modified by interactions with the environment. Certain characteristics of behavior and temperament appear to be associated with enhanced risk for alcoholism: hyperactivity, impulsivity, aggression, short attention span, quickly changing emotions, slowed ability to calm oneself following stress, thrill-seeking behavior, and inability to delay gratification.

Brain Effects When a person drinks alcoholic beverages, various behavioral changes occur that are commonly called **intoxication**, impairment of the functioning of the central nervous system (the brain and spinal cord). **Table 8.3** lists the changes that characteristically take place as a person consumes more and more alcohol. In this table, alcohol consumption and blood alcohol concentrations (BACs) are listed as ranges because the number of drinks as related to body weight determines the concentration of alcohol in the blood. That is, in general, the larger the person, the greater the amount of alcohol that must be consumed for a specific blood alcohol concentration. Blood alcohol concentrations also rise more quickly in women than in men. One of the reasons for this occurrence is that women have proportionately more fat and less water in their bodies than do men. Alcohol is more soluble in water than in fat; therefore, if a woman drinks the same amount as a man, her generally smaller size and lower water content result in a higher concentration of alcohol in watery body tissues such as the blood. In addition, the stomach enzyme that breaks down alcohol before it reaches the bloodstream is less active in women than it is in men.

Why do certain changes take place in the body when a person consumes alcoholic beverages? The answer has to do with how alcohol affects interactions among nerve cells in the brain. Psychoactive drugs (including alcohol) act at communication points among nerve cells. Psychoactive drugs interfere with the normal activity of the chemicals that carry nerve impulses from one nerve cell to another. The manner of this interference varies among drugs.

Table 8.3

Effects of Various Levels of Alcohol Consumption on Inexperienced Drinkers

Number of Standard Drinks	Blood Alcohol Concentration (BAC)*	Effects
1–2	0.02 to 0.06%	Euphoria; reduction in anxiety
3–5	0.08 to 0.15%	Impairment of judgment, motor coordination, and emotional control; involuntary rapid eye movements; double vision; speech disorders; may be accompanied by aggressive behavior as alcohol level rises
7–8	0.20 to 0.25%	Sedation; impairment of ability to learn and remember information
12–18	0.40 to 0.50%	Loss of adequate respiration; dangerously low blood pressure; dangerously low internal body temperature; coma or death may result

*Blood alcohol concentration is expressed in percentages: A BAC of 0.05% means an alcohol concentration of 5 milliliters (ml) for every 10,000 ml of blood.

tolerance A physiologic response in chronic users of drugs in which increased amounts of the drug are required to achieve effects previously produced by lower amounts.

Alcohol acts on parts of the brain that are responsible for drives and emotions, as well as the part of the brain that coordinates skeletal muscle movements. It also affects the "thinking" part and reward centers in the brain.

Many people drink alcohol to "get drunk," but other factors often contribute to excessive alcohol consumption. Anxious people, for example, may use alcohol to relieve their anxieties. Researchers think that persons with a family history of alcoholism are more likely to be motivated to drink alcohol to get "high," whereas persons with no family history of alcoholism are more likely to be motivated by anxiety.

At high doses, alcohol also has effects that are aversive; that is, they are sufficiently unpleasant (such as nausea and vomiting) that people often lose their desire to drink. Severe aversive effects, such as unconsciousness, result in a person's inability to continue drinking. Therefore, aversive effects help curb excessive alcohol consumption.

Chronic drug users develop **tolerance** to the drug; that is, increased amounts of alcohol are required to achieve effects previously produced by lower amounts. Tolerance develops because the chronic use of the drug stimulates liver enzymes to break down the drug with increasing swiftness. Also, brain cells become less responsive to the drug over time. Tolerance develops for both the pleasant and unpleasant effects of alcohol consumption, so chronic drinkers do not experience the aversive effects as quickly as do occasional drinkers. Therefore, their alcohol consumption is not curbed as quickly.

Psychological, Social, and Developmental Factors People drink for reasons other than to experience the "brain effects" of feeling good or reducing anxiety. Similarly, people curb their drinking or abstain from drinking for reasons other than aversive brain effects that may stimulate nausea and vomiting. Many of these reasons are *psychological*, having to do with thoughts, feelings, attitudes, and expectations about alcohol. Some of the reasons are *social*, relating to interactions with friends, relatives, and coworkers. Still other reasons are *developmental*, relating to the psychological, social, and biological changes in individuals over time and as they mature.

People often consume alcoholic beverages because they expect positive psychological effects from their drinking, such as enhancing social interactions, feeling pleasurable effects, or producing sedation. People develop their expectations concerning alcohol from experience, observation, and what they are told. In fact, a person's beliefs about alcohol can be predictive of their future drinking habits: Heavy drinkers tend to view the positive effects of alcohol as arousing, whereas light drinkers tend to view the positive effects as sedating.

Individuals often consume alcohol to ease their social interactions or because it's the thing to do in a particular social setting. With adolescents and young adults, peers may pressure one another to drink alcohol. The section titled "Alcohol and College Students," which follows, explores the role of peer pressure in the drinking patterns of college students. Cultural factors are additional important social reasons for drinking alcohol. In many cultures, people consume alcohol with meals or as a part of other traditional social activities.

Abusive and alcohol-dependent drinking patterns often begin in adolescence. A wide variety of factors affects children as they mature and influences the development of patterns of drinking alcoholic beverages. The biggest early risk factor for alcohol abuse and dependence is having a parent who is an alcoholic or who abuses alcohol. Children of alcoholics are 4 to 10 times more likely to become alcoholics than are children of nonalcoholics. A child reared in an alcoholic family has a greater risk of developing alcoholism than a child who is not reared in such an environment.[7,8]

Another way in which parents influence their children is by their parenting practices. Teenagers who report receiving high levels of nurturing and support from their parents also report fewer alcohol-related problems than teenagers who report little parental nurturing and support. Teenagers who report feeling close to their parents drink alcoholic beverages less frequently than teenagers who report that they do not feel close to their parents. Children are more likely to use alcohol if their parents are not involved in their activities, there is a lack of, or inconsistent, discipline, and the parents have low educational aspirations for the children. Positive family relationships, involvement, and attachment appear to discourage youths' initiation into alcohol use.

Psychological, social, and developmental factors all interact with genetic factors to result in a certain kind of behavior. These interactions explain why not all alcoholics have a family history of alcoholism, and why not all persons with a family history of alcoholism become alcoholics. These dynamic interactions occur throughout life, with varying contributions from genes and environment at different times.

Alcohol and College Students

Alcohol abuse is a serious problem that often appears to begin or accelerate during the college years. In fact, the most abused drug among college students is alcohol. Most studies of alcohol use by college students examine psychological and social issues; those issues are discussed here. However, there are also economic, political, and ecological factors of college alcohol use, such as the alcohol environment on college campuses and their surrounding communities.

Studies show that college students drink alcohol for a variety of reasons. **Table 8.4** lists the primary reasons that students give to explain why they drink. However, there are differences between moderate and heavy drinkers with regard to their reasons for drinking.

Moderate drinkers who do not abuse alcohol do not cite many reasons for their drinking. They drink to feel more comfortable in social situations or to relieve stress. They do not drink with any goal in mind such as getting drunk.

Heavy drinkers who abuse alcohol, however, often state many reasons for their drinking, including the reasons listed in Table 8.4, but their drinking tends to be escapist and goal oriented. They often drink to get drunk. Results of studies show that college students who drink heavily believe that drinking is part of the college experience and that it is something they are entitled to do as undergraduates. College men are more likely to think this way than women. In addition, college students who are heavy drinkers tend to have been drinkers in high school and have friends who drink.[9]

Additional student characteristics correlate with alcohol abuse as well. Although any student may abuse alcohol, abusers are more likely to be younger students with low self-esteem, high levels of anxiety, a mildly assertive personality, and at least one alcoholic parent. The freshman and sophomore years are the most likely times for students to exhibit alcohol abuse. Additionally, students who are fraternity/sorority members and who are athletes are more likely than nonfraternity/sorority members or nonathletes to abuse alcohol.[9,10]

Drinking alcohol during the college years poses many risks for students, including driving after drinking, getting behind in schoolwork, and getting into trouble with campus or local police. In fact, many students who abstain from alcohol do so because they want to avoid such risks. Alcohol can also be a vehicle for date-rape drugs. The Managing

Table 8.4

College Students: Major Reasons for Drinking

Reason	Category
It makes them feel good	Enhancement
They want to get drunk	Enhancement
It helps them feel more comfortable in social situations	Social
It helps them relax	Coping
It puts them in a better mood	Coping
It helps relieve tension and stress	Coping
It helps them feel more accepted by their peers	Conformity

Data from Patrick, M. E., et al. (2011). Drinking motives, protective behavioral strategies, and experienced consequences: Identifying students at risk. *Addictive Behaviors*, 36, 270–273.; LaBrie, J. W., et al. (2007). Reasons for drinking in the college student context: The differential role and risk of the social motivator. *Journal of Studies on Alcohol and Drugs*, 68, 393–398.; Ham, L. S., & Hope, D. A. (2003). College students and problematic drinking: A review of the literature. *Clinical Psychology Review*, 23, 719–759.

Table 8.5

College Students: Major Reasons for Not Drinking

College students report that they abstain from drinking alcohol because of:

- Disapproval/Lack of interest (against religious/moral convictions)
- Risks and negative effects (hangovers/alcoholism/medication interactions)
- Social responsibility (might interfere with job/family/school/relationships)
- Loss of control (negatively affects mood/effects unpleasant)
- Lack of availability (expense/hard to obtain)
- Health concerns (in training/fattening/bad for health)

Adapted from Johnson, T. J., & Chen, E. A. (2004). College students' reasons for not drinking and not playing drinking games. *Substance Use and Misuse*, 39, 1139–1162.

Your Health box "Drinking and Date-Rape Drugs: Safety Tips for Women" provides guidelines to help women avoid ingesting these dangerous substances in alcoholic beverages. **Table 8.5** lists the primary reasons some students abstain from drinking alcohol.

Binge Drinking and Drinking Games College men who belong to fraternities, especially those who live in fraternity houses, make up a large proportion of students who drink heavily. Drinking in fraternities, as in other campus social groups including many sororities, is perceived as promoting a feeling of unity and cohesiveness among their members. A Harvard School of Public Health survey found that about 75% of college students who lived in fraternities and sororities binge drank versus about 55% of students who lived in off-campus housing alone or with a roommate, 45% who lived in residence halls, 30% who lived off campus with parents, and 27% who lived off campus with a spouse.[11]

Table 8.6 shows binge drinking prevalence, frequency, and intensity by sex and age group in 2011. Those aged 18–24 years, including those attending and those not attending college, had the highest overall prevalence of binge drinking at 30.0%. That is, one out of every four people in this age group who responded to the binge drinking telephone survey reported at least one binge drinking episode during the preceding month. The table shows that the prevalence of binge drinking decreases as age increases. Although those aged 18–24 years did not have the highest number of binge drinking episodes during the preceding month (frequency), they did have the highest average number of drinks consumed by binge drinkers on any occasion during the preceding month (intensity).

Binge drinking is often accompanied by drinking games. There is a high prevalence of drinking games on college campuses, with approximately two-thirds of college students engaging in these activities.[12] **Table 8.7** lists specific motives for playing drinking games. Compare this table with Table 8.4 and you will see some similarities. Although some motives for playing drinking games seem specific to the games (e.g., competition), current research has not conclusively established that the motives for playing drinking games are separate from the general motives for drinking.

In drinking games, participants follow rules that specify when and how much they must drink and that mandate certain verbal, physical, or memory skills. When players make mistakes or are cued by game rules, they are required to drink. The more game players drink, the more they make mistakes, and the amount of alcohol they consume increases. The danger of unconsciousness, coma, and death increases as alcohol consumption increases.

What can you do to help an intoxicated person avoid serious medical consequences or death? A person who has slurred speech, a staggering walk, double vision, and is not alert (but is able to be aroused by voice) should be stopped from drinking and taken away from the source of the alcohol. A person with signs of more severe intoxication, such as not making sense, urinating on himself or herself, breathing irregularly, vomiting repeatedly, and not being able to be aroused with a strong stimulus like a slap, should be taken to an emergency room immediately.

Alcohol-Related Injury Deaths in College Students One sobering statistic is that more than 5,000 alcohol-related deaths occur each year among those aged 18 to 24 years (including college and noncollege individuals), which is more than the number of U.S. soldiers killed in the Iraq war. Ralph Hingson and colleagues of the National Institute on Alcohol Abuse and Alcoholism made this comparison. The researchers also determined that among college students aged 18 to 24 years, approximately 1,600 are

Managing Your Health

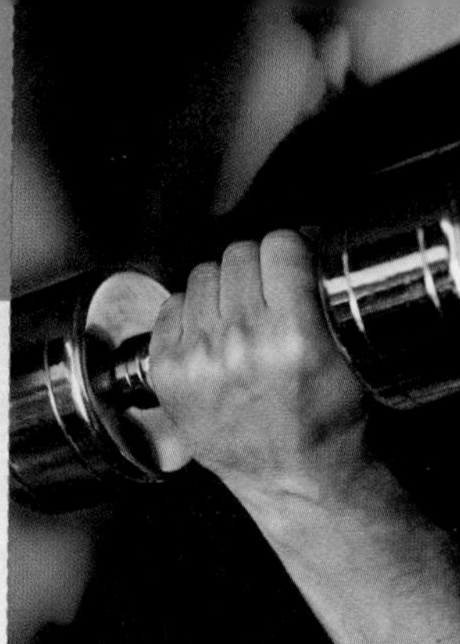

© Kzenon/ShutterStock

Drinking and Date-Rape Drugs: Safety Tips for Women

- When you can, drink from tamper-proof bottles or cans and open them yourself.
- If at a bar or club, accept drinks only from the bartender or server. Try to watch your drink being prepared.
- Always keep your drink with you, even in the restroom.
- If you leave your drink or lose sight of it for any reason, discard it and get a fresh drink.
- Don't trust someone to watch your drink. Even a friend can get distracted.
- Don't share or exchange drinks.
- Don't take a drink from a punch bowl or container that is passed around.
- Don't drink anything that has an unusual taste or appearance, although a date-rape drug dissolved in alcohol may not change the taste of your drink.
- If your drink changes color, suddenly becomes "fizzy," or appears to have something floating in it, discard it. Someone likely tried to drug you.
- Don't mix drugs with alcohol.
- Limit your drinking to one to two drinks to remain aware and able to follow safety procedures.
- If you feel ill or lightheaded while drinking away from home, tell a friend, call a cab, and return home. If you feel extremely ill, go to an emergency room.

Table 8.6

Binge Drinking Prevalence, Frequency, and Intensity, by Sex and Age Group—United States, 2011*

	Prevalence		Frequency†		Intensity§	
Sex/Age Group	No.	%	No.	No. of Episodes	No.	No. of Drinks
Sex						
Men	154,834	20.8	25,212	4.6	23,409	8.5
Women	254,011	10.0	18,703	3.1	17,687	5.7
Age group (yrs)						
18–24	12,312	25.6	2,950	4.1	2,713	9.1
25–34	35,441	22.5	7,415	3.9	6,983	8.0
35–44	57,057	17.8	9,891	3.9	9,375	7.3
45–64	173,869	12.1	19,464	4.2	18,233	6.5
≥65	130,166	3.8	4,195	5.4	3,792	5.5
Total	408,845	15.2	43,915	4.1	41,096	7.5

*Respondents were from all 50 states and the District of Columbia.
†Average number of binge drinking episodes during the preceding 30 days.
§Average largest number of drinks consumed by binge drinkers on any occasion during the preceding 30 days.
Reproduced from Centers for Disease Control and Prevention. Kanny, D., et al. (January 14, 2011). Binge drinking—United States, 2009. *Morbidity and Mortality Weekly Report*, 60, 101–104.

Table 8.7

College Students: Major Reasons for Playing Drinking Games

Competition and thrills
Conformity (to fit in)
Novelty (to try something different)
Fun and celebration
Social lubrication
Sexual manipulation (in order to have sex with someone or get a date)
Boredom
Coping (to forget about problems)

Adapted from Johnson, T. J., & Sheets, V. L. (2004). Measuring college students' motives for playing drinking games. *Psychology of Addictive Behaviors*, 18(2), 91–99.

killed each year as a result of alcohol-related injuries. About three-fourths of these deaths are from alcohol-related car crashes and one-fourth from other alcohol-related causes, such as drownings, falls, gunshots, and alcohol/drug poisonings.[13]

How the Body Processes Alcohol

When an alcoholic beverage is consumed, the alcohol in the drink is absorbed into the bloodstream from the stomach and intestinal tract. The blood transports alcohol to the "detoxification center" of the body—the liver. The liver breaks down harmful substances such as drugs, changing them into compounds that are safer or easier to excrete.

The liver can break down only a certain amount of alcohol per hour, no matter how much has been consumed. That rate depends, in part, on the concentration of enzymes that break down alcohol in the liver, and this concentration varies among individuals. Nevertheless, alcohol is absorbed into the bloodstream more quickly than it can be broken down by the liver, and the excess alcohol stays in the blood. Therefore, the intake of alcohol needs to be controlled to prevent its accumulation in the blood, resulting in an increase in the blood alcohol level.

The stomach also breaks down some alcohol. Eating food while drinking alcoholic beverages results in the alcohol being held in the stomach for a longer time with the food. Therefore, more of it gets broken down in the stomach, and less alcohol enters the bloodstream. A person who drinks while eating will have a slower rise in the blood alcohol level than will a person who drinks on an empty stomach. Conversely, aspirin and cimetidine (an ulcer drug) inhibit the breakdown of alcohol in the stomach. A person who takes either of these drugs along with alcohol will have a quicker rise in the blood alcohol level than will a person who does not take these drugs when drinking alcohol.

Consequences of Alcohol Abuse and Dependence

Diseases and Conditions The harmful use and abuse of alcohol result in multiple effects on the body that are serious threats to health. Alcohol consumption does not affect all individuals in the same way; various effects result from differences among abusers' genetic makeup, general health, and drinking patterns. Despite these differences, however, excessive alcohol consumption exerts its most serious effects on the liver, cardiovascular system, immune system, reproductive system, and brain. It also affects how vitamins are used by the body and can result in vitamin deficiencies. In pregnant women, it has devastating effects on the fetus.

Diseases of the Liver Because the liver is the major detoxification site for alcohol, it is particularly prone to harm by chronic alcohol consumption. Years of drinking can result in three types of liver disease: fatty liver, alcoholic hepatitis, and cirrhosis of the liver. The symptoms of each may overlap, and a person can have more than one of these conditions simultaneously. Women tend to develop these conditions at lower levels of alcohol intake than men do (see "Factors Related to Alcohol Abuse and Dependence" in this chapter).

Nearly 90% of heavy drinkers develop a *fatty liver* because alcohol stimulates the buildup of fat in liver cells. This process begins immediately upon drinking: Fat accumulation has been found in the livers of young men after only one night of heavy drinking. Most liver cells are not specialized for fat storage, and their ability to perform their normal functions declines when they store fat. These liver cells eventually die; the scar tissue that remains produces cirrhosis.

Analyzing Health-Related Information

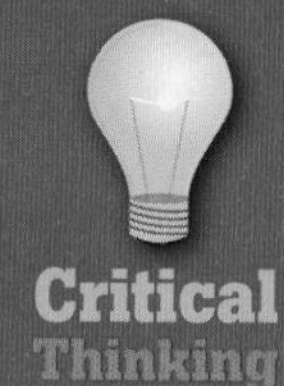

Critical Thinking

© tele52/ShutterStock

The following news release appeared on the website of the National Institute on Alcohol Abuse and Alcoholism. It was posted on January 14, 2014. Read the news release and explain why you think it is a reliable or an unreliable source of information. Use the model for analyzing health information to guide your thinking; the main points of the model are noted here.

1. Which statements are verifiable facts, and which are unverified statements or value claims?
2. What are the credentials of the person (in this case press office) who makes health-related claims? Does this press office have the appropriate background and education in the topic area? What can you do to check the credentials of this press office?
3. What might be the motives and biases of the press office making the claims?
4. What is the main point of the article? Which information is relevant to the issue, main point, product, or service? Which information is irrelevant?
5. Is the source reliable? What evidence supports your conclusion that the source is reliable or unreliable? Does the source of information present the pros and cons of the topic or the benefits and risks of the product?
6. Does the source of information attack the credibility of conventional scientists or medical authorities?

Based on your analysis, do you think that this article is a reliable source of health-related information? Summarize your reasons for coming to this conclusion.

NIH Study—Research-Based Strategies Help Reduce Underage Drinking

by NIAAA Press Office

Strategies recommended by the Surgeon General to reduce underage drinking have shown promise when put into practice, according to scientists at the National Institute on Alcohol Abuse and Alcoholism (NIAAA), part of the National Institutes of Health. These approaches include nighttime restrictions on young drivers and strict license suspension policies, interventions focused on partnerships between college campuses and the community, and routine screening by physicians to identify and counsel underage drinkers.

NIAAA researchers Ralph Hingson, Sc.D., and Aaron White, Ph.D., evaluated studies conducted since the 2007 "Call to Action to Prevent and Reduce Underage Drinking." A report of their findings appears in the January issue of the *Journal of Studies on Alcohol and Drugs*.

"The downward trend in underage drinking and alcohol-related traffic deaths indicates that certain policies and programs put in place at the federal, state, and local levels have had an impact," said NIAAA Acting Director Kenneth R. Warren, Ph.D.

Since 2007, alcohol use and heavy drinking have shown appreciable declines in national surveys of middle and high school students. One study found that 12th-grade alcohol use declined from 66.4% to 62% in 2013, with a similar downward trend seen in eighth- and tenth-graders.

The researchers' analysis of recent studies on driving policies found that certain driving laws affecting underage drivers deter drunk driving and reduce fatal crashes. Graduated driver licensing laws for underage drivers, which include nighttime restrictions, and use/lose laws that lead to license suspension for an alcohol violation, have been effective, the review said. Individuals under the age of 21 are half as likely to drive after drinking in states with the strongest use/lose and graduated licensing laws, based on a national study.

The Surgeon General's Call to Action also recommended addressing college drinking by increasingly involving the surrounding community in intervention efforts. Studies since 2007 have shown the effectiveness of this approach, with successful programs implemented on campuses in North Carolina, West Virginia, Rhode Island, California, and Washington state. These programs focused on addressing alcohol availability, alcohol pricing and marketing, and enforcement of existing laws. Many campuses saw reductions in drunk driving and other alcohol-related harms.

Since the Call to Action, progress has also been made in establishing the effectiveness of screening and brief motivational interventions. In these types of short counseling sessions, individuals get feedback about their drinking patterns, and counselors work with clients to set goals and provide ideas for helping to make a change.

While studies show that brief motivational interventions can reduce alcohol consumption, only a small proportion of individuals under 21 are screened for alcohol use and advised of the risks. Among the 62 percent of 18- to 20-year-olds who saw a doctor in the past year, only 25 percent were asked about driving and only 12 percent were advised of health risks.

"An evaluation of the recommendations in the Call to Action reveals that certain strategies show promising results," said first author Dr. Hingson, director of NIAAA's Division of Epidemiology and Prevention Research. "While progress has been made in addressing underage drinking, the consequences still remain unacceptably high. We must continue research to develop new interventions and implement existing strategies that have been shown to be effective."

Drs. Hingson and White say expanded studies of the effects of alcohol on the developing brain, legal penalties for providing alcohol to minors, and parent-family alcohol interventions are among the research opportunities that could lead to further reductions in underage drinking.

Recent studies show that interventions aimed at strengthening family relationships in the middle-school years can have a lasting effect on students' drinking behavior, but more studies are needed to build on this finding, say the authors.

Underage drinking is linked to 5,000 injury deaths per year, poor academic performance, potential damage to the developing brain, and risky sexual behavior.

Reproduced from National Institute on Alcohol Abuse and Alcoholism. Retrieved February 25, 2014 from http://www.niaaa.nih.gov/news-events/news-releases/nih-study-research-based-strategies-help-reduce-underage-drinking

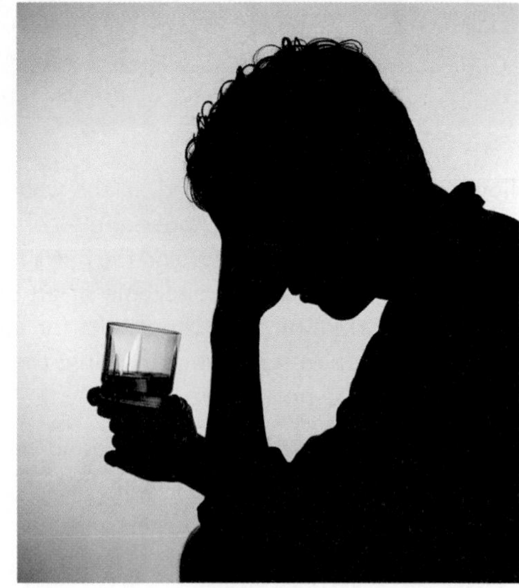

Approximately 15% to 30% of alcoholics develop liver cirrhosis (**Figure 8.2**). This disease develops as alcohol begins to kill liver cells. Liver cells have the ability to regenerate, much like skin heals from a small cut. However, if cell damage is extensive, the liver cannot produce new cells quickly enough to replace destroyed ones. Connective tissue cells fill the spaces left by the dead cells, similar to the way scar tissue may fill the gap of tissue caused by a severe cut. However, connective tissue is not functional liver tissue, and the liver's ability to perform its many important functions declines. Eventually the person must have a liver transplant or he or she will die.

Approximately 40% of chronic abusers develop *alcoholic hepatitis*. Hepatitis is an inflammation of the liver, which can be caused by hepatitis viruses or by toxic chemicals such as alcohol. A severe case of hepatitis can result in death.

The majority of individuals who develop cirrhosis of the liver have been drinking heavily for 10 to 20 years. Women, however, are more at risk than men for liver disease. Because women detoxify alcohol less efficiently than men do, the concentration of alcohol in their blood rises more quickly than in men when both consume the same number of drinks. Therefore, serious forms of alcoholic liver disease occur more frequently in women than in men. Additionally, women are more likely than

Figure 8.2

A Healthy and Unhealthy Liver (with Cirrhosis).
(a) Healthy liver tissue is smooth and dark red/brown. (b) The liver with cirrhosis develops scar tissue and nodules (bumps) as it works to repair damage.

(a and b) Courtesy of Leonard V. Crowley, MD, Century College.

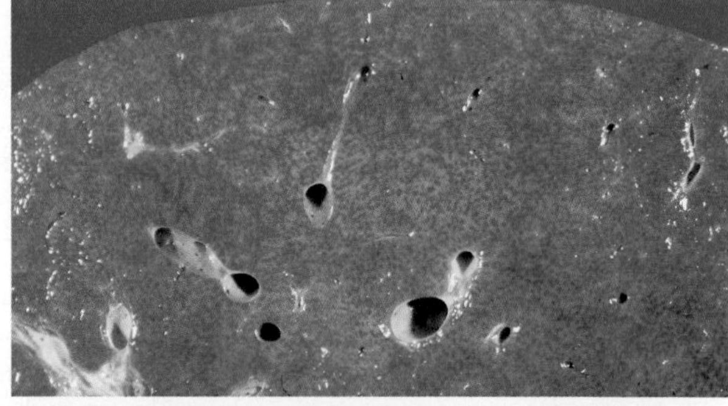

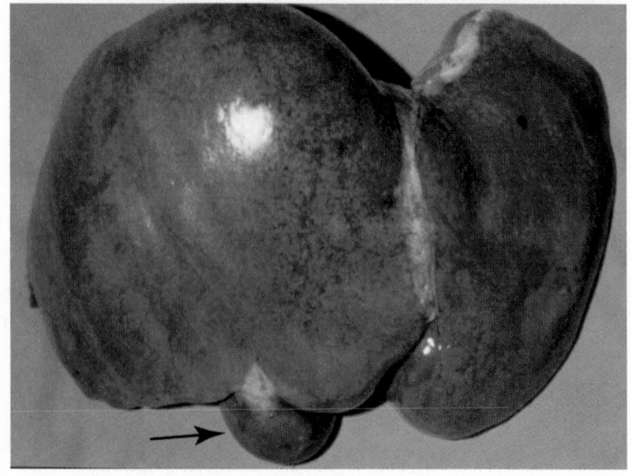

men to develop these conditions at lower levels of alcohol consumption and after shorter periods of alcohol dependence. Hereditary factors and body weight, as well as sex, appear to play a role in susceptibility to liver disease. Obese alcoholics have a higher risk of having alcoholic liver disease than nonobese alcoholics, and heavy alcohol consumption increases the severity of liver disease associated with obesity.[14]

Cardiovascular Disease and Cancer There is considerable evidence that limiting alcohol consumption to 1 oz or less of ethanol per day (two drinks or less) decreases the risk of death from coronary artery disease and stroke. However, heavier drinking is associated with cardiovascular diseases such as cardiomyopathy (heart muscle disease), hypertension (high blood pressure), arrhythmias (disturbances in heart rhythm), and stroke.[15]

Alcohol abuse is a risk factor for certain cancers. The heavy consumption of alcohol can cause cancers of the esophagus and liver. It is also associated with the development of stomach cancer and increases the likelihood of larynx and mouth cancer. People who smoke cigarettes and drink alcohol, even in moderate amounts, multiply their risk of cancer of the esophagus because together these drugs have a multiplier effect. That is, when people take both drugs routinely, their risk of cancer is much higher than if the risk of each was added.[16]

Even when not abused, alcohol can raise the risk of cancer. Consuming three-quarters to one drink per day raises a woman's risk of developing breast cancer by 9%. The risk increases as consumption increases. Consuming two to three drinks per day raises breast cancer risk by 43%. Data also suggest that women who drink alcohol while taking estrogen in postmenopausal estrogen replacement therapy may increase their breast cancer risk more than if they used either one alone.[17,18]

Immune System Suppression The immune system, which protects the body from invasion by pathogens, also suffers as a result of chronic alcohol abuse. This behavior impairs the functioning of the immune system, predisposing the drinker to infectious diseases such as colds, pneumonia, and tuberculosis. Chronic alcohol abuse even suppresses the activity of certain immune system cells that defend the body against the spread of cancer.

Detrimental Effects on the Reproductive System Alcohol affects the reproductive systems of both men and women. It affects the functioning of the testes, decreasing the amount of the sex hormone, testosterone, these organs produce. Alcoholic men often experience shrinking of the testicles, impotence, and loss of libido, or sex drive. In women, alcohol affects the functioning of the ovaries. The menstrual periods of alcoholic women are often irregular or cease altogether. As a result, alcoholic women often have difficulty becoming pregnant. Alcoholic women also have a higher rate of early menopause than nonalcoholic women. During pregnancy, alcohol consumption can have devastating effects on the fetus. This topic is discussed in the Across the Life Span section of this chapter.

Detrimental Effects on the Brain Alcohol consumption has multiple effects on the brain. Chronic alcoholics may experience brain disorders. One of the most serious is the Wernicke-Korsakoff syndrome. This syndrome includes mental confusion, abnormal eye movements, and an inability to coordinate skeletal muscles, which results in abnormal posture and a staggering walk. Scientists have discovered that this syndrome may be to the result of the alcoholic's inability to use the B vitamin thiamin properly. Some alcoholics are deficient in this vitamin (and many other nutrients) because their diets consist primarily of alcohol rather than food. In either case, if given thiamin, the alcoholic can be cured of the abnormal eye movements, posture, and gait if he or she stops drinking. However, the person is left with anterograde amnesia—the inability to remember new information for more than a few seconds.

Another effect of alcohol on the brain is intoxication, the impairment of the central nervous system (see Table 8.3). *Withdrawal* is also a brain effect of alcohol but only in alcohol-dependent individuals who stop drinking or reduce their alcohol intake. Withdrawal symptoms usually occur about 24 to 36 hours after an alcoholic stops drinking. Typically, the alcoholic experiences mild agitation, shaking, anxiety, loss of appetite, restlessness, and insomnia. Five percent to 15% of alcoholics experience grand mal seizures (convulsions) during withdrawal. Additionally, a small percentage of alcoholics have severe withdrawal symptoms that include hyperactivity, hallucinations, disorientation, and confusion. This severe withdrawal syndrome is called *delirium tremens*, or *DTs*.

Some researchers suggest that a *hangover* is a mild form of withdrawal that can occur in anyone who consumes alcoholic beverages heavily during a session of drinking. The signs of a hangover can include headache, mental slowness, dry mouth, fatigue, diarrhea, anxiety, stomach pains, and tremors. If the "mild withdrawal" explanation is true, it explains why consuming additional alcohol temporarily relieves hangover effects.

In addition to alcohol causing hangovers, other substances in alcoholic beverages may cause hangovers too. Alcoholic beverages contain certain acidic compounds that have toxic effects on the body. These compounds differ among types of alcoholic beverages and affect whether someone will experience a hangover. Another compound called formaldehyde (a preservative of dead animals) is produced by the body when it cannot keep up with the breakdown of alcohol being consumed. The buildup of formaldehyde contributes to a hangover. Alcohol causes the body to lose water. This dehydration occurs in brain cells as well as other body cells. Pain accompanies their rehydration.

Whatever the causes of a hangover, home remedies such as taking vitamins, getting in a cold shower, or drinking coffee will not cure the "morning-after" pain of drinking too much. Time alone will cure a hangover.

Effects on Behavior and Safety

Serious and Fatal Injuries Statistics show that alcohol use and abuse are related to serious and even fatal injuries. Alcohol frequently contributes to water-related accidents, motor vehicle accidents, general aviation crashes, domestic and nondomestic violence including sexual assault and rape, suicides, and homicides.

Data show that 31% of all fatal motor vehicle crashes in 2012 were alcohol-related.[19] Other types of injury fatalities are also more likely for current drinkers as compared to abstainers and prior drinkers, including unintentional falls, fires, drownings, and poisonings. Current drinkers are also more likely to commit suicide or to be intentionally killed by another person.

Automobile Accidents Drinking and driving are potentially deadly because alcohol impairs the perceptual, intellectual, and motor skills needed to operate motor vehicles safely. Traffic accidents are the leading cause of death among people aged 5 to 24 years, the second leading cause of death after other unintentional injuries in children aged 1 to 4 years, and the fifth leading cause of death after cancer, heart disease, other unintentional injuries, and suicide in adults aged 25 to 44 years.[20] In all states, the District of Columbia, and Puerto Rico, the legal blood alcohol concentration (BAC) limit for operating an automobile is 0.08%. It is a criminal offense to operate a motor vehicle at or above that limit. All states have a lower unlawful BAC threshold for youth younger than 21 years, and in some cases, younger than 18 years. **Figure 8.3** shows approximate BAC by body weight and the time from the first drink. Note the number of drinks a person can have over a period of time before he or she is considered legally drunk. Also realize that some impairment occurs after a person consumes only one drink.

Alcohol-related fatal automobile accidents occur more frequently at certain times of the day and during certain days of the week than others. For example, in 2011, the rate of alcohol-related driving fatalities was 4.5 times higher at night than during the day. Furthermore, 41% of 2011 alcohol-related fatalities occurred on weekend nights in comparison to 7% on weekend days. The National Highway Transportation Safety Administration (NHTSA) notes that a BAC of 0.08 g/dL or higher indicates alcohol-impaired driving.[21]

Figure 8.4 shows that the percentage of traffic fatalities resulting from alcohol-related crashes peaks between midnight and 3 A.M. A comparatively low percentage of traffic fatalities are alcohol-related between 6 A.M. and 3 P.M., but the percentage rises throughout the late afternoon and evening until the midnight-to-3 A.M. peak. A significant percentage occurs from 3 A.M. to 6 A.M. as well. The statistics in the previous paragraph, together with these, show that a person driving at night and in the early morning hours, especially on weekends, is more likely to be involved in a fatal alcohol-related motor vehicle accident than when driving during the day and during the week. Using the subway system in safe areas, walking in safe areas away from the street, or staying at home during these peak alcohol-related traffic fatality times are strategies to consider to help lower your risk of being involved in an alcohol-related car crash.

Alcohol-impaired driving fatalities declined 27% over the past 10 years from 13,472 in 2002 to 9,878 in 2011. The drivers with the highest percentage of intoxication in fatal crashes (0.08% BAC or higher) were young adults aged 21 to 24 years (32% of this group), followed closely by those aged 25 to 34 years (30%) and 35 to 44 years (24%).[21]

For safety, women who drink and drive must remember that their BACs rise more quickly than the BACs of males who consume the same number of drinks. Both sexes must also remember that the risk

Figure 8.3

Blood Alcohol Concentration (BAC) by Weight and Gender. These graphs show the approximate BACs of men and women in various weight ranges. All states have set 0.08% as the legal BAC limit while driving for those 21 years and older. All states have lower thresholds for those younger than 21 years of age. However, you may be convicted of driving under the influence (DUI) of alcohol if evidence exists that your driving is impaired. Commercial drivers may be convicted of a DUI at a BAC of 0.04%.

Reproduced from "Alcohol Impairment Chart" from "Blood Alcohol Concentration by Weight and Gender". University of Wisconsin Center for Health Sciences, 1988, and U.S. Dept. of Transportation, National Highway Traffic Safety Administration, 1992. Formulation and compilation by the Pennsylvania Liquor Control Board, Bureau of Alcohol Education. Used by permission.

ALCOHOL IMPAIRMENT CHART

NEVER DRINK AND DRIVE

APPROXIMATE BLOOD ALCOHOL PERCENTAGE

FEMALE

Drinks	Body Weight in Pounds								
	100	**120**	**140**	**160**	**180**	**200**	**220**	**240**	
0	.00	.00	00	00	00	.00	00	.00	ONLY SAFE DRIVING LIMIT
1	.05	.04	.03	.03	.03	.02	.02	.02	Impairment Begins
2	.09	.08	.07	.06	.05	.05	.04	.04	Driving Skills Affected
3	.14	.11	.10	.09	.08	.07	.06	.06	Possible Criminal Penalties
4	.18	.15	.13	.11	.10	.09	.08	.08	
5	.23	.19	.16	.14	.13	.11	.10	.09	
6	.27	.23	.19	.17	.15	.14	.12	.11	Legally Intoxicated
7	.32	.27	.23	.20	.18	.16	.14	.13	Criminal Penalties
8	.36	.30	.26	.23	.20	.18	.17	.15	
9	.41	.34	.29	.26	.23	.20	.19	.17	
10	.45	.38	.32	.28	.25	.23	.21	.19	

Your body can get rid of one drink per hour.
Each 1.5 oz. of 80 proof liquor, 12 oz. of beer or 5 oz. of table wine = 1 drink.

ALCOHOL IMPAIRMENT CHART

NEVER DRINK AND DRIVE

APPROXIMATE BLOOD ALCOHOL PERCENTAGE

MALE

Drinks	Body Weight in Pounds								
	140	**160**	**180**	**200**	**220**	**240**	**260**	**280**	
0	.00	.00	00	00	00	.00	00	.00	ONLY SAFE DRIVING LIMIT
1	.03	.02	.02	.02	.02	.02	.01	.01	Impairment Begins
2	.05	.05	.04	.04	.03	.03	.02	.02	
3	.08	.07	.06	.06	.05	.05	.04	.04	Driving Skills Affected
4	.11	.09	.08	.08	.07	.06	.06	.05	Possible Criminal Penalties
5	.13	.12	.11	.09	.09	.08	.08	.07	
6	.16	.14	.13	.11	.10	.09	.09	.09	
7	.19	.16	.15	.13	.12	.11	.11	.10	Legally Intoxicated
8	.21	.19	.18	.17	.15	.13	.13	.12	Criminal Penalties
9	.24	.21	.20	.19	.17	.16	.15	.14	
10	.27	.23	.21	.19	.17	.16	.16	.15	

Your body can get rid of one drink per hour.
Each 1.5 oz. of 80 proof liquor, 12 oz. of beer or 5 oz. of table wine = 1 drink.

THIS CHART IS INTENDED FOR INDIVIDUALS 21 YEARS OF AGE OR OLDER.
IT IS A GUIDE, NOT A GUARANTEE.

Alcohol can affect each person in a different way. The way your body reacts to alcohol depends on your gender, how much you weigh, how quickly you drink, and whether or not you have eaten. You also need to remember that drinks may contain different amounts of alcohol.

This chart uses 1.5 oz of 80 proof liquor, 12 oz of beer, or 5 oz of table wine as one drink.

Females reach a higher BAC level faster than males. A woman should use the female version on the chart that is highlighted in pink on the other side.

Pennsylvania has set .08% BAC as the legal limit for a Driving Under the Influence (DUI) conviction. You may be convicted of DUI at .05 % and above if there is supporting evidence of driving impairment. Commercial drivers can be convicted of DUI nationwide with a BAC level of .04%. A BAC reading is not necessary for an individual to be convicted of DUI. You may be convicted of DUI if there is circumstantial evidence that you imbibed a sufficient amount of alcohol such that you are incapable of safe driving.

The Zero Tolerance Law (Section 3802(e) of the PA Vehicle Code, Title 75) lowered the Blood Alcohol Content (BAC) for minors (persons under 21) to .02%.

REMEMBER:

- **A person must be 21 years of age or** older to legally purchase, attempt to purchase, possess, consume, or transport any alcohol, liquor, malt or brewed beverages.
- Impairment begins with the first drink - the only safe driving limit is .00%.
- For safety's sake, never drive after drinking!
[Source: Refer to www.lcb.state.pa.us]

REFERENCES:

http://www.wikihow.com/Calculate-Blood-Alcohol-Content-(Widmark-Formula)
http://www.alcohol.vt.edu/Students/alcoholEffects/estimatingBAC/index.htm
http://www.ehow.com/how_7315381_calculate-estimated-blood-alcohol-content.html
http://www.ctduiattorney.com/dui_information/calculating_bac.html

LCB-79 09/13
Reorder Item #0079

PA pennsylvania LIQUOR CONTROL BOARD

of fatal crashes rises rapidly with increasing BAC. As **Figure 8.5** shows, compared to persons with no alcohol in their blood, drivers with BACs between 0.050% and 0.079% have a 5-fold increased risk of having a fatal car crash, whereas males aged 16–20 years have a 10-fold increased risk at this same BAC level. Male and female drivers aged 21–34 years with BAC levels between 0.80% and 0.99% (legally drunk) have a 13-fold increased risk, and those aged 35 years and older have a 6-fold risk. However, while driving at this BAC level, young men aged 16–20 years have a 24-fold risk of being killed in a car crash, and that increases to an 83-fold risk at a BAC level of 0.100% to 0.149%. At the same BAC level, others have about an 11- to 13-fold increased risk of killing themselves in a car crash. Not shown in Figure 8.5 is the fact that young men aged 16–20 years have more than a 2,000-fold increase of being killed while driving with a BAC level of 0.150% and over. Others have an 84- to 88-fold increased risk.

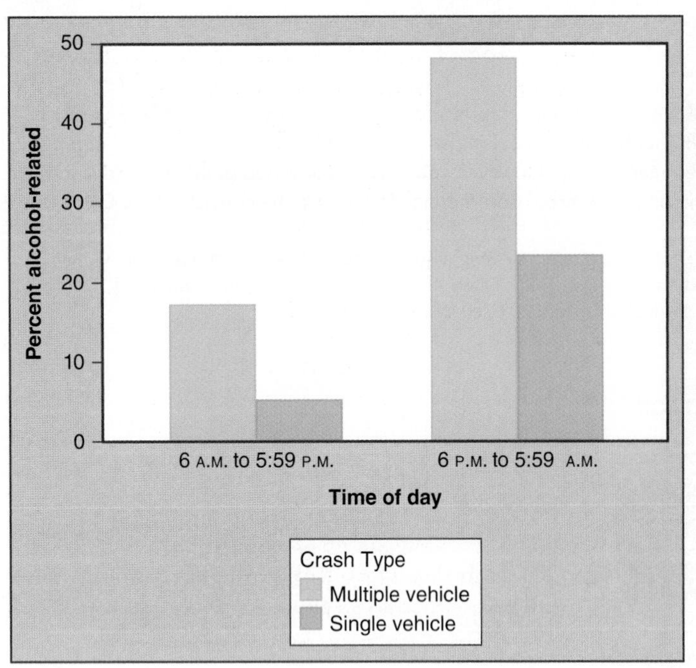

Figure 8.4

Percentage of Traffic Fatalities Resulting from Alcohol-Related Crashes, by Time of Day.
Data from National Highway Transportation Safety Administration. (2012). Traffic safety facts 2011 Data (U.S. Department of Transportation DOT HS 811 700). Retrieved from: http://www-nrd.nhtsa.dot.gov/Pubs/811700.pdf

Airplane Accidents Alcohol also impairs the ability of pilots to fly aircraft. Alcohol has not been directly implicated in U.S. commercial airline crashes; however, it appears to play a more prominent role in general aviation crashes. Alcohol has been shown to impair flight performance in pilots when they drink and up to 8 hours after drinking.[22] Canfield and colleagues from the Federal Aviation Administration Aerospace Medical Institute found that 92 pilots (7%) out of the 1353 pilots killed in the aviation accidents they studied had alcohol in their blood at the time of the crash.[23]

Water-Related Accidents Alcohol is also a significant factor in water-related accidents. Researchers estimate that alcohol consumption is associated with between 30% and 70% of adult drownings.[24,25] The highest percentages are associated with males older than 25 years. Most alcohol-related drownings are associated with motor vehicle accidents, but alcohol is also present in the blood of more than half the drowning victims who were swimming, boating, or rafting when they died. Alcohol also contributes to diving accidents that leave victims with serious spinal cord injuries.

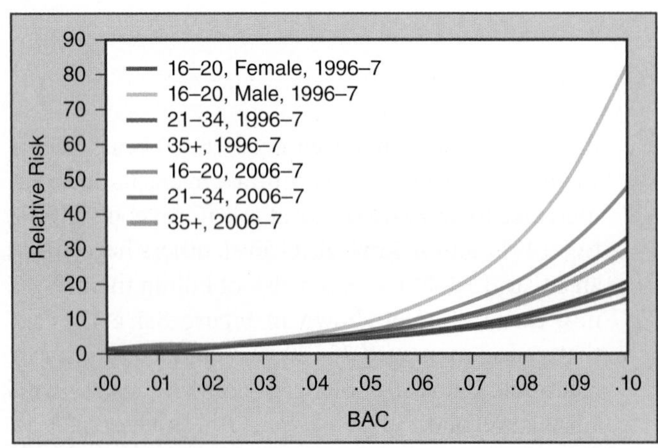

Figure 8.5

Fatality Risk at Various Levels of Blood Alcohol Concentration by Age and Sex. This graph shows that as the BAC rises, the likelihood of being killed while driving a car increases. The risk rises dramatically for males aged 16–20 years, well beyond that for females or for older males.
Reproduced from Voas, R. B., et al. (2012). Alcohol-related risk of driver fatalities: An update using 2007 data. *Journal of Studies on Alcohol and Drugs*, 73(3), 341–350.; permission conveyed through Copyright Clearance Center, Inc.

Prevention

Because many people begin drinking alcoholic beverages during adolescence, prevention programs often target younger children to educate them about alcohol before they reach their teenage years. Prevention efforts include school-based programs for children in grades 5 through 10, but most target fifth and sixth graders. Because this time is developmentally critical as students move from elementary school to middle school or junior high, those who have experimented with alcohol may begin to misuse it at this time.

There is a variety of school-based programs. *Affective education* seeks to influence students' beliefs about alcohol by helping them develop problem-solving and refusal skills as well as decision-making abilities. In addition, these programs promote an understanding of how alcohol use can interfere with personal values and goals. Results of research show that such programs have limited effectiveness. *Life skills programs* emphasize the development of communication, conflict resolution, and assertiveness skills to help students cope with peer pressure to drink alcohol, smoke cigarettes, or take other drugs. Results of research show that life skills programs reduce alcohol use primarily among females. *Resistance training*—the "Just say no" approach—shows mixed results. *Normative education* aims to correct erroneous beliefs about the prevalence and acceptability of alcohol use among peers. (Results of survey research show that young people believe that alcohol use among their peers is more common than it really is.) Adding normative components to alcohol education programs for adolescents appears useful. In fact, normative education is a recent trend in adolescent alcohol education. Current normative programs include teaching students how to resist peer influence and often incorporate activities and events outside of the classroom.

Prevention efforts that focus on the entire population of drinkers are called *environmental approaches.* Such approaches are important because 52.1% of Americans aged 12 years or older were current alcohol users in 2012,[4] and many drinkers experience moderate to severe alcohol-induced impairment at least occasionally. These drinkers are all at risk for alcohol-related injuries and health problems.

Beginning in 1989, one prevention strategy for the general population was the requirement by the U.S. government to place warnings on alcoholic beverage containers; however, survey data show that only about one-fourth of adults realize that the labels exist. Researchers have not found evidence that warning labels reduce alcohol consumption. Another prevention strategy was the establishment of 21 as the minimum age for purchase and consumption of alcohol. Evidence shows that this strategy significantly reduced youth drinking and related problems such as alcohol-related traffic accidents in those younger than age 21 years.[26]

In 2007, in response to the finding that alcohol was the number one abused substance by America's youth, the acting Surgeon General of the United States, Kenneth P. Moritsugu, issued *The Surgeon General's Call to Action to Prevent and Reduce Underage Drinking.*[27] This report notes that parents of adolescents do not recognize how widespread alcohol use is in this population and how the brains of adolescents are particularly susceptible to the negative effects of alcohol use. Noting that alcohol use by America's youth is influenced by many factors, the report develops six goals, including fostering changes in society that facilitate healthy adolescent development, engaging not only adolescents but also the social systems that interact with adolescents in a coordinated effort to prevent and reduce underage drinking, and conducting additional research on adolescent alcohol use and its relationship to development.

How to Control Alcohol Consumption

Studies show that light drinkers have certain behavior patterns that help them curb their drinking. These attributes are listed in the Managing Your Health box "Guidelines for Safer Drinking" and are effective rules for controlling alcohol consumption.

Diagnosis and Treatment of Alcoholism and Alcohol Abuse

According to the 2012 National Survey on Drug Use and Health, approximately 2.5 million Americans received treatment for alcohol abuse during the year prior to the survey.[4] Various types of treatments are available for those who need help. Screening techniques help identify those persons who need treatment.

The CAGE screening test is considered one of the most effective screening devices for alcohol abuse or alcoholism. A variety of other screening instruments is available also.

Healthcare professionals who determine that their patients are alcohol dependent refer them to substance abuse specialists for evaluation and possible treatment. Patients that show nondependent problem drinking are often encouraged to participate in brief intervention programs.

In the past, physicians and substance abuse practitioners thought that an alcoholic could not be helped until he or she "hit bottom" and then asked for help. A person who did not ask for help was considered to be denying his or her alcoholism and lacking motivation to change. Current thinking regards motivation as a process of behavioral change rather than a trait that people have or do not have.

Before treatment, the role of clinical intervention is to help the patient understand the serious dangers inherent in his or her abusive or dependent drinking behavior. Once the alcoholic realizes the need to change his or her behavior, he or she tries to decide what course of action to take. The clinician helps the patient select a course of action or treatment program that best suits his or her needs.

Both inpatient and outpatient programs exist. *Inpatient treatment*, in which the alcoholic resides at a treatment facility, is sometimes used for the early phases of treatment, particularly acute detoxification. During this time, the patient abstains from alcohol and experiences withdrawal symptoms (see "Detrimental Effects on the Brain" in this chapter). Approximately 10% to 13% of patients need medication during this time to help them reduce potentially life-threatening effects of withdrawal. During the detoxification period, patients participate in group therapy and alcohol education sessions for several hours daily. Recovering alcoholics usually live with patients to help them through the process. Such programs usually last 28 days. Near the end of this process the alcoholic's family is usually asked to participate in treatment.

Because of rising medical costs, acute detoxification, as well as further treatment, may take place in outpatient programs. Such programs, developed over the past 25 years, have been extremely successful. Approximately 90% of patients are now treated in outpatient facilities. In these programs, the patient spends a specific amount of time at the treatment facility but lives at home.

After a person has sought treatment for alcohol abuse or dependence, the next stage in behavior change is *maintenance*. For long-term maintenance treatment, recovering alcoholics take part in group meetings and attend individual counseling sessions once or twice a week at outpatient facilities, participate in self-help group meetings, and sometimes participate in family therapy. The maintenance period usually lasts 1 year.

Sometimes *relapse* occurs. During a relapse, a recovering alcoholic returns to his or her drinking habits. Relapse can be triggered by a variety of factors such as stress, depression, alcohol craving, negative life events, and interpersonal tensions. To recover once again, the patient goes through the stages of behavior change. Treatment to prevent an initial or repeated relapse often involves self-help groups.

Alcoholics Anonymous (AA) is the best known and most widely available of the self-help groups. Governed by its members, the organization's philosophy is that alcoholism is a physical, emotional, and spiritual disease for which there is no cure. Recovery is a lifelong process that involves attention to AA's Twelve Steps, which are listed in **Table 8.8**. AA also has related support groups for family members and friends of alcoholics, such as Alateen and Al-Anon.

Although not as well known, other self-help groups exist. The Secular Organization for Sobriety (SOS) is a group similar to AA, except its program does not include spiritual aspects. The Rational Recovery (RR) program is also a secular organization and emphasizes the importance of alcoholics becoming aware of their irrational beliefs, self-perceptions, and expectancies to be successful in changing their behavior. These groups suggest abstinence as a preferred drinking goal but emphasize personal choice. One self-help approach for women is Women for Sobriety. This group emphasizes women's issues such as assertiveness, self-confidence, and autonomy as part of the change process.

Tobacco

Types of Tobacco Products

Cigarettes are the most prevalent tobacco product in the United States. In 2012, an estimated 7.5 million Americans smoked cigarettes, representing 22.1% of the population age 12 years and older.[4]

Smoking rates increase with age to the early 20s, and then generally decline with age. In 2012 6.6% of youths aged 12 to 17 years were current cigarette smokers, 28.2% of young adults aged 18 to 20 years were current smokers, and 34.1% of those aged 21 to 25 were current smokers. Use then declined with age:

Managing Your Health

Guidelines for Safer Drinking

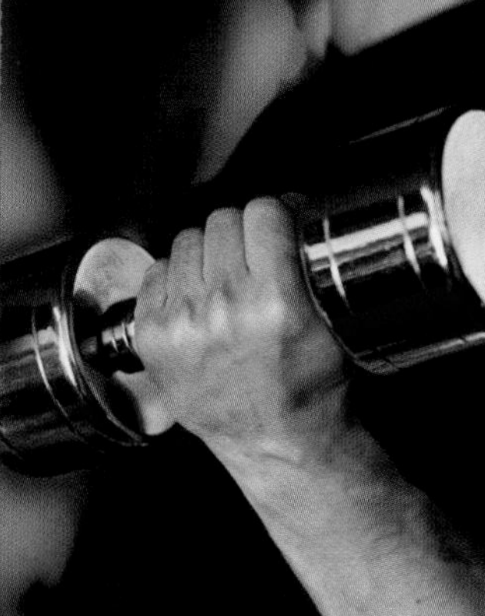
© Kzenon/ShutterStock

1. If you choose to drink, plan ways to drink that promote safety behind the wheel and safety for health. Considering some of the following points should help.
2. Eat before you drink and while you are drinking.
3. Drink alcoholic beverages slowly. Consider watering down your drinks or alternating alcoholic drinks with nonalcoholic drinks.
4. For safety behind the wheel, set a limit on the amount of alcohol you can drink per hour. Use the chart in Figure 8.3 to determine how many drinks you can have per hour and still maintain a BAC of 0.05% or below. If you are a 120-pound woman, for example, you can have only one drink per hour to stay below a BAC of 0.05%. Count drinks to stay within your limit.
5. For health safety, men should consume no more than 2 drinks per day/14 drinks per week, and women should consume no more than 1 drink per day/7 drinks per week.
6. Refuse drinks you do not want and that do not fit within your plan.
7. Cultivate alternatives to drinking to help you relax, such as meditating.
8. Learn to socialize without drinking. For example, use fun venues or fun foods as a social lubricant instead of alcohol.

33.4% of those aged 26 to 29 years were current smokers, as were 31.9% of those aged 30 to 34 years. By age 35 years and older, the percentage of those who were current smokers dropped to 20.1%.[4] **Figure 8.6** shows the proportion of current smokers in each age group, with the younger and older groups broken down in more detail.

The prevalence of smoking is high in college students. In 1991, 35.6% of college students smoked at least once during the past year. This percentage rose throughout the 1990s to a peak of 44.5% in 1999. The percentage has fallen since then to 29.8% in 2012, which is below 1991 levels.[28]

The prevalence of smoking in high school students is lower than in college students. However, the Consumer Health box "Kreteks and Bidis: Unwrapping the Facts" describes types of cigarettes that were becoming popular particularly with high school students, so much so that University of Michigan Monitoring the Future researchers, who track drug, alcohol, and tobacco use among the nation's youth, added a question about these products in 2001. The popularity of kreteks (clove cigarettes) and bidis (small, strong, flavored cigarettes) declined between 2001 and 2012; however, in 2012 3.0% of high school seniors smoked kreteks and 1.4% smoked bidis.[26]

Smoking cigars and pipes is not as popular in the American population as is smoking cigarettes. Most cigar and pipe smokers are male. In 2012, 8.5% of males were current cigar smokers versus 2.0% of females, and 1.6% of males were current pipe smokers versus 0.4% of females.[4]

Smokeless tobacco, which includes *snuff* and *chewing tobacco*, is not very popular in the American population either. Snuff, the most popular form of smokeless tobacco, is powdered or finely cut tobacco. It may be used loose or wrapped in a paper pouch. Although snuff can be inhaled, most users in the United States today place snuff between the cheek and gum. This practice is called *dipping*.

Chewing tobacco is loose-leaf tobacco or a plug of compressed tobacco, which is sometimes called a *quid*. It is placed in the cheek. It can be chewed, as its name suggests, or, more often, it is sucked. During the time that snuff or chewing tobacco remains in the mouth, it forms a liquid that smokeless tobacco users usually spit out. For this reason, smokeless tobacco is often called spitting tobacco. In 2012, 6.7% of males currently used smokeless tobacco versus 0.4% of females.[4]

Worldwide, a variety of other tobacco products exists besides those mentioned here. Additionally, methods of tobacco use vary among cultures. The Diversity in Health essay "Tobacco Drinking?" describes a few tobacco-related practices of various South American cultures.

Who Uses Tobacco and Why?

As mentioned earlier, most people who smoke cigarettes began this habit when they were adolescents, primarily in high school. **Figure 8.7** shows the ages at

nicotine An addictive psychoactive drug found in tobacco.

Table 8.8

The Twelve Steps of Alcoholics Anonymous

1. We admitted we were powerless over alcohol—that our lives had become unmanageable.
2. Came to believe that a Power greater than ourselves could restore us to sanity.
3. Made a decision to turn our will and our lives over to the care of God as we understood Him.
4. Made a searching and fearless moral inventory of ourselves.
5. Admitted to God, to ourselves, and to another human being the exact nature of our wrongs.
6. Were entirely ready to have God remove all these defects of character.
7. Humbly asked Him to remove our shortcomings.
8. Made a list of all persons we had harmed, and became willing to make amends to them all.
9. Made direct amends to such people wherever possible, except when to do so would injure them or others.
10. Continued to take personal inventory and when we were wrong promptly admitted it.
11. Sought through prayer and meditation to improve our conscious contact with God, as we understood Him, praying only for knowledge of His will for us and the power to carry that out.
12. Having had a spiritual awakening as the result of these Steps, we tried to carry this message to alcoholics, and to practice these principles in all our affairs.

which adults say they started smoking. Only 11% of adult smokers started this habit after age 18. Smokeless tobacco use usually begins in early adolescence or in childhood also.

Data show that during the early 1990s through 1996/1997 there was an increase in the percentage of high school students who smoked cigarettes daily, after a decrease had been seen in the prevalence of smoking by high school seniors from 1976 through 1992. However, those percentages have declined steadily through 2011 (**Figure 8.8**). Nevertheless, 18.1% of high school students responded that they were current cigarette smokers on the national Youth Risk Behavior Survey in 2011.[29]

Psychosocial Reasons for Using Tobacco Products Adolescents initially try tobacco products for a variety of reasons. Adolescents who have family members or friends who smoke cigarettes or use smokeless tobacco are more likely to begin these habits than teenagers who do not observe these behaviors in people close to them. Many adolescents try smoking, chewing, or dipping simply to experiment. Others use tobacco as a way to feel older and more independent, as a response to advertising, or as a response to social pressure.

Certain characteristics are associated with increased tobacco use among adolescents, including susceptibility to peer pressure, a sensation-seeking nature, a rebellious personality, depression or anxiety, low academic achievement, and a low level of knowledge about the immediate health risks of smoking. Additionally, adolescents who think that their parents do not care about them or adolescents who are alone much of the time are more likely to try smoking. Girls are significantly less likely to begin smoking if they are involved in an organized sport; however, participation in sports is not associated with decreased smoking among boys.

Nicotine Addiction

Why do teenagers and adults continue smoking and using smokeless tobacco? Most people continue because they are addicted to **nicotine**. Nicotine is a psychoactive drug that acts at communication points among nerve cells in the brain, as do other psychoactive drugs. It becomes addicting during the first few years of use.

The many reasons that people say they continue to smoke (other than craving or being addicted to cigarettes) include the following:

- It is arousing and gives them energy.
- It helps concentration.

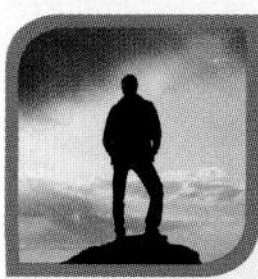

© djgis/ShutterStock

Healthy Living Practices

- Responsible drinking includes limiting consumption to reduce negative impact on your health, while not endangering the safety of others or interfering with business or personal relationships.
- If drinking alcohol is damaging your physical and/or psychological health, you should seek medical help.
- If you use alcohol in physically dangerous situations, have developed a tolerance to alcohol, exhibit withdrawal symptoms when you are not drinking, and compulsively use alcohol, you are probably alcohol dependent and should seek medical help.
- Be sure to eat while drinking alcoholic beverages so that less alcohol will enter the bloodstream.
- If you consume alcohol and are male, drink only 1 oz of ethanol per day (two drinks) or less to decrease the risk of coronary artery disease and stroke. The safest alcohol consumption level for women is 0.5 oz of ethanol per day (one1 drink). Heavier alcohol consumption is associated with a variety of conditions and diseases.
- Do not drive after consuming alcoholic beverages. Alcohol impairs many of the skills needed to operate motor vehicles safely. As your blood alcohol concentration increases, your risk of having a car crash increases significantly.

- It lifts the mood.
- It reduces anger, tension, depression, and stress.
- It is a habit.
- It is a pleasurable activity.

However, some of the pleasure of smoking (as well as using smokeless tobacco) is really the relief of the symptoms of nicotine withdrawal. During the day, as a person smokes, he or she builds up tolerance to nicotine. Nicotine withdrawal symptoms become more pronounced between each successive cigarette. To relieve these symptoms (**Table 8.9**), most cigarette addicts smoke more as the day goes on. Overnight, the level of nicotine in the blood drops and tolerance decreases; thus, the smoker is resensitized to the effects of nicotine. The first cigarette of the day is usually quite satisfying to the smoker as the cycle of tolerance and then resensitization begins once again.

The Health Effects of Tobacco Use

In 1964, U.S. Surgeon General Luther Terry issued a landmark report that linked cigarette smoking with the development of lung cancer and other diseases. Since that famous report, scientists have learned a great deal about the health consequences of smoking and smokeless tobacco use, and the Surgeon General's Office has issued 30 more tobacco-related reports. In these reports, cigarette smoking is recognized as the leading source of preventable illness and death in the United States. Every year, approximately 443,000 people die in the United States as a result of using tobacco products.[30] **Figure 8.9** shows the cancers and chronic diseases to which smoking has a causal link.

Immediate Effects of Nicotine and Carbon Monoxide After entering the body, nicotine produces a variety of effects. It increases the heart rate and the amount of blood that the heart pumps in a single beat. However, nicotine also constricts, or narrows, the blood vessels. As a result, the blood pressure rises. Nicotine also increases the metabolic rate—the speed at which all the chemical reactions of the body take place. These effects increase the body's demand for oxygen. However, the carbon monoxide in cigarette smoke binds to hemoglobin in the red blood cells, reducing its ability to carry oxygen.

Nicotine and carbon monoxide are not the only components of cigarette smoke that affect the body. There are more than 4,000 chemical compounds in the gases and particles that make up cigarette smoke. Some are poisonous, such as hydrogen cyanide; some are irritating to the lungs and mucous membranes, such as particulate matter; and some cause cancer, such as the tars—sticky substances similar to road tar. The rest of this section describes specific health effects of smoking tobacco and using smokeless tobacco products.

Respiratory Illnesses The windpipe and its major subdivisions are lined with microscopic hairlike structures called *cilia*, which are embedded in a layer of sticky mucus. This mucus traps inhaled particles and microbes. As the cilia beat, the mucus moves upward, sweeping this debris up and out of the air passageways.

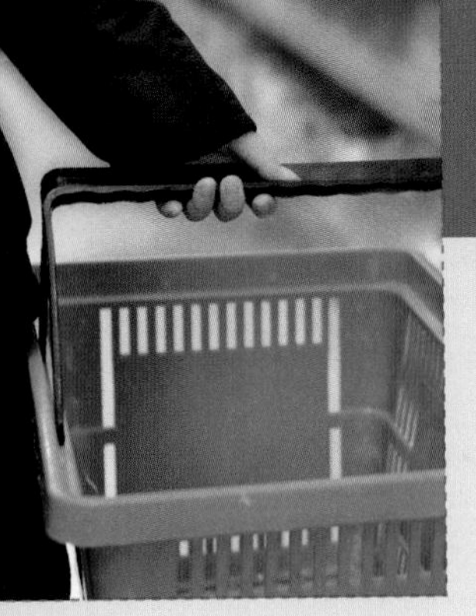

© sevenke/ShutterStock

Consumer Health

Kreteks and Bidis: Unwrapping the Facts

Kreteks (clove cigarettes) and bidi cigarettes (small, strong-smelling brown cigarettes) appeared to be popular with American youth in the late 1990s, but their use by high school seniors declined from 10.1% in 2001 to 3.0% in 2012. Clove cigarettes, developed in Indonesia in the early 1900s and presently manufactured there, have been imported into the United States since 1968. Bidis, manufactured primarily in India and other Southeast Asian countries, were not widely used in the United States until the mid-1990s. In 2000, 9.2% of high school seniors smoked bidis, but by 2012 that figure had fallen to 1.4%.

Clove cigarettes look much like tobacco cigarettes and are made with or without filter tips. Most are wrapped with white paper, but some have brown or black coverings. Clove cigarettes contain approximately 40% ground cloves and 60% tobacco, although the specific amount varies among manufacturers and brands. Clove oil is added as well, often discoloring the cigarette paper. As these cigarettes burn, the cloves make a crackling sound. (Kretek means "crackle.")

Many users of clove cigarettes think that they are less dangerous to smoke than regular cigarettes because 40% of their content is cloves rather than tobacco. However, they are making an incorrect assumption. Clove cigarettes are rolled tighter than regular cigarettes, resulting in a denser product. Put simply, there is less air in clove cigarettes than in regular cigarettes, so the tobacco content of kreteks is similar to that of regular cigarettes. Additionally, tests show that clove cigarettes deliver, on average, twice as much tar, nicotine, and carbon monoxide as do moderate tar-containing American cigarettes.

Clove cigarettes also contain an anesthetic called eugenol (a natural component of the cloves), which can cause allergic reactions in some. This anesthetic numbs the backs of smokers' throats and windpipes. Researchers think that this numbing effect is the reason that smokers inhale kretek smoke more deeply and retain it in their lungs longer than when smoking regular cigarettes. They also suspect that this numbing effect may encourage smoking by people who might otherwise find smoking cigarettes harsh and distasteful.

Bidis are wrapped in leaves (much like cigars) and tied with a string. They are smaller and thinner than regular cigarettes and come in flavors such as cherry, mango, chocolate, and strawberry. Young people smoke bidis because they like the flavor and find bidis cheaper and easier to buy than regular cigarettes. In addition, they perceive bidis to be safer than smoking regular cigarettes. As with clove cigarettes, however, this assumption is false. Tests show that bidis produce approximately three times the amount of carbon monoxide and nicotine as American cigarettes and about five times the amount of tar. Smokers inhale more often and more deeply when smoking bidis than when smoking regular cigarettes because the leaf wrapper does not burn well.

Are smoking kreteks and bidis safe alternatives to smoking regular cigarettes? The answer is an emphatic no! In fact, the data show that these alternative smoking products pose even greater health risks than regular cigarettes do.

Data from Johnston, L. D., et al. (2013). *Monitoring the future: National survey results on drug use, 1975–2012: Vol. 1. Secondary school students.* Bethesda, MD: National Institute on Drug Abuse. Retrieved from http://www.monitoringthefuture.org/pubs/monographs/mtf-vol1_2012.pdf

Inhaled cigarette smoke paralyzes the cilia. With continued smoking, the cilia are damaged. Cigarette smoke also irritates the airways and tar builds up on the cilia, causing excess mucus to be produced. The chronic cough of smokers, usually called *smoker's cough*, is a result of the body's attempt to remove this excess, stationary mucus.

Acute bronchitis is an inflammation of the mucous membranes of the bronchi, which is usually caused by a viral infection. However, smokers are more susceptible than nonsmokers to acute bronchitis because of their impaired and irritated bronchi. The signs and symptoms of this disease are soreness or tightness in the chest, slight fever, cough, chills, and a vague feeling of weakness or discomfort. Bronchitis with accompanying high fever, breathlessness, and yellow, gray, green, or bloody sputum is serious and the person should seek medical attention immediately.

Chronic bronchitis is usually caused by cigarette smoking, but cigar and pipe smoking may also be causes. Chronic bronchitis is a persistent

Diversity in Health

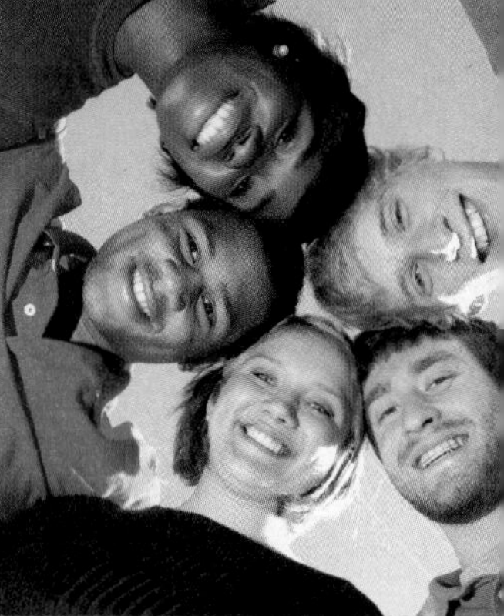

© PhotoEdit/Alamy Images

Tobacco Drinking?

To North Americans, the phrase "using tobacco" usually means smoking cigarettes, cigars, or pipes. Occasionally, we might envision a person using chewing tobacco or placing a pinch of snuff between the gums and cheek. But various cultures use tobacco in other ways—including some ways that may be new to you.

Drinking liquid tobacco is one of the oldest methods of tobacco use. The members of certain tribal populations in South America, particularly those living in Guiana, the upper Amazon, and the mountainous regions of Ecuador and Peru, drink tobacco juice. The drinking of tobacco has also been reported in other South American regions, including northwestern coastal Venezuela, northwestern Colombia, and a few scattered places in Bolivia and Brazil.

The various groups of people who drink tobacco juice prepare it in different ways. The leaves may be first pounded, chewed, or shredded. Sometimes they are left untreated. Then, the tobacco leaves are placed in water; sometimes other ingredients are added such as salt, pepper, or plant materials such as tree bark. The mixture is boiled and then strained to obtain the liquid. Usually it is then set aside to allow much of the water to evaporate. The remaining material has the consistency of a paste, syrup, or jelly. The syrups and jellies are usually liquid enough to drink by mouth or pour in the nose. People from some areas squirt the juice from one person's mouth to another.

Various tribes of the northernmost extension of the Andes in Colombia and Venezuela and in parts of the northwest Amazon make a thick extract of tobacco called ambil that they rub across their teeth, gums, or tongue. This thick black gelatin is made by boiling tobacco leaves for hours or days and then thickening the extract with starch. Recipes vary; some tribes add pepper, avocado seeds, sugar, or tapioca. Ambil is sometimes ingested with other tobacco products or hallucinogenic drugs.

Using chewing tobacco is practiced by about 2% to 3% of the population in the United States. It is more widely practiced in South America and the West Indies. A person who uses tobacco in this way usually sucks or sometimes chews tobacco quids, which are simply pieces of tobacco made for this purpose. However, the South American and West Indian practices of preparing quids may seem unusual to North Americans. South American and West Indian recipes may include soil, ashes, salt, or honey with the finely crushed tobacco leaves. (North American quids are also flavored in various ways.) South American Indians generally swallow the juices from the tobacco, rather than spit them out.

Another practice among South American Indians that may seem unusual to North Americans is the use of tobacco as an enema or suppository. Generally, these native people use tobacco in this manner to treat constipation or worm infestations. Various tribes of Indians who reside in the mountains of Peru also use tobacco in this way during certain rituals.

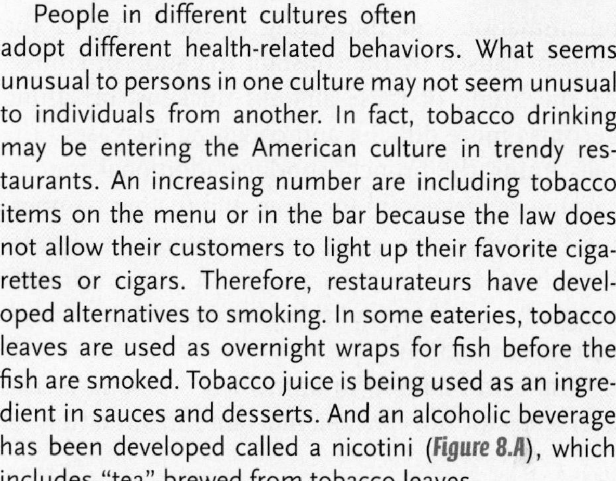

People in different cultures often adopt different health-related behaviors. What seems unusual to persons in one culture may not seem unusual to individuals from another. In fact, tobacco drinking may be entering the American culture in trendy restaurants. An increasing number are including tobacco items on the menu or in the bar because the law does not allow their customers to light up their favorite cigarettes or cigars. Therefore, restaurateurs have developed alternatives to smoking. In some eateries, tobacco leaves are used as overnight wraps for fish before the fish are smoked. Tobacco juice is being used as an ingredient in sauces and desserts. And an alcoholic beverage has been developed called a nicotini (**Figure 8.A**), which includes "tea" brewed from tobacco leaves.

Tobacco drinking? It may be happening at the table next to yours, and its health effects are still to be determined.

Data from Kuntzman, G. (2003, May 19). Tobacco in your tiramisu? Newsweek. Available at http://gershkuntzman.homestead.com/files/tobacco_in_Your_Tiramisu.htm; U.S. Department of Health and Human Services. (1992). Smoking and health in the Americas: A 1992 report of the Surgeon General, in collaboration with the Pan American Health Organization (DHHS Publication No. CDC 92-8419). Atlanta, GA: U.S. Department of Health and Human Services, pp. 19–31.

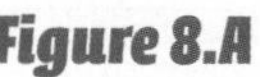

Figure 8.A

The Nicotini. Nicknamed the liquid cigarette, the nicotini is made by soaking tobacco leaves overnight in vodka or other spirits. Nicotine is a powerful, toxic drug, and the amount served in nicotinis is not regulated. Drinking a nicotini may result in unpleasant and harmful side effects.

© PhotoEdit/Alamy Images

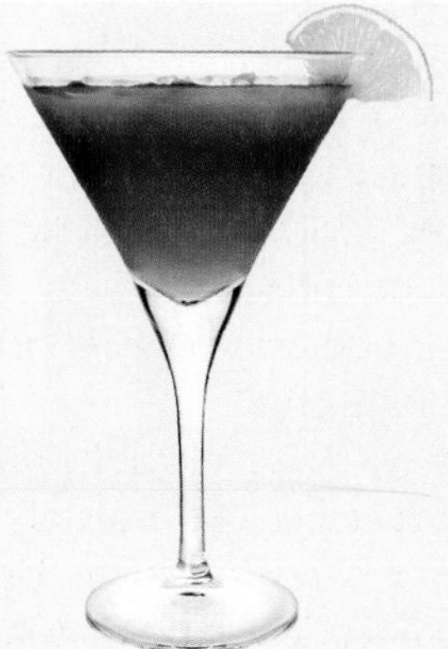

acute bronchitis A temporary inflammation of the mucous membranes of the bronchi.

chronic bronchitis A persistent inflammation and thickening of the lining of the bronchi.

emphysema (EM-fih-SEE-mah) A chronic condition in which the air sacs of the lungs lose their normal elasticity, impairing respiration.

inflammation and thickening of the lining of the bronchi caused by the constant irritation of smoke. As the lining of these airways thickens, breathing becomes more difficult and coughing increases. The cells lining the bronchi produce additional mucus, causing congestion in the lungs and further hampering breathing. The signs and symptoms of chronic bronchitis are shortness of breath and a chronic cough that produces considerable amounts of mucus. Chronic bronchitis is a serious disease that can result in death. In addition to bronchitis, smoking is also a risk factor for *pneumonia*, an inflammation of the lungs that is caused by a variety of bacteria and viruses.

Smoking is also the main cause of **emphysema** (**Figure 8.10**), a condition in which the air sacs of the lungs lose their normal elasticity. Some air sacs become overstretched and eventually rupture, resulting in larger air sacs with less surface area over which gas exchange can take place. Under these conditions, the lungs can no longer accommodate normal amounts of air. Also, without the normal elasticity of the lungs, a person can no longer inhale and exhale normally. Breathing becomes a continual effort.

The lung damage of emphysema can never be repaired. As the disease progresses, the heart becomes increasingly overworked. Because the blood it is pumping is oxygen poor, the body sends signals to the heart to pump more blood more quickly. Eventually the person with extensive lung damage dies, usually from heart failure. However, if emphysema is detected early (especially before symptoms develop), its destructive effects can be halted by stopping smoking.

Figure 8.6

Past Month Cigarette Use Among Persons Aged 12 Years or Older, by Age: 2012. This graph shows that persons aged 21–25 years had the highest prevalence of current smoking in 2012. In general, smoking prevalence declined as age decreased and increased from that peak. There was a slight increase in smoking prevalence in those aged 45 to 54 years from those aged 40 to 44 years, however.

Reproduced from Substance Abuse and Mental Health Services Administration. (2013). Results from the 2012 National Survey on drug use and health: Summary of national findings (HHS Publication No. SMA 13-4795). Retrieved from http://www.samhsa.gov/data/NSDUH/2012SummNatFindDetTables/NationalFindings/NSDUHresults2012.pdf

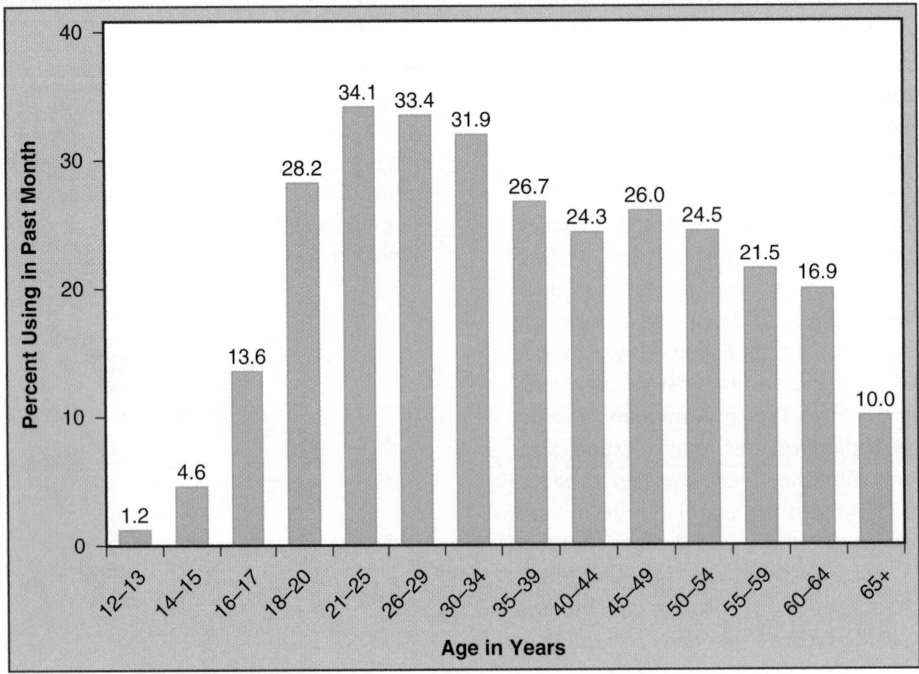

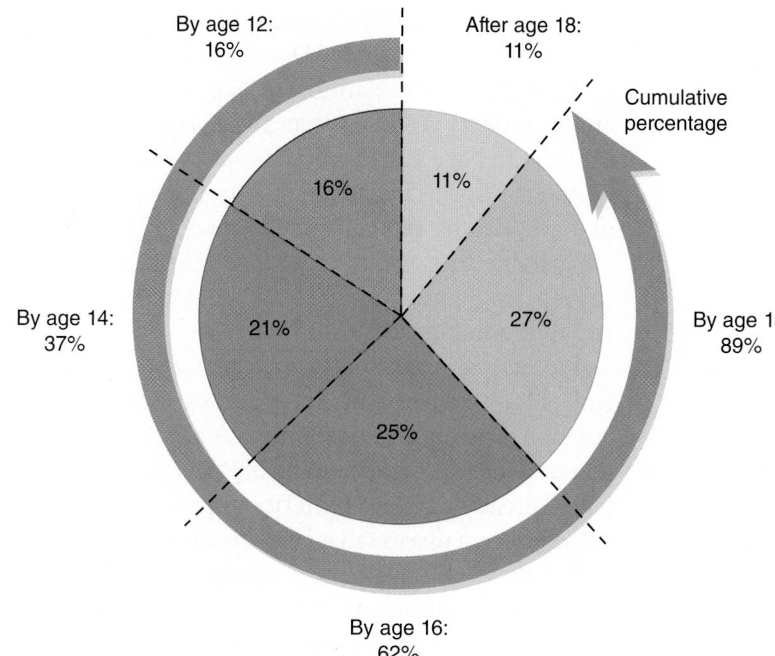

Figure 8.7

Age at Which Adults Say They Started Smoking. Most smokers started this habit when they were in their teens or preteens.
Data from Substance Abuse and Mental Health Services Administration. Office on Smoking and Health, Centers for Disease Control and Prevention.

Figure 8.8

Cigarettes: Trends in Daily Use by Eighth, Tenth, and Twelfth Graders.
Reproduced from Johnston, L. D., et al. (2013). Monitoring the future: National survey results on drug use, 1975–2012: Volume 1, secondary school students. Bethesda, MD: National Institute on Drug Abuse. Retrieved from http://www.monitoringthefuture.org/pubs/monographs/mtf-vol1_2012.pdf

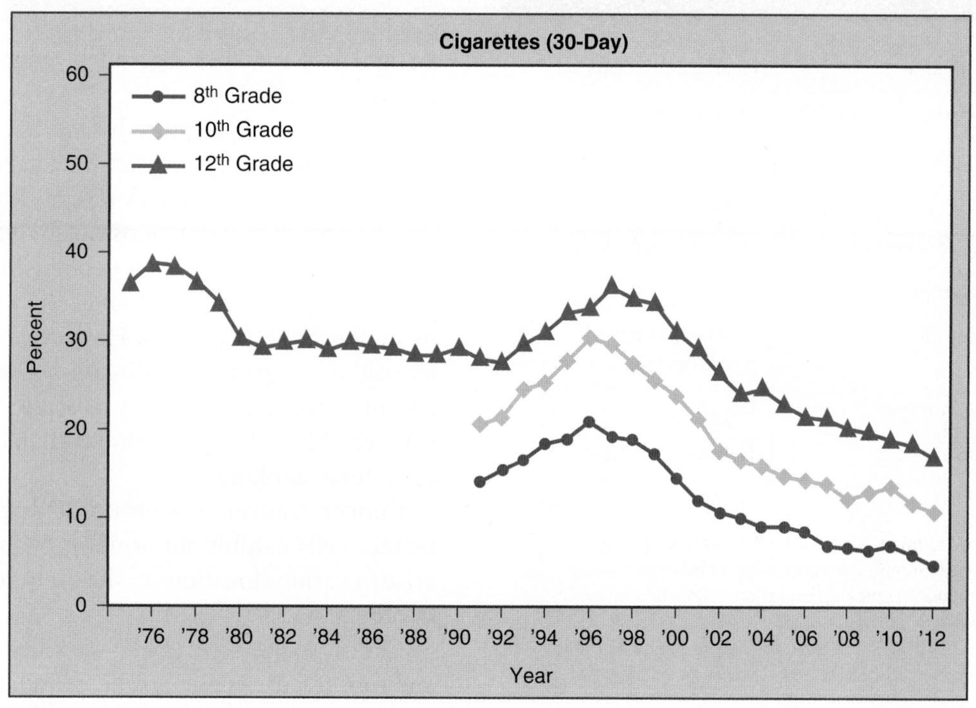

chronic obstructive pulmonary disease (COPD) A syndrome that includes chronic bronchitis, asthma, and emphysema and that is characterized by extreme difficulty in breathing.

cardiovascular disease (CVD) Disorders of the heart and blood vessels.

People with chronic bronchitis and emphysema are said to have **chronic obstructive pulmonary disease (COPD)**. Cigarette smoking is the major cause of COPD; it would probably be a minor health problem if people did not smoke. Smoking is thought to be responsible for approximately 108,000 deaths from COPD per year, or 85% to 90% of all COPD deaths.[31]

Cardiovascular Disease Thirty-one percent of people who die from smoking-related causes die from **cardiovascular disease (CVD)**, or dysfunction of the heart and blood vessels.[32] There is a variety of cardiovascular diseases, including *coronary artery disease (CAD)*, *hypertension* (chronic high blood pressure), and stroke (blood vessel disease of the brain). *Atherosclerosis*, the buildup of fatty deposits in the arteries, is an important cardiovascular disease process that is an underlying cause in CAD and stroke.

According to the National Stroke Association, cigarette smokers are more than twice as likely as nonsmokers to have a stroke because of smoking's effects on the cardiovascular system. As many as one-third of CVD deaths in the United States each year are attributable to cigarette smoking.[30] Using smokeless tobacco is a significant CVD risk factor also, but cigar and pipe smoking are less significant.

Women who take oral contraceptives (birth control pills) and who smoke cigarettes increase their risk of heart attack several times. Oral contraceptives increase the risk of developing blood clots, which can block already narrowed arteries in persons with atherosclerosis, a disease that smokers have an increased risk of developing. For these reasons, smoking while taking oral contraceptives also increases the risk of peripheral vascular disease and stroke.

Smokers often think that smoking low-yield ("light") cigarettes poses fewer health risks than smoking regular-strength cigarettes. Light cigarettes, which began to be marketed in the 1960s in response to health concerns, are lower in tar and nicotine. However, research data show that smokers generally puff on these cigarettes longer and inhale more deeply than when smoking regular cigarettes. Also, they often smoke more light cigarettes than they would regular cigarettes, so they may take in as much tar, nicotine, and other noxious and cancer-causing compounds than if they smoked regular cigarettes. Scientists have found no evidence that smoking low-tar and low-nicotine cigarettes reduces the risk of coronary heart disease.[30]

When a smoker quits, his or her risk of heart disease begins dropping immediately. The time it takes for a former smoker's risk of death from heart attack to reach that of a nonsmoker's varies from 3 to 9 years. The recovery time depends on the number of years a person smoked and how many cigarettes he or she smoked per day. However, if a smoker has already developed heart disease before quitting, the risk of heart attack will not return to that of a nonsmoker, although it will be lower than if he or she had continued smoking.

Cancer Cancer is a group of diseases in which certain cells exhibit abnormal growth. Cancers can arise in various locations in the body and then spread to others.

Cancer is the second biggest killer of Americans, and tobacco use is responsible for about 30% of cancer deaths and 87% of lung cancer deaths annually in

Table 8.9

Typical Symptoms of Nicotine Withdrawal

Anxiety/tension	Heart palpitations
Cough/dry mouth/nasal drip	Impatience
Craving cigarettes	Insomnia
Depression	Irritability
Difficulty concentrating	Loss of energy/fatigue
Disorientation	Restlessness
Dizziness	Stomach or bowel problems/nausea
Excessive hunger	Sweating
Frustration	Tightness in chest
Headaches	Tremors

Data from Shiffman, S., West, R., & Gilbert, D. (2004). Recommendation for the assessment of tobacco craving and withdrawal in smoking cessation trials. *Nicotine and Tobacco Research*, 6, 599–614.; Gritz, E. R., Carr, C. R., & Marcus, A. C. (1991). The tobacco withdrawal syndrome in unaided quitters. *British Journal of Addiction*, 86(1), 57–69.

periodontal (PER-ee-oh-DON-tal) disease A disorder of the tissues that support the teeth.

the United States.[33] Tobacco use causes or is related to cancers of the lungs, larynx, oral cavity, esophagus, kidneys, bladder, pancreas, stomach, and cervix (see Figure 8.9). Lung cancer is the most prevalent form of cancer caused by tobacco use.

Periodontal Disease Smoking tobacco and using smokeless tobacco can have serious effects on the oral cavity. These effects can range from embarrassing problems such as bad breath and stained teeth to life-threatening conditions such as oral cancer (**Figure 8.11**).

People who use tobacco products regularly, often develop **periodontal disease,** commonly known as gum disease. Periodontal disease is actually more than just disease of the gums. It is a disease of all the supporting tissues around the teeth, which include the gums, the bone in which the teeth are embedded, and the ligaments that hold the teeth to the bone.

People can develop periodontal disease for a variety of reasons, such as poor dental hygiene, overzealous brushing that damages the gums, and clenching and grinding of the teeth. Using tobacco products is especially destructive to the gums and often is a cause of severe periodontal disease. Nicotine narrows the blood vessels in the gums, reducing the amount of oxygen that reaches these tissues. As a result, the gum tissue becomes less resistant to infection. Additionally, good oral hygiene and proper periodontal treatment are often ineffective when a person with periodontal disease continues to use tobacco.

Young people who use smokeless tobacco products often develop periodontal disease. Gum recession most often occurs at places where smokeless tobacco is held in the mouth. *Leukoplakia*, a disease characterized by precancerous white patches that develop on the mucous membranes of the mouth (**Figure 8.12**), is common in adolescents who use these products. Approximately 5% of these lesions become cancerous within 5 years. However, if a smokeless tobacco user discontinues use, the leukoplakia regresses and may disappear.

Osteoporosis Smoking cigarettes can lead to lower bone density, or osteoporosis, which occurs most frequently in postmenopausal white women. This disease is serious because it places women at risk for bone fractures, back pain, and other accompanying problems. Hip fractures are particularly serious; the death rate for people who sustain hip fractures is 20% to 24% higher in the year following the fracture than for people of the same age who did not sustain this injury.[34]

Environmental Tobacco Smoke

In the past 3 decades, nonsmokers have become increasingly aware that smoke in their indoor environments could pose a health risk. This smoke,

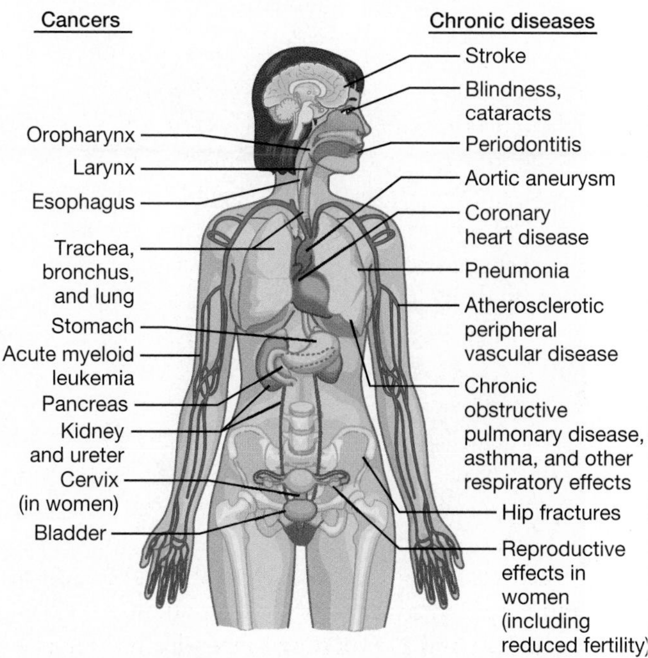

Figure 8.9

Smoking Cigarettes Can Cause These Cancers and Chronic Diseases.

Reproduced from U.S. Department of Health and Human Services. (2010). How Tobacco Smoke Causes Disease: The Biology and Behavioral Basis for Smoking-AttribuTable Disease: A Report of the Surgeon General. Atlanta, GA: U.S. Department of Health and Human Services. Retrieved April 3, 2011 from http://www.surgeongeneral.gov/library/tobaccosmoke/report/full_report.pdf

environmental tobacco smoke (ETS) The smoke emitted from a lit cigarette, cigar, or pipe and the smoke exhaled by smokers.

termed **environmental tobacco smoke (ETS)** or *secondhand smoke*, is made up of the sidestream smoke emitted from a lit cigarette, cigar, or pipe and the smoke exhaled by smokers.

In 1986, the National Research Council (NRC) and the United States Surgeon General's Office compiled research data to assess the health effects of exposure to ETS[35,36] Both landmark reports conclude that ETS can cause lung cancer in adult nonsmokers. In 2006, the Surgeon General's Office released another report on secondhand smoke: *The Health Consequences of Involuntary Exposure to Tobacco Smoke*.[37] At the press release of the report, Surgeon General Richard H. Carmona stated, "The debate is over. The science is clear: secondhand smoke is not a mere annoyance, but a serious health hazard that causes premature death and disease in children and nonsmoking adults."

Conclusions from these reports prompted the designation of governmental and other public buildings, many workplaces, and restaurants in many states as smoke-free environments to reduce the effects of ETS on the public. By 1993, nearly 82% of indoor workers were restricted from smoking in their workplaces.[38] By 2006, almost all workplaces, governmental buildings, and public places in the United States were smoke free.[37] However, if a "smoke-free" area is

Figure 8.10

A Healthy Lung and a Lung from a Person with Emphysema. (a) The healthy lung is smooth, a deep pink, and relatively uniform in color. (b) Due to emphysema, some of the alveoli have ruptured, creating tiny craters within the lung, which are difficult to see in this picture. Note the blackened tissue as a result of years of smoking.

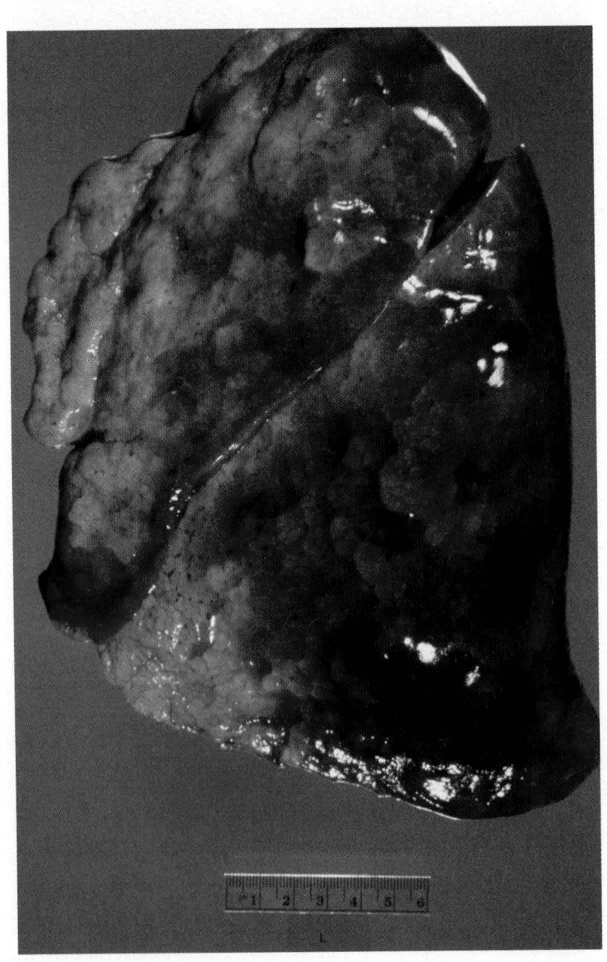

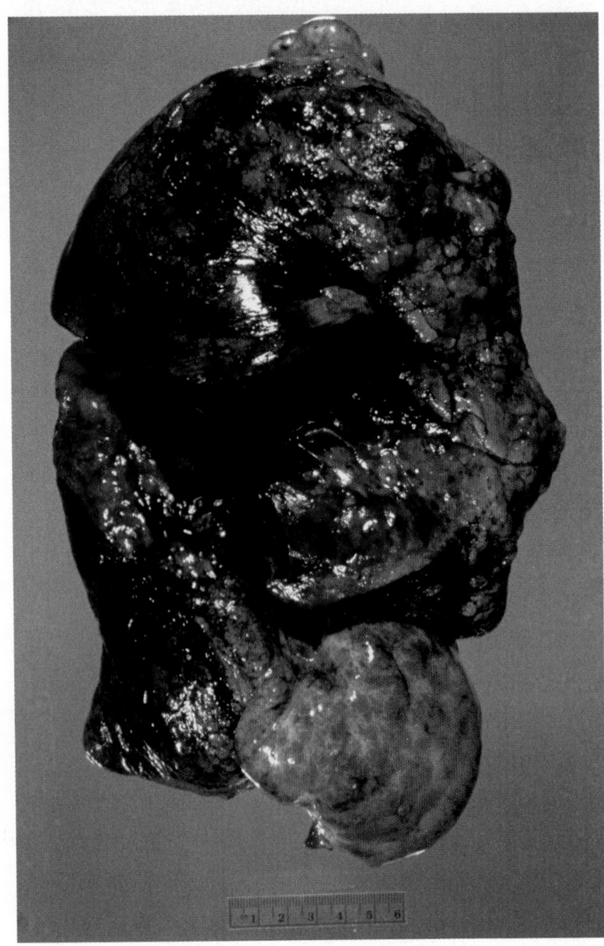

Figure 8.11

Gruen Von Behrens, After Using Smokeless Tobacco. Gruen began using smokeless (spit) tobacco at age 13, and by age 17 he had oral cancer and a 25% chance of survival. Formerly a star baseball player, Gruen can no longer play sports, and after 40 operations he is still missing his lower teeth and jawbone. His body rejected a bone transplant that would have created a new jaw. Gruen is now a spokesperson for Oral Health America's National Spit Tobacco Education Program (NSTEP), warning audiences of the dangers of using smokeless tobacco.

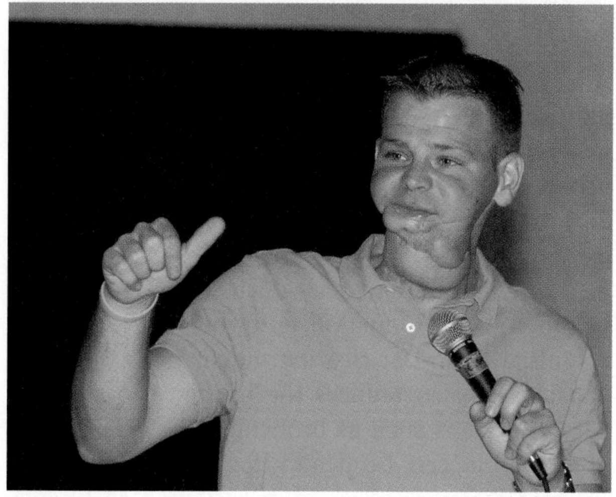

Figure 8.12

Advanced Leukoplakia. This precancerous condition often develops on the mucous membranes of the mouths of those who use smokeless tobacco products.

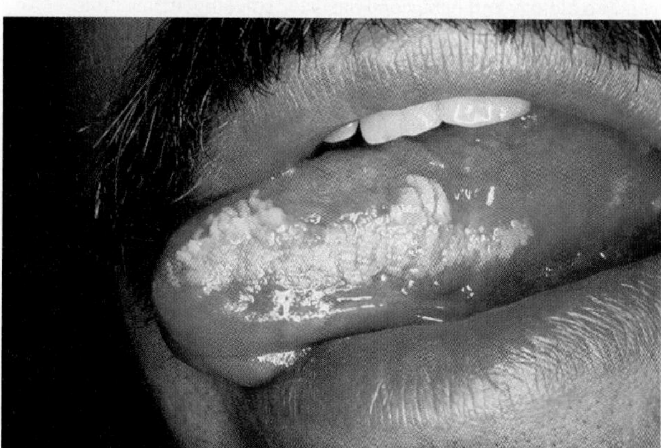

adjacent to a smoking area it will contain unacceptable levels of airborne pollutants unless the two areas have separate ventilation systems.

Figure 8.13 shows the health consequences of repeated exposure to secondhand smoke for both children and adults. Avoiding secondhand smoke will help you stay healthier. The Managing Your Health box includes tips on how to say no to secondhand smoke.

Quitting

Most smokers want to quit. In a 2013 Gallup poll, 74% of smokers told Gallup interviewers that they would like to give up cigarettes. Eighty-six percent of smokers said that they think secondhand smoke is very or somewhat harmful to health, and 95% of smokers reported that they think smoking is very or somewhat harmful to health.[39]

Benefits of Quitting At any age, there are many reasons to stop smoking cigarettes. Some of those reasons are to lower your risk of various diseases and conditions including certain cancers, heart attack, stroke, and chronic lung disease; in pregnant women, to reduce the risk of having a low-birth-weight baby; to stop exposing your family and other people around you to secondhand smoke; to rid yourself of a stale cigarette odor on your body and breath; and to rid yourself of an expensive addiction to nicotine.

On quitting, an addicted smoker experiences some or all of the nicotine withdrawal symptoms listed in Table 8.9. These unpleasant psychological and physiologic conditions peak 1 to 2 days following quitting but subside during the following weeks. The two withdrawal symptoms that last the longest are the urge to smoke and an increased appetite. However, using a nicotine replacement therapy product, such as the nicotine patch, nicotine gum, or nicotine inhaler; buproprion (an antidepressant used to treat nicotine dependence); or varenicline (Chantix) during the early cessation period may help reduce these symptoms and make quitting easier. Varenicline eases withdrawal symptoms by providing some nicotine effects to the brain while simultaneously blocking the effects of nicotine from cigarettes. Of these therapies, varenicline appears to be the most effective.[40]

Electronic cigarettes, or *e-cigarettes*, which are marketed as an alternative cigarette and as a quitting aid, have been cited by the FDA for "unsubstantiated claims and poor manufacturing practices."[41] For example, the FDA found nicotine in e-cigarettes labeled as having no nicotine and similarly labeled e-cigarettes as delivering differing amounts of nicotine.[42] Most e-cigarettes are manufactured to look

Figure 8.13

The Health Consequences of Repeated Exposure to Secondhand Smoke.

Reproduced from U.S. Department of Health and Human Services. (2010). How tobacco smoke causes disease: The biology and behavioral basis for smoking-attribuTable disease: A report of the surgeon general. Atlanta, GA: U.S. DepArtment of Health and Human Services. Retrieved on April 3, 2011, from http://www.surgeongeneral.gov/library/tobaccosmoke/report/full_report.pdf

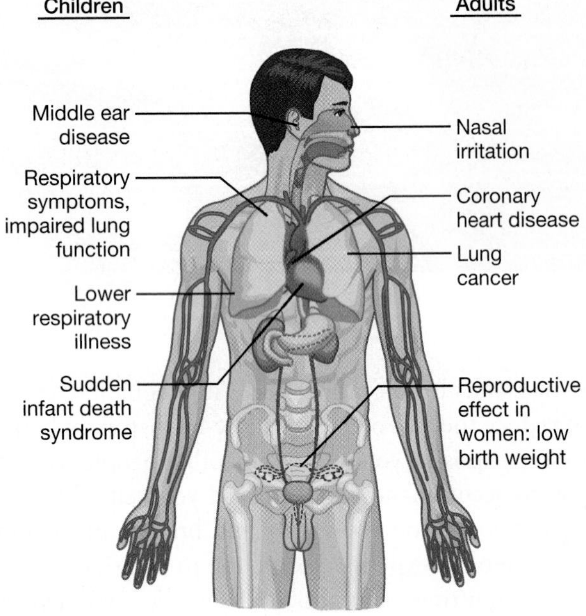

like cigarettes and contain a stainless steel shell encasing a heating element, a chemical-containing cartridge, and an atomizer that vapo rizes the chemicals when heated (**Figure 8.14**). The vapor is inhaled. Only e-cigarettes marketed for therapeutic purposes are regulated by the FDA.

Availability of e-cigarettes could also create potential health risks for nonsmokers. Some researchers have warned that cheap pricing, availability of many flavors, and celebrity promotional activities, which are clearly targeted at adolescents, will increase use and lead to higher rates of nicotine addiction among young people.[43] Results from the 2012 National Youth Tobacco Survey indicated 20.3% of high school students have tried e-cigarettes, and 7.2% who have tried e-cigarettes reported never smoking conventional cigarettes.[44] These data suggest that "vaping" is becoming more popular among adolescents. Because e-cigarettes are relatively new, it is important to note that short- and long-term impact of e-cigarette use on health is unclear.

A promising quitting aid is the nicotine addiction vaccine, which was in late-stage clinical trials in early 2011. The vaccine, called NicVAX, works by stimulating the body to produce antibodies against nicotine so that the drug cannot get to the brain, stimulate pleasure centers, and reinforce the craving for nicotine. In an early trial of 1,000 smokers who wanted to quit, NicVax did spur production of antibodies against nicotine as expected; however, no significant improvement in smoking cessation rate was found over the placebo group. Researchers are currently studying whether vaccines, such as NicVax, along with evidence-based smoking cessation programs can increase the rate or quitting.

During the quitting process, as withdrawal symptoms subside, former smokers report that favorable psychological changes occur over time, such as enhanced self-esteem and an increased sense of self-control. Because smoking cigarettes has negative effects on the respiratory system, a person who quits notices that it is easier to breathe. Smoking cessation reduces the rate at which symptoms such as cough, mucus production, and wheezing occur after an initial period of clearing mucus from the lungs subsides. It also reduces the incidence of respiratory infections such as bronchitis and pneumonia. (Pneumonia can be deadly for people who have chronic diseases.) Also, after sustained abstinence from smoking cigarettes, persons with COPD have less chance of dying from this disease than they did before they quit.

Quitting also has positive effects on the cardiovascular system. Data show that the smoker who quits cuts his or her elevated risk of coronary heart disease in half only 1 year after quitting. The degree of risk that remains then declines gradually. At 15 years, a former smoker reaches the risk level of a nonsmoker for coronary heart disease and death.[45] The more cigarettes a person smoked and the earlier a person started to smoke, the longer the recovery time. Because the risk of cardiovascular disease increases as the number of cigarettes smoked increases, smoking fewer cigarettes can be a way to lower CVD risk if an individual has little success quitting. However, smoking low-yield (low tar and nicotine) cigarettes does not appear to reduce risk. Among persons diagnosed with cardiovascular disease, smoking cessation markedly reduces the risk of additional heart attacks and cardiovascular death. The benefits of quitting exist for people of all ages. Older individuals should not think that it is "too late" to quit.

Managing Your Health

How to Say No to Secondhand Smoke

If you live with a smoker:

- Ask him or her not to smoke in your home. Discuss how his or her habit puts you and others living there at risk.
- If he or she is unwilling to go outside, suggest ways to limit the exposure to smoke for you and others. Maybe a room could be set aside for smoking—one that is seldom used by other members of the household. Some smokers protect others at home by smoking near an open window or when no one is around.
- Keep rooms well ventilated. Open windows.
- Support smokers who decide to quit.

When visitors come:

- Ask all smokers who visit not to smoke in your house or apartment, but to please smoke outside.
- Do not keep ashtrays around.

In others' homes or in vehicles:

- Tell friends and relatives politely that you would appreciate their not smoking while you are there.
- Let people know when their smoke is causing immediate problems. If it is making your allergies worse, making you cough or wheeze, or making your eyes sting, say so. Some smokers put their cigarettes away when they see the discomfort it causes.

If you have children:

- Insist that babysitters, grandparents, and other caregivers not smoke around your children.
- Help children avoid secondhand smoke if smokers do use tobacco around them. Have them leave the room or play outside while an adult is smoking. Air rooms out after smoking occurs.
- Keep smokers away from places in which children sleep.

When smoking is allowed at the workplace:

- Talk to your employer about the company's smoking policy. Give your employer copies of the Environmental Protection Agency (EPA) report on the harmful effects of environmental tobacco smoke. Call 1-800-438-4318 to obtain this report.
- Ask to work near other nonsmokers and as far away from smokers as possible.
- Ask smokers if they would not smoke around you.
- Use a fan and open windows (if possible) to keep air moving.
- Hang a Thank You for Not Smoking sign in your work area.
- Volunteer to help develop a fair company policy that protects nonsmokers.
- Contact the local Lung Association, the American Cancer Society, or the National Cancer Institute (1-800-4-CANCER) for information concerning smoking cessation programs that can be conducted at your workplace.

When you are in public places:

- Always take the nonsmoking options that are available in rental cars, hotels, and restaurants.
- If a restaurant puts you at a table near smokers (even if you are in a nonsmoking section), ask to move.
- Keep children out of smoking areas.

Adapted from National Cancer Institute. (n.d.). I mind very much if you smoke. Retrieved from http://dccps.nci.nih.gov/tcrb/i_mind_if_you_smoke/mindsmo.html

Quitting reduces cancer risk. In 5 years after quitting, the excess risk has been cut in half of developing mouth, throat, esophagus, and bladder cancers, and the excess risk of cervical cancer has been eliminated. In 10 years after quitting, the excess risk of dying from lung cancer is cut in half and the risk of cancer of the larynx and pancreas decreases.[45] **Figure 8.15** is a visual summary of the health benefits of quitting smoking.

The Process of Quitting Cigarette smoking is an addiction, and an addicted smoker who is quitting goes through the same process of behavioral change as does anyone addicted to any drug. For a smoker to contemplate quitting, he or she must understand and accept that cigarette smoking is dangerous or must have other reasons for quitting that are important to him or her. Then, the smoker begins to see the potential benefits and negative effects associated with quitting. For example, the smoker may realize that nicotine is a drug and that he or she is addicted to this drug. Quitting will stop the addiction. However, along with this positive behavior (stopping the

Figure 8.14

The Anatomy of an E-cigarette. An electronic cigarette has a stainless steel casing that is often manufactured to look like a filter-tipped cigarette, but may look like a pen or a thumb drive for those who wish to conceal their use of the product. Internally, the e-cigarette contains a heating element, a chemical-containing cartridge, and a vaporizing unit.

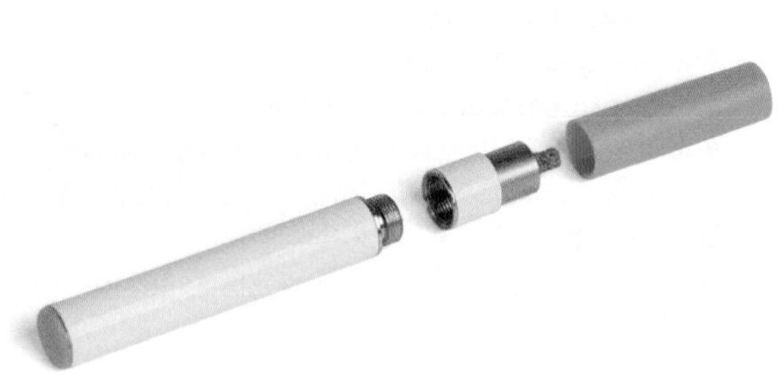

addiction) comes negative consequences: withdrawal symptoms. To be prepared to quit, the smoker should analyze both the negative and positive aspects of change and prepare to deal with the negative aspects. Often, discussion with a medical practitioner is helpful. Also, if a smoker analyzes the reasons he or she smokes (see "Why Do You Smoke?" in the Student Workbook pages at the end of this text), the smoker will be better equipped to handle the consequences of quitting (see the Managing Your Health box "Tips for Quitters").

Once the smoker realizes the need to quit, he or she should decide what course of action to take. Should it be quitting "cold turkey" or cutting down at first? (If a person is addicted to nicotine, stopping "cold turkey" may be best. The assessment activity "Why Do You Smoke?" can help identify addiction.) Will the smoker join a smoking cessation program or stop without group support? Again, the advice of a medical practitioner may be helpful at this stage. A smoker can also call the American Lung Association, the American Heart Association, the American Cancer Society, or the National Cancer Institute for free literature on quitting and information on smoking cessation programs. Many programs are available, and the smoker needs to select the program that suits his or her needs best. Medication may also be helpful at this stage, such as a nicotine replacement product, buproprion, or varenicline to lessen the withdrawal symptoms from nicotine. Also, the smoker may enlist the support of family and friends through the quitting process.

After the first 6 months, which is considered the *quitting period*, the former smoker enters the period of *maintenance*, which lasts 6 months also. Some quitters who join smoking cessation programs continue to attend group meetings for support. Others get continued support from friends, family members, or other former smokers.

As with other addictions, sometimes *relapse* occurs. During a relapse, a former smoker returns to smoking habits. Relapse can be triggered by a variety of factors such as stress, depression, a craving for cigarettes, negative life events, and interpersonal tensions. To quit, the relapsed smoker goes through the stages of behavior change once again.

One barrier to quitting is the smoker's fear of gaining weight. In fact, about 25% of smokers cite this possibility as the reason for not quitting. Likewise, about 25% of people who quit relapse because they begin to gain weight and are afraid of gaining more. This fear is not unfounded—80% of persons who quit smoking gain weight. Data show, however, that the average weight gain is only 6 to 9 pounds and the risk of large weight gain is extremely low. Individuals who smoked heavily gain the most weight after quitting.

People gain weight when they stop smoking for two reasons: They eat more (often to put something other than a cigarette into their mouths) and their metabolism slows slightly. To combat this effect, as part of your smoking cessation plan be sure to include an exercise program to maintain your metabolic rate. Also, keep fat-free, low-calorie snacks handy, such as slices of vegetables with low-fat dip, fruits, pretzels, and sugar-free gelatin.

Prevention

Prevention programs developed in the 1980s reflect an understanding that smoking begins in early adolescence and that young people go through stages in the development of smoking behavior (see the section titled "Psychosocial Reasons for Using Tobacco Products" earlier in this chapter). Today's programs also recognize that a child's social environment is the most important determinant of whether he or she will smoke. Therefore, prevention programs now target seventh and eighth graders, reaching children before most start smoking. Their focus is on helping

Figure 8.15

The Health Benefits of Quitting Smoking. The risks of developing many diseases and conditions drop dramatically, in varied lengths of time, after a person quits smoking.
Modified from Centers for Disease Control and Prevention. (2004). The benefits of quitting. Retrieved April 4, 2011, from http://www.cdc.gov/tobacco/data_statistics/sgr/2004/posters/benefits/index.htm

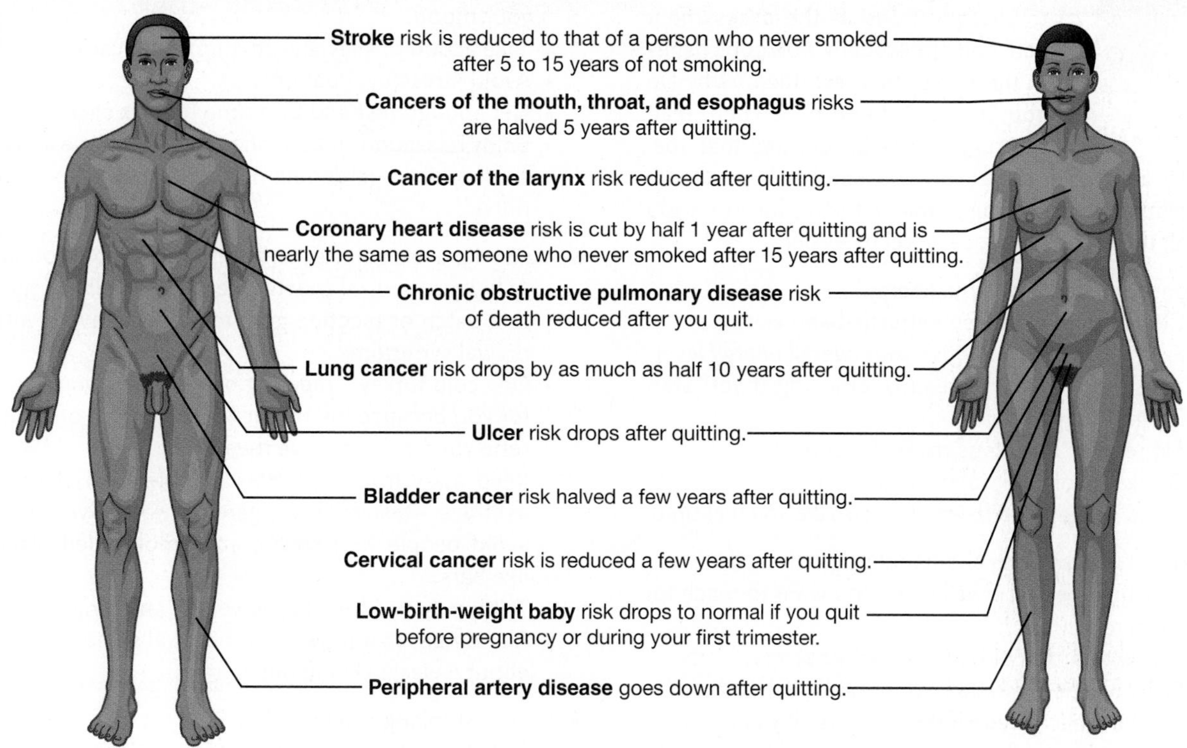

young people develop skills to identify and resist social influences to smoke, such as advertising and peer pressure. Additionally, they educate adolescents about the short-term negative effects of tobacco use. Understanding short-term consequences positively affects adolescent behavior more than knowledge of long-term effects. Data show that several types of prevention programs delay or reduce youth tobacco use for periods of 1 to 5 years and more. Effective prevention programs engage the school, parents, and media.

Stroke risk is reduced to that of a person who never smoked after 5 to 15 years of not smoking.
Cancers of the mouth, throat, and esophagus risks are halved 5 years after quitting.
Cancer of the larynx risk reduced after quitting.
Coronary heart disease risk is cut by half 1 year after quitting and is nearly the same as someone who never smoked after 15 years after quitting.
Chronic obstructive pulmonary disease risk of death reduced after you quit.
Lung cancer risk drops by as much as half 10 years after quitting.
Ulcer risk drops after quitting.
Bladder cancer risk halved a few years after quitting.
Cervical cancer risk is reduced a few years after quitting.
Low-birth-weight baby risk drops to normal if you quit before pregnancy or during your first trimester.
Peripheral artery disease goes down after quitting.

Other programs have been developed that focus on smokeless tobacco use. The goal of these programs is to counter the perception that smokeless tobacco is a safe alternative to smoking cigarettes.

Reducing the availability of cigarettes to adolescents is another prevention measure. Unfortunately, adolescents can get cigarettes quite easily even though the sale of tobacco products to minors is illegal in all states and the District of Columbia. One of the goals of *Healthy People 2020* is to enforce laws that prohibit sales to minors to reduce the percentage of minors who successfully purchase cigarettes to 5%.

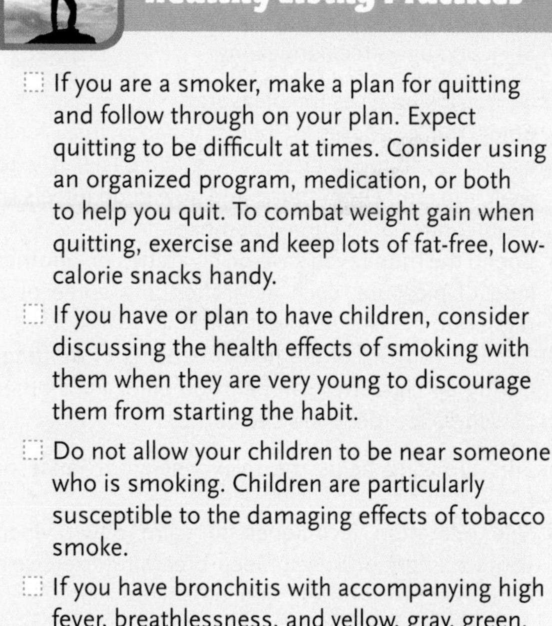

© djgis/ShutterStock

Healthy Living Practices

- If you are a smoker, make a plan for quitting and follow through on your plan. Expect quitting to be difficult at times. Consider using an organized program, medication, or both to help you quit. To combat weight gain when quitting, exercise and keep lots of fat-free, low-calorie snacks handy.
- If you have or plan to have children, consider discussing the health effects of smoking with them when they are very young to discourage them from starting the habit.
- Do not allow your children to be near someone who is smoking. Children are particularly susceptible to the damaging effects of tobacco smoke.
- If you have bronchitis with accompanying high fever, breathlessness, and yellow, gray, green, or bloody sputum, seek medical attention immediately.

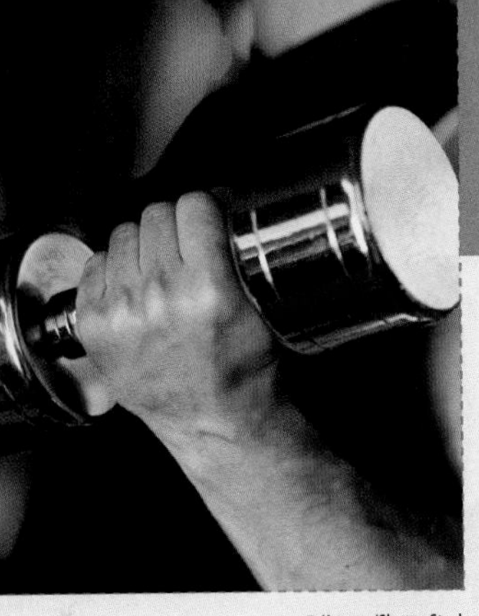
© Kzenon/ShutterStock

Managing Your Health

Tips for Quitters

If you smoke and have not responded to the questions in the assessment activity in the Student Workbook pages at the end of this text titled "Why Do You Smoke?" do so now. Then, read the suggestions for quitting that specifically address each reason you smoke. If you tailor your plan to quit smoking to match the reasons that you smoke, the cessation process will be easier.

Reason: "Smoking gives me energy."

- Get enough rest to feel refreshed and alert.
- Exercise regularly to raise your overall energy level.
- Take a brisk walk instead of smoking if you start feeling sluggish.
- Eat regular, nutritious meals for energy.
- Drink lots of cold water to refresh you.
- Avoid getting bored, which can make you feel tired.

Reason: "I like to touch and handle cigarettes."

- Pick up a pen or pencil when you want to reach for a cigarette.
- Play with a coin or handle nearby objects.
- Put a plastic cigarette in your hand or mouth.
- Hold a real cigarette if the touch is all you miss.
- Eat regular meals to avoid confusing the desire to eat with the desire to put a cigarette in your mouth.
- Take up a hobby such as knitting or carpentry that keeps your hands busy.
- Eat low-fat, low-sugar snacks such as carrot sticks or bread sticks.
- Suck on sugar-free hard candy.

Reason: "Smoking gives me pleasure."

- Enjoy the pleasures of being tobacco free, such as how good foods taste; how much easier it is to walk, run, and climb stairs; and how good it feels to be in control of the urge to smoke.
- Spend the money you save on cigarettes on another kind of pleasure, such as a shopping spree or a night out.
- Remind yourself of the health benefits of quitting. Giving up cigarettes can help you enjoy life's other pleasures for many years to come.

Reason: "Smoking helps me relax when I'm tense or upset."

- Use relaxation techniques to calm down when you are angry or upset. Deep breathing exercises, muscle relaxation, and imagining yourself in a peaceful setting can make you feel less stressed.
- Exercise regularly to relieve tension and improve your mood.
- Take action to alleviate situations that cause stress.
- Avoid stressful situations.
- Get enough rest and take time to relax each day.
- Enjoy relaxation. Take a long, hot bath. Have a massage. Lie in a garden hammock. Listen to soothing music.

Reason: "I crave cigarettes and am addicted to nicotine."

- Ask your medical practitioner about using a nicotine patch or nicotine gum to help you avoid withdrawal symptoms.
- Go "cold turkey." Tapering off probably won't work for you because the moment you put out one cigarette you begin to crave the next.
- Keep away from cigarettes completely. Get rid of ashtrays. Destroy any cigarettes you have. Try to avoid people who smoke and smoke-filled places like bars.
- Tell family and friends you've quit smoking.
- Remember that physical withdrawal symptoms last about 2 weeks. Hang on!

Reason: "Smoking is a habit."

- Cut down gradually. Smoke fewer cigarettes each day or only smoke them halfway down. Inhale less often and less deeply. After several months it should be easier to stop completely.
- Change your smoking routines. Keep your cigarettes in a different place. Smoke with your opposite hand. Do not do anything else while smoking. Limit smoking to certain places, such as outside or in one room at home.
- When you want a cigarette, wait 1 minute. Do something else instead of smoking.
- Be aware of every cigarette you smoke. Ask yourself, "Do I really want this cigarette?" You may be surprised at how many you can easily pass up.
- Set a date for giving up smoking altogether and stick to it.

Adapted from National Cancer Institute. (1993). *Learning why you smoke can teach you how to quit*. Washington, DC: U.S. Department of Health and Human Services.

- If you have a smoker's cough that produces considerable amounts of mucus and shortness of breath, seek medical attention immediately because you may have chronic bronchitis, a serious disease.
- See your healthcare provider regularly for an evaluation of your respiratory system.
- If you are a nonsmoker, avoid areas where cigarette smoke is present. Breathing in this smoke increases your risk of developing heart disease, lung cancer, and various respiratory diseases and conditions.
- If you use tobacco products, you can reduce your risk of developing various cancers, cardiovascular disease, and periodontal disease by quitting.
- If you are female and smoke cigarettes, you have a higher risk of developing osteoporosis than nonsmoking women. To reduce this risk, stop smoking.

fetal alcohol spectrum disorders (FASDs) A variety of incurable conditions and birth defects caused by alcohol exposure during prenatal development.

fetal alcohol syndrome (FAS) The most severe FASD. Children born with FAS may suffer mental retardation and have characteristic facial anomalies, growth deficiency, and central nervous system abnormalities.

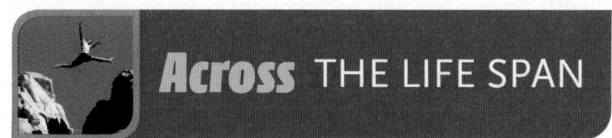

THE EFFECTS OF ALCOHOL AND TOBACCO USE

Fetuses and infants are significantly affected by the alcohol and tobacco use of their mothers. Babies of women who consume alcohol while pregnant may be born with certain incurable birth defects caused by alcohol exposure during prenatal development. These disorders range in their severity and effects; the phrase **fetal alcohol spectrum disorders (FASDs)** refers to the entire group of disorders. The various effects seen in FASDs include growth deficiencies, brain dysfunctions, distinctive facial features, and structural birth defects. One of the most severe of these disorders is **fetal alcohol syndrome (FAS)**.

The predominant feature of FAS is brain effects and may include mental retardation. This syndrome is also characterized by slowed growth both before and after birth; other central nervous system defects, such as behavioral problems, and skull or brain malformations; and characteristic facial features that include small eye openings, a broad thin upper lip, and a flattened nose bridge and midface (**Figure 8.16**).

Researchers have not determined an exact relationship between the amount and timing of drinking during pregnancy and the effects on the fetus. Thus, *there is no identified safe level of alcohol consumption during pregnancy*. Women who are pregnant, who are trying to get pregnant, or who are of childbearing age, sexually active, and not using contraception consistently and well should refrain from drinking to avoid exposing their fetus to alcohol in the womb. In 2012, the prevalence of current alcohol consumption in pregnant women aged 15 to 44 years was 8.5%, and the prevalence of binge drinking was 2.7%. Heavy alcohol use was rare (0.3%).[4]

Figure 8.16

Garrison Lee, a Victim of Fetal Alcohol Syndrome, Who Has Lived on the Streets of Gallup, N.M., for 11 Years. Garrison exhibits features characteristic of FAS: small eye openings, a broad, thin upper lip, and a flattened nose bridge and mid-face.

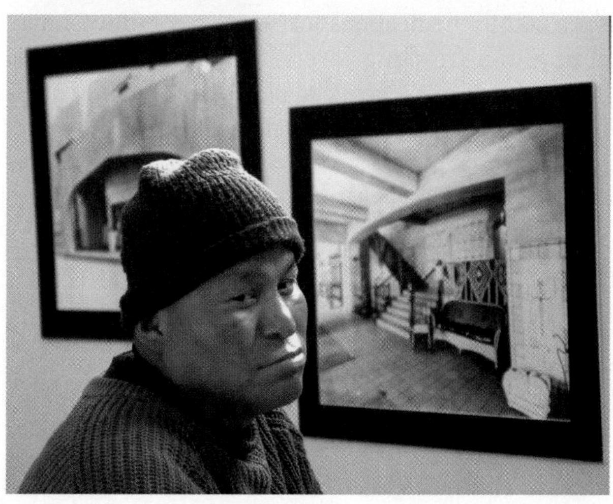

Maternal smoking during pregnancy can harm not only the fetus, but the pregnant woman as well. Abruptio placentae occurs when the placenta separates from the uterus, resulting in hemorrhage (life-threatening bleeding). (The placenta is an organ shared with the mother through which the fetus obtains nutrients and oxygen, and excretes wastes.) Maternal smoking is associated not only with abruptio placentae but also with placenta previa, in which the placenta implants abnormally and covers the opening of the cervical canal. As this opening dilates at the beginning of the birth process, bleeding and severe hemorrhage can occur.

Smoking during pregnancy also reduces the flow of blood in the placenta, limits the nutrients that reach the fetus, and causes an average reduction in birth weight.[46] Additionally, the fetuses or infants of women who smoke during pregnancy are 25% to 30% more likely to die between 28 weeks of gestation and 4 weeks after birth than those of women who do not smoke. Babies born of mothers who smoke also have a higher than average incidence of death from *sudden infant death syndrome (SIDS)* and from respiratory diseases. The sudden, unexpected death of an apparently healthy infant, SIDS occurs while the baby is sleeping. It is the most common cause of death of children between the ages of 2 weeks and 1 year.

During 2011–2012, the percentage of women who smoked during pregnancy was 15.9%. Pregnant young women 18 to 25 years old had the highest rate of smoking among pregnant women—20.9%.[4]

Another age group of persons strongly affected by alcohol and tobacco use is the elderly. Because older adults are more physically vulnerable to the effects of alcohol, they may develop alcohol problems even though their formerly unproblematic patterns of drinking have not changed. Alcohol also reacts adversely with many medications. Elderly persons taking medications for various conditions may appear to be reacting adversely to their medications rather than experiencing an alcohol problem. If alcohol worsens their health, their healthcare providers may prescribe additional or different medications. A vicious cycle of drug interactions and health complications may continue until the healthcare practitioner recognizes that the patient has an alcohol problem.

Older adults face special harm from smoking because most people older than 65 years of age who smoke have been doing so for 30, 40, or 50 years. As a result, a disproportionate number of elderly persons develop life-threatening diseases such as cancer and emphysema because these diseases usually take decades to develop.

Among those older than 65 years, the death rate of current smokers is twice that of people who never smoked. Smoking is associated with a variety of other ailments that are often seen in older adults, such as cataracts (a loss of transparency of the lens of the eye), delayed healing of broken bones, periodontal problems, ulcers, high blood pressure, brain hemorrhages, and skin wrinkles. Additionally, heavy smoking in middle age more than doubles the risk of Alzheimer's disease and other dementias later in life.[47]

From prenatal development to the elderly years, no one who uses alcohol or tobacco products, or breathes in smoke from others' use, can escape their health effects. Except in pregnant women, one drink per day for women and two drinks per day for men may confer health advantages, however.

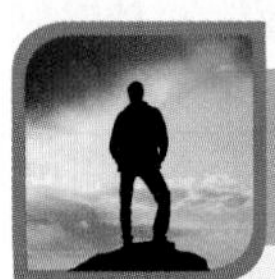

© djgis/ShutterStock

Healthy Living Practices

- Do not consume alcoholic beverages when pregnant because alcohol exposure can result in incurable lifelong disabilities in the fetus.
- Smoking during pregnancy is associated with serious, and possibly deadly, health effects in both the mother and the fetus.

CHAPTER REVIEW

Summary

Drinking alcohol and smoking cigarettes are behaviors that often begin in adolescence. Alcohol use is quite prevalent in the United States; 52.1% of Americans use alcohol. Some people use alcohol responsibly, not allowing their drinking to threaten their health or interfere with their relationships. In contrast, the harmful user drinks alcoholic beverages while knowingly damaging his or her health. The alcohol-dependent person, or alcoholic, additionally develops tolerance to the drug, exhibits withdrawal symptoms when not drinking, compulsively uses alcohol, and may exhibit other behaviors that are a part of the alcohol dependence syndrome.

The cause of alcoholism is unknown. However, alcoholism has a genetic (hereditary) component. People abuse alcoholic beverages and become alcohol dependent for psychological, social, and developmental reasons as well.

When a person drinks alcoholic beverages, various behavioral changes that are commonly called intoxication result from impairment of the central nervous system. The harmful use and abuse of alcohol results in multiple effects on the body that are significant threats to health. Excessive alcohol consumption exerts its most dangerous effects on the liver, cardiovascular system, immune system, reproductive system, and brain. Alcohol use and abuse are also related to serious and even fatal injuries.

Approximately 2.5 million Americans were treated for alcohol abuse and dependence in 2012. Alcohol abuse and dependence are often detected by the use of screening tests. Healthcare professionals who determine that their patients are alcohol dependent refer them to substance abuse specialists for evaluation and possibly treatment. Patients who show nondependent problem drinking are often encouraged to participate in brief intervention programs. Self-help groups support the alcoholic on a long-term basis to help prevent relapse into abusive or dependent behaviors.

Cigarettes are the most prevalent type of tobacco product used in the United States today. Approximately 22% of Americans smoked cigarettes regularly in 2012. Most people who smoke cigarettes and use smokeless tobacco began this habit when they were adolescents. Adolescents initially try tobacco products for a variety of reasons: to do what parents or peers do, to experiment, to feel older and more independent, or to join certain social groups. Adolescents most likely to use tobacco have particular characteristics such as low self-esteem, high susceptibility to peer pressure, and a sensation-seeking nature.

Most teenagers and adults continue to smoke and use smokeless tobacco because they are addicted to the psychoactive drug nicotine. Nicotine, like all psychoactive drugs, acts on certain communication points among nerve cells in the brain.

Cigarette smoking is the leading source of preventable illness and death in the United States because many of the 4,000 chemical compounds in cigarette smoke affect the body adversely. Every year, approximately 443,000 people die in the United States as a result of using tobacco products.

Inhaled cigarette smoke affects the airways by damaging the cilia that sweep debris from this region, by causing the airways to secrete excess mucus, and by irritating and inflaming the airways. As a result, smokers suffer chronic cough and are at high risk for a variety of respiratory infections, such as acute and chronic bronchitis and pneumonia. Smoking is also the main cause of emphysema, a condition in which the air sacs of the lungs have lost their usual elasticity so that a person cannot inhale and exhale normally.

CHAPTER REVIEW

Thirty-one percent of people who die from smoking-related causes die from cardiovascular disease. Scientists have found no evidence that smoking low-tar and low-nicotine cigarettes reduces the risk of coronary heart disease.

Cancer is the second-biggest killer of Americans, and tobacco use is responsible for about 30% of cancer deaths annually in the United States. Lung cancer is the most prevalent form of cancer caused by tobacco use. Smokeless tobacco use does not cause lung cancer, but it does cause cancers of the larynx, oral cavity, and esophagus. These cancers are also caused by smoking cigarettes, cigars, and pipes.

People who use tobacco products regularly often develop periodontal disease, which is a disease of the supporting structures of the teeth. Eventually, if periodontal disease is not treated and controlled, the teeth become loose and fall out.

Smoking cigarettes causes a loss of bone density in women. This condition is serious because it places women at risk for bone fractures, back pain, and other accompanying problems.

Environmental tobacco smoke (ETS), the sidestream smoke emitted from a lit cigarette, cigar, or pipe and the smoke exhaled by smokers, can cause lung cancer in adult nonsmokers. Chronic ETS exposure is also a risk factor for cardiovascular disease and heart attack. Children of parents who smoke have an increased frequency of respiratory symptoms such as coughing and wheezing, and lower respiratory tract infections such as bronchitis and pneumonia.

Seventy-five percent of smokers say they would like to quit smoking. Quitting has major and immediate health benefits for people of all ages.

Cigarette smoking is an addiction, and an addicted smoker who is trying to quit goes through the same process of behavioral change as does anyone addicted to any drug. Quitting is easier if the smoker analyzes why he or she smokes and develops or chooses a method of quitting that addresses these reasons.

Successful smoking-prevention programs reflect an understanding that smoking begins in early adolescence and that a child's social environment is the most important determinant of whether he or she will smoke. Prevention programs help young people develop the skills to identify and resist social influences to smoke.

Fetuses and infants are significantly affected by the alcohol and tobacco use of their mothers. The syndrome of fetal effects from alcohol consumption during pregnancy is called fetal alcohol spectrum disorders (FASDs). One of the most severe of these disorders is fetal alcohol syndrome. Children born with FAS may suffer mental retardation and have characteristic facial anomalies, growth deficiency, and central nervous system abnormalities. Maternal smoking during pregnancy can harm the pregnant woman and her fetus, placing both at risk for developing several serious conditions.

Another age group of persons strongly affected by alcohol and tobacco use is the elderly. Older adults are more physically vulnerable to the effects of alcohol and are more likely to be taking a variety of medications that may interact negatively with alcohol.

Smoking is associated with a variety of ailments in older adults. Among those older than 65 years, the death rate of current smokers is twice that of people who have never smoked.

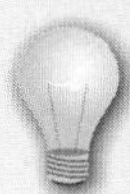

Applying What You Have Learned

1. Using the information in this chapter, write a paragraph that would describe what you might say to a friend to discourage him or her from abusing alcohol. **Application**
2. Analyze your reasons for smoking or those of a smoking friend or relative by using the assessment "Why Do You Smoke?" located in the Student Workbook section. Then, list the elements of a smoking cessation program that would be most helpful for you or for that individual. **Synthesis**
3. For the past 2 decades or so, researchers have viewed alcoholism from a "biomedical" point of view. Many researchers thought that it was only a matter of time before a gene for alcoholism would be found. Recently, many researchers have agreed that biology plays a role in addiction but suggest that biology is only one factor in the development of alcoholism. Based on what we know to date, discuss factors associated with alcoholism. Then, determine which factors programs such as Alcoholics Anonymous address in its 12 steps to recovery. Based on your findings, do you think the 12-step program is an effective method for alcoholism treatment? **Evaluation**
4. List all the places where you are regularly exposed to environmental tobacco smoke. Decide whether you should change any of your activities to reduce your exposure to ETS. Explain what you may lose by no longer attending these places or events. Discuss whether or not these places or activities are worth being exposure to ETS. **Evaluation**

Key

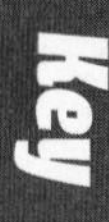

Application using information in a new situation.

Synthesis putting together information from different sources.

Evaluation making informed decisions.

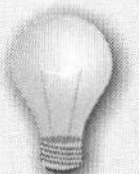

Reflecting on Your Health

1. Describe your attitudes toward alcoholics before reading this chapter. Have your attitudes changed after reading this chapter? Why or why not?
2. If you drink alcohol, what motivates your use of this drug? Are you comfortable with your patterns of drinking and reasons for doing so? Why or why not? If you are uncomfortable with your drinking patterns, what can you do to change them?
3. If you were out with friends who were drinking, would you attempt to stop someone from driving who was clearly unfit to get behind the wheel? If not, why not? If so, what strategy might be successful? Why do you think this strategy would work?
4. If you are a smoker, what do you do to avoid having others breathe your secondhand smoke? If nothing, what might you do in the future? If you are a nonsmoker, what do you do to avoid breathing others' secondhand smoke? If nothing, what might you do in the future?
5. Do you smoke bidis or clove cigarettes? If so, why did you start smoking these products? After reading the Consumer Health feature in this chapter, do you think you will continue this practice? Why or why not?

CHAPTER REVIEW

References

1. O'Hegarty, M., et al. (2007, April). Young adults' perceptions of cigarette warning labels in the United States and Canada. *Preventing Chronic Disease, 4*(2), A27. Retrieved March 22, 2011, from http://www.cdc.gov/pcd/issues/2007/apr/06_0024.htm
2. Pierce, J. P., et al. (2010). Camel No. 9 cigarette-marketing campaign targeted young teenage girls. *Pediatrics, 125*(4), 619–626.
3. Hanewinkel, R., et al. (2011). Cigarette advertising and teen smoking initiation. *Pediatrics, 127*(2), e271–e278.
4. Substance Abuse and Mental Health Services Administration. (2013). *Results from the 2012 National Survey on Drug Use and Health: Summary of National Findings* (HHS Publication No. SMA 13-4795). Retrieved from http://www.samhsa.gov/data/NSDUH/2012SummNatFindDetTables/NationalFindings/NSDUHresults2012.htm#ch3
5. Centers for Disease Control and Prevention. (2010, October 5). Vital signs: Binge drinking among high school students and adults—United States, 2009. *Morbidity and Mortality Weekly Report*, 59, 1–6.
6. van der Zwaluw, C. S., & Engels, R. C. M. E. (2009). Gene–environment interactions and alcohol use and dependence: Current status and future challenges. *Addiction, 104*, 907–914.
7. Enoch, M. A. (2006). Genetic and environmental influences on the development of alcoholism: Resilience vs. risk. *Annals of the New York Academy of Sciences, 1094*, 193–201.
8. Schuckit, M.A. (2009). An overview of genetic influences in alcoholism. *Journal of Substance Abuse Treatment, 36*(1), S5–14.
9. Wechsler, H., & Nelson, T. F. (2008). What we have learned from the Harvard School of Public Health College Alcohol Study: Focusing attention on college student alcohol consumption and the environmental conditions that promote it. *Journal of Studies on Alcohol and Drugs, 69*, 481–490.
10. Turrisi, R., et al. (2006). Heavy drinking in college students: Who is at risk and what is being done about it? *Journal of General Psychology, 133*, 401–420.
11. Wechsler, H., et al. (2002). Trends in college binge drinking during a period of increased prevention efforts: Findings from 4 Harvard School of Public Health college alcohol study surveys: 1993–2001. *Journal of American College Health, 50*, 203–217.
12. Ahern, N. R., & Sole, M. L. (2010). Drinking games and college students part 1: Problem description. *Journal of Psychosocial Nursing, 48*(2), 17–20.
13. Hingson, R. W., et al. (2009, July). Magnitude of and trend in alcohol-related mortality and morbidity among U.S. college students ages 18–24, 1998–2005. *Journal of Studies on Alcohol and Drugs,* (Suppl 16), 12–20.
14. Addolorato, G., et al. (2006). Understanding and treating patients with alcoholic cirrhosis: An update. *Alcoholism: Clinical and Experimental Research, 33*(7), 1136–1144.
15. Klatsy, A. L. (2010). Alcohol and cardiovascular health. *Physiology and Behavior, 100*(1), 76–81.
16. Khan, N., et al. (2010). Lifestyle as risk factor for cancer: Evidence from human studies. *Cancer Letters, 293*(2), 133–143.
17. Zhang, S. M., et al. (2007). Alcohol consumption and breast cancer risk in the Women's Health Study. *American Journal of Epidemiology, 165*, 667–676.
18. Li, Y., et al. (2009). Wine, liquor, beer and risk of breast cancer in a large population. *European Journal of Cancer, 45*(5), 843–850.
19. U.S. Department of Transportation, National Highway Transportation Safety Administration. (2013). *Traffic safety facts: Alcohol-impaired driving, 2012 Data* (DOT HS 811 870). Retrieved from http://www-nrd.nhtsa.dot.gov/Pubs/811870.pdf
20. Hoyert, D. L., et al. (2011). Deaths: Preliminary data for 2011. *National Vital Statistics Reports, 61*(6), 1–52. Retrieved from http://www.cdc.gov/nchs/data/nvsr/nvsr61/nvsr61_06.pdf
21. U.S. Department of Transportation, National Highway Transportation Safety Administration. (2012). *Traffic safety facts 2011 Data* (DOT HS 811 700). Retrieved from http://www-nrd.nhtsa.dot.gov/Pubs/811700.pdf
22. Mumenthaler, M. S., et al. (2003). Psychoactive drugs and pilot performance: A comparison of nicotine, donepezil, and alcohol effects. *Neuropsychopharmacology, 28*, 1366–1373.
23. Canfield, D. V., et al. (September, 2011). *Drugs and alcohol in civil aviation accident pilot fatalities from 2004–2008.* (Federal Aviation Administration DOT/FAA/AM11/13). Retrieved from http://www.faa.gov/data_research/research/med_humanfacs/oamtechreports/2010s/media/201113.pdf
24. Driscoll, T. R., et al. (2004). Review of the role of alcohol in drowning associated with recreational aquatic activity. *Injury Prevention, 10*(2), 107–113.
25. Laosee, O. C., Gilchrist, J., & Rudd, R. (2012). Drowning 2005–2009. *Morbidity and Mortality Weekly Report, 61*(19), 344–347. Retrieved from http://www.cdc.gov/mmwr/preview/mmwrhtml/mm6119a4.htm
26. Wagenaar, A. C., & Toomey, T. L. (2010). The effects of minimum legal drinking age 21 laws on alcohol-related driving in the United States. *Journal of Safety Research, 41*(2), 173–181.
27. U.S. Department of Health and Human Services. (2007). *The Surgeon General's call to action to prevent and reduce underage drinking.* Atlanta, GA: Author.
28. Johnston, L. D., et al. (2013). *Monitoring the future: National survey results on drug use, 1975–2012: Vol. 1. Secondary school students.* Bethesda, MD: National Institute on Drug Abuse. Retrieved from http://www.monitoringthefuture.org/pubs/monographs/mtf-vol1_2012.pdf
29. Centers for Disease Control and Prevention. (2012). Youth risk behavior surveillance—United States, 2011. *Morbidity and Mortality Weekly Report*, 61(4). Retrieved from http://www.cdc.gov/mmwr/pdf/ss/ss6104.pdf
30. U.S. Department of Health and Human Services. (2010). *How tobacco smoke causes disease: The biology and behavioral basis for smoking-attributable disease: A report of the Surgeon General.* Atlanta, GA: Author. Retrieved April 3, 2011, from http://www.surgeongeneral.gov/library/tobaccosmoke/report/full_report.pdf
31. American Lung Association. (2013). *Chronic obstructive pulmonary disease (COPD) fact sheet.* Retrieved from http://www.lung.org/lung-disease/copd/resources/facts-figures/COPD-Fact-Sheet.html

32. American Heart Association. (2014). *Smoking and cardiovascular disease.* Retrieved from http://www.heart.org/HEARTORG/GettingHealthy/QuitSmoking/QuittingResources/Smoking-Cardiovascular-Disease_UCM_305187_Article.jsp
33. American Cancer Society. (2010). *Cancer facts and figures 2010.* Atlanta, GA: Author. Retrieved April 3, 2011, from http://www.cancer.org/acs/groups/content/@epidemiologysurveilance/documents/document/acspc-026238.pdf
34. International Osteoporosis Foundation. (2014). *Facts and statistics about osteoporosis and its impact.* Retrieved from http://www.iofbonehealth.org/facts-statistics
35. Centers for Disease Control and Prevention. (1986). *The health consequences of involuntary smoking—A report of the Surgeon General* (DHHS Publication No. [CDC] 87–8398). Rockville, MD: U.S. Department of Health and Human Services, Public Health Service.
36. National Research Council. (1986). *Environmental tobacco smoke: Measuring exposure and assessing health effects.* Washington, DC: National Academy Press.
37. U.S. Department of Health and Human Services. (2006). *The health consequences of involuntary exposure to tobacco smoke: A report of the Surgeon General.* Atlanta, GA: Author.
38. Farrelly, M. C., Evans, W. N., & Sfekas, A. E. (1999). Impact of workplace smoking bans: Results from a national survey. *Tobacco Control, 8,* 272–277.
39. Gallup Organization. (2010). *Tobacco and smoking.* Retrieved from http://www.gallup.com/poll/1717/tobacco-smoking.aspx
40. McNeil, J. J., et al. (2010). Smoking cessation—recent advances. *Cardiovascular Drugs and Therapy, 24*(4), 359–367.
41. U.S. Food and Drug Administration. (2010, September 9). *FDA acts against 5 electronic cigarette distributors.* Retrieved April 4, 2011, from http://www.fda.gov/NewsEvents/Newsroom/PressAnnouncements/2010/ucm225224.htm
42. U.S. Food and Drug Administration. (2014). *E-cigarettes: Questions and answers.* Retrieved from http://www.fda.gov/ForConsumers/ConsumerUpdates/ucm225210.htm
43. Polosa, R., & Maziak, W. (2014). Harm reduction and e-cigarettes: not evidence-based. *The Lancet Oncology, 15*(3), e104.
44. Centers for Disease Control and Prevention (2013). Notes from the field: Electronic cigarette use among middle and high school students—United States, 2011-2012. *Morbidity and Mortality Weekly Report, 62*(35), 729–730.
45. American Cancer Society. (2013). *When smokers quit—what are the benefits over time?* Retrieved from http://www.cancer.org/healthy/stayawayfromtobacco/guidetoquittingsmoking/guide-to-quitting-smoking-benefits
46. Andersen, M. R., et al. (2009). Smoking cessation early in pregnancy and birth weight, length, head circumference, and endothelial nitric oxide synthase activity in umbilical and chorionic vessels: An observational study of healthy singleton pregnancies. *Circulation, 119,* 857–864.
47. Rusanen, M., et al. (2011). Heavy smoking in midlife and long-term risk of Alzheimer disease and vascular dementia. *Archives of Internal Medicine,* 171(4), 333–339.

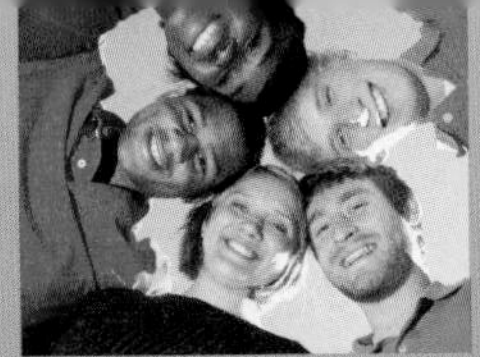

Diversity in Health
Asian American Food

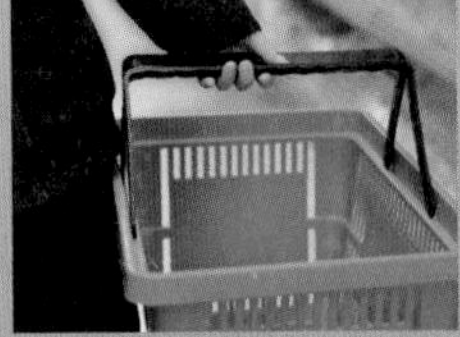

Consumer Health
Dietary Supplements

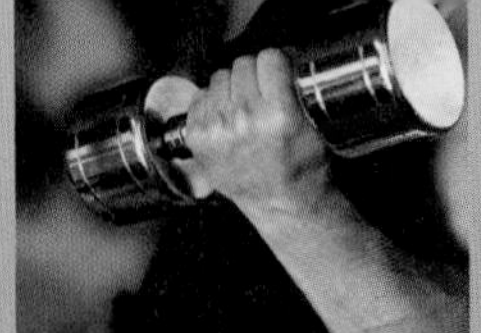

Managing Your Health
Trimming Unhealthy Fats from Your Diet

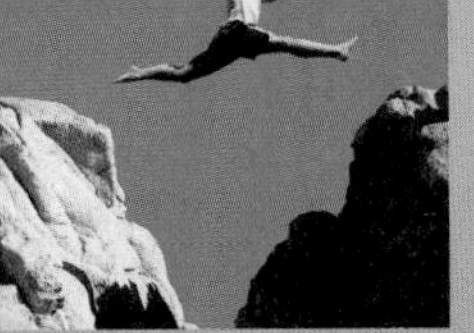

Across the Life Span
Nutrition

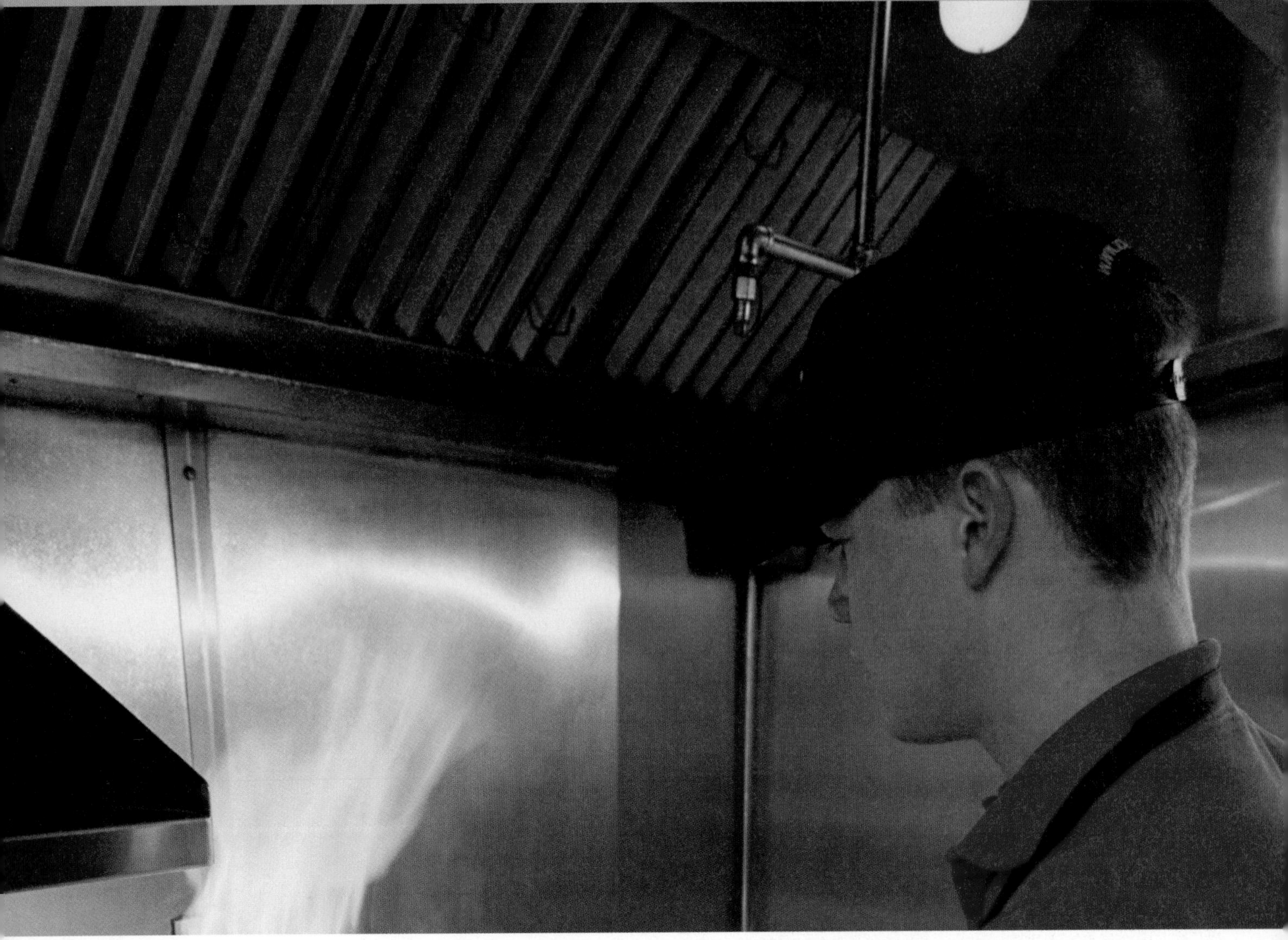

Chapter Overview

The basic principles of nutrition

How your body digests and uses the food you eat

The functions and sources of nutrients

How to plan a nutritious diet

How malnutrition affects health

Student Workbook

Self-Assessment: Assessing the Nutritional Quality of Your Diet | Diabetes Risk Test | Using MyPlate

Changing Health Habits: Are You Ready to Improve Your Diet?

Do You Know?

Which foods might help prevent cancer?

How to judge the nutritional adequacy of your diet?

If any vitamins are poisonous?

CHAPTER 9

Nutrition

Learning Objectives

"Why do you eat certain foods and not others?"

After studying this chapter, you should be able to:

1. List the six classes of nutrients, including micronutrients and macronutrients.
2. Identify major roles and food sources for each class of nutrients.
3. Identify sources of unsaturated fat, saturated fat, and cholesterol.
4. Describe how a person can reduce fat intake.
5. Differentiate between complete and incomplete proteins.
6. Describe characteristics and benefits of well-balanced and plant-based diets.
7. Use resources and interactive tools at www.choosemyplate.gov.
8. Use Nutrition Facts panel and other food labeling to make informed food choices.
9. Describe health problems associated with nutritional deficiencies or excesses.
10. Discuss varying nutritional needs of young, middle-aged, and older populations.

diet One's usual pattern of food choices.

nutrients Substances in food that are necessary for growth, repair, maintenance of tissues.

Hamburger, cola, french fries, pizza, potato chips, tofu, yogurt, olive oil, nonfat milk, mango, and wheat germ—which of these foods do you eat regularly? Have you eaten chutney, trifle, black beans, calamari, sushi, or hummus? How often do you buy soft drinks and snacks from vending machines? During the past week, how many times did you eat at fast-food restaurants? Why do you eat certain foods and not others? Before deciding what to eat, do you consider the nutritional value of food? When asked if they care about what they eat, three students who were enrolled in a college health class responded as follows:

Do I care about what I eat? Well, it depends on how hungry I am. If I am hungry enough, I'll eat anything, except some processed meats. I don't care about the amount of fat, calories, or nutritional value in foods. All I care about is how much the food costs and how much it takes to fill me up. I'm young and healthy and have hardly any body fat—I've been eating greasy, cheap, fast foods for years.

I care about what I eat, but my diet doesn't show it. When I wake up, I don't have time to eat. After class I eat burritos or pizza rolls before going to work. After work, I usually stop at a fast-food place. ... I eat lots of french fries. I do want to eat better, but it's hard when you're always on the go.

I'm not concerned about what I eat. People call me the "fast-food queen" because that's all I eat. I know fast food is not always healthy, but I'm going to school full-time and working. It's hard finding time to buy food and cook it.

If you are like these students, taste, cost, and convenience are the most important factors that influence your food choices. You may not be aware, however, that many other factors, including food advertising and moods, can also influence your diet. Although people usually associate **diet** with losing weight, the term actually refers to one's usual pattern of food choices. A healthful diet provides substances that are necessary for life, but most people do not eat simply to satisfy their nutritional needs.

Your diet reflects not only your food likes and dislikes but also your lifestyle, financial status, and educational, cultural, religious, and ethnic backgrounds. Additionally, certain foods have social significance. When you watch a major sports event at a friend's apartment with a group of people, do you help share the cost of pizzas that are delivered?

Some foods have personal emotional meanings. People often use such foods, especially sweets, to lift their mood when they are feeling sad or distressed. Do you head for the kitchen not because you are hungry, but because you are bored or lonely? At other times, do you reward yourself for achieving a desired goal by eating a favorite food? Eating food to feel better, substitute for social activity, or reward yourself can result in a nutritionally inadequate diet and unwanted weight gain.

For many young adults, selecting a nutritionally inadequate diet has a major effect on their current and future health. Poor diet can reduce the effectiveness of the *immune system*, the body's defense against many acute illnesses, including the common cold and other infectious diseases. Poor food choices can result in *anemia*, a group of conditions characterized by an insufficient number of properly formed red blood cells. People who have anemia lack the energy to carry out their normal activities and exercise without tiring easily. For women, unhealthy diets can increase the risk of having a baby born too early or with birth defects. Poor diet is also a major risk factor for serious chronic diseases that are the major killers of Americans: cardiovascular disease (CVD), which includes heart disease and stroke; diabetes; obesity; Alzheimer's disease; kidney disease; and possibly, certain cancers (**Figure 9.1**). Sensible lifelong eating and physical activity habits play important roles in maintaining good health and preventing these chronic diseases. By making specific dietary changes, people can improve their chances of enjoying good health now and later in life.

This chapter highlights the nutrients, their major food sources and roles in the body, and the benefits of choosing a nutritious diet. The information in this chapter will help you evaluate the nutritional adequacy of your diet and plan nutritious menus.

Basic Nutrition Principles

What Are Nutrients?

Nutrition is the study of the way the body processes and uses **nutrients**, substances in food that are needed for growth, repair, and maintenance of cells. In addition to these functions, some nutrients regulate cellular activity or supply energy. **Table 9.1** lists the

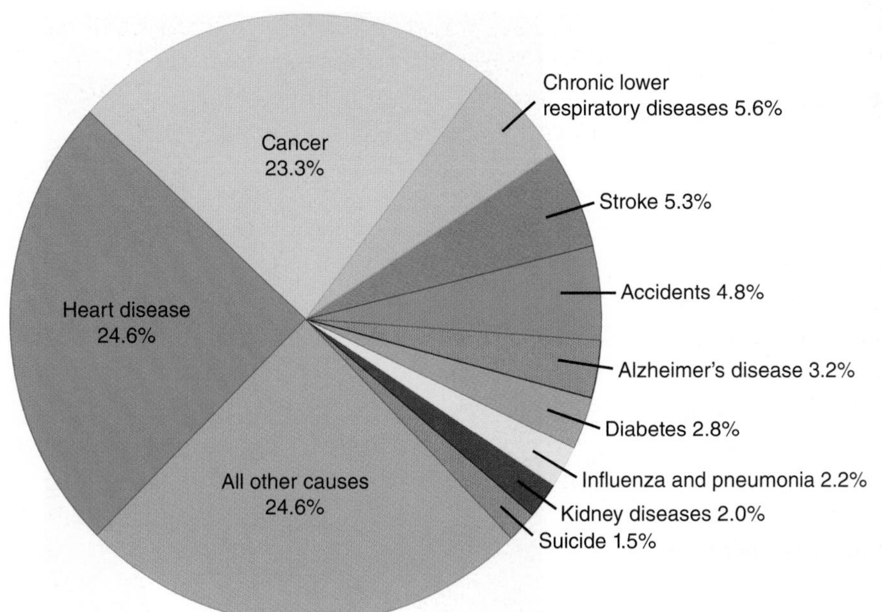

Figure 9.1

Diet and Causes of Death (U.S., 2009). In the United States, diet contributes to several of the leading causes of death, especially heart disease, certain cancers, stroke, diabetes, Alzheimer's disease, and kidney disease.

Table 9.1

The Six Classes of Nutrients

Nutrient Class	Major Roles in the Body	Rich Food Sources
Carbohydrates	Energy	Grain products, beans, vegetables, fruits, honey, sugar-sweetened soft drinks, and candy
Lipids	Triglycerides: energy Cholesterol: most steroid hormones, bile production, skin maintenance, vitamin D synthesis, and nerve function	Vegetable oils, nuts, margarines, fatty meats, cheeses, cream, butter, and fried foods
Proteins	Growth, repair, and maintenance of all cells; production of enzymes, antibodies, and certain hormones	Dried beans, peas, nuts, soy products, meats, shellfish, fish, poultry, eggs, and dairy products (except cream and butter)
Vitamins	Metabolism, reproduction, development, and growth	Widespread in foods: nuts, beans, peas, fruits and vegetables, whole grains, meats, enriched breads and cereals, fortified milk
Minerals	Metabolism, development, and growth	Widespread in foods: nuts and whole grains; meats, fish, and poultry; dairy products; vegetables and fruits; enriched breads and cereals
Water	Essential for life: many chemical reactions require water; helps maintain normal body temperature; dissolves and transports nutrients	Water, nonalcoholic and caffeine-free beverages, fruits, vegetables, and milk (nearly every food contributes water to the diet)

phytochemicals A group of nonnutrients that are produced by plants and may have beneficial effects on the body.

antioxidants Compounds that protect cells from free-radical damage.

six classes of nutrients, describes some of their roles in the body, and identifies their major food sources. In general, carbohydrates and fats supply energy; vitamins and minerals participate in chemical reactions that regulate body processes; and proteins provide the material for tissue (cellular) growth, repair, and maintenance. Water transports materials in the body and also participates in numerous chemical reactions.

The human body can *synthesize* (produce) certain nutrients. For example, exposing skin to sunlight enables the body to make vitamin D. Other nutrients are essential; that is, the diet must supply nutrients that the body does not make or does not make in the amounts needed for good health. Nutritional deficiency diseases can develop when diets contain inadequate amounts of essential nutrients. These diseases are uncommon in the United States because we have a wide variety of foods available to eat. Additionally, many commonly eaten foods and certain beverages are *enriched* or *fortified* with vitamins and minerals. Enriched bread, for example, has iron and certain B vitamins added to it. Milk is usually fortified with vitamins A and D, and you can purchase orange juiced that has been fortified with calcium.

What Are Nonnutrients?

Some foods contain substances that you can live without. Many of these *nonnutrients* are naturally found in plants and have beneficial effects on the body. Other nonnutrient substances, such as pesticide residues or lead, enter food unintentionally and can be hazardous to health.

Plants produce **phytochemicals**, a large group of nonnutrients that may provide health benefits. Many phytochemicals, including beta-carotene, lutein, and anthocyanin, are antioxidants. **Antioxidants** prevent or reduce the formation of *free radicals*, unstable and highly reactive atoms or compounds that can cause cellular damage. Such damage may contribute to heart disease, certain cancers, and the aging process. There is no scientific evidence, however, that people benefit from taking pills that contain phytochemicals.

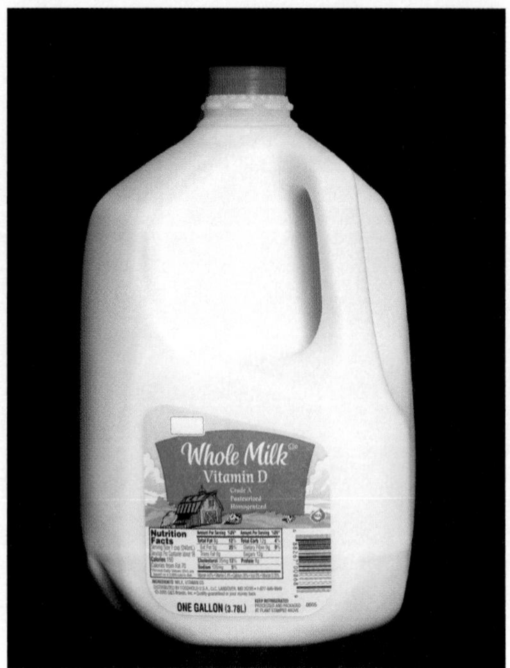

Vitamin-D fortified milk.

Therefore, nutrition experts recommend that people eat a variety of fruits, vegetables, and whole grains daily to obtain a natural array of these substances. Dark green, yellow, orange, red, and purple fruits and vegetables tend to have the most antioxidant phytochemicals, so let color be your key to selecting the richest food sources of antioxidants (**Figure 9.2**). **Table 9.2** lists some phytochemicals as well as their food sources and possible effects on the body.

Natural, Health, Organic, and Functional Foods

Food manufacturers can label their products as *natural* if they are minimally processed and contain no artificial additives such as synthetic colors or flavors. So-called natural foods are not necessarily more nutritious than foods that do not carry this description. Many consumers think natural foods such as honey, herbal teas, and cider vinegar are *health foods* because they have medicinal benefits. Although these foods provide nutrients, there is little or no scientific evidence to support claims that they prevent or treat various health conditions. Regardless of whether it is natural or manufactured, a "healthy" food contributes to your nutrient needs and is safe to eat. Herbs, for example, may contain beneficial phytochemicals, but some are natural sources of toxic substances and should be avoided.

Food producers can label their fruits, vegetables, and meat and poultry products as *organic* if they meet

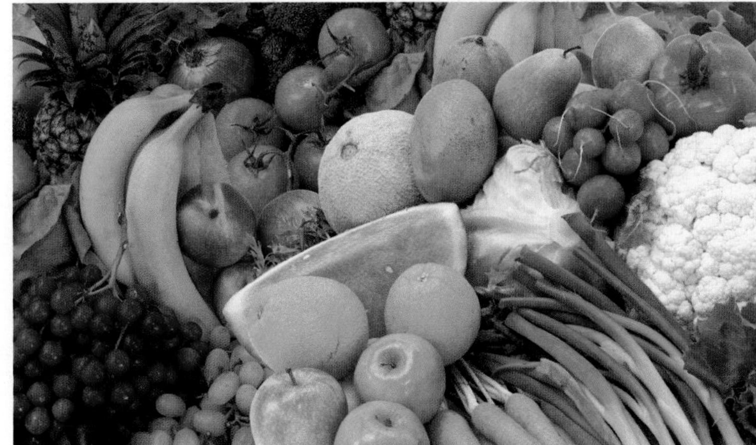

Figure 9.2

Color Palette for Good Health. Add colorful fruits and vegetables to your meals and snacks to boost your intake of antioxidant phytochemicals.

certain standards. Fruits and vegetables, for example, must be grown without the use of synthetic pesticides and fertilizers. Advertisers sometimes refer to their products as organic to imply that these items are superior. Although organically grown foods may contain less pesticide residue, they are not more nutritious than similar foods that have been grown using conventional farming methods. Chemists classify compounds as organic if they contain carbon. Carbohydrates, fats, proteins, and vitamins contain carbon; therefore, they are organic compounds. Because most foods naturally consist of these nutrients, all foods are organic.

Table 9.2

Phytochemicals

Phytochemicals	Major Plant Sources	Possible Disease-Fighting Properties
Allium	Garlic, onions, leeks	Enhances immune function; may reduce risk of certain cancers
Indoles, isothiocyanates (includes sulforaphane)	Broccoli, cabbage, watercress, kale, cauliflower, bok choy, collard and mustard greens, brussels sprouts	May inhibit cancer tumor growth
Ellargic acid	Nuts (especially walnuts), grapes, apples, berries	Has antioxidant activity; may inhibit tumor growth
Flavonoids (includes anthocyanin)	Soy products, apples, artichokes, red grapes and wines, tea, onions, berries, red cabbage	Have antioxidant activity; may reduce risk of heart disease and certain cancers
Polyphenols	Black and green tea, red wine	Inhibit tumor growth; may reduce risk of heart disease
Monoterpenes	Citrus peel oils, citrus fruits, cherries	Anticancer agents
Carotenoids (includes beta-carotene, lutein, and lycopene)	Dark orange, yellow, and green fruits and vegetables; tomatoes	May reduce risk of cancer, but more research is needed
Phytic acid	Whole wheat (bran and germ)	May reduce risk of certain cancers and heart disease

Data from Heiner, et al. (2012). Critical review: Vegetables and fruit in the prevention of chronic diseases; Dietary flavonoids and risk of coronary heart disease. (1994). *Nutrition Reviews*, 52(2), 59–68.; Marwick, C. (1995). Learning how phytochemicals help fight disease. *Journal of the American Medical Association*, 274, 1328–1330.; A garden of phytochemicals. (1995). University of California of Berkeley Wellness Letter, 12(1), 6–7.

probiotics Microorganisms that may provide healthful benefits when consumed

digestion The process of breaking down large food molecules into smaller molecules that the intestinal tract can absorb.

absorption The passage of nutrients through the walls of the intestinal tract.

Functional foods, sometimes called *nutraceuticals*, are defined by the Academy of Nutrition and Dietetics as "whole foods along with fortified, enriched, or enhanced food that have a potentially beneficial effect on health when consumed as part of a varied diet on a regular basis at effective levels." Based on this definition, functional foods include conventional foods such whole grains, fruits and vegetables, modified foods such as yogurt, cereal and orange juice, and foods for special dietary needs such as infant formula or hypoallergenic foods. A person must eat a certain amount of these foods regularly to obtain the desired effects. For example, a phytochemical that can lower blood cholesterol levels has been added to certain margarines and salad dressings. Another example is food containing **probiotics**, live bacteria, which are often considered functional foods because that may benefit digestive health. Many different kinds of bacteria naturally reside in the large intestine. If certain bacteria overpopulate this region, diarrhea and serious infections can result. Eating foods that contain certain kinds of microbes (*probiotics*) regularly may help maintain or regain the normal balance of bacteria in the large intestine. Some brands of yogurt contain probiotics. *Prebiotics* are substances in certain foods that support probiotics.

In the future, a variety of other specially formulated or fortified foods with advertised health benefits will be available in supermarkets, including those that claim to reduce appetite or risk of heart disease. In many cases, much larger portions of formulated or fortified foods are necessary to ingest the amount of a phytochemical found in whole foods; therefore, nutrition experts recommend using whole foods, rather than fortified foods or dietary supplements, as primary sources of nutrition.

It is also important note that there is no current legal definition for functional foods. The United States Food and Drug Administration (FDA) only regulates claims manufacturers make about functional foods' nutrient content and effects on disease, health, or body function. The Academy of Nutrition and Dietetics' position statement on functional foods indicates that many nutrition professionals consider the term *functional food* a marketing term and that all food is functional because it provides energy and nutrients necessary for sustained life.[1]

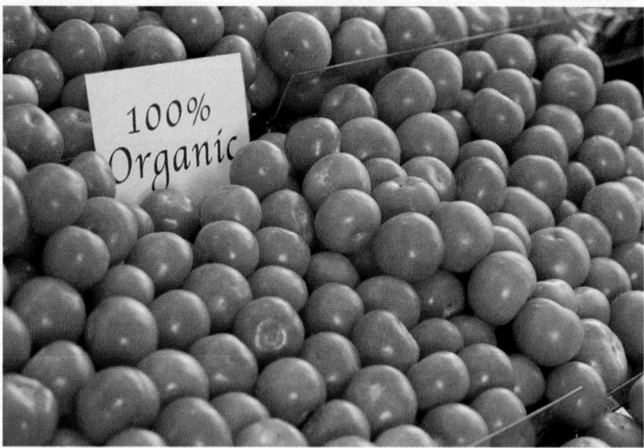

What Happens to the Food You Eat?

Humans eat a wide variety of plants, animals, and animal products to obtain nutrients and other beneficial substances. In their natural state, many nutrients are in complex forms that the body cannot use. During the process of **digestion**, the gastrointestinal tract (digestive system) breaks down complex food substances into nutrients (**Figure 9.3**). Various *enzymes*, compounds that speed up chemical changes, participate in the process of digestion.

Absorption is the passage of nutrients through the walls of the intestinal tract and eventually into the blood. After nutrients enter the bloodstream, many are transported to the liver, where they are processed or stored.

By the time any remaining food material enters the colon (the major segment of the large intestine), most of its nutrients have been absorbed. This residue, which makes up some of the *feces* or *stool*, remains in the rectum until the individual has a bowel movement to eliminate the waste. The entire process of digesting the food, absorbing its nutrients, and eliminating fecal residue generally takes about 1 to 3 days.

The kidneys play an important role in maintaining the body's normal nutrient levels by filtering excess *water-soluble* nutrients from the blood so that they can be eliminated in the urine. A water-soluble nutrient dissolves in water. Many nutrients, such as proteins, B vitamins, and vitamin C, are water soluble. *Fat-soluble* nutrients such as cholesterol and vitamin

metabolism Chemical reactions that take place in the body.

calorie A unit of energy.

A do not dissolve in water, and the kidneys cannot eliminate them as easily. Fat-soluble nutrients generally circulate until the liver or fat cells remove them for storage.

Nutrient toxicities occur when the body cannot use or store excess nutrients, especially minerals and fat-soluble vitamins. For example, signs of vitamin A toxicity include nausea, vomiting, headaches, bone pain, hair loss, liver damage, birth defects, and, even, death (see Table 9-7 later in this chapter). People rarely eat enough food to obtain excessive amounts of nutrients. Nutrient toxicities, however, are more likely to occur from taking too many pills (*dietary supplements*) that contain the substances.

Energy from Foods **Metabolism** refers to all of the chemical reactions that take place in the body. These reactions are necessary to power muscular movements, synthesize and repair tissues, release and use energy, and produce enzymes and hormones. To carry out metabolic activities, cells need the energy stored in fat, certain carbohydrates, and to a small extent, protein. Oxygen, which enters the body from the lungs, is needed to release the stored energy. This energy powers cell activities and helps maintain body temperature.

Figure 9.3

The Digestive System. The stomach and small intestine break down large compounds in foods into smaller molecules that can be absorbed through the intestinal walls.

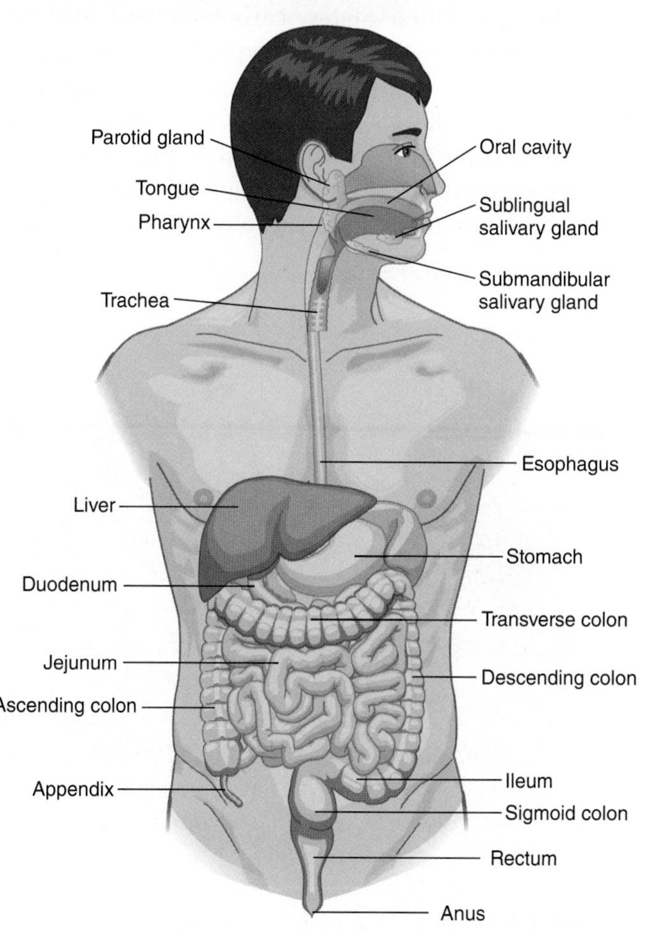

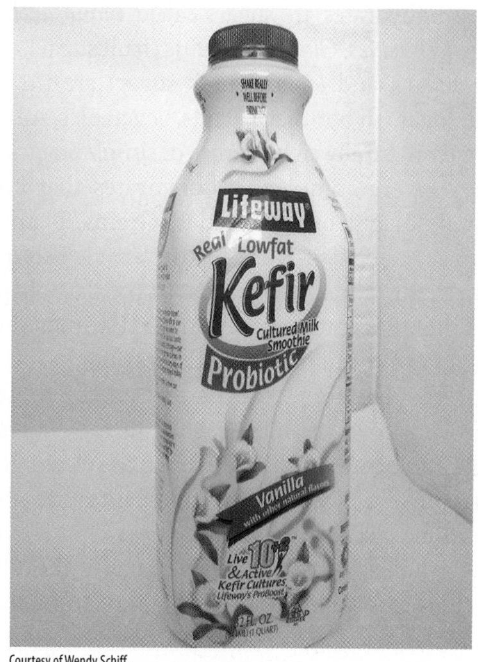

Courtesy of Wendy Schiff.

The amount of energy in foods is expressed as a number of *kilocalories*, commonly referred to as "calories." A **calorie** is a unit of energy. Foods containing carbohydrates, fats, proteins, and the nonnutrient alcohol provide calories. Proteins and most carbohydrates supply 4 calories per gram, alcohol provides 7 calories per gram, and fat provides 9 calories per gram. The body cannot extract energy from water, vitamins, and minerals; therefore, these nutrients do not provide calories. The following sections provide some basic information about the six major classes of nutrients.

carbohydrates A class of nutrients that includes sugars and starches.

glucose The most important monosaccharide in the human body.

dietary fiber Indigestible substances produced by plants.

Energy-Supplying Nutrients

Carbohydrates

Carbohydrates include sugars and starches. The simplest carbohydrates are sugars called *monosaccharides* and *disaccharides*. *Glucose*, *fructose* (fruit sugar), *sucrose* (table sugar), and *lactose* (milk sugar) are the major simple sugars in our diets. Fruits, vegetables, milk, and honey are naturally rich sources of simple sugars.

Starches are complex carbohydrates that contain hundreds of glucose molecules. Grains, beans, and certain vegetables such as potatoes are rich sources of starch. Plant foods supply most of the carbohydrates in the diet. Except for honey and milk, most animal foods do not contain carbohydrates.

During digestion, the large starch molecules are broken down to release glucose molecules, and sucrose molecules are broken down to release glucose and fructose molecules. The small intestine absorbs these monosaccharides, and the liver converts much of the fructose to glucose. Eventually, the glucose molecules enter the bloodstream and can be used by cells.

Glucose, commonly referred to as "blood sugar," is the most important monosaccharide in the human body. All cells, especially nerves, metabolize glucose for energy. A healthy body carefully maintains a normal blood glucose level.

Plants make lignin and certain carbohydrates that the human small intestine cannot digest. This material is called **dietary fiber**, or simply fiber. Soluble forms of fiber swell or dissolve in water; insoluble forms remain relatively unchanged in water. Apples, bananas, citrus fruits, carrots, kidney beans, psyllium seeds, and oats are rich sources of *soluble fiber*. Brown rice, wheat bran, and whole-grain wheat products are rich sources of *insoluble fiber*. Plants usually contain mixtures of these forms of fiber. **Table 9.3** lists fiber-rich foods; note that none are from animal sources.

Table 9.3

Fiber-Rich Foods

Whole-grain products	Whole-wheat flour, high-fiber wheat bran cereals, psyllium,* oat bran,* oatmeal,* brown rice, whole-grain crackers, buckwheat groats, barley,* wheat germ
Dried beans and peas	Lentils, pinto beans, lima beans, kidney beans,*navy beans, split peas
Fruits	Bananas,* berries, oranges,* figs, grapefruits,* fruits with edible peels (e.g., apples,* peaches, pears)
Vegetables	Vegetables with edible peels (e.g., potatoes), brussels sprouts, broccoli, okra, cabbage, peas, turnips, spinach, sweet potatoes, carrots*

*Rich source of soluble fiber.

In the United States, carbohydrates constitute about 44% to 47% of the typical person's caloric intake. The *Dietary Guidelines for Americans 2010,* however, indicates 45–65% of our daily calories should come from carbohydrates, primarily complex carbohydrates that are high in fiber.[2] Recommendations for simple carbohydrate intake range

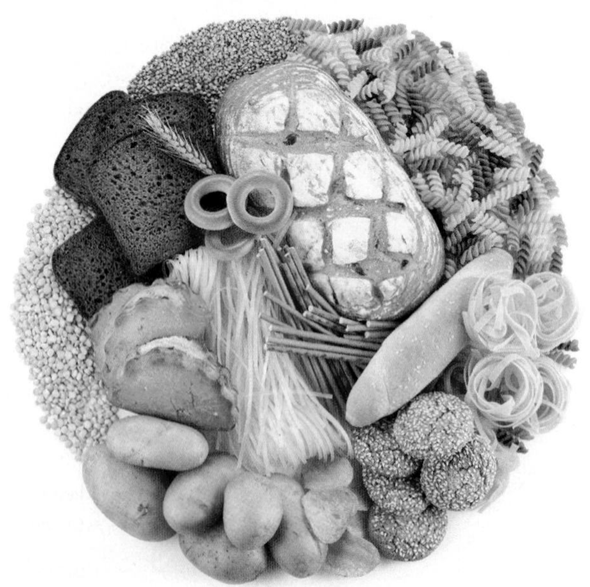

Table 9.4

Other Names for Sugars

Sucrose
Table sugar, raw sugar, turbinado sugar
Granulated cane juice or evaporated cane juice
Confectioner's or powdered sugar
Brown sugar
Invert sugar
Maple syrup
Molasses or blackstrap molasses
Honey
Date sugar
Corn syrup, cultured corn syrup, or high-fructose corn syrup
Fruit sugar
Levulose
Fruit juice concentrate
Concentrated fruit juice sweetener
Glucose or dextrose
Polydextrose
Maltose
Maltodextrin

from 10% to 25% of calories. Foods that contain high amounts of the simple carbohydrate sucrose and another form of sugar called high fructose corn syrup (HFCS) are often poor sources of vitamins and minerals. Thus, eating a lot of sugary foods can displace more nutritious foods from a person's diet. It can be difficult to identify sugars in foods by the ingredients listed on the label. **Table 9.4** lists names for various sugars.

Most nutrition experts recommend that Americans reduce their intake of sucrose and high fructose corn syrup by consuming fewer regular soft drinks, candies, and bakery items. Sugar substitutes such as rebaudiana (a form of stevia), aspartame (Nutrasweet), sucralose, and saccharin are available in packets for consumers to use. Food manufacturers may also use sugar substitutes to sweeten sugar-free gums, candies, and diet soft drinks. When consumed in normal amounts by healthy people, these sweeteners are safe and contribute few or no calories to diets.[3]

Carbohydrates and Health Recent data from the National Center for Health Statistics indicated the average American consumed 11% to 14% of their total calories from sucrose and other caloric sweeteners between 2005 and 2010.[4] Women consumed a larger portion of their total calories from added sugars and Americans 20–39 years of age consumed the most sugar. High fructose corn syrup (HFCS) and sucrose are the primary caloric sweeteners in soft drinks, candies, desserts, and many processed foods. These simple carbohydrates are blamed for numerous health problems, including diabetes, hyperactivity, mental illness, and criminal behavior. Does scientific evidence support these claims?

Despite popular beliefs, there is no scientific evidence that sucrose or other sugars cause or contribute to hyperactivity, mental illness, or criminal behavior. Sucrose cannot be absorbed by the intestinal tract. During digestion, the sugar is broken down into glucose and fructose, which are sources of energy for the body. However, recent research indicates eating less sugar is better for long-term health. Recent research indicates added sugar intake increases risk of obesity, type 2 diabetes, and death from cardiovascular disease.[5,6,7]

Tooth decay is also directly related to carbohydrate consumption. Carbohydrates can stick to teeth, providing food for bacteria in the mouth. As the bacteria metabolize carbohydrates, they produce acids that destroy the enamel of teeth, and decay results. Good oral hygiene practices, including brushing and flossing after meals and snacks, can reduce the risk of dental decay.

Some people avoid eating table sugar, which is made from sugar beets or sugar cane, but will use honey as a sweetener because they think it is more "natural" and nutritious than sugar. Although honey contains very small amounts of phytochemicals, it has essentially the same nutritional value as other sugars.

Honey should not be added to baby foods because it may contain spores of *Clostridium botulinum*, a bacterium that produces a dangerous toxin. This toxin affects nerves, causing loss of muscle functioning, which can be life threatening when it impairs breathing. Infants who eat contaminated honey are at risk of developing infantile botulism because their stomachs do not produce enough acid to kill the bacterial spores. Children older than 1 year and adults produce sufficient amounts of stomach acid, so they can eat honey safely.

diabetes mellitus ("diabetes") A group of chronic diseases characterized by the inability to metabolize carbohydrates properly.

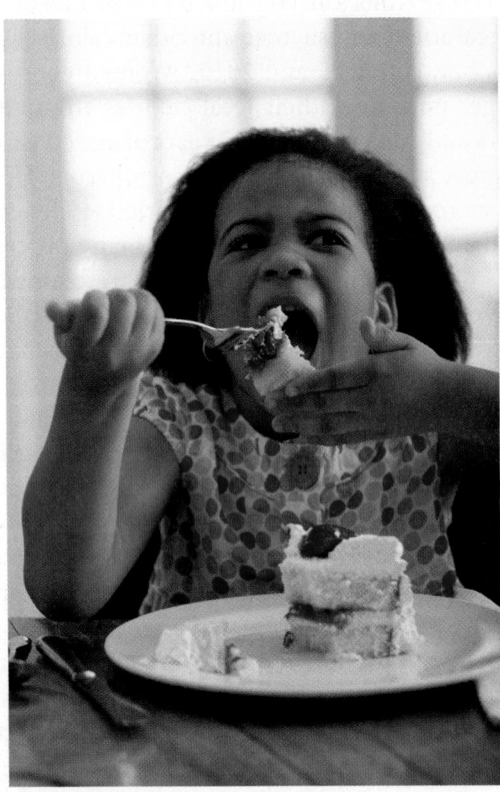

Contrary to popular myth, eating sugar does not make children hyperactive.

© Thomas Northcut/Digital Vision/Thinkstock

Diabetes Mellitus **Diabetes mellitus**, often simply called diabetes, is a group of chronic diseases characterized by an inability to metabolize carbohydrates properly. This abnormality also affects metabolism of proteins and fats. A person with diabetes produces no insulin or insufficient amounts of insulin or has cells that do not respond normally to insulin. *Insulin*, a hormone that is produced in the pancreas (see Figure 9.3), helps glucose enter cells. Without the normal action of insulin, the cells cannot carry out their metabolic activities properly, and glucose builds up in the blood. High blood glucose levels can lead to serious chronic health disorders, including hypertension, loss of vision, and nerve damage. In the United States, poorly controlled diabetes is a major cause of kidney failure, blindness, and lower limb amputations. Furthermore, having diabetes greatly increases one's risk of heart disease and stroke. Each year, thousands of people die as a result of diabetes. In 2009, diabetes was the seventh leading cause of death in the United States.[8]

Table 9.5

Common Signs and Symptoms of Diabetes Mellitus

Type 1 Diabetes

(Generally develops in childhood and young adulthood)

- Lack of energy
- Listlessness
- Frequent urination
- Excessive thirst
- "Fruity" odor in breath
- Increased appetite with weight loss
- Vision problems

Type 2 Diabetes

Usually few symptoms, but when they exist:

- Excessive thirst
- Frequent urination
- Vision problems
- In women, recurrent vaginal infections
- Skin sores that do not heal

Nearly 26 million Americans have diabetes; 7 million of these people were unaware that they had the disease.[9] The two most prevalent forms of diabetes are *type 1 diabetes* and *type 2 diabetes*. Most people with diabetes have type 2. **Table 9.5** lists the common signs and symptoms of each type.

Type 1 diabetes is caused by an inappropriate immune system response to an infection (autoimmune disease) that damages the cells of the pancreas that make insulin. People with this condition require daily injections of insulin because the pancreas does not produce the hormone. Some people with type 1 diabetes wear a small device that pumps insulin into their bodies. Although type 1 diabetes is often called juvenile diabetes, the label is misleading because type 1 can strike at any age. The majority of cases, however, are diagnosed in childhood.

People with type 2 diabetes are usually older than 40 years and have excess body fat (*obesity*) and a family history of diabetes. Since 1997, the prevalence of type 2 diabetes has increased dramatically in the United States, particularly among black and Hispanic Americans.[10] Moreover, this form of the disease is becoming more common among children and adolescents, as rates of obesity increase among younger members of the population.

adipose cells Cells that store fat.

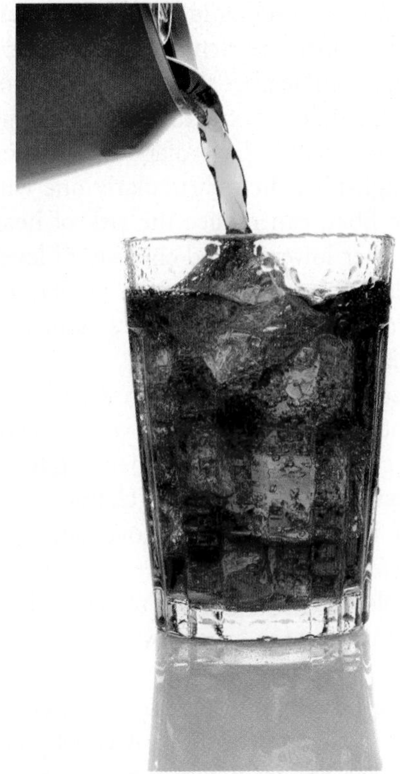

© Steve Cukrov/ShutterStock

Obesity contributes to type 2 diabetes, especially when one has a family history of the disorder. In many instances, people with type 2 diabetes can improve their blood glucose levels by losing their excess body fat. Regular physical activity can also reduce high blood glucose levels, and adopting a physically active lifestyle helps people achieve and maintain healthy body weights.

Poor diet also contributes to the development of type 2 diabetes. When too much glucose enters the bloodstream after a high-carbohydrate snack or meal, the pancreas may respond by releasing an excess of insulin. High blood insulin levels may increase the risk of heart disease, obesity, and type 2 diabetes. Scientists have measured the intestinal absorption rates of many commonly eaten carbohydrate-rich foods and assigned *glycemic index* (*GI*) values to them. Foods with high GIs (over 70), such as white, short-grained rice, increase blood glucose levels more than foods with low GIs (under 55), such as kidney beans. People may reduce their risk of type 2 diabetes by eating diets that contain more low-GI than high-GI foods. Among nutrition experts, however, the contribution of a high-GI diet to the development of type 2 diabetes is controversial.

Poor diets often contain high amounts of *added sugars*, such as sucrose or HFCS. Although added sugars make foods and beverages more appealing to some people, they supply few vitamins and minerals. As a result, sugary foods displace more nutritious foods from meals and snacks. Americans' high intake of products sweetened with HFCS may contribute to the rising prevalence of obesity and type 2 diabetes in the United States.[6] Soft drinks sweetened with HFCS such as colas, fruit drinks, and energy drinks are the primary source of sugar in the typical American's diet.[11] In the United States, soft drink consumption has increased dramatically since 1970. During this same period, the percentage of Americans who are obese and have diabetes increased as well. It is difficult to prove that sugar-sweetened soft drinks cause excess weight gain and diabetes; more research is needed to support these findings. Nevertheless, you may want to analyze your sugar-sweetened soft drink consumption. Instead of satisfying your thirst with sugary soft drinks, consider drinking plain water.

Type 2 diabetes can often be controlled by dietary modifications and regular exercise. Many affected persons, however, need to take medications, some of which increase the production of insulin by the pancreas. Some people with type 2 diabetes need daily insulin injections. By carefully controlling their blood sugar levels through diet, exercise, and, if necessary, medication, people with diabetes can often lessen the long-term damaging effects of the disease.

You may be able to reduce your risk of type 2 diabetes by losing excess weight and increasing physical activity.[12,13] It is also important to have routine health checkups that include diabetes testing because many people with type 2 diabetes are not aware that they have the disorder. You may want to take the diabetes quiz in the Student Workbook at the end of this text to assess your risk of developing this disease.

Metabolic Syndrome About one-fourth of American adults have *metabolic syndrome*, a condition that increases the risk of CVD and type 2 diabetes.[14] People with metabolic syndrome have excess abdominal fat and at least two of the following health problems: hypertension (chronically elevated blood pressure), high blood glucose, high blood triglycerides (fat), and low HDL ("good") cholesterol levels. People who have large waistline measurements generally have excess *visceral* fat, deposits of **adipose cells** that are located deep within the abdomen. Adipose cells store fat, but the tissue also secretes substances that have important immune functions. Storing too

constipation A condition characterized by having fewer than three bowel movements per week.

hemorrhoids Painfully swollen veins in the rectal and anal areas.

diverticulosis An intestinal disorder that occurs when the colon lining forms small pouches that protrude through the outer wall of the colon.

much fat disrupts the normal functioning of visceral fat cells. As a result, these cells secrete *C-reactive protein* and other factors that are thought to contribute to systemic inflammation—inflammation that occurs throughout the body. Systemic inflammation may be partially responsible for heart disease, hypertension, and type 2 diabetes. Losing excess body fat can reduce levels of inflammatory substances and lower the risk of these chronic conditions.

Poor dietary habits such as eating a diet that lacks fruits, vegetables, and other fiber-rich foods contribute to metabolic syndrome. By exercising regularly, maintaining a healthy body weight, and eating plenty of fiber-rich foods, people may be able to avoid this common condition.

Lactose Intolerance *Lactose* (milk sugar) is composed of two monosaccharides. During digestion, lactose is broken down, releasing its component simple sugars. Many older children and adults, however, cannot digest lactose. Such lactose-intolerant people may experience intestinal bloating, cramps, and diarrhea if they consume milk or other products that contain the sugar. Lactose intolerance affects millions of Americans. Members of certain minority groups, especially people with Asian or African ancestry, are more likely to be affected than Caucasians.[15]

Because milk is an excellent source of the mineral nutrient calcium, it is important that lactose-intolerant people consume alternative calcium-rich foods, such as cheese, yogurt, broccoli, turnip and mustard greens, and some types of tofu. People with this condition can add a special enzyme to milk and other foods that contain lactose before consuming them. The enzyme breaks down lactose, reducing the risk of unpleasant side effects. Also, supermarkets often sell fresh milk that has been treated with the enzyme. Affected individuals, however, can often consume small amounts of lactose-containing foods without experiencing discomfort.

Fiber and Health Fiber provides some important health benefits. By eating more high-fiber cereals, people may reduce their risk of developing metabolic syndrome, a condition that often precedes type 2 diabetes. Table 9.3 lists some foods that contain fiber and indicates which are rich sources of *soluble* and *insoluble* fiber. Soluble fiber slows the absorption of glucose from the digestive tract, which is beneficial for people who already have diabetes. Furthermore, eating a high-fiber diet, particularly one with plenty of soluble fiber, can reduce the risk of heart disease. Soluble fiber lowers blood cholesterol levels by reducing cholesterol absorption in the small intestine. Elevated blood cholesterol levels are associated with increased risk of CVD.

Many Americans are concerned with their bowel habits; they spend millions of dollars a year on laxatives that promise "regularity." Eating fiber-rich foods can prevent **constipation**, a condition characterized by having fewer than three bowel movements per week.[16] *Insoluble fiber* contributes to the formation of softer, larger stools that stimulate the muscles of the colon, producing the urge to have bowel movements more frequently.

Constipation results when stools are too small and hard to stimulate the colon regularly. A constipated individual often has to strain while having bowel movements, increasing the pressure on veins in the rectum. This pressure can result in **hemorrhoids**, which are painfully swollen veins in the rectal and anal areas. Straining during bowel movements causes **diverticulosis**, a chronic condition in which the lining of the colon forms small pouches called *diverticula* (**Figure 9.4**). Fecal material that becomes lodged in some of these little pouches can cause serious bleeding and inflammation (diverticulitis). Diverticulitis can be life threatening if an inflamed pouch ruptures and spills fecal material into the abdominal cavity. Diverticulosis commonly occurs in Americans older than 50 years, but the condition often produces no serious symptoms.

In addition to eating more fiber-rich foods, you may prevent constipation by consuming adequate amounts of water. Regular exercise may also improve bowel functioning.[16] If constipation persists, or if you have intestinal pain, blood in your stools, or rectal bleeding, check with a physician to rule out serious health problems.

Can eating a high-fiber diet reduce your chances of developing certain cancers of the intestinal tract? Over the past few years, several population studies have provided conflicting findings concerning fiber intake and the risk of colon and rectal cancer. Some medical researchers have found no association between high-fiber diets and risk of these cancers, but others have determined that eating such diets

Figure 9.4

Diverticula. Diverticula are small pockets of the large intestine's inner lining that protrude through the outer wall of the large intestine. Diverticula can become infected and rupture.

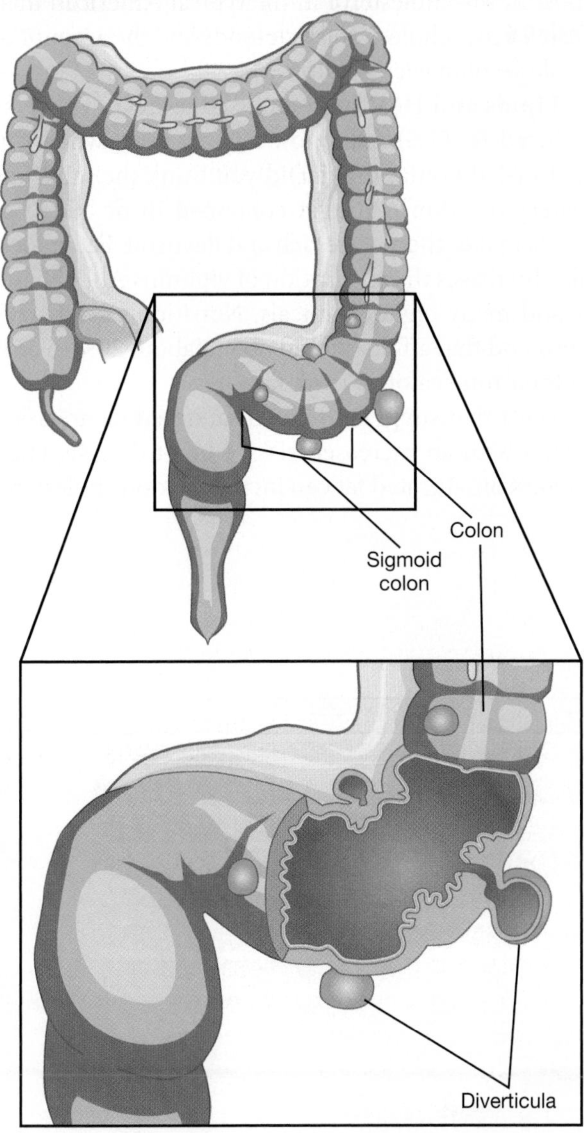

lowers the risk. More research is needed to clarify the role of dietary fiber in gastrointestinal health.

The typical American consumes less than 20 g of fiber a day. Medical experts think individuals should consume at least 25 g of fiber by eating more fruits, vegetables, beans, and whole-grain cereal products each day. During processing, grains often lose their vitamin, mineral, and fiber-rich parts. White flour, for example, is a refined grain product made from wheat kernels. Compared to whole-wheat flour, white flour contains very little fiber. Replacing refined flour products, such as white bread, with whole-grain foods is an easy way to increase the fiber content of your diet. Some "100% wheat" breads contain little fiber; use the nutrient label to compare the fiber content of breads.

lipids A class of nutrients that includes triglycerides and cholesterol.

triglycerides The most prevalent form of lipids in foods; often called fat.

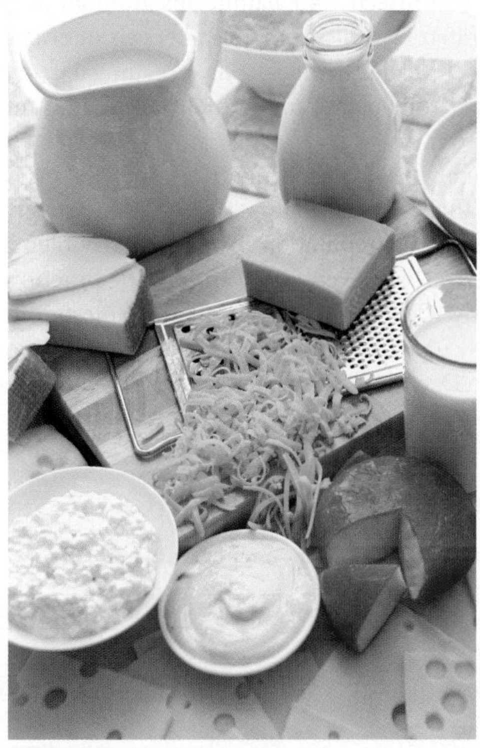

Dairy foods are often sources of lactose.

Lipids

Dietary **lipids** include cholesterol and triglycerides. About 95% of the lipid content in foods are **triglycerides**, commonly called *fats* and *oils*. Because each cell contains triglycerides, it is not surprising that a small amount of fat is necessary for health. Compared to carbohydrates, fat is a more concentrated source of calories. The body stores energy in its fat deposits, which insulate the body from cold temperatures, give the body shape, and protect internal organs from jarring movements.

Each triglyceride has three fatty acids. Scientists classify fatty acids into three types—*saturated*, *monounsaturated*, and *polyunsaturated*—according to their chemical structures. Although the triglycerides found in foods contain mixtures of these three types of fatty acids, one type usually predominates. **Figure 9.5** indicates the amounts of lipid as well as

cholesterol A type of lipid found only in animals.

the percentages of saturated, monounsaturated, and polyunsaturated fatty acids in a tablespoon of various fats and oils.

Animal foods generally contain more saturated fat than do plant foods. Olive, peanut, and canola oils are rich sources of monounsaturated fat; corn, safflower, cottonseed, and walnut oils are high in polyunsaturated fat. Oils from palm kernels or coconuts, commonly called tropical oils, are unusual in that they are from plants but contain large amounts of saturated fat.

Animal foods also contain **cholesterol**, a compound that is structurally different from a triglyceride. Despite its reputation for being a troublemaker, cholesterol has several very important functions in the body. Cell membranes contain cholesterol, and the body uses this lipid to produce steroid hormones, vitamin D, and bile, a substance needed for proper fat digestion. Even if you could avoid eating foods that contain cholesterol, your liver and small intestine would make this essential compound.

Only animals produce cholesterol; therefore, the compound is found in animal and not plant foods. Meats, whole-milk products, and egg yolks supply most of the cholesterol in the typical American diet. **Table 9.6** lists cholesterol-rich foods and the amount of cholesterol in each serving.

Lipids and Health If you used to drink whole or reduced-fat (2%) milk, how did you react when you first tasted nonfat milk? Did you think the milk was watery or "thin"? The fat contained in or added to foods makes them taste rich and flavorful. Fat in food also increases the absorption of vitamins A, D, E, and K and many phytochemicals. Nutrition experts recommend that adults should obtain about 20% to 35% of their total calories from fat.[2]

Diets that supply too much saturated fat are associated with an increased risk of heart disease. High intakes of saturated fat can increase blood cholesterol

Figure 9.5

Fatty Acid Content of Common Fats and Oils.

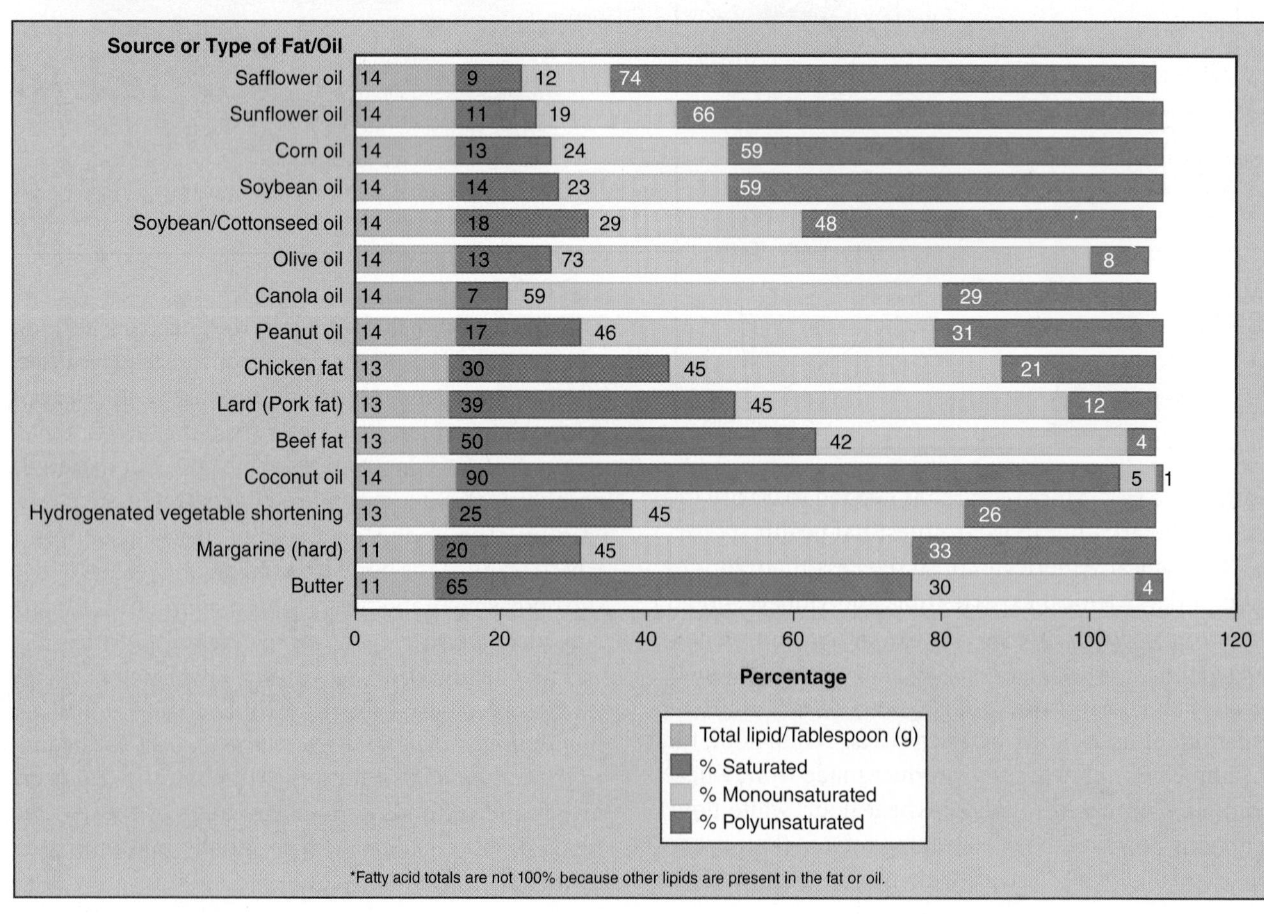

Table 9.6

Cholesterol in Foods

Food	Serving Size	Cholesterol (mg)
Beef liver	4 oz	545
Egg	1 large	212
Yolk		212
White		0
Shrimp	3 oz	167
Turkey, ground cooked	4 oz	116
Beefsteak	4 oz	94
Ice cream (rich = 16% fat)	1 cup	90
Sherbet (2% fat)	1 cup	10
Yogurt, plain low-fat	1 cup	14
Whole milk	1 cup	33
Reduced-fat (2%) milk	1 cup	18
Nonfat milk	1 cup	4
Butter	1 tablespoon	31
Swiss cheese	1 oz	26
Cream cheese	1 oz	10
Bacon	3 slices	16

levels. Although eating foods that contain cholesterol may also raise blood levels of this lipid, saturated fat tends to increase blood cholesterol levels to a much greater extent.

Diets that contain an adequate amount of unsaturated fatty acids, particularly *omega-3 fatty acids*, may reduce inflammation in the body and reduce risk for some chronic diseases.[17] The American Heart Association reports diets rich in foods containing omega-3 fatty acids have been shown to decrease risk of arrhythmias (irregular heartbeats), decrease blood fat levels, slow growth of plaque in arteries, and lower blood pressure.[7] Other studies indicated foods rich in omega-3 fatty acids slow aging and may reduce Alzheimer's disease risk. *Omega-6* fatty acids are also essential fatty acids. Along with *omega-3* fatty acids, *omega-6* fatty acids are necessary for brain functions; however, some studies indicate diets high in *omega-6* fatty acids, such as the typical American diet, tend to increase inflammation and may play in a role in increased pain associated with arthritis.[18] Although there is currently no recommended dietary intake for *omega-3* and *omega-6* fatty acids, nutrition experts recommend consuming more *omega-3* fatty acids than *omega-6* fatty acids by eating several servings of fish, plants, and nuts each week.

Rich food sources of omega-3 fatty acids include fatty fish and shellfish from cold water, such as wild salmon, herring, tuna, mackerel, and shrimp. Plant foods such as canola and soybean oils, walnuts, and flax and pumpkin seeds also contain omega-3 fat. The body, however, can convert only a small amount of the plant form of omega-3 fat into the types that are more effectively used by human cells. Therefore, it is best to rely on fish and shellfish for omega-3 fats.

Fish is not a staple of the typical American (Western) diet; therefore, some people take fish oil supplements to obtain the omega-3 fats. Consuming too many fish oil supplements, however, may interfere with blood clotting, making excessive bleeding likely. Instead of relying on fish oil supplements, try to include cold-water fish and shellfish in your meals a couple of times each week.

Unlike the typical American diet that contains large amounts of red meat and few fruits and vegetables, traditional food choices of Mediterranean populations supply smaller amounts of meat, fried foods, and sweets and larger amounts of plant foods, fish, and olive oil. The risk of heart disease is lower for individuals who consume the traditional Mediterranean diet.[19] Unlike the traditional American diet, fruits, vegetables, legumes, nuts, fish, and other seafood are primary sources of nutrients in the Mediterranean. Poultry and dairy are consumed less, and meat and sweets are rarely eaten. The Diversity in Health essay discusses the traditional Asian diet, which also contains less animal protein and saturated fat than Western diets do.

Trans Fats Not all foods made with vegetable oil have healthful properties. *Hydrogenation* is a food processing technique that partially hardens the oil so that it can be made into shortening and sticks of margarine. This process alters the natural chemical structure of some unsaturated fatty acids in vegetable oils, forming *trans fatty acids*. In the body, trans fatty acids behave like saturated fats, raising unhealthy forms of cholesterol in blood.[17] To reduce your intake of trans fatty acids, use soft or liquid margarines, eat less

proteins A class of nutrients that build, maintain, and repair cells.

amino acids The chemical units that compose proteins.

commercial cake frostings, and avoid baked goods and fried foods, which are often made with hydrogenated fats. In response to consumer concerns, many restaurant chains and food manufacturers have eliminated trans fats from their products. Other factors besides dietary lipids contribute to heart disease.

Fat Substitutes Engineered compounds such as Olestra, Oatrim, and Simplesse are used to replace some or all of the fat in certain processed foods. Olestra, for example, supplies no calories because it cannot be digested and absorbed. A 1-oz serving of regular tortilla chips supplies 130 calories and contains 6 g of fat; the same amount of chips fried in Olestra contains 76 calories and no fat. For consumers demanding a variety of fat-free snack foods that taste good, Olestra seems to be a good fat substitute. However, eating foods made with Olestra may produce some unpleasant side effects. Additionally, the substance interferes with the absorption of certain vitamins. Food scientists are currently developing fat replacers that taste good, do not cause side effects, and are chemically stable when heated.

Setting Limits The typical American diet contains too much fat, especially the unhealthy kinds of fat (saturated and trans fats) from dairy products, meats, baked goods, and processed snack foods. College students and other busy people often consume more fat than is necessary by eating greasy snacks and fast foods regularly. Popular fast foods, such as cheeseburgers, pizza, fried chicken and fish, french fries, and milk shakes, contain large amounts of saturated fat. Many fast-food restaurants, however, offer less fatty items such as roast chicken, low-fat yogurt, bean burritos, and meatless salads. The Managing Your Health feature "Trimming the Unhealthy Fats from Your Diet" provides some practical ways to reduce your intake of saturated and trans fats.

Most food labels provide nutrition information concerning the amounts of total fat, saturated fat, trans fat, and cholesterol in food products. A later section of this chapter describes how to use this information to control the amount and type of fat in your diet.

Proteins

Your body needs **proteins** to build, maintain, and repair cells; to form structural components such as hair and nails; and to make enzymes, antibodies, and numerous hormones. Although carbohydrates and fats are its primary fuels, the body derives a small amount of energy from protein. Proteins consist of **amino acids**. During digestion, proteins in plant or animal foods are broken down, releasing amino acids for absorption. Human cells use about 20 different amino acids to synthesize the thousands of proteins in the body. The cells can make 11 of these amino acids; the other 9 amino acids are essential and must be supplied by the diet. If the diet lacks the essential amino acids, the body is unable to grow properly or carry out vital functions.

Most foods, even plant foods, contain some protein. Animal foods generally contain adequate amounts of

Figure 9.6

Soybean Products. Tofu and other processed soybean products are excellent plant sources of protein.

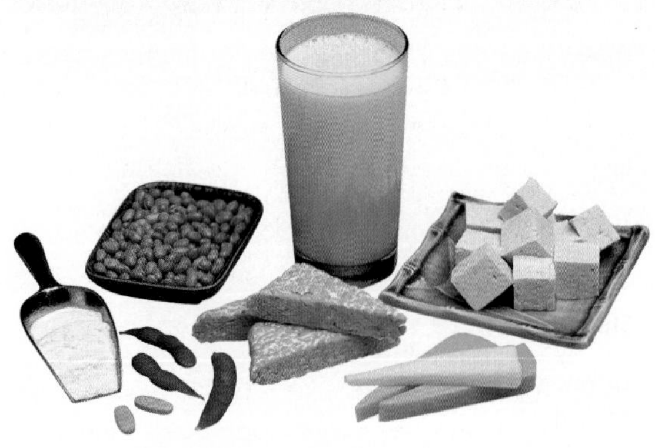

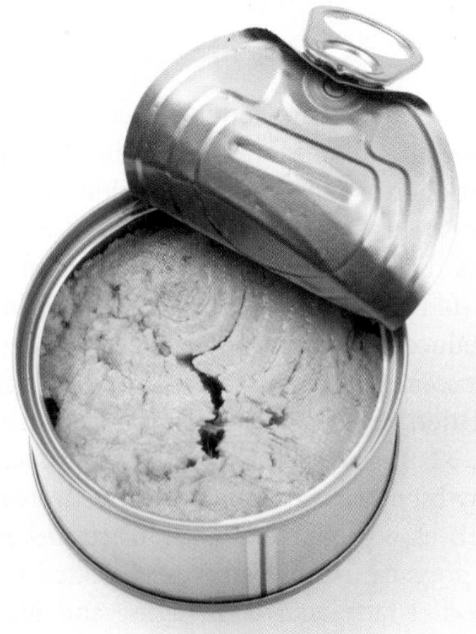

Tuna is an excellent source of omega-3 fat.

Diversity in Health

Asian American Food

Asian populations consume large quantities of rice, wheat noodles, and vegetables combined with eggs or a small amount of meat (usually seafood, poultry, fish, or pork). The traditional Asian diet is high in starch and fiber and usually low in fat, especially saturated fat. Stir-frying vegetables and meats in a lightly oiled wok and steaming foods are popular Asian cooking methods that add fewer calories than deep-fat frying and preserve more vitamins and minerals than boiling. To season their foods, most Asian cooks use low-fat items such as garlic, ginger, and sauces made from mustard and soybeans.

Not all features of the traditional Asian diet are healthful. Asian meals contain little or no dairy products; therefore, the amount of calcium in these diets is usually low. Among the residents of northern Japan, the consumption of soy sauce as well as fermented and pickled foods adds excessive amounts of sodium to diets and may contribute to the relatively high incidence of certain cancers and hypertension. After immigrating to the United States, many Asians adopt Western food preferences and preparation practices. For example, American-style Chinese meals often include larger portions of meat and breaded, deep-fat fried foods.

Some people experience an adverse reaction when they eat Asian or other foods to which the flavor enhancer *monosodium glutamate* (*MSG*) has been added. After eating food that contains MSG, persons who are sensitive to the compound may report a "tight" sensation in the face and chest, headache, and pain and reddening of skin, especially on the face. Results of clinical studies, however, fail to show consistently that MSG causes adverse reactions in most people.[20]

© Mike Flippo/ShutterStock

When you eat at Chinese, Japanese, Thai, and other Asian American restaurants, select menu items carefully. Choose plenty of steamed vegetables and rice or noodles to accompany the entrée. Avoid dishes containing foods that have been dipped in batter and fried, avoid or limit your intake of fried wontons and egg rolls, and do not add soy sauce to your food. If you react adversely to MSG, many cooks, upon request, will prepare your food without it.

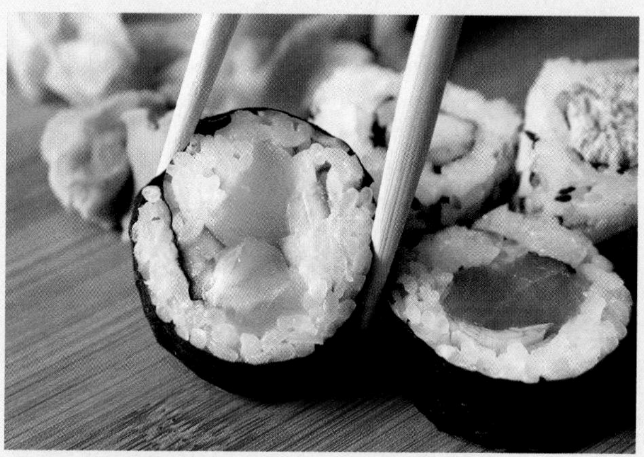

© tkemot/ShutterStock

each essential amino acid; these foods are *complete* or high-quality protein sources. Most plants are sources of *incomplete* or low-quality protein because they either contain insufficient amounts or lack one or more of the essential amino acids. The best plant sources of essential amino acids are soybeans, quinoa, whole grains, seeds, nuts, peas, and lentils (**Figure 9.6**). Fruits do not contain appreciable amounts of essential amino acids.

Proteins and Health Animal products, especially meat, fish, poultry, eggs, milk, and milk products, contribute almost two-thirds of the protein in the typical American's diet.[21] Although consuming more that the recommended amount of protein does not harm most healthy individuals, generous portions of animal foods contribute excessive amounts of saturated fat to the diet. Diets that contain high amounts of saturated fat are associated with increased risk of heart disease, the number one killer of Americans. Diets very high in protein are associated with increased risk for stroke, diabetes, and several types of cancer.[22]

Many athletes and bodybuilders think it is necessary to consume large quantities of animal foods and protein supplements to increase their muscle mass. This practice does not build bigger muscles; instead, the body must metabolize the extra amino acids for energy or convert them into body fat. Additionally, the kidneys need more water to eliminate the excess amino acid by-products. The most effective way to enhance muscle mass is to combine a nutritionally adequate diet with a program of muscle-strengthening exercises.

Animal foods are among the most expensive items on the typical American's grocery list. You can reduce your food costs and decrease your saturated fat intake by substituting certain plant foods for meat and other animal protein sources. The following section discusses vegetarianism, a way to reduce your animal protein intake without sacrificing the nutritional adequacy of your diet.

Vegetarianism A growing number of Americans are consuming plant-based, or *vegetarian*, diets that

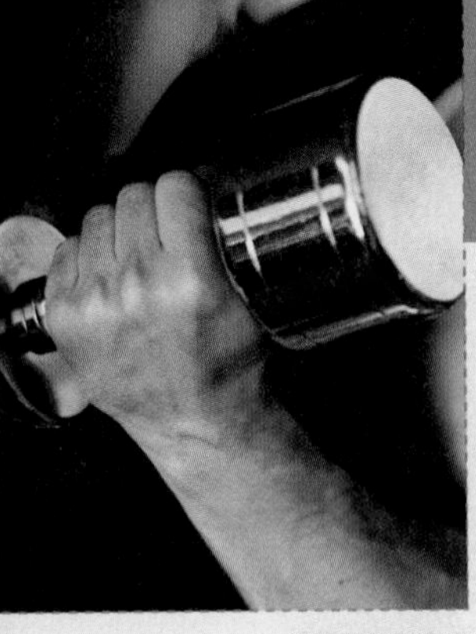

© Kzenon/ShutterStock

Managing Your Health

Trimming Unhealthy Fats from Your Diet

Americans can reduce the amount of unhealthy fats in their diets by changing the ways they select and prepare their food. The following tips can help you trim unwanted fat from your diet.

- Avoid breaded and fried vegetables, chicken, fish, and meats.
- Eat less red meat and more poultry and fish.
- Avoid sausage, bacon, and fatty luncheon meats.
- Eat boiled or baked instead of fried potatoes.
- Trim all visible fat from meats before cooking them.
- Chill cooked chili, stews, soups, sauces, and gravies. Then, skim off the fat before reheating and serving these foods.
- Substitute fat-free ("skim") milk for whole or reduced-fat (2%) milk.
- Substitute reconstituted, nonfat dry milk in recipes that use milk or cream.
- Eat low-fat or fat-free frozen yogurt and ice milk.
- Replace hard cheeses with part-skim or low-fat cheeses.
- Substitute fat-reduced cream cheese for regular cream cheese.
- Substitute plain low-fat or fat-free yogurt for sour cream in recipes.
- Skim frostings from cakes; commercial frostings are often made with hydrogenated shortening, which is 100% fat and contains trans fats.
- When eating two-crust pies, eat the filling and only one crust; discard the remaining crust.
- Replace shortening in recipes with oil or margarine.

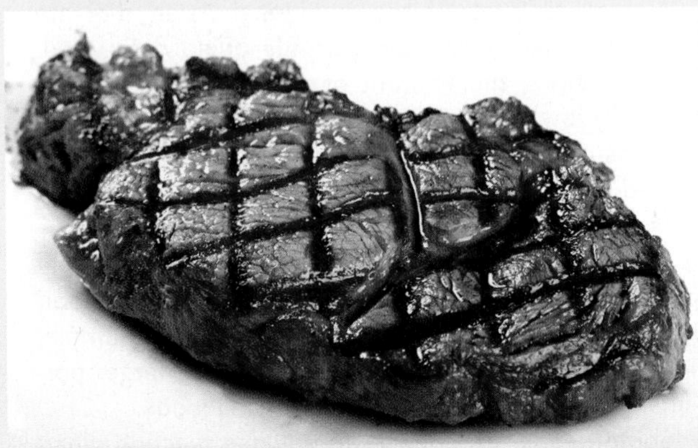

© Dan Peretz/ShutterStock

contain little or no animal foods. Many people associate meat with protein, but processed soybean foods, such as tofu, soymilk, and soy nut butter; quinoa; various beans, peas, and lentils; nuts; seeds; and foods made from cereal grains (for example, wheat and oats) are among the best sources of protein from plants.

There are several types of vegetarian diets. The vegan, or total vegetarian, diet consists of plant foods only. Other vegetarian diets include some animal foods. For example, the *lacto-vegetarian* diet contains dairy products, and the *lacto-ovo-vegetarian diet* includes eggs as well as dairy products. Some people who eat fish or poultry still call themselves vegetarians because they do not eat *red* meats. There are so many different plant-based diets it is difficult to estimate the number of Americans practicing some form of vegetarianism.

Are vegetarian diets nutritious? Plant-based diets may promote good health because they contain more fiber, antioxidants, and phytochemicals and less saturated fat and cholesterol than the traditional meat-rich Western diet. Generally, the nutritional adequacy of a vegetarian diet varies according to the degree of its dietary restrictions. Animal foods are rich sources of essential amino acids as well as certain minerals and vitamins. Plant foods, on the other hand, generally lack one or more essential amino acids.

In the past, nutrition experts advised vegans to consume mixtures of plant foods that supplied all the essential amino acids in one meal because it was believed the body did not save essential amino acids and was unable to make proteins unless all of them were available at one time. Now it is known that the body can conserve essential amino acids after a meal or snack and use them for protein production later in the day. Although it is not necessary to combine plant foods to obtain the proper mix of amino acids, combinations such as peanut butter on toast or red beans and rice make vegetarian meals nutritious, inexpensive, and easy to prepare. Most vegetarians can obtain adequate amounts of essential amino acids and other nutrients by eating a variety of plant foods, consuming dairy products, and taking a multiple vitamin/mineral supplement.

Thus, with careful planning, most plant-based diets can be nutritionally adequate.[23] If you are interested in learning specific details about vegetarian cookery and menu planning, you can obtain this information from registered dietitians (RDs) or University Outreach Extension nutritionists in your area.

Food Allergies A 3-year-old child develops hives—small, itchy, swollen, reddened areas on her skin—soon after she eats eggs. Her older brother must avoid peanuts and foods that may contain peanuts because he can experience *shock*, a drop in blood pressure and loss of consciousness that can be deadly if not treated immediately. These reactions are the result of food allergies, the immune system's inappropriate response to harmless proteins (*allergens*) in certain foods. In the United States, 5% of children and about 4% of adults are allergic to one or more foods.[24] Proteins in cows' milk, eggs, peanuts, tree nuts (such as cashews and walnuts), wheat, soybeans, fish, and shellfish are most likely to cause allergic reactions in susceptible people. Food manufacturers must identify ingredients that are common food allergens on labels (**Figure 9.7**).

Hives are the most common sign of food allergy; other signs include *eczema*, a scaly skin rash; asthma symptoms, such as wheezing and difficulty breathing; and vomiting and diarrhea. Shock (anaphylaxis) occurs when the entire body reacts to the allergen. As mentioned earlier, shock can be fatal.

If you think you or someone you know has a food allergy, consult an allergist/immunologist, a physician who specializes in the diagnosis and treatment of allergies. Special skin and blood tests are used to identify food allergies (**Figure 9.8**). Alternative medical procedures to diagnose allergies, such as food specific IgG tests, leukocyte cytotoxic tests, sublingual and intradermal provocation tests, electrodermal (VEGA) testing, and applied kinesiology, are inappropriate and unproven.[25]

In the case of a true food allergy, the best treatment is to avoid the offending food. Additionally, the allergic person should be prepared to treat shock by taking antihistamines or administering injectable *epinephrine*, a naturally produced substance that raises blood pressure. Parents of children with food allergies must read labels carefully to check ingredients for allergens. They should inform their children's adult caregivers, teachers, and the parents of their children's friends about the allergy and the importance of not offering foods that may contain allergens to their children. Although most children outgrow milk, egg, and wheat allergies, they are likely to

Figure 9.7

Labeling Food Allergens. The Food Allergen Labeling and Consumer Protection Act requires food manufacturers to identify common food allergens that may be in packaged foods on their products' labels.

Courtesy of Wendy Schiff.

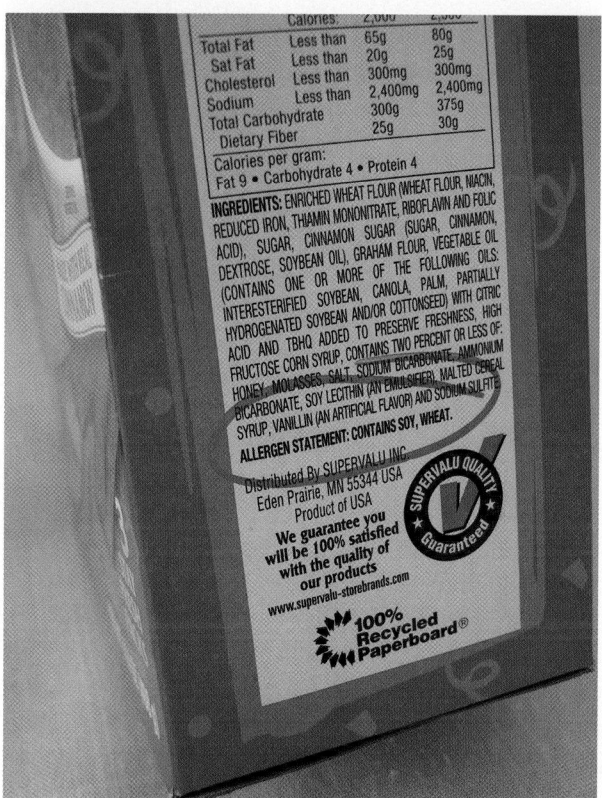

Figure 9.8

Skin Testing for Food Allergies. Skin testing that is performed by a physician is an effective method of diagnosing food allergies.

© Andy Lidstone/ShutterStock

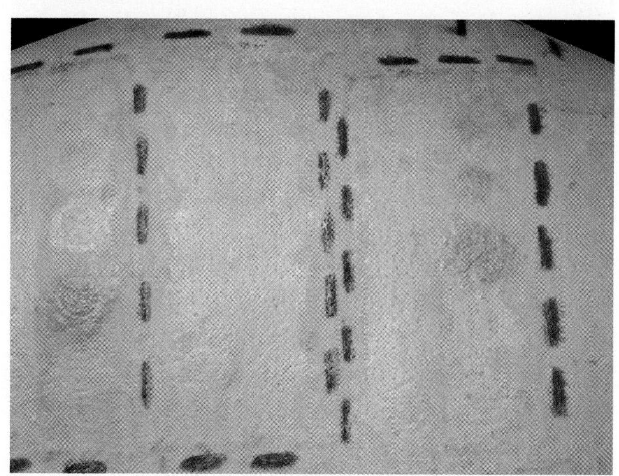

celiac disease A condition characterized by hypersensitivity to gluten.

vitamins A class of organic nutrients that help regulate growth; release energy from carbohydrates, fats, and proteins; and maintain tissues.

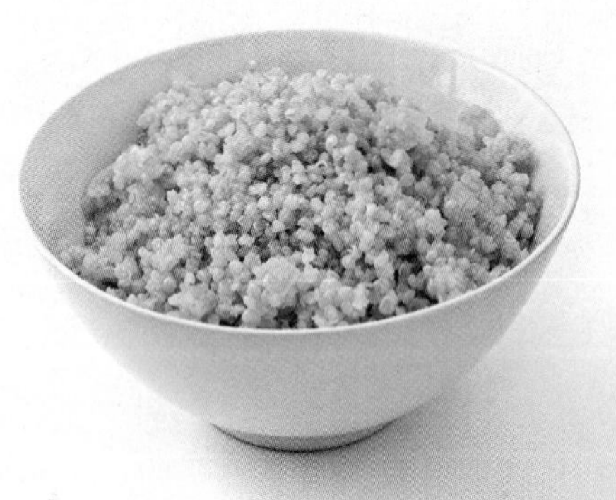

Quinoa (keen'-wah) is a vegetable that is often prepared like cooked cereal.

© Noam Armonn/ShutterStock

remain allergic to peanuts, tree nuts, fish, and shellfish throughout their lives.

Celiac Disease People with **celiac disease** are hypersensitive to *gluten*, a protein in wheat, rye, and barley. When a person with the disease consumes gluten, his or her immune system responds by causing an inflammation of the lining of the small intestine. The inflammation damages the lining, and the body cannot absorb nutrients from food as a result.

Celiac disease affects about 1 in 141 people in the United States.[26] Signs and symptoms of celiac disease include malnutrition; fatigue; arthritis; skin rash; abdominal bloating and pain; chronic diarrhea; vomiting; pale, foul-smelling stools; and weight loss. Children with the disease are irritable and fail to grow properly.

Celiac disease is an *autoimmune disorder*. People with this chronic condition are also likely to have other autoimmune diseases, such as type 1 diabetes, rheumatoid arthritis, and Sjögren's syndrome.[27] Celiac disease has a genetic basis, so people who have family members with the condition are more likely to develop the disease.

The only cure for celiac disease is the complete avoidance of gluten-containing foods and products, such as lipstick, that may contain gluten. Many supermarkets have sections devoted to gluten-free foods, and in major urban areas, some restaurants have chefs that prepare meals in gluten-free kitchens for their customers with celiac disease. For people with celiac disease, a gluten-free diet is critical for maintaining good health. Gluten-free foods are not necessarily "low-calorie" or useful for people who do not have the condition but want to lose weight. For more information about celiac disease, visit the website of the American Celiac Disease Alliance at http://www.americanceliac.org.

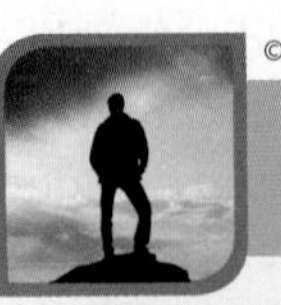

© djgis/ShutterStock

Healthy Living Practices

- To reduce your risk of obesity, heart disease, type 2 diabetes, and certain digestive tract disorders, exercise regularly and consume at least 25 g of fiber each day by eating more fruits, vegetables, beans, and whole-grain cereal products.
- To lower your risk of diabetes and heart disease consume 20% to 35% of your daily calories from fat, limit your intake of saturated fat, avoid trans fat, and consume less than 300 or fewer milligrams of cholesterol per day.
- Dietary cholesterol and saturated and trans fat can be limited by consuming low-fat yogurt and nonfat milk and by eating less cheese, fatty meat, fried food, and fat-laden bakery goods and snack foods.
- Many fast foods are high in saturated fat. If you eat at fast-food restaurants regularly, reduce your intake of meat and fried foods by selecting salads or grilled chicken or fish items.
- If you eat large amounts of red meat and other animal foods, consider eating less and consuming more fatty, cold-water fish; beans; nuts; and whole-grain cereals instead.

Non-Energy-Supplying Nutrients

Vitamins

Vitamins are organic compounds that have numerous functions in the body. Vitamins help regulate growth; release energy from carbohydrates, fats, and proteins; and maintain tissues. Although many vitamins participate in the chemical reactions that release energy, they do not provide calories.

Scientists classify vitamins according to their ability to dissolve in water or fat. Vitamin C and the eight

Table 9.7

Major Vitamins

Vitamin	Major Functions	Rich Food Sources	Deficiency Signs/ Symptoms	Toxicity Signs/ Symptoms
A and provitamin A (beta-carotene)	Vision in dim light, growth, reproduction, maintains immune system and skin, antioxidant	Liver, milk, dark green and leafy vegetables; carrot, sweet potato, mango, oatmeal, broccoli, apricot, peach, and romaine lettuce	Poor vision in dim light, dry skin, blindness, poor growth, respiratory infections	Intestinal upset, liver damage, hair loss, headache, birth defects, death (betacarotene has low toxicity)
D	Bone and tooth development and growth; immune system functioning	Few good food sources other than eggs, fortified milk, and orange juice	Weak, deformed bones (rickets)	Growth failure, loss of appetite, weight loss, death
E	Antioxidant: protects cell membranes	Vegetable oils, whole grains, wheat germ, sunflower seeds, almonds	Anemia (rarely occurs)	Intestinal upsets, bleeding problems
C	Scar formation and maintenance, immune system functioning, antioxidant	Citrus fruits, berries, potatoes, broccoli, peppers, cabbage, tomatoes, fortified fruit drinks	Frequent infections, bleeding gums, bruises, poor wound healing, depression (scurvy)	Diarrhea, nosebleeds, headache, weakness, kidney stones, excess iron absorption and storage
Thiamin	Energy metabolism	Pork, liver, nuts, dried beans and peas, whole-grain and enriched breads and cereals	Heart failure, mental confusion, depression, paralysis (beriberi)	No toxicity has been reported
Riboflavin	Energy metabolism	Milk and yogurt, eggs and poultry, meat, liver, wholegrain and enriched breads and cereals	Enlarged, purple tongue; fatigue; oily skin; cracks in the corners of the mouth	No toxicity has been reported
Niacin	Energy metabolism	Protein-rich foods, peanut butter, whole-grain and enriched breads and cereals	Skin rash, diarrhea, weakness, dementia, death (pellagra)	Painful skin flushing, intestinal upsets, liver damage
Vitamin B_6	Protein and fat metabolism	Liver, oatmeal, bananas, meat, fish, poultry, whole grains, fortified cereals	Anemia, skin rash, irritability, elevated homocysteine levels	Weakness, depression, permanent nerve damage
Folate (folic acid)	DNA production	Leafy vegetables, oranges, nuts, liver, enriched breads and cereals	Anemia, depression, spina bifida in developing embryo, elevated homocysteine levels	Hides signs of B_{12} deficiency; may cause allergic response
B_{12}	DNA production	Animal products	Pernicious anemia, fatigue, paralysis, elevated homocysteine levels	No toxicity has been reported

B vitamins are water soluble; vitamins A, D, E, and K are fat soluble. The body does not store most water-soluble vitamins to any appreciable extent, whereas fat-soluble vitamins are stored in the liver and body fat and can accumulate to toxic levels. **Table 9.7** lists most of the vitamins as well as their major roles in the body and rich food sources.

Compared to the energy-supplying nutrients and water, the body requires very small amounts of vitamins. Diets that include a wide variety of foods can meet the vitamin needs of healthy individuals. Some persons, however, take nutrient supplements that provide several times the recommended levels of vitamins to treat or prevent illness. Taking more of a nutrient than the body needs is not necessarily better. Cells use limited amounts of each vitamin daily. In many instances, excessive amounts of these nutrients accumulate in the body and cause harmful side effects. Vitamins A, B6, and niacin are very toxic when taken in large doses. Table 9.7 provides information concerning the signs and symptoms of vitamin toxicity disorders.

Antioxidants The chemical structures of certain compounds, particularly polyunsaturated fatty acids, make them vulnerable to damage by free radicals. Free radical formation produces chemical changes in cells that may contribute to the development of cardiovascular disease (diseases of the heart and blood vessels), certain cancers, degenerative changes in the eye, and other chronic health conditions.

Many foods contain antioxidants that can protect cells by preventing or reducing the formation of free radicals. These antioxidants include vitamins E and C and a variety of phytochemicals such as beta-carotene, a yellow-orange pigment in plants that the body converts to vitamin A. Table 9.2 lists some phytochemicals that have antioxidant activity and their major food sources; **Table 9.8** lists foods commonly consumed in the United States that have high antioxidant activity per serving.

Since the 1980s, scientists have been investigating the possible risks and benefits of eating diets rich in antioxidants or taking antioxidant supplements. No strong scientific data support the popular belief that vitamin C prevents the common cold, but taking the vitamin may shorten the duration of the infection.[28] Vitamin C may also reduce the risk of developing heart disease, but its usefulness in preventing diabetes, cancer, and Alzheimer's disease is not supported by scientific evidence.[28]

Should you take large doses of vitamins, especially antioxidant vitamins, to prevent disease? Nutrition experts are divided over the issue of antioxidant vitamin supplementation. The cells in your body make antioxidants. Some scientists think modern humans are exposed to much higher levels of environmental hazards, such as air pollution and pesticide residues, than their ancestors. These conditions may increase the body's need for antioxidants beyond the amounts that are made or can be obtained from food, making supplementation necessary. Other scientists think plant foods are the best source of antioxidants. Unlike nutrient supplements, plant foods contain mixtures of vitamins and phytochemicals that collectively may provide healthful benefits. Taking large doses of antioxidant vitamins may have harmful side effects, including promoting the growth of cancer cells.

Between 2003 and 2006, 33% of adult Americans reported taking multiple vitamin supplements that contain three or more vitamins.[29] Unless medically

Table 9.8

Antioxidant-Rich Foods

Blackberries	Cranberries	Blueberries	Cranberry juice	Pineapple juice
Walnuts	Coffee	Cloves, ground	Cherries, sour	Guava nectar (beverage)
Strawberries	Raspberries	Grape juice	Wine, red	
Artichokes (cooked)	Pecans	Chocolate, baking, unsweetened	Power bar, chocolate	

Data from Halvorsen, B. L., et al. (2006). Content of redox-active compounds (i.e., antioxidants) in foods consumed in the United States. *American Journal of Clinical Nutrition*, 84(1), 95–135.

necessary, taking dietary supplements is often an economically wasteful and risky practice. By eating a variety of whole-grain products, fruits, and vegetables daily, you are less likely to encounter toxicity problems because these foods naturally supply vitamins in smaller quantities.

Minerals

Minerals are a group of elements such as calcium, iron, and sodium. Several minerals are nutrients that have a wide variety of roles in the body. For example, the mineral nutrient magnesium regulates chemical reactions; other mineral nutrients are structural components of certain organic molecules, like the iron in red blood cells and calcium in bones. The body needs very small amounts of minerals, compared to the energy-supplying nutrients and water. Excesses of any mineral can create imbalances with other minerals or can be toxic.

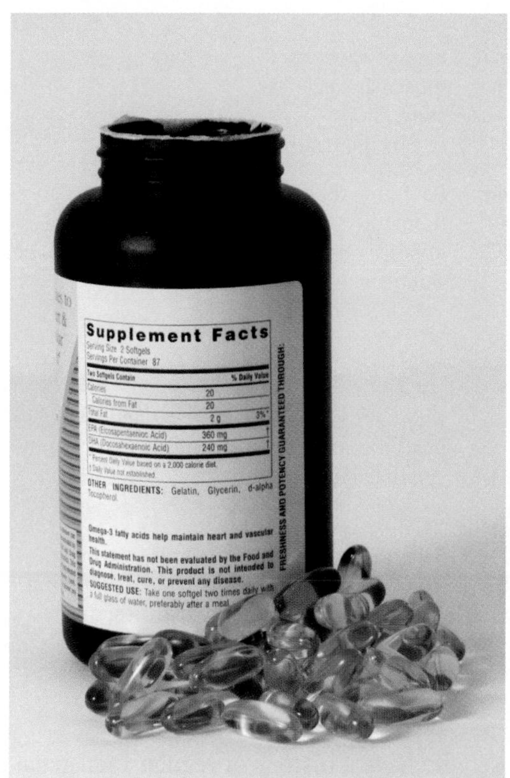

Table 9.9 lists some essential minerals, describes their major roles, and identifies common foods that contain high amounts of these substances. The following section provides information about calcium and iron, two minerals that have considerable health importance for Americans.

minerals A class of inorganic nutrients that includes several elements, such as iron, calcium, and zinc.

osteoporosis An age-related condition in which bones lose density, becoming weak and breaking easily.

Calcium Calcium is the most plentiful mineral in the body. You may be aware that calcium is necessary for the development of strong bones and teeth, but this mineral has other important roles as well, such as regulating blood pressure and participating in muscular movements. The body carefully maintains the level of calcium in the blood within a specific range. When the level is too high, the bones can remove and store the excess. If the amount of calcium in the blood begins to drop below normal levels, the bones release some of the mineral from storage, returning the level to normal.

As it adjusts to the demands of bearing the body's weight, bone tissue undergoes a continual process of being built, torn down, and rebuilt. After about 40 years of age, the bones of most people begin to break down at a faster rate than they rebuild. As bones gradually lose mineral density, they become weak and brittle. Fragile bones break easily and sometimes shatter because they cannot support the body. Although any bone can be affected, bones in the hip, spine, and wrist are most likely to break. This condition, **osteoporosis**, threatens the health of millions of aging Americans, especially older adult women. In the United States, 40 million Americans either have osteoporosis or are at risk of the disorder; most of these persons are older women.[30] Men usually have denser bones than women, which may explain why most aging men are not affected by osteoporosis to the same extent as aging women are.

Fractures are associated with an increased risk of permanent disability or death, particularly if the fracture immobilizes the person; immobility increases the likelihood that fatal blood clots or pneumonia will develop. A painful and disabling condition known as "dowager's hump" can occur when bones in the upper spine are so weak that they experience small compression fractures over time while trying to support the weight of the skull. As these bones heal into wedge shapes, the upper spine assumes an abnormal curvature (**Figure 9.9**). As a result, people with osteoporosis often "shrink"—they lose some of their height.

As one ages, a calcium-rich diet and weight-bearing physical activity help build and maintain strong bones. After *menopause*, however, such practices may

Table 9.9

Some Essential Minerals

Mineral	Roles	Rich Food Sources	Deficiency Signs/ Symptoms	Toxicity Signs/ Symptoms
Calcium	Builds and maintains bones and teeth, regulates muscle and nerve function, regulates blood pressure and blood clotting	Milk products; fortified orange juice, tofu, and soy milk; fish with edible small bones such as sardines and salmon; broccoli; hard water	Poor bone growth, weak bones, muscle spasms, convulsions	Kidney stones, calcium deposits in organs, mineral imbalances
Potassium	Maintains fluid balance, necessary for nerve function	Whole grains, fruits, and vegetables, yogurt, milk	Muscular weakness, confusion, death	Heart failure
Sodium	Maintains fluid balance, necessary for nerve function	Salt, soy sauce, luncheon meats, processed cheeses, pickled foods, snack foods, canned and dried soups	Muscle cramping, headache, confusion, coma	Hypertension
Magnesium	Regulation of enzyme activity, necessary for nerve function	Green leafy vegetables, nuts, whole grains, peanut butter	Loss of appetite, muscular weakness, convulsions, confusion, death	Rare
Zinc	Component of many enzymes and the hormone insulin, maintains immune function, necessary for sexual maturation and reproduction	Meats, fish, poultry, whole grains, vegetables	Poor growth, failure to mature sexually, improper healing of wounds	Mineral imbalances, gastrointestinal upsets, anemia, heart disease
Selenium	Component of a group of antioxidant enzymes, immune system function	Seafood, liver, and vegetables and grains grown in selenium-rich soil	May increase risk of heart disease and certain cancers	Hair and nail loss
Iron	Oxygen transport involved in the release of energy	Clams, oysters, liver, red meats, and enriched breads and cereals	Fatigue, weakness, iron-deficiency anemia	Iron poisoning, nausea, vomiting, diarrhea, death

not be enough to prevent osteoporosis or slow its progress. Within the first 5 to 10 years after menopause, even healthy women are susceptible to losing a large percentage of their bone mass. Why?

The hormone *estrogen* stimulates bones to maintain their mass and retain calcium. A sign of normal estrogen production is regular menstrual cycles. A woman has reached menopause when her estrogen levels drop dramatically and her menstrual cycles have ceased. As women approach this time of life, those who have a history of regular menstrual cycles are more likely to maintain their bone mass than those who had irregular or absent menstrual cycles.

Besides being a postmenopausal woman, other characteristics increase one's risk of osteoporosis. The condition may be inherited, and members of certain racial groups are more susceptible to osteoporosis than others. African Americans tend to have larger bone masses that afford some protection against osteoporosis. On the other hand, slender, small-boned people

Figure 9.9

Dowager's Hump. In people with osteoporosis, the bones in the upper spine develop small compression fractures. These bones heal into wedge shapes, and the upper spine assumes a deformed, curved shape known as "Dowager's hump."

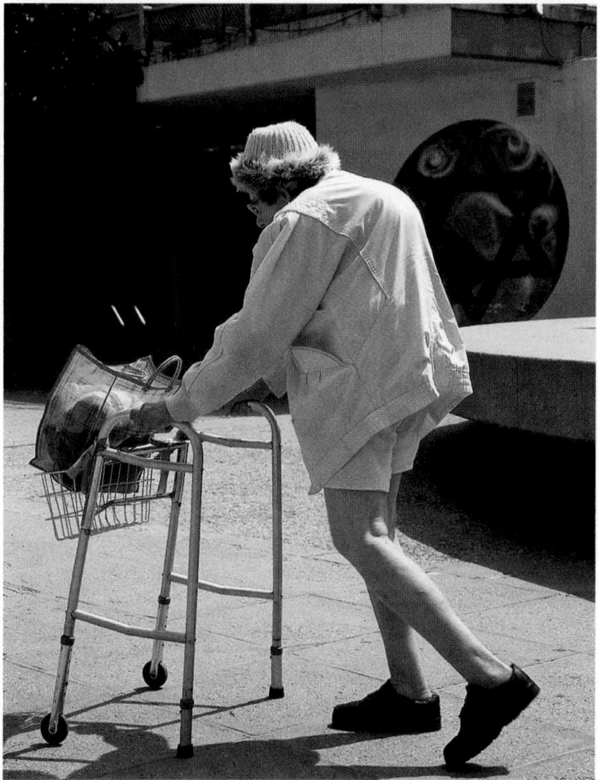

Figure 9.10

Calcium-Rich Foods. Some of the richest food sources of calcium are low-fat milk and yogurt, and greens. Although most cheeses are high in saturated fat, they are good sources of calcium.

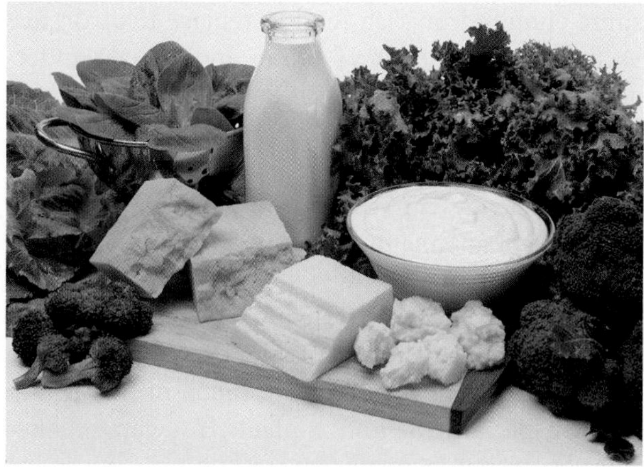

of European and Asian ancestry are more likely than people with large bones to develop osteoporosis.

Certain lifestyle choices can increase a person's risk of osteoporosis. Young people with low-calcium diets are likely to have less-dense bones that are susceptible to osteoporosis as they grow older. Cigarette smoking and alcohol consumption can accelerate bone loss. Furthermore, young women who exercise excessively may disrupt their body's normal estrogen production and menstrual cycles. This reduction in estrogen levels can lead to premature bone loss. Special X-rays are used to diagnose bone loss clinically.

To treat menopausal women who are at risk of osteoporosis, physicians often prescribe hormone replacement therapy, that is, synthetic hormones that contain estrogen or a combination of estrogen and progesterone. Nonhormonal treatments are available also. Women who are approaching menopause should consult their physicians about their risks of developing osteoporosis and their treatment options.

Most medical experts recommend that young men and women adopt behaviors that maximize their bone mass. If you are concerned about your risk of developing osteoporosis, consume foods that supply calcium such as those shown in **Figure 9.10**.

If you do not consume dairy products or foods fortified with calcium, ask your physician about alternative ways to obtain this mineral, such as calcium-containing supplements or antacids. In addition to calcium, vitamin D and the mineral magnesium are important for bone health. Adopting healthful lifestyles, such as refraining from smoking, reducing alcohol consumption, and engaging in physical activities that place stress on your bones, such as walking, weight lifting, or jogging, can help maintain your skeleton's structural integrity.

Osteoporosis can occur at any age. If you think your risk of developing this condition is high, ask your doctor to perform a bone density test. By treating osteoporosis in its early stages, substantial bone loss can be prevented.

Iron Most of the body's iron is found in the hemoglobin molecules within the red blood cells. Hemoglobin combines with oxygen in the lungs and transports it to cells throughout the body. Oxygen is necessary to release the energy stored in glucose.

Anemia results when the body produces abnormal red blood cells. In cases of iron-deficiency anemia, the bone marrow forms red blood cells that are smaller and contain less hemoglobin than normal cells.

Without sufficient hemoglobin, the red blood cells carry less oxygen than usual as they circulate. Anemic individuals often report feeling tired because their cells are unable to obtain adequate amounts of energy.

Iron deficiency is one of the most prevalent nutritional disorders in the United States. Many individuals, especially premenopausal women, are at risk of becoming iron deficient because they do not consume enough iron-rich food to replace the iron lost each month in menstrual blood. Individuals undergoing rapid growth, such as infants, children, teenagers, and pregnant women, have high needs for iron and are at risk of iron deficiency. If untreated, severe iron deficiency can cause iron-deficiency anemia. This type of anemia often occurs in people who lose a lot of blood.

To ensure adequate iron intake, you can eat the iron-rich foods listed in Table 9.9. Normally, the small intestine does not absorb much of the iron in foods, especially the iron in plants. You can enhance the absorption of plant sources of iron by eating them with meat or vitamin C–rich foods. In addition to eating more foods that contain iron, people with iron-deficiency anemia may need to take iron supplements.

Annually, thousands of young children unintentionally poison themselves, a few of them fatally, after ingesting toxic amounts of iron-containing supplements. Many of these cases involve unsupervised young children who take overdoses of flavored vitamin/mineral supplements, thinking they are candy. To prevent such tragedies, store nutrient and other dietary supplements like other medications, making them inaccessible to children.

Hemochromatosis An estimated 5 in 1,000 white Americans have *hemochromatosis*, a genetic condition that increases the intestinal absorption of dietary iron.[31] The iron accumulates in their organs and reaches toxic levels by the time they are middle-aged. These people are often unaware that they have the potentially fatal condition until it causes serious conditions such as diabetes, liver damage, and heart disease. A simple blood test can detect this treatable disorder. People with hemochromatosis should not take supplements that contain iron and should limit their intake of iron-rich foods.

Water

Water is essential for life on earth. You can survive weeks, months, and even years without one of the other nutrients, but you cannot survive for more than a few days without water. Water has many functions in the body: dissolving and transporting materials, eliminating wastes, lubricating joints, and participating in numerous chemical reactions.

About 60% of an adult's body is water. To function properly, the body maintains its fluid levels within specific limits, generally by increasing or decreasing urine production. Although it carefully conserves water, the body loses water when one perspires, urinates, exhales, and defecates. Drinking plain water and fluids such as milk, juices, and soft drinks replenishes the body's water. Most foods, especially fruits and vegetables, also supply water.

Advertisements often promote beer as a thirst quencher; however, drinking alcoholic beverages does not replace body water. Alcohol acts as a diuretic, a compound that increases urinary losses of water. Caffeine is also a diuretic, but its effects are less than alcohol's. The amount of caffeine contained in coffee, energy drinks, energy and weight loss pills and soda vary; however, some popular brands contain as much as 400 milligrams per serving. Too much regular caffeine intake can result in *caffeinism*, which includes nervous irritability, occasional muscle twitching, heart palpitations, rapid heartbeat, and gastrointestinal irritability.[32] Nutrition experts recommend consuming no more than 300 milligram of caffeine each day, or about two cups of regular coffee.

According to a report issued by an expert panel of the National Institute of Medicine, the daily recommended amounts of water from food and beverages are about 16 cups for men and 11 cups for women.[33] In general, Americans' water intake is adequate. Dehydration occurs when the normal level of body water declines and the affected individual does not consume replenishing fluids. The symptoms of dehydration include weakness, confusion, and irritability. During prolonged fevers or bouts of diarrhea or vomiting, the body can lose substantial amounts of water, causing dehydration. These conditions cause the loss of minerals such as sodium and potassium as well. If untreated, severe dehydration is usually fatal.

Healthy people can become dehydrated while working or exercising in hot conditions. Is it helpful to consume sports drinks under these situations? In addition to water and glucose, sports drinks contain small amounts of the minerals sodium and potassium; therefore, these beverages may be beneficial for individuals engaging in prolonged strenuous physical activities during which considerable sweating occurs. Most people, however, can maintain their fluid and mineral balance by eating a variety of foods and by drinking water before and during the activity.

nutrient requirement The minimum amount of a nutrient that prevents that nutrient's deficiency disease.

Dietary Reference Intakes (DRIs) A set of standards for evaluating the nutritional quality of diets.

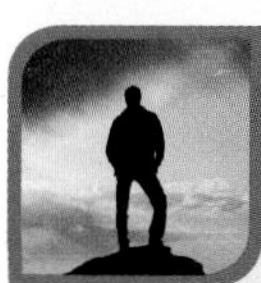
© djgis/ShutterStock

Healthy Living Practices

- To obtain all of the vitamins and minerals you need, eat a wide variety of foods each day; include whole grains, dairy products, fruits, and vegetables.
- Store dietary supplements like other medications, making them inaccessible to children.
- If you are hot or exercising heavily, to prevent dehydration, drink plenty of water and other beverages that do not contain caffeine or alcohol.
- To increase the likelihood that you will maintain your bone mass as you age, consume adequate amounts of calcium-rich foods, drink less alcohol, do not smoke, and engage in weight-bearing exercise regularly.

The Basics of a Healthful Diet

When you eat a milk-chocolate candy bar or some french-fried potatoes, you probably know that these foods contain carbohydrate and fat, but you may be surprised to learn that they also supply some protein, water, and even vitamins and minerals. Most foods are mixtures of nutrients that contain relatively large quantities of water, carbohydrate, fat, or protein, with much smaller quantities of vitamins and minerals. Candy bars and french fries are commonly called "junk" foods because they contain considerable calories from fat and sugar. Dietitians, however, generally refer to such foods as "empty-calorie" rather than junk foods.

A nutritious diet has two key features: *nutrient adequacy* and *nutrient balance.* The foods in a nutritionally adequate and balanced diet contain all essential nutrients in the proper proportions. By selecting a wide variety of foods, you can usually obtain all essential nutrients. Many people upset the nutritional balance of their diets by consuming more food than they need, by making poor food choices, or by taking massive doses of nutrient supplements. Eating too much food can make one overweight; eating too much salty food may raise one's blood pressure; ingesting too many supplements can cause nutrient toxicity disorders. Consuming mostly foods with high-quality nutrients, such as lean proteins, fruits, and vegetables and limiting foods associated with increased health risk, such as refined grains, saturated fats, and trans fats is the best approach to planning nutritionally adequate and well-balanced diets.

How much of each nutrient do you need for optimal health? How can you be certain that your diet is nutritionally adequate? The following information provides answers to these questions.

Nutrient Requirements and Recommendations

A **nutrient requirement** can be defined as the minimum amount that prevents an average person from developing the nutrient's deficiency disease. A required level of a nutrient, however, is not necessarily an optimal amount. By obtaining only the required levels of most vitamins, for example, the body does not have amounts to store in various tissues. The body relies on its nutrient reserves if nutritious food becomes unavailable. Thus, nutrition experts recommend that people consume more than just the required amounts of many nutrients.

To determine whether a diet supplies adequate amounts of certain nutrients that can prevent deficiency diseases, nutritionists now use a complex set of standards called the **Dietary Reference Intakes (DRIs)**. The DRIs are composed of four different recommendations for nutrient and energy intake levels, including the *Recommended Dietary Allowances* (*RDAs*), which at one time were the only standards for planning nutritious diets and analyzing the nutritional adequacy of diets. To establish the RDA for a nutrient, scientists take the required level and add a certain amount to provide a margin of safety. For example, the current RDA for vitamin C is 90 mg/day for men and 75 mg/day for women (nonsmokers). The average person, however, requires only about 8 to 10 mg of vitamin C each day to prevent scurvy, the vitamin's deficiency disease. Therefore, most people will not develop scurvy even if their intake does not meet 100% of the RDA.

The DRIs include a set of values called the "Tolerable Upper Intake Level" or simply "UL." The UL is the maximum average daily intake amount for a nutrient that is unlikely to be harmful. Therefore, regularly consuming amounts of a nutrient that exceed its UL is likely to cause toxicity signs and symptoms. The adult UL for vitamin C, for example, is 2,000 milligrams per day. Tables 9.7 and 9.9 indicate toxicity signs and symptoms for certain vitamins and minerals, respectively.

You can evaluate the nutritional adequacy of your diet by using the RDAs or other DRI values. A brief version of the DRI tables is shown in Appendix C. Complete the activity "Assessing the Nutritional Quality of Your Diet" in the Student Workbook section at the end of this text. If your usual intake of a nutrient is between 75% and 100% of the recommended amount, you probably are not at risk of developing that nutrient's deficiency disease. If you need to increase your intake of one or more nutrients, you can identify foods that are rich sources of the nutrient by using food composition tables, such as those on this text's accompanying website, and eat more of these foods.

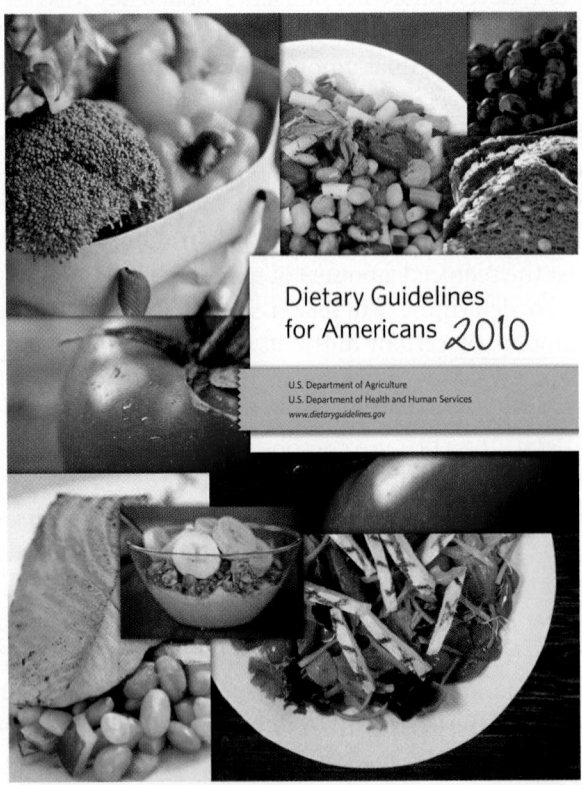

Courtesy of U.S. Department of Agriculture and U.S. Department of Health and Human Services. *Dietary Guidelines for Americans, 2010*, 7th Edition. Washington, DC: U.S. Government Printing Office, December 2010.

The Dietary Guidelines

Every 5 years, the U.S. Department of Agriculture (USDA) and the U.S. Department of Health and Human Services issue the *Dietary Guidelines for Americans*, a publication that provides general recommendations for a healthful diet. The *Guidelines* focus attention on the association between diet and chronic diseases, such as type 2 diabetes and cardiovascular disease. These guidelines provide basic advice concerning lifestyle behaviors that relate to nutritional health, such as choosing nutrient-dense foods, being more physically active, and following food safety practices. The key recommendations of the 2010 *Dietary Guidelines* are described here.

Balance calories with physical activity to achieve and maintain healthy weight.

1. Prevent and/or reduce excess body fat by improving dietary practices and increasing physical activity.
   - Focus on the total number of calories consumed.
   - Monitor food intake by recording what you eat.
   - Consume smaller sized portions or low-calorie options.
   - Eat a nutrient-dense breakfast.
   - Limit the amount of time spent sitting.
2. Control total calorie intake to manage body weight. For people who are overweight or obese, consume fewer calories.
   - Increase intake of plant foods, such as whole grains, vegetables, and fruits.
   - Reduce intake of sugar-sweetened beverages, such as regular soft drinks, fruit drinks, and energy drinks.
   - Monitor the 100% fruit juice intake of children, especially those who are overweight or obese.
   - Avoid excess intake of alcoholic beverages.
3. Increase physical activity and reduce time spent being inactive (sedentary).
   - Balance calorie intake with calorie needs throughout the life span.

Foods and food components to reduce.

1. Limit sodium intake to less than 2,300 mg/day. People older than 50 years of age or who are African American or have hypertension, diabetes, or chronic kidney disease should limit their sodium intake to 1,500 mg/day.
2. Consume less than 10% of calories from unhealthy saturated fats by replacing them with foods that are rich sources of healthy monounsaturated and polyunsaturated fats.
3. Consume less than 300 mg of cholesterol daily.
4. Avoid foods that contain trans fatty acids, such as solid fats and foods that are made with partially hydrogenated oils.

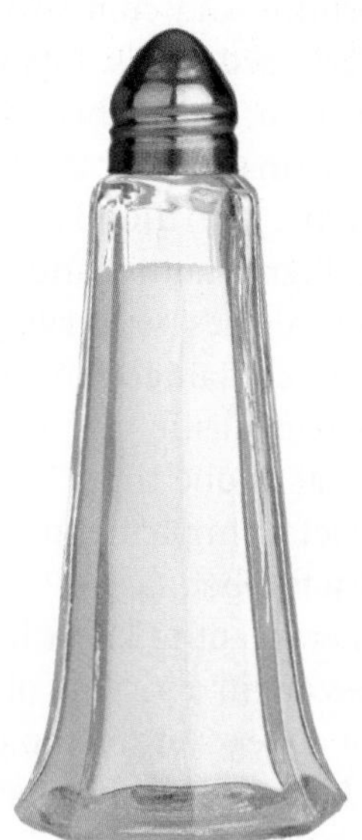

© Picsfive/ShutterStock

5. Reduce intake of calories from foods that contain solid fats and added sugars, such as cakes, cookies, and pastries.
6. Limit consumption of refined grains, especially those with added solid fat, sugar, and sodium.
7. If alcohol is consumed, limit intake to up to one drink per day (women) and two drinks per day (men). Only adults of legal age should consume alcohol.

Foods and nutrients to increase.

1. Increase vegetable and fruit intake.
2. Eat a variety of colorful vegetables, especially dark green, red, and orange vegetables, and beans and peas.
3. Consume at least half of all grain products as whole grains. Replace foods made with refined grains with those made from whole grains.
4. Increase intake of fat-free or low-fat milk and milk products or substitutes, such as yogurt, cheese, or fortified soy beverages.
5. Choose protein foods from a variety of sources, including seafood, lean meat and poultry, eggs, beans and peas, soy products, and unsalted nuts and seeds.
6. Increase the amount and variety of fish and shellfish in your diet by replacing some meat and poultry with such foods.
7. Replace solid fats with vegetable oils.
8. Choose foods that provide more potassium, dietary fiber, calcium, vitamin D. These foods include vegetables, dried beans and peas, fruit, whole grains, and milk and milk products.

Build healthy eating patterns.

1. Select an eating pattern that meets nutrient and energy needs over time.
2. Account for all foods and beverages consumed and evaluate the nutritional quality of your eating pattern.
3. Prepare, eat, and store foods by following food safety recommendations to reduce risk of foodborne illnesses.

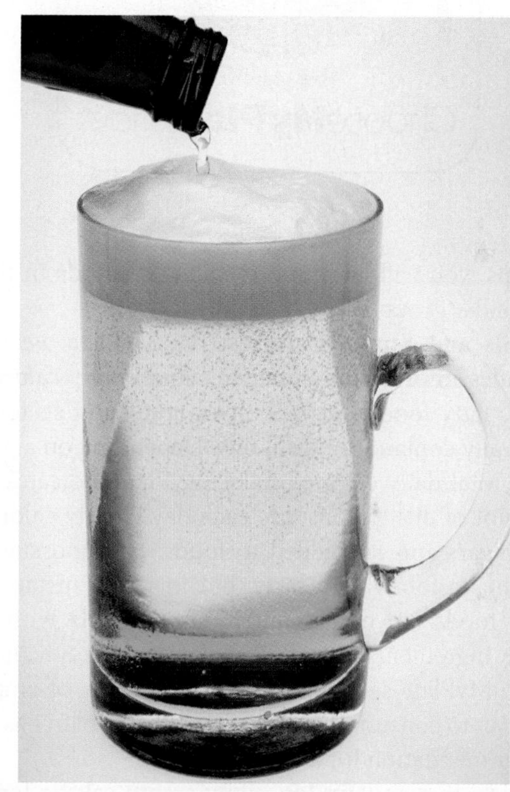

© AbleStock

MyPlate

In spring 2011, the USDA introduced **MyPlate**, a practical guide for planning healthful diets that incorporates recommendations from the 2010 *Dietary Guidelines*. MyPlate has five primary food groups: grains, vegetables, fruits, dairy, and protein foods (**Figure 9.11**).

To obtain more information about MyPlate, access the USDA's interactive website (www.choosemyplate.gov/index.html). By clicking on the glass or section of the plate that represents one of the five major food

Figure 9.11

Choose MyPlate. The USDAs Choose MyPlate interactive tool at www.choosemyplate.gov can be used to plan nutritious menus and evaluate the nutritional quality of a person's diet.

Courtesy of the USDA.

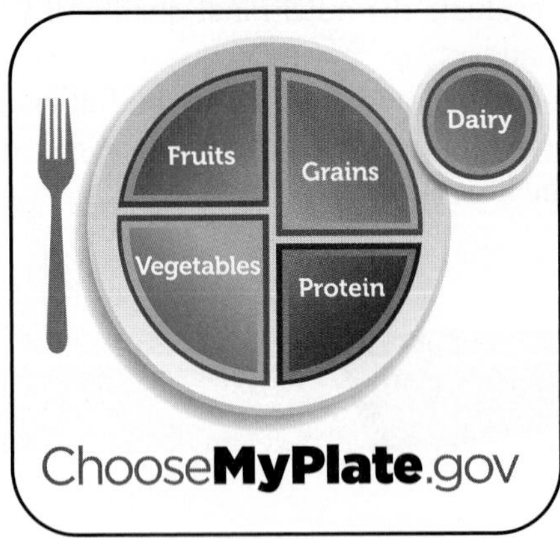

groups, you will learn more about the foods in that particular group.

Oils and Empty Calories The MyPlate website includes information about oils and *empty calories.* Some fatty foods, such as olives, nuts, and seafood, naturally contain healthful oils. Depending on a person's total daily caloric intake, MyPlate indicates an amount of oils to consume each day. Empty calories are sugars and fats added to foods. Fats and sugars can make foods very tasty, but in many instances, such foods are not as nutritious as foods without these ingredients. Alcohol is also an empty-calorie food. MyPlate sets a limit for the number of empty calories to consume each day. The dietary plan has no recommendation for alcohol intake.

Diets that contain too many empty-calorie foods may contribute to excess body fat, heart disease, diabetes, and alcoholism. Additionally, these items can displace more nutrient-dense foods from your diet. Consuming a reasonable amount of empty-calorie foods may be acceptable if your diet is nutritionally adequate and you are physically active and need the extra calories to fuel physical activity. The Student Workbook section at the end of this text includes an activity that enables you to use MyPlate to evaluate the nutritional adequacy of your daily food choices.

Using Nutritional Labeling

The FDA requires nearly every packaged food to have nutritional labeling. Consumers can use food labeling to determine and compare the nutritional value of most packaged foods. **Figure 9.12** illustrates the current Nutrition Facts label and provides tips for using this information. In 2014, the FDA proposed changes to the Nutrition Facts label found on food packaging. Significant changes include larger print to highlight calories per serving and the number of servings per container. Furthermore, serving sizes will be more realistic and reflect how much people typically eat at one time.[34] As of April 2014, there is no projected implementation date for the new Nutrition Facts label.

Many consumers want to know how many grams of fat and calories are in a serving of packaged food. This information appears at the top of the Nutrition Facts label (see Figure 9.12). People can also monitor the amounts of cholesterol, sodium, and fiber in packaged foods. The Nutrition Facts label indicates these amounts by weight and as percentages of established nutrient labeling standards called the *Daily Values (DVs).*

Health officials at the FDA used various sources of nutritional information to determine the DVs for many nutrients and for fiber. As you can see in Figure 9.11, the lower part of the Nutrition Facts label shows two sets of DVs. One set of DVs is for people who consume 2,000 calories each day; the other set is for those who consume 2,500 calories daily. The DVs for total fat, saturated fat, cholesterol, and sodium are maximum amounts. Most Americans should keep their daily intake of these nutrients below these amounts.

Specific information concerning the nutritional content per serving of the food product appears on the upper half of the label. In addition to showing amounts of fat, saturated fat, cholesterol, sodium, total carbohydrate, fiber, sugar, and protein by weight, the Nutrition Facts label displays most of this information as percentages of the DVs for a 2,000-calorie diet. Percentages of the DVs for key vitamins and minerals are shown below the second bold line.

According to the information near the top of the Nutrition Facts label shown in Figure 9.12, a serving of the product supplies 250 calories, 110 of which are from fat. To determine the percentage of calories from fat, divide the calories from fat (110) by the number of calories in the serving (250), and multiply the figure by 100. Forty-four percent of the calories in this food are from fat. Because most health experts recommend that healthy Americans eat no more than 35% of their total calories from fat, you might decide to purchase other food

Figure 9.12

Nutrition Facts. Most packaged foods have nutrient facts on their labels. People can use this information to evaluate the nutritional quality of their food. In 2014, the government proposed changes to Nutrition Facts label format.

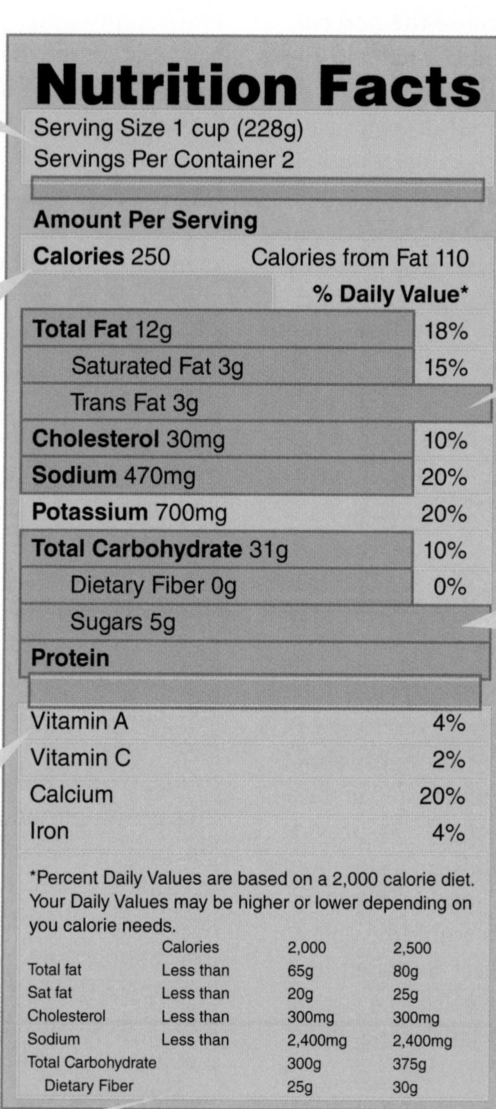

products that contain lower percentages of calories from fat.

1. **Serving Size** This section shows how many servings are in the package. *Remember*: all nutrition information on the label is based on one serving.
2. **Amount of Calories** The calories listed are for one serving. "Calories from fat" are also for one serving.
3. **Consume Adequate Amounts of These Nutrients** Get the most nutrition for your calories—compare the calories to the nutrients to make a healthier food choice.
4. **Limit These Nutrients** Too much total fat (especially saturated fat and trans fat), cholesterol, and sodium may increase your risk of certain chronic diseases.
5. **Choose "Healthy" Carbohydrates** Fiber and sugars are types of carbohydrates. Healthy sources like fruits, vegetables, beans, and whole grains can reduce the risk of heart disease and improve digestive functioning. Limit foods with added sugars (sucrose, glucose, fructose, corn or maple syrup) which add calories but not other nutrients such as vitamins and minerals.
6. **The Daily Value is a Key to a Balanced Diet** The % DV is a general guide to help you link nutrients in a serving of food to their contribution to your total daily diet. It can help you determine if a food is high or low in a nutrient—5% or less is low, 20% or more is high. The % DV is based on a 2,000-calorie diet.
Nutrition Facts
Serving Size 1 cup (228g)
Servings Per Container 2
Amount Per Serving
Calories 250 Calories from Fat 110
% Daily Value*
Total Fat 12g 18%
Saturated Fat 3g 15%
Trans Fat 3g
Cholesterol 30mg 10%
Sodium 470mg 20%
Potassium 700mg 20%
Total Carbohydrate 31g 10%
Dietary Fiber 0g 0%
Sugars 5g
Protein
Vitamin A 4%
Vitamin C 2%
Calcium 20%
Iron 4%
*Percent Daily Values are based on a 2,000 calorie diet. Your Daily Values may be higher or lower depending on you calorie needs.
Calories 2,000 2,500
Total fat Less than 65g 80g
Sat fat Less than 20g 25g
Cholesterol Less than 300mg 300mg
Sodium Less than 2,400mg 2,400mg
Total Carbohydrate 300g 375g
Dietary Fiber 25g 30g

Another approach to controlling your fat intake is to eat foods with a variety of fat contents, but your intake should not exceed 65 g of fat per day, the DV for a 2,000-calorie diet. For example, you might eat a 1-oz. serving of corn chips that contains 6 g of fat and supplies 40% of its calories from fat. The other foods

malnutrition Overnutrition or undernutrition that results when diets supply improper amounts of nutrients.

eaten on this day should provide no more than 59 grams of fat (65 – 6 = 59).

Not everyone thinks that the Nutrition Facts label is easy to use or helpful. Because the percentage of total calories from fat is not listed, people cannot easily compare the fat content of packaged food products. Additionally, many adult Americans need to consume lower amounts of calories and fat than the DVs. Furthermore, most people eat a variety of foods, some of which is fresh or prepared in restaurants. As a result, these people will probably underestimate the amounts of calories and nutrients in their diet if they rely only on the information provided by food labels.

You can learn more about the calories and nutrients in your foods and beverages by using the "What's in the Food You Eat" search tool at www.ars.usda.gov/Services/docs.htm?docid=17032.

What About Foods Sold in Restaurants?

In 2010, the U.S. federal government passed legislation that required restaurants and food vendors with more than 20 locations to inform consumers about caloric and nutrient contents of products sold at these outlets. The goal of the legislation was to provide accurate and easy-to-understand information about the nutritional value of prepared foods. By considering this information, consumers would be able to make more educated decisions concerning their food choices when purchasing meals and snacks. At the time of this writing, the specific details of the guidelines had not been established.

In response to consumer demand and government regulation, some restaurants, including fast-food establishments, have developed "health option" menus. It is important to note, however, that not all items on "healthy options" menus are actually healthy choices. For example, some salads served at fast-food restaurants contain added sugar and excessive amounts of salt. In some cases items on healthy options menus contain more fat or calories than other options. To determine food content before ordering, it is best to review nutrition facts labels, which are now provided on menus or nutrition facts sheets in most restaurants.

Do You Need Vitamin or Mineral Supplements?

Do you buy dietary supplements such as the ones listed in **Table 9.10**? If your answer is yes, why do you take them? Millions of Americans purchase dietary supplements, especially multivitamin/multimineral products that contain mixtures of vitamins and minerals. Approximately 40% of adult Americans take at least one multivitamin/multimineral supplement.[35] In 2011, sales of dietary supplements, which include vitamin and mineral pills, herbal products, and certain hormones, were estimated to be almost $30 *billion* in the United States.[36]

Many people take vitamin and mineral supplements to reduce the risk of heart disease, osteoporosis, and other serious chronic diseases. By carefully selecting a variety of foods and eating recommended amounts from the major food groups, healthy adults should be able to obtain enough nutrients without supplementation. Some people, however, need to supplement their diets with certain nutrients. Pregnant and breastfeeding women need more iron, calcium, and folic acid than what is available in foods. Some vegetarians need more calcium, iron, zinc, and vitamins B12 and D. Elderly persons may benefit from extra vitamins D and B12.

Nutrient supplements do not contain all of the substances found in food that benefit health; therefore, they are not substitutes for nutrient-dense foods. If your diet is nutritious and you still want to take a multiple vitamin and mineral supplement as an "insurance policy," choose a reasonably priced product that contains no more than 100% of the DV for each of the vitamins and minerals listed on the label. The supplement should meet United States Pharmacopeia (USP) standards for strength, purity, and ability to dissolve. Vague advertising statements or labeling declarations, such as "meets laboratory standards for quality," do not guarantee product quality. Vitamin and mineral pills are dietary supplements. The Consumer Health feature "Dietary Supplements" provides information about claims made for dietary supplements.

Malnutrition: Undernutrition and Overnutrition

Malnutrition results when a person's usual food intake supplies inadequate or excessive amounts of nutrients. *Under*nutrition occurs when a diet does not contain enough nutrients; *over*nutrition results

Table 9.10

Nutritional Dietary Supplements

Supplement	Major Claims	Health Risks/Benefits
Apple cider vinegar	Cures arthritis, promotes weight loss, reduces blood cholesterol level	No scientific evidence to support claims.
Beta-carotene	Reduces risk of cancer and heart disease; antioxidant	Acts as antioxidant, but supplements may stimulate cancer cell growth.
Choline	Improves memory	No scientific evidence to support claim.
Chondroitin sulfate	Treats arthritis (often combined with glucosamine)	No scientific evidence to support claims.
Coenzyme Q-10	Reverses signs of aging and disease; antioxidant	Helps cells generate energy and may have medicinal benefits, but more research is needed.
DHEA	Slows aging process, increases muscular strength, and cures numerous ailments	Does not slow rate of aging or cure ailments; long-term effects of taking this naturally occurring hormone are unknown.
Fish oil	Prevents heart disease and stroke, cures rheumatoid arthritis, reduces risk of disease	Reduces inflammation by suppressing the body's immune response and lowers elevated triglyceride levels. May interfere with blood clotting, increasing the risk of hemorrhagic stroke. Cod liver oil contains vitamins A and D, which are toxic when taken in large doses.
Garlic	Lowers blood cholesterol levels	Does not lower cholesterol consistently, and can cause allergic reaction and unpleasant body odor and interfere with prescription blood thinners.
Glucosamine sulfate	Treats arthritis	May slow the destruction of cartilage in knee joint.
Lysine	Prevents herpes simplex viral outbreaks from recurring	No scientific evidence to support claim.
Melatonin	Treats insomnia and jet lag	Scientific evidence suggests this hormone can treat certain sleep disorders, but information about its long-term safety is lacking.
SAM-e	Relieves pain and depression	More research is needed to support claims and determine health risks; may increase risk of heart disease.
Yogurt (containing live bacterial cultures)	Slows aging process, prevents and cures vaginal yeast infections	No scientific evidence to support these claims, but may improve intestinal health

from consuming excessive amounts of nutrients. Undernutrition can be especially devastating for children. Undernourished youngsters often develop nutritional deficiency diseases; as a result, they may not grow properly or perform physical and mental tasks optimally. In parts of the world where many babies are not vaccinated against common childhood diseases, undernourished children often die from infections such as measles.

Undernutrition also occurs in the United States. During 2012, the people living in about 14.5% of U.S. households were uncertain about having or unable to obtain enough food for all members because of lack of resources.[37] Even some people with adequate incomes are marginally nourished because they choose diets that supply barely enough vitamins and minerals. Such individuals may experience more frequent infections and take longer to recover from

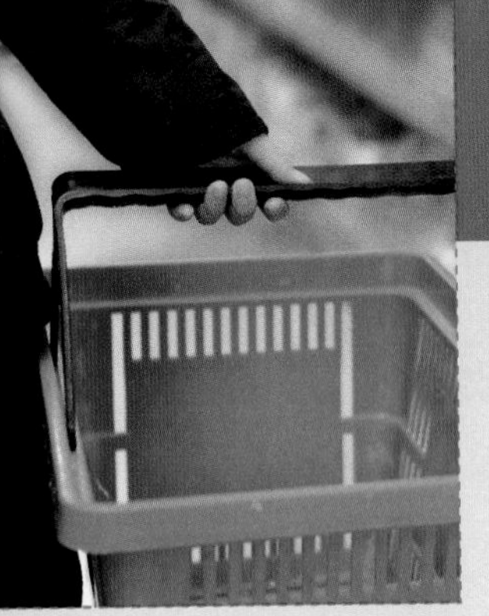

© sevenke/ShutterStock

Consumer Health

Dietary Supplements

Provisions of the 1994 Supplement and Health Education Act allow manufacturers to classify vitamin and mineral pills, protein or amino acid preparations, and certain hormones as "dietary supplements." The FDA does not regulate dietary supplements as extensively as it regulates medicinal drugs. For example, a pharmaceutical company that is developing a new drug to treat diabetes must submit the medication to thorough testing and provide scientific evidence of its safety and effectiveness as a treatment before the drug can be introduced into the marketplace. Thus, the process of approving a new medication generally takes several years. When the medication finally becomes available, purchasing it is likely to require a physician's prescription.

Dietary supplement manufacturers do not need to provide the FDA with scientific evidence that a supplement is safe for humans or provides measurable health benefits before they can market the product. As a result, many supplements contain ingredients that have not been scientifically tested for safety or effectiveness. Even if an ingredient in a dietary supplement is known to cause serious side effects, the product can still be sold through Internet outlets or in health food stores, pharmacies, and supermarkets without a prescription. If the FDA collects enough convincing evidence that a dietary supplement is dangerous, then the agency can ask manufacturers to remove the product from the marketplace voluntarily or require them to stop distributing it. Table 9.10 lists popular nutritional dietary supplements and their claimed health benefits and notes their potential risks.

The FDA requires manufacturers to provide certain information on dietary supplement labels. The label must show the product's name, state that it is a supplement, provide a list of ingredients, and indicate the net weight of the product's contents. The label also needs to display the name and address of the product's packer, distributor, or manufacturer. Supplements must have a Supplement Facts label that lists the product's ingredients and includes other information, such as the suggested daily dose.

The FDA allows manufacturers to make certain claims about a dietary supplement's nutrient content, health benefits, and structure/function usefulness. If manufacturers indicate that a dietary supplement treats a specific nutritional deficiency, supports health in some manner, or reduces the risk of a health condition, such claims must be followed by the disclaimer "This statement has not been evaluated by the Food and Drug Administration. This product is not intended to diagnose, treat, cure, or prevent any disease." To learn which kinds of health-related claims have been approved by the FDA, visit http://www.fda.gov/Food/GuidanceRegulation/GuidanceDocumentsRegulatoryInformation/DietarySupplements/ucm179018.htm.

According to the FDA, many consumers of dietary supplements want to know if health claims for these products on labels or in advertisements and printed material are truthful. Such claims do not require FDA approval before they can be used, but manufacturers are supposed to provide evidence to support the claims if the agency asks them to do so. The FDA, however, lacks sufficient funding and personnel to investigate all questionable or misleading claims.

illnesses than those who are well nourished. Alcoholics, people with anorexia nervosa, and individuals with chronic digestive system diseases are also at risk for undernutrition.

People living in countries with high standards of living are more likely to suffer from the ill effects of *over*nutrition rather than undernutrition. Individuals who eat too much sugar and fat may develop obesity, which increases their risk of diabetes, hypertension, and heart disease.

Many elderly persons are unable to shop for groceries or prepare foods because of arthritis and strokes. Older individuals who are psychologically depressed, socially isolated, or financially impoverished often lack the interest or the resources to prepare nutritious meals. These people are at risk of becoming malnourished. Many communities offer federally subsidized nutrition programs such as Meals-on-Wheels and congregate meals for those who are at least 60 years old. The Meals-on-Wheels program relies on community volunteers to deliver a hot meal, milk, and fresh fruit to homebound people as often as five days a week. More mobile aged individuals can participate in congregate meal programs in which they visit community centers where hot meals are served 5 days a week (**Figure 9.13**). Besides providing a nourishing meal, these sites enable elderly participants to interact socially. Frequent contact with other people can reduce an elderly person's risk of depression, a health problem that often affects isolated aged people.

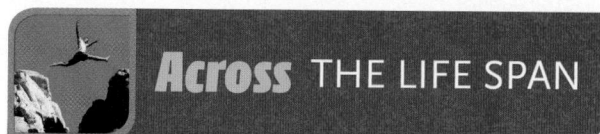

© Galina Barskaya/ShutterStock

NUTRITION

From conception until birth, the developing embryo/fetus depends on its mother to supply the nutrients it needs for development and growth. Women often become more health conscious during pregnancy, and as a result, they may select more nutritious diets. A woman's nutritional status prior to conception, however, has a significant impact on the health of her baby. By consuming a nutritious diet before becoming pregnant, a woman can build optimal nutrient reserves that prepare her body for the nutritional demands of pregnancy. During pregnancy, malnourished women have a higher risk than well-nourished mothers-to-be of miscarrying, having premature or underweight infants, and delivering babies with birth defects.

Consuming diets that supply adequate folate (a B vitamin) is critical, especially during the first 4 weeks of pregnancy when the *neural tube*, the embryonic region that forms the brain and spinal cord, develops. Occasionally, the neural tube fails to develop properly, resulting in *spina bifida* and related defects. Spina bifida occurs when a section of the spine does not fuse to form the channel that encases and protects the spinal cord. In severe cases, the spinal cord protrudes from the infant's back, seriously impairing the child's ability to control the lower part of its body.

Many pregnant women are not even aware of their pregnancy when the neural tube is forming. To maximize the amount of folate in their tissues, women should eat plenty of folate-rich foods, especially enriched breads and cereals, lentils, fruits, and green leafy vegetables (see Table 9.7), *before* pregnancy. During pregnancy, women should eat nutritious diets, obtain medical care, and take their prescribed doses of prenatal vitamin and mineral supplements. Before taking other supplemental nutrients, pregnant women should always check with their physicians. Consuming excessive amounts of nutrient supplements during pregnancy increases the risk of certain birth defects.

Current infant feeding recommendations include the following: provide breastmilk and a supplement that contains vitamin D and iron for at least the first 12 months of life. Iron-fortified infant formulas are acceptable alternatives, but every healthy pregnant woman should consider the benefits of breastfeeding her baby. Breastmilk is the most suitable food for infants. Caregivers should not feed fresh whole or reduced-fat cows' milk to babies before their first birthday. Furthermore, babies should not be fed solid foods before they are 4 months of age.

Breastmilk offers many health benefits to infants and their mothers. Babies who consume breastmilk have reduced risks for sudden infant death syndrome,

© djgis/ShutterStock

Healthy Living Practices

- To plan well-balanced, nutritious daily menus, you can follow the recommendations of the latest dietary guidelines and MyPlate.
- Use the Nutrition Facts on food labels to compare the nutritional content of packaged foods and plan nutritious meals and snacks.
- If you want to take a multiple vitamin and mineral supplement, choose a product that meets United States Pharmacopeia (USP) standards and supplies no more than 100% of each nutrient's DV.

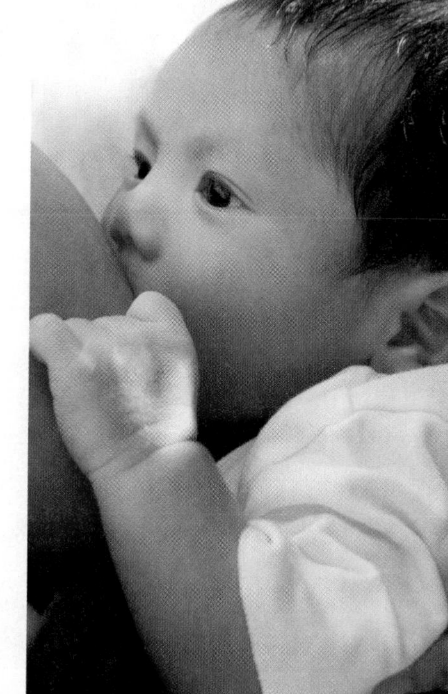

© iStockphoto/Thinkstock

childhood leukemia, ear infections, asthma, childhood obesity, and diabetes.[38] The proteins in human milk will not cause allergies like those in formulas do. Women who breastfeed can also obtain important health benefits—they have lower risks of type 2 diabetes, breast cancer, and ovarian cancer than do women who do not breastfeed.

Breastfeeding is economical and convenient; mothers can breastfeed anywhere they feel comfortable doing so. Individuals who are interested in breastfeeding can obtain educational materials and advice from members of the La Leche League, an organization with groups in many U.S. communities.

Many women do not breastfeed because they want to return to a job, they lack the support of family and friends, or they are uncomfortable with this practice. These women should follow their pediatrician's advice concerning the use of commercially prepared infant formulas.

Parents often describe their preschool-aged children as picky eaters because they do not seem to be as hungry or interested in eating as when they were infants. However, most children eat enough calories to maintain their normal growth pattern. During this period, children often establish their food preferences and eating habits; well-informed, responsible adults can serve as role models, teaching youngsters how to choose nutrient-dense foods.

Eating a nutritious breakfast is an important habit to develop early in life. The child who routinely skips breakfast and eats too many sugary snacks can develop borderline or overt nutritional deficiencies. This child often lacks energy, has difficulty concentrating on school work, and experiences behavioral problems. In severe cases, a malnourished child fails to grow properly.

Adolescents experience rapid growth during puberty, and their appetites increase accordingly. Teenagers often become overly concerned with their body size and shape. As a result, boys may experiment with dietary supplements to increase muscle mass. To lose weight, girls may skip meals or choose diets that limit nutritious foods, such as calcium-rich dairy products. Growing adolescents require plenty of calcium to maximize bone mass. An obsession with body size can foster poor eating practices and eating disorders that last into adulthood.

Older adults who consumed a nutritious diet and have exercised regularly since their youth are more likely to enjoy good health than those who ate poor diets and were inactive. However, physical, psychological, social, and economic factors often influence the quality and quantity of the elderly person's food intake. As one ages, production of acid and other stomach secretions decreases, reducing the ability of the small intestine to absorb calcium, iron, and vitamins D and B12. Therefore, older adults should ask their physicians about the need to take certain nutrient supplements.

Figure 9.13

Nutrition for Older Adults. Many older adult Americans participate in congregate meal programs within their community.

© michaeljung/iStockphoto.com

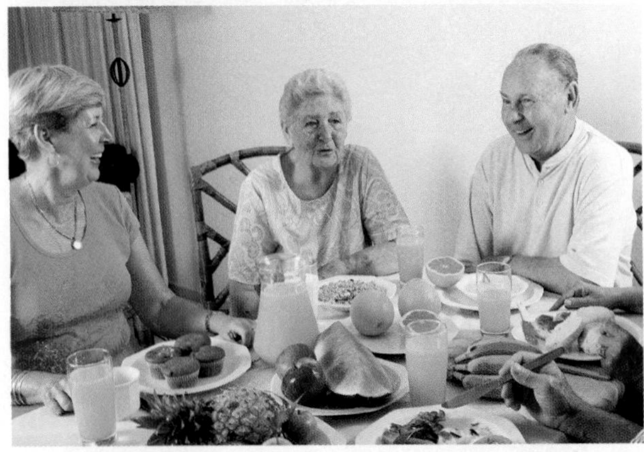

© djgis/ShutterStock

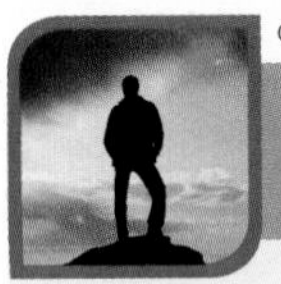

Healthy Living Practices

- To increase your chances of having a healthy baby, improve the quality of your diet *before* you become pregnant.
- Excesses of certain nutrients can produce birth defects, so ask your physician for advice before you take nutrient supplements during pregnancy.
- If you are a woman who plans to have children, consider the benefits of breastfeeding, especially during their first 12 months of life.

Analyzing Health-Related Information

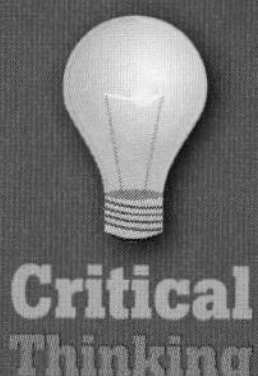

Critical Thinking

© tele52/ShutterStock

The following advertisement promotes a dietary supplement, garlic oil tablets, to relieve fatigue. Read the ad and evaluate it using the model for analyzing health-related information. The main points of the model are noted here.

1. Which statements are verifiable facts, and which are unverified statements or value claims?
2. What are the credentials of the person who makes the health-related claims? Does this person have the appropriate background and education in the topic area? What can you do to check the person's credentials?
3. What might be the motives and biases of the person making the claims?
4. What is the main point of the ad? Which information is relevant to the product? Which information is irrelevant?
5. Is the source reliable? What evidence supports your conclusion that the source is reliable or unreliable? Does the source of information present the pros and cons of the topic or the benefits and risks of the product?
6. Does the source of information attack the credibility of conventional scientists or medical authorities?

Based on your analysis, do you think that this ad is a reliable source of health-related information? Summarize your reasons for coming to this conclusion.

RUSSIAN SCIENTISTS DISCOVER NEW TREATMENT FOR FATIGUE!

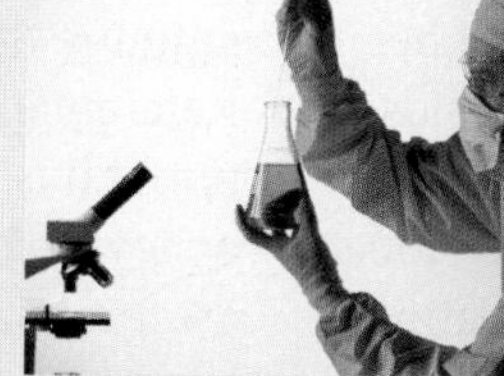

Kiev, Russia—Russian researchers working under the direction of famed doctor Igor X. Ivanamiraculsky of Minsk have discovered that Russian garlic oil is a safe and effective treatment for chronic fatigue. In hundreds of double-blind studies performed at the Minsk Institute of Food Research, college students, athletes, and even elderly persons who took the garlic oil capsules reported having 25% more energy than those persons taking placebos. These results are nothing short of amazing!

Now, you can benefit from Dr. Ivanamiraculsky's discovery. For the first time, the doctor's energy-boosting garlic oil pills are available in the United States. No prescription is needed for this 100% completely natural energizer. Just ask for odor-free GARGOIL at your local pharmacy or health-food store. Satisfaction guaranteed! If you are not completely satisfied after taking GARGOIL, return the unused portion to the place of purchase for a refund. Remember to be careful and follow the label's instructions; some people report feeling too energized after taking GARGOIL! Accept no garlic oil substitutes—ask for GARGOIL.

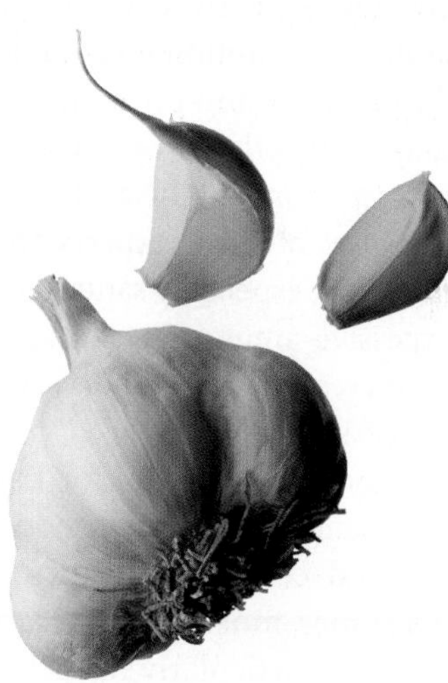

© Photodisc

© Photodisc

CHAPTER REVIEW

Summary

Nutrients are substances in foods that supply energy; regulate body processes; and provide material for growth, maintenance, and repair of tissues. The six classes of nutrients are carbohydrates, lipids, proteins, vitamins, minerals, and water. Many foods also contain nonnutrients, substances that are not essential but may have healthful benefits. Phytochemicals may prevent various chronic diseases, including certain cancers.

During digestion, food is broken down into nutrients that can be absorbed. Cells metabolize carbohydrates, fats, and proteins for energy. The amount of energy stored in food is measured in calories. Cells cannot release energy from water, vitamins, and minerals.

Carbohydrates, the sugars and starches, are a major source of energy for the body. The only disorder that is clearly associated with excessive carbohydrate consumption is tooth decay. Plant foods supply dietary fiber and phytochemicals. Diets rich in fiber may reduce the risks of diverticulosis, hemorrhoids, constipation, and heart disease.

Many medical experts think Americans eat too much fat, especially saturated fat and trans fat. Eating excessive amounts of these lipids is associated with an increased risk of obesity, heart disease, and certain cancers.

Protein is essential for tissue growth, repair, and maintenance and for producing enzymes, antibodies, and certain hormones. The average American consumes more than twice the amount of protein needed, particularly from animal foods. One way to reduce the amount of animal foods in the diet is to eat more protein from plants. Vegetarian diets are associated with lower risks of chronic conditions such as heart disease.

Vitamins and minerals regulate body processes; some minerals are structural components of tissues. Overdoses of many vitamins and most minerals can cause nutritional imbalances and be toxic; therefore, unless medically indicated, people should avoid taking high doses of nutrient supplements.

A lifetime of inadequate calcium intake coupled with low estrogen levels after menopause increases a woman's risk of osteoporosis. Iron deficiency is a common nutritional problem, especially among women of childbearing age. Dehydration is a serious condition that results when water intake is inadequate or water losses are excessive.

The key features of a nutritious diet are nutrient adequacy and nutrient balance. By selecting a variety of foods and by avoiding the indiscriminate use of nutrient supplements, one's diet can be nutritionally adequate and balanced.

A requirement for a nutrient is the smallest amount that prevents a deficiency disease. Dietary Reference Intakes (DRIs) are standards for planning nutritious diets and determining the nutritional adequacy of diets. MyPlate and the *Dietary Guidelines* are practical daily menu-planning guides. Nutrient labeling can help consumers select nutritious foods. Malnutrition occurs when diets supply too little or too many nutrients.

The quality of a woman's diet before and during pregnancy has an impact on the health of her developing child. During the first year of life, human milk is the best food for infants; solid foods should not be fed to babies until they are 4 months old. Without proper supervision, children and teenagers may skip meals or select inadequate diets. Physical, psychological, economic, and social factors contribute to the risk of malnutrition among older adults.

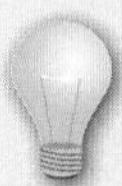

Applying What You Have Learned

1. Locate the nutrition label on three foods you often eat. View each label and explain how you would use nutrient labeling information to determine the amount of complex carbohydrates, sugar, protein, total fat, saturated fat, and trans fat. **Application**
2. Keep a food record for one day by writing down all foods and beverages you consume during a 24-hour period. Analyze this day's food choices by using the "Tracker" at the MyPlate website (http://www.choosemyplate.gov/). **Analysis**
3. Consider the results of your food record. For which foods should you reduce consumption. Which foods can be added to your diet to improve the nutritional value of your food intake? **Evaluation**
4. Plan a menu for a day (meals, snacks, and beverages) that meets MyPlate's recommended amounts of foods for a person of your age, sex, weight, height, and physical activity level. You'll need to visit www.choosemyplate.gov to do this activity. **Synthesis**

Key

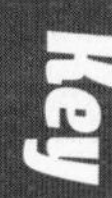

Application	Analysis	Synthesis	Evaluation
using information in a new situation.	breaking down information into component parts.	putting together information from different sources.	making informed decisions.

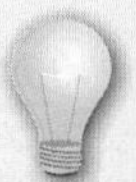

Reflecting on Your Health

1. After reading this chapter, what changes can you make to improve your diet? How is your present diet different from what you ate as a child or while in high school? Why do you think your present diet is better or worse than your past diet?
2. What factors influence your food choices? Factors may include personal preference, family/social norms, economics, or food availability. How willing are you to try new healthy foods? Have you tried any new healthy foods in the past year? Did you continue to eat the new foods? Why or why not?
3. Do you use nutrition labels? If you do, which information do you think is most important? How does nutritional labeling help you be a better consumer? If you do not use nutrition labels, why not? What do you think you might gain or lose by using nutrition labels?
4. Do you take dietary supplements? If you do, which supplements do you take? Why do you take them? Do you know if the supplement ingredients have been tested for safety or effectiveness?
5. Females: Would you or did you breastfeed your children? Explain why you would or did breastfeed your children. Males: Would you want or did the mother of your children breastfeed them? Why or why not?

CHAPTER REVIEW

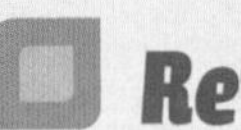

References

1. U.S. Department of Agriculture and U.S. Department of Health and Human Services. (2010) *Dietary guidelines for Americans, 2010*. Washington DC: U.S. Government Printing Office.
2. American Diabetes Association. (2014). *Sugar and desserts: The hype about sugar*. Retrieved from http://www.diabetes.org/food-and-fitness/food/what-can-i-eat/understanding-carbohydrates/sugar-and-desserts.html
3. American Dietetic Association. (2012). Position of the Academy of Nutrition and Dietetics: Use of nutritive and nonnutritive sweeteners. *Journal of the Academy of Nutrition and Dietetics, 112*(5), 739–785.
4. Ervin, R. B., & Ogden, C. L. (2013). *Consumption of added sugars among U.S. adults, 2005–2010* (NCHS Data Brief No. 122). Hyattsville, MD: National Center for Health Statistics.
5. Yang, Q., et al. (2014). Added sugar intake and cardiovascular disease mortality among U.S. adults. *Journal of the American Medical Association Internal Medicine, 174*(4), 516–524.
6. Lichtenstein, A. H., et al. (2006). Diet and lifestyle recommendations revision 2006: A scientific statement from the American Heart Association nutrition committee. *Circulation, 114*(1), 82–96
7. American Heart Association. (2014). *Fish and omega-3 fatty acids*. Retrieved from http://www.heart.org/HEARTORG/GettingHealthy/NutritionCenter/HealthyDietGoals/Fish-and-Omega-3-Fatty-Acids_UCM_303248_Article.jsp
8. Heron, M. (2013). Deaths: Leading causes for 2010. *National Vital Statistics Reports*, 62(6). Hyattsville, MD: National Center for Health Statistics. Retrieved from http://www.cdc.gov/nchs/data/nvsr/nvsr62/nvsr62_06.pdf
9. American Diabetes Association. (2014). *Fast facts: Data and statistics about diabetes*. Retrieved from http://professional.diabetes.org/admin/UserFiles/0%20-%20Sean/14_fast_facts_june2014_final3.pdf
10. Centers for Disease Control and Prevention. (2014). *National Diabetes Statistics Report: Estimates of diabetes and its burden on the U.S., 2014*. Atlanta, GA: U.S. Department of Health and Human Services. Retrieved from: http://www.cdc.gov/diabetes/pubs/statsreport14/national-diabetes-report-web.pdf
11. Centers for Disease Control and Prevention, National Center for Chronic Disease Prevention and Health Promotion. (2011, January). Age-adjusted incidence of diagnosed diabetes per 1,000 population aged 18–79 years, by race/ethnicity, United States, 1997–2009. *Data and trends, National Diabetes Surveillance System*. Retrieved from http://www.cdc.gov/diabetes/statistics/incidence/fig6.htm
12. Malik, V. S., & Hu, F. B. (2012). Sweeteners and risk of obesity and type 2 diabetes: The role of sugar-sweetened beverages. *Current Diabetes Care, 12*(2), 195–203.
13. U.S. Centers for Disease Control and Prevention. (2012). *Diabetes Public Health Resource: Prevent diabetes*. Retrieved from http://www.cdc.gov/diabetes/consumer/prevent.htm
14. U.S. National Institutes of Health, National Heart Lung and Blood Institute. (2011). *What is metabolic syndrome?* Retrieved from http://www.nhlbi.nih.gov/health/dci/Diseases/ms/ms_whatis.html
15. National Institutes of Health, National Digestive Diseases Information Clearinghouse. (2009). *Lactose intolerance*. Retrieved from http://digestive.niddk.nih.gov/ddiseases/pubs/lactoseintolerance/
16. American Gastroenterological Association. (2013). *Patient center: Understanding constipation*. Retrieved from http://www.gastro.org/patient-center/digestive-conditions/constipation
17. Clifton, P. (2009). Dietary fatty acids and inflammation. *Nutrition & Dietetics, 66*(1), 7-11.
18. Wall, R., et al. (2010). Fatty acids from fish: The anti-inflammatory potential of long-chain omega-3 fatty acids. *Nutrition Reviews, 68*(5), 280–289.
19. Buckland, G., et al. (2009). Adherence to the Mediterranean diet and risk of coronary heart disease in the Spanish EPIC Cohort Study. *American Journal of Epidemiology, 170*(12), 1518–1529.
20. Williams, A. N., & Woessner, K. M. (2009). Monosodium glutamate "allergy": Menace or myth? *Clinical and Experimental Allergy, 39*(5), 640–646.
21. U.S. Department of Agriculture, Center for Nutrition Policy and Promotion. (2011). *Nutrient content of the U.S. food supply: Developments between 2000–2006*. Retrieved from http://www.cnpp.usda.gov/sites/default/files/nutrient_content_of_the_us_food_supply/Final_FoodSupplyReport_2006.pdf
22. American Heart Association. (2014). *High protein diets*. Retrieved from http://www.heart.org/HEARTORG/GettingHealthy/NutritionCenter/High-Protein-Diets_UCM_305989_Article.jsp
23. American Dietetic Association. (2009). Position of the American Dietetic Association: Vegetarian diets. *Journal of the American Dietetic Association, 109*(7), 1266–1282.
24. National Institutes of Health, National Institute of Allergy and Infectious Diseases. (2013). *Food allergy*. Retrieved from http://www.niaid.nih.gov/topics/foodallergy/Pages/default.aspx
25. Gerez, I. F. A., et al. (2010). Diagnostic tests for food allergy. *Singapore Medical Journal, 51*(1), 4–9.
26. Rubio-Tapia, et al. (2012). The prevalence of celiac disease in the United States. *American Journal of Gastroenterology, 107*, 1538–1544.
27. National Institutes of Health, National Digestive Diseases Information Clearinghouse. (2012). *Celiac disease*. Retrieved from http://digestive.niddk.nih.gov/ddiseases/pubs/celiac/index.aspx
28. U.S. National Institutes of Health. (2011). Vitamin C (ascorbic acid). *Medline Plus*. Retrieved from http://www.nlm.nih.gov/medlineplus/druginfo/natural/1001.html
29. Bailey, R. L., et al. (2011). Dietary supplement use in the United States: 2003–2006. *Journal of Nutrition, 141*(2), 261–266.
30. National Institutes of Health, National Institute of Arthritis and Musculoskeletal and Skin Diseases. (2011). *What is osteoporosis?* Retrieved from http://www.niams.nih.gov/Health_Info/Bone/Osteoporosis/osteoporosis_ff.asp
31. National Institutes of Health, National Digestive Diseases Information Clearinghouse. (2014). *Hemochromatosis* (NIH Pub No. 14-4621). Retrieved from http://digestive.niddk.nih.gov/ddiseases/pubs/hemochromatosis/index.htm
32. Mayo Clinic. (2011). *Caffeine: How much is too much?* Retrieved from http://www.mayoclinic.org/healthy-living/nutrition-and-healthy-eating/in-depth/caffeine/art-20045678
33. Food and Nutrition Board, National Institute of Medicine. (2004). *Dietary reference intakes for water, potassium, sodium, chloride, and sulfate*. Washington, DC: National Academy Press.

34. U.S. Food and Drug Administration. (2014). *Proposed changes to the nutrition facts label*. Retrieved from http://www.fda.gov/Food/GuidanceRegulation/GuidanceDocumentsRegulatoryInformation/LabelingNutrition/ucm385663.htm#Summary

35. Gahche, J., et al. (2011). Dietary supplement use among U.S. adults has increased since NHANES III (1988–1994). *NCHS Data Brief*, No. 61. Retrieved from http://www.cdc.gov/nchs/data/databriefs/db61.htm

36. National Institutes of Health, Office of Dietary Supplements. (2013). *Multivitamin/mineral supplements*. Retrieved from http://ods.od.nih.gov/factsheets/MVMS-HealthProfessional/

37. Nord, M., et al. (2010). *Household food security in the United States, 2012* (Economic Research Report No. ERR-155). Retrieved from http://www.ers.usda.gov/publications/err-economic-research-report/err155.aspx#.Uz2AzfldXHU

38. U.S. Department of Health and Human Services, Office of Women's Health. (2013). *Breastfeeding fact sheet*. Retrieved from https://www.womenshealth.gov/publications/our-publications/fact-sheet/breastfeeding.html

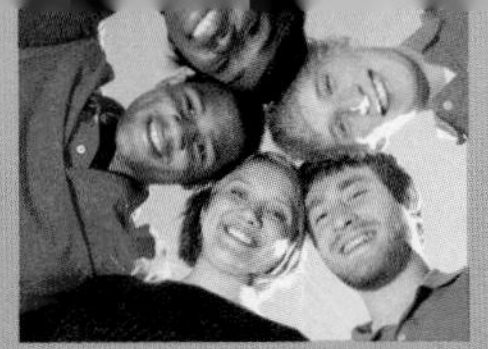

Diversity in Health
The Plight of the Pima

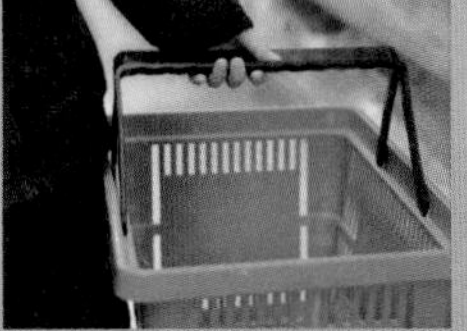

Consumer Health
Dietary Supplements: Weight Loss Aids

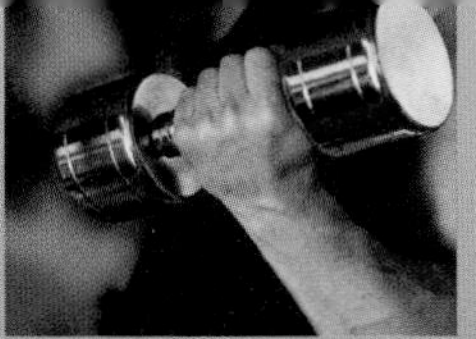

Managing Your Health
General Features of Reliable Weight Reduction Plans

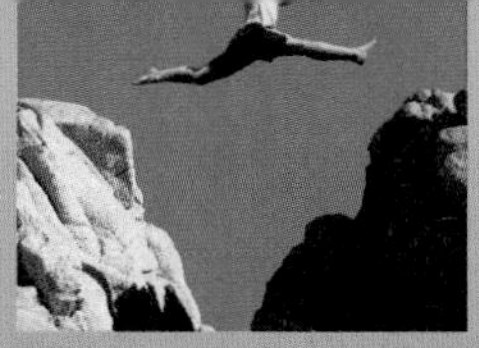

Across the Life Span
Weight Management

Obesity Trends* Among U.S. Adults
BRFSS, 2010
(*BMI ≥30, or ~ 30 lbs. overweight for 5′ 4″ person)

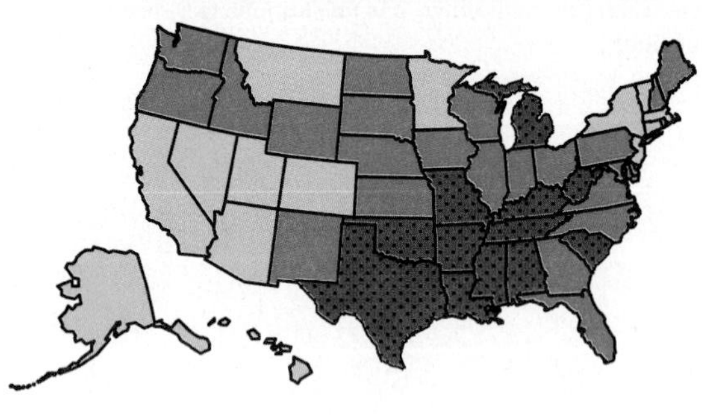

No Data | <10% | 10%–14% | 15%–19% | 20%–24% | 25%–29% | ≥30%

Source: Behavioral Risk Factor Surveillance System, CDC.

Obesity Trends* Among U.S. Adults
BRFSS, 2000
(*BMI ≥30, or ~ 30 lbs. overweight for 5′ 4″ person)

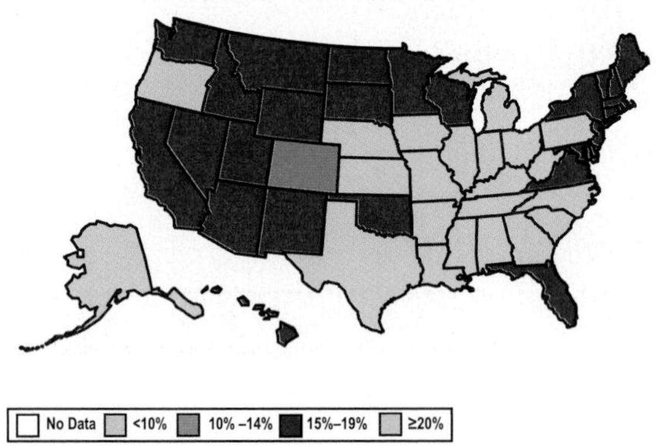

No Data | <10% | 10%–14% | 15%–19% | ≥20%

Source: Behavioral Risk Factor Surveillance System, CDC.

Chapter Overview

The definitions of weight categories

How your body uses the energy from foods

How to determine your percentage of body fat

The causes of obesity

How to manage your weight

Student Workbook

Self-Assessment: How Much Energy Do You Use Daily?

Changing Health Habits: Altering Caloric Intake and Physical Activity

Do You Know?

How to shed fat and gain muscle?

What causes "middle-age spread"?

How to lose weight and keep it off?

CHAPTER 10

Body Weight and Its Management

Learning Objectives

> "In 2012, about 63% of American adults were overweight or obese."

After studying this chapter, you should be able to:

1. Identify major health problems that are associated with excess body fat.
2. Explain how the body mass index (BMI) is used to define degrees of overweight and obesity.
3. List the three major ways the body expends energy.
4. Explain the concept of energy balance and how it relates to body weight.
5. Compare various methods of determining body composition.
6. Explain how biological, environmental, and psychological factors influence the development of excess body weight.
7. Compare and contrast various weight loss methods.
8. Describe the typical features of fad diets.
9. List characteristics of safe and reasonable weight reduction programs.
10. Describe steps a person can take to gain lean body weight safely.
11. Explain the importance of weight gain during pregnancy.
12. Describe how obesity affects the health of children and the elderly.

overweight A condition in which the body has more fat, muscle, bone, and/or body water than a person whose weight is healthy. Overweight is classified as having a BMI of 25.0–29.9.

obesity A condition in which the body has an excessive and unhealthy amount of fat. Obesity is classified as having a BMI of 30.0 or higher.

adipose cells Specialized cells that store extra food energy as fat.

body mass index (BMI) A standard that correlates body weight with the risk of developing chronic health conditions associated with obesity. BMIs are calculated with a person's height and weight.

In 2012, about 63% of American adults were overweight or obese.[1] A person who is **overweight** has more fat, muscle, bone, and/or body water than a person whose weight is classified as normal (e.g., healthy). Being overweight is not necessarily unhealthy, but people who are overweight and have too much body fat are at risk of becoming *obese*. In this chapter, we use the term overweight to refer to *overfat*. **Obesity** is a condition characterized by excessive and unhealthy amounts of body fat. As these maps indicate, the prevalence of obesity in the United States rose rapidly between 2000 and 2010. In 2000, 20% or more of the adult population in 22 states was obese. Ten years later, 20% or more of adults in every state was obese. The obesity rates remained consistent for 2010–2012 (the most recent data available) at 27.5%, 27.8%, and 27.6%, respectively. What is the prevalence of obesity in your state?

Overweight and obesity are the most common nutritional disorders in the United States.[2] These conditions often result from a combination of two behavioral risk factors—poor diet and physical inactivity. In this country, an increasing number of people are dying of causes related to these risk factors.[3]

There is a widespread misperception that persons who are overweight or obese lack the willpower to control their eating and weight. It is true that a person gains body fat by eating more food energy (calories) than needed and that losing the excess weight involves a considerable amount of motivation and commitment. However, overweight and obesity result from a complex combination of biological, psychological, environmental, cultural, and socioeconomic influences. Thus, shedding excess fat to achieve a healthy body weight is not an easy task. According to most medical experts, obesity is a chronic metabolic disease that is extremely difficult to treat.

This chapter examines factors that contribute to the development of excess body fat, identifies health problems associated with this condition, and discusses various weight loss methods. Some individuals are underweight and want to increase their muscle mass; therefore, this chapter also provides information concerning healthy ways to gain weight.

Overweight and Obesity

A healthy body is not fat free; a small amount of fat is essential for the normal functioning of all cells. Additionally, the body has specialized cells called **adipose cells** that store the extra energy from food as triglyceride (fat). If a person eats more food energy than is needed, his or her fat cells continue storing fat and increasing in size. Under certain conditions, additional fat cells can develop, further enlarging the fat mass, and this person soon notices that his belts are too small or her slacks are too tight as a result.

Body Mass Index

How much extra fat must a person have to be considered overweight? At what point does a person who is overweight become obese? Most health experts use the **body mass index (BMI)** instead of height/weight tables to determine whether an individual weighs too much. BMI is calculated by dividing weight (kilograms) by height (meters squared): kg/m^2. BMI correlates body weight with the risk of developing chronic health conditions associated with excess body fat.

To estimate your BMI, multiply your weight in pounds by 705. Then, divide that number by your height in inches squared. For example, if you weigh 150 lb and your height is 6'7", multiplying your weight times 705 equals 105,750 and squaring your height equals 4,489. Dividing 105,750 by 4,489 produces approximately 23.56. Thus, your BMI is 23.56. You can also determine your BMI by using the interactive BMI calculator at the National Heart Lung and Blood Institute's website (http://www.nhlbi.nih.gov/guidelines/obesity/BMI/bmicalc.htm) or the adult and child BMI calculators available on the Centers for Disease Control and Prevention's website (http://www.cdc.gov/healthyweight/assessing/bmi/index.html).

Table 10.1 indicates weight classifications according to BMIs. Adults with BMIs below 18.5 are classified as *underweight*. Healthy BMIs are between 18.5 and 24.9. Adults with BMIs between 25.0 and 29.9 are *overweight*; those with BMIs of between 30.0 and

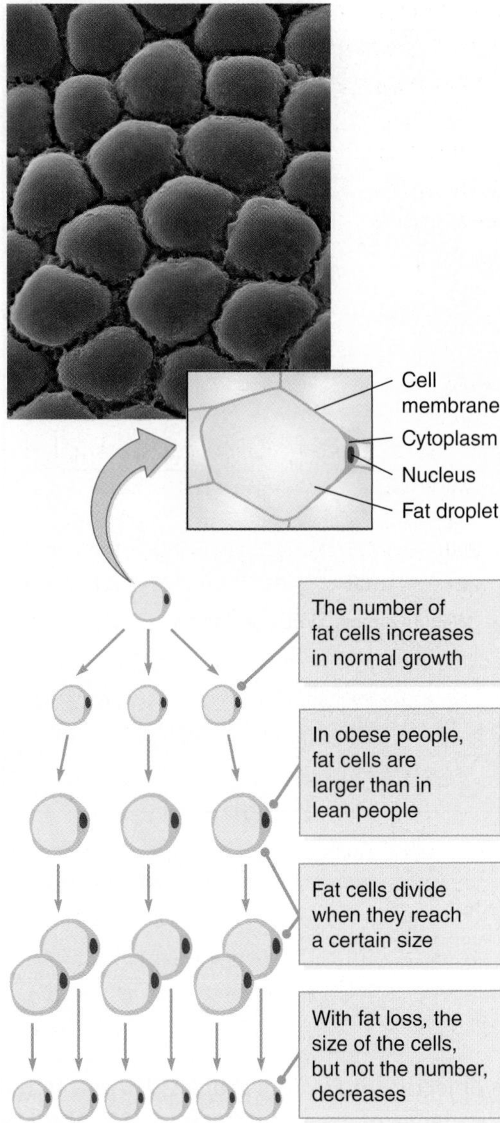
Cell membrane
Cytoplasm
Nucleus
Fat droplet
The number of fat cells increases in normal growth
In obese people, fat cells are larger than in lean people
Fat cells divide when they reach a certain size
With fat loss, the size of the cells, but not the number, decreases
Adipose (fat) cells.
Photo: © Dr. Dennis Kunkel/Visuals Unlimited

Table 10.1

Weight Classifications

BMI	Weight Classification
Below 18.5	Underweight
18.5–24.9	Healthy
25.0–29.9	Overweight
30–39.0	Obese
40.0 and higher	Morbidly or extremely obese

39.9 are *obese*. People who have BMIs of 40 or more are often referred to as morbidly, extremely, or super obese.

By using your BMI as a guide, you can determine whether your weight is in the overweight or obese range for your height (**Table 10.2**).

You can also use the graph shown in **Figure 10.1** to determine if your weight is within the healthy BMI range. Find your height, without shoes, on the left-hand side of the graph and place your left index finger on that point. Then, find your weight, without clothing, on the bottom line of the graph, and place your right index finger on that point. Move your left finger

Table 10.2

Classifying Body Weight Based on BMI

Height (in.)	Overweight (BMI 25.0 to 29.9) Lower Limit (lb)	Obese (BMI 30 or more) Lower Limit (lb)
58	119	143
59	124	148
60	128	153
61	132	158
62	136	164
63	141	169
64	145	174
65	150	180
66	155	186
67	159	191
68	164	197
69	169	203
70	174	207
71	179	215
72	184	221
73	189	227

Reproduced from National Institutes of Health, National Heart, Lung, and Blood Institute. (1998). Clinical guidelines on the identification, evaluation, and treatment of overweight and obesity in adults. Bethesda, MD: Author.

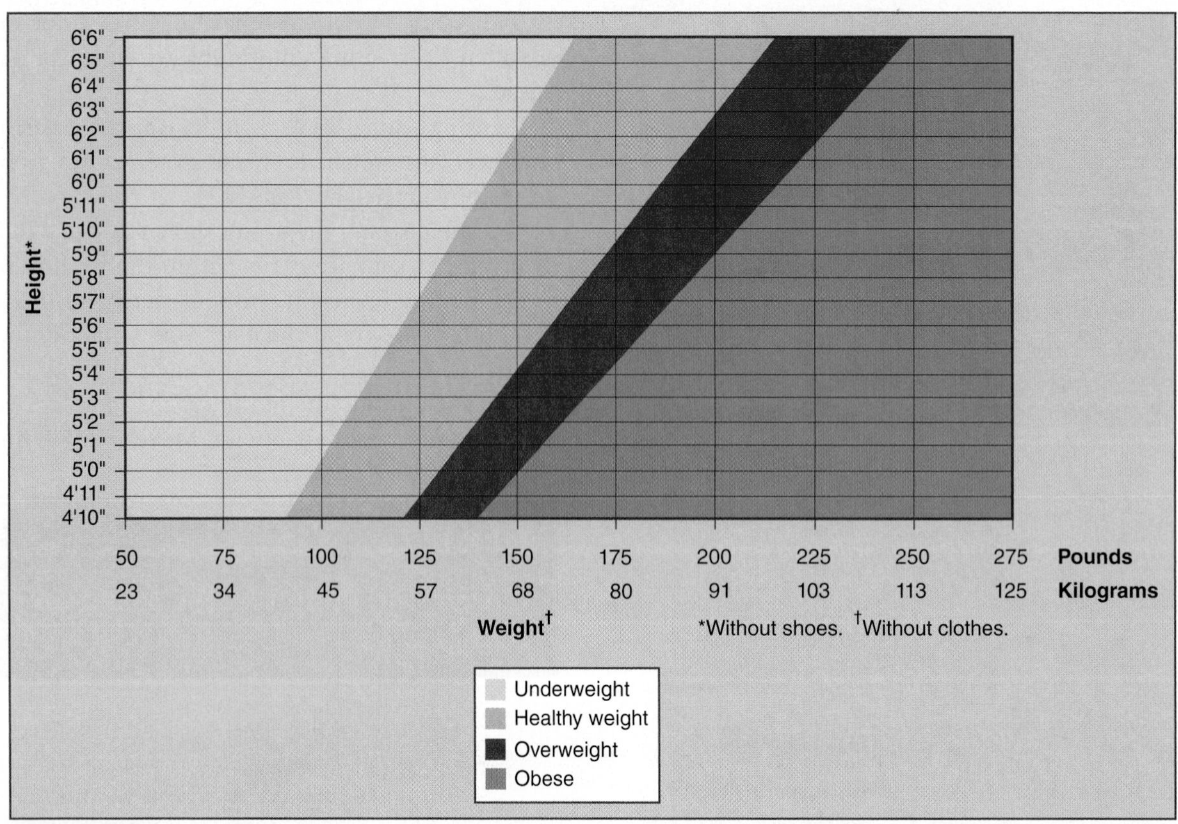

Figure 10.1

BMI Graph. Find your BMI by following the instructions provided in the text.

Modified from National Heart Lung and Blood Institute. (n.d.). Body mass index table 1. Retrieved on September 17, 2011, from http://www.nhlbi.nih.gov/guidelines/obesity/bmi_tbl.htm

to the right and your right finger up until they meet. Note which range that point is in. Is your weight in the healthy BMI range?

Defining overweight and obese as certain BMIs can produce inaccurate conclusions, especially for very muscular people. For example, athletic individuals may have a BMI of 26 and be overweight according to Figure 10.1. Because muscle is denser than fat, an athletic, muscular person can be heavier but healthier than a physically inactive (sedentary) individual who is the same height and weighs less.

The Prevalence of Obesity

The prevalence of obesity has reached epidemic proportions in the United States. Since 1980, obesity rates have doubled for American adults and nearly tripled among children and adolescents who are 2–19 years of age. In 2009, approximately 17% of American children and adolescents were obese.[4] More American infants and preschool children are also overweight than in the past.[5]

An objective of *Healthy People 2010* was to reduce the prevalence of excess body fat to 40% of the adult American population.[6] However, Americans did not meet this objective by 2010. A later section of this chapter discusses factors that contribute to the rising prevalence of overweight in the United States. *Healthy People 2020* includes two objectives related to obesity: (1) reducing the proportion of adults who are considered obese and, (2) reducing the proportion of children and adolescents who are obese.[7] Do you believe these objectives will be met?

The United States is not the only country experiencing a rapid increase in the prevalence of obesity. The World Health Organization (WHO) recognizes obesity as a global health problem. The worldwide prevalence of obesity (*globesity*) is rising rapidly, especially in nations with developed market economies such as those in western Europe. Globally, an estimated 500 million people, or more than 1 in 10 adults, were obese in 2008 (the most recent data available mid-2014).[8]

How Does Excess Body Fat Affect Health?

Excess body fat, particularly obesity, contributes to many serious and disabling health problems. Obesity increases one's risk of developing *gout*, a condition that affect joints; *carpal tunnel syndrome*, a painful nerve disorder involving the wrist and hand; and *sleep apnea*, a condition in which one stops breathing periodically while sleeping. Those with obesity are also more likely to suffer from metabolic syndrome, gallbladder disease, hypertension, diabetes, and heart disease. Obesity significantly increases the risk of cancers of the large intestine (colon), breast (postmenopausal women), uterus, kidney, and esophagus.[9] Compared to people who have healthy body weights, people who are obese are more likely to die prematurely.[10] In the United States, excess body fat contributes to more than 90,000 cancer deaths each year.[11]

Surgery is riskier for people who are obese because physicians have more difficulty estimating the amount of anesthesia needed. Obese men and women are more likely to experience fertility problems than people whose weights are in the healthy range. Pregnant overweight or obese women have greater risks of developing diabetes (gestational diabetes), a form of severe hypertension during pregnancy, as well as giving birth to babies with birth defects and/or babies who do not survive.[12] Furthermore, being too fat can interfere with one's ability to perform daily activities that require walking, carrying, kneeling, and stooping.

Many physical health problems result from being overweight or obese. Excess body weight can stress joints, especially weight-bearing joints in the knees and hips, so they wear out sooner. People who are obese often have breathing problems because the excess fat interferes with lung expansion when they inhale.

When fat cells become too large, they lose their ability to respond to the hormone insulin, which leads to the development of diabetes. Fat tissue also contains cells called *macrophages*. Although these cells play a role in immune system processes that protect an individual from disease, they may multiply excessively and malfunction in people who have too much body fat. Macrophages found in fat tissue produce chemicals that cause inflammation, resulting in damage to the heart and blood vessels, which sets the stage for heart disease.[13]

A person who is obese does not have to become slim to reap some benefits of losing weight. By losing 10% of body weight and maintaining that loss, people who are obese can reduce their risks of obesity-related health problems such as heart disease and stroke.[14] Additionally, this weight loss can save thousands of dollars that would have been spent on treating medical conditions related to excess body fat.

metabolism All chemical reactions that take place in the body.

Besides affecting physical health, excess body fat can have a negative impact on psychological health. People who are obese, particularly women who seek weight loss treatment, often suffer from depression and low self-esteem.[12] Some people may develop these psychological conditions after being discriminated against or having humiliating and embarrassing experiences. Some people perceive individuals who are obese as physically unattractive, lacking willpower, and/or lazy. Not surprisingly, many people who are overweight or obese are dissatisfied and preoccupied with their body image.[15]

What are the factors that contribute to the development of excess body fat? Why are so many Americans overweight? Is it possible to control one's weight?

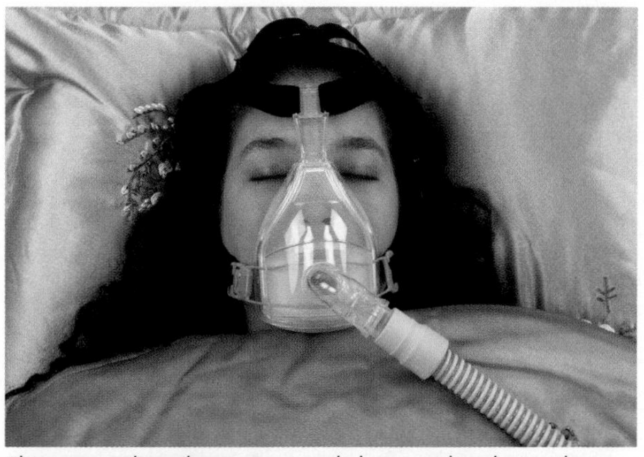

This person has sleep apnea and sleeps with a device that regulates her breathing.

The Caloric Cost of Living

Energy for Basal (Vital) Metabolism

Metabolism refers to all chemical changes that take place in cells. Human cells use energy (calories) from food to perform vital activities such as building and repairing tissues, circulating and filtering blood, and producing and transporting substances. Nevertheless, cells release much of the calories from food as heat,

metabolic rate The amount of energy the body requires to fuel cellular activities during a specified time.

which is necessary for maintaining one's body temperature. Every day the body expends the largest portion of calories (50% to 70%) to carry out these vital activities. The **metabolic rate** is the amount of energy required to fuel cellular activities within a specified time.

Metabolic rates vary; genetic factors probably play a major role in setting these rates. Hormones, especially thyroid hormone produced in the thyroid gland, regulate metabolism (**Figure 10.2**). In some people, the thyroid gland does not function properly, and as a result the organ produces too much (hyperthyroidism) or too little thyroid hormone (hypothyroidism). An individual who produces too much thyroid hormone has a higher than normal metabolic rate. This person may feel warm, be nervous and shaky, have chronic diarrhea, and lose weight despite eating large amounts of food. People with overactive thyroid glands can take medication or have surgery to reduce the amount of hormone produced by the organ. A person who suffers from lack of thyroid hormone has a lower than normal metabolic rate. This individual may feel cold, have little energy, be constipated, and gain weight easily. People suffering from underactive thyroid glands can increase their metabolic rates by taking thyroid hormone pills. The vast majority of people who have excess body fat, however, have normal thyroid hormone levels and normal metabolic rates.

Figure 10.2

The Thyroid Gland. The thyroid gland produces hormones that control the metabolic rate.

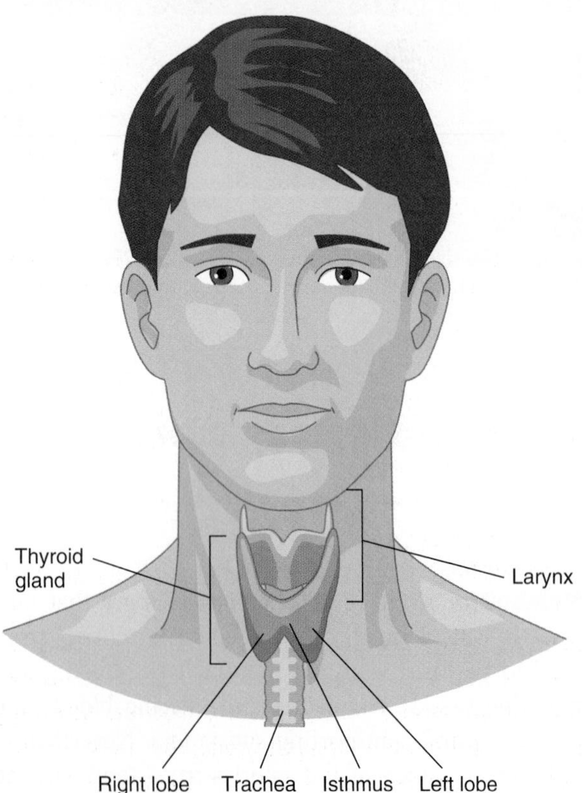

The proportion of muscle and fat tissue also influences the metabolic rate. Muscle cells use more energy than fat cells; therefore, people with greater amounts of muscle mass have higher metabolic rates than those with more fat tissue. *Testosterone* is a hormone that stimulates muscle mass development. Because men normally produce more testosterone than women do, they usually have more muscle and less fat. On average, men have higher metabolic rates than women.

Age also influences the metabolic rate. Infants and children have higher metabolic rates than adults, because they are growing rapidly. After 20 years of age, metabolic rates decline about 1% to 2% each decade. As a result of this gradual slowdown, people need less energy as they age. Thus, if people continue to eat the same amount of food as their age increases, they gain weight (assuming consistent activity levels). Although the declining metabolic rate is a contributing factor, many health experts think physical inactivity is more responsible for "middle-age spread" than is overeating. As one grows older, exercising regularly can help retain muscle, which slows the metabolic rate decline.

Energy for Physical Activity

In addition to the caloric cost of vital metabolic activities, the body expends energy to contract skeletal muscles. The amount of energy needed for physical activity depends on the type of activity, the time spent performing the activity (its duration), and the intensity at which it is performed. Although it is not related directly to physical activity, a person's body size influences the amount of physical effort needed to move. For example, a person who weighs 120 pounds and another who weighs 175 pounds might spend the same amount of time playing a game of tennis. If both of them play tennis with the same intensity, the muscles of the heavier person require more energy to move than those of the lighter person.

According to the 2008 Physical Activity Guidelines for Americans, adults need 150 minutes of moderate-intensity aerobic activities each week.[16] However, less than half of adults report meeting this guideline in 2012.[17]

People can increase the amount of energy expended during physical activity by increasing its duration or intensity. Furthermore, the metabolic rate often remains elevated for several hours after one discontinues vigorous physical activity. This elevation may result from an increase in the metabolic activity of muscle cells that occurs after physical exertion. Therefore, individuals who engage in regular vigorous activity may be able to raise their resting metabolic rates.

Some health experts classify physical activities as sports types of exercise, movement for daily living, or spontaneous muscular movements. *Sports types* of exercise are physical activities that are planned and carried out for the purpose of improving health and well-being. Swimming, brisk walking, and lifting weights are sports types of exercises. *Movement for daily living* includes various unstructured physical activities such as housework, gardening, walking, and leisure-time physical activities that are not associated with sports, eating, or sleeping.[18] Each day, the typical American expends more energy for physical activities associated with daily living than for sports types of exercise. *Spontaneous muscular movement* includes fidgeting and maintaining balance and body posture. Movements for daily living and spontaneous muscular movements are sometimes referred to as *nonexercise activity thermogenesis* (*NEAT*). As a result of NEAT, people can reduce the risk of gaining body fat by being restless and busy because they will metabolize far more energy each day than people who spend much of their day engaging in sedentary activities such as lying down or sitting still. Nevertheless, more research is needed to determine the role of NEAT in weight maintenance.

Table 10.3 lists some common physical activities and the number of calories people expend per minute of performing each activity. Note that the number of calories used for an activity varies according to body weight. For most people, the total number of calories expended daily for physical activity is less than the number expended for basal metabolism. To assess your daily energy expenditure, visit http://www.choosemyplate.gov/supertracker-tools/supertracker.html.

Energy for the Thermic Effect of Food

Together, metabolic and physical activity energy needs constitute more than 90% of a person's energy expenditure. After eating a meal, the body requires a small amount of energy to digest, absorb, and process the nutrients from food. This use of energy, the **thermic effect of food (TEF)**, accounts for a very small portion, less than 10%, of one's total energy expenditures.

thermic effect of food (TEF) The small amount of energy that the body uses to digest, absorb, and process the nutrients from foods.

How many calories does your body need daily? To estimate your daily caloric expenditures, you can add the number of calories needed for basal metabolism, physical activity, and TEF. The assessment activity in the Student Workbook section at the end of this text can help you estimate the number of calories you expend in a day.

The Basics of Energy Balance

In general, people maintain, gain, or lose body weight according to the basic principles of energy balance, as illustrated in **Figure 10.3**. When the caloric intake from food equals the number of calories expended for energy needs, no change in body weight occurs. When caloric intake is less than caloric expenditures, the body loses weight as cells burn stored fat. If caloric intake is more than caloric expenditures, the body conserves much of the excess calories as fat, and weight gain occurs. Each pound of body fat represents about 3,500 calories of potential energy; therefore, consuming as little as 100 extra calories per day for a year can result in a 10-pound weight gain.

Body Composition

How Much Body Fat Is Healthy?

When you step on a scale, you can determine your body weight as a number of pounds or kilograms. That weight, however, does not specify how much water, muscle, or fat is in your body. Fat-free body weight consists of water, proteins, and minerals found in the bones, muscles, and organs (*lean tissues*). About 60% of a healthy adult's weight is water, 6% to 22% is protein, and 3% is minerals. Most of the remaining weight is fat.

Many health experts use the percentage of body fat to determine if a person is overfat. The average healthy young woman has more body fat than the average healthy young man because the fat is needed for hormonal and reproductive purposes. Although people tend to gain fat as they age, the increase does not necessarily cause health problems. **Table 10.4**

Table 10.3

Approximate Energy Costs of Various Physical Activities

Physical Activity	Calories per Pound of Body Weight per Minute	
	Range for Women	Range for Men
Sedentary	up to 0.017	up to 0.017
Sitting quietly, playing a musical instrument		
Light	0.017 to 0.033	0.017 to 0.035
Playing pool, bowling, golf, volleyball, walking (3 mph)		
Moderate	0.033 to 0.050	0.035 to 0.052
Badminton, canoeing, gymnastics, hockey, cycling, swimming, dancing, tennis, skiing		
Vigorous/Heavy	0.050+	0.052+
Basketball, climbing, cross-country running, rowing		

To estimate the number of calories you expend while performing a particular physical activity, multiply the calories per pound per minute by your weight. Use the figures in the left-hand column if you are a woman, and in the right-hand column if you are a man. Then, multiply that number by the number of minutes spent performing the activity. For example, if you are a woman who weighs 120 lb, and you spent 40 minutes cycling: $0.033 \times 120 = 3.96$ calories per minute; 3.96×40 minutes = about 158 calories spent. (The rates of caloric expenditure per minute are given as ranges. For example, if you cycled intensely, use a rate at the high end of the range.)

Adapted from Durnin, J. V. G. A., & Passmore, R. (1967). *Energy, Work, and Leisure*. London, England: Heinemann.

Figure 10.3

Energy Balance. (a) When energy expenditure equals energy intake, the body maintains its weight; (b) when energy expenditure is greater than energy intake, the body loses weight; (c) when energy expenditure is less than energy intake, the body gains weight.

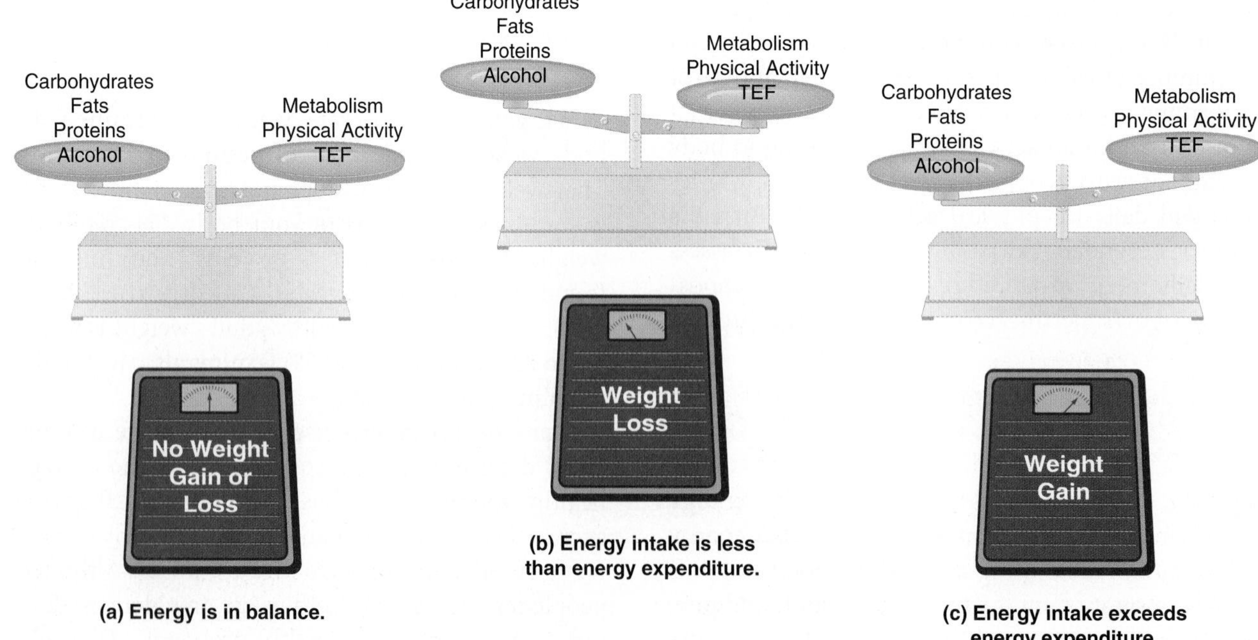

Table 10.4

Classifying Adult Weight by Percentage of Body Fat

Classification	Body Fat (%) Men	Women
Healthy	13–20	23–30
Overweight	21–24	31–36
Obese	≥ 25	≥ 37

Data from Food and Nutrition Board. (2005). Dietary Reference Intakes for energy, carbohydrate, fiber, fat, fatty acids, cholesterol, protein, and amino acids (macronutrients). Washington, DC: National Academies Press. Table 5.5, p. 126.

indicates percentages of body fat that are healthy, overweight, and obese.

About one-half of an average healthy person's body fat is located in a layer under the skin (*subcutaneous fat*). Small amounts of fat are stored in muscles, which rely on the fat for energy. Besides subcutaneous and muscle fat, regions of the abdomen, thighs, hips, and buttocks store considerable amounts of fat.

Every year Americans spend money on ineffective treatments to eliminate "cellulite." Many people think cellulite is an abnormal type of fat that appears as lumpy, dimpled skin on the buttocks and thighs. Cellulite fat, however, does not exist. There is no difference between the fat cells in so-called cellulite and those in subcutaneous fat.[19] Strands of connective tissue hold subcutaneous fat in place. If these strands hold the fat in an irregular pattern, the fat tissue can extend into layers of skin, giving the skin a lumpy appearance. Women are more likely than men to have irregular connective tissue under their skin. The best way to improve the appearance of thighs and buttocks is to exercise and lose excess weight.

Fat Cells Obesity can begin at any age. However, the number and size of fat cells increase dramatically when this condition occurs during childhood and other periods of rapid growth.[20] People who become overweight in adulthood usually have normal numbers of fat cells, but their fat cells are larger than normal. The number of fat cells, however, can increase when extreme obesity occurs during the adult years.

Once fat cells form, there is little evidence that they can disappear with short-term weight reduction efforts. Under these conditions, most fat cells shrink as they release stored fat to meet the energy needs of other tissues. After shrinking, fat cells may send chemical signals to the nervous system that stimulate the urge to eat, making it difficult for people to maintain their reduced body weights.

Estimating Body Fat

A variety of methods is used to determine one's percentage of body fat, including hydrostatic weighing, bioelectrical impedance, dual-energy X-ray absorptiometry, air-displacement plethysmography, and skinfold thicknesses. The following sections discuss these techniques.

Hydrostatic Weighing Hydrostatic weighing (underwater weighing) is one of the most reliable methods to estimate an individual's percentage of body fat (**Figure 10.4**). Body fat is less dense than lean tissues or water; therefore, extra fat makes the body more

Figure 10.4

Hydrostatic (Underwater) Weighing. Hydrostatic weighing is one of the most reliable methods to estimate an individual's percentage of body fat.

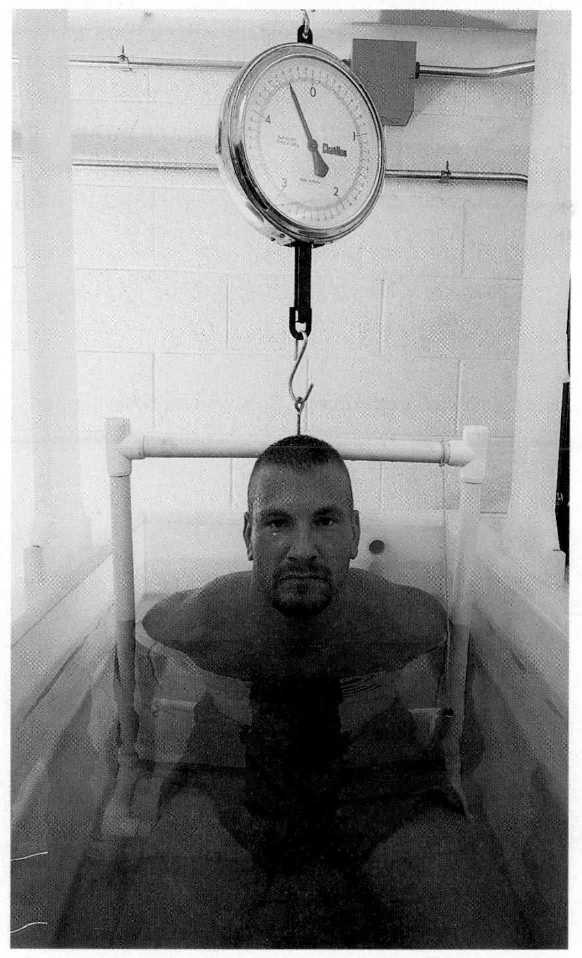

buoyant. Because the equipment needed to perform hydrostatic weighing is not widely available, the method is not a practical or convenient way to determine a person's percentage of body fat.

Bioelectrical Impedance Bioelectrical impedance uses electrical currents to estimate the percentage of body fat. Water and certain mineral elements conduct electrical currents, whereas fat is a poor conductor of electricity. The equipment shown in **Figure 10.5** safely measures the body's electrical conductivity to determine the percentage of body fat. When subjects have normal amounts of body water (i.e., are adequately hydrated), bioelectrical impedance provides reliable estimates of their percentage of body fat.

Dual-Energy X-ray Absorptiometry Dual-energy X-ray absorptiometry (DEXA or DXA) is often used in clinical studies to measure body fat as well as bone density, which is useful for diagnosing osteoporosis (**Figure 10.6**). Although the technique is very accurate for measuring body composition, the equipment is very expensive and requires trained X-ray technicians to use it.

Air-Displacement Plethysmography The air-displacement plethysmography technique uses a special chamber (BOD POD) to measure a person's body volume (**Figure 10.7**). The BOD POD determines the volume of air that a body displaces while sitting in the device. After information about the air displacement has been obtained, the person's fat mass can be calculated. Air-displacement plethysmography

Figure 10.5

Bioelectrical Impedance. This woman is having her percentage of body fat determined by the bioelectrical impedance method

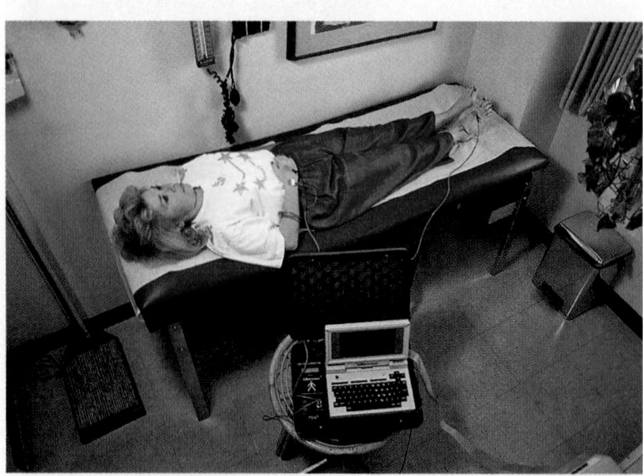

Figure 10.6

Dual-Energy X-ray Absorptiometry. DEXA is often used in clinical studies to measure body fat as well as bone density.

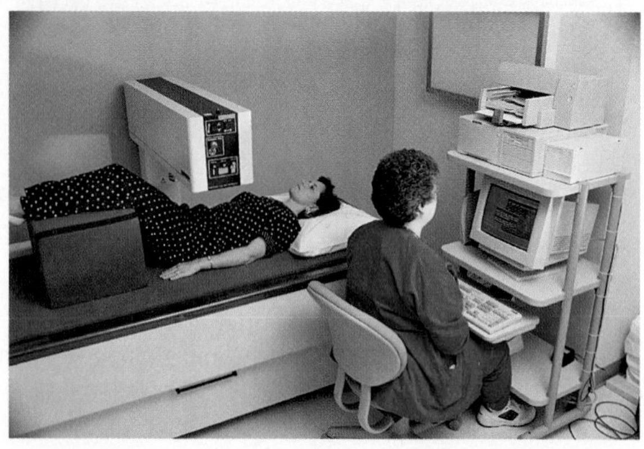

Figure 10.7

Air-Displacement Plethysmography. The technique uses a special chamber to measure a person's body volume.

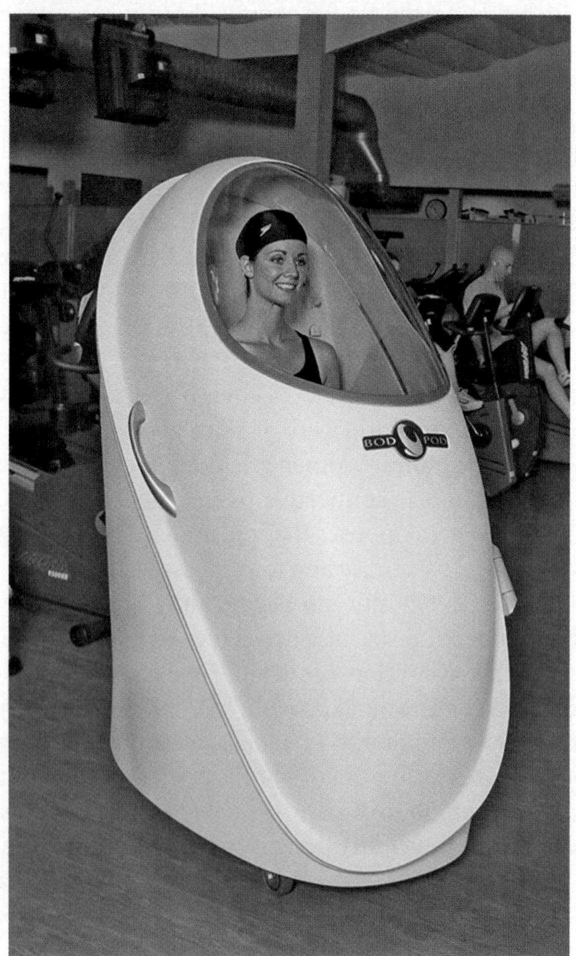

is a quick and reliable way to measure fat mass and involves no exposure to radiation as does DEXA.[21]

Skinfold Thicknesses Many years ago, advertisements for a breakfast cereal asked people to "pinch an inch" as a method of determining their amount of body fat. If people could pinch a fold of abdominal skin that was more than an inch wide, according to the advertisement, they were too fat. This crude technique of measuring skinfold thicknesses relied on the principle that one-half of a person's fat is located beneath the skin, if the person has a healthy BMI.

Using skinfold thicknesses to assess body composition is not as accurate as the underwater weighing and bioelectrical impedance techniques, but it is more practical and less costly. Instead of using fingers to pinch a section of skin and its underlying layer of fat, a trained person uses special calipers to measure skinfold thickness more precisely (**Figure 10.8**). Skinfold measurements should be taken at three or more select body sites; averaging these measurements accounts for individual differences in body fat distribution.

The reliability of using skinfolds to estimate the percentage of body fat depends on the accuracy of the calipers, the number of skinfolds measured, and the skill of the person performing the measurements. Although measuring skinfolds is a popular technique, some health experts challenge the value of skinfold thicknesses to determine the degree of body fat in individuals who are overweight or obese. Unlike persons with healthy weights, individuals who are obese have less than half of their body fat under their skin, because they store considerable amounts of fat in their abdomens.

Figure 10.8

Skinfold Thickness Measurements. A trained person uses special calipers to measure skinfold thickness at three or more body sites. This person is having her triceps skinfold measured.

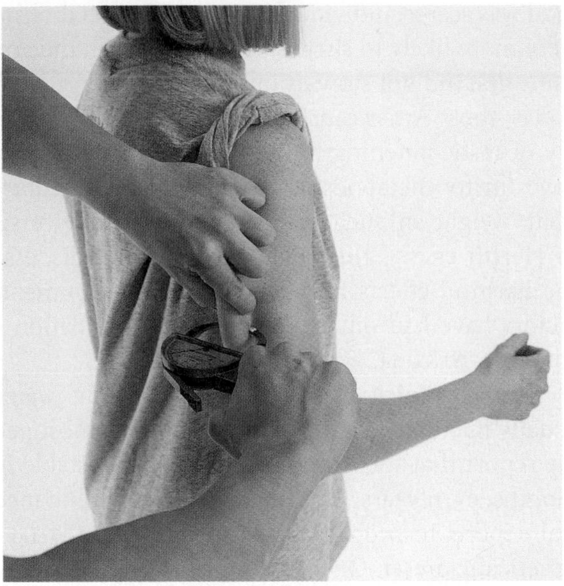

Waist Circumference Waist circumference measurements determine the distribution—rather than percentage—of body fat. The distribution of body fat may be more important than body fat percentage for determining risk factors for the health conditions that are associated with excess body fat. Men and women who have large body fat deposits centrally located deep within their abdomens tend to have higher blood cholesterol levels and a greater risk of developing diabetes, hypertension, and heart disease than individuals with the same amount of fat located below the waist.[22] Why? Certain obese abdominal fat cells (*visceral fat*) may be more likely to release inflammatory compounds into the blood than subcutaneous fat cells found in the hips and thighs. Excessive amounts of these substances in the blood increase the risk of cardiovascular disease and type 2 diabetes.[23] More research is needed, however, to determine the link between abdominal fat and these chronic diseases.

As both men and women grow older, they usually add body fat in their abdominal regions, which often increases their waist circumference to unhealthy levels. **Figure 10.9** shows a man with central obesity ("apple-shaped") and a woman whose excess body fat is located primarily below the waistline ("pear-shaped").

The only equipment you need to determine your waist circumference is a flexible but nonstretchable tape measure. **Figure 10.10** illustrates where to place the tape measure. To measure your waistline, place the tape around your body just below the rib-cage and at the top of the hipbone. What is your waist circumference? Men who have waistlines greater than 40 inches and women with waist circumferences greater than 35 inches have increased risks of developing the health problems associated with excess body fat.[24]

What Causes Obesity?

In most cases, there is no single cause for obesity. According to the principles of energy balance, the body gains fat when it has an excess of food energy; the body loses weight when energy intake does not meet its needs. However, biological, environmental,

Figure 10.9

Typical Fat Distribution in Persons Who Are Obese. Men and women who have large body fat deposits centrally located deep within their abdomens tend to have a higher risk of chronic health problems than do individuals with the same amount of fat located below the waist. (a) Men who are obese typically have central fat deposits ("apple-shaped bodies"). (b) Women who are obese often have excess body fat below the waist ("pear-shaped bodies").

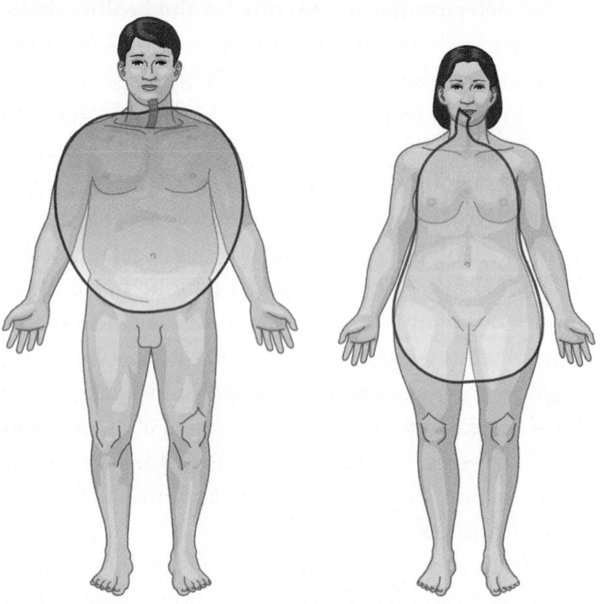

Figure 10.10

Measuring Waist Circumference. To determine one's waist circumference, measure the waist directly above the hipbone.

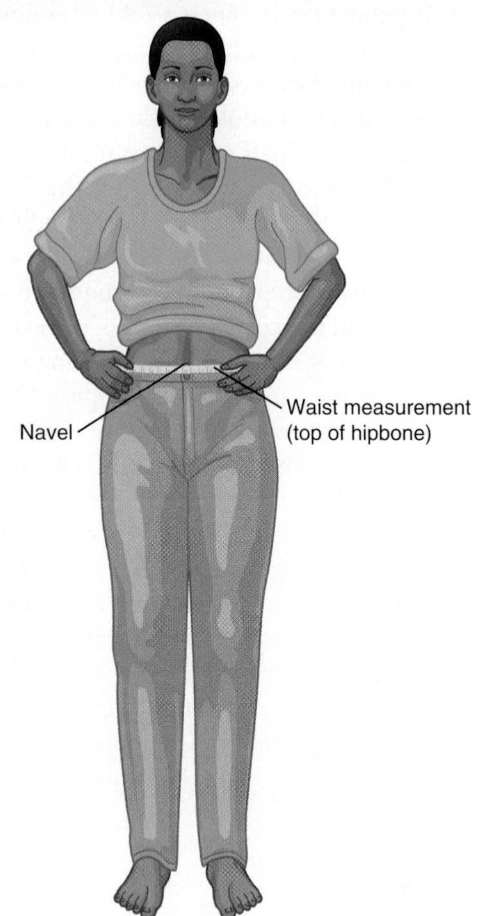

social, and emotional factors contribute to weight gain by influencing food intake. The following section examines these factors.

Biological Influences

Genes control the development of many physical characteristics, including height, fat distribution, and body frame size. Genes may also code for weight gain by determining the production of hormones that regulate one's metabolic rate and interest in eating tasty foods. As a result, cases of obesity are more likely to occur in certain families. When one or both parents are obese, they are more likely to have offspring who gain excessive amounts of body fat than do two parents of normal weights. Could a person benefit from inheriting genes that code for gaining weight easily?

Thousands of years ago, "fat" genes were vital to human survival. Our early ancestors probably endured long periods of fasting, interrupted by shorter periods of feasting. When food was plentiful, our ancestors thrived on the bounty. Some members of the population may have inherited metabolisms that "burned off" the excess food energy as body heat. Others had "thrifty" metabolisms that enabled them to store much of the excess energy as body fat. When food was scarce, individuals with thrifty metabolisms were more likely to survive than those with metabolisms that did not store as much excess energy as fat. Today, most Americans have access to a steady supply of tasty, fattening food. Therefore, persons who have thrifty metabolisms find it difficult to control their weight in such environments. The Diversity in Health essay "The Plight of the Pima" discusses the harmful effects that genetic and environmental factors have had on the Pima Indian population of southern Arizona.

The Set Point Theory Although body weight usually fluctuates slightly from day to day, most people report that their weight remains fairly stable for months, even years. This observation led some medical experts to propose that the level of body fat is genetically preset. Once the level of body fat reaches

Diversity in Health

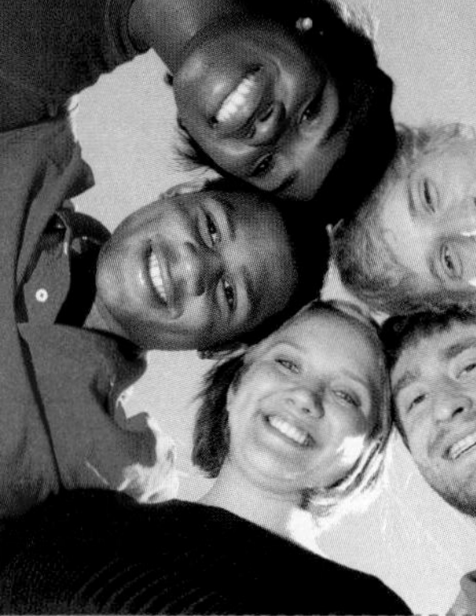
© Mike Flippo/ShutterStock

The Plight of the Pima

After the July rains, the Sonora Desert of southwestern Arizona becomes transformed for a brief time into a natural fast-food restaurant. For hundreds of years, the Pima Indians residing in this harsh environment harvested the seasonal bounty of mesquite pods, acorns, wolfberries, prickly pears, tepary beans, and cholla blossoms to supplement their regular diet of hunted animals and cultivated maize (corn) and lima beans. The Pima were slim, but they flourished while enduring this cycle of feast and famine.

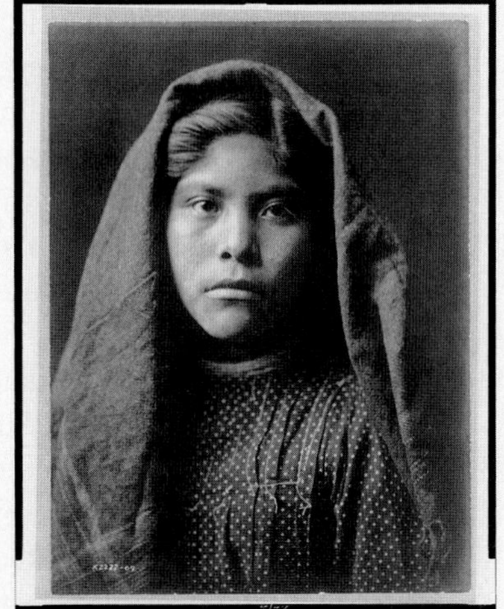
Courtesy of Library of Congress, Prints & Photographs Division, Curtis (Edward S.) Collection [Reproduction Number LC-USZ62-112212].

By the 1930s, the Arizona Pima had discontinued eating most of their ancient fare and adopted Western foods that provided generous amounts of lard (pork fat), refined starches, and sweets. Within a couple of decades, an alarming number of U.S. Pima had become obese and developed type 2 diabetes. According to one study, about 64% of U.S. Pima males and 75% of U.S. Pima females were obese. Among the U.S. Pima, about one-third of the men and almost half of the women had type 2 diabetes. Rates of obesity and diabetes are much higher in the U.S. Pima population than in the Mexican Pima Indians. U.S. Pima have the highest known incidence of type 2 diabetes in the world. Why are the U.S. Pima so severely affected by obesity and type 2 diabetes?

Medical experts suspect certain biological and environmental factors influence the development of obesity and diabetes in this population. Experts think the Pima have thrifty metabolisms that allow them to survive their harsh desert environment with its natural cycles of feast and famine. Although their current dietary habits have made the need for such metabolisms obsolete, the Pima are still genetically programmed to conserve a major share of their food intake as fat. Additionally, most Arizona Pima lead more sedentary lives than their ancestors did or relatives living in Mexico do. The typical Mexican Pima Indian has fewer labor-saving devices and performs more physical work than the typical Arizona Pima.

The abandonment of ancient dietary practices may contribute to the current health problems of the Arizona Pima. Besides being lower in fat, traditional Pima foods provide more complex carbohydrates than typical modern menus do. Furthermore, the ancestral diet supplied substances that may have protected the Pima from diabetes. Many desert plants contain significant amounts of amylose, a digestible carbohydrate, as well as gums and mucilages, two forms of soluble fiber. Eating foods rich in these substances slows digestion and delays the absorption of glucose from the small intestine. This delay prevents sharp increases in blood levels of insulin, the hormone that signals cells to remove glucose (blood sugar) from the blood. Under normal circumstances, the body can prevent sharp increases or decreases of blood glucose. However, individuals who suffer from type 2 diabetes are unable to avoid dramatic fluctuations in blood glucose or insulin levels, which can damage the body.

Today medical experts are studying the U.S. Pima to determine what steps can be taken to reduce their prevalence of obesity and diabetes. Some scientists think tribal members should return to their former dietary practices; many of these ancestral foods are still available. By eating desert plant foods rich in amylose and soluble fibers, the Pima may reduce their risk of developing type 2 diabetes. If the U.S. Pima are to survive as a population, they may need to recover their traditional "roots."

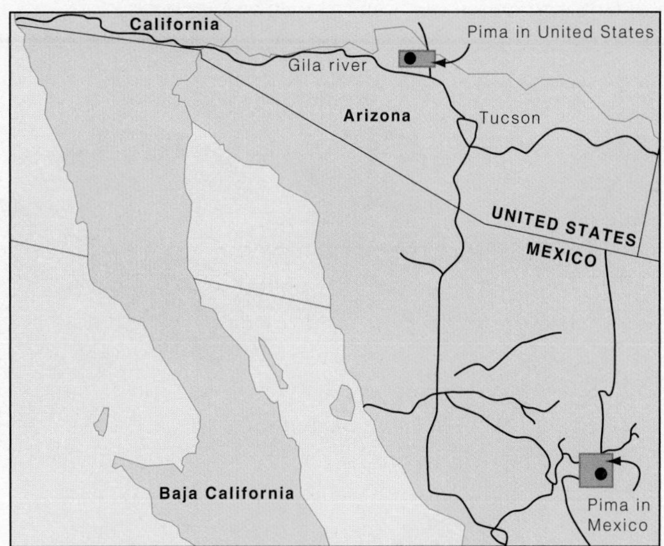

Data from Boyce, V. L., & Swinburn, B. A. (1993). The traditional Pima Indian diet: Composition and adaptation for use in a dietary intervention study. Diabetes Care, 16(51):369–371.; Cowen, R. (1990). Seeds of protection: Ancestral menus may hold a message for diabetes-prone descendants. Science News, 137:350–351.; Valencia, M. E., Bennett, P. H., Ravussin, E., Esparza, J., Fox, C., & Schultz, L. O. (1999). The Pima Indians of Sonora, Mexico. Nutrition Reviews, 57(5):S55–S58.

set point A theoretical level of body fat that resists weight loss efforts.

hunger The physiological drive to seek and eat food.

appetite The psychological desire to eat foods that are appealing.

satiety The feeling that enough food has been eaten to relieve hunger and turn off appetite.

this **set point**, the metabolic rate and other internal mechanisms maintain the degree of fatness, like a thermostat can be set to maintain the temperature of a room. Persons who are lean may have lower set points than do persons who are obese. For example, when people who are lean deliberately overeat to gain weight, they usually lose the extra weight after resuming their normal eating habits.

Although having a high set point may result in an unhealthy percentage of body fat, that amount of fat may be normal for that person. As a result, the person's fat cells may resist efforts to lose storage fat. Furthermore, when a person who is obese loses weight, she/he is likely to regain some or all of it within a few years. Why? Some scientists think "slimmed down" fat cells send messages to the brain that are interpreted as hunger. As a result, the person overeats and his or her fat cells expand again.

Appetite Regulation Nearly everyone knows what it feels like to be hungry. **Hunger** is the physiologic drive to seek and eat food. **Appetite** is the psychological desire to eat specific foods, which is not the same as being hungry. **Satiety** is the feeling that enough food has been eaten to relieve hunger and turn off appetite.

The digestive system, brain, and fat cells play important roles in controlling hunger and satiety. While a person is eating, the intestinal tract releases several chemicals that signal the brain to eat less food. The sensation of stomach fullness results in termination of eating. *Leptin*, a hormone produced by fat cells, and *insulin*, the pancreatic hormone that lowers blood sugar levels, affect the *hypothalamus*, a region of the brain that regulates eating behavior (**Figure 10.11**). Leptin and insulin play important roles in regulating eating behavior, but in people who are obese, these hormones seem to lose their effectiveness.[25]

Composition of the Diet An excess of calories from carbohydrate, protein, fat, and alcohol can result in weight gain. Foods that are rich sources of simple carbohydrates (sugars) contribute to overconsumption of calories. Sugar-sweetened soft drinks ("liquid candy") are convenient to purchase from vending machines and convenient stores. However, high-fat diets are associated with overeating and gaining body fat.[26] An ounce of fat supplies more than twice the number of calories as an ounce of carbohydrate or protein. Furthermore, the body stores more fat when the excess of calories is supplied by dietary fat rather than carbohydrate or protein.[27]

No specific calorie-restricted diet enhances long-term weight loss and maintenance. However, people who are overweight often lose weight when following

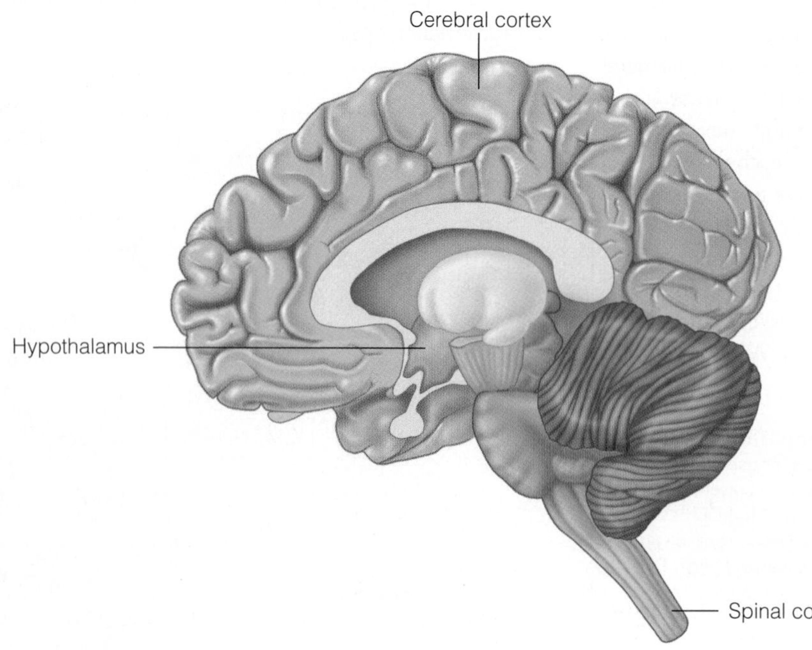

Figure 10.11

Hypothalamus. Research indicates that regions of the hypothalamus in the brain control hunger and satiety.

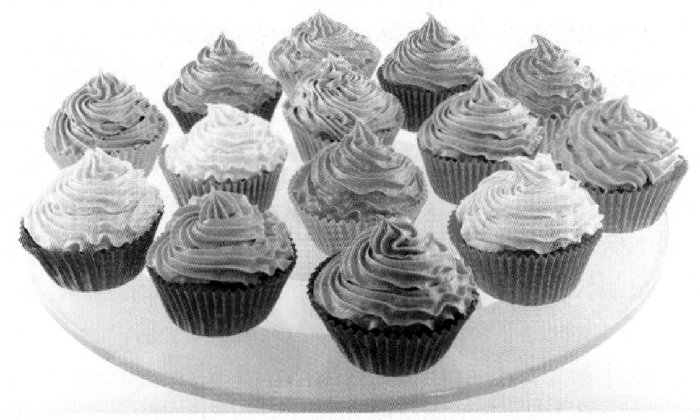

© Sander Crombeen/ShutterStock

a low-fat, high-complex carbohydrate diet because the food plan includes generous servings of fruits, vegetables, beans, and whole-grain cereals. These nutrient-dense, high-fiber foods are quite filling, and dieters may fail to eat enough to meet their total permissible number of calories.

Carbohydrate-rich foods often taste better when they are fried or when fats such as butter, sour cream, or gravy are added to them. Most desserts and snack foods contain refined carbohydrates and fat; mixtures of sugar and fat are almost irresistible. Thus, the typical American diet promotes overeating because it provides an interesting, tasty, and enjoyable variety of fatty, sweet foods.

People who are obese often claim that they gain weight by eating small amounts of food. Underreporting caloric intake, however, is common, especially by persons who are obese.[26] Many people are unaware of or they underestimate the number of calories that are in their snacks and meals. Calorie and fat-counting guides are helpful if you are trying to control your weight. Keeping a record of everything you eat and drink each day can also be useful for identifying problem foods and poor eating habits. By eating more fruits and vegetables and fewer sugary and fatty foods, you can control your caloric intake.

Environmental, Social, and Psychological Influences

A variety of environmental, social, and psychological factors promotes overeating in the United States. Since the early 1900s, typical portion sizes of many popular foods have increased.[28] When the Hershey chocolate bar was introduced in 1906, it weighed a little over half an ounce; today a regular-sized Hershey bar weighs 1.6 ounces. Compared with original bakery bagels, an average bakery bagel now weighs three times as much and provides three times the amount of energy. Fast-food hamburgers and standard servings of french fries and soft drinks are often considerably larger than those served when these popular restaurants first opened in the 1950s and 1960s. Many fast food and family-style restaurants promote their "super-size" portions as being bargains. Such food production practices encourage overeating and excess caloric intake.

Advertisers know the value of making foods look appealing. To stimulate sales, for example, fast-food restaurants show hamburgers topped with crisp lettuce and bacon extending beyond the bun. Actors in food ads appear to be happy and satisfied with their food choices.

Today, it is easier to obtain meals and snacks when you are not at home than in the past. Many fast-food restaurants, convenience stores, and supermarkets are open 24 hours. Supermarkets often have a deli section that offers cooked or fried chicken, baked macaroni and cheese, a variety of potato salads, and other ready-to-eat foods. You do not even have to leave home to buy food; pizza, Chinese, and other food can be delivered to your front door.

Many people respond to certain social situations by overeating. For example, you may be "stuffed" after eating a Thanksgiving dinner, but when you see pumpkin pie topped with whipped cream, you can find "room" in your stomach for dessert. Events that mark important milestones of life usually include big meals and special foods. Imagine a birthday party or wedding celebration that does not include a frosted layer cake!

Work and home environments often do not provide opportunities for Americans to be physically active. Modern technology enables machines, instead of our muscles, to do much of our work. As a result, we tend to spend more time sitting than walking around during the day. At home, many people spend their leisure time engaged in sedentary activities such as watching television or using a computer.

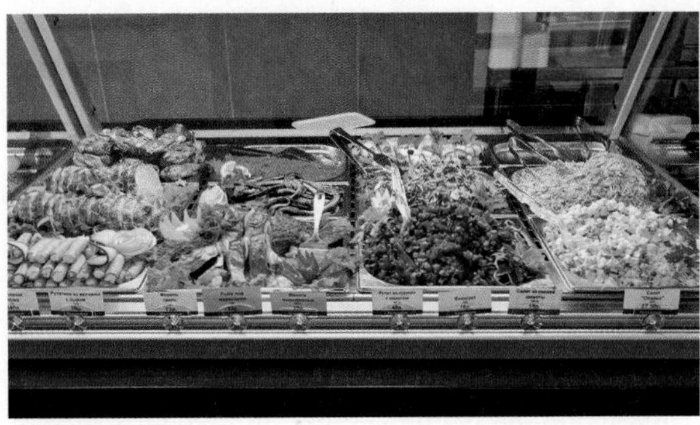

Deli sections of supermarkets usually offer a variety of appealing prepared foods.
© karamysh/ShutterStock

fad diets Eating plans that are popular for a time, then quickly lose their widespread appeal.

People who are physically inactive are likely to gain weight unless they restrict their food intake.

Psychological state can influence eating behavior. Some people eat long after satisfying their hunger because they are excited, anxious, or bored. Many people seek comfort from eating, especially foods that are fatty and sugary, when they are distressed or depressed. The following personal reflection written by a young woman who is overweight illustrates how emotions can affect eating behavior:

I gained 20 pounds between the ages of 16 and 18. At the time I was in an abusive relationship with my boyfriend. I felt like dirt and the only thing that made me feel good was food. I was totally devastated when he was killed in a car accident when I was 18. I ate even more. I went to a nutritionist for a diet. I tried to stay on it but failed. Looking back, every time I gained weight it was due to stress. When I am stressed, I need to get out of the house, take my mind off things.

In developed nations, eating disorders such as bulimia nervosa and binge eating affect considerable numbers of people, especially girls and women. These conditions are associated with serious psychological disturbances.

Because families share environments as well as genes—and both the environment and genes affect obesity—obesity is classified as a genomic disease. Not only do families share common eating and exercise practices, they often adopt similar perspectives regarding body weight and health. For example, some cultures view excess body fat favorably, as a sign of financial security, and may not perceive overweightness as a health risk. Such a perspective could contribute to the incidence of obesity.

Weight Management

According to a recent survey, the majority of American adults who were overweight or obese were trying to lose weight.[29] Improving one's appearance and health were among the reasons subjects gave for deciding to reduce their excess weight. The majority of the people who wanted to lose weight used calorie reduction as their primary method.

Dissatisfaction with body size is common, particularly among young women. In a 2009 survey of American high school students, about 60% of females and 30% of males reported that they were attempting to lose weight at the time of the survey.[30]

Even though they may have gained the weight gradually, individuals who are overweight or obese who want to lose weight often seek methods that promise quick and dramatic results. When people are desperate to lose weight, they are more likely to believe advertisement promises for rapid weight loss without dietary or physical activity changes. Each year, Americans spend billions of dollars on various weight loss products and services. These efforts include joining weight loss programs or spas and buying special foods, books, pills, and gadgets. Do these products and services enable people to lose weight? How can you judge the value of a weight loss method? The following sections answer these questions.

Weight Reduction Diets

As mentioned earlier, the body loses weight when its caloric intake is less than its energy needs. In this situation, the body relies primarily on stored fat for energy. To lose weight, individuals should eat fewer calories than they need or expend more calories than they eat via physical activity. Most reliable weight reduction regimens incorporate both of these features by combining a low-calorie diet with a plan that increases physical activity.

Fad Diets Some of the more popular weight loss diets of the last 3 decades have included a variety of recommendations such as fasting, counting calories, not counting calories, avoiding certain food combinations, eating plenty of protein and little carbohydrate, or eating only a few foods. Such diets are often referred to as **fad diets** because they remain popular for a period of time and then quickly lose their widespread appeal. The low-carbohydrate "Atkins diet," for example, gained many followers when it was first

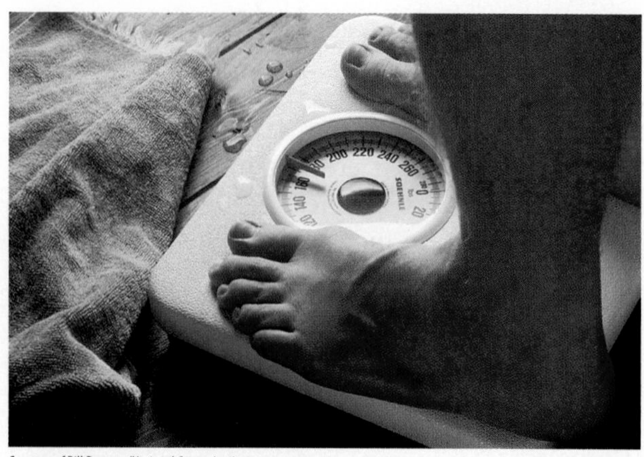

Courtesy of Bill Branson/National Cancer Institute.

introduced in 1973, but dieters soon lost interest in its restrictive food choices. When the Atkins diet was reintroduced about 25 years later, its renewed popularity resulted in the marketing of a wide array of "low-carb" foods.

Fad diets usually have a few common features—gimmicks and caloric restriction. A gimmick is a promotional feature that makes a fad weight loss diet appear to be new, unique, and more effective than other diet plans. Some fad diets, including the Atkins diet, use carbohydrate restriction as a gimmick. Other fad diets use gimmicks such as prescribed food combinations based on your blood type, dietary supplements that "melt fat while you sleep," and "secret" food ingredients that allow you to eat all your favorite foods or retain fat in desirable places (the breasts of women, for example) while shedding it from the hips, abdomen, and thighs. Although such claims are untrue and not based on scientific evidence, they attract people who are seeking quick and easy ways to lose their excess body fat.

People who are overweight can lose weight while following fad diets because the diet plans that accompany the gimmicks usually provide fewer calories than the level of energy supplied by typical American diets. Regardless of the type of diet they used to lose excess fat, the majority of persons who were formerly overweight find it difficult to maintain their reduced body weights.

Very Low-Calorie Diets Very low-calorie diets may provide fewer than 800 calories per day and be nutritionally inadequate because they limit food choices. Diets that provide 400 or fewer calories daily are often called fasts. Fasts are essentially starvation regimens. Some fasts permit only fruit juices and nutrient supplements. Fasting accelerates the loss of fat and lean body tissue, creating unhealthy metabolic by-products. Healthy individuals should not fast for more than a day without medical supervision.

Initially, people who are obese typically lose substantial amounts of weight while following a low-calorie diet or fast. When caloric intake is very low, the body burns fat as well as lean tissue for energy. Because fat and lean tissue store water, using these tissues for energy creates a surplus of water in the body. The kidneys eliminate the excess water, causing a dramatic loss of weight that often encourages dieters during the early phase of their weight reduction efforts. Within a few weeks, however, the body regains its normal water balance, and the rate of weight loss slows.

Very low-calorie diets or fasts trigger energy-conserving mechanisms in the body that are designed to help people survive starvation. The metabolic rate decreases with caloric restriction, especially when individuals consume fewer than 800 calories a day. Thus, dieters must cut their caloric intakes even further to continue losing weight, which often makes adhering to their diets even more difficult.

Despite their efforts, most individuals experience a decline in their rate of weight loss after several weeks of following a calorie-reduced diet. Some of this slowdown occurs because the body expends fewer calories to maintain the new weight. As the body adjusts to the reduced caloric intake, it metabolizes less fat and lean tissue for energy, slowing the rate of weight loss. Additionally, dieters who follow restrictive diet plans for more than a few weeks often become bored with the regimens and gradually return to their old eating habits.

Most people who have lost weight regain some or all of it—and often, even more weight—after a period of caloric restriction. Frustrated dieters often blame themselves for lack of self-control. Episodes of losing and regaining weight are referred to as "yo-yo" dieting or weight cycling. Results of studies do not provide consistent evidence that weight cycling is associated with increased disease or death.[32] Although more research is needed, obesity appears to pose more health risks than does weight cycling. Rather than endure periodic fad dieting, people who have excess body fat should consider other, more successful methods of losing weight—namely, changing eating and exercise patterns for life.

In 2014, *U.S. News & World Report* published new rankings of 32 popular U.S. diets.[31] A panel of nationally recognized experts in nutrition, obesity, food psychology, diabetes, and heart disease was assembled to evaluate the selected diets. Some of these diets can be classified as fad diets; others are roadmaps of health nutritional plans that could be sustained over a lifetime. The specialists ranked each diet on a scale of 1 to 5 on seven measures: short-term weight loss, long-term weight loss, ease of following, nutrition, safety, performance as a diabetes diet, and performance as a heart diet. U.S. News used scores on all seven measures (not all measures were weighed equally) to compute an overall score for each diet, and subsequently ranked the diets from highest (best) to lowest. The following diets were identified as the best diets overall, and won a best diets Gold Medal: DASH Diet (with an overall score of 4.1 out of 5.0), TLC Diet (score of 4.0), Mayo Clinic Diet (3.9), Mediterranean Diet (3.9), Weight

Watchers (3.9), Flexitarian Diet (3.8), and Volumetics (3.8). Full results, including rankings, overall scores, and scores on the aforementioned seven measures are published on U.S. News' website: http://health.usnews.com/best-diet/best-overall-diets/data.

In addition to ranking these diets by best overall scores, six other rankings were derived from the data from five measures evaluated by the expert panel, including best weight-loss diets. The best diets for overall weight loss were computed using the short-term weight loss and long-term weight loss measures previously identified. The following diets were identified as the best weight-loss diets and won a best weight-loss diet Gold Medal: Weight Watchers (with an overall weight loss score of 3.8), Biggest Loser Diet (score of 3.5), Jenny Craig (3.5), and Raw Food Diet (3.5), Volumetrics (3.4), Atkins (3.3), Flexitarian Diet (3.3), Slim-Fast (3.3), Spark Solution Diet (3.3), and Vegan Diet (3.3). Full results for overweight weight loss diets can be located on U.S. News' website: http://health.usnews.com/best-diet/best-weight-loss-diets/data.

Although the U.S. News diet rankings provide comparison data between the diets, it is important to note that these data are not from clinical trials. As such, they should be interpreted as subjective—if expert—opinions and not as objective fact. Persons wishing to lose weight should always consult with their physician before embarking on a new eating plan to ensure it meets their nutritional needs.

Physical Activity

Many American adults are less active physically than when they were younger, partly because they have occupations that require little physical effort. Men who had trim, athletic builds during adolescence often develop bulging waistlines by the time they are 40 years old. As they reach middle age, women often blame "gravity" or pregnancy for the expanding dimensions of their waists, hips, and thighs. Can adopting more physically active lifestyles reverse these changes?

I gained 20 pounds before my wedding. My husband bought me a stepper for a wedding present (that's what I wanted), and I use it with an exercise video. Now, I exercise more than ever, but I haven't lost much weight.

This student has discovered that exercising to lose body fat often does not produce the desired change in body weight. Physical activity alone is not as effective as low-calorie diets for treating obesity because most individuals who are overweight cannot perform enough exercise to create a significant deficit of calories. However, this does not mean that they should abandon physical activity as a means of losing excess body fat. Exercise retains lean tissue and builds muscle mass, which may stabilize or even increase one's body weight. Thus, what appears to be a lack of progress while restricting food intake and exercising may be the result of a healthy increase in muscle mass. (This is one reason why measuring one's body fat percentage or waist circumference is more insightful than measuring weight, alone.)

In addition to tracking weekly changes in body weight, physically active people who are overweight can keep weekly records of waist circumferences. People who become more physically active while dieting often report that their clothing fits better, or they can wear smaller sizes, even though they have not lost much weight. Besides improving physical appearance, exercise reduces elevated blood pressures and lipid levels. Furthermore, individuals who exercise for at least 250 minutes per week may be more likely to maintain their weight loss than those who are less active.[33]

Most individuals who are overweight can safely increase their physical activity by walking, bicycling, or swimming for at least 30 minutes, preferably on a daily basis. Regardless of the activity, it should be enjoyable and practical to perform on a year-round basis. Before beginning a vigorous physical activity program, inactive people over 40 years of age should obtain the approval of their personal physicians.

Surgical Procedures

Individuals who are morbidly obese generally experience little success following low-calorie diet plans

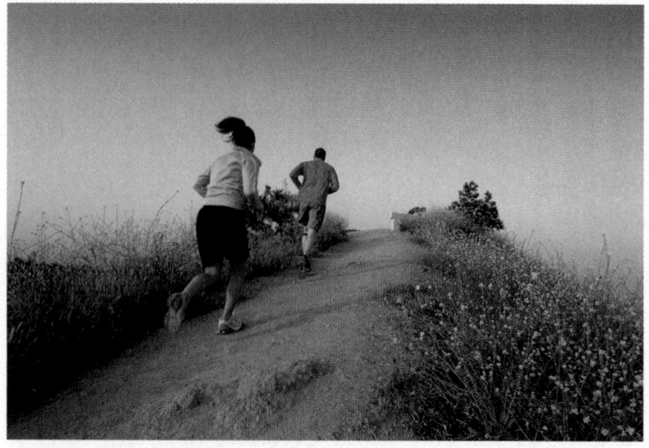

Exercise may result in a healthy increase in muscle mass.

Figure 10.12

Gastric Bypass Surgery. Gastric bypass is a procedure used to treat severe obesity. After surgery, the obese person exerpiences discomfort after overeating and is less likely to overeat.

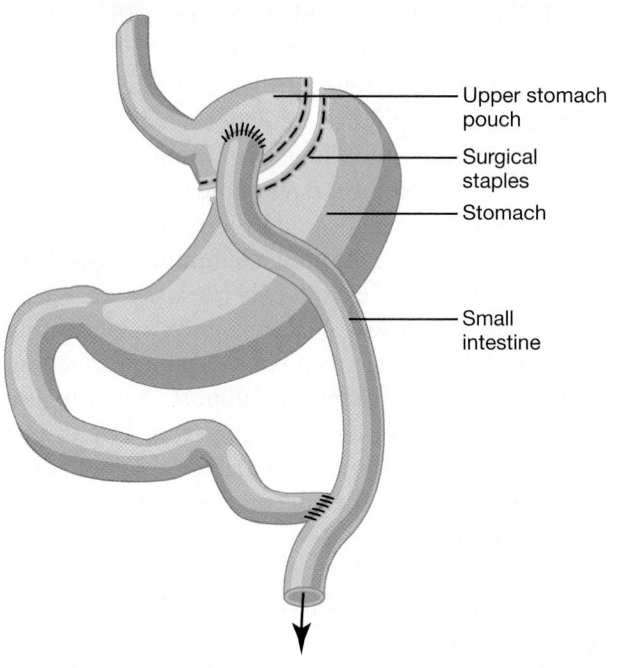

Figure 10.13

Liposuction. Liposuction is a medical procedure in which a special instrument is inserted into body fat through an incision made in the skin, and the fat is vacuumed from the body.

© Girish Menon/ShutterStock

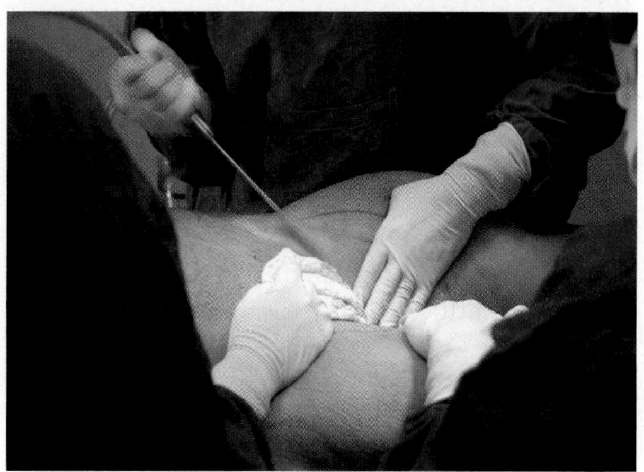

and exercising to lose weight. In such cases, *bariatric surgeries*, particularly *gastric bypass* procedures, may be used. **Figure 10.12** illustrates the appearance of the stomach and small intestine after one type of gastric bypass surgery. A surgeon drastically reduces the capacity of the stomach by creating a small pouch in the upper part of the stomach for food to enter. After having this procedure, the patient loses weight rapidly because he or she can no longer eat large portions of food without vomiting or experiencing uncomfortable feelings of fullness. On average, people who have had gastric bypasses can lose about 60% of their presurgery weight, improving their overall health.[34]

Liposuction, a surgical procedure that involves vacuuming subcutaneous fat out of the body, is the most common type of cosmetic surgery in the United States. Before removing the fat, the area is injected with an anesthetic-containing fluid or treated with ultrasound (*ultrasound-assisted lipoplasty*). This technique has cosmetic value when used to remove small areas of fat that create unsightly bulges such as "saddlebag thighs" or double chins (**Figure 10.13**). Liposuction can be hazardous; infections, blood clots, disfigurement, and even death can result. For most individuals who are overweight, liposuction is not a suitable weight loss method.

Medications

People who are trying to follow low-calorie diets often lose control over their appetites and—as a result—overeat. For decades, medical researchers have been testing various compounds to determine whether they can help people adhere to their diet plans more easily or lose weight faster.

Orlistat (Xenical), approved in 1999, was the only prescription drug for weight loss approved by the Food and Drug Administration (FDA) for more than a decade. Orlistat does not suppress appetite but interferes with fat digestion. As a result, some of the fat in foods is not digested and is eliminated in feces. Fat-soluble vitamins are generally found in fats and oils, so a person taking orlistat will not absorb as many of these nutrients from foods, and therefore should take a vitamin supplement. An over-the-counter version of orlistat (Alli) became available in 2007.[35]

In 2012, the FDA approved a second prescription drug for weight loss, Belviq. Belviq activates the serotonin 2C receptor in the brain, which may help one successfully eat less and feel full after consuming smaller food portions. Belviq was approved for use in conjunction with a reduced-calorie diet and exercise plan, in adults who are obese (i.e., have a BMI of 30 or greater) or who have a BMI of 27 or greater and have at least one weight-related health condition (e.g., type 2 diabetes, high cholesterol, hypertension).[36]

Alternative Therapies

People who are overweight may turn to alternative therapies to lose weight, especially if they have had no success with conventional medical weight loss practices that include calorie restriction and increased physical activity. Acupressure, a therapy that is based on ancient Chinese medicine, is a popular alternative therapy for weight, but there is a lack of scientific evidence to support its long-term effectiveness.[37]

Dietary supplements such as those containing chitosan, green tea, chromium picolinate, and hoodia are promoted for weight loss. Medical experts, however, do not recommend these products because reports of their safety and effectiveness are not based on well-designed clinical studies. Manufacturers of weight loss products often recommend that dieters also follow a calorie-reduced diet and an exercise regimen. Therefore, any significant weight loss can be attributable to the calorie-restricted diet and increased physical activity—not the product. People who have lost weight with the help of "diet drugs" usually regain it when they discontinue using the products and following the diet and exercise plan. The Consumer Health feature "Dietary Supplements: Weight Loss Aids" provides information about some popular over-the-counter weight loss products. The Analyzing Health-Related Information feature in this chapter includes an advertisement for a dietary supplement that is marketed for weight loss.

Strategies for Successful Weight Loss

Individuals who are overweight can lose body fat and maintain their new weight by following sensible and safe weight loss plans, which have four major characteristics:

1. They are medically and nutritionally sound.
2. They include practical ways to engage in regular physical activity.
3. They are adaptable to one's psychological and social needs.
4. They can be followed for a lifetime.

Nutritionally sound weight reduction diets emphasize nutrient-dense foods, and they are nutritionally well balanced and adequate. Without being overly restrictive, such diets supply fewer calories than one needs. No special foods are necessary; the recommendations of the U.S. *Dietary Guidelines* and MyPlate (www.choosemyplate.gov) form the basis of nutritious calorie-reduced daily menus.

Reasonable and reliable diet plans recommend ways to increase physical activity such as by adding 30 to 90 minutes of walking, swimming, or bicycling to one's routine on most days of the week. Additionally, weight loss plans should meet the psychological and social needs of those attempting weight loss. A reliable plan, for example, helps a person set an achievable weight loss goal, recognize faulty eating habits, build self-esteem and body shape satisfaction, and obtain family or group support. You can use the criteria listed in the Managing Your Health tips titled "General Features of Reliable Weight Reduction Plans" to judge the effectiveness of most weight reduction methods.

Effective weight loss plans usually emphasize behavior modification. Behavior modification involves learning to identify behaviors that contribute to one's inability to lose weight, such as eating too much fatty food and not engaging in enough physical activity. The person learns to modify inappropriate behaviors so that weight loss and its maintenance are possible. **Table 10.5** lists key behaviors, such as not watching television while eating, that can help people achieve their weight loss goals. By identifying and modifying behaviors that resulted in weight gain, a person can develop a weight loss and maintenance plan that works best for his or her specific needs.

To avoid regaining weight, successful dieters must make lifestyle changes they can follow throughout their lifetimes, such as exercising regularly and controlling caloric intake. Small incremental changes that are implemented gradually are easier to adopt than extreme exercise regimens and overly restrictive diets. Most fad diets do not focus on behavior modification. However, even reliable weight loss programs that promote behavior modification do not offer guarantees for long-term success. The process of changing behaviors takes education, practice, time, and perseverance.

The majority of people who have lost weight through nonsurgical methods experience relapse, regaining some or all of the weight within 4 years.[34] Relapses occur when one fails to modify eating behaviors and physical activity patterns permanently

Table 10.5

Examples of Behavior Modification for Weight Management

Behavior	Actions to Modify Behavior
Identify faulty eating behaviors and eliminate or ignore improper eating cues.	• Keep daily food records to identify problem foods. • Use a shopping list and do not buy problem foods. • Eat fruit or a meal before shopping for food. • Discard problem foods. • While at home, restrict eating to the kitchen or dining room. • Do not eat while watching TV, reading, or talking on the phone. • Avoid places with vending machines. • Avoid fast-food restaurants that do not sell low-fat foods.
Reduce caloric intake.	• Serve meals on smaller plates. • Prepare smaller amounts of foods to reduce the likelihood of "seconds." • Avoid buffet-style or all-you-can-eat restaurants. • Eat a low-fat, high-fiber snack such as a piece of fruit or vegetable before a meal. • Keep fruit and vegetables on hand to snack on when hungry. • Ask for salad dressing "on the side" at restaurants. • Prepare low-calorie lunches and snacks to take to work or school. • Substitute fresh fruit or yogurt for rich desserts. • Read nutrition labels to identify high-calorie foods. • Learn to leave some food on your plate.
Stay focused on weight loss goal.	• Set reasonable incremental goals, such as losing 5 pounds in 5 weeks. • Place a picture of yourself on the refrigerator, pantry door, or bedroom mirror. • Measure your waistline once a week. • Place exercise equipment and walking shoes where you can see them. • Buy new pants that are one size smaller and hang them where you can see them. • Ask your friends and family to support your efforts. Give them examples of how they can help.
Practice appropriate behaviors.	• Find ways to move around while at work, school, or home. For example, take the stairs instead of the elevator. • If you relapse, tell yourself that this is normal. Do not label yourself a failure. Ask yourself what you can learn from the experience so it is less likely to affect your eating again. Minor occasional indulgences will not affect your weight. Continue to focus on your weight loss goal. • Set aside at least 30 minutes each day to engage in an enjoyable physical activity. Gradually increase the duration of the activity to 45 to 60 minutes daily.
Use nonfood rewards for behaviors.	• Praise yourself frequently for exercising or taking smaller servings of high-calorie appropriate foods. • Buy a desired item such as a new CD, DVD, or an item of clothing. • Take a walk or ride a bike through a park.

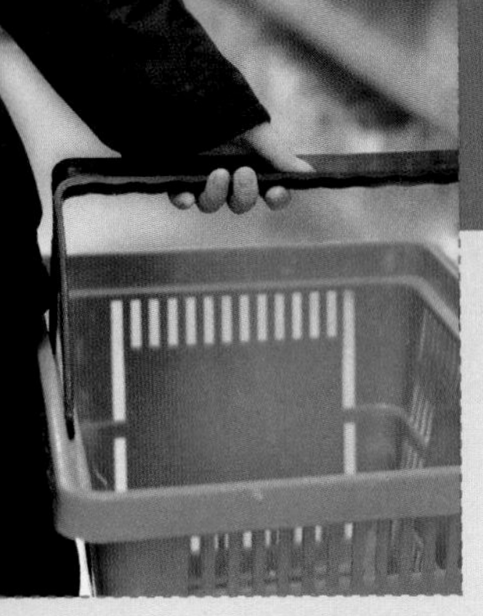

© sevenke/ShutterStock

Consumer Health

Dietary Supplements: Weight Loss Aids

Anyone who has tried to lose weight knows it can be a frustrating effort. Hunger seems to be a constant companion. For years, people attempting to lose weight have taken various pills and dietary supplements sold over the counter to promote weight loss and prevent hunger. **Table 10.A** includes several of the more popular supplements that people take to lose weight and provides information concerning the scientific support for health-related claims associated with the product.

Consumers need to be wary of weight loss products that are marketed on websites. Such products often include misleading or untruthful claims such as the following:

"Eat all you want without gaining weight."
"Lose weight by blocking starch."
"Clinically tested fat inhibitor instantly prevents weight gain."
"Prevents carbs from being converted into fat."
"Burns fat without increasing your metabolic rate."

Claims about a supplement's effect on the structure or function of the body must be supported by scientific evidence, and not be misleading or dishonest.

Taking certain weight loss products may be dangerous. In 2011, the Food and Drug Administration determined that "Slim Xtreme Herbal Slimming Capsules," which were available at various online websites, contained an undeclared drug ingredient (*sibutramine*). The agency warned consumers to stop using the capsules and discard them because the product posed a threat to health. Sibutramine is known to increase blood pressure in some people and could be harmful for patients with heart disease and stroke.

Individuals should not use any dietary supplement for weight loss without the advice and monitoring of their physician. If you experience any side effects while taking such products, report the problem to the FDA's MedWatch hotline by calling 1-800-332-1088 or the agency's online reporting site at https://www.accessdata.fda.gov/scripts/medwatch/medwatch-online.htm.

Table 10.A

Dietary Supplements: Weight Loss

Dietary Supplement	Claims	Scientific Findings
Garcinia	Reduces body fat	The evidence to support the claim is weak.
Bitter orange	Enhances weight loss	Bitter orange can increase heart rate and blood pressure; therefore, its use is risky.
Blue-green algae (spirulina)	Promotes weight loss, boosts immune system functioning, and treats asthma, depression, and several other common disorders	No evidence to support claims. Algae may be contaminated with toxins that are in their environment.
Chitosan (chitin)	Enhances weight loss, reduces blood lipid levels	No evidence to support weight loss claim. Chitosan may reduce cholesterol levels, but the effect is minimal.
Chromium picolinate	Increases metabolic rate, facilitates weight loss	May result in slight reduction in body weight, but the loss is not impressive.
Glucomannan	Enhances weight loss	Some evidence to support claim, but more research is needed.
Yerba maté	Enhances weight loss	Results of one study suggest that a combination of yerba maté, guarana, and damiana may assist weight loss, but more research is needed.
Hoodia	Suppresses appetite	No human studies support claims of hoodia's effectiveness or safety.

Data from Swartzberg, J. E., et al. (2001). *The Complete Home Wellness Handbook*. New York, NY: Health Letter Associates.; Pittler, M. H., & Ernst, E. (2004). Dietary supplements for body-weight reduction: A systematic review. *American Journal of Clinical Nutrition*, 79(4), 529–536.; and Hollarnder, J. M., & Mechanick, J. I. (2008). Complementary and alternative medicine and the management of the metabolic syndrome. *Journal of the American Dietetic Association*, 108(3), 495–509.

Analyzing Health-Related Information

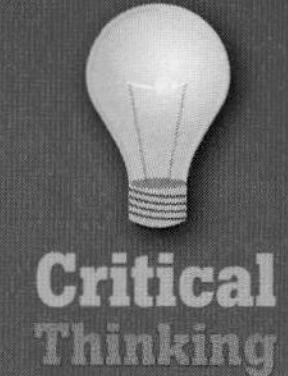

Critical Thinking

© tele52/ShutterStock

This advertisement promotes a weight loss product. Read the ad and evaluate it using the model for analyzing health-related information. The main points of the model are noted here

1. Which statements are verifiable facts, and which are unverified statements or value claims?
2. What are the credentials of the person who makes the health-related claims? Does this person have the appropriate background and education in the topic area? What can you do to check the person's credentials?
3. What might be the motives and biases of the person making the claims?
4. What is the main point of the ad? Which information is relevant to the product? Which information is irrelevant?
5. Is the source reliable? What evidence supports your conclusion that the source is reliable or unreliable? Does the source of information present the pros and cons of the topic or the benefits and risks of the product?
6. Does the source of information attack the credibility of conventional scientists or medical authorities?

Based on your analysis, do you think that this ad is a reliable source of health-related information? Summarize your reasons for coming to this conclusion.

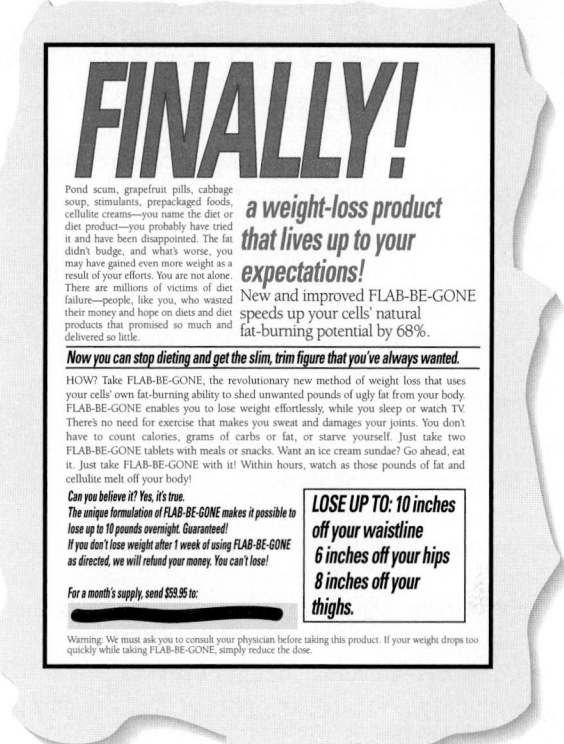

---

and have unrealistic weight loss expectations. Individuals who lose weight while following fad diets are prone to relapse when they return to their usual food habits.

Presently, there is no safe or effective treatment that "cures" being overweight. Therefore, one should strive to prevent excessive weight gain by making permanent lifestyle changes that include reducing the size of food portions, especially fatty foods, and increasing physical activity.

Weight Gain

Although it may seem that nearly everyone is on a diet to lose weight, some people are underweight and trying to gain weight. Many health experts think underweight individuals should avoid gaining body fat unless their condition is the result of chronic illness. Nevertheless, individuals who are thin are often just as dissatisfied with their body sizes as those who are overweight.

To gain lean tissue, persons who are underweight need to consume at least 700 to 1,000 more calories per day than they usually eat and perform muscle-building exercises. To obtain the extra calories, people who are underweight can eat more than three meals a day and snack on nutrient-dense foods such as dried fruit, whole-wheat muffins, granola bars, yogurt and fruit smoothies, peanut butter, and nuts. You can find other nutritious foods that are high in food energy by consulting food composition tables.

Because fatty foods are a source of considerable calories, physically active individuals can eat

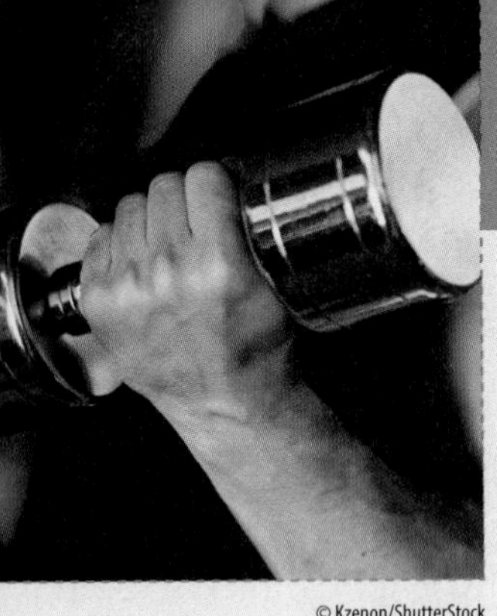
© Kzenon/ShutterStock

Managing Your Health

General Features of Reliable Weight Reduction Plans

Use the following features to judge the quality of weight loss programs.

The diet plan is medically sound if it

- Provides recommendations that are safe and supported by scientific evidence
- Suggests receiving a physician's approval prior to initiating the plan
- Encourages gradual weight loss

The diet is nutritionally sound if it

- Meets nutritional needs
- Includes foods from each food group
- Encourages eating smaller portions of nutritious foods
- Encourages self-control over problem foods such as sweets
- Considers individual food preferences
- Includes reasonable amounts of fiber and complex carbohydrates
- Reduces caloric intake to no lower than 1,000 calories per day
- Recommends losing 0.5 lb to 2 lb per week
- Avoids requiring special or costly supplements and foods
- Avoids claims about the superiority of the plan
- Avoids guarantees concerning weight loss

The diet plan considers physical fitness needs if it

- Recommends an exercise plan that is tailored to the individual's needs, time constraints, interests, and capabilities
- Includes practical suggestions for altering sedentary behaviors
- Encourages daily aerobic activities that last at least half an hour
- Avoids promoting costly exercise equipment, joining exercise clubs, or buying special gadgets to shed pounds
- Recommends physical activities that are safe and enjoyable
- Considers special health concerns of the individual

The diet plan meets psychological and social needs if it

- Provides practical suggestions for modifying food-related attitudes and behaviors
- Educates about the need to set realistic weight loss goals
- Includes techniques to monitor progress (such as weekly recording of waist circumference)
- Builds self-esteem
- Includes tips to control eating in social situations
- Includes foods that family and friends eat
- Provides strategies for coping with setbacks, difficult situations, and unsupportive people
- Offers opportunities for group support

Source: Adapted from Dwyer, J. T. (1992). Treatment of obesity: Conventional programs and fad diets. In P. Björntorp & B. N. Brodoff (Eds.), *Obesity* (pp. 662–676). Philadelphia, PA: Lippincott.

as much as 35% of their caloric intake from these items. Because of the association with cardiovascular disease, people trying to gain weight should avoid eating excessive amounts of saturated fats. Avocados, olives, and nuts are high in unsaturated fat, which is healthier than saturated fat. For people trying to gain weight, the effort must be maintained over the long term, just as it is for people trying to lose weight.

Childhood and adolescent obesity often becomes a problem that affects the entire family. Children who are obese may develop eating disorders and low self-esteem when parents, other adults, or peers treat them negatively. An effective program that helps children lose weight should not interfere with their normal physical development and should not encourage the development of eating disorders. Successful treatment involves teaching children and their parents how to make appropriate dietary modifications, increase physical activity, and resolve conflicts that may involve eating habits.

By 65 years of age, most people have experienced a decline in their lean mass and an increase in their fat mass. This change occurs to a lesser extent in individuals who maintain a high degree of physical activity as they age. Even modest increases in physical activity, such as walking, swimming, or light exercise, can benefit most elderly people.

Obese older adults who have chronic health problems that are associated with excess body fat can follow the same recommendations for losing weight as do younger individuals: Select nutrient-dense foods, reduce intakes of fatty and sugary foods, and become more physically active.

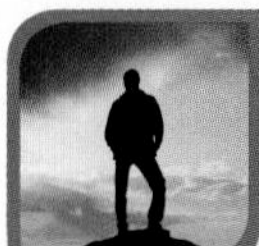
© djgis/ShutterStock

Healthy Living Practices

- If you want to lose weight, modify your lifestyle. For example, eat less fatty sugary foods by replacing them with more nutrient-dense foods.
- To decrease or control your body weight, engage in vigorous physical activity such as jogging, brisk walking, cycling, or swimming for at least 30 minutes, preferably every day.
- To judge whether a weight loss plan or program is sensible and safe, determine whether it is medically and nutritionally sound, includes a plan to increase regular physical activity, is adaptable to your psychological and social needs, and can be followed for a lifetime.
- If you want to gain weight, add at least 700 to 1,000 calories to your usual daily intake and exercise to build muscle mass. To boost the caloric content of meals and snacks, eat more nutrient-dense foods such as dried fruit, whole-wheat muffins, granola bars, peanut butter, and nuts.

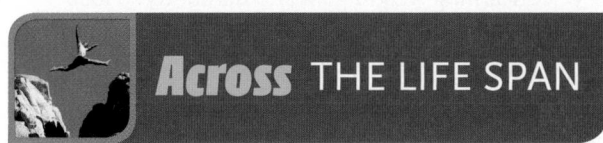

© Galina Barskaya/ShutterStock

WEIGHT MANAGEMENT

The amount of weight a woman gains during pregnancy affects the health of her baby. Women who begin pregnancy at a healthy weight should gain about 25 to 35 pounds during the following 9 months.[38] This weight gain includes not only the fetus's weight but also the weight of the pregnant woman's additional body fluids, fat stores, and breast and uterine tissues. Women who are underweight when they become pregnant can expect to gain more weight; those who are overweight may gain less. **Table 10.6** indicates suggested ranges of weight gain for pregnant women based on their prepregnancy BMIs.

In 2006, 21% of pregnant women gained more than 40 pounds during their pregnancies.[39] Some pregnant women restrict their food intake to limit their weight gain because they do not want to struggle with losing the extra pounds after the baby arrives. However, caloric restriction during pregnancy may be hazardous to the developing fetus. The time to lose weight is *before* or *after* pregnancy and not during this period.

Table 10.6

Suggested Weight Gain During Pregnancy

Weight Classification (prior to pregnancy)	BMI	Range of Weight Gain (pounds)
Underweight	< 18.5	28–40
Healthy	18.5–24.9	25–35
Overweight	25.0–29.9	15–25
Obese	30.0 and up	11–20

Data from March of Dimes. (2009). Weight gain during pregnancy. Retrieved September 14, 2011, from http://www.marchofdimes.com/pregnancy/yourbody_weightgain.html

Nevertheless, within 2 years of giving birth, many women remain several pounds heavier than those who have not been pregnant.

Infancy is a period characterized by rapid gains in both weight and height. According to the rule of thumb, a healthy baby doubles its birth weight by the time it is 6 months of age and triples its birth weight by its first birthday. A 7-pound newborn, for example, should weigh about 14 pounds at 6 months of age and 21 pounds when it is 12 months of age.

Many babies who are overweight at their first birthday slim down by the time they enter school. However, rapid weight gain during the first 2 years of life is associated with increased blood pressure, BMI, and waist circumference in adulthood.[40] Women who smoke cigarettes or gain too much weight during their pregnancies are more likely to have infants and young children who are overweight and obese.[39] On the other hand, babies who are breastfed, particularly for the recommended length of time, are less likely to develop obesity in adulthood.

As mentioned in the beginning of this chapter, the percentage of school-age children who are overweight is increasing in the United States (**Figure 10.14**). Children and adolescents need adequate amounts of energy for physical development and activity, but they often eat more calories than recommended by dietitians. Besides dietary factors, preoccupation with sedentary activities such as playing computer

Figure 10.14

Childhood Obesity. The percentage of overweight children is increasing in the United States

© Goga/ShutterStock

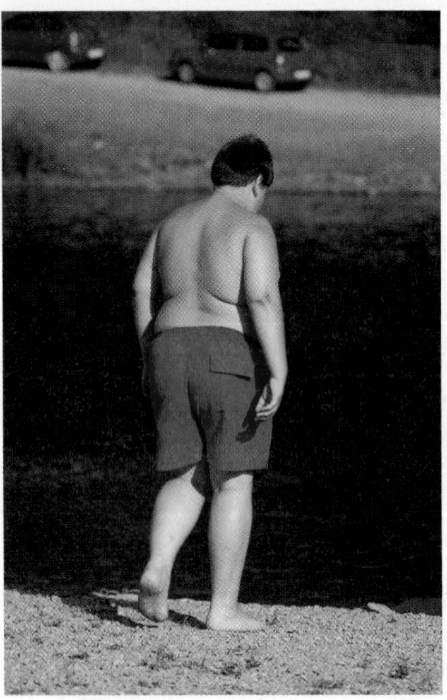

games and watching television contributes to the increase of childhood obesity.[41]

No one can predict whether a child who is obese will become an adult who is obese. However, children and adolescents who are obese are more likely to remain obese into adulthood.[40] Thus, preventing childhood obesity has become a national health priority. What are the consequences of childhood obesity?

According to the Centers for Disease Control and Prevention,[42] childhood obesity is linked with the following disorders:

- High blood pressure and high cholesterol (risk factors for heart disease and stroke)
- Type 2 diabetes
- Breathing problems, such as sleep apnea and asthma
- Joint problems
- Fatty liver disease, gallstones, and heartburn
- Poor self-esteem

© djgis/ShutterStock

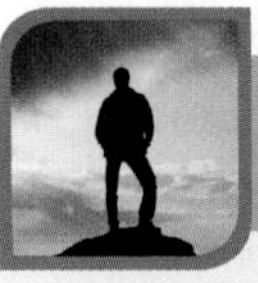

Healthy Living Practices

- Weight gain is necessary during pregnancy, so if you are pregnant, follow recommendations concerning weight gain and do not try to lose weight at this time.
- Encourage your children to be physically active.
- To avoid becoming too fat as you age, select nutrient-dense, low-fat foods and maintain moderate to high degrees of physical activity.

CHAPTER REVIEW

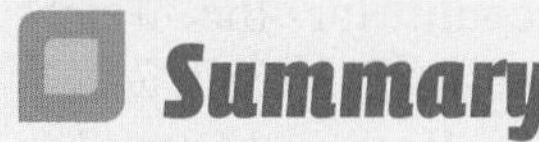

Summary

Recent health surveys indicate that more Americans are overweight or obese than in previous decades. More than 65% of the adult U.S. population is overweight. Excess body fat is associated with low self-esteem and increased risks of chronic health conditions such as osteoarthritis, sleep apnea, gallbladder disease, gout, hypertension, diabetes, certain cancers, and heart disease.

The body uses the energy in foods to power vital metabolic activity, to move skeletal muscles, and to process nutrients after meals. According to the principles of energy balance, the body requires a certain number of calories to maintain its weight. When one consumes more calories than needed, weight gain occurs; when one ingests fewer calories than needed, weight loss occurs. Because each pound of body fat represents about 3,500 calories, consuming 500 fewer calories a day than needed should result in a weight loss of about 1 lb per week.

Methods of determining the percentage of body fat include measuring subcutaneous fat (skinfold thicknesses), hydrostatic weighing, and bioelectrical impedance. To determine whether they are overfat, many people rely on waist circumference measurements and body mass indices (BMIs). Risks of chronic health problems and death increase as the waist circumference and BMI increase.

Obesity is not simply the result of a lack of willpower. The development of obesity is a complex process involving interactions among biological, psychological, social, and environmental factors. These factors include genetics, responses to social situations, food availability and composition, and levels of physical activity.

Obesity is a chronic disease. Most people who have lost weight will regain much or all of it within a few years. To lose weight and maintain the loss, individuals need to decrease their caloric intake by eating less food and increase their caloric expenditures by increasing their levels of physical activity. A reliable weight loss regimen should include a well-balanced, nutritionally adequate but calorie-reduced diet and an exercise regimen that can be followed for life.

To increase her chances of having healthy babies, a healthy woman needs to gain about 25 to 35 pounds during pregnancy. While pregnant, women should not consume low-calorie diets because caloric restriction may harm the fetus. Children and adolescents need adequate amounts of energy for physical development and activity. In the United States, the percentage of children and teenagers who are obese is growing. Experts think that this increase is primarily the result of sedentary lifestyles and poor eating habits. Children who are obese are at risk of being obese when they are adults. Many older adults benefit from having some extra body fat.

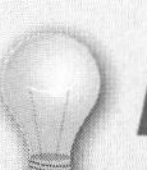

Applying What You Have Learned

1. Develop a day's menu, including meals and snacks, for a nutritionally adequate weight loss plan. Your plan should include foods from all major food groups. **Application**
2. You see an advertisement for a special drink that is supposed to eliminate excess body fat while you sleep. According to the ad, this product helps you lose weight "fast" by increasing your metabolic rate; there is no need to eat less food or exercise more often. Explain why you think this ad is a source of reliable or unreliable health-related information. **Synthesis**
3. A man has been maintaining his weight by consuming 2,500 calories a day. If he does not alter his physical activity level, how many calories should he consume daily to lose 4 lb in a month? **Application**

CHAPTER REVIEW

4. Compare your present weight to your weight of 2 years ago. If you have gained or lost weight over the past couple of years, explain how you reached your present weight by evaluating your lifestyle. What factors might account for the weight change? If you have not gained or lost weight during this period, explain why this situation has occurred. **Evaluation**

Key

Application using information in a new situation.

Synthesis putting together information from different sources.

Evaluation making informed decisions.

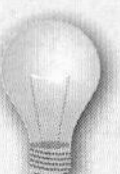

Reflecting on Your Health

1. "Fat people could lose weight if they would just push themselves away from the dinner table." After reading this chapter, what have you learned about obesity and weight control that might cause you to react differently to this statement than you might have prior to reading this chapter?
2. As mentioned in this chapter, some people have negative feelings toward individuals who are obese. What were your feelings about people who are obese before you read this chapter? After reading this chapter, have your feelings changed? If so, describe how your feelings changed.
3. How would you respond if a close friend or relative told you that you needed to lose weight? If someone you know is trying to lose weight, what would you do to help with his or her weight loss efforts?
4. The U.S. National Transportation Safety Board (NTSB) proposed reducing the weight limit of each airline passenger and his or her luggage because of concern that the excess load could result in plane crashes. Explain your reaction to this proposal.
5. How does the media influence your satisfaction with your body size and shape? Do you think the media should encourage people to be more satisfied with their body sizes and shapes? If you think the media should take such steps, how could this affect people's health?

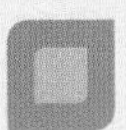

References

1. Centers for Disease Control and Prevention. Office of Surveillance, Epidemiology, and Laboratory Services. (n.d.). *Behavioral Risk Factor Surveillance System: Prevalence and trends data. Overweight and obesity (BMI)—2012.* Retrieved July 23, 2014, from http://apps.nccd.cdc.gov/brfss/list.asp?cat=OB&yr=2012&qkey=8261&state=All
2. Yanovski, S. Z., & Yanovski, J. A. (2002). Obesity. *New England Journal of Medicine, 346*(8), 591–601.
3. Mokdad, A. H., et al. (2005). Correction: Actual causes of death in the United States, 2000. *Journal of the American Medical Association, 293*(3), 293–294.
4. Centers for Disease Control and Prevention. (2011, April). *Overweight and obesity, data and statistics, obesity rates among all children in the United States.* Retrieved May 19, 2011, from http://www.cdc.gov/obesity/childhood/data.html
5. Ogden, C. L., et al. (2008). High body mass index for age among U.S. children and adolescents, 2003–2006. *Journal of the American Medical Association, 299*(20), 2401–2405.
6. U.S. Department of Health and Human Services, National Center for Health Statistics, Public Health Service. (2000). *Healthy People 2010.* Washington, DC: Government Printing Office.
7. U.S. Department of Health and Human Services, National Center for Health Statistics, Public Health Service. (2010). *Healthy People 2020.* Washington, D.C. Government Printing Office.
8. World Health Organization. (2014, May). *Obesity and overweight.* Geneva, Switzerland. Retrieved July 23, 2014 http://www.who.int/mediacentre/factsheets/fs311/en/
9. Olver, I. N., & Grogan, P. B. (2008). Cancer adds further urgency to prioritising obesity control. *Medical Journal of Australia, 189*(4), 191–192.

10. Flegal, K. M., et al. (2005). Excess deaths associated with underweight, overweight, and obesity. *Journal of the American Medical Association, 293*(15), 1861–1867.
11. Calle, E. E., et al. (2003). Overweight, obesity, and mortality from cancer in a prospective studied cohort of U.S. adults. *New England Journal of Medicine, 348*(17), 1625–1638.
12. Kulie, T., et al. (2011). Obesity and women's health: An evidence-based review. *Journal of the American Board of Family Medicine, 24*(1), 75–85.
13. Zhang, H., et al. (2010). Emerging role of adipokines as mediators in atherosclerosis. *World Journal of Cardiology, 2*(11), 370–376.
14. Wee, C. C., et al. (2004). Assessing the value of weight loss among primary care patients. *Journal of General Internal Medicine, 19*(12), 1206–1211.
15. Kim, K. Y., et al. (2007). The impacts of obesity on psychological well-being: A cross-sectional study about depressive mood and quality of life. *Journal of Preventive Medicine and Public Health, 40*(2), 191–195.
16. Centers for Disease Control and Prevention. (2011, March). *How much physical activity do adults need?* Retrieved May 19, 2011, from http://www.cdc.gov/physicalactivity/everyone/guidelines/adults.html
17. Centers for Disease Control and Prevention, National Center for Chronic Disease Prevention and Health Promotion. (2014, May). *Facts about physical activity*. Retrieved July 23, 2014, from http://www.cdc.gov/physicalactivity/data/facts.html
18. Levine, J. A. (2007). Nonexercise activity thermogenesis—Liberating the life-force. *Journal of Internal Medicine, 262*(3), 273–287.
19. Smalls, L. K., et al. (2005). Quantitative model of cellulite: Three-dimensional skin surface topography, biophysical characterization, and relationship to human perception. *Journal of Cosmetic Science, 56*(2), 105–120.
20. Robertson, S. M., et al. (1999). Factors related to adiposity among children aged 3 to 7 years. *Journal of the American Dietetic Association, 99*(8), 938–943.
21. Lee, S. Y., & Gallagher, D. (2008). Assessment methods in human body composition. *Current Opinion in Clinical Nutrition & Metabolic Care, 11*(5), 566–572.
22. Leitzmann, M. F., et al. (2011). Waist circumference as compared with body-mass index in predicting mortality from specific causes. *PLoS ONE, 6*(4), e18582. doi:10.1371/journal.pone.0018582
23. Barnett, A. H. (2008). The importance of treating cardiometabolic risk factors in patients with type 2 diabetes. *Diabetes & Vascular Disease Research, 5*(1), 9–14.
24. National Heart Lung and Blood Institute. (2000). *The practical guide: Identification, evaluation, and treatment of overweight and obesity in adults* (NIH Publication No. 00-4084). Retrieved May 20, 2011, from http://www.nhlbi.nih.gov/files/docs/guidelines/prctgd_c.pdf
25. Yamada, T., & Katagiri, H. (2007). Avenues of communication between the brain and tissues/organs involved in energy homeostasis. *Endocrinology Journal, 54*(4), 497–505.
26. Goris, A. H., & Westerterp, K. R. (2008). Physical activity, fat intake and body fat. *Physiology & Behavior, 94*(2), 164–168.
27. Little, T. L., et al. (2007). Modulation of high-fat diets of gastrointestinal function and hormones associated with the regulation of energy intake: Implications for the pathophysiology of obesity. *American Journal of Clinical Nutrition, 86*(3), 531–541.
28. Young, L. R., & Nestle, M. (2003). Expanding portion sizes in the U.S. marketplace: Implications for nutrition counseling. *Journal of the American Dietetic Association, 103*(2), 231–234.
29. Bish, C. L., et al. (2007). Health-related quality of life and weight loss practices among overweight and obese U.S. adults, 2003 Behavioral Risk Factor Surveillance System. *Medscape General Medicine, 9*(2), 35.
30. Eaton, D. K., et al. (2010). Youth risk behavior surveillance—United States, 2009. *Morbidity and Mortality Weekly Report, 59*(SS-5), 1–141.
31. Field, A. E., et al. (2009). Weight cycling and mortality among middle-aged and older women. *Archives of Internal Medicine, 169*(9), 881–886.
32. *U.S. News & World Report*. (2014). *U.S. News best diets: How we rated 32 eating plans*. Retrieved July 24, 2014 from http://health.usnews.com/health-news/health-wellness/articles/2014/01/07/us-news-best-diets-how-we-rated-32-eating-plans
33. Donnelly, J. E., et al. (2009). American College of Sports Medicine position stand: Appropriate physical activity intervention strategies for weight loss and prevention of weight regain for adults. *Medicine & Science in Sports & Exercise, 41*(2), 459–471.
34. Shafipour, P., et al. (2009). What do I do with my morbidly obese patient? A detailed case study of bariatric surgery in Kaiser Permanente Southern California. *Permanente Journal, 13*(4), 56–63.
35. U.S. Food and Drug Administration (2013, June 17). *Orlistat (marketed as Alli and Xenical) information*. Retrieved July 24, 2014 from http://www.fda.gov/drugs/drugsafety/postmarketdrugsafetyinformationforpatientsandproviders/ucm180076.htm
36. U.S. Food and Drug Administration. (2012, June 27). *FDA news release: FDA approves Belviq to treat some overweight or obese adults*. Retrieved July 24, 2014 from http://www.fda.gov/newsevents/newsroom/pressannouncements/ucm309993.htm
37. Turk, M. W., et al. (2009). Randomized clinical trials of weight-loss maintenance: A review. *Journal of Cardiovascular Nursing, 24*(1), 58–80.
38. March of Dimes. (2009). *Weight gain during pregnancy*. Retrieved May 22, 2011, from http://www.marchofdimes.com/Pregnancy/yourbody_weightgain.html
39. Wojcicki, J. M., & Heyman, M. B. (2010). Let's move—Childhood obesity prevention from pregnancy and infancy onward. *New England Journal of Medicine, 362*(16), 1457–1459.
40. Tzoulaki, I., et al. (2010). Relation of immediate postnatal growth with obesity and related metabolic risk factors in adulthood. *American Journal of Epidemiology, 171*(9), 989–998.
41. Speiser, P. W., et al., on behalf of the Obesity Consensus Working Group. (2005). Consensus statement: Childhood obesity. *Journal of Clinical Endocrinology and Metabolism, 90*(3), 1871–1887.
42. Centers for Disease Control and Prevention. (2011, April). *Overweight and obesity: Basics about childhood obesity*. Retrieved May 23, 2011, from http://www.cdc.gov/obesity/childhood/basics.html

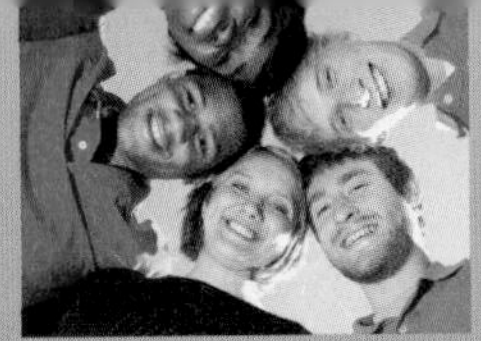

Diversity in Health
New Interest in an Ancient Approach to Fitness

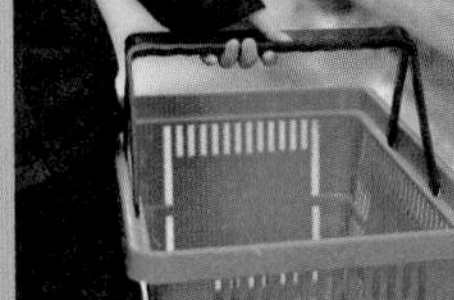

Consumer Health
Choosing a Fitness Center

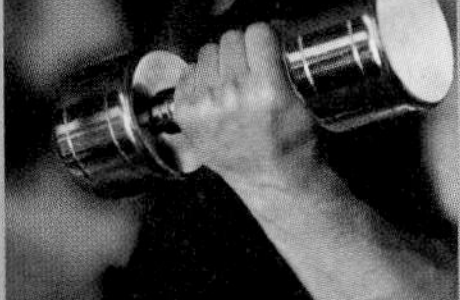

Managing Your Health
Assessing the Intensity of Your Workout: Target Heart Rates

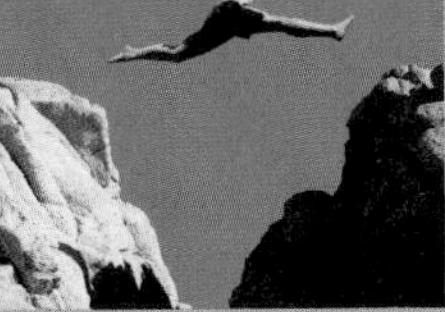

Across the Life Span
Physical Fitness

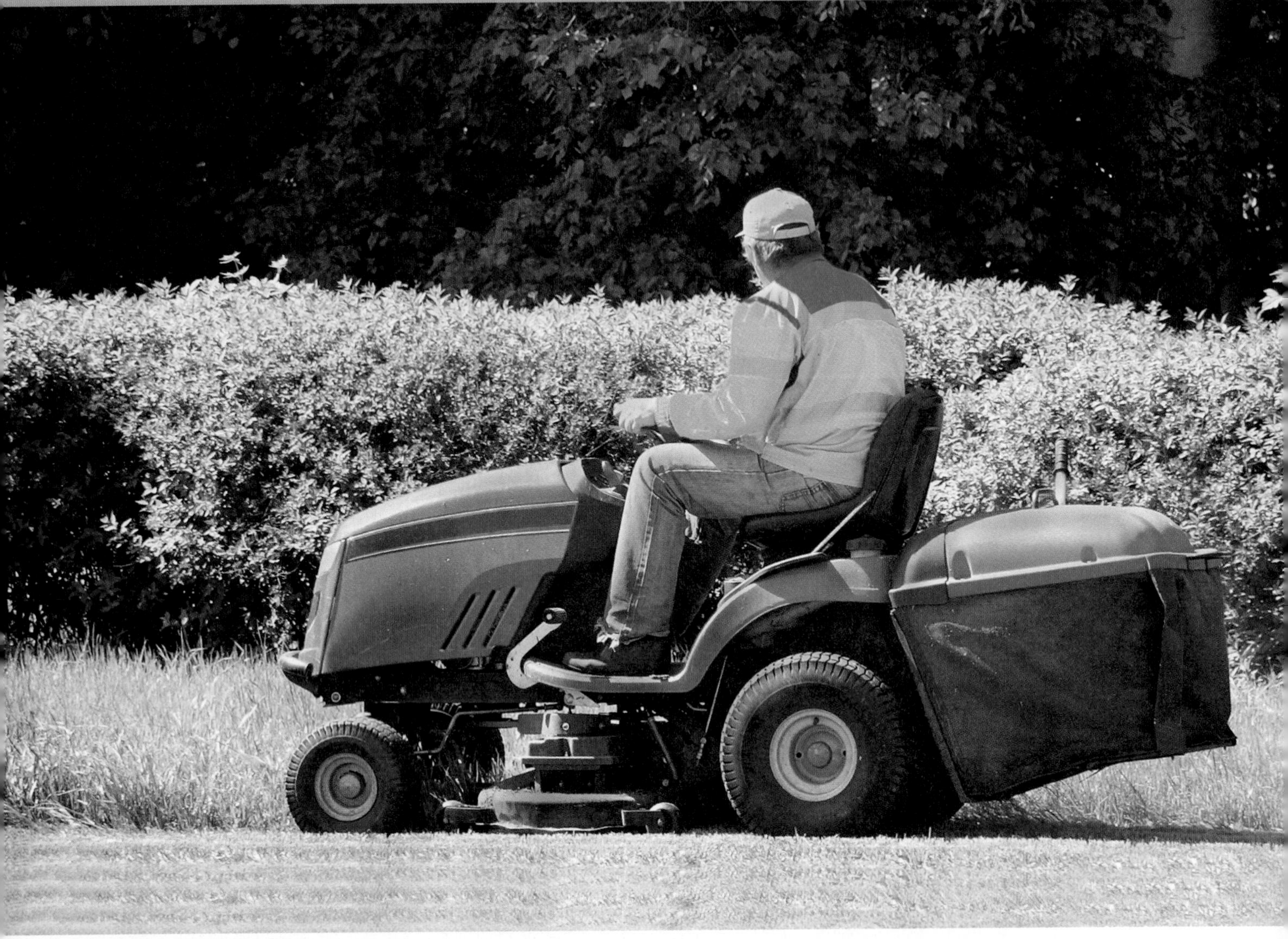

Chapter Overview
The principles of physical fitness

The health-related components of fitness

Exercising for optimal health

Preventing and managing exercise injuries

Developing your own exercise program

Student Workbook
Self-Assessment: Cardiorespiratory Fitness: The Rockport Fitness Walking Test | Push-Up Test for Muscular Endurance | Sit-and-Reach Test for Flexibility Assessment | Check Your Physical Activity and Heart Disease IQ

Changing Health Habits: Do You Want to Be More Physically Active?

Do You Know?
How to calculate your target heart rate?

How to bulk up safely?

If muscles can turn into fat?

Circle of People: © SergeBertasiusPhotography/ShutterStock; Consumer: © sevenke/ShutterStock; Weight Training: © Kzenon/ShutterStock; Rock Climbing: © Galina Barskaya/ShutterStock; Chapter opener: © Vereshchagin Dmitry/ShutterStock

CHAPTER 11

Physical Fitness

Learning Objectives

After studying this chapter, you should be able to:

1. Define physical activity and exercise.
2. Identify benefits of engaging in regular physical activity.
3. List health-related components of fitness.
4. Define aerobic exercise and list examples of aerobic activity.
5. Calculate your target heart rate.
6. Differentiate between isometric and isotonic exercises.
7. Identify effects of anabolic steroids.
8. Develop a workout using the FITT principle.
9. Explain how to use RICE for exercise-related injuries.
10. Describe exercise considerations for various stages of life.

"Most people can derive important health benefits by exercising regularly."

tendons Tough bands of tissue that connect many skeletal muscles to bones.

joints The places where two or more bones come together.

ligaments Tough bands of connective tissue that hold bones together at joints.

If you look around your home, you will see many devices and products that make your life easier: electric can openers, microwave ovens, dishwashers, garage-door openers, remote controls and tables (e.g., iPad). Outside of your home, there are more labor-saving machines. You can ride a lawn mower instead of push one, drive a car rather than walk to places, use elevators and escalators rather than climb stairs, and take moving walkways rather than walk through some of the larger airports. You can even make your leisure time less physically demanding by using a motorized cart to get around a golf course or a motorboat to get around a lake. Besides using labor-saving products, you can have other people perform your physical work. For example, you can pay a team of people to mow your grass, wash your car, or clean your house.

A hundred years ago Americans often performed hard physical work at home and on the job. By the beginning of this century, a variety of machines, products, and services had become available that made our daily lives less physically demanding. Today, we generally have more leisure time than our great-grandparents did, but many of us spend it performing activities that do not contribute to our physical health.

Most people can derive important health benefits by exercising regularly and becoming more physically active. Healthy adults under age 65 years should perform moderate-intensity physical activity for 150 minutes per week.[1] Healthy adults can obtain similar health benefits by engaging in vigorous-intensity physical activity for 75 minutes a week. Moderate to vigorous activities should be performed in episodes that last at least 10 minutes, preferably spread throughout the week. Moderate-intensity physical activities include brisk walking, bicycling, housework, or other actions that cause small but noticeable increases in breathing or heart rates. Vigorous-intensity physical activities, such as running, performing aerobic exercise, or doing heavy yard work, cause relatively large increases in breathing or heart rates.

Each year, lack of regular physical activity (a *sedentary* lifestyle) contributes to thousands of American deaths, primarily from heart disease, stroke, and diabetes. In 2012, approximately 77% of adult Americans reported engaging in physical activity; however, less than 25% of adults meet physical activity guidelines.[2,3] A *physically fit* person has the physical strength, endurance, flexibility, and balance as well as energy to perform various daily living activities, including typical occupational responsibilities and recreational interests that require physical movement. This chapter discusses the basic principles of fitness, including the health benefits of exercise and a physically active lifestyle, and how to design a basic fitness program that you can follow for the rest of your life.

Principles of Physical Fitness

The Body in Motion

Physical movement involves the interrelated functioning of the muscular and skeletal systems. The functioning of the muscular system is so closely associated with the skeletal system that the two are often referred to as the musculoskeletal system.

The skeletal muscles provide shape, support, and movement for your body. Most skeletal muscles are attached to bones of the skeleton. **Figure 11.1** identifies the major skeletal muscle groups of the human body. A typical skeletal muscle consists of hundreds of muscle cells called muscle fibers. Movement occurs when the muscle fibers contract, shortening the length of the muscle. Skeletal muscles can contract voluntarily, which means the muscles contract when a nervous impulse from the brain signals them. Thus, a healthy person can choose when and how intensely to move a muscle.

Tendons, tough bands of fibrous tissue, connect skeletal muscles to bones or other muscles and play an important role in muscular movement. **Joints** are places where two or more bones come together. Most joints are movable; therefore, such joints permit the movement between bones. **Ligaments** are tough bands of connective tissue that hold bones together at the joints.

The Circulatory and Respiratory Systems

Optimal functioning of the circulatory and respiratory systems (sometimes referred to as the cardiorespiratory system) is necessary to achieve a high degree of physical fitness. The circulatory system includes the heart, blood, and blood vessels. The lungs

Figure 11.1

Major Skeletal Muscles of the Human Body. (a) Front view. (b) Back view.

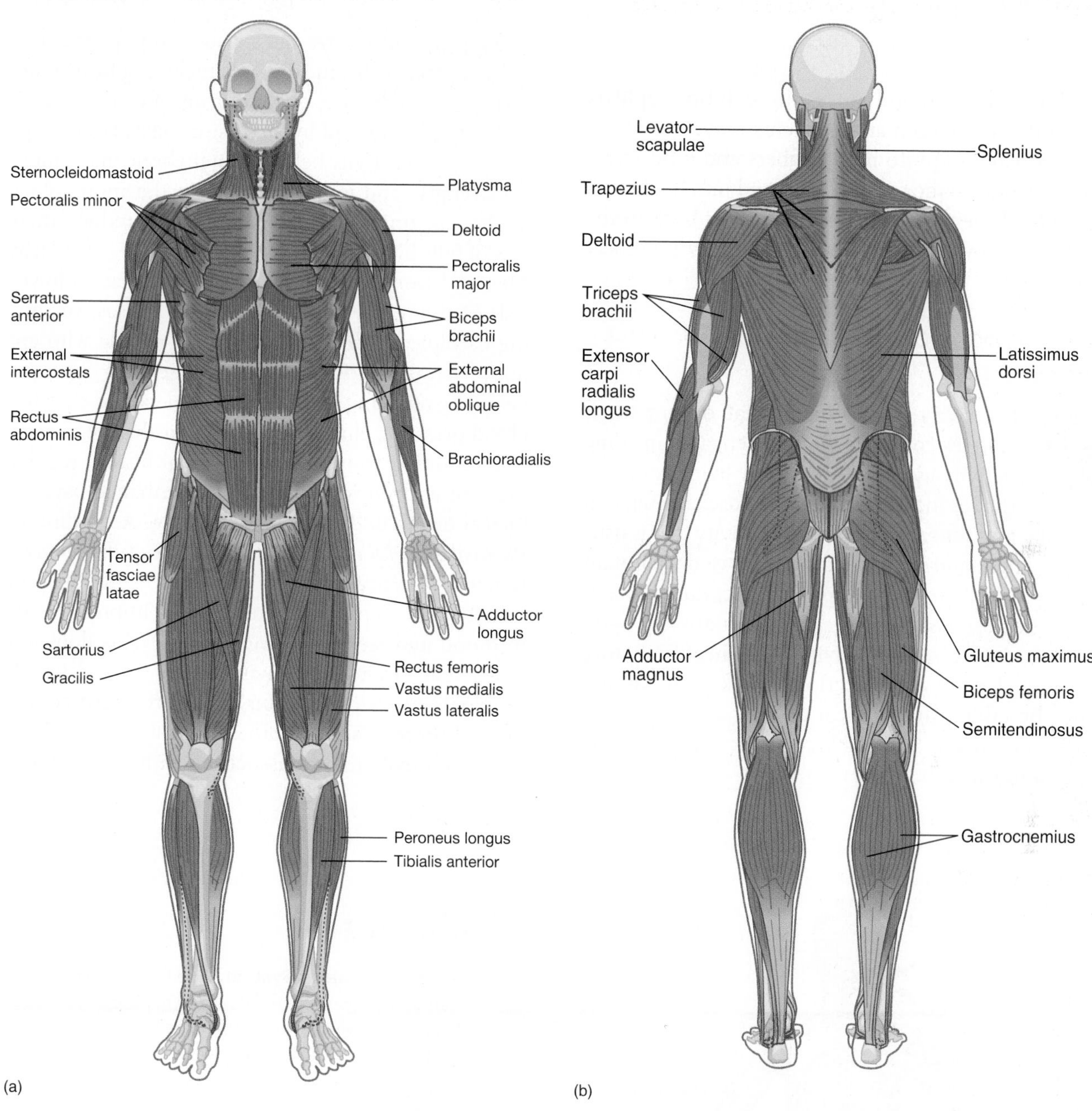

are the major structures of the respiratory system. As **Figure 11.2** illustrates, the functioning of the heart and lungs is interrelated.

The heart is a muscular pump that usually beats about 70 to 80 times each minute on average; however, some people may have slower or faster heart rates. Its job is to circulate blood throughout the body's vast network of blood vessels: the arteries, veins, and capillaries. Blood transports oxygen and nutrients to cells and carries waste products such as carbon dioxide away from them.

Cells need oxygen to release the energy stored in glucose and fats. As the heart pumps blood through microscopic blood vessels in the lungs, carbon dioxide leaves the blood and is exhaled. While in the lungs, hemoglobin in the red blood cells picks up oxygen from the inhaled air. The oxygen-rich blood returns to the heart, which pumps it to the rest of

physical activity Movement that occurs when skeletal muscles contract.

exercise Physical activity that is usually planned and performed to improve or maintain one's physical condition.

the body. As the blood moves through tiny capillaries in tissues, oxygen and nutrients move out of the bloodstream and into muscle fibers and other cells. Waste products move out of cells and into the blood. The blood then circulates through veins back to the heart. This cycle repeats itself with every heartbeat and breath.

Defining Physical Activity and Exercise

Physical activity is movement that occurs when skeletal muscles contract; everyone engages in some physical activity as part of their daily living routines. These activities include shopping, housekeeping, and walking pets. **Exercise** is physical activity that is usually planned and performed to improve or maintain one's physical condition. For example, doing biceps curls is an exercise that develops upper arm strength.

How does physical activity affect health? Before reading the following section, check your knowledge by taking the physical activity and heart disease quiz in the Student Workbook section at the end of this text.

Physical Activity and Health

Being physically active can substantially reduce your risks of serious chronic diseases including heart (coronary artery) disease, certain forms of cancer, type 2 diabetes, obesity, and hypertension (**Table 11.1**).[4] Regular physical activity helps maintain bone mass, muscle strength, and joint function. Furthermore, older adults can improve their balance and reduce their risk of falls by performing certain exercises regularly. Men and women who are physically fit have a lower risk of dying prematurely from all causes, including cardiovascular disease, than do people who are not physically fit. Regular physical activity improves health by reducing excess abdominal fat and elevated blood pressure, glucose, and triglyceride levels.

In addition to improving physical health, regular exercise and physical activity can enhance psychological health and sense of well-being. According to *Physical Activity and Health: A Report of the Surgeon General*, physical activity "reduces symptoms of anxiety and depression and fosters improvements in mood and feelings of well-being."[5] This does not mean that physical inactivity causes mental health problems or that exercising will cure these conditions; however, some studies indicate that lack of physical activity may be associated with development

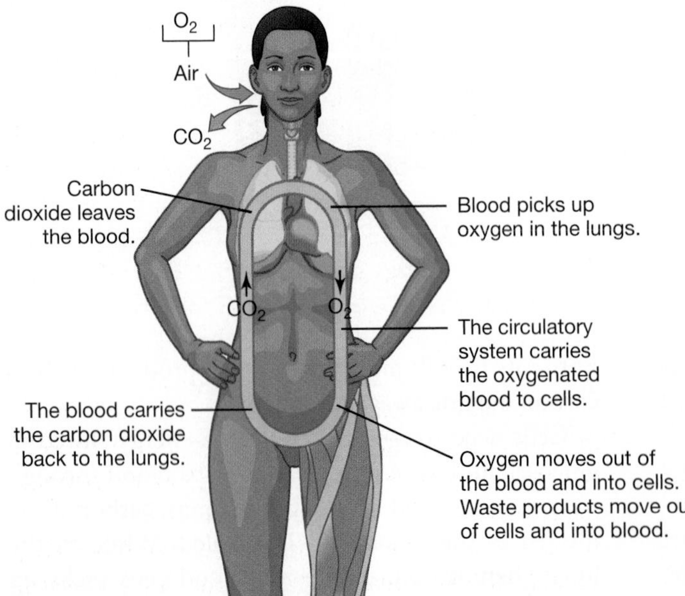
O_2
Air
CO_2
Carbon dioxide leaves the blood.
Blood picks up oxygen in the lungs.
CO_2
O_2
The circulatory system carries the oxygenated blood to cells.
The blood carries the carbon dioxide back to the lungs.
Oxygen moves out of the blood and into cells. Waste products move out of cells and into blood.

Figure 11.2

Cardiorespiratory System. The functioning of the heart and lungs is interrelated. The heart pumps blood to the lungs, where it picks up oxygen. The oxygenated blood returns to the heart, which pumps it throughout the body.

Table 11.1

Health Benefits of Physical Activity (Adults)

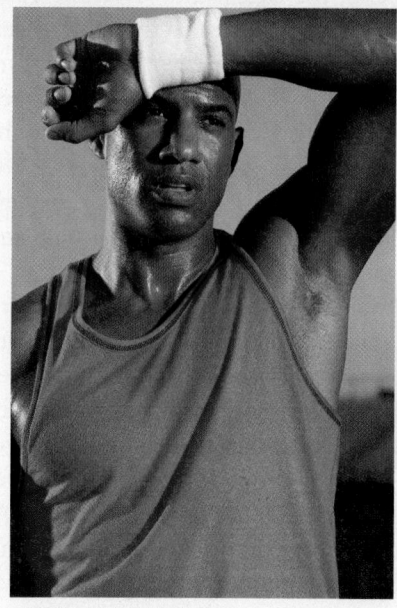
© Wendy Hope/Stockbyte/Thinkstock

Physical activity can lower the risk of:

- Early death
- Heart disease
- Stroke
- High blood pressure
- Type 2 diabetes
- Metabolic syndrome
- Colon cancer
- Breast cancer
- Hip fracture

A physically active lifestyle:

- Prevents weight gain
- Aids weight loss, particularly when combined with reduced calorie intake
- Improves cardiorespiratory and muscular fitness
- Prevents falls
- Reduces depression
- Improves cognitive function (for older adults)
- Improves bone density

Reproduced from U.S. Department of Health and Human Services. (2008). Chapter 2: Physical activity has many health benefits. In Physical activity guidelines for Americans. Retrieved May 25, 2011, from http://www.health.gov/paguidlines/guidelines/chapter2.aspx

of mental disorders.[6] Additionally, regular physical activity can improve the quality of sleep, which benefits psychological health.[7,8,9]

Many people experience short-term psychological benefits during or immediately after exercising. Strenuous physical activity produces chemical changes in the body that can improve psychological health. For example, the central nervous system releases beta-endorphins during exercise. Beta-endorphins are pain-killing substances that may provide natural relaxing and mood-elevating effects. Also, exercise can divert a person's attention away from distressing thoughts and negative emotions, which relieves anxiety. Long-term psychological benefits of exercise may include boosting self-esteem.[10] People who exercise with others can experience psychological benefits from the social interaction.

Physical activity can be measured in terms of caloric use per minute, physical activity level (PAL) or metabolic equivalents (METS). A calorie is defined as the amount of heat required to raise the temperature of one gram of water one degree Celsius. Energy is generated within muscle cells, which creates movement; therefore, then number of calories burned during physical activity is a good indicator of exercise intensity.

Physical activity level (PAL) can also be used to determine energy expenditure during physical activity. PAL represents the amount of energy used each day over energy needs for our basal (resting) metabolism. Basal metabolism is our daily energy requirement to fuel life functions, such as brain function, food digestions, and breathing. A person with a PAL of less than 1.4 is considered sedentary. A PAL between 1.4 and 1.7 indicated moderate physical activity, whereas a PAL greater than 1.7 indicates a vigorous level of activity. For example, assume Sarah has a basal metabolic rate of 1,800 calories per day and her average daily energy expenditure is 2,200 calories per day. We calculate Sarah's PAL by dividing her daily energy expenditure (2,200 calories per day) by her basal metabolic rate of 1,800 calories per day for a PAL of 1.2, which indicates a sedentary lifestyle.

Metabolic equivalents, or METS, are multiples of the energy used while sitting or lying still per minute, which is defined as one MET. Physical activity that requires 3–6 METS is considered moderate activity, whereas movement requiring more than 6 METS is considered vigorous. **Table 11.2** lists some physical activities classified as moderate and vigorous by calories per minute and METS.

cardiorespiratory fitness The ability to perform muscular movements intensely and for long periods without tiring.

aerobic Refers to oxygen-requiring activities.

The Health-Related Components of Physical Fitness

Cardiorespiratory fitness, muscular strength, muscular endurance, flexibility, and body composition are the health-related components of physical fitness. These physical characteristics provide support for the body, sustain its effective and efficient movement, and influence overall health and well-being.

Table 11.2

Physical Activities by Level of Intensity

Moderate Activity (3.5 to 7 kcal/min)	Intense/Vigorous Activity (more than 7 kcal/min)
Walking at a brisk pace (3–4.5 mph)	Racewalking (5 mph or faster)
Hiking	Jogging or running
Cycling on level terrain (5 to 9 mph)	Cycling (more than 10 mph) or uphill
Yoga	Karate, tae kwan do, jujitsu
Table tennis	Tennis—singles
Coaching a children's sports team	Most competitive sports (e.g., football, soccer)
Weight training	Circuit weight training
Skateboarding	Long-distance running
Dancing (most kinds)	Running up stairs
Gardening and yard work	Shoveling heavy snow
Scrubbing a floor	Pushing a lawnmower

Modified from U. S. Centers for Disease Control and Prevention. (2010). *General physical activities defined by level of intensity*. Retrieved from http://www.cdc.gov/nccdphp/dnpa/physical/pdf/PA_Intensity_table_2_1.pdf

Cardiorespiratory Fitness

During intense physical activity, skeletal muscles need large quantities of oxygen to release enough energy to sustain movement. To supply more oxygen for working muscles, the heart and breathing rates increase as the intensity of physical activity increases. However, the lungs and heart have a maximum capacity to distribute an adequate supply of oxygen throughout the body within a certain time. Once the lungs and heart reach this maximum capacity, the skeletal muscles cannot obtain the additional oxygen needed to sustain their intense level of activity, and they become fatigued.

Individuals with high degrees of **cardiorespiratory fitness** (or endurance) can perform muscular work more intensely and longer without becoming fatigued than persons with low levels of cardiorespiratory fitness can. Young, healthy 20-year-old individuals can raise their heart rates to about 190 to 200 beats per minute while engaging in intense aerobic activities. As people grow older, their maximum heart rates decline. In addition to physical condition and age, other personal characteristics, including heredity, sex and body composition, influence the maximum degree to which a person's lungs and heart can function.

During vigorous physical activity, the heart of a physically fit person pumps more blood with each beat. When the activity ceases, the fit person's heart and breathing rates rapidly return to normal. Even while resting, a fit individual's heart is efficient; each minute, it can pump the same amount of blood with fewer heartbeats than the heart of an unfit person can.

Developing cardiorespiratory fitness requires **aerobic** (oxygen-requiring) activities that use our *oxidative* energy system. The oxidative (aerobic) energy system, which requires oxygen to make energy, is used for physical activity that lasts longer than 2 minutes. Aerobic activity increases heart and breathing rates and involves prolonged movement of large muscle groups, such as quadriceps and hamstrings. Examples of aerobic activities include running, jogging, race-walking, swimming, cycling, stair-stepping, aerobic dancing and cross-country skiing When you engage in vigorous physical activities, your heart and breathing rates increase considerably above resting values, and you may sweat excessively.

While performing aerobic activities, people can use their heart rates to determine whether the intensity of the activities is high enough to provide cardiorespiratory benefits. To be very effective, a

Managing Your Health

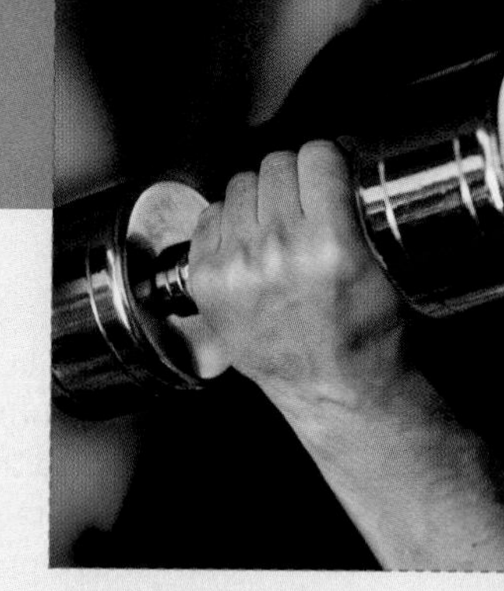

© Kzenon/ShutterStock

Assessing the Intensity of Your Workout: Target Heart Rates

To maximize the cardiorespiratory benefits of aerobic activity, you should work out at the level of intensity that raises your heart rate to within your target heart rate zone. To estimate your target heart rate zone, you need to take your pulse. Figure 11-A illustrates where you can feel your pulse using the carotid artery in your neck or radial artery in your wrist. Although locating the carotid artery pulse can be easier than the radial pulse, applying pressure to the carotid artery can reduce the heart rate, which interferes with obtaining a reliable measurement. For some people with cardiovascular disease, applying pressure to the carotid artery can be dangerous. Many medical experts advise using gentle pressure on your carotid artery to measure your pulse. Practice finding your radial pulse so that you can take it quickly while exercising.

To obtain the most accurate heart rate, measure your pulse while you are still engaging in the physical activity or within 10 seconds after discontinuing the muscular movement. This timing is necessary because your pulse declines rapidly when you stop exercising. Count your pulse for 10 seconds, and then multiply that number by 6 to obtain your heart rate per minute.

To estimate your target heart rate zone, obtain your *age-predicted maximum heart rate* by subtracting your age from 220. For example, if you are 20 years old and healthy, your age-predicted maximum heart rate is 200 beats per minute. Recently, a team of heart experts proposed a different formula for healthy women.[11] According to their formula, a woman should multiply her age in years by 0.88 and then subtract that figure from 206. For example, a 20-year-old woman would multiply her age (20) by 0.88, which equals 17.6. By subtracting 17.6 from 206, she would determine her maximum heart rate to be about 188 beats per minute.

Figure 11.A

Taking Your Pulse. (a) Carotid site. (b) Radial site.

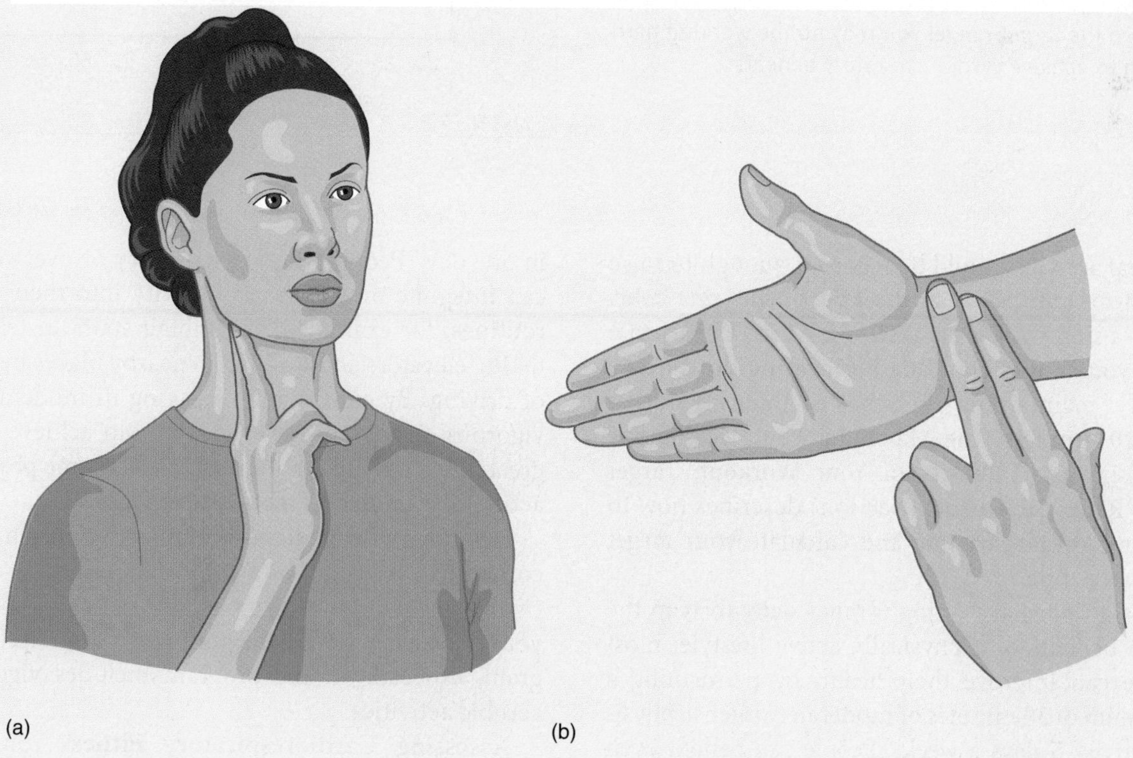

Exercising at your age-predicted maximum heart rate is undesirable and uncomfortable; this extreme level of intensity is unnecessary for achieving cardiorespiratory fitness. Healthy people should exercise with enough intensity to raise their heart rates to within 65% to 90% of their age-predicted maximum heart rates. This interval is the *target heart rate zone* (**Figure 11-B**). People in excellent physical condition may calculate their target heart rates at the 85% to 90% intensity level. Most experts do not recommend that individuals raise their heart rates more than 90% of their age-predicted maximum levels.

If you are sedentary and just starting an exercise program, strive for a maximum heart rate at the low end of your target zone. As your physical condition improves, you will need to recalculate your target heart rate so that it is in "the zone."

While exercising, if you can raise your heart rate to a value in your target zone and maintain this rate for 30 to 60 minutes, you are giving your heart and lungs a beneficial aerobic workout. During aerobic activity, you should measure your pulse about every 10 minutes without stopping the activity. If your heart rate is higher than the maximum value of your target heart rate zone, it is possible that you underestimated your zone, or you may be overexerting yourself at your present level of fitness. You may need to reduce your muscular workload. On the other hand, if your heart rate during aerobic exercise is less than the target range, you may not be working hard enough to achieve cardiorespiratory benefits.

Figure 11.B

Target Heart Rate Zones. The shaded areas include pulse rates within the 65% to 90% intensity ranges.

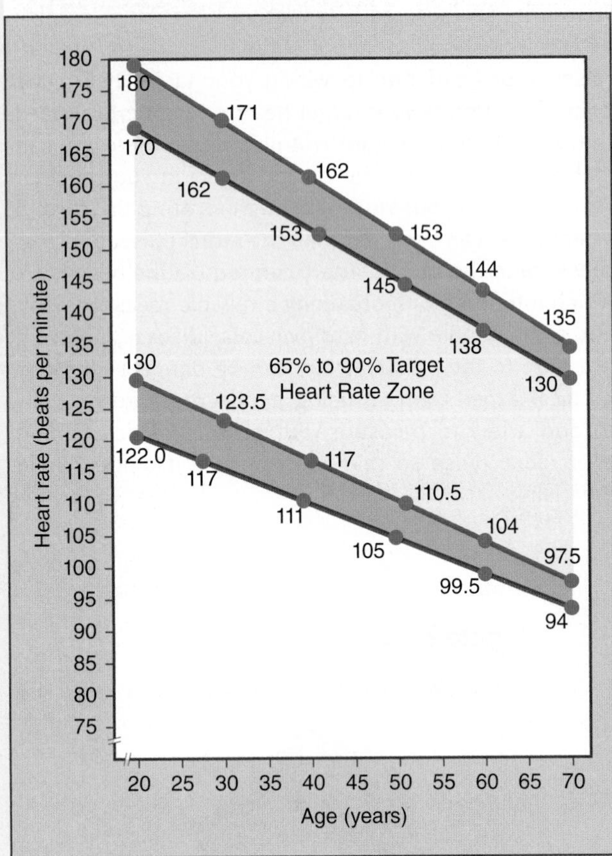

physical activity should be vigorous enough to raise your heart rate to reach the *target heart rate zone*. After raising your heart rate to the target heart rate zone, you should continue performing the aerobic activity, maintaining the level of intensity for at least 20 minutes. The Managing Your Health box "Assessing the Intensity of Your Workout: Target Heart Rates" (in the next section) describes how to measure your heart rate and calculate your target heart rate zone.

You do not have to jog 6 miles daily to reap the health benefits of a physically active lifestyle; most people can improve their health by performing a minimum of 30 minutes of moderately intense physical activity 5 days a week.[1] People can benefit even from intermittent episodes of aerobic activity that last 10 minutes and accumulate to at least 30 minutes in one day.[1] People who are sedentary or overweight can integrate more physical activity into their daily routines; for example, by climbing stairs instead of taking elevators and walking to nearby places instead of driving. By consistently engaging in moderate to vigorous activity, however, people can achieve even greater health benefits. Table 11.2 lists some physical activities classified as moderate or vigorous.

If you have heart disease or other serious chronic conditions, are unfit, or are 40 years of age or older (male) or 50 years of age or older (female), consult your physician before beginning an exercise program, especially if the program includes vigorous aerobic activities.

Assessing Cardiorespiratory Fitness You can judge your level of cardiorespiratory fitness by answering the following questions. While engaging in strenuous exercise, can you carry on a conversation with others, or are you panting for air and unable to talk? How long does it take you to catch your breath or for your heart to stop racing after you stop the activity? If you are unable to talk while exercising and it takes you a long time to recover your normal breathing and heart rates when you finish the physical activity, you probably have a relatively low degree of cardiorespiratory fitness. The first assessment activity for this chapter involves a simple test that you can perform to determine your level of cardiorespiratory fitness (see the Student Workbook section at the end of the book).

After a few months of regular aerobic exercise, it is common for your resting heart rate to decrease. Observing such a decline in resting heart rate not long after beginning a regular aerobic exercise program is usually an indication that cardiorespiratory fitness has improved.

To track your aerobic fitness progress, record your resting heart rates before and after initiating an exercise regimen. Determine your resting heart rate by measuring your pulse when you first wake up, before getting out of bed, on 3 consecutive days. Calculate your average resting heart rate over this 3-day period, and record it and the date. After a few months of engaging in a vigorous exercise program, repeat the procedure to determine your resting heart rate and compare the before and after measurements.

Muscular Strength

Muscular strength is an important aspect of muscular fitness. **Muscular strength** is the ability of muscles to apply maximum force against an object that is resisting this force. Many individuals perform specific resistance training exercises to increase muscular strength because they want to lift heavy objects with ease or improve their appearance (**Figure 11.3**). Other people are interested in developing larger, stronger muscles because they want to compete in sporting events that require strength. How do the strength and size of a muscle increase?

Resistance training is an effective methods for developing muscular strength. To develop muscular strength, muscles must be *progressively overloaded* by moving heavy objects repeatedly. For example, using a weight-lifting machine regularly can increase the size and strength of the biceps muscle in the upper arm. This response is called the *training effect*. Under these conditions, the individual fibers of the biceps muscle can enlarge, or **hypertrophy**, making the entire muscle stronger and larger. Engaging in resistance training regularly helps maintain their size and strength.

muscular strength The ability to apply maximum force against an object that is resisting this force.

hypertrophy A condition in which muscles become larger and stronger.

atrophy A condition in which muscles lose size and strength.

detraining A condition characterized by atrophied and weak muscles, which occurs when skeletal muscles are not used regularly.

The saying "Use it or lose it" generally applies to skeletal muscles. Muscular **atrophy**, a condition of a muscle that has lost size and strength, results from a few weeks of **detraining**. If you have ever had a broken arm or leg, you may recall that after the cast was removed, the muscles of the recovered limb were atrophied and weak. When you first used the limb, the weakened muscles ached for a brief time,

Figure 11.3

Muscular Strength. Many individuals perform specific exercises to improve their appearance or to develop larger, more well-defined muscle groups.

© LiquidLibrary

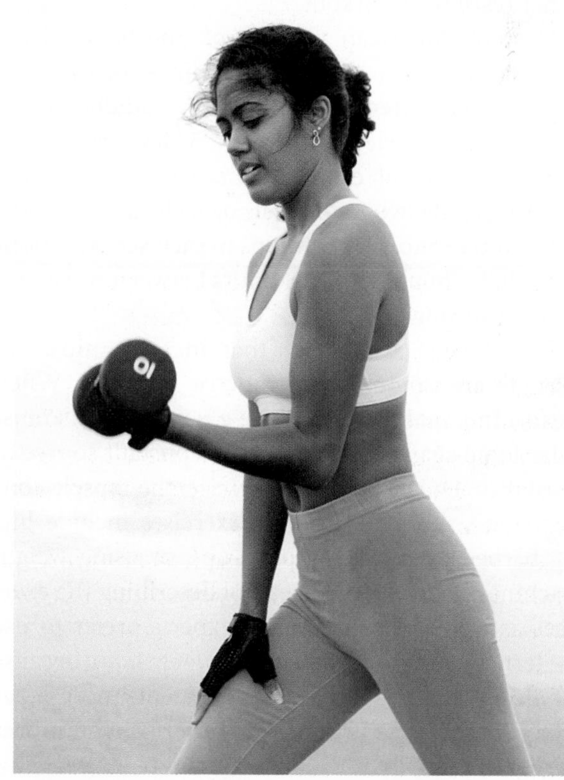

isotonic A type of exercise in which the individual exerts muscular force against a movable but constant source of resistance.

isometric A type of exercise in which the individual exerts muscular force against a fixed, immovable object.

muscular endurance A muscle's ability to contract repeatedly without becoming fatigued.

but within days they became stronger. Eventually, using these muscles enabled them to regain their full strength and original size. The degree of detraining or atrophy, however, is associated with fitness level. The rate of detraining and atrophy in people who are fit, especially highly trained athletes, is generally much slower than the rate for those who are less fit.[12] The rate of detraining also inc reases with age.

Exercising for Muscular Strength A safe and effective way to increase muscle strength and size is to perform repetitive exercises that overload a particular muscle group, such as lifting weights. A repetition is the completion of a particular exercise, for example, lifting a handheld weight and returning to the resting position. A set involves performing the same resistance exercise movement usually 8 to 12 times. Healthy people can begin to train their major muscle groups by performing a single set of exercises for each group of muscles.[13] Over time, the individual should develop enough muscular strength to perform multiple sets (generally three) during his or her resistance workout.[14]

Current American College of Sports Medicine (ACSM) resistance training guidelines for developing muscular strength indicate that adults should train major muscle groups 2 or 3 days each week using a variety of exercises. Each exercise session should include two to four sets of each exercise and a minimum of 8 to 12 repetitions in each set. Additionally, adults should allow 48 hours between resistance training sessions.

Two forms of exercise that increase muscular strength are isotonic and isometric exercises. When performing **isotonic** exercises, a person exerts muscular force against a movable but constant source of resistance. During isotonic exercise, the muscle contracts and shortens. Isotonic exercises include lifting barbells, performing push-ups, or using weight machines (**Figure 11.4**). Instead of describing the exercises as isotonic, some fitness experts prefer to use the term *dynamic constant external resistance* because it reflects the nature of these movements more accurately. An exercise is dynamic if the skeleton moves during the activity.

Figure 11.4

Isotonic Contraction. While performing isotonic exercise, the muscle contracts, shortening in length.

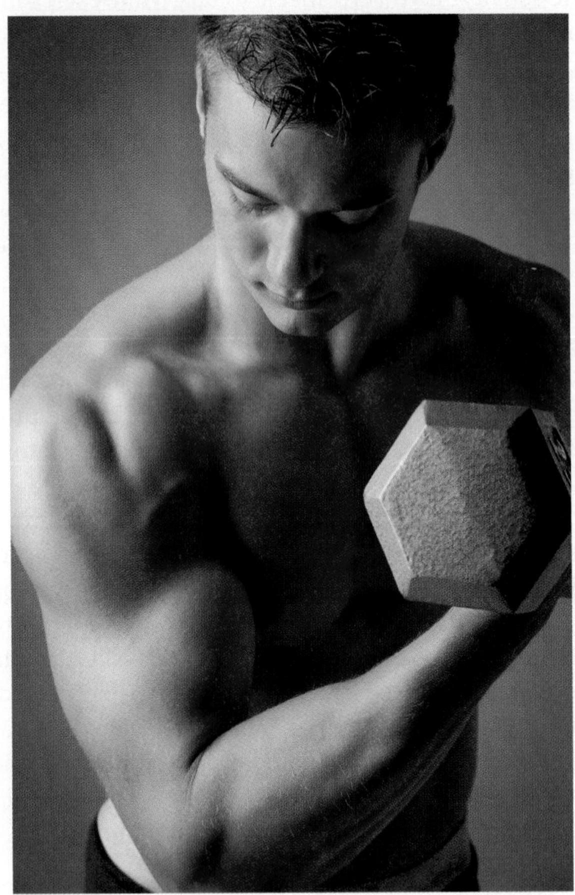

In an **isometric** exercise an individual exerts muscular force against a fixed, immovable object of resistance. For example, applying a constant amount of force while pushing against an immovable door frame is an isometric exercise. During isometric contraction, the muscle does not shorten. Although isometric exercises can increase muscular strength, they do not increase muscular endurance or flexibility effectively. Furthermore, muscles can apply excessive pressure on certain arteries during isometric contractions, raising blood pressure. Therefore, many physicians do not recommend isometric exercises for people older than 35 years or those suffering from cardiovascular disease.

Muscular Endurance

Muscular endurance is another important aspect of muscular fitness. **Muscular endurance** is the ability of a muscle to contract repeatedly without becoming

flexibility The ability to move a muscle to any position in its normal range of motion.

fatigued easily. For example, many people perform lunges to strengthen their leg muscles. A sedentary person will likely experience muscular fatigue after only a few repetitions; however, if she continues to perform lunges two or three times a week for several weeks or months, she will gradually develop muscular endurance in her legs and be able to perform more lunges in each exercise session. As she develops muscular endurance, the effort required to perform lunges will also decrease. Current ACSM resistance training guidelines for developing muscular endurance are the same as for muscular strength: 2 or 3 days each week, two to four sets of each exercise per session, and a minimum of 15 to 20 repetitions in each set. You can assess your muscular endurance by taking the push-up test in the Student Workbook section at the end of this book.

Furthermore, the ability to sustain muscular contractions over a relatively long period requires a constant source of energy. Glucose is skeletal muscles' preferred fuel for high-intensity endurance exercise. Muscles metabolize glucose derived from the bloodstream or from glycogen that is stored in muscle tissue. Muscle fibers can use fatty acids and amino acids for energy.

Flexibility

A third aspect of muscular fitness is flexibility. Movement is limited if joints are damaged or muscles cannot extend themselves fully. **Flexibility** refers to the ability to extend muscles, enabling a person to position a movable joint anywhere in its normal range of motion. Flexibility allows people to perform a variety of skeletal movements with ease, including bending, gliding, rotating, and twisting. Many daily tasks require the ability to extend muscles and move joints easily: reaching for an item stored on a high shelf, stretching to pull up a back zipper, or bending to pick up a tennis ball. Having fully extendable muscles and flexible joints enables you to care for yourself and to participate in enjoyable activities. You can assess your flexibility by taking the sit-and-reach test in the Student Workbook.

Flexibility can be developed and maintained by engaging in activities such as yoga, Pilates, or stretching exercises like those displayed in **Figure 11.5**. *Static stretching* involves slowly and fully extending the muscle and nearby joints throughout their natural ranges of motion. When performing a static stretch, gently extend the muscle until you feel tension; if you feel discomfort, relax the stretch slightly. While stretching, breathe normally; do not hold your breath. The ACSM recommends engaging in flexibility exercises 2 to 3 times a week for each muscle group. Each stretch should be held for 10–30 seconds to the point of tightness in the muscle. Flexibility exercises should be repeated 2 to 4 times each session. Stretching is most effective when muscles are warm; therefore, stretching should be performed following a light aerobic warm up.

Dynamic stretching is performed by moving through a challenging but comfortable range of motion repeatedly in a controlled, smooth, and deliberate motion. Swinging your leg forward and backward to stretch your hamstrings and quadriceps several times, while deliberately swing your leg higher or further back each repetition, is an example of dynamic stretching. Dynamic stretching should not be confused with *ballistic stretching,* which involves uncontrolled jerking or bouncing. Dynamic stretching has been shown to be beneficial for sport performance and is commonly used by competitive athletes. Although the ACSM states that all forms of stretching can be effective, there are no specific recommendations for dynamic stretching.

Proprioceptive Neuromuscular Facilitation (PNF) Although sources of fitness information often recommend static stretching for 15 to 30 seconds, a review of scientific literature indicates that a variety of stretching techniques, durations, and positions are effective means of increasing hamstring muscle flexibility.[15]

Most fitness experts do not recommend *ballistic stretching* activities that involve bouncing. Additionally, you should not use unnatural stretching motions that injure muscles and tendons or extend joints beyond their normal ranges of motion. If pain occurs while stretching, discontinue the activity immediately. The Analyzing Health-Related Information activity in this chapter describes safe alternatives to outdated stretching exercises.

Low Back Pain The majority of Americans encounter low back pain during their lives.[16] As its name implies, low back pain occurs in the lumbar region of the spine (the lower back, above the hips), and it can be disabling (**Figure 11.6**). People with this condition are unable to perform activities essential to daily living comfortably, if at all. Furthermore, low back pain is responsible for a significant percentage of worker absenteeism and workers' medical compensation claims.

Figure 11.5

Stretching to Improve Flexibility. Flexible muscles enable one to make a variety of skeletal movements occur with ease. People can develop flexibility by performing stretching exercises such as the (a) low back stretch, (b) calf stretch, (c) modified hurdle, (d) lunge, (e) supine hamstring stretch, and (f) groin stretch.

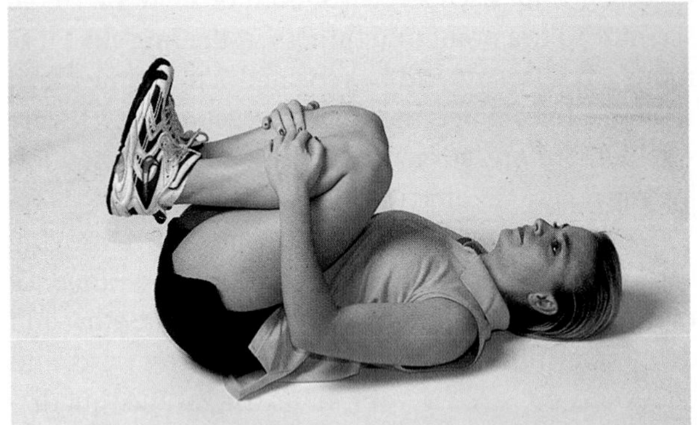

(a)

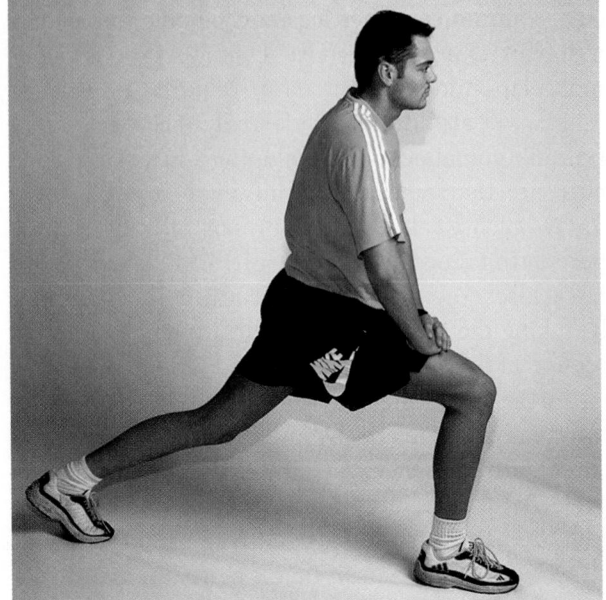

(d)

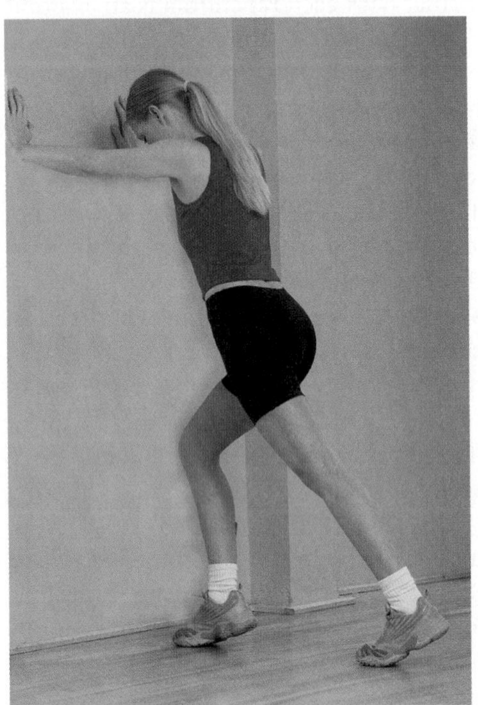

(b) © Photos.com

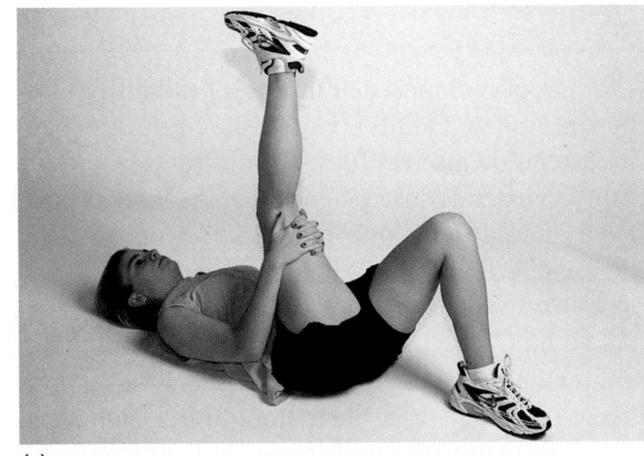

(e)

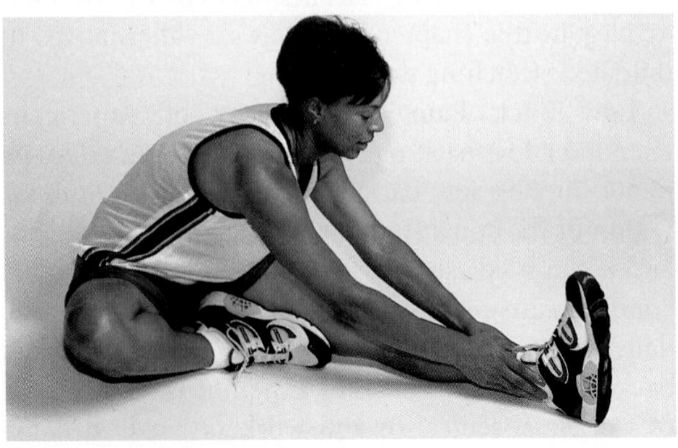

(c)

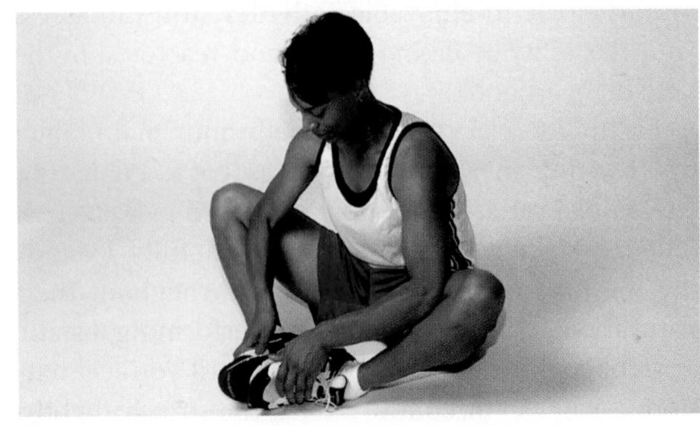

(f)

Figure 11.6

Spinal Discs. (a) Normal disc position. (b) Bulging disc pressing on spinal cord.

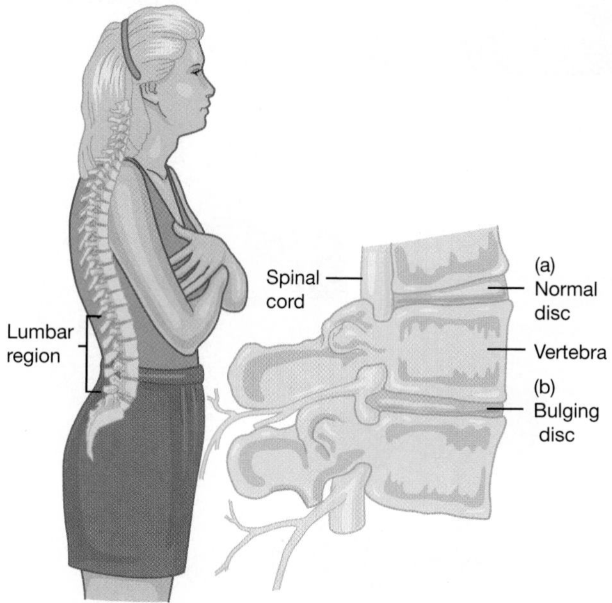

Weak abdominal, back, and leg muscles as well as worn lumbar *spinal discs* often contribute to the development of low back pain. The spinal discs are flexible pads that separate the bones of the spine and act as shock absorbers, protecting the bones from striking each other. As people age, their spinal discs become worn and sometimes bulge out of their normal position. Pounding, twisting, and lifting place physical stress on the lumbar spine and are likely responsible for displacing or damaging some discs. Such movements include jogging on a sidewalk, swinging a golf club, carrying a heavy backpack, and picking up a heavy box or a child. In addition, people who have poor posture, sit for hours in awkward positions, wear high-heeled shoes, or have too much body fat are susceptible to low back pain, especially if they have weak abdominal muscles.

Although medical experts agree that exercising to strengthen the abdominal, hip, upper leg, and back muscles can prevent or treat many cases of low back pain, they do not agree on which exercises to recommend. Some physicians recommend aerobic exercises; others promote various stretching activities. **Figure 11.7** shows various exercises designed to strengthen the weak muscles that contribute to low back pain and improve the flexibility of the spinal joints.

You can reduce your risk of developing low back pain by practicing prevention behaviors, for example, exercising regularly, wearing shoes with low or no heels, and avoiding sitting for long periods of time.[17] You can often prevent low back pain by following the lifting and sitting practices recommended in **Figure 11.8**.

Over-the-counter pain medicines and heat treatments can often relieve low back pain. After the discomfort subsides, people should perform exercises that strengthen the lower back, hip, and abdominal muscles. If the pain is intense or persists, however, the person should obtain a complete medical evaluation to determine the source of the pain. In some cases, surgery may be necessary.

Body Composition

A healthy body contains large quantities of water and smaller amounts of fat and lean tissues (bones, muscles, and organs). Body composition, the percentages of body weight contributed by lean tissue and fat mass, is a major factor in health. Although a small amount of body fat (about 4% in men and 10% in women) is essential, too much fat contributes to a variety of chronic diseases, including cardiovascular disease, hypertension, and diabetes. Regular exercise builds and maintains muscle mass and helps keep the amount of body fat at healthy levels.

The cells that comprise lean tissues, particularly muscle cells, are more metabolically active than fat cells are. Therefore, muscle cells burn more calories than fat cells do. By exercising and increasing muscle mass, you can increase your metabolic rate.[18]

Aging muscle cells eventually wear out and die. Unfortunately, the body does not replace these cells. As a result, people usually lose muscle mass and gain fat as they age. Some people believe unused or dying muscle cells can "turn into" fat cells; however, muscle cells are not able to transform themselves into fat cells. Muscle and fat cells have specific structures and functions; nevertheless, you can preserve more of your muscle mass as you get older by engaging in a regular exercise program.

Although regular physical activity can help a person maintain muscle mass while maintaining or losing body fat, "spot" reducing is not effective. For example, performing 100 crunches daily does not reduce the amount of fat stored in the abdominal area. During physical activity, fat deposits throughout the body release fatty acids into the bloodstream to supply energy for the vigorously moving muscles. Exercising a specific muscle group, however, can

Figure 11.7

Exercises to Prevent Lower Back Pain.

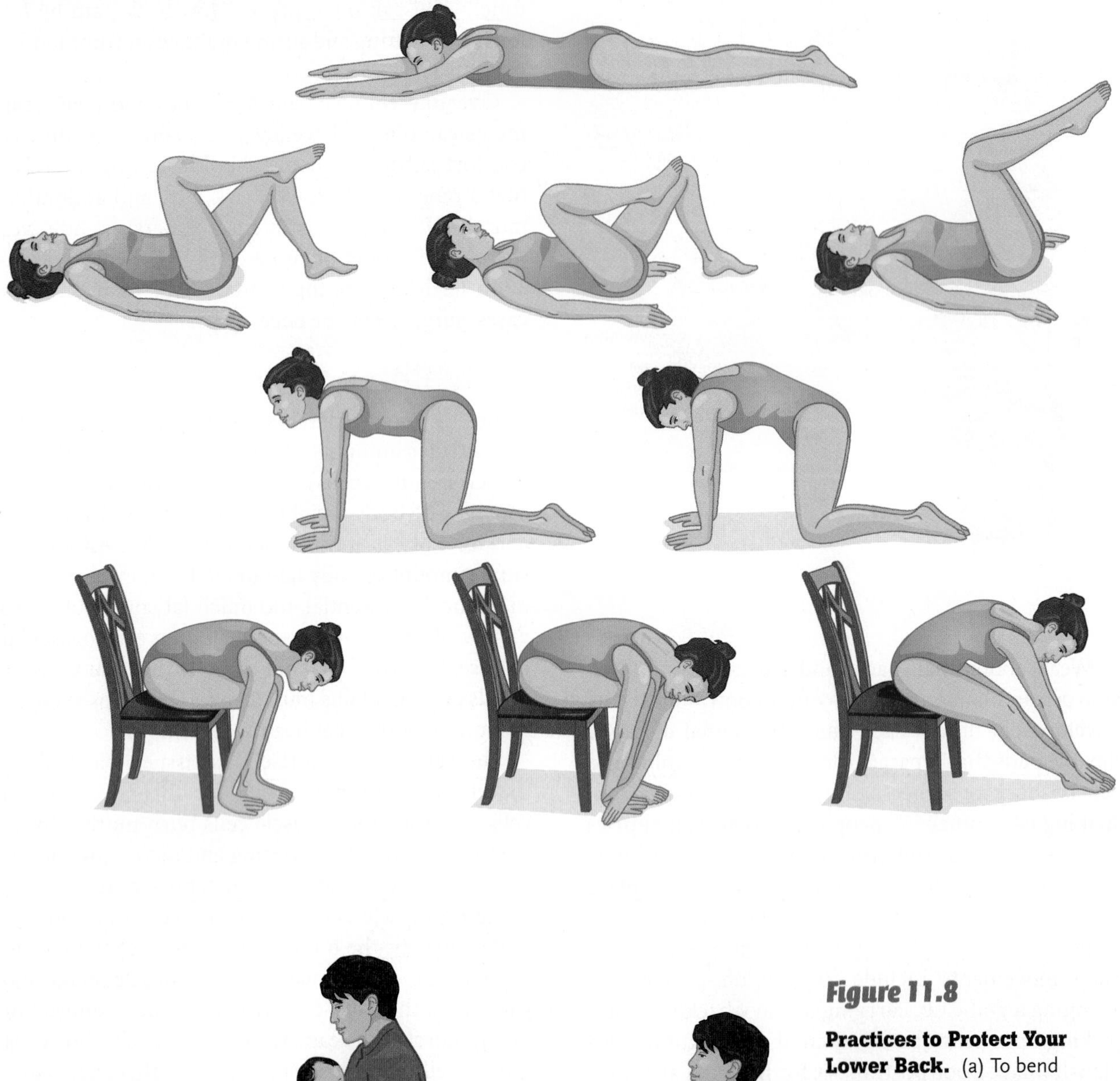

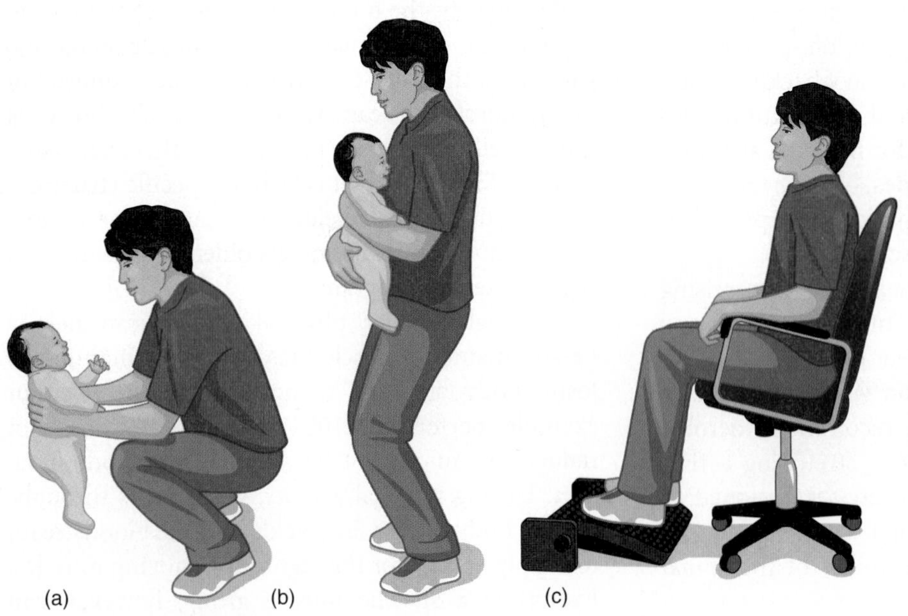

Figure 11.8

Practices to Protect Your Lower Back. (a) To bend safely, bend your knees, not your back. (b) When lifting a child or heavy object, hold it close to your body, at chest level, and do not make twisting motions. (c) To protect your lower back while sitting, rest your lower back against the chair's back and avoid bending forward. Use and adjustable seat and prop up your feet so that you sit with your hips slightly lower than your knees.

Analyzing Health-Related Information

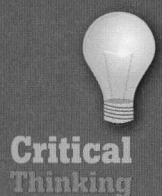

© tele52/ShutterStock

The accompanying article describes safe alternatives to outdated exercises. Read the article and evaluate it using the model for analyzing health-related information. The main points of the model are noted here.

1. Which statements are verifiable facts, and which are unverified statements or value claims?
2. What are the credentials of the person who wrote the article? Does this person have the appropriate background and education in the topic area? What can you do to check the person's credentials?
3. What might be the motives and biases of the person who wrote the article?
4. What is the main point of the article? Which information is relevant to the main point? Which information is irrelevant?
5. Is the source reliable? What evidence supports your conclusion that the source is reliable or unreliable? Does the source of information present the pros and cons of the topic?
6. Does the source of information attack the credibility of conventional scientists or medical authorities?

Based on your analysis, do you think this article is a reliable source of health-related information? Explain why you would or would not use the information. Summarize your reasons for coming to this conclusion.

Safe Alternatives for Outdated Exercises

by Bryant Stamford, PhD

Stretching and strengthening exercises are, of course, good for you. As a part of a complete fitness program, they help you stay flexible and avoid injury.

Not all exercises, though, are good for all people. Healthy young people can do almost any exercise with little risk. And older people who have exercised all their lives can exercise safely under most circumstances. But middle-aged and older people who have been inactive need to know that some of the old standbys—such as sit-ups and toe touches—can result in injury.

So how do you get the important benefits of stretching and strengthening but avoid the injuries? You need to choose exercises carefully, especially if you are getting up in years and haven't exercised regularly. To help you, potentially troublesome exercises are cited below, with recommended alternatives.

If you aren't very flexible or have had back problems, it's best to consult a doctor before starting an exercise program. You may be more susceptible to injury because of a number of factors, including past injuries, fitness, body type, flexibility, technique, and age.

Regardless of the exercises you select, apply the following principles for maximum safety:

- Use strict technique. Stop using an exercise when physical limitation prevents you from performing it well. Also stop when you are tired.
- Use a slow, deliberate approach. Never bounce: The momentum can make a safe exercise dangerous.
- Hold stretches at least 6 seconds initially, building gradually to 30 seconds, then to 2 minutes. Holding a stretched position is more effective than doing many repetitions.
- Reject the "no pain, no gain" philosophy. Pain means something is wrong, so stop immediately.

Many popular exercises stress the lower back. High on the list is the standing toe touch, which stretches the hamstring muscles at the back of your thighs. This is a bad exercise even if done slowly, but it's even worse if you bounce. A safer option is the one-legged stretch (**Figure 1**).

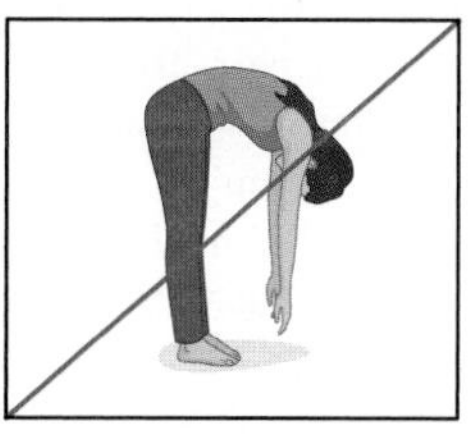

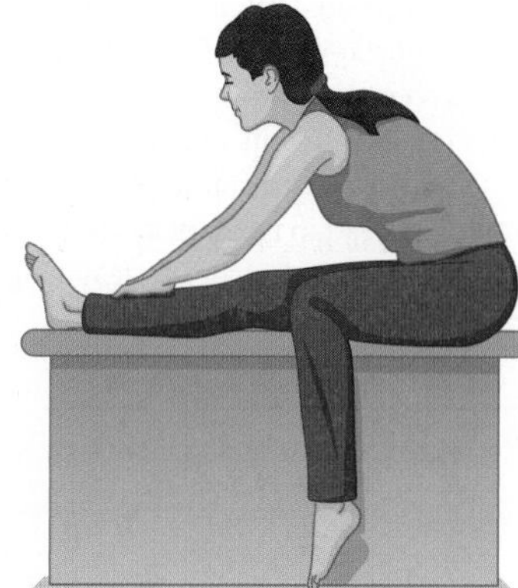

Figure 1 One-legged stretch.

Sit-ups are popular, supposedly for stomach toning. But full sit-ups stress the lower back, and they work the hip muscles more than the abdominal muscles. The "crunch" is better (**Figure 2**).

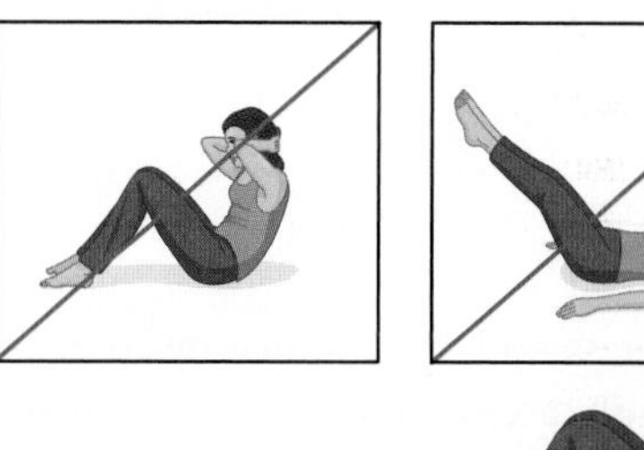

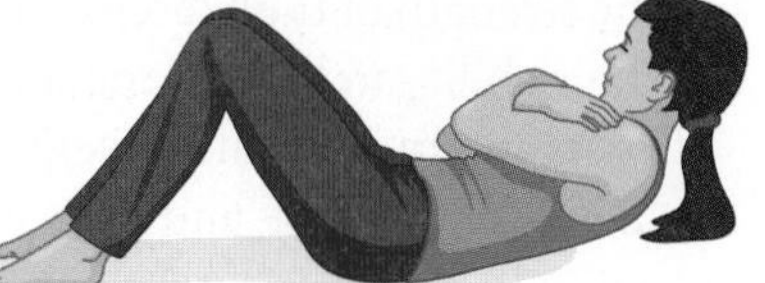

Figure 2 The Crunch.

The donkey kick can also be dangerous, especially to your neck and lower back. It involves being on all fours and lifting one leg as high as possible in a kicking fashion. An alternative to the donkey kick is the rear-thigh lift (**Figure 3**).

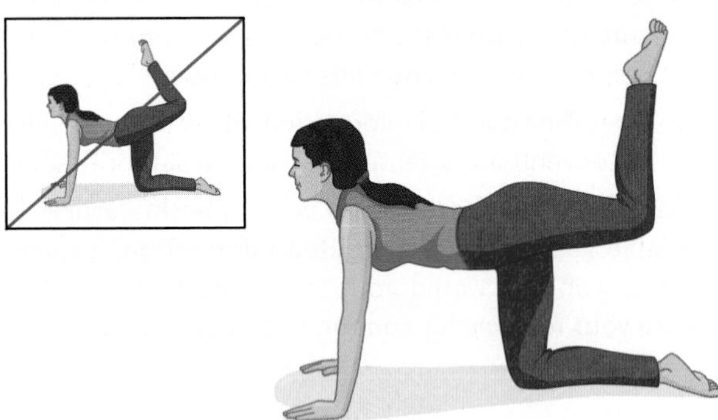

Figure 3 Rear-thigh lift.

Exercises that involve twisting can be especially dangerous. Windmills, in which you bend over and try to touch one hand to the opposite foot, are very stressful on the lower back. But in some sports—like golf—twisting plays a major part. Therefore, when recovering from a low-back injury, perform mild, pain-free twisting movements under professional supervision.

Some exercises can harm the neck. Head rolls, in which you roll your head in a complete circle, are very stressful to the upper spine. Do neck stretches instead (**Figure 4**).

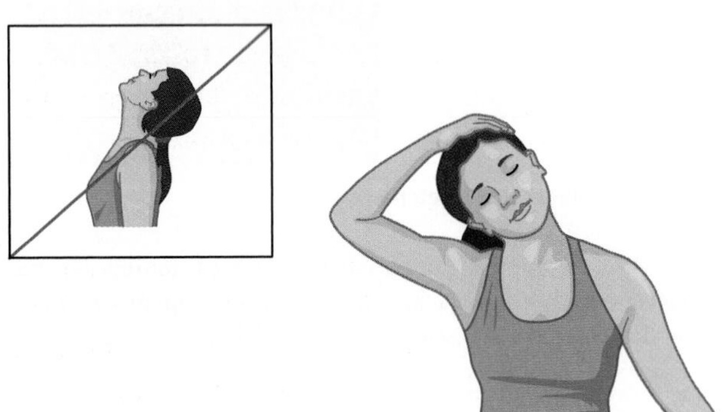

Figure 4 Neck stretch.

People do the yoga plow to stretch upper and lower back muscles by lying on their back and bringing their feet up and over until they touch the floor beyond their head. Unfortunately, this forces the discs in the neck to bulge, risking injury. For the same reason, avoid the "bicycle," in which you lie on your back, raise your hips, and "pedal" your feet. An excellent alternative is the fold-up stretch (**Figure 5**).

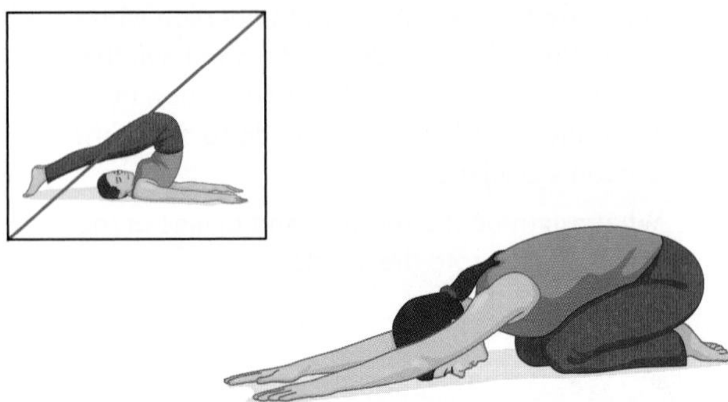

Figure 5 Fold-up stretch.

Full squats or deep knee bends can damage your knees, especially when you bounce out of the squat. Partial squats done slowly and under control are safer.

Jumping jacks involve considerable forces on your legs, particularly the knees. If you land on your toes, the Achilles tendons at the back of your heels bear a major load and could rupture if your legs aren't in the best of shape. Gently running in place provides a lower-impact way to warm up.

Less Risky Business

No matter what your age or physical condition, choosing safer exercise options will lower your risk of injury. And remember that whatever the exercise, good technique is essential.

Remember: This information is not intended as a substitute for medical treatment. Before starting an exercise program, consult a physician.

Adapted from Stamford, B. (1995). Safer alternatives to outdated exercises. *The Physician and Sportsmedicine, 23*(6), 87–88.

This article was written when Dr. Stamford was director of the Health Promotion and Wellness Center and Professor of Allied Health in the School of Medicine at the University of Louisville, Kentucky.

improve physical fitness and appearance by increasing the strength of the exercised muscles and improving their ability to hold in the underlying fat mass.

To maintain a healthy weight, the U.S. Centers for Disease Control and Prevention recommends engaging in moderate- to vigorous-intensity aerobic activities for at least 150 minutes each week, which is approximately 30 minutes a day, 5 days a week. To reduce body fat, 60 to 90 minutes of moderate-intensity physical activity daily may be necessary. Additionally, engaging in muscle-strengthening activities focused on major muscle groups, including legs, hips, back, chest, and shoulders should also be performed at least 2 days a week. An appropriate level of physical activity, along with a sensible diet, is the most effective way to control weight.

ergogenic aids Products or devices that enhance physical development or performance.

© djgis/ShutterStock

Healthy Living Practices

- Engaging in intense aerobic activity regularly can improve your cardiorespiratory fitness and burn excess body fat.
- Engaging in regular resistance exercises, such as lifting weights, can increase the size and strength of your muscles.
- Stretching muscles can improve their flexibility.

Athletic Performance

The Sports-Related Components of Fitness

Although genetic factors contribute to cardiorespiratory fitness, training is essential for athletes to develop their inborn physical capabilities and compete successfully in sports. The sports-related components of fitness include *speed*, *power*, *coordination*, *agility*, *balance*, and *reaction time*. Speed is the rate of movement; power is the ability to concentrate a considerable amount of force, usually from a particular group of muscles, when performing work. Coordination is the ability to perform a series of complicated muscular movements in a continuous manner. Agility enables a person to make quick precise movements, such as changing direction, with ease. Balance enables one to maintain a poised upright body position. Reaction time is the time it takes a person to adjust his or her body position to a changing environment. Although athletes often focus on improving the sports-related components of fitness that are associated with their specific sports, they also need to develop the health-related components of fitness.

Diet and Performance

Most athletes are on the lookout for something—a diet, supplement, or drug—that may give them the competitive edge. The best advice for all athletes is to drink adequate amounts of water and choose a well-balanced diet composed of a variety of foods. By eating more servings of fruits and vegetables, athletes can obtain safe quantities of vitamins and minerals without taking supplements. There is no scientific evidence that protein-rich diets build bigger muscles, so eating large servings of meat or taking protein supplements is unnecessary. High protein intakes may cause dehydration and accelerate the loss of calcium from bones. Furthermore, protein-rich foods often contain a lot of fat, especially saturated fat. Protein supplements are often consumed to help build muscle and for quicker recovery; however, recent research indicated protein supplementation yielded no significant increase in muscle size and reduction in soreness when protein supplementation was used prior to, during, or after a workout.[19]

Carbohydrate is the preferred fuel of the body, and a diet that supplies plenty of complex carbohydrates from starchy foods is recommended. Starchy foods usually contain more vitamins and minerals than sugary foods do. Some athletes practice "carbohydrate loading" to maximize the amount of carbohydrate stored in their muscles. A few days before an event, for example, the athlete gradually increases the amount of carbohydrate eaten to about 70% of calories and gradually decreases the amount of time working out. Two to 4 hours before the competitive event, the athlete eats a light meal composed of starchy foods such as bagels, pasta, or breads and cereals. Not all athletes find that carbohydrate loading helps their performance. Thus, one should test the effects of the diet when not preparing for competition.

Ergogenic Aids

Ergogenic (work-producing) **aids** include a variety of products such as dietary supplements, stimulant drugs, and mechanical devices that supposedly enhance physical development or performance. Some of these aids are beneficial and harmless, but others are dangerous and illegal. *Chromium picolinate*, for example, is a popular dietary supplement that some people use to build lean body mass. Although results of some studies indicate chromium picolinate may provide some health benefits, more research is needed. Furthermore, information about the long-term safety of chromium picolinate supplementation is lacking.

Another popular ergogenic aid is *creatine*, a compound that is naturally in muscle tissue. According to research, creatine can be effective in increasing

Table 11.3

Dietary Supplements as Ergogenic Aids

Aid	Claim	Current Scientific Findings
Caffeine	Improves strength; enhances fat metabolism	Increases alertness, but at high doses causes nervousness; raises free fatty acid levels during exercise; might provide modest improvement of performance.
Creatine	Enhances release of energy during exercise	May enhance performance during short bouts of intense exercise; more research is needed.
Carnitine	Enhances fat metabolism	No significant improvement in performance, but more research is needed.
Wheat-germ oil	Increases oxygen uptake by cells, improving stamina	Results of well-designed studies do not support ergogenic claims.
Lecithin and choline	Increases production of a neurotransmitter, resulting in more muscular strength	Results of well-designed studies do not support ergogenic claims.
Omega-3 fatty acids	Makes blood flow better, stimulates muscle growth	Results of well-designed studies do not support ergogenic claims; large doses may increase the risk of stroke.
Amino acids, brewer's yeast, enzymes, and DNA supplements	General performance-enhancing effects	Results of well-designed studies do not support ergogenic claims; large doses of amino acids can inhibit amino acid absorption and increase water requirement.
CoQ-10 (coenzyme Q or ubiquinone)	Improves heart function	Results of well-designed studies do not show consistent improvement in performance; more research is needed. Long-term safety is unknown.
Bee pollen	Shortens recovery time	Results of well-designed studies do not support ergogenic claims; may cause allergic responses in some individuals.
CLA (conjugated linoleic acid)	Increases lean body mass	Results of well-designed studies do not support ergogenic claims. Long-term safety is unknown.

strength, especially for short bouts of high-intensity physical activities such as sprinting and jumping.[20] Although creatine supplementation appears to be safe, more research is needed to determine the safety of taking creatine supplements over the long term. **Table 11.3** lists some dietary supplements, claims about their ergogenic effects, and information concerning whether scientific studies support these claims. In many instances, more research is needed to support or refute claims.

For more than 4 decades, the outstanding physical accomplishments of many athletes have been tainted by reports of athletes relying on "doping," the use of foreign substances to enhance performance. For example, Danish cyclist Knud Enemark Jensen crashed his bike and fractured his skull while competing in the 1960 Summer Olympics. The young man died a few hours later. The autopsy of the cyclist's body revealed he had used amphetamines, a class of stimulant drugs. By the late 1960s, the International Olympic Committee (IOC) and some other sports federations had established lists of banned substances and required their athletes to be tested for these chemicals. In January 2008, a judge sentenced track star Marion Jones to several months in jail after she admitted lying to federal investigators about her use of performance-enhancing drugs and her involvement in a check-fraud scheme (**Figure 11.9**). As a result of her admission, the IOC disqualified Jones from the five track events in which she won medals at the 2000 Summer Olympic Games. Shortly before being disqualified, Jones returned her Olympic medals to the committee. Most recently, Lance Armstrong, seven-time winner of the Tour de France, admitted to using ergogenic aids.

anabolic steroids A group of drugs that can have muscle-building effects on the body.

Figure 11.9

Fallen Star. In January 2013, Lance Armstrong admitted to doping and received a lifetime ban from the World Anti-Doping Agency. Because of his admission, he was stripped of all seven of his Tour de France titles.

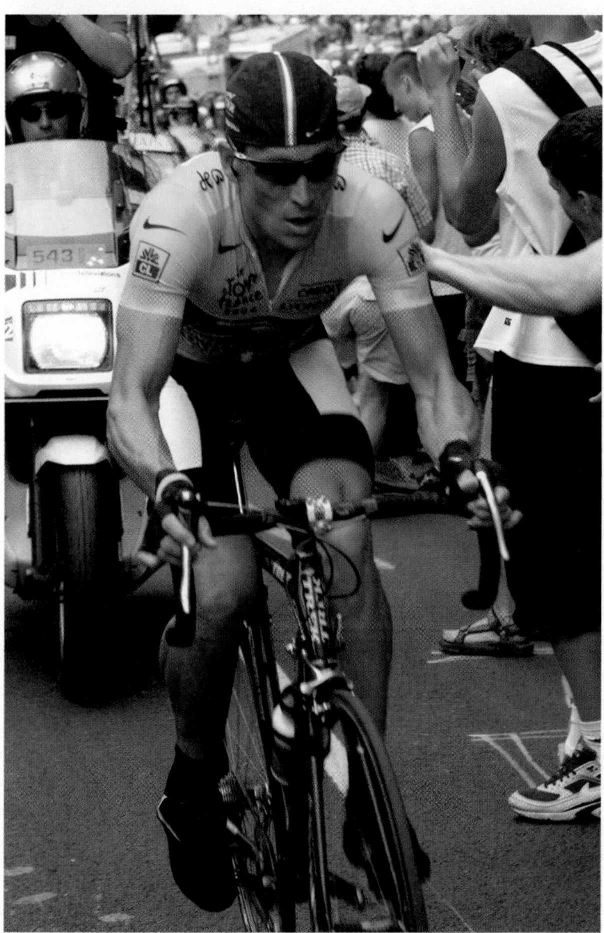

Armstrong was banned from competition for life by the World Anti-Doping Agency and stripped of all seven Tour de France titles. Nike, among other sponsors, cut all ties with Livestrong, Lance Armstrong's foundation.

Athletes in other sports also use banned substances to improve their physical abilities. According to the 2007 Mitchell Report, doping is widespread among professional baseball players.[21] The report includes the names of several Major League Baseball players who allegedly purchased illegal substances, particularly *anabolic steroids*, to enhance their performance. In the report, former U.S. Senator George Mitchell recommends that the players and the management of Major League Baseball teams work together to rid the sport of doping.

Anabolic Steroids Both men and women may lift weights during their workout sessions to build stronger, more well-defined muscles. Men, however, are capable of developing larger muscles and having greater overall strength because their testosterone levels are higher than those of women. Testosterone is an anabolic (tissue-building) hormone.

Anabolic steroids are a group of synthetic and natural substances that are chemically related to testosterone and may have muscle-building properties. Although certain anabolic steroids are classified as controlled substances, they can be prescribed by physicians for legitimate medical uses. These drugs, however, are often illegally obtained and abused by athletes and others who want to enhance their physical performance or muscle development or both. In the United States, it is difficult to estimate the prevalence of anabolic steroid abuse because people are often unwilling to admit to taking the substances.

Medical experts are especially concerned about anabolic steroid use among adolescents because of the long-term serious health consequences. In 2010, 2% of American high school seniors reported using steroids at some point in their lives.[22]

Why is there so much concern over the abuse of anabolic steroids? Athletes who abuse these drugs to improve their physical strength can have an unfair competitive advantage over athletes who choose not to use them. Anabolic steroids can have serious irreversible effects on the body (**Figure 11.10**). Male anabolic steroid abusers often experience shrunken testicles and infertility. Women who abuse these drugs may become bald, grow facial hair, and experience menstrual irregularities. Anabolic steroid abuse increases the risks of developing heart and kidney diseases, certain cancers, and liver tumors. In some cases, damage to the liver or kidneys is so severe that death occurs. Additionally, anabolic steroids can affect personality. People who abuse anabolic steroids may act more aggressive, hostile, and irritable than usual. Regular resistance exercise is the only safe way to increase the size and strength of a muscle.

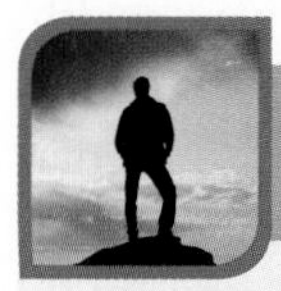

Healthy Living Practices

- Do not use anabolic steroids to build your muscles; they can be very harmful.

Figure 11.10

Possible Effects of Anabolic Steroids on the Body. To increase their muscle mass, some men and women abuse anabolic steroids or other chemicals that are promoted for their muscle-building properties. These drugs can have serious irreversible effects on the body.

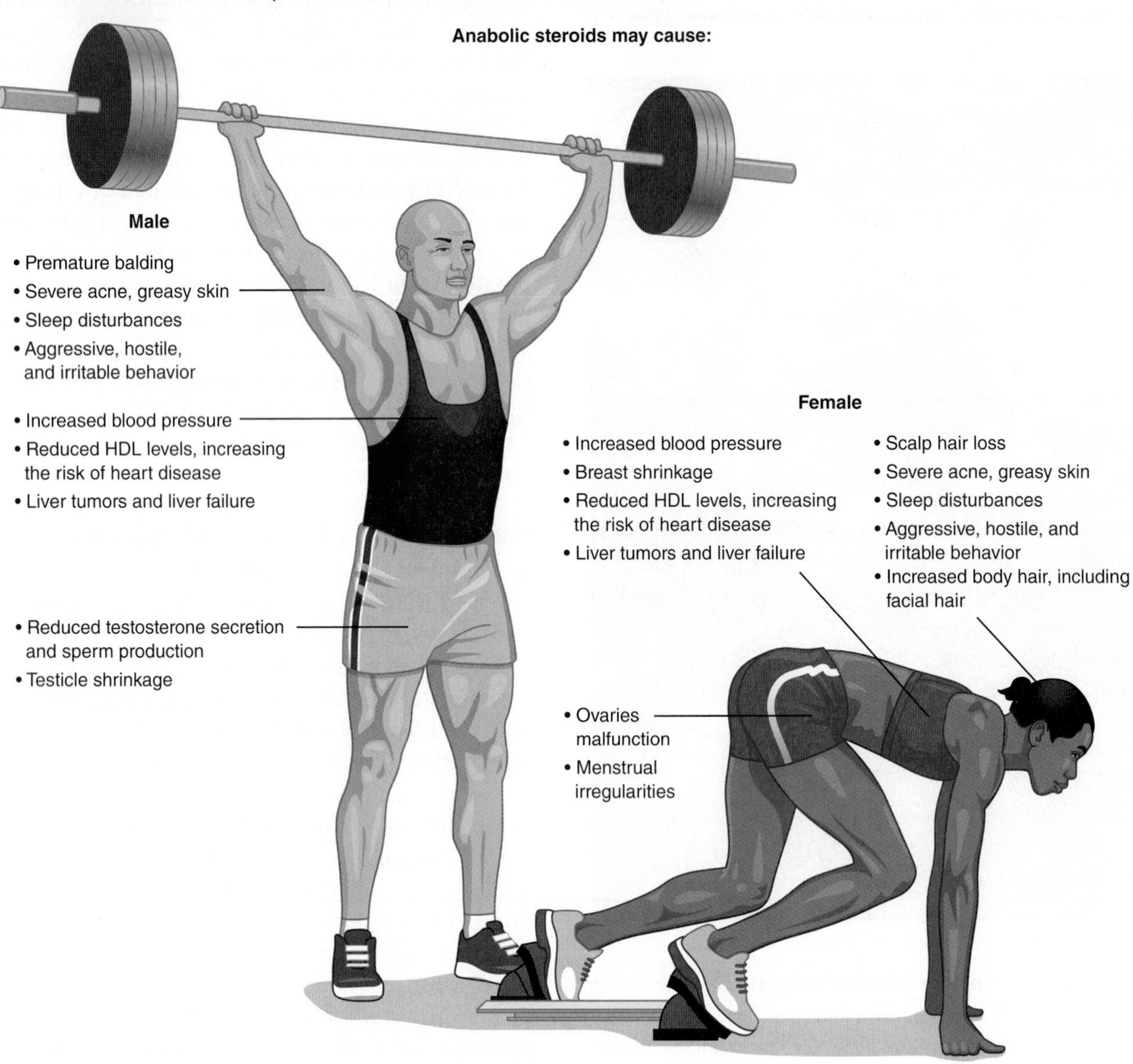

Anabolic steroids may cause:
Male
• Premature balding
• Severe acne, greasy skin
• Sleep disturbances
• Aggressive, hostile, and irritable behavior
• Increased blood pressure
• Reduced HDL levels, increasing the risk of heart disease
• Liver tumors and liver failure
• Reduced testosterone secretion and sperm production
• Testicle shrinkage
Female
• Increased blood pressure
• Breast shrinkage
• Reduced HDL levels, increasing the risk of heart disease
• Liver tumors and liver failure
• Scalp hair loss
• Severe acne, greasy skin
• Sleep disturbances
• Aggressive, hostile, and irritable behavior
• Increased body hair, including facial hair
• Ovaries malfunction
• Menstrual irregularities

Exercising for Health

Regular exercise is important for long-term health and is associated with better cardiovascular health, among other health benefits. Aerobic activities increase cardiorespiratory fitness and muscular endurance. Performing high-impact aerobic activities, including basketball and jogging, can build stronger bones. Although isometric and isotonic exercises develop muscular strength, these activities may not increase cardiorespiratory fitness significantly. Many people combine aerobic and muscle-strengthening activities in their daily workouts to improve their overall physical condition; others perform isotonic and aerobic workouts on alternate days. For example, one day's workout session would be devoted to weightlifting; the following day's session would involve race-walking. The American College of Sport Medicine recommends waiting 48 to 72 hours between strength training sessions using the same muscle groups.

The FITT principle can be used to develop exercise programs to enhance health-related components of fitness. FITT is an acronym for frequency, intensity, time, and type components of exercise that influence the degree of health benefits a person derives from it. Using the FITT principle allows you to manipulate your program for continued improvement. For example, it is common to reach a plateau in weight loss or muscular strength improvement when the same program is repeated for an extended period of time. Increasing exercising intensity or time can help break plateaus for continued improvement.

Exercise *frequency* is the number of times an individual exercises, usually reported as the number of days or exercise sessions in a week. People who exercise at least three times a week generally experience more rapid improvements to their overall fitness than do people who exercise less often. The *intensity* of an exercise reflects the amount of physical exertion a person uses while performing the activity. Fitness experts use several methods to estimate the intensity of exercise, including the rate of oxygen consumption during exercise, heart rate, and personal perceptions of physical exertion. For the average person, playing nine holes of golf while using a power golf cart or bowling for 30 minutes are light activities; playing tennis or walking briskly for a half-hour are moderate activities; and running for 6 miles or playing racquetball for 30 minutes are intense activities (see Table 11.2).

Time refers to the total time the person is physically active during each exercise session. For example, people who jog for 40 minutes, 3 days a week experience more cardiorespiratory benefits than do those who jog for 10 minutes, 3 days a week.[23,24] People who are currently sedentary can develop cardiorespiratory fitness if they engage in an aerobic exercise program that gradually increases the duration of the activity, usually over several weeks. The *type* of exercise, sometimes called mode, refers to the kind of exercise you choose. For example, to improve flexibility, one person may choose to engage in static stretching, and another may choose to practice yoga. It is important to match the type of exercise chosen with desired abilities and goals.

Many tools are available to help you assess your level of activity. A relatively easy way to assess and increase your physical activity level is to measure the number of steps you take in a day. You will need to purchase a pedometer; inexpensive ones sell for under $30 (**Figure 11.11**). Before you begin a typical day's activities, place the pedometer on your belt or waistband. Then, check the pedometer before going to bed and record the number of steps you took that day. If you have a sedentary lifestyle, you probably will have taken fewer than 3,000 steps. Gradually increase the number of steps you take by making a conscious effort to be more active. A brisk walking routine, for example, can increase the number of steps you take daily and increase your cardiorespiratory fitness level. Your goal should be to record at least 8,000 steps each day.

Figure 11.11

Examples of Pedometers. A pedometer is a relatively easy way to assess your physical activity level.

(a) © Andrew Haddon/ShutterStock; (b) © Coprid/ShutterStock

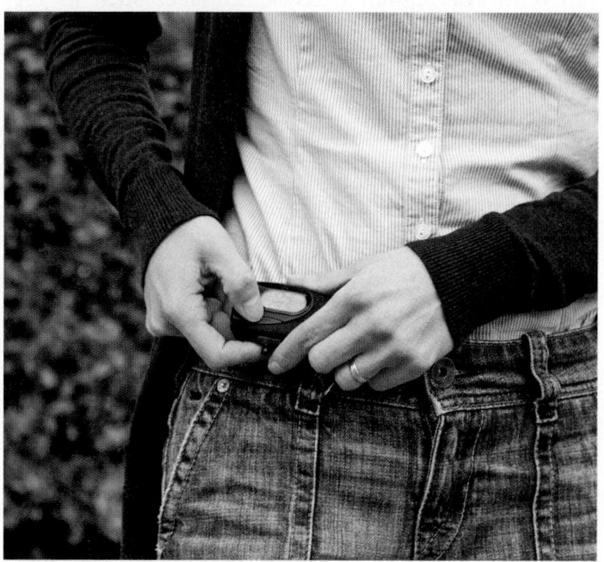

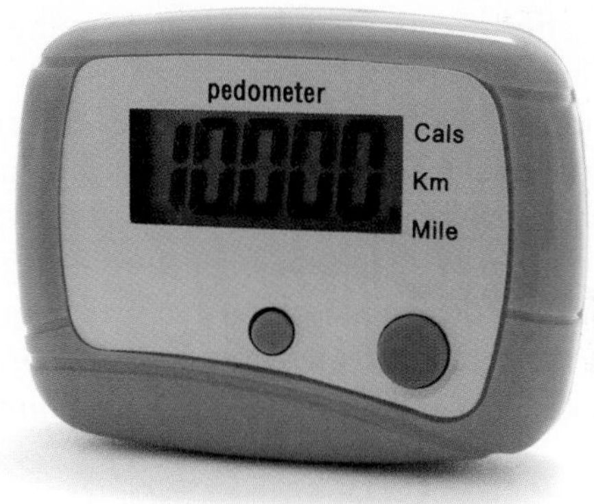

Other, more interactive tools, such as FitBit and Body Bugg, can also help you track the number of steps you take daily, while serving several other functions. FitBit also tracks distance traveled, calories burned, and activity minutes. The Body Bugg system performs similar functions and also monitoring and displaying your heart rate. Additionally, the Body

Bugg Web-based system and app provide a means to track data over time, which allows you see progress and adapt your exercise sessions as you become more fit. Research indicates immediate feedback during exercise, as well as feedback on long-term goals, can reinforce regular exercise. Devices such as FitBit and Body Bugg are, however, more costly than a pedometer.

The frequency, intensity, time, and type of aerobic physical activities influence fitness. For example, you can exercise intensely for 20 minutes or moderately for 30 minutes and achieve similar cardiorespiratory benefits. Using the FITT principle allows you to individualize a workout program that works best for your particular needs and abilities.

The Exercise Session

People should *warm up* before and *cool down* ("warm down") after intense exercise. Warming up reduces the physical stress that vigorous exercise can place on the body. The person's skeletal muscles become warm and extend easily, joints become more flexible, and heart and breathing rates increase gradually. Some studies indicate warming up can reduce the extent of muscle soreness after exercise[25] and may reduce the likelihood of injuries.[26] More research is needed to support these findings. Cooling down facilitates the circulation of blood, especially in the leg muscles, enabling the body to recover from intense physical activity.

To warm up the entire body before engaging in a vigorous physical activity, you can walk at an easy pace and then gradually increase your speed until you have walked for 5 to 10 minutes. At this point, your muscles should be warm enough to perform stretching exercises such as those shown in Figure 11.5. Stretching muscles before the warm-up session is usually not recommended because extending "cold" muscles may injure them. Stretching, however, does not protect against sports injuries.[27,28]

After stretching, many persons perform active, task-specific activities to warm up specific muscles. For example, a jogger would jog slowly for a few minutes, gradually increasing the pace until reaching his or her usual training speed. Before playing a sport, it can be helpful to perform sport-specific movements at a slower pace prior to the game. A recent study indicated a soccer-specific warm-up reduced injury rate and severity among collegiate male soccer players.[29]

Warming up before exercising is essential for people with heart disease. Abnormal functioning of the heart may occur when sedentary, middle-aged people begin to exercise suddenly without warming up. Warm-up activities increase the blood flow to the heart gradually, reducing the risk of heart attack during physical exertion.

After exercising vigorously, people should cool down by gradually reducing the intensity of their activity and by stretching. Many types of strenuous exercise increase the blood supply to the leg muscles; suddenly stopping these intense muscular movements can cause blood to accumulate in the leg veins, which can reduce the blood flow to the brain, causing dizziness, faintness, or loss of consciousness. Cooling down by engaging in 5 to 10 minutes of light exercise gradually decreases the blood flow to the leg muscles. **Figure 11-12** illustrates a 50-minute workout session

Figure 11.12

A Suggested Workout Session. A reasonable 50-minute workout session may consist of 10 minutes of warm-up activities, 30 minutes of jogging, and 10 minutes of cool-down exercises.

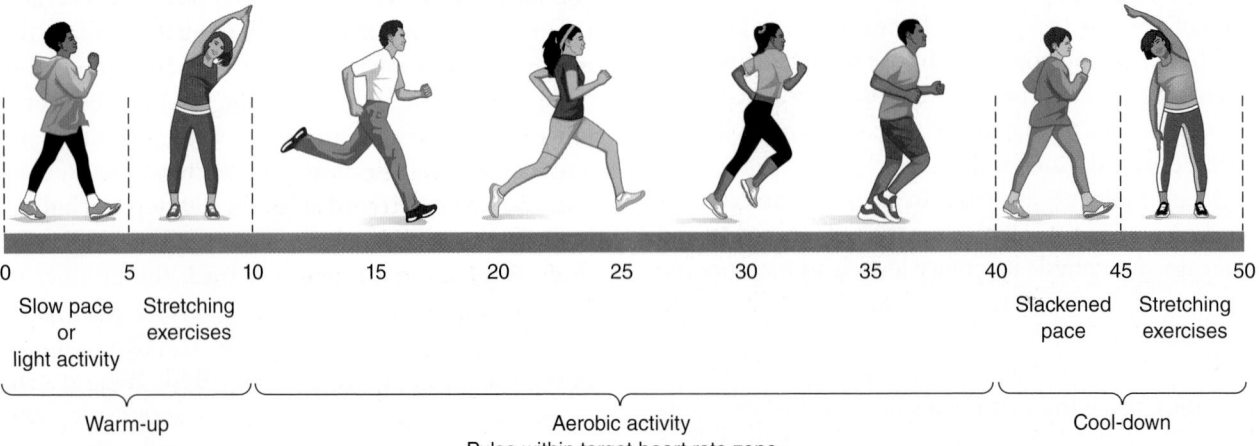

that consists of 10 minutes of warm-up activities, 30 minutes of jogging, and 10 minutes of cool-down exercises.

strain Generally refers to an injured muscle or tendon.

sprain Generally refers to an injured ligament.

Exercise Danger Signs

Exercise improves the functioning of the heart and reduces the risk of heart disease. Sudden and intense physical exertion, however, can strain the heart, especially the heart of an unfit individual or someone with cardiovascular disease.

To reduce the risk of overtaxing your cardiovascular system during vigorous exercise, warm up first, and then exercise at a reduced intensity level for about 10 to 15 minutes. Keep records of your activity level and any discomfort that you experience. Discontinue the activity and consult a physician if any of the following signs or symptoms of heart disease occur during or after exercising:

- Heart abnormalities, such as irregular rhythms, a feeling that your heart is pounding in your throat, or fluttering in your chest
- Pain or pressure in your chest, throat, or arms
- Shortness of breath, dizziness, sudden loss of coordination, cold sweating, or fainting

Preventing and Managing Common Exercise Injuries

Everyone should be concerned about personal safety while exercising. People should check their exercise equipment for defects and wear the proper clothing, shoes, and protective gear for the activity. Bicyclists and joggers, for example, should obey traffic signals and avoid busy roads that have narrow or rocky shoulders. Engaging in physical activity outdoors at night, or in very hot or very cold conditions, is especially dangerous; wearing clothing with reflective strips can also help you be more visible.

Although engaging in regular physical activity is essential for optimal health, some activities are likely to result in musculoskeletal injuries. Suddenly raising the intensity level or duration of a physical activity may damage muscles or supportive tissues or aggravate existing injuries, so gradual changes are recommended. Using some general exercise precautions can help minimize the risk of musculoskeletal injury. Sudden, awkward movements are likely to injure muscles, tendons, and joints; therefore, avoiding physical activities that involve exaggerated twisting can reduce the risk of injury.

Strains and Sprains

Almost everyone who is physically active has experienced muscle soreness or musculoskeletal injuries such as *strains* and *sprains*. Although there are no clear clinical definitions for strain or sprain, a **strain** generally refers to the damage that a muscle or tendon sustains when overextended rapidly. A **sprain** usually refers to a damaged ligament. Although these two types of injuries often occur together, a sprain tends to be more serious than a strain is. The sprained ligament may be partially or completely torn, and the nearby muscle, joint, or bones may be damaged; therefore, severe sprains generally require immediate medical attention.

RICE, the acronym for rest, ice, compression, and elevation, is often effective for treating strains and sprains:

Rest can reduce the pain, but light exercise or activity that uses the injured muscles is usually recommended, as long as the discomfort is tolerable.

Ice treatments should be limited to 20-minute sessions and can be repeated every 2 hours (while the injured person is awake) for 2 to 3 days. Do not place ice directly on the skin; instead, place a thin towel or wrap between the ice and your skin.

Compression, an external source of pressure, can prevent swelling. Apply a pressure bandage on the injury to produce compression. Make sure the bandage is not tight enough to interfere with circulation.

Elevation also reduces swelling. When an injured limb is elevated, g ravity helps the veins of the limb return blood to the heart, reducing the amount of blood and other fluids that accumulates in the damaged tissue.

With RICE and over-the-counter pain medicines, muscle soreness usually disappears within a day or two. If an injured area does not improve with RICE and the pain persists or worsens, consult a physician.

hyperthermia A condition that occurs when body temperature rises above the normal range.

heat cramps In a dehydrated and hot person, the signs and symptoms of heat cramps include muscular tightening and pain in the limbs or abdomen.

heat exhaustion The extreme fatigue that results from exercise or work in hot temperatures.

heatstroke A life-threatening condition that can occur when people exercise or work in hot temperatures.

Dislocation

Healthy joints control the ability of muscles to move bones. Joints are susceptible to *dislocation*, that is, becoming displaced by force. Dislocation can result when joints and their supportive tissues are torn or worn after engaging in certain strenuous physical activities. When a joint becomes damaged, the injury reduces its normal range of motion, and movement often becomes painful. Although involvement in certain sports, such as American football, increases the risk that the participants will damage their joints, any physically active person can experience joint injuries. A later section of this chapter describes steps for designing personal fitness programs that can reduce the risk of such injuries.

Temperature-Related Injuries

When exercising in hot weather, the body gains heat from the environment and from its active muscles. To cool itself, the body perspires heavily, transferring heat to the environment. *Dehydration* (lack of body water) can occur if a person does not replace the fluid lost by perspiration. Signs of dehydration include weight loss immediately after exercising and reduced urine production.[30] The muscles of a person suffering from dehydration are less able to work efficiently. It is essential that people replace the water lost in sweat by consuming adequate amounts of fluids, especially plain water. Soups, fruits, vegetables, and nonalcoholic drinks contribute water to the diet also.

Hyperthermia **Hyperthermia**, higher than normal body temperature, can result from dehydration. If a person becomes hot and dehydrated, heat cramps, heat exhaustion, or heatstroke may occur. The signs and symptoms of **heat cramps** include muscular tightening and pain in the limbs or abdomen. The affected individual usually recovers after stopping the activity, resting in a shady area, stretching the cramped muscles, and drinking several ounces of water. After recovering, this person should not exercise for the remainder of the day.

Heat exhaustion and **heatstroke** are more serious conditions than heat cramps. People suffering from heat exhaustion have pale and clammy skin; sweat profusely; and feel nauseated, tired, and weak. They need to move to a cooler area and drink plenty of cool water. If heat exhaustion is not recognized and treated, heatstroke can develop. The signs and symptoms of heatstroke include hot, dry, reddened skin; rapid pulse; fever; and loss of consciousness. Heatstroke is a life-threatening emergency; victims should be removed from the heat and receive immediate medical attention.

When the weather is hot and humid, avoid exerting yourself outdoors during the hottest time of the day. If you must be outdoors when it is hot, follow a few precautions to reduce the likelihood of heat-related injury. Several hours before exercising or performing intense physical activity, especially in warm conditions, slowly drink water or other acceptable fluids and eat salty foods or snacks to achieve adequate hydration.[30] Alcoholic beverages are not acceptable fluids for hydration because alcohol is a *diuretic*. A diuretic increases urine production; therefore, people lose some body water when they drink alcohol-containing beverages. Although caffeine is also a diuretic, drinking caffeinated beverages does not stimulate excess urine production by the body.[30] Consuming large amounts of caffeine can increase the risk of heat-related injury.

During and after engaging in activities that make you perspire heavily, consume enough fluids to replace the amount of weight lost by sweating. Drinking too much fluid before, during, or after physical activities should be avoided because the practice may cause *overhydration*, a potentially deadly condition. A rule of thumb is to drink about 1.5 L (approximately 6.25 cups) of water or other acceptable beverage for every kilogram (2.2 lb) of body weight lost during the activity.[30] When the weather first becomes hot, individuals should begin working or exercising outdoors at a reduced intensity and then gradually increase the intensity over a 2-week period to become *acclimatized*, that is, physically adjusted to the extreme temperature change. Wearing light-colored, loose clothing in sunny, hot, and humid weather helps people stay comfortable because light colors reflect sunlight and loose clothing allows perspiration to evaporate more easily. When environmental temperature and humidity are very high, most individuals should consider reducing the intensity and duration of their outdoor workouts to reduce the risk of heat-related illness.

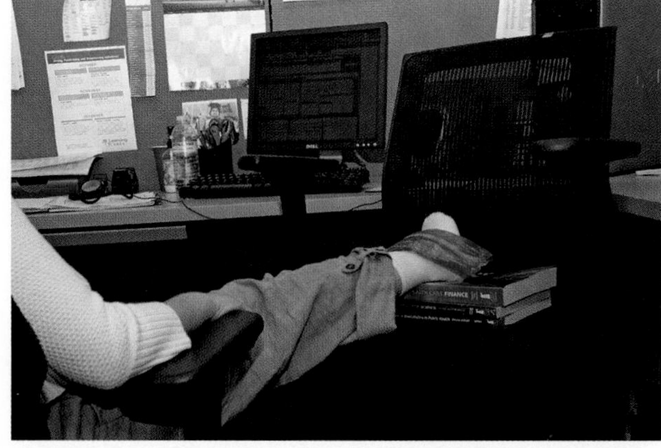

Elevation and ice treatments can reduce swelling of a sprain or strain.

People who perspire excessively can lose considerable amounts of sodium chloride in their sweat. Most of these individuals can drink more water and fruit juices and consume foods to replace the lost nutrients. While engaging in strenuous exercise that lasts an hour or more, people can also consume sports drinks for fluid replacement.[31] In addition to water, these drinks contain sodium chloride and energy-supplying carbohydrate (e.g., sports drinks and gels). Salt (sodium chloride) tablets are typically not needed.[32]

Frostbite and Hypothermia Participating in outdoor activities during the winter months increases the risk of cold injury. Exposed to cold temperatures, the body reduces its blood flow to the skin, conserving body heat. The chilled person shivers and feels tingling, numbness, or burning in exposed skin or body parts. *Frostbite* occurs when ice crystals form in the deeper tissues of the skin, damaging them. Blood flow to the affected area slows, causing clots to form. Unable to obtain oxygen and nutrients, the tissue dies. The damage may be so extensive that the frostbitten areas must be amputated. A person's fingers, toes, nose, ears, and face are most susceptible to frostbite, but any exposed skin can become frostbitten. Frostbite requires immediate and proper medical treatment. Avoid rubbing frostbitten skin because it can further damage cold tissues. To prevent frostbite, people need to wear gloves or mittens, thick socks, hats that can be pulled down over the ears, and scarves when outdoors in cold weather.

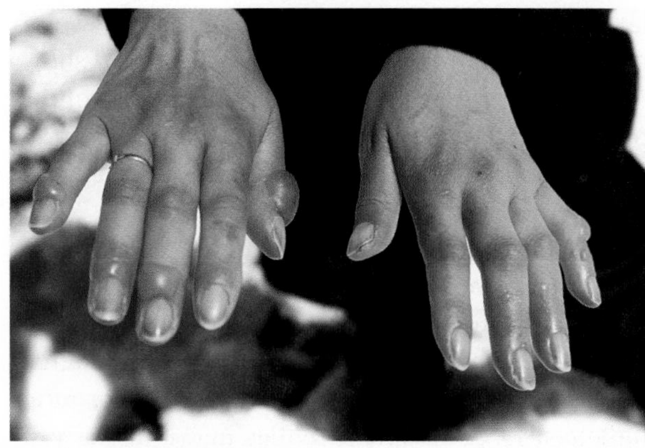

Frostbite.
Courtesy of Neil Malcom Winkelmann.

hypothermia A condition that occurs when the body's core temperature drops below 95°F.

Hypothermia occurs when the body's core temperature drops below 95°F.[33] (A rectal thermometer is used to measure core body temperature.) As body temperature declines, the person shivers, feels tired, displays poor judgment, acts disoriented, and eventually loses consciousness. Death can occur when the core temperature falls below 82°F, and breathing and circulation are too weak to support life.

As in cases of frostbite, hypothermia requires prompt medical treatment. It is important to shelter people suffering from hypothermia from the cold and remove their wet clothing. Covering them in dry blankets keeps them warm until they can be taken to a hospital. To protect against hypothermia, wear a hat and layers of warm, dry clothing when you are in cold environments.

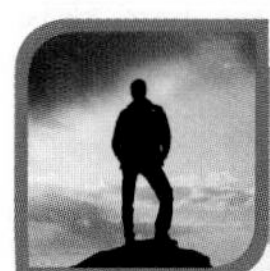

© djgis/ShutterStock

Healthy Living Practices

- ☐ If you have musculoskeletal injuries as a result of exercise, use RICE as treatment. If pain and swelling persist, contact your personal physician.
- ☐ If you develop heat cramps or heat exhaustion while working or exercising, stop the activity immediately, get out of the heat, and drink plenty of water.
- ☐ If you plan to exercise or work in hot conditions, wear loose, light clothing and take an ample supply of water, fruit juices, or sports drinks with you.
- ☐ When you exercise or work in cold conditions, protect yourself against hypothermia and frostbite by wearing layers of warm, dry clothing, a hat or ski mask, gloves or mittens, and thick socks.
- ☐ Avoid drinking beverages that contain alcohol to replace body water that is lost by sweating.

cross-training Incorporating a variety of aerobic activities into a fitness program.

Developing a Personal Fitness Program

A basic personal physical fitness program should include activities that enhance cardiorespiratory fitness, muscular strength and endurance, and flexibility. To develop an effective program, determine your needs, interests, and limitations. Answering the following questions can help you accomplish this step:

- How can I schedule my day's activities so that I have time to exercise?
- Which physical activities am I most likely to enjoy and practice regularly for the rest of my life?
- Do I want to develop or enhance specific sports-related skills?
- Would I rather work out alone or with others?
- Where will I exercise?
- Do I have physical limitations that require special equipment or rule out certain activities?

The "Changing Health Habits" activity for this chapter can help you determine whether you are ready to improve your level of physical fitness (see the Student Workbook section at the end of this text).

After completing the first step, make a list of your general fitness goals. One of them should be to enhance the health-related components of fitness, for example, improving your cardiorespiratory fitness or flexibility. Other goals may be changing your appearance or building agility. Although your list may include several goals, choose one or two to work on at a time.

At this point, you need to choose enjoyable physical activities that will help you meet your fitness goals. As mentioned earlier, aerobic exercise is necessary for achieving cardiorespiratory fitness. Resistance training is important for increasing lean body mass and maintaining muscular strength and endurance. Warm-up and cool-down stretching exercises can improve range of motion. Faculty who conduct personal fitness classes in the physical education department at your college can answer your questions concerning the need for special equipment or how to perform activities safely.

If you are overweight or have been sedentary, give your body time to adapt to the fitness program. For the first 2 to 3 weeks, do not try to exercise at a high intensity level or for more than 15 minutes. Keep an exercise log or diary detailing exercises performed can help you track your progress. Making note of exercise frequency, intensity, time, and type (FITT), as well as how you felt during your workout, can help you make adjustments as needed. Stop when you experience signs of exercise intolerance, such as pain or breathlessness, and note this in your log. A common problem encountered by enthusiastic but out-of-shape people is trying to do too much too soon.

When you do not experience fatigue or discomfort as a result of the activity, you are ready to move on to the improvement stage of the program. By gradually increasing the intensity and duration of your physical activity, you can progressively overload your muscles and achieve your fitness goals. For example, add 5 minutes to the time of your aerobic workout session each week, until you are exercising for 45 to 90 minutes most days of the week. If you are walking at 2 mph, gradually increase the pace until you are able to walk between 3 and 4 mph without effort. To acquire the fitness benefits of aerobic exercise, a person must engage in the activity for at least 30 minutes most days of the week. Engaging in aerobic exercise more often, for longer periods, or at higher intensity can help develop higher degrees of fitness; however, more is not always better for long-term health

You can enhance muscular size and strength with a weightlifting program that gradually overcomes the resistance of progressively heavier weights. As your muscles adapt to the workload, you should be able to develop strength by adding resistance while performing fewer repetitions. After each bout of heavy training, muscles engaged in resistance exercises need at least 48 hours to recover, to repair themselves, and to grow. Thus, experts often recommend alternating the days of the week in which you perform cardiorespiratory and strength training activities. **Table 11.4** shows a sample aerobic and weight resistance program that includes stretching exercises. By the end of 6 months, you should be ready to move on to the maintenance stage of the program.

A major feature of the maintenance stage of your fitness program is sustaining your fitness level and interest. Adding new activities prevents boredom with the workout program and develops different muscle groups or skills. **Cross-training**, incorporating a variety of aerobic activities into a fitness program, is an excellent way to maintain enthusiasm

Table 11.4

A Sample 4-Week Combined Workout Program

Week 1	Warm-Up* (min)	Workout	Cool-Down* (min)
Monday	5 to 10	Brisk walking 15 min.	5 to 10
Tuesday	5 to 10	Resistance training, beginning load Reps: 5, Sets: 4	5 to 10
Wednesday	5 to 10	Brisk walking 15 min.	5 to 10
Thursday	5 to 10	Resistance training, beginning load Reps: 5, Sets: 4	5 to 10
Friday	5 to 10	Brisk walking 15 min.	5 to 10
Saturday	5 to 10	Resistance training, beginning load Reps: 5, Sets: 4	5 to 10
Sunday	5 to 10	Brisk walking 15 min.	5 to 10
Week 2	**Warm-Up* (min)**	**Workout**	**Cool-Down* (min)**
Monday	5 to 10	Brisk walking 20 min.	5 to 10
Tuesday	5 to 10	Resistance training, beginning load Reps: 5, Sets: 4	5 to 10
Wednesday	5 to 10	Brisk walking 20 min.	5 to 10
Thursday	5 to 10	Resistance training, beginning load Reps: 5, Sets: 4	5 to 10
Friday	5 to 10	Brisk walking 20 min.	5 to 10
Saturday	5 to 10	Resistance training, beginning load Reps: 5, Sets: 4	5 to 10
Sunday	5 to 10	Brisk walking 20 min.	5 to 10
Week 3	**Warm-Up* (min)**	**Workout**	**Cool-Down* (min)**
Monday	5 to 10	Brisk walking 25 min.	5 to 10
Tuesday	5 to 10	Resistance training, beginning load Reps: 5, Sets: 4	5 to 10
Wednesday	5 to 10	Brisk walking 25 min.	5 to 10
Thursday	5 to 10	Resistance training, beginning load Reps: 5, Sets: 4	5 to 10
Friday	5 to 10	Brisk walking 25 min.	5 to 10
Saturday	5 to 10	Resistance training, beginning load Reps: 5, Sets: 4	5 to 10
Sunday	5 to 10	Brisk walking 25 min.	to 10
Week 4	**Warm-Up* (min)**	**Workout**	**Cool-Down* (min)**
Monday	5 to 10	Brisk walking 30 min.	5 to 10
Tuesday	5 to 10	Resistance training, beginning load Reps: 10, Sets: 4	5 to 10
Wednesday	5 to 10	Brisk walking 30 min.	5 to 10
Thursday	5 to 10	Resistance training, beginning load Reps: 10, Sets: 4	5 to 10
Friday	5 to 10	Brisk walking 30 min.	5 to 10
Saturday	5 to 10	Resistance training, beginning load Reps: 10, Sets: 4	5 to 10
Sunday	5 to 10	Brisk walking 30 min.	5 to 10

and interest. Working out in different environments can also add interest. Walking in parks or hiking on trails, for example, can be more interesting than walking around indoor tracks. By working out with friends or family members, you can enhance your physical as well as social health.

Once people achieve high degrees of physical fitness, continued regular exercise is needed to maintain the healthful benefits gained during training. Sometimes physically fit individuals discontinue intensive regular exercise regimens for a variety of reasons, such as experiencing injuries or losing motivation. Detraining can occur within a couple of weeks after exercise sessions are discontinued. The rate of detraining is influence by current fitness level. A very fit person will detrain at a slower rate than a less fit person. Even if they have to reduce the frequency of their exercise sessions, people can usually maintain their high level of physical fitness as long as they do not stop working out.

Active for a Lifetime

People are more likely to engage in physical activity regularly if they enjoy it, recognize the health benefits, and make it a priority. Some people dislike vigorous exercise because they do not feel competent performing the activity; others may associate the activity with sweating, strain, and pain. Adults who enjoy being active are more likely to make exercise and physical movement integral parts of their daily routines.

Many people find it easier to be physically active while in college than when they are out of school and working full time. Most college and university campuses have physical education departments that offer a variety of sports and fitness courses; some of these departments have well-equipped fitness centers. Additionally, the staff of the physical education department may conduct intramural athletic programs that are open to students, and at certain times, they may open the college's gyms and athletic fields to all students. While in school, students should take advantage of the fitness opportunities available on their college or university campus.

After leaving college, individuals can continue to build or maintain their fitness level by exercising at home or by joining fitness centers or clubs. Although large resistance exercise machines are highly effective for building muscular strength, their expense and size make them unlikely to be found in most homes. However, you can buy barbells and smaller handheld weights at most department or sporting goods stores for use at home. To improve cardiorespiratory fitness, rowing machines, stationary bikes, and cross-country skiing machines can be purchased for home fitness centers. Before buying any large piece of fitness equipment, you should visit a gym or fitness club to test the machine and discuss its value with qualified fitness experts. For additional information, check popular consumer magazines that occasionally rate exercise equipment.

Building or maintaining physical fitness does not require a long-term commitment with a gym or fitness club, but many people enjoy the social aspects of exercising at these facilities. The quality and cost of gyms and fitness clubs vary, so you may want to consider the points listed in the Consumer Health feature "Choosing a Fitness Center" before joining one.

Unless you have a job that requires physical exertion or you work at a company that provides a worksite fitness center for its employees, you need to find ways to be more physically active at work. If your office building has stairways, climb the stairs rather than ride the elevators. Instead of eating lunches in restaurants, bring your lunches from home to eat at your desk, and use the remaining time to go outside and walk. You might consider buying two pairs of athletic shoes—one for your office and one for home. You may like walking with others better than walking alone; ask someone to walk with you. Colleagues, spouses, or friends can provide the valuable social support you may need to maintain your motivation to exercise at work or home. In addition to increasing your physical activity at work, you can move around more at home. Child care, housework, and gardening chores often require contracting large muscle groups, which expends energy and strengthens the muscles. How many times a week do you go up and down steps, walk a pet, or go shopping? What lifestyle changes can you make to increase your physical activity?

Like many people, you may want to be more active, but you cannot seem to find the time to exercise. It is important to remember that you do not have to spend hours each day engaging in strenuous exercises to improve your health. Even 10 to 20 minutes of vigorous aerobic activity can boost your fitness level. Determine how you spend your leisure time. Each day, how much time do you spend engaging in sedentary activities such as watching TV, communicating with others in a chat room, or playing computer games? Can you set aside at least 30 minutes each day to engage in some moderately intense physical activities? **Figure 11.13** illustrates physical activity

Figure 11.13

The Activity Pyramid. This physical activity pyramid includes recommendations for healthy lifestyles.

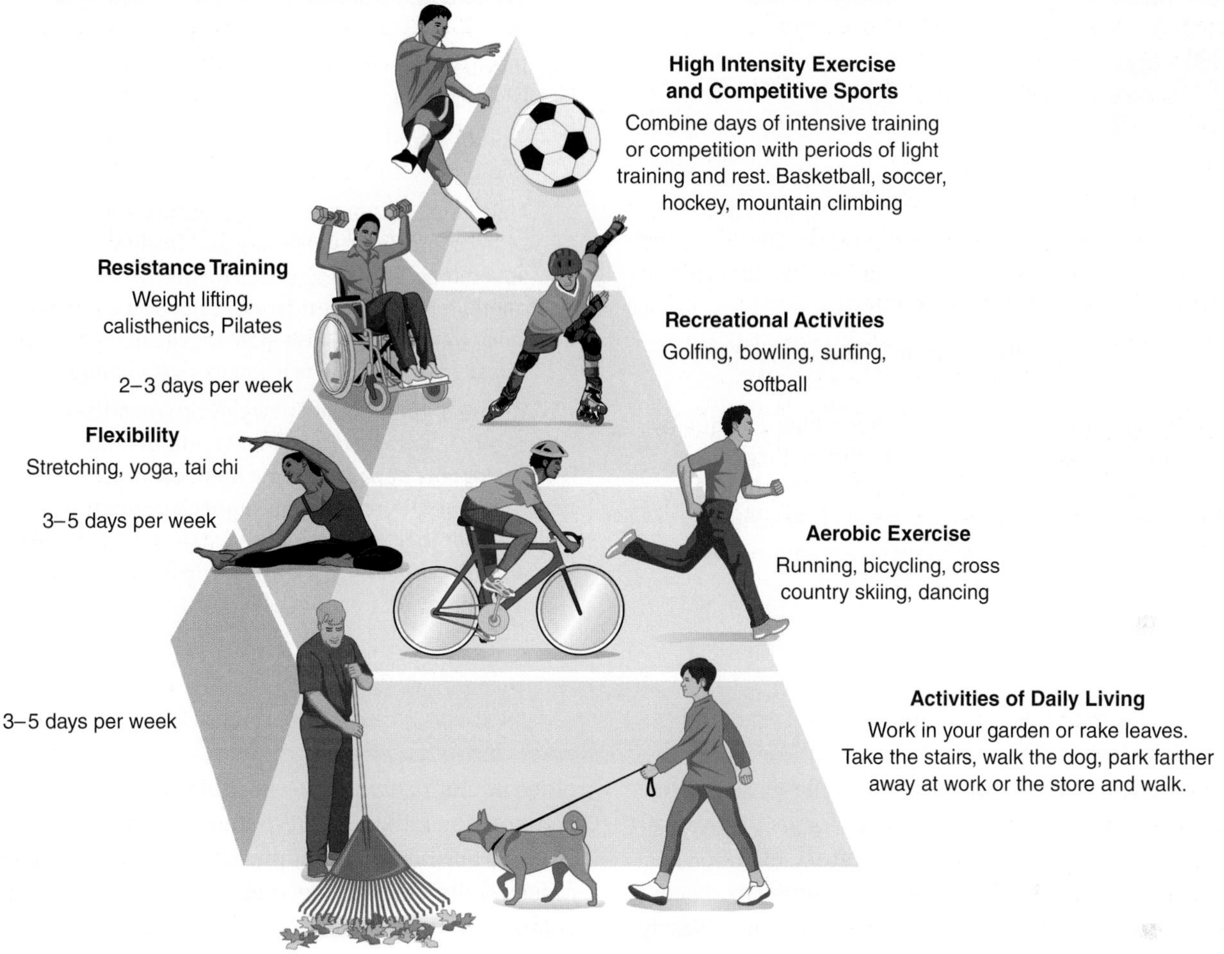

High Intensity Exercise and Competitive Sports
Combine days of intensive training or competition with periods of light training and rest. Basketball, soccer, hockey, mountain climbing

Resistance Training
Weight lifting, calisthenics, Pilates
2–3 days per week

Recreational Activities
Golfing, bowling, surfing, softball

Flexibility
Stretching, yoga, tai chi
3–5 days per week

Aerobic Exercise
Running, bicycling, cross country skiing, dancing

3–5 days per week

Activities of Daily Living
Work in your garden or rake leaves. Take the stairs, walk the dog, park farther away at work or the store and walk.

recommendations for healthy lifestyles. To track your physical activity, visit http://www.choosemyplate.gov/supertracker-tools.html.

Many aerobic and resistance activities do not require extensive time, complex skills, or special and costly equipment. For example, people can exercise by dancing to music or videos or by performing tai chi in the privacy of their homes. The main objective is to select physical activities that you enjoy and can perform regularly for the rest of your life.

As mentioned earlier, if you are unfit or older than 40 years (males) or 50 years (females), consult a physician before beginning a physical fitness program, especially one that includes vigorous-intensity activities. This precautionary measure can determine whether you have serious health problems. If you have a chronic condition, consult your physician for an exercise prescription. Most adults can begin a

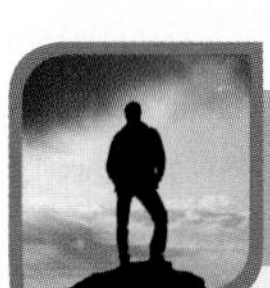

Healthy Living Practices

- Perform isometric or isotonic exercises to increase your muscular strength, and also engage in aerobic exercises to enhance your cardiorespiratory fitness.
- You can enhance your muscular strength, muscular endurance, and flexibility by increasing the frequency, duration, and intensity of your exercise sessions.
- If you have heart disease or other serious chronic conditions, are unfit, or are older than 40 years (males) or 50 years (females), obtain your physician's approval before beginning an exercise program, especially if the program includes vigorous aerobic activities.

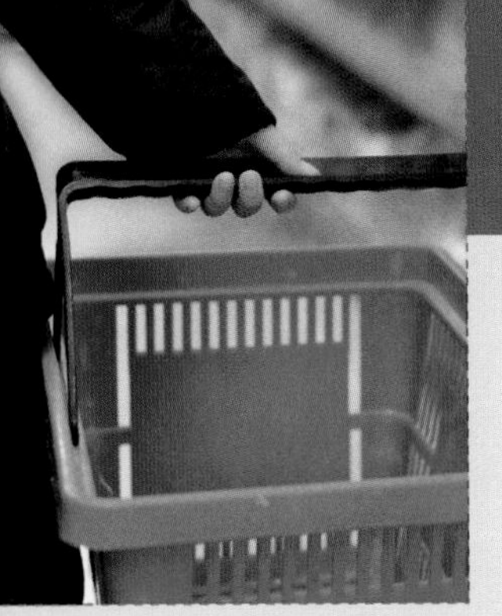

© sevenke/ShutterStock

Consumer Health

Choosing a Fitness Center

Every year millions of Americans join health clubs, gyms, and exercise and fitness centers. Thousands of these people complain about their membership to states' attorneys general, Better Business Bureaus, and other consumer protection groups. The following tips can help you avoid becoming another dissatisfied health and fitness center consumer:

- Determine whether you can afford to join the center.
- Inspect the center for cleanliness, type and quality of equipment, and especially staff qualifications. Ask if staff are certified as aerobics instructors, weight trainers, or athletic trainers. Are they trained in cardiopulmonary resuscitation (CPR) and first aid?
- Ask current members about their satisfaction with the center's facilities.
- Ask your local Better Business Bureau about the number and nature of complaints against the organization.
- Ask for a trial period to use the facilities before joining.
- Never sign a contract under pressure at the center. Many centers use confusing and misleading advertising, including prizes or special short-term offers, to spark your interest. Once you are in the facility, aggressive sales staff engage in high-pressure sales tactics to convince you to sign a contract.
- Before signing, take a few days to read the contract carefully. Make certain that you understand the details concerning payment options, membership restrictions, cancelation terms, and the membership period. If a staff member makes additional promises, have the individual record it in writing, on the contract.

regular walking program to get into shape; after a few weeks, they can add more intense forms of physical activity to boost their cardiorespiratory fitness.

It is a good idea for pregnant women to discuss their exercise plans with their physicians. Nearly all pregnant women can safely walk, swim, or ride a stationary bicycle (**Figure 11.14**). Healthy pregnant women should engage in at least 30 minutes of moderate-intensity exercise daily on most or all days of the week.[35,36] Those who are obese or severely underweight, are sedentary, or have histories of health problems should consult their physicians before following an exercise program.

As people age, they experience numerous changes that indicate a decline in their physical conditions. For example, the maximum age-predicted heart rates of older adults are lower during exercise, and their hearts pump less blood with each beat. Compared to when they were young adults, most aged persons have more body fat. Although exercise training of older adults does not prevent these physical changes, it can limit the extent of the decline.

Most Americans become less active as they age. Less than half (48%) of all U.S. adults meet physical activity guidelines.[37] It is important for people to continue exercising as they age (**Figure 11.15**). Physically fit older adults usually have healthier hearts and body compositions than unfit people of the same age. Even by performing light physical activities regularly, older adults can reduce their risk of heart disease, colon cancer, diabetes, obesity, and hypertension.[38]

Figure 11.14

Exercising During Pregnancy. Nearly all pregnant women can safely stretch, walk, swim, or ride a stationary bicycle.

© Photodisc

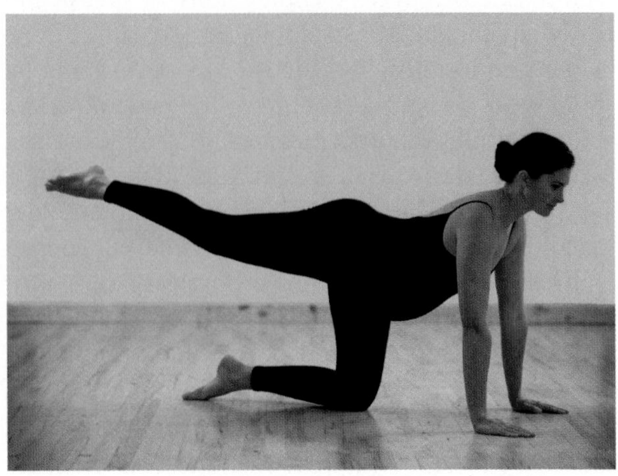

Figure 11.15

Exercise Is for Everyone. It is important for people to continue exercising as they age.

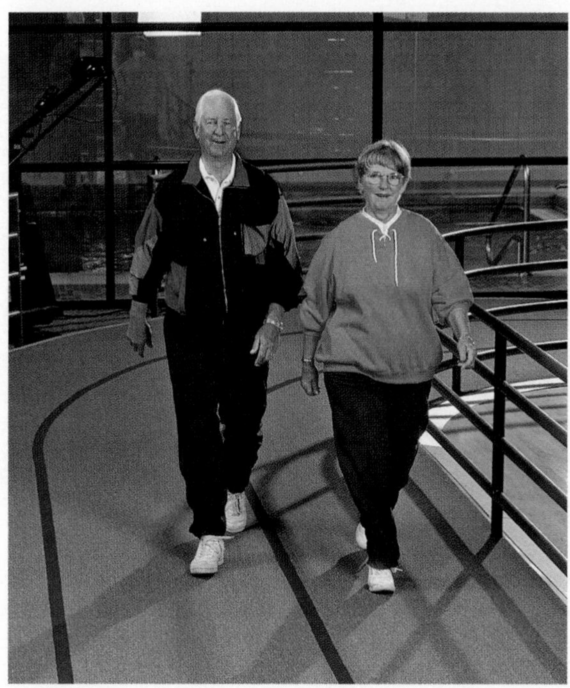

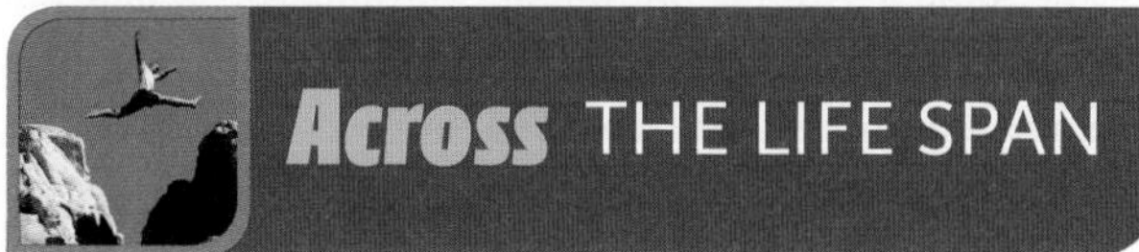

Across THE LIFE SPAN

PHYSICAL FITNESS

The health habits that a person adopts in childhood, including physical and sports activities, are likely to be practiced and enjoyed for a lifetime. Children who are physically active have better measures of all health-related fitness components than those who are sedentary. Because sedentary lifestyles are associated with heart disease in adults, many pediatricians are concerned that children may begin to develop this disease, especially if they do not engage in physical activities regularly. To improve the overall health and well-being of children, parents and schools need to find ways to encourage youngsters who are physically unfit to increase their fitness levels.

Another major concern of health and fitness experts is the proportion of American children and adolescents who spend a considerable amount of time engaged in sedentary activities, such as playing computer games or viewing television. In 2013, about 29% of American high school students attended physical education (PE) classes 5 days a week.[34] More research is needed to determine the long-term effects of childhood and adolescent activity habits on their future health.

Regular exercise is just as important during pregnancy as in the other times of a woman's life. Healthy, physically fit women can continue engaging in a program of mild to moderate physical activity throughout their pregnancies.[35] However, performing strenuous exercise (e.g., jogging) five or more times per week may increase the risk of having a low-birth-weight baby.[36] The ability to engage comfortably and safely in many physical activities often becomes limited in the latter stage of pregnancy. During this time, a woman's weight usually increases dramatically, especially in the center and front part of her body. As a result, she often feels awkward while engaging in many physical activities, and her risk of injury increases.

A pregnant woman should avoid activities if they pose a risk to her health and that of her developing fetus. Physical activities that might result in falls or injuries to the abdominal area and exhaustive exercises such as contact sports, heavy weightlifting, or training and participating in competitive events are generally not recommended for pregnant women. Additionally, exercising while lying down may interfere with blood flow to the uterus and is not recommended. It is important for pregnant women to be well hydrated before, during, and after exercise and to avoid overheating. Physicians do not recommend that pregnant women exercise in hot, humid conditions or use hot tubs and saunas because these activities can raise the woman's body temperature, endangering the fetus.

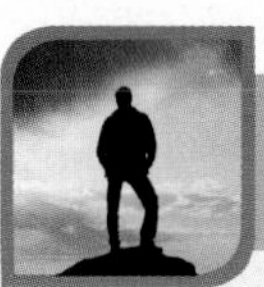

Healthy Living Practices

- ☐ To become physically fit or to maintain a high degree of fitness, design a personal fitness program that includes activities that you enjoy and can perform regularly while you are in college and throughout your lifetime.
- ☐ If you have a sedentary lifestyle, find ways to become more physically active at work and home, such as walking some of the way to work, using the stairs instead of elevators, doing housework, and walking during your leisure time.

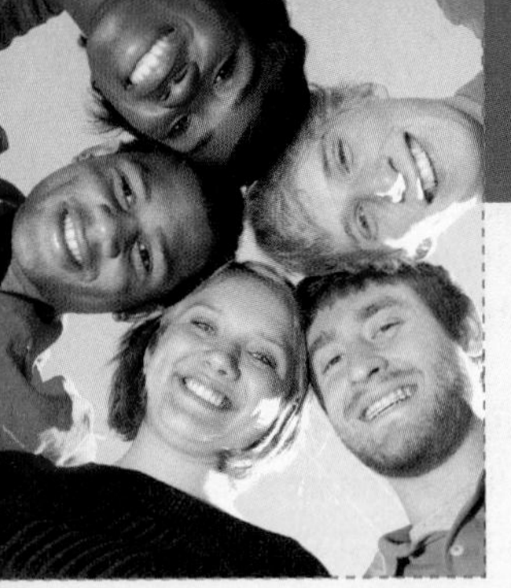

© Mike Flippo/ShutterStock

Diversity in Health

New Interest in an Ancient Approach to Fitness

In motion
all parts of the body must be
light,
nimble,
and strung together.

From T'ai chi ch'uan
by Chang San-feng (1279–1386)

To people outside of China, it may seem difficult to believe that the graceful dancelike movements of t'ai chi ch'uan (tie-jee-chwahn), commonly called "tai chi," are a form of exercise. Unlike Western physical activities that often require rapid, forceful, and extensive motions, tai chi involves gentle gliding muscular movements that do not overextend body parts. According to its promoters, tai chi promotes good health, physical fitness, and longevity.

The exact origins of traditional tai chi are unknown. For more than 2,000 years, the Chinese have practiced *qigong* (*ch'i-kung*), a series of simple exercises that focus on breathing, maintaining certain body postures, and relaxing. These features are also emphasized in tai chi. In fact, the word *chi* means "breath energy." Thus, the ancient practice of qigong may have set the stage for the development of tai chi.

In addition to qigong, the Chinese martial arts probably contributed to the development of tai chi ch'uan. *Ch'uan* means "the joy of fighting with bare fists." Originally tai chi ch'uan may have been used for self-defense or boxing. However, a major principle of tai chi ch'uan is to overcome brute force and harshness with softness, gentleness, and smoothness.

Chang San-feng, the 13th-century Taoist priest whose writing appears here, is usually credited with creating tai chi. Taoism is an ancient Chinese religion and philosophy that emphasizes living in harmony with nature. To Taoists, the harmonious functioning of the body is important if one is to achieve good health and live a long life. Today, tai chi is growing in popularity with Western exercise enthusiasts who are interested in achieving its potential health benefits (**Figure 11.C**). Promoters of tai chi claim that the physical exercises improve digestion and circulation, as well as increase alertness. People who practice tai chi often report that the exercises reduce stress.

While performing the specific sequential exercises, the upper part of the body remains loose; the knees are slightly bent but firmly supporting the weight of the body. Movements flow from one to another. Opposing arms and legs move in harmony; for example, as one arm gracefully arches upward, the other moves down in the same fashion. According to those who teach tai chi, if one body part does not follow another, the body is not in harmony. The series of vertical and horizontal movements continues until the sequence of exercises has been completed.

Figure 11.C

Tai Chi. Practicing tai chi improves flexibility, muscular strength, and balance.

© Thomas Barrat/ShutterStock

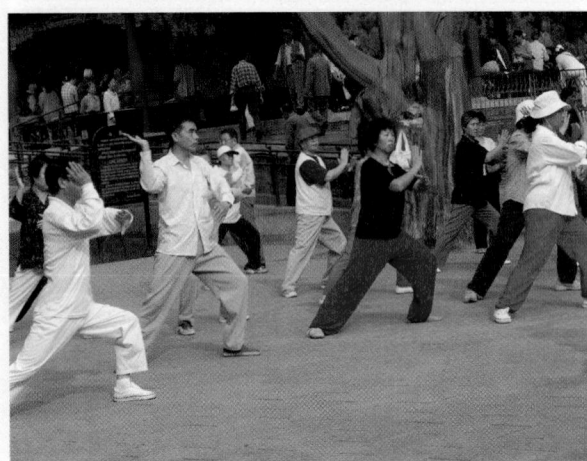

An important aspect of tai chi is mental concentration. As individuals engage in these exercises, they focus their attention on the sensations associated with the sequential movements; such attention requires silence.

As with other physical activities, practicing tai chi every day improves flexibility, muscular strength, and balance. Because tai chi does not require rapid, forceful muscular movements, it is a beneficial form of physical activity for elderly people or anyone who cannot engage in aerobic exercises.

A specially trained instructor is necessary to teach the proper posture, sequences of coordinated movements, and breathing technique of tai chi. Therefore, if you are interested in learning the exercises, check with the physical education department at your college or university to see if it offers tai chi instruction. Fitness centers in your community, such as the YMCA, might also offer tai chi classes.

Additionally, physical activity helps maintain or improve the flexibility of joints as well as the strength and endurance of muscles. Regular exercise improves the mood of elderly people and increases their ability to live independently.[38] Older adults can enjoy the social aspects of exercising by joining mall-walking, dancing, or fitness classes that are designed for older adults.

People lose their ability to maintain their balance as they age, which increases their risk of falling. A minor fall that would not injure a healthy 23-year-old person can have dire consequences for a frail 85-year-old one. An elderly person who falls is more likely to suffer a disabling bone fracture or die from the injury than a younger person is. Aged people who survive falls often experience some degree of immobility and pain that limits their ability to care for themselves and interact socially. By participating in exercise classes that improve balance and muscular strength, older adults can reduce their risk of falls.[39] The Diversity in Health essay in this chapter describes the benefits of tai chi, a form of martial arts that helps some elderly people become healthier.

It is never too late to become physically fit. By increasing physical activity, even very old people can gain healthful benefits such as improved muscular strength and endurance, flexibility, and psychological well-being. To achieve these benefits, participation in strenuous formal exercise programs is not necessary; most elderly people can improve their overall health by engaging in light to moderate physical activities regularly such as walking, gardening, or mall-walking every day.

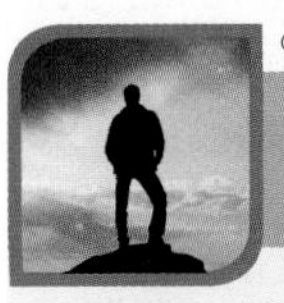

Healthy Living Practices

- ☐ If you have children, consider limiting the amount of time they spend watching television or playing computer games. Encourage your children to be physically active.
- ☐ If you are pregnant, consult your physician to determine which physical activities are safe to perform during this time.
- ☐ As you age, exercise regularly and be physically active.

CHAPTER REVIEW

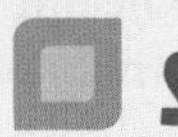

Summary

Regardless of age and physical condition, nearly everyone can achieve numerous health benefits by engaging in physical activity and exercise. Performing regular, vigorous exercise and physical activity can build, maintain, and preserve skeletal muscles; improve the circulation and functioning of the heart; and regulate the amount of body fat. Weight-bearing exercises such as walking, dancing, and jogging strengthen bones, which can prevent or delay the development of osteoporosis. Healthy adults younger than 65 years should perform moderate-intensity physical activity for 30 minutes a day, 5 days a week.

Besides improving physical health, exercise can have short-term and long-term psychological benefits. Physical activity can reduce symptoms of anxiety and depression and improve mood and well-being.

The health-related components of physical fitness are cardiorespiratory fitness, muscular strength, muscular endurance, flexibility, and body composition. Many fitness experts consider cardiorespiratory fitness the most important health-related element of physical fitness.

Regular aerobic exercise enhances cardiorespiratory fitness, increasing the stroke volume of the heart and reducing the resting heart rate. Examples of popular aerobic activities include running, jogging, race-walking, lap swimming, cycling, stair-stepping, aerobic dancing, cross-country skiing, and rope skipping.

To develop muscular strength, muscles need to be overloaded by repeatedly moving objects that become progressively heavier. When muscles are overloaded, they hypertrophy; when muscles are not used, they atrophy or detrain. Detraining can occur within a couple of weeks after people discontinue their exercise training regimen. Thus, people must maintain their exercise programs to avoid detraining.

Immediate first aid for most musculoskeletal injuries includes RICE, the combination of rest, ice, compression, and elevation. Hypothermia and hyperthermia are serious temperature-related injuries that can occur when the body is unable to maintain its temperature in the normal range. Exercising in hot weather can produce heat cramps, heat exhaustion, or heatstroke. If untreated, heat cramps or heat exhaustion can lead to heatstroke, which can be fatal. Maintaining adequate hydration and avoiding overexertion in hot and humid conditions can reduce the risk of heat-related illnesses. To avoid frostbite or hypothermia, people should dress warmly while outdoors in cold and windy conditions, keeping their skin well covered.

When planning an effective overall fitness regimen, people need to consider the type, frequency, duration, and intensity of their exercise activities. Individuals should design personal fitness programs that provide health benefits, satisfy their needs and interests, and can be followed for a lifetime. Before beginning fitness regimens that include aerobic activities, people with heart disease or other serious chronic conditions and people who are out of shape or older than 40 years should obtain the approval of their physicians.

Regular physical activity is just as important for youngsters as for adults. Performing certain activities may be risky during pregnancy; therefore, pregnant women should discuss their physical activity with their physicians. In most cases, it is never too late for people to begin fitness programs. By engaging in light to moderate physical activities regularly, such as walking or gardening every day, older adults can improve their overall health.

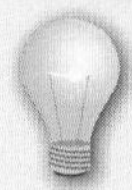

Applying What You Have Learned

1. Calculate your target heart rate zone. **Application**
2. For 3 days, record the amount of time you spend engaging in various physical activities, such as walking to class, playing racquetball, or riding a bike. Use Table 11-2 to classify your physical activities as being light, moderate, or intense. **Analysis**
3. Plan an exercise program. **Synthesis**
4. Evaluate your current level of cardiorespiratory fitness. **Evaluation**

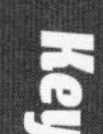

Key

Application using information in a new situation.

Analysis breaking down information into component parts.

Synthesis putting together information from different sources.

Evaluation making informed decisions.

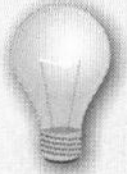

Reflecting on Your Health

1. Are you satisfied with your level of physical fitness? Why or why not? If you are dissatisfied, what ideas did you get from reading this chapter that will help you improve your fitness? If you are satisfied, how will you maintain your fitness?
2. What benefits would you derive from adopting a more physically active lifestyle? What factors interfere with and what factors reinforce your efforts to become more physically fit?
3. Before reading this chapter, how did you feel about ergogenic aids such as dietary supplements or anabolic steroids to enhance athletic performance? Based on what you have read in this chapter, has your attitude changed? Why or why not?
4. If you have children or are thinking about having children, how would you encourage them to maintain a balance between the time they spend engaging in sedentary activities such as watching TV and in activities that develop physical fitness?
5. Which labor-saving devices would you be willing to stop using so that you could use your muscles to do the work? Why did you choose these devices or machines? Describe practical steps you can take to increase your physical activity level.

CHAPTER REVIEW

References

1. U.S. Department of Health and Human Services. (2008). *Physical activity guidelines for Americans.* Retrieved from http://www.health.gov/PAGuidelines/factsheetprof.aspx
2. Centers for Disease Control and Prevention. (2012). *Behavioral Risk Factor Surveillance System: Exercise—2012.* Retrieved from http://apps.nccd.cdc.gov/brfss/list.asp?cat=EX&yr=2012&qkey=8041&state=All
3. Centers for Disease Control and Prevention. (2014). *Facts about physical activity.* Retrieved from http://www.cdc.gov/physicalactivity/data/facts.html
4. U.S. Department of Health and Human Services. (2008). Chapter 2: Physical activity has many health benefits. In *Physical activity guidelines for Americans.* Retrieved from http://www.health.gov/paguidelines/guidelines/chapter2.aspx
5. U.S. Department of Health and Human Services. (1996). *Physical activity and health: A report of the Surgeon General.* Atlanta, GA: Centers for Disease Control and Prevention, National Center for Chronic Disease Prevention and Health Promotion.
6. Ströhle, A. (2009). Physical activity, exercise, depression and anxiety disorders. *Journal of Neural Transmission, 116*(6), 777–784.
7. Youngstedt, S. D. (2005). Effects of exercise on sleep. *Clinics in Sports Medicine, 24*(2), 355–365.
8. Lang, C., et al. (2013). Increased self-reported and objectively assessed physical activity predict sleep quality among adolescents. *Physiology & Behavior, 120*, 46–53.
9. Josefsson, T., Lindwall, M., & Archer, T. Physical exercise intervention in depressive disorders: Meta-analysis and systematic review. *Scandinavian Journal of Medicine & Science in Sports, 24*(2), 259–273.
10. Anners, L., Hannevig, C. E., & Pederson, G. (2013). Prescribed exercise: A prospective study of health-related quality of life and physical fitness among participants in an officially sponsored municipal physical training program. *Journal of Physical Activity & Health, 10*(7), 1016–1015.
11. Gulati, M., et al. (2010). Heart rate response to exercise stress testing in asymptomatic women: The St. James Women Take Heart Project. *Circulation, 122*(2), 130–137.
12. Bosquet, L., et al. (2013). Effect of training cessation of muscular performance: A meta-analysis. *Scandinavian Journal of Medicine & Science in Sports, 23*(3), 140–149.
13. Feigenbaum, M. S., & Pollock, M. L. (1999). Prescription of resistance training for health and disease. *Medicine & Science in Sports & Exercise, 31*(1), 38–45.
14. Garber, C. E., et al. (2011). Quantity and quality of exercise for developing and maintaining cardiorespiratory, musculoskeletal, and neuromotor fitness in apparently healthy adults: Guidance for prescribing exercise. *Medicine & Science in Sports & Exercise, 43*(7), 1334–1359.
15. Behm, D., & Chaouachi, A. (2011). A review of acute effects of static and dynamic stretching on performance. *European Journal of Applied Physiology, 111*, 2633–2651.
16. Hoy, D., et al. (2010). The epidemiology of low back pain. *Best Practices in Research Clinical Rheumatology, 24*(6), 769–781.
17. McGill, S. (2007). *Low back disorders: Evidence-based prevention and rehabilitation* (2nd ed.). Champaign, IL: Human Kinetics.
18. Potteiger, J. A., et al. (2008). Changes in resting metabolic rate and substrate oxidation after 16 months of exercise training in overweight adults. *International Journal of Sport Nutrition and Exercise Metabolism, 18*, 79–95.
19. Pasiakos, S., Harris, L., & McLellan, T. (2014). Effects of protein supplements on muscle damage, soreness and recovery of muscle function and physical performance: A systematic review. *Sports Medicine, 44*(5), 655–670.
20. Schoch, R. D., et al. (2006). The regulation and expression of the creatine transporter: A brief review of creatine supplementation in humans and animals. *Journal of International Society of Sports Nutrition, 3*, 60–66.
21. Mitchell, G. J. (2007). *Report to the commissioner of baseball of an independent investigation into the illegal use of steroids and other performance enhancing substances by players of Major League Baseball.* Retrieved May 25, 2011, from http://files.mlb.com/mitchrpt.pdf
22. National Institute on Drug Abuse. (2010, August). *NIDA infofacts: High school and youth trends.* Retrieved May 25, 2011, from http://www.nida.nih.gov/infofacts/hsyouthtrends.html
23. Yu, S., et al. (2003). What level of physical activity protects against premature cardiovascular death? The Caerphilly study. *Heart, 89*(5), 502–506.
24. Sundquist, K., et al. (2005). The long-term effect of physical activity on incidence of coronary heart disease: A 12-year follow-up study. *Preventive Medicine, 41*(1), 219–225.
25. Law, R. Y., & Herbert, R. D. (2007). Warm-up reduces delayed onset muscle soreness but cool-down does not: A randomised controlled trial. *Australian Journal of Physiotherapy, 53*(2), 91–95.
26. Fradkin, A. J., et al. (2006). Does warming up prevent injury in sport? The evidence from randomised controlled trials. *Journal of Science and Medicine in Sport, 9*(3), 214–220.
27. Lepanen, M., et al. (2014). Interventions to prevent sport related injuries: A systematic review and meta-analysis of randomized controlled trials. *Sports Medicine, 44*(4), 473–486.
28. Hart, L. (2005). Effect of stretching on sport injury risk: A review. *Clinical Journal of Sport Medicine, 15*(2), 113.
29. Grooms, D., et al. (2013). Soccer-specific warm-up and lower extremity injury rates in collegiate male soccer players. *Journal of Athletic Training, 48*(6), 782–788.
30. American College of Sports Medicine, Sawka, M. N., et al. (2007). American College of Sports Medicine position stand: Exercise and fluid replacement. *Medicine & Science in Sports & Exercise, 39*(2), 377–390.
31. Kenefick, R., & Cheuvront, S. N. (2012). Hydration for recreational sport and physical activity. *Nutrition Reviews, 70*(ps137), 6.
32. Williams, M. H. (2007). *Nutrition for health, fitness, and sport* (8th ed.). New York, NY: WCB McGraw-Hill.
33. National Library of Medicine, National Institutes of Health. (2011, May 18). Hypothermia. Retrieved May 25, 2011, from http://www.nlm.nih.gov/medlineplus/hypothermia.html

34. Centers for Disease Control and Prevention. (2014). Youth risk behavior surveillance: United States, 2013. *Morbidity and Mortality Weekly Report, 63*(SS-4).

35. American College of Obstetricians and Gynecologists. (2002; reaffirmed 2009). ACOG committee opinion: Exercise during pregnancy and the postpartum period. *International Journal of Gynaecology and Obstetrics, 77*(1), 79–81.

36. Campbell, M. K., & Mottola, M. F. (2001). Recreational exercise and occupational activity during pregnancy and birth weight: A case-control study. *American Journal of Obstetrics and Gynecology, 184*(3), 403–408.

37. Centers for Disease Control and Prevention. (2014). *Facts about physical activity*. Retrieved from http://www.cdc.gov/physicalactivity/data/facts.html

38. Agency for Healthcare Research and Quality, Centers for Disease Control and Prevention, U.S. Department of Health and Human Services. (2002). *Physical activity and older Americans: Benefits and strategies*. Retrieved September 22, 2014 from http://www.innovations.ahrq.gov/content.aspx?id=991

39. Liu, H., & Frank, A. (2010). Tai chi as a balance improvement exercise for older adults: A systematic review. *Journal of Geriatric Physical Therapy, 33*(3), 103–109.

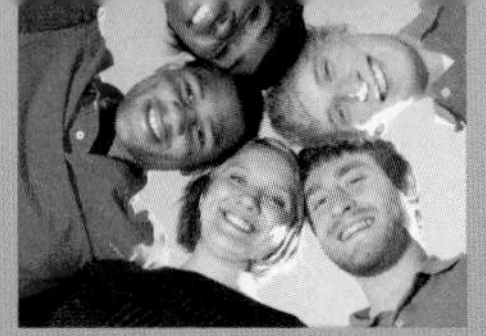

Diversity in Health
The Italian Gene: A Hope for Reversing Atherosclerosis?

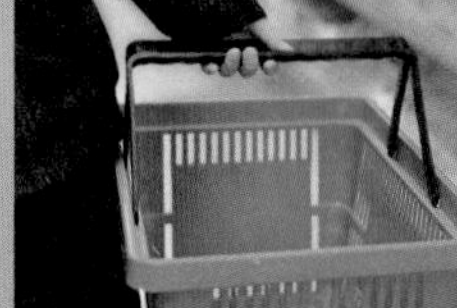

Consumer Health
Vitamin Pills for a Healthier Heart?

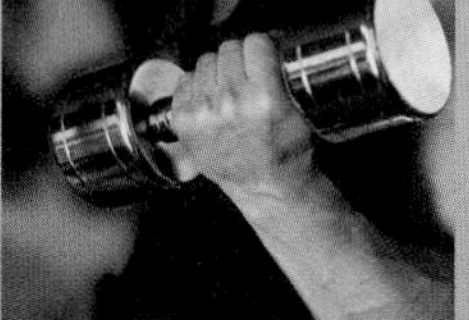

Managing Your Health
Heart Attack and Stroke (Brain Attack) Symptoms: What to Do in an Emergency

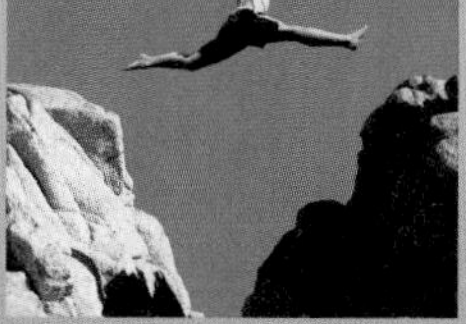

Across the Life Span
Cardiovascular Health

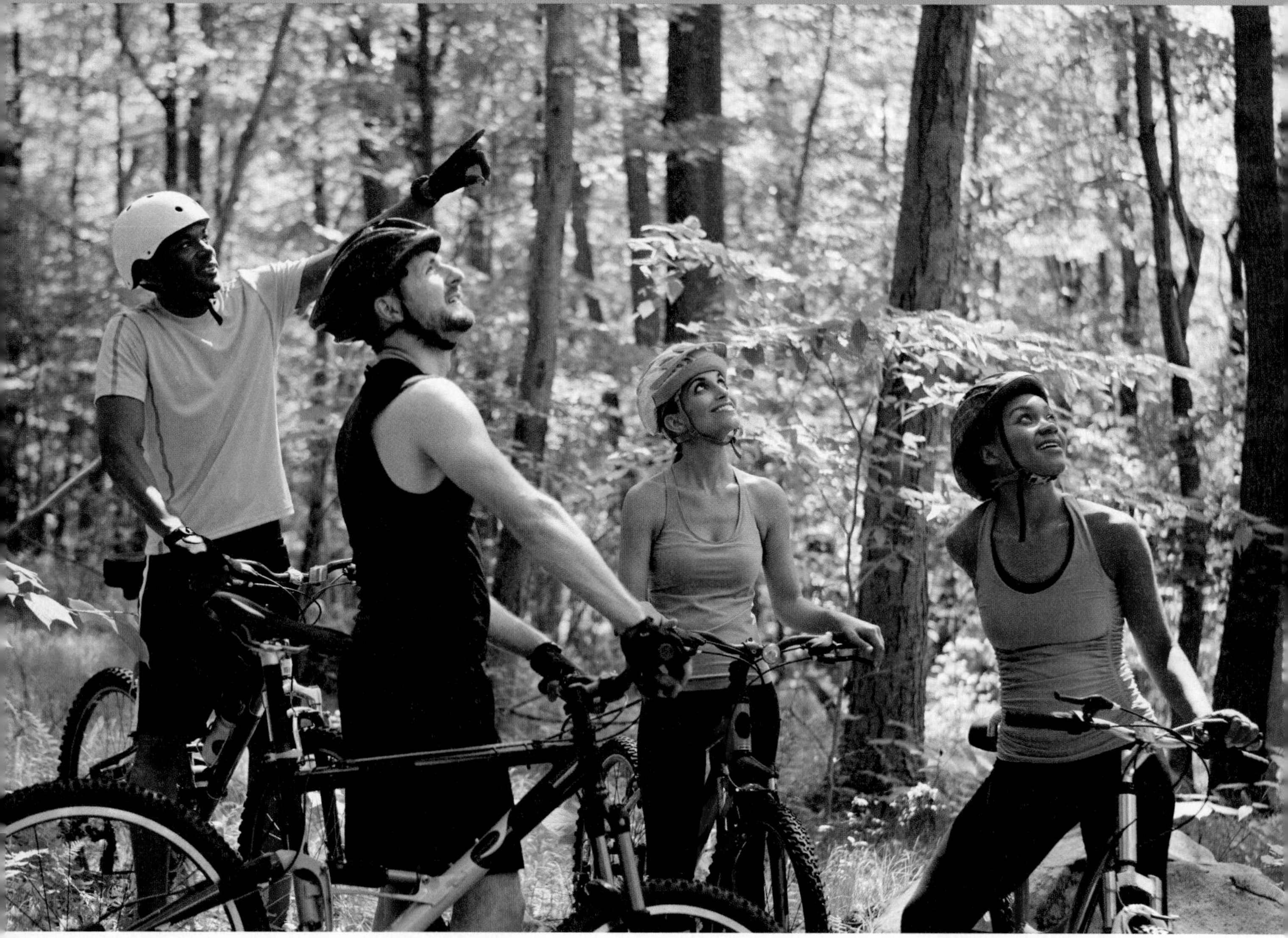

Chapter Overview

How the cardiovascular system works

Symptoms of and treatments for cardiovascular disease

Risk factors for cardiovascular disease

How to maintain your cardiovascular health

Student Workbook

Self-Assessment: What Is Your Risk of Developing Heart Disease or Having a Heart Attack?

Changing Health Habits: Reducing Your Risk of Cardiovascular Disease

Do You Know?

What to do to keep your heart and blood vessels healthy?

What to do if you or someone you know is having a heart attack?

If you are likely to have a heart attack or stroke?

CHAPTER 12

Cardiovascular Health

Learning Objectives

After studying this chapter, you should be able to:

1. Describe functions of the cardiovascular system.
2. Define atherosclerosis and explain how this process results in cardiovascular disease.
3. Identify major risk factors for cardiovascular disease.
4. Identify recommendations for cholesterol and blood pressure levels.
5. Differentiate between HDL and LDL and identify healthy levels of each.
6. Explain the significance of HDL or LDL levels on cardiovascular disease risk.
7. Describe the signs and symptoms of angina, heart attack, and stroke.
8. Describe actions that can reduce cardiovascular disease risk.
9. Discuss modern methods of treating cardiovascular disease.

"... reducing the likelihood of developing cardiovascular disease later in life involves controlling risk factors early in life."

Do you think that you are immune from cardiovascular disease—dysfunction of the heart and blood vessels—because you are young? If so, think again! Even though cardiovascular disease (CVD) does not normally occur in young adults, unhealthy lifestyle patterns practiced and ingrained during this stage of life predispose a person to cardiovascular disease. Metabolic processes leading to cardiovascular disease *can* begin in childhood and accelerate at adolescence.[1]

In one large multicenter study, medical researchers examined the relationship of the risk factors for cardiovascular disease (such as smoking, obesity, poor diet, and lack of exercise) to the development of fatty deposits in the arteries, which is one process that occurs in the development of this condition.[2] They studied nearly 3,000 persons aged 15 to 34 years who died from accidents, homicides, and suicides. The results of the study revealed that young persons with risk factors for CVD began developing fatty streaks within their arteries in their teenage years. By age 25, young persons with risk factors also had developed raised lesions in the major blood vessels of the heart. The results of this and other studies show that reducing the likelihood of developing cardiovascular disease later in life involves controlling risk factors early in life.[3] Behaviors in adolescence and young adulthood *do* matter: They can influence your health for years to come and can affect your life span.

Research results also show that college students are aware of cardiovascular risk factors, but many do not put this knowledge into practice. In other words, their understandings of heart-healthy behaviors and their lifestyles do not match.[4,5]

One reason for this disconnection may be rooted in emotions and psychology; how people feel about what they know has an effect on their actions. For example, if you know smoking causes many types of cancers, but you love to smoke, it may affect how you respond to that knowledge. For some, the pleasure derived from smoking may outweigh their concerns about cancer risk. The disconnection between knowledge and actions may also be explained by misconceptions about heart disease.[4] For example, some college students may think that heart disease is a significant health concern only for men, when it is the leading cause of death in both genders. College-aged women holding this misconception may think that practicing heart-healthy behaviors is not important for them. Some college students may also think people who are White are most affected by heart disease; however, Americans who are Black or Pacific Islanders have higher death rates from heart disease in the United States.. Thus, some Blacks and Pacific Islanders may perceive a lower level of risk for heart disease.

The "Changing Health Habits" feature "Reducing Your Risk of Cardiovascular Disease" in the Student Workbook pages at the end of this text can help you understand the impact of your current lifestyle beahviors on your risk for developing cardiovascular disease, and may motivate you to implement heart-healthy lifestyle changes. But first, this chapter explores the cardiovascular system and how it works. It then describes the causes of cardiovascular diseases and hypertension—noninfectious diseases in which hereditary, environmental, and lifestyle factors interact to create an individual's risk level for developing any one of them. It also describes the interrelatedness of these diseases and how the development of one affects the development of another. Last, it explores the factors critical to maintaining cardiovascular health, to help you preserve the fitness of your heart and blood vessels throughout your lifetime.

The Cardiovascular System and How It Works

You may have heard the cardiovascular system also referred to as the circulatory system. These terms are often used interchangeably. The term *cardiovascular* refers to the heart (*cardio-*) and blood vessels (*vascular*). The term *circulatory* refers to the circulation of the blood. In practical use, both terms describe a body system that pumps blood enclosed in blood vessels to all parts of the body.

Blood is a somewhat viscous fluid made up of cells suspended in a liquid. Blood performs many functions:

- It contains red blood cells and fluid (plasma) that transport the respiratory gases (oxygen and carbon dioxide), nutrients, hormones, enzymes, and waste products.
- It helps regulate body temperature by distributing the heat generated by chemical reactions in the body.
- It contains blood clotting factors (including pieces of cells called *platelets*) that protect the blood supply from excessive losses and help in tissue repair.
- It contains white blood cells (including the lymphocytes of the immune system) that help protect the body from infection.

The blood is pumped by the heart, a muscular, fist-sized organ that lies in the chest cavity about midway between the shoulders and the waist, and slightly to the left of the midline (**Figure 12.1**). The heart consists of four chambers: two upper chambers called *atria* and two lower chambers called *ventricles*. The upper chambers receive blood and then push it into the lower chambers, which pump blood to the lungs and the rest of the body.

Figure 12.1

The Major Arteries of the Body. The heart is located to the left of the midline in the chest cavity. The arteries take blood away from the heart and are shown in red. Veins return blood to the heart and are shown in blue.

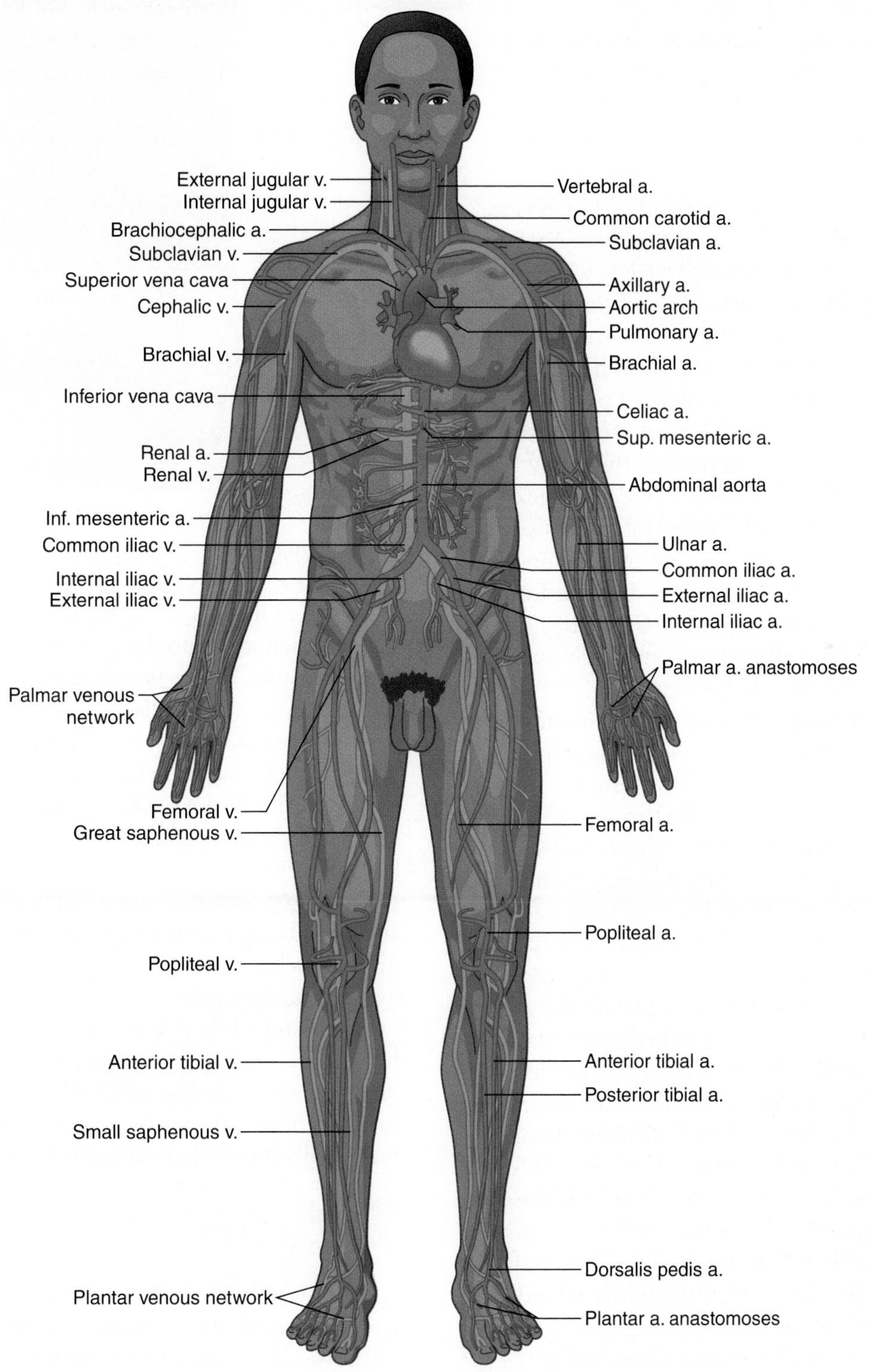

arteries Blood vessels that carry blood away from the heart.

capillaries (KAP-ih-LAIR-eez) Microscopic blood vessels that permeate tissues, connecting small arteries to small veins.

veins Blood vessels that return blood to the heart.

coronary arteries Blood vessels that arise from the base of the aorta and bring freshly oxygenated blood to the heart muscle.

coronary artery disease (CAD) A condition in which the coronary vessels are blocked partially or completely by fatty deposits, blood clots, or both. Also commonly called coronary heart disease (CHD).

Blood flows within a vast network of blood vessels. **Arteries** carry blood away from the heart. They have muscular, elastic walls that bulge slightly when the left ventricle contracts and pushes blood through them, and they recoil at the end of the beat. Arteries branch into smaller vessels called *arterioles*. When these vessels become so small that they allow the passage of only one blood cell at a time, they are called **capillaries**.

The capillaries permeate tissues. These tiny blood vessels have walls that are only one cell thick. The thinness of capillary walls allows substances such as nutrients and oxygen to move out of the blood, and other substances such as waste products and carbon dioxide to move into the blood. Capillaries join to form larger vessels called *venules*, which in turn join to form still larger vessels, the veins.

Veins return blood to the heart. By the time the blood reaches the veins, it has lost most of the force (pressure) of its push from the heart. Therefore, veins have thinner walls than do arteries; they contain less muscle and elastic tissue. In addition, veins have one-way valves along their length, which help prevent the backflow of blood. Blood returning to the heart from the head, neck, and shoulders is helped along by the force of gravity. Blood returning to the heart from the arms, legs, and torso combats the force of gravity but is pushed along as the skeletal muscles squeeze the veins in these areas.

If the walls of the veins in the arms, legs, and torso are weak, or if the valves are stretched or damaged, blood may not be returned to the heart efficiently. Blood may collect in the veins and may flow backward. This situation puts additional pressure on the walls of the veins and contributes to a condition called *venous disease*. Venous disease includes varicose veins (distended or stretched veins), deep vein thrombosis (blood clots in the deep veins), and chronic venous insufficiency (swollen legs). **Figure 12.2** shows varicose veins.

Figure 12.2

Close-up of Varicose Veins on a Man's Leg.

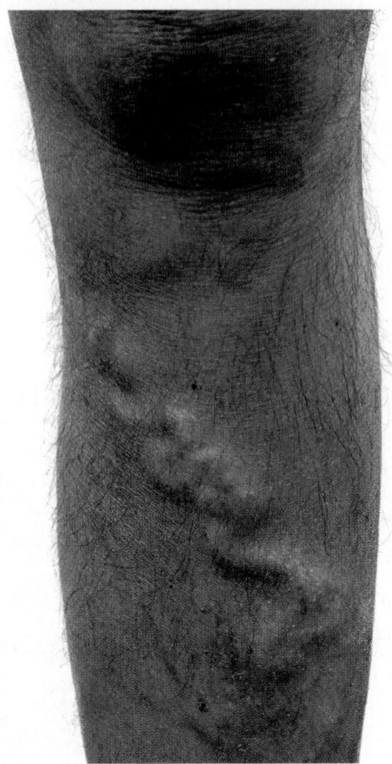

The incidence of both moderate and severe venous disease increases with age. Although women are twice as likely as men to have moderate venous disease, men are more likely to have severe disease. Non-Hispanic White people are much more likely to have severe venous disease compared to Hispanic, African American, and Asian people, in the United States. Other risk factors for venous disease include family health history, obesity, having borne more than one child, and consistently standing for prolonged periods.[6]

Coronary arteries arise from the base of the aorta and bring freshly oxygenated blood to the heart muscle itself. (Although blood flows in and out of the heart's chambers, the heart muscle is not nourished by the blood while it is in the chambers.) There are two main coronary arteries: the left and the right coronary arteries (see Figure 12.8 later in this chapter). Both of these arteries branch into multiple vessels that supply the entire heart with blood.

Cardiovascular Diseases

A person with blocked coronary arteries is said to have **coronary artery disease (CAD)**, one type of cardiovascular disease. (Coronary artery disease is also commonly called coronary heart disease [CHD].) Coronary artery disease may result in a heart attack in which a portion of the heart muscle dies or in **angina pectoris** (chest pain).

Coronary artery disease is only one type of **cardiovascular disease (CVD)**, or dysfunction of the heart and blood vessels. Other major cardiovascular diseases are hypertension (chronic high blood pressure), stroke (blood vessel disease of the brain), and rheumatic heart disease (a complication of strep throat). Atherosclerosis (blood vessel disease) is an important cardiovascular disease process that is an underlying cause of CAD and stroke. Other cardiovascular diseases are described throughout this chapter. More than 82 million Americans (more than 1 in 3) are estimated to have one or more forms of CVD.[7] As **Figure 12.3** shows, cardiovascular disease kills more people in the United States than does any other disease.

Of the cardiovascular diseases, coronary artery disease is the number one killer, accounting for about half of all CVD deaths each year. Stroke is the next biggest CVD killer.[7] Coronary artery disease and stroke result from the development of yet another cardiovascular disease: atherosclerosis.

angina pectoris (an-JEYE-nah PECK-tor-iss) Chest pain caused by insufficient oxygen in a portion of the heart.

cardiovascular disease (CVD) (KAR-dee-oh-VAS-ku-lar) Disorders of the heart and blood vessels.

plaques (plaks) Fatty deposits in artery walls.

atherosclerosis (ATH-er-oh-skle-ROW-sis) Disease of large and medium-sized arteries in which the inner lining has areas that are deteriorated, thickened, and inelastic.

Atherosclerosis

In many CAD cases, the blood supply to portions of the heart is reduced because the coronary arteries are blocked by fatty deposits. These fatty deposits, or **plaques**, develop as part of a disease of the arteries called **atherosclerosis**. (Arterial plaque is not the same as dental plaque.) An *atheroma* is a deteriorated, thickened area on the inner lining of a large or medium-sized artery. *Sclerosis* refers to loss of elasticity, or hardening of these arteries. *Atherosclerosis* is one form of arteriosclerosis (hardening of the arteries).

Figure 12.3

Leading Causes of Death, United States, 2010. This graph shows that cardiovascular disease is the number one cause of death for both men and women (all races, all ages).

Reproduced from Heron, M. (2013, December). Deaths: Leading causes for 2010. *National Vital Statistics Reports*, 62(6). Retrieved from http://www.cdc.gov/nchs/data/nvsr/nvsr62/nvsr62_06.pdf

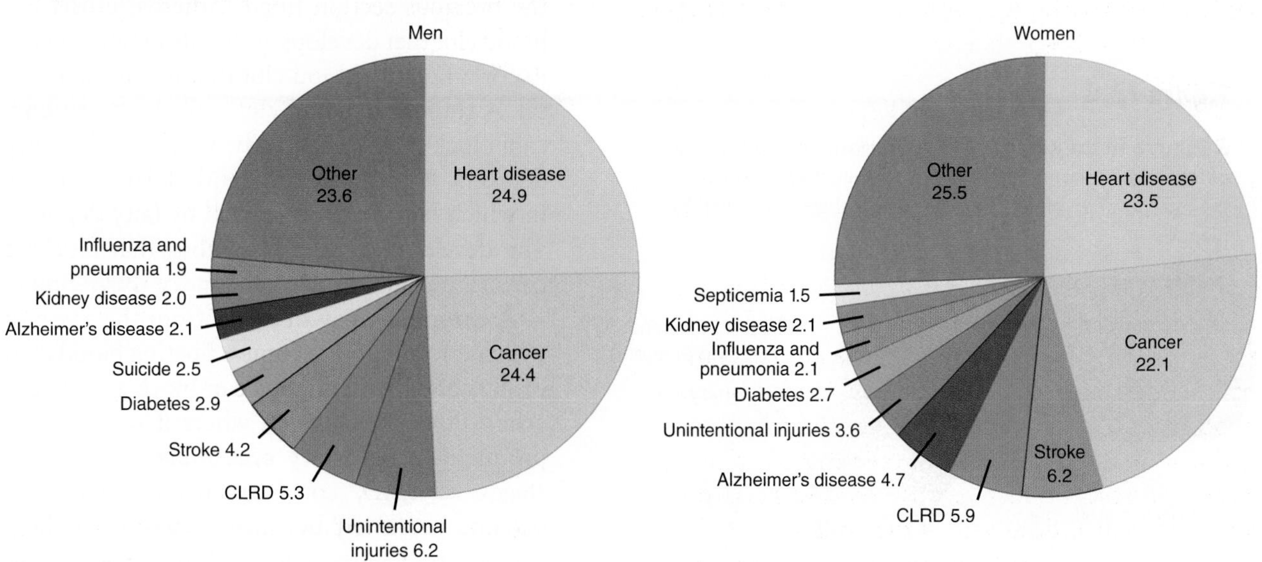

Notes: CLRD is Chronic lower respiratory diseases. Values show percentage of total deaths.

peripheral vascular disease Any blockage of vessels other than those to the heart.

thrombus (THROM-bus) A stationary blood clot.

coronary thrombosis (throm-BOW-sis) The development of a stationary blood clot that blocks blood flow in an artery that brings blood to the heart muscle.

embolus (EM-bow-lus) A floating blood clot.

coronary embolism (EM-bow-lizm) A floating blood clot that lodges in an artery that brings blood to the heart muscle, blocking blood flow.

Atherosclerosis may begin with an injury to the lining of a blood vessel. Factors such as high blood pressure, for example, can damage this lining, or the immune system may play a role. Lipids, especially cholesterol, accumulate at injury sites and cling to the interior of blood vessel walls. These plaques thicken blood vessel walls, which narrows the interiors of arteries (**Figure 12.4**) and interferes with arterial cells' ability to obtain nutrients. Eventually, the wall beneath a plaque degenerates. Scar tissue forms and calcium is often deposited there, "hardening" the artery. Blood clots sometimes develop there, too, and may be the ultimate cause of a heart attack or stroke.

Although the incidence of atherosclerosis increases with age, not all elderly people have extensive plaques. Conversely, *some young people do* (see this chapter's opening section).

Atherosclerosis occurs most often in the aorta and in the coronary, femoral, iliac, internal carotid, and cerebral arteries. Most of these vessels are labeled on Figure 12.1. As you can see, these arteries supply blood to the heart, torso, legs, and head. The cerebral arteries, not shown in the diagram, branch from the carotid arteries and other vessels to supply large portions of the brain with blood. Atherosclerosis is most serious when it develops in the vessels that supply the heart, which can lead to heart attacks, and in the vessels that supply the brain, which can result in strokes.

Heart attacks can also be caused by *coronary microvascular dysfunction*. Heart disease in women is often the result of this dysfunction, alone or in addition to plaques that block blood flow in the large coronary arteries. In coronary microvascular dysfunction, the small blood vessels of the heart do not dilate (widen) properly to supply sufficient blood to the heart muscle. Because of differences in the sizes of vessels that may be blocked or that do not function properly in their hearts, men and women often experience different symptoms when suffering heart attacks (see the section titled "Heart Attack" later in this chapter).[8]

Any blockage of vessels other than those to the heart is often referred to as **peripheral vascular disease**. This disease affects the organs and tissues that blocked vessels serve. One result of peripheral vascular disease, for example, can be erectile dysfunction (impotence) in men.

Figure 12.4

A Plaque in an Artery. A plaque is formed by a buildup of fatty material on an artery wall. This illustration shows the interior of an affected artery that has been narrowed by plaque.

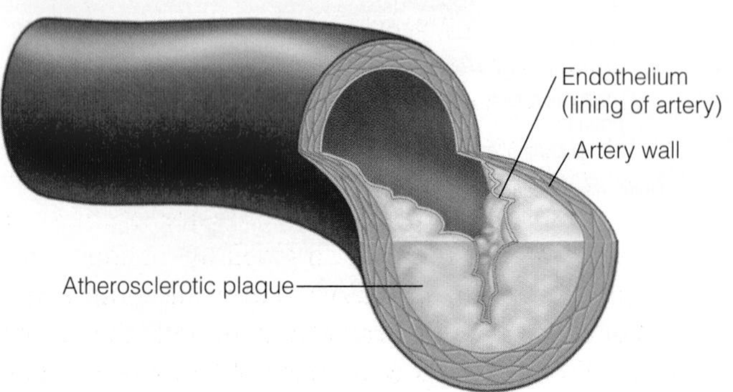

Coronary Artery Disease

In CAD, coronary vessels may become partially or completely blocked by one or more of the following: fatty deposits, which narrow blood vessels (see the previous section titled "Atherosclerosis"); a blood clot that develops at the site of fatty deposits; or a floating blood clot that lodges in a vessel. A stationary blood clot, called a **thrombus**, can block a vessel already narrowed by fatty deposits. Blood clots frequently form in vessels in which blood flow is slowed by fatty deposits. The development of a thrombus that blocks a coronary artery is called **coronary thrombosis**.

A thrombus may dislodge from the place in which it forms and become a floating blood clot, or **embolus**. An embolus can block a coronary artery downstream from where it was formed, producing a **coronary embolism**. In the early stages of CAD, coronary arteries may also become narrowed by muscle spasms of these vessels, frequently triggered by exposure to cold, physical exertion, or anxiety. Usually such muscle spasms are short lived and do not damage the heart muscle.

Angina Pectoris Spasms, partial blockage, or complete blockage of one or more of the coronary vessels can cause insufficient blood to reach part of the heart, which is called **ischemia**. When this happens, the heart does not receive sufficient oxygen and a person experiences angina pectoris, or chest pain. Angina is felt beneath the breastbone and extends to the left shoulder and down the left arm. (Pain in the arm may help you distinguish between angina and heartburn or other gastric distress.) Angina pain may also be felt in the jaw and neck and, infrequently, in the back. The pain is described as aching, squeezing, burning, heaviness, or pressure. Some people experience *silent* (painless) *angina*, which consists of strange feelings at angina sites without pain. Silent angina can be diagnosed by exercise testing or by wearing a portable device that monitors the electrical activity of the heart during a 24-hour period.

Angina attacks may come and go, brought on by physical exertion or by mental or emotional stress, but they are signs of serious coronary artery disease. Angina should not be ignored; a person experiencing angina attacks should seek medical attention immediately. Rest and drugs that dilate, or widen, the blood vessels (such as nitroglycerin) relieve attacks of angina. Other drugs used to treat angina include those to reduce blood pressure or those that slow the heart rate. Both types of drugs reduce the workload of the heart and its need for oxygen.

Diagnosis To diagnose whether chest pain is heart-related and to find out how well the heart handles work, a physician may begin testing the heart with a *stress test*. During this test, the patient walks on a treadmill while hooked up to equipment that monitors the heart. The physician notes the patient's heart rate and electrical activity along with breathing and blood pressure as the conditions of the stress test change. The physician may also suggest an *echocardiogram*, in which the chambers of the beating heart are visualized using ultrasound (sound waves) at the same time as the heart's electrical activity is measured. In this way a physician can examine the structure of the heart and its pumping function.

If the physician suspects that one or more blood vessels of the heart are blocked, he or she may suggest a *coronary angiography* to visualize the coronary blood vessels. This test can determine the degree and location of vessel blockage to help assess whether further treatment is necessary to reduce symptoms and avoid a heart attack.

ischemia (is-KI-me-ah) Insufficient blood in part of the heart.

angioplasty (AN-jee-oh-PLAS-tee) The reconstruction of damaged blood vessels.

stent A springlike mesh device that is implanted within an artery to cover compressed plaque, support the artery, and smooth the artery wall.

An *angiogram* is an X-ray image of blood vessels after they have been injected with a fluid called a *contrast medium*. The contrast medium used in angiography is composed primarily of iodine because it absorbs X-rays, making visible the interiors of blood vessels. To perform coronary angiography, physicians first thread a thin plastic tube called a *catheter* through an artery in the arm or the groin until it reaches the coronary arteries. After injecting the contrast medium into the catheter, they take high-speed X-ray movies of blood flowing through the arteries. **Figure 12.5** shows frames of such a movie and indicates where physicians are able to detect irregularities and narrowing of the coronary arteries.

Other tests such as magnetic resonance imaging (MRI) are also performed at many medical centers to create images of the heart and its vessels for various diagnostic purposes. MRI uses magnetic fields and radio waves to visualize structures.

Unclogging Arteries If a patient has atherosclerosis in many coronary vessels, a physician may recommend coronary artery bypass graft surgery. If only one of a patient's coronary arteries is narrowed significantly, a physician may recommend widening the interior of the artery with a type of **angioplasty**, the reconstruction of damaged blood vessels. In balloon angioplasty, the physician threads a catheter through an artery in the arm or the groin until it reaches the coronary arteries, as done when performing an angiogram. However, instead of injecting dye into the catheter, the physician threads a second, balloon-tipped catheter through the first. When the second catheter reaches the area of blockage, the balloon is inflated, breaking up the plaque while compressing it against the arterial wall (**Figure 12.6**). This balloon technique also stretches the artery somewhat. In almost all balloon angioplasties, a stent is also used.

A **stent** is a springlike mesh device (**Figure 12.7**) that is mounted on an angioplasty balloon and implanted within an artery to cover the compressed plaque, support the artery, and smooth the artery wall. The first stents were made of bare metal. After

atherectomy (ATH-er-EK-toe-me) The removal of plaque from the interior of an artery.

coronary artery bypass graft (CABG) surgery A surgical procedure in which healthy blood vessels are used to redirect blood flow around blocked vessels of the heart.

a time, tissue frequently grew around the stent, increasing the risk of the artery reclogging. Newer types of stents are coated with drugs that inhibit reclogging, but improvements are still needed.[9] Biodegradable stents are in development that support the artery as it heals from angioplasty, and then the stent dissolves.[10]

Atherectomy refers to methods that remove plaque from the interior of an artery. The procedure is performed like balloon angioplasty, but the second catheter contains a rotating cutting device (burr tip) or a laser instead of a balloon tip.

One technique that is used frequently to treat coronary artery disease is bypass surgery. In the United States in 2010 an estimated 395,000 of these procedures were performed.[7]

The phrase *bypass surgery* usually means **coronary artery bypass graft (CABG) surgery**. The coronary arteries are blood vessels that supply oxygen-rich blood to the heart muscle. When these vessels become blocked, blood flow is slowed and the heart muscle does not get enough oxygen.

People who have chronic angina, blockage in the vessels that supply the left side of the heart (the side that pumps blood to the body), or blockage in multiple coronary arteries are often candidates for bypass surgery. To perform this operation, surgeons first open the chest cavity. Using a blood vessel taken from another part of the patient's body (usually the leg), they graft one end of the new vessel to the aorta, the major artery that carries blood away from the heart and to the body. Heart surgeons graft the other end of the new vessel to the damaged coronary artery, past the area of blockage (**Figure 12.8**). The grafted vessel thus bypasses the blocked portion of the diseased vessel.

A therapy aimed at increasing blood flow to the heart muscle is transmyocardial laser revascularization (TMLR), which has been used for more than 2 decades. In TMLR, surgeons use a laser to bore narrow channels from the heart chamber into the heart muscle. Although TMLR does not help a heart patient live longer, it reduces the frequency of recurrent heart pain and increases the quality of life. In addition, TMLR is being used in conjunction with CABG. Together, these procedures appear to provide results superior to CABG alone or to TMLR alone.[11]

Heart Attack Victims of coronary artery disease are often unaware that the arteries supplying their heart with blood have become blocked. They may have no signs or symptoms of CAD or may not notice any. For this reason, one-third to one-half of persons with CAD are stricken suddenly and unexpectedly

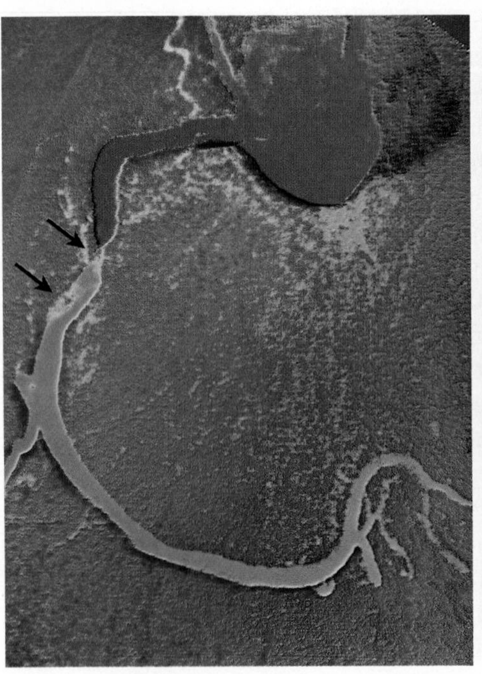
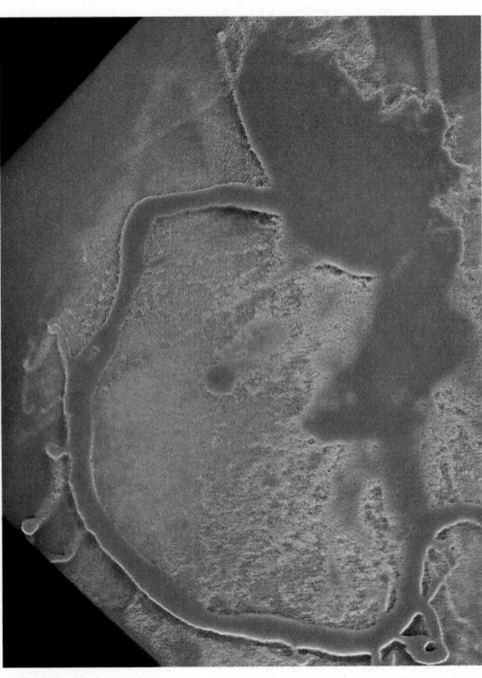

Figure 12.5

Angiogram. The arrows on the left angiogram point out some of the irregularities and areas of narrowing of this coronary artery. This same vessel is shown in the image on the right, taken minutes after balloon angioplasty.

heart attack Myocardial infarction (MI); an area of heart muscle that dies because it does not receive enough oxygen as a result of insufficient blood supply.

arrhythmias (uh-RITH-me-uhs) Abnormal heartbeats.

heart failure Ineffective pumping of the heart, which results in the overfilling of the veins that bring blood to the heart.

Figure 12.6

Balloon Angioplasty. In balloon angioplasty, a thin tube containing a balloon is threaded through an artery until it reaches the area of plaque that is narrowing the vessel. The balloon is inflated, compressing the plaque against the artery wall and stretching the artery.

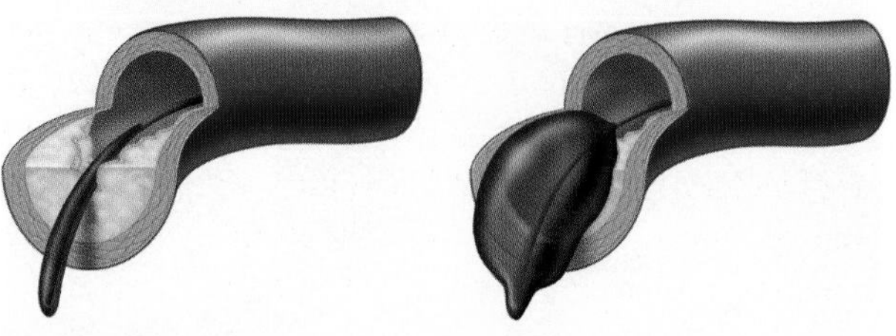

with a **heart attack**, which healthcare practitioners call a *myocardial infarction (MI)*. *Myocardial* simply means heart (*cardium*) muscle (*myo-*). An infarction is an area of heart muscle that dies because it does not receive enough oxygen because of insufficient blood. As heart muscle dies, it may trigger abnormal electrical activity that causes the ventricles to beat irregularly. Abnormal heartbeats are called **arrhythmias**. Heart failure, cardiac arrest, and death may occur during ventricular arrhythmia.

Heart failure is sometimes called *congestive* heart failure because the veins bringing blood to the heart become congested, or overfilled, with blood when the heart cannot pump effectively. Heart failure

Figure 12.7

An Arterial Stent. This springlike mesh device is implanted in an artery after balloon angioplasty procedure to cover the compressed plaque, smooth the artery wall, and support the vessel.

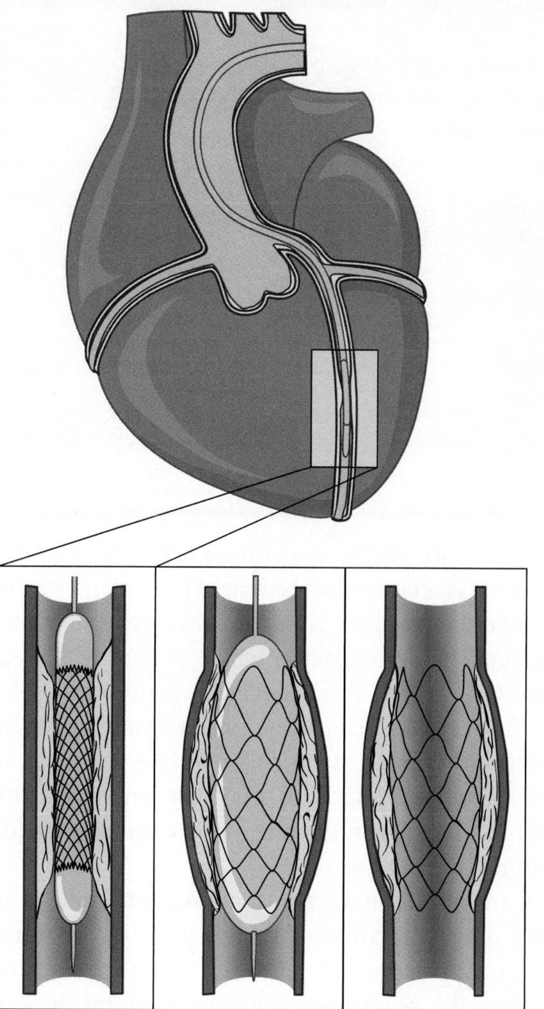

Figure 12.8

Vessel Position in a Coronary Artery Bypass Graft. In a coronary artery bypass graft, blood vessels taken from another part of the body are grafted to the aorta, the large artery emerging from the heart. The other ends of these vessels are grafted to the coronary arteries (those that serve the heart) beyond the area of blockage.

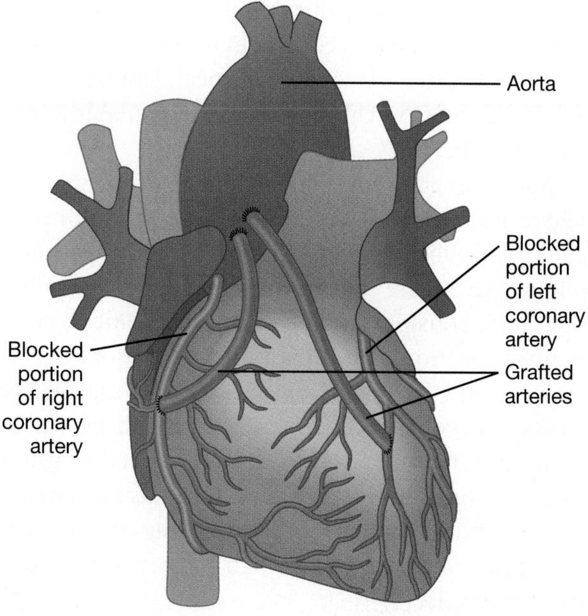

sudden cardiac arrest Cessation of the heartbeat.

(ineffective pumping) may be the result of all forms of cardiac disease, including CAD, structural heart defects, and rheumatic heart disease, and may also be a chronic condition, resulting in shortness of breath, retention of fluid, congestion of the lungs, and fatigue. A person experiencing severe cardiac failure may be a candidate for a heart transplant or the implantation of a left ventricular assist device (which has replaced the artificial heart) while waiting for a donor heart. The pump is implanted in the abdomen and is connected to the main pumping chamber of the heart, the left ventricle. The power source for the pump is located outside of the patient's body on a rolling cart or is a portable battery that hangs by a strap from the shoulder (**Figure 12.9**).

Sudden cardiac arrest (sudden cardiac death) may also occur as a result of a heart attack. During cardiac arrest, the heart suddenly stops beating. Getting immediate medical care is crucial in such a situation because the heart must be *defibrillated* (given electric shock) within a few minutes of its stopping to cause it to begin beating again and avoid heart, lung, kidney, and brain damage and to avoid death. Sudden cardiac death is the result of an unresuscitated cardiac arrest, usually the result of ventricular fibrillation, the rapid, erratic contraction of the lower chambers of the heart. On March 10, 2014, Dallas Stars player Rich Peverley collapsed on the bench after exiting the ice. Medical staff at the American Airlines Center responded quickly by providing oxygen and using a defibrillator located near the benches to shock his heart back into rhythm. Peverley survived and continues to recover after surgery to correct an irregular heartbeat. Unfortunately, a defibrillator is not always as readily available as one was when Peverley collapsed.

Approximately 80% of heart attacks occur at home, where most Americans do not have an automated external defibrillator, or AED. On the other hand, public AEDs are increasingly available in public buildings, transportation centers, large offices, commercial locations, and many other locations where large groups of people gather. The American Red Cross believes that all Americans should be within 4 minutes of an AED and someone trained to use it. A recent study, however, revealed that access remains limited and is further restricted during the evening, nighttime, and weekends, when the majority of cardiac arrests occur.[12]

Figure 12.9

The Left Ventricular Assist Device (LVAD). Billy Bean has an LVAD implanted in his body. A tube from the LVAD exits his body at the abdomen and connects to a power source that Billy keeps on a rolling cart (not shown).

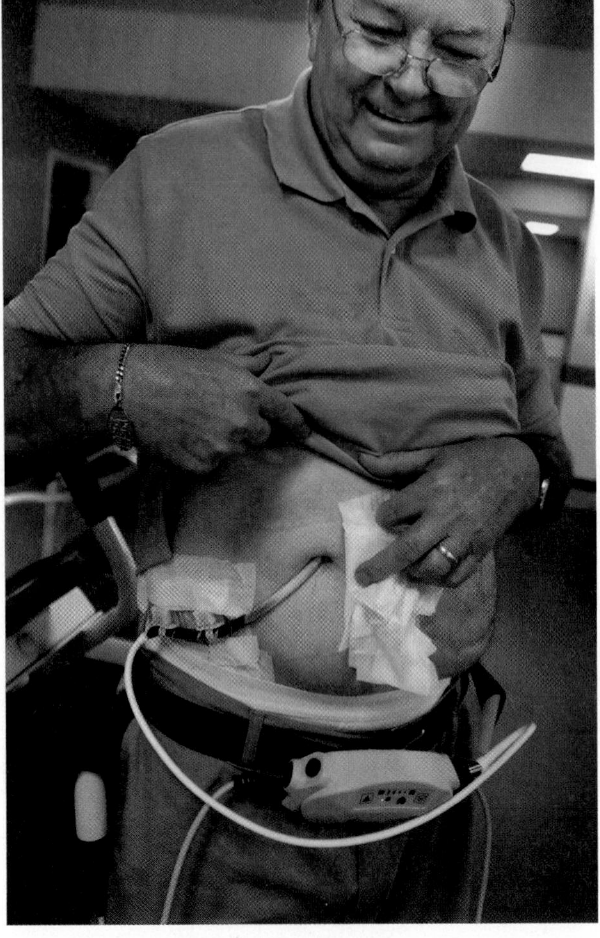

Although AEDs are automated, the American Heart Association states that AED operators must be able to recognize signs of cardiac arrest, when to activate the emergency medical system (EMS), and how to do CPR. Also, because various models of AEDs exist, the user must understand how to successfully operate the specific devise they will use. Therefore, anyone who may use an AED, either as a medical professional or bystander, should be trained in AED use.

Cardiopulmonary resuscitation, or CPR, is also used during a cardiac event such as sudden cardiac arrest. Approximately 92% of sudden cardiac arrest victims die before reaching the hospital; however, administering CPR immediately can double or triple a victim's chance of survival. The American Heart Association lists *Two Steps for Staying Alive with Hands-Only CPR*: (1) call 9-1-1 and, when asked, be specific about your location, and (2) push hard and fast in the center of the chest to the beat of the classic Bee Gees' disco song "Stayin' Alive." If you are unfamiliar with the song, you can hear it by going to www.youtube.com and using the search term "Bee Gees Stayin' Alive."

For more information about CPR and AEDs, including how to use and AED, AED cost, and AED and CPR training, visit www.heart.org. From 250,000 to 350,000 persons in the United States die each year from sudden cardiac arrest. In the United States, the average age for a man to have his first heart attack (but not necessarily die from it) is 66 years and for women it is 70 years. Most of the time the underlying cause of a heart attack and cardiac arrest is coronary artery disease, although medical researchers now realize that heart attacks in women often may be caused by *coronary microvascular dysfunction* (see the section titled "Atherosclerosis"). Other causes of heart attacks include conditions such as an inflammation of the heart caused by infection, rheumatic fever, or medications; heart muscle disorders having unknown causes; congenital heart defects; and drug abuse (**Figure 12.10**). (Rheumatic fever is a disorder that sometimes occurs as a result of strep throat. It affects the heart.) One of these conditions is often the reason a young, physically fit person such as an athlete dies suddenly on the basketball court, track, or skating rink.

Figure 12.10

A Heart Attack Prematurely Ended the Life of Professional Surfer Andy Irons. Irons died of a heart attack in 2010 at age 32. Following his death, Irons' family acknowledged his use of prescription drugs to treat anxiety and insomnia, as well as his recreational drug use.

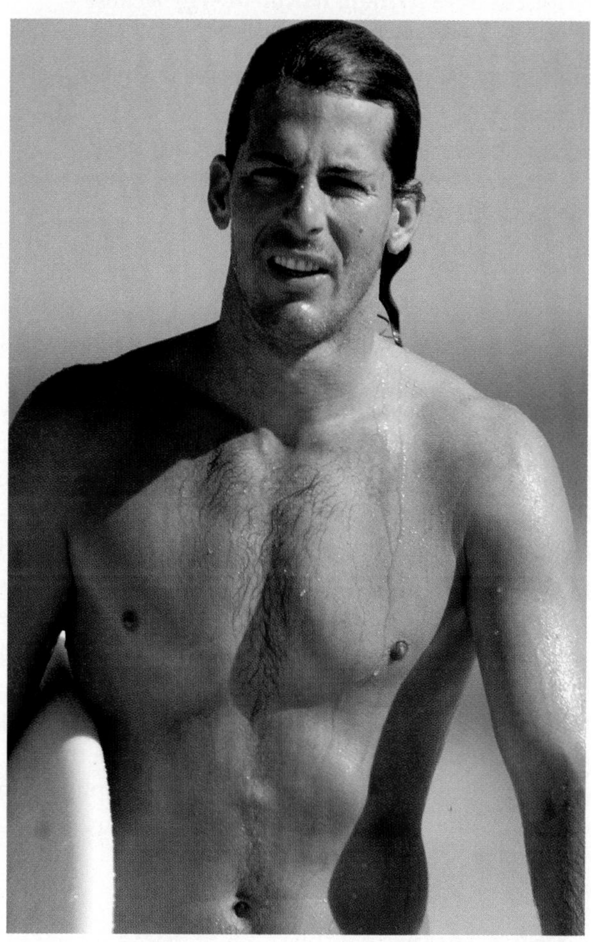

Learn the warning signs of a heart attack and what to do if you or someone you are with experiences them (see the Managing Your Health feature). You can distinguish a heart attack from angina by the severity of the pain: Heart attack pain is much more severe and lasts longer than that of angina. The pain of a heart attack is usually described as pressure (heaviness), burning, aching, and tightness, which is felt in the same locations as angina pain. The person suffering a heart attack may also experience shortness of breath, profuse sweating, weakness, anxiety, or nausea. Women may have these symptoms or may have more subtle symptoms: discomfort spread over a wide chest area, exhaustion, depression, and shortness of breath. In addition, women are more likely than men to have nausea, vomiting, back or jaw pain, and shortness of breath with chest pain.

If you experience some or all of these signs and symptoms or are with someone who does, obtain emergency medical care *immediately*. Many heart attack victims die because they do not seek medical attention quickly, denying that they are having a heart attack; however, if you call for help quickly, an emergency response team trained to provide prompt medical care can keep a heart attack victim alive and help reduce damage to the heart while transporting him or her to the hospital.

Most heart attacks are results of coronary artery thrombosis. Blood clots often form suddenly when the plaque in an artery breaks apart and blood platelets clump at that site (**Figure 12.11**). Therefore, in the emergency room, heart attack patients are quickly given clot-dissolving drugs intravenously.

stroke A brain injury that occurs when arteries that supply the brain become blocked and prevent blood flow or become damaged and leak blood onto or into the brain.

cerebral thrombosis A stroke caused by a stationary blood clot.

cerebral embolism A stroke caused by a floating blood clot that becomes lodged in a cerebral artery, blocking blood flow.

cerebral hemorrhage (HEM-ah-rij) A stroke caused by a burst artery that supplies the brain.

aneurysm (AN-you-rizm) A swollen, weakened blood vessel.

atrial fibrillation (fih-brih-LAY-shun) A type of arrhythmia in which the upper chambers of the heart contract with no set pattern.

Most patients who survive a heart attack do not experience complications after the attack if they receive appropriate medical treatment. Some may not even have detectable heart abnormalities if their heart attack involved only a small portion of the heart muscle; unfortunately, some patients do experience life-threatening complications. If a substantial portion of the heart was involved, the heart attack victim may develop cardiogenic shock, in which the left ventricle of the heart does not pump sufficient blood to sustain the body. Although physicians can treat this condition with angioplasty or surgery, cardiogenic shock is fatal more than 50% of the time.[13]

After diagnosing a heart attack, the physician evaluates the health of the patient's heart. Using measurements of enzymes released from the heart and techniques to visualize the heart and blood vessels, such as an angiogram or MRI, the physician assesses cell damage and ventricular function (the ability of the heart to pump blood to the body) to select a patient's therapy. Such therapy may include surgical procedures, medications, and lifestyle changes.

Figure 12.11

An Occluded (Blocked) Vessel. This coronary artery is totally blocked with plaque and a blood clot (dark area).

© W. Ober/Visuals Unlimited

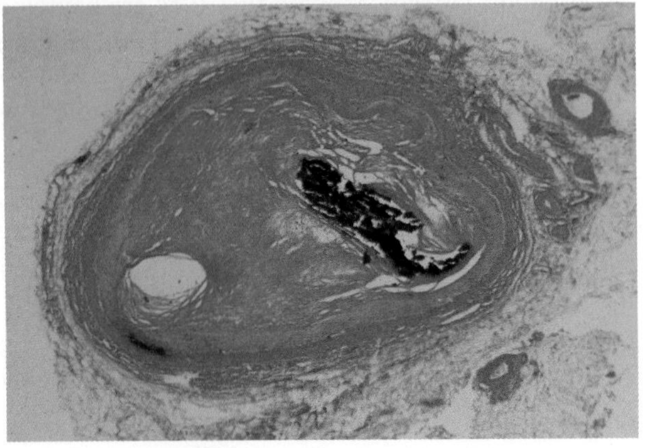

Stroke

A **stroke** (brain attack) occurs when arteries that supply the brain with blood become blocked, preventing blood flow. The primary cause of stroke is the same as that for heart attacks or angina pectoris: atherosclerosis—the buildup of plaque or a blood clot that blocks arteries bringing blood to the organ. Blood clots are a common cause of a stroke. If the stroke is caused by a stationary clot, the condition is called a **cerebral thrombosis**. If the blood clot was formed elsewhere and becomes lodged in a cerebral artery, blocking flow, it is called a **cerebral embolism**.

A stroke may also occur if an artery supplying the brain bursts. This situation is called a **cerebral hemorrhage** and may occur when atherosclerosis and high blood pressure are present. Cerebral hemorrhage may also occur from a head injury or from a burst **aneurysm** (a swollen, weakened blood vessel).

During a stroke, the brain cells normally supplied by the blocked or burst vessel do not receive oxygen. Brain cells, like heart cells, die when they do not receive the oxygen they need. A cerebral hemorrhage affects the brain in an additional way: Pressure builds in the brain as a result of blood that has leaked out of the burst vessel. When this blood clots, it can damage brain tissue, causing physical disability.

The signs and symptoms of a stroke vary (see Managing Your Health), depending on the location of the damage. In most cases, one side of the body becomes weak, numb, or paralyzed.

One group at highest risk for a stroke is people with **atrial fibrillation**. Atrial fibrillation is a type of arrhythmia. During atrial fibrillation, the upper chambers of the heart contract with no set pattern, which upsets the normal rhythm of the heartbeat. This arrhythmia can result in the formation of floating blood clots (emboli) that can travel to the brain, block a blood vessel, and result in a stroke.

More than 1 million Americans have atrial fibrillation. Its incidence increases with age because its primary underlying causes, hypertension and coronary artery disease, also increase with age.

Managing Your Health

Heart Attack and Stroke (Brain Attack) Symptoms: What to Do in an Emergency

IF YOU NOTICE ONE OR MORE OF THESE SIGNS IN ANOTHER PERSON (OR IF YOU HAVE THEM YOURSELF), DO NOT WAIT. CALL 9-1-1 OR YOUR EMERGENCY MEDICAL SERVICES AND GET TO A HOSPITAL RIGHT AWAY!

Common or "classic" signs of heart attack:

- Uncomfortable pressure, fullness, squeezing, or pain in the center of the chest that lasts more than a few minutes or goes away and comes back
- Pain that spreads to the shoulders, neck, or arms
- Chest discomfort with light-headedness, fainting, sweating, nausea, or shortness of breath

Less common warning signs of heart attack:

- Atypical chest, stomach, or abdominal pain
- Nausea or dizziness (without chest pain)
- Shortness of breath and difficulty breathing (without chest pain)
- Unexplained anxiety, weakness, or fatigue
- Palpitations, cold sweat, or paleness

Not all of these signs occur in every heart attack. Sometimes they go away and return. If some occur, get help fast.

Some or all of these signs accompany a stroke:

- Weakness, numbness, or paralysis on one side of the body
- Loss or dimming of vision, particularly in one eye
- Loss of speech, or difficulty speaking or understanding speech
- Sudden, severe headache
- Sudden dizziness, unsteadiness, or episodes of falling

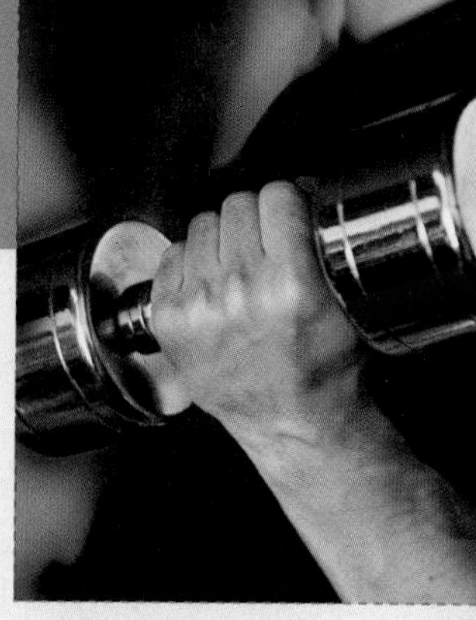
© Kzenon/ShutterStock

Be prepared:

- Keep a list of emergency rescue service numbers next to the telephone and in your pocket, wallet, or purse.
- Find out which area hospitals have 24-hour emergency cardiovascular care.
- Know (in advance) which hospital or medical facility is nearest your home or office.

Take action:

- If you have heart attack or stroke symptoms that last more than a few minutes, don't delay! Immediately call 9-1-1 or the emergency medical services (EMS) number so that an ambulance (ideally with Advanced Life Support) can quickly be sent for you.
- If ambulance service isn't available in your area, immediately have someone drive you to the nearest hospital emergency room (or another facility offering 24-hour life support).
- If you're with someone who may be having heart attack or stroke symptoms, immediately call 9-1-1 or EMS. Expect the person to protest—denial is common. Don't take "no" for an answer. Insist on taking prompt action.
- Give cardiopulmonary resuscitation (CPR—mouth-to-mouth breathing and chest compressions) if it's needed and you're properly trained.

Another group at high risk for strokes is persons with *stenosis* (narrowing) of one or both of the carotid arteries. The right and left carotid arteries branch off major vessels leaving the heart and bring blood up the neck to the brain (see Figure 12.1). Physicians diagnose carotid artery stenosis by using ultrasound (a technique that uses sound waves to visualize soft tissues of the body) or angiography.

Physicians often recommend *carotid endarterectomy* to reduce significantly the risk of stroke in patients with carotid artery stenosis. In this procedure, surgeons remove the inner lining of the partially blocked carotid artery along with the plaque. Also, physicians may prescribe long-term aspirin therapy or anticoagulant drugs for treatment of either carotid artery stenosis or atrial fibrillation.

In the hospital, physicians usually perform computed tomography (CT) scans (detailed X-rays of cross-sectional slices of body structures) or MRI scans of the brain of the stroke victim to confirm the

transient ischemic (is-KI-mik) attacks (TIAs) Minor strokes that usually cause no permanent damage and have signs that last for only a short time.

diagnosis and determine the location and extent of injury (**Figure 12.12**). The standard therapy for stroke is a clot-dissolving drug called tissue plasminogen activator (tPA). If given within 3 hours of a stroke's onset, it raises the chances that no permanent brain damage will occur. Researchers are exploring ways to lengthen the window of time during which this drug can be administered.[14] Poststroke rehabilitation focuses on helping patients redevelop skills that may have been lost as a result of damage to part of the brain. These skills may involve movement, language, thinking, and memory. Mental health professionals work with stroke patients who may have had personality changes or who may have developed emotional disturbances, such as depression.

Just as heart attacks may be preceded by smaller angina attacks, major strokes may be preceded by minor strokes called **transient ischemic attacks (TIAs)**. Ischemic attacks are similar to strokes, usually cause no permanent damage, and have signs that last only a short time. A TIA is a serious warning that a stroke may occur within weeks or months. Persons experiencing a TIA should see their physicians immediately. Often, blood-thinning drugs such as aspirin are prescribed to lessen the possibility of a stroke.

The Incidence of Strokes Is Rising Among Young Americans Analyzing more than 100 studies from 1990 to 2010, stroke researchers found the rate of stroke has increased by 25% in people aged 20 to 64 years and that those patients make up nearly 33% of all stroke cases, worldwide.[15] At an American Stroke Association conference in early 2011, researchers reported that the incidence of strokes rose 51% among men and 17% among women aged 15 through 34 years between 1994–1995 and 2006–2007. The incidence of strokes also rose 47% in males aged 35 to 44 years and 36% in females in the same age group. Researchers hypothesize that the obesity epidemic is a major factor in the increase in the stroke incidence in these age groups.

While the occurrence of strokes was rising in young adults, it was declining in older adults. The incidence of strokes dropped 25% among men and 28% in women aged 65 years and older between 1994–1995 and 2006–2007. Researchers suggest that this decline is caused in part by better treatment of risk factors in older adults and better prevention efforts.[16]

Figure 12.12

CT Scan of a Stroke Victim. The darkened area on the left side of the brain scan reveals dead tissue due to a lack of oxygen during a stroke.

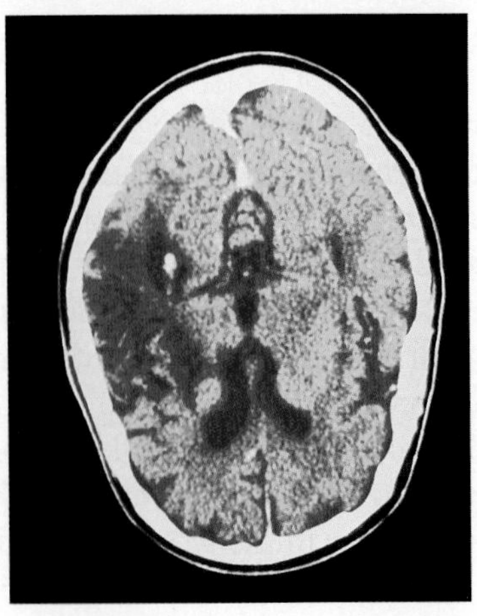

Risk Factors for Cardiovascular Disease

Medical researchers have identified several risk factors for cardiovascular disease, traits that have been shown to be associated with the incidence of CVD. In general, people with more than one of these traits, which are listed in **Table 12.1**, have a greater probability of developing atherosclerosis and suffering a heart attack or stroke than do people with one or none of these risk factors. Many of these risk factors are modifiable; in other words, people can often reduce their risk of cardiovascular disease by changing one or more health-related behaviors.

The major risk factors for the development of CVD are male gender (comparable rates of a first major cardiovascular event occur 10 years later in women than in men), increasing age (the incidence of coronary artery disease rises in both men and women with each decade from age 40 to age 79 years), family health history of cardiovascular disease, cigarette smoking, obesity, hypertension (chronic high blood pressure), abnormal blood lipid levels, and lack of physical activity. All these risk factors are important in the development of CAD; however, hypertension is the most important risk factor for stroke.

Family Health History

A family health history of atherosclerosis, stroke, or coronary artery disease indicates a genetic

© djgis/ShutterStock

Healthy Living Practices

- Any person who experiences chest pain, especially pain beneath the breastbone that extends to the neck, shoulders, and/or arms, should seek medical attention immediately.
- Any person experiencing weakness, numbness, or paralysis on one side of the body; loss or dimming of vision; loss of speech, or difficulty speaking or understanding speech; a sudden, severe headache; or sudden dizziness or unsteadiness should seek medical attention immediately.

high-density lipoproteins (HDL) (LIP-oh-PRO-teenz or LIE-poe-PRO-teenz) "Good" cholesterol that carries cholesterol from the cells and to the liver for removal from the body.

low-density lipoproteins (LDL) "Bad" cholesterol that carries cholesterol to the cells, including the cells that line the blood vessel walls.

predisposition to these conditions or reflects similar diets, stresses, and lifestyles among family members. A person with a family health history of premature CAD is twice as likely to suffer a heart attack as a person with no family health history. A family health history of premature atherosclerosis, heart attack or sudden death among males before 55 years of age or females before the age of 65, especially in a first-degree relative (e.g. father, mother, or sibling), is more meaningful than having relatives who developed atherosclerosis in the elderly years. The genetic effect decreases at older ages. Unfortunately, you cannot change your family health history, but you can monitor other factors to reduce your risk in other ways.

Table 12.1

Risk Factors for Cardiovascular Disease

- Cigarette smoking
- Diabetes mellitus
- Blood cholesterol above 200 mg/dl
- A ratio of total cholesterol to high-density lipoprotein (HDL) cholesterol above 5:1 (optimum ratio is 3.5:1)
- High levels of low-density lipoprotein (LDL) cholesterol
- Physical inactivity
- Family history of cardiovascular disease
- Obesity
- Uncontrolled, persistent high blood pressure
- Heavy alcohol use
- Gender (women are at lower risk of heart attack until menopause)
- Age (risk increases with age)
- Anxiety disorders (increased risk of fatal heart attack in men)
- Elevated C-reactive protein*

*Elevated C-reactive protein is an indicator of inflammation and is not specific to coronary artery disease.

Abnormal Blood Lipid Levels

Another major risk factor in the development of atherosclerosis, coronary artery disease, and stroke is abnormal blood lipid levels, including elevated blood cholesterol levels (also called serum cholesterol). The American Heart Association states that the desirable range of total blood cholesterol is less than 200 milligrams per deciliter (200 mg/dl). A cholesterol level of 200 to 239 mg/dl is considered borderline high, and a total cholesterol level of 240 mg/dl and higher is considered high. In 2010, 13% of U.S. adults had high total cholesterol, which represents a 27% decrease from 1999 (**Table 12.2**).[17]

What is cholesterol? This substance is a *steroid*, a type of lipid. The most abundant steroid in the human body, cholesterol is used to make the sex hormones and composes part of the membranes of the body's cells. Some cholesterol is essential for health but a high blood cholesterol level is associated with development of cardiovascular disease. We take in cholesterol when consuming most animal foods, such as egg yolks, fatty meats, and butter, but our bodies can also produce cholesterol.

Cholesterol circulates in the blood as part of particles called lipoproteins, which consist primarily of triglycerides, protein, and cholesterol, and are also critical to cardiovascular health. The major lipoproteins are **high-density lipoproteins (HDL)** and **low-density lipoproteins (LDL)**. HDL carries cholesterol from the cells and to the liver for removal from the body. LDL carries cholesterol to the cells, including the cells that line the blood vessel walls. You may have heard these molecules referred to as "good" cholesterol and "bad" cholesterol, respectively.

Table 12.2

Classification of Total, HDL, and LDL Cholesterol Levels and Triglyceride Levels (mg/dl)

Total Cholesterol Levels	
Less than 200 mg/dl	Desirable level that puts you at lower risk for heart d isease. A cholesterol level of 200 mg/dl or greater increases your risk.
200–239 mg/dl	Borderline high.
240 mg/dl and above	High blood cholesterol. A person with this level has more than twice the risk of heart disease compared with someone whose cholesterol is below 200 mg/dl.
HDL Cholesterol Levels	
Less than 40 mg/dl	A major risk factor for heart disease.
40–59 mg/dl	The higher your HDL, the better.
60 mg/dl and above	An HDL of 60 mg/dl and above is considered protective against heart disease.
LDL Cholesterol Levels	
Less than 100 mg/dl	Optimal.
100–129 mg/dl	Near optimal/above optimal.
130–159 mg/dl	Borderline high.
160–189 mg/dl	High.
190 mg/dl and above	Very high.
Triglyceride Levels	
Less than 150 mg/dl	Normal.
150–199 mg/dl	Borderline high.
200–499 mg/dl	High.
500 mg/dl or above	Very high.

Reproduced with permission, Third Report of the NCEP Expert Panel on Detection, Evaluation, and Treatment of High Blood Cholesterol in Adults (*Circulation*. 2002;106:3237). © 2002 American Heart Association, Inc. Lippincott Williams & Wilkins.

It is firmly established that the level of bad cholesterol, or LDL, is of major importance in the development of atherosclerosis and coronary artery disease. As the level of LDL rises, the risk of coronary artery disease and atherosclerosis rises because LDL is related to the formation and growth of plaques.

The level of good cholesterol, or HDL, is very important too. As the level of HDL rises, the risk of coronary artery disease and atherosclerosis falls (Table 12.2 lists the classification levels for HDL and LDL.) HDL cholesterol reduces and recycles LDL cholesterol by transporting it to the level; thus, higher levels of HDL cholesterol help control the level and LDL cholesterol. Furthermore, HDL cholesterol helps "clean" arterial walls to prevent damage to inner arterial walls, which is the first step in development of atherosclerosis. By performing these functions, HDL cholesterol helps reduce the risk of cardiovascular disease. High HDL levels are also the key to why premenopausal women, in general, do not experience heart attacks at as young an age as men; the female sex hormone estrogen raises women's HDL levels by about 20%. As noted in Table 12.2, desirable levels of HDL cholesterol are above 40 mg/dl. Women are encouraged, however, to maintain an HDL cholesterol level above 50 mg/dl.[18]

A primary component of HDL is apolipoprotein A-I (apoA-I), which has been shown to reverse atherosclerosis and is therefore a potentially powerful treatment for vascular diseases. The Diversity in Health essay describes how a mutant form of this cholesterol-lowering protein found in a certain Italian family (apoA-I [Milano]) protects them against vascular disease. ApoA-1 (Milano) has a more effective cholesterol-removing function than apoA-1 and may therefore prove to be a more effective treatment.[19]

Triglycerides, which are plasma lipids different from cholesterol, are also important in cardiovascular health. When the body does not immediately use all the energy-supplying nutrients consumed, it converts them to triglycerides and transports them to fat cells for storage. Excess triglycerides in the plasma are linked to CAD in some people. Additionally, researchers have linked high levels of triglycerides to an increased risk of stroke. A normal, fasting triglyceride level is less than 150 mg/dl (see Table 12-2).

Cigarette Smoking

Smoking cigarettes significantly increases the risk of heart attack and stroke. Cigarette smokers are 2 to 4 times more likely than nonsmokers to develop CAD and over 10 times more likely to develop peripheral vascular disease.[17] In addition, smoking interacts with other risk factors, multiplying its negative health effects. Even more alarming is that cigarette smoking is directly responsible for the majority of heart disease in women under the age of 50 years.[20,21] These figures show that premenopausal women, who are generally protected from heart attacks by estrogen, raise their risk of heart disease significantly when they smoke.

Research results show that cigarette smokers tend to have reduced HDL levels, increased LDL levels, and increased levels of blood clotting factors. In addition, evidence suggests that compounds in cigarette smoke enter the bloodstream and may damage blood vessel linings directly, leading to the formation of plaques.[22] Chewing tobacco is a significant CVD risk factor also, but cigar and pipe smoking appear to be less important because cigar and pipe smokers are less likely than cigarette smokers to inhale the smoke.[23]

Passive smoking, breathing in other people's smoke, has also been identified as an important risk factor for cardiovascular disease. The American Heart Association (AHA) estimates that approximately 40,000 people die each year from heart and blood vessel disease caused by passive smoking.[23] Results of research show a harmful effect of passive smoking on the circulation of blood within the heart tissue itself.[24]

hypertension Persistently high arterial blood pressure.

systolic (sis-TOL-ik) pressure The higher number in the blood pressure reading, which is the pressure exerted by the blood on the artery walls when the left ventricle contracts.

diastolic (DIE-as-TOL-ik) pressure The lower number in the blood pressure reading, which is the pressure exerted by the blood on the artery walls when the left ventricle relaxes.

High Blood Pressure

Blood pressure becomes elevated during periods of excitement or exertion; however, in healthy individuals it returns to normal levels when the activity stops. **Hypertension**, persistently high arterial blood pressure, is a major risk factor for heart attack and the most important risk factor for stroke. Data show that nearly one-third of Americans age 20 years and older are hypertensive; furthermore, nearly 47% of Americans with hypertension had uncontrolled hypertension in between 2009 and 2012.[25]

The cause of most cases of high blood pressure is unknown. It has been shown, however, that hypertension may have a genetic link; it runs in families. There are also racial genetic links in hypertension. African Americans and Latinos are more likely to have hypertension than Whites and, as a result, suffer strokes at an earlier age and with greater severity. Nongenetic, modifiable factors that contribute to hypertension include obesity, lack of physical activity, cigarette smoking, stress, and long-term intake of excessive amounts of salt. Other identifiable causes of hypertension include increasing age, enzyme deficiencies, sleep apnea, drugs, chronic kidney disease, and thyroid or parathyroid disease.[26] Social and psychological factors, although not fully understood, may also increase blood pressure. When the sympathetic nervous system is activated by stress, fear, anxiety, or other emotions, blood vessels constrict, which increases blood pressure. This may explain why people with low incomes or educational achievement, who generally suffer from more distress, are at increased risk for developing hypertension.[27,28]

You may know your blood pressure reading, such as 120/75 mm Hg (millimeters of mercury). The first (higher) number is the **systolic pressure**, which is the pressure exerted by the blood on the artery walls when the left ventricle contracts and is able to move blood through the constricted artery (***Figure 12.13***). The second (lower) number is the **diastolic pressure**, which is the pressure exerted by the blood on

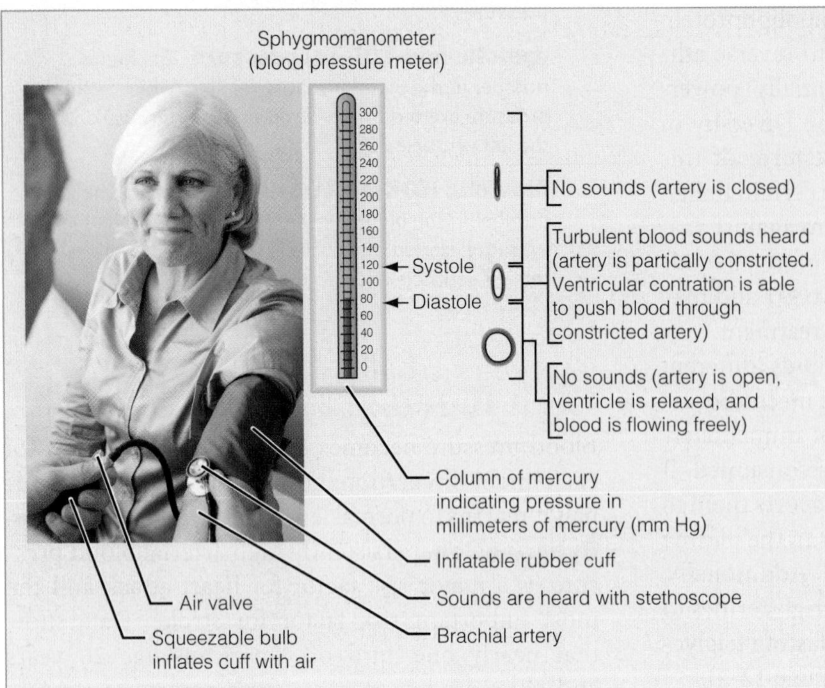

Figure 12.13

Blood Pressure. The inflatable cuff, which is wrapped around the upper arm, squeezes the brachial artery tightly so that blood cannot pass. The systolic reading is taken when turbulent blood sounds can first be heard in this artery, indicating the strength of the pressure against the artery wall when the ventricle contracts and can push the blood through the constricted artery. If the blood pressure is high, it will force the blood vessel open sooner (at a higher reading) than if the blood pressure is low. The diastolic reading is taken when the turbulent blood sounds stop, indicating the strength of the pressure against the artery wall when the ventricle relaxes, the artery is no longer constricted, and the blood is flowing freely.

the artery walls when the left ventricle relaxes. The units, mm Hg, refer to the force needed to push a column of mercury to a particular height, such as 120 mm or 75 mm. The normal blood pressure level for people older than 18 years is less than 120/80 mm Hg. *Prehypertension* is indicated by a systolic blood pressure between 120 and 139 mm Hg, or a diastolic pressure between 80 and 89 mm Hg. *Stage 1 hypertension* is indicated by a systolic reading between 140 and 159, or a diastolic reading of 90 to 99. *Stage 2 hypertension* is indicated by a systolic reading of 160 or more or a diastolic reading of 100 or more.

Persistently high arterial blood pressure contributes to the development of atherosclerosis in two ways. First, high blood pressure may injure the lining of artery walls, triggering plaque formation. In addition, the increased pressure enhances the amount of lipid added to plaques, especially if serum LDL cholesterol levels are elevated. These factors combined increase risk for development of atherosclerosis and, over time, narrowing of the arteries. This narrowing limits or blocks blood flow to the heart and deprives heart muscle of needed oxygen. When the heart's oxygen supply is depleted, a heart attack can occur.

Physical Inactivity

Within the past 2 decades, physical inactivity has been shown to be a major risk factor for developing cardiovascular disease, although research results have linked physical activity and health for more than 60 years. People who are physically inactive are about twice as likely as active people to develop coronary artery disease. This risk extends to people who sit for a large portion of the day rather than stand and move about, independent of exercising. Results of research studies show that sitting for extended periods raises the risk of dying from cardiovascular disease, and the longer one sits, the higher the mortality risk.[29,30]

The 1996 Surgeon General's report on physical activity and health recommends that persons of all ages obtain "a minimum of 30 minutes of physical activity of moderate intensity (e.g., brisk walking) on most, if not all, days of the week."[31] In 2011, the Centers for Disease Control and Prevention (CDC) suggests at least 150 minutes per week of physical activity of moderate intensity to lower the risk of heart disease and stroke.[32] However, as a group, Americans are relatively sedentary; more than 50% of American adults do not get enough physical activity to provide health benefits, and 25% are not active at all during leisure time.[33]

In addition to its direct cardiovascular benefits, routine exercise helps alleviate stress, reduce body weight, and control diabetes—other CVD risk factors.

Obesity

Most medical researchers agree that obesity increases the risk of cardiovascular disease. The risk of developing coronary artery disease is nearly double for people who have a BMI over 30. Being moderately

Diversity in Health

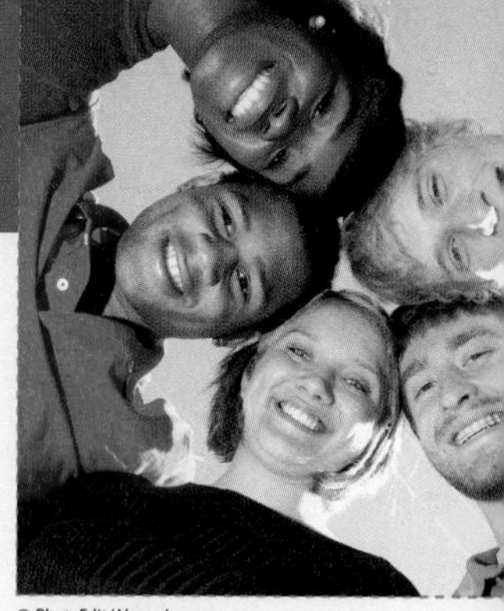
© PhotoEdit/Alamy Images

The Italian Gene: A Hope for Reversing Atherosclerosis?

The University of Milan's Dr. Cesare Sirtori could hardly believe it: Thirty-eight members of one Italian family had no atherosclerosis. If that was not surprising enough, many of them smoked cigarettes and ate high amounts of fat in their diets. What was protecting them from developing plaques in their blood vessels? The answer to that question is a mutation in the gene that directs the production of a cholesterol-lowering protein.

We all have this cholesterol-lowering protein in our bodies: apolipoprotein A-I (apoA-I). ApoA-I is a primary component of high-density lipoprotein (HDL), so-called good cholesterol. HDL helps bring excess cholesterol to the liver for transport out of the body. (Researchers do not fully understand the exact mechanism of this action.) In women, estrogen increases the body's production of apoA-I and is thought to be one reason that premenopausal women have a greater protection than men of the same age from the development of atherosclerosis and heart attacks.

Apolipoprotein A-I (Milano) (apoA-IM) is a mutant apoA-I protein produced by the mutated Italian gene. The change in the molecular structure of apoA-IM from the nonmutant form makes this HDL molecule more stable and alters its properties so that it works even better than its normal counterpart. Those who carry the apoA-IM gene—the members of the Italian family that Sirtori studied—are protected against vascular disease.

Researchers have been able to make apoA-IM in the laboratory. They have used this synthetic molecule in animal models to study its potential as a treatment to reverse atherosclerosis and cardiovascular disease. Results showed a rapid regression of atherosclerosis in the treated animals. Similar studies have been performed with humans and have shown similar results. In recent studies, scientists have begun testing effectiveness of intravenous injection of various forms of apoA-IM and have seen significant reduction in arterial plaque in rabbits and mice. Scientists are currently conducting larger clinical trials. If successful, scientists and generations of one Italian family will have made a medical breakthrough in slowing the death rate from the United States' number one killer.

Data from Tian, F., et al. (2014). Comparative antiatherogenic effects of intravenous AAV8- and AAV2-mediated ApoA-IMilano gene transfer in hypercholesterolemic mice; Chowdhury M. A. U., et al. (2012). High-density lipoprotein as a therapeutic target: Treatment strategies. *Cardiovascular Journal*, 5(1), 73–80.; Speidl, W. S., et al. (2010). Recombinant apolipoprotein A-I Milano rapidly reverses aortic valve stenosis and decreases leaflet inflammation in an experimental rabbit model. *European Heart Journal*, 31(16), 2049–2057.; Spillmann, F., et al. (2010). High-density lipoprotein-raising strategies: Update 2010. *Current Pharmaceutical Design*, 16(13), 1517–1530.

overweight also increases cardiovascular disease risk. Studies show a strong positive association between weight and heart disease in both men and women. In addition to heart disease, obesity also increases risk for type 2 diabetes, some cancers, and osteoarthritis. Are you within the desirable weight range for your age and height? Do you have a body mass index (BMI) of less than 25?

Diabetes Mellitus

Diabetes mellitus is a group of diseases in which glucose is not metabolized properly. Affected individuals are at a higher risk of developing cardiovascular disease because of their elevated blood glucose levels, which damage heart muscle, small coronary vessels, and major arteries. Therefore, atherosclerosis occurs more frequently and at an earlier age in diabetic patients, particularly women. Unfortunately, people with diabetes mellitus are about five times as likely to develop cardiovascular disease as are persons without this disease.

Anxiety and Stress

As mentioned previously, stress can result in spasms of the coronary arteries, which can contribute to angina attacks. In addition, research studies link anxiety disorders (such as phobias and panic disorders) to an increased risk of fatal CAD and particularly to sudden, fatal heart attacks in men.[34] Persons with anxiety disorders are from two to six times as likely to die from a heart attack as persons without anxiety disorders.

Elevated C-Reactive Protein

Results of research show that elevated blood levels of C-reactive protein (CRP) can be a positive risk

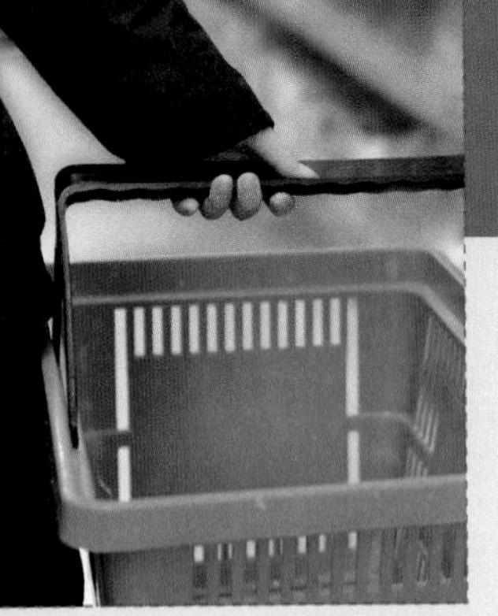

© sevenke/ShutterStock

Consumer Health

Vitamin Pills for a Healthier Heart?

Vitamins A, C, E, B_6, B_{12}, folate, and the nonnutrient beta-carotene . . . what do they have to do with cardiovascular health? Should you be rushing to the store for vitamin supplements to keep your blood vessels healthy?

Vitamins play many roles in cardiovascular health. For example, our bodies use vitamins B_6, B_{12}, and folate in the metabolism of amino acids, including the essential amino acid methionine. In the process of metabolizing methionine, cells produce homocysteine (ho-mo-SIS-teen), another amino acid. High blood levels of this amino acid can damage artery walls and encourage the formation of blood clots and plaques. However, if the cells have enough folate, B_6, and B_{12}, then methionine is metabolized normally and the blood level of homocysteine does not rise.

Methionine intake also affects homocysteine levels. In general, the more methionine people eat, the higher their blood levels of homocysteine. Diets rich in animal protein contain high amounts of methionine and may elevate blood homocysteine levels. Conversely, diets rich in plant protein may lower homocysteine levels because plant foods are relatively low in methionine yet rich in folate and vitamin B_6.

Other factors also influence homocysteine blood levels. Smoking cigarettes, drinking coffee, and a sedentary lifestyle are all associated with decreased B_6 activity, and therefore higher homocysteine levels. The use of oral contraceptives and hormone replacement therapy lowers homocysteine blood levels in women. Homocysteine levels also depend on age, gender, kidney function, genetics, and general health.

So, do you need to take vitamin pills to lower your blood homocysteine levels? The answer is not simple, and only your physician can advise you based on your health. If you show evidence of B_6 or B_{12} deficiency (more likely in elderly than in younger populations) or evidence of folate deficiency (more likely in younger than in elderly populations), your physician may suggest testing. Also, if you are experiencing kidney failure, are on a special metabolic diet, have cancer, or have a strong family health history of heart attack, stroke, or abnormal blood clotting, your physician may recommend that your homocysteine levels be checked. The determination of homocysteine levels is complex, and interpretation of the finding is not simple.

So, what about vitamins A, C, E, and beta-carotene? (Beta-carotene is a yellow pigment in plants that the body converts to vitamin A.) Vitamins E and C and beta-carotene are antioxidants, substances that can protect cells by preventing or reducing the formation of free radicals. Studies have consistently shown that the more antioxidants a population consumes in its food, the lower the rate of cardiovascular disease. But what about vitamin supplements? In general, vitamin supplements, including vitamins B, C, D, and E, and supplements of beta-carotene, calcium, and folic acid have not been found to lower the risk of cardiovascular diseases. In addition, the AHA does not recommend taking antioxidant vitamin supplements or other supplements such as selenium to prevent coronary artery disease. The AHA also notes that consuming soy protein products instead of dairy or other proteins does not show a direct cardiovascular health benefit.

So . . . should you take vitamin pills to reduce your risk of CVD? Only your physician can advise you properly because the answer depends on the status of various facets of your health, family health history, and lifestyle. The best advice at this time is to get your vitamins in the food you eat—be sure to have at least 2½ cups of fruits and vegetables every day, including dark, leafy greens and members of the cabbage family. Consult your physician to determine whether you might also need to take vitamin pills because of possible vitamin deficiencies for a healthier heart and blood vessels.

Data from American Heart Association Nutrition Committee. (2006). AHA scientific statement: Diet and lifestyle recommendations revision 2006. *Circulation, 114*, 82–96.; Debreceni, B., et al. (2014). The role of homocysteine-lowering B-vitamins in the primary prevention of cardiovascular disease. *Cardiovascular Therapeutics, 32*(3), 130–138.; Clarke, R., et al. (2011). Homocysteine and vascular disease: Review of published results of the homocysteine-lowing trials. *Journal of Inherited Metabolic Disease, 34*(1), 83–91.; Clarke, R., et al. (2010). Effects of lowering homocysteine levels with B vitamins on cardiovascular disease, cancer, and cause-specific mortality: Meta-analysis of 8 randomized trials involving 37,485 individuals. *Archives of Internal Medicine, 170*(18), 1622–1631.; Fortmann, S. P., et al. (2013). Vitamin and mineral supplements in the primary prevention of cardiovascular disease and cancer: An updated systematic review for the U.S. preventive services task force. *Annals of Internal Medicine, 159*(12), 824–834.; Lichtenstein, A. H., et al. (2009). Nutrient supplements and cardiovascular disease: A heartbreaking story. *Journal of Lipid Research, 50*(Suppl), S429–433.; Wang, L., et al. (2010). Systematic review: Vitamin D and calcium supplementation in prevention of cardiovascular events. *Annals of Internal Medicine, 152*(5), 315–323.

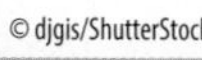

© djgis/ShutterStock

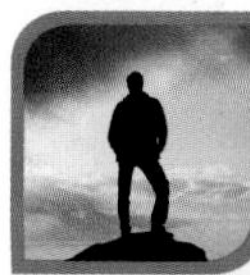

Healthy Living Practices

- If any of your male first-degree relatives had a heart attack before age 55, or female first-degree relatives before age 65, you may be genetically predisposed to heart disease. See your physician for an evaluation and advice.
- If you are a healthy adult, you should have your serum cholesterol level and HDL level measured once every 5 years.

factor for coronary artery disease.[35] C-reactive protein is produced by the liver during acute inflammation. Inflammation may be present at the site of plaques in CAD, but it may also be present in other diseases such as rheumatoid arthritis. Therefore, it is not a test specific to CAD and cannot identify where, exactly, the inflammation is occurring. In addition, a low CRP value does not mean that inflammation is absent. In some cases, a doctor may choose to perform a high-sensitivity C-reactive protein (hs-CRP) test to determine a person's risk for heart disease. Although CRP is considered a risk factor for heart disease, whether CRP is a sign of heart disease or a cause remains unclear. Regardless, several clinical trials are currently ongoing to determine effectiveness of medications to lower CRP levels in people with elevated CRP levels.[36]

Maintaining Cardiovascular Health

Table 12.3 presents a summary of recommendations to help you maintain cardiovascular health and lower your risk of cardiovascular disease. As you can see, there are many factors to consider. You cannot control heredity, gender, and age. However, you can stop smoking, exercise regularly, lose weight, eat less fat, learn to relax, and reduce your salt intake. Results of research reveal that adopting a healthy lifestyle (at least 2½ cups of fruits and vegetables daily,[37] exercising regularly, maintaining a BMI of 18.5 to 29.9, and not smoking) is extremely important to cardiovascular health and a long life. When middle-aged adults (45 to 64 years) who were not following this healthy lifestyle changed their behavior to adopt these healthy habits, they reduced their risk of dying during the next 4 years by 40% and their risk of cardiovascular disease by 35% compared to those who did not change. Only 8% of middle-aged adults practice these healthy lifestyle behaviors.[38,39] Adopting a healthy lifestyle while you are young not only promotes immediate health but also increases the chances that you will continue these behaviors throughout your life, thereby increasing your chances of living a longer, heart-healthy life.

In addition to adopting healthy lifestyle behaviors, you can enhance your cardiovascular health by managing stress properly. Emotional stress contributes to hypertension and the incidence of angina attacks.

If you have diabetes mellitus, work with your primary diabetes physician, such as an endocrinologist,

Table 12.3

How to Reduce Your Risk of Cardiovascular Disease

- Get regular medical checkups.
- Do not smoke cigarettes.
- Manage diabetes mellitus properly.
- Exercise regularly.
- Maintain an intake of dietary cholesterol of less than 300 mg per day, or less than 200 mg per day if you have high LDL levels.
- Maintain an intake of dietary fat of between 20% and 35% of daily calories.
- Maintain an intake of saturated fats of 7% or less* and trans fat of less than 1% of daily calories.
- Eat foods rich in soluble fiber, such as fruits, beans, and oats.
- Eat a diet rich in fruits, vegetables, and low-fat dairy products.
- Maintain an appropriate weight for your height.
- Limit alcohol consumption to 1 drink per day for women and 2 drinks per day for men.
- Maintain salt intake at approximately two-thirds teaspoon or 1,500 mg of sodium per day.*
- Reduce your stress level.

*This recommendation is from the American Heart Association. See: American Heart Association. (2011, January 31). American Heart Association supports the new USDA/HHS dietary guidelines and encourages adherence. AHA also expresses disappointment that sodium, saturated fat guidance is weak. Retrieved on October 4, 2011, from http://newsroom.heart.org/pr/aha/1243.aspx. Also see: U.S. Department of Agriculture and U.S. Department of Health and Human Services. (2010, December). Dietary guidelines for Americans, 2010 (7th ed.). Washington, DC: U.S. Government Printing Office. Retrieved on April 11, 2011, from http://www.health.gov/dietaryguidelines/dga2010/DietaryGuidelines2010.pdf

to develop a diabetes management plan that is specific for you; diabetics who conscientiously manage their disease and their blood sugar level lower their risk of cardiovascular disease.

Getting regular medical checkups (the frequency of which should be determined by your physician) can help you assess your CVD risk factors. Your physician may recommend other steps to lower CVD risks. The following sections describe actions that physicians often recommend for reducing CVD risk and maintaining cardiovascular health.

Smoking Cessation

If you smoke, stop now. If you do not smoke, avoid breathing in secondhand (other people's) smoke. Approximately 150,000 cardiovascular deaths could be avoided each year if people did not smoke cigarettes.[22] Studies suggest that when someone quits smoking, his or her elevated risk of CAD is cut in half only 1 year after quitting. Within 15 years, the elevated risk of a former smoker declines to the level of a nonsmoker.[40] According to the National Stroke Association, the risk of stroke may revert to that of nonsmokers within 5 years after quitting. The more cigarettes a person smokes and the earlier a person started to smoke, the longer the recovery time. In addition, the risk of cardiovascular disease increases as the number of cigarettes smoked increases. Therefore, smoke fewer cigarettes if you cannot quit. Smoking "low-yield" (low tar and nicotine) cigarettes does not appear to reduce CVD risk.

Maintaining a Healthy Weight

Maintaining a healthy weight, a BMI measurement of 20 to 24.9, reduces your risk of heart disease. If your BMI is 25 or more, then losing weight will reduce your risk of cardiovascular disease. In general, a regular exercise program coupled with a low-calorie diet will reduce body fat. Weight reduction lowers total blood cholesterol levels, raises HDL levels, and lowers LDL levels. It also helps maintain proper blood glucose levels.

Regular Exercise

In the late 1980s, a review of 43 studies about the relationship between physical activity and the risk of CAD and atherosclerosis was conducted.[41] Two-thirds of these studies documented a substantial inverse relationship between physical activity and risk for these two related diseases: As the level of physical activity rose, the risk of CAD and atherosclerosis declined and vice versa. These findings have been upheld by more recent studies.[33] Research results also show that exercise is associated with a decreased risk of stroke.[42]

Exercise has been shown to lower blood pressure and boost HDL levels. The AHA recommends that healthy people perform any moderate- to vigorous-intensity aerobic activity, such as brisk walking, hiking, stair-climbing, jogging, bicycling, and swimming, for at least 30 minutes per day, 5 days per week.[43] (Aerobic activities are those that raise the heart rate for a sustained period of time.) The AHA notes that regular physical activity for longer periods or at greater intensity will likely provide greater health benefits. Even moderate-intensity activities, such as slow walking, gardening, housework, and recreational activities, can have some long-term health benefits when performed daily and can help lower the risk of cardiovascular disease.

Lowering Blood Pressure

Nearly one of every three American adults has hypertension. In 90–95% of cases, hypertension can be controlled. Doing so reduces the risk of both stroke and heart attack. The American Heart Association recommends having your blood pressure checked every 2 years and more often if it is high.

To lower blood pressure, the AHA suggests decreasing sodium intake to a maximum of 1,500 mg per day, which is about two-thirds of a teaspoon of salt.[44] Nutritionists suggest checking the amount of sodium that you consume in prepackaged, processed foods and not salting your food. The sodium in salt causes the body to retain fluids and may contribute to hypertension in some people.

Other dietary factors, in addition to sodium, also affect blood pressure. The DASH diet (Dietary Approaches to Stop Hypertension) has been shown to lower blood pressure in diverse subgroups of the U.S. population. This diet is low in total and saturated fat compared to a more typical U.S. diet, and is rich in fruits, vegetables, and low-fat dairy foods. Researchers also studied decreased sodium intake with both the DASH diet and the typical U.S. diet. Data show highly significant decreases in blood pressure with either diet. Researchers conclude that the DASH diet plus reduced sodium intake is effective in controlling blood pressure.[45]

The blood pressure of overweight individuals often drops when they lose weight. If you are overweight and have high blood pressure, weight reduction is the most important action you can take to lower your blood pressure and risk of CVD. Regular aerobic exercise lowers blood pressure and will also help control weight. Reducing the intake of dietary saturated fat and cholesterol will promote overall cardiovascular health and will also help reduce caloric intake, which is important for weight control.

The heavy consumption of alcoholic beverages has also been shown to lead to high blood pressure, increasing the risk of heart attack, stroke, and death from CAD. Limiting consumption to 1 oz of alcohol (ethanol) per day (two drinks or fewer) for men and 0.5 oz (one drink) for women may help lower blood pressure and may reduce your risk of cardiovascular disease. One ounce of ethanol is equivalent to 2 oz of 100-proof whiskey, 8 to 10 oz of wine (the alcohol content in wines varies), or two 12-oz cans of beer.

If none of these lifestyle changes lowers the blood pressure sufficiently, hypertension can be treated with a wide array of antihypertensive drugs. These drugs are not suitable or appropriate for all hypertensive individuals but may be essential therapy for many.

Reducing Blood Cholesterol

Decades of scientific research show that a high level of cholesterol in the blood is a major risk factor for cardiovascular disease. Eating saturated fats (found in foods such as red meat, cream, and whole milk), trans fats (found in many baked goods and french fries), and dietary cholesterol (found in foods such as meats, egg yolks, and dairy products) tends to raise blood cholesterol. Therefore, the American Heart Association recommends that healthy Americans older than age 2 years should limit their saturated fat intake (primarily animal fats and tropical oils) to less than 7% and their trans fat intake to less than 1%.[46] The AHA also recommends that Americans restrict dietary cholesterol intake to 300 mg per day. (One large egg, for example, has slightly more than 200 mg, and a quarter-pound cheeseburger has slightly more than 100 mg.

Polyunsaturated fats (found in nuts, seeds, and certain plant oils, such as canola, safflower, and sesame oil) and monounsaturated fats (found in avocados and olive, canola, and peanut oil) tend to lower blood cholesterol levels. Omega-3 fatty acids, which are found in certain fish such as salmon, tuna, cod, and sole, appear to lower the risk of CAD and stroke. The American Heart Association suggests that individuals should adjust their total fat intake to meet their caloric needs. People who are overweight or obese should limit their overall fat intake to less than 30% of their daily intake of calories and replace saturated and trans fats in their diet with poly- and monounsaturated fats.[46]

Studies show that, on average, people can achieve a 10% reduction in cholesterol levels by following these dietary guidelines. Each 1% reduction in the blood cholesterol level reduces the risk of CAD by 2% to 3%, so a 10% reduction reduces your risk of CAD by 20% to 30%. If you are at high risk for cardiovascular disease, your physician will likely place you on a diet that has cholesterol and other fat intake recommendations different from those mentioned here, which are for the general population.

Eating whole grains and foods rich in soluble fiber (such as fruits, beans, oats, and barley) can help reduce your LDL and total cholesterol levels (**Figure 12.14**).[47] Soluble fiber, which dissolves in water, makes its way into your bloodstream during digestion where it interferes with the absorption of cholesterol. By doing so, soluble fiber helps decrease cardiovascular disease risk. The American Heart Association notes that insoluble dietary fiber, found in many foods such as green leafy vegetables, fruit skins, seeds, and nuts, also appears to decrease cardiovascular risk and slows progression of cardiovascular disease in high-risk individuals. The AHA suggests a total dietary fiber intake of 25 g from foods, not supplements, to ensure enough nutrients in the diet.[39] Currently, most Americans take in only half that amount.

Figure 12.14

Foods High in Soluble Fiber. Soluble fiber helps lower LDL cholesterol. The foods shown here include whole wheat bread, oatmeal, broccoli, navel oranges, beans, avocado, and pitted prunes.

Courtesy of Wendy Schiff.

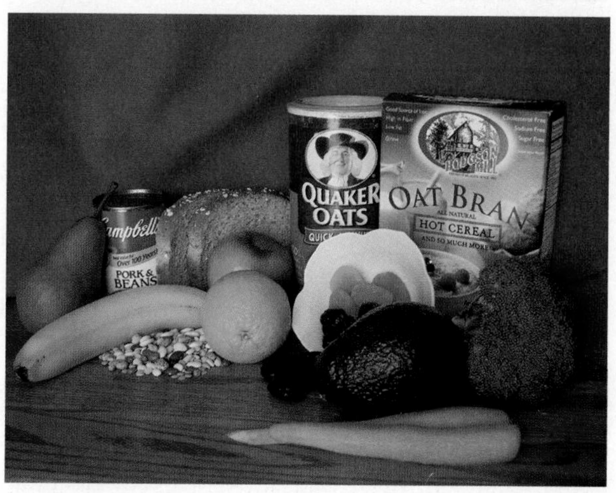

If eating a heart-healthy diet and exercising regularly do not significantly reduce elevated blood cholesterol levels, cholesterol-lowering medications called "statins" are available by prescription. Research results have shown that statins are safe, reduce CAD deaths, reduce total cholesterol and LDL cholesterol, and appear to reduce the risk of stroke.[48]

Aspirin Therapy

A treatment to reduce the risk of cardiovascular disease that has gained attention in recent years is long-term use of aspirin in a dosage no greater than a baby aspirin (80 mg). The benefit of aspirin therapy increases with increasing cardiovascular risk; it reduces the risk for heart attack in men and strokes in women.[49] Aspirin can have damaging effects on the gastrointestinal system and reduces the blood's ability to clot; therefore, long-term aspirin therapy should be undertaken only on the advice of a physician.

Hormone Replacement Therapy

Hormone replacement therapy (HRT) is the use of estrogen plus progestin in postmenopausal women or the use of estrogen alone in postmenopausal women with prior hysterectomy (surgical removal of the uterus). Analysis of data from the Women's Health Initiative (WHI) 15-year research program, which addresses the most common causes of death, disability, and poor quality of life in postmenopausal women, suggests that cardiovascular risk is neither increased nor decreased in women who begin hormone therapy less than 10 years after menopause.[50–52] Cardiovascular risk increases in women beginning hormone therapy after that time. Women who are between 50 and 59 years of age when they begin postmenopausal hormone therapy appear to have a lower risk of death from any cause than women who do not take postmenopausal hormones or who begin taking hormones later in life. Researchers caution, however, that HRT is not without risk and do not recommend postmenopausal hormone therapy for the prevention of heart attacks. Women nearing menopause should talk with their physicians to determine whether HRT is appropriate for them.

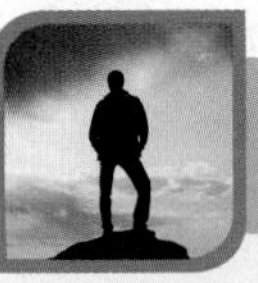

Healthy Living Practices

- One of the most important things you can do to lower your risk of coronary artery disease and stroke is to reduce your modifiable risk factors, which include quitting smoking, maintaining a healthy body weight, and maintaining an active lifestyle that includes regular aerobic exercise.
- To lower your blood pressure, engage in regular aerobic exercise, lose weight if you are overweight, limit your alcohol consumption to 1 oz of ethanol per day for men and 0.5 oz per day for women, and limit your daily sodium intake to 1,500 mg.
- To reduce your total cholesterol level, raise your HDL level, and lower your LDL level, eat no more than 20% to 35% of your daily intake of calories from fat and no more than 7% from saturated fat and less than 1% from trans fat. Also, eat foods rich in soluble fiber, such as fruits, beans, and oats.

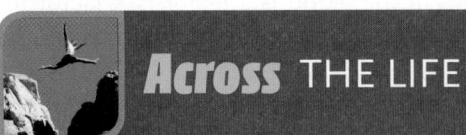

Across THE LIFE SPAN

CARDIOVASCULAR HEALTH

The American Heart Association estimates that approximately 1% of babies are born each year with a variety of heart and blood vessel structural and functional abnormalities.[53] Many congenital defects (those present at birth) can now be diagnosed before birth with the use of echocardiography, or ultrasound of the heart. Sound waves are directed through the heart of the fetus; as they pass through different types of tissues (such as heart muscle and blood), they are reflected, or echoed, producing an image of the movements of the heart structures. This technique can also be used with infants, children, and adults. Such early diagnostic techniques have helped surgeons correct infants' cardiovascular defects within the first few weeks of life. This approach helps avoid complications from cardiovascular defects in older children and adults. Presently, about 1 million Americans have congenital heart defects.

The Bogalusa Heart Study, a long-term study of the development of coronary artery disease, showed that cardiovascular disease caused by atherosclerosis is a process that begins in childhood.[54] Habits of diet and lifestyle develop at an early age and often continue into adulthood, affecting this disease process. Data from the Bogalusa Heart Study show that the average diet of children and adolescents consisted of 14% of their total daily calories from protein, 50% from carbohydrate, and 36% from fat.[55] The more recent School Nutrition Dietary Assessment Study found that most children and adolescents had nutritionally adequate diets, but 80% had diets too high in saturated fat and 92% had diets too high in sodium.[56] Such diets do not meet the recommendations of the American Heart Association and can lead to the development of atherosclerosis and obesity, both risk factors for coronary artery disease and stroke.

In the Bogalusa study, school breakfasts and lunches had a major impact on the diets of children, providing approximately half of the day's total caloric intake and about 49% of daily total fat intake—too high a proportion. Many school lunch programs have reduced their percentages of total fat, saturated fat, and sodium. In addition, several innovative "heart-healthy" school lunch programs such as Healthy Edge, Lunch Power, and Heart Smart have been developed in schools across the nation.

The results of studies show that older adults should be treated with lipid-lowering therapy when needed because it will help prevent the progression of CVD and other diseases common in this age group.[57] Treating hypertension in older adults is also recommended because it reduces the risk of cardiovascular events. However, treating hypertension in the very elderly (those older than 80 years) may have more risks than benefits.[58]

Analyzing Health-Related Information

Critical Thinking

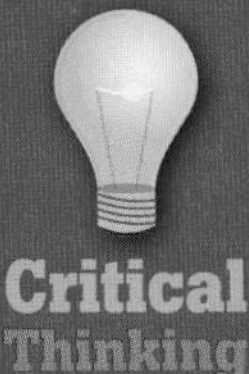

This article focuses on claims that manufacturers make on food labels. Explain why you think this article is a reliable or an unreliable source of information. Use the model for analyzing health information to guide your thinking; the main points of the model are noted here.

1. Which statements are verifiable facts, and which are unverified statements or value claims?
2. What are the credentials of the source making these health-related claims? Does the source have the appropriate background and education in the topic area? What can you do to check the credentials of this source?
3. What might be the motives and biases of the source making the claims?
4. What is the main point of the article? Which information is relevant to the issue, main point, product, or service? Which information is irrelevant?
5. Is the source reliable? What evidence supports your conclusion that the source is reliable or unreliable? Does the source of information present the pros and cons of the topic or the benefits and risks of the product?
6. Does the source of information attack the credibility of conventional scientists or medical authorities?

Based on your analysis, do you think that this article is a reliable source of health-related information? Summarize your reasons for coming to this conclusion.

Trans Fat Now Listed with Saturated Fat and Cholesterol on the Nutrition Facts Label

Trans Fat Coming to a Label Near You!

The Food and Drug Administration (FDA) now requires food manufacturers to list trans fat (i.e., trans fatty acids) on Nutrition Facts and some Supplement Facts panels. Scientific evidence shows that consumption of saturated fat, trans fat, and dietary cholesterol raises low-density lipoprotein (LDL or "bad") cholesterol levels that increase the risk of coronary heart disease (CHD). According to the National Heart, Lung, and Blood Institute of the National Institutes of Health, over 12.5 million Americans suffer from CHD, and more than 500,000 die each year. This makes CHD one of the leading causes of death in the United States today.

Since 1993, the FDA has required that saturated fat and dietary cholesterol be listed on the food label. By adding trans fat on the Nutrition Facts panel (required as of January 1, 2006), consumers now know for the first time how much of all three—saturated fat, trans fat, and cholesterol—are in the foods they choose. Identifying saturated fat, trans fat, and cholesterol on the food label gives consumers information to make heart-healthy food choices that help them reduce their risk of CHD. This revised label, which includes information on trans fat as well as saturated fat and cholesterol, will be of particular interest to people concerned about high blood cholesterol and heart disease.

However, all Americans should be aware of the risk posed by consuming too much saturated fat, trans fat, and cholesterol. But what is trans fat, and how can you limit the amount of this fat in your diet?

Nutrition Facts

Serving Size 1 cup (228g)
Servings Per Container 2

Amount Per Serving	
Calories 250	Calories from Fat 110
Total Fat 12g	
Saturated Fat 3g	
Trans Fat 1.5g	
Cholesterol 30mg	10%
Sodium 470mg	20%
Total Carbohydrate 31g	10%
Dietary Fiber 0g	0%
Sugars 5g	
Protein 5g	
Vitamin A	4%
Vitamin C	2%
Calcium	20%
Iron	4%

Appearing on product labels as of January 2006

* Percent Daily Values are based on a 2,000 calorie diet. Your Daily Values may be higher or lower depending on your calorie needs:

	Calories:	2,000	2,500
Total Fat	Less than	65g	80g
Sat Fat	Less than	20g	25g
Cholesterol	Less than	300mg	300mg
Sodium	Less than	2,400mg	2,400mg
Total Carbohydrate		300g	375g
Dietary Fiber		25g	30g

Reproduced from Food and Drug Administration. (2011, June 24). Available at http://www.accessdata.fda.gov/videos/cfsan/hwm/hwmres.cfm

What Is Trans Fat? Where Will I Find Trans Fat?

Vegetable shortenings, some margarines, crackers, cookies, snack foods, and other foods made with or fried in partially hydrogenated oils.

Unlike other fats, the majority of trans fat is formed when liquid oils are made into solid fats like shortening and hard margarine. However, a small amount of trans fat is found naturally, primarily in some animal-based foods. Essentially, trans fat is made when hydrogen is added to vegetable oil—a process called hydrogenation. Hydrogenation increases the shelf life and flavor stability of foods containing these fats.

Trans fat, like saturated fat and dietary cholesterol, raises the LDL (or "bad") cholesterol that increases your risk for CHD. On average, Americans consume four to five times as much saturated fat as trans fat in their diet.

Although saturated fat is the main dietary culprit that raises LDL, trans fat and dietary cholesterol also contribute significantly. Trans fat can often be found in processed foods made with partially hydrogenated vegetable oils such as vegetable shortenings, some margarines (especially margarines that are harder), crackers, candies, cookies, snack foods, fried foods, and baked goods.

Are All Fats the Same?

Simply put: no. Fat is a major source of energy for the body and aids in the absorption of vitamins A, D, E, and K, and carotenoids. Both animal- and plant-derived food products contain fat, and when eaten in moderation, fat is important for proper growth, development, and maintenance of good health. As a food ingredient, fat provides taste, consistency, and stability and helps us feel full. In addition, parents should be aware that fats are an especially important source of calories and nutrients for infants and toddlers (up to 2 years of age), who have the highest energy needs per unit of body weight of any age group.

Saturated and trans fats raise LDL (or "bad") cholesterol levels in the blood, thereby increasing the risk of heart disease. Dietary cholesterol also contributes to heart disease. Unsaturated fats, such as monounsaturated and polyunsaturated, do not raise LDL cholesterol and are beneficial when consumed in moderation. Therefore, it is advisable to choose foods low in saturated fat, trans fat, and cholesterol as part of a healthful diet.

What Can I Do About Saturated Fat, Trans Fat, and Cholesterol?

When comparing foods, look at the Nutrition Facts panel, and choose the food with the lower amounts of saturated fat, trans fat, and cholesterol. Health experts recommend that you keep your intake of these nutrients as low as possible while consuming a nutritionally adequate diet. However, these experts recognize that eliminating these three components entirely from your diet is not practical because they are unavoidable in ordinary diets.

Where Can I Find Trans Fat on the Food Label?

Take a look at the Nutrition Facts panel accompanying this article. Consumers can find trans fat listed on the Nutrition Facts panel directly under the line for saturated fat. If trans fat is not declared on the label and you are curious about the trans fat content of a product, contact the manufacturer listed on the label.

How Do Your Choices Stack Up?

With the addition of trans fat to the Nutrition Facts panel, you can review your food choices and see how they stack up. The following labels illustrate total fat, saturated fat, trans fat, and cholesterol content per serving for selected food products.

Don't assume similar products are the same. Be sure to check the Nutrition Facts panel (NFP) when comparing products because even similar foods can vary in calories, ingredients, nutrients, and the size and number of servings in the package. When buying the same brand product, also check the NFP frequently because ingredients can change at any time and any change could affect the NFP information.

Look at the highlighted items on the sample labels. Combine the grams (g) of saturated fat and trans fat and look for the lowest combined amount. Also, look for the lowest percent (%) Daily Value for cholesterol. Check all three nutrients to make the best choice for a healthful diet.

Note: The following label examples do not represent a single product or an entire product category. In general, the nutrient values were combined for several products and the average values were used for these label examples.

How Can I Use the Label to Make Heart-Healthy Food Choices?

The Nutrition Facts panel can help you choose foods lower in saturated fat, trans fat, and cholesterol. To lower your intake of saturated fat, trans fat, and cholesterol, compare similar foods and choose the food with the lower combined saturated and trans fats and the lower amount of cholesterol.

Data from Food and Drug Administration. (2014, June 13). Retrieved from http://www.fda.gov/food/ingredientspackaginglabeling/labelingnutrition/ucm20026097.htm

Compare Spreads![*]

Keep an eye on saturated fat, trans fat, and cholesterol!

Butter[**]

Nutrition Facts	
Serving Size 1 Tbsp (14g)	
Servings Per Container 32	
Amount Per Serving	
Calories 100	Calories from Fat 100
	% Daily Value*
Total Fat 11g	17%
Saturated Fat 7g ←	35%
Trans Fat 0g ←	
Cholesterol 30mg →	10%

Saturated Fat : 7 g
+ *Trans* Fat : 0 g
Combined Amt. : 7 g
Cholesterol : 10 % DV

Margarine, stick[†]

Nutrition Facts	
Serving Size 1 Tbsp (14g)	
Servings Per Container 32	
Amount Per Serving	
Calories 100	Calories from Fat 100
	% Daily Value*
Total Fat 11g	17%
Saturated Fat 2g ←	10%
Trans Fat 3g ←	
Cholesterol 0mg →	0%

Saturated Fat : 2 g
+ *Trans* Fat : 3 g
Combined Amt. : 5 g
Cholesterol : 0 % DV

Margarine, tub[†]

Nutrition Facts	
Serving Size 1 Tbsp (14g)	
Servings Per Container 32	
Amount Per Serving	
Calories 60	Calories from Fat 60
	% Daily Value*
Total Fat 7g	11%
Saturated Fat 1g ←	5%
Trans Fat 0.5g ←	
Cholesterol 0mg →	0%

Saturated Fat : 1 g
+ *Trans* Fat : 0.5 g
Combined Amt. : 1.5 g
Cholesterol : 0 % DV

*Nutrient values rounded based on FDA's nutrition labeling regulations. Calorie and cholesterol content estimated.
**Butter values from FDA Table of Trans Values, 1/30/95.
†Values derived from 2002 USDA National Nutrient Database for Standard Reference, Release 15.

Compare Desserts![*]

Keep an eye on saturated fat, trans fat, and cholesterol!

Granola Bar[±]

Nutrition Facts	
Serving Size 1 bar (33g)	
Servings Per Container 10	
Amount Per Serving	
Calories 140	Calories from Fat 45
	% Daily Value*
Total Fat 5g	8%
Saturated Fat 1g ←	5%
Trans Fat 0g ←	
Cholesterol 0mg →	0%

Saturated Fat : 1 g
+ *Trans* Fat : 0 g
Combined Amt. : 1 g
Cholesterol : 0 % DV

Sandwich Cookies[±]

Nutrition Facts	
Serving Size 2 cookies (28g)	
Servings Per Container 19	
Amount Per Serving	
Calories 130	Calories from Fat 45
	% Daily Value*
Total Fat 5g	8%
Saturated Fat 1g ←	5%
Trans Fat 1.5g ←	
Cholesterol 0mg →	0%

Saturated Fat : 1 g
+ *Trans* Fat : 1.5 g
Combined Amt. : 2.5 g
Cholesterol : 0 % DV

Cake, Iced and Filled[±]

Nutrition Facts	
Serving Size 2 cakes (66g)	
Servings Per Container 6	
Amount Per Serving	
Calories 280	Calories from Fat 140
	% Daily Value*
Total Fat 16g	25%
Saturated Fat 3.5g ←	18%
Trans Fat 4.5g ←	
Cholesterol 10mg →	3%

Saturated Fat : 3.5 g
+ *Trans* Fat : 4.5 g
Combined Amt. : 8 g
Cholesterol : 3 % DV

*Nutrient values rounded based on FDA's nutrition labeling regulations.
±Values for total fat, saturated fat, and trans fat were based on the means of analytical data for several food samples from Subramaniam, S., et al., "Trans, saturated, and unsaturated fat in foods in the United States prior to mandatory trans-fat labeling," *Lipids* 39, 11–18, 2004. Other information and values were derived from food labels in the marketplace.

Compare Snacks!*

Keep an eye on saturated fat, trans fat, and cholesterol!

	Frozen Potatoes± (e.g., French Fries)	Potato Chips±	Mini-Sandwich Crackers±
Nutrition Facts			
Serving Size	3 oz (84g/ about 12 pieces)	1 oz (28g/ about 20 chips)	14 pieces (31g)
Servings Per Container	11	12	10
Amount Per Serving			
Calories	160	150	160
Calories from Fat	50	90	70
% Daily Value*			
Total Fat	6g — 9%	10g — 15%	8g — 12%
Saturated Fat ←	1g — 5%	2g — 10%	2g — 10%
Trans Fat ←	1.5g	0g	2g
Cholesterol →	0mg — 0%	0mg — 0%	< 5mg — 1%
Saturated Fat :	1 g	2 g	2 g
+ *Trans* Fat :	1.5 g	0 g	2 g
Combined Amt. :	2.5 g	2 g	4 g
Cholesterol :	0 % DV	0 % DV	1 % DV

*Nutrient values rounded based on FDA's nutrition labeling regulations.

±Values for total fat, saturated fat, and trans fat were based on the means of analytical data for several food samples from Subramaniam, S., et al., "Trans, saturated, and unsaturated fat in foods in the United States prior to mandatory trans-fat labeling," *Lipids* 39, 11–18, 2004. Other information and values were derived from food labels in the marketplace.

CHAPTER REVIEW

Summary

The leading cause of death in the United States is a noninfectious disease: coronary artery disease (CAD). In CAD, the arteries that supply blood to the heart become blocked, restricting blood flow. CAD is only one disease of the cardiovascular system; hypertension, stroke, and rheumatic heart disease are three other prominent cardiovascular diseases. Atherosclerosis is an important cardiovascular disease process that is an underlying cause of CAD and stroke.

The cardiovascular system includes the heart and blood vessels. The heart, a muscular, fist-sized organ, pumps blood to the body. The blood performs many functions, such as bringing nutrients and oxygen to the tissues and removing wastes, including the waste gas carbon dioxide. Blood vessels called arteries bring blood away from the heart; veins return blood to the heart. Microscopic vessels called capillaries join the two and allow the exchange of nutrients, gases, and wastes at the tissues.

Fatty deposits develop in arteries as part of a disease called atherosclerosis. Atherosclerosis occurs most frequently in the arteries supplying blood to the heart, brain, and legs. In coronary artery disease, the coronary arteries, which supply the heart muscle with blood, become blocked by fatty deposits, a blood clot, or both. When the heart is deprived of the blood (and therefore the oxygen) that it needs, chest pain (angina pectoris) or a heart attack results. A physician usually performs diagnostic tests to assess the degree and location of blockage. Medication can help widen blood vessels and reduce symptoms.

During a heart attack, part of the heart muscle dies. As the muscle dies, it may trigger electrical activity that causes the ventricles to stop beating properly, possibly resulting in heart failure, cardiac arrest, and death. A heart attack victim needs immediate medical care.

A stroke occurs when arteries that supply blood to the brain become blocked by fatty deposits or by a blood clot. A stroke may cause a loss or dimming of vision, difficulty in speaking or understanding speech, headache, dizziness, unsteadiness, and even death.

The major risk factors for developing cardiovascular disease are family health history, abnormal blood lipid levels, cigarette smoking, high blood pressure, physical inactivity, obesity, diabetes mellitus, and stress. Behaviors that may lower the risk of cardiovascular disease are stopping smoking, maintaining a healthy weight, exercising regularly, maintaining healthy blood pressure levels, maintaining favorable blood lipid levels, managing diabetes mellitus to stabilize the blood glucose level, and coping effectively with stress.

Infants may be born with a wide variety of heart and blood vessel structural and functional abnormalities. Many of these congenital defects can now be diagnosed before birth and treated during the first few weeks of life.

Cardiovascular disease caused by atherosclerosis may begin in childhood. American children are still consuming diets that promote cardiovascular disease. Healthy school meal programs can help change this fact, and education can promote healthy lifestyles.

Data suggest that physicians should treat abnormal lipid levels and high blood pressure in older adults.

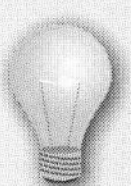

Applying What You Have Learned

1. If a family member experienced a transient ischemic attack, how would you recognize it? What would you do? What long-term action might this family member take to avoid the onset of a stroke? **Analysis**
2. Analyze your lifestyle to determine which modifiable risk factors are raising your probability of developing cardiovascular disease. List these risk factors and explain how each increases your risk for developing cardiovascular disease. **Analysis**
3. Using the list you developed by answering question 2, describe how you could modify your behavior to lower your risk of developing cardiovascular disease. **Synthesis**
4. List all of your risk factors for developing cardiovascular disease, both those you can change and those you cannot. Using the information from answer 3, evaluate your course of action. Which changes do you realistically expect to make and which do you expect not to make? What can you do to offset uncontrollable risk factors (e.g., family health history)? Give rationales for your answers. If you follow this plan, do you think that you will substantially reduce your risk of developing CVD? Why or why not? **Evaluation**

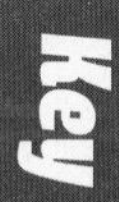

Analysis	Synthesis	Evaluation
breaking down information into component parts.	putting together information from different sources.	making informed decisions.

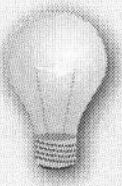

Reflecting on Your Health

1. If you are a parent or plan to be a parent some day, what are you doing (or will you do) to encourage your child's heart-healthy lifestyle?
2. If you are a cigarette smoker, identify your reasons or motivations for smoking. After learning about the effects of smoking on cardiovascular health, do you want to quit? If so, what steps might you take to reduce the amount you smoke or to stop smoking? Be sure to include things you can do as an individual, as well as sources of help to assist you in the process. If you are a nonsmoker, list the situations in which you regularly breathe secondhand smoke. Reflect on what you believe to be your increased risk of cardiovascular disease because of your exposure. What can you do to lessen your exposure?
3. Do you feel confident that you would be able to recognize when another person is having a stroke, TIA, or heart attack and help him or her? Visit helpful websites, such as the American Heart Association (www.heart.org) and review warning signs of stroke and/or TIA. Then, reflect on what you would do to handle such an emergency?
4. Rate your lifestyle on a scale of 1 to 10, with 1 being an extremely heart-unhealthy lifestyle and 10 being an extremely heart-healthy lifestyle. Discuss why you rated your lifestyle as you did. Based on what you read in this chapter, what changes can you make to move closer to a 10 if you're not already there?
5. Do you think medical researchers are able to assess accurately the factors that are detrimental or helpful to cardiovascular health? Why do you feel this way? How do you think your attitudes concerning medical research affect your behavior? Have your attitudes about medical research and cardiovascular health changed since reading this chapter? Why or why not?

CHAPTER REVIEW

References

1. Tailor, A. M., et al. (2010). An update on the prevalence of the metabolic syndrome in children and adolescents. *International Journal of Pediatric Obesity, 5*(3), 202–213.
2. Zieske, A. W., et al. (2002). Natural history and risk factors of atherosclerosis in children and youth: The PDAY study. *Pediatric Pathology and Molecular Medicine, 21*, 213–237.
3. Roberts, C. K., et al. (2007). Effect of a short-term diet and exercise intervention in youth on atherosclerotic risk factors. *Atherosclerosis, 191*, 98–106.
4. Collins, K. M., et al. (2004). Heart disease awareness among college students. *Journal of Community Health, 29*(5), 405–420.
5. Munoz, L. R., et al. (2010). Awareness of heart disease among female college students. *Journal of Women's Health, 19*(12), 2253–2259.
6. Kostas, T. I., et al. (2010). Chronic venous disease progression and modification of predisposing factors. *Journal of Vascular Surgery, 51*(4), 900–907.
7. American Heart Association. (2014). Heart disease and stroke statistics—2014 update. *Circulation, 129*, e28–e292. Retrieved from http://circ.ahajournals.org/content/129/3/e28.full.pdf+html
8. Leuzzi, C., & Modena, M. G. (2010). Coronary artery disease: Clinical presentation, diagnosis and prognosis in women. *Nutrition, Metabolism, and Cardiovascular Diseases, 20*(6), 426–435.
9. Garg, S., Bourantas, C., & Serruys, P. W. (2013). New concepts in the design of drug-eluting coronary stents. *Nature Reviews Cardiology, 10*(5), 248–260.
10. Garg, S., & Serruys, P. (2009). Biodegradable stents and non-biodegradable stents. *Minerva Cardioangiologica, 57*(5), 537–565.
11. Pratali, S., et al. (2010). Transmyocardial laser revascularization 12 years later. *Interactive Cardiovascular and Thoracic Surgery, 11*(4), 480–481.
12. American Red Cross. (n.d.). *Learn about automatic external defibrillators.* Retrieved from: http://www.redcross.org/prepare/location/workplace/easy-as-aed
13. National Institutes of Health. (2011). *Cardiogenic shock.* Retrieved from http://www.nhlbi.nih.gov/health/health-topics/topics/shock/
14. Elijovich, L., & Chong, J. Y. (2010). Current and future use of intravenous thrombolysis for acute ischemic stroke. *Current Atherosclerosis Reports, 12*(5), 316–321.
15. Associated Press. (2013, October 23). *Study: Strokes affecting more younger people.* Retrieved from http://bigstory.ap.org/article/study-strokes-affecting-more-younger-people
16. Associated Press. (2011, February 9). *Strokes are rising fast among young, middle-aged.* Retrieved from http://cnsnews.com/news/article/strokes-are-rising-fast-among-young-middle-aged
17. Carroll, M. D., Kit, B. K., & Lacher, D. A. (2012). Total and high-density lipoprotein cholesterol in adults, 2009–2010. *NCHS Data Brief* (No. 92). Hyattsville, MD: National Center for Health Statistics.
18. Mosca, L., et al. (2007). Evidence-based guidelines for cardiovascular disease prevention in women: 2007 update. *Circulation, 115*, 1481–1501.
19. Spillmann, F., et al. (2010). High-density lipoprotein-raising strategies: Update 2010. *Current Pharmaceutical Design, 16*(13), 1517–1530.
20. U.S. Department of Health and Human Services. (2001). *Women and smoking: A report of the Surgeon General.* Atlanta, GA: U.S. Department of Health and Human Services, Centers for Disease Control and Prevention, National Center for Chronic Disease Prevention and Health Promotion. Retrieved from http://www.cdc.gov/tobacco/data_statistics/sgr/2001/
21. U.S. Department of Health and Human Services. (2014). *The health consequences of smoking—50 years of progress.* Rockville, MD: Public Health Service, Office of the Surgeon General. Retrieved from http://www.surgeongeneral.gov/library/reports/50-years-of-progress/full-report.pdf
22. U.S. Department of Health and Human Services. (2010). *How tobacco smoke causes disease: The biology and behavioral basis for smoking-attributable disease: A report of the Surgeon General.* Atlanta, GA: Author. Retrieved from http://www.ncbi.nlm.nih.gov/books/NBK53017/
23. American Heart Association. (2014). *Smoking and cardiovascular disease.* Retrieved from http://www.heart.org/HEARTORG/GettingHealthy/QuitSmoking/QuittingResources/Smoking-Cardiovascular-Disease_UCM_305187_Article.jsp
24. U.S. Department of Health and Human Services. (2006). *The health consequences of involuntary exposure to tobacco smoke: A report of the Surgeon General.* Atlanta, GA: Centers for Disease Control and Prevention, National Center for Chronic Disease Prevention and Health Promotion, Office on Smoking and Health. Retrieved from http://www.ncbi.nlm.nih.gov/books/NBK44324/
25. National Center for Health Statistics. (2014). *Health, United States, 2013.* Hyattsville, MD: Author. Retrieved from http://www.cdc.gov/nchs/data/hus/hus13.pdf
26. Mayo Clinic Staff. (2014). *High blood pressure (hypertension): Risk factors.* Retrieved from http://www.mayoclinic.com/health/high-blood-pressure/DS00100/DSECTION=risk-factors
27. Roux, D., & Ana, V. (2014). The foreclosure crisis and cardiovascular disease. *Circulation, 129*(22), 2248–2249.
28. Trudel-Fitzgerald, C., Boehm, J. K., Kivimaki, M., & Kubzansky, L. D. (2014). Taking the tension out of hypertension: A prospective study on psychological well being and hypertension. *Journal of Hypertension, 32*(6), 1222–1228.
29. Katzmarzyk, P. T., et al. (2009). Sitting time and mortality from all causes, cardiovascular disease, and cancer. *Medicine & Science in Sports & Exercise, 41*(5), 998–1005.
30. Petersen, C. B., et al. (2014). Total sitting time and risk of myocardial infarction, coronary heart disease and all-cause mortality in a prospective study of Danish adults. *International Journal of Behavioral Nutrition and Physical Activity, 11*(1), 843–853.
31. U.S. Department of Health and Human Services. (1996). *Physical activity and health: A report of the Surgeon General.* Atlanta, GA: U.S. Department of Health and Human Services, Centers for Disease Control and Prevention, National Center for Chronic Disease Prevention and Health Promotion. Retrieved from http://www.cdc.gov/NCCDPHP/sgr/pdf/sgrfull.pdf
32. Centers for Disease Control and Prevention. (2011). *Physical activity for everyone.* Retrieved from http://www.cdc.gov/physicalactivity/everyone/health/index.html#ReduceCardiovascularDisease

33. U.S. Department of Health and Human Services. (2008). *Physical activity and good nutrition: Essential elements to prevent chronic diseases and obesity 2008.* Atlanta, GA: Centers for Disease Control and Prevention, National Center for Chronic Disease Prevention and Health Promotion. Retrieved from http://www.cdc.gov/nccdphp/publications/aag/pdf/dnpa.pdf
34. Katerndahl, D. A. (2008). The association between panic disorder and coronary artery disease among primary care patients presenting with chest pain: An updated literature review. *Primary Care Companion to the Journal of Clinical Psychiatry, 10*, 276–285.
35. Zakynthinos, E., & Pappa, N. (2009). Inflammatory biomarkers in coronary artery disease. *Journal of Cardiology, 53*(3), 317–333.
36. Buckley, D., et al. (2009). C-reactive protein as a risk factor for coronary heart disease: a systematic review and meta-analyses for the U.S. Preventive Services Task Force. *Annals Of Internal Medicine, 151*(7), 483–495.
37. U.S. Department of Agriculture and U.S. Department of Health and Human Services. (2010, December). *Dietary guidelines for Americans, 2010* (7th ed.). Washington, DC: U.S. Government Printing Office. Retrieved from http://www.health.gov/dietaryguidelines/dga2010/DietaryGuidelines2010.pdf
38. King, D. E., et al. (2007). Turning back the clock: Adopting a healthy lifestyle in middle age. *American Journal of Medicine, 120*, 598–603.
39. King, D. E., et al. (2009). Adherence to healthy lifestyle habits in U.S. adults, 1988–2006. *American Journal of Medicine, 122*(6), 528–534.
40. American Heart Association. (2014, May 30). *Smoke-free living: Benefits and milestones.* Retrieved from http://www.heart.org/HEARTORG/GettingHealthy/QuitSmoking/YourNon-SmokingLife/Smoke-free-Living-Benefits-Milestones_UCM_322711_Article.jsp
41. Powell, K., et al. (1987). Physical activity and the incidence of coronary heart disease. *Annual Review of Public Health, 8*, 253–287.
42. Galimanis, A., et al. (2009). Lifestyle and stroke risk: A review. *Current Opinion in Neurology, 22*, 60–68.
43. American Heart Association. (2014, May 16). *American Heart Association guidelines.* Retrieved from http://www.heart.org/HEARTORG/GettingHealthy/PhysicalActivity/GettingActive/American-Heart-Association-Guidelines_UCM_307976_Article.jsp
44. American Heart Association. (2011, January 31). *American Heart Association supports the new USDA/HHS dietary guidelines and encourages adherence. AHA also expresses disappointment that sodium, saturated fat guidance is weak.* Retrieved from http://newsroom.heart.org/pr/aha/1243.aspx
45. Appel, L. J., et al. (2006). Dietary approaches to prevent and treat hypertension: A scientific statement from the American Heart Association. *Hypertension, 47*, 291–308.
46. American Heart Association. (2014). *Know your fats.* Retrieved from http://www.heart.org/HEARTORG/Conditions/Cholesterol/PreventionTreatmentofHighCholesterol/Know-Your-Fats_UCM_305628_Article.jsp
47. American Heart Association. (2014, February 19). *Whole grains and fiber.* Retrieved from http://www.heart.org/HEARTORG/GettingHealthy/NutritionCenter/HealthyDietGoals/Whole-Grains-and-Fiber_UCM_303249_Article.jsp
48. Ebrahim, S., Taylor, F., & Brindle, P. (2014). Statins for the primary prevention of cardiovascular disease. *British Medical Journal, 348*(7944), 32–35.
49. Wolff, T., et al. (2009). Aspirin for the primary prevention of cardiovascular events: An update of the evidence for the U.S. Preventive Services Task Force. *Annals of Internal Medicine, 150*(6), 405–410.
50. Writing Group for the Women's Health Initiative Investigators. (2011). Health outcomes after stopping conjugated equine estrogens among postmenopausal women with prior hysterectomy. *Journal of the American Medical Association, 305*(13), 1305–1314.
51. Writing Group for the Women's Health Initiative Investigators. (2008). Health risks and benefits 3 years after stopping randomized treatment with estrogen and progestin. *Journal of the American Medical Association, 299*(9), 1036–1045.
52. Women's Health Initiative Participant Website. (2007, April). *Postmenopausal hormone therapy and risk of cardiovascular disease by age and years since menopause.* Retrieved from https://www.whi.org/participants/findings/Pages/ht_cvd.aspx
53. American Heart Association. (2014, May 6). *About congenital cardiovascular defects.* Retrieved from http://www.heart.org/HEARTORG/Conditions/CongenitalHeartDefects/About-CongenitalHeartDefects/About-Congenital-Heart-Defects_UCM_001217_Article.jsp
54. Tulane University School of Medicine, Center for Cardiovascular Health. (n.d.). *The Bogalusa Heart Study.* Retrieved from http://tulane.edu/som/cardiohealth/index.cfm
55. Nicklas, T. A., et al. (2001). Trends in nutrient intake of 10-year-old children over two decades (1973–1994): The Bogalusa Heart Study. *American Journal of Epidemiology, 153*, 969–977.
56. Clark, M. A., & Fox, M. K. (2009). Nutritional quality of the diets of U.S. public school children and the role of the school meal programs. *Journal of the American Dietetic Association, 109*(2 Suppl), S44–56.
57. Petersen, L. K., Christensen, K., & Kragstrup, J. (2010). Lipid-lowering treatment to the end? A review of observational studies and RCTs on cholesterol and mortality in 80+-year olds. *Age & Ageing, 39*(6), 674–680.
58. Pinto, E. (2007). Blood pressure and aging. *Postgraduate Medical Journal, 83*, 109–114.

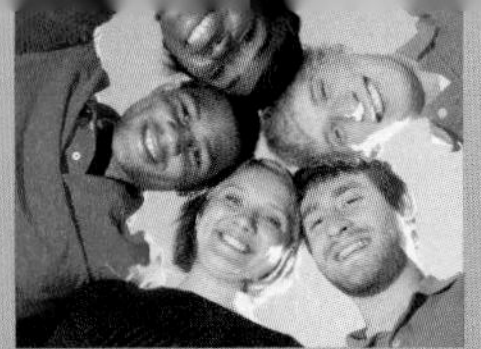

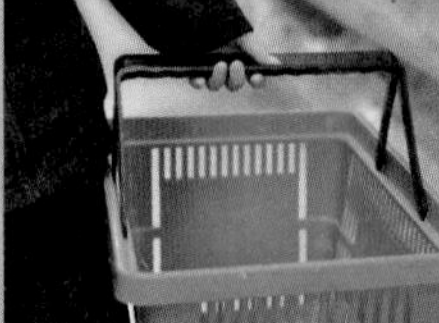

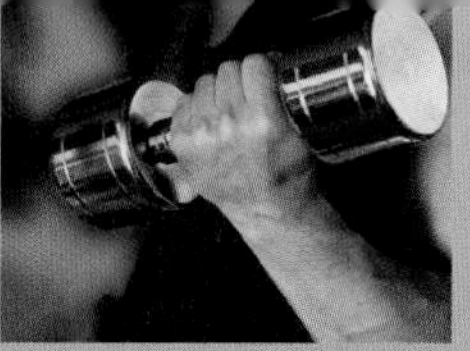

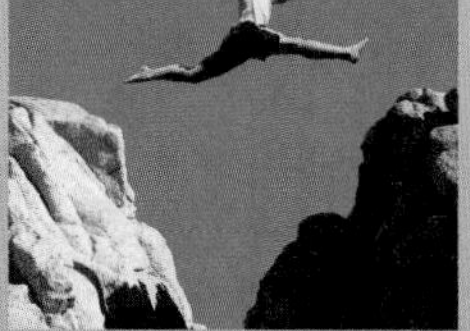

Diversity in Health
Stomach Cancer: Variation in Mortality Among Countries

Consumer Health
Alternative Cancer Therapies

Managing Your Health
Screening Guidelines for the Early Detection of Cancer in Average-Risk Asymptomatic People | Breast Self-Examination | Testicular Self-Examination | Reducing Your Risk for Cancer | Cancer's Seven Warning Signs

Across the Life Span
Cancer

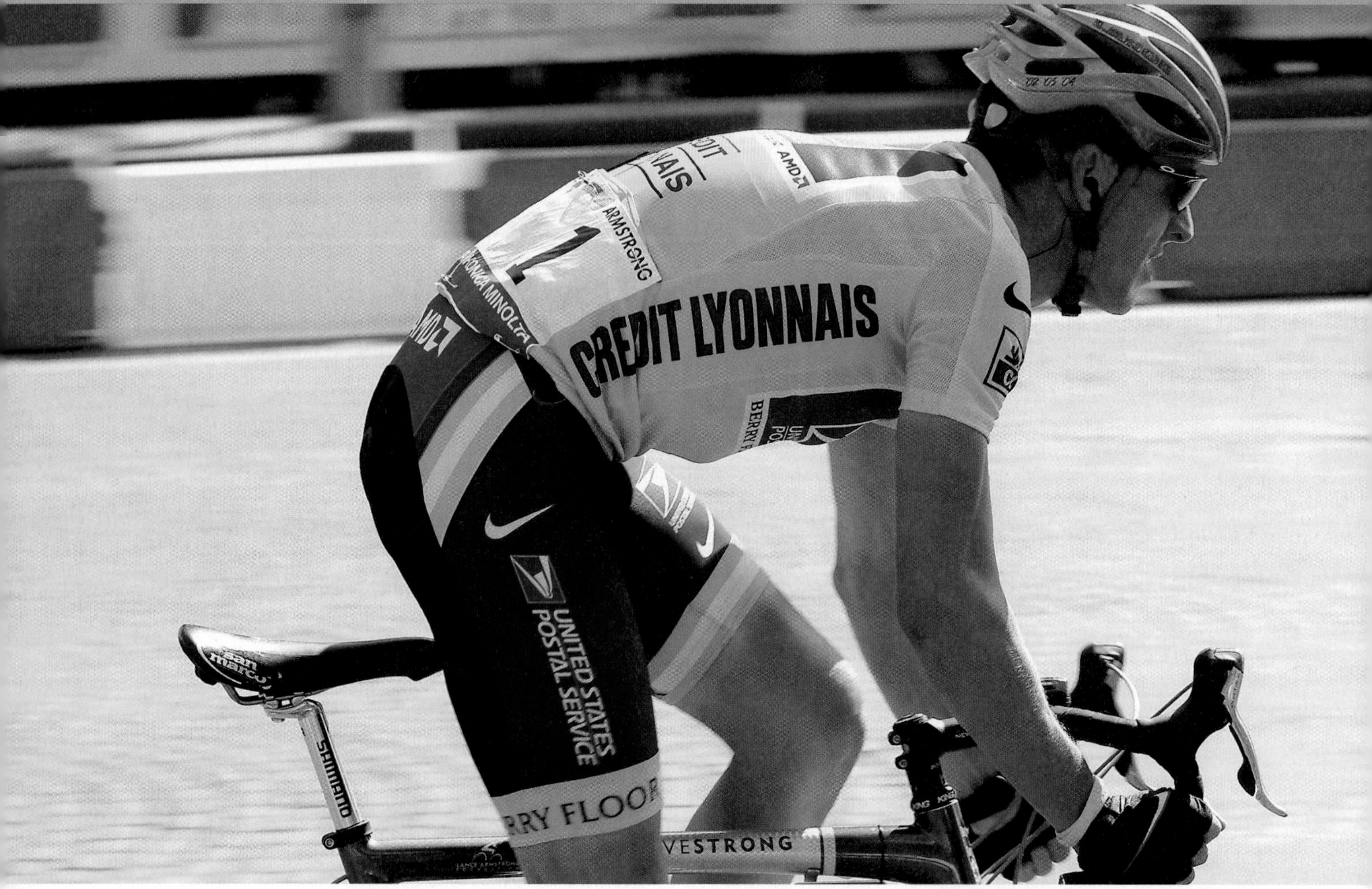

Chapter Overview

What is cancer?

How cancers develop and spread

How physicians detect cancer

How cancer is treated

Which cancers are the most prevalent in the United States

How you can reduce your risk for cancer

Student Workbook

Self-Assessment: What Are Your Cancer Risks?

Changing Health Habits: Modifying Behavior to Reduce Cancer Risk

Do You Know?

What the most prevalent cancer is for your age group?

What you can do to lower your risk of cancer?

Which cancers are on the rise?

CHAPTER 13

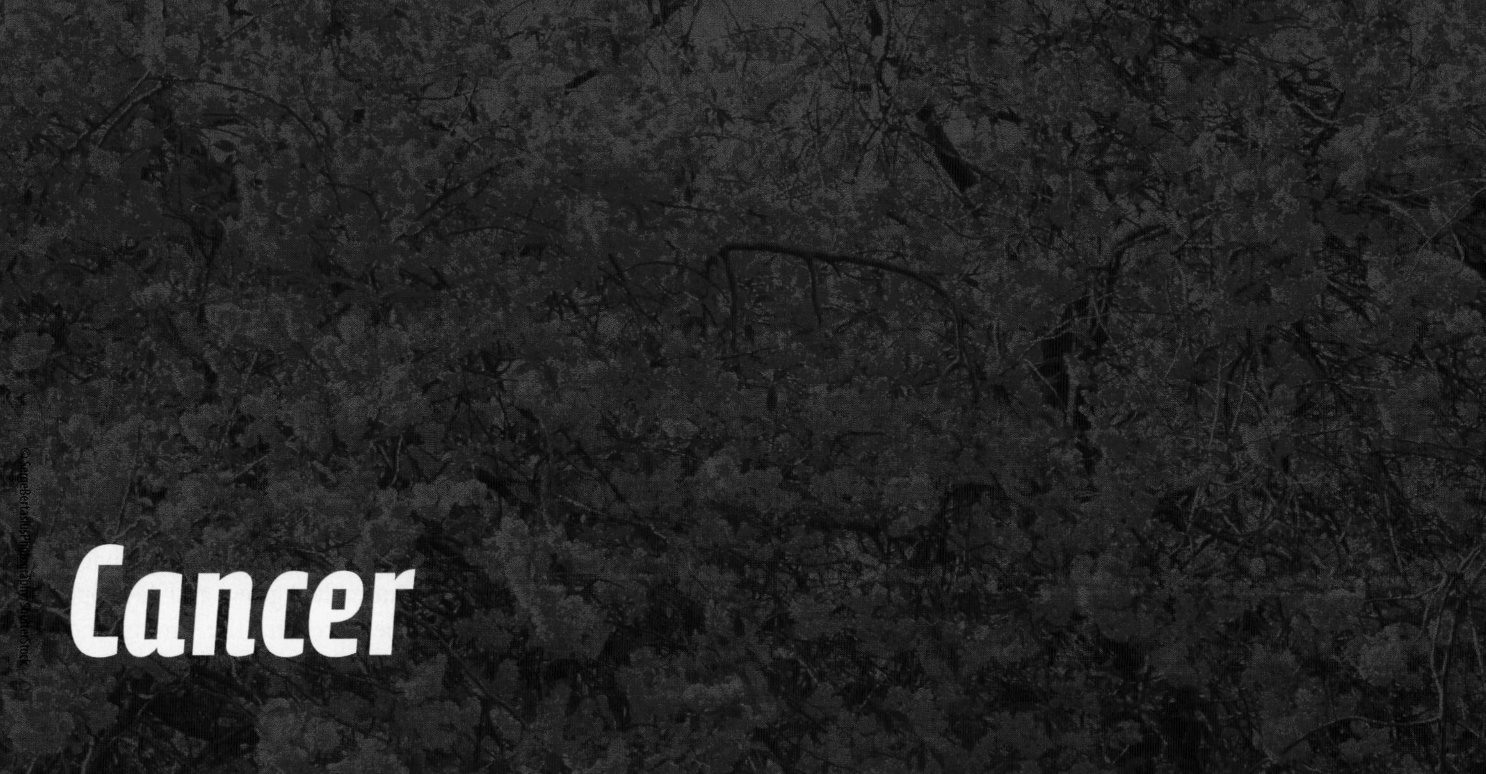

Cancer

Learning Objectives

After studying this chapter, you should be able to:

1. List three traits of cancer cells that make them different from normal cells.
2. Name four factors that can cause mutations in human cells.
3. Describe at least two important differences between a benign and a malignant tumor.
4. List risk factors for major cancers including cancers of the skin, breast, prostate, lung, cervix, uterus, ovary, and oral cavity.
5. Identify which types of cancer are responsible for most deaths in America.
6. Describe lifestyle factors that contribute to the development of cancers.
7. Identify tests or examinations used to identify major forms of cancer.
8. List the seven warning signs of cancer.
9. List three cancer risk factors over which a person has no control.
10. Describe steps that can be taken to reduce cancer risk.

"Many cancers can be cured, especially those detected early."

metastasize (meh-TAS-tah-size) The ability of cancer cells to spread from where they develop to another part of the body.

malignant (mah-LIG-nant) tumors Masses of cancer cells that invade body tissues and interfere with the normal functioning of tissues and organs.

mutations (myou-TAY-shunz) Changes in genes or chromosomes; damaged genes.

"By winning the Tour, you stick in the minds and hearts of the cycling public. You can win every classic and the world championship, but the Tour is everything. It's a global event."[1]

These words were uttered to newspaper reporters by Lance Armstrong, the second American to win the Tour de France and the only person to win the Tour seven times. Armstrong officially retired from competitive cycling in February 2011, but on that clear sunny day in July 1999, he won more than this most rigorous and prestigious 3-week cycling race. He showed the world that he had truly won his battle with testicular cancer—a battle that had nearly cost him not only his career but also his life. His cancer, diagnosed in 1996, had spread to his lungs and brain, but aggressive chemotherapy helped his body win the war against this dreaded disease.

For years, questions about Armstrong's use of performance-enhancing drugs cast a shadow of doubt over his wins. In January 2013, Armstrong finally admitted to using performance enhancers during competition. Despite this revelation, Armstrong's story highlights the ability of humans to be healthy and productive after recovering from cancer.

Armstrong won the Tour de France each year from 1999 through 2005. Then at age 37, after a 4-year hiatus from biking competition, Armstrong entered the 2009 Tour to promote his cancer-support foundation Livestrong. He finished third on the Tour. At the time of Armstrong's retirement in 2011, International Cycling Union President Pat McQuaid referred to Armstrong as "the global icon for cycling."[2]

Although it is still the nation's second biggest killer (cardiovascular disease is the first), cancer is not an automatic death sentence. Armstrong and other cancer survivors, such as former Major League Baseball pitcher Dave Dravecky, pro football Hall of Famer Len Dawson, and American figure skater and gold-medal Olympian Peggy Fleming are living testimony to that fact. Many cancers can be cured, especially those detected early. Even cancers in advanced stages, as was Armstrong's, may respond to therapies available today.

Cancer researchers are making discoveries daily that help win the war against cancer. A tremendous body of research is available that provides guidelines to help people avoid cancer, and people can take many actions to lessen their risk of developing certain cancers. This chapter discusses such preventive measures.

What Is Cancer?

People often talk about cancer as if it were a single disease. However, cancer is many diseases. Lung cancer, for example, is a very different disease from leukemia (cancer of the blood) or skin cancer. Although different, all cancers have common characteristics: Their cells exhibit abnormal growth, division, and differentiation. Differentiation is the process by which cells develop into certain types, such as liver cells or muscle cells. In addition, cancer cells have the potential to **metastasize**, or spread from where they develop to another part of the body.

Cells are the building blocks of all organisms; they are the smallest unit of living material. In any multicelled organism such as humans, cells divide and differentiate as an individual grows and develops and when its tissues need repair. The timing and events of cell division, growth, and differentiation are highly controlled by regulatory proteins. Cells make regulatory proteins in response to the instructions of the hereditary material, or genes. Normal cells are programmed to grow and divide, and to stop growing and dividing at appropriate times.

Unlike normal cells, cancer cells do not stop growing and dividing at appropriate times. Additionally, cancer cells do not differentiate normally and tend to spread. These cells may form masses called **malignant tumors** that invade body tissues and interfere with the normal functioning of tissues and organs. Tumors often cause pain as they invade nerves or press on nerves. Why do cancer cells behave differently from noncancer cells? The answer lies in the genetic material in the cell.

How Cancers Develop and Spread

Cancer develops only in cells that have **mutations**, that is, damaged genes. Mutations can be inherited or can occur from exposure to low-dose radiation, drugs, or toxic chemicals. Infection with certain viruses can also cause changes in genes. Excluding inheritance, then, cancer is determined largely by environmental factors, including components of lifestyle. Lifestyle factors play a major role in cancer prevention.

oncogenes (ONG-ko-geenz) Tumor genes that manufacture altered proteins that speed cell growth and decrease the level of cell differentiation.

tumor-suppressor genes Pieces of hereditary material that slow cell growth; antioncogenes.

carcinogens (kar-SIN-oh-jenz) Cancer-causing substances.

benign (be-NINE) tumors Encapsulated masses of abnormal cells that remain in one location and do not invade surrounding tissues.

Genes and Cancer Development

Oncogenes are "on" switches that speed cell growth. Successive mutations to the hereditary material of particular body cells produce oncogenes. **Tumor-suppressor genes** are "off" switches that slow cell growth. If tumor-suppressor genes mutate or are lost from the hereditary makeup of a cell, they will no longer restrict cell growth.

The activation of oncogenes and deactivation of tumor-suppressor genes (and, therefore, the development of cancer) is a multistage process. In other words, successive genetic changes must take place for a normal cell to change into a cancer cell. These changes take place over time as various environmental factors affect cells and cause mutations. Therefore, the chances of developing cancer generally increase with age and with exposure to cancer-causing substances, or **carcinogens**. Of course, many factors determine an individual's risk for developing cancers. These factors, discussed throughout this chapter, modify this generalization.

Cells that begin to grow abnormally, although not yet cancer cells, may form growths called **benign tumors**. Surrounded by a fibrous capsule, benign tumors remain in one location; they do not invade surrounding tissues. Usually these growths are not life threatening unless their presence interferes with a vital function. For example, a benign brain tumor may be life threatening if it compresses blood vessels serving a vital center in the brain. In most cases benign tumors can be removed completely by surgery.

Some benign tumor cells exhibit traits that are characteristic of the development of cancer cells. These cells are said to exhibit dysplasia. Notice that the dysplastic cells in **Figure 13.1a** vary in size, shape, and the appearance of their nuclei. They are not differentiating properly into a specific type of cell. The normal cells, however, are somewhat regular in these same characteristics (**Figure 13.1b**). Dysplastic cells have the potential to develop into cancer cells.

Metastasis

One of the characteristics of cancer cells is their ability to spread, or metastasize, from where they initially developed to other places in the body. Cells with the ability to metastasize are *malignant*. As a cancer develops, metastasis does not take place immediately. As cancer cells grow and divide, they often

Figure 13.1

A Comparison of Dysplastic and Normal Cells. (a) Dysplastic cells. These cells (stained differently from those in [b]) are irregular in size and the appearance of their nuclei. (b) Normal cells. These cells are all approximately the same size and have nuclei that look similar.

(a and b) © Visuals Unlimited

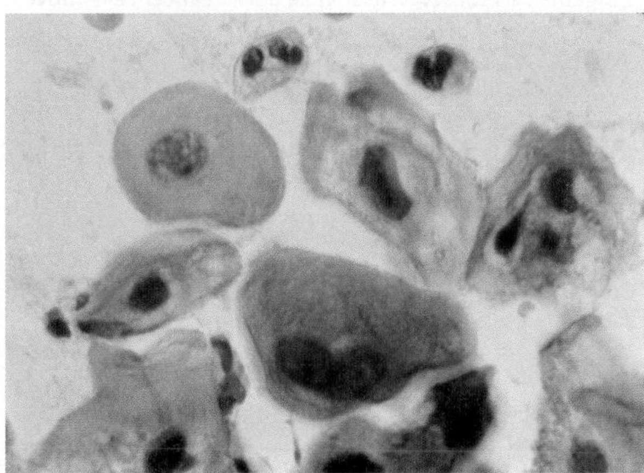

(a)

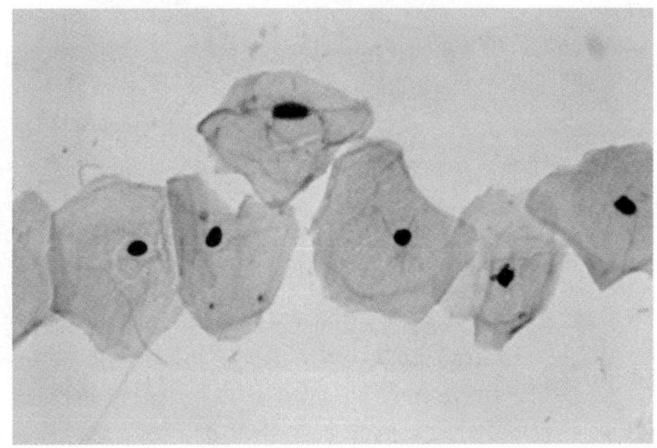

(b)

carcinomas (KAR-si-NO-mahz) Cancers that arise from epithelial tissues.

sarcomas (sar-KO-mahz) Cancers that arise from connective or muscle tissue.

leukemias (lew-KEY-me-ahz) Cancers of the blood and related cells.

lymphomas (lim-FOE-mahz) Cancers of the lymphatic system.

form a malignant tumor. At this stage the cancer is in situ (in place) because it has not invaded other tissues. However, these localized cancer cells begin to secrete chemicals that destroy the substances that hold the surrounding tissues together. When this occurs, cancer cells enter blood and lymph vessels and travel to other parts of the body. Cancerous cells can move out of the blood vessels at a distant location, enter the tissues there, and divide to form new masses of malignant cells. **Figure 13.2** shows this process of cancer cell division and metastasis. Once metastasis occurs, the cancer becomes much more difficult to control.

Cancers are named according to the type of tissue from which they develop. **Carcinomas** (which comprise most adult cancers) arise from epithelial tissue, which lines and covers internal and external body surfaces. Lung, oral, stomach, skin, breast, colon, and ovarian cancers are carcinomas. **Sarcomas** are cancers that arise from connective or muscle tissue. **Leukemias** are cancers of the blood and related cells. **Lymphomas** are cancers of the lymphatic system, the network of vessels and nodes that transports and filters tissue fluid. Cancers of the nervous system have a variety of names.

Figure 13.3 shows death rates (the number of persons dying per year per 100,000 people) of various cancers in the United States. Overall cancer death rates have decreased since the early 1990s.[3] Continued declines for overall cancer death rates and for many of the top cancers (see Figure 13.3) reflect progress in the prevention, early detection, and treatment of cancer.

Figure 13.2

How Cancer Cells Multiply and Spread. Cancer cells secrete chemicals that destroy the substances holding tissues together. As these tissues break down, cancer cells move from their original site, enter the blood and lymph, and travel to other parts of the body.

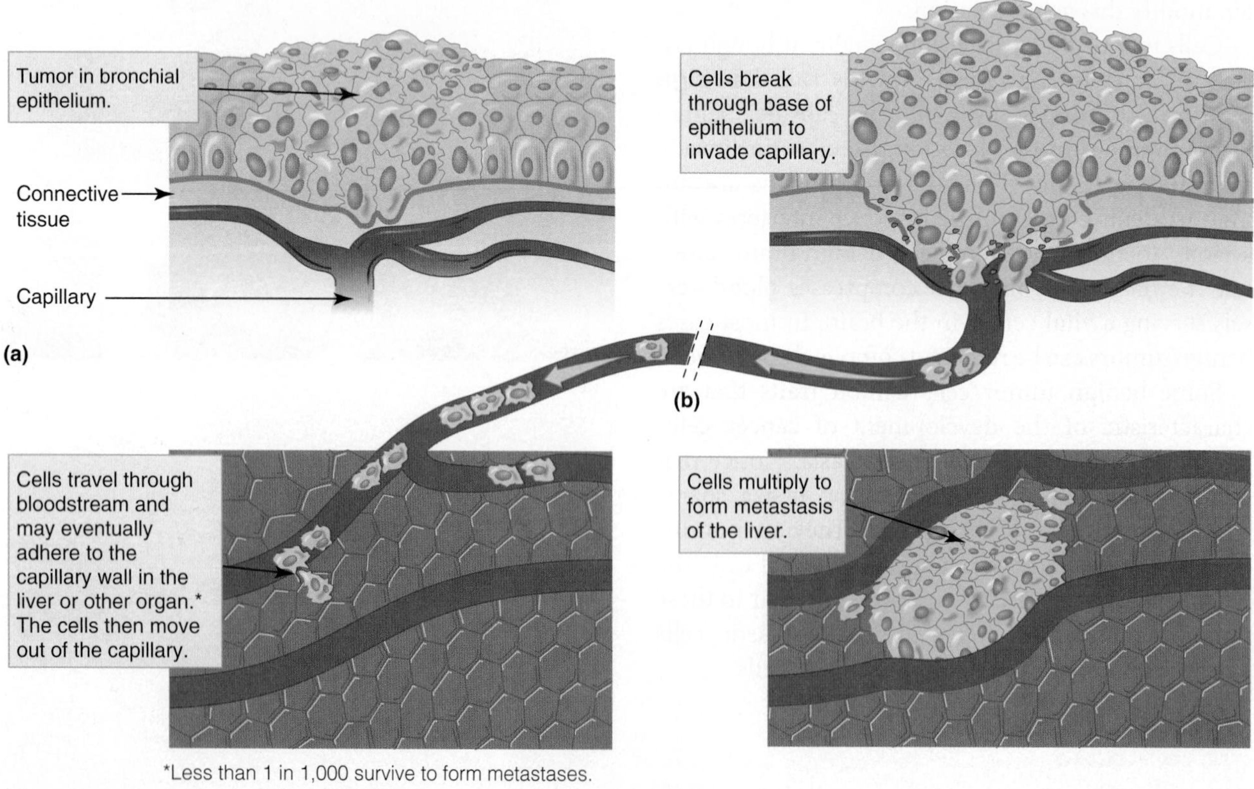
Tumor in bronchial epithelium.
Connective tissue
Capillary
(a)
Cells break through base of epithelium to invade capillary.
(b)
Cells travel through bloodstream and may eventually adhere to the capillary wall in the liver or other organ.* The cells then move out of the capillary.
*Less than 1 in 1,000 survive to form metastases.
(c)
Cells multiply to form metastasis of the liver.
(d)

Figure 13.3

Cancer Death Rates, 1930–2011. (a) Male. (b) Female.

Reproduced from American Cancer Society. Cancer Facts and Figures 2015. Atlanta: American Cancer Society, Inc.

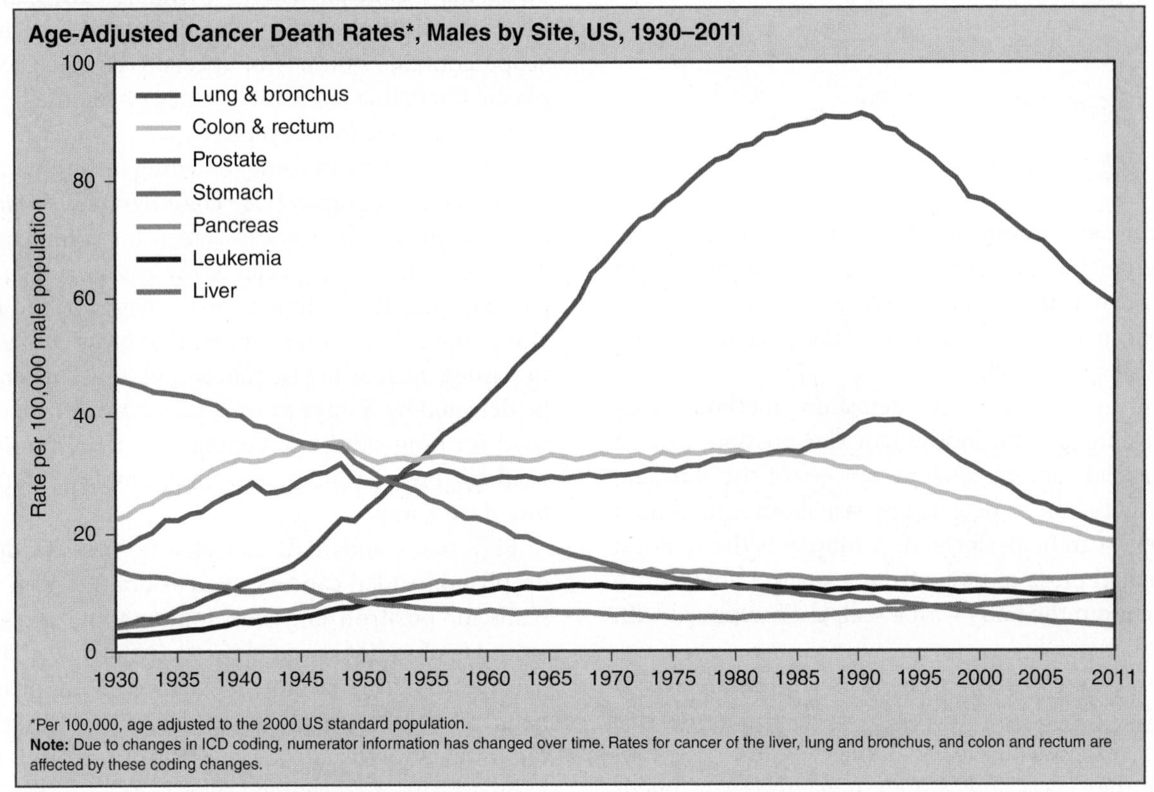

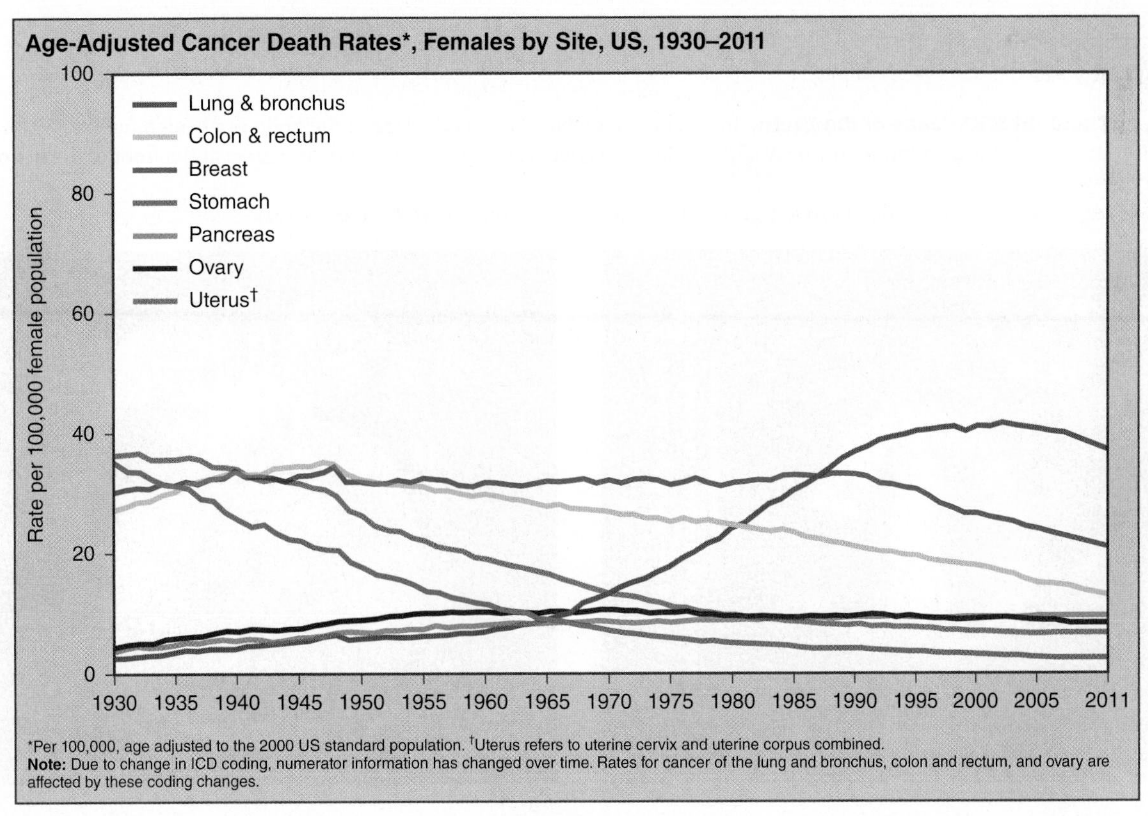

cancer screening An examination to detect malignancies in a person who has no symptoms.

biopsy (BI-op-see) A small piece of tissue that is taken from a growth so that the cells can be studied and a diagnosis confirmed.

Cancer Detection and Staging

Cancer screening is an examination to detect malignancies in a person who has no symptoms. The American Cancer Society (ACS) recommends the screening procedures listed in the Managing Your Health box that follows.

Cancer screening or detection methods vary depending on the location of the possible cancer. Superficial cancers, such as cancers of the skin and oral cavity, can be detected by visual examination, or a biopsy can be performed. A **biopsy** is the removal of a small piece of tissue from a suspect area. It can be cut from the body with a scalpel or removed with a needle.

Some cancers in internal areas can be detected by collecting cells for microscopic examination. This process is possible, for example, for detecting cancer of the cervix and of the esophagus. Even mucus coughed up from the lungs can be analyzed for the presence of cancer. Some cancers, such as colon cancer and stomach cancer, can be detected by fiberoptic examination. To see these internal areas of the body, the physician inserts a flexible tube called a fiberscope into the area to be examined. The fiberscope contains bundles of specially coated glass or plastic fibers that transmit an image from the lighted end of the scope to an eyepiece.

X-rays are used in some screening techniques. The computed tomography (CT) colonography, or *virtual colonoscopy*, can be used to screen for colon cancer. This technique uses special X-ray equipment to create two- and three-dimensional images of the interior of the colon. Other cancers that grow embedded in tissues, such as breast cancer and lung cancer, can be detected by X-rays as well. Chest X-rays are often used for lung cancer screening, and mammograms, used for breast cancer screening, employ a type of low-dose X-ray.

PET scans and MRI can also be used to detect deeply embedded cancers, such as brain cancer. PET scans, or positron emission tomography, use small amounts of radioactive positrons (positively charged particles) to visualize body structures. MRI, or magnetic resonance imaging, uses magnetic fields and radio waves for visualization. MRI is sometimes used in breast cancer screening (**Figure 13.4**).

Figure 13.4

(a) PET and (b) MRI Scans of the Brain. In (a), the round blue area on the side of the brain is a benign tumor. In (b), the round blue area toward the back of the brain is a cancerous tumor. The round structures at the front of the brain are the eyes.

(a) Courtesy of Dr. Giovanni Dichiro, Neuroimaging Section, National Institute of Neurologic Disorders and Stroke/National Cancer Institute; (b) © National Cancer Institute/Photodisc/Getty Images

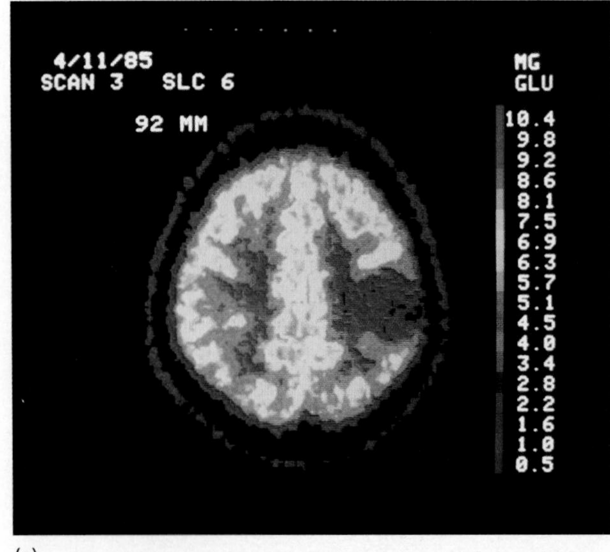

(a)

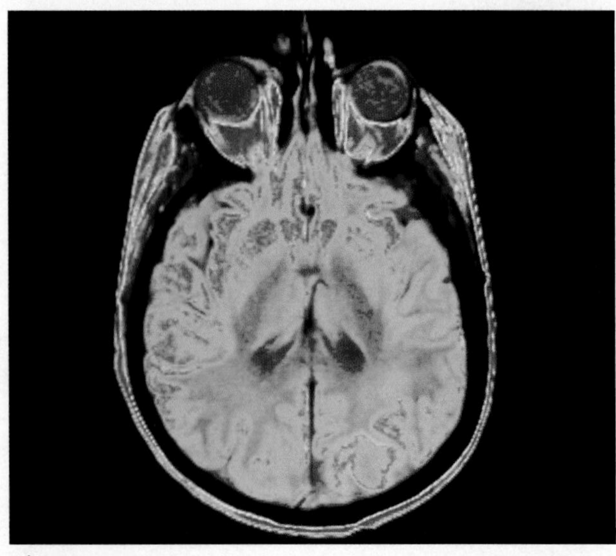

(b)

Ultrasound, an imaging technique that uses sound waves, is used occasionally to detect cancerous growths.

Cancer staging describes the extent of the growth and metastasis of the cancer so that physicians can determine appropriate therapy and provide a prognosis (outlook) for the patient. To stage a cancer, physicians usually use the TNM system first. T describes the original tumor, N describes whether the cancer has reached nearby lymph nodes, and M describes whether the cancer has metastasized (spread) to distant body parts. Once the T, N, and M are determined, they are combined for an overall stage. These overall stages are I, II, III, and IV, with stage I cancer being the least advanced and stage IV cancer being the most advanced. Sometimes stages are subdivided (such as stage IIB), and sometimes other staging systems are used.

The 5-year survival rate is the percentage of persons who are alive 5 years after their cancer is diagnosed, whether they are disease free, under treatment, or in remission (having a partial or complete disappearance of the signs and symptoms of the cancer). The overall 5-year survival rate for all cancers diagnosed between 1999 and 2005 was 68%, up from 50% in the 1970s.[3] **Table 13.1** shows the 5-year survival rate for cancers discussed in this chapter.

cancer staging A description of the extent of the growth and metastasis of a cancer to determine appropriate therapy and prognosis.

Cancer Treatment

The principal forms of cancer treatment are surgery, radiation, and chemotherapy. Newer modes of treatment are biomodulation (immunotherapy),

Table 13.1

Five-Year Relative Survival Rates* (%) by Stage at Diagnosis, 2004-2010

	All Stages	Local	Regional	Distant		All Stages	Local	Regional	Distant
Breast (female)	89	99	85	25	Ovary	45	92	72	27
Colon & rectum	65	90	71	13	Pancreas	7	26	10	2
Esophagus	18	40	21	4	Prostate	99	>99	>99	28
Kidney†	72	92	65	12	Stomach	28	64	29	4
Larynx	60	75	43	35	Testis	95	99	96	73
Liver‡	17	30	11	3	Thyroid	98	>99	98	55
Lung and bronchus	17	54	27	4	Urinary bladder§	77	69	34	6
Melanoma of the skin	91	98	63	16	Uterine cervix	68	91	57	16
Oral cavity and pharynx	63	83	61	37	Uterine corpus	82	95	68	18

*Rates are adjusted for normal life expectancy and are based on cases diagnosed in the SEER 18 areas from 2004-2010, all followed through 2011.

†Includes renal pelvis.

‡Includes intrahepatic bile duct.

§Rate for in situ cases is 96%.

Local: an invasive malignant cancer confined entirely to the organ of origin. **Regional:** a malignant cancer that 1) has extended beyond the limits of the organ of origin directly into surrounding organs or tissues: 2) involves regional lymph nodes; or 3) has both regional extension and involvement of regional lymph nodes.

Distant: a malignant cancer that has spread to parts of the body remote from the primary tumor either by direct extension or by discontinuous metastasis to distant organs, tissues, or via the lymphatic system to distant lymph nodes.

Reproduced from American Cancer Society. *Cancer Facts and Figures 2015*. Atlanta: American Cancer Society, Inc. with data from Howlader N, Noone AM, Krapcho M, et al. (eds). *SEER Cancer Statistics Review, 1975–2011*. National Cancer Institute, Bethesda, MD, http://seer.cancer.gov/csr/1975–2011/, based on November 2013 SEER data submission

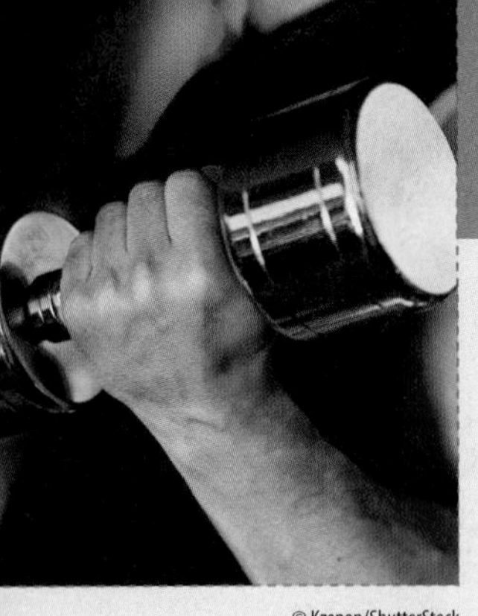
© Kzenon/ShutterStock

Managing Your Health

Screening Guidelines for the Early Detection of Cancer in Average-Risk Asymptomatic People

Cancer Site	Population	Test or Procedure	Frequency
Breast	Women, ages 20+	Breast self-examination (BSE)	It is acceptable for women to choose not to do BSE or to do BSE regularly (monthly) or irregularly. Beginning in their early 20s, women should be told about the benefits and limitations of BSE. Whether or not a woman ever performs BSE, the importance of prompt reporting of any new breast symptoms to a health professional should be emphasized. Women who choose to do BSE should receive instruction and have their technique reviewed on the occasion of a periodic health examination.
		Clinical breast examination(CBE)	For women in their 20s and 30s, it is recommended that CBE be part of a periodic health examination, preferably at least every 3 years. Asymptomatic women ages 40 and over should continue to receive a CBE as part of a periodic health examination, preferably annually.
		Mammography	Begin annual mammography at age 40.*
Cervix†	Women, ages 21-65	Pap test and HPV DNA test	Cervical cancer screening should begin at age 21. For women ages 21-29, screening should be done every 3 years with conventional or liquid-based Pap tests. For women ages 30-65, screening should be done every 5 years with both the HPV test and the Pap test (preferred), or every 3 years with the Pap test alone (acceptable). Women ages 65+ who have had ≥3 consecutive negative Pap tests or ≥2 consecutive negative HPV and Pap tests within the past 10 years, with the most recent test occurring within 5 years, and women who have had a total hysterectomy should stop cervical cancer screening. Women should not be screened annually by any method at any age.
Colorectal	Men and women, ages 50+	Fecal occult blood test (FOBT) with at least 50% test sensitivity for cancer, or fecal immunochemical test (FIT) with at least 50% test sensitivity for cancer, **or**	Annual, starting at age 50. Testing at home with adherence to manufacturer's recommendation for collection techniques and number of samples is recommended. FOBT with the single stool sample collected on the clinician's fingertip during a digital rectal examination is not recommended. Guaiac-based toilet bowl FOBT tests also are not recommended. In comparison with guaiac-based tests for the detection of occult blood, immunochemical tests are more patient-friendly, and are likely to be equal or better in sensitivity and specificity. There is no justification for repeating FOBT in response to an initial positive finding.
		Stool DNA test, **or**	Every 3 years, starting at age 50

Reproduced from American Cancer Society. *Cancer Facts and Figures 2015*. Atlanta: American Cancer Society, Inc.

Cancer Site	Population	Test or Procedure	Frequency
		Flexible sigmoidoscopy (FSIG), **or**	Every 5 years, starting at age 50. FSIG can be performed alone, or consideration can be given to combining FSIG performed every 5 years with a highly sensitive gFOBT or FIT performed annually.
		Double contrast barium enema (DCBE), **or**	Every 5 years, starting at age 50
		Colonoscopy	Every 10 years, starting at age 50
		CT Colonography	Every 5 years, starting at age 50
Endometrial	Women, at menopause	At the time of menopause, women at average risk should be informed about risks and symptoms of endometrial cancer and strongly encouraged to report any unexpected bleeding or spotting to their physicians.	
Lung	Current or former smokers ages 55-74 in good health with at least a 30 pack-year history	Low-dose helical CT (LDCT)	Clinicians with access to high-volume, high-quality lung cancer screening and treatment centers should initiate a discussion about lung cancer screening with apparently healthy patients ages 55-74 who have at least a 30 pack-year smoking history, and who currently smoke or have quit within the past 15 years. A process of informed and shared decision making with a clinician related to the potential benefits, limitations, and harms associated with screening for lung cancer with LDCT should occur before any decision is made to initiate lung cancer screening. Smoking cessation counseling remains a high priority for clinical attention in discussions with current smokers, who should be informed of their continuing risk of lung cancer. Screening should not be viewed as an alternative to smoking cessation.
Prostate	Men, ages 50+	Digital rectal examination (DRE) and prostate-specific antigen test (PSA)	Men who have at least a 10-year life expectancy should have an opportunity to make an informed decision with their healthcare provider about whether to be screened for prostate cancer, after receiving information about the potential benefits, risks, and uncertainties associated with prostate cancer screening. Prostate cancer screening should not occur without an informed decision-making process.
Cancer-related checkup	Men and women, ages 20+		On the occasion of a periodic health examination, the cancer-related checkup should include examination for cancers of the thyroid, testicles, ovaries, lymph nodes, oral cavity, and skin, as well as health counseling about tobacco, sun exposure, diet and nutrition, risk factors, sexual practices, and environmental and occupational exposures.

*Beginning at age 40, annual clinical breast examination should be performed prior to mammography.

Reproduced from American Cancer Society. *Cancer Facts and Figures 2015*. Atlanta: American Cancer Society, Inc.

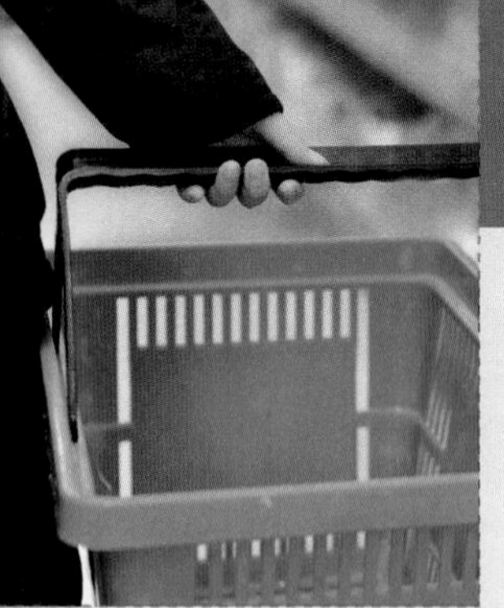

© sevenke/ShutterStock

Consumer Health

Alternative Cancer Therapies

Modern medicine has its limitations; not every condition can be prevented, managed, or cured. It is not surprising, therefore, that some individuals who are diagnosed with incurable conditions seek help from anyone who offers a cure. Cancer patients who seek alternative therapies also hope to find a "softer" treatment with fewer side effects. Many want to use a holistic approach or take charge of their health when conventional medicine offers no more options. When faced with a potentially life-threatening illness such as cancer, most people feel the need to do everything possible to survive.

Most users of alternative cancer therapies expect their treatments to boost their immune system or slow the progression of or cure their cancer. However, the effectiveness of most alternative therapies in cancer treatment has not been established in scientific studies. Additionally, cancer patients erroneously perceive alternative therapies as safe because they are "natural," but therapies such as herbal and vitamin supplements may interact in dangerous ways with drugs or therapies being used in conventional cancer treatment. Many have serious side effects of their own. And if cancer patients delay conventional treatment in favor of unconventional treatment, they may diminish their chances of survival, spend money needlessly, and lower their quality of life.

Herbal therapies, plant extracts, and therapeutic vitamins are the most common alternative therapies in cancer treatment today, and up to 50% of cancer patients use some form of alternative treatment. The greatest danger with the use of substances not controlled by the Food and Drug Administration (FDA) in cancer treatment is the risk of contamination, misidentification, or substitution with a harmful substance because of lack of quality control.

If you or someone you know is thinking about using alternative therapies for cancer treatment, remember that it is important to evaluate all evidence about these methods carefully and make decisions with a cancer physician (oncologist). At the least, informing the physician about other therapies being used can help avoid adverse drug interactions. Also, in evaluating therapies, remember that any remedy used by a large number of people will, by chance, be used by a long-term survivor. In many cases, the patient used conventional treatments as well as alternative ones. However, the alternative method often gets the credit even though there is no evidence to show that it played a role in the patient's long-term survival.

Data from Wilkinson, J. M., et al. (2014). Use of complementary and alternative medical therapies (CAM) by patients attending a regional comprehensive cancer care centre. *Journal of Complementary & Integrative Medicine, 11*(2), 139–147.; Wilson, M. K., et al. (2014). Review of high-dose intravenous vitamin C as an anticancer agent. *Asia Pacific Journal of Clinical Oncology, 10*(1), 22–37.; Ulbricht, C., et al. (2009). Essiac: Systematic review by the Natural Standard Research Collaboration. *Journal of the Society for Integrative Oncology, 7*, 73–80.; Yang, A. K., et al. (2010). Herbal interactions with anticancer drugs: Mechanistic and clinical considerations. *Current Medicinal Chemistry, 17*(16), 1635–1678.; Yang, C. S., & Wang, X. (2010). Green tea and cancer prevention. *Nutrition and Cancer, 62*(7), 931–937.

Figure 13.A

Plant Extracts Are a Common Type of Alternative Cancer Therapy. (a) *Astragalus membranaceus*. An extract of this plant is used to produce Huang ch'i. (b) *Camellia sinensis*. Green tea is made from the dried leaves and leaf buds of this shrub.

(a) Courtesy of John Martin (http://www.geocities.com/herbalogic2001/index.html); (b) © Tracing Tea/ShutterStock

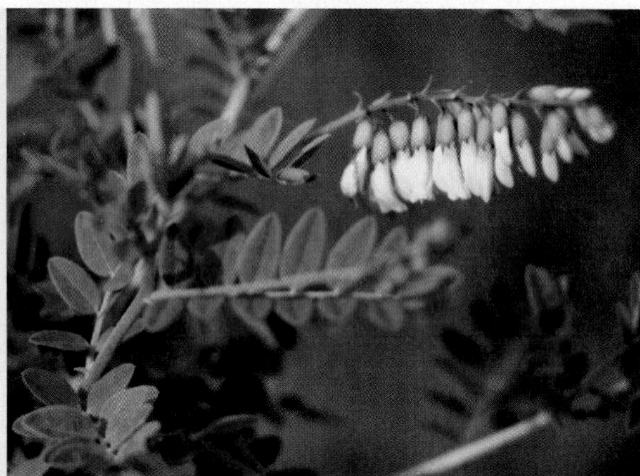

(A)

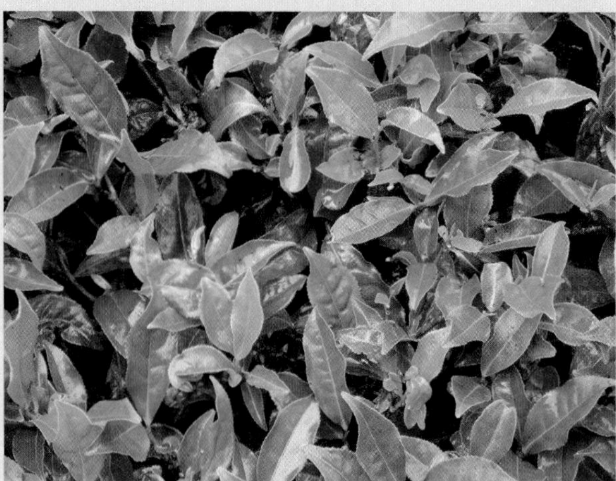

(B)

photodynamic therapy, antiangiogenesis therapy, and bone marrow and peripheral blood stem cell transplants. In the past, physicians referred to a cancer as "cured" if the patient survived for 5 years with no sign of the cancer returning. This is no longer the case, however, because some cancers grow after extended periods and others recur after they seem to have been eliminated. Today, the term *cure* means that all traces of a localized tumor have been removed from the body and the former cancer patient has the same life expectancy as a person who never had cancer.

Surgery

During surgery, physicians remove a localized cancer by cutting it away from noncancerous tissue. Microscopic extensions of cancerous tissue may not be easy to detect during surgical procedures, so a physician usually removes tissue beyond the obvious cancer to increase the probability that all the cancerous tissue is removed. Although surgery is often a life-saving treatment, one drawback is that removal of healthy tissue with unhealthy tissue may impair the body's functioning or cause disfigurement. The other drawback is that surgery is futile if the cancer has spread to multiple sites in the body.

Radiation

Radiation is also used to treat localized cancers, either alone or in conjunction with surgery. Radiation is energy or particles emitted from the nucleus of an atom. The energy of any high-dose radiation interferes with the molecular structures of cells, killing them. Healthy cells recover more quickly and easily from radiation treatment than do cancer cells, so the healthy tissue surrounding a cancer usually survives while the cancer dies. For this reason, a physician may recommend radiation over surgery in particular instances. Preserving healthy tissue surrounding a cancer is extremely important, especially with cancers such as laryngeal cancer (cancer of the voice box), in which it may mean the difference between a patient's retaining or losing the ability to speak. Physicians also choose radiation over surgery for treatment of cancers that respond well to radiation therapy, such as cervical cancer, prostate cancer, and Hodgkin's disease. Physicians often use radiation treatment with elderly patients because their chances of recovering from it may be higher than that of recovering from surgery.

High-dose X-ray and gamma-ray irradiation are widely used today. Patients may undergo one of two methods of radiation treatment. One method is to focus a beam of radiation on the cancerous tissue from an outside source. The machine delivering the beam of radiation rotates around the patient while continually targeting the tumor so that various areas of healthy tissue receive minimal doses of radiation but the tumor receives high doses. Another method is to implant tiny radioactive "beads" in the cancerous tissue for a specific time and then remove them. With either approach, cancer patients usually undergo numerous treatments over a 5- to 8-week period.

Figure 13.5

Proton Therapy. This patient at the James M. Slater, M.D. Proton Treatment and Research Center at Loma Linda University Medical Center is ready to receive proton therapy to treat cancer of the brain. The mask immobilizes the head to ensure that the beam will hit its target.

Courtesy of the James M. Slater, M.D. Proton Treatment and Research Center, Loma Linda University Medical Center

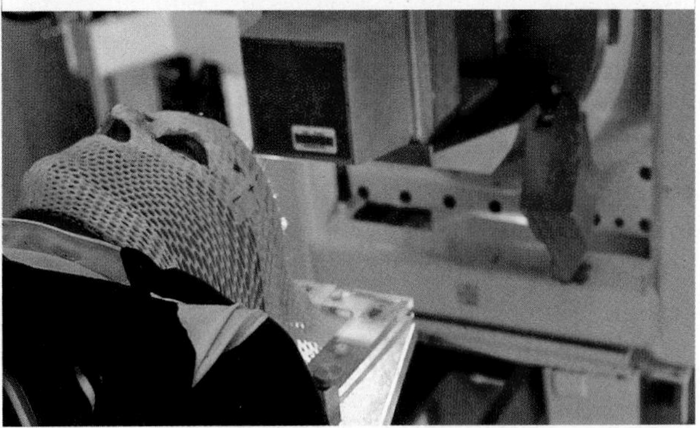

Figure 13.5 shows a highly effective treatment against cancer called *proton therapy*. In this treatment, a patient's cancer is bombarded with a stream of positively charged subatomic particles called protons.

At high doses, proton irradiation kills cells, as does any type of high-dose radiation. Proton radiation, however, can be focused more precisely on the cancer than can other forms of radiation. Therefore, a higher dose of radiation can be used with less radiation affecting surrounding cells. Nonetheless, proton therapy is still not in widespread use because it is about three times as costly as traditional radiation therapies, and few treatment facilities in the United States offer proton irradiation.

Chemotherapy

Chemotherapy is the use of anticancer drugs to inhibit cancer cell reproduction or to destroy cancer cells. Chemotherapy is used most often when cancer has spread to various regions of the body. As with radiation therapy, chemotherapy may be used in

targeted therapies Drugs or other substances that block the growth and spread of cancer by interfering with specific molecules involved in tumor growth and progression.

immunotherapy Manipulation of the body's immune system to rid the body of cancer.

conjunction with surgery. In certain cases, physicians combine all three approaches to cancer treatment.

Radiation and chemotherapy treatments also kill and damage healthy cells and may cause serious side effects such as severe nausea and hair loss. In addition, these treatments do not always destroy cancers completely because their doses are not high enough to do so. Doses sufficiently high to kill all cancer cells often cause too much damage to normal tissue. Also, certain tumors are drug resistant or develop drug resistance during therapy.

Laser and Photodynamic Therapy

Lasers are high-intensity lights that can be focused with great precision. A few types of lasers are used in cancer treatment, and they shrink and destroy tumors. Lasers can be used not only to remove superficial cancers, such as some skin cancers, but they also can be used with an endoscope to deliver the laser light to interior body locations, such as the uterus, esophagus, and colon.

In photodynamic therapy, a chemical called a photosensitizer, which is administered to the patient, reacts with laser or other types of special light, killing tumor cells. The treatment is specific to tumors because they take up the photosensitizer better than do normal tissues, and physicians target the light at the tumors. Therefore, this type of treatment does not significantly damage normal tissues. Death of the tumor cells results from the interaction of the light and the chemical.[4] In addition, as the tumor cells become inflamed before dying, they trigger an immune response that not only acts on the treated cells but also on the same type of tumor cells that may be elsewhere in the body.[5]

Targeted Therapies

The National Cancer Institute defines **targeted therapies** as "drugs or other substances that block the growth and spread of cancer by interfering with specific molecules involved in tumor growth and progression."[6] Targeted therapies are also called "molecularly targeted drugs" and "molecularly targeted therapies." Because these therapies target specific molecules in specific cancers, they are often more effective than general types of treatments and harm only the cancer, not surrounding tissues. One major limitation of targeted therapies, however, is that the cancer cells may develop mutations (changes) that no longer allow the therapy to work. Therefore, targeted therapies are often used alongside other targeted therapies and conventional treatments, such as surgery and radiation.

The two primary types of targeted therapies are small-molecule drugs and immunotherapy.

Small-Molecule Drugs Small-molecule drugs are tiny enough to pass through pores in the cell membrane and do their work from within the cancer cell. An array of small-molecule drugs for targeted cancer therapy has been developed and approved by the U.S. Food and Drug Administration (FDA) for use. Some are not yet approved but are in clinical trials.

Small-molecule drugs each do a specific job, such as blocking certain enzymes and growth factor receptors that cancer cells use as they grow and multiply, modifying the function of proteins that regulate cancer cell functions, and stopping cancerous tumors from developing new blood vessels.

Immunotherapy Some targeted therapies help the immune system destroy cancer cells. The umbrella term for these methods is *biomodulation* (biological response modification), or **immunotherapy**.

Key to the working of the immune system is its ability to recognize an intruder as foreign. The immune system does this by recognizing foreign antigens (certain foreign proteins) on intruders as nonself. However, tumor cells appear to contain antigens that evoke only a weak response from the immune system. As a result, the immune system has difficulty detecting and identifying malignant tumors, so it does a poor job destroying these abnormal cells.

Immunotherapies involve a variety of techniques that help boost the immune system response. For example, injecting tumor antigens into the patient's bloodstream can increase the numbers of tumor-fighting immune system cells in the body. This procedure is similar to the way in which a vaccine works to boost the body's immune response against an infectious disease. For this reason, such cancer-fighting products are called *cancer vaccines*. However, cancer vaccines are given to patients who already have cancer to help rid them of their disease, not to cancer-free persons to prevent cancer. Some medical facilities involved in cancer vaccine research are using a patient's own tumor cells to develop personalized cancer vaccines that hold promise for boosting immune system function higher than can vaccines developed from tumor antigens from other sources.[7]

Examples of other immunotherapies are drugs that decrease the suppressor mechanisms of the immune system, thus increasing the host's immune response. Another approach is to augment the patient's immune system by bone marrow transplants (tissue that produces immune system cells; see next subsection) or transfusions of particular immune system cells. Other immunotherapies are chemicals that act on tumor cells by making them more recognizable by the body or more susceptible to dying as a result of immune system processes.

Bone Marrow and Peripheral Blood Stem Cell Transplants

Stem cells are undifferentiated cells whose daughter cells can develop into a variety of cell types. Bone marrow cells are stem cells that continually give rise to a variety of types of blood cells. Peripheral blood (blood in the bloodstream) can be used as a source of blood stem cells too, but donors must be treated with growth factors (hormone-like substances) a few days before the donation, which causes their stem cells to grow and enter their bloodstream. Their harvested blood is processed by a machine that separates out the stem cells; the rest of the blood is returned to the donor.

Bone marrow and peripheral blood stem cell transplants are used in two primary ways in cancer treatment: (1) to resupply the bone marrow when it has been destroyed by chemotherapy or radiation, or (2) to supply healthy stem cells to a person who has cancer of the blood-forming tissue, such as leukemia. In the first situation, a patient's own stem cells are harvested before chemotherapy or radiation, and the stem cells are given back to the patient after the treatment. In the second instance, the stem cells come not from the patient but from a healthy donor whose tissue type best matches the patient. The healthy stem cells are transplanted into the patient, and these cells produce healthy blood cells.

Patients receive stem cell transplants (whether the stem cells are their own or those of a donor) in a process much like a blood transfusion. The stem cells take up residence in the bone marrow, grow, and send out new blood cells.

This section discusses many types of cancer treatments. Although these useful and amazing treatments can be life saving, prevention and early detection are still the best ways to live a healthy, long, cancer-free life.

Prevalent Cancers in the United States

Over decades of research, scientists have learned what causes certain cancers. In some cases, scientists are unsure of the cause but know which factors are related to cancer development. These factors, when present, increase the chances that a person will develop a particular cancer and thus are called risk factors. Although heredity influences cancer risk, it explains only a fraction of all cancers and variations in cancer risk. Behavioral factors such as cigarette smoking, dietary patterns, physical activity, and weight control, however, *substantially* affect the risk of developing cancer.[8]

This chapter organizes the discussion of cancers according to factors that appear to be significant in the development of particular cancers, most of which are prevalent in the United States. Advanced age is a significant risk factor for most cancers except certain childhood cancers, testicular cancer, cervical cancer, and, in part, breast cancer.

Before reading this section, take the self-assessment "What Are Your Cancer Risks?" found in the Student Workbook section at the end of this text.

Cancers Caused by or Related to Tobacco

In 2004, U.S. Surgeon General Richard Carmona issued a report on smoking and health that listed tobacco smoking as a cause of various cancers.[9] **Table 13.2** lists these cancers. In 2010, U.S. Surgeon General Regina Benjamin expanded on the information in the 2004 report by issuing a new report on how tobacco smoke causes disease.[10] Thirty percent of all cancer deaths, including 87% of lung cancer deaths, can be attributed to tobacco use.[11]

This section explores the first seven cancers in Table 13-2 because they are all caused primarily by this preventable risk. Stomach cancer and cancer of the cervix are discussed in other sections of this chapter because their primary causes relate to factors other than tobacco use. Pancreatic cancer has a variety of risk factors.

Lung Cancer Looking at **Table 13.3**, you can see that lung cancer is the leading cause of cancer deaths

Table 13.2

Cancers Caused by Cigarette Smoking

Bladder
Esophagus
Kidney
Larynx (voice box)
Acute myeloid leukemia
Lung
Mouth and throat
Pancreas
Stomach
Cervix

Data from U.S. Department of Health and Human Services. (2004). The health consequences of smoking: A report of the Surgeon General. Washington, DC: U.S. Government Printing Office.

in both men and women in the United States. Death rates resulting from lung cancer have risen dramatically in men since the 1930s through the 1980s and in women since the 1960s through the early 1990s (see Figure 13-3). Estimates put tobacco use as the main cause of 90% of male lung cancers and 79% of female lung cancers; about 90% of lung cancer deaths overall can be attributed to smoking cigarettes.[12]

The increases in lung cancer death rates shown in Figure 13-3 are because of increases in the percentage of the population who smoked tobacco in the decades prior to the 1960s. Lung cancer, like most cancers, takes years to develop, so a rise in lung cancer death rates occurs decades after a rise in the percentage of the population who smoke.

Incidence rates of lung cancer (the number of people diagnosed per 100,000 population) have begun to stabilize in women and drop in men (see **Figure 13.3**). This stabilization and drop reflect the beginning of a predicted decline in incidence rates resulting from the steady decline in cigarette smoking in the U.S. population since 1964. In that year, U.S. Surgeon General Luther Terry issued a report that linked cigarette smoking to the development of lung cancer and other diseases.[13]

Signs and Symptoms In the early stages of disease, the signs and symptoms of lung cancer may be hard to detect. Cigarette smokers often have chronic cough, chronic bronchitis, or excess sputum (saliva and mucus) production. Tumors growing in the bronchioles (small airways in the lungs) also cause a cough and sputum production; they may also cause blood to appear in the sputum as they disrupt airway tissues. A lung cancer victim may also wheeze when breathing if the airways become substantially narrowed by tumor growth. In addition, the air sacs in that part of the lung may collapse and cease to function; infection may develop. The patient may experience pain in the chest, shoulder, and arm if the cancer spreads to the chest wall and affects certain nerves there.

Physicians use chest X-rays and other imaging techniques, including MRI and CT scans; analyses of the types of cells in the sputum; and fiber-optic examination of the bronchial passageways to assist in their diagnoses.

Risk Factors and Prevention Malignant growths develop in the lungs and airways in many persons as they inhale cancer-causing substances such as tobacco smoke over long periods of time. The risk of lung cancer rises proportionately with the number of cigarettes (or cigars or pipes) a person smokes per day, the number of years a person smokes, and how deeply he or she inhales. Persons who smoke low-tar cigarettes have a lower risk of lung cancer than those who smoke high-tar cigarettes.[9] (Smoking "low-yield" cigarettes does not lower cardiovascular disease risk.) Likewise, those who smoke filter-tipped cigarettes have a lower risk of lung cancer than those who smoke unfiltered cigarettes. However, results of research show that people who smoke filter-tipped or "low-yield" cigarettes are at increased risk for developing deep lung tumors because, when smoking, they inhale more deeply and forcefully than people who smoke non-filter-tipped or "regular-yield" cigarettes.[9]

If you smoke, giving up cigarette smoking will slowly lower your risk of developing lung cancer, several other cancers, and cardiovascular disease as well. Your risk of developing lung cancer will never return to that of a lifetime nonsmoker, but after 10 years it will be about half that of a person who continued to smoke.[9] However, your risk of developing cardiovascular disease will lower considerably in only 1 year and return to that of a nonsmoker in 3 to 15 years, depending on how much and how long you smoked.

Other lifestyle factors that appear to raise the risk of lung cancer are regular, high consumption of alcoholic beverages and obesity. Combined estrogen and progestin postmenopausal hormone therapy does not increase the incidence of lung

Table 13.3

Leading New Cancer Cases and Deaths—2015 Estimates

Estimated New Cases*		Estimated Deaths	
Male	**Female**	**Male**	**Female**
Prostate 220,800 (26%)	Breast 231,840 (29%)	Lung and bronchus 86,380 (28%)	Lung and bronchus 71,660 (26%)
Lung and bronchus 115,610 (14%)	Lung and bronchus 105,590 (13%)	Prostate 27,540 (9%)	Breast 40,290 (15%)
Colon and rectum 69,090 (8%)	Colon and rectum 63,610 (8%)	Colon and rectum 26,100 (8%)	Colon and rectum 23,600 (9%)
Urinary bladder 56,320 (7%)	Uterine corpus 54,870 (7%)	Pancreas 20,710 (7%)	Pancreas 19,850 (7%)
Melanoma of the skin 42,670 (5%)	Thyroid 47,230 (6%)	Liver and intrahepatic bile duct 17,030 (5%)	Ovary 14,180 (5%)
Kidney and renal pelvis 38,270 (5%)	Non-Hodgkin lymphoma 32,000 (4%)	Leukemia 14,210 (5%)	Leukemia 10,240 (4%)
Non-Hodgkin lymphoma 39,850 (5%)	Melanoma of the skin 31,200 (4%)	Esophagus 12,600 (4%)	Uterine corpus 10,170 (4%)
Oral cavity and pharynx 32,670 (4%)	Kidney and renal pelvis 23,290 (3%)	Urinary bladder 11,510 (4%)	Non-Hodgkin lymphoma 8,310 (3%)
Leukemia 30,900 (4%)	Pancreas 24,120 (3%)	Non-Hodgkin lymphoma 11,480 (4%)	Liver and intrahepatic bile duct 7,520 (3%)
Liver and intrahepatic bile duct 25,510 (3%)	Leukemia 23,370 (3%)	Kidney and renal pelvis 9,070 (3%)	Brain and other nervous system 6,380 (2%)
All sites 848,200 (100%)	All sites 810,170 (100%)	All sites 312,150 (100%)	All sites 277,280 (100%)

*Excludes basal and squamous cell skin cancers and in situ carcinoma except urinary bladder.

Reproduced from American Cancer Society. *Cancer Facts and Figures 2015*. Atlanta: American Cancer Society, Inc.

cancer, but it does appear to increase the risk of death from lung cancer.[14] The relationships between various dietary factors and lung cancer is controversial;[11,15] more research is needed to determine clear associations.

Scientists have been unable to show that lung cancer is inherited. Nonetheless, correlational studies show that relatives of lung cancer patients have a higher risk of developing lung cancer if they smoke than do smokers with no relatives who have lung cancer. Scientists speculate that relatives of lung cancer patients may inherit a defect in their cells' ability to resist genetic damage by the carcinogens in cigarette smoke.

passive smoking The inhalation, by nonsmokers, of tobacco smoke in the air.

asbestos (as-BES-tose) A fiber-like mineral found in rocks that, when inhaled, can cause lung cancer or other lung conditions.

radon gas A colorless, odorless, radioactive gas present in the rocks and soils in many areas in the United States that, when inhaled, can cause mutations in cells.

In the early 1970s, medical researchers began investigating the effects of passive smoking on the development of lung cancer. **Passive smoking** is the inhalation by nonsmokers of environmental tobacco smoke (ETS; secondhand smoke) present in the air from others who smoke. Environmental tobacco smoke has been associated with a 20–30% increase in lung cancer risk for persons who live with a smoker. The following are a few of the many conclusions regarding the effects of secondhand smoke in the 2006 Surgeon General's report *The Health Consequences of Involuntary Exposure to Tobacco Smoke*: "Secondhand smoke causes premature death and disease in children and in adults who do not smoke," "More than 50 carcinogens have been identified in sidestream and secondhand smoke," and "The evidence is sufficient to infer a causal relationship between secondhand smoke exposure and lung cancer among lifetime nonsmokers."[16]

Substances other than those in tobacco smoke have also been linked to lung cancer. For example, certain metals, listed in **Table 13.4**, are carcinogenic. Only people in certain occupations encounter most of these substances.

Two substances significantly associated with the development of lung cancer and often encountered in the environment are asbestos and radon. **Asbestos** is a fiber-like mineral found in rocks that resists damage by fire or other natural processes. Because of these properties, asbestos has been used in the manufacture of a variety of products and is used in the construction, shipbuilding, and railroad industries. People in these industries as well as those who mine asbestos are at risk of developing lung cancer if they inhale asbestos particles. Additionally, the effects of inhaling asbestos particles multiply the effects of smoking tobacco and therefore greatly increases risk.

Exposure to radon gas also appears to multiply the carcinogenic effect of tobacco smoke. **Radon gas** is colorless and odorless and is produced as the radioactive element uranium decays, emitting subatomic particles and energy. When inhaled, radon can cause mutations in cells because it is radioactive also. Radon is present in the rocks and soils in many areas in the United States (**Figure 13.6**). People who live in these regions may be exposed to radon gas if it leaks through cracks in basement walls and collects in their homes. Home radon detectors can ascertain the presence of this gas. If radon is present, specialists in radon abatement can advise a homeowner on procedures to prevent this gas from leaking into and accumulating in the house (**Figure 13.7**).

Treatment Physicians treat lung cancer primarily with surgery, radiation, and chemotherapy. Surgeons often remove the lobe of the cancerous lung. They may combine therapies if the cancer has spread, using radiation or chemotherapy with surgery, targeted therapies, and/or laser therapy.

Cancers of the Larynx, Oral Cavity, and Esophagus Although these cancers are not as prevalent as others, they have preventable causes: tobacco use, which includes the use of cigarettes, cigars, pipes, and smokeless (chewing) tobacco of all types, and excessive alcohol consumption. Heavy consumption of alcohol is often a causal factor in cancers of the esophagus and liver, but if a heavy drinker is also a smoker, the effects of both substances multiply the risk of developing cancer of the larynx, oral cavity, and esophagus.

Results of recent research show that an increasing percentage of oral cancers are associated with the human papillomavirus (HPV), which enters the mouth during oral sex with an infected person. The primary population developing HPV-related oral cancers is White men between the ages of 40 and 55 years.[17]

Cancers of the larynx, or voice box, are usually detected early if they involve the vocal cords because the voice quickly becomes hoarse. However, cancers of the larynx that do not involve the vocal cords are more difficult to discover early. Their symptoms may include a sore throat, difficulty swallowing, or a visible lump in the neck.

The esophagus is the tube that carries food and drink from the mouth to the stomach. Difficulty swallowing is also a symptom of esophageal cancer. In addition, people who have recurrent heartburn or a burning sensation while swallowing should be checked for possible esophageal carcinoma.

In oral cancer, malignant or benign growths are often visible (**Figure 13.8**). Malignancies may appear as sores that bleed easily and do not heal, red or white patches that do not go away, or thickened areas

Table 13.4
Carcinogenic Metals Found in the Workplace

Metal	Cancers	Present in	Human Carcinogen?	Workers Exposed
Arsenic	Skin, lung, bladder, kidney, liver	Wood preservatives, glass, pesticides	Yes	Smelting of ores containing arsenic, pesticide application, and wood preservation
Beryllium	Lung	Nuclear weapons, rocket fuel, ceramics, glass, plastic, fiberoptic products	Yes	Beryllium ore miners and alloy makers, phosphor manufacturers, ceramic workers, missile technicians, nuclear reactor workers, electric and electronic equipment workers, and jewelers
Cadmium	Lung	Metal coatings, plastic products, batteries, fungicides	Yes	Smelting of zinc and lead ores; producing, processing, and handling cadmium powders; welding or remelting of cadmium-coated steel; and working with solders that contain cadmium
Chromium	Lung	Automotive parts, floor covering, paper, cement, asphalt roofing, anticorrosivemetal plating	Yes	Stainless steel production and welding, chromate production, chrome plating, ferrochrome alloys, chrome pigment, and tanning industries
Lead	Kidney, brain	Cotton dyes; metal coating; drier in paints, varnishes, and pigment inks; certain plastics; specialty glass	Probable carcinogen	Construction work that involves welding, cutting, brazing, or blasting on lead paint surfaces; most smelter workers, including lead smelters where lead is recovered from batteries; radiator repair shops
Nickel	Nasal cavity, lung	Steel, dental fillings, copper and brass, permanent magnets, storage batteries, glazes	Nickel metal: Probable carcinogen Nickel compounds: Yes	Battery makers, ceramic makers, electroplaters, enamellers, glass workers, jewelers, metal workers, nickel mine workers, refiners and smelters, paint related workers and welders

Reproduced from National Cancer Institute. (2003). Cancer and the environment. Retrieved October 11, 2011, from http://www.cancer.gov/newscenter/Cancer-and-the-Environment

of tissue. Oral cancer metastasizes relatively quickly; over half of cases are diagnosed in advanced stages. To detect oral cancer early, persons older than age 50 years should have complete oral examinations as part of their annual physical checkups. Dentists should routinely screen all of their patients for oral cancer.

Cancers of the Kidney and Bladder The kidneys and bladder are organs of the urinary system, yet tobacco smoking is a causal factor in cancers of these organs. These organs come in contact with inhaled carcinogens in tobacco smoke (or other inhaled carcinogens) after they enter the bloodstream at the lungs. The kidneys filter the carcinogens into the urine, which exposes the kidneys and bladder to these substances before urination.

Most signs and symptoms of kidney and bladder cancer are the same as those of several other conditions, so experiencing any of them is not a sure sign of cancer. One such sign of both cancers is blood in the

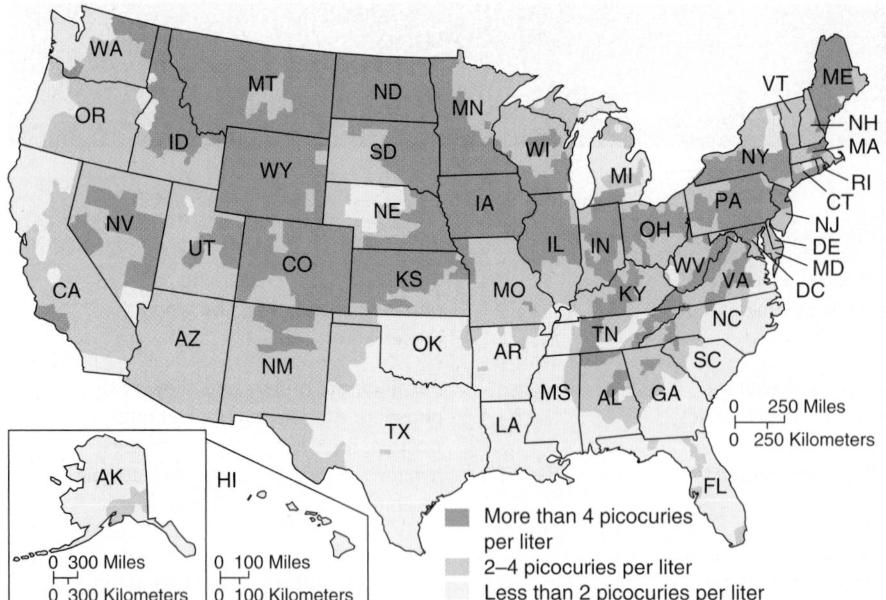

Figure 13.6

Areas of the United States in Which Radon Gas Is Most Prevalent.

urine. Frequent, urgent, or difficult urination is also a sign of bladder cancer. Additional signs and symptoms of kidney cancer include a fever of unknown origin, weight loss, and anemia (a decrease in the hemoglobin in the blood).

Most people who get bladder or kidney cancer are men older than 50 years of age who are heavy smokers. Cigarette smokers have 2 to 10 times the risk of developing bladder or kidney cancer as do nonsmokers. As with lung cancer, the risk increases with the number of cigarettes smoked per day and the number of years a person has been a smoker. People lessen their risk when they decrease the number of cigarettes they smoke or stop smoking. Obesity is another known risk factor for kidney cancer.[18]

Cancer of the Pancreas A long, slender gland, the pancreas lies near the stomach. As an accessory organ of the digestive system, the pancreas secretes digestive enzymes that enter the small intestine by means of a duct. As an endocrine gland, the pancreas secretes the hormones insulin and glucagon, which help regulate blood levels of glucose.

Pancreatic cancer is a particularly deadly form of cancer, striking men and women fairly equally. The fourth most common cause of cancer death in men and women (see Table 13.3), pancreatic cancer is often called a silent cancer because the early symptoms, which include nausea, vomiting, weakness, and discomfort in the abdomen, are vague and nonspecific. The more specific signs and symptoms of pancreatic

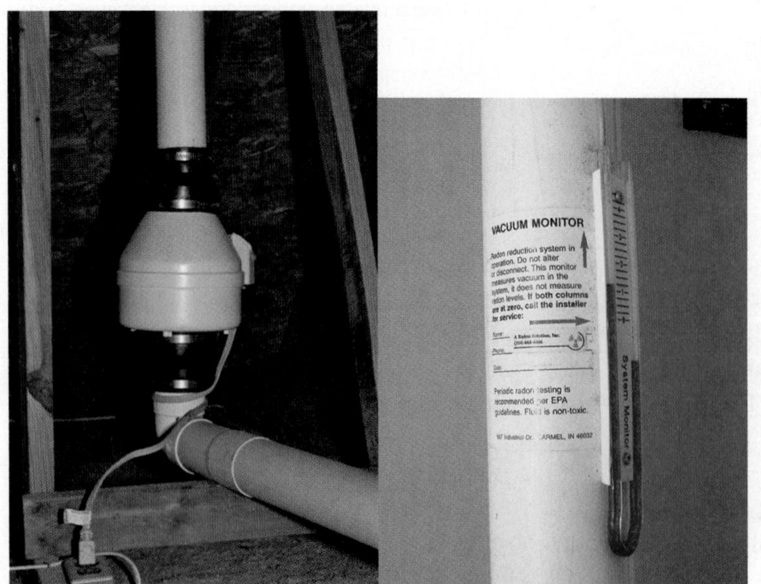

Figure 13.7

Radon Gas Abatement. Although many types of radon gas abatement exist for homes, one of the most common and reliable is active sub-slab suction. This technique is used in homes with basements or built on slabs. One or more pipes is inserted through the floor slab into the crushed rock or soil below. The pipe travels up the wall to the attic, where the gas is vented. (a) The part of the pipe in the attic houses a radon exhaust fan. The fan draws the radon up the pipe while simultaneously creating a vacuum beneath the slab. The radon gas is vented to the outside. (b) Somewhere along its length, the pipe has a vacuum monitor so that the homeowner can see that the system is operating.

(a) Courtesy of Robert Fingland; (b) Courtesy of Wendy Schiff

Diversity in Health

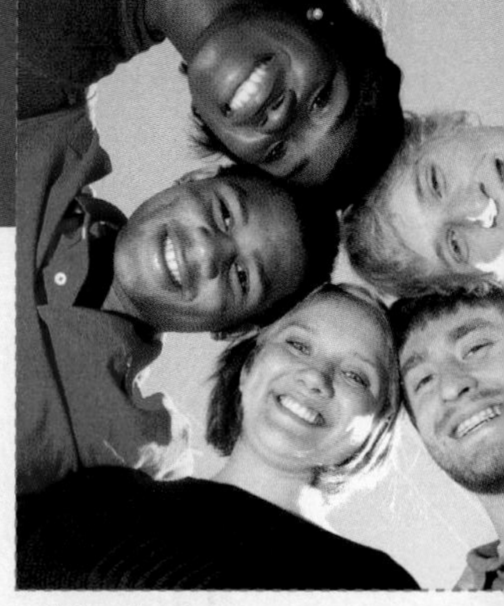
© Mike Flippo/ShutterStock

Stomach Cancer: Variation in Mortality Among Countries

More Americans died of stomach cancer in 1930 than of any other type of cancer. In the United States, the death rate resulting from this cancer has fallen dramatically since then (see Figure 13.3). However, the International Agency for Research on Cancer at the World Health Organization reports that stomach cancer is still the number two cancer killer worldwide. (Lung cancer is number one.) Why has the death rate from this cancer fallen in the United States? Why is this cancer so prevalent in other parts of the world?

As scientists studied worldwide patterns of mortality from stomach cancer, they noticed high mortality rates in Central and South American countries such as Brazil, Chile, Colombia, Costa Rica, and Venezuela. They also noticed large differences in death rates from stomach cancer in some of these countries. In Colombia, for example, death rates from this disease differ dramatically in populations living in the mountains compared with populations living along the coast. A similar situation exists in central and eastern European countries. There are high mortality rates from stomach cancer in these countries; however, the death rates between countries and within countries in this part of the world vary. In addition, countries in Eastern Asia, which includes China, Taiwan, Japan, North Korea, South Korea, and Mongolia, have extremely high mortality rates from stomach cancer. Why are some countries' rates of death resulting from stomach cancer dramatically higher than others? (You can research incidence and mortality rates for various cancers in countries around the world at www-dep.iarc.fr/.)

Scientists have determined that differences in worldwide stomach cancer death rates are related to diet and environment rather than to race or country of origin. Likewise, the reduction in stomach cancer deaths in the United States is the result primarily of these factors.

Regarding diet, methods of food processing and preservation affect the incidence of stomach cancer. In the early 1900s in the United States, methods of food processing and preservation changed dramatically. By midcentury, refrigeration and freezing replaced salting, pickling, and smoking as the primary methods of food preservation. Scientists have since discovered that the regular consumption of highly salted foods (including pickled foods) increases the risk of developing stomach cancer. Foods that are smoke cured, charbroiled, or grilled contain high quantities of polycyclic aromatic hydrocarbons (PAHs), which are carcinogenic and mutagenic. These compounds are also found in cigarette smoke and air pollution because they are the products of the incomplete combustion of fossil fuels such as charcoal and gasoline. Although many Americans enjoy eating grilled foods, their consumption of smoked, salted, and pickled foods has decreased since the early 1900s, reducing Americans' risk of developing and dying from stomach cancer. However, peoples of various cultures still use salting and smoking to preserve meats and pickling to preserve vegetables, thereby increasing their risk of stomach cancer.

Another dietary factor with an environmental link plays a role in the development of this disease. Ingesting nitrosamines, which are found in nitrite-cured foods (such as bacon, cold cuts, and some hot dogs) and in water supplies in some parts of the world (such as Colombia and South America), appears to increase the risk of stomach cancer. Nitrosamines are also found in cigarette smoke. Chemical reactions that occur in the stomach produce nitrosamines from other compounds. For example, substances in certain fish consumed in Japan and in fava beans consumed in Colombia are converted in the stomach to nitrosamines.

(*Continues*)

cancer—jaundice (yellowing of the eyeballs and skin), pain, and weight loss—do not usually occur until the disease is advanced and then may be confused with many other diseases, such as gallbladder or liver disease.

The risk of pancreatic cancer increases after age 50; most cases occur in persons aged 65 to 79 years. The incidence of pancreatic cancer for smokers is more than twice as high as for nonsmokers. Other persons at risk for developing pancreatic cancer are chemists and those in occupations that involve close exposure to gasoline and dry cleaning agents. Inhaled carcinogens appear to reach the pancreas via the bloodstream. Risk also appears to increase with obesity, physical inactivity, chronic inflammation of the pancreas, diabetes, and cirrhosis of the liver. In addition, rates of pancreatic cancer appear to be higher in those who use smokeless tobacco.

Only 6% of people who have pancreatic cancer survive beyond 5 years.[3] Late detection and

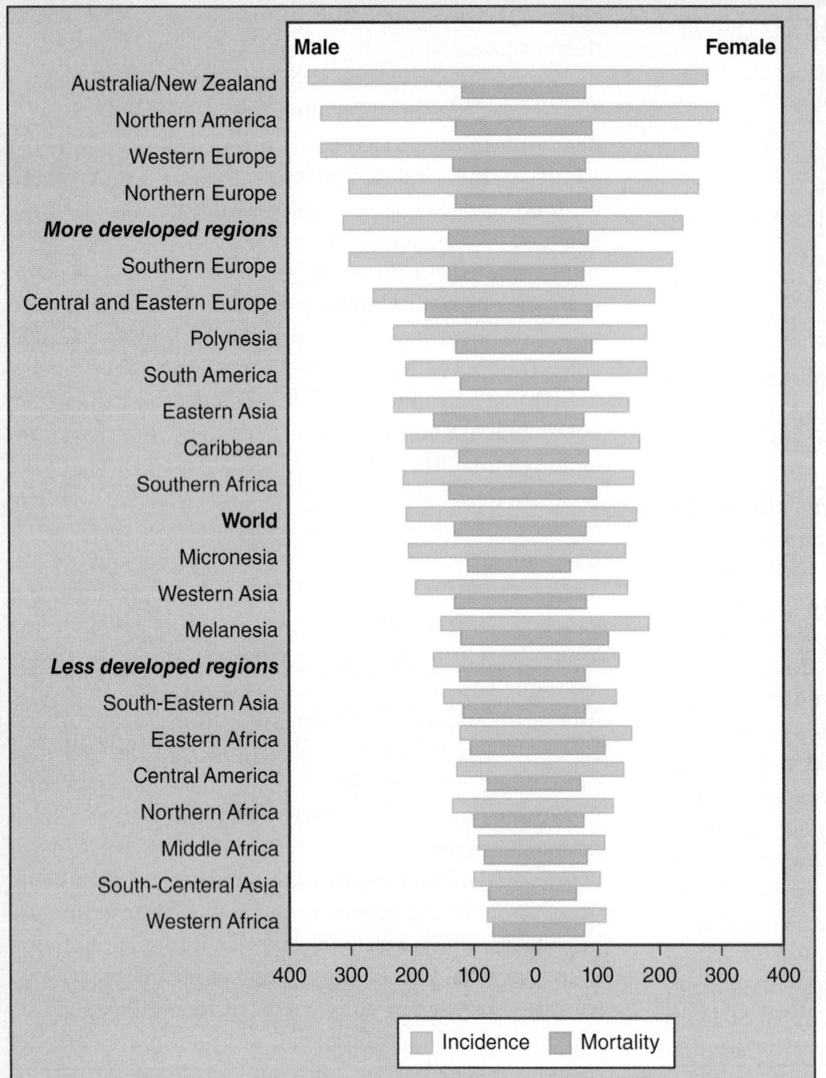

Figure 13.B

Estimated Rates of Stomach Cancer Around the World, 2012.

Reproduced from Ferlay J., Soerjomataram I., Ervik M., Dikshit R., Eser S., Mathers C., Rebelo M., Parkin D.M., Forman D., Bray, F. (2013). The GLOBOCAN 2012 v1.0, Cancer Incidence and Mortality Worldwide: IARC CancerBase No. 11, 2013. Unit of Descriptive Epidemiology at the International Agency for Research on Cancer. Available at http://globocan.iarc.fr/Pages/fact_sheets_cancer.aspx

Eating fruits and vegetables appears to inhibit the reactions in the stomach that form nitrosamines. In addition, they appear to protect the stomach from the effects of carcinogens. Populations who consume large quantities of fruit and vegetables generally have a low risk of stomach cancer.

In addition to dietary factors, infection with the bacterium *Helicobacter pylori* has been found to be associated with the development of stomach cancer. *H. pylori*, which also increases the risk of digestive system ulcers, is highly prevalent in Asian countries. Persons with *H. pylori* can be treated with antibiotics to eradicate the stomach infection. Although killing this microorganism is an effective treatment for ulcers, it results in only a slowing of the precancerous process and does not prevent all stomach cancers.

metastasis reduce survival. For the rare patients who discover their cancer in its early stages, surgery is a primary treatment that may lead to a cure and long-term relief of symptoms. In patients diagnosed in later stages of the disease, surgery, radiation, chemotherapy, and certain targeted cancer therapies may extend survival.

Acute Myeloid Leukemia Acute myeloid leukemia (AML) affects blood-producing cells in the bone marrow. In AML, white blood cells that combat bacterial infection (neutrophils) are primarily affected, but occasionally red blood cells or platelets are affected as well. These cells do not differentiate properly from stem cells in the bone marrow (see the

Figure 13.8

Tongue Cancer. This close-up of a cancer patient's mouth shows a malignant tumor on the edge of the tongue. This type of cancer spreads rapidly. The survival rate is low. Tongue cancer may be related to smoking cigarettes or to the use of smokeless tobacco.

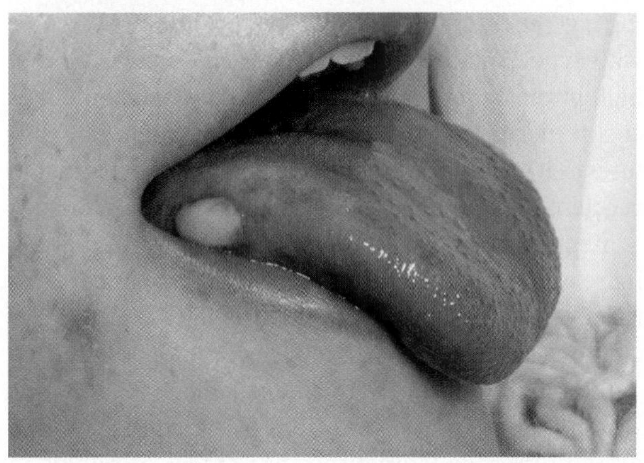

section titled "Bone Marrow and Peripheral Blood Stem Cell Transplants" in this chapter), resulting in fewer than normal numbers of these cells in the bloodstream. AML is a serious disease and is likely fatal if not treated. Chemotherapy and stem cell transplantation are standard treatments.

The primary known causes of AML are exposure to benzene and ionizing radiation. Cigarette smoke contains benzene and substances that emit ionizing radiation, along with other substances thought to cause AML. Data from human and experimental animal studies show a causal relationship between smoking and acute myeloid leukemia. The risk for AML increases with the number of cigarettes smoked and with the duration of smoking.[9]

Cancers Related to Diet

Research results suggest that about one-third of the cancer deaths that occur annually in the United States result from nutrition and physical activity factors, including obesity.[8] For Americans who do not use tobacco (to which another one-third of cancer deaths are attributed annually), dietary choices and physical activity are *the most important* modifiable determinants of cancer risk. Along with adopting a physically active lifestyle and maintaining a healthful weight, the American Cancer Society recommends eating a variety of healthful foods, with an emphasis on plant sources. ***Table 13.5*** lists the ACS's dietary recommendations.

Table 13.5

Dietary Recommendations for Reducing Cancer Risk

- Eat five or more servings of fruits and vegetables per day.
- Eat whole-grain foods rather than processed (refined) grain foods.
- Limit consumption of red meats and processed meats.
- Choose foods that help maintain a healthy weight.
- Drink no more than one alcoholic beverage per day (women) or two per day (men).

Adapted from American Cancer Society. (2010). *Cancer facts and figures, 2010*. Atlanta, GA: Author.

As you can see from Table 13.5, diet has both a positive and a negative effect on the development of cancer. There are dietary components that raise the risk of certain cancers and others that lower the risk of certain cancers. One cancer strongly related to diet is stomach cancer. The other cancer related to diet—colorectal cancer—can be affected significantly by one's heredity. Other cancers, such as breast cancer, have risk factors related to diet but are related to other risk factors as well.

Cancer of the Stomach The incidence of and mortality from stomach cancer has declined dramatically over the past 75 years in the United States. In the early part of the 20th century, stomach cancer, not lung cancer, was the number one cancer killer of Americans. (See the Diversity in Health essay titled "Stomach Cancer: Variation in Mortality Among Countries" for an explanation of this decline.)

Stomach cancer is another of the silent cancers because no signs and symptoms appear early in its course. As the disease progresses, a person may experience mild stomach discomfort with gas pains or vague sensations of fullness. Suspecting minor digestive problems, a person with these symptoms may take antacid tablets, and the symptoms disappear. As the cancer continues to grow, the malignancy causes more severe pain that is less responsive to antacids. The stomach cancer victim may then experience a decreased appetite, a feeling of fullness after just beginning to eat, pain on eating, nausea and vomiting, weight loss, excessive burping, and weakness.

The risk of stomach cancer increases with age and doubles each decade over the age of 55. However,

colon The large intestine.

rectum The lower part of the large intestine.

fecal occult (FEE-kle ok-KULT) blood test (FOBT) Home test that detects hidden blood in the stool.

the primary risk factors for cancer of the stomach are dietary factors. Diets high in salt-cured, nitrate-cured, or smoked food increase the risk of stomach cancer. Cigarette smoking and consuming large quantities of alcoholic beverages are also risk factors. The Diversity in Health essay discusses the risk factors for stomach cancer in greater detail.

Stomach cancer is easily diagnosed with barium studies. During this procedure, the patient swallows a milky fluid called barium sulfate. As this material reaches the stomach, a series of X-rays is taken that show the movement of this fluid through the stomach, while visualizing obstructions and other growths. Physicians often obtain stomach cells by the use of a fiber-optic tube, which can be fitted with instruments for such procedures. If a tumor is found, a biopsy is taken of the growth so that the cells can be studied and the diagnosis confirmed.

In the United States, stomach cancer is no longer a major killer; therefore, routine screening is not performed as it is in high-risk populations such as Japan. Thus, most stomach cancers are not diagnosed early in the United States. If found early, however, stomach cancer can be treated with surgery to remove the tumor. Chemotherapy and radiation are also used to treat stomach cancer and may be used in conjunction with surgery.

Cancer of the Colon and Rectum The **colon**, or large intestine, is an organ of the digestive system that reabsorbs water and certain chemicals from waste materials (feces). Bacteria in the colon decompose materials that the human body cannot digest. The **rectum** is the lower part of the large intestine; it terminates at the anus.

Cancer of the colon and rectum, jointly referred to as *colorectal cancer*, is the third most deadly cancer in the United States (see Table 13.3). The signs and symptoms of colorectal cancer depend on the location of the tumor. A person may have no symptoms or few symptoms at first. Some persons first experience vague or crampy abdominal pain that may be mistaken for an ulcer. Other indications may be a change in bowel habits, such as constipation alternating with diarrhea. Blood may be visible in the stool (feces) or on screening a person may have a positive occult (hidden) blood test. As the cancer worsens, a person with colorectal cancer may have a complete obstruction of the colon that requires emergency surgery.

The primary risk factors for developing colorectal cancer are advanced age, heredity, personal or family history of colorectal polyps (small growths) or inflammatory bowel disease, physical inactivity, obesity, smoking cigarettes, and heavy alcohol consumption. People with type 2 diabetes are at higher risk as well. A diet high in red or processed meat (hot dogs and some luncheon meats) and meat cooked at very high temperatures as in grilling and an inadequate intake of fruits and vegetables might raise colorectal cancer risk.[19]

Beginning at age 40, both men and women are at increased risk for developing colorectal cancer; this risk doubles with each decade after age 50 and peaks at about age 70. More than 90% of people diagnosed with colorectal cancer are older than age 50.[19] People who have hereditary conditions in which they tend to grow numerous (sometimes hundreds) of polyps in their gastrointestinal tracts have very high incidences of colorectal malignancies. In addition, people who have a first-degree relative (parent or sibling) with colon cancer are three to five times more likely to develop colorectal cancer than are people with no such family history of this disease.

Aspirin has been found to have a protective effect against colorectal cancer when taken daily at a dose of at least 75 mg, about one baby aspirin, for 5 years or more.[20] In addition, exercising moderately and consistently reduces the risk of colon cancer. Consuming a diet that contains adequate amounts of fruits, vegetables, and whole grains; replaces red and processed meats with chicken and fish; and replaces most saturated fats with unsaturated fats can reduce the risk of colorectal cancer. Postmenopausal hormone replacement and calcium reduce colorectal cancer risk as well.[11,21]

Early detection of colorectal cancer usually results in a high chance of survival. Although colorectal cancer may have no easily recognizable early symptoms, tests are available to screen for this cancer. Common tests are the fecal occult blood test, digital rectal examination, sigmoidoscopy, and colonoscopy. Less common tests are the double-contrast barium enema, the CT colonography (virtual colonoscopy), and the stool DNA test (sDNA).

The **fecal occult blood test (FOBT)** detects hidden blood in the stool. The patient performs the simple test at home by smearing stool onto a piece of paper that has been sensitized to detect occult blood. Often, the test papers can be mailed to a laboratory or

digital rectal exam A test in which a physician uses a gloved finger to feel the rectum or the prostate for abnormal growths.

sigmoidoscopy (SIG-moid-OS-ko-pee) A procedure in which a physician views the lower portion of the colon via a flexible fiber-optic tube.

colonoscopy (KO-lon-OS-ko-pee) A procedure in which a physician views the entire length of the colon using a flexible fiber-optic tube.

to the physician for interpretation. This test will not detect all colorectal cancers, however, because not all colorectal cancers bleed. Also, positive tests may indicate conditions other than colorectal cancer.

A stool DNA test for colorectal cancer screening was developed recently and is endorsed by the American Cancer Society. Using extremely sensitive laboratory methods, the sDNA test detects cells shed into the stool from precancerous or cancerous polyps, which have recognizable changes in their DNA. Research results show sDNA tests to be more effective than FOBT in detecting colorectal cancer.[22]

To perform the **digital rectal exam**, a physician uses a gloved finger to feel the rectum for abnormal growths. **Sigmoidoscopy** is a procedure in which the physician views the lower portion of the colon (the sigmoid [S-shaped] colon) with a flexible fiber-optic tube. During a similar procedure called a **colonoscopy**, the fiber-optic tube is threaded through the entire length of the colon. The sigmoidoscope or colonoscope can also be used to remove or biopsy polyps or other growths.

The double-contrast barium enema is an X-ray examination of the colon when it is filled with a barium solution. Additional X-rays are taken after the patient expels the solution. The barium provides a contrast medium that helps visualize polyps or other growths. Another method to visualize the entire length of the colon is the *virtual colonoscopy*. This test is a type of CT or MRI scan that produces both two- and three-dimensional images of the colon. Although expensive and not as sensitive as the colonoscopy, the virtual colonoscopy could become an option for patients who want a test that is less invasive than a colonoscopy.

See the Managing Your Health box titled "Screening Guidelines for the Early Detection of Cancer in Average-Risk Asymptomatic People" earlier in this chapter for information on early detection of colorectal cancer. When colorectal cancer is detected early, surgery is the primary treatment. Physicians often use chemotherapy and radiation therapy after surgery to kill any metastasized cancer that was not detected or removed by surgery. If surgery is not possible, a physician may treat the cancer with chemotherapy or radiation therapy alone. Targeted therapies may also be used.

Cancers Related to Hormone Function

Breast Cancer From the mid-1950s until 1985 in the United States, breast cancer was the number one cancer killer of women. Lung cancer then usurped the top position because the death rate from lung cancer in women continued to rise while the death rate from breast cancer began to decline.

The incidence of breast cancer in women has remained stable for decades, but its incidence increased nearly 4% per year between 1980 and 1987 when mammography screening came into widespread use. More cancers in earlier stages were detected than previously, which showed up as in increase in the incidence rate. The incidence rate held steady from 1987 to 1994 but rose 1.6% from 1994 to 1999. The American Cancer Society suggests that this increase was because of rising rates of obesity and an increased use of postmenopausal combined estrogen plus progestin hormone replacement therapy (HRT). Combined HRT has since been shown to increase the risk of breast cancer, with the cancer risk rising with increasing length of use of HRT. From 1999 to 2006, incidence rates fell 2%, which may be the result of a decrease in mammography screening and a decrease in the use of HRT following the publication of the Women's Health Initiative study revealing the link between combined HRT and breast cancer in 2002.[23,24] The rate of breast cancer continued to decline through 2013, although an estimated 232,000 new cases of invasive breast cancer were diagnosed in 2013.[25] Breast cancer is rare in men; it accounts for 1% of U.S. cases. Even so, men should report any changes in their breast tissue to their doctor.

Signs and Symptoms The signs and symptoms of breast cancer involve changes in the breast tissue, including lumps in the breast; dimpling, thickening, discoloration, irritation, or scaling of the breast skin; tenderness of the nipple or nipple discharge; and swelling or distortion of the breast. Pain is not usually a sign of breast cancer; most breast cancers are painless in their early development. Breast pain is usually caused by cyclic hormonal changes and related breast swelling.

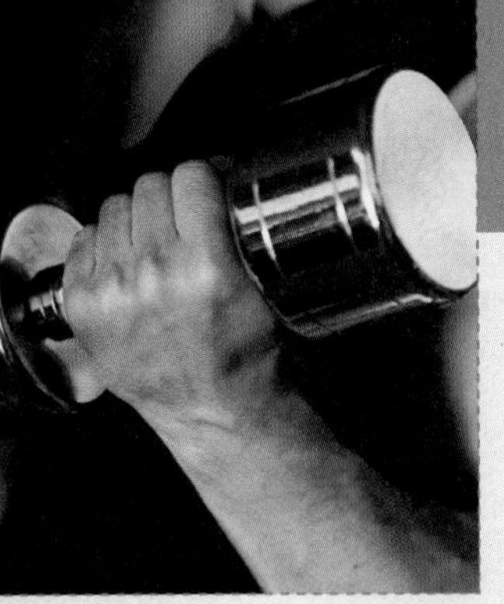

© Stockbyte/Thinkstock

Managing Your Health

Breast Self-Examination

Breast self-examination should be done once a month so you become familiar with the usual appearance and feel of your breasts. Familiarity makes it easier to notice any changes in the breast from month to month. Early discovery of a change from what is "normal" is the main idea behind BSE. The outlook is much better if you detect cancer in an early stage.

If you menstruate, the best time to do BSE is 2 or 3 days after your period ends, when your breasts are least likely to be tender or swollen. If you no longer menstruate, pick a day such as the first day of the month to remind yourself it is time to do BSE.

Here is one way to do BSE:

1. Stand before a mirror. Inspect both breasts for anything unusual such as any discharge from the nipples or puckering, dimpling, or scaling of the skin.

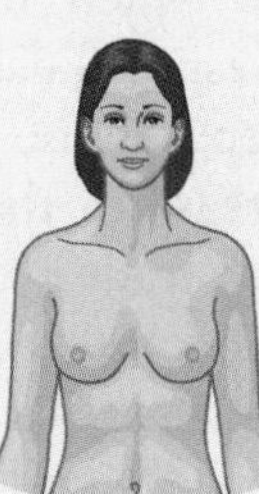

The next two steps are designed to emphasize any change in the shape or contour of your breasts. As you do them, you should be able to feel your chest muscles tighten

2. Watching closely in the mirror, clasp your hands behind your head and press your hands forward.

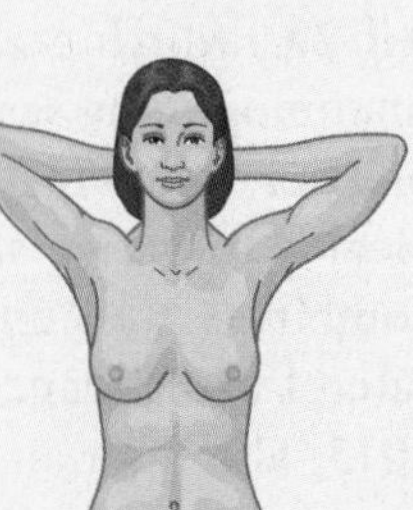

3. Next, press your hands firmly on your hips and bow slightly toward your mirror as you pull your shoulders and elbows forward.

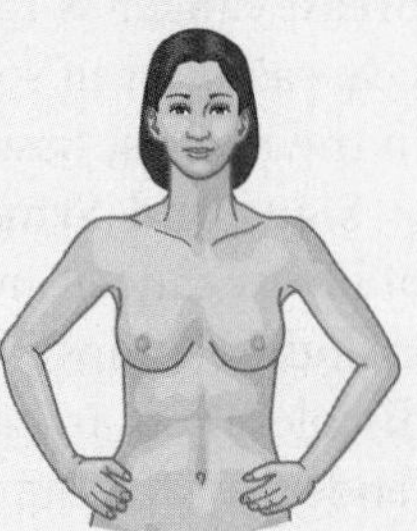

Some women do the next part of the exam in the shower because fingers glide over soapy skin, making it easy to concentrate on the texture underneath.

4. Raise your left arm. Use three or four fingers of your right hand to explore your left breast firmly, carefully, and thoroughly. Beginning at the outer edge, press the flat part of your fingers in small circles, moving the circles slowly around the breast. Gradually work toward the nipple. Be sure to cover the entire breast. Pay special attention to the area between the breast and the underarm, including the underarm itself. Feel for any unusual lump or mass under the skin.

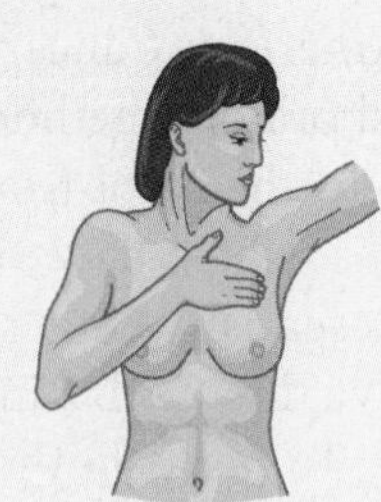

5. Gently squeeze the nipple and look for discharge. (If you have any discharge during the month—whether or not it is during BSE—see your doctor.) Repeat steps 4 and 5 on your right breast.

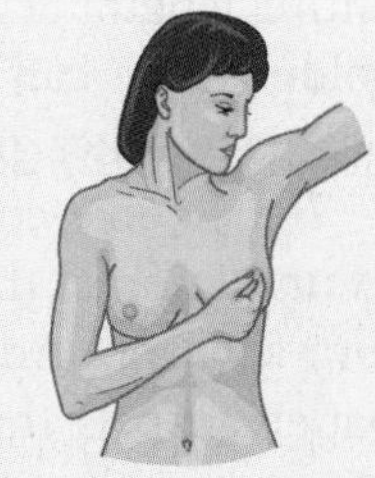

6. Steps 4 and 5 should be repeated lying down. Lie flat on your back with your left arm over your head and a pillow or folded towel under your left shoulder. This position flattens the breast and makes it easier to examine. Use the same circular motion described earlier. Repeat the exam on your right breast.

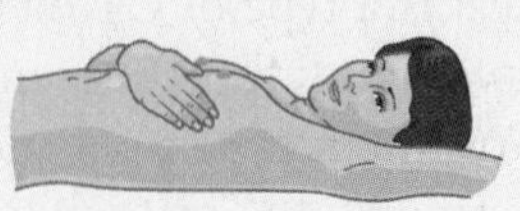

Figure 13.9

Breast Cancer: Incidence and Mortality Rates by Age and Race, U.S., 2006–2010

Reproduced from American Cancer Society. Breast Cancer Facts and Figures 2013-2014. Atlanta: American Cancer Society, Inc.

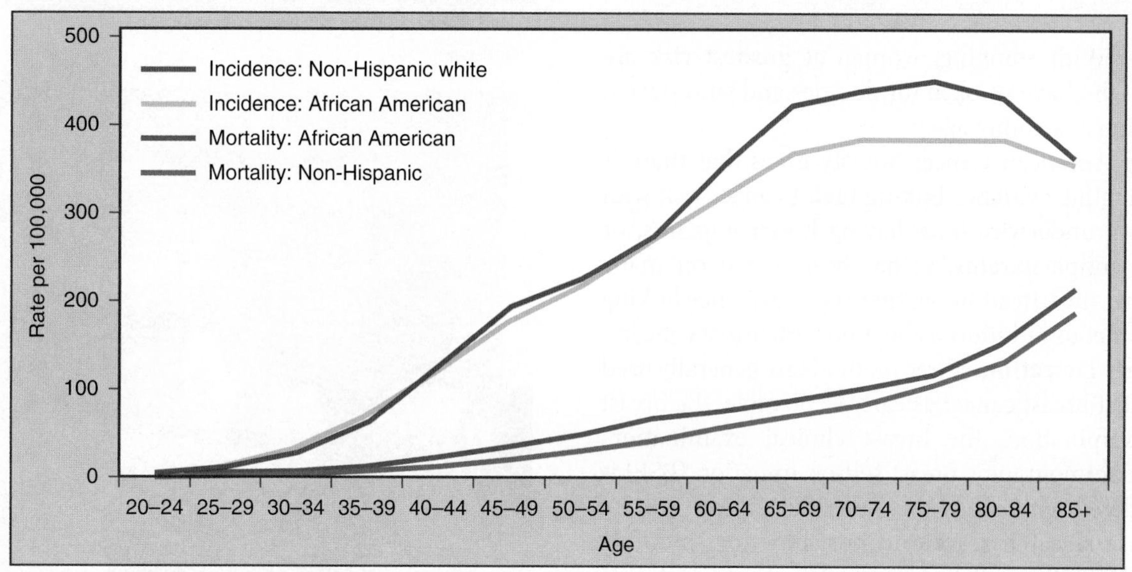

Risk Factors and Prevention Approximately 5–10% of breast cancers are the result of the inheritance of mutations in the breast cancer susceptibility genes *BRCA1* and *BRCA2*.[25] In addition, women with first-degree relatives (mothers, sisters, daughters) who have breast cancer are at increased risk for developing the disease. Men are at very low risk for developing breast cancer. Genetic testing is available for people whose family history suggests that they carry breast cancer susceptibility genes.

Another major risk factor for the development of breast cancer in women is age. Breast cancer is rare in women younger than 20 years, but the incidence begins to climb throughout the 20s, rises dramatically during the 30s through the mid-70s, and then drops significantly (**Figure 13.9**). Researchers at the American Cancer Society estimated that 90% of new breast cancer cases and 93% of breast cancer deaths occurred in women aged 45 years and older in 2009. Incidence and death rates from breast cancer are generally highest among White and African American women.[25]

In addition to age and heredity, a third major group of breast cancer risk factors are those that increase a woman's cumulative exposure to ovarian hormones, particularly estrogen. Evidence suggests that having a high number of menstrual cycles is a breast cancer risk factor. For example, early menarche (younger than age 12) and late menopause (older than age 55) are risk factors for breast cancer. Also, women who did not have a full-term pregnancy (therefore did not have their cycles interrupted) are at a higher risk than those who have. Women who did not have a full-term pregnancy until after age 30 are also at higher risk.[25]

Breast cancer risk is slightly elevated in women currently taking oral contraceptives and remains slightly elevated until about 10 years after use is discontinued. Recent use of hormone replacement therapy (HRT) that combines estrogen and progestin increases breast cancer risk as well. The longer HRT is taken, the greater the increase in risk.

Overweight and obesity are other risk factors for breast cancer because fat tissue produces estrogen. Therefore, overweight and obese women have higher circulating levels of estrogen than do nonoverweight and nonobese women. Postmenopausal obesity is thought to increase the risk of breast cancer threefold;[12] overweight and obese women can lower their risk of breast cancer by exercising and losing weight. Regular exercise not only helps a person maintain a healthy weight but also appears to have an effect on hormones and energy balance in a way that lowers breast cancer risk.

Smoking cigarettes and drinking alcohol are also associated with breast cancer risk. Drinking more than one alcoholic drink per day raises the risk of breast cancer, so to lower risk, minimize alcohol

lumpectomy (lum-PECK-toe-me) Surgical removal of a breast tumor, including a layer of surrounding tissue.

intake. With smoking, women at greatest risk are those who have smoked for decades and who started smoking at a young age.[26]

The American Cancer Society notes that there is no scientific evidence linking breast cancer risk with wearing underwire bras, having breast implants, or using antiperspirants, as has been stated on many Internet sites. In addition, there is no evidence linking spontaneous or induced abortion with breast cancer.[23]

Early Detection Three methods are generally used to detect breast cancer as early as possible: the breast self-examination, the breast clinical examination, and mammography. Breast self-examination (BSE) is considered optional by the American Cancer Society because research results do not show that monthly BSE saves lives. Research results also reveal that when women find changes or lumps in their breasts, it is usually not during structured breast self-examinations but during the normal course of dressing, bathing, or other similar activities.[25] However, women should become aware of how their breasts normally feel and report any breast change to a healthcare professional immediately. The Managing Your Health box titled "Breast Self-Examination" shows how to perform the BSE should you choose to do so. The breast clinical examination is performed by a healthcare professional. The ACS recommends that a clinical examination be performed every 3 years for women from ages 20 to 39 and every year thereafter.

Mammography is the process of taking X-rays of breast tissue to detect benign and malignant growths. As you can see in ***Figure 13.10***, each breast is placed over a plate containing X-ray film, and the tissue is compressed. The ACS recommends that women aged 40 years and older have a mammogram every year. Women at high risk for breast cancer, such as those with a strong family history of the disease, should consult their physicians regarding the need for mammograms on a different schedule (e.g., at an earlier age, or more often).

If screening reveals a suspicious mass in the breast tissue, a physician usually performs a biopsy. To perform this procedure, a physician inserts a fine needle into the mass and withdraws cells. An individual trained to detect cancer studies the cells to determine if the growth is malignant. Fine-needle biopsy is relatively painless and is about 90% accurate.

Figure 13.10

Mammography. Each breast is placed on a platform, and the tissue is compressed while the X-ray is taken.

© Photodisc

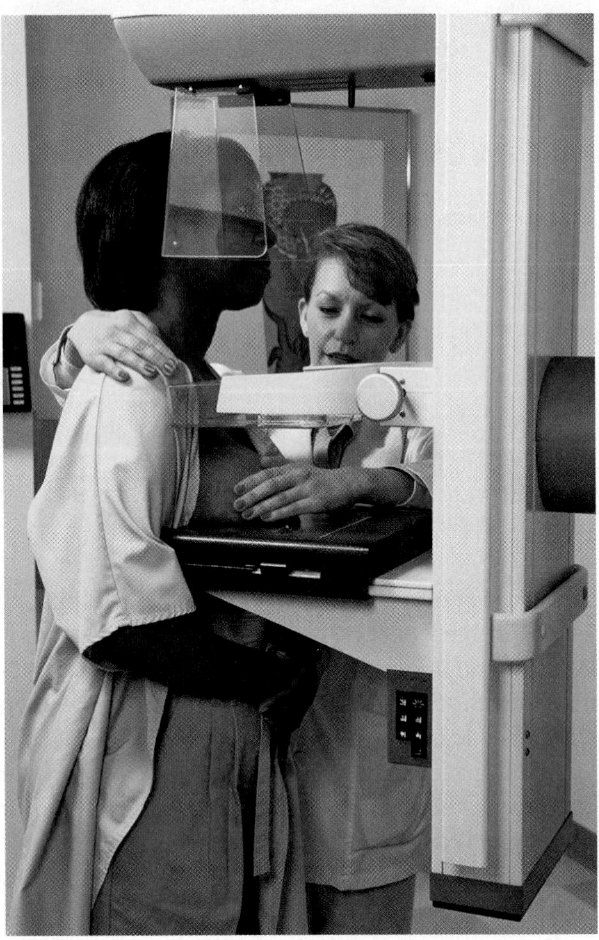

Treatment Stage 0, I, or II breast cancer is usually treated with **lumpectomy**, surgical removal of the tumor, followed by breast irradiation. (Stage 0 in breast cancer is often a precancerous condition.) The surgeon also removes a layer of normal tissue surrounding the tumor so that it is less likely that cancer tissue is left in the breast. He or she also removes some lymph nodes under the nearby armpit to determine if the cancer has spread. About 6 weeks of radiation therapy typically follows lumpectomy. Clinical trials are under way to determine whether irradiating only the part of the breast with the excised tumor might be a better postsurgical approach than irradiating the entire breast, which is the current approach.

Accelerated partial-breast irradiation (APBI) might reduce the amount of radiation absorbed by normal breast tissue and increase the percentage of

total mastectomy (mas-TEK-toe-me) Surgical removal of a breast and involved lymph nodes for the treatment of breast cancer.

radical mastectomy Surgical removal of a breast, underlying muscle, and underarm fat and lymph nodes as a treatment for breast cancer.

lumpectomy patients who choose radiation therapy. APBI would be a shorter course of treatment—only 1 to 2 weeks—but the doses of radiation would be higher than in whole-breast irradiation.[27]

Women with advanced breast cancer may need more aggressive surgery than a lumpectomy. **Total mastectomy** is removal of the entire breast and involved lymph nodes. A **radical mastectomy** is removal of the entire breast and underlying muscle as well as the underarm lymph nodes and fat. In a *modified radical mastectomy*, underlying muscle is not removed.

Immunotherapy, hormonal therapy, and chemotherapy are also used in breast cancer treatment in addition to surgery and radiation. Herceptin (trastuzumab) is a drug used in targeted immunotherapy. Women with late-stage recurring cancer are often treated with this monoclonal antibody. Antibodies are receptor proteins that recognize foreign substances (antigens) in the body and bind to them. Monoclonal antibodies are made in the laboratory from a single type of antibody. In this case, Herceptin is an antibody that targets a particular breast tumor protein. After binding to this protein, the antibody works in various ways to shrink breast cancer tumors and stop tumor cells from multiplying. Women treated with both Herceptin and chemotherapy have been found to be less likely to experience a recurrence of their cancer than women treated with chemotherapy alone.[25]

The primary drug used in hormonal therapy is tamoxifen, an antiestrogen. Antiestrogens counteract the effects of estrogen on breast cancers that depend on estrogen for their growth. Tamoxifen has few serious side effects compared to other anticancer drugs, reduces the annual recurrence rate by 41%, and reduces the death rate by 33%.[25]

Chemotherapy is also used to treat breast cancer, sometimes in conjunction with tamoxifen. Compounds have been discovered that have demonstrated good antitumor activity in breast cancer treatment. Taxol was the first to be discovered. (Taxol is found in the bark of the Pacific yew tree [*Taxus brevifolia*].) Today a variety of drugs is used in breast cancer chemotherapy, with combinations of drugs providing more effective results than single drugs.[25]

Endometrial Cancer The endometrium is the lining of the uterus, the organ in which a fetus develops until birth. Endometrial cancer most often occurs in postmenopausal women; only 5% of endometrial cancers occur in women younger than 40 years.[28] The primary symptom of this cancer is abnormal uterine bleeding. Premenopausal women usually experience symptoms of irregular, heavy, or prolonged uterine bleeding during menstrual periods or bleeding between periods. Postmenopausal women experience uterine bleeding although they no longer have menstrual periods.

Most endometrial cancer is diagnosed at an early stage because of postmenopausal bleeding. The Pap test for cervical cancer does not detect cancer in the body of the uterus. (This test is discussed shortly.) However, if the physician suspects that a patient has endometrial cancer, he or she usually performs an endometrial biopsy, in which a sample of tissue is removed from the endometrium and examined microscopically.

Although the cause of endometrial cancer is unknown, it is associated with prolonged exposure to estrogen. Therefore, the risk factors for endometrial cancer are similar to those for breast cancer: early menarche, late menopause, not bearing children, and delaying pregnancy. Additionally, women who are more than 50 lbs overweight, especially postmenopausal women, have a 10-fold greater risk for developing endometrial cancer than women who are not overweight. As with breast cancer, exercising reduces risk.[3] Using oral contraceptives that combine estrogen and progesterone reduces risk as well, but estrogen replacement therapy without progesterone (unopposed ERT) is a risk factor.[14] Infertility and diabetes are possible risk factors for endometrial cancer as well.[3]

Many women diagnosed with endometrial cancer undergo total hysterectomy: removal of the uterus, fallopian tubes, and ovaries. Radiation, hormones, and/or chemotherapy are sometimes used after surgery. The outlook for survival after treatment for endometrial cancer is good: The 1-year and 5-year survival rates are 92% and 82%, respectively.[3]

Cancers Related to Viral Infection: Cervical Cancer

Certain viruses are implicated in the development of a variety of cancers; **Table 13.6** lists these viruses and the cancers to which they are related. However, viruses alone do not appear to cause cancer. Scientists think

Papanicolaou (PAP-eh-nik-eh-LOUW) test (Pap test) A screening procedure for cervical cancer in which cells from the cervical canal are removed and then smeared on a glass slide for microscopic examination.

that interactions between these viruses and other agents, or cocarcinogens, result in the development of cancer. For example, the high incidence of liver cancer in certain regions of Africa and Asia appears to be caused by interactions between the hepatitis B virus and aflatoxins. Aflatoxins are a group of carcinogens produced by a mold that grows on improperly stored peanuts and grains. Many people in these regions eat these moldy foods.

The virally related cancer most prevalent in the United States is cervical cancer. Since 1960, the incidence of cervical cancer has declined dramatically, primarily because of the widespread routine use of the **Papanicolaou test (Pap test)** to screen women for cervical cancer. To perform the Pap test, a physician or other specially trained healthcare professional takes a sample of cells from the cervical canal. These cells are examined under a microscope. A newer method of collecting and analyzing samples is the liquid-based thin-layer slide preparation, which appears to be more sensitive than standard Pap tests. In addition, computer-automated readers improve the analysis of Pap tests.

Most women who are diagnosed with cervical cancer have no symptoms; their cancers are discovered at an early stage during their annual gynecologic examination and Pap test. If undiagnosed, the cancer may cause symptoms of abnormal vaginal bleeding (the most common symptom), pelvic pressure or pain, and/or a foul-smelling vaginal discharge.

Table 13.6

Viruses and Cancers to Which They Are Related

Virus	Cancer Type
Hepatitis B virus (HBV)	Primary liver cancer
Human T-cell lymphotropic/leukemia virus (HTLV)	Adult T-cell lymphoma/leukemia
Cytomegalovirus (CMV)	Kaposi's sarcoma
Human papillomavirus (HPV)	Cervical cancer, penile cancer, oropharyngeal cancer
Epstein-Barr virus (EBV)	Burkitt's lymphoma, nasopharyngeal cancer

Cervical cancer most often develops in young and middle-aged women, generally between the ages of 35 and 54 years, with a median age at diagnosis of 48. Fourteen percent of cervical cancer cases are diagnosed in women between the ages of 20 and 34 years.[29] If untreated, cervical cancer can invade surrounding tissues and metastasize. Having regular screening tests can reduce the risk of developing invasive cancer of the cervix.

A causal association exists between infection with human papillomavirus (HPV) and cervical cancer. HPV is transmitted by infected men to their female partners during sexual intercourse and vice versa. Therefore, the greater the number of male sexual partners a woman has over time, the greater are her chances of becoming infected with HPV. If a woman is monogamous but her male sex partner is not, her risk rises because he is more likely to become infected than if he were monogamous. Also, women who had their first sexual intercourse before age 17 are at increased risk because they are more likely to have a greater number of sexual partners over time than those women who became sexually active at an older age. In addition, long-term use of oral contraceptives is associated with an increased risk of cervical cancer.[3]

At low risk for cervical cancer are women who are celibate or who are monogamous with a monogamous partner over many years. Sexually active women with multiple partners or with nonmonogamous partners can lower their risk by using male or female condoms to protect themselves against infection with HPV.

In 2006, the U.S. Food and Drug Administration approved the first vaccine developed to prevent cervical cancer (Gardasil) and in 2009 approved a second (Cervarix). Gardasil is highly effective in preventing infection by four types of HPV. Two types (HPV-16 and HPV-18) cause approximately 70% of cervical cancers,[8] and the other two types (HPV-6 and HPV-11) cause about 90% of all genital warts. The FDA in 2009 expanded the approval of Gardasil for use in boys and young men to prevent genital warts. Cervarix acts against HPV-16 and HPV-18 only. The American Cancer Society recommends routine HPV vaccination for females aged 11 and 12 years, and for females aged 13 to 18 years "to catch up on missed vaccine or complete the vaccination series."[8]

HPV vaccines do not prevent infection with all types of HPV, so vaccinated women should still have regular Pap tests. In addition, neither vaccine protects nor treats women already infected with HPV, so it is important for girls and young women to be vaccinated before they become sexually active.

The American Cancer Society recommends that all women should have annual conventional Pap tests or biannual liquid-based Pap tests 3 years after their first vaginal intercourse but no later than age 21. The ACS suggests that after three consecutive normal Pap tests, women older than 30 years may have this test performed every 2 to 3 years or at the discretion of their physicians.

If the Pap test shows that cervical cancer may be present, a physician usually performs a *colposcopy*. Using a specially designed microscope, the physician examines the cervix. If the physician observes abnormal cervical tissue during this procedure, he or she usually performs a biopsy to confirm the diagnosis.

Physicians treat dysplasia or cervical cancers in situ with surgery, electrocoagulation, cryotherapy, and carbon dioxide (CO_2) laser surgery. Laser energy destroys the tissue. Cryotherapy is the use of extreme cold to destroy cells. Usually solid carbon dioxide or liquid nitrogen is applied briefly to the abnormal tissue with a sterile cotton-tipped applicator. A blister forms and the tissue dies. Electrocoagulation kills the tissue through intense heat by electric current.

With invasive cervical cancers, surgeons may perform a simple hysterectomy (removal of just the uterus) or a total hysterectomy (removal of the uterus and ovaries). With certain cervical cancers, radiation is the treatment of choice. Detected early, cervical cancer is highly survivable.

Cancers Related to Ultraviolet Radiation: Skin Cancers

Lying on the beach or on a tanning bed to develop a tanned "healthy" look is anything but healthy! When skin tans it is a sign of skin damage. Certain skin cells produce a pigment called *melanin* to protect the skin from the damaging rays of the sun. Melanin is a built-in sun protector for dark-skinned people and is produced in response to sun damage in light-skinned people. In addition to causing the skin to wrinkle and age prematurely, the ultraviolet (UV) radiation in sunlight can result in the development of skin cancer. In fact, UV light exposure is the most important factor (other than heredity and age) that influences the development of skin cancer. In addition to tanning (UV rays) causing skin damage in general, sunburns during childhood and intense intermittent sun exposure increase the risk of melanoma and other skin cancers later in life.[8]

There are three types of ultraviolet radiation: UVA, UVB, and UVC. All three types are harmful and have the potential to cause skin cancer. Claims by tanning parlors that using only UVB rays will protect you from the effects of UV radiation are false. This type of ultraviolet radiation is associated with sunburn and skin cancer formation, as is UVA radiation. UVA radiation is also strongly associated with premature aging effects. Artificial UV sources, such as sun lamps and tanning beds, may also generate UVC rays. UVC radiation is a highly potent cancer-causing radiation. Although a danger from artificial sources, these rays are filtered out by the Earth's atmosphere and pose little danger from environmental sources.

There are three main types of skin cancer: basal cell carcinoma, squamous cell carcinoma, and malignant melanoma. Approximately 60% of skin cancers are basal cell carcinomas and approximately 30% are squamous cell carcinomas. Although malignant melanoma makes up less than 10% of skin cancers, this fast-growing, metastasizing cancer results in the most deaths. Malignant melanoma spreads quickly via the blood and lymph. Death is usually the result of either respiratory failure or brain or spinal cord complications. **Table 13.7** lists steps for preventing skin cancer.

Table 13.7

Steps to Reduce the Risk of Melanoma and Other Skin Cancers

- Do not use tanning beds.
- Avoid exposure to the sun (particularly sunbathing), especially between 10 a.m. and 4 p.m. when UV radiation is highest.
- When in the sun, wear sunglasses that block at least 99% of UVA and UVB radiation. Larger glasses and wraparounds provide the best protection.
- When in the sun, wear wide-brimmed hats and clothing that covers as much as possible of the arms, legs, and torso.
- Use sunscreens with a sun protection factor (SPF) of 15 or higher regularly on sun-exposed skin.

basal (BAY-sl) cell carcinoma The most common cancer of the skin, which frequently develops on portions of the skin exposed to the sun.

squamous (SKWAY-muss) cell carcinoma A common form of skin cancer that develops from exposure to noxious chemicals and high levels of X-rays, as well as from trauma.

malignant melanoma (MEL-ah-NO-mah) A deadly form of skin cancer that develops most often in persons who have been exposed to the sun in short, intense sessions, have had severe sunburn and extensive sun exposure in childhood, or have first-degree relatives who had the disease.

Basal cell carcinoma, the most common cancer of the skin, often affects persons older than 40 years. A slow-growing cancer that rarely metastasizes, basal cell carcinoma frequently develops on portions of the skin exposed to the sun: the face, head, neck, and arms. Lesions may look like moles or chronic pimples with pearl-like borders. They often become crusty and scaly and may ulcerate and bleed (**Figure 13.11a**). Basal cell carcinoma tumors are usually removed by surgery and cryotherapy, freezing with liquid nitrogen. The cure rate for basal cell carcinoma is high.

Squamous cell carcinoma is the second most common skin cancer in light-skinned persons; it develops in the same sun-exposed areas as does basal cell carcinoma. However, people with darker skin can develop this type of cancer, not from sunlight exposure, but from exposure to noxious chemicals and high levels of X-rays, as well as from trauma (burns and chronic ulcers). The skin lesions of squamous cell carcinoma look flat, red, scaly, and may be slightly elevated (**Figure 13.11b**). These tumors are removed by the same methods as basal cell carcinoma.

Both basal and squamous cell carcinomas develop from prolonged, repeated exposures to the sun. At risk are persons who are outdoors much of the time, such as construction workers, farmers, and people who regularly sunbathe and use tanning beds.

Malignant melanoma is a deadly skin cancer that affects men at a 50% higher rate than women and usually occurs in people who are White. The incidence of melanoma has been rising over the last 30 years, most notably in young women aged 15 to 39 years who are White. Additionally, an increase has been seen in both sexes aged 65 years and older.[3]

The risk for developing malignant melanoma and other skin cancers is higher the closer a person lives to the equator because of the increasing intensity of UV rays. Fair-skinned people are at greater risk than those who have darker skin. At highest risk are persons with light blue eyes, very light hair, and skin that burns easily and freckles rather than tans. Malignant melanoma develops more often in persons who are exposed to the sun in short intense sessions, such

Figure 13.11

Skin Cancers. (a) This basal cell carcinoma is a raised lesion with central depressions that bleed and crust over. (b) Squamous cell carcinoma looks like a red rounded mass or a flat sore as shown in the photo. (c) Lesions of malignant melanoma are usually characterized by irregular borders with red, white, blue, or blue-black spots. Some portions may be raised.

Courtesy of National Cancer Institute.

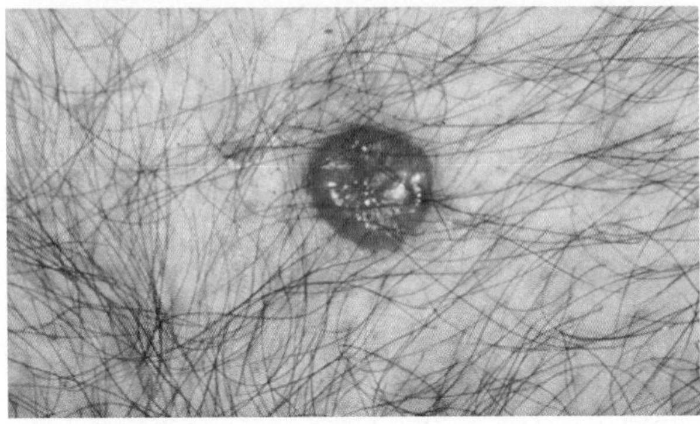

(a)

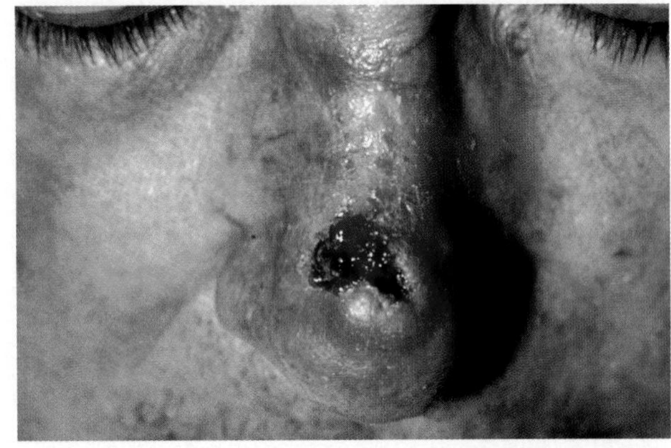

(b)

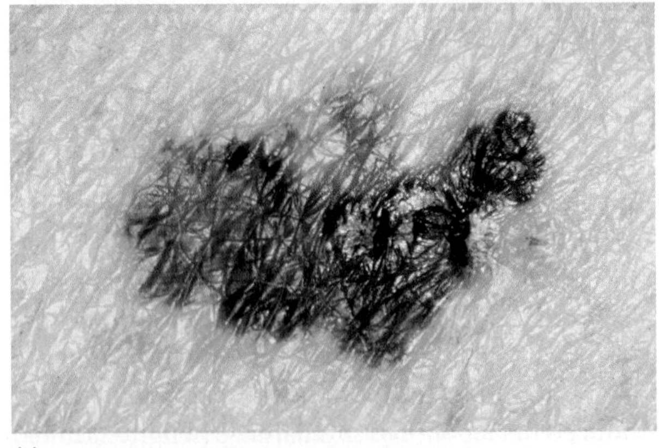

(c)

Analyzing Health-Related Information

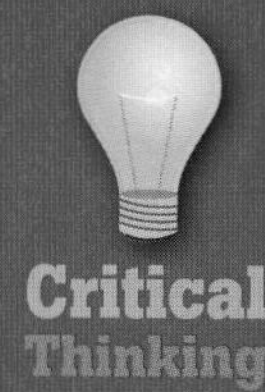

Critical Thinking

© tele52/ShutterStock

This article focuses on the use of tanning beds and the link to malignant melanoma. Explain why you think this article is a reliable or an unreliable source of information. Use the model for analyzing health information to guide your thinking; the main points of the model are noted here.

1. Which statements are verifiable facts, and which are unverified statements or value claims?
2. What are the credentials of the source making these health-related claims? Does the source have the appropriate background and education in the topic area? What can you do to check the credentials of this source?
3. What might be the motives and biases of the source making the claims?
4. What is the main point of the article? Which information is relevant to the issue, main point, product, or service? Which information is irrelevant?
5. Is the source reliable? What evidence supports your conclusion that the source is reliable or unreliable? Does the source of information present the pros and cons of the topic or the benefits and risks of the product?
6. Does the source of information attack the credibility of conventional scientists or medical authorities?

Based on your analysis, do you think that this article is a reliable source of health-related information? Summarize your reasons for coming to this conclusion.

Study Links Tanning Bed Use to Increased Risk of Melanoma

People who use tanning beds are more likely to develop melanoma, the deadliest form of skin cancer, than never users, according to a new study from the University of Minnesota. The more regularly a person frequents tanning salons, the greater the risk, the study shows.

In July 2009, after a comprehensive review of the available research, the International Agency for Research on Cancer (IARC) elevated tanning devices to its highest cancer risk category—"carcinogenic to humans" (Group 1). Despite this risk, approximately 30 million Americans still visit indoor tanning salons each year. That may be at least in part because the tanning industry has pointed to limitations in previous studies and continues to tout the purported health benefits of tanning, including vitamin D production.

The new study, funded by the National Cancer Institute and the American Cancer Society, was designed to help answer more definitively whether tanning bed use is linked to skin cancer.

"Most reports were not able to adjust for sun exposure, confirm a dose-response, or examine specific tanning devices," said study author DeAnn Lazovich, PhD, professor of epidemiology, University of Minnesota School of Publishing and co-leader of the Masonic Cancer Center's Prevention and Etiology Research Program. "Our population-based, case-control study was conducted to address these limitations."

What This Study Found

The researchers, led by Lazovich, collected detailed information on the tanning habits of more than 1,100 Minnesotans aged 25 to 59 who had been diagnosed with melanoma between July 2004 and December 2007, as well as a matched group of more than 1,100 people without melanoma.

The researchers gathered data on tanning bed use, including years of use, age at which use began, and the specific devices used, as well as other factors such as age, sunscreen use, and family history of melanoma.

According to their findings, people who had ever used an indoor tanning device were about 75% more likely to have developed melanoma. Frequent users—defined as using a tanning device for at least 50 hours, at least 100 sessions, or at least 10 years—were 2.5 to 3 times more likely to develop melanoma than those who had never used them. The risk went up with increasing tanning bed use, the study showed, and was elevated regardless of the type of device.

"We found that it didn't matter the type of tanning device used; there was no safe tanning device," Lazovich said. "We also found—and this is new data—that the risk of getting melanoma is associated more with how much a person tans and not the age at which a person starts using tanning devices. Risk rises with frequency of use, regardless of age, gender, or device."

Lazovich and her team's findings are published in *Cancer Epidemiology, Biomarkers and Prevention*, a journal of the American Association for Cancer Research.

Melanoma on the Rise

The number of new cases of melanoma in the United States has been increasing for at least 30 years. The American Cancer Society estimates that about 68,720 new melanomas will be diagnosed in the United States during 2009. Melanoma is 10 times more common in Whites than in African Americans. It is slightly more common in men than in women.

More than 2 million skin cancers are diagnosed each year in the United States. That's more than cancers of the prostate, breast, lung, colon, uterus, ovaries, and pancreas combined.

Most skin cancers are caused by too much exposure to ultraviolet (UV) rays. Much of this exposure comes from the sun, but it also comes from manmade sources, such as tanning beds.

Because of the popularity of tanning among young people, both the World Health Organization and the International Commission on Non-ionizing Radiation Protection recommend that the use of indoor tanning should be restricted in anyone under the age of 18. On May 29, 2014, the U.S. Food and Drug Administration announced that tanning beds must now carry a visible warning explicitly stating that the device should not be used by people under age 18. The mandate was spurred by building evidence that tanning in childhood and early adulthood significantly increases a person's risk of melanoma later in life.

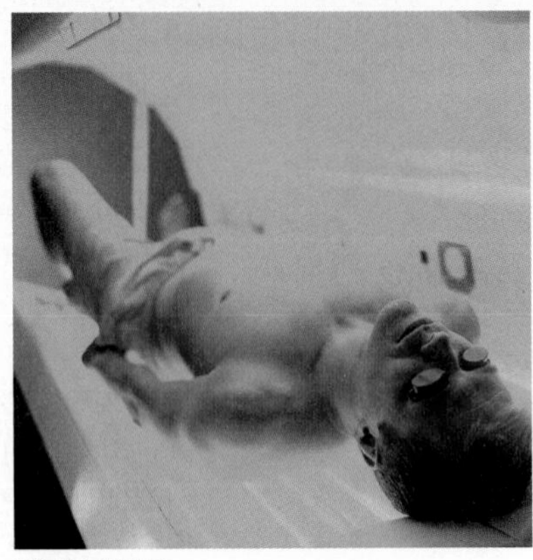

The American Cancer Society recommends people avoid tanning beds altogether. For information on how you can lower your risk of skin cancer, see *Skin Cancer Prevention and Early Detection*.

Data from Snowden, R. V. (2010, May 27). Study links tanning bed use to increased risk of melanoma. American Cancer Society. Retrieved April 25, 2011, from http://www.cancer.org/Cancer/news/News/study-links-tanning-bed-use-to-increased-risk-of-melanoma

as persons who work indoors and then vacation in a sunny climate. Severe sunburn and extensive sun exposure in childhood also increase the risk for developing malignant melanoma in adulthood. First-degree relatives of people with melanoma have a two- to eightfold increase in their risk of developing this cancer. Individuals who have two or more relatives with a history of melanoma may be at substantially higher risk.

Malignant melanoma can develop on any skin surface as well as in the eye and on mucous membranes. In men, the trunk is the most common site; in women, the legs are a common site. If you are in a high-risk group for skin cancer, especially melanoma, examine your skin regularly. Early detection is key to curing this disease. Typically, melanoma tumors are asymmetrical, have irregular borders, multiple colors (such as blue, black, red, or gray), and have a diameter greater than a pencil eraser (**Figure 13-11c**). An easy way to remember these signs is ABCD: asymmetry, border, color, and diameter. Medical researchers recently determined, however, that very rapidly growing melanomas do not necessarily show the ABCD signs. These melanomas, most often found in men and women older than age 65 years, may be red and raised with regular borders. They often itch and bleed.[30]

Healthy People 2020 is a program to improve the health of all Americans by guiding individuals to make healthy choices and monitoring progress made. A *Healthy People 2020* objective is to reduce the death rate from malignant melanoma from 2.7 deaths per 100,000 population (baseline in 2007) to 2.4 deaths per 100,000. One way to achieve this objective is to increase to at least 80.1% the proportion of persons age 18 years or older who follow protective measures that may reduce the risk of skin cancer, such as limiting sun exposure and using sunscreens and protective clothing when exposed to sunlight. Baseline data from *Healthy People 2020* show that 72.8% of U.S. adults followed sun-protective measures in 2008. Another objective is to increase the proportion of high school students who follow sun-protective measures from 9.3% (baseline in 2009) to 11.2%.[31]

Reducing the proportion of adults and high school students who use tanning beds and lights is another *Healthy People 2020* cancer-reduction objective. For high school students, the baseline was 15.6% who used tanning beds and lights in 2009; the target is a decrease to 14%. For adults, the baseline was 15.2% in 2008; the target is a decrease to 13.7%.[31]

Cancers with Unknown Causes

Prostate Cancer The prostate is a walnut-sized accessory sex organ in men. It lies beneath the bladder, surrounding the urethra, and secretes part of the seminal fluid.

Prostate cancer is the most prevalent cancer in men, and the second most prevalent cause of cancer deaths in men (see Table 13.3). (Lung cancer is the most prevalent cause of cancer death in men.) The signs and symptoms of prostate cancer mimic those of benign prostatic hypertrophy (BPH) and other noncancerous conditions of the prostate. Therefore, experiencing symptoms that include uneven flow of urine while urinating, incomplete emptying of the bladder, reduced urine flow, and urinating more frequently at night does not necessarily mean a man has prostate cancer. However, serious signs and symptoms that are more likely to be related to prostate cancer are pain in the floor of the pelvis, sudden development of impotence, and presence of blood in the urine.

In the United States, African Americans have the highest prostate cancer incidence rate, followed by Whites, Hispanics, Native Americans, and Asian/Pacific Islanders, in that order. Advanced age and heredity are strong risk factors for prostate cancer. Along with family history of prostate cancer, having certain genetic mutations, such as *BRCA2*, increase risk. This disease is rare in men younger than 45 years, but its incidence rises as men age. The median age of death from prostate cancer is 80 years.[3]

The American Cancer Society suggests that maintaining a healthy body weight and being physically active may reduce the risk of developing aggressive prostate cancer. Statins—cholesterol-lowering drugs—may reduce the risk of advanced prostate cancer. Long-term low-dose aspirin therapy may reduce prostate cancer risk as well, but taking aspirin for prostate cancer prevention is not recommended by the ACS.[3] Substituting fish for red meat in the diet may lower prostate cancer risk.[12]

For early detection of prostate cancer, the American Cancer Society recommends that all men 50 years and older have an annual prostate-specific antigen (PSA) test, with or without a digital rectal exam. During the digital rectal exam, a physician inserts a gloved finger into the rectum to feel the prostate gland The PSA is a blood test that detects a protein secreted by the prostate. If the protein concentration in the blood is elevated, it indicates that the prostate may be abnormal but not necessarily cancerous and should be checked further. The topic of prostate screening and the use of the PSA test is controversial. The United States Preventive Services Task Force recommends that healthy men not be screened for prostate cancer using the PSA because the test has been shown to not save lives. The American Cancer Society suggests that men make this decision with their physician after being fully informed of the risks and benefits of test results.[32]

testicular (tes-TIK-you-lar) self-examination (TSE) A self-screening test that males can perform to detect cancer of the testicles.

Physicians may treat localized prostate cancer by surgically removing the prostate and some surrounding tissue. However, this treatment can result in impotence, incontinence, and other complications. New surgical techniques with fewer side effects have been developed, leading to a resurgence of prostate surgery as a treatment. Advanced prostate cancer is sometimes treated with drug/hormone therapy or by removal of the testicles to reduce male sex hormone levels, which may influence the progression of this cancer. Chemotherapy, radiation, or a combination of therapies may be used if the cancer has metastasized.[3]

Prostate cancer is, in many cases, a slow-growing cancer. Many prostate cancer patients die *with* prostate cancer rather than *of* it. Because the side effects of prostate cancer treatment can be quite serious, physicians carefully consider "watchful waiting" as the treatment of choice for this cancer.[3]

Testicular Cancer The testicles, or testes, are the organs in which sperm develop and are located in the scrotal sac beneath the penis. Cancer of the testicles is a rare and highly curable cancer. Only 1% of cancers in men occur in the testicles.

The signs and symptoms of testicular cancer are a painless, swollen testis and a sensation of heaviness or aching in the testis. Men who perform testicular self-examination might feel a small lump in one testis.

Youth is a risk factor for testicular cancer. This cancer strikes primarily men between the ages of 20 and 54 years. Another risk factor for testicular cancer is the failure of one or both of the testicles to descend into the scrotum by age 1 year. White males have the highest risk, Latino males have less risk, and African American men have the least risk. Men with a family history of testicular cancer are at increased risk as are men who are infected with HIV or have AIDS. Men who have had testicular cancer in one testicle may develop it in the other.[33]

To detect testicular cancer early, the American Cancer Society recommends that men perform a **testicular self-examination (TSE)** once a month after a warm bath or shower (see the Managing Your Health box titled "Testicular Self-Exam"). The heat relaxes the scrotal skin, making tumors easier to detect. If detected and treated early, testicular cancer is one of the most curable cancers. Surgery is most often used, frequently in conjunction with radiation or chemotherapy.

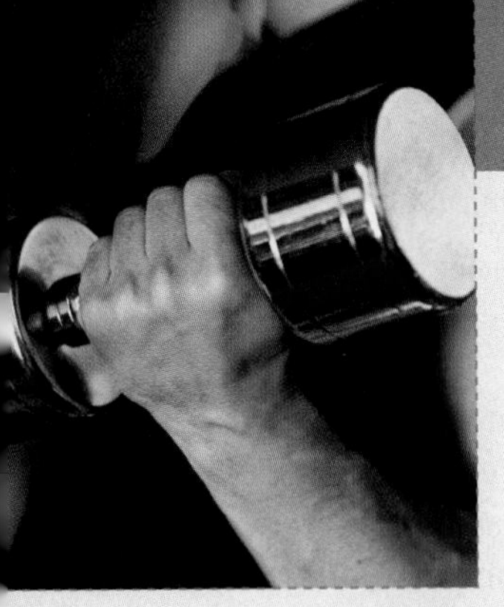
© Kzenon/ShutterStock

Managing Your Health

Testicular Self-Examination

How the Test Is Performed

Perform this test during or after a shower. This way, the scrotal skin is warm and relaxed. It's best to do the test while standing.

1. Gently feel your scrotal sac to locate a testicle.
2. Hold the testicle with one hand while firmly but gently rolling the fingers of the other hand over the testicle to examine the entire surface.
3. Repeat the procedure with the other testicle.

Why the Test Is Performed

A testicular self-exam is done to check for testicular cancer. Normal testicles contain blood vessels and other structures that can make the exam confusing. Performing a self-exam monthly allows you to become familiar with your normal anatomy. Then, if you notice any changes from the previous exam, you'll know to contact your doctor.

You should perform a testicular self-exam every month if you have or have had any of the following risk factors:

1. Family history of testicular cancer
2. Previous testicular tumor
3. Undescended testicle
4. Are a teenager or young adult (to about 35 years old)

Normal Results

Each testicle should feel firm but not rock hard. One testicle may or may not be lower or slightly larger than the other.

Always ask your doctor if you have any doubts or questions.

What Abnormal Results Mean

If you find a small hard lump (like a pea), have an enlarged testicle, or notice any other concerning differences from your last self-exam, see your doctor as soon as you can.

Consult your doctor if:

- You can't find one or both testicles—the testicles may not have descended properly in the scrotum.
- There is a soft collection of thin tubes above the testicle—it may be a collection of dilated veins (varicocele).
- There is pain or swelling in the scrotum—it may be an infection or a fluid-filled sac (hydrocele), causing blockage of blood flow to the area.

Sudden, severe (acute) pain in the scrotum or testicle is an emergency. If you experience such pain, seek immediate medical attention.

Considerations

A lump on the testicle is often the first sign of testicular cancer. Therefore, if you find a lump, see a doctor immediately. Keep in mind that some cases of testicular cancer do not show symptoms until they reach an advanced stage.

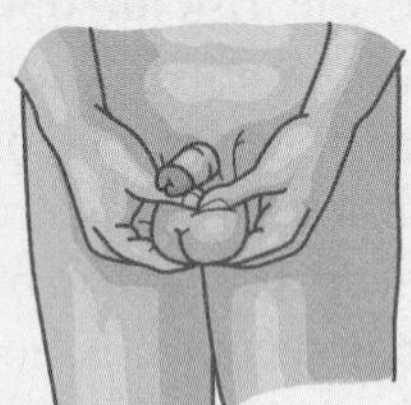

Repdoduced from MedlinePlus Medical Encyclopedia. (updated September 2009). Testicular self-examination. Retrieved April 21, 2011, from http://www.nlm.nih.gov/medlineplus/ency/article/003909.htm

Ovarian Cancer The ovaries are female organs in which eggs mature and are ovulated each month. Ovaries also produce the female sex hormones estrogen and progesterone. Cancer of the ovaries is difficult to detect, especially in its early stages when most women have no symptoms. However, as the cancer progresses and the ovarian tumor enlarges, many women develop symptoms such as frequent urination or bloating and pressure in the abdomen. Thus, advanced ovarian cancer is confused frequently with other urinary and gastrointestinal tract disorders. Postmenopausal women may experience vaginal bleeding, and premenopausal women may have irregular or heavy menses.

Advancing age is a risk factor for ovarian cancer. Most deaths from this disease occur in women 55 years and older. Other than advanced age, the risk factors for ovarian cancer are similar to those of breast and endometrial cancer: early menarche, late menopause, and not bearing children. The links between these risk factors and ovarian cancer, however, are not as well defined as they are in breast and endometrial cancer. Additional risk factors include having had breast cancer, having a family member who had breast or ovarian cancer, and having mutations in the *BRCA1* or *BRCA2* breast cancer genes.[34]

Research results show that the use of oral contraceptives that contain both estrogen and progesterone lower a woman's risk of developing ovarian cancer. Estrogen replacement therapy without progesterone increases a woman's risk of this cancer.[34]

No accurate routine screening test for women at average risk for ovarian cancer is available. However, screening techniques are available for women who have symptoms of or are at high risk for ovarian cancer. Screening techniques include a thorough pelvic examination, transvaginal ultrasound, a blood test for tumor marker CA125, and a CT or MRI scan of the pelvic area. Ovarian cancer is treated with surgery, chemotherapy, and, rarely, radiation.[34]

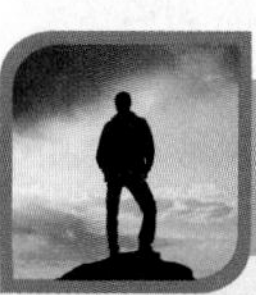

Healthy Living Practices

- To lower your risk of developing lung cancer, do not smoke cigarettes, avoid inhaling airborne asbestos fibers, and avoid exposure to radon gas.
- If you are exposed to lung carcinogens at your place of work, explore ways to avoid future exposure.
- To prevent the development of larynx, mouth, and esophagus cancers, avoid smoking and chewing tobacco and excessive drinking of alcoholic beverages.
- Have a complete oral examination annually for early cancer detection.
- To lower your risk of developing cancer of the bladder and kidney, avoid smoking cigarettes.
- To lower your risk of pancreatic cancer, avoid smoking cigarettes and inhaling chemical fumes.
- To lower your risk of developing stomach cancer, avoid eating salt-cured, nitrate-cured, or smoked foods. Also avoid smoking cigarettes and drinking excessive amounts of alcoholic beverages.
- To reduce your risk of developing colorectal cancer, follow the American Cancer Society's screening guidelines and remove precancerous polyps.
- If you are female, you can reduce your risk of breast cancer by exercising and avoiding alcoholic beverages.
- To detect breast cancer in its early stages, follow the ACS guidelines for breast clinical examination and mammography. Be aware of any changes in your breasts.
- If you are female, you can reduce your risk of developing endometrial cancer by losing weight if you are overweight and by controlling diabetes mellitus if you have this disease.
- Discuss the impact of estrogen replacement therapy on the development of endometrial cancer with your healthcare provider if you are considering or are taking this medication.
- If you are female and older than 40 years, have annual pelvic examinations for early detection of endometrial cancer.
- If you are a sexually active woman with multiple partners or with nonmonogamous partners, you can lower your risk of cervical cancer by using male or female condoms to protect yourself against HPV. Young women can be vaccinated against certain types of HPV.
- All women can lower their risk of cervical cancer by avoiding cigarette smoking.
- If you have been sexually active and are age 21 years or older, the American Cancer Society recommends that you have annual Pap tests to screen for cervical cancer. See the ACS guidelines for detailed recommendations.
- To protect against skin cancer, stay out of the sun, wear sunscreen when outdoors, and do not use tanning beds or lights.
- Detect melanoma early by checking your skin for growths that exhibit these warning signs: asymmetry, irregular border, multiple colors, and large diameter. Be aware that fast-growing melanomas may be red, raised, and itchy with symmetrical borders.
- If you are male and older than 50, talk to your healthcare provider about annual digital rectal exams and PSA tests for the early detection of prostate cancer.
- If you are male, perform a testicular self-examination once every month to detect this cancer early.

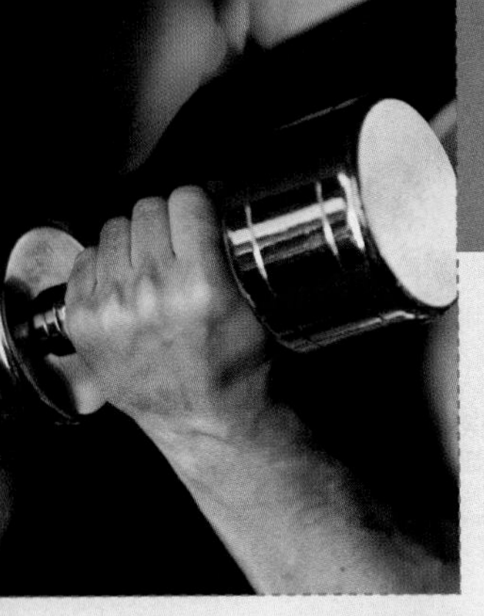
© Kzenon/ShutterStock

Managing Your Health

Reducing Your Risk for Cancer

DO'S

- Eat a diet low in red meats, especially high-fat and processed meats.
- Eat a variety of fruits and vegetables daily.
- Follow the American Cancer Society's recommendations for screening tests to detect cancer in its early stages.
- Men should perform monthly testicular self-examinations.
- Know the warning signs of cancer and see your healthcare provider immediately if you detect any of them.
- Sexually active women with multiple partners or with nonmonogamous partners should use male or female condoms during sexual intercourse to protect themselves against infection with human papillomavirus.
- Maintain a healthy weight.
- Women should consult their healthcare providers regarding the use of oral contraceptives and estrogen replacement therapy with respect to cancer prevention and risk.
- Exercise most days of the week.
- When in the sun, wear wide-brimmed hats and sunglasses that block UV radiation.
- Wear sunscreen on sun-exposed skin.

DON'TS

- Avoid cigarette use. If you already smoke and can't quit, try to smoke less.
- Avoid breathing environmental tobacco smoke.
- Don't chew tobacco products.
- Don't drink excessive amounts of alcoholic beverages.
- Women should avoid drinking alcoholic beverages to reduce the risk of breast cancer.
- Avoid unnecessary exposure to ionizing radiation, such as X-rays and ultraviolet light.
- Don't lie in the sun or in tanning beds.
- Avoid direct sun exposure between 10 A.M. and 4 P.M.
- Avoid exposure to toxic chemicals, such as certain occupational carcinogens.
- Avoid inhaling chemical fumes, such as gasoline fumes.
- Avoid breathing asbestos dust and radon gas.
- Avoid eating salt-cured, nitrate-cured, or smoked foods.

Reducing Your Risk for Cancer

You cannot change some of your cancer risk factors: heredity, age, ethnicity, lifelong exposure to naturally produced estrogen (in women), and the nondescent of testes (in male children). However, you can avoid many risk factors, thereby reducing your risk of developing one or more cancers. The Managing Your Health box titled "Reducing Your Risk for Cancer" lists modifiable cancer risks and actions you can take to lower your risk.

A summary of the American Cancer Society's recommendations for the early detection of cancer is listed in the Managing Your Health box titled "Screening Guidelines for the Early Detection of Cancer in Average-Risk Asymptomatic People" earlier in this chapter. Finally, the next Managing Your Health box lists cancer's seven warning signs. In addition to being aware of these signs, you can learn the more detailed early warning signs for the various cancers described in this chapter. If you have concerns about your risk of developing cancer, discuss them with your healthcare provider. Early detection and treatment are critical to winning the war against cancer.

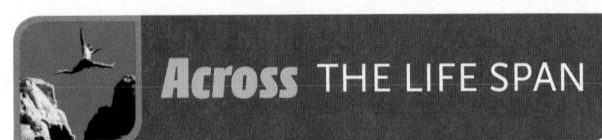

© Galina Barskaya/ShutterStock

CANCER

Most cancers arise in people older than 50 years, and the risk continues to rise as people grow older. The only cancers described in this chapter that are prevalent in young adults are malignant melanoma, testicular cancer, cervical cancer, and breast cancer. Only 1% of cancers occur in children. However, cancer

Managing Your Health

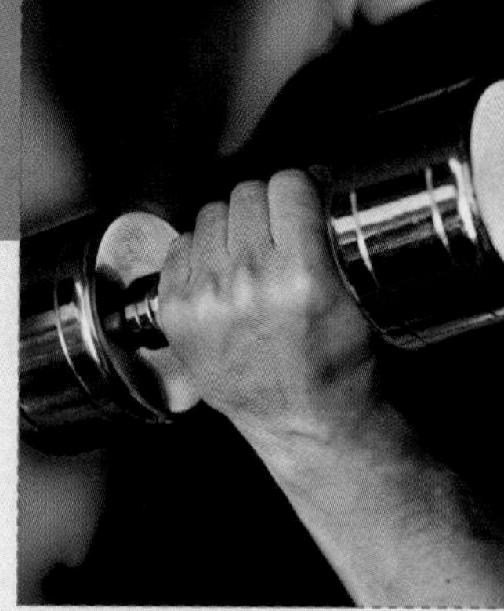

© Kzenon/ShutterStock

Cancer's Seven Warning Signs

You can remember the following signs easily by knowing that they are a CAUTION: These signs do not necessarily mean you have cancer but that you should see your healthcare provider to evaluate the sign.

Change in bowel or bladder habits

A sore that does not heal

Unusual bleeding or discharge

Thickening or lump in breast or elsewhere

Indigestion or difficulty in swallowing

Obvious change in a wart or mole

Nagging cough or hoarseness

is the most frequent cause of death from disease in American children older than 1 year of age. The most prevalent cancers of children up to 5 years old are listed in ***Table 13.8***.

Adult cancers rarely occur in children. These cancers are largely related to the effects of cancer-causing agents acting on cells over a lifetime, whereas children's cancers seem more often related to genetic factors.

Although pediatric cancers usually grow more rapidly than adult cancers do, they are, in general, more responsive to anticancer drugs than are adult cancers. For this reason chemotherapy is the treatment of choice for most childhood cancers, while surgery and radiation are the primary treatments for adult cancers. Effective cancer chemotherapy has produced a remarkable decline in childhood deaths resulting from cancer over the past 30 years.

Table 13.8

The Most Prevalent Cancers of Children up to Age 5 Years

Leukemia (cancer of the blood)
Central nervous system cancers
Lymphomas (cancer of the lymph nodes)
Nervous system tumors (often in adrenal glands)
Wilms' tumor (cancer of the kidney)
Bone cancer
Retinoblastoma (cancer of the eye)
Liver cancer

CHAPTER REVIEW

Summary

Cancer is a variety of diseases that have common characteristics: Their cells exhibit abnormal growth, division, and differentiation and have the potential to spread from where they develop. These cells form masses called malignant tumors that interfere with normal body processes.

Cancer develops in cells that have damaged or mutated genes. Mutations can be inherited or can occur from exposure to low-dose radiation, drugs, toxic chemicals, or certain viruses. Successive genetic changes must take place for a normal cell to change into a cancer cell. Therefore, the probability of developing cancer generally increases with age and with exposure to cancer-causing substances.

This chapter organizes the discussion of cancers according to factors that appear to be most significant in their development. Advanced age is a risk factor for most cancers; heredity is a significant risk factor in some cancers.

Tobacco use causes cancers of the lung, larynx, oral cavity, esophagus, kidney, bladder, pancreas, stomach, blood, and cervix. To lower the risk of developing any of these cancers, avoid smoking and chewing tobacco products. Additionally, avoid drinking excessive amounts of alcoholic beverages to lower the risk of developing larynx, oral, and esophageal cancer. Have a complete oral examination annually for early cancer detection in this area.

Diet accounts for a significant number of cancers and has both a positive and a negative effect on the development of cancer. A primary risk factor in the development of stomach cancer is eating salt-cured, nitrate-cured, or smoked foods. To lower the risk of developing this cancer, avoid eating these foods. To reduce the risk of developing colorectal cancer, avoid having more than one alcoholic drink per day and eat a diet adequate in vegetables and fruits. Refer to the ACS recommendations for screening recommendations for colon cancer in persons over the age of 50.

The cancers related to hormone function are breast cancer and endometrial cancer. These cancers are associated significantly with prolonged exposure to estrogen. Risk factors associated with these cancers are early menarche, late menopause, not bearing children, and delaying pregnancy. Exercising helps reduce breast cancer risk in women. Avoiding alcoholic beverages also reduces the risk. For early cancer detection, women aged 20 to 39 years should have a breast clinical examination every 3 years, and every year at age 40 and after. Women should become aware of the normal condition of their breasts and seek medical attention if they notice any changes. Women aged 40 and older should have mammography every year. For early detection of endometrial cancer, women at menopause should report any unexpected bleeding or spotting to their physician.

Certain viruses are implicated in the development of a variety of cancers. The virally related cancer most prevalent in the United States is cervical cancer. The virus implicated in this disease, human papillomavirus (HPV), is transmitted by infected men to their female partners during sexual intercourse, and vice versa. Sexually active women with multiple partners or with nonmonogamous partners can lower their risk of cervical cancer by using male or female condoms to protect themselves against HPV. Women can also lower their risk by avoiding cigarette smoking. Young women can be vaccinated against certain types of HPV.

The ultraviolet radiation in sunlight is the most important factor that influences the development of cancer of the skin. There are three main types of skin cancer: basal cell carcinoma, squamous cell carcinoma, and malignant melanoma. Of these cancers malignant melanoma results in the most deaths because it is a fast-growing metastatic cancer. Light-skinned, fair-haired Whites are a high-risk group for developing skin cancer. To protect against skin cancer, stay out of the sun and wear sunscreen when outdoors. Detect melanoma early by checking your skin for growths exhibiting these warning signs: asymmetry, irregular border, multiple colors, and large diameter. Seek medical attention for any suspicious lesions that do not heal.

Cancers with unknown causes include prostate cancer, testicular cancer, and ovarian cancer. The risk factors for prostate cancer are age and heredity. For early detection of this cancer, men older than 50 should have annual prostate-specific antigen blood tests with or without a digital prostate exam. Men between the ages of 20 and 54 years are at the highest risk for testicular cancer. For early detection of this disease, all males 15 years and older should perform monthly testicular self-examinations. Ovarian cancer is primarily a disease of postmenopausal women.

Childhood cancers, although rare, are the most frequent cause of death from disease in American children older than 1 year. Children develop cancers as a result of hereditary or developmental reasons. Occasionally, environmental agents are the cause. Treatment for childhood cancers is highly effective.

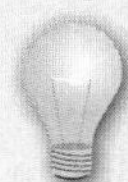

Applying What You Have Learned

1. Imagine that you or a female friend had an annual Pap test. The report from the lab stated that cells exhibiting dysplasia were seen in the smear. What does this statement mean? How would these cells look different from normal cells? What would be your or your friend's next course of action? **Application**
2. List three cancer risk factors over which a person has no control. Suppose that at least one of them was a risk factor for you. List this hypothetical (or real) factor and the cancer(s) related to this risk. What might you do regarding cancer prevention if you are aware of this (these) factor(s)? **Application**
3. Your good friend is a heavy drinker, eats lots of spicy food, and experiences heartburn regularly. He takes antacids, but recently they have not helped. He also tells you that he seems to have some difficulty swallowing, but he's not quite sure. He thinks it's "all in his head." What would you advise your friend to do? Might cancer be causing his problems? If so, which type? Which symptoms led you to this conclusion? **Application**
4. List two dietary factors related to the development of cancer and two dietary factors related to lowering the risk of cancer. Name the cancers to which these dietary factors relate. Now list, as best you can remember, the foods you ate for the past 2 days. What is your intake of the types of foods related to cancer development and prevention? Based on this analysis, should you make changes in your diet to lower your risk of certain cancers? **Evaluation**
5. With respect to the cancers discussed in this chapter, which cancer(s) are you at least risk for developing? Why? Which cancers are you at highest risk for developing? Why? **Synthesis**
6. Referring to your answer to question 5, what can you do to lower your risk of developing the cancers for which you are at high risk? State rationales for each suggestion. Why will these lifestyle changes lower your risk? **Evaluation**

Application	**Synthesis**	**Evaluation**
using information in a new situation.	putting together information from different sources.	making informed decisions.

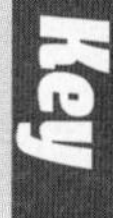

CHAPTER REVIEW

© SergeBertasiusPhotography/ShutterStock

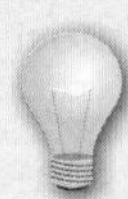

Reflecting on Your Health

© tele52/ShutterStock

1. Have your attitudes about cancer changed since reading this chapter? If so, explain how your attitude has changed and discuss why.
2. Were you aware of all the ACS recommendations for the early detection of cancer prior to reading this chapter? If you were not, which recommendations were new to you? Will you follow these recommendations? Why or why not? If you were aware of all the ACS recommendations, do you follow those recommendations for your sex and age group? Why or why not?
3. Do you know anyone who has or has had cancer, or have you read stories written by cancer patients about their disease? Did you learn about cancer from them that affected your life? Did you make any changes to your lifestyle based on these individuals' experiences?
4. Complete the assessment "What Are Your Cancer Risks?" in the Student Workbook pages at the end of this text. Do your cancer risks match your self-perception of your risks? Did the self-assessment identify cancer risks of which you were unaware? After reading this chapter, develop a list of things you could do to reduce your cancer risks.

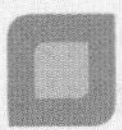

References

1. Abt, S. (1999, July 26). Armstrong wins tour and journey. *The New York Times.*
2. BBC News. (2011, February 16). *Lance Armstrong confirms retirement from cycling.* Retrieved from http://news.bbc.co.uk/sport2/hi/other_sports/cycling/9399280.stm
3. American Cancer Society. (2014). *Cancer facts and figures, 2014.* Atlanta, GA: Author. Retrieved from http://www.cancer.org/acs/groups/content/@research/documents/webcontent/acspc-042151.pdf
4. Davila, M. L. (2011). Photodynamic therapy. *Gastrointestinal Endoscopy Clinics of North America, 21*(1), 67–79.
5. Mroz, P., et al. (2011). Stimulation of anti-tumor immunity by photodynamic therapy. *Expert Review in Clinical Immunology, 7*(1), 75–91.
6. National Cancer Institute. (2014, April 25). *Targeted cancer therapies.* Retrieved from http://www.cancer.gov/cancertopics/factsheet/Therapy/targeted
7. Noguchi, M., Sasada, T., & Itoh, K. (2013). Personalized peptide vaccination: A new approach for advanced cancer as therapeutic cancer vaccine. *Cancer Immunology, Immunotherapy, 62*(5), 919–929.
8. American Cancer Society. (2014). *Cancer prevention and early detection facts and figures, 2014.* Atlanta, GA: Author. Retrieved from http://www.cancer.org/acs/groups/content/@research/documents/document/acspc-042924.pdf
9. U.S. Department of Health and Human Services. (2004). *The health consequences of smoking: A report of the Surgeon General.* Washington, DC: U.S. Government Printing Office. Retrieved from http://www.cdc.gov/tobacco/data_statistics/sgr/2004/index.htm
10. U.S. Department of Health and Human Services. (2010). *How tobacco smoke causes disease: The biology and behavioral basis for smoking-attributable disease.* Washington, DC: U.S. Government Printing Office. Retrieved from http://www.ncbi.nlm.nih.gov/books/NBK53017/
11. U.S. Department of Health and Human Services. (2014). *The health consequences of smoking—50 years of progress: A report of the Surgeon General, 2014.* Washington, DC: U.S. Government Printing Office. Retrieved from http://www.surgeongeneral.gov/library/reports/50-years-of-progress/full-report.pdf
12. Khan, N., et al. (2010). Lifestyle as risk factor for cancer: Evidence from human studies. *Cancer Letters, 293*(2), 133–143.
13. U.S. Public Health Service. (1964). *Smoking and health: Report of the advisory committee to the Surgeon General of the Public Health Service* (PHS Publication No. 1103). Atlanta, GA: U.S. Department of Health, Education, and Welfare, Public Health Service, CDC. Retrieved from http://profiles.nlm.nih.gov/ps/access/NNBBMQ.pdf
14. Taylor, H. S., & Manson, J. E. (2011). Update in hormone therapy use in menopause. *Journal of Clinical Endocrinology and Metabolism, 96*(2), 255–264.
15. Bradbury, K. E., Appleby, P. N., & Key, T. J. (2014). Fruit, vegetable, and fiber intake in relation to cancer risk: Findings from the European prospective investigation into cancer and nutrition (EPIC). *American Journal of Clinical Nutrition, 100*(Suppl.), 394S–8S.
16. U.S. Department of Health and Human Services. (2006). *The health consequences of involuntary exposure to tobacco smoke: A report of the Surgeon General.* Atlanta, GA: U.S. Department of Health and Human Services. Retrieved from http://www.surgeongeneral.gov/library/reports/secondhand-smoke-consumer.pdf
17. Cole, L., Polfus, L., & Peters, E. S. (2012). Examining the incidence of human papillomavirus-associated health and neck cancers by race and ethnicity in the U.S., 1995–2005. *PLoS ONE, 7*(3), 1011.
18. Lowrance, W. T., et al. (2010). Obesity is associated with a higher risk of clear-cell renal cell carcinoma than with other histologies. *BJU International, 105*(1), 16–20.
19. American Cancer Society. (2011, March 11). *Colorectal cancer early detection.* Retrieved from http://www.cancer.org/acs/groups/cid/documents/webcontent/003170-pdf.pdf

20. Rothwell, P. M., et al. (2010). Long-term effect of aspirin on colorectal cancer incidence and mortality: 20-year follow-up of five randomized trials. *Lancet, 376*(9754), 1741–1750.

21. Chan, A. T., & Giovannucci, E. L (2010). Primary prevention of colorectal cancer. *Gastroenterology, 138*(6), 2029–2043.

22. Mayo Clinic staff. (2011, January 18). *Stool DNA test.* Retrieved from http://www.mayoclinic.com/health/dna-stool-test/MY00623

23. American Cancer Society. (2009). *Breast cancer facts and figures, 2009–2010.* Atlanta, GA: Author. Retrieved April 20, 2011, from http://www.cancer.org/acs/groups/content/@nho/documents/document/f861009final90809pdf.pdf

24. Li, C. I. (2003). Relationship between long durations and different regimens of hormone therapy and risk of breast cancer. *Journal of the American Medical Association, 289*(24), 3254–3263.

25. American Cancer Society. (2014). *Breast cancer facts and figures, 2013–2014.* Atlanta, GA: Author. Retrieved from http://www.cancer.org/acs/groups/content/@research/documents/document/acspc-042725.pdf

26. Luo, J., et al. (2011). Association of active and passive smoking with risk of breast cancer among postmenopausal women: A prospective cohort study. *British Medical Journal, 342,* d1016.

27. Shaitelman, S. F., Khan, A. J., Atif, J., et al. (2014). Shortened radiation therapy schedules for early-stage breast cancer: A review of hypofractionated whole-breast irradiation and accelerated partial breast irradiation. *Breast Journal, 20*(2), 131–146.

28. Srikantia, N., et al. (2009). Endometrioid endometrial adenocarcinoma in a premenopausal woman with multiple organ metastases. *Indian Journal of Medical and Paediatric Oncology, 30*(2), 80–83.

29. National Cancer Institute. (2010). *Surveillance, Epidemiology and End Results (SEER) stat fact sheets: Cervix uteri.* Retrieved from http://www.seer.cancer.gov/statfacts/html/cervix.html

30. Martorell-Calatayud, A., et al. (2011). Defining fast-growing melanomas: Reappraisal of epidemiological, clinical, and histological features. *Melanoma Research, 12*(2), 131–138.

31. HealthyPeople.gov. (2014, July 9). *Healthy People 2020 topics and objectives: Cancer.* Retrieved from http://www.healthypeople.gov/2020/topicsobjectives2020/overview.aspx?topicid=5

32. American Cancer Society. (2014, February, 25). *Prostate cancer; Early detection.* Retrieved from http://www.cancer.org/cancer/prostatecancer/moreinformation/prostatecancerearlydetection/prostate-cancer-early-detection-acs-recommendations

33. American Cancer Society. (2014, February, 11). *Testicular cancer.* Retrieved from http://www.cancer.org/cancer/testicularcancer/detailedguide/testicular-cancer-risk-factors

34. MedlinePlus. (2012, November, 17). *Ovarian cancer.* Retrieved from http://www.nlm.nih.gov/medlineplus/ency/article/000889.htm

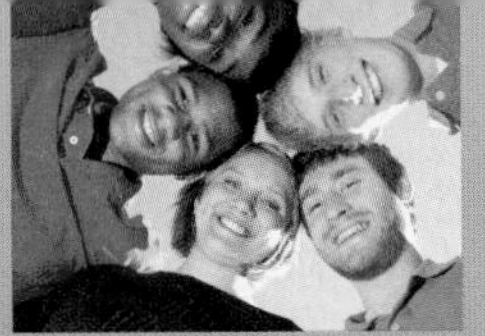

Diversity in Health

Sickle Cell Disease: Why Does This Deleterious Gene Persist?

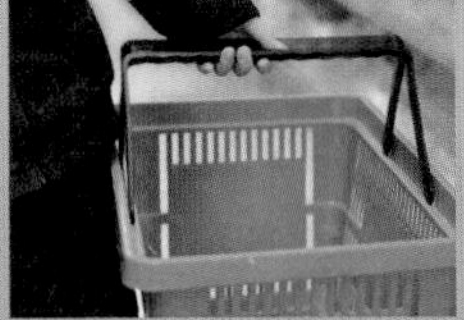

Consumer Health

CAM Products and Colds

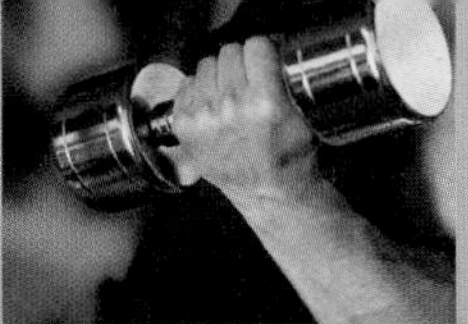

Managing Your Health

Eliminating or Reducing Your Risk of HIV Infection and Other STIs

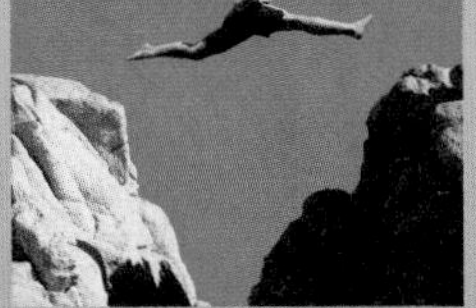

Across the Life Span

Infectious and Noninfectious Diseases

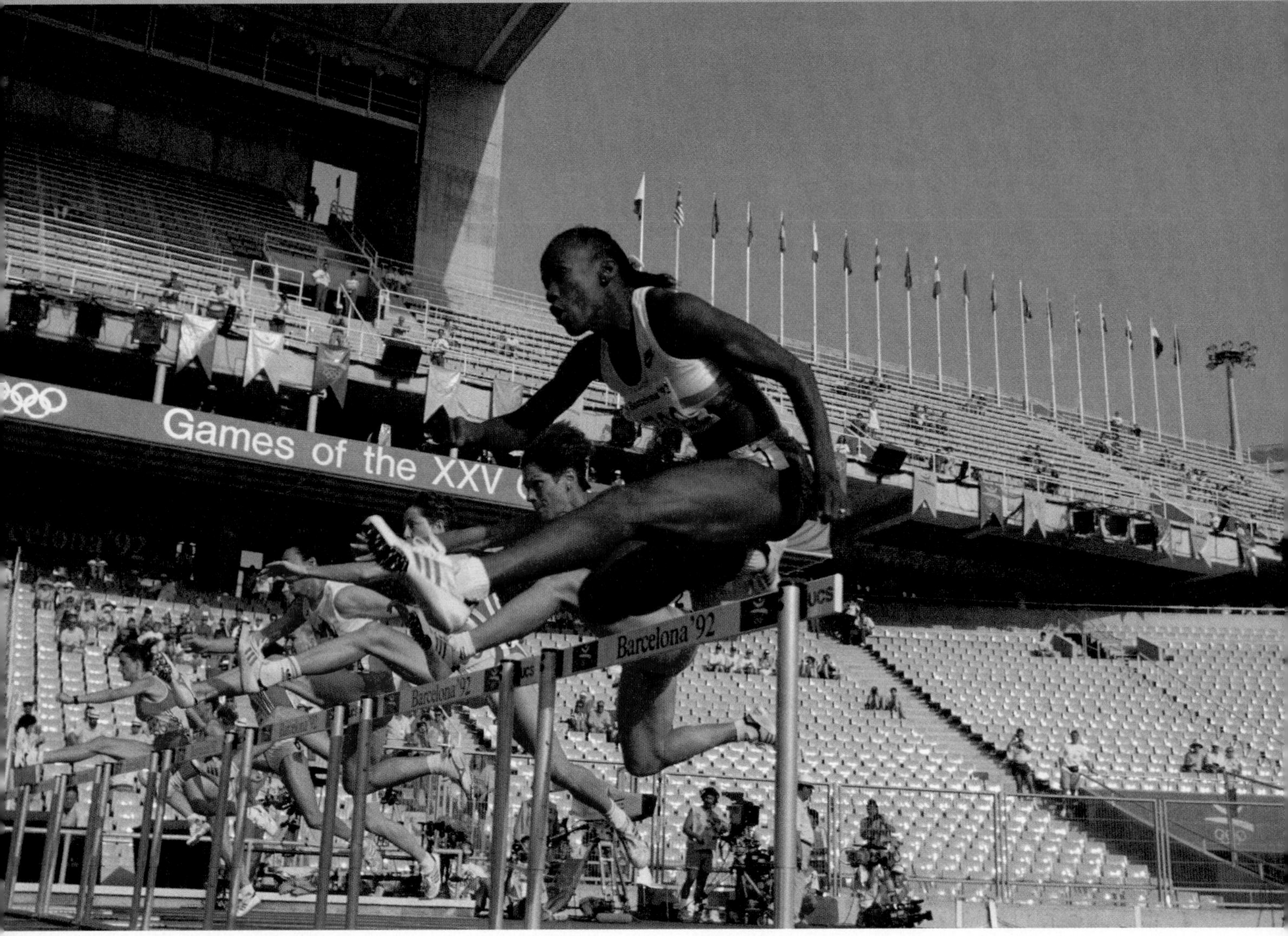

Chapter Overview

Causes of noninfectious diseases

Symptoms of and treatments for noninfectious diseases

Trends in infectious diseases since 1900

How the chain of infection works

How nonspecific and specific immunity work

How to protect yourself against infectious disease

Symptoms of sexually transmitted infections

Treatments and prevention methods for sexually transmitted infections

Student Workbook

Self-Assessment: STI Attitude Scale

Changing Health Habits: Reducing Your Risk of Contracting an STI

Do You Know?

How to protect yourself from sexually transmitted infections?

If over-the-counter cold remedies really work?

Which types of diseases you can catch and which you cannot?

CHAPTER 14

Infection, Immunity, and Noninfectious Disease

Learning Objectives

After studying this chapter, you should be able to:

1. Distinguish between infectious and noninfectious disease.
2. Distinguish between communicable and noncommunicable transmission of infectious disease.
3. Explain the process of infection.
4. Describe the chain of infection.
5. Discuss the body's specific and nonspecific defenses against pathogens.
6. Explain the transmission of sexually transmitted infections (STIs).
7. Explain risk factors for contracting HIV and describe how HIV is transmitted.
8. Describe steps you can take to reduce your risk of contracting STIs.
9. Describe long-term health effects of genital herpes, HPV, HIV, syphilis, gonorrhea, and chlamydial infection.

"Exercise-induced asthma has not deterred this outstanding athlete from making her indelible mark in the world of sports..."

disease A process that affects the proper functioning of the body and is usually accompanied by characteristic signs and symptoms.

infectious (in-FEK-shus) disease A disease caused by bacteria, rickettsias, viruses, fungi, protozoans, or parasitic worms.

pathogen (PATH-oh-jen) A disease-causing agent of infection; the first link in the chain of infection.

noninfectious (NON-in-FEK-shus) disease Illness caused by genetic abnormalities, by interactions between hereditary and environmental factors, or solely by environmental factors.

inherited disease A genetic disease transmitted solely by gene transfer from parents to offspring.

mutation (mew-TAY-shun) In reference to human biology, a change in a gene or a chromosome.

Jackie Joyner-Kersee: Olympian gold, silver, and bronze medalist. The photo shows Kersee leading her competitors in the 100 meter hurdle portion of the women's heptathlon. Some consider Joyner-Kersee the greatest woman athlete ever. At this writing, she is the heptathlon world record holder and the American record holder in the indoor long jump. She has won six Olympic medals, more than any woman in track and field history. Joyner-Kersee officially retired from track and field in 2001.

In late 2004, Joyner-Kersee was honored by USA Track & Field, the national governing body for track and field, long-distance running, and race walking in the United States. They cited Joyner-Kersee's breaking of her own women's heptathlon world record at the 1988 Olympic Games as the ninth greatest moment in U.S. track and field history in the last 25 years. In mid-2007, Joyner-Kersee was named one of six "women of power" by the National Urban League. In 2010, she was one of the first inducted into the new St. Louis Sports Hall of Fame, which honors achievements of St. Louis teams and athletes past and present. Clearly, exercise-induced asthma has not deterred this outstanding athlete from making her indelible mark in the world of sports, nor has it deterred other athletes.

Exercise-induced asthma is a condition in which the airways narrow after sustained exertion, making it more difficult than usual for a person to breathe. What triggers this problem is the cooling and reheating of the airways as a person exercises. As exercise begins, a person begins to breathe deeply and rapidly. During this deep and rapid inhalation, more air is moistened and warmed in the respiratory passageways than before exercise began, which draws moisture and heat from the airways. After a person is warmed up, the breathing rate falls, and the airways return to their normal temperature. Health scientists do not know how airway cooling and reheating triggers asthma attacks.

Asthma is one of a variety of noninfectious diseases. **Diseases** are processes that affect the proper functioning of the body and are usually accompanied by characteristic signs and symptoms. **Infectious diseases**, such as colds or the flu, are caused by **pathogens**, which are agents of infection: bacteria, rickettsias, viruses, fungi, protozoans, and parasitic worms. (Infectious diseases are discussed later in this chapter.) **Noninfectious diseases** are caused by abnormalities in the hereditary material (genetic diseases), interactions between heredity and environmental factors (especially those related to lifestyle, such as asthma), or environmental factors alone, as in repetitive-use injuries or lead poisoning.

Noninfectious Diseases

Genetic Diseases

There are two types of genetic diseases: inherited diseases and diseases caused by errors in cell division when gametes (sex cells) are formed.

Inherited Diseases **Inherited diseases** are transmitted solely by gene transfer from parents to offspring. They occur more frequently among close relatives than in the general population and show patterns in their transmission. An inherited disease may strike only males, for example.

Inherited diseases are caused by disorders of *genes*, the physical and functional units of heredity. Genes are segments of *DNA*, a complex chemical compound that codes for the production of proteins. Genes carry information about every aspect of an organism and may carry normal instructions for a particular characteristic in one person and defective instructions in another. A defective gene in the eggs or sperm of an individual can be passed on to a child unless the person dies before reaching reproductive age.

Defective genes arise through mutation. A **mutation** is a change in a gene or a chromosome. A chromosome is a strand of DNA with associated protein; humans have 23 pairs of chromosomes. One member of each pair is inherited from the mother and one pair from the father.

A mutation can be inherited from a parent and passed on to children, or it can arise suddenly in a

Diversity in Health

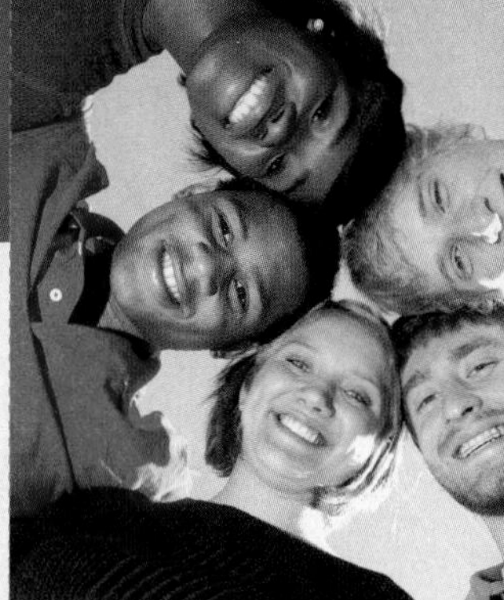

© Mike Flippo/ShutterStock

Sickle Cell Disease: Why Does This Deleterious Gene Persist?

Sickle cell disease is one of the most common genetic disorders among African Americans, having arisen in their African ancestors. It has also been observed in people whose ancestors came from the Mediterranean basin, the Indian subcontinent, the Caribbean, and parts of Central and South America (particularly Brazil). The sickle cell gene has persisted in these populations—even though the disease eventually kills its victims—because of a curious interaction between this disease and another disease prevalent in these regions. Today, an estimated 70,000 to 100,000 Americans of African and Hispanic origins have the disease. Medical researchers estimate that 1 out of 10 African Americans and 1 out of 100 Hispanic Americans carry the trait.

Sickle cell disease gets its name from the curved (sickle) shape of the red blood cells of individuals with this disease (**Figure 14.A**). Anemia, or a low number of red blood cells, results from the short life of these abnormal cells. An error in the gene that codes for hemoglobin, the oxygen-carrying molecule in red blood cells, is responsible for the signs and symptoms of sickle cell disease.

These sickle-shaped cells cause pain when they become trapped in the small blood vessels of the body. This condition results in oxygen depletion to the tissues surrounding the blocked vessels, which damages tissues and causes infections. Most sickle cell patients die in their 40s or 50s from conditions such as stroke, infection, kidney failure, or congestive heart failure.

Figure 14.A

Normal and Sickled Red Blood Cells. The red blood cell on the left has a normal, rounded shape. The one the right has the curved shape of sickle cell disease, which results in its becoming trapped in the small blood vessels of the body.

© Dr. Stanley Flegler/Visuals Unlimited

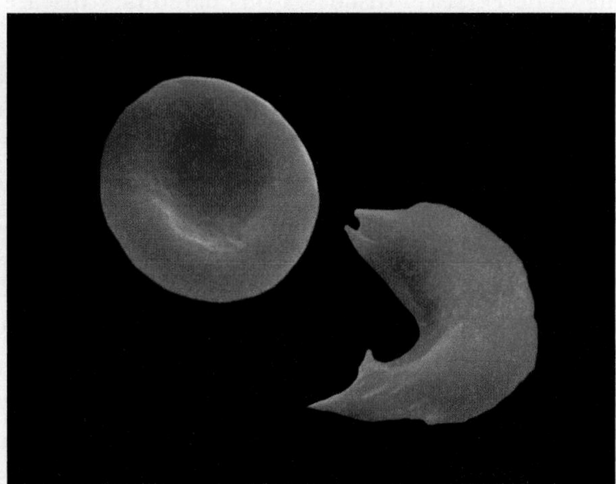

To have sickle cell disease, a person must inherit two defective hemoglobin genes—one from each parent. A person who inherits a single defective gene is a carrier and is said to have *sickle cell trait*. People with sickle cell trait do not have sickle cell disease, but they do have something in common with sufferers of sickle cell disease—resistance to malaria.

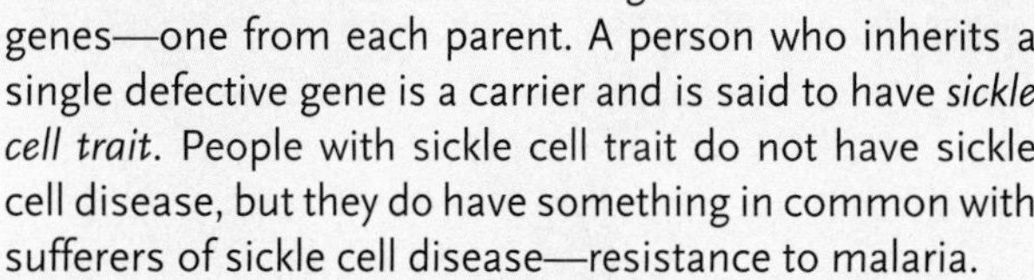

Those with the sickle cell gene have a survival advantage in regions of the world in which malaria is prevalent. The map in **Figure 14.B** shows where malaria is widespread; notice from the listing of affected populations in the first paragraph that sickle cell disease is prevalent in these areas as well. Although many of these peoples have since migrated from these areas, this ancestral gene persists in their populations.

How does a defective hemoglobin gene protect against malaria? In sickle cell trait, red blood cells sickle under a variety of conditions, such as when the oxygen tension is low (at high altitudes, for example) and if these cells become acidic. Results of research show that infection of the red blood cells by malaria parasites causes the infected cells to become acidic as a result of the metabolism of the parasite. This change induces the red blood cells to sickle, which interrupts multiplication of the parasite. The spleen, an organ that destroys worn-out red blood cells, traps the sickled cells. Under these conditions, the parasites die and malaria does not develop. For populations who live in regions where malaria is prevalent, the sickle cell gene persists because people who harbor the gene are more likely to live to reproductive age than those who do not have the gene and die from malaria. Therefore, this "deleterious" gene is beneficial to those with sickle cell trait living in malaria-infested areas and is passed from generation to generation. Unfortunately, some offspring inherit sickle cell disease and not simply sickle cell trait.

Healthcare providers alleviate symptoms in those with worsening anemia and sickle cell complications by administering painkillers and blood transfusions. Those receiving transfusions to prevent stroke must continue transfusions indefinitely or the risk of stroke returns. Penicillin is given to children aged 1 to 5 years to ward off infection. The drug hydroxyurea reduces the frequency of pain, hospital admissions, and life-threatening complications by about 50%. Bone marrow stem cell trans plantation is also used to treat sickle cell disease. Bone marrow stem cells are undifferentiated cells that give rise to all types of blood cells.

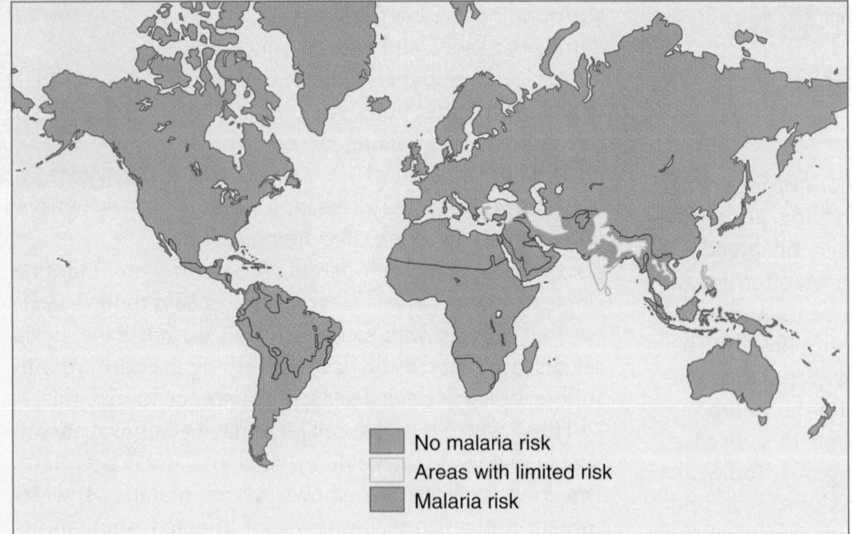

Figure 14.B

Areas of the World in Which Malaria Is Prevalent. Malaria is a serious infectious disease in the tropical and subtropical regions of the world. Sickle cell disease is prevalent in these regions as well.

The Sickle Cell Treatment Act of 2003 helps expand services for patients with this blood disorder. The federal government provides states with funding for patient counseling, educational initiatives, and community outreach programs and provides patients with federal matching funds for sickle cell disease-related services under Medicaid. In addition, this law has initiated the development of sickle cell treatment centers across the country and has established a National Coordinating and Evaluation Center Sickle Cell Disease and Newborn Screening Program.

Couples can be screened to detect if they are carriers of the trait to help them in their family planning decisions. Researchers are studying new medications and treatments for sickle cell anemia, and eventually, medical experts may discover a way to weed out this life-threatening gene in populations no longer living in malaria-prone areas.

Data from Centers for Disease Control and Prevention. (2014, March 31). Sickle cell disease. Retrieved from http://www.cdc.gov/ncbddd/sicklecell/index.html; St. Jude Children's Research Hospital. (2014). Disease information: Hematologic disorders: Sickle cell disease. Retrieved from http://www.stjude.org/stjude/v/index.jsp?vgnextoid=0f3c061585f7011oVgnVCM1000001e0215acRCRD&vgnextchannel=bc4fbfe82e118010VgnVCM1000000e2015acRCRD

person and be passed on to children. Mutations in eggs and sperm can occur for no apparent reason or from exposure to a variety of environmental sources. One source is ionizing radiation such as X-rays, which is the reason the dentist places a protective lead shield over your pelvic area when taking X-rays of your teeth. Another source of damage to genes is drugs such as lysergic acid diethylamide (lysergide, LSD) or marijuana (*Cannabis sativa*). Exposure to toxic chemicals, which can lead to poisoning, are a third source of genetic damage. People often come into contact with toxic chemicals in the workplace and do not realize the danger because they feel no ill effects.

Three hereditary diseases that are common in the United States are sickle cell disease, cystic fibrosis, and muscular dystrophy. The Diversity in Health essay "Sickle Cell Disease: Why Does This Deleterious Gene Persist?" discusses this hereditary disease, which is common among African Americans.

Cystic fibrosis (CF) is the most common lethal genetic disease in the White population. (It seldom affects African Americans, Asians, or Jews.) Cystic fibrosis affects the glands that secrete mucus and sweat. In CF patients, the sweat glands produce an abnormally salty secretion and the mucous glands produce an exceptionally thick and sticky secretion that builds up and plugs the ducts of glands and other passageways. Although the pancreas (an organ that secretes digestive juices) is often seriously affected, lung disease accounts for most of the illness and nearly all deaths from CF. Multiple disorders of the lungs arise when mucus blocks the airways. Infections result and breathing becomes impaired. According to the Cystic Fibrosis Foundation, in 2009 the median predicted age of survival with CF was in the mid-30s, which means that half of those with CF would be expected to live to that age.[1]

Duchenne/Becker muscular dystrophy (DBMD) is the most common type of muscular dystrophy (*dys* means "abnormal"; *trophy* means "growth"). DBMD is a disease in which the muscles gradually weaken and degenerate. The two versions of the disease are similar, but Becker muscular dystrophy has a later onset than Duchenne and a slower progression of symptoms. Recent estimates by the Centers for Disease Control and Prevention (CDC) reveal that DBMD occurs in 1.3 to 2.6 newborn males in the United States per 10,000, usually striking before the age of 5 years, which is the average age at diagnosis.[2]

Children with DBMD are usually slow to walk and talk. Their thigh and pelvic muscles gradually deteriorate, resulting in unsteadiness in standing, walking, climbing stairs, and getting up from a seated position. As the muscles of the shoulder, trunk, and back weaken, the child's spine begins to curve and the posture becomes swayback. This abnormal body posture interferes with the functioning of internal organs, especially the lungs. Although heart problems sometimes cause sudden death in DBMD patients, these children and young adults usually die in their teens or 20s of respiratory infections or respiratory failure when the diaphragm (a sheetlike muscle that forms the floor of the chest cavity and that is essential to breathing) becomes affected. Survival of patients with DBMD is enhanced by the use of noninvasive mechanical ventilation at night along with the use of assisted coughing techniques and medications that protect the heart.[3]

Diseases Caused by Errors in Sex Cell Division Gametes, or sex cells, are produced in the ovaries or testes. Sometimes eggs or sperm are made that have too many or too few chromosomes. Other times gametes may be formed in which parts of chromosomes have been lost, gained, or moved to new positions. If conception takes place with a gamete that has a severe defect, the usual result is a spontaneous abortion. However, some genetic defects result in a fertilized egg that is capable of developing into a full-term baby. The child may be born with structural or functional problems, or both.

Down syndrome, which affects approximately 1 in 1,000 newborns,[4] is a common genetic disorder caused by improper cell division in gametes. Cell division problems occur more often in eggs than in sperm because men produce new sperm throughout their lives, whereas women are born with all the potential eggs they will ever have. Therefore, a woman's eggs age as she ages. Each month, a single egg reaches maturity. During this maturation process, a division of the potential egg takes place. The division may result in an error in the number of chromosomes in the mature egg. The majority of Down syndrome children have three number 21 chromosomes instead of the usual pair (**Figure 14.1**). For this reason, Down syndrome is also called *trisomy 21*. As the graph in **Figure 14.2** shows, the risk of bearing a child with Down syndrome or another chromosomal abnormality rises dramatically after the maternal age of 30. This association between the incidence of Down syndrome and increasing age is not observed in fathers.[5] Various screening methods have been developed to detect whether a fetus is affected with trisomy 21 or other chromosomal problems.

cystic fibrosis (SIS-tik fie-BROH-sis) (CF) A common, lethal, inherited disease that affects the glands that secrete mucus and sweat, resulting in multiple disorders of the lungs and pancreas.

Duchenne/Becker muscular dystrophy (do-SHAYN BECK-er MUSS-ku-lar DIS-tro-fee)(DBMD) An inherited disease in which the muscles gradually weaken and degenerate. It usually strikes boys before the age of 6 years.

Down syndrome A genetic disease usually caused by the presence of three (rather than two) number 21 chromosomes; the child is usually mentally retarded, with a short body and a broad, flat face.

Noninfectious Disease and the Interaction of Genetic Factors with the Environment

The genetic diseases just discussed have simple and predictable inheritance patterns. They involve a change in a single gene or an error in sex cell division. Other noninfectious diseases have no simple and predictable inheritance patterns like genetic diseases do, but their development involves interplay between genetic and environmental factors. For example, a person with a family health history of type 2 diabetes is more likely to develop this disease if he or she becomes overweight or obese than is a person without the genetic link. Moreover, even in those genetically predisposed, type 2 diabetes can be

Figure 14.1

Down Syndrome. (a) This girl has Down syndrome. She exhibits the stocky build, short hands, and flattened facial features characteristic of this genetic condition. (b) Down syndrome is called trisomy 21 because it is caused by the presence of an extra chromosome 21, as shown in the karyotype, the array of chromosomes in a cell. In addition, Down syndrome individuals experience delays in physical and intellectual development. Although some Down syndrome individuals function in the low average range of intellectual capability, the majority function in the mild to moderate range of mental retardation.

(a) © PhotoCreate/ShutterStock; (b) Courtesy of Viola Freeman, Associate Professor, Faculty of Health Sciences, Dept. of Pathology and Molecular Medicine, McMaster University

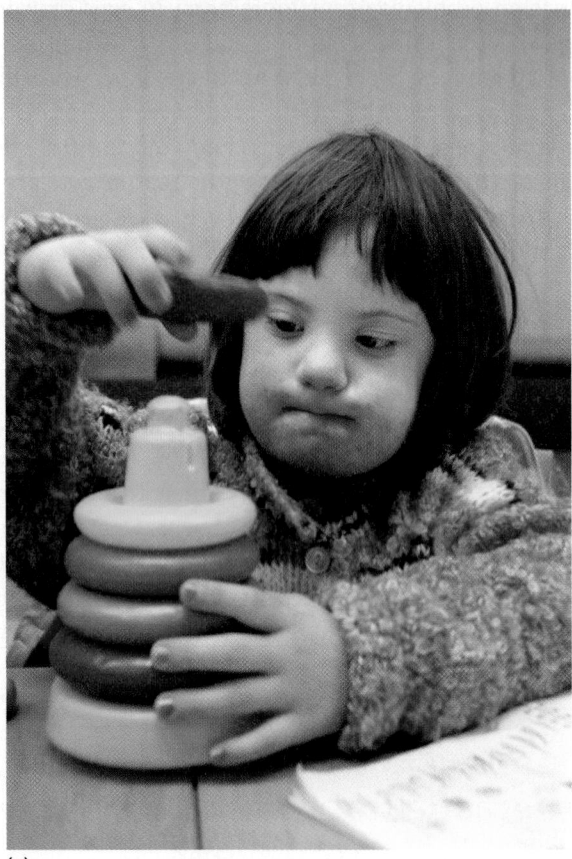

(a)

(b)

Figure 14.2

The Effect of Maternal Age on the Incidence of Down Syndrome. As maternal age increases, the age of a woman's eggs also increases, and genetic abnormalities become more common. The graph shows that the incidence of Down syndrome rises significantly as maternal age increases beyond 30 years.

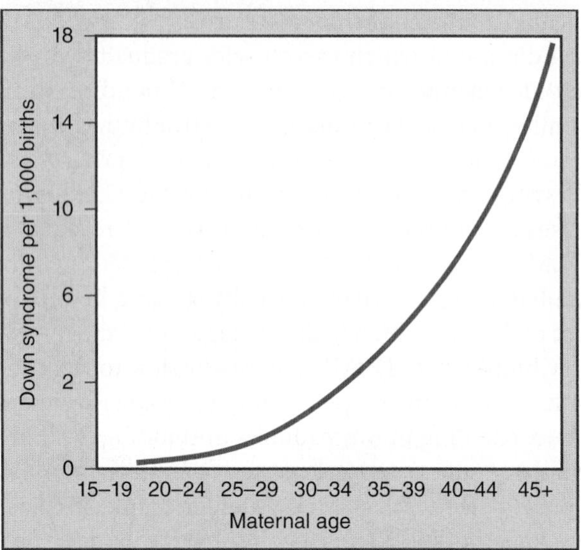

prevented or managed with weight loss and regular physical activity.

Until recently, scientists were able to look at genetics only in a limited way when studying disease. They did not have the tools to identify genetic factors and the roles they play in diseases with complex genetic links, such as type 2 diabetes, heart disease, and cancer. However, in 1989 an international effort began that would change this narrow view of genetics and health. Research scientists around the world set out to map the entire set of human genes—the human genome—determining its complete DNA sequence. With this endeavor, called the Human Genome Project, a new branch of molecular biology was born: *genomics*. This science focuses on understanding the structure and function of the genome. By 2003, researchers had mapped the entire human genome, revealing the "genetic code" of humans.

Genomics holds promise for helping researchers understand how genetic factors interact with environmental factors, resulting in health or disease. Researchers can now look for genetic variations that increase the risk of certain diseases and may, in turn, be able to develop more effective approaches to prevention and treatment of those diseases. In the future, diagnosis and treatment could be based on an individual's unique genetic makeup.

Asthma, ulcers, diabetes, migraine headaches, cardiovascular disease, and cancer are common noninfectious diseases that have both genetic and environmental causes. Ulcers are sores in the lining of the esophagus, stomach, or duodenum. Diabetes is a group of diseases in which a person does not metabolize carbohydrates properly. Migraine headaches are thought to be an inherited disorder that can be triggered by a variety of environmental factors. The nation's number one killers are cardiovascular disease and cancer.

Asthma, the most common chronic illness in childhood, is a disease of the airways. The bronchioles of people with asthma narrow in response to certain stimuli much more easily than do the bronchioles of those who do not have asthma. (Bronchioles are air passageways, about the diameter of a pencil lead, that lead to the air sacs of the lungs [**Figure 14.3**].) When these airways become narrowed, airflow to and from the lungs is blocked. As a result, asthmatic people have trouble breathing and begin to wheeze, which people refer to as having an asthma attack.

Environmental factors such as air pollution, respiratory infections, tobacco smoke, and allergens such as dust mites often trigger asthma attacks. (Dust mites are microscopic organisms that live in carpets, mattresses, pillows, and curtains.) As mentioned in the opening paragraphs of this chapter, exercise may also stimulate asthma attacks. Breathing warm, moist air is best for the athlete with exercise-induced asthma. For example, swimming in a warm pool will usually cause fewer problems than snow skiing. Also, warming up before exercise reduces the likelihood of an exercise-induced asthma attack. With other types of asthma, the key to management is discovering what stimulates attacks and avoiding these factors. For example, if a trigger is house dust mites, exposure can be reduced by not using carpeting or draperies and washing bedding often in hot water. Medication is another important tool for asthma management.

asthma (AZ-mah) A common, chronic, childhood illness characterized by sensitive airways.

carpal tunnel syndrome Numbness, pain, or pins-and-needles sensations in either of the hands that extends down the fingers, resulting from improper alignment of the wrist while engaging in repetitive-use activities.

Figure 14.3

The Respiratory System. The bronchioles are the narrow air passageways that branch from the bronchi and lead to the air sacs of the lungs. The bronchioles are covered with muscle tissue that constricts during asthma attacks, narrowing these passageways and making it difficult to breathe.

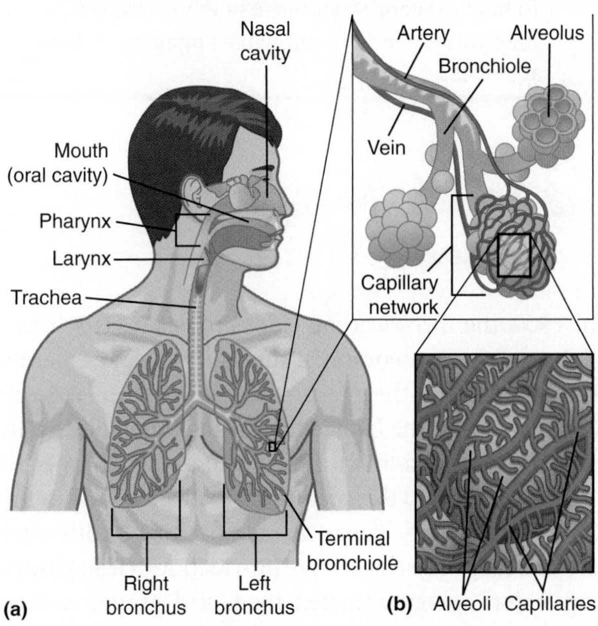

Noninfectious Conditions with Environmental or Unknown Causes

Many conditions are caused by exposure to various substances in the environment. In general, environmental factors that are the sole cause of disease are toxic chemicals. Not only are toxic chemicals present in the home, workplace, and environment, they are also used and abused in ways that seriously affect health.

A few noninfectious conditions are caused by the ways in which people use their bodies. Temporomandibular disorder is characterized by pain in the jaw and chewing muscles that often results from grinding or clenching the teeth. **Carpal tunnel syndrome**, a painful condition of the hands and fingers, results from improper positioning of the wrist while engaging in repetitive activities that use the hands, wrists, and arms. Ten percent of the population experiences occasional symptoms of this syndrome.

Carpal tunnel syndrome is usually the result of repetitive use. Activities such as using power tools frequently, typing for a long time, and playing piano or guitar often result in such injuries because people hold the wrist in a bent position rather than holding it straight. The injury causes inflammation and

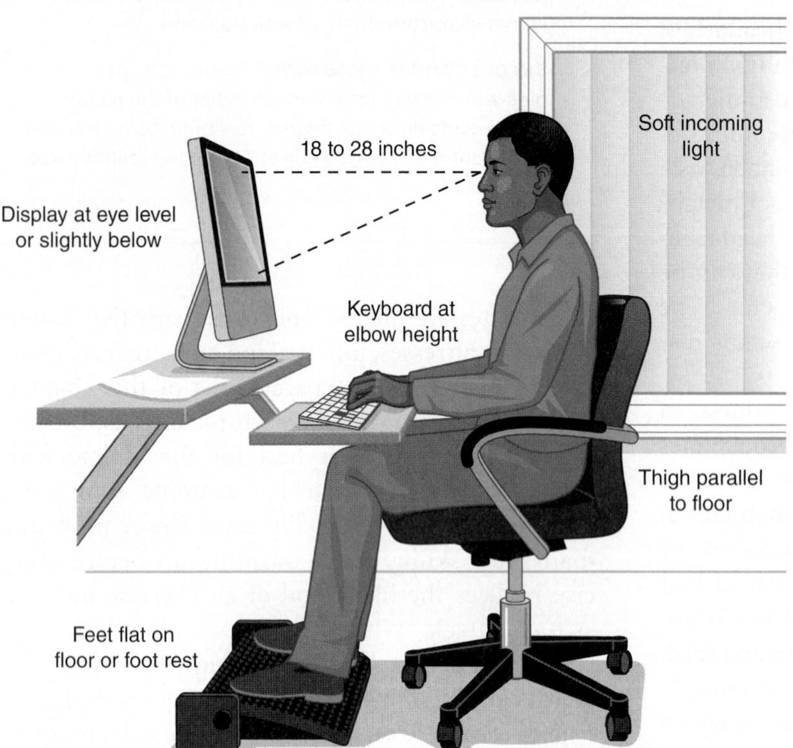

Figure 14.4

The Proper Sitting Position for Typing at the Computer. The screen should be at eye level or slightly lower. The keyboard should be at elbow height, the forearms parallel to the floor, the back supported, the thighs parallel to the floor, and the feet flat on the floor or foot rest.

a buildup of fluid in a tunnel that runs through the bones of the wrist, or carpals. The fluid presses on the nerves and blood vessels in the tunnel. Other conditions such as arthritis, diabetes, and pregnancy may also contribute to pressure in the carpal tunnel. To help avoid injury when typing for a long time, place your computer keyboard at elbow height and keep your wrists unbent as shown in **Figure 14-4**. Use wrist rests and arm rests only when you are resting, not when you are typing.

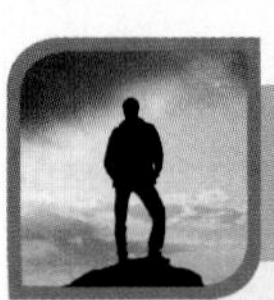

© djgis/ShutterStock

Healthy Living Practices

- The risk of chromosomal abnormalities in a woman's eggs increases significantly after her 30th birthday. Therefore, if you and your partner are considering a pregnancy at or beyond this age, consult your healthcare provider for advice regarding options to increase your chances of having a healthy infant.
- If you have asthma, learn your asthma triggers and avoid them. If you have exercise-induced asthma, consider restricting your activity on cold days or when the pollen count or air pollution levels are high.
- Abusing drugs, or living and working under toxic conditions, can damage the hereditary material of your cells, particularly the sex cells. Therefore, to protect your health and possibly that of your offspring, avoid exposure to toxic substances.
- Carpal tunnel syndrome often results from bending the wrists while engaging in a repetitive activity such as typing, using hand tools, or completing various household chores. To help prevent repetitive-use injury, always keep your wrists unbent while engaging in such activities.

Trends in Infectious Disease

In 1900, the three leading causes of death were infectious diseases: pneumonia, tuberculosis, and enteritis (inflammation of the intestine, causing severe diarrhea). Since that time, the United States (and other industrialized countries) has made achievements in public health that have changed this picture dramatically. Early in the 20th century, U.S. departments of public health were established, whose activities provided for clean drinking water, uncontaminated food, and proper sewage disposal and treatment. These actions have reduced the transmission of pathogens tremendously. *Antibiotics*, which are medications that kill bacteria, and *vaccines*, which are preparations that boost the immune system to help it ward off infection from specific pathogens, combat infection as well. Additionally, new treatments for certain viral illnesses such as influenza have been developed. As a result, after a century, the three leading causes of death in 2010 were no longer infectious diseases but were noninfectious diseases: heart disease, cancer, and stroke. The only infectious diseases in the "top 15" were pneumonia and influenza, together ranked as the ninth leading cause of death.[6]

Although infectious diseases are less significant contributors to death in the United States at this time, the worldwide picture is much different. Infectious diseases are the leading cause of death in the world. At least 30 new diseases have emerged in the past 30 years, including HIV infection and a new strain of hepatitis—hepatitis C. Additionally, many bacterial diseases once easily cured with antibiotics are appearing as incurable diseases, resistant to the variety of antibiotics available at this time. "Old" diseases that once seemed under control, such as diphtheria and tuberculosis, are making a comeback as well.

Ebola, a viral hemorrhagic fever, causes severe internal hemorrhaging and can decrease kidney and liver function. For many, contracting Ebola results in death. The largest outbreak of Ebola occurred in 2014 in western African nations of Guinea, Sierra Leone, and Liberia. As of mid-July 2014, this Ebola outbreak was responsible for 539 deaths, with many new cases of Ebola being reported each day.

With international travel commonplace, transmission of infection is a worldwide concern, not just a concern in our own country, state, or city. The resistance of many strains of bacteria to antibiotics and the reemergence of serious diseases once thought conquered make complacency to infection a dangerous attitude. In this time of increasing illness and death from infectious disease in the global community, it is important to understand how infectious diseases are transmitted and how pathogens interact with the body. This knowledge is key to avoiding infection and staying healthy.

The Chain of Infection

Infection results from the interaction between a pathogen (also called an agent of infection), a **host** (the organism that supports the growth of the pathogen), and the environment surrounding the host. The **chain of infection** illustrates how an infection spreads from an infected person to an uninfected person. A pathogen leaves the host through the portal of exit. Disease **transmission** can be direct or indirect, with a pathogen entering a susceptible host through the portal of entry to establish a new infection. For example, let's examine transmission of the influenza (the flu) virus through the chain of infection. The pathogen (influenza virus) leaves the reservoir (nose, throat, bronchial tubes, and lungs) through the portals of exit (mouth and nose) when the host sneezes. Transmission can occur directly, if the expelled droplets enter a susceptible host's mouth or nose (portals of entry), or indirectly, if the expelled droplet dry and become airborne. If either direct or indirect transmission occurs, a new infection is established. **Figure 14.5** depicts the chain of infection,

host In reference to disease, an organism that supports the growth of a pathogen; the third, and last, link in the chain of infection.

chain of infection The relationship among the factors important in the development of infectious diseases: the pathogen, transmission, and the host.

transmission In reference to disease, the means by which a pathogen gets to a host; the second link in the chain of infection.

Figure 14.5

The Chain of Infection. Infection is the invasion of the body by disease-causing organisms, or pathogens. Infection results when the pathogen is transmitted to a host. The host is the organism that supports the growth of the pathogen.

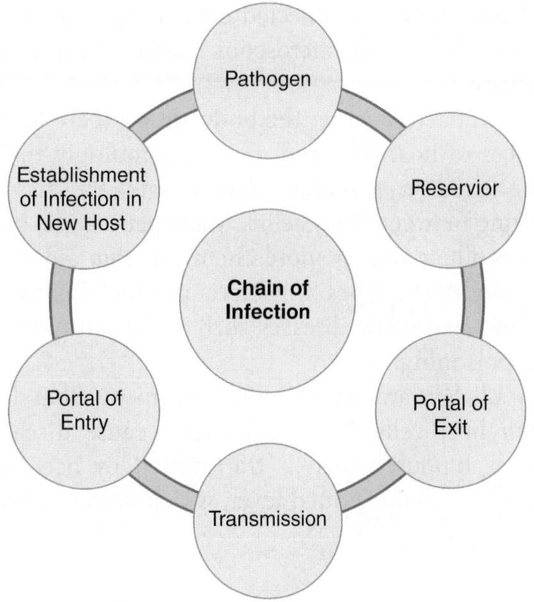

bacteria Unicellular, microscopic organisms with a simple cell structure; some are pathogenic to humans and produce infections such as strep throat, bacterial pneumonia, food poisoning, and infected cuts.

virus Hereditary material surrounded by a coat of protein; some viruses are pathogenic to humans and produce infections such as the common cold, influenza, mumps, measles, chicken pox, hepatitis, and AIDS.

acquired immune deficiency syndrome (AIDS) A set of certain diseases and conditions that results from infection by the human immunodeficiency virus (HIV).

including the relationship among factors important for contraction and spread of infectious diseases.

Pathogens

The severity of an infectious disease depends on a variety of factors:

- The type of pathogen (such as a bacterium or virus)
- Its virulence (how easily it causes disease)
- Its ability to multiply and spread within the body
- Its ability to combat the defense mechanisms of the body
- The body's reaction to this invader

This chapter first describes pathogens that cause infectious diseases. A later section focuses on the host's defense mechanisms.

Bacteria and Rickettsias **Bacteria** produce infections such as strep throat, bacterial pneumonia, food poisoning, and infected cuts. These organisms are unicellular and microscopic, with a simple cell structure.

When bacteria enter the body, they adhere to the surfaces of host cells and grow and multiply there. Some bacteria penetrate deeply into the tissues (moving between body cells). Many pathogenic bacteria produce one or more chemicals that aid their invasion. A few types of bacteria produce toxins, or poisons, that cause diseases such as certain types of food poisoning.

Rickettsias are bacteria-like organisms that live *within* host cells. These organisms cause diseases such as typhus, which is transmitted by lice, and Rocky Mountain spotted fever, which is transmitted by ticks.

Viruses **Viruses** cause many diseases with which you are familiar: the common cold, influenza (the flu), mumps, measles (**Figure 14.6**), chicken pox, hepatitis, and **acquired immune deficiency syndrome (AIDS)**. Viruses are very different from bacteria and, in fact, are very different from any organism: They do not have a cellular structure. Because the basis of life is the cell, viruses are not considered living organisms. They are simply hereditary material surrounded by a coat of protein.

Like bacteria, viruses cause disease by adhering to host cells, but unlike bacteria, viruses enter the cells of the body and use those cells to make more virus particles. The new virus particles break open the infected cell, killing it, and are then ready to infect additional body cells. The death of body cells causes many of the signs and symptoms of viral disease.

Certain types of viruses invade cells but enter a *latent state* during which time infective virus particles

Figure 14.6

Child with the Typical Rash of Measles. This highly contagious viral disease is characterized by a spreading rash. The rash consists of small, red spots; some of the spots may be raised.

Courtesy of CDC

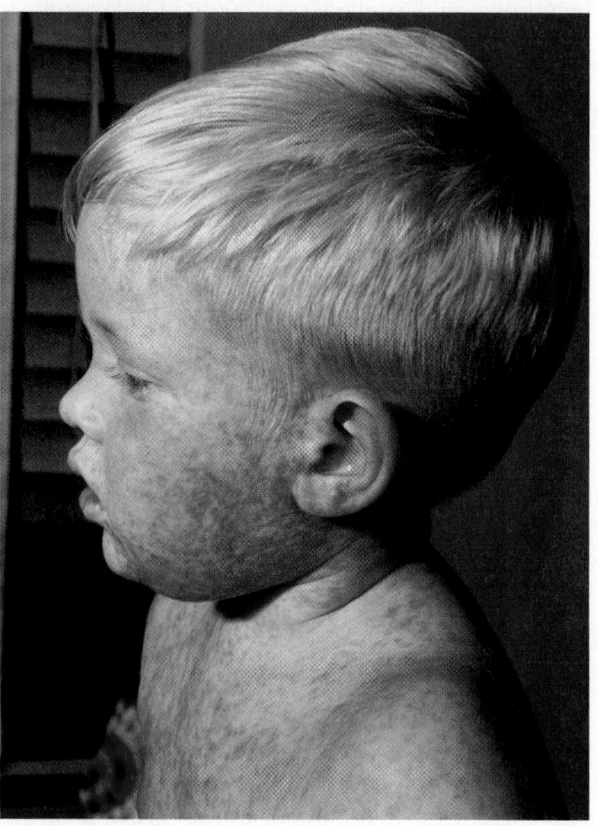

are not produced. Although no signs or symptoms of the viral infection are apparent, latency may cause changes in a cell that lead to cancer. In many instances, the latent viral hereditary material can become reactivated and replicate once again, causing disease.

Some infections are characterized by a cycling of latent and actively replicating periods, such as the sexually transmitted infection (STI) genital herpes. During the usual course of this disease (discussed later in this chapter), a person suffers active episodes when he or she can transmit this disease to others. The infection then subsides (latency) only to reappear at another time, often triggered by stress or other factors.

Fungi You have probably heard of, or may have experienced, yeast infections or athlete's foot (**Figure 14.7**), which is a type of ringworm (a fungal infection of the skin, hair, or nails). These diseases are caused by **fungi**, more commonly known as molds and yeasts. Fungi cannot make their own food and, therefore, grow on a wide range of organisms that they use as food sources, such as rotting logs, spoiling fruit, and the human body. Most human fungal infections, with the exception of yeast infections, are caused by molds.

fungi (FUN-jeye) Cellular organisms that cannot make their own food; some are pathogenic to humans and produce infections such as athlete's foot, ringworm, and yeast infections. *Fungus* is the singular term.

Medical researchers know less about how fungi cause disease in humans than they know about the other agents of infection. However, fungi appear to invade humans in much the same way as do bacteria. Humans have a high degree of resistance to fungi, which may explain why humans become infected with fungi less often than with bacteria or viruses. Fungi are considered *opportunistic* organisms; that is, they invade the human body when the host has another disease or condition that diminishes its ability to combat fungal infection. People with diabetes or AIDS, for example, are more likely to contract fungal infections than people with no underlying illness.

Figure 14.7

Athlete's Foot. Athlete's foot, or *tinea pedis*, is a fungal infection that usually arises between the toes or on the soles of the feet. This condition often develops when a person wears enclosed footwear without socks or stockings, and the feet become moist for long periods. To help avoid athlete's foot, dry the feet between the toes after bathing or showering and use powder to help keep the feet dry.

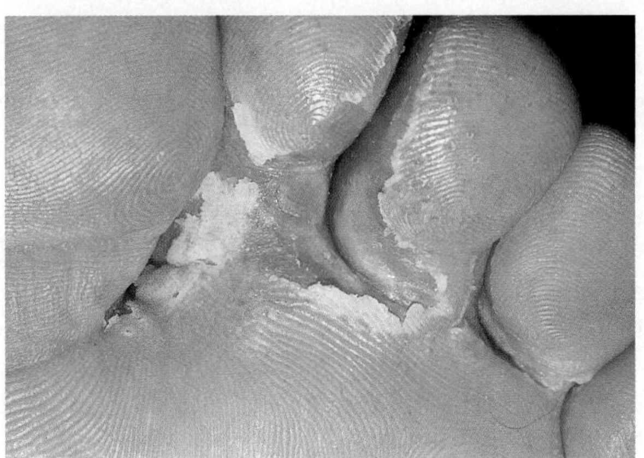

Other Types of Pathogens Two additional groups of organisms cause infections in humans: *protozoans* and *worms*. Protozoans cause diseases such as malaria (a tropical disease transmitted by mosquitoes) and trichomonas urogenital infections, or "trich" infections. All protozoans that cause infectious diseases in humans are single-celled organisms, but they differ from one another in the ways they cause disease.

The other group of infectious organisms is the parasitic worms: certain types of roundworms, flatworms (tapeworms), and flukes. Tapeworms are contracted by eating infected pork or beef; these worms live in the intestines, producing digestive disturbances. Adult roundworms also inhabit the intestinal tract and cause digestive disorders; they enter the body in various ways depending on the species of worm. Flukes differ in that they can inhabit the intestine, the liver, the lungs, or the veins depending on the species; they are contracted from water infected with human feces and are not prevalent in the United States.

One other group of organisms important to mention is the *arthropods*. Certain species of this group live on or in the skin of humans, a condition usually referred to as *infestation* rather than infection. Arthropods are organisms such as lice, fleas, mites, and ticks. Some STIs are caused by certain lice and mites (discussed later in this chapter). Ticks only occasionally infest humans but may transmit other pathogens to humans, as can mosquitoes, lice, and flies.

communicable (ka-MYOO-ni-kah-bl) Transmissible from person to person.

noncommunicable Not transmissible from person to person.

Transmission

Some infectious diseases are passed from person to person and others are not. Those that are spread from person to person, such as colds, flu, strep throat, and STIs, are **communicable** diseases. Diseases that are not transmitted from person to person, including both infectious and noninfectious diseases, are **noncommunicable**.

Noncommunicable Infectious Diseases Noncommunicable infectious diseases can be caused in various ways: by the growth of bacteria that normally inhabit the body, the ingestion of poisons produced by some bacteria, or infection with pathogens from environmental or animal sources.

Many species of bacteria normally reside on and in the human body. However, these beneficial bacteria can cause occasional problems. For example, *Staphylococcus* bacteria normally present on the skin can multiply and cause skin infections, especially in persons with chronic diseases such as diabetes.

Noncommunicable infections can also be caused by the ingestion of *toxins*, or poisons, produced by some bacteria. Staphylococcal food poisoning (formerly called ptomaine poisoning), for example, is caused by taking in a toxin that certain staphylococcal bacteria produce when they grow on foods. Dairy products and poultry are the foods most commonly contaminated with staphylococcal bacteria from their animal sources or from infected food handlers. The staphylococcal bacteria grow well in high-protein, high-carbohydrate foods. Most often, staphylococcal food poisoning occurs when people eat foods such as potato salad, chicken salad, custard, or cream pies that have not been refrigerated properly after preparation. Picnics are a common time of infection because such foods are left out under warm conditions for long periods of time, which allows the bacteria to grow and produce toxin. Because the bacteria grow on the food and not in the body, this type of noncommunicable infection is more properly called *intoxication* (poisoning) rather than infection. Staphylococcal food poisoning should not be confused with *Salmonella* food infection, in which the bacteria are taken in with food and multiply in the small intestine.

Botulism is another type of food poisoning, caused by a powerful toxin produced by the bacterium *Clostridium botulinum*. This organism most often grows in improperly home-canned, low-acid foods such as green beans and green peppers. Boiling home-canned foods for 10 to 15 minutes inactivates the toxin. (Infants can contract botulism from raw honey.)

A third type of noncommunicable infection is caused by pathogens that infect people via environmental or animal sources. Legionnaire's disease, caused by the bacterium *Legionella pneumophila*, is an infectious disease contracted from an environmental source. Under favorable conditions, this pathogen can grow in and be dispersed by any apparatus that provides a water aerosol or mist, such as air conditioners, whirlpool spas, humidifiers, decorative fountains, showerheads, and water faucets. When this water mist is inhaled, these microbes lodge in the lungs and multiply, producing a pneumonia-like disease that includes high fever, cough, chest pain, and diarrhea. This disease is quite serious; 5% to 30% of its victims die, but victims are often those who are older (65 years and older), people who smoke, have a compromised immune system, and/or have chronic lung disease. To reduce the growth of this organism and protect against infection, periodically clean and thoroughly disinfect mist-creating items, such as those mentioned previously, and maintain an appropriate concentration of chlorine in home spas.[7]

Lyme disease is an example of a noncommunicable infection contracted from an animal source. Named for the small community of Lyme, Connecticut, where the disease was first recognized in 1975, this bacterial disease is transmitted by ticks that infest animals such as white-footed mice and white-tailed deer. The ticks ingest the bacterial pathogen that causes Lyme disease from infected animals. When a tick harboring this bacterium bites a human, it injects the bacterium into the bloodstream. Usually a painless but large rash (sometimes looking like a bull's-eye) appears at the site of the bite from a few days to 1 month after being bitten (**Figure 14-8**). This rash is generally accompanied by severe headaches, fatigue, chills, and fever. If the disease is not treated with antibiotics at this early stage, it may develop into severe inflammation of the heart muscle or nervous system weeks to months later. Within 2 years, if untreated, arthritic attacks develop (inflammation of the joints) that can become chronic.

In the United States, Lyme disease is found primarily in the Northeast, the mid-Atlantic (Virginia and North Carolina area), and the upper Midwest. It has also been reported in several areas in northwestern

Figure 14.8

The "Classic" Rash That Develops at the Site of a Tick Bite in Lyme Disease. Not everyone who contracts Lyme disease will develop this type of rash.

Courtesy of James Gathany/CDC

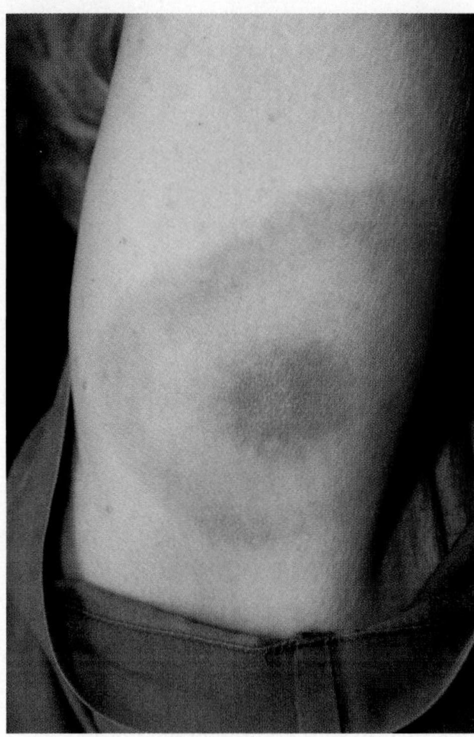

Figure 14.9

Deer ticks transmit the bacterium that causes Lyme disease from infected animals to humans.

(a) © iStockphoto/Thinkstock; (b) Courtesy of Jim Gathany/CDC.

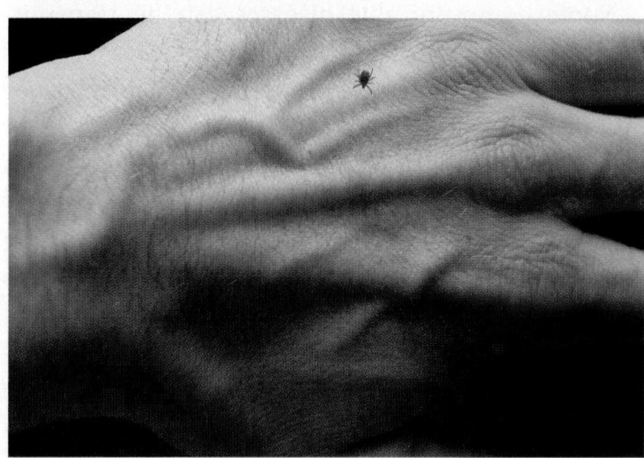

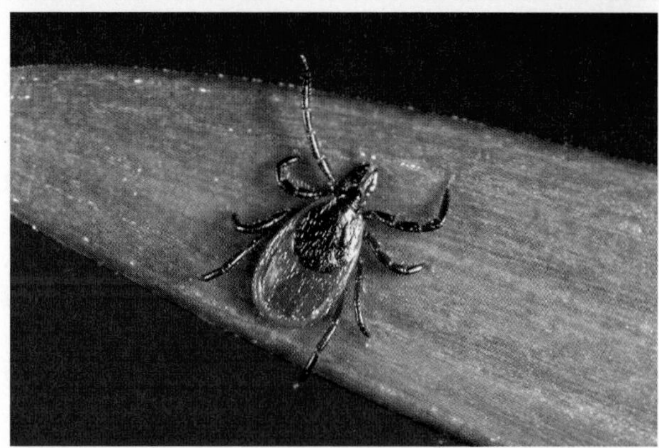

California. Deer ticks favor a moist, shaded environment, particularly areas of woods, brush, or tall grass. If you are walking, gardening, or engaging in other activities in these types of areas and in which deer and mice live (and therefore deer ticks [**Figure 14.9**]), wear long pants and a long-sleeved shirt. Tuck your pant legs into your socks or boots. Spray insect repellent containing at least 30% DEET on your clothing and exposed skin. (Do not spray it on your face.)

Spray it on your hands and pat that on your face. Use products with no more than 10% DEET on children.) Check yourself carefully for ticks, removing any you find with tweezers.

A Lyme disease vaccine was introduced in 1999, but the manufacturer withdrew the vaccine from the market in 2002, citing poor sales. Moreover, the public was concerned about possible serious side effects of the vaccine even though preliminary evidence showed the vaccine was safe. As of mid-2014, there was no vaccine available to prevent Lyme disease in humans.[8]

Communicable Infectious Diseases Communicable diseases are transmitted from person to person by direct or indirect contact, by means of a common vehicle, through the air, and by means of vectors such as mosquitoes.

Some infectious diseases, such as STIs, are passed from person to person by close physical (direct) contact. In the case of STIs, of course, the close contact is usually vaginal intercourse, anal intercourse, genital contact without intercourse, or oral sex. Other diseases such as colds and the flu are often transmitted by direct contact also, such as shaking hands. Therefore, it is important to wash your hands well and frequently to help avoid transmitting or contracting such communicable diseases. These diseases can also be transmitted indirectly by means of an object, such as a shared drinking glass, or through close contact with droplets sneezed or coughed by a person. Strep throat and measles are spread in this way.

Frequently, a source contaminated with pathogens from humans may transmit an infectious disease to many people. Examples of common sources of infection are a blood supply contaminated with human immunodeficiency virus, food contaminated with the hepatitis virus by an infected food handler, and water contaminated by the feces of a person infected with typhoid fever. A variety of infectious diseases are transmitted via food or water.

Some communicable diseases can be transmitted from infected persons to noninfected persons through the air on microscopic water droplets or on dust particles. Certain disease-causing organisms of the respiratory tract, such as the bacterium that causes tuberculosis, can be transmitted in this way, propelled into the air when an infected person coughs or sneezes. When not in isolation, persons with communicable tuberculosis should wear surgical or other types of masks to help prevent transmission of their disease.

Other communicable diseases are spread indirectly by means of vectors. A *vector* is an organism (other than a human) that transmits a pathogen from one person to another. Usually a part of the life cycle of the pathogen takes place in or on the vector. For example, the malaria organism is a protozoan that carries out part of its life cycle in humans and another part in the gut of *Anopheles* mosquitoes. When a mosquito bites an infected person, it ingests blood that contains the protozoan. After the organism undergoes sexual reproduction in the mosquito, its progeny can infect new hosts when the mosquito bites them.

The Host

Why do you remain healthy sometimes, yet get sick at other times? How did you avoid getting the cold that everyone else seems to have? Why didn't your spouse come down with the flu like the rest of the family? So far we've seen that some of the answers to these questions have to do with the pathogen and certain of its characteristics, such as its virulence. Transmission may also mean the difference between infection and health. Persons exposed frequently to pathogens are likely to become infected more often than those exposed less frequently. The other answers to these questions have to do with your body's resistance to the invading microbe.

Stress can be one factor that reduces your resistance to infection. High-intensity or exhaustive exercise, such as running more than 60 miles per week or for 3 or more hours per session, also suppresses the immune system. Moderate exercise, however, such as running fewer than 20 miles per week or walking for 45 minutes per day for 5 days per week, stimulates the immune system. Exercising when you are sick lowers the body's defenses.

Race and age affect an individual's resistance or susceptibility to certain diseases. Africans or people

Healthy Living Practices

- Refrigerate cold starchy and protein-rich foods and cold foods made with dairy products or poultry immediately after preparation. At picnics, keep these foods chilled until it is time to eat.
- Boil all low-acid home-canned foods before eating or avoid eating home-canned foods.
- Periodically clean and thoroughly disinfect mist-creating items such as humidifiers and maintain an appropriate concentration of chlorine in home spas.
- Avoid close contact with people who have communicable diseases.
- Wash your hands well and frequently to help avoid contracting communicable diseases, such as colds and the flu.
- Do not share drinking glasses and eating utensils with others.
- Do not share hypodermic needles with others because they may be contaminated with pathogens such as the hepatitis B virus or the AIDS virus.
- Use a condom when engaging in sex unless you are in a long-term, mutually monogamous relationship with an uninfected partner. Infectious bodily secretions can be passed from one partner to another during sexual activity.
- Use insect repellents formulated to repel ticks and flying insects that may be carriers of disease-producing organisms.
- Do not drink the water when traveling in developing countries. Also avoid raw fruits, vegetables, and salads because they may have been washed with contaminated water.
- Avoid the following hazardous foods when traveling in developing countries: uncooked or poorly cooked beef, pork, fish, and seafood and unpasteurized milk and other local dairy products.
- Avoid or limit stress; high levels of stress reduce your resistance to infection.
- Avoid high-intensity or exhaustive exercise because it reduces your resistance to infection.
- Engage in moderate exercise to boost the immune system.

with African ancestry, for example, have a higher resistance to tropical diseases such as malaria and yellow fever than do non-Africans. People of Asian ancestry are more resistant to the sexually transmitted infection syphilis than are non-Asians. Children are more likely to contract certain "childhood" infectious diseases such as measles and chicken pox, whereas older adults are more susceptible to pneumonia and influenza. And, as mentioned earlier, people with other diseases, such as AIDS, diabetes, and cancer, have weakened defense mechanisms.

Your body has two main types of defenses against infectious agents: mechanisms of nonspecific resistance, which are a variety of defenses that combat any foreign invader, and the immune system, which is a specific defense system that combats the particular invading pathogen. The following sections describe these two major defense mechanisms.

immunity (im-MYOU-nih-tea) Resistance to disease.

nonspecific immunity A variety of defense mechanisms that combat any type of damage to the body, including the invasion of infectious agents.

specific immunity Defense mechanism carried out by the immune system.

immune system A collection of cells and organs of the body that recognizes and combats pathogens and other foreign substances with cells and proteins that are specific for particular invaders. The immune system has two branches: antibody-mediated immunity and cell-mediated immunity.

portal of entry Site on or in the body where pathogens enter.

Immunity

Immunity is protection from disease, particularly infectious disease. You have two types of immunity: nonspecific and specific. **Nonspecific immunity** comprises a variety of defense mechanisms that combat any type of damage to the body, including the invasion of infectious agents. **Specific immunity** is carried out by the immune system. The **immune system** recognizes and combats pathogens and other foreign cells (such as cancer cells or tissue transplants) with cells and proteins that are specific for particular invaders. The immune system is discussed later in this chapter.

Nonspecific Immunity

Pathogens can enter the body at sites called **portals of entry** (**Figure 14.10**). The mucous membranes lining the respiratory, digestive, urinary, and reproductive systems are all portals of entry. Whether resulting from a cut, insect bite, burn, or injection, broken skin is a portal of entry. The placenta may be a portal of entry for a fetus, which may become infected with pathogens (mostly viruses) from an infected mother. Unbroken skin is a portal of entry only for some fungi and the larvae of certain parasitic worms.

The Skin and Mucous Membranes The skin provides a *mechanical barrier* to pathogens. The hardened cells at the surface of the skin provide a waterproof barrier that most infective agents cannot penetrate. In addition, acidic skin oils and sweat help make the skin an inhospitable environment for most organisms.

Body openings, such as the eyes, and tubes that open to the outside, such as the digestive and respiratory tracts, are lined with tissue called *mucous membranes*. Most mucous membranes have a thin layer of cells that produces a sticky, viscous secretion called mucus. Mucus keeps the membrane moist and traps foreign particles and organisms.

Another defense mechanism that works with the mucous membranes is *cilia*. These short, hairlike structures project from the surfaces of the cells lining the

Figure 14.10

Portals of Entry of the Human Body. Portals of entry are areas of the body where pathogens can intrude: the skin and mucous membranes lining the respiratory, digestive, urinary, and reproductive systems; the placenta; broken skin; and unbroken skin (only for some fungi and the larvae of certain parasitic worms).

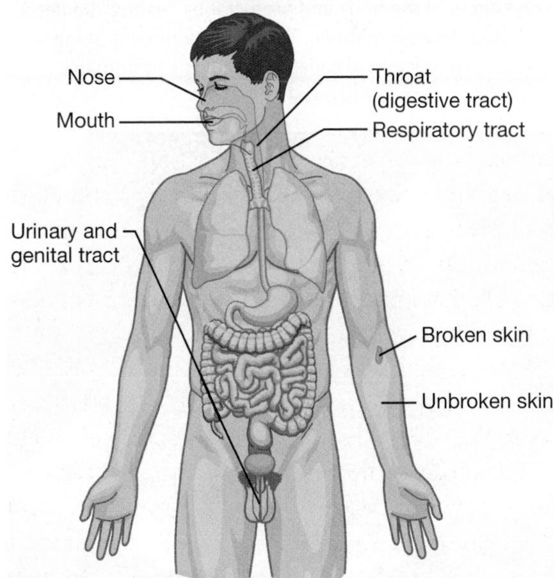

leukocytes (LEWK-oh-sites) White blood cells; active in both specific and nonspecific defenses of the body.

phagocytosis (FAG-oh-sigh-TOE-sis) The process of white blood cells ingesting foreign cells and debris, such as the dirt or dead cells in a cut.

lymph (limf) Tissue fluid.

upper respiratory tract. As they beat in wavelike fashion, they move mucus that contains trapped foreign material such as dust and bacteria up toward the back of the mouth where it can be swallowed, keeping it away from lower respiratory structures, especially the lungs.

Other tissues have a *chemical defense* mechanism. The lacrimal glands (located above the upper, outer corners of the eyes) produce tears that wash away foreign material on the eyes and also contain a chemical called *lysozyme* that kills certain bacteria. Lysozyme is also found in saliva. Another structure that provides a nonspecific chemical defense is the stomach. Stomach acid kills most of the microorganisms ingested with food.

White Blood Cells and Phagocytosis Another nonspecific line of defense is the action of certain white blood cells, or **leukocytes**, that ingest foreign cells and debris, such as the dirt or dead cells in a cut. This process is **phagocytosis** (literally, *phago*, "eating," and *cyto*, "cell") and is shown in **Figure 14.11**.

Figure 14.11

White Blood Cell Ingesting Bacteria. This is a highly magnified, colorized photo of a white blood cell called a macrophage (yellow/orange). Macrophages are the scavengers of the body and protect it by "eating" bacteria and other foreign material. The bacteria (green) being ingested in this image cause tuberculosis in humans.

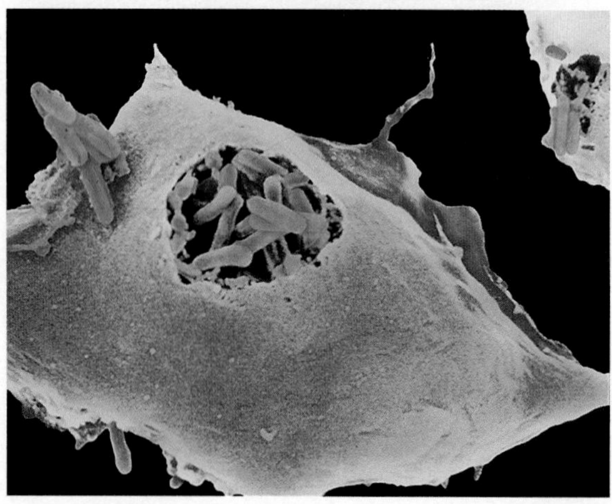

Two types of leukocytes—the neutrophils and the macrophages—are important phagocytes in the human body. Other white blood cells called *lymphocytes* help protect the body against infection and are part of the immune system.

The Lymphatic System The lymphatic system, another key player in nonspecific immunity, is composed of vessels and nodes through which tissue fluid, or **lymph**, flows. Pictured in **Figure 14.12**, the lymphatic system also consists of lymphocytes and three lymphatic organs: the tonsils, the spleen, and the thymus (which is active only until puberty). The lymphatic system removes microorganisms and other foreign substances from the tissue fluid, the fluid surrounding the cells that is derived from the blood.

Lymph nodes are located at many points along the lymphatic vessels. Lymphatic vessels enter and exit each lymph node, which is a mesh of tissue containing lymphocytes and macrophages. The nodes cleanse tissue fluid by trapping microorganisms and other foreign substances in their weblike structures; macrophages in the nodes phagocytize this material.

The tonsils are large groups of lymph nodes located at the back of the oral cavity; they rid the nose and mouth area of bacteria and other debris. The spleen, located in the upper left corner of the abdominal cavity (see Figure 14.12), not only performs the function of a lymph node but also destroys worn-out red blood cells and stores red blood cells to provide an emergency supply in the case of severe loss. The thymus, located just above the heart at the midline of the chest, is the place where the lymphocytes destined to be T cells mature during fetal life and early childhood (see the section titled "Specific Immunity" later in this chapter). These T cells then reside in the lymphatic tissue and produce new T cells when the thymus is no longer active.

Inflammation Can you remember the last time you got a splinter or a cut? If so, you can probably remember (quite well!) your body's response. The inflammatory response is a series of events that takes place when the body is harmed by occurrences such as bacterial or viral invasion (infection), cuts, chemical damage, and burns. This response can be *local*, as in the case of getting a splinter in your finger, or *systemic* (affecting the whole body), as in the case of contracting a cold. Inflammation involves a variety of defense mechanisms that isolate and destroy the pathogens or other injurious agents and then remove the foreign materials and damaged cells so that the body can repair itself.

The presence of infectious agents or damage to the body triggers the inflammatory response. As a result, many chemicals are released. Some of these chemicals,

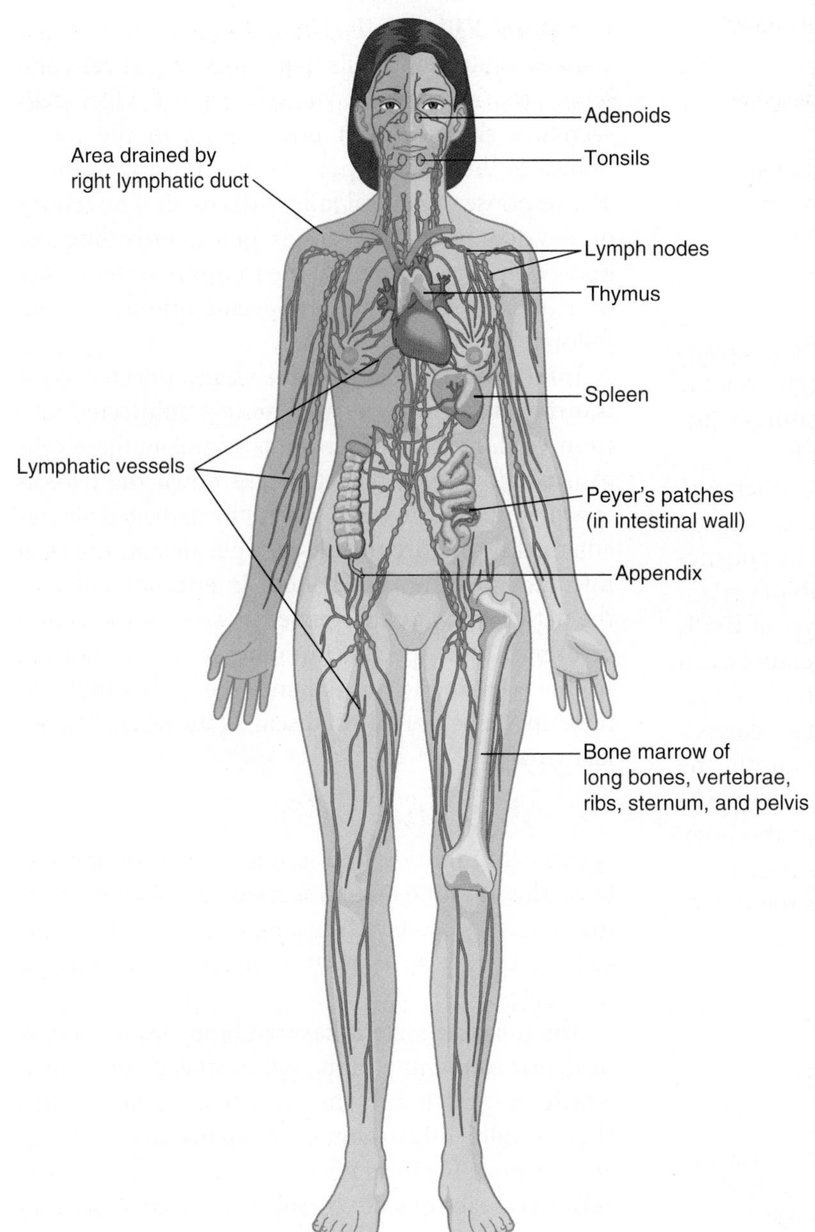

Figure 14.12

The Lymphatic System. The lymphatic system is made up of blind-ended vessels, nodes, and a few organs. Tissue fluid, derived from the blood, flows through the lymphatic vessels and is cleansed of debris and microorganisms by white blood cells that reside in the nodes. The fluid eventually returns to the blood.

such as histamine, cause an increase of blood flow to the affected area, which brings phagocytes and other white blood cells to ingest microorganisms and debris—pieces of a splinter, for example. In addition, other chemicals stimulate phagocytes to move to the affected area, where they leave the blood and enter the damaged tissues. Yet other chemicals allow the surrounding blood vessel walls to leak, permitting phagocytes, certain blood-clotting factors, and other chemicals that enhance the inflammatory response to enter the tissues. The blood-clotting factors wall off the infected area, which prevents the spread of the infection. **Figure 14.13** illustrates the inflammatory process.

The signs and symptoms of local inflammation are redness, heat, swelling, pain, and a loss of function. The redness, heat, and swelling are results of increased blood flow to the affected area, including movement of fluids into surrounding tissues. Pain results as nerves are stimulated by the swelling and the chemicals released during inflammation. The pain, tissue damage, and swelling may contribute to a temporary loss of function of the affected body part.

Systemic inflammation occurs when you have a widespread infection such as a cold, the flu, strep throat, or pneumonia. Systemic inflammation has the same signs as local inflammation, but additional processes occur that result in more significant signs. The red bone marrow, located in the ends of certain bones, produces and releases large

Interferons (IN-ter-FEAR-onz) Proteins produced by the body during a viral infection that protect uninfected cells from viral invasion.

antigens (AN-tih-jenz) Proteins that are foreign or recognized as "nonself" by the body.

autoimmune diseases Diseases in which the body perceives its own cells as foreign, attacking them and causing localized and systemic (whole-body) reactions.

numbers of white blood cells. In addition, invading microorganisms and white blood cells release chemicals that affect the body's temperature-regulating system in the brain, resulting in a fever.

A *fever* is a rise in the internal body temperature from the human average of about 98.6°F. A fever lower than 104°F helps the body fight infection by enhancing phagocytosis and inhibiting the growth of certain microorganisms. However, a prolonged fever of 104°F, or a fever higher than 104°F, is dangerous because it can destroy proteins in the body. Other symptoms of systemic inflammation are fatigue, aches, and weakness.

The inflammatory process continues until the pathogens are killed or inactivated, or other injurious agents are walled off from the rest of the body and no longer pose a threat. Phagocytes ingest cellular debris and other organic material as the tissues recover from the infection.

Figure 14.13

The Inflammatory Process. (a) A splinter damages the skin, thrusting bacteria deep into the wound. Injured cells release chemicals such as histamine that cause the blood vessels to widen, bringing more blood to the area. (b) White blood cells squeeze through vessel walls and migrate to the bacteria, where they phagocytize them. Blood clots and connective tissue wall off the area.

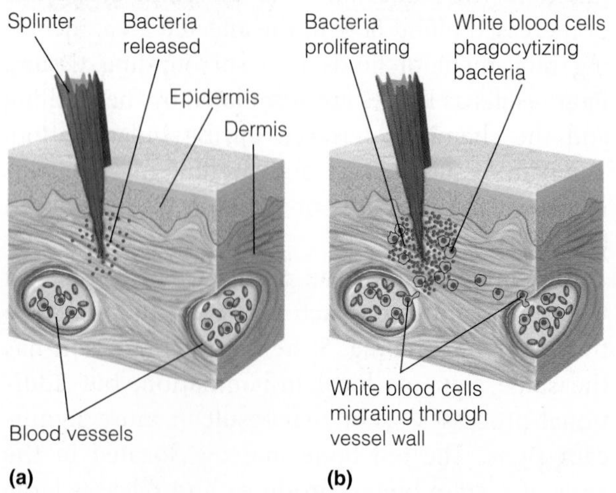

Natural Killer Cells Natural killer cells are specialized white blood cells that attack cancer cells and body cells invaded by viruses. Natural killer cells secrete a chemical that pokes holes in the membranes of these two types of cells, destroying them. The response of natural killer cells to viral infections or developing cancer cells is quick, providing the body with protection until the immune system takes over (see the section titled "Specific Immunity" that follows).

Interferons Released from virally infected cells, **interferons** are proteins that protect uninfected cells from viral invasion. Interferons stimulate these cells to produce a protein that breaks down the hereditary material of the virus. When the damaged viruses enter cells, they are unable to replicate and the viral infection is eventually halted. Interferons enhance the activity of the phagocytes as well as the action of other, more specific immune system responses. In this role, interferons enhance the body's ability to fight invasions from most disease-causing agents, not just viruses.

Specific Immunity

Specific immunity is a function of the immune system. The immune system is made up of cells residing in tissues scattered throughout the body. These cells can react to specific pathogens and foreign molecules.

The immune system has two branches: *antibody-mediated immunity* and *cell-mediated immunity*, which are discussed shortly. Each branch works slightly differently to attack foreign invaders and stop an infection. The immune system also has a memory: cells that react quickly to subsequent attacks by an invader.

Antigens: The Triggers of Specific Immunity **Antigens** are usually foreign, or "nonself," proteins. Sometimes, entire infectious agents act as antigens. In other instances, parts of pathogens or the poisons they may secrete act as antigens. Noninfectious agents such as plant pollens, blood transfusions, or tissue transplants are antigenic, although the response to these antigens may differ from person to person. Unfortunately, the body sometimes perceives its own cells as foreign, attacking them and causing localized and systemic reactions, as in the case of **autoimmune diseases** such as *rheumatoid arthritis*. In this disease, the reactions include inflammation and deformity of the joints. The following sections describe how the immune system reacts to antigens that enter the body.

Antibody-Mediated Immunity The antibody-mediated portion of the immune system reacts to *extracellular* antigens, that is, antigens that reside outside of body cells, such as most bacteria and any toxins they produce. **Antibodies** are proteins that interact in a lock-and-key fashion with antigens. When they bind with an antigen, antibodies interfere with the normal functioning of the antigen. Antigen–antibody binding also stimulates the inflammatory response and promotes phagocytosis of the antigen.

The workhorses of antibody-mediated immunity (the cells that produce antibodies) are specialized white blood cells called *B lymphocytes*, or **B cells**. Each B cell has receptors on its membrane that bind to a specific antigen. When a foreign antigen enters the body, B cells bind to it. After stimulation by lymphocytes called helper T cells, the B cells reproduce in large numbers and become plasma cells, which produce antibodies. **Figure 14-14** illustrates the antibody-mediated immune response.

Some of the stimulated B cells do not differentiate into plasma cells. These cells circulate as *memory B cells*, which respond more rapidly and forcefully whenever the antigen is encountered in the future. Memory cells confer immunity (resistance) to a disease. Many infections stimulate lifelong immunity (measles and chicken pox, for example); others, such as diphtheria, confer immunity for only a few years. Unfortunately, not all infectious agents stimulate the formation of memory cells, so no immunity is produced as a result of their infection. Examples of such infections are strep throat and gonorrhea (an STI).

Cell-Mediated Immunity The cell-mediated portion of the immune system reacts to *intracellular* antigens; that is, antigens that reside inside our body cells, such as viruses, fungi, a few types of bacteria, and parasites. It also acts against foreign tissues such as organ transplants and controls the growth of tumor cells.

Lymphocytes called **T cells** function in cell-mediated immunity. T cells reside in lymphoid tissues and in the bloodstream with the B cells. The body contains thousands of different T cells. Upon binding to antigens, T cells reproduce and differentiate into four types: cytotoxic T cells, helper T cells, suppressor T cells, and memory T cells.

Cytotoxic T cells destroy invading intracellular pathogens (primarily viruses) by secreting chemicals that break apart infected host cells. By destroying host cells, the cytotoxic T cells take away what a virus or any other intracellular infective agent needs to reproduce or replicate. Cytotoxic T cells destroy nonself tissue transplants or tumorous growths in much the same way (**Figure 14-15**).

Helper T cells and *suppressor T cells* regulate the activities of both branches of the immune system.

antibodies Proteins that interact in a lock-and-key fashion with antigens, interfering with the normal functioning of the antigen.

B cells Specialized white blood cells (lymphocytes) that function in antibody-mediated immunity and produce antibodies.

T cells Specialized white blood cells (lymphocytes) that function in cell-mediated immunity; there are four types of T cells.

Figure 14.14

The Antibody-Mediated Immune Response. White blood cells called macrophages ingest invading microbes and display their antigenic parts. Helper T cells and B cells specific to the antigens attach to them, which activates both types of cells. The helper T cells produce a chemical that stimulates the growth of the B cells. These B cells, now called plasma cells, secrete proteins called antibodies. Antibodies attach to and promote the death of the invading microbes.

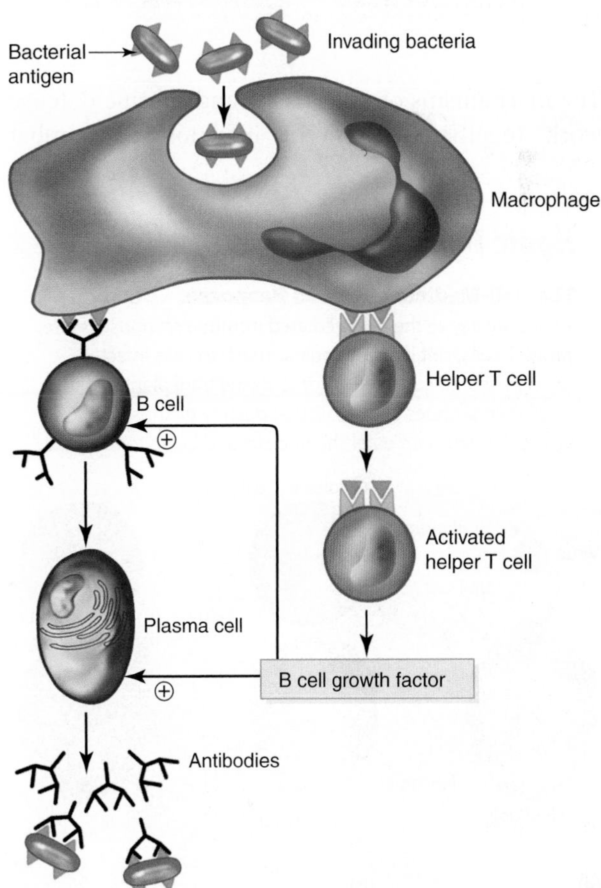

acquired immunity Specific resistance to infection that is not inherited but develops during a person's lifetime.

vaccine A preparation of a killed or weakened pathogen or its antigenic parts to be administered to a person to induce immunity and thereby prevent infectious disease.

Helper T cells secrete various chemicals that enhance the activity of cytotoxic T cells and suppressor T cells and attract phagocytes to the area. Some helper T cells secrete chemicals that enhance the development and reproduction of B cells.

When the infection has subsided, suppressor T cells shut down the immune system. Although these cells inhibit the activity of various immune system cells, they increase in number more slowly than do other T cells. Therefore, suppressor T cells shut down the immune response only after it has successfully done its job.

A group of stimulated T cells circulates as *memory T cells*. Like memory B cells, memory T cells respond rapidly and forcefully during subsequent encounters with antigens, resulting in immunity to a disease.

Interactions Between Nonspecific and Specific Immunity

The mechanisms of nonspecific and specific defense work together to prevent infection or combat infection when it occurs. For example, the intact skin, mucous membranes, and chemicals in body fluids are effective barriers against viral invasion. However, if viruses gain entry to the body, macrophages phagocytize them before they can enter body cells. Activated helper T cells secrete chemicals that stimulate the B cells to become antibody-producing cells.

If some of the virus particles enter body cells despite these defenses, the infected cells produce interferons, which protect uninfected cells. Natural killer cells poke holes in the infected cells, killing them, thus destroying the virus's host. After binding to infected cells, cytotoxic T cells reproduce, developing large populations specific for this viral infection. As armies of cytotoxic T cells break apart infected cells, the freed viruses are phagocytized by macrophages and inactivated by antibodies. Usually this complex process stops the viral infection. The memory B cells and T cells continue to circulate and recognize this same virus quickly if it reenters the body. Most likely, the virus will never again cause infection because it will have been stopped before it could gain a foothold in the cells.

Figure 14.15

The Cell-Mediated Immune Response. Cytotoxic T cells are key to the cell-mediated immune response. Here, whole T cells, not just antibodies, attach to cells infected with viruses, to cancer cells, or to tissue transplants. The T cell then secretes chemicals that destroy the host cell before the virus can enter the nucleus and begin to replicate.

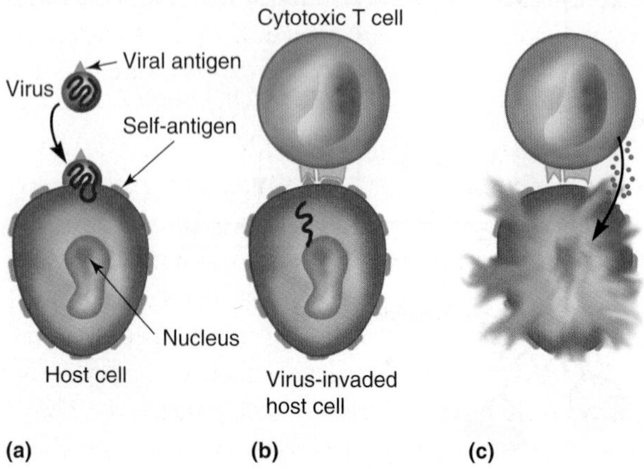

Protection Against Infectious Diseases

A variety of factors determine whether a person develops an infectious disease. In general, to prevent infectious disease, you must break the chain of infection. This chapter offers many tips on breaking the chain of infection and preventing disease. However, one of the best ways to protect yourself against infection is to increase your resistance.

Specific immunity is either inborn or acquired. *Inborn immunity* is inherited, such as immunity to infectious diseases that attack other organisms (your cat or dog, for example) but not humans. **Acquired immunity** is not inherited; it develops during a person's lifetime. Acquired immunity develops in a variety of ways: either actively or passively and by natural or artificial means.

Active acquired immunity is an immune system response developed as a result of contact with a pathogen, which includes development of memory B cells or T cells. Contact with the pathogen can occur naturally, during day-to-day life. It can also occur artificially, by a **vaccine** prepared from a killed or weakened pathogen or its antigenic parts. Depending on how the vaccine is prepared, it may have long- or short-term effects. That is why people need booster vaccinations every few years against some infectious diseases.

Children develop active acquired immunity to many serious childhood diseases by being vaccinated according to a schedule recommended by the American Academy of Pediatrics and the American Academy of Family Physicians. The CDC, at www.cdc.gov/vaccines, lists the current childhood and adolescent immunization schedule. In addition, immunization of adults and children prior to travel to foreign countries leads to active acquired immunity to diseases not generally found in the United States. If you are traveling outside the United States, consult your physician 4 to 6 weeks prior to your trip for the required and recommended immunizations. The CDC provides health-related travel information at www.cdc.gov/travel.

Passive acquired immunity is conferred when a person is given antibodies. Passive immunity can be acquired naturally when antibodies from a mother cross the placenta and enter the bloodstream of a developing fetus. After birth, a breast-fed infant passively acquires antibodies from its mother's milk. These antibodies help a newborn resist disease for the first month of life until its own immune system becomes functional. Passive immunity can also be acquired artificially, when a person receives an injection of antibodies after exposure to a serious infection (such as hepatitis A or rabies) or a lethal poison (such as certain snake venoms).

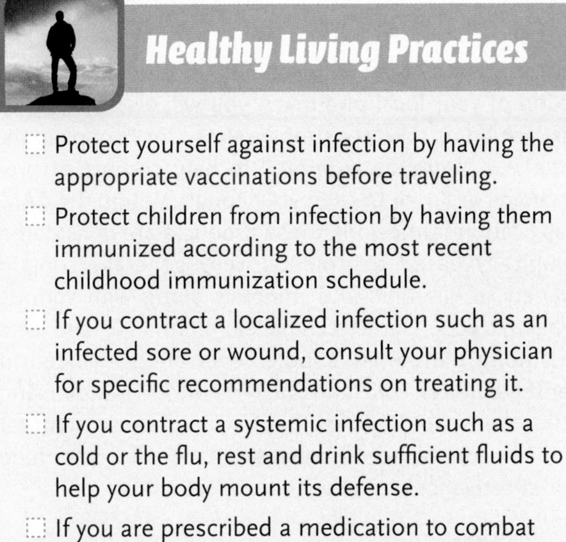

Healthy Living Practices

- Protect yourself against infection by having the appropriate vaccinations before traveling.
- Protect children from infection by having them immunized according to the most recent childhood immunization schedule.
- If you contract a localized infection such as an infected sore or wound, consult your physician for specific recommendations on treating it.
- If you contract a systemic infection such as a cold or the flu, rest and drink sufficient fluids to help your body mount its defense.
- If you are prescribed a medication to combat an infection, follow all instructions and take the prescribed amount.

antibiotics (AN-tie-by-OT-iks) A group of chemicals that kill bacteria or inhibit their growth.

Drugs That Combat Infection

Once a person has an infection like the common cold, what can he or she do to combat it? Most often, getting rest and drinking sufficient fluids helps the body as it mounts its defense. Sometimes over-the-counter cold medications such as decongestants, antihistamines, and cough medicines can help relieve symptoms. Many products are also available that are considered part of complementary and alternative medicine (CAM). See the Consumer Health feature "CAM Products and Colds" for more information. For other infections, individuals can obtain specific recommendations from a physician. These medical practitioners often prescribe medicines to inhibit the growth of or inactivate the infectious agent.

Antibiotics are a group of chemicals that kill bacteria or inhibit their growth. Antibiotics work by attacking parts of bacterial cells or bacterial processes that differ from human cells. When taking an antibiotic, it is important to finish the medication your physician prescribed, even though your symptoms may be gone prior to that time. All the bacteria may not have been killed, and the infection could return.

Antibiotics do nothing to combat viral infections and may kill some of the body's normal bacterial inhabitants. These bacteria control the growth of troublesome microorganisms; when they are gone, it is easier for unwanted disease-causing bacteria to multiply and cause a secondary bacterial infection. Therefore, *taking antibiotics when they are unnecessary can be harmful.* Furthermore, the unnecessary use of antibiotics provides additional opportunities for antibiotic-resistant strains of bacteria to develop.

Various topical antibiotics (those applied to the skin, such as bacitracin) are available without prescription to treat or prevent minor skin infections. Over-the-counter topical antifungal drugs are also available to treat fungal infections of the skin, such as athlete's foot and ringworm, and vaginal yeast infections. Antifungal drugs that must be taken orally for more serious fungal infections require a prescription.

Progress in the production of effective antiviral drugs has been slow because viruses reside inside the body's cells. Therefore, a drug must inactivate the virus without

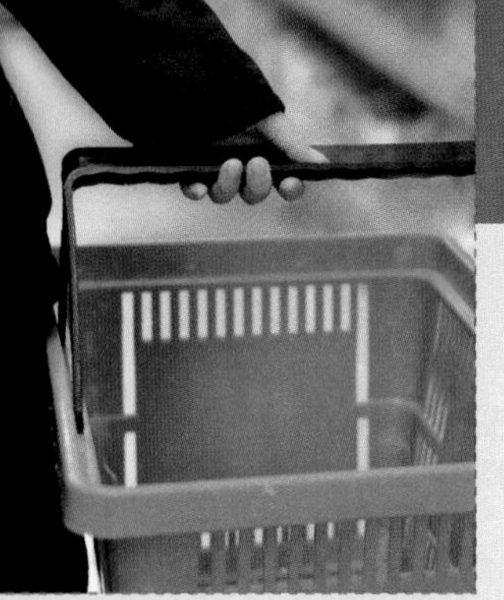
© sevenke/ShutterStock

Consumer Health

CAM Products and Colds

Adults have an average of two to four colds per year, and children have more—about six to eight. Each year Americans experience many colds, making the market for cold/cough/flu remedies huge and manufacturers anxious to tap into it. The last time you had a cold or the flu, you likely roamed the aisles of your local pharmacy trying to find a product to shorten the duration of your illness and lessen its symptoms.

Pharmacy shelves are stocked with the usual over-the-counter kinds of decongestants, cough suppressants, and antihistamines. However, you might have noticed other products packaged as cold or flu treatments and labeled "homeopathic medicine" or "dietary supplement." These are two types of *alternative* cold products. Complementary and alternative medicine (CAM) is a diverse group of healthcare systems, treatments, and products that differ from conventional (scientific or evidence-based) medicine. Can the alternative cold treatments available on pharmacy shelves help support your immune system, quiet your cough, shorten the duration of your cold or flu infection, relieve your sinus pain and pressure, or dry up your nasal congestion as they claim?

Homeopathic Products

Within the CAM classification framework, homeopathic (ho-me-oh-PAH-thick) "medicine," or *homeopathy* (ho-me-AH-pah-thee), is a type of alternative medical system. Developed in Germany more than 200 years ago, homeopathy operates on the principle of "similar" or "like cures like." Proponents believe that a disease or condition can be cured by using small amounts of a substance that in much larger amounts causes those same symptoms in healthy people. For example, homeopaths use substances from onions to stop the watery eyes and runny nose of a cold—the same substances that cause tears when an onion is cut during food preparation.

To prepare homeopathic products, the "principle of dilutions" is used, which states that the lowest dosage possible has the greatest effect. Therefore substances are diluted with water in a stepwise fashion, with a special and specific type of shaking occurring after each dilution. Scientific and mathematical analyses have determined that no molecules of the original substance are present in most preparations after the dilution process. However, homeopaths believe that the "essence" of the original substance remains because the water used in the dilutions has a "memory" of it and can therefore stimulate the body to heal itself. These basic principles, beliefs, and methods of homeopathy oppose the basic principles, understandings, and methods of science and evidence-based medicine.

A variety of products labeled "homeopathic medicine" can be found on drugstore shelves claiming "to reduce the duration and severity of flulike symptoms," "to shorten the duration of the common cold," or "for sinus pain, nasal congestion, sinus pressure, and headache pain." The "active ingredients" listed on the package are the substances used at the beginning of the dilution process and can be a single item, a few, or a long list. These substances come from plants, animals, or minerals.

Are these products safe, and are they effective? The National Center for Complementary and Alternative Medicine (NCCAM) of the National Institutes of Health (NIH) states that "there is little evidence to support homeopathy as an effective treatment for any specific condition." Edzard Ernst, physician and director of the Complementary Medicine Peninsula Medical School at the Universities of Exeter in the United Kingdom, agrees with this NCCAM assessment and notes, "Today, about 200 clinical trials of homeopathy are available. Collectively these data fail to provide good evidence that the clinical effects of homeopathic remedies are different from those of placebos." Placebos are sugar pills or sham therapies that often make patients feel better solely because of their belief that they are being given a helpful treatment.

Although the NCCAM notes that the side effects and risks of homeopathic products have not been well researched, it adds that most homeopathic products contain little to no active ingredients. Therefore, the NCCAM concludes that these products are likely safe but ineffective.

Dietary Supplements and Supplement Drops

Alongside homeopathic products in the cough/cold section of your local pharmacy, you will also find products labeled as "dietary supplements," or "supplement drops" for "immune support," to help combat or prevent colds or flu, or to calm your cough. Within the CAM classification framework, these products are considered biologically based treatments. They generally contain a variety of vitamins and minerals along with various herbal extracts. Garlic, echinacea, vitamin C, and zinc are among the dietary supplements often included in over-the-counter cold and flu remedies. The following sections describe the results of scientific research that has been conducted on these substances to determine their effectiveness to prevent and treat colds.

Garlic (Allium sativum)

Garlic is touted to have many and varied health benefits, including clearing acne, reducing high blood cholesterol, preventing cancer, and repelling mosquitoes. It is also said to have antimicrobial, antiviral, and anti-inflammatory properties, which work to relieve colds. Garlic contains various substances, such as sulfur-containing compounds, that could result in positive health effects when ingested.

Laboratory studies show that garlic appears to have some antiviral and antimicrobial properties. Few studies have been conducted on the effects of garlic on human health, however. Weak evidence shows that garlic may prevent occurrences of colds, but much more evidence is needed.

Echinacea

Extracts of the flowering plant *Echinacea* (eh-kih-NAY-sha) are used to make over-the-counter products claiming to reduce the severity and duration of colds and flu and prevent these upper respiratory infections when taken regularly. Results of studies with mice show that various compounds from echinacea appear to stimulate white blood cells, act against viruses, and help reduce inflammation, which lends credence to these claims. However, it is difficult to study the effects of echinacea products in humans because over-the-counter echinacea products differ greatly. Products are formulated from different species and parts of the plant, by using differing extraction processes, and by combining echinacea with other substances.

There is some evidence that echinacea preparations made of the above-ground parts of *Echinacea purpurea* (**Figure 14.C**) might shorten the duration or decrease the severity of symptoms of a cold when taken as soon as symptoms appear. There is no evidence to support its prolonged use for cold prevention, and its long-term safety has not been established. Side effects are reported infrequently. Well-designed studies are needed to confirm the effects of echinacea in humans and to characterize its active ingredients and mechanism of action.

Figure 14.C

Echinacea purpurea.

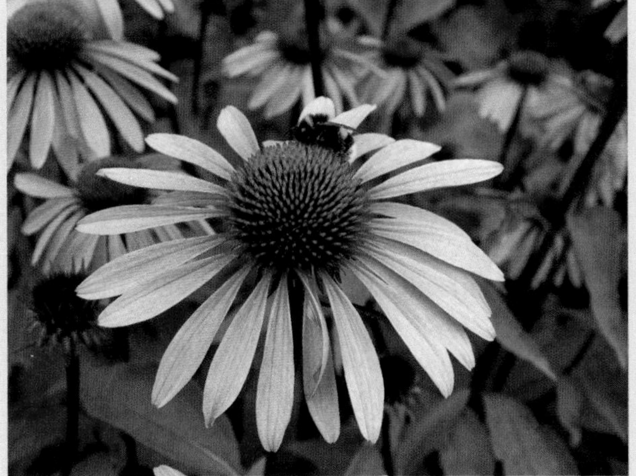

Vitamin C

Vitamin C is essential for good health, and most balanced diets provide a sufficient quantity. Eating a citrus fruit or drinking its juice along with having a serving of another vitamin-C-containing vegetable or fruit, such as broccoli, butternut squash, pineapple, or strawberries, is adequate to achieve the recommended dietary allowance. The tolerable upper limit to avoid side effects or toxicity is 2,000 milligrams (mg) per day. Although it is a water-soluble vitamin, which means that it dissolves in bodily fluids and the excess is flushed out in the urine, vitamin C can cause a variety of side effects, including diarrhea, heartburn, cramps, headache, and kidney stones if too much is ingested.

Among the many jobs it performs in the body, vitamin C enhances various functions of the immune system. Therefore, it has been used for the treatment of a variety of ills, including treating and preventing colds. Although taking vitamin C does not appear to prevent colds, regular vitamin C ingestion (200 mg/day, for example) might reduce the duration, and possibly the severity, of cold symptoms.

Zinc

Zinc is a mineral that is an essential part of the diet. It plays a variety of roles in metabolism and is involved in proper immune function. Zinc is stored in bone and skeletal muscle, but infection can cause a drop in normal blood levels of the mineral.

Zinc is sold in various forms including lozenges, tablets, capsules, and nasal sprays for the treatment of colds. Scientists hypothesize that zinc may compete for cold virus receptors in the lining of the nose, and this is the reasoning behind zinc nasal sprays. Put simply, if the cold virus receptors in the nose are saturated with zinc, the viruses cannot gain entry into the body.

According to results of recent studies, zinc-containing nasal sprays appear to shorten the duration of cold symptoms and lessen symptoms. However, a loss of smell—possibly a permanent loss—has been reported and appears to be a major roadblock to the study and use of zinc nasal sprays.

Along with competing for cold virus receptors in the lining of the nose, zinc also appears to inhibit the replication of the cold virus, which makes it an excellent candidate as a cold treatment when taken orally. A review of decades of scientific studies on the use of zinc as a treatment for colds concludes that zinc reduced the duration and severity of cold symptoms when taken within 24 hours of the onset of symptoms. Supplementation of the diet with zinc over a 5-month period also reduced the incidence of colds. Zinc lozenges, however, can produce undesirable side effects, such as stomach disturbances and diarrhea. Scientists are unable to make recommendations concerning which formulation of zinc might be used and how much might be taken and for how long for the possible prevention and treatment of colds.

Complementary and alternative products for the prevention and treatment of colds can differ dramatically from one another. In addition, the scientific evidence supporting their usefulness is often weak or absent. When evidence supporting the usefulness of a therapy becomes strong, it usually becomes accepted by the scientifically based (conventional) medical community and is no longer considered "alternative." Being an informed consumer will help you make the best choices for your health. Always check with your physician before taking any new medications or other treatments, including CAM products; they can react with medications you are already taking or have adverse effects of which you are unaware.

Reproduced from Sultan, M. T., et al. (2014). Immunity: Plants as effective mediators. *Critical Reviews in Food Science and Nutrition, 54*, 1298–1308.; Barrett, B., et al., & CRD. (2011). *Echinacea* for upper respiratory infection (structured abstract). *Cochrane Library Database of Abstracts of Reviews of Effects*, no. 2.; Dass, R. R., et al. (2014). Oral zinc for the common cold. *Journal of the American Medical Association, 311*(14), 1440–1441.; Ernst, E. (2011). Pharmacists and homeopathic remedies. *American Journal of Health-System Pharmacy, 68*, 478.; Hemila, H., et al. (2013). Vitamin C for preventing and treating the common cold. *Cochran Database Systematic Reviews, Cochrane Library*, no. 1.; Heimer, K. A., et al. (2009). Examining the evidence for the use of vitamin C in the prophylaxis and treatment of the common cold. *Journal of the American Academy of Nurse Practitioners, 21*, 295–300.; Allan, G., et al. (2014). Prevention and treatment of the common cold: Making sense of the evidence. *Canadian Medical Association Journal, 186*(3), 190–199.; National Center for Complementary and Alternative Medicine. (2013, May). Homeopathy: An introduction. National Institutes of Health. Retrieved April 29, 2011, from http://nccam.nih.gov/health/homeopathy/

harming its host. A few antiviral drugs treat infections caused by the herpesvirus (such as genital herpes, cold sores, and chicken pox) and others treat diseases associated with AIDS. Antiviral medications have been developed to control influenza (flu) infection.

Specific medications have also been developed to treat protozoal diseases such as malaria, amebic dysentery, and trichomoniasis. Likewise, prescription medicines are available to treat infestations of worms such as tapeworms and pinworms.

Sexually Transmitted Infections

Sexually transmitted infections (STIs), which are also called sexually transmitted diseases (STDs), are spread from person to person by the intimate contact that occurs during sexual activity, primarily vaginal intercourse and anal intercourse. In general, the pathogens that cause STIs are passed from the sores, secretions, or tissues of an infected individual's reproductive system to the mucous membranes or broken skin of the reproductive system and surrounding tissue of another. Infectious organisms can also be transferred from the mouth to the genitals and vice versa during oral sex.

Contracting a sexually transmitted infection is more likely when other STIs are present. For example, infection with the herpes simplex virus (HSV) or with syphilis has been shown to increase the risk of human immunodeficiency virus (HIV) transmission by as much as 10- to 100-fold for a single act of intercourse. Both HSV and syphilis cause sores on the genitals, which apparently facilitate the transfer of the human immunodeficiency virus.

Most pathogens that cause STIs cannot survive long (or at all) outside the human body. Therefore, most STIs cannot be contracted by genital contact with contaminated toilet seats or bed linens. Most STIs are passed directly from one person to another.

Some sexually transmitted infections are caused by yeasts, protozoans, mites (organisms closely related to spiders), and lice (organisms closely related to fleas). Most STIs are caused by bacteria and viruses.

Before you read more of this chapter, complete the "STI Attitude Scale" self-assessment in the Student Workbook pages at the end of this text. A high score on this assessment indicates a predisposition toward high-risk STI behavior. A low score indicates a predisposition toward low-risk STI behavior. This chapter can help you develop low-risk behaviors.

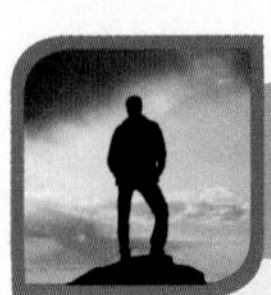

Healthy Living Practices

- To protect yourself and others against the transmission of sexually transmitted infections, use latex condoms during sexual intercourse.

Sexually Transmitted Infections Caused by Viruses

Sexually transmitted infections caused by viruses are extremely serious because they cannot be cured. Certain medications ease the discomfort of viral STI symptoms, but virus particles remain in the tissues and can cause recurrent symptoms. Also, the virus can be passed continually from chronically infected individuals to others during sexual activity.

In addition to causing STIs, three sexually transmitted viruses have been implicated in the development of particular cancers: HIV, human papillomavirus (HPV), and **hepatitis B virus (HBV)**. Therefore, contracting any one of these viruses not only results in an incurable infectious disease but also increases the risk of developing particular types of cancers. HPV is discussed later in this chapter. HBV causes a serious inflammation of the liver and can result in liver cancer. Although hepatitis is caused by a variety of hepatitis viruses (such as A, B, C, and D), hepatitis B virus is the one most commonly transmitted by sexual contact. Although hepatitis B is a serious and long-term disease, people can recover from it.

Human immunodeficiency virus is the most serious viral sexually transmitted pathogen. HIV infection not only raises the risk of developing the cancer Kaposi's sarcoma, but the virus also attacks the immune system, disabling the body's defenses. Eventually, the immune system of an HIV-infected individual becomes so weakened that he or she succumbs to an array of illnesses (the syndrome known as AIDS) that lead to death.

sexually transmitted infection (STI) Infection spread from person to person by intimate sexual contact, primarily anal or vaginal intercourse and oral sex.

hepatitis B virus (HBV) A serious infectious disease of the liver transmitted via blood or blood products.

Human Immunodeficiency Virus

As of January 1995, AIDS became the leading cause of death among Americans aged 25 to 44 years. By 1996 death rates from AIDS began to decline, by 1997 AIDS had dropped to the fifth leading cause of death in this age group, and by 2001 it was the sixth leading cause of death (**Figure 14.16**). In the United States, about three-fourths of new HIV infections each year occur in men.[9]

Since AIDS was first recognized in the early 1980s, the number of known deaths in all age groups in the United States increased annually through 1995.

Then, with the introduction of antiretroviral therapy, deaths declined from 1996 through 1998. Antiretroviral therapy uses combinations of medications to slow the replication (copying) of the AIDS virus and reduce its levels in the bloodstream. Deaths have leveled off since the decline (**Figure 14.17**).

The annual number of new AIDS cases increased steadily from 1984 until its dramatic increase in 1993. Much of the 1993 increase is to the result of a change in the definition of AIDS, which broadened the list of conditions reportable as AIDS and included measures of immune system function. Beginning in 1994, the annual number of new AIDS cases declined steadily through 2001. This decrease reflects, in part, the waning effect of the 1993 definition change. A slight decline occurred beginning in 2006 and extending through 2011.

Globally, HIV infection is a widespread epidemic disease. Approximately 35.3 million people were living with HIV in 2012. In that same year, approximately 2.3 million people became newly infected, and about 1.8 million died from HIV/AIDS.[10] The majority of new HIV infections occur in sub-Saharan Africa, a poor, developing part of the continent. Although

Figure 14.16

Leading Causes of Death Among Persons 25–44 Years of Age: United States, 1997–2007. Although AIDS was the leading cause of death in this age group in 1995, the graph shows that by 1997 AIDS had dropped to the fifth leading cause of death. By 2008, AIDS dropped to the seventh leading cause of death through 2011.

Reproduced from Centers for Disease Control and Prevention, National Center for Health Statistics. (2011, February). *Health, United States, 2011 With Special Feature on Death and Dying*. Retrieved from http://www.cdc.gov/nchs/data/hus/hus10.pdf

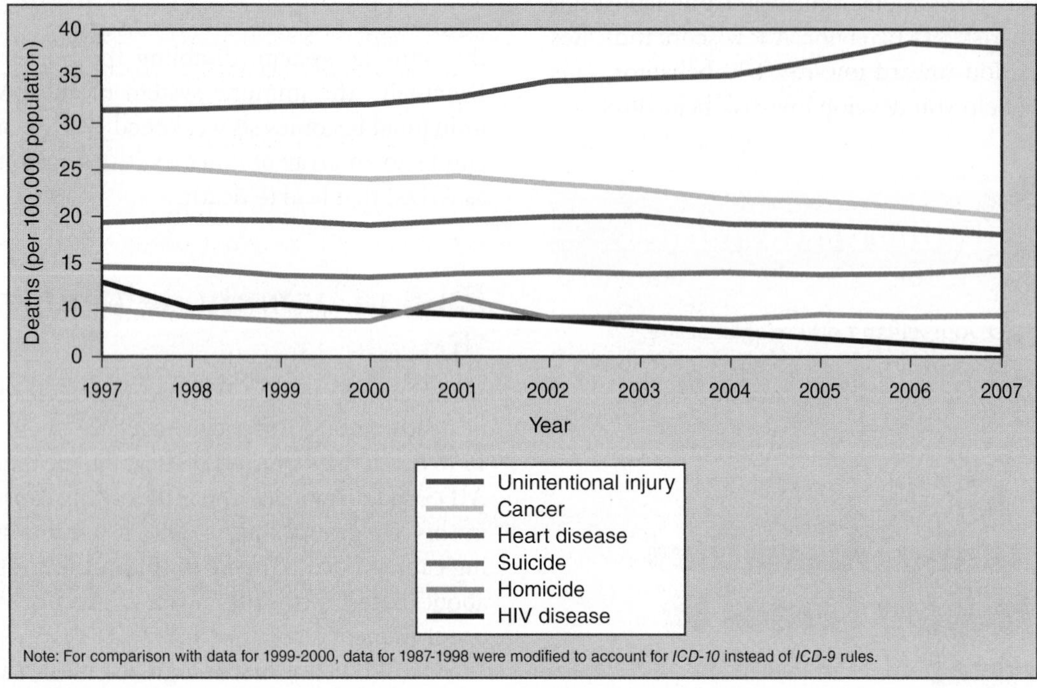

Figure 14.17

Reported Cases and Known Deaths from AIDS, United States, 1984–2010/11. The extreme rise in reported cases in 1993 is the result of a change in the definition of AIDS, which broadened the list of conditions reportable as AIDS and included measures of immune system function.

Data from National Center for Health Statistics, National Vital Statistics System. U.S. Department of Health and Human Services, Centers for Disease Control and Prevention.

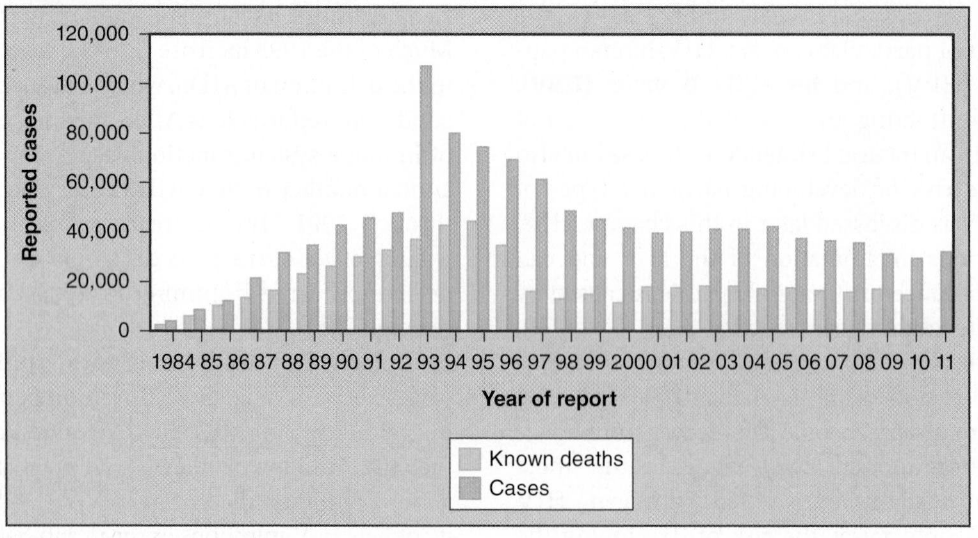

death rates from AIDS have not fallen as dramatically in developing regions of the world as they have in industrialized countries, they are falling somewhat because of antiretroviral therapy, which has finally become more available and affordable.

Overall, United Nations Programme on HIV/AIDS (UNAIDS) reports that the global AIDS epidemic has stabilized and the annual number of new HIV infections has been declining worldwide.

The Progression of the Disease: HIV Infection and AIDS Although medical researchers realized in 1981 that AIDS was a new disease, its cause (infection with human immunodeficiency virus) was not discovered until 1983. AIDS is a *syndrome*, a set of signs and symptoms occurring together. Being infected with HIV does not mean that a person has AIDS; infection leads to AIDS. Current data suggest that all infected individuals will develop AIDS eventually because HIV infection results in a continuous, prolonged, and ongoing disease process that still cannot be cured.

Approximately 1 to 3 weeks after becoming infected with HIV, most people experience a brief flulike illness that lasts for 1 to 2 weeks. During this stage of infection, people usually do not know that they are infected with HIV and think that they have a particularly bad case of the flu. When this initial illness subsides, the HIV-infected person seems to be healthy but is in the *asymptomatic phase* of HIV disease, which usually lasts about 8 to 10 years. (*Asymptomatic* means that no disease symptoms are apparent.) This time varies widely among individuals; it can be as short as a few months or longer than 10 years. During this time, many HIV-infected individuals do not realize that they are infected and may pass the virus on to others.

Although people with asymptomatic HIV infection may feel well, the virus is actively killing helper T cells in their bodies. Gradually, the number of helper T cells declines.

Although various laboratory tests can detect abnormalities in infected asymptomatic patients, these persons remain relatively symptom-free until they enter the *symptomatic phase* of HIV disease. The symptomatic phase usually begins when mature helper T cells (also called CD4 cells) have declined to about 500 cells (or fewer) per cubic millimeter of blood (500 cells/mm^3). The normal level is 800 to 1,200 helper T cells/mm^3. When the T cell count drops to 500/mm^3, the body begins to have trouble warding off infections that a normal, healthy body resists. These infections are called *opportunistic infections* because they are caused by organisms that normally cannot produce infections except in people with lowered resistance.

During this phase of disease, the HIV-infected individual experiences a tremendous array of signs and symptoms. Some of these are nonspecific; that is, they are not in response to any opportunistic infection. These nonspecific signs and symptoms include fever, night sweats, headache, and fatigue. Chronic diarrhea usually occurs as opportunistic organisms infect the digestive system. Also, the HIV-infected individual often contracts minor oral infections such as thrush, caused by the yeast *Candida albicans* (KAN-de-dah AL-bih-kanz) (**Figure 14.18**). These symptoms and infections of the symptomatic phase are not usually life threatening, but the infected individual has trouble maintaining the normal pace of his or her lifestyle.

As the helper T cell count declines further to about 200/mm^3, the rate of contracting serious opportunistic diseases increases. Common infections at this stage include *Pneumocystis carinii* pneumonia (a fungal infection of the lungs), *Cryptococcus* meningitis (a fungal infection of the coverings that surround the brain), toxoplasmosis (a protozoal infection of

Figure 14.18

Thrush, or Oral Candidiasis. This oral infection is caused by the yeast *Candida albicans* and is a common infection of the symptomatic stage of HIV infection. It can also occur in persons taking broad-spectrum drugs or medications that suppress the immune system. Infants can acquire the disease during birth from mothers with vaginal candidiasis.

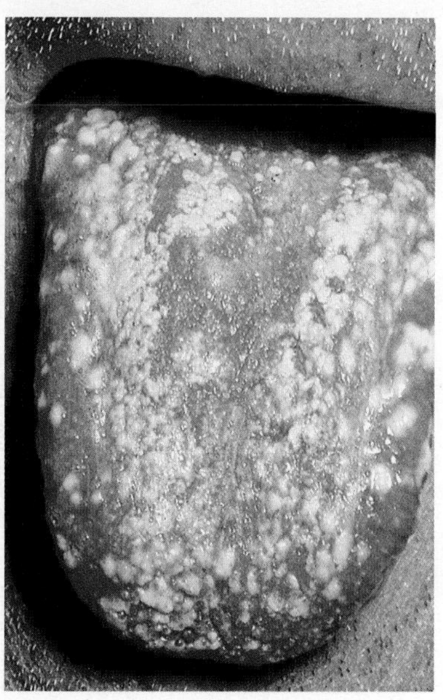

the brain, heart, and/or lungs), Kaposi's sarcoma (a type of cancer; **Figure 14.19**), and cytomegalovirus retinitis (a viral infection of the retina). A condition called *wasting syndrome* can also occur at this stage, which includes a marked loss of weight and a decrease in physical stamina, appetite, and mental activity. A person with HIV infection is usually diagnosed as having AIDS when the helper T cell count falls below 200/mm^3 and one of these conditions (or another condition typical of this stage) is present.

On average, if treated with antiretroviral therapy, people live about 22 years from their initial HIV diagnosis[11] and about 5 years with AIDS.[12] Again, the amount of time varies tremendously from individual to individual. But as the T cell count falls below 50/mm^3, the risk of death increases dramatically.

Figure 14.19

Kaposi's Sarcoma. Named after an Austrian dermatologist, this cancer is a serious, opportunistic disease of the HIV-infected person. It begins in the skin and metastasizes to the lymph nodes and body organs.

Courtesy of National Cancer Institute

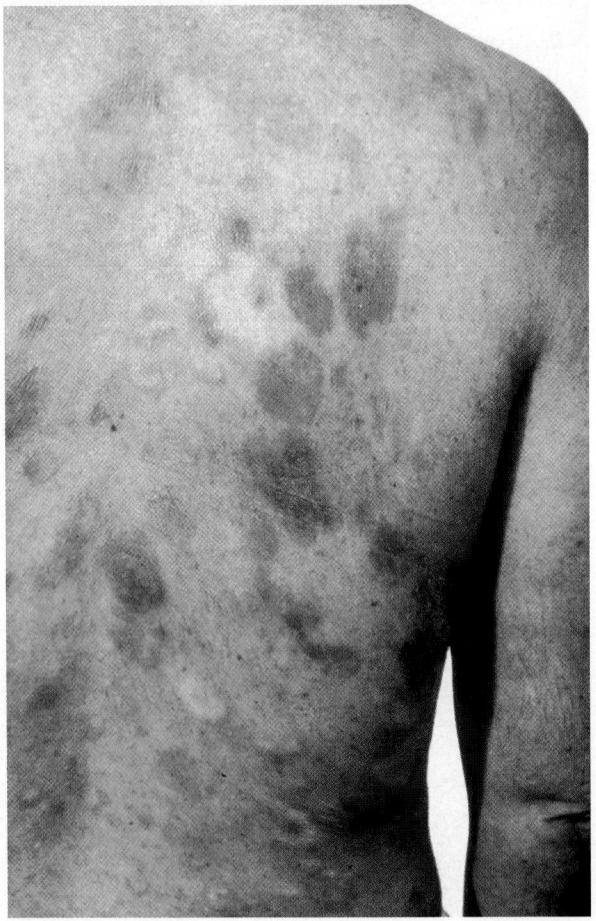

How HIV Is Transmitted Human immunodeficiency virus is transmitted in three ways: sexual contact with an infected person; exposure to infected blood or blood products; and placental transfer during fetal development, during labor and delivery, and during breastfeeding. These transmission routes are related in that, with the exception of breastfeeding, they all require the blood of the uninfected person to come into direct contact (or close contact, as in the case of placental transfer) with the blood, semen, or vaginal secretions of an infected person.

In 2011, approximately 56% of all HIV/AIDS cases diagnosed were men who had sex with men. One-fifth (13%) of cases were both men and women exposed through heterosexual sex.[13] Between 2008 and 2010, gay and bisexual men and adolescents accounted for 72% of new HIV infections for all people aged 13 to 24 years. Sexual behaviors that carry risk of HIV infection are unprotected anal intercourse between men and unprotected anal or vaginal intercourse between a man and a woman. However, any sexual behavior that results in the contact of infected blood, semen, or vaginal secretions with the blood of an uninfected individual is risky because it may result in HIV transmission. Because minor abrasions or tears in the skin and mucous membranes of the genitals often occur during sex without partners being aware of it, such contact may take place much more readily than might be thought. Another primary route of HIV transmission is the sharing of contaminated needles and syringes among injecting drug abusers.

Some children and adults with AIDS acquired the disease by receiving contaminated blood during blood transfusions. These incidents occurred before blood banks instituted HIV antibody testing. However, staff at U.S. blood banks use new, sterile needles and syringes with each person who donates blood so that donating blood never has been a risk and is not a risk now.

Most children with AIDS contracted it during the birth process from their infected mothers. The fetus is thought to become infected during labor contractions, after the rupture of the membranes, or while in the birth canal. Elective cesarean section is one way to prevent mother-to-child transfer of the virus during the birth process and does not always present higher risk than vaginal delivery for the mother.[14] An HIV-infected pregnant woman can also take the drug zidovudine (AZT) to decrease the chance of HIV being transmitted to her fetus.

Transmission of HIV also occurs via breastmilk. Therefore, women with HIV who live in industrialized countries such as the United States, where infant formula is available and safe, should not breastfeed their children.

How HIV Is Not Transmitted There is no need to worry about contracting HIV disease if you work, go to school, and come into casual contact with a person who is infected with HIV. People in certain professions, such as health professionals and police officers, are at some risk of HIV infection because they may come into contact with HIV-infected blood. The results of numerous studies show that HIV is not transmitted by sharing such things as telephones or drinking fountains. Likewise, living with an HIV-infected person and sharing personal items such as combs, towels, eating utensils, and dishes do not transmit the virus.

Although HIV has been detected in saliva, it does not appear to be transmitted by kissing, except in the remote chance of transfer during open-mouth, deep kissing with an infected person who has bleeding gums or other spots in the mouth.[15] HIV transmission can take place through oral sex, but the level of risk is lower than with vaginal or anal intercourse.[16] Transmission of the virus by mosquitoes or other insects does not occur.[17]

Protecting Yourself Against HIV Infection The primary means of protecting yourself against becoming infected with HIV is to avoid behaviors that put your blood in contact with the blood, semen, or vaginal secretions of an infected person. Abstaining from sex with infected individuals eliminates that particular risk of HIV infection. Engaging in sex in a mutually monogamous relationship in which neither partner is infected also eliminates that risk. HIV testing before engaging in sex can assure both of you that there is no risk of contracting the disease. Of course, both partners must *remain* monogamous throughout the relationship.

Unfortunately, sexual partners do not always know if a potential sexual partner is infected; also, the partner may be unaware of his or her own infection. Therefore, to reduce your risk of HIV infection, reduce your number of sexual partners. **Table 14.1** lists the characteristics of high-risk partners. Avoid casual sexual encounters (having sex with people you do not know well) so that you have time to evaluate whether potential partners have any of these characteristics.

Always use a latex condom or a polyurethane vaginal pouch (female condom) during each act of sexual intercourse. Both types of condoms provide a barrier between you and the body fluids of another. Never use a male condom and a female condom at the same time. The two materials may tear as they rub against one another and the condoms may not stay in place. Also, do not use contraceptives that contain the spermicide nonoxynol-9. Some contraceptives containing this chemical might increase the risk of transmission of HIV and other STIs.[18] Using a cut-open condom or a dental dam (a rectangular sheet of latex used in dentistry) as a physical barrier between the mouth and the genitals or anus during oral sex can reduce the likelihood of HIV or other STI transmission.[16]

Another risk factor for HIV infection is drug abuse of both injecting and noninjecting drugs. Eliminate this risk by abstaining from using drugs. Injecting drug abusers are primarily at risk because HIV-contaminated needles transmit the virus to anyone who shares the contaminated needles. Noninjecting drug abusers are also at an increased risk of contracting HIV because drug abusers engage in risky sexual behaviors while under the influence of drugs.

If you use drugs, you can reduce your risk of HIV infection by never sharing needles or syringes. If you do share needles and syringes, cleaning this equipment with bleach and then rinsing it with water will reduce your risk of infection. It is also best to avoid having sex while under the influence of drugs.

In summary, medical researchers have discovered the ways in which HIV is transmitted and the ways in

Table 14.1

People at High Risk for HIV Infection (United States)

People at High Risk for HIV Infection (United States)
Injecting drug users
People who have had sex with injecting drug users
Homosexual or bisexual men
Women who have had sex with bisexual men
People who received blood transfusions between 1978 and 1985
People with hemophilia
People who have another STI, particularly syphilis or herpes
Women from countries where heterosexual transmission is common (Latin America, the Caribbean, and Africa)

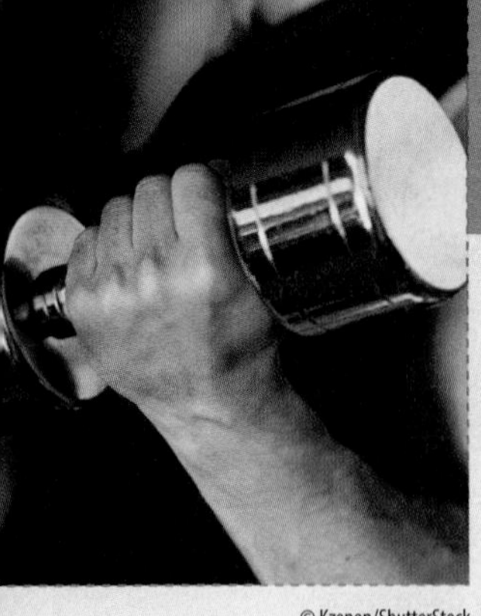
© Kzenon/ShutterStock

Managing Your Health

Eliminating or Reducing Your Risk of HIV Infection and Other STIs

How to Eliminate Your Risk of Becoming Infected with HIV or Other STIs

Abstain from sex. If that is not an option:

- Avoid having sex with HIV-infected individuals or those infected with any STI.
- Engage in sex only in a monogamous relationship in which it is certain that neither partner is infected.
- Abstain from using drugs.

Note: People in certain professions, such as healthcare workers and police officers, have additional risks of infection because of the nature of their work. Such risks are not eliminated by these practices. These people can become infected with hepatitis B virus or HIV if their blood mixes with the blood or bodily secretions of an infected person.

How to Reduce Your Risk of Becoming Infected with HIV or Other STIs

- Limit your number of sexual partners.
- Avoid having sex with high-risk partners.
- Avoid having sex with people you do not know well.
- Avoid having sex while under the influence of drugs, including alcohol.
- Use a new latex condom during each act of anal or vaginal intercourse.
- Never share needles or syringes.
- Do not use contraceptives containing the spermicide nonoxynol-9.
- Use a cut-open condom or a dental dam during oral sex.

which it is not. This information was used to develop the lists shown in the Managing Your Health box "Eliminating or Reducing Your Risk of HIV Infection and Other STIs." One list summarizes the behaviors that virtually eliminate your risk of HIV infection and the other summarizes the behaviors that reduce your risk.

Treatment of HIV Infection There is no cure for HIV infection and AIDS. Thus far, attempts to develop an effective vaccine to protect against HIV infection have been unsuccessful. Because of the variability of the virus, developing an effective HIV vaccine is extremely difficult. It is unlikely that a vaccine will be available before 2020.[19]

Researchers are continually working on ways to treat HIV infection by boosting the immune system, inactivating the virus, or protecting immune system cells from infection. All approved anti-HIV drugs interfere with viral replication. However, the virus becomes immune to the drugs quite quickly as it mutates. Therefore, combinations of drugs appear to work best to retard HIV.

AIDS researchers consider a lifelong drug regimen referred to as ART (antiretroviral therapy; also called HAART [highly active antiretroviral therapy]) as the best treatment for HIV/AIDS. ART combines three or more HIV drugs that suppress HIV replication. Researchers have found that the concentration of HIV in the bloodstream of some patients declines to undetectable levels with ART treatment. When HIV is suppressed, the concentration of mature helper T cells (CD4 cells) rises. HIV-infected patients who respond in this way to ART treatment may have their CD4 cell concentrations return to normal levels with long-term ART treatment. Although ART is extending the lives of AIDS patients, it has serious side effects with long-term use, including cardiovascular problems and bone demineralization.

ART may be used to prevent HIV; it appears to reduce susceptibility to infection in HIV-uninfected individuals. A vaginal gel incorporating the antiretroviral drug tenofovir has also shown promising results in reducing the rate of HIV transmission. The gel is still under study and not yet approved for use in the United States.[20]

Another promising area of research in the treatment of HIV/AIDS is *gene therapy*. In this approach, the HIV-infected cells of an AIDS patient are replaced with cells engineered to resist virus replication. Progress has been slow, but the results of clinical trials suggest that this approach may be useful.[21]

genital herpes An STI caused by the herpes simplex virus that results in sores in the genital and anal areas.

Genital Herpes

Genital herpes (herpes simplex virus-2; HSV-2) is another STI that many people fear contracting because it is painful and incurable. When asked, "Do you worry about contracting an STI?" one health student responded: "I am really worried about getting herpes. Once you have it, you can't get rid of it. That's scary!"

The herpes "scare" began in the United States in the 1970s, and the number of initial visits to doctors' offices for concerns about HSV-2 has increased since then as **Figure 14.20** shows. Because HSV-2 is not a disease that must be reported to the CDC, epidemiologists (medical researchers who study such topics as the spread of disease) use data such as visits to doctors' offices and the results of blood tests to estimate its prevalence. (Reportable STIs are gonorrhea, syphilis, chlamydia, and chanchroid, a disease that is rare in most parts of the United States and is not discussed in this chapter.) CDC data show that the prevalence of HSV-2 based on the number of the persons aged 14–49 years who tested positive for the virus has decreased in the past 2 decades or so, from 21% in years 1988–1994 to 16.2% in years 2009–2012. The CDC notes, however, that "most persons with HSV-2 have not received a diagnosis," and that the increase in the number of doctor visits "may indicate increased recognition of infection."[22]

Like all STIs, HSV-2 is contracted through vaginal and anal intercourse with an infected individual. In addition, HSV-1 (which causes cold sores/fever blisters in the mouth) can infect the genital and anal areas during oral sex, and HSV-2 can infect the mouth. Either virus gains a foothold in the body by first infecting the skin cells in the immediate area of contact and spreading to surrounding cells. During an incubation period (the time between exposure to the pathogen and the onset of symptoms) that lasts about a week, the virus begins to replicate and destroy skin cells. The patient may experience irritation at these sites of infection prior to the eruption of skin lesions. The first lesions appear as groups of tiny, raised, solid bumps that turn clear or yellowish and become filled with fluid. These blisters eventually break open, oozing fluid containing viruses, and then develop into painful sores. The sores turn gray, crust over, and heal usually in 5 to 10 days. With this initial infection, the patient often experiences a headache, fever, weakness, and muscle pain.

HSV-2 usually infects the labia, vagina, and cervix in women and the penis in males, but it can also infect tissues in the genital/anal area that are not protected by a condom. Therefore, the use of latex condoms can only *reduce* the risk of herpes transmission; it does not eliminate the risk for neighboring tissues. The tenofovir vaginal gel being tested to reduce HIV transmission has been shown to reduce transmission of HSV as well.[20] Follow the practices outlined in the section "Protecting Yourself Against STIs" (later in this chapter).

Transmission of HSV occurs when the infected tissues of a person who is shedding virus come in contact with the mucous membranes or with small cracks in the skin in the genital, anal, or oral areas of another. A person sheds virus when the virus is present in the skin cells, usually just prior to the appearance of sores and when they first appear. Often, a person shedding virus is unaware of this danger; he or she may have no symptoms of disease at the time. The sexual partners of a person shedding virus may

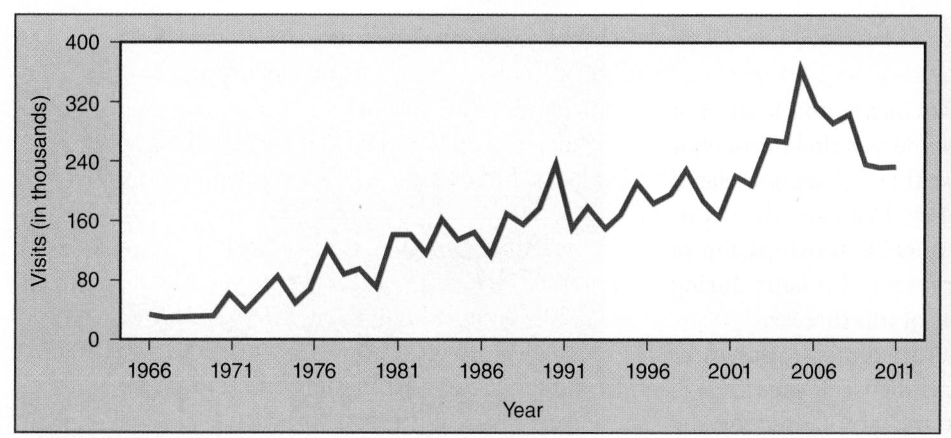

Figure 14.20

Genital Herpes—Initial Visits to Physicians' Offices, United States, 1966–2012.

Reproduced from Centers for Disease Control and Prevention. (2014, January). Sexually transmitted disease surveillance 2012. Retrieved from http://www.cdc.gov/sTD/stats12/Surv2012.pdf

genital warts An STI caused by the human papillomavirus that results in noncancerous skin tumors of the genital area.

not see sores or other indications that their partner is infected.

When the sores heal, the herpes infection is not cured—the virus is establishing itself in the nervous system for life. The virus particles enter the nerve endings in the area of infection and move up these nerves until they are close to the base of the spinal cord. There, the virus particles lie dormant. During the dormant phase, the infected person shows no signs or symptoms of herpes and is not shedding the virus.

From time to time, the virus becomes reactivated. Researchers are unsure about the exact mechanisms of reactivation, but infected individuals appear to have triggers that initiate a recurrence of infection. Common triggers are stress, lack of sleep, and menstruation. During a recurrence, the virus descends along the nerves close to the areas of original infection. No symptoms may be present, but the person sheds virus and can infect others during this time. Often, skin lesions appear, but these sores are not usually as painful nor do they last as long as during the initial infection. Most individuals experience five to eight recurrences per year. However, treatment with the drug acyclovir reduces the recurrence rate dramatically. Some persons have no recurrences for as long as 2 years. No vaccine is currently available to protect against HSV-2. A recent vaccine trial failed; however, two clinical trials are currently in progress with positive initial results.[23,24]

Herpesvirus can also infect newborns as they pass through the cervical opening and vagina of a mother with an active infection. Infected newborns may die or suffer damage to their nervous systems. In cases of active maternal infection, cesarean section (delivering the baby surgically, by cutting through the abdominal wall and the uterus) is often recommended.

Genital Warts

Genital warts (*Condylomata acuminata*) are not painful, unlike the sores of herpes infection, but some of the viruses that cause this STI are associated with the development of cervical cancer. This association with cancer and the possible transmission of this disease to the respiratory tract of infants during birth are the gravest concerns of this disease.

Warts are noncancerous skin tumors, masses of cells that result from uncontrolled cell growth. All warts are called *papillomas* and are caused by the *human papillomavirus* (PAP-ih-LOW-mah-vigh-rus) (HPV). However, there are more than 60 types of papillomaviruses (named HPV-1, HPV-2, and so on); each affects only certain areas of the body.

About 40 types of HPV can infect the genital tract, but visible genital warts are usually caused by HPV-6 and HPV-11. These viruses cause warts particularly in the cervical, vaginal, and vulvar areas in women and various parts of the penis in men. They can also infect the urethra and anal areas in both sexes (**Figure 14.21**). The HPV types that infect the genital area but do not result in the growth of warts cause tissue changes that a physician usually can see by using special techniques. Some of these viruses, particularly HPV-16 and HPV-18, are associated with cancer of the cervix and less often with cancer of the vulva and penis. The American Cancer Society recommends that women have regular Papanicolaou tests (Pap smears) to detect atypical, precancerous, or cancerous cells within the cervix and that men consider having any abnormal tissue growth in the genital area microscopically examined for the presence of cancer. In addition, the HPV DNA test, which is used along with the Pap test, can determine whether a woman is infected with one of the 13 high-risk types of HPV.

Healthcare professionals are not required to report cases of genital warts to the CDC, so data are collected on initial visits to physicians' offices to receive medical care for this STI, as shown in **Figure 14.22**. The number of initial visits for warts fell from 1987 to 1997 but has been rising since then. In 2012, the number of initial visits to physicians' offices for genital warts was slightly above that for herpes.

Figure 14.21

***Condylomata acuminata* (Genital Warts).** These warts are growing around the anus of a man, nearly obscuring that opening.

Courtesy Dr. Wiesner/CDC

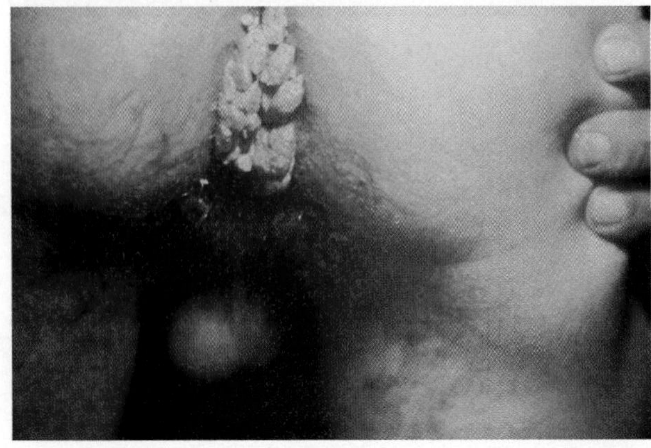

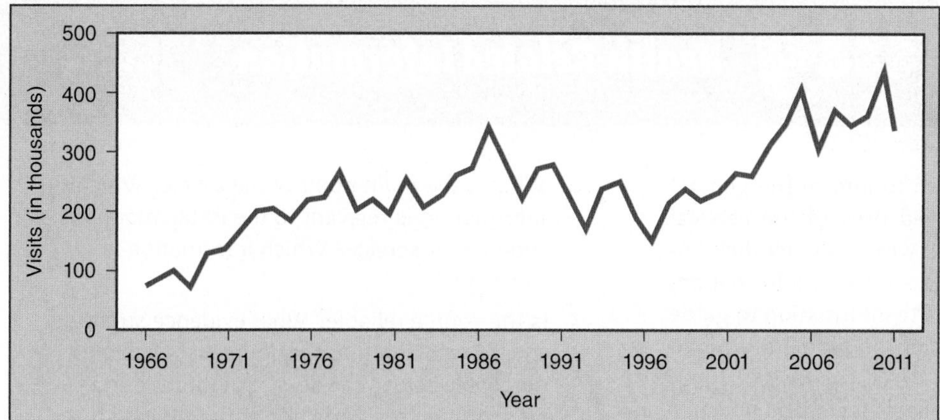

Figure 14.22

Genital Warts—Initial Visits to Physicians' Offices, United States, 1966–2012.

Reproduced from Centers for Disease Control and Prevention. (2014, January). Sexually transmitted disease surveillance 2012. Retrieved from http://www.cdc.gov/sTD/stats12/Surv2012.pdf

To avoid infection with this cancer-causing virus, follow the precautions in "Protecting Yourself Against STIs." Remember, however, that HPV, like genital herpes, can infect genital and anal tissue that is not protected by a condom. Additionally, because skin-to-skin contact can transmit HPV, infection can occur even if anal or vaginal intercourse does not take place. Transmission is also possible during oral sex, so a person with genital HPV could infect the lips, tongue, or palate of an uninfected sexual partner.

Adults as well as infants can develop warts on the larynx, or voice box, if the virus is breathed in. Furthermore, infants may acquire such infections from an infected mother during the birth process.

Although genital warts may go away on their own, the virus particles may remain in the tissue and can reactivate and infect others. These warts may also persist, grow larger, and spread. The removal of genital warts involves applying medications to the skin that break down the wart tissue, freezing them with liquid nitrogen, cauterizing (burning) them, or treating them with carbon dioxide lasers. Treatment for hard-to-remove warts involves the injection of the antiviral agent alpha-interferon directly into the tumorous growths. If you contract genital warts, you may want to discuss the benefits and drawbacks of various treatments with your physician. Many treatments are far more painful than the warts, interferon treatments can be costly, and medical researchers are unsure whether treatment to remove warts reduces the risk of transmission.

In June 2006, the U.S. Food and Drug Administration (FDA) approved a new vaccine (Gardasil) that protects against four major types of HPV: HPV-16 and HPV-18 that cause about 70% of cervical cancers and HPV-6 and HPV-11 that cause about 90% of genital warts. The vaccine is recommended for adolescent girls who have not yet had sex because they have not yet been exposed to HPV. Once infection with a type of HPV occurs, the vaccine cannot protect against it. A girl's or young woman's physician is the best person to determine whether she should be vaccinated. In 2009, the FDA expanded the approval of Gardasil for use in boys and young men to prevent genital warts and approved a second HPV vaccine (Cervarix), which acts against HPV-16 and HPV-18 only.[25] See the following Analyzing Health-Related Information feature for more information on another approved use of Gardasil.

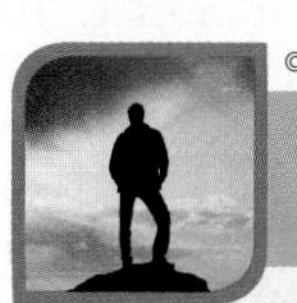

Healthy Living Practices

- To virtually eliminate your risk of contracting HIV infection, do not have sex with infected persons or share needles and syringes.
- To reduce your risk of contracting HIV, use a new latex condom with each act of sexual intercourse.
- Adolescent girls and young women, and boys and young men, should consult with their physician to determine whether they should receive an HPV vaccine.

Sexually Transmitted Infections Caused by Bacteria

In contrast to viral STIs, bacterial STIs can be cured with treatment. Nevertheless, bacterial infections can be quite serious. If not treated, or not treated promptly and properly, bacterial STIs can damage

Analyzing Health-Related Information

Critical Thinking

© tele52/ShutterStock

The following article was written to inform the general public about additional approved uses of the cervical cancer vaccine Gardasil. Explain why you think this article is a reliable or an unreliable source of information. Use the model for analyzing health information to guide your thinking; the main points of the model are noted here.

1. Which statements are verifiable facts, and which are unverified statements or value claims?
2. What are the credentials of the source making these health-related claims? Does the source have the appropriate background and education in the topic area? What can you do to check the credentials of this source?
3. What might be the motives and biases of the source making the claims?
4. What is the main point of the article? Which information is relevant to the issue, main point, product, or service? Which information is irrelevant?
5. Is the source reliable? What evidence supports your conclusion that the source is reliable or unreliable? Does the source of information present the pros and cons of the topic or the benefits and risks of the product?
6. Does the source of information attack the credibility of conventional scientists or medical authorities?

Based on your analysis, do you think that this article is a reliable source of health-related information? Summarize your reasons for coming to this conclusion.

Gardasil Approved to Prevent Anal Cancer

FDA Press Office

The U.S. Food and Drug Administration today approved the vaccine Gardasil for the prevention of anal cancer and associated precancerous lesions due to human papillomavirus (HPV) types 6, 11, 16, and 18 in people ages 9 through 26 years.

Gardasil is already approved for the same age population for the prevention of cervical, vulvar, and vaginal cancer and the associated precancerous lesions caused by HPV types 6, 11, 16, and 18 in females. It is also approved for the prevention of genital warts caused by types 6 and 11 in both males and females.

"Treatment for anal cancer is challenging; the use of Gardasil as a method of prevention is important as it may result in fewer diagnoses and the subsequent surgery, radiation or chemotherapy that individuals need to endure," said Karen Midthun, M.D., director of the FDA's Center for Biologics Evaluation and Research.

Although anal cancer is uncommon in the general population, the incidence is increasing. HPV is associated with approximately 90% of anal cancer. The American Cancer Society estimates that about 5,300 people are diagnosed with anal cancer each year in the United States, with more women diagnosed than men.

Gardasil's ability to prevent anal cancer and the associated precancerous lesions [anal intraepithelial neoplasia (AIN) grades 1, 2, and 3] caused by anal HPV-16/18 infection was studied in a randomized, controlled trial of men who self-identified as having sex with men (MSM). This population was studied because it has the highest incidence of anal cancer. At the end of the study period, Gardasil was shown to be 78% effective in the prevention of HPV 16– and 18–related AIN. Because anal cancer is the same disease in both males and females, the effectiveness data was used to support the indication in females as well.

Gardasil will not prevent the development of anal precancerous lesions associated with HPV infections already present at the time of vaccination. For all of the indications for use approved by the FDA, Gardasil's full potential for benefit is obtained by those who are vaccinated prior to becoming infected with the HPV strains contained in the vaccine.

Individuals recommended for anal cancer screening by their healthcare provider should not discontinue screening after receiving Gardasil.

As of May 31, 2010, more than 65 million doses of Gardasil had been distributed worldwide, since its approval in 2006 according to the manufacturer, Merck and Co. Inc, of Whitehouse Station, N.J. The most commonly reported adverse events include fainting, pain at the injection site, headache, nausea, and fever. Fainting is common after injections and vaccinations, especially in adolescents. Falls after fainting may sometimes cause serious injuries, such as head injuries. This can be prevented by keeping the vaccinated person seated for up to 15 minutes after vaccination. This observation period is also recommended to watch for severe allergic reactions, which can occur after any immunization.

Source: Food and Drug Administration. (2010, December 22). FDA news release. Retrieved October 13, 2011, from http://www.fda.gov/NewsEvents/Newsroom/PressAnnouncements/ucm237941.htm

the reproductive system, possibly resulting in infertility. Some diseases such as syphilis can cause even more devastating health effects. Therefore, it is crucial to seek medical attention immediately if you suspect that you are infected and to refrain from sex to avoid transmitting the disease to others.

syphilis (SIF-ih-lis) An STI that can progress from skin sores to more generalized symptoms (e.g., weight loss and muscle pain) to life-threatening, tissue-destroying skin abnormalities.

Syphilis

For centuries, **syphilis**, a serious STI caused by the bacterium *Treponema pallidum* (TREP-oh-NEE-mah PAL-ih-dum), has been a dreaded disease. Historically, the infection rate of syphilis reached a peak in the United States at the end of World War II. Physicians were soon able to demonstrate the effectiveness of the antibiotic penicillin against the syphilis bacterium. Although syphilis is not as prevalent as it once was, its incidence increased in the late 1980s, declined dramatically through 2000, and increased overall from 2001 to 2009, as **Figure 14-23** shows. The increases between 2001 and 2009 were primarily among men who have sex with men. Female infection rates dropped from 2001 to 2003 and then remained relatively steady through 2009. The male-to-female rate ratio (see Figure 14-23) was about 6 to 1 in 2009. Syphilis remains an important problem in the South and in some urban areas in other regions of the country.[22]

An individual can contract syphilis by having sex with a person who has sores caused by *T. pallidum*. These bacteria enter the body through a break in the skin of an uninfected person. Some syphilis bacteria remain in the skin at the site of entry, where a dime-sized sore called a chancre forms. Some of these bacteria move to the lymph nodes.

The incubation period for syphilis is about 3 weeks. The first sign of the disease is a chancre, which is characteristic of the first stage of syphilis, *primary syphilis*. Most often this sore appears in the genital or anal areas, but it can occur on the lips, tongue, breast, or fingers. The chancre first appears as a dull, red, flat spot, but becomes raised and then ulcerates. **Figure 14-24** is a photograph of a chancre on the penis. Although it looks as though it would be extremely painful, a chancre does not hurt. If untreated, a chancre usually heals in 3 to 6 weeks. During that time, however, *T. pallidum* is multiplying in the body; the disease is not gone.

After the chancre heals, the signs and symptoms of *secondary syphilis* appear. These symptoms are throughout the body because the bloodstream has distributed the bacteria to most of the tissues. Common symptoms of secondary syphilis are sore throat, weakness, headache, weight loss, fever, and muscle pain. In some patients, wartlike growths develop in moist areas of the body such as the genital region and under the arms. Most persons develop a rash that covers the body—even the soles of the feet. Although the appearance of this rash varies from person to person, it is often scaly.

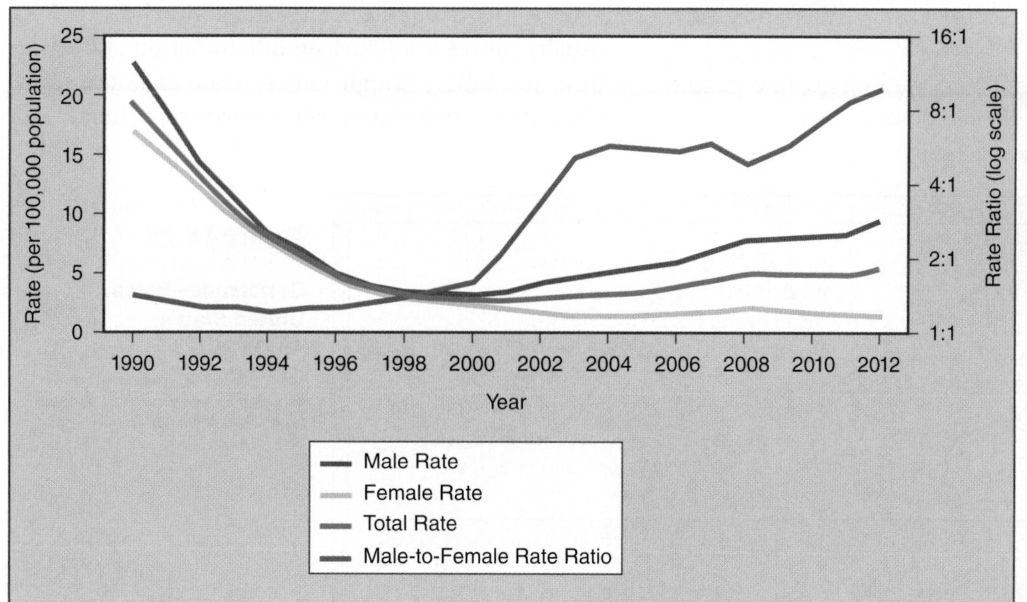

Figure 14.23

Primary and Secondary Syphilis—Rates by Sex and Male-to-Female Rate Ratios, United States, 1990–2012.

Reproduced from Centers for Disease Control and Prevention. (2014, January). Sexually transmitted disease surveillance 2012. Retrieved from http://www.cdc.gov/sTD/stats12/Surv2012.pdf

gonorrhea (GON-ah-REE-ah) An STI characterized by infection of the urethra in men and the cervix in women, usually resulting in a thick discharge from the penis or vagina.

Figure 14.24

A Syphilitic Chancre of the Penis. These painless sores can occur on the genital or anal areas, lips, tongue, breast, or fingers. They are characteristic of the first stage of syphilis.

Courtesy of Dr. N. J. Fiumara/CDC.

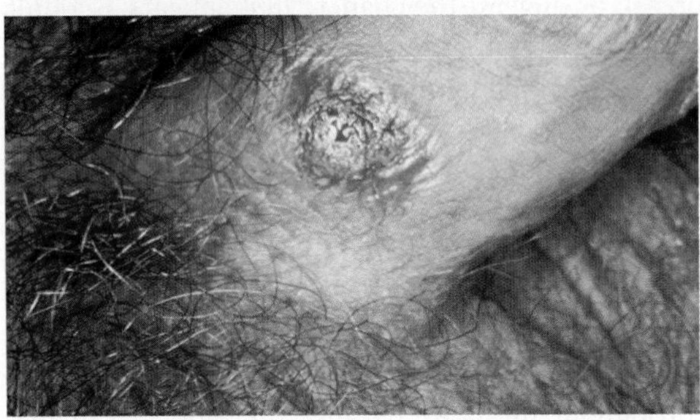

When the symptoms of secondary syphilis subside, the infected person is said to be in *latent syphilis*. He or she has no outward signs of disease but is still infected. This stage may last a lifetime, or the infected individual may enter *tertiary syphilis*. During the tertiary stage of infection, tissue-destroying lesions called *gummas* develop. Gummas not only affect the skin but can destroy any type of tissue in the body—even bones. This stage of syphilis is, therefore, often disfiguring. If the tissues of the heart, major blood vessels, or brain are destroyed, paralysis and death can result.

Since the introduction of antibiotics, few people with syphilis in the United States reach this stage of the disease. Most people are given antibiotics for various infectious diseases over a period of years; even if they are not treated specifically for syphilis, the administration of penicillin for any reason will kill *T. pallidum*. Nevertheless, approximately 40–50 people each year die in the United States as a result of untreated tertiary syphilis.

Unfortunately, the syphilis bacterium can cross the placenta during pregnancy, infecting the fetus. Infants infected with *T. pallidum* are born with a wide variety of serious conditions, such as bone deformities, low birth weight, lung damage, brain damage, deafness, and blindness. In addition, the infant can be infected during birth or after birth by coming into contact with the mother's lesions.

Gonorrhea

The incidence of gonorrhea declined dramatically between 1975 and 1996, remained relatively stable through 2006, and declined through 2009; however, a slight increase was seen between 2009 and 2012 (**Figure 14.25**). In 2012, the age group with the highest prevalence of gonorrhea infection was young men and women aged 15 to 29 years.[22] This fact is worrisome to health officials because gonorrhea can cause irreversible damage to the reproductive tract.

Gonorrhea is caused by tiny, spherical bacteria called *Neisseria gonorrhoeae* (neye-SEE-ree-ah GON-ah-REE-ah) that enter the body via the mucous membranes. The bacteria infect primarily the urethra in men and the cervix in women. Therefore, condoms are an excellent measure to prevent gonorrhea because they protect these areas well.

The incubation period of gonorrhea is from 2 to 8 days. In men, infection with gonorrhea bacteria usually causes urethritis, an inflammation of the urethra, the tube through which urine exits the body. Urethritis is also commonly known as a urinary tract

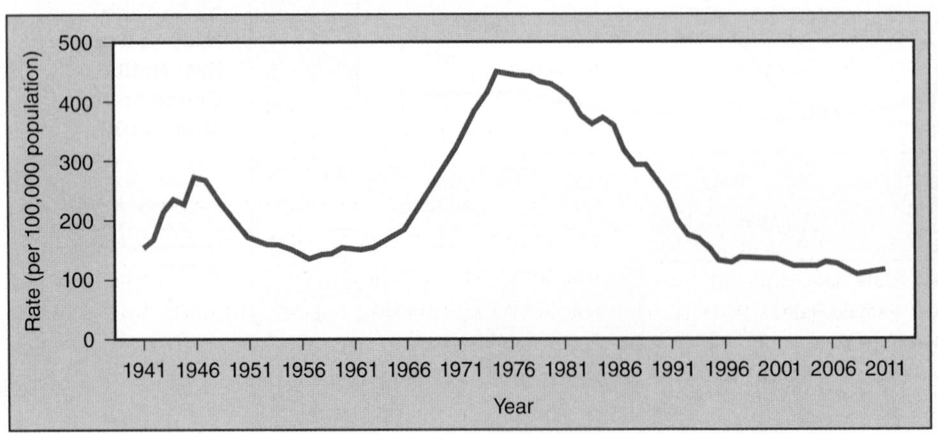

Figure 14.25

Gonorrhea—Rates, United States, 1941–2012.

Reproduced from Centers for Disease Control and Prevention. (2014, January). Sexually transmitted disease surveillance 2012. Retrieved from http://www.cdc.gov/sTD/stats12/Surv2012.pdf

chlamydial (klah-MID-dee-ahl) infection An STI that results in gonorrhea-like symptoms.

Figure 14.26

Pus-Containing Discharge from the Penis as a Result of Gonorrhea.

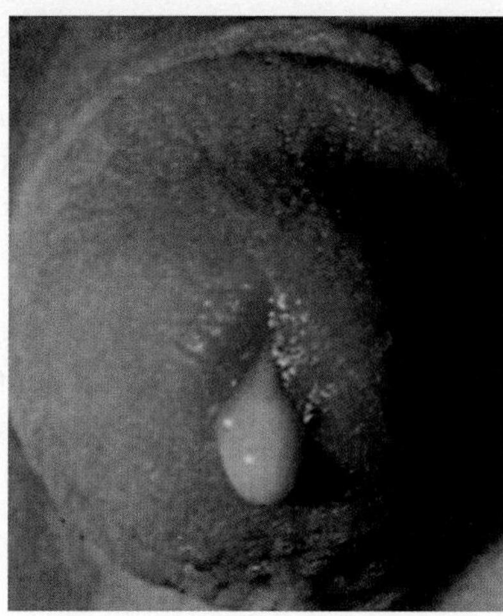

infection (UTI). A UTI caused by the gonorrhea bacterium results in a pus-containing discharge from the urethra (**Figure 14.26**). (Pus is a thick fluid made up of tissue fluid, white blood cells, dead microorganisms, and dead body cells.) The infected male then experiences painful urination and an urgency to urinate. Most men seek attention quickly because of these symptoms, but if untreated, within several weeks to several months their body's natural defenses will suppress the infection. Until an infection is suppressed, however, a man can spread it to his sexual partners.

Gonorrhea infection in females may cause urethritis, but it more commonly causes inflammation of the cervix and uterus, resulting in a pus-containing vaginal discharge, uterine bleeding, and abnormally long and heavy menstrual periods.

The bacteria can infect the prostate, epididymis, and seminal vesicles in males. Although infection of these male reproductive structures is rare, it does occur and can result in sterility. Women are more prone to widespread infection of the reproductive tract than are men. Infection of the uterine (fallopian) tubes or other female reproductive organs is called *pelvic inflammatory disease (PID)*.

Gonorrhea is the most common cause of PID, a serious, painful condition. Its symptoms are lower abdominal pain, pain during sexual intercourse, abnormal menstrual periods, bleeding between periods, and sometimes fever. Often, the uterine tubes become constricted from infection, resulting in sterility or in ectopic pregnancy. An *ectopic pregnancy* occurs when a fertilized egg implants outside of the uterus, most often in a uterine tube. Ectopic pregnancies are extremely serious situations. Abscesses (collections of pus) on the pelvic organs are also complications of PID and may require a hysterectomy, an operation to remove some or all of a woman's reproductive organs.

Another complication of gonorrhea is that the eyes of newborns can become infected with *N. gonorrhoeae* during birth if the mother is infected. If untreated, blindness may occur. For this reason, the eyes of all newborns in the United States are treated with antibiotic ointment or silver nitrate immediately after birth.

Gonorrhea can be treated with a variety of antibiotics. In recent years, many antibiotic-resistant strains of bacteria have emerged, sometimes making treatment difficult. However, laboratory testing of the particular strain can determine the most effective antibiotic to administer. Although gonorrhea is curable, reinfections are possible.

Chlamydial Infections

Chlamydia trachomatis (klah-MID-dee-ah trah-ko-MA-tiss) causes **chlamydial infections**, which are similar to gonorrhea. The bacteria that cause both STIs infect mucous membranes in the genital area, primarily infecting the urethra in males and the urethra and cervix in females. The symptoms of both infections are similar, and both organisms can travel throughout the reproductive tract to spread infection. Both can cause PID in women. One difference is that the incubation period for gonorrhea is from 2 to 8 days and that of chlamydial infections is from 2 to 3 weeks.

Chlamydia is the most frequently reported STI in the United States and its rate is increasing, as **Figure 14.27** shows. One reason for its prevalence is that infection with the organism causes only mild symptoms or no symptoms in most people. Therefore, many infected people transmit the disease unknowingly to their sexual partners. This disease is important to diagnose, however, because women with silent chlamydial infections are at a high risk for developing more serious illness such as PID, and they can transmit the infection to their children during birth. Men rarely develop serious disease from *C. trachomatis* infection, but men with undiagnosed infection continue to transmit the organism to women.

***T. vaginalis* infection** An STI caused by a protozoan, resulting in infection of the urethra in men and of the urethra and walls of the vagina in women.

The symptoms of chlamydial infection in men are painful urination and a whitish or clear discharge from the urethra. The amount of discharge and the level of pain are usually much milder than with gonorrheal infections, so men tend to wait longer to seek treatment than with gonorrheal infections. Occasionally, *C. trachomatis* travels to other parts of the male reproductive tract and causes epididymitis, an inflammation of the epididymides, tubules located on the back of the testes in which sperm mature. This bacterium also infects the rectum in people who engage in anal sex.

Some women develop urethritis when they are infected with *C. trachomatis*. Most often, the main site of female infection is the cervix, and a vaginal discharge may occur.

One of the most serious consequences of infection with chlamydia is pelvic inflammatory disease. No matter which organism causes it, PID has similar symptoms and can result in sterility or ectopic pregnancy, even though chlamydia causes less painful infection than other organisms such as *N. gonorrhoeae*.

Babies born to mothers with chlamydial infections not only can develop serious eye infections but their lungs can become infected also. Chlamydial pneumonia in a newborn can cause long-term damage to the lungs, which affects lung function throughout childhood.

Chlamydia trachomatis infections are treated with various antibiotics. The CDC suggests using latex condoms to reduce the risk of contracting chlamydial infections and following suggestions such as those in the section entitled "Protecting Yourself Against STIs."

Other Sexually Transmitted Infections

Organisms other than bacteria and viruses also cause sexually transmitted infections. The itch mite (a close relative of spiders) and the pubic louse (a close relative of fleas) cause sexually transmitted *infestations*, conditions in which these organisms live on the skin in the genital area. The yeast *Candida albicans* causes an infection of the genital tract, primarily in women, that can be acquired sexually or in nonsexual ways. *Trichomonas vaginalis*, a protozoan (a single-celled organism much more complex than a bacterium), causes an infection of the lower genital tract of both men and women.

Trichomonas Vaginalis Infections

As the name of this organism implies, ***T. vaginalis* infections** (trichomoniasis) are more of a problem for women than for men. Women are 20 times more likely to contract trichomoniasis than are men. The reason for higher infection rates in women is that *T. vaginalis* lives on the surface tissues of the reproductive tract, such as the walls of the vagina, and uses glucose (a sugar) as a principal nutrient. This nutrient is more abundant in the reproductive tract of women than men. However, *Trichomonas* does not grow well in acidic conditions, which is the normal environment of the vagina (and of the male urethra). If the acid environment of the vagina changes, such as when a woman has another genital infection, is taking antibiotics, or is pregnant, the organism will grow easily if she becomes infected.

According to the CDC, an estimated 3.7 million women and men in the United States are infected annually with *Trichomonas*. Men usually contract the

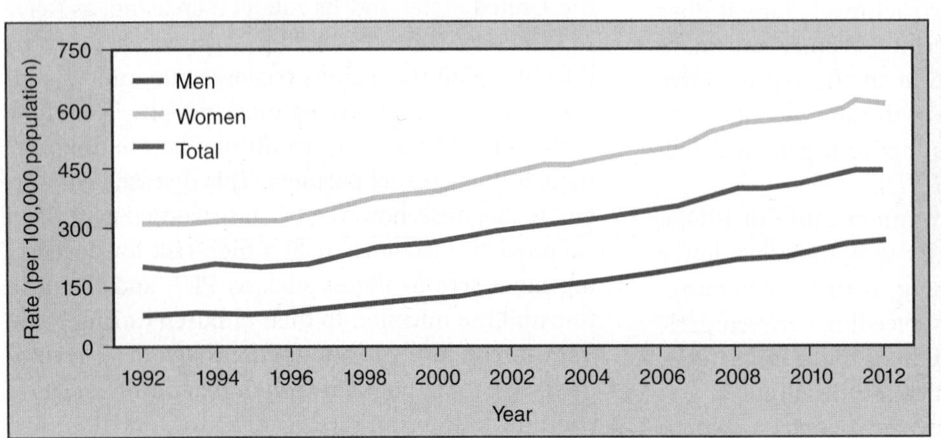

Figure 14.27

Chlamydia—Rates by Sex, United States, 1990–2012.

Reproduced from Centers for Disease Control and Prevention. (2014, January). Sexually transmitted disease surveillance 2012. Retrieved from http://www.cdc.gov/sTD/stats12/Surv2012.pdf

disease by having sexual intercourse with an infected woman, but women can contract it not only from sexual intercourse with an infected man but also from genital contact with an infected woman.

The symptoms of this STI in men are that of a mild infection of the urethra: mildly painful urination and urgency to urinate. The symptoms in women are more extensive and serious: an abnormal, bad-smelling vaginal discharge, which may be thin and foamy, along with itching, burning, swelling, redness, and tenderness of the vulva. These symptoms vary in their severity among patients. *Trichomonas* infections are treated with a specific drug that kills the organism.

Yeast Infections

Yeast infections (candidiasis) are common among women and are acquired in a variety of ways, including sexual intercourse. *Candida albicans* is the organism most commonly responsible for yeast infections. (These infections are *not* caused by the yeasts used to make certain baked products or beer.) These organisms are thought to be always present in the genital-anal area (as are a variety of bacteria) because they are present in fecal material. The bacteria that normally inhabit the vagina in high numbers keep yeast and other bacteria from growing because they produce acids and outcompete other organisms for nutrients and space. However, under certain conditions, yeast may grow in the vagina.

Yeast may begin to grow and produce a vaginal infection during antibiotic use or pregnancy. Women who have poorly controlled diabetes or other STIs are also prone to yeast infections. Yeast grows best under warm and moist conditions, so clothing that is tight and poorly ventilated in the crotch may also contribute to the development of yeast infections. All these factors change the vaginal environment, allowing the yeast to grow.

The most common symptom of yeast infections in women is itching in the genital area. Other symptoms are soreness, burning, irritation, swelling, and a vaginal discharge that is white and looks somewhat like cottage cheese. Although numerous over-the-counter preparations are available to treat yeast infections, women should report symptoms to their healthcare providers before self-treatment.

Women infected with *Candida* can pass the infection to their male partners during sexual intercourse. Typically, the penis becomes infected; parts of this organ, the scrotum, and the groin may become irritated and swollen and may develop a rash, white patches, or both. Infected men may also experience the symptoms of a mild urethritis.

yeast infection A condition in which the fungus *Candida albicans* grows in the vagina or on the penis; also known as candidiasis or moniliasis.

pubic louse A close relative of fleas that causes sexually transmitted infestation; also called crabs.

Pubic Lice

Phthirus pubis (THIR-us PEW-bis) is a **pubic louse**, often called a crab louse because it has crablike claws (**Figure 14.28**). Therefore, infestation with pubic lice is often referred to as "having crabs." Pubic lice are closely related to head lice but are not found in the scalp or on head hair. Crab lice can also attach to underarm hair and eyelashes and occasionally infest these body areas.

Pubic lice are transmitted primarily by sexual contact and are rarely spread via contaminated toilet seats and bed linens, although these routes of infestation are possible. They move from the pubic hairs of an infected individual to a partner when the genital areas touch. The lice then anchor themselves by grasping pubic hairs. For nourishment, pubic lice pierce the host's skin with their mouthparts and suck the blood of their host. When a person contracts pubic lice, he or she may notice tiny droplets of blood on the underwear before the symptoms of itching, swelling, redness, and irritation begin.

Pubic lice also reproduce in the pubic area. Female lice lay their eggs and then glue them to pubic hairs,

Figure 14.28

The Pubic Louse. This color-enhanced scanning electron microscope image shows two pubic lice, one adult and one juvenile, magnified about 40 times. They are hanging from pubic hair by their massive, crablike claws.

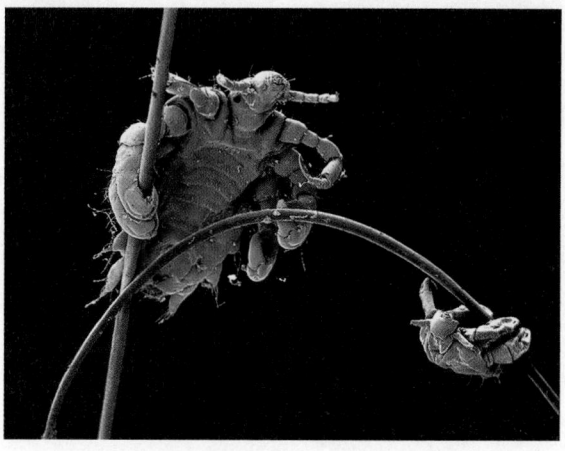

scabies (SKAY-beez) An infestation of the pubic area in which a spider-like organism burrows into the skin and lays eggs there.

where they eventually hatch and mature. Unless the infestation is treated, the lice will continue to reproduce and infest their host.

Both nonprescription and prescription medications are available to treat infestations of pubic lice, but a healthcare provider should be consulted to confirm the diagnosis. Bed linens and clothing should be washed in hot water and dried to kill any eggs or lice. Sexual partners must also be treated at the same time, as with all STIs, so that reinfestation (or reinfection) does not occur.

Scabies

Scabies (*Sarcoptes scabiei*) (sar-COP-tees SKAY-bee-ee) produce infestations of the pubic area similar to those of the pubic louse. These spider-like organisms (often called *itch mites*) burrow into the skin and lay eggs there. Therefore, one sign of infestation with scabies is thin, red lines or bumps in the skin, which result from burrowing and egg laying. In addition to the pubic region, these organisms infest other areas of the body (**Figure 14.29**).

Itch mites are transmitted by prolonged, close, personal contact, including sexual intercourse. However, if one member of a family becomes infested, the infestation can spread to other family members via infected bed linens, towels, or other household items. Outbreaks also occur in institutional settings such as hospitals and nursing homes. Scabies is treated with prescription medications that are applied to the skin and sometimes with accompanying oral medications.

Protecting Yourself Against STIs

The first step in protecting yourself against sexually transmitted infections is to realize that STIs can strike anyone who is sexually active. Regardless of your age, gender, ethnicity, or socioeconomic status, if you are sexually active, you can contract an STI.

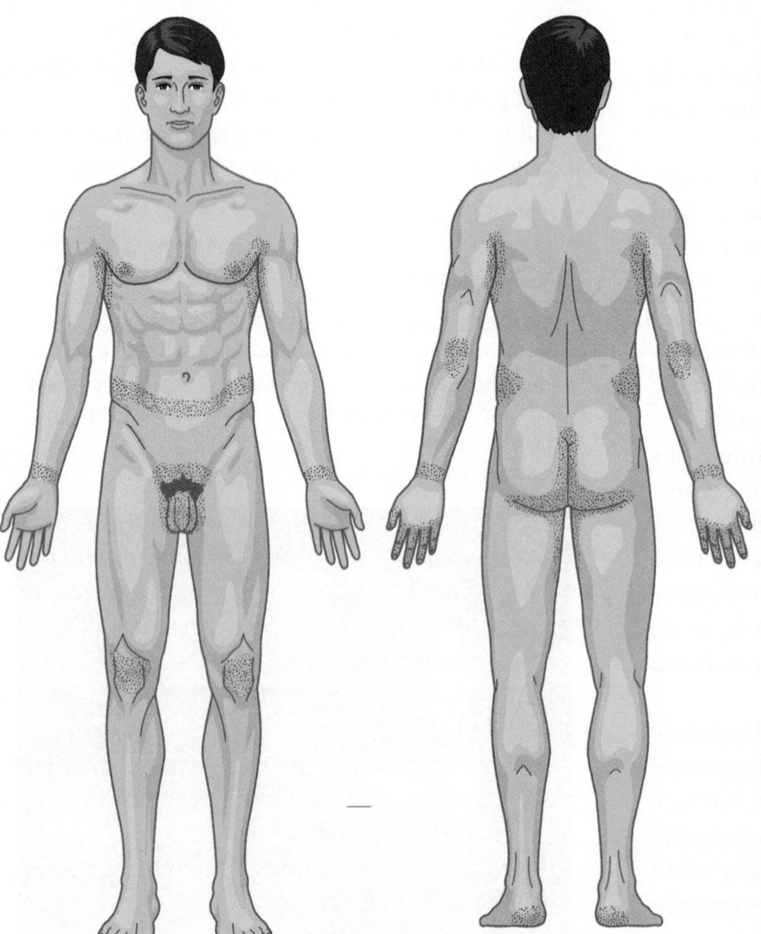

Figure 14.29

The Distribution of Scabies Skin Lesions. The red dotted areas show where infestation usually occurs. The areas without dots are rarely affected.

The Managing Your Health box in this chapter lists behaviors that will help protect you from infection with HIV and other STIs. Of course, you may choose to abstain from sexual activity and drug use, which virtually eliminates your risk of contracting a sexually transmitted infection. If you choose not to abstain from sex, having sex with noninfected individuals also eliminates your risk. How do you know if your partner is infected?

The best way to know if you are having sex with an uninfected partner is to be in a long-term, monogamous relationship in which you and your partner have been tested for STIs. A monogamous relationship is one in which a person has only one mate or partner at any one time. Unfortunately, monogamy is not foolproof. You must be absolutely certain that your partner is not having sex with anyone else. Consider the comment by a health student when asked, "Do you know someone who has a sexually transmitted infection? What was their reaction when they found out?":

A married friend of mine went to the doctor right away after she suspected she had a sexually transmitted infection. The doctor said she had herpes. She was so upset with her husband; she later divorced him.

Apparently, this "monogamous" relationship was one sided. It obviously did not eliminate this woman's risk of contracting an STI. Also, don't equate *serial monogamy* with elimination of risk. Having sex with only one person for a short period and then having sex only with a new partner, and so on, does not eliminate your risk of contracting a sexually transmitted infection.

Because it is difficult to eliminate your risk of contracting an STI (or to be certain that you have no risk), it is prudent to adhere to behaviors that reduce your chances of becoming infected.

Limiting your number of sexual partners statistically reduces your chances of contracting any STI. With regard to the partners you have, you will lower your risk if you delay having sex with people until you know them well enough to assess their risk as sexual partners. Although you may question your partner about his or her previous sexual experiences, history of STIs, and drug use habits, be aware that people often conceal this information. Avoid having sex with individuals who consistently have sex with multiple partners. Also avoid having sex with individuals who are in the high-risk categories listed in Table 14-1. If you choose to have sex with a person in one or more of these categories, avoid penetrating activities: anal, vaginal, and oral sex. Also, do not use contraceptives that contain nonoxynol-9, which might increase the risk of transmission of STIs.

If you use drugs, you are putting yourself in jeopardy of contracting an STI. To avoid contracting STIs, never share needles and syringes if you are an injecting drug user, and never have sex while under the influence of drugs or alcohol. While under the influence, you are more likely to engage in sexually risky and dangerous behaviors.

The most effective strategy to prevent HIV and other STIs is to refrain from anal and vaginal intercourse as well as oral sex with infected partners. The second most effective strategy is to use latex condoms during sexual activity. According to the CDC, condom use substantially reduces the risk for contracting the following STIs: gonorrhea, HSV infection, syphilis, HIV infection, hepatitis B, and chlamydial infection. By reducing the risk of gonorrheal and chlamydial infections in women, condoms also reduce their risk of contracting pelvic inflammatory disease.

Although the use of synthetic condoms will reduce your risk of becoming infected, they do not provide a guarantee against transmission because they may tear or slip (although with proper use, this is unlikely) and they do not cover the entire genital area. Condoms made of natural membranes such as sheep intestine are not effective barriers. HIV and other sexually transmitted viruses can penetrate this type of condom, so use latex ones. When using latex condoms, however, do not use oil-based lubricants such as petroleum jelly, mineral oil, vegetable oils, massage oils, and body lotions, which can weaken the latex. Apply only water-based lubricants such as K-Y Jelly.

Another practice to avoid is storing condoms in hot cars or wallets for extended periods of time; keep them in a cool, dry place and out of direct sunlight. Do not use them after the expiration date, or if the packaging on the condom shows signs of damage or deterioration, such as brittleness, stickiness, or discoloration.

It is important to use condoms consistently (a new one for each act of intercourse) and properly for them to be effective in reducing your risk against STIs. As you use a condom, handle it carefully, being sure not to damage it with your fingernails, teeth, or other sharp objects.

Female polyurethane condoms are also available. Laboratory tests show that viruses such as HIV cannot pass through the polyurethane; studies with actual use show the female condom to be effective in preventing transmission of STIs. In 2009, the FDA approved the "second-generation" female condom (FC2).[26]

The female condom is a plastic sheath that covers the cervix much like a diaphragm, lines the vagina, and covers the labia. The same precautions and care regarding the use of male condoms should be followed when using female condoms. Female condoms can also be used as protection during anal intercourse.

Condoms can be slit open and used flat to cover the genital areas during oral sex to help prevent STI transmission. Dental dams (flat pieces of latex) are useful for this purpose as well.

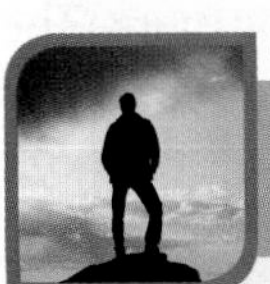

© djgis/ShutterStock

Healthy Living Practices

- If you are sexually active, you are at risk for contracting sexually transmitted infections. You can reduce your risk by abstaining from sex or by engaging in sex only within a mutually monogamous relationship in which you and your partner are free of disease.
- You can reduce your risk by limiting your number of sexual partners, never sharing needles and syringes during drug use, and not engaging in sex while under the influence of alcohol or drugs.
- Another way to reduce your STI risk is by using synthetic condoms for each act of anal or vaginal intercourse. In addition, you can use a flat piece of latex to cover the genital areas during oral sex. If you choose not to use condoms, you can reduce STI risk by having both yourself and your partner screened for STIs before engaging in sex.

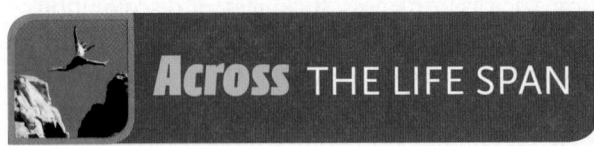

© Galina Barskaya/ShutterStock

INFECTIOUS AND NONINFECTIOUS DISEASES

Noninfectious diseases and conditions that are present at birth are termed *birth defects*. According to the CDC, 1 in 33 babies in the United States are born with a birth defect, and more than 5,500 of these children die.[27]

Some birth defects are caused by environmental influences such as fetal exposure to teratogens—drugs, alcohol, viruses, or other substances that directly damage the tissues of the embryo (during weeks 3 to 8 of pregnancy) or fetus (during week 9 of pregnancy through birth). Dietary deficiencies during pregnancy can also cause birth defects.

Metabolic diseases are also types of birth defects. An infant born with a metabolic disease lacks an enzyme necessary for normal metabolism. Such problems are genetic and result in an infant's cells being unable to make a necessary body compound. Sometimes abnormal substances are made that build up in the blood and urine; these substances can damage tissues in the body such as the liver, brain, and kidney.

Most metabolic diseases are rare; two of the more well-known are Tay-Sachs disease and phenylketonuria. In Tay-Sachs disease, which occurs predominantly among Ashkenazi Jews (the descendants of Jews who settled in eastern and central Europe), certain fatlike molecules accumulate in the brain and other tissues, retarding development and causing death by the age of 3 to 4 years. In phenylketonuria (PKU), cells are unable to convert the amino acid phenylalanine to other needed compounds. Phenylalanine and related chemicals build up in the blood and damage tissues, causing intellectual disability. Because the ill effects of this disease can be avoided by restricting the amount of phenylalanine in the diet, most newborn infants are tested for this disorder.

Although many genetic diseases claim the lives of infants and children, genetic disorders persist in those children who survive to become adolescents or young adults. Down syndrome, cystic fibrosis, and Duchenne muscular dystrophy are all noninfectious diseases, discussed earlier in this chapter, that affect children. The hope for curing these and other genetic diseases is *gene therapy*, in which corrected copies of defective genes are inserted into the hereditary material of infected individuals. A preventive measure is genetic counseling, in which prospective parents seek advice regarding the probability that they will have a child with particular genetic disorders. Couples can use this information to make family planning decisions.

Most genetic diseases strike early in life. However, one disease, Huntington's chorea (also called Huntington's disease), does not become evident until approximately age 40. By this time, victims may have already passed on the genes for this disease to their children. In Huntington's chorea, the individual makes involuntary, purposeless, rapid motions such as flexing and extending the fingers or raising and lowering the shoulders. (*Chorea* refers to involuntary muscle twitching.) The mental faculties of the person also deteriorate. Fifteen years or so after the onset of the disease, the individual dies. Although there is no cure or effective treatment for this disease, certain medications can relieve or lessen some of the symptoms. Genetic testing is available so that young adults who have affected parents can learn whether they carry the lethal gene. The gene is dominant, which means that if you inherit one gene from either parent, you will develop this disease. This information allows people at risk for this disease to make informed reproductive choices.

Other than heart disease, cancer, and stroke, one of the most well-known noninfectious diseases of older adults is Alzheimer's disease. This disease has a strong genetic link.

Infectious diseases also have a variety of effects across the life span. As life begins, infection can do harm. Viral infections can be dangerous to a pregnant woman because many viruses can cross the placenta, the organ through which the fetus absorbs nutrients and excretes wastes. Certain viruses, such as the German measles virus, can cause birth defects, including deafness, heart defects, and intellectual disability. Other viruses, such as the human immunodeficiency virus (HIV), can infect the fetus, resulting in an infected newborn. Most bacteria cannot cross the placenta, but if bacteria infect the birth canal at the time of delivery, the baby can become infected as it passes through, as in the case of gonorrhea (discussed earlier).

In the past, certain bacterial diseases (e.g., diphtheria and whooping cough) and viral diseases (e.g., measles, mumps, and German measles) were common childhood infectious diseases in the United States. However, vaccines for these diseases have been developed, and most children are immunized routinely in the United States according to a schedule. Occasionally, serious outbreaks of these diseases occur in people who are not immunized. These childhood diseases are still prevalent in developing countries.

Other than contracting common infections such as colds and the flu, sexually active adolescents, teens, and young adults are at highest risk for contracting STIs because they frequently have unprotected intercourse. The one nonsexually transmitted infectious disease prevalent in adolescents and young adults is infectious mononucleosis. "Mono" primarily strikes young adults ranging in age from 15 to 25 years (although some suggest this age range extends from 10 to 35).

Infectious mononucleosis has been nicknamed the "kissing disease" because it is spread via infectious saliva. However, it is also contracted by inhaling infectious droplets sneezed or coughed into the air by an infected person or by drinking from an infected person's glass. This disease is usually not serious, but the Epstein-Barr (EB) virus (a herpesvirus), which causes mononucleosis, has been associated with the subsequent development of two forms of cancers: Burkitt lymphoma in certain African populations and nasopharyngeal (nose and throat) carcinoma in Asian populations. Furthermore, infection with EB virus can cause a prolonged period of exhaustion, lasting up to 2 to 3 months. Rest is the primary treatment.

The most common symptoms of infectious mononucleosis are a sore throat; low-grade, long-term fever; swollen lymph nodes and spleen (which may result in pain in the upper left side of the abdomen); fatigue; and weakness. However, the symptoms can vary and may include a rash, headache, or nausea. Previously, mono was difficult to diagnose in some cases, but healthcare practitioners can now test for mono in their offices.

Infections are a major cause of illness and death among older adults; respiratory infections are the sixth leading cause of death in persons 85 years and older, and the seventh leading cause of death for those aged 75–84 years. Bacterial pneumonia and influenza, for example, together have well more than 100 times the fatality rate for persons 75–84 years than for those between the ages of 25 and 34 years and nearly 600 times the fatality rate for persons 85 years and older.[6]

Older adults are more susceptible to infections and have a more difficult time recovering from them than do younger persons for a variety of reasons. The cell-mediated component of the immune system functions less well as people age. Also, the respiratory tract changes during the aging process, resulting in decreased elasticity of the lungs and a diminished cough reflex, making elderly people more susceptible to respiratory infections. Other organ systems may also experience structural and degenerative changes that predispose elderly persons to infection. Many elderly people have chronic diseases too, which lower their organs' functional reserves and contribute to their decreased resistance to infection. However, older adults are in a low-risk category for contracting STIs because they usually have fewer sexual partners than younger people do.

CHAPTER REVIEW

Summary

Noninfectious diseases are processes that affect the proper functioning of the body, are usually accompanied by characteristic signs and symptoms, and are not caused by pathogens, but rather, abnormalities in the hereditary material, factors in the environment, or an interaction of the two cause noninfectious diseases.

Genetic factors are the sole cause of some noninfectious diseases; such genetic diseases are inherited or are caused by mistakes during cell division when gametes are formed. Inherited diseases are caused by disorders of the hereditary material, or genes. Two inherited diseases that are prevalent in the United States are cystic fibrosis and Duchenne/Becker muscular dystrophy. Down syndrome is a genetic disease caused by errors during gamete formation.

Some diseases are caused by an interaction of genetic and environmental factors. Genetic factors can predispose a person to a disease. Diseases having both genetic and environmental causes include asthma, ulcers, diabetes mellitus, and migraine headaches.

Some noninfectious conditions have environmental or unknown causes. A few noninfectious conditions are caused by improperly performing certain activities. Carpal tunnel syndrome, for example, is a painful condition of the hands and fingers that results from improper positioning of the wrist while engaging in repetitive activities that use the hands, wrists, and arms.

Birth defects are noninfectious conditions present at birth that affect either the body's structures or how it functions. Anatomic defects can be caused by genetic or environmental factors or a combination of both. Metabolic defects are genetic and affect a person throughout life. Alzheimer's disease is a prominent noninfectious disease of older adults.

Infectious diseases affect the proper functioning of the body, are usually accompanied by characteristic signs and symptoms, and are caused by disease-producing (pathogenic) bacteria, viruses, fungi, protozoans, or worms. Some infectious diseases are communicable; that is, they are spread from person to person either directly or by means of an intermediary organism called a vector. Other infectious diseases are noncommunicable; they are caused by organisms such as bacteria that normally (and usually harmlessly) reside on a person's body, by the ingestion of toxins produced by pathogens, or by pathogens from environmental or animal sources.

The severity of a disease's symptoms depends on a variety of factors: the type of organism; its virulence; the manner in which it enters, multiplies, and spreads in or on the body; the chemicals it produces, if any; its ability to combat the defense mechanisms of the body; and the body's reaction to the invading microbe.

Two primary causes of infectious diseases are bacteria and viruses. Bacteria, microscopic organisms that have a simple cell structure, cause disease by first adhering to the surfaces of cells. Some penetrate more deeply into tissues, and many bacteria produce chemicals that break down the connections between cells, aiding their invasion. Viruses are noncellular, nonliving, protein-coated pieces of hereditary material. They cause infection by adhering to cells also, but then enter cells and use them to make more viruses, killing the cells in the process.

The human body has two main types of immunity, or defense against disease: nonspecific and specific immunity. Nonspecific immunity combats any foreign invader. Mechanisms of nonspecific immunity include the skin and mucous membranes, white blood cells and their phagocytic properties, the lymphatic system, the inflammatory response, natural killer cells, and interferons.

Specific immunity combats each specific invading pathogen and is carried out by the immune system. The immune system has two branches: antibody-mediated immunity and cell-mediated immunity. Antibody-mediated immunity reacts to antigens (foreign proteins) that reside outside of the body cells, such as most bacteria and the toxic products they produce.

Cell-mediated immunity reacts to antigens that reside inside body cells, such as viruses, fungi, a few types of bacteria, and parasites. It also acts against foreign (nonself) tissues such as transplanted organs and controls the growth of tumor cells.

Immunity is either inborn or acquired. Inborn immunity is inherited, such as immunity to infectious diseases that attack other organisms but not humans. Acquired immunity develops during a person's lifetime. Immunity is acquired either actively or passively and by natural or artificial means.

Many drugs have been developed to combat infection. Antibiotics kill or inhibit the growth of bacteria and are in wide use. Antiviral drugs are limited in availability and scope. Specific medications have been developed to treat protozoal diseases and infections caused by worms.

Sexually transmitted infections (STIs) are infectious diseases spread from one person to another during sexual activity, primarily sexual intercourse. Most pathogens that cause STIs can survive for only a short time outside of the body; therefore, transmission of these diseases from objects, such as toilet seats, is either impossible or rare, depending on the STI. Sexually transmitted infections are caused primarily by viruses and bacteria, but some infections and infestations are caused by yeast, protozoans, mites, and lice. The transmission of STIs is often facilitated in persons infected with other STIs.

Sexually transmitted infections caused by viruses are incurable, although the body may clear itself of some human papillomavirus (HPV) infections. In addition to causing STIs, three sexually transmitted viruses have been implicated in the development of particular cancers: human immunodeficiency virus (HIV), HPV, and hepatitis B virus (HBV).

The most serious viral STI is HIV infection because it not only raises the risk of developing a particular type of cancer, but also the virus attacks the immune system, disabling the body's defenses. Eventually, the immune system of an HIV-infected individual becomes so weakened that he or she succumbs to an array of illnesses that lead to death. This stage in HIV infection is called acquired immunodeficiency syndrome (AIDS). The best ways to protect yourself against contracting this deadly disease or any STI are to refrain from having sex with infected individuals, reduce your number of sexual partners, avoid sex with high-risk partners, and use a latex condom with each act of sexual intercourse.

Sexually transmitted infections caused by bacteria are curable with antibiotics. Three prevalent bacterial STIs are syphilis, gonorrhea, and chlamydial infections.

One protozoan, *Trichomonas vaginalis*, causes a sexually transmitted infection primarily in women. The yeast *Candida albicans* may cause troublesome, itchy infections in women that can be transmitted sexually. The crab louse, *Phthirus pubis*, and itch mite, *Sarcoptes scabiei*, both can cause sexually transmitted infestations of the genital area.

Adolescents and young adults are in the age category at highest risk for contracting sexually transmitted infections. Infants are at risk of infection from infected mothers. Middle-aged and older people are less likely to contract sexually transmitted infections because they are less likely to have multiple sex partners. However, anyone who practices high-risk behaviors or who has sex with an infected person can contract a sexually transmitted infection.

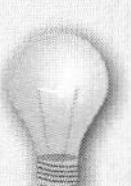

Applying What You Have Learned

1. Based on the information in this chapter, describe two ways in which you can lower your or your unborn children's risk of contracting noninfectious diseases. **Analysis**
2. The human immunodeficiency virus (HIV) attacks helper T cells. How does this affect the body's ability to resist disease? **Application**
3. Think about the last infectious disease you contracted (e.g., common cold, influenza). Outline what you think might have been the chain of infection for this disease. What could you have done to break the chain of infection and avoid becoming infected? **Analysis**
4. Analyze your behaviors regarding your risk for contracting STIs (e.g., having multiple sex partners, drug use). What can you do to lower your risk of contracting a sexually transmitted infection? **Analysis**

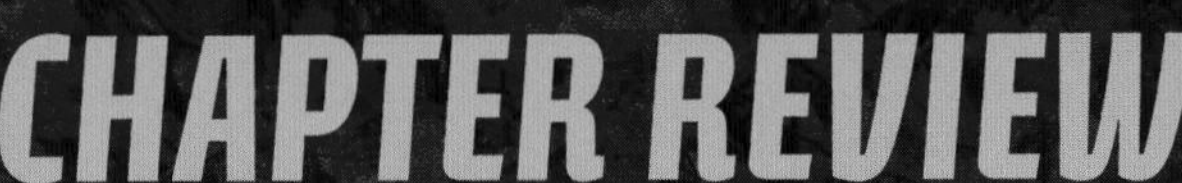

CHAPTER REVIEW

5. A man develops a sore on his genitals but is too busy to go to his healthcare provider. The sore heals, so he decides that he "got better" on his own. State two reasons why his reasoning is faulty and dangerous. With which STI(s) might this man be infected? Support your answer with evidence. **Synthesis**

6. State a behavior or behaviors that you could adopt or change to help you become more resistant to infection in general. How would this behavioral change increase your resistance to infection? **Evaluation**

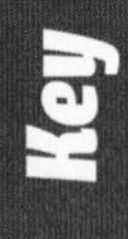

Key

Application	**Analysis**	**Synthesis**	**Evaluation**
using information in a new situation.	breaking down information into component parts.	putting together information from different sources.	making informed decisions.

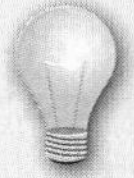

Reflecting on Your Health

1. Think back to a time when you dated a person you'd only recently met. What did you do to be sure that you would not catch an STI from this person? What did you do to reduce your risk of infection? After reading this chapter, would you behave any differently now to protect yourself? Why or why not? If so, what would you do differently?
2. When you have a common communicable infectious disease like a cold or the flu, do you do anything to protect others, such as members of your family, from catching your illness? If so, what? Would you do anything differently after reading this chapter? If so, what? Would you use CAM to help "cure" your cold? Why or why not?
3. Have you ever traveled outside the United States? If so, to what countries did you travel? Think back to your trip(s) and describe what you did before departing to protect yourself from infection. What did you do to protect yourself while you were there? Has reading this chapter alerted you to additional steps you should take to protect yourself from infection? If so, what? If you have never traveled outside of the country, pick a country to which you would like to travel and explain what steps you would take before you left to protect yourself from infection. What steps would you take while you were there?
4. Do any hereditary diseases run in your family? If you are not sure, ask your family members, including parents, grandparents, uncles, aunts, and cousins, if possible. What steps can you take to protect your future children from a hereditary disease? Include specifics about diseases that run in your family, if any.
5. Many strains of bacteria are becoming resistant to the antibiotics used to treat them. One reason for this is that people pressure their healthcare providers for antibiotics when they do not have bacterial illnesses. Also, some people stop taking antibiotics before their physician says they should. Both these situations provide an opportunity for resistant strains of bacteria to develop and replicate. Do you practice either of these behaviors? If so, why? What have you learned in this chapter that may cause you to change those behaviors?

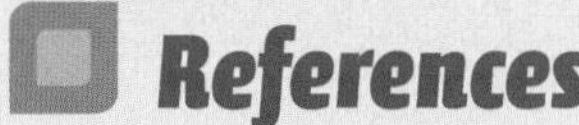

References

1. Cystic Fibrosis Foundation. (2014, March 12). *About cystic fibrosis: Frequently asked questions*. Retrieved from http://www.cff.org/AboutCF/Faqs/
2. Centers for Disease Control and Prevention. (2009, October 16). Prevalence of Duchenne/Becker muscular dystrophy among males aged 5–24 years—four states, 2007. *Morbidity and Mortality Weekly Report, 58*(40), 1119–1122.
3. Ishikawa, Y., et al. (2011). Duchenne muscular dystrophy: Survival by cardio-respiratory interventions. *Neuromuscular Disorders, 21*(1), 47–51.
4. University of California San Francisco Medical Center. (2014). *Down syndrome*. Retrieved from http://www.ucsfhealth.org/education/down_syndrome/
5. Allen, E. G., et al. (2009). Maternal age and risk for trisomy 21 assessed by the origin of chromosome nondisjunction: A report from the Atlanta and National Down Syndrome Projects. *Human Genetics, 125*, 41–52.
6. Murphy, S. L., Xu, J., & Kochanek, K. D. (2013, May 8). Deaths: Final data for 2010. *National Vital Statistics Reports, 61*(4), 1–118. Retrieved from http://www.cdc.gov/nchs/data/nvsr/nvsr61/nvsr61_04.pdf
7. Mayo Clinic staff. (2014). *Legionnaires' disease: Risk factors*. Retrieved from http://www.mayoclinic.com/health/legionnaires-disease/DS00853/DSECTION=risk-factors
8. Centers for Disease Control and Prevention. (2012, April 2). *Vaccinations and immunizations: Lyme disease vaccination*. Retrieved from http://www.cdc.gov/VACCINES/vpd-vac/lyme/default.htm
9. Centers for Disease Control and Prevention. (2014, June 16). *HIV surveillance—epidemiology of HIV infection (through 2011)*. Retrieved May 4, 2011, from http://www.cdc.gov/hiv/topics/surveillance/resources/slides/general/index.htm
10. United Nations Programme on HIV/AIDS (UNAIDS). (2010). *UNAIDS report on the global AIDS epidemic*. Retrieved from http://www.unaids.org/en/media/unaids/contentassets/documents/epidemiology/2013/gr2013/unaids_global_report_2013_en.pdf
11. Harrison, K. M., et al. (2010). Life expectancy after HIV diagnosis is based on national HIV surveillance data from 25 states, United States. *Journal of Acquired Immune Deficiency Syndrome, 53*(1), 124–130.
12. Schneider, M. F., et al. (2005). Patterns of the hazard of death after AIDS through the evolution of antiretroviral therapy: 1984–2004. *AIDS, 19*(17), 2009–2018.
13. Centers for Disease Control and Prevention. (2014, May 1). *HIV Surveillance Report, Diagnoses of HIV infection and AIDS in the United States and dependent areas, 2011*.
14. Chama, C. M., & Morrupa, J. Y. (2008). The safety of elective caesarean section for the prevention of mother-to-child transmission of HIV-1. *Journal of Obstetrics and Gynaecology, 2*, 194–197.
15. Centers for Disease Control and Prevention. (2014, May 14). *Basic information about HIV and AIDS*. Retrieved from http://www.cdc.gov/hiv/basics/index.html
16. Centers for Disease Control and Prevention. (2014, May 21). *Oral sex and HIV risk*. Retrieved from http://www.cdc.gov/hiv/risk/behavior/oralsex.html
17. Crans, W. J. (2014, July 15). *Why mosquitoes cannot transmit AIDS*. Rutgers Center for Vector Biology. Retrieved from http://www.rci.rutgers.edu/~insects/aids.htm
18. Moscicki, A.-B. (2008). Vaginal microbicides: Where are we and where are we going? *Journal of Infection and Chemotherapy, 14*, 337–341.
19. Willyard, C. (2010, July 15). Tiny steps toward an HIV vaccine. *Nature, 466*(7304), S8.
20. Centers for Disease Control and Prevention. (2010, December 17). Sexually transmitted diseases treatment guidelines, 2010. *Morbidity and Mortality Weekly Report, 59*(RR-12), 1–110. Retrieved from http://www.cdc.gov/std/treatment/2010/STD-Treatment-2010-RR5912.pdf
21. Zhou, J., & Rossi, J. J. (2011). Current progress in development of RNA-based therapeutics for HIV-1. *Gene Therapy, 18*, 1134–1138.
22. Centers for Disease Control and Prevention. (2014, January). *Sexually transmitted disease surveillance 2012*. Retrieved from http://www.cdc.gov/std/stats12/Surv2012.pdf
23. Cohen, J. (2010). Immunology. Painful failure of promising genital herpes vaccine. *Science, 330*(6002), 304.
24. Reuters. (2013, November, 7). *Genital herpes vaccine succeeds in mid-stage trial*. Retrieved from http://www.foxnews.com/health/2013/11/07/genital-herpes-vaccine-succeeds-in-mid-stage-trial/
25. American Cancer Society. (2013). *Cancer prevention and early -detection facts and figures, 2013*. Atlanta, GA. Retrieved from http://www.cancer.org/acs/groups/content/@epidemiologysurveilance/documents/document/acspc-037535.pdf
26. Witte, S. S., et al. (2010). Can Medicaid reimbursement help give female condoms a second chance in the United States? *American Journal of Public Health, 100*(10), 1835–1840.
27. Centers for Disease Control and Prevention. (2014, June 9). *National Center for Birth Defects and Developmental Disabilities: About us*. Retrieved from http://www.cdc.gov/ncbddd/AboutUs/index.html

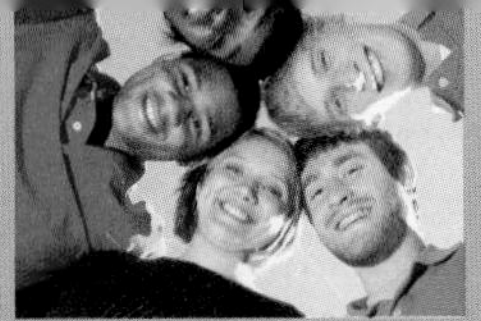

Diversity in Health
Hunting for Supercentenarians

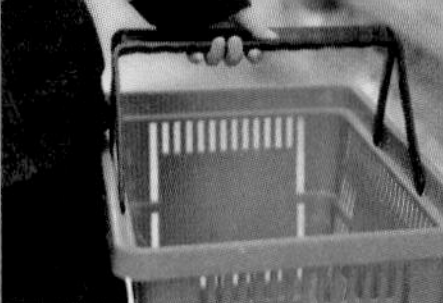

Consumer Health
Choosing a Long-Term Care Facility

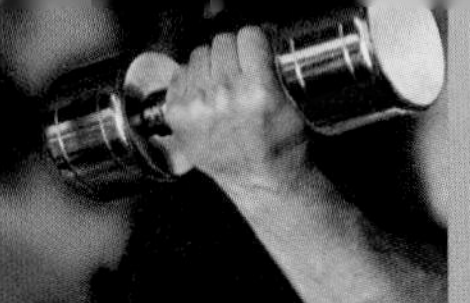

Managing Your Health
After the Death of a Loved One

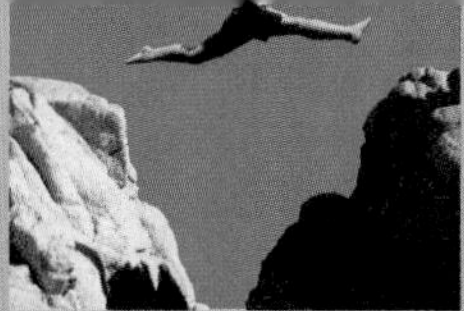

Across the Life Span
Dying and Death

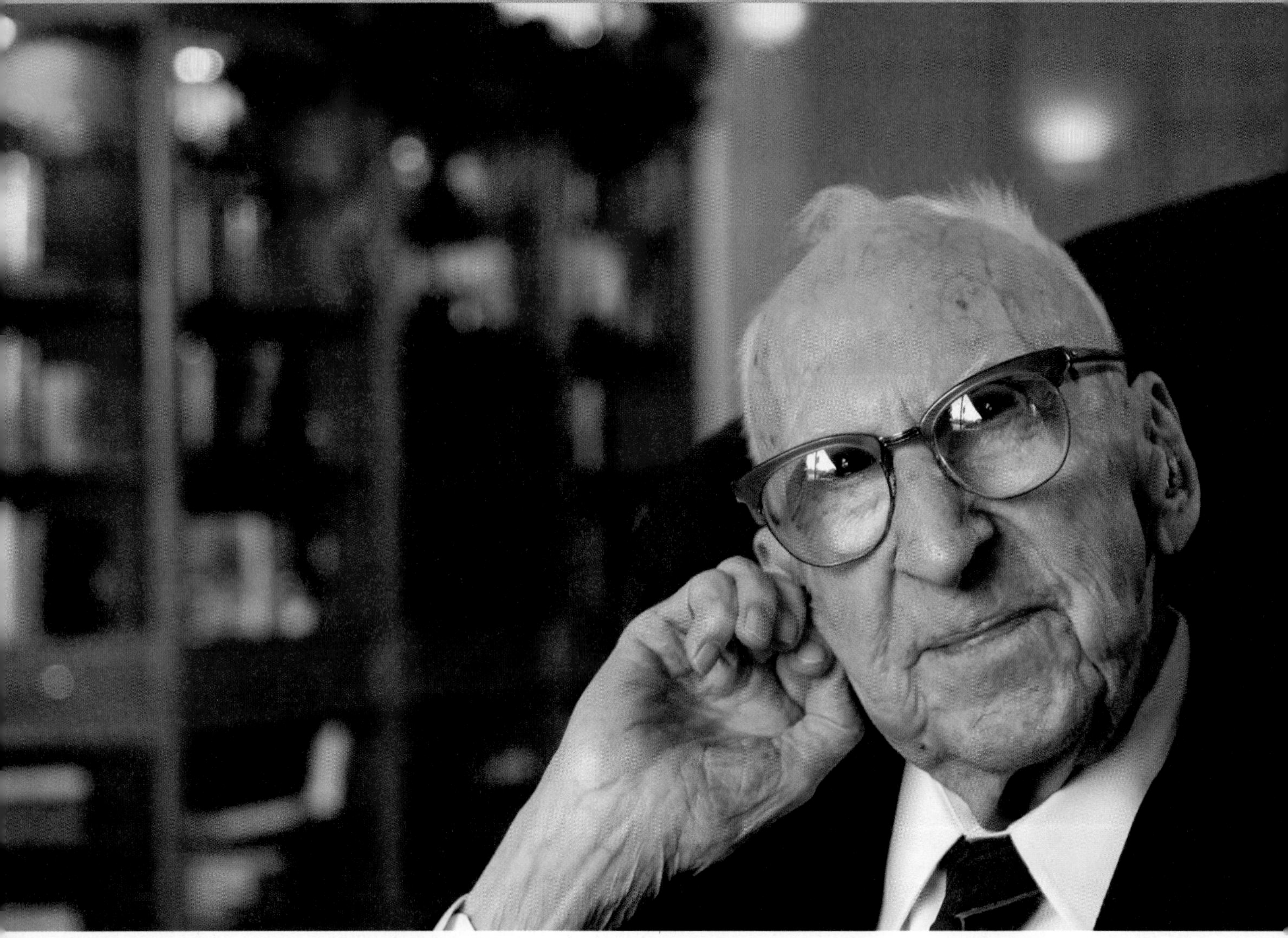

Chapter Overview

The status of aging Americans

Why we age

The effects of aging on health and well-being

The spiritual and emotional aspects of dying

The options for terminal care

The definition of death

How to prepare for death

Student Workbook

Self-Assessment: Preparing for Aging and Death

Changing Health Habits: Can Changing a Health Habit Extend Your Life?

Do You Know?

Who was the oldest person to ever live?

What happens to your body as you age?

How to increase your chances of living a long and healthy life?

CHAPTER 15

Aging, Dying, and Death

© Sergej Petrakov/Photography/Shutterstock

Learning Objectives

"Take care of your mind and body."

After studying this chapter, you should be able to:

1. Define aging, senescence, life span, life expectancy, and ageism.
2. Discuss the effects of ageism.
3. Describe physical and psychological changes associated with the normal aging process.
4. Explain aging theories.
5. Explain what is meant by "successful aging" and a "good death."
6. Discuss Kübler-Ross's five stages of emotional responses of dying persons.
7. Differentiate between active and passive forms of euthanasia.
8. Explain the benefits of advance directives.
9. Differentiate between normal and abnormal grieving.

gerontologists Scientists who study aging.

aging The sum of all changes that occur in an organism during its life.

life span The maximum number of years that members of a species can expect to live when conditions are optimal.

senescence (seh-NES-ens) The stage of life that begins at age 65 years and ends with death.

On April 15, 2011, Walter Breuning died in Montana. You might be thinking, "So what?" When Walter died of natural causes, he was *114* years of age—the oldest man in the world. Walter's recipe for living more than 100 years included the following recommendations:

- Accept change. "Every change is good."
- Take care of your mind and body.
- Eat two meals a day.
- Work as long as possible.
- Help others.
- Accept death. "You're born to die."[1,2]

Centenarians are people who are older than 100 years of age; people who are at least 110 are *super*centenarians. Why are centenarians able to live such long lives? Lifestyle, environmental, and social factors are known to influence *longevity*, but genetic differences play a major role in determining whether a person lives to be at least 100 years of age.[3]

In December 2010, nearly 53,364 Americans were 100 or more years of age.[4] Today in the United States, more people are living to be 100 years old than in past decades. According to the U.S. Census Bureau, more than 600,000 Americans will be centenarians by 2060.[5]

Gerontologists, scientists who study aging, note that individuals who have the genetic potential to live longer than average often eliminate this advantage by adopting unhealthy lifestyles, such as using tobacco and being physically inactive.[6] Therefore, an important key to enjoying a long and healthy life is taking actions now to improve your health and well-being.

For humans, growing old is a natural and universal process. The prospect of aging and dying, however, has troubled people for centuries. Instead of dreading this time of life, many older adult Americans are busy pursuing a variety of enjoyable and rewarding activities. Healthy people do not let the aging process interfere with their active lifestyles.

This chapter provides more detailed information concerning the aging process, including ways to enjoy good health and a positive sense of well-being while growing old. Additionally, this chapter examines dying and death as well as ways of coping with loss and grief. The assessment activity for this chapter in the Student Workbook can help you examine your current beliefs about aging and death.

Aging

We can define **aging** as the sum of all changes that occur in an organism during its life. The **life span** is the maximum number of years that members of a species can live when conditions are optimal. The life span of an adult mayfly is a few days; the life span of a human is 122 years. In 1997, Jeanne Calment of Marseilles, France, died at the age of 122. According to official records, Ms. Calment lived longer than any other person (**Figure 15.1**). However, very few people live longer than 105 years. Contrary to popular belief, there are no regions of the world where populations usually live more than 100 years (see the Diversity in Health feature "Hunting for Supercentenarians" that follows).

Figure 15.1

Jeanne Calment.

© Launette/AP Images

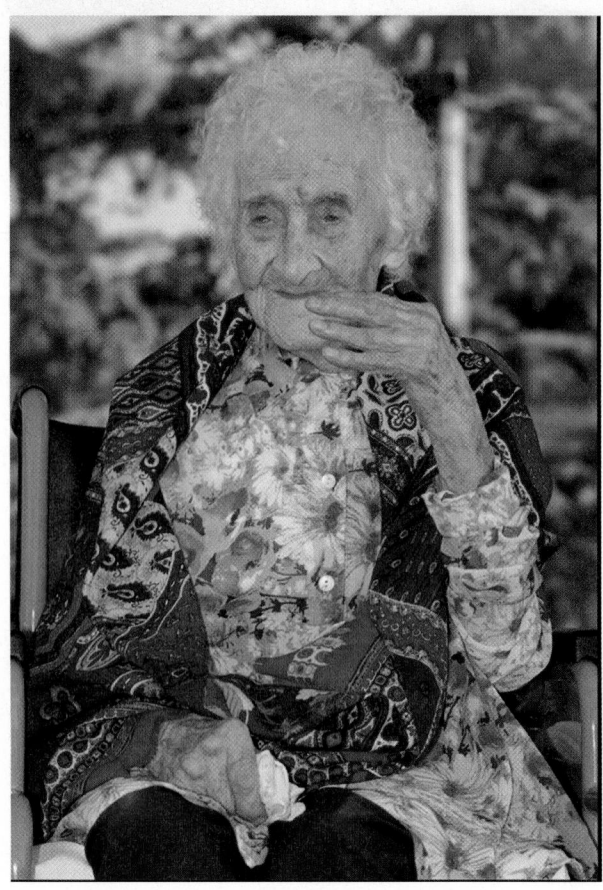

Diversity in Health

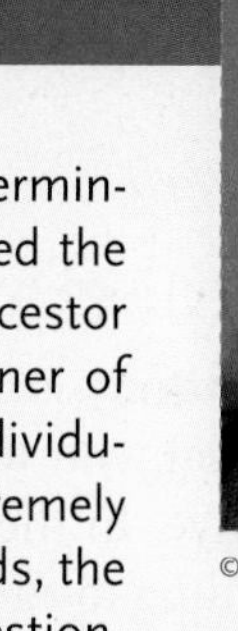

© Mike Flippo/ShutterStock

Hunting for Supercentenarians

Despite the high standard of living and excellent quality of medical care in the United States, few Americans live to be 100 years old. According to verifiable records, no one in the United States has lived longer than 120 years. Yet in certain isolated parts of the world, hundreds of people claim to be more than 120 years old (supercentenarians). Do people who live in these places actually live longer than Americans or the rest of the world's population?

In the first half of the 20th century, reports emerged concerning the extreme longevity of people living in the Hunza area of northern Pakistan, in the village of Vilcabamba in Ecuador, and in the Caucasus region in the eastern European country of Georgia. Scientists visited these regions to question the very old people and determine factors that were associated with their extreme longevity. After interviewing the oldest people in these regions, some experts concluded that living in an isolated and unpolluted rural environment, eating a simple nutritious diet, avoiding the use of alcohol and tobacco, and maintaining an active daily schedule were the keys to superlongevity.

By the 1970s, however, the real story began to unfold concerning the existence of the so-called supercentenarians. As some investigators returned to locate and interview the same old people that they had met previously, their elderly subjects gave ages that did not match. For example, if 5 years had lapsed since the first interview, instead of being 5 years older, the old person reported being 7 or 10 years older. It did not take researchers long to realize that these elderly people typically inflated their ages. How could so many people have been fooled into believing that supercentenarians existed?

It is difficult to verify the ages of very old individuals who live in rural, undeveloped places. During the 1800s, birth records that could document the ages of very elderly persons were not kept, or they were destroyed. In some cases, investigators initially believed the authenticity of an extremely old individual's birth record, but later rejected it after determining that the person shared the name of a long-dead ancestor who was the rightful owner of the document. Even if individuals who claim to be extremely old have their birth records, the documents' value is questionable because birth dates can be altered.

Why would elderly people add years to their actual ages? In many isolated and impoverished places, conditions are not ideal for enjoying a lengthy life. Aged members of these populations know that the longer they live, the more fame, respect, and status they can expect to receive from younger members of the population. Government officials often do little to refute citizens' astounding superlongevity claims because the notoriety attracts a steady stream of curious international visitors whose money supports the local economy.

Scientists who study individuals who claim to be supercentenarians think that their subjects are old but not that old. They may be older than 80 years of age, but few are older than age 90. Thus, no convincing evidence exists that supports the amazing longevity claims of supercentenarians. Many people, however, persistently believe stories that there are concentrations of extremely old people living in certain regions of the world.

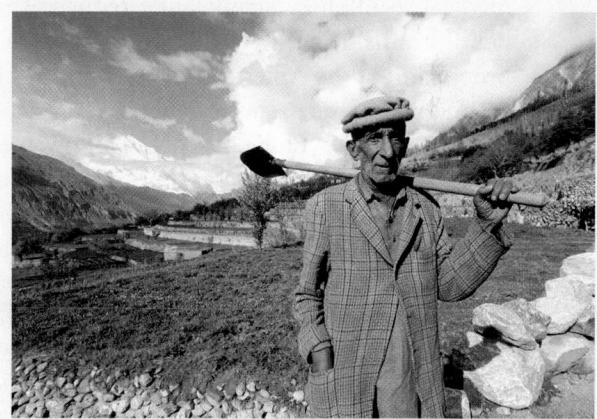

© Martin Puddy/age footstock

Medical experts customarily divide the human life span into stages or periods. Most people reach physical maturity or adulthood by the time they are 25 years old, but *adulthood* usually refers to the period spanning 21 through 65 years of age. Older adulthood, or **senescence**, is the stage of life that begins at 65 years of age and ends with death. In this chapter, the terms *older adulthood*, *old*, *aging*, *older adult*, and *elderly* are interchangeable with *senescence*. The ages that define these life stages are arbitrary; there are no obvious physical signs that indicate the precise ages when one passes from young adulthood into middle age or from middle age into senescence.

life expectancy The average number of years that an individual who was born in a particular year can expect to live.

Life Expectancy

Life expectancy is the average number of years that an individual who was born in a particular year can expect to live. In the United States, life expectancies vary according to age, sex, and socioeconomic status. Overall, American females outlive American males by about 5 years.[7] As a result, the older adult population consists of about one-third more women than men. The reasons for these differences are unclear, but hormonal, genetic, and socioeconomic factors are thought to influence life expectancy.

Life expectancies increased dramatically during the 20th century, especially for people who live in developed countries. In the United States, for example, individuals born in 1900 could expect to live 47 years; individuals born in 2009 can expect to live 78.7 years.[7] An increase in life expectancy generally occurs when fewer people die during the earlier stages of life rather than in the later ones.

In the first part of the 20th century, people lived past 65 years of age, but so many younger individuals died from serious injuries, infections, and in childbirth that these statistics lowered overall life expectancy. By the 1950s advances in scientific and medical technology significantly reduced the number of deaths from these conditions. Today, a greater proportion of the American population lives beyond age 65 than in the past.

In 2012, 13.7% of the U.S. population was 65 years of age and older.[4] Between the mid-1940s and the mid-1960s, the birthrate was unusually high in the United States. As a result, experts estimate that about 23.3% of the U.S. population will be 65 years and older by the year 2030.[5] **Figure 15.2** shows estimates of the number of Americans who are or will be 65 or more years of age in 2020, 2040, and 2060.

Scientists are learning more about the causes of aging and are seeking ways to extend life expectancy. Their efforts have led to the development and testing of new therapies for today's major killers: cancer and cardiovascular disease. Advances in genetic engineering offer ways to prevent and treat inherited disorders that can lead to disability and premature death. Additionally, organ transplantation gives thousands of dying individuals the opportunity to survive by replacing their failing organs with healthy ones. Living longer, however, does not necessarily mean living better.

Preserving the quality of life becomes increasingly important as people grow older. By the time Americans reach 65 years of age, chronic illnesses and disabilities often reduce their quality of life. A measurement called "years of healthy life" estimates the negative impact that quality of life can have on life expectancy. Two broad goals of *Healthy People 2020* include attaining high-quality, longer lives free of preventable disease, disability, injury, and premature death and promoting quality of life, healthy development, and health behaviors across all life stages. Presently, Americans males and females can still expect to live in good health for 65 and 68 years, respectively.[8]

The Characteristics of Aged Americans

The majority of Americans older than 65 years of age own their homes or live with family members, and they can handle their financial matters and manage various daily living activities such as bathing, dressing, and cooking. Most older adults suffer from at least one chronic health problem, particularly hypertension, heart disease, arthritis, cancer, and diabetes.[9] Many older adults with mild physical disabilities live independently by making some adaptations to their homes. For example, installing elevated toilets, grab bars, and shower seats makes it easier for people with physical conditions such as arthritis to take care of their personal hygiene (**Figure 15.3**).

In July 2012, approximately 5.9 million Americans were 85 years or older.[4] This population is increasing so rapidly that experts think about 21 million people will be in this age group by 2060. People who are 85 years old and older, the "oldest of the old," are more likely to be severely disabled and unable to live independently than the "young old" who are 65 to 74 years. In 2012, 3.6% of Americans 65 years and older lived in institutional settings, such as extended-care or long-term care facilities ("nursing homes").[10] However, more than 11% of people 85 years or older lived in these places.

A significant number of older adults are independent and financially secure, often because they planned for their retirement needs when they were young. Today, fewer older Americans live in poverty than in the late 1960s, thanks largely to federal programs such as Social Security, Medicaid, and Medicare. Nevertheless, many older Americans must live on lower incomes than when they were younger. In 2012, 8.7% of older adults had incomes that were less

Figure 15.2

Estimates of the U.S. Population 65 Years of Age and Older in 2020, 2040, and 2060. The number of older adults in the United States is expected to increase significantly in the next 40 years.

Data from U.S. Census Bureau. (n.d.). U.S. population projections. Retrieved from http://www.census.gov/population/projections/data/national/2012.html

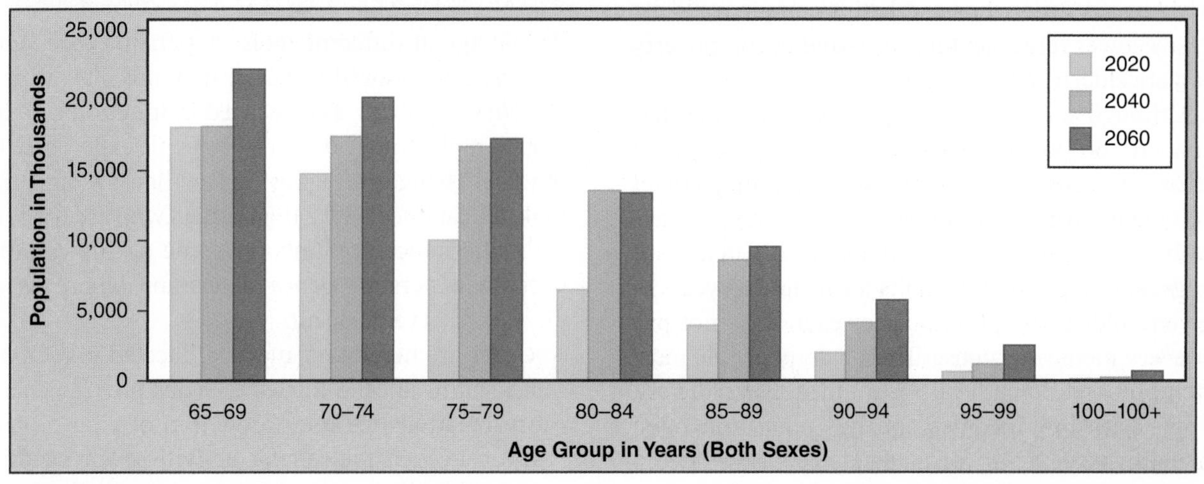

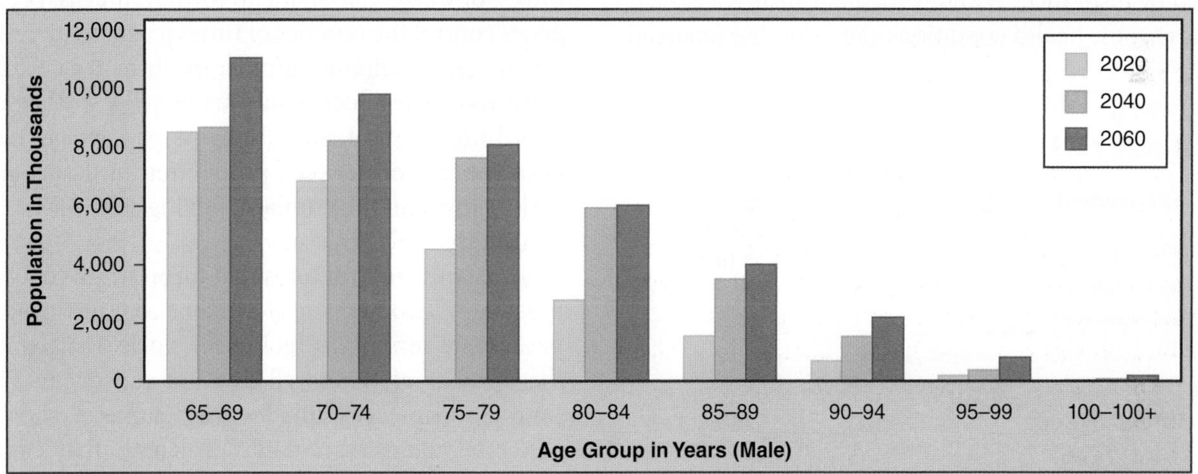

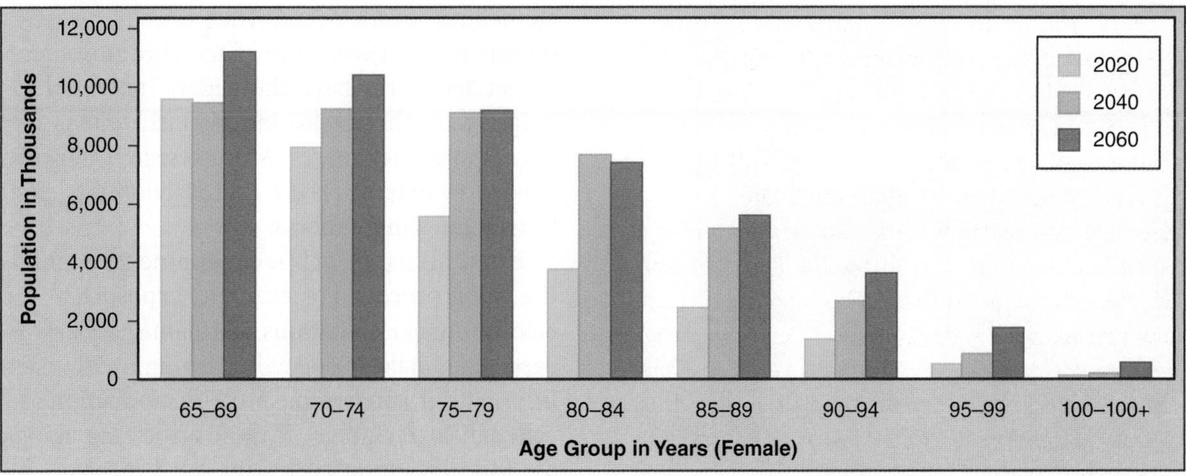

Medicare A federal health insurance program that provides benefits for people 65 years of age and older.

than the federal government's poverty level.[10] Older adults who are members of minority groups, particularly African Americans and Latinos, are more likely to have lower retirement incomes and live in poverty than are elderly White people.

Although some of their expenses are less because they are no longer working, healthcare costs of retirees are generally higher than those of younger individuals. Almost all older American adults have **Medicare**. Medicare is a federal health insurance program that provides benefits for people 65 years of age and older. The program, however, does not pay for every medical expense. Thus, elderly people must often buy additional health insurance. Nevertheless, people with low incomes and less education often have difficulty paying for medical expenses not covered by insurance. Without adequate insurance, serious chronic health conditions can drain the financial resources of older adults and their families. Many older adults continue working beyond the usual retirement age to help pay for health insurance and other expenses.

Figure 15.3

Independent Living. Adding certain features to homes, such as "grab bars" in and next to the shower stall and supportive arms around the toilet, can help older adults with physical disabilities live independently.

Courtesy of Wendy Schiff

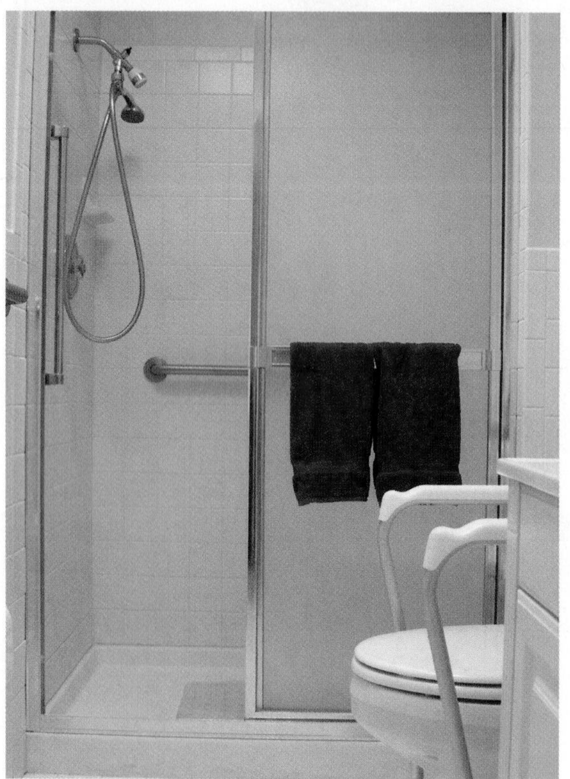

Why Do We Age?

People age at different rates. A person's *chronological age*, as measured in years, may not match his or her *physiologic age*, as measured in functional ability. For example, some 50-year-old people experience the physical changes of aging earlier than average; they look, act, and feel older than others who are the same age. Inheritance accounts for some of this variation because a person's genes determine when certain physiologic events occur.

Genes are hereditary material located on *chromosomes* within a cell's nucleus. Genes provide chemical instructions for the production of vital proteins that are needed for cellular activities. For example, most body cells can divide to form new cells. A cell's genes control the number of times it can divide. After dividing its maximum number of times, the cell dies. Most tissues produce a surplus of cells, so they can afford the death of some cells. As people age, however, the rate of new cell production in tissues normally slows and the number of living cells declines as existing cells die.

Telomeres are structures that form the tips of chromosomes. Telomeres play a major role in the aging process by serving as biological clocks that control the number of times cell division can occur. Each time a normal cell divides, its telomeres shorten. When telomeres reach a certain length, they cannot become shorter and chemical processes that initiate cellular death occur. Theoretically, people who inherit instructions to produce chromosomes with longer telomeres have the genetic potential to live longer than those who inherit instructions to produce shorter telomeres. More research, however, is needed to determine the role of telomere length in the human aging process.

External factors such as environment also influence the aging process. For example, exposure to certain environmental conditions can damage genes. Damaged genes make mistakes in copying and transferring information concerning protein production. Young cells can correct many of these errors, but aging cells are less efficient at correcting such mistakes. When the parts of cells that manufacture proteins receive faulty instructions from the genes, they are unable to produce these compounds. Without an adequate supply of proteins, the affected cells eventually die.

An organ fails if it does not contain enough functioning cells. The systems of the body are interrelated, so when the organs of one system fail, the organs of the other systems soon lose their functional capacities. For example, when a heart that has been weakened by disease cannot pump blood efficiently, the lungs and kidneys are not able to function properly. As a result, other organs fail to perform their jobs, and death occurs.

Radiation, pollution, and some drugs and viruses may damage genes, thereby accelerating the rate of aging and shortening life expectancy. By limiting contact or exposure to these agents, you may be able to lengthen your life expectancy.

Furthermore, adopting a lifestyle that includes regular exercise and a diet high in fruits and vegetables, as well as avoiding smoking, can significantly reduce your risk of common chronic diseases (e.g., heart disease, cancer). The "Changing Health Habits" feature of this chapter can help you identify and change unhealthy practices.

The Effects of Aging on Physical Health

People begin to experience a gradual and irreversible decline in the functioning of their bodies when they are about 30 years old. Even healthy people experience this progressive decline as they grow older. Some common signs of aging, such as menopause, delayed sexual responsiveness, graying and thinning hair, loss of height, and *presbyopia*, the inability to see close objects clearly, reflect normal changes associated with growing old. **Table 15.1** describes some significant physical changes that are associated with normal senescence. As you can see, growing old affects every system of the body.

Table 15.1

Biological Effects of Normal Aging

System	Normal Changes
Cardiovascular	Heart function remains normal, but the heart muscle thickens; arterial walls thicken; pulse rate declines
Skeletal	Bone loss occurs, which can be abnormal if excessive (osteoporosis)
Nervous	Brain weight decreases, especially in the cerebral cortex; neurotransmitter levels decline, nervous message transmission and muscular responses slow; short-term memory becomes less efficient; visual and hearing ability decreases; the ability to taste bitter and salty foods declines; sleep disturbances, such as taking longer to fall asleep and frequent awakening during the night, often occur
Immune	Immune response against pathogens or developing cancer cells declines
Endocrine	Many hormone levels decline, including insulin (regulates carbohydrate metabolism), aldosterone (regulates sodium metabolism), thyroid, estrogen, and growth hormones
Digestive	Tooth loss becomes more likely as gums recede; levels of stomach acid drop; intestinal absorption of calcium is less efficient; constipation can occur, often the result of medications or poor diet
Muscular	Muscle mass declines, resulting in less strength; stamina reduction occurs
Reproductive	Menopause occurs in women, resulting in thinning of vaginal lining, less vaginal lubrication, and shrinkage of reproductive organs; breast tissue shrinks; prostate gland enlarges in men; sexual responsiveness slows so that it takes longer for erections to occur; orgasms are shorter and less intense
Urinary	Kidneys become less efficient at filtering wastes from the blood
Skin (integument)	Skin becomes drier and less elastic, resulting in wrinkles; scalp hair growth slows, and its loss increases; hair growth in the nose and ears increases; fingernails often become yellow, develop ridges, and split

macular degeneration A leading cause of vision loss for people age 60 years and older.

cataracts A chronic condition in which the lens of the eye becomes cloudy and opaque, impairing vision.

glaucoma (glaw-KO-mah) A chronic ailment that occurs when fluid pressure increases in the eye.

Aging is an individual process. There is no timetable that specifies at what age people can expect a particular physical change to occur. The rate at which these alterations occur, however, accelerates after 65 years of age. As a result of these normal changes, the aging body is less able to adapt to stress, repair itself, and resist or fight infection. Infections and accidents that were minor health problems when a person was young can become disabling or deadly experiences when a person is old.

Compared to young adults, elderly people are more likely to develop nutritional deficiencies, especially of vitamins D and B12, because aging bodies are less able to absorb or use certain nutrients. The serious health problems that often affect older adults, such as heart disease and hypertension, are associated with lifestyle and are preventable to some extent.

Although certain chronic conditions such as arthritis commonly affect elderly people, they are not normal aspects of aging. These ailments may not be life threatening, but they frequently reduce the quality of life.

Age-Related Macular Degeneration In the United States, **macular degeneration** is a leading cause of vision loss for people age 60 and older.[11] The macula is a small region in the eye that enables you to see objects in your central line of vision clearly. As many people age, the light-sensitive cells in the macula gradually die, resulting in distorted, blurry, or lost central vision. People with macular degeneration have difficulty reading, driving, and viewing television or a computer monitor. To test your vision for macular degeneration, visit www.amd.org/living-with-amd/resources-and-tools/31-amsler-grid.html.

In about 10% of cases, tiny blood vessels form under the macula and leak fluid and bleed, causing severe vision loss ("wet" or advanced macular degeneration). Medication and laser surgery can stop the bleeding in early stages of wet macular degeneration, but these treatments cannot restore lost vision. There is no effective treatment for the "dry" form of macular degeneration, and this condition can lead to the "wet" form.

Preventing macular degeneration is important. Aging people who smoke and have a family history of macular degeneration have a high risk of developing the condition. Other risk factors include age, obesity, and female sex. Eating a diet that contains plenty of dark green leafy vegetables, such as spinach, collards, and mustard greens, may protect against macular degeneration. For people who have been diagnosed with the disease, zinc and antioxidant supplements may slow the deterioration of the macula. However, these dietary substances can be toxic and should not be taken without consulting a physician.

Cataracts Although the reasons for their occurrence are unclear, **cataracts** are common in people older than 50 years of age. A cataract forms when the normally transparent lens of the eye becomes cloudy and opaque with aging. Clouded lenses scatter light as it enters the eyes, making it difficult to see images clearly. Symptoms of cataracts include blurry and double vision, sensitivity to bright light, and seeing halos around objects. Without surgery to remove damaged lenses, cataracts can lead to blindness. In many cases, surgeons can replace natural lenses with artificial ones; in others, they remove the damaged lenses and prescribe eyeglasses or contact lenses.

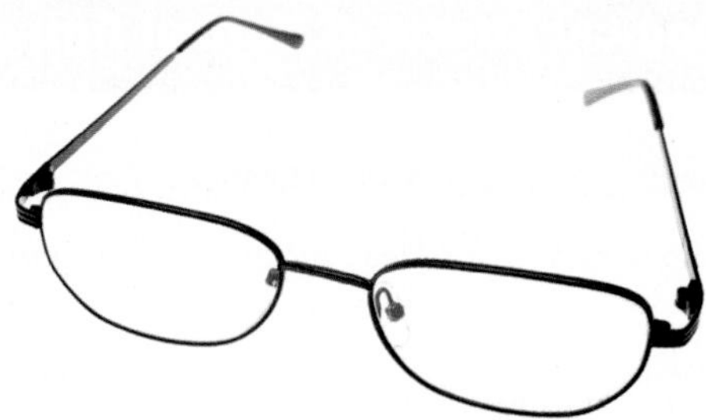

Some medical experts think that exposure to ultraviolet light can cause cataracts. You may be able to reduce your risk of cataracts by wearing sunglasses to shield your eyes, when you are outdoors.

Glaucoma **Glaucoma** is another ailment that frequently affects the vision of aged people. In this condition, an abnormal amount of fluid accumulates in the eyeball. Over time, the high fluid pressure causes vision loss by permanently damaging the optic nerve, the nerve that transmits visual information to the brain. Eye pain, headache, and loss of peripheral vision are symptoms of glaucoma. Risk factors for developing glaucoma include family history, African ancestry, diabetes, and cardiovascular disease. In most cases, placing medicinal drops into the eyes can control the condition. In severe cases of glaucoma, surgery is necessary to reduce the fluid pressure within the eyeball.

Glaucoma may not produce noticeable symptoms; therefore, early detection is the best way to control the effects of the disorder. A simple, painless screening test is available that can identify the disease before serious damage to the optic nerve occurs. Thus, you can prevent the irreversible effects of glaucoma by having a physician or optometrist perform periodic screenings.

Arthritis **Arthritis** is a broad group of chronic joint diseases characterized by inflammation, pain, swelling, and loss of mobility ("stiffness") of affected joints. Rheumatoid arthritis, osteoarthritis, "lupus," fibromyalgia, and gout are forms of arthritis. Rheumatoid arthritis and lupus can affect multiple organs and cause a wide variety of symptoms (**Figure 15.4**).

According to the Centers for Disease Control and Prevention, an estimated 50 million adult Americans suffer from doctor-diagnosed arthritis.[12] Regardless of age, arthritis is the leading cause of disability among Americans.[12] In *osteoarthritis*, the cartilage that protects the ends of bones and keeps them from rubbing together at joints wears away and breaks down. As a result, tiny bits of cartilage or bone float in the fluid that fills the joint and the joint becomes misshapen (**Figure 15.5**). People often confuse osteoarthritis with osteoporosis, a different condition that affects older adults.

Older adults are more likely to develop osteoarthritis than young persons are.[12] Joints simply wear out as a person ages. Other contributing factors include heredity, overuse, injury, and obesity. Overuse and injury of joints can occur when performing sports or jobs that place excessive stress on joints. Obese older adults have a high risk of developing osteoarthritis because carrying around extra weight stresses joints, especially the knees.

Figure 15.4

Effects of Arthritis on the Hands. Arthritis damages joint tissue, resulting in deformities and the loss of flexibility.

© Dr. Ken Greet/Visuals Unlimited

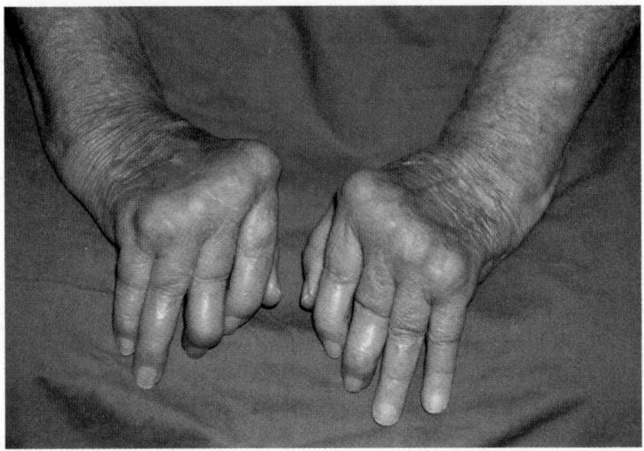

arthritis A group of diseases characterized by inflammation of the joints.

Although arthritis is a chronic disease, symptoms tend to come and go. Treatment for osteoarthritis includes medications to relieve inflammation and pain and exercises to strengthen muscles and improve or maintain joint mobility. Losing weight reduces

Figure 15.5

Effects of Osteoarthritis. (a) In a healthy joint, such as the knee joint, the ends of bones are encased in smooth cartilage. The bone ends are protected by a joint capsule lined with a synovial membrane that produces synovial fluid. The capsule and fluid protect the cartilage, muscles, and connective tissues. (b) This illustration shows a knee joint severely affected by osteoarthritis. Note that the cartilage has worn away. Spurs grow out from the edge of the bone, and synovial fluid within the joint increases. As a result, the joint is difficult to move and it is sore.

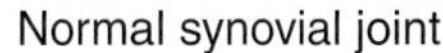

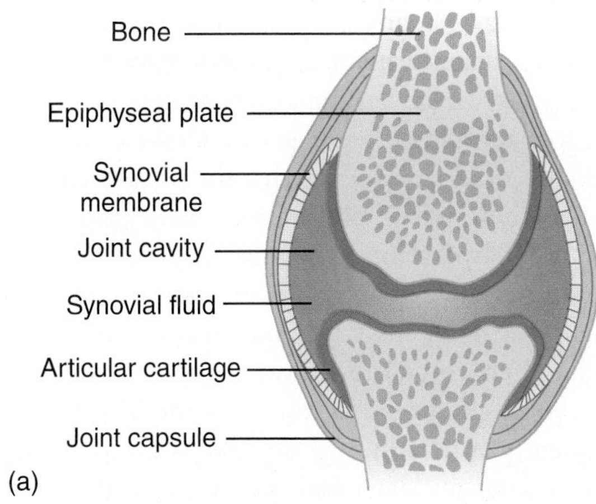

Pathologic changes in osteoarthritis

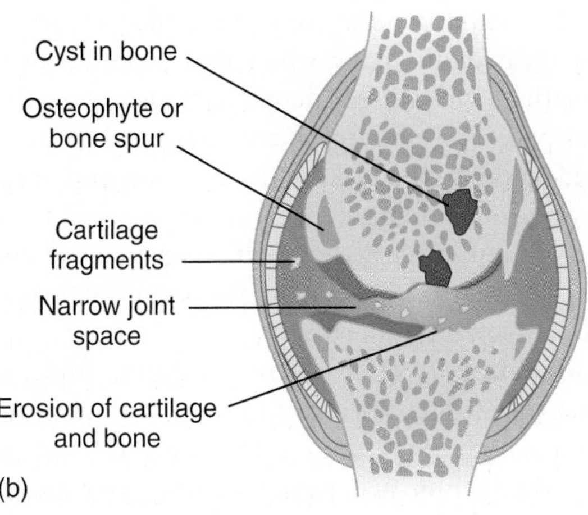

urinary incontinence The inability to control the flow of urine from the bladder.

Alzheimer's disease (AD) An incurable, progressive, degenerative disease that affects the functioning of the brain.

dementia A brain disorder that seriously affects normal cognitive abilities.

stress on weight-bearing joints in obese people. In some cases, surgery is necessary to replace damaged joints with artificial implants.

Urinary Incontinence **Urinary incontinence**, the inability to control the flow of urine from the bladder, is an embarrassing and costly problem for millions of Americans. As people age, the muscles that control bladder emptying weaken, making it easier for urine to leak out when people move, sneeze, cough, or lift heavy things. Many older adults experience involuntary contractions of their bladders that cause some urine to be eliminated unexpectedly. Medications, infections, strokes, tumors, history of childbirth in women, and enlargement of the prostate gland in men can contribute to urinary incontinence.

The fear of leaking urine accidentally while in public often makes many incontinent people avoid social situations. If family members cannot manage an incontinent elderly relative at home, they often find it necessary to place him or her in an extended-care facility.

Many older adults restrict their fluid intake to reduce their urine production. This practice can lead to dehydration. The majority of individuals who experience urinary incontinence can benefit from treatment, such as behavioral techniques that enable them to be more aware of the bladder's state of fullness. By learning to empty the bladder more frequently, a person may be able to avoid the leakage. People can learn and practice a series of exercises that strengthen the pelvic muscles that control urination. These exercises, called *Kegel* exercises, involve imitating the same muscular movements that individuals make when they voluntarily stop urinating. Incontinent people can also wear absorbent pads and undergarments designed to prevent incidents of urine leakage. Medication and surgery may alleviate incontinence. Embarrassment or concerns about surgery, however, keep many incontinent people from discussing this common problem with personal physicians.

Alzheimer's Disease You cannot find your keys; you forget an appointment; you sometimes call your child by your cat's name. Do you ever have the feeling that you are losing your mind? It may be reassuring to know that everyone has these and other similar annoying experiences from time to time, but many middle-aged Americans worry that instances of forgetfulness are early symptoms of **Alzheimer's disease (AD)**. According to the Alzheimer's Association, the most common early sign of the disease is difficulty recalling newly learned information.[13]

AD is an incurable, progressive, degenerative disease that affects the functioning of the brain. People with AD have abnormal amounts of a protein that forms clumps between cells in the brain. These clumps interfere with brain cells' ability to communicate with each other. Furthermore, tangled bundles of useless protein fibers form within the brain cells, disrupting cell function. As an increasing number of brain cells die, the signs and symptoms of AD become more apparent.

Experts with the Alzheimer's Association estimate that more than 5 million Americans, mostly elderly persons, currently live with AD.[14] As the baby boom generation ages, 10 million more people will be added to this number. By the year 2050, three times as many Americans will suffer from this dreaded disease.

AD is the most common form of **dementia**, a brain disorder that seriously affects normal *cognitive* (thinking) abilities, such as recalling information and solving problems. Strokes and Parkinson's disease also are major causes of dementia. Common features of AD include memory loss, mental confusion, and loss of control over behavior and body functions. Although AD is incurable, a few medications can be prescribed to slow the decline in cognitive functioning, control certain inappropriate behaviors of patients, and improve patients' moods.

Age and family history are major risk factors for AD. Although the disease is common among older adults, it is not a normal feature of growing old. What are the signs of AD? Is it preventable?

In the early stages of Alzheimer's, affected people may notice lapses in their memories and cognitive abilities. For example, they may have unusual difficulty remembering events that happened recently, learning new information, and using information to make reasonable conclusions. These symptoms typically begin between 40 and 60 years of age. Over time, people with the disease become increasingly forgetful, confused, disoriented, restless, and moody. Communicating becomes difficult as their speech deteriorates; depression is common. These changes are distressing to patients with AD, their family members, and their associates. One woman recalls her affected mother-in-law's gradual loss of cognitive functioning:

The first time I had a feeling that my elderly mother-in-law might have a serious problem with her memory occurred in April when she got lost while driving to our house. We live close to her and she had made the short trip dozens of times. When I told my husband that this was unusual behavior for her and could be a sign of a memory problem, he disagreed and said it was "easy" to make a wrong turn on the way to our house. A few months later, I was driving Mother to a store when she insisted that I should be making a right turn instead of a left one at a familiar intersection in our town. When I told her she was wrong, she became angry and argued with me about the directions to the store. When I finally reached the store, she recognized the place but didn't apologize for her behavior. At Christmas, Mother was very quiet and seemed to be in a fog. My husband and his sister finally recognized that she was "not herself," and they took her to the doctor's for an evaluation. After a series of medical tests to rule out minor strokes and other causes of brain damage, her condition was diagnosed as mild-to-moderate Alzheimer's disease.

Mother now takes two medications that seem to help her memory a little. At this point, she is not supposed to drive and she needs help with housework. She still cooks, but I'm concerned she'll forget that she's making something and she'll start a fire in her kitchen. My husband and his sister are thinking about selling Mother's house and placing her in a special group home for people with this terrible disease. I dread the day when my husband greets his mother and she doesn't recognize him.

As AD progresses, its victims neglect their personal hygiene; their facial expressions become "flat" (emotionless); and they exhibit inappropriate and unpredictable behaviors such as undressing in public and attacking caregivers. In the terminal stages, individuals with this devastating illness require constant care. They are bedridden and unable to talk and eat. Nothing can be done to stop the relentless progression of the disease. After diagnosis, the average person can expect to survive about 8 years. Some people with AD live only 4 years after diagnosis, whereas others are able to live for 20 years with the disease.[14] Death often results from pneumonia and starvation as the degenerating brain is unable to control vital functions such as breathing, swallowing, and digestion. In 2011, about 84,691 Americans died of AD, making it the sixth leading cause of death.[7]

Physicians often diagnose AD when patients cannot answer questions like those listed in **Table 15.2**.

Table 15.2

Simple Memory Test for Identifying Dementia

Ask the person:

1. His or her age
2. His or her date of birth
3. The time to the nearest hour
4. His or her address
5. The current year
6. Where he or she is
7. The names of two people who are pictured in family photos
8. The years of World War II
9. The name of the current president of the United States
10. To count backwards from 100 to 1
11. His or her phone number

Adapted from Wattis, J. (1996). What an old age psychiatrist does. *British Medical Journal*, 313, 101–104.

Until recently, the only way to confirm the diagnosis was by examining the patient's brain after death. Brain imaging techniques such as magnetic resonance imaging (MRI) scans can now detect shrinkage in areas of the cerebral cortex, the thinking part of the brain. Such brain shrinkage is a sign of AD.

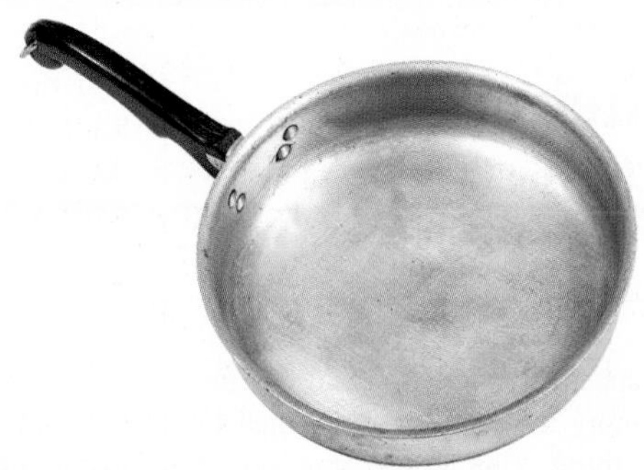

Using aluminum cookware does not increase the risk of Alzheimer's disease.

The factors that cause AD are unclear. At least two forms of the disorder are inherited. Although genetic testing is available to determine whether relatives of patients with AD have the genes associated with the condition, many people who test positive do not develop the disease. Other forms of AD may be

Analyzing Health-Related Information

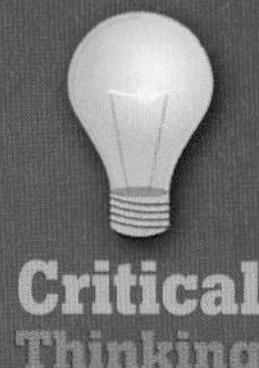

Critical Thinking

The following article is an abbreviated version of "Alzheimer's: Few Clues on the Mysteries of Memory" that appeared in *FDA Consumer* magazine. Read the article and evaluate it using the model for analyzing health-related information. The main points of the model are noted here.

1. Which statements are verifiable facts, and which are unverified statements or value claims?
2. What are the credentials of the person who wrote the article? Does this person have the appropriate background and education in the topic area? What can you do to check the person's credentials?
3. What might be the motives and biases of the person who wrote the article?
4. What is the main point of the article? Which information is relevant to the issue, main point? Which information is irrelevant?
5. Is the source reliable? What evidence supports your conclusion that the source is reliable or unreliable? Does the source of information present the pros and cons of the topic?
6. Does the source of information attack the credibility of conventional scientists or medical authorities?

Based on your analysis, do you think that this article is a reliable source of health-related information? Explain why you think it is or is not. Summarize your reasons for coming to this conclusion.

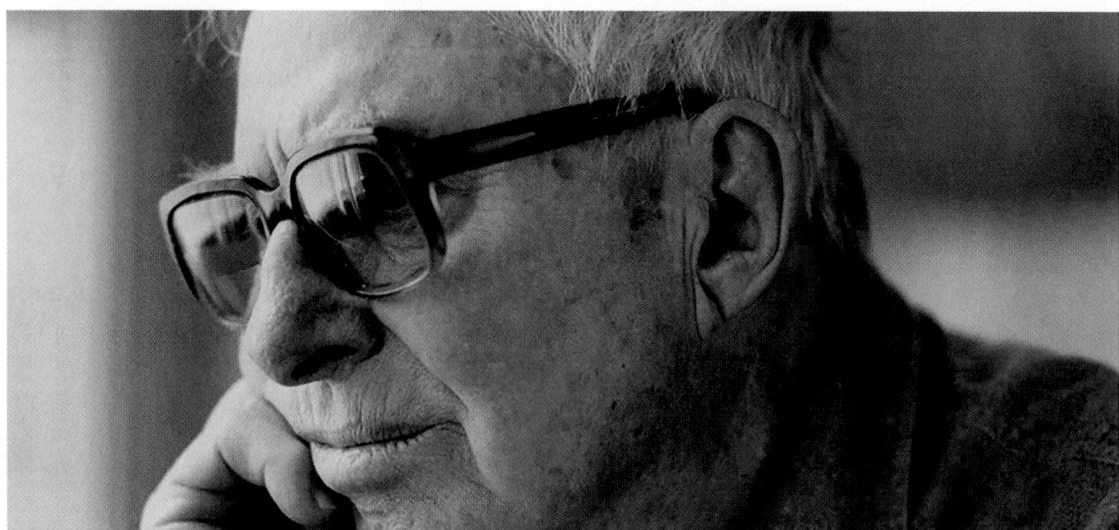

Alzheimer's

Few Clues on the Mysteries of Memory

by Audrey T. Hingley

It happened some years ago but the memory is still firmly implanted in my mind. One sunny afternoon I heard the sound of a car pulling into our driveway, peered out of my living room window, and saw one of my father's friends, Sam (not his real name), then in his early 80s. Sam got out of his car and walked just a few steps. I watched as he stood for a few moments, gazing at our house with an expressionless face. Then he silently returned to his car, got in, and drove away, without ever knocking on our door or communicating with us in any way.

I thought the incident puzzling, but it wasn't until months later that I learned the reason for it. Sam had Alzheimer's, a progressive disease in which nerve cells in the brain degenerate and brain substance shrinks.

A widower living alone, Sam clearly was in a dangerous position. Once he was followed home by a police officer, who told his grown children he had found Sam stopped by the side of the road, not able to remember how to get home by himself.

Sam's story is being played out in the lives of up to 4 million Americans who suffer from Alzheimer's disease. The disease plays no favorites, attacking rich and poor, famous and ordinary. Among its most famous sufferers: former President Ronald Reagan.

With an average lifetime cost of care per patient of $174,000, it is the third most expensive disease in America, following only heart disease and cancer. But perhaps even more staggering than the monetary costs are the emotional and psychological costs borne by both patients and their families.

"People are very frightened of the possibilities because they know it represents a loss of one's self," says Steven T. DeKosky, M.D., director of the Alzheimer's Disease Research Center at the University of Pittsburgh and a practicing neurologist. "It's a very frightening prospect to see a loved one who looks the same but doesn't talk or act the same."

"I Have Lost Myself"

Alzheimer's disease, a progressive, degenerative disease attacking the brain and resulting in impaired thinking, behavior and memory, was first described by

Alois Alzheimer, M.D., in 1906. German researchers recently found an important set of notes from Alzheimer's journal of the world's first documented case of the disease. The patient exhibited many of the symptoms seen in Alzheimer's patients today. But perhaps most poignant of all is the patient's own description of the disease: "I have lost myself."

In Alzheimer's, nerve cells in the part of the brain responsible for memory and other thought processes degenerate for still-unknown reasons. Some of the most severely affected cells normally use acetylcholine, a brain chemical, to communicate. Tacrine (brand name Cognex, also called THA), the first drug approved by the Food and Drug Administration specifically to treat Alzheimer's disease, works by slowing the breakdown of acetylcholine. This results in relieving some memory impairment.

Tacrine does not cure Alzheimer's or slow the disease's progression. It has only been studied in those with mild to moderate Alzheimer's disease who were otherwise in generally good health. Because tacrine can increase the blood levels of a liver enzyme that can indicate liver damage, regular monitoring is necessary. Other side effects include nausea, vomiting, diarrhea, abdominal pain, skin rash, and indigestion.

Aricept (generic name donepezil hydrochloride, also called E2020), approved by the Food and Drug Administration (FDA) in 1996, is by far the most used drug for Alzheimer's treatment. Like tacrine, Aricept inhibits the breakdown of acetylcholine but does not cause the kind of increase in liver enzymes that tacrine does. It can also cause diarrhea, vomiting, nausea, fatigue, insomnia, and anorexia, but in most cases, such side effects are mild and decline with continued use of the drug. Again, the drug helps only those patients with mild to moderate symptoms of Alzheimer's and does not stop or slow the disease's progression.

Forgetfulness or Alzheimer's?

Although most people understand at least some of the horrifying aspects of Alzheimer's disease, DeKosky says a big challenge is educating people regarding the widely held assumption that people are supposed to have memory impairment as they age.

"There's this huge prejudice where we think people should have severe mental impairment as they get older," he says. Memory loss, disorientation, and confusion are not part of the normal aging process, he explains. They are symptoms of dementia, and the most common form of dementia is Alzheimer's.

"You need to look at the functional consequences of what someone cannot remember," DeKosky says. "If mom forgets where she put her car in the parking lot at the mall, that's not abnormal. But if she walks home from the mall because she forgot she took her car, that's not normal. Memory is the first and worst change, but you will also see social withdrawal and less willingness to interact with others."

The Need for Answers

Although no cure for Alzheimer's is available now, planning and medical/social management can help ease the burden on both patient and family members. Physical exercise, good nutrition, and social activities are important. A calm, structured environment may also help the person to continue functioning.

At some point, however, people with Alzheimer's require 24-hour care. The financing of such care, including diagnosis costs, treatment, and paid care, is estimated to be $100 billion annually, according to the Alzheimer's Association. The federal government covers $4.4 billion and the states another $4.1 billion, with much of the remaining costs borne by patients and their families.

"It's a national imperative to find effective means to diagnose, treat and prevent this disease," says David Banks, R.Ph., a public health specialist in the FDA's Office of Special Health Issues. "When you look at it demographically, the nearly 80 million baby boomers living in the United States . . . now have an average life expectancy of approximately 78 years. One in five Americans could be age 65 or older by 2030, and tens of millions of baby boomers will live into their 80s. The Alzheimer's Association projects that as many as 14 million Americans could have Alzheimer's disease in 2050. When viewed in the context of accelerating Social Security and Medicare costs . . . , the future monetary costs of Alzheimer's disease may be unsustainable. The human costs could be even greater."

Note: Audrey T. Hingley is a freelance writer in Mechanicsville, Virginia.

the result of slow-acting brain viruses, brain injury, or exposure to pollutants. At one time, scientists thought that aluminum poisoning caused the disease because higher than normal amounts of this metal are found in the brains of patients who died of AD. Many people are concerned about the safety of using aluminum cookware and the natural presence of this element in drinking water. However, most experts think that the unusual concentration of aluminum in the brains of persons with AD is a result, not a cause, of the disorder. Nevertheless, scientists are investigating whether environmental factors, such as exposure to other minerals, may contribute to AD.

Can Alzheimer's disease be prevented? Lifestyle factors appear to play a role in reducing the risk of AD. Keeping physically active, being involved in a variety of intellectually stimulating activities, and maintaining an extensive social network are associated with a lower risk of AD.[15] Making certain dietary changes may also help. Results of one study indicated that people who eat high amounts of salad dressing, fruit, nuts, fish, tomatoes, cruciferous vegetables (broccoli and cabbage, for example), dark green and leafy vegetables, and low amounts of high-fat milk products, red meat, and butter have lower risk of AD than people who did not eat this dietary pattern.[16]

More research is needed to determine whether a particular dietary pattern protects against AD.

Elevated blood cholesterol levels, particularly LDL cholesterol, are associated with increased risk of AD.[17] Results of recent studies, however, do not support taking cholesterol-lowering medications, such as certain *statins*, to reduce the risk of AD.[17,18] Nevertheless, more research is needed to confirm these findings.

Inflammation and the effects of excess oxidation in the body, especially in the brain, may increase the risk of AD.[19] Thus, herbal preparations and substances in foods that have anti-inflammatory and antioxidant activity may protect against AD. *Curcumin*, a chemical with anti-inflammatory and antioxidant activity, may help prevent the disease.[20,21] The spice and food coloring agent turmeric contains curcumin. *EGb 761*, an extract made from leaves of the ginkgo biloba tree, has antioxidant activity. Promoters of dietary supplements that contain ginkgo claim their products can treat memory loss, confusion, depression, and other conditions associated with Alzheimer's disease.[22]

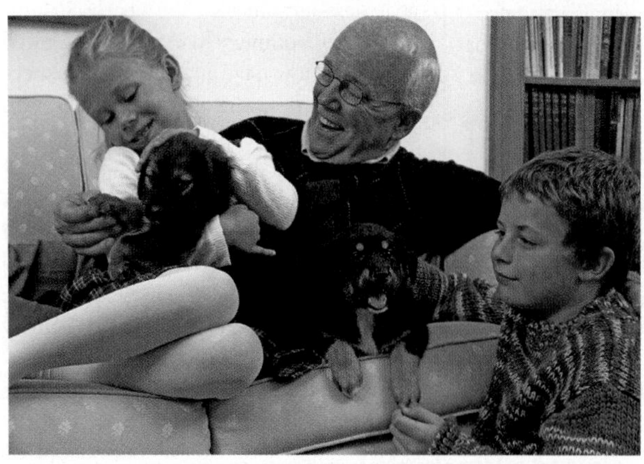

Older adults often enjoy caring for their grandchildren.

Although a review of several scientific studies indicated EGb 761 can improve cognitive functioning, the extract's beneficial effects were slight.[23] Results of the Ginkgo Evaluation Memory Study indicate ginkgo had no effect on memory loss or AD.[24]

Vitamins E and C have antioxidant effects. According to results of certain studies, populations that consume vitamin E–rich diets have lower risk of Alzheimer's disease.[25] No such benefit, however, was observed in groups of people taking high amounts of vitamin E, multivitamin, or other vitamin supplements.[24] Researchers continue to investigate the association between dietary sources of antioxidants, such as fruits, vegetables, and vegetable oils, and the risk of Alzheimer's disease. At present, there is no conclusive scientific evidence that supports the effectiveness of any specific dietary supplement in preventing the disease.[24]

Patients with Alzheimer's often live at home until they reach the terminal stage and require the care provided in a skilled nursing care facility. Living with an affected loved one can be emotionally stressful and physically demanding. While caring for a patient with this disease, family members must try to maintain their own health and well-being. To provide assistance, many communities have special "adult day care" centers where persons with AD can spend a few hours during the day before returning to their homes. Not every community offers this service, so if you need help caring for someone with AD, check with your local mental health association or Alzheimer's Association for information about adult day care centers in your area.

The Effects of Aging on Psychological Health

As they approach the end of middle age, most employed people face retirement, and many aging parents have grown children with families who have moved away. If older adults equate retirement from jobs and separation from their families with being old and useless, they may experience serious psychological distress. Additionally, the dramatic reduction of financial resources that often accompanies retirement can mean a serious loss of economic stability.

On the other hand, many older adults approach retirement age with a positive outlook and look forward to this time of life. Some find pleasure from traveling, volunteering in their communities, spending time with their grandchildren, and exploring new interests. Others choose to continue working, especially if they enjoy what they do and their work is intellectually stimulating and personally fulfilling. Older adults often have a wealth of knowledge and experience that they can share with younger members of society.

Older adults, especially those older than 85 years of age, can experience deteriorating health, difficult social circumstances, and poor economic conditions. Deaths of spouses and friends, separations from family, and reductions in financial resources create emotional stress. As a result, elderly persons often suffer depression.

Regardless of one's age, depression is associated with an increased risk of suicide. In the United States, older adults are twice as likely to commit suicide when compared to people who are 10–24 years of age.[26] Older adults who are divorced or widowed are more likely to commit suicide than married older adults.[27] Poor health is another risk factor for suicide. Older adults suffering from chronic conditions, particularly mental illness, heart failure, obstructive lung disease, and pain, are more likely to commit suicide than older adults who did not have these conditions.[28]

Like younger people, older people who are depressed or isolated can benefit from participation in social and physical activities. In addition, antidepressant medications or psychotherapy can help people regain and maintain their emotional balance.

The Effects of Aging on Social Health

Although a large segment of the U.S. population is older than 65 years, our society is highly youth oriented. Not surprisingly, middle-age Americans often worry that aging will mean losing their jobs to younger people, being forced into early retirement, becoming widowed, and suffering from debilitating illnesses. Growing old in America can have serious social impacts on older adults; they may be ignored, neglected, and abused by younger members of the population.

Some people in our society have negative attitudes toward older adults and stereotype older people as poor, sick, useless, and dependent. Some young adults believe that older adults demand too much from the rest of society. **Ageism** is a bias against older adults. Ageism creates conflict between the generations because the old do not trust the young and vice versa. Realizing that growing older does not always mean having poor health, living in an institution, depending on public support, or being useless can help combat ageism.

Older adults represent a valuable social asset that is not well used. Aging parents and grandparents often have experience and wisdom that they can share with younger family members. Additionally, many retirees have a variety of talents and special organizational skills that enable them to serve as consultants, managers, or advisors in business, governmental, or educational settings. Although many younger people think they can find any information needed by "Googling it," older people have a wealth of knowledge and social, relationship, and employment experiences to share. Both young and old benefit when each accepts, values, and trusts the other.

Successful Aging

Many people would like to believe that it is possible to prevent aging or delay the process. Restricting caloric intakes without creating nutritional deficiencies may slow the rate of aging.[29] The modern search for a "fountain of youth" has resulted in the promotion of pills, potions, diets, or treatments that are touted as having "antiaging" or "life-extending" capabilities. Contrary to the claims of advertisers, none of these substances or regimens prevents or slows aging.[30]

ageism A bias against elderly people.

Instead of searching for magic formulas to extend your life, you can engage in lifestyle choices while you are young to increase your chances of aging successfully. Although there is no generally agreed upon definition for "successful aging," people who age successfully have good physical functioning.[29] Other characteristics of such healthy older adults include having positive attitudes toward themselves and the future and being connected socially with others.

To increase your chances of aging successfully, evaluate your health status and lifestyle, identify specific unhealthy or risky behaviors, and then work at changing those behaviors. Although modifying all unhealthy behaviors is commendable, certain practices are associated more closely with lengthening one's life span than others are.

Physically active people live longer, have higher quality of life, and report being happier than people who are sedentary.[31] Engaging in regular exercise throughout your life will help you control your body weight as well as improve your circulation, strengthen your heart, and maintain your muscle and bone mass. People older than 65 years of age who perform regular exercise improve their physical strength and flexibility, features that can enhance their quality of life.[31] Exercise may improve some cognitive abilities of aging adults, such as memory, and delay the onset of Alzheimer's disease.[32] More research, however, is needed to further support these findings.

The U.S. Centers for Disease Control and Prevention guidelines indicate that older adults should exercise, at a moderate intensity, for at least 150 minutes a week; for greater health benefits, 300 minutes of moderate-intensity exercise is recommended each week. Aerobic exercises, including walking, jogging, water aerobics, cycling, hiking, and exercise machines (stationary bike, elliptical), help maintain cardiovascular health, weight management, and mental/emotional stress relief.

Strength training exercise is recommended for all adults, and it an important part of health maintenance as we age. The U.S. Centers for Disease Control and Prevention recommends older adults engage in strength training at least 2 days a week. Maintaining strength in major muscle groups, especially around important joints (i.e., hips, shoulders, knees) can help us avoid accidents and injuries that become more common as we age (e.g., falling). Weight-bearing exercises are also important for maintaining bone mass and avoiding osteoporosis. Lifting weights, using resistance bands, yoga, and body weight exercise (e.g., pushups) are all appropriate exercises for older people.

Flexibility exercises (e.g., stretching) are also an important aspect of maintaining health as we age. As with strength training, engaging in flexibility exercise regularly helps us maintain range of motion in our hips, shoulders, and backs. Scientific evidence suggests maintaining strength and flexibility helps us maintain healthy circulation and reduces our risk of injury as we age. The American College of Sports Medicine recommends engaging in flexibility exercises at least twice a week, although doing so more often can lead to better results. Flexibility can be gained or maintained through static stretching or engaging in exercises such as yoga or Pilates.

Maintaining social and psychological health is also important of healthy aging. Social isolation is associated with physical and psychological health problems, injuries, and hospitalization. On the other hand, older adults who maintain or develop social networks tend to be happier and have better health.[33] Older adults who engage in social activities display better cognitive, psychological and emotional health and are more likely to adhere to any necessary medical treatment plans. Institutionalization is also less common among older adults who have active social networks. Organized events, such as game nights or dances, and transportation services are available in many areas and can help facilitate social connections among older people. Although we can maintain our social network as we age, it is also important for family members to actively maintain connections with older family members.

As previously stated, engaging in regular exercise and socialization are associated with positive health outcomes as we age. These activities have also been shown to reduce our risk of cognitive decline, which has become more common over past decades. Brain training, or mind games, has also been suggested as a means for maintaining cognitive function. Early studies on rodents demonstrated positive effects on brain function; however, few human studies have shown significant brain function improvement in participants.[34] The effectiveness of brain training remains unclear; however, continued learning, reading and engaging in social activities appears to help us maintain brain function as we age.

Table 15.3 lists some basic recommendations for enhancing your health and quality of life as you age, such as managing stress, maintaining relationships, and developing a positive attitude. It is worth remembering the words of Eubie Blake, a jazz musician who died in 1983 at the age of 100, "If I had known that I was going to live this long, I would have taken better care of myself."

Table 15.3

Tips for Successful Aging

Taking the following actions now, while you are still young, may help you enjoy a healthier, longer life:
• Maintain a healthy weight and eat a nutritious, low-fat diet that includes plenty of whole grains, fruits, and vegetables.
• Be physically active; exercise daily.
• Do not smoke, drink too much alcohol, or abuse other drugs.
• Manage stress; take time to relax daily.
• Have regular physical examinations.
• Adopt safer sex practices.
• Do not drive while under the influence of alcohol or other drugs; always wear a seat belt in vehicles.
• Protect your skin and eyes from sunlight.
• Obtain enough sleep.
• Be concerned about your safety at home, work, or play.
• Maintain social networks with your family and friends.
• Be flexible; expect changes.
• Develop a positive attitude; have a sense of humor.
• Find opportunities to learn new skills or information.
• Get involved with living while accepting your mortality.

Data from Kerschner, H., & Pegues, J. A. (1998). Productive aging: A quality of life agenda. *Journal of the American Dietetic Association*, 98, 1445–1448.; and Turner, L. W., Sizer, F. S., Whitney, E. N., & Wilks, B. B. (1992). *Life Choices: Health Concepts and Strategies*. Minneapolis, MN: West Publishing.

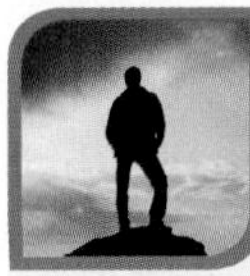

Healthy Living Practices

- Planning for your future financial needs while you are still young can help you enjoy your retirement years.
- To age successfully, evaluate your present health and lifestyle, identify risky behaviors, and then consider changing those behaviors.

Dying

Many Americans, including health professionals, fear dying and death, especially the possibility that dying will be premature and painful. Fearing death makes it difficult to be around someone who is dying. One reason many Americans may fear dying and death is that few have had contact with dying persons or dead bodies. Usually an ambulance rushes the critically injured or terminally ill person to a hospital, where he or she is connected to a variety of life-support machines and placed in an intensive care unit (**Figure 15.6**). Most hospitals permit family members to visit the seriously ill patient for only a few minutes each hour. In other instances, elderly or incurably ill patients die in long-term care facilities with few or no family members present. In the United States, dying often becomes a mechanized, isolated, and depersonalized process.

Dying was very different a hundred years ago. In that era, nearly everyone died at home, surrounded by family and friends. Shortly after death, the body was cooled, and it often remained in the home for the funeral ceremony. It was even customary for people to have photographs taken of their deceased loved ones to remember them (**Figure 15.7**). These practices helped survivors accept dying and death as a part of life.

Figure 15.6

Intensive Care. Treatment of a critically injured or terminally ill person may include being connected to a variety of life-support machines in a hospital's intensive care unit.

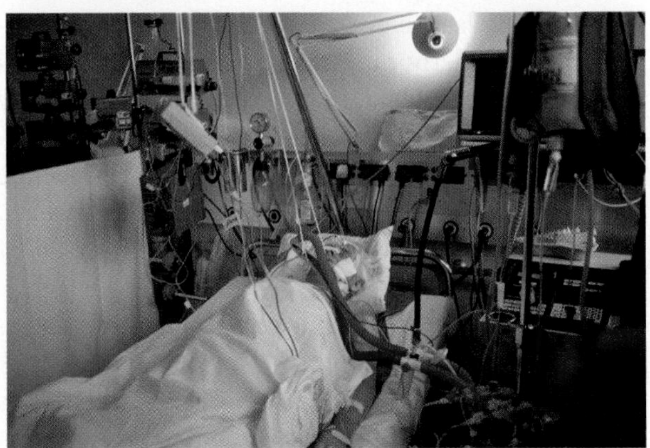

Figure 15.7

Remembrance Photo, Circa 1895. A hundred years ago, nearly everyone died at home, surrounded by their families and friends. It was customary for people to have photographs taken of their deceased loved ones to remember them.

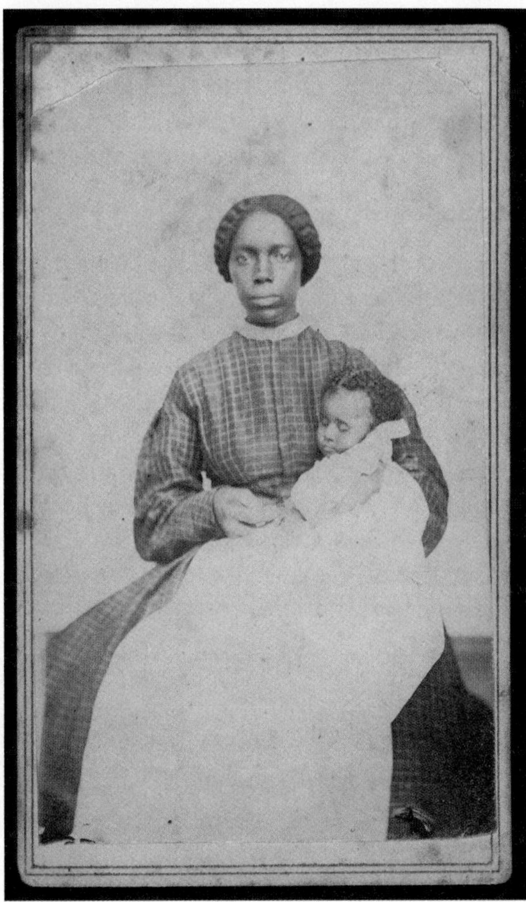

The Spiritual Aspects of Dying

Some people who have been revived after being unresponsive describe "near-death" experiences and relate them as spiritually uplifting events. They report that they were aware of what was happening before they recovered consciousness. They often recall feeling temporarily disengaged from their bodies and having unusual but peaceful sensations. Accounts of near-death experiences often include some features of the person's spiritual or religious beliefs. People who have been in these situations are often profoundly affected by their experiences, but scientists have no ways of verifying their stories.

People who believe in an afterlife may have less fear of dying and death. Many people believe that a soul exists, which leaves the body after death and goes to heaven or hell. Others believe in reincarnation, coming back to life as another person or organism after death. Some individuals are not concerned with what happens to them after death. In many instances, cultural and religious backgrounds provide the foundation for a person's feelings about life after death.

The Emotional Aspects of Dying

Although coping with the death of a beloved person is one of life's most difficult experiences, knowing that your own death is near is especially difficult. In the late 1960s, Elisabeth Kübler-Ross, a psychiatrist at the University of Chicago Billings Hospital, pioneered efforts to understand the psychological processes of dying and death.[35] After interviewing more than 200 terminally ill patients, she formulated a five-stage model to describe the emotional responses that people often experience as they face their deaths (**Table 15.4**).

Table 15.4

Kübler-Ross's Stages of Emotional Responses to Dying

Stage	Typical Responses
Denial	Feels emotionally numb, avoids thinking about his or her condition, ignores the reality of his or her condition
Anger	Lashes out at healthcare providers and loved ones
Bargaining	Makes deals with healthcare providers, loved ones, or God to live long enough to do special things or experience certain events
Depression	Mourns his or her impending death, withdraws socially
Acceptance	Realizes that his or her condition is terminal, gives away cherished items, makes funeral plans

Data from Kübler-Ross, E. (1969). *On Death and Dying*. New York: Macmillan.

The first stage of this coping process is denial. People in denial may act shocked after receiving news of their terminal condition. Frequently, they do not believe their physician's prognosis. While in denial, dying individuals may ignore their troublesome symptoms or seek more optimistic outlooks from other physicians. Some dying patients completely lose faith in the value of conventional medical care; some maintain hope of "beating this thing" by using untested alternative treatments.

As the dying begin to accept their situation, they may enter the second stage, anger. In this stage, dying people are provoked easily; they may lash out at loved ones, medical staff, and anything or anybody. They often demand to know "Why me? Why not someone else?" It is important for people who care for or visit dying individuals to expect this reaction and not take such anger personally.

The third emotional stage of dying is bargaining. Incurably ill individuals may make deals with medical staff or God, promising to exchange exceptionally good behavior for a few more years of life or a painless death. In the fourth stage, depression, dying people become increasingly aware that their condition will not improve. Terminally ill individuals mourn for themselves after realizing that they will not live long enough to enjoy experiences such as watching their children mature or playing with their grandchildren.

The final emotional stage of dying is acceptance. Although terminally ill people continue to hope for cures, they accept the possibility that nothing can be done to save them. Friends, family members, and caregivers can help maintain the self-esteem and dignity of the dying by visiting and touching them, as well as by listening to their concerns.

Critics of Kübler-Ross's research charge that she focused on people who were dying prematurely of chronic illnesses and had time to experience each stage. Therefore, her findings may have been different if she had studied people who were dying of acute illnesses or very sick elderly persons. Some people, particularly the elderly, may not experience all five stages of dying. In addition, aged people who are terminally ill may accept their impending deaths more readily than people who face the prospect of dying while they are still young. The Kübler-Ross model, however, is useful for understanding the complex emotions of dying people.

Dying people are usually under extreme emotional distress. They often feel helpless and hopeless, and they have difficulty relaxing. Treatments such as surgery, chemotherapy, or radiation add to

hospice Health care specifically designed to give emotional support and pain relief to terminally ill people in the final stage of life.

their discomfort. Some terminally ill people fight the prospect of dying; others accept what is happening to them and choose to make the most out of the time they have remaining. In modern societies, death can be the final stage of personal fulfillment if dying people have opportunities to satisfy their social and emotional needs. Thus, some terminally ill people choose to spend more time with their friends and families; others travel far from home.

As the end of life nears, some terminally ill people may become more detached from others and the environment. They may sleep more often and may lapse in and out of consciousness. When awake or conscious, dying persons may not want to talk as much as they did before reaching this stage. According to Kübler-Ross, dying individuals are almost without feelings; most die without fear.

When you know that a beloved person is dying, you may experience a variety of intense emotions. You may be afraid of enduring the emotional pain of watching a close friend or relative die. You may be angry at the dying person, physicians, or God because you feel they are responsible for the impending death, or they are unable or unwilling to prevent it. You may feel guilty about your feelings toward the dying individual. Recognizing that someone is terminally ill forces us to face the reality that we will someday die.

Family and friends of a dying person typically feel helpless and intensely sad. As a result, they may avoid the person because such feelings are difficult to hide and uncomfortable to bear. This reaction does little to boost the dying person's dignity and sense of well-being. Being avoided makes the dying person feel isolated and rejected at a time when he or she usually has a high need for the compassionate support and comfort of others.

Physicians and family members have become increasingly aware that positive thinking, including hopefulness, can improve one's well being while dying. Meeting the emotional and spiritual needs of terminally ill persons can help them live better while dying. Many physicians actively seek the participation of their seriously ill patients and their families in decisions concerning treatment. Medical practitioners can enhance the dignity and self-worth of dying patients by discussing the serious nature of their conditions with them, listening carefully to their concerns, and allowing them to make decisions regarding their medical care.

Terminal Care: The Options

The majority of Americans die in hospitals or extended-care facilities such as nursing homes. The goal of hospital-based health care is to provide technologically sophisticated medical care that enables sick people to become well. Because hospital care is costly, elderly patients who are too ill or frail to return home often move into extended-care facilities (e.g., nursing homes). These extended-care facilities offer less comprehensive medical care than hospitals, but they are designed and equipped to manage the long-term care of people recovering from surgery or illness. Not every condition is curable; many chronically ill patients die while residing in these care centers.

Choosing to place an aged parent or relative into a nursing home is often an emotionally difficult decision. Family members may have to select an available facility quickly and without researching their options. The Consumer Health feature "Choosing a Long-Term Care Facility" lists some important questions to answer when selecting a residential facility that provides long-term and/or skilled nursing care.

When patients have only a few months to live, their personal physicians may refer them to hospice. **Hospice** is health care specifically designed to give emotional support and pain relief to terminally ill people in the final stage of life, where patients receive palliative care. Palliative care, specialized medical care for people with serious illness, often occurs in hospice; however, it is not limited to older adults. Any patient with a serious illness may receive palliative care, at any age. For those with a terminal illness, care may be provided in the patient's home or in a hospice center. The primary goal of hospice care is not to save dying patients with aggressive treatments but to relieve their discomfort. Hospice physicians often prescribe powerful medications to keep terminally ill patients as free from pain as possible. Freedom from extreme pain permits the dying person to manage his or her activities more effectively and die with dignity.

Hospice staff receive specialized training to work closely with and to provide emotional and spiritual support to dying patients and their families. Staff encourage patients and their relatives to participate in decision making regarding care. Most terminally ill people and their families can obtain hospice services in their homes from a team of medical professionals. Family members are taught simple medical procedures such as care of surgical wounds or maintenance of feeding tubes. Hospice nurses make home visits to check patients' conditions and are available

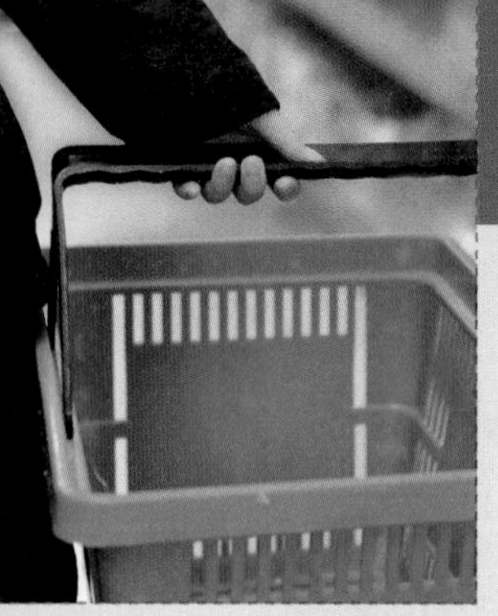

© sevenke/ShutterStock

Consumer Health

Choosing a Long-Term Care Facility

The most important feature to consider when choosing a residential facility is the quality of medical care that it provides. Before making this decision for a loved one, visit a few facilities, observe the condition of the buildings, its rooms, and residents, and answer the following questions:

1. Is the facility licensed by the state?
2. Is the facility clean, well maintained, and free of objectionable odors?
3. Are staff members friendly, helpful, and respectful to visitors and residents?
4. Does the family member's physician provide services at the facility?
5. Are the rooms clean, comfortably furnished, well lit, and cheerful?
6. Do the residents appear to be appropriately dressed, clean, and well groomed? Do they appear to be alert?
7. Are there enough staff members to take care of the number of residents?
8. Are there handrails along the hallways and grab bars in the bathrooms?
9. Does the facility have rehabilitation and exercise areas, a quiet place with reading material, and a chapel?
10. Does the facility have an activities director and scheduled social events that are appropriate for elderly people?
11. Are the dining room and kitchen clean?
12. Are menus nutritious? Do menus indicate that a variety of foods is offered? Can you sample a meal? How are the special dietary needs of patients handled?
13. If you have an opportunity, ask some residents and staff (privately) what they like and dislike about the facility.
14. What are the monthly fees? Can you afford this facility? Does the facility accept Medicaid or other forms of insurance?
15. Contact your state's division of aging to obtain information about the facility's inspection reports.
16. Using the Eldercare Locator found at www.eldercare.gov (or 1-800-677-1116) can also help you locate an appropriate facility.

Before making a final decision, visit the facility at least one additional unscheduled time to make another set of observations.

Adapted from Goldsmith, S. B. (1990). *Choosing a nursing home.* New York: Prentice Hall.; Centers for Medicare and Medicaid Services. (2013). *Your guide to choosing a nursing home or other long-term care facility.* Baltimore, MD: U.S. Department of Health and Human Services.

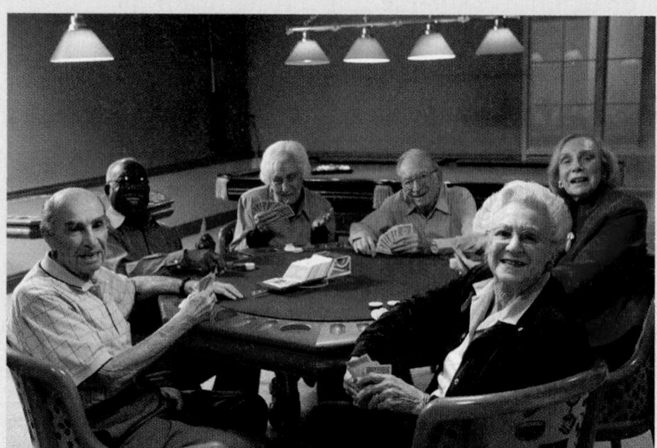

Older adults enjoying a social activity at a long-term care facility.

© Monkey Business Images/Dreamstime.com

to answer questions concerning their care. Dying at home allows patients to remain in a comfortable and familiar environment where they can participate in holiday and other family-oriented events.

Some dying patients receive hospice care in clinical settings that have rooms designed to look more like patients' homes than hospitals. The staff encourage patients to decorate their rooms with favorite possessions to foster a homelike environment. Visiting family and friends provide additional social, emotional, and spiritual support and often participate in caring for their ill loved ones. Regardless of whether the terminally ill person dies at home or in a hospice center, hospice staff provide grief counseling services for survivors.

Many nursing homes and hospitals offer hospice services that are covered by health insurance plans. To find such resources in your community, contact local hospitals or check the Yellow Pages under Hospice. Social workers in these facilities can provide information about local support groups for the terminally ill and their families. The National Hospice and Palliative Care Organization can also provide information about hospice programs in your area; this group's toll-free phone number is 1-800-658-8898.

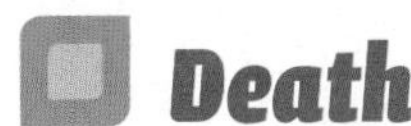 Death

death The cessation of life, which occurs soon after a person's heart or lungs stop functioning.

autopsy The various medical examinations and tests that usually can determine the cause of death.

comatose The condition in which a person is unresponsive to the environment and in a coma.

persistent vegetative state The condition in which a person has a nonfunctioning cerebral cortex and is in an irreversible coma.

Some people have a difficult time thinking about and discussing death. For example, they may avoid using the term *died*, preferring to use euphemisms such as *passed away*. Whether people believe in an afterlife or not, most are reluctant to handle matters concerning their own dying and death, such as preparing a will or signing an organ donor card.

What Is Death?

Death, the cessation of life, occurs when the heart or lungs stop functioning. When this happens, no oxygen is available for metabolism, and brain cells begin to die. Within 4 to 5 minutes, the dying person loses consciousness. As remaining body cells die, other signs of death become obvious.

When a person dies, the muscles that control voluntary and involuntary movements no longer function. As a result, the body eliminates the contents of the bladder and rectum, and reflexes are absent. *Reflexes* are neuromuscular responses that do not require thinking, such as eye blinking. Gradually, skeletal muscles become rigid, and body temperature cools until it matches that of the environment. Unless the body is chilled or treated with embalming chemicals, it decomposes rapidly. Decomposition occurs because the immune system no longer prevents bacteria and other microorganisms from breaking down the organic material of the body.

The physician who attended the dying patient is usually responsible for certifying that the patient has died. Then, the medical staff informs family members. In most cases, they deliver the body to a funeral home or medical school, according to the deceased person's wishes. If there are any questions or suspicions about the cause of death, the family, physicians, or coroner can request an **autopsy**. During an autopsy, a specially trained physician conducts various medical examinations and tests that usually determine the cause of death.

In 1968, a team of experts at the Harvard Medical School defined death according to four irreversible physical criteria:

- The absence of electrical activity in the brain
- No spontaneous muscular movements, including breathing
- No reflexes
- No responses to the environment

These criteria define what is commonly referred to as *brain death*. The majority of state laws recognize these criteria as the basis for defining death. A legal definition of death is important for criminal cases that involve murder. Defining death is necessary for physicians who need to establish that patients are dead before removing tissues or organs for transplantation.

Since the 1980s, advances in medical technology have made it necessary for medical experts to reconsider the traditional definition of death. By using *cardiopulmonary resuscitation* (CPR), *respirators* (devices that assist breathing), and feeding machines, physicians can often save the lives of certain seriously ill persons and, in some instances, may sustain patients who have virtually no chance of recovering.

Cerebral Death The cerebral cortex of the brain controls thoughts, interprets sensory information, and integrates voluntary muscular activities. An individual who experiences severe damage to his or her cerebral cortex is **comatose**, that is, unresponsive to the environment and in a *coma*. If the damage is irreversible, it is unlikely that the person will regain consciousness. In some comatose patients, the areas of the brain that control and regulate vital activities, including digestion and breathing, continue to function. Although their conditions do not meet the standard criteria for brain death, such individuals have experienced *cerebral death*. With specialized care, a person with a nonfunctioning cerebral cortex can exist in an irreversible coma, a **persistent vegetative state**, for years.

The level of care required to maintain patients in persistent vegetative states is stressful for their families, as well as expensive. Under what circumstances can physicians remove life-sustaining care from a patient in an irreversible coma? The U.S. Supreme Court decision in the Quinlan case provides an answer.

In 1975, Karen Ann Quinlan, a 21-year-old New Jersey woman, was hospitalized in an unconscious state after allegedly consuming a combination of alcohol and tranquilizers. After realizing that she would not recover, Ms. Quinlan's parents requested that the medical staff and hospital administrators allow their daughter to die by disconnecting her respirator. However, the administrators and attending physicians denied the parents' request, noting that the young woman was not dead according to established criteria.

After lower state courts supported the hospital's position, the Quinlans took their daughter's case to the New Jersey Supreme Court. In 1976, this court ruled that because Karen had previously told her mother and some friends that she would not want to live in a persistent vegetative state, her parents had the right to ask physicians to remove her respirator. After being removed gradually from the ventilation device, Karen was able to breathe without the machine's assistance, but she continued to be fed through tubes. The Quinlans moved their comatose daughter to a nursing home, where she died 10 years later.

Since the Quinlan case, several states have passed laws that establish steps for withholding or removing life-sustaining care in similar cases involving the terminally ill. A later section of this chapter describes how you can inform other people in advance about your wishes concerning such medical care.

Euthanasia and the Right to Die

Euthanasia is the practice of allowing permanently comatose or incurably ill persons to die. In cases of active euthanasia, physicians hasten the deaths of dying people by giving them large doses of pain-relieving medications that can completely suppress breathing. Passive euthanasia involves cases in which terminally ill people die because physicians do not provide life-sustaining treatments, or they withdraw such care.

Since the Quinlan case, the courts have decided several right-to-die cases, particularly those involving people who were seriously ill but not dying. Some chronically ill individuals decide that life is not worth living or that they are tired of living in pain. To hasten death, these people may refuse life-prolonging medical treatment, demand that it be withdrawn, or remove it themselves. In recent years, the courts often have made or upheld decisions that give such seriously ill people the right to die. After physicians discontinued their life support, many of these patients died naturally within a couple of weeks.

In some instances, the seriously ill person is too physically or mentally incapacitated to actively end his or her life. Concerned relatives, friends, or caregivers risk criminal prosecution by helping people commit suicide. Although most physicians strive to preserve life, some assist in the suicides of dying patients by prescribing overdoses of certain drugs. In the 1990s, retired physician Jack Kevorkian focused national attention on the controversial practice of physician-assisted suicide by helping more than 125 people end their lives. In 1999, a judge sentenced Kevorkian to prison for injecting a deadly dose of drugs into a man who was suffering from an incurable deadly disease. Kevorkian spent about 8 years in prison before being paroled. In 2011, Kevorkian died after a brief illness.

Oregon, Montana, Washington, Vermont, and New Mexico are the only states that allow physicians to prescribe drugs to terminally ill patients so that they can end their lives. On January 14, 2014, New Mexico became the latest state to allow physicians to prescribe lethal drugs to dying patients. Oregon and Washington maintain records concerning the number of deaths attributed to physician-assisted suicide each year. Between 1998 and 2013, 752 Oregonian patients chose to end their lives by taking a prescribed dose of deadly medications.[36]

The latest, highly publicized "right to die" debate involved began in 1990, when 26-year-old Terri Schiavo's heart failed and the young woman's body entered a persistent vegetative state after a significant number of her brain cells died from the lack of nutrients and oxygen (**Figure 15.8**). For several years, Terri's parents fought legal battles with her husband over their desire to keep her alive in a long-term care facility by providing nourishment through tube feedings. Terri's husband contended that her life-supporting care should be withdrawn, because before her heart attack, she had indicated to him that she would not want to be kept alive in such a manner if she were incapacitated. By spring of 2005, the parents' legal options were exhausted after courts ruled consistently in Terri's husband's favor. When the comatose woman's feeding tube was removed, the tragic case made headline news in the United States and around the world, rekindling debate over euthanasia. Terri died almost 2 weeks after her feeding tube was withdrawn.

Preparing for Death

Young adults may see the need to plan for a comfortable retirement, but planning for a good death may seem too morbid to consider (see **Table 5.5**). When a person dies while maintaining a high degree of dignity and experiences little physical and emotional pain during the dying process, it is considered a good death. A good death also causes minimal amounts of emotional trauma for the person's survivors.

Not everyone has time to prepare for a good death; death can be premature and unexpected, such as in cases of homicides, fatal accidents, or sudden, unexpected disease. Healthy people, however, can

Figure 15.8

Terri Schiavo. These photographs show Terri before and after a heart attack deprived her brain of oxygen and resulted in a persistent vegetative state.

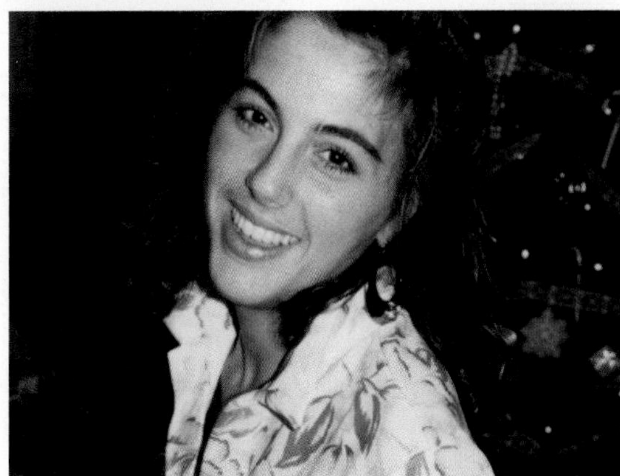

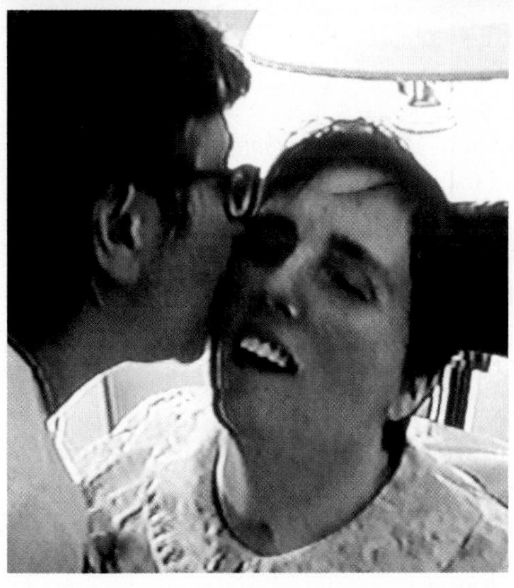

Table 15.5

Planning for Death

Advance Directive	Indicates a person's wishes about treatment should they become incapacitated.
Living Will	A legal document that specifies how you want your property and assets to be distributed after death. Guardiansfor minor children can also be designated. The document must be signed and witnessed by at least two people.
Executor	A person appointed to manage your estate after death. Executors use existing resources to pay your debts and funeral costs.
Organ Donation	Receiving donated organs can allow people who are seriously ill to live normal lives. You can choose to donate your organs by completing an organ donation card or signing the back of your driver's license.
Funeral Arrangements	Funerals can be costly and difficult for grieving survivors to attend. Having adequate life insurance allows the executor to pay for the funeral and protects survivors' assets.

make various legal, financial, emotional, and spiritual preparations for their deaths. Such planning can reduce their survivors' confusion and anxiety.

Advance Directives The Patient Self-Determination Act gives people the right to prepare advance directives that indicate their wishes concerning treatment if they become incapacitated. The act also allows physicians and administrators of certain medical facilities to withhold or remove life-support care from comatose patients who have no hope of regaining consciousness and who would not want to be kept alive in such conditions.

A living will or a durable power of attorney document can specify your wishes concerning your medical care in the event that you become permanently incapacitated. **Figure 15.9** shows a sample living will. Not every state honors such documents. For example, your state may exclude the right to have artificial feeding and hydration (water) tubes removed, regardless of your wishes.

Although some states do not sanction living wills, they allow other advance directives such as a durable power of attorney. In this document, you identify a mentally competent individual to serve as a healthcare surrogate or proxy. A healthcare proxy will make decisions concerning your care if you become unable to do so. Additionally, you may indicate which life-prolonging medical actions are acceptable or necessary under certain circumstances. The results of surveys indicate that most Americans would want limited care if they became incapacitated. Few Americans, however, have prepared living wills or other advance directives.

Before preparing an advance directive, it is a good idea to discuss your wishes with family and address their concerns. Your physician can probably answer questions that you or your family may have about life-support care. Family members or the person who agrees to serve as your healthcare surrogate and your personal physician will need copies of these documents. It is a good idea to store your copy along with your other important documents in a safety deposit box.

Figure 15.9

A Living Will. While still able, a person can sign a living will to specify wishes concerning medical care in the event that he or she becomes permanently incapacitated. This advance directive is for the District of Columbia.

DISTRICT OF COLUMBIA DECLARATION – PAGE 1 OF 2

INSTRUCTIONS

PRINT THE DATE

Declaration made this ________ day of ________________.
(date) (month, year)

PRINT YOUR NAME

I,
________________________________,
(name)

being of sound mind, willfully and voluntarily make known my desires that my dying shall not be artificially prolonged under the circumstances set forth below, do declare:

If at any time I should have an incurable injury, disease or illness certified to be a terminal condition by two physicians who have personally examined me, one of whom shall be my attending physician, and the physicians have determined that my death will occur whether or not life-sustaining procedures are utilized and where the application of life-sustaining procedures would serve only to artificially prolong the dying process, I direct that such procedures be withheld or withdrawn, and that I be permitted to die naturally with only the administration of medication or the performance of any medical procedure deemed necessary to provide me with comfort care or to alleviate pain.

ADD OTHER INSTRUCTIONS, IF ANY, REGARDING YOUR ADVANCE CARE PLANS

THESE INSTRUCTIONS CAN FURTHER ADDRESS YOUR HEALTH CARE PLANS, SUCH AS YOUR WISHES REGARDING HOSPICE TREATMENT, BUT CAN ALSO ADDRESS OTHER ADVANCE PLANNING ISSUES, SUCH AS YOUR BURIAL WISHES

ATTACH ADDITIONAL PAGES IF NEEDED

Other directions:

____

DISTRICT OF COLUMBIA DECLARATION — PAGE 2 OF 2

In the absence of my ability to give directions regarding the use of such life-sustaining procedures, it is my intention that this declaration shall be honored by my family and physician(s) as the final expression of my legal right to refuse medical or surgical treatment and accept the consequences from such refusal.

SIGN AND DATE THE DOCUMENT AND PRINT YOUR ADDRESS

I understand the full importance of this declaration and I am emotionally and mentally competent to make this declaration.

Signed ________________________ Date__________

Address ________________________________

WITNESSING PROCEDURE

I believe the declarant to be of sound mind. I did not sign the declarant's signature above for or at the direction of the declarant. I am at least eighteen years of age and am not related to the declarant by blood, marriage, or domestic partnership, entitled to any portion of the estate of the declarant according to the laws of intestate succession of the District of Columbia or under any will of the declarant or codicil thereto, or directly financially responsible for declarant's medical care. I am not the declarant's attending physician, an employee of the attending physician, or an employee of the health facility in which the declarant is a patient.

TWO WITNESSES MUST SIGN AND DATE HERE

Witness ________________________ Date__________

Witness ________________________ Date__________

Estate Management In addition to an advance directive, it is important to have a will, a legal document that specifies how you want your property to be distributed after your death. To prepare a formal will, it is a good idea to consult an attorney, preferably one who specializes in estate administration. For the will to be valid, you must be of "sound mind" (aware of your actions) when you write and sign your will, and the document must be signed and witnessed by at least two people.

Most Americans die without having a will. When this happens, probate courts follow state laws concerning the division and distribution of the deceased person's estate. An estate includes the individual's sources of money, such as checking and savings accounts, life insurance policies, and retirement plans. In addition, possessions that can be sold, such as jewelry, real estate, furniture, and collectibles, are part of one's estate. A carefully constructed will can ensure that these assets go to whomever you want and not to whom the courts choose. Furthermore, a will can eliminate much unhappiness, stress, and confusion among your survivors. If family members feel that provisions stated in your will unfairly distribute the estate, they can contest it in court.

In addition to making a will, it is a good idea to appoint an executor to manage your estate after your death. The executor uses income from the estate to pay your debts and funeral costs. If you have young children, it is important to identify and ask a person who will act as their legal guardian in case they become orphans. Most people choose a guardian who is a close relative or friend to whom they can entrust the care of their children.

In addition to having a will and an executor, you can protect your survivors' assets by having enough health and life insurance to cover your final medical and funeral expenses. The best time to buy life and health insurance is while you are young and healthy.

Organ Donation In dying, people can make a priceless contribution to the living by donating their tissues or organs. Soon after death, a donor's kidneys, liver, skin, heart, and corneas can be removed and transplanted into people whose organs or tissues are failing. Many seriously ill patients who would have died without receiving donated organs are able to live nearly normal lives after having the procedures.

As of July 2014, more than 123,000 people in the United States were on waiting lists to receive organ transplants.[37] Patients are more likely to need kidneys and/or livers than other organs. Unfortunately, the demand for organs is greater than the supply. In 2013, more than 6,880 Americans died while waiting for matching organs to become available for transplantation.[38] Although people may express an interest in having their organs donated when they die, they often do not make their wishes known to others nor do they document them formally. For example, potential donors may fail to inform family members of their decision or sign organ donor cards. In most states, family members can override the deceased person's wishes concerning organ donation.

People can help those who need healthy tissues and organs by completing and signing uniform donor cards like the one shown in **Figure 15.10**. This card should be kept in a person's wallet. Additionally, people have their desire to be an organ donor designated on their driver's license. The process for having "donor" identified on your driver's license may vary by state. Individuals who would like to become organ donors when they die should inform their relatives of their wishes. Although there are no guarantees that surgeons will be able to transplant a person's tissues after death, it may be reassuring for some people to know that, even after death, they might be able to help others.

Figure 15.10

A Uniform Donor Card. By completing and signing a donor card like this one, people can help others who need healthy tissues and organs.

Reproduced with permission from the National Kidney Foundation, Inc.

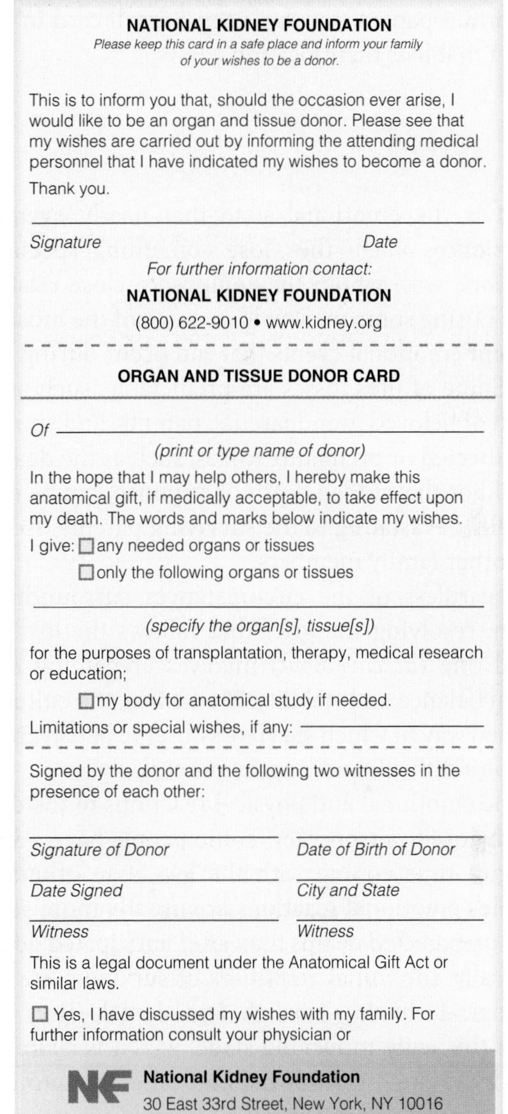

NATIONAL KIDNEY FOUNDATION

Please keep this card in a safe place and inform your family of your wishes to be a donor.

This is to inform you that, should the occasion ever arise, I would like to be an organ and tissue donor. Please see that my wishes are carried out by informing the attending medical personnel that I have indicated my wishes to become a donor.

Thank you.

Signature *Date*

For further information contact:

NATIONAL KIDNEY FOUNDATION

(800) 622-9010 • www.kidney.org

ORGAN AND TISSUE DONOR CARD

Of ______

(print or type name of donor)

In the hope that I may help others, I hereby make this anatomical gift, if medically acceptable, to take effect upon my death. The words and marks below indicate my wishes.

I give: ☐ any needed organs or tissues

☐ only the following organs or tissues

(specify the organ[s], tissue[s])

for the purposes of transplantation, therapy, medical research or education;

☐ my body for anatomical study if needed.

Limitations or special wishes, if any: ______

Signed by the donor and the following two witnesses in the presence of each other:

Signature of Donor *Date of Birth of Donor*

Date Signed *City and State*

Witness *Witness*

This is a legal document under the Anatomical Gift Act or similar laws.

☐ Yes, I have discussed my wishes with my family. For further information consult your physician or

NKF National Kidney Foundation

30 East 33rd Street, New York, NY 10016

Some Final Thoughts on Death

Funeral and memorial services can help friends and family members deal with the loss of a loved one. You can ease some of the emotional and financial burdens of your survivors by planning your funeral arrangements. A funeral can be very costly, and it is often a difficult emotional task for families to make such arrangements when a loved one dies.

Many mortuaries offer prearranged funerals that enable you to specify the kind of funeral you want and the most affordable services. For example, you could choose to have a simple memorial service, your body *cremated* (burned), and your ashes placed in a container and given to your survivors. You can contact mortuaries in your area for more information about making funeral and burial prearrangements.

In addition to making funeral and burial arrangements, you can prepare spiritually for your death. One spiritual arrangement you can make in preparation for death is to write your own obituary or death notice. Many obituaries include a brief biography. If you prepare these documents, you can give copies of them to your survivors and let them know where to send them. Newspapers, college alumni associations, and professional organizations usually print death notices.

After a beloved person dies, survivors often experience confusion and distress because they cannot locate the deceased person's will and other important documents. To reduce the likelihood that this situation will occur after your death, share copies of these personal papers with your spouse, adult children, the executor, and the individual who has the power of

grief An emotional state that usually occurs after the loss of something or someone special.

mourning The culturally defined way in which survivors resolve the grief surrounding a death.

attorney. A safety deposit box is a safe place to store such documents. To help your survivors find these important papers, you can keep a small card in your wallet that lists their location.

Grief

Grief is the emotional state that nearly everyone experiences when they lose something special or someone with whom they enjoyed a close relationship. Losing someone you love is one of the most significant emotional events that can occur during your life. Some of life's losses are predictable, such as the death of beloved grandparents, parents, and spouses. Unexpected or premature losses, such as the death of a child or the sudden death of a spouse, can be emotionally devastating to the surviving parents, spouse, and other family members.

Regardless of the circumstances surrounding a death, resolving the grief that follows the loss of a loved one (*bereavement*) involves regaining emotional balance and stability. **Mourning**, the culturally defined way in which survivors observe bereavement, can be a difficult and lengthy process.

The emotional and physical reactions to the death of a beloved person vary; some people have a more difficult time coping with the loss than others do. People's emotional reactions are usually more severe after unexpected deaths than after anticipated deaths. Typically, the initial responses of survivors are psychological shock, disbelief, and denial. They next enter the acute mourning stage, which is characterized by crying, withdrawal, and other symptoms of depression. In many societies, people in mourning are expected to display their grief, for example, by crying and by wearing somber clothing. After mourning, survivors are often able to accept the death of their loved one, recognize that they have grieved, and regain a sense of emotional balance.

The most intense period of grieving normally lasts about 4 to 6 weeks after the death. It is not uncommon for people to continue mourning for a year or longer after the loss. Some people experience psychological and physical problems if they are unable to resolve their feelings of grief.

Much of the research that examines the impact of grieving on health involves people whose spouses have recently died. Most widowed people experience some signs and symptoms of depression, such as sadness, withdrawal, and sleep disorders. With the support of family and friends, however, people who are grieving can often regain their emotional balance within a few months. Survivors may become saddened again over the loss of a spouse, especially on anniversaries, on holidays, and during family reunions. An estimated 10% to 20% of widowed people suffer severe depression that lasts a year or more after their spouses die. The Managing Your Health feature "After the Death of a Loved One" contains some suggestions that can help people endure the first year after the death of a spouse or other beloved individual.

In addition to affecting emotional health, bereavement often influences the physical health of survivors. Most people who are grieving are emotionally distressed, and such stress often has a negative impact on their immune systems. Individuals who have weakened immune systems are at risk of developing frequent infections and chronic health problems such as cardiovascular disease. Additionally, grieving people may not take good care of themselves; for example, they may not eat nutritious foods or exercise, and some may abuse drugs, including alcohol.

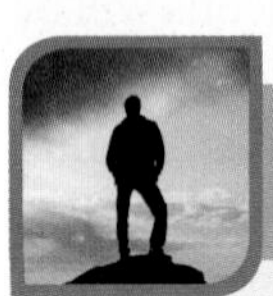

© djgis/ShutterStock

Healthy Living Practices

- If you would like to be an organ donor when you die, complete a uniform donor card or sign the declaration on the back of your driver's license. Inform your relatives of this decision.
- Preparing a will can help your survivors manage your estate.
- To convey your wishes concerning treatment in case you become severely disabled and cannot communicate, consider preparing an advance directive.

People who undergo an abnormal grieving process may have had a poor relationship with the deceased person. According to Kübler-Ross, grief includes some degree of anger that is directed toward the dead individual. Survivors may hide their anger; others may express it by lashing out at someone else or by grieving for an unusually long period. **Table 15.6** lists the signs of abnormal grieving. People with these signs may need professional counseling.

Managing Your Health

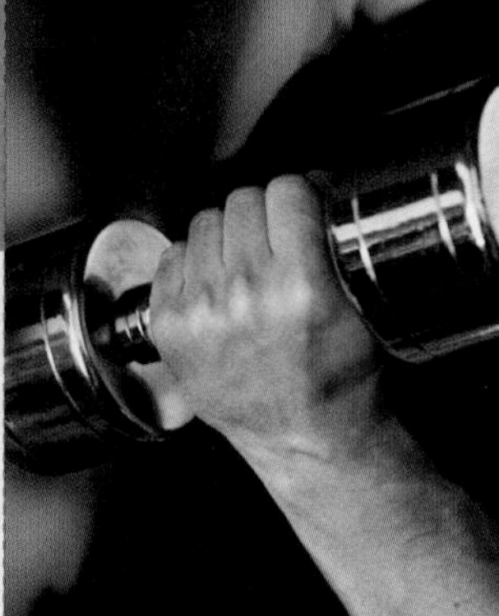
© Kzenon/ShutterStock

After the Death of a Loved One

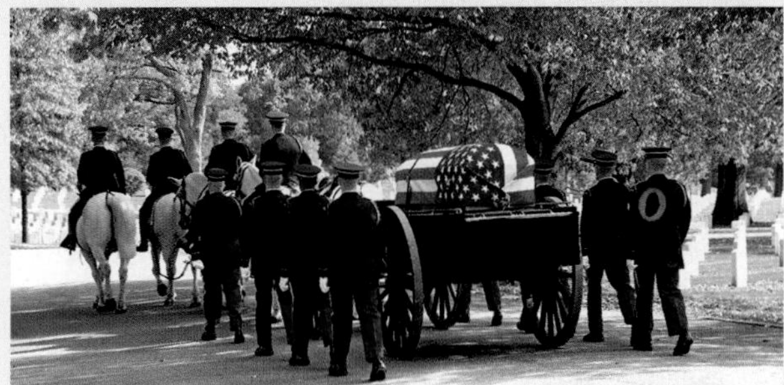
© David Kay/ShutterStock

The "Managing Grief" sections of this box provide some suggestions that may help you cope with the death of a beloved individual. The "Managing Legal, Social, and Financial Concerns" sections provide some actions that you can take to manage various concerns that often arise after the death of a spouse or other beloved person.

Immediate Actions and Concerns

Managing Grief

- Resolve to survive the first few days of the sorrowful event.
- Accept the support and company of friends, family, professionals (e.g., counselors, clergy).
- Permit yourself to vent your feelings, for example, to cry or to feel anger.

Managing Legal, Social, and Financial Concerns

- Notify your attorney; obtain the deceased person's will and make several photocopies of it.
- Order several copies of the death certificate; the funeral director may do this for you.

Within the First 4 Weeks

Managing Grief

- Acknowledge those who sent food or flowers or who made memorial donations. Consider responding to those who visited or sent cards. This is an emotionally difficult task, but the process may be beneficial in itself.
- Anticipate feelings of grief: the tears, anger, guilt, and blame. Delayed or prolonged absence of grief may lead to negative physical and psychological consequences.
- If troubled by sleeplessness, nightmares, agitation, headaches, and even skin rashes, consult your physician for help to alleviate these conditions.
- Note changes in your appetite.

Managing Legal, Social, and Financial Concerns

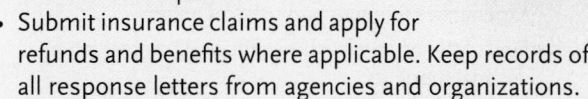

- Notify relevant government agencies and other organizations of the death, such as the Social Security Administration, Veterans Administration, and insurance companies.
- Submit insurance claims and apply for refunds and benefits where applicable. Keep records of all response letters from agencies and organizations.
- Notify the deceased person's banks, credit card accounts, custodians of mutual funds and annuities, and accountant of the death.

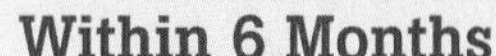

Within 6 Months

Managing Grief

- Join a grief support group. For information concerning support groups in your area, contact social workers at a local hospital or hospice or your local United Way.
- Adapt to lifestyle changes. You may need to learn how to do unfamiliar chores such as maintaining the house, tracking investments, cooking meals, or paying bills.
- Continue previous activities such as participating in hobbies or clubs if they are satisfying.
- Participate in healthful physical activities such as walking, swimming, or golfing. Join a health spa or similar organization.

Managing Legal, Social, and Financial Concerns

- Share meals with friends and accept the invitations of others to dine out with them.
- Update your will: change beneficiaries, trustees, or executors if necessary.
- Consult your accountant; your tax situation may have changed.

Long Term

Managing Grief

- Establish your own identity to function independently. Your degree of dependence and attachment to the deceased may determine the time needed for adjustment.
- Establish new relationships; continue existing relationships.
- Consider participating in activities or organizations that help others.

Managing Legal, Social, and Financial Concerns

- Plan for the future. Do not rush into making major changes or decisions.

Table 15.6

Grieving Danger Signs

Professional counseling to handle grief may be necessary if the grieving person:
• Doubts that his or her grieving is normal
• Experiences frequent outbursts of anger
• Finds little or no pleasure in life and has persistent suicidal thoughts
• Is preoccupied with thinking about the deceased loved one, or has hostile or guilty feelings that persist for more than a couple of years
• Experiences significant weight loss, weight gain, or persistent insomnia
• Begins engaging in risky behaviors such as abusing drugs or practicing unsafe sex
• Loses interest in taking care of personal hygiene for more than 2 weeks

Adapted from Kouri, M. K. (1991). *Keys to Dealing with the Loss of a Loved One*. Hauppauge, NY: Barrons Educational Series.

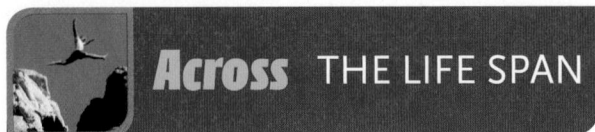

© Galina Barskaya/ShutterStock

DYING AND DEATH

In the United States, parents often find it difficult to discuss death with their children until someone or something, such as a pet, is dying or has died. Young children have difficulty grasping the concepts of dying and death (**Figure 15.11**). For example, if a 4-year-old child attends a funeral and views a loved one's body, the youngster may think this person is asleep.

Children as young as 2 years old miss a familiar person who has died, especially if the deceased was a parent. Preschool-aged children, however, do not express grief as older children or adults do. At this age, children typically grieve differently from how adults grieve; they may act unconcerned about the death and become intensely involved in play activities or misbehave.

School-age children are able to understand that dead things do not come back to life, and they respond to the loss much like adults: crying, withdrawing, or being angry. Older children often associate death with being old, particularly if they have experienced the death of a grandparent. Thus, they may have a great deal of difficulty coping when a peer dies.

Figure 15.11

Children's Responses to End-of-Life Concepts. Young children have difficulty grasping the concepts of dying and death. When faced with the loss of a loved one, preschool children typically grieve differently from how adults grieve.

© Cheryl Casey/ShutterStock

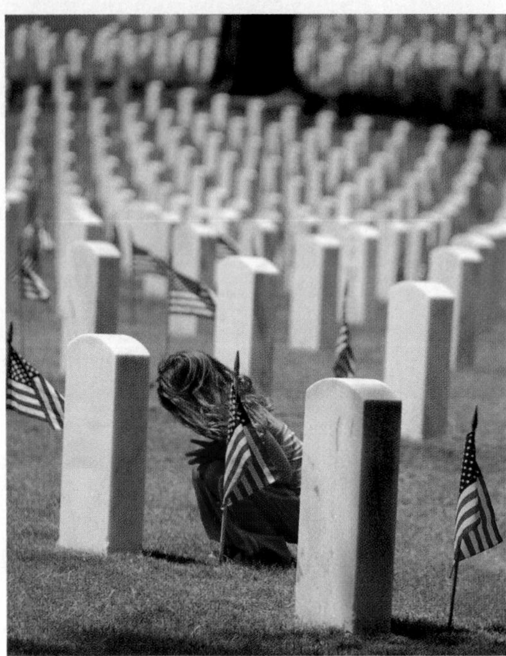

Experts suggest being honest and straightforward when discussing terminal illness and death with children, while also considering the child's ability to understand the meaning of death. Frequently, children begin to understand and accept death when caring people share what is happening with them. It is important to allow grieving children to express their concerns and feelings about dying and death. Professional counseling may be necessary if the child's responses are excessive, if the young person becomes preoccupied with death, or if the child becomes depressed.

© djgis/ShutterStock

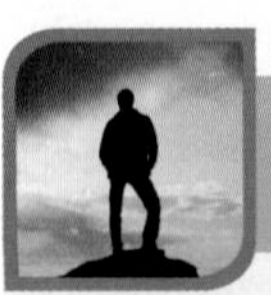

Healthy Living Practices

- ☐ Consider seeking professional counseling if your grief is severe or does not subside over time after the death of a loved one.
- ☐ If your child becomes preoccupied with death or depressed after someone or something has died, professional counseling can help him or her deal with the loss.

CHAPTER REVIEW

Summary

Aging is the sum of all changes that occur in an organism over its life span. The human life span is divided into stages. The final stage, senescence, generally refers to the stage of life that begins at 65 years of age.

The overall life expectancy of Americans has increased since 1900. In the United States, a person born in 2009 can expect to live for about 78.7 years. Life expectancies, however, vary according to age, sex, and socioeconomic status. For example, American females outlive American males by about 5 years.

As of 2012, 13.7% of the U.S. population was 65 years of age and older. By the year 2030, nearly 23% of Americans will be in this age group. This segment of the American population is increasing at a rapid rate.

Aged people must often live on incomes that are lower than when they were younger. In the United States, older adult members of certain minority groups are more likely to have lower retirement incomes and live in poverty than are White aged persons. With appropriate financial planning, Americans who have adequate incomes when they are young may be able to maintain adequate incomes during their retirement years.

A gradual and irreversible decline in the functioning of the human body begins to occur around 30 years of age. However, people age at different rates. Genetic, environmental, and lifestyle factors influence the rate of aging.

Some of the physical changes associated with the aging process, such as gray hair, presbyopia, and menopause, are normal and inevitable. Other age-related physical changes such as heart disease, cancer, and osteoporosis are not normal and are signs of disease processes. People who modify their lifestyles while they are young may be able to prevent or delay such conditions.

According to Kübler-Ross, the typical emotional responses to dying include denial, anger, bargaining, depression, and acceptance. However, death can be the final stage of personal fulfillment if dying people have opportunities to satisfy their social and emotional needs. Family, friends, and medical care providers can help terminally ill individuals live better while dying by taking steps to enhance their dignity and self-worth.

Death occurs when the heart or lungs cease functioning and cells in the brain do not receive oxygen. The criteria for brain death include no brain waves, no spontaneous muscular movements, no reflexes, and no responses to the environment. A brain-dead person can exist in a persistent coma for years as long as the heart is functioning, nutritional needs are met, and the supply of oxygen to the heart is maintained by the use of a respirator. Euthanasia is the practice of allowing a permanently comatose or an incurably ill person to die.

The Patient Self-Determination Act gives people the right to prepare advance directives, documents that indicate a person's wishes concerning life-support measures if the individual becomes incapable of making such decisions.

Nearly everyone experiences grief with the loss of something special or someone with whom he or she enjoyed a close relationship. Although it is normal to grieve after such a loss, grief can have negative effects on health. To resolve grief, a person accepts the death of a loved one, recognizes that he or she has grieved for this person, and regains a sense of emotional balance. An individual who grieves for a prolonged period may require professional counseling.

Preschool children do not understand the concept of death, yet they still experience distress over the missing loved one. At this age, children may mourn by acting uninterested about the death or by misbehaving. Older children often grieve like adults by crying, withdrawing, and being angry. Grieving youngsters need to express their concerns and feelings about death. Like adults, children may need professional counseling if their emotional responses to death are severe or prolonged.

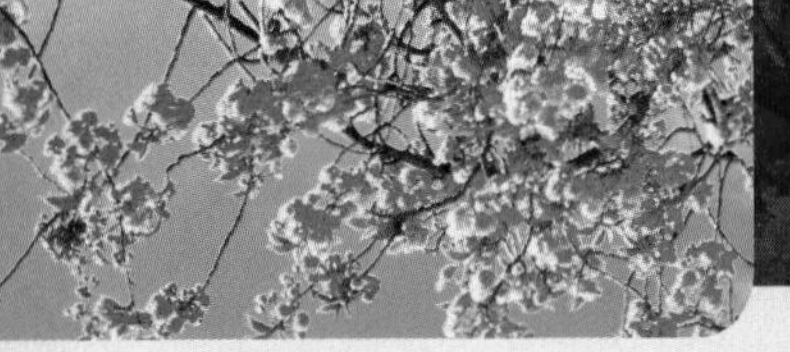

CHAPTER REVIEW

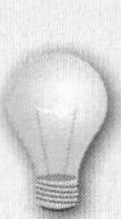

Applying What You Have Learned

1. Using the sample will provided in Figure 15.9, develop a will that reflects your wishes concerning the distribution of your assets after death. **Application**
2. Analyze how your present lifestyle may affect your life span. **Analysis**
3. Propose a program to reduce ageism by promoting understanding and cooperation between young and old members of your community. **Synthesis**
4. Choose a position concerning the issue of euthanasia. How would you defend your position? **Evaluation**

Key

Application	Analysis	Synthesis	Evaluation
using information in a new situation.	breaking down information into component parts.	putting together information from different sources.	making informed decisions.

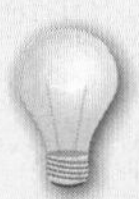

Reflecting on Your Health

1. How do you feel about aging? Are you undergoing the age-related changes that Table 15.1 describes? Which age-related changes trouble you the most? Are you making any lifestyle changes that will increase your chances of living a long and healthy life? If you answered yes to the previous question, what changes are you making, and how do you think they will affect your longevity?
2. If you suffered severe brain damage in an accident, would you want to be maintained in a persistent vegetative state? Why or why not? If so, for how long would you want to be kept alive? Why?
3. Do you intend to donate your organs if you die in an accident? Why or why not? Have you signed an organ donor card or the back of your driver's license, enabling survivors to donate your organs when you die? If you have not signed an organ donor card on the back of your license, explain why.
4. Have you ever known someone who knew he or she was dying? If so, describe any stages of Kübler-Ross's emotional responses to dying that you observed in that person.
5. If someone you loved has died, how did the grieving process affect your psychological, social, and spiritual health? What did you do to overcome the grief?

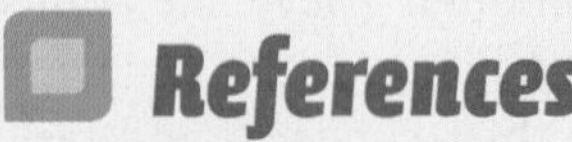

References

1. Volz, M. (2011). World's oldest man dies in Montana at 114. *Associated Press.* Retrieved from http://www.foxnews.com/us/2011/04/14/worlds-oldest-man-dies-age-114/
2. Colton, A. (2011, April). Survival skills: World's oldest man. *Men's Journal*, p. 126.
3. Flachsbart, F., et al. (2009). Association with *FOXO3A* variation with human longevity confirmed in German centenarians. *Proceedings of the National Academy of Sciences*, 106(8), 2700–2705.
4. U.S. Census Bureau. (2014, March). *Older Americans Month: May 2011.* Retrieved from http://www.census.gov/newsroom/releases/archives/facts_for_features_special_editions/cb14-ff07.html
5. U.S. Census Bureau. (n.d.). *U.S. population projections.* Retrieved from http://www.census.gov/population/projections/data/national/2012.html
6. Kahana, E., et al. (2002). Long-term impact of preventive proactivity on quality of life of the old-old. *Psychosomatic Medicine*, 64(3), 382–394.

7. Kochanek, K. D., et al. (2011). Deaths: Preliminary data for 2011. *National Vital Statistics Reports*, 61(6), 1–52. Retrieved from http://www.cdc.gov/nchs/data/nvsr/nvsr61/nvsr61_06.pdf
8. U.S. Department of Health and Human Services. (2014, June 30). *Healthy People 2020: About Healthy People*. Retrieved from http://www.healthypeople.gov/2020/about/default.aspx
9. Centers for Disease Control and Prevention. (2013, November 22). Life expectancy free of chronic condition-induced activity limitations—United States, 1999–2008. *Vital and Health Statistics*, 62(3). Retrieved from http://www.cdc.gov/mmwr/preview/mmwrhtml/su6203a15.htm
10. U.S. Department of Health and Human Services, Administration on Aging. (2014). *A profile of older Americans: 2013*. Retrieved from http://www.aoa.gov/Aging_Statistics/Profile/2013/docs/2013_Profile.pdf
11. U.S. National Library of Medicine, National Eye Institute. (2013, July). *Facts about age-related macular degeneration*. Retrieved from http://www.nei.nih.gov/health/maculardegen/armd_facts.asp
12. Centers for Disease Control and Prevention, Chronic Disease Prevention and Health Promotion. (2013, July 18). Arthritis: Meeting the challenge. *At a Glance*. Retrieved from http://www.cdc.gov/chronicdisease/resources/publications/aag/arthritis.htm
13. Alzheimer's Association. (2014). *What is Alzheimer's?* Retrieved from http://www.alz.org/alzheimers_disease_what_is_alzheimers.asp#basics
14. Alzheimer's Association. (2014). 2014 Alzheimer's disease facts and figures. *Alzheimer's and Dementia*, 7(2), 208–244. Retrieved from http://www.alz.org/alzheimers_disease_facts_and_figures.asp
15. National Institute on Aging. (2014, March 20). *Looking for the causes of AD*. Retrieved from http://www.nia.nih.gov/alzheimers/publication/part-3-ad-research-better-questions-new-answers/looking-causes-ad
16. Otaegui-Arrazola, A., et al. (2014). Diet, cognition, and Alzheimer's disease: Food for thought. *European Journal of Nutrition*, 53(1), 1–23.
17. Wood, G. W., et al. (2014). Cholesterol as a causative factor in Alzheimer's disease: A debatable hypothesis. *Journal of Neurochemistry*, 129(4), 559–572.
18. Ligthart, S. A., et al. (2010). Treatment of cardiovascular risk factors to prevent cognitive decline and dementia: A systematic review. *Vascular Health and Risk Management*, 6, 775–785.
19. Lau, F. C., et al. (2007). Nutritional intervention in brain aging: Reducing the effects of inflammation and oxidative stress. *Subcellular Biochemistry*, 42, 299–318.
20. Shah, R. (2013). The role of nutrition and diet in Alzheimer disease: A systematic review. *Journal of the American Medical Directors Association*, 14(6), 398–402.
21. Wang, Y., et al. (2013). Curcumin as a potential treatment for Alzheimer's disease: A study of the effects of curcumin on hippocampal expression of glial fibrillary acidic protein. *American Journal of Chinese Medicine*, 41(1), 59–70.
22. Evans, J. G., et al. (2004). Evidence-based pharmacotherapy of Alzheimer's disease. *International Journal of Neuro-psychopharmacology*, 7(3), 351–369.
23. O'Brien, J. T., & Burns, A. (2011). Clinical practice with anti-dementia drugs: A revised (second) consensus statement from British Association for Psychopharmacology. *Journal of Psychopharmacology*, 25(8), 997–1019.
24. Dwyer, J., & Donoghue, M. D. (2010). Is risk of Alzheimer disease a reason to use dietary supplements? *American Journal of Clinical Nutrition*, 91(5), 1155–1156.
25. Usoro, O. B., & Mousa, S. A. (2010). Vitamin E forms in Alzheimer's disease: A review of controversial and clinical experiences. *Critical Reviews in Food Science & Nutrition*, 50(5), 414–416.
26. Centers for Disease Control and Prevention. (2014, January 2). *National suicide statistics at a glance: Trends in suicide rates among both sexes, by age group, United States, 1991–2009*. Retrieved from http://www.cdc.gov/violenceprevention/suicide/statistics/trends02.html
27. Podgorski, C. A., et al. (2010). Suicide prevention for older adults in residential communities: Implications for policy and practice. *PLoS Medicine*, 7(5), e10000254.
28. LeFevre, M. L. (2014). Screening for suicide risk in adolescents, adults, and older adults in primary care: U.S. preventive services task force recommendation statement. *Annals of Internal Medicine*, 160(10), 719–726.
29. Jeste, D. V., et al. (2010). Successful cognitive and emotional aging. *World Psychiatry*, 9(2), 78–84.
30. Perls, T. T. (2010). Antiaging medicine: What should we tell our patients? *Aging Health*, 6(2), 149–154.
31. Warburton, D. E., et al. (2006). Health benefits of physical activity: The evidence. *Canadian Medical Association Journal*, 174(6), 801–809.
32. Larson, E. B., et al. (2006). Exercise is associated with reduced risk for incident dementia among persons 65 years of age and older. *Annals of Internal Medicine*, 144(2), 73–81.
33. Nicholson, N. R. (2012). A review of social isolation: An important but underassessed condition in older adults. *Journal of Primary Prevention*, 33, 137–152
34. Nouchi, R., et al. (2012). Brain training game improves executive functions and processing speed in the elderly: A randomized controlled trial. *PLOS ONE*, 7(1), e29676
35. Kübler-Ross, E. (1969). *On death and dying*. New York: Macmillan.
36. Oregon Department of Human Services. (2014). *Death with Dignity Act annual reports*. 2013 Summary. Retrieved from http://public.health.oregon.gov/ProviderPartnerResources/EvaluationResearch/DeathwithDignityAct/Documents/year16.pdf
37. United Network for Organ Sharing. (2014, July 18). *Data: Waiting list candidates*. Retrieved from http://www.unos.org
38. U.S. Department of Health and Human Services, Health Resources and Services Administration, Organ Procurement and Transplant Network. (2014, July 18). *Death removals by region by year*. Retrieved from http://optn.transplant.hrsa.gov/converge/latestData/viewDataReports.asp

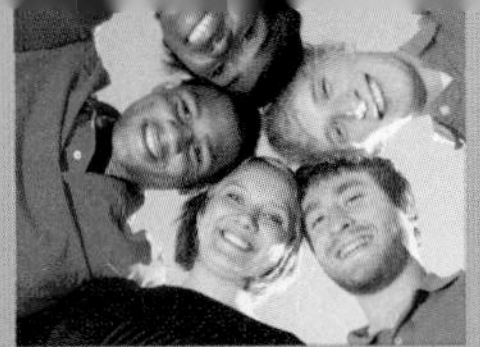

Diversity in Health

Hunger, the Environment, and the World's Population

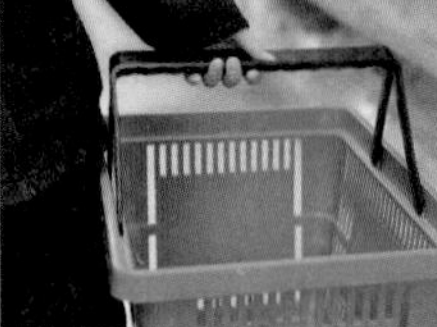

Consumer Health

Carbon Monoxide Detectors: Are They Reliable?

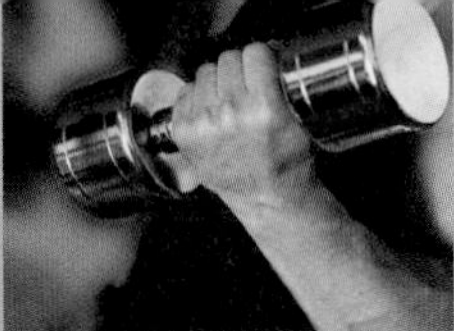

Managing Your Health

Tips to Prevent Poisonings | Avoiding ELF Radiation | Reducing Pesticide Levels in the Food You Eat

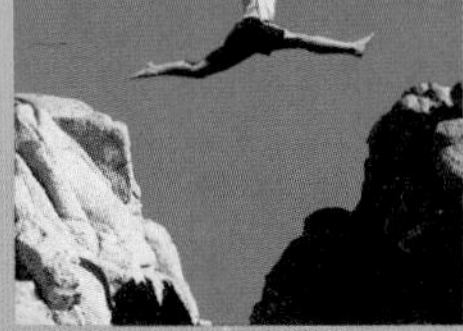

Across the Life Span

Environmental Health

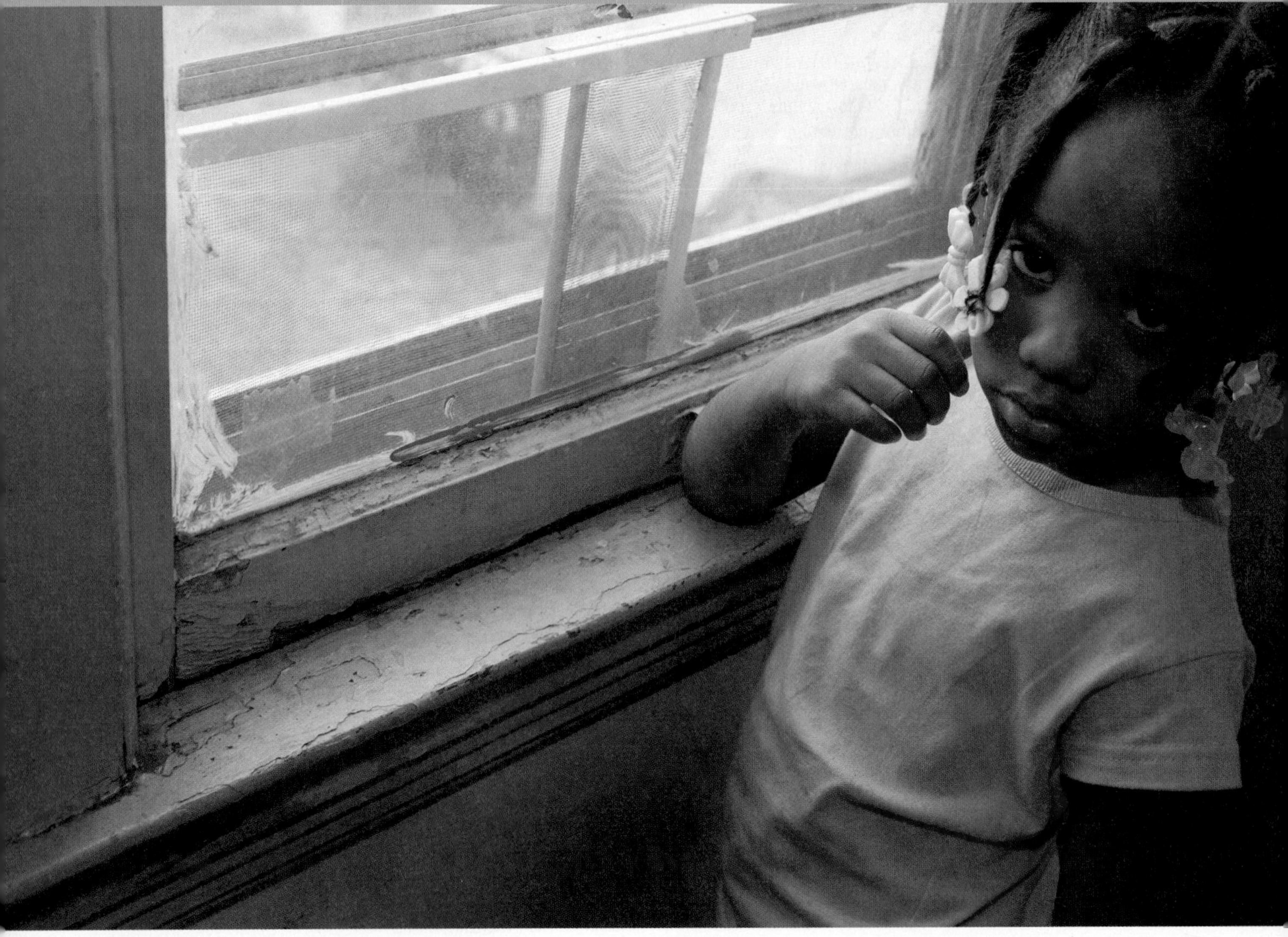

Chapter Overview

Which types of poisoning are prevalent in the United States?

How to avoid poisoning in the home

Which toxic chemicals are prevalent in the workplace?

What factors contribute to indoor air pollution?

How water supplies become contaminated

Why air pollution is a threat to health

How noise pollution affects hearing

Student Workbook

Self-Assessments: Poison Lookout Checklist | Checklist for the Prevention of Carbon Monoxide Poisoning

Changing Health Habits: Can You Reduce Environmental Threats to Your Health?

Do You Know?

If you work or go to school in a "sick" building?

If you are in danger of pesticide poisoning?

If your house or apartment is painted with lead-based products?

CHAPTER 16

Environmental Health

Learning Objectives

After studying this chapter, you should be able to:

1. Describe ways to reduce the risk of accidental poisoning in the home.
2. Identify common environmental health hazards and their sources.
3. Identify federal legislation intended to protect consumers from being harmed by toxic chemicals and products.
4. Describe the negative effects that air pollution, water pollution, and loud sounds have on health.
5. Distinguish between gray-air and brown-air cities.
6. Take practical steps to reduce exposure to environmental health hazards.
7. Relate the effects of overpopulation on world health.

"[One way] in which U.S. children are poisoned by lead . . . by eating lead-based paint chips . . ."

environmental health The effects of environmental factors on humans and the effects of humans on their environments.

ozone holes Depleted areas of the ozone (O_3) layer in the upper atmosphere.

municipal solid waste Nonhazardous refuse generally collected from homes and offices.

toxic chemicals Poisonous substances present in the home, workplace, or outdoor environments that affect human health.

toxicity (tok-SIH-si-tea) Poisonous quality.

Azarcon, greta, litargirio, and pay-loo-ah . . . if you have Hispanic or Asian ancestry, the names of one or more of these traditional ethnic remedies may be familiar to you. Greta and azarcon are Mexican remedies for empacho, a colicky digestive disorder. Pay-loo-ah is a Southeast Asian tonic for rash or fever. All three are fine powders and may be given as a tea, or a pinch may be added to a baby's bottle. They also can be mixed with milk or sugar and administered by teaspoon. Litargirio is used as an antiperspirant/deodorant and as a folk remedy for burns and fungal infections of the feet. Family members who rely on folk medicine give these remedies regularly to children.

Many folk remedies contain substances that are useful in medical practice. In fact, pharmaceutical companies often start looking for new drugs by chemically analyzing the herbs and other plants used in many traditional folk remedies that have been part of a culture for generations. However, some remedies, like those mentioned here, can cause harm. Azarcon, greta, litargirio, and pay-loo-ah all contain high levels of lead. Even seemingly harmless over-the-counter herbal dietary supplements have been found to be associated with high lead levels in women. Some Ayurvedic "medications" contain lead as well.[1–4] Ayurveda (AH-yer-VAY-da) is a type of traditional or folk medicine practiced in India and other South Asian countries.

Lead is only one of the many substances in our environment that can cause serious illness. The major ways in which U.S. children are poisoned by lead are by eating lead-based paint chips and by inhaling lead particles in contaminated dust or soil.[5] In adults in the United States, about 95% of lead poisoning occurs from occupational exposure, such as the mining and smelting of lead ore, the manufacture of batteries, and construction work involving lead-based products.[6] Nonetheless, folk remedies containing lead, and lead-based paints and other products in the home, pose a serious health risk for both children and adults.

The study of the effects of environmental factors on humans and the effects of humans on their environments is called **environmental health**. People often affect the environment in ways that later influence their health. For example, people emitted chlorofluorocarbons (CFCs) into the atmosphere when they used certain spray can propellants prior to their being banned in 1979. CFCs contribute to the depletion of the ozone layer in the upper atmosphere. These depleted areas are commonly referred to as **ozone holes**. The upper atmospheric ozone layer protects people from some of the sun's harmful ultraviolet (UV) radiation, which can cause skin cancer. Many automobile air conditioners still contain chemicals harmful to the ozone layer. In another example, people in industrialized countries such as the United States produce millions of tons of **municipal solid waste** per year—all of those items that trash collectors pick up from homes and offices each week. This waste is usually placed in landfills. Along with running out of space for this trash, a problem with landfills is that chemicals may seep into the ground from these massive waste sites and pollute water supplies. We discuss water pollution from various sources later in this chapter.

Many **toxic chemicals** present in the home, workplace, or outdoor environments affect human health. They may be in the form of dusts, fumes, particles, or liquids and are found in a wide variety of substances, such as household products, plants, products manufactured or used in the workplace, and prescription and illegal drugs. Toxic chemicals are also present in the air we breathe and the water we drink.

Toxic chemicals result in poisoning, or **toxicity**, which damages body tissues and affects bodily functioning in various ways. Toxins may affect chemical reactions of the body. They may also hinder the normal functioning of body cells. Additionally, toxins may cause cells in the body to release chemicals that may have an adverse effect on certain body structures. The consequences of these effects are a variety of conditions such as dermatitis (inflammation of the skin), asthma, lung disease, and immune system disorders.

Environmental Health in and Around the Home

Poisoning

The Toxic Exposure Surveillance System (TESS) is composed of participating poison centers that report on human poisoning incidents. Begun in

1983, TESS grew from 16 participating centers to a high of 73 centers in 1991; in 2009, TESS was made up of 60 centers. TESS data are compiled by the American Association of Poison Control Centers (AAPCC). Because the number of centers composing TESS has changed from year to year, the data from 1983 to the present cannot be used to determine a trend in human poisoning incidents. TESS reported that there were nearly 2.4 million human poisonings in 2011, which is a 9% decrease from 2010.[7]

Most human poisonings in 2011 occurred in the home. About 1.5% occurred in workplaces and 1.3% in schools. Poisoning in healthcare facilities increased by 4.8%. Most poisonings were unintentional, which included medication errors, bites and stings, food poisonings, and occupational mishaps. Approximately 14% were intentional and included suicides and drug abuse. The remaining cases were the result of causes such as malicious intent and adverse reactions to drugs or food.[7]

Only about 1.8% of all human poisoning incidents in 2012 were fatal. Ninety-three percent of poisoning fatalities occurred in adults aged 20 years and older.[7] Nonfatal poisonings are most often caused by the ingestion of household products and over-the-counter or prescription drugs. In 2012, they occurred in children younger than the age of 6 years approximately 44% of the time.[7] **Table 16.1** lists the substances most frequently involved in the poisoning of children younger than 6 years. **Table 16.2** lists substances that are usually not toxic.

Unless a child or adult is observed ingesting a toxic substance, it may be difficult to determine whether he or she is poisoned. Poisoning does not always start the moment exposure occurs. Also, symptoms vary depending on the substance and how it entered the body, which can occur by ingestion, inhalation, or skin contact (**Figure 16.1**).

Suspect poisoning in a person who becomes suddenly ill with symptoms that affect many systems of the body, appears drowsy and indifferent, or exhibits bizarre behavior. Also, consider poisoning as a possibility in children or young adults with chest pain; they may have ingested poison or an overdose of drugs. If poisoning may have occurred, call the local poison control center immediately. If the suspected poisoning victim is experiencing severe symptoms such as unconsciousness, seizures, intense chest pain, or repeated vomiting, he or she should be rushed to the emergency room of the closest hospital. Follow the tips in the following Managing Your Health box titled "Tips to Prevent Poisonings" to lessen the chances of being accidentally poisoned.

Toxic Plants Toxic (poisonous) plants can be the source of poisoning emergencies, especially in children. A wide variety of plants have parts that are poisonous and parts that are not. For example, tomatoes are not poisonous, but the stems and leaves of tomato plants are. Some common plant parts that are poisonous include holly berries, morning glory seeds, narcissus and daffodil bulbs, rhubarb leaves, and sweet pea seeds. The entire hemlock, jimson weed, dieffenbachia, philodendron, and mountain laurel plants are poisonous. Some plants are so poisonous that drinking the water from a vase in which their cut flowers were kept can result in poisoning.

Although many plants are not poisonous—including the poinsettia, which for years has been inaccurately reported to be toxic—house plants and cut flowers should be kept out of reach of children younger than 5 years old, and all children should be instructed that eating house and yard plants can make them sick. Many plants, such as the poinsettia, may be highly irritating when ingested, even if they are not poisonous. If a child ingests a plant, call the local poison control center and describe the plant, where it was growing, and what part of the plant the child ate. If possible, take a leaf from the plant for identification when seeking emergency medical treatment. Only plant experts should rely on their knowledge of whether the plant is poisonous.

In addition to plants, approximately 1% to 2% of mushroom species are poisonous. (Mushrooms are not plants, but fungi.) One type of mushroom is so poisonous that eating one-third of its cap can be lethal.

Symptoms of mushroom poisoning may occur immediately after ingestion and may include increased salivation, tearing, increased urination, diarrhea, difficulty breathing, and an abnormal heartbeat. Other mushroom species have toxins that produce symptoms 12 to 24 hours after ingestion that include headache, jaundice (a yellowish cast to the skin), confusion, convulsions, and possible coma. Because poisonous mushrooms can be lethal or cause severe poisoning, do not eat any mushrooms that you find growing wild. Only a person trained in mushroom identification should attempt to distinguish between mushrooms that are safe to eat and those that are not.

Ingestion of Household Cleaning Aids, Medications, and Vitamins Children younger than the age of 5 years are most in danger of being poisoned from

Table 16.1

Substance Categories Most Frequently Involved in Pediatric (≤ 5 years) Exposures (Top 25)[a]

Substance (Major Generic Category)	All Substances	Percentage[b]
Cosmetics/personal care products	159,970	13.94
Analgesics	113,975	9.93
Cleaning substances (household)	111,148	9.68
Foreign bodies/toys/miscellaneous	79,738	6.95
Topical preparations	72,638	6.33
Vitamins	49,086	4.28
Antihistamines	44,521	3.88
Pesticides	37,035	3.23
Plants	31,920	2.78
Antimicrobials	30,623	2.67
Gastrointestinal preparations	29,946	2.61
Cold and cough preparations	28,837	2.51
Cardiovascular drugs	25,025	2.18
Dietary supplements/herbals/homeopathic	23,736	2.07
Hormones and hormone antagonists	22,147	1.93
Arts/crafts/office supplies	21,721	1.89
Electrolytes and minerals	21,558	1.88
Deodorizers	19,351	1.69
Other/unknown nondrug substances	15,181	1.32
Sedative/hypnotics/antipsychotics	13,641	1.19
Antidepressants	12,299	1.07
Alcohols	11,726	1.02
Information calls	11,195	0.98
Hydrocarbons	10,890	0.95
Asthma therapies	10,863	0.95

[a]Includes all children with actual or estimated ages ≤ 5 years old. Results do not include "Unknown Child" or "Unknown Age"

[b]Percentages are based on total number of substances reported in pediatric exposure.

Reproduced from Bronstein, A.C., et al. (2010, December). 2009 annual report of the American Association of Poison Control Centers' National Poison Data System (NPDS): 27th annual report. *Clinical Toxicology*, 48, 979–1178.

Table 16.2

Frequently Ingested Products by Children (≤ 5 years) That Are Usually Nontoxic

Antacids	Hand dishwashing detergents
Antibiotics	Hydrogen peroxide (3%)
Baby oil	Lotions
Ballpoint pen ink	Noncoloring shampoos
Bath oil	Paint (latex)
Bubble bath	Pencil graphite
Calamine lotion	Perfume
Candles	Petroleum jelly
Chalk	Play-Doh
Clay (modeling)	Poinsettia (*Euphorbia pulcherrima*)
Conditioners	Shaving cream
Cosmetics	Silica or charcoal dehumidifying packets
Crayons	Soaps
Deodorants	Toothpaste
Deodorizers	Topical steroids (e.g., hydrocortisone cream)
Diaper rash products	Vitamins
Etch-A-Sketch	Water colors
Fabric softener	Water-based paints
Furniture polish	White glue

Note: Some of these products, although considered nontoxic, may present a choking hazard.

Data from Muller, A. A. (2005). Common nontoxic pediatric ingestions. *Journal of Emergency Nursing*, 31(5), 494–496.; Mofenson, H. C., et al. (1984). Ingestions considered nontoxic. *Clinics in Laboratory Medicine*, 4(3), 587–602

Figure 16.1

The Path of Toxic Substances Through the Body. The body absorbs toxic substances via the digestive system if they are ingested or via the respiratory system if they are inhaled. Some toxic substances can be absorbed through the skin. Once in the body, toxic substances reach the blood and lymph, which brings them to all the cells. Body cells (principally the liver) metabolize toxins; the products of metabolism are stored or excreted.

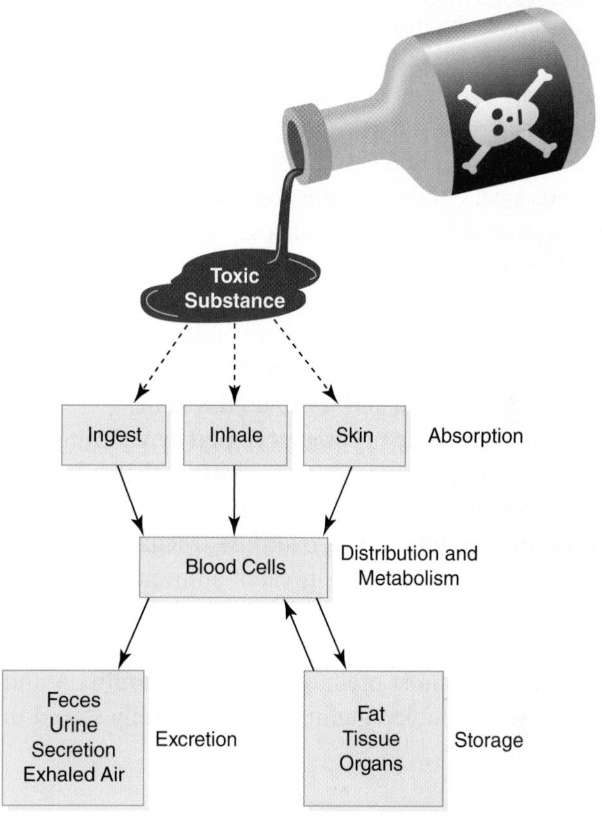

household cleaning aids and from over-the-counter and prescription drugs and vitamins. The Federal Hazardous Substances Act, passed into law by the Consumer Product Safety Commission in 1966, has been helpful in lowering the incidence of poisoning in children by controlling the concentration of toxic chemicals in household products. The Poison Prevention Packaging Act of 1972 established standards for the packaging of potentially harmful household products and medications by requiring child-resistant caps and packaging on products that present a serious danger to children. The intent of this packaging is to make it difficult for children to open toxic substances so that adults will discover their attempts before they are successful. The use of blister packs in which pills are individually encased is another approach to lessen a child's ability to remove pills from packaging.

Although warning stickers such as Mr. Yuk (**Figure 16.2**) are available for placing on hazardous substances, the results of research suggest that their use does not lower the incidence of poisoning in children.[8] Additionally, children and adults do not view the facial expression of disgust, which Mr. Yuk portrays, as precautionary; a facial expression of fear

lead poisoning A toxic condition that affects the central nervous system, caused by the ingestion or inhalation of the metallic element lead.

might be more appropriate as a deterrent.[9] Because child-resistant packaging can be opened by children (although with difficulty) and because warning stickers do not appear to discourage children from investigating package contents, all dangerous household substances, including medications and cleaning aids, should be locked in cabinets. Special child-proof locks are available that enable an adult to open a cabinet easily but bar the child from doing so. Placing items on high shelves is not a good substitute and is not safe; children easily stack items and climb on them to reach these substances.

Never suggest to a child that any medication or vitamin pill is candy because the child will seek out the pills at another time. Never take medication or vitamins in front of a young child who may think that it is candy or food and try to do the same.

Children rarely become poisoned by vitamins and mineral supplements in the amounts they accidentally consume (see Table 16.2), but adults become poisoned by intentional overdose. Megadosing with vitamins (taking much greater amounts than that recommended per day) has become a popular practice but may cause health problems. Vitamin overdosing in adults most often occurs with vitamins A and D, two fat-soluble vitamins that are readily stored in the body. Daily overdoses of most fat-soluble vitamins build up, resulting in chronic intoxication. Daily doses of 3 to 10 times the recommended amount of vitamin A over a few months to a few years produce toxic symptoms. Accutane, a form of vitamin A taken to treat skin conditions, can cause vitamin A toxicity when taken by mouth. Daily doses of 10 times the recommended amount of vitamin D over 6 months to a year produce toxic symptoms as well. Minerals that most commonly cause poisoning are iron, selenium, and zinc.

Lead Poisoning **Lead poisoning** is still a health problem in children in the United States even though many sources of lead poisoning have been eliminated in this country: leaded gasoline, leaded solder in food and soft drink cans, and leaded paint. (Solder is a metal that is heated and then used, when soft, to join other metals. It hardens on cooling and makes the joint solid.)

Even though many sources of lead have been removed from the environment, leaded dangers still exist. Ceramicware that is poorly made can have very high levels of leaching lead (that is, lead that dissolves out of the dishes and passes into food). Car batteries contain lead and should be brought to collection centers for proper disposal or recycling. Some pipes that bring water to homes contain lead-based solder. Additionally, the soil surrounding roads and highways often contains lead from years-past auto emissions.

Houses and apartments built before 1978 were often painted with lead-based paint. Although layers of nonleaded paint may cover leaded paint, the top coats of paint can chip. The exposed leaded paint creates leaded dust that may be inhaled, or the leaded paint may chip and children may eat it. Leaded paint on the exterior of homes and apartments often contaminates the surrounding soil in which children may play.

Decorating techniques that use old, salvaged building components, such as old doors, and old decorative items, such as distressed-looking old furniture, old dishes, and old toys, can be a lead health hazard.[10] Many cases of lead poisoning occur when older homes are remodeled without attention to the containment of leaded dust and paint chips. When doing such work, use a high-efficiency particulate air filter–equipped vacuum cleaner, properly fitted respirators, wet sanding equipment, and protective clothing (**Figure 16.3**). Seal off work areas with heavy-duty polyethylene plastic sheeting, and keep all nonworkers away from the area.

Figure 16.2

Poison Prevention Symbols. The skull and crossbones used to be the traditional warning symbol of poison, but the symbol was and is used to denote fun things like pirates and adventure. Therefore, Mr. Yuk (left) was developed as a warning label in the early 1970s. The image on the right is the updated skull and crossbones figure for poisons. Using these labels on toxic substances are unreliable deterrents, however. Lock all toxic substances in cabinets, away from children.

Managing Your Health

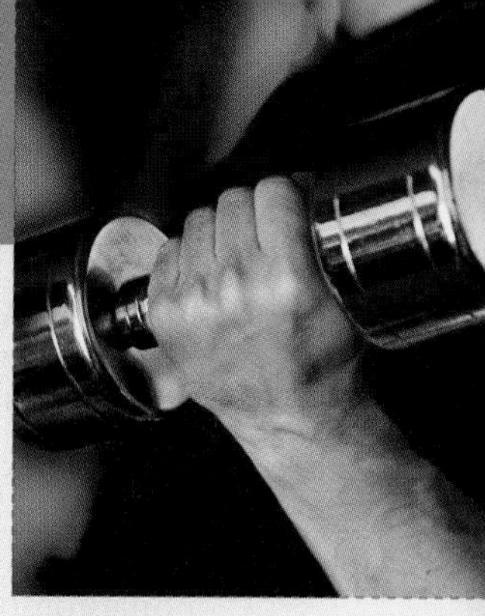
© Kzenon/ShutterStock

Tips to Prevent Poisonings

Keep Young Children Safe

- Keep all drugs in medicine cabinets or other childproof cabinets that young children cannot reach.
- Never call medicine "candy" when giving medicine to children.
- Be aware of any legal or illegal drugs that guests may bring into your home. Do not let guests leave drugs where children can find them, for example, in a pillbox, purse, backpack, or coat pocket.
- When you take medicines yourself, do not put your next dose on the counter or table where children can reach them.
- Never leave children alone with household products or drugs. If you have to do something else while using chemical products or taking medicine, such as answer the phone, take any young children with you.
- Do not leave household products out after using them. Return the products to a childproof cabinet as soon as you are done with them.
- Identify poisonous plants in your house and yard and place them out of reach of children or remove them.

Drugs and Medicines

- Follow directions on the label when you give or take medicines. Read all warning labels. Some medicines cannot be taken safely when you take other medicines or drink alcohol.
- Turn on a light when you give or take medicines at night so that you know you have the correct amount of the right medicine.
- Keep medicines in their original bottles or containers.
- Never share or sell your prescription drugs.
- Keep opioid pain medications, such as methadone, hydrocodone, and oxycodone, in a safe place that can be reached only by people who take or give them.

Household Chemicals

- Always read the label before using a product that may be poisonous.
- Keep chemical products in their original bottles or containers. Do not use food containers to store chemical products.
- Never mix household products together. For example, mixing bleach and ammonia can result in toxic gases.
- Wear protective clothing (gloves, long sleeves, long pants, socks, shoes) if you spray pesticides or other chemicals.
- Turn on the fan and open windows when using chemical products such as household cleaners.

Adapted from Department of Health and Human Services, Centers for Disease Control and Prevention. (2013, July). Tips to prevent poisonings. Retrieved from http://www.cdc.gov/homeandrecreationalsafety/poisoning/preventiontips.htm

Lead poisoning is serious because it affects the central nervous system and can cause coma, convulsions, and even death. Today, deaths resulting from lead poisoning are rare in the United States. Nonetheless, many children are severely affected by this toxin. Whereas adults absorb about 11% of lead reaching the digestive tract, children absorb from 30% to 75%. When lead is inhaled, up to 50% is absorbed.[11]

Low levels of lead in the blood (10 micrograms per deciliter [mg/dl]) are associated with decreased intelligence, learning disabilities, impaired development of the nervous system, and delayed or stunted growth. Behavioral disorders also have been linked to lead poisoning. At slightly higher levels of lead poisoning, the body does not metabolize certain vitamins properly or manufacture red blood cells correctly.

A child with high blood levels of lead (70 mg/dl) will show some of the following symptoms: decreased appetite, vomiting, abdominal pain, constipation, drowsiness, and indifference. Children who have even higher blood levels will exhibit some of the signs and symptoms of degenerative brain disease: coma, seizures, bizarre behavior, impaired muscular coordination, and vomiting. Either situation is a medical emergency and the child should be hospitalized. Tests should be performed to determine the child's lead blood level, and medications will be administered to reduce that level. However, the most important therapy is removing sources of lead from the child's environment. Call the National Lead Information Center at 1-800-424-LEAD for more information on how to avoid lead poisoning or visit its website at www.epa.gov/lead/.

Carbon Monoxide Poisoning Carbon monoxide (CO) is a colorless, odorless, tasteless gas that can kill. In fact, unintentional CO poisoning from

carbon monoxide poisoning A toxic condition that affects red blood cells' ability to carry oxygen, caused by the inhalation of the gas carbon monoxide.

asbestosis (AS-bes-TOE-sis) A condition in which scar tissue forms in the lungs as a response to irritation by asbestos.

nonautomotive sources causes about 170 deaths in the United States per year.[12] Carbon monoxide is produced by the incomplete combustion of carbon-containing fuels such as oil, coal, wood, natural gas, charcoal, and gasoline. Fires are a major source of **carbon monoxide poisoning**; persons caught in a fire often die from inhaling carbon monoxide and other toxic gases rather than from the fire. Firefighters also are at risk for carbon monoxide poisoning. Other primary sources of carbon monoxide poisoning are automobile exhaust, malfunctioning furnaces, charcoal fires, gasoline-powered tools, wood stoves, fireplaces, unvented kerosene and gas space heaters, gas cooking stoves and ovens, and tobacco smoking. See the self-assessment "Checklist for the Prevention of Carbon Monoxide Poisoning" in the Student Workbook pages at the end of this text to determine whether your home, auto, cabin, or camper is as safe as it can be.

Figure 16.3

Lead Paint Removal. These experts are removing lead paint from an old home in Providence, Rhode Island. They are using a specialized vacuum cleaner and are wearing protective clothing and respirators.

© Chitose Suzuki/AP Images

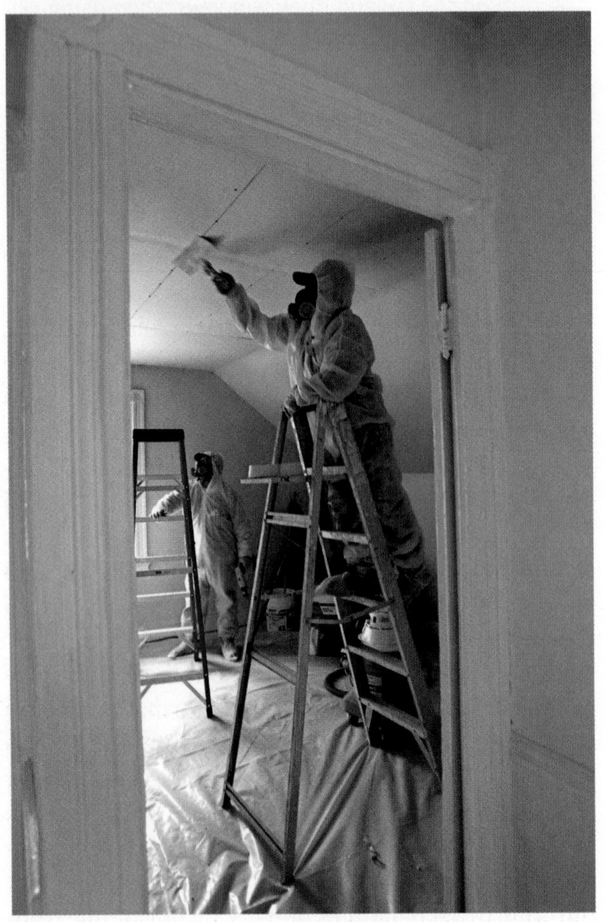

The proper maintenance and use of tools and appliances that burn fuel cuts down on the amount of CO they produce; these levels are usually not hazardous. Improper maintenance and incorrect use often result in dangerous levels of CO. To protect against these dangers, be certain that home heating stoves or furnaces are vented properly and are inspected regularly for carbon monoxide leakage. Use charcoal grills and gas-powered tools only in well-ventilated areas. (Don't use your charcoal grill in your garage or in a tent while camping.) Do not leave a car running in an attached garage where fumes can leak into the house. Run the car engine outdoors only. Carbon monoxide can also leak into a car if the exhaust system is faulty.

Carbon monoxide sensors are available for home use. These products are designed to sound an alarm when indoor air contains dangerously high levels of this toxin. Research results show that the use of carbon monoxide detectors could reduce by half the number of unintentional deaths by CO poisoning in the home. (See the Consumer Health box "Carbon Monoxide Detectors: Are They Reliable?")

Carbon monoxide kills because it binds to the oxygen-carrying molecule hemoglobin in the bloodstream. When CO is bound to hemoglobin, oxygen cannot bind and the person dies of suffocation. Before carbon monoxide poisoning kills, however, it produces signs and symptoms that become more severe as blood levels of this gas increase. At first, a person may have a slight headache that worsens as blood levels rise. (This level of poisoning can even occur if you jog near rush-hour traffic.) Fatigue sets in and the poison victim may become dizzy. As the poisoning continues, nausea, vomiting, a cherry-red skin color, and blurry vision result. Eventually the person collapses, may have convulsions, and dies.

Carbon monoxide poisoning is an emergency; immediately get the victim to fresh air and seek medical help. Healthcare practitioners treat CO poisoning victims with oxygen and test them for other medical problems that may have occurred at the time of the poisoning (such as a blow to the head in a fall).

Consumer Health

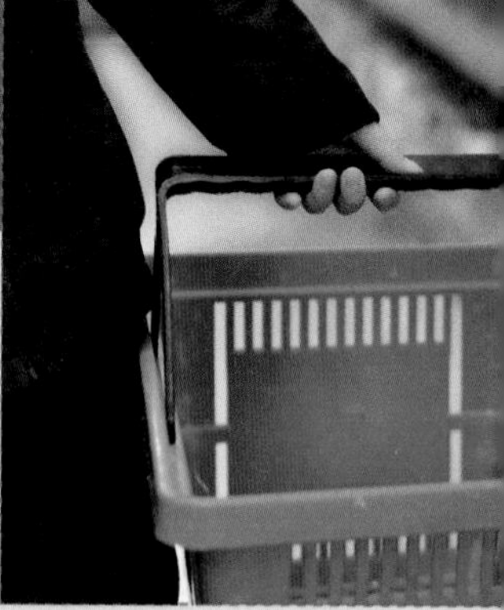
© sevenke/ShutterStock

Carbon Monoxide Detectors: Are They Reliable?

Carbon monoxide (CO) detectors should be thought of only as a backup to proper use and maintenance of fuel-burning appliances. The technology of these detectors is still developing, and a variety of types is available for home use. However, none is considered to be as reliable as home smoke detectors.

The U.S. Environmental Protection Agency reports that CO detectors have been laboratory tested with varying results. Some performed well, others failed to alarm at high CO levels, and still others alarmed at low levels that do not pose an immediate health risk. Because CO is invisible and odorless, it is hard to tell if an alarm is false or a real emergency.

When purchasing a CO detector, research the features of various models and brands and use this knowledge, not the price, as your basis for selection. Carefully follow the manufacturer's instructions for its placement, use, and maintenance. CO detectors have an average life span of approximately 2 years, after which they should be replaced. If your CO detector goes off:

- Make certain it is the CO detector alarm and not the smoke detector alarm.
- Seek medical help for anyone experiencing CO poisoning symptoms.
- Ventilate the home with fresh air and turn off all potential sources of CO.
- Have a qualified technician inspect all fuel-burning appliances and chimneys to make sure they are operating correctly and that there is nothing blocking fumes from being vented.

Adapted from U.S. Environmental Protection Agency, Indoor Environments Division, Office of Air and Radiation. (2014, May). Protect your family and yourself from carbon monoxide poisoning (EPA-402-F-96-005). Retrieved from http://www.epa.gov/iaq/pubs/coftsht.html.

In some circumstances, the poisoning victim is placed in a hyperbaric (pressure) chamber and administered oxygen.

Inhalation of Asbestos Fibers

Asbestos is a fiber-like mineral that resists damage by fire and other natural processes. Because of these qualities, asbestos has been used in the manufacture of products exposed to fire, such as stoves, furnaces, and appliances; insulation in walls and ceilings; insulation surrounding pipes; patching compounds and textured paints (as a binding compound and texturizer); roofing and siding materials; and vinyl flooring (as a strengthener).

Asbestos-containing products came into use beginning in the 1920s, but by the early 1970s scientists discovered that long-term inhalation of microscopic asbestos fibers can result in asbestosis as well as cancer of the lungs and stomach. When **asbestosis** occurs, scar tissue forms in the lungs as a response to irritation by asbestos fibers. The patient experiences shortness of breath, which progresses to a fatal lack of oxygen or heart failure. Because of the danger that asbestos exposure poses to humans, the U.S. Environmental Protection Agency (EPA) banned the use of various asbestos-containing products during the 1970s and 1980s. In 1989, the EPA announced a ban on all asbestos products by 1996.

Aside from the danger to those who mine asbestos, those in primary danger of asbestos exposure are people who live in houses built between 1920 and 1978. Various asbestos products were developed at different times during those years and were used in home construction. Asbestos was also widely used in schools built between 1950 and 1973. Intact asbestos products do not pose a hazard. Danger exists when asbestos fibers are released from the products of which they were a part and become airborne. Asbestos fibers are released from products that are deteriorating; banged, rubbed, or handled frequently; or disturbed during home remodeling. Asbestos fibers are also released when asbestos-containing flooring is sanded or seriously damaged.

To protect against the inhalation of asbestos fibers, avoid disturbing this material. Do not vacuum particles that may be asbestos laden; vacuuming them releases microscopic asbestos fibers that are inhaled. If possible, contact the contractor who built the house to determine whether asbestos was used. If this is not possible, contact a certified professional trained in asbestos removal and repair to determine whether the house contains asbestos. Sometimes materials must be sent to a laboratory to assess their content. If so, use a laboratory accredited to perform asbestos analysis. If removal, repair, or sealing of the material is necessary, hire only trained, certified personnel who can do this job safely and properly.

Electromagnetic Radiation

Are computer screens, television sets, electric blankets, microwave ovens, cell phones, or electric appliances health hazards? Are people putting their health at risk if they live near high-power electric lines or electrical distribution substations? A variety of studies has been conducted regarding the effects on the body of extremely low frequency (ELF) radiation, which is emitted by some of these sources. ELF radiation has been associated with negative effects such as risk of cancer, DNA damage, and changes in human brain electrical activity. So far, however, most scientists see no major negative effects and no reason to recommend extreme caution.[13,14] However, taking reasonable preventive measures against undue exposure may be prudent.

Extremely low frequency radiation is a type of *electromagnetic radiation*—electric and magnetic fields of energy that travel at the speed of light through the atmosphere. Sunlight, for example, is electromagnetic energy. Other forms of electromagnetic radiation include X-rays, ultraviolet light, infrared light, and radio waves.

The electric fields of extremely low frequency radiation are not as potentially problematic as are their magnetic fields. Although the strength of both the electric and magnetic fields decreases dramatically and quickly as a person moves away from the source, magnetic fields penetrate the walls of buildings that electric fields cannot.

Cathode ray tube (CRT) televisions and computer monitors produce radiation that spans the electromagnetic spectrum from X-rays to radio waves. However, they were manufactured with protective shielding to prevent most of the radiation from escaping. The small amount that does escape results in electric and magnetic fields in the atmosphere surrounding the user, but the level of radiation where the user sits is well below occupational and exposure limits recommended by governmental and industrial safety standards. CRT televisions and computer monitors are no longer manufactured. Liquid-crystal displays (LCDs) and plasma screens do not emit ELF radiation.

Cell phones and microwave ovens emit a form of electromagnetic radiation called nonionizing radiofrequency (RF) energy. RF energy is not able to break bonds in DNA—the hereditary material—so it cannot cause cancer in that way. However, at high enough levels, RF energy can heat living tissue; this is the principle used in microwave cooking. A person using a microwave often stands away from the oven, and results of studies show that radiation exposure from microwaves during regular use is unlikely to be harmful.

The heat generated by cell phones is small in comparison to that generated by microwave ovens. A cell phone's main source of RF energy is its antenna, which is part of the body of the phone. The closer the phone (and therefore the antenna) is to the user's head, the higher the user's exposure to the phone's RF energy. Cell phones (and lower energy cordless home phones) with antennas mounted away from the user are considered safe.

In recent years, many studies and reviews have been conducted regarding cell phone use and an increased risk of cancer or other adverse health effects.

The American Cancer Society has summarized research results with this statement:

> *Most studies published so far have not found a link between cell phone use and the development of tumors. However, these studies have had some important limitations that make them unlikely to end the controversy about whether cell phone use affects cancer risk.*[15]

The World Health Organization's International Agency for Research on Cancer (IARC) in a May 31, 2011, press release revealed that it had "classified radiofrequency electromagnetic fields as possibly carcinogenic [cancer-causing] to humans . . . based on an increased risk for glioma, a malignant type of brain cancer, associated with wireless phone use." The many sources of data that the IARC reviewed suggest a 40% increase in risk for glioma in heavy cell phone users, defined as an average of 30 minutes per day for 10 years. The IARC concludes that further research was needed to clarify links between cancer risk and cell phone use.[16]

To decrease your risk of these adverse health effects, put distance between yourself and your cell phone; RF exposure decreases rapidly with increasing distance from the source. Thus, use a headset or earpieces and carry the phone away from your body, or use a cell phone connected to a remote antenna. Household cordless phones operate at lower power

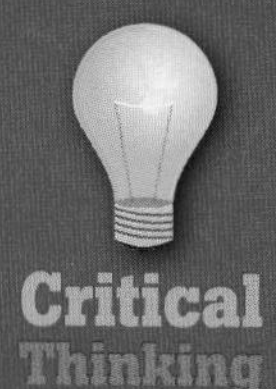

The following abstract is from an online environmental health journal, written to inform the general public about research and current thinking on cell phone use and cancer. Explain why you think this abstract is a reliable or an unreliable source of information. Use the model for analyzing health information to guide your thinking; the main points of the model are noted at the end of this abstract.

Mobile Phones, Brain Tumors, and the Interphone Study: Where Are We Now?

Anthony J. Swerdlow[1], Maria Feychting[2], Adele C. Green[3,4], Leeka Kheifets[5], and David A. Savitz[6,7], International Commission for Non-Ionizing Radiation Protection Standing Committee on Epidemiology

[1]Section of Epidemiology, Institute of Cancer Research, Sutton, United Kingdom
[2]Karolinska Institutet, Institute of Environmental Medicine, Stockholm, Sweden
[3]Cancer and Population Studies Unit, Queensland Institute of Medical Research, Brisbane, Australia
[4]School of Translational Medicine, University of Manchester, Manchester, United Kingdom
[5]Department of Epidemiology, University of California at Los Angeles, Los Angeles, California, USA
[6]Department of Community Health
[7]Department of Obstetrics and Gynecology, Brown University, Providence, Rhode Island, USA

Abstract

Background

In the past 15 years, mobile telephone use has evolved from an uncommon activity to one with > 4.6 billion subscriptions worldwide. However, there is public concern about the possibility that mobile phones might cause cancer, especially brain tumors.

Objectives

We reviewed the evidence on whether mobile phone use raises the risk of the main types of brain tumor—glioma and meningioma—with a particular focus on the recent publication of the largest epidemiologic study yet: the 13-country Interphone Study.

Discussion

Methodological deficits limit the conclusions that can be drawn from the Interphone study, but its results, along with those from other epidemiologic, biological, and animal studies and brain tumor incidence trends, suggest that within about 10–15 years after first use of mobile phones there is unlikely to be a material increase in the risk of brain tumors in adults. Data for childhood tumors and for periods beyond 15 years are currently lacking.

Conclusions

Although there remains some uncertainty, the trend in the accumulating evidence is increasingly against the hypothesis that mobile phone use can cause brain tumors in adults.

1. Which statements are verifiable facts, and which are unverified statements or value claims?
2. What are the credentials of the researchers/journal abstract making these health-related claims? Do the researchers/journal abstract have the appropriate background and education in the topic area? What can you do to check the credentials of this source?
3. What might be the motives and biases of the researchers/journal abstract making the claims?
4. What is the main point of the abstract? Which information is relevant to the issue, main point, product, or service? Which information is irrelevant?
5. Are the researchers/journal abstract reliable? What evidence supports your conclusion that the source is reliable or unreliable? Do the researchers/journal abstract present the pros and cons of the topic or the benefits and risks of the product?
6. Do the researchers/journal abstract attack the credibility of conventional scientists or medical authorities?

Based on your analysis, do you think that this abstract is a reliable source of health-related information? Summarize your reasons for coming to this conclusion.

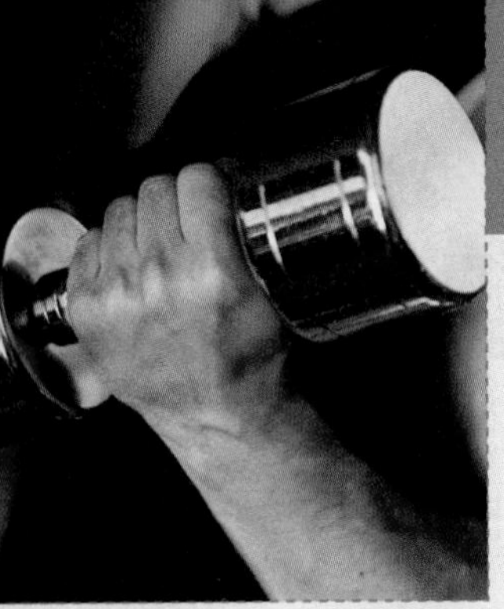
© Kzenon/ShutterStock

Managing Your Health

Avoiding ELF Radiation

- Do not sleep or sit for a long time near electric devices, particularly those with motors.
- Sit a minimum of 18 inches (at arm's length) from your CRT computer screen.
- Turn off your CRT computer monitor when it is not being used.
- Sit several feet away from the back or sides of a CRT computer monitor or television. Follow this rule even if the TV or monitor is in another room; magnetic fields travel through walls.
- Adults and especially children should sit several feet away from a CRT television screen.
- Turn on your waterbed heater or electric blanket before going to bed. Unplug them when you get into bed.
- Use a mobile phone in the car with an antenna located outside the vehicle, or use a cell phone with a headset.

levels and do not appear to have these adverse health effects. The Analyzing Health-Related Information activity in this chapter contains an article that discusses the results of research on the cancer–cell phone link.

Regarding exposure to ELF radiation of all types, medical researchers have adopted the position of "prudent avoidance" until research data indicate that another course of action should be taken. The Managing Your Health box titled "Avoiding ELF Radiation" gives some tips.

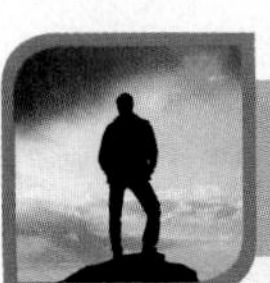
© djgis/ShutterStock

Healthy Living Practices

- Teach children not to ingest house or yard plants because they may be poisonous. In homes with young children, substitute safe plants for poisonous ones.
- Eat only mushrooms that you are certain are nonpoisonous.
- In homes with small children, store all dangerous household substances, including medications and cleaning aids, in locked cabinets.
- Never suggest to a child that medications or vitamin pills are candy.
- Do not take large doses of fat-soluble vitamins except under the direction of a physician.
- If you live in a house or apartment built before 1978, be certain that children do not ingest peeling paint. Consult a professional to test for lead, and, if lead is present, to minimize its release into the home.
- To avoid carbon monoxide poisoning, maintain and use fuel-burning tools and appliances properly, be certain that heating stoves and furnaces are correctly vented, and warm up the car outside rather than in the garage.
- Seek medical assistance immediately for anyone who exhibits symptoms of carbon monoxide poisoning.
- Do not disturb asbestos that is deteriorating.
- Seek professional help for asbestos cleanup.
- Avoid exposure to ELF radiation.

Irradiation of Food

Many types of organisms contaminate the food supply. *E. coli* (a common intestinal bacterium) can be found in such foods as hamburger and unpasteurized apple juice. A particularly deadly strain of *E. coli* (O157:H7) has caused illness and death. *Salmonella* bacteria are common contaminants of poultry. Certain insects and their larvae contaminate wheat and wheat flour. A wide range of organisms cause not only foodborne illness but the spoilage of food.

One method of killing organisms in food is irradiation; that is, treating food with radiation. Radiation is the emission of energy by the unstable nuclei of certain atoms in the form of rays or waves. Food is irradiated in its packaging by exposing it either to gamma (g) rays (a form of electromagnetic radiation similar to X-rays) or to high-energy electron beams produced by electron accelerators. Radiation is harmful to living tissue, so it kills living organisms in the food as the energy passes through it, much like microwaves pass through food in a microwave oven.

pesticides Chemicals that kill plant and animal pests and that can cause poisoning when ingested.

And just as a dentist's X-ray does not make your teeth radioactive, irradiation does not make food radioactive.

Food irradiation is a process that was patented in the United States in 1921 but was not approved for use on the first food products (wheat, wheat flour, and white potatoes) by the Food and Drug Administration (FDA) until the early 1960s. Since then, whether to irradiate food in the United States has been a contentious issue. Approximately 50 years after its approval, irradiation remains in limited use, although the FDA has since approved the use of irradiation on fresh produce, herbs, spices, pork, poultry, and red meat.

Numerous national and international organizations (such as the American Medical Association and the World Health Organization) as well as many university-based research institutes endorse the irradiation of food. Irradiation has been shown to be the only way to rid ground beef of *E. coli* O157:H7 before cooking. (Cooking ground beef thoroughly also kills this pathogen.) Irradiation also kills other bacteria, as well as insects and fungi that can make people sick or spoil food. Additionally, irradiating food inhibits the sprouting of vegetables and delays the ripening of fruits. Using this process makes the food supply safer, provides a better quality of food, and extends the "shelf life" of food.

Environmental Health in the Workplace

Exposures to some toxins can occur both at home and at work, depending on one's occupation. Accidental carbon monoxide poisoning, for example, is certainly a hazard for automobile mechanics if car exhaust is not properly vented, but carbon monoxide poisoning more frequently occurs in the home. Pesticides are another group of toxic substances that persons may accidentally ingest at home if these chemicals are placed in unlabeled containers. However, pesticide poisoning more frequently occurs on the job in people who manufacture or apply pesticides. Poisoning by exposure to certain solvents, metals, plastics, and adhesives generally occurs only during their manufacture.

Pesticide Poisoning

Pesticides are chemicals that kill plant and animal pests; they are used on farms and in homes and businesses to control insects, rodents, and weeds. People rarely become poisoned from spraying pesticides in their homes or yards; however, they should be cautious, spray downwind, and protect their skin and eyes. Occasionally, people accidentally drink or eat pesticides (or other toxic chemicals) stored in unmarked food containers in storage areas. For this reason, pesticides always should be kept in clearly marked containers. A person who has ingested pesticides should receive immediate medical attention.

People also ingest pesticides in the food they eat. These pesticides are not simply what is sprayed on fruits and vegetables but are found in fish, seafood, and meat. Animals often ingest foods sprayed with pesticides. Marine and freshwater organisms also eat food contaminated with pesticides when rain washes chemicals from the land into the water. Animals store certain pesticides they eat (and other toxic chemicals such as heavy metals) in their tissues, especially in fat.

Although many harmful pesticides, such as DDT, have been banned in the United States, these toxic chemicals, as well as pesticides being manufactured today, persist in the food chain. In addition, certain harmful pesticides such as DDT are still used in other countries on crops that are imported to the United States. However, pesticide levels in humans from eating supermarket produce are not considered toxic. The FDA, EPA, and Food Safety and Inspection Service of the U.S. Department of Agriculture together ensure that the levels of pesticides in food are not hazardous to the health of consumers. Data collected by the FDA over a 7-year period show that pesticide residues on infant foods and adult foods that infants and children eat are almost always *well below* the highest levels legally allowed by the EPA (and that includes testing foods such as bananas without washing and peeling them). See the Managing Your Health feature for tips on reducing the level of pesticides in your food.

Most often, pesticide poisoning occurs in workers who manufacture or apply pesticides (**Figure 16.4**). Such workers inhale or have their skin exposed to toxic chemicals over a period of time if their skin and respiratory passageways are not properly protected. The signs and symptoms of poisoning in such cases may be vague and nonspecific at first: headache, intermittent dizziness, and general discomfort.

sick building syndrome A variety of vague health-related problems reported by many occupants of large buildings.

formaldehyde (form-AL-de-hide) A chemical used in the manufacture of certain building materials and furnishings; may cause health problems when released into indoor air.

As the poisoning worsens, the symptoms progress to include insomnia, nausea, increased sweating, involuntary eye movements, double or blurred vision, ringing in the ears, and involuntary body movements. If exposure continues, the poisoning victim may have convulsions. Treatment of chronic pesticide poisoning requires careful medical evaluation and is individualized for each patient.

The relationship of high-level exposure to pesticides and cancer has been studied by many researchers. Determining whether a causal link exists between pesticide exposure and cancer is difficult in that occupational exposure may include a variety of pesticides and cancer can have many causes. Cancers that have been associated with heavy pesticide exposure include non-Hodgkin's lymphoma (cancer of the lymphoid tissue), leukemia (cancer of the blood), multiple myeloma (cancer of antibody-producing cells of the bone marrow), as well as cancers of the following organs: brain, breast, prostate, colon, rectum, lung, and skin. Continued research is needed to clarify these associations.[17,18]

Figure 16.4

Protection Against Pesticides. This worker is using proper protection for his skin and respiratory passageways.

Courtesy of Tim McCabe/USDA NRCS

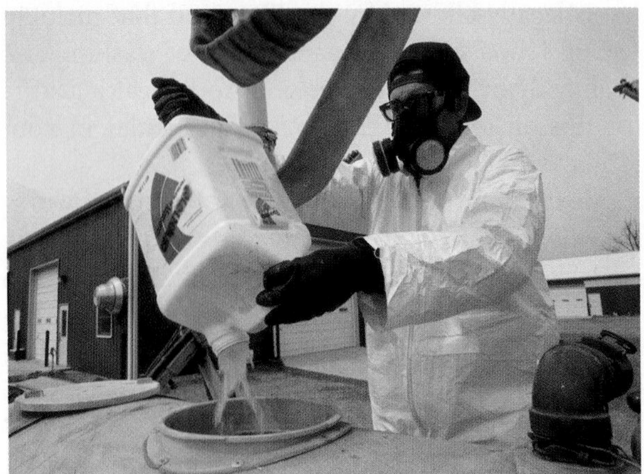

Exposure to and Inhalation of Other Toxic Chemicals

A *solvent* is a liquid in which another substance is dissolved. Solvents are varied and perform a broad range of tasks in business and industry, such as removing unwanted substances (e.g., dry-cleaning solvents remove stains from clothing) or adding coatings such as paints and sealers to surfaces. (In the latter case, the coating is dissolved in the solvent, which then evaporates upon drying.)

Exposure to most solvents slows nerve transmission in the brain and spinal cord, resulting in slowed movements and thought processes. Continued solvent exposure can lead to unconsciousness. Some solvents are irritants that can cause fluid to collect in the lungs or cause the skin to redden. Chronic exposure to solvents can also cause cracking or scaling of the skin.

Metals (such as aluminum, tin, copper, and iron) are elements that are usually shiny, are good conductors of heat and electricity, and can be melted, fused, hammered into thin sheets, or drawn into wires. Metals are extracted from ores by various processes.

During these processes, ores are crushed, melted, and poured, which results in the production of metal dusts and vapors (**Figure 16.5**). Processing metal ores sometimes uses toxic and caustic chemicals such as sulfuric acid or cyanide and often produces other toxic gases such as carbon monoxide and sulfur dioxide (discussed later in this chapter). Various industries use metals in the manufacture of products such

Figure 16.5

Processing Steel. This factory worker in east China is working at the furnace of a steel plant. He is wearing an asbestos suit for protection as he takes a sample of the molten ore with a long tool. In the process, he is exposed to metal vapor.

© Imagechina/AP Images

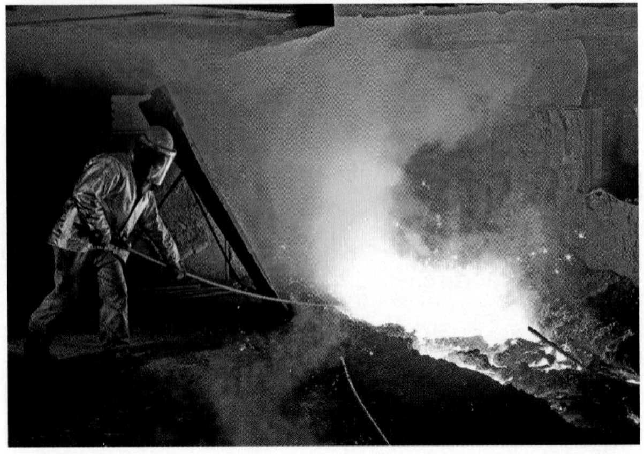

Managing Your Health

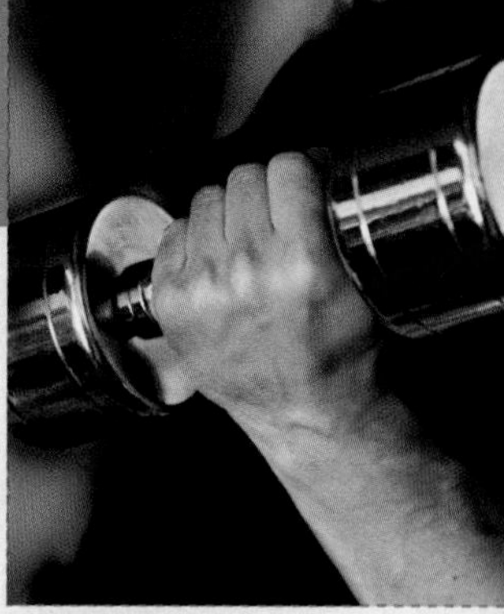
© Kzenon/ShutterStock

Reducing Pesticide Levels in the Food You Eat

- Scrub all fruits and vegetables with water for at least 20 seconds.
- Remove and discard the outer leaves of leafy vegetables.
- Trim the fat from red meats.
- Remove the skin and underlying fat from fish and poultry.
- Discard pan drippings and broths from animal products.

as bearings, solder, batteries, cutting tools, plumbing, cookware, and roofing materials.

Exposure to heavy metals results in a variety of signs and symptoms depending on the metal and how it enters the body. Inhaling metal dusts or fumes, for example, can cause a variety of lung disorders such as lung scarring, fluid in the lungs, and emphysema (a lung disease in which the air sacs break apart and breathing is difficult). Inhaling fumes of heavy metals can also irritate the eyes and mouth, damage the kidneys, and damage the brain and spinal cord, especially with exposure to lead, mercury, or manganese. Skin contact with fumes can cause burns, rashes, reddening, swelling, and itching. Exposure to many heavy metals also causes cancer.

Adhesives are used to join substances during assembly operations. In order to join parts, other processes may also be used, such as etching, roughening, or solvent cleaning. Each of these processes may introduce its own specific hazards.

In most cases, the U.S. Occupational Safety and Health Administration (OSHA) of the U.S. Department of Labor regulates procedures in industries to protect the health of workers. However, many small companies, such as auto repair shops, are not regulated by OSHA.

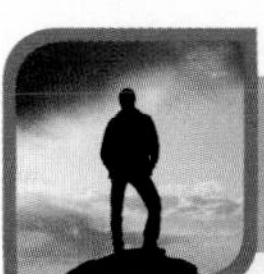
© djgis/ShutterStock

Healthy Living Practices

- ☐ Always keep pesticides and other chemicals away from children and stored in sealed, marked containers.
- ☐ When working with pesticides, wear clothing that protects your skin, eyes, nose, and mouth.
- ☐ If you work with toxic chemicals, take measures to protect yourself from damage to skin and eyes, assess the danger from toxic fumes that may be created as a result of your work, and contact OSHA for more information.

Indoor Air Pollution

As people became concerned about the excessive use of energy in the 1970s and started creating "tighter" buildings to conserve energy in heating and cooling, they also became concerned about the quality of indoor air. Numerous studies have been conducted during the past 2 decades to address this concern and determine the cause of "sick building syndrome."

Sick building syndrome refers to a variety of symptoms reported by occupants of large buildings. These symptoms are attributed to the physical environments of the buildings. Buildings are identified as problems when a large proportion (sometimes as many as 30%) of their occupants complain about the same vague health-related problems, such as headaches; unusual fatigue; eye, nose, and throat irritation; and shortness of breath.

The results of studies of sick buildings show the predominant problem to be inadequate ventilation. Another cause of health problems is chemical contamination from a variety of sources such as building materials, carpets, paints, adhesives, and furniture. In addition, if the building moisture level is too high, it can promote the growth of mold and cause symptoms in those allergic to mold.[19] Other sources of contamination of indoor air include asbestos and combustion-generated pollutants (discussed earlier in this chapter), radon, and formaldehyde. Authors of a study in England, however, conclude that poor psychosocial conditions in a workplace may far outweigh poor physical conditions of a building in causing symptoms of sick building syndrome.[20]

Formaldehyde is a chemical used in the manufacture of many building materials and furnishings, which then release formaldehyde into the air. Specific products that are most frequently responsible for high levels of formaldehyde in indoor air are pressed wood products such as fiberboard, particleboard, and

radon gas A substance present in the rocks and soils in many areas in the United States; may seep through cracks in basements and cause health problems.

hazardous waste Toxic chemical refuse.

hardwood plywood paneling and urea-formaldehyde foam, which is usually used to insulate walls.

Formaldehyde irritates the eyes, nose, and sinuses; people who inhale formaldehyde may have difficulty breathing, experience chest pain, and begin to wheeze. Some people experience headaches, fatigue, nausea, and have difficulty sleeping, whereas others exhibit gastrointestinal disturbances such as vomiting and diarrhea. Formaldehyde's role in the development of asthma and cancer is controversial.

If formaldehyde contamination occurs in a home or public building (as noted by occupants' symptoms), the source must be determined and removed, or other measures must be taken to reduce the level of this gas in the indoor air. This process may be difficult and expensive. Removing urea-formaldehyde foam insulation from walls is costly and damages the walls. (However, urea-formaldehyde foam insulation installed 5 to 10 years ago is unlikely to still release formaldehyde.) Paneling may need to be removed or furniture discarded. Alternatives are to install an air ventilation system designed to remove toxic substances such as formaldehyde from the air, bring large amounts of fresh air into the building, or seal the surfaces of the formaldehyde-containing products.

Radon gas may also contaminate indoor air. Radon is present in the rocks and soils in many areas in the United States. People who live in these regions may be exposed to radon gas if it leaks through cracks in basement walls and collects in their homes

Homes that were built or remodeled between 2001 and 2008 may have been constructed with defective imported drywall (often called Chinese drywall) that emits various sulfur-containing compounds. Along with causing corrosion in the homes' plumbing and electrical systems, the drywall emissions have been linked to negative health effects in some sensitive individuals.[21]

Environmental Health in the Outdoors

Water Pollution

People get the water they drink from underground reservoirs called aquifers and from above-ground sources: lakes, rivers, and human-made reservoirs. Both sources of water can become contaminated with toxic chemicals. Surface water, however, can also become contaminated with pathogens, plant fertilizers, sediments (soil), radioactivity, and heat.

In developed countries, waterborne pathogens are infrequently a cause of disease because sewage plants treat wastewater so that it will not contaminate water supplies. Additionally, public drinking water is chlorinated to kill pathogens. However, infection can occur when water purification and supply systems break down. Waterborne infectious disease is a widespread problem in developing countries, which have no water purification systems.

Plant fertilizers, sediments, and heat, which often contaminate surface waters, do not generally harm humans. The radioactivity emitted by nuclear power plants that enters the water supply is thought to be so low as to be harmless to humans. However, chemical contaminants such as toxic chemical compounds (including pesticides), heavy metals (such as mercury and lead), and acids (from acid precipitation; see the section titled "Air Pollution" later in this chapter) can cause noninfectious diseases and poisoning.

Chemical contaminants pollute both groundwater (aquifers) and surface water. Such pollutants enter surface water when industries spill waste chemicals into waterways, mining wastes flow into rivers, pesticides wash into rivers and lakes during a rain, and salt used to de-ice roads washes into rivers and streams during spring rains.

Heavy metals can also contaminate surface water. Metals enter the water when they are dumped into rivers and streams from industrial sources. However, the Clean Water Act of 1972 and the Federal Water Pollution Control Act of 1972 and their amendments have all been instrumental in prohibiting industry from discharging such toxic chemicals into surface water. Metals also get into drinking water on its way to homes by leaching from lead solder in water pipes. (Leaching is the removal of the dissolvable parts of a substance as water moves through or over it.) The Safe Drinking Water Act and its 1986 amendments authorize the EPA to monitor the safety of drinking water and requires the use of lead-free solder in plumbing pipes.

Groundwater becomes polluted from deteriorating underground petroleum storage tanks at gasoline stations, chemicals from road salting, or agricultural chemicals that leach into the ground. However, **hazardous waste** (toxic chemical waste) is the primary source of groundwater pollution as toxic chemicals leach into aquifers.

In 1980, Congress passed a toxic waste cleanup bill and allocated funds to clean up hazardous substances. Known as the Superfund, it provides money to find the parties guilty of dumping toxic waste at specific sites and forces them to pay cleanup costs. If the government cannot find the guilty parties, it pays to have the sites cleaned up. Since 1980, the Superfund program has fostered the cleanup of hundreds of hazardous waste sites nationwide. Sites are continually being deleted and added to the National Priorities List (NPL), which is the list of hazardous waste sites eligible for cleanup under Superfund.

To ensure the safety of drinking water, purification methods in the United States often involve chlorination to kill unwanted pathogens. In fact, 75% of the nation's drinking water is treated with chlorine. In 1974, however, scientists realized that this chemical interacts with other chemicals in drinking water to form new compounds such as chloroform. Since this discovery, scientists have been studying whether these compounds are associated with the incidence of cancer. At normal levels of consumption, compounds formed from chlorine in drinking water are not likely to produce cancer, miscarriages, or birth defects.

Becoming aware of the potential for water pollution is only the first step in protecting against the short-term and long-term health effects of drinking contaminated water. Tap water can be tested to be sure that it does not contain toxic or other unwanted chemicals. If it does, it can be treated using various methods such as carbon filtration. Carbon filters remove many carbon-containing compounds and chlorine from the water, improving its taste, odor, and color. The filters are not useful for all water-treatment needs. Some persons choose to use only bottled water for cooking and drinking. However, bottled water is not necessarily better than tap water. To judge its purity, have your bottled water tested for the presence of toxic chemicals, or write to the International Bottled Water Association (IBWA), 1700 Diagonal Road, Suite 650, Alexandria, VA 22314 for information regarding a specific bottler. Their information hotline is 1-800-WATER-11.

Air Pollution

Air pollution is also a threat to health. The primary substances in the air that harm humans are sulfur dioxide (SO_2), nitrogen dioxide (NO_2), carbon monoxide (CO), ozone (O_3), and particulates. These substances are formed when fossil fuels are burned. Fossil fuels are carbon-containing substances formed over time and under pressure from once-living organisms (both plants and animals). Gasoline, coal, natural gas, and oil are all fossil fuels.

acid precipitation Rain, snow, or fog combined with sulfur dioxide from fossil fuel emissions.

smog (smoke plus fog) A haze in the atmosphere formed by various pollutants.

The two main contributors to air pollution are automobiles and coal-fired power plants. The use of small gasoline-powered machines such as leaf blowers, chainsaws, weed cutters, and snow blowers also contributes to air pollution.

Coal-fired power plants generate particulates and sulfur dioxide as their primary pollutants. People who live downwind of such power plants experience the greatest impact from these pollutants. Sulfur dioxide combines with water in the atmosphere to produce sulfuric acid, the major component of **acid precipitation**. Acid precipitation (rain, snow, and fog) damages both living and nonliving things and acidifies surface water. When it falls in cities, it can harm vegetation as well as damage stone statues and buildings, as shown in **Figure 16.6**. Acid water in reservoirs leaches metals from pipes carrying the water into the drinking water supplies. The regions of the United States affected most heavily by acid precipitation are the Great Lakes area and New England. Southern Canada also experiences the effects of U.S. power plant emissions.

Sulfur oxides and particulates also combine with atmospheric moisture to form a grayish haze called **smog** (smoke plus fog). Smog can harm the lungs. Cities with sulfur oxide smog (called *gray-air cities*) are usually located in cold, moist climates and rely on coal and oil for electricity and home heating. The smog in gray-air cities, such as New York City and Paris, France, is worst during cold, wet winters (**Figure 16.7a**).

Of the sulfur oxides and particulates in smog, particulates do the most damage to the lungs. *Particulates* are small particles that are dispersed in the air. Although nasal hairs and mucus in the nose and throat trap large particles, particulates reach the lungs and accumulate over time. Eventually, this material irritates the lungs and blocks their microscopic air sacs, making breathing more difficult. Particulates in the air passageways and lungs can also be a factor in the development of respiratory diseases such as bronchitis, emphysema, and asthma. They also make existing respiratory illness worse.

Sulfur dioxide in the air irritates the mucous lining of the eyes and lungs. Like particulates, sulfur

Air Quality Index (AQI) A guide to air quality that uses levels of various pollutants to determine its values.

dioxide worsens respiratory illness. Together, particulates and sulfur dioxide have a greater effect on respiratory problems than if only one of these pollutants were present. At highest risk are older adults and people with chronic lung and/or heart disease.

Cities located in the warm, dry climates of the southwestern United States are plagued by smog too, but the smog of these *brown-air cities* is created primarily by the emissions of automobiles. Photochemical smog comprises carbon monoxide (discussed earlier in this chapter), nitrogen dioxide, and ozone. Nitrogen dioxide is formed when nitrogen gas in the air chemically combines with oxygen during the combustion of fuel. This compound irritates the eyes, lungs, and other mucous membranes. It also reacts with hydrocarbons (the hydrogen and carbon in fuel) in the presence of sunlight to produce a secondary pollutant—ozone. In the upper atmosphere, ozone protects us from the sun's damaging ultraviolet rays. But when it is in the air we breathe, ozone is irritating to the lungs. The smog in brown-air cities, such as Los Angeles and Phoenix, is worst during the summer months (**Figure 16.7 b**).

The **Air Quality Index (AQI)** is a means by which the public is informed of air quality. Levels of five major air pollutants (CO, NO_2, O_3, SO_2, and particulates) are monitored and used to determine AQI values (**Figure 16.8**). The descriptor for air quality (good, moderate, unhealthful, and so forth) is determined by the highest concentration of each pollutant in

Figure 16.6

The Effects of Acid Rain. This stone statue is located on the side of a church in England. The pitting of the stone is due to the effects of acid rain.

© Peter Clark/ShutterStock

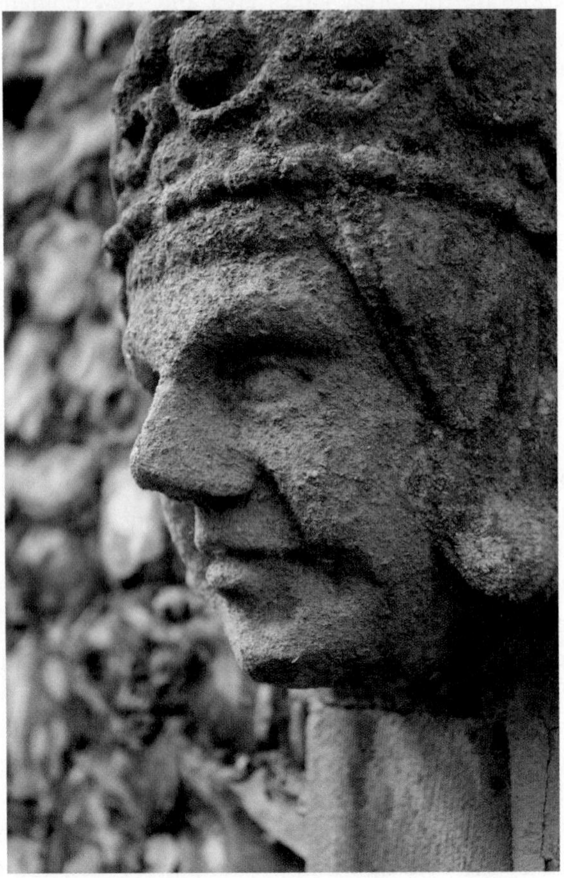

Figure 16.7

Two Forms of Smog Created in Two Ways.
(a) New York City exhibits the gray haze of a gray-air city. Its smog is formed from the byproducts of coal and oil combustion mixing with moisture in the air.
(b) Los Angeles exhibits the brown haze of a brown-air city. Its smog is formed from the byproducts of vehicle emissions that react with sunlight.

(a) © Jupiterimages/Photos.com/Thinkstock; (b) © Chad Littlejohn/ShutterStock

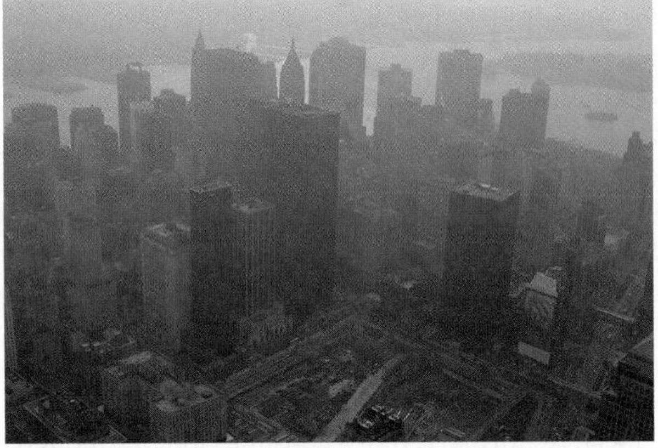

(a)

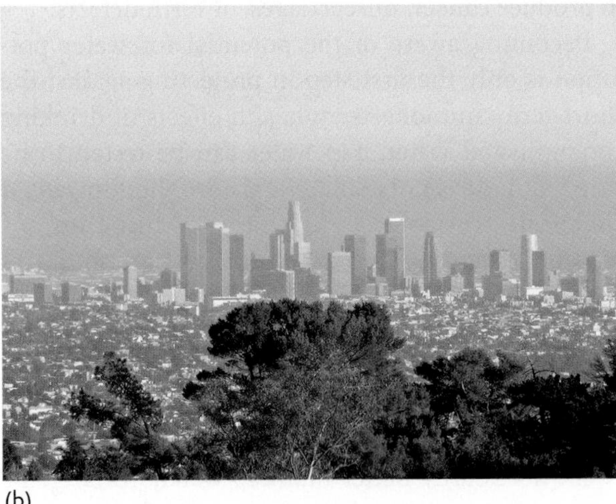

(b)

Figure 16.8

The Air Quality Index (AQI).

Reproduced from United States Environmental Protection Agency. (2014, May 22). Air Quality Index: A guide to air quality and your health. Retrieved on May 12, 2011, from http://www.airnow.gov/index.cfm?action=aqibasics.aqi

Air Quality Index (AQI) Values	Levels of Health Concern	Colors
When the AQI is in this range:	*...air quality conditions are:*	*...as symbolized by this color:*
0 to 50	Good	Green
51 to 100	Moderate	Yellow
101 to 150	Unhealthy for Sensitive Groups	Orange
151 to 200	Unhealthy	Red
201 to 300	Very Unhealthy	Purple
301 to 500	Hazardous	Maroon

the air. When the air is unhealthful or worse, the AQI cautionary statements should be heeded; many elderly persons and those with chronic lung or heart conditions can die during times of unhealthful and hazardous air quality. Since strict amendments to the Clean Air Act were passed in 1970 and even tougher standards were set with the passage of amendments in 1990, the quality of the air in the United States has improved greatly, but many cities and areas of the country still have high levels of pollution.

Noise Pollution

Noise pollution can have a negative effect on health, but it is unlike any of the environmental dusts, fumes, vapors, gases, and liquids discussed previously. Noise is composed of sound waves. If sound waves were visible, they would look much like ripples on water—areas of compressed air molecules followed by areas in which the molecules are more spread out. These waves in the air are the result of the vibration of an object disturbing the air around it.

The human ear detects these sound vibrations in the air as they hit the eardrum, causing it to vibrate. The vibrating eardrum moves the tiny bones of the middle ear, which, in turn, cause the fluid of the inner ear to move across delicate hairs. The hairs of the inner ear are connected to nerves that send messages to the brain. These messages are interpreted as sound. The fragile hairs, however, can be permanently injured by sound waves that are too loud.

How loud are everyday sounds? **Table 16.3** lists some everyday sounds and their loudness. Sound intensity, or loudness, is expressed in decibels (dB). The faintest sound a human can hear is considered zero (0) dB. As the intensity of sound increases on the decibel scale, each 10-dB increase means a 10-fold increase in the intensity of the sound. Therefore, a 50-dB sound is 10 times louder than a 40-dB sound.

Table 16.3

Loudness of Some Everyday Sounds

Sounds	dB
Rustling leaves	10
Normal conversation	50
Suburban neighborhood noise	52
Vacuum cleaner	70
City noise; busy traffic	80
Inside a passenger jet (takeoff)	78–83
Heavy trucks at 50 feet	76–88
Home shop tools	65–110
Subway noise	80–114
Nearby jet airplane	150
Shooting a gun	150–170

Sounds that are considered quiet or soft are 50 dB or less. The National Institute on Deafness and Other Communication Disorders (NIDCD) states that sounds of less than 75 dB are unlikely to cause hearing loss. When sounds get as loud as 80 dB, they begin to be annoying and can be harmful over time. At 85 dB, hearing is at risk of permanent damage. Pain sets in at 120 dB.

The EPA estimates that 40% of the U.S. population is exposed to enough noise to cause permanent hearing loss. The average person can damage his or her hearing if he or she

- Uses a power lawn mower (90 dB) for 8 hours
- Is at a loud party (90 dB) for 6 to 8 hours
- Uses a chain saw (100 dB) for 2 hours
- Uses a gasoline-powered leaf blower (110 dB) for 30 minutes
- Is at a dance club or rock concert (115 dB) for 15 minutes

Although you may not be at one party for 8 hours, damage to hearing from loud sounds is cumulative.

That is, the effects add up. These effects can be devastating; the National Institutes of Health have determined that permanent hearing loss will result from years of exposure, 8 hours per day, to 85-dB and louder sounds. Permanent deafness may result from such continual exposure and can also result from a single exposure, such as being close to an explosion of 140 dB.

How do people know if they are losing their hearing? First, a person may lose the ability to hear high-frequency sounds. He or she may be unable to hear occasional words in conversation or have difficulty hearing on the telephone. Additionally, people with partial hearing loss often experience ringing or roaring in their ears, called tinnitus. Tinnitus makes hearing even more difficult. Hearing aids may be helpful to the person with partial hearing loss but cannot totally compensate for the problem.

Total or partial hearing loss is only one of the effects of listening to sounds that are too loud. Parts of the body other than the ear react to noise. Researchers have shown that exposure to 70-dB noise results in an increase in the heart rate and a rise in blood pressure; muscles tighten and breathing patterns change. Exposure to noise also increases the rate at which stress-related hormones are secreted into the bloodstream. Even moderate daytime noise levels have been shown to increase anxiety and hostile behavior in some persons. Environmental noise exposure has also been linked to impaired learning ability and performance in school.

Paying attention to the noise in your environment will help save your hearing. For example, many health clubs blast loud music as an aerobics instructor yells commands. Often, these sounds top 110 dB. Request that the volume be turned down. If you wear ear protection, use only materials and items manufactured to reduce sound; placing cotton or tissue in your ears does not do an adequate job of protecting your ears.

If you attend loud concerts, check your hearing when you leave. Set your car or home radio to a level at which you can barely hear the words. Then, as soon after the concert as possible, turn on the radio. Can you hear the words? If not, you have sustained short-term hearing loss from the loudness of the music. Frequently listening to such loud music could result in a permanent hearing problem.

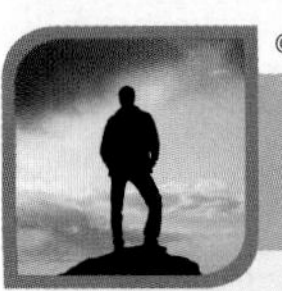

Healthy Living Practices

- To avoid hearing loss and the other effects of noise pollution, avoid situations in which the sound is over 80 dB. Pay attention to noise levels and complain if they are too high.

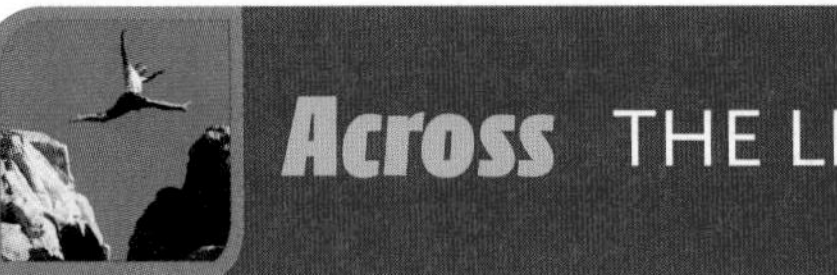

Across THE LIFE SPAN

ENVIRONMENTAL HEALTH

Environmental health hazards are a risk for all segments of the population. However, young children are most at risk for unintentional poisoning by ingestion of toxic substances because they lack understanding that these materials are harmful and they put most things in their mouths; this is a normal exploratory behavior for small children. Carbon monoxide and lead are particularly injurious to fetuses and young children because their brains and nervous systems are still developing. Also extremely susceptible to carbon monoxide poisoning or air pollutants are older adults and persons with chronic lung or heart disease, whose lung function may be impaired.

Diversity in Health

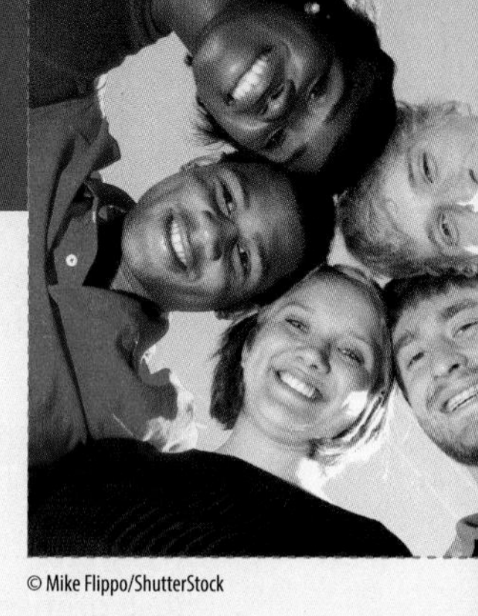

© Mike Flippo/ShutterStock

Hunger, the Environment, and the World's Population

Nearly one of six people in the world suffers from acute or chronic hunger. Hunger is more than appetite, the psychological desire for food, or feeling hungry after not eating for a few hours. Acute hunger, or starvation, is a condition in which a person has not eaten for a prolonged period and will eventually die from lack of food. *Chronic hunger* refers to a long-term condition in which food intake is inadequate. People who experience chronic hunger are undernourished and do not have the nutrients they need for proper growth, development, and body function.

Although many of the factors that lead to hunger are political, social, and economic, environmental conditions play a role in the many perceived causes of world hunger. Overpopulation, environmental limits to food production, and land use problems are factors that scientists debate with regard to their roles in hunger. In fact, many scientists assert that there is no global hunger problem. Instead, they assert, regional hunger problems exist, each with diverse causes.

The world population reached 7.2 billion people in December 2013. The *2012 Revision of World Population Prospects* issued by the United Nations (UN) in May 2011 projects that the world population will reach 9.6 billion by 2050 and 10.9 billion by 2100. By the turn of the century, projects the UN, only high-fertility countries such as those in Africa will have populations on the increase. The populations of medium-fertility countries, such as India and the United States, will peak in about 2060 and then very slowly start to decline. Populations in low-fertility countries, such as most countries in Europe, will peak in 2030 and decline more quickly than the populations of medium-fertility countries.

Various experts predict that the world population will level off, reaching its carrying capacity between 12.4 billion and 14 billion people. The carrying capacity is the maximum number of individuals that can be supported by the available resources. However, scientists disagree as to whether the global food output can support that many individuals. Many scientists calculate that even with the use of the best agricultural technologies, the carrying capacity of the Earth will be limited to 7.5 billion people.

Scientists disagree as to whether the increase in food production during the 1980s kept up with the need for food worldwide. They also disagree as to whether technological advances in various areas of agriculture, such as changes in machinery, seed varieties, fertilizers, pesticides, and management practices, as well as the genetic engineering of plants to resist certain crop pests, will allow the world's farmers to produce greater and greater crop yields. Many scientists assert that to increase sufficiently the amount of food produced around the world, farmers must increase the amount of land they cultivate. However, using marginal land (land not well suited for cultivation) may increase the danger of erosion, landslides, and floods. Marginal land is also likely to produce lower crop yields than land already in cultivation. Additionally, the limited availability of water in many regions may constrain agricultural expansion.

Many parts of the Earth cannot support the population that now exists on their lands. A country is overpopulated when its natural resources cannot sustain its people. An example of such overpopulation is Africa, the continent with the fastest population growth in the world. According to the UN's *Revision of World Population Prospects*, in 2010 62% of the African population was younger than age 25 years. Therefore, the size of this population will increase in the next decade and beyond because a large proportion of the population is and will be in its reproductive years. Much of the land in Africa has a low natural carrying capacity. Its climate is highly changeable and therefore unreliable for growing crops.

The problem of world or regional hunger is serious. Environmental issues such as overpopulation, methods of food production, and approaches to land use interact with political, cultural, social, and economic issues to create situations that can affect the health of many peoples throughout the world.

CHAPTER REVIEW

Summary

In general, environmental factors that are the sole cause of disease are toxic chemicals. Such substances damage body tissues and affect bodily functioning; they are present in the home, workplace, and environment. Toxic chemicals are found in a wide variety of substances, such as household products, plants, products used in the workplace, and prescription and illegal drugs.

Toxic (poisonous) plants can be the source of poisoning emergencies, especially in children. Although many plants are not poisonous, house plants and cut flowers should be kept out of reach of children younger than 5 years old. In addition to plants, approximately 1% to 2% of mushroom species are poisonous.

Children younger than the age of 5 years are those most in danger of being poisoned from household cleaning aids and from over-the-counter and prescription drugs and vitamins. Special packaging that makes it difficult for young children to open hazardous products has lowered the incidence of poisoning in this age group. Nevertheless, such substances should be locked in cabinets in homes in which young children reside or visit often.

Lead poisoning is still a health problem in children in the United States even though many sources of lead poisoning have been eliminated in this country. Lead poisoning is serious because it affects the central nervous system and can cause coma, convulsions, and death. Children can exhibit a wide range of symptoms of lead poisoning, depending on the level of lead in the blood. It is extremely important to remove sources of lead, such as lead-based paint, from a child's environment.

Carbon monoxide poisoning can occur when levels of this gas build up in an enclosed environment. Major sources of carbon monoxide poisoning are fires, automobile exhaust, malfunctioning furnaces, charcoal fires, gasoline-powered tools, woodstoves, fireplaces, unvented kerosene and gas space heaters, gas cooking stoves and ovens, and tobacco smoke. To avoid this hazard, properly maintain and use tools and appliances that burn fuel, avoid running the car in the garage, vent home heating stoves and furnaces properly, and use charcoal grills and gas-powered tools only in well-ventilated areas.

Extremely low frequency (ELF) radiation is emitted by computer screens, microwave ovens, cell phones, television sets, electric blankets, electric appliances, high-power electric lines, and electrical distribution substations. ELF radiation has been associated with negative effects such as risk of cancer, DNA damage, and changes in human brain electrical activity. Nonetheless, scientists have seen no major negative effects in most situations and with most products and see no reason to recommend extreme caution. Medical researchers suggest, however, that people avoid being unnecessarily close to products and power lines that emit ELF radiation. Additional caution is needed with cell phones. It is recommended that cell phones be used with a headset or earpieces or that a cell phone be connected to a remote antenna.

Many types of environmental hazards exist in the workplace. Common workplace hazards include exposure to pesticides while manufacturing or applying them and exposure to toxins in the industrial manufacture and use of certain solvents, metals, plastics, and adhesives. People who work with toxic chemicals should protect themselves from damage to their skin and eyes and should assess the danger from toxic fumes that may be created as a result of their work.

Indoor air may be contaminated with pollutants such as formaldehyde, asbestos, and combustion-generated products. Some buildings have poor ventilation systems, which appear to be a primary cause of vague health-related symptoms in building occupants.

The air we breathe and the water we drink are also contaminated with toxins to a greater or lesser degree in various parts of the United States. Contaminated drinking water can result in both short-term and long-term health effects. The air is contaminated with emissions from coal-fired power plants and vehicles. When the air is unhealthful, older adults and those with respiratory illness are most at risk for further damage to their health.

Noise pollution can have a negative effect on health. Sounds of less than 75 dB are unlikely to cause hearing loss. To avoid hearing loss and other negative health effects of noise pollution, avoid situations in which the sound is over 80 dB or wear specially designed ear protection in such situations.

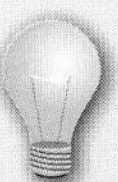

Applying What You Have Learned

1. Your 4-year-old cousin is coming to visit for the summer. What steps would you take to make your house or apartment safe for your cousin? **Application**
2. List and then analyze your interactions with your environment in the last 24 hours. Develop a list of potential environmental threats to your health from these interactions. **Analysis**
3. You have just moved to a part of the country that is new to you. Develop a plan to assess whether you are being exposed to hazardous chemicals and toxins and to evaluate which health hazards might be present, if any. **Synthesis**
4. Develop a fictitious set of at least three outcomes based on question 3. What will be your course of action to diminish or eliminate these threats to your health? **Evaluation**
5. Gather the chemicals that you use in your home, such as cleaning products. Many such products have warnings on their labels about physical hazards, storage, and disposal. Read the labels of the products you have gathered and list the types of warnings you see. State what you learned about safeguarding not only your health but also the health of the environment when using these chemicals. **Synthesis**

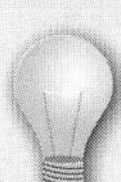

Reflecting on Your Health

1. Do you take steps to protect your hearing? If so, what do you do? Do you think about possible hearing loss when you are in noisy environments? Describe three situations in which you regularly are exposed to harmful noise levels and discuss what you can do to avoid hearing loss in these situations.
2. Go through your house or apartment and identify environmental health risks. What can you do to reduce these risks to health?
3. Do you ever put yourself or others at risk for carbon monoxide poisoning? If so, describe your behaviors that increase risk and what you can do to reduce or eliminate the risk. If not, identify

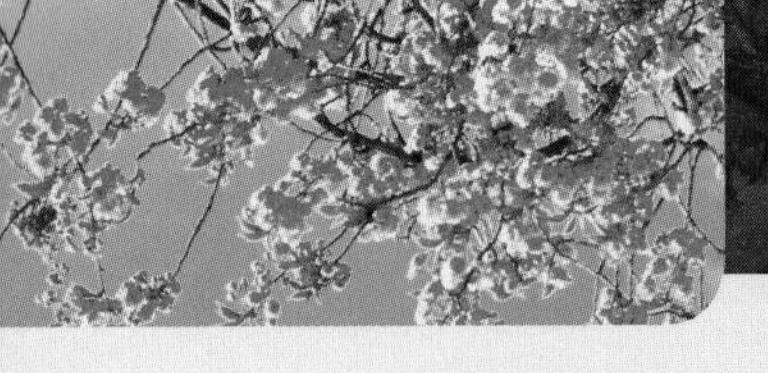

© SergeBertasiusPhotography/Shutterstock

behaviors in others that you have observed that put people at risk for carbon monoxide poisoning. How might you help others avoid such risks?

4. Find out about environmental risks in your area. For example, is your tap water chlorinated to levels that are worrisome? Do you live in a region of the country in which water comes to your home in lead pipes? What might you do in either of these situations to reduce or eliminate your health risks from water? Investigate air pollution in your area. How can you protect your respiratory health in the region in which you live? Describe any environmental health risks that affect your community and suggest what you might do to reduce health risks to yourself and your family.
5. Do you ever discard toxic waste improperly, such as putting old batteries (especially car batteries), solvents, or paints in the trash? If so, describe the proper disposal methods for these substances in your city or town.

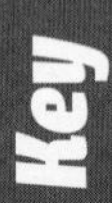

Key

Application	Analysis	Synthesis	Evaluation
using information in a new situation.	breaking down information into component parts.	putting together information from different sources.	making informed decisions.

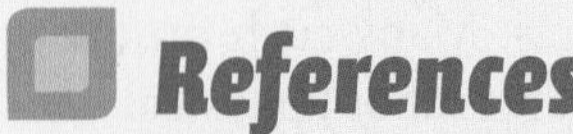

References

1. Gupta, N., et al. (2011). Lead poisoning associated with Ayurvedic drug presenting as intestinal obstruction: A case report. *Clinica Chimica Acta, 412*(1–2), 213–214.
2. Saper, R. B., et al. (2008). Lead, mercury, and arsenic in US- and Indian-manufactured Ayurvedic medicines sold via the Internet. *Journal of the American Medical Association, 8*, 915–923.
3. Centers for Disease Control and Prevention. (2005). Lead poisoning associated with use of litargirio—Rhode Island, 2003. *Morbidity and Mortality Weekly Report, 54*(9), 227–229.
4. Buettner, C., et al. (2009). Herbal supplement use and blood lead levels of United States adults. *Journal of General Internal Medicine, 24*(11), 1175–1182.
5. Gaitens, J. M., et al. (2009). Exposure of U.S. children to residential dust lead, 1999–2004: I. Housing and demographic factors. *Environmental Health Perspectives, 117*, 461–467.
6. Centers for Disease Control and Prevention. (2011). Adult blood lead epidemiology and surveillance—United States, 2008–2009. *Morbidity and Mortality Weekly Report, 60*(25), 841–845.
7. Mowry, J. B., et al. (2013, December). 2012 annual report of the American Association of Poison Control Centers' National Poison Data System (NPDS). *Clinical Toxicology, 51*, 911–1164. Retrieved from https://aapcc.s3.amazonaws.com/pdfs/annual_reports/2012_NPDS_Annual_Report.pdf
8. Vernberg, K., Culver-Dickinson, P., & Spyker, D. A. (1984). The deterrent effect of poison-warning stickers. *American Journal of Diseases of Children, 138*, 1018–1020.
9. Pooley, A. J., & Fiddick, L. (2010). Social referencing "Mr. Yuk": The use of emotion in a poison prevention program. *Journal of Pediatric Psychology, 35*(4), 327–339.
10. Sharmer, L., et al. (2010, December). A potential new health risk from lead used in consumer products purchased in the United States. *Journal of Environmental Health, 73*(5), 8–12.
11. Farley, D. (1998). Dangers of lead still linger. *FDA Consumer, 32*(1), 16–21.
12. U.S. Consumer Product Safety Commission. (2014). Carbon monoxide: The invisible killer. Retrieved from http://www.cpsc.gov//PageFiles/121843/464.pdf
13. Kheifets, L., et al. (2010). A pooled analysis of extremely low-frequency magnetic fields and childhood brain tumors. *American Journal of Epidemiology, 172*(7), 752–761.
14. Kheifets, L., et al. (2010). Extremely low frequency electric fields and cancer: Assessing the evidence. *Bioelectromagnetics, 31*(2), 89–101.
15. American Cancer Society. (2012). Learn about cancer: Cellular phones. Retrieved from http://www.cancer.org/Cancer/CancerCauses/OtherCarcinogens/AtHome/cellular-phones
16. International Agency for Research on Cancer. (2011, May 31). IARC classifies radiofrequency electromagnetic fields as possibly carcinogenic to humans [Press Release No. 208]. Geneva: World Health Organization. Retrieved from http://www.iarc.fr/en/media-centre/pr/2011/pdfs/pr208_E.pdf

17. Weichenthal, S., et al. (2010). A review of pesticide exposure and cancer incidence in the Agricultural Health study cohort. *Environmental Health Perspectives, 118*(8), 1117–1125.

18. Clapp, R. W., et al. (2008). Environmental and occupational causes of cancer: New evidence 2005–2007. *Reviews on Environmental Health, 23*(1), 1–37.

19. Buckmaster, P. K. (2009). Sustaining acceptable indoor environmental quality. *Occupational Health and Safety, 78*(10), 48, 50.

20. Norbäck, D. (2009). An update on sick building syndrome. *Current Opinion in Allergy and Immunology, 9*, 55–59.

21. Centers for Disease Control and Prevention. (2011, March). Imported drywall and your home. Retrieved from http://www.cdc.gov/nceh/drywall/imported_drywall_and_your_home.html

APPENDIX A

The Mission, Vision, and Goals of *Healthy People 2020*

Vision—A society in which all people live long, healthy lives.

Mission—Healthy People 2020 strives to:

- Identify nationwide health improvement priorities
- Increase public awareness and understanding of the determinants of health, disease, and disability, and the opportunities for progress
- Provide measurable objectives and goals that are applicable at the national, state, and local levels
- Engage multiple sectors to take actions to strengthen policies and improve practices that are driven by the best available evidence and knowledge
- Identify critical research, evaluation, and data collection needs

Foundation Health Measures

Healthy People 2020 includes broad, cross-cutting measures without targets that will be used to assess progress toward achieving the four overarching goals.

Overarching Goals of *Healthy People 2020*	Foundation Measures Category	Measures of Progress
Attain high quality, longer lives free of preventable disease, disability, injury, and premature death	General Health Status	Life expectancy Healthy life expectancy Physical and mental unhealthy days Self-assessed health status Limitation of activity Chronic disease prevalence International comparisons *(where available)*
Achieve health equity, eliminate disparities, and improve the health of all groups	Disparities and Inequity	Disparities/inequity to be assessed by: Race/ethnicity Gender Socioeconomic status Disability status Lesbian, gay, bisexual, and transgender status Geography
Create social and physical environments that promote good health for all	Social Determinants of Health	Determinants can include: Social and economic factors Natural and built environments Policies and programs
Promote quality of life, healthy development, and healthy behaviors across all life stages	Health-Related Quality of Life and Well-Being	Well-being/satisfaction Physical, mental, and social health-related quality of life Participation in common activities

Reproduced from U.S. Department of Health and Human Services. Office of Disease Prevention and Health Promotion. *Healthy People 2020*. Washington, DC.

Topic Areas

The Topic Areas of *Healthy People 2020* identify and group objectives of related content, highlighting specific issues and populations. Each Topic Area is assigned to one or more lead agencies within the federal government that is responsible for developing, tracking, monitoring, and periodically reporting on objectives.

1. Access to Health Services	22. HIV
2. Adolescent Health	23. Immunization and Infectious Diseases
3. Arthritis, Osteoporosis, and Chronic Back Conditions	24. Injury and Violence Prevention
4. Blood Disorders and Blood Safety	25. Lesbian, Gay, Bisexual, and Transgender Health
5. Cancer	26. Maternal, Infant, and Child Health
6. Chronic Kidney Disease	27. Medical Product Safety
7. Dementias, Including Alzheimer's Disease	28. Mental Health and Mental Disorders
8. Diabetes	29. Nutrition and Weight Status
9. Disability and Health	30. Occupational Safety and Health
10. Early and Middle Childhood	31. Older Adults
11. Educational and Community-Based Programs	32. Oral Health
12. Environmental Health	33. Physical Activity
13. Family Planning	34. Preparedness
14. Food Safety	35. Public Health Infrastructure
15. Genomics	36. Respiratory Diseases
16. Global Health	37. Sexually Transmitted Diseases
17. Healthcare-Associated Infections	38. Sleep Health
18. Health Communication and Health Information Technology	39. Social Determinants of Health
19. Health-Related Quality of Life and Well-Being	40. Substance Abuse
20. Hearing and Other Sensory or Communication Disorders	41. Tobacco Use
21. Heart Disease and Stroke	42. Vision

Reproduced from U.S. Department of Health and Human Services. Office of Disease Prevention and Health Promotion. *Healthy People 2020*. Washington, DC.

APPENDIX B

Injury Prevention and Emergency Care

Injury Prevention

During the next hour, at least 11 people will die in the United States from unintentional injuries. The causes will be diverse, including automobile crashes, drownings, poisonings and fires. Some of those who die this hour will probably be children because unintentional, preventable injury is the number one killer of children (through young adulthood, from 1 through 21 years old) in the United States. In fact, unintentional injuries kill more children than all childhood diseases combined.

Until recently, the number of fatal unintentional injuries had been steadily declining, reaching a 68-year low of approximately 89,000 in 1994. However, that number has been rising annually since then. In 2011, approximately 126,500 people died from unintentional injuries. This Appendix alerts you to the most prevalent types of unintentional injuries and deaths in the United States today and discusses their causes, prevention, and emergency treatment.

Automobile Safety

Motor vehicle crashes are the greatest cause of preventable death resulting from injuries, but the number of deaths has been dropping. In 2011, 33,783 people died on U.S. roads and highways, resulting in the lowest highway fatality rate ever recorded. Approximately 30% of the fatalities involved alcohol. In addition to deaths, motor vehicle accidents are the leading cause of unintentional injury in the United States. To keep yourself and others safe while riding in automobiles, heed the following recommendations. For general vehicle safety:

- Never drink and drive or take other drugs that impair your ability to drive.
- Always wear your seat belt; this practice reduces by half your chance of injury or death in a motor vehicle crash.
- Slow down and prepare to stop as you approach yellow lights. Many people cause automobile crashes because they try to "beat" the light.
- Yield the right of way at intersections.
- Don't tailgate; allow at least one car length for each 10 mph (e.g., stay four car lengths behind the car ahead if you are traveling at 40 mph).
- Know the traffic laws of the state in which you are driving and obey these laws.
- Read and heed traffic signs, especially railroad warning signals and gates. Always proceed cautiously across railroad tracks. Not all railroad crossings have gates or sound warnings to signal oncoming trains.
- Obey the speed limit.

Children and Automobile Safety To protect children while they are passengers in automobiles, follow these safety recommendations:

- Place infants and toddlers in properly secured rear-facing safety seats until they are 2 years of age or until they reach the highest weight or height allowed by their car safety seat's manufacturer.
- Always put rear-facing child safety seats in the back seat. Deploying passenger-side air bags in the front seat can injure or kill infants and toddlers in rear-facing seats.
- Children older than age 2, or those children who have outgrown the rear-facing seat before age 2, should be restrained in a forward-facing car seat with a harness *in the back seat* until they reach the highest weight and height allowed by the manufacturer.
- When children outgrow the forward-facing car seat, and until the vehicle seat belt fits properly, they should be restrained in a belt-positioning booster seat *in the back seat*. The vehicle seat belt typically fits properly when the child reaches a height of 4 feet 9 inches and they are between 8 and 12 years old.
- When adolescents reach age 13 they can ride in the front seat. Push the seat back as far as possible to create distance between the child and the air bag.
- An infant's or child's car seat needs to be secured so tightly that it will not move more than 1 in. from side to side. Locate a certified Child Passenger Safety Seat Technician in your area to check the installation of your child's safety seat.
- Never leave a child alone in the car.

Pedestrian Safety

Pedestrians accounted for 12% of preventable deaths involving motor vehicles in the United States and approximately 3% of motor vehicle–related injuries in 2009. Not only are drunk drivers often a cause of these injuries and deaths, but intoxicated pedestrians put themselves at increased risk. Other high-risk groups for sustaining unintentional pedestrian–automobile injuries and deaths are older adults and young children. Children are most frequently hit when they dart into traffic from between parked cars. Children younger than 10 years old do not have fully developed cognitive, developmental, behavioral, physical, and sensory abilities to be safe pedestrians on their own. To help prevent pedestrian injuries, practice these safety steps:

- Help children develop injury-prevention skills by modeling proper safety behaviors such as those listed here.
- Be sure that children younger than 10 years of age are accompanied by an older person when they cross the street.
- Cross at marked crosswalks and at corners whenever possible. Do not assume that drivers will stop because you are in a crosswalk.
- Stop, look both ways, and listen before deciding that it is safe to cross. Continue to look and listen as you cross.
- Cross only on a green light or a "walk" signal.
- Never cross between parked cars.
- Never run into the street.
- Walk on sidewalks whenever possible. If you must walk in the street, walk to the left facing traffic.
- When walking at dusk or at night, wear light colors and some type of reflective device. Walk with someone, not alone.
- Do not allow children to play in driveways, in adjacent unfenced yards, in streets, or in parking lots.

Water Safety

Between 2005 and 2009, an average of 3,533 people died from drowning, not including those involved in boat-related incidents. Drowning is the second leading cause of injury-related death for children aged 1 through 14 years, the highest rates being for children aged 1 through 4 years. (Fatalities involving automobiles are the leading cause of injury-related death for children.) Children younger than 1 year of age most often drown in bathtubs, buckets, or toilets. Children older than 1 year of age most often drown in pools, hot tubs, or spas owned by their parents, relatives, or friends, and they happen within 5 minutes of the child's being missing from sight. Children usually drown silently, so don't think that splashing or screaming will alert you to the danger.

Safety for Small Children To protect small children from drowning in residential pools or other accessible bodies of water, follow these safety practices:

- Provide barriers to water, such as fences and walls. If the house is part of the barrier, install door alarms so that you know when the child has gone outside, and install a power safety cover over the pool, hot tub, or spa.
- Fence gates should be self-closing and self-latching. The latch should be out of a child's reach.
- Never prop open the fence gate.
- Instruct baby-sitters about pool hazards for young children.
- If a young child is missing, check the pool first.
- Do not assume that children will not drown because they know how to swim.
- Never leave a child unsupervised near a pool, and while at the pool, watch small children continuously; do not become preoccupied with something else.
- Never leave children alone, even for a minute, when they are in or near any type of water.
- Safety for Swimmers Even good swimmers have accidents in the water and drown. For safety in the water, follow these guidelines:
- Never swim alone.
- Don't push or jump on others.
- Check water depth before you dive or jump into the water.
- Never swim in unsupervised areas such as quarries, canals, or ponds.
- Don't swim or use a hot tub or spa while drinking alcoholic beverages or taking other drugs that could impair your judgment, impair your ability to swim, or make you drowsy. (Alcohol is involved in 25–50% of adolescent and adult deaths associated with water recreation.)

Bicycle Safety

In 2009 in the United States, 630 people died in traffic-related bicycle crashes. Seventy-five percent of such deaths are usually caused by head injuries. Supporters of wearing bicycle helmets contend that 40–75% of head-injury deaths could be prevented if riders wore helmets. Opponents suggest that these statistics are unreliable and that most bicycle fatalities involve a crash with an automobile, a situation in which a helmet cannot protect the bicyclist. Those who take a middle stance suggest that it is prudent to wear helmets because they protect the head in many types of falls and make bicyclists more visible to automobile drivers.

As of August 2014, 22 states, the District of Columbia, and approximately 201 local governments had enacted legislation about bicycle helmets. Most of these laws pertain to children and adolescents. In 1999, the U.S. Consumer Product Safety Commission issued a new safety standard for bike helmets.

Bicycle helmets are designed to absorb much of the impact when the head hits another object like a car or the road. Often, a cyclist hits a car and then the road, so the helmet needs a strap to ensure that it stays on during multiple hits. Also, it should not be covered with any material that can catch on something during a fall and twist the cyclist's head. When purchasing a helmet, make sure that it is level on the head, covers the top of the forehead, touches all around, and is comfortably snug. Many sellers and manufacturers of helmets offer instructions about the proper fit of helmets.

Bicycle injuries are a leading cause of preventable death in children, exceeding the death rate from poisonings, falls, and firearm injuries combined. Most bicycle-related deaths occur from head trauma and are not caused by colliding with cars. Rather, children fall from their bikes or lose control of their bikes and collide with objects such as curbs and trees. Therefore, all children benefit from wearing helmets while bicycling. They should also wear helmets while being carried as passengers on adults' bikes. Have a pediatrician check a toddler's helmet, however, because the neck muscles of toddlers are weak and may be unable to properly support a helmeted head.

Bicycle Safety Rules For bicycling safety, follow these simple rules:

- Make yourself or your children visible with light-colored clothing and reflective tape.
- Be certain that your bicycle horn or bell is working properly.
- Drive on the right-hand side of the road in single file, obeying all traffic signs and signals. Small children should ride their bikes on the sidewalk.
- When cycling in the road, leave a distance of about 3 ft between you and parked cars. You will be more noticeable to drivers and will not be knocked off your bike by the opening doors of parked cars.
- Walk your bike at busy street corners in pedestrian crosswalks.
- Never carry a passenger on your bicycle unless you have a tandem bike or are carrying a child in a properly mounted child seat.
- When exiting a driveway into a lane of traffic, stop, look both ways, and listen to determine that it is safe to enter.
- Before turning, use hand signals and look in all directions.
- Don't ride your bike on rainy nights. Your chances of being involved in a crash are 30 times greater than on a dry night because roads are slippery, wet bicycle brakes do not work well, and automobile drivers cannot see bicyclists well in the rain.
- If you are falling off your bike, tuck and roll rather than extending an arm to break your fall.
- Children should not ride in the street until they are 10 years old, demonstrate good riding skills, and are able to observe the basic rules of the road.

Fire Prevention

Although the number of residential fires has declined since 1980, there were 365,000 residential fires in 2012 in which 2,380 people died, not including firefighters. Most home fires are started by cooking. Lit cigarettes, cigarette lighters, or matches cause the least number of residential fires but result in the most fire-related deaths. A fewer number of fires are ignited by faulty electrical wiring or supplemental home heating devices such as wood stoves, kerosene heaters, gas-fired space heaters, and portable electric heaters than by cooking but a greater number than by cigarette-related causes.

The number of supplemental home heaters has decreased in recent years, as has the number of fires associated with them. However, supplemental heaters still cause about 13% of residential fires. Additionally, thousands of people are burned each year by coming into contact with the hot surfaces of these devices, and hundreds are poisoned by their carbon monoxide emissions.

Home Heaters Some safety recommendations for the use of supplemental home heaters include the following:

- Be certain that any supplemental heater is properly installed and meets building codes.
- Inspect wood stoves according to the manufacturer's directions (usually twice monthly) and have chimneys inspected and cleaned by a professional chimney sweep.
- Use a floor protector designed for use under the type of supplemental heater you have. It should extend 18 inches beyond the heater on all sides.
- Follow directions regarding how far the heater must be from combustible walls and other materials such as draperies.
- Never burn trash in a wood-burning stove because this practice could cause overheating.
- Never use gasoline to start a wood fire.
- Use only the fuel(s) the manufacturer has designated as safe in the heater.
- If using a liquid fuel, be certain that its container is well marked and is out of the reach of children.
- Place kerosene heaters out of the path of traffic and where they cannot be knocked over.
- Always fill a kerosene heater outdoors and when the heater is not operating.
- Kerosene heaters are not usually vented; therefore, keep a window ajar for ventilation.
- Use unvented gas heaters only in large, open areas that are well ventilated; do not operate vented styles unvented.
- Do not use supplemental heating devices while you are sleeping or not at home; many

fires and deaths occur at these times from the unsupervised use of supplemental heaters.

- With electric heaters, follow the manufacturer's recommendations regarding the type of power cord to use. Avoid using extension cords, but if you do, be certain that it is marked with a power rating at least as high as that of the heater itself. Keep the cord stretched out and do not place anything on top of the cord.

General Fire Prevention Many residential fires could have been prevented with little trouble. To decrease your risk of fire, take the following precautions:

- Keep matches and cigarette lighters away from children.
- Do not store food items such as candy or other items attractive to children above the stove.
- Always check ashtrays to be certain that cigarettes are out. After a party or other gathering, check under and between the cushions of upholstered furniture to make sure that no smoldering ashes are present.
- Never place ashtrays on the arms of furniture, especially upholstered furniture that is likely to ignite from lit cigarettes or their ashes.
- Avoid placing lit candles near draperies or other flammable materials. Be certain that they do not tip easily and are not positioned where they can be easily knocked over.
- Consider purchasing clothes made out of fabrics that are difficult to ignite and tend to self-extinguish, such as 100% polyester, nylon, wool, and silk. Cotton, cotton/polyester blends, rayon, and acrylic ignite easily and burn rapidly.
- Store flammable liquids, such as gasoline and paint thinners, outside the house. They produce invisible explosive vapors.
- Install at least one smoke detector on each floor of your home and near the bedrooms. Replace the batteries annually or when they make a chirping sound.
- Plan an escape route from each room in the house. Have each family member rehearse the plan often. Designate a safe place to meet if you have to escape a fire in your home. This helps firefighters determine whether there are people in a burning building.

Source of statistics for injury prevention: American Academy of Pediatrics; Bicycle Safety Helmet Institute; Centers for Disease Control and Prevention, National Center for Injury Prevention and Control; Department of Transportation, National Highway Traffic Safety Administration; and the U.S. Fire Administration.

Emergency Care

When to Call for Help

Know the emergency number in your area; in most areas that number is 9-1-1. Calling for help in a medical emergency is important and may save a person's life. When a serious situation occurs, call for emergency medical help first. Do not call your doctor, the hospital, a friend, relatives, or neighbors. Calling anyone else first only wastes time.

Call for emergency help in the following situations:

- Fainting
- Chest or abdominal pain or pressure
- Sudden dizziness, weakness, or change in vision
- Difficulty breathing, shortness of breath
- Severe or persistent vomiting
- Sudden, severe pain anywhere in the body
- Suicidal or homicidal feelings
- Bleeding that does not stop after 10 to 15 minutes of pressure
- A gaping wound with edges that do not come together
- Problems with movement or sensation following an injury
- Cuts on the hand or face
- Puncture wounds
- The possibility that foreign bodies such as glass or metal may have entered a wound
- Most animal bites and all human bites
- Hallucinations and clouding of thoughts
- A stiff neck in association with a fever or a headache
- A bulging or abnormally depressed fontanel (soft spot) in infants
- Stupor or dazed behavior accompanying a high fever that is not alleviated by acetaminophen or aspirin

- Unequal pupil size, loss of consciousness, blindness, staggering, or repeated vomiting after a head injury
- Spinal injuries
- Severe burns
- Poisoning
- Drug overdose
- When in doubt, CALL.

Good Samaritan Laws

States have enacted laws to protect physicians and other medical personnel from legal actions that may arise from emergency treatment they give while not on duty. Although Good Samaritan laws cover medical personnel primarily, several states have expanded them to include laypersons who, in good faith, help others in emergency situations. Unless a person acts in a reckless or wantonly negligent manner when trying to voluntarily assist another, he or she is usually immune from conviction in a legal action. These laws vary from state to state; find out about your state's Good Samaritan laws by contacting a legal professional or checking with your local library.

Heart Attack

For information on recognizing the signs of a possible heart attack and on how to respond, see Chapter 12.

Poisoning

For information on preventing poisonings and how to treat a person who has been poisoned, see Chapter 16, especially the section titled "Environmental Health in and Around the Home."

Bleeding

If a person is bleeding heavily from a wound, it is important to stop the bleeding as quickly as possible. First, take the following action, and then call for help or take the person to an emergency room.

- Protect yourself from disease by wearing medical exam gloves.
- Expose the wound by removing or cutting the clothing to see where the blood is coming from.
- Place a sterile gauze pad or a clean cloth (such as a washcloth or towel) over the entire wound and apply direct pressure with your fingers or the palm of your hand.
- If the bleeding is from an arm or leg, while still applying pressure, elevate the injured area above heart level to reduce blood flow.
- When the bleeding stops, wrap a roller gauze bandage tightly over the dressing to hold it in place and prevent further bleeding.

Breathing Emergencies

Signs of inadequate breathing include a rate of breathing significantly less than 12 times per minute (for adults), skin that is pale or bluish and cool, and nasal flaring, especially in children. Ask someone to call for emergency care, and then if the person is not breathing:

- Tilt the head back and lift the chin to open the airway.
- Pinch the victim's nose shut, take a deep breath, and make a tight seal around the victim's mouth with your mouth.
- Slowly blow air into the victim's mouth until you see the chest rise.
- Remove your mouth to allow the air to come out, and turn your head away as you take another breath.
- Repeat one more breath.
- Check the victim for signs of circulation (breathing, coughing, or movement). If the victim is not breathing and has signs of circulation:
    - Give one breath about every 4 to 5 seconds for an adult.
    - Recheck for signs of circulation about every minute.
    - Continue this process as long as the person has signs of circulation, until help arrives.

If the first breath does not go in, retilt the victim's head and try a second breath. If the second breath does not go in, use the procedure to aid a choking victim.

Choking

You can tell if a person is choking if he or she is unable to speak, breathe, or cough or breathes with a high-pitched wheezing. A choking victim may instinctively reach up and clutch his or her neck. To help, first tell someone to call for emergency care. Then, do the following:

- Stand behind the choking person.
- Wrap your arms around the victim's waist. (Do not allow your forearms to touch the ribs.)
- Make a fist with one hand and place the thumb side just above the victim's navel.
- Grasp your fist with your other hand.
- Press your fist into the victim's abdomen with quick inward and upward thrusts.
- Continue thrusts until the object is removed or the victim becomes unresponsive.

Each thrust should be a separate and distinct effort to dislodge the object.

Burns

If a person is burned by fire and his or her clothing is on fire, have the victim roll on the ground using the "stop, drop, and roll" method. You can also smother the flames with a blanket or douse the victim with water. Ask someone to call for emergency help. Then, do the following:

- Remove jewelry and hot or burned clothing immediately, but do not remove clothing stuck to the skin.
- Cool the burn. Use large amounts of cool water, not ice. Immerse the burn in cool water if possible.
- Apply a thin layer of antibiotic ointment and cover the burn with dry, sterile dressings or clean cloths.
- Wait for help or transport the person to the emergency room of the local hospital.

Heat-Related Emergencies

Everyone is susceptible to heat illness if environmental conditions overwhelm the body's temperature-regulating mechanisms. Such illnesses are progressive conditions and could become life threatening. Therefore, it is important to recognize heat-related illness early and treat it immediately.

Heat cramps are painful muscular spasms that happen suddenly, usually in the legs and abdomen. If someone has heat cramps, have him or her do the following:

- Rest in a cool place.
- Drink lightly salted cool water ($^1/_4$ tsp. salt per quart of water) or a commercial sports drink diluted to half strength.
- Lightly stretch and gently massage the cramped muscle.

Heat exhaustion is another heat-related emergency. It is characterized by heavy perspiration with normal or slightly above normal body temperatures and is caused by water or salt depletion or both. To help a person with heat exhaustion, have him or her do the following:

- Rest in a cool place.
- Drink lightly salted cool water ($^1/_4$ tsp. salt per quart of water) or a commercial sports drink diluted to half strength.
- Remove excess clothing.
- Lie down and raise the legs 8 to 12 inches, while keeping them straight.

Sponge the victim with cool water and fan him or her. If no improvement occurs within 30 minutes, seek medical attention.

In its advanced stages, heat exhaustion is called heatstroke and can cause death. It must be treated rapidly. Heatstroke is characterized by red, hot, dry skin and an altered mental state ranging from slight confusion and disorientation to coma. To treat heatstroke, send someone for emergency care and do the following:

- Have the person rest in a cool place.
- Remove clothing down to the victim's underwear.
- Keep the victim's head and shoulders slightly elevated.
- Cool the person by placing ice bags wrapped in wet towels on the wrists, ankles, groin, and neck, and in the armpits.
- Fan the person.

APPENDIX C

Dietary Reference Intakes for Certain Nutrients

Food and Nutrition Board, National Academy of Sciences—National Research Council Dietary Reference Intakes for Certain Nutrients* (Abridged)

Life Group Stage	Protein (g)	Vitamin A (mg RE)	Vitamin E (mg a-TE)	Vitamin D (mg)	Vitamin C (mg)	Thiamin (mg)	Niacin (mg)	Vitamin B_6 (mg)	Vitamin B_{12} (mg)	Folate (mg)	Iron (mg)	Calcium (mg)	Zinc (mg)	Selenium (mg)
Infants														
0–6 mo	9.1	400	4	10	40	0.2	2	0.1	0.4	65	0.27	200	2	15
7–12 mo	11.0	500	5	10	50	0.3	4	0.3	0.5	80	11	260	3	20
Children														
1–3 y	13	300	6	15	15	0.5	6	0.5	0.9	150	7	700	3	20
4–8 y	19	400	7	15	25	0.6	8	0.6	1.2	200	10	1,000	5	30
Males														
9–13 y	34	600	11	15	45	0.9	12	1.0	1.8	300	8	1,300	8	40
14–18 y	52	900	15	15	75	1.2	16	1.3	2.4	400	11	1,300	11	55
19–30 y	56	900	15	15	90	1.2	16	1.3	2.4	400	8	1,000	11	55
31–50 y	56	900	15	15	90	1.2	16	1.3	2.4	400	8	1,000	11	55
51–70 y	56	900	15	15	90	1.2	16	1.7	2.4	400	8	1,000	11	55
>70 y	56	900	15	20	90	1.2	16	1.7	2.4	400	8	1,200	11	55
Females														
9–13 y	34	600	11	15	45	0.9	12	1.0	1.8	300	8	1,300	8	40
14–18 y	46	700	15	15	65	1.0	14	1.2	2.4	400	15	1,300	9	55
19–30 y	46	700	15	15	75	1.1	14	1.3	2.4	400	18	1,000	8	55
31–50 y	46	700	15	15	75	1.1	14	1.3	2.4	400	18	1,000	8	55
51–70 y	46	700	15	15	75	1.1	14	1.5	2.4	400	8	1,200	8	55
>70 y	46	700	15	20	75	1.1	14	1.5	2.4	400	8	1,200	8	55
Pregnant														
19–50 y	71	770	15	15	85	1.4	18	1.9	2.6	600	27	1,000	11	60
Lactating														
19–50 y	71	1,300	19	15	120	1.4	17	2.0	2.8	500	9	1,000	12	70

*Daily intakes. For more information about the DRIs, go to http://ods.od.nih.gov/Health_Information/Dietary_Reference_Intakes.aspx.

Reproduced from Food and Nutrition Board, Institute of Medicine, National Academies. (2011). Dietary reference intakes (DRIs): Recommended Dietary Allowance and Adequate Intake Values, Vitamins and Elements. Available at http://www.iom.edu/Activities/Nutrition/SummaryDRIs/DRI-Tables.aspx

APPENDIX D

Food Intake Patterns Based on MyPlate Recommendations

The following table indicates suggested amounts of food to consume from the basic food groups, to meet recommended nutrient intakes at 12 different calorie levels. Nutrient and energy contributions from each group are calculated according to the nutrient-dense forms of foods in each group (e.g., lean meats and fat-free milk). This appendix also includes a sample seven day menu guide for a 2000 Calorie/day food pattern.

Daily Amount of Food from Each Group

Calorie Level[1]	1,000	1,200	1,400	1,600	1,800	2,000	2,200	2,400	2,600	2,800	3,000	3,200
Fruits[2]	1 cup	1 cup	1.5 cups	1.5 cups	1.5 cups	2 cups	2 cups	2 cups	2 cups	2.5 cups	2.5 cups	2.5 cups
Vegetables[3]	1 cup	1.5 cups	1.5 cups	2 cups	2.5 cups	2.5 cups	3 cups	3 cups	3.5 cups	3.5 cups	4 cups	4 cups
Grains[4]	3 oz-eq	4 oz-eq	5 oz-eq	5 oz-eq	6 oz-eq	6 oz-eq	7 oz-eq	8 oz-eq	9 oz-eq	10 oz-eq	10 oz-eq	10 oz-eq
Protein foods[5]	2 oz-eq	3 oz-eq	4 oz-eq	5 oz-eq	5 oz-eq	5.5 oz-eq	6oz-eq	6.5 oz-eq	6.5 oz-eq	7 oz-eq	7 oz-eq	7 oz-eq
Dairy[6]	2 cups	2 cups	2 cups	3 cups	3 cups	3 cups	3 cups	3 cups	3 cups	3 cups	3 cups	3 cups

[1]**Calorie Levels** are set across a wide range to accommodate the needs of different individuals. The table "Estimated Daily Calorie Needs" can be used to help assign individuals to the food intake pattern at a particular calorie level.

[2]**Fruit Group** includes all fresh, frozen, canned, and dried fruits, and may be whole, cut-up or pureed. Any 100% fruit juice created as a form of fruit. In general, 1 cup of fruit or 100% fruit juice, or 1/2 cup of dried fruit can be considered as 1 cup from the fruit group.

[3]**Vegetable Group** includes all fresh, frozen, canned, and dried vegetables and vegetable juices. In general, 1 cup of raw or cooked vegetables or vegetable juice, or 2 cups of raw leafy greens can be considered as 1 cup from the vegetable group.

[4]**Grains Group** includes all foods made from wheat, rice, oats, cornmeal, barley, such as bread, pasta, oatmeal, breakfast cereals, tortillas, and grits. In general, 1 slice of bread, 1 cup of ready-to-eat cereal, or 1/2 cup of cooked rice, pasta, or cooked cereal can be considered as 1 ounce equivalent from the grains group. At least half of all grains consumed should be whole grains.

[5]**Protein Foods Group** in general, 1 ounce of lean meat, poultry, or fish, 1 egg, 1 Tbsp. peanut butter, 1/4 cup cooked dry beans, or 1/2 ounce of nuts or seeds can be considered as 1 ounce equivalent from the meat and beans group.

[6]**Dairy Group** includes all fluid milk products and foods made from milk that retain their calcium content, such as yogurt and cheese. Foods made from milk that have little to no calcium, such as cream cheese, cream, and butter, are not part of the group. Most dairy group choices should be fat-free or low-fat. In general, 1 cup of milk or yogurt, 1 1/2 ounces of natural cheese, or 2 ounces of processed cheese can be considered as 1 cup from the dairy group.

Although MyPlate does not include an "oils" group, some fat is essential for good health. Oils include fats from many different plants and from fish that are liquid at room temperature, such as canola, corn, olive, soybean, and sunflower oil. Some foods are naturally high in oils, like nuts, olives, some fish, and avocados. Foods that are mainly oil include mayonnaise, certain salad dressings, and soft margarine.

Estimated Daily Calorie Needs

To determine which food intake pattern to use for an individual, the following chart gives an estimate of individual calorie needs. The calorie range for each age/sex group is based on physical activity level, from sedentary to active.

	Calorie Range		
Children	**Sedentary***	**Æ**	**Active†**
2–3 years	1,000	Æ	1,400
Females			
4–8 years	1,200	Æ	1,800
9–13	1,600	Æ	2,200
14–18	1,800	Æ	2,400
19–30	2,000	Æ	2,400
31–50	1,800	Æ	2,200
51+	1,600	Æ	2,200
Males			
4–8 years	1,400	Æ	2,000
9–13	1,800	Æ	2,600
14–18	2,200	Æ	3,200
19–30	2,400	Æ	3,000
31–50	2,200	Æ	3,000
51+	2,000	Æ	2,800

*Sedentary means a lifestyle that includes only the light physical activity associated with typical day-to-day life.

†Active means a lifestyle that includes physical activity equivalent to walking more than 3 miles per day at 3 to 4 miles per hour, in addition to the light physical activity associated with typical day-to-day life.

Sample Menus for a 2000 Calorie Food Pattern

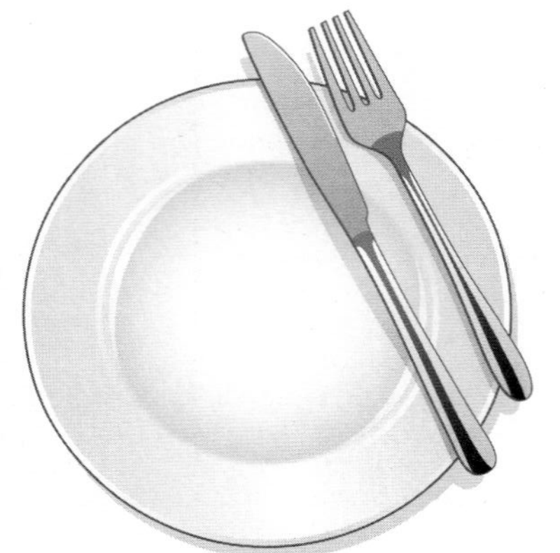

Use this 7-day menu as a motivational tool to help put a healthy eating pattern into practice, and to identify creative new ideas for healthy meals. Averaged over a week, this menu provides the recommended amounts of key nutrients and foods from each food group. The menus feature a large number of different foods to inspire ideas for adding variety to food choices. They are not intended to be followed day-by-day as a specific prescription for what to eat.

Spices and herbs can be used to taste. Try spices such as chili powder, cinnamon, cumin, curry powder, ginger, nutmeg, mustard, garlic powder, onion powder, or pepper. Try fresh or dried herbs such as basil, parsley, cilantro, chives, dill, mint, oregano, rosemary, thyme, or tarragon. Also try salt-free spice or herb blends.

While this 7-day menu provides the recommended amounts of foods and key nutrients, it does so at a moderate cost. Based on national average food costs, adjusted for inflation to March 2011 prices, the cost of this menu is less than the average amount spent for food, per person, in a 4-person family.

DAY 1	DAY 2	DAY 3
BREAKFAST Creamy oatmeal (cooked in milk): *½ cup uncooked oatmeal* *1 cup fat-free milk* *2 Tbsp raisins* *2 tsp brown sugar* Beverage: 1 cup orange juice **LUNCH** Taco salad: *2 ounces tortilla chips* *2 ounces cooked ground turkey* *2 tsp corn/canola oil (to cook turkey)* *¼ cup kidney beans** *½ ounce low-fat cheddar cheese* *½ cup chopped lettuce* *½ cup avocado* *1 tsp lime juice (on avocado)* *2 Tbsp salsa* Beverage: 1 cup water, coffee, or tea** **DINNER** Spinach lasagna roll-ups: *1 cup lasagna noodles(2 oz dry)* *½ cup cooked spinach* *½ cup ricotta cheese* *1 ounce part-skim mozzarella cheese* *½ cup tomato sauce** 1 ounce whole wheat roll *1 tsp tub margarine* Beverage: 1 cup fat-free milk **SNACKS** 2 Tbsp raisins 1 ounce unsalted almonds	**BREAKFAST** Breakfast burrito: *1 flour tortilla (8" diameter)* *1 scrambled egg* *⅓ cup black beans** *2 Tbsp salsa* ½ large grapefruit Beverage: 1 cup water, coffee, or tea** **LUNCH** Roast beef sandwich: *1 small whole grain hoagie bun* *2 ounces lean roast beef* *1 slice part-skim mozzarella cheese* *2 slices tomato* *¼ cup mushrooms* *1 tsp corn/canola oil (to cook mushrooms)* *1 tsp mustard* Baked potato wedges: *1 cup potato wedges* *1 tsp corn/canola oil (to cook potato)* *1 Tbsp ketchup* Beverage: 1 cup fat-free milk **DINNER** Baked salmon on beet greens: *4 ounce salmon filet* *1 tsp olive oil* *2 tsp lemon juice* *⅓ cup cooked beet greens (sauteed in 2 tsp corn/canola oil)* Quinoa with almonds: *½ cup quinoa* *½ ounce slivered almonds* Beverage: 1 cup fat-free milk **SNACKS** 1 cup cantaloupe balls	**BREAKFAST** Cold cereal: *1 cup ready-to-eat oat cereal* *1 medium banana* *½ cup fat-free milk* 1 slice whole wheat toast *1 tsp tub margarine* Beverage: 1 cup prune juice **LUNCH** Tuna salad sandwich: *2 slices rye bread* *2 ounces tuna* *1 Tbsp mayonnaise* *1 Tbsp chopped celery* *½ cup shredded lettuce* 1 medium peach Beverage: 1 cup fat-free milk **DINNER** Roasted chicken: *3 ounces cooked chicken breast* 1 large sweet potato, roasted ½ cup succotash (limas & corn) *1 tsp tub margarine* 1 ounce whole wheat roll *1 tsp tub margarine* Beverage: 1 cup water, coffee, or tea** **SNACKS** ¼ cup dried apricots 1 cup flavored yogurt (chocolate)

Sample Menus for a 2000 Calorie Food Pattern (Cont'd)

DAY 4	DAY 5	DAY 6	DAY 7
BREAKFAST 1 whole wheat English muffin *1 Tbsp all-fruit preserves* 1 hard-cooked egg Beverage: 1 cup water, coffee, or tea** **LUNCH** White bean-vegetable soup: *1 ¼ cup chunky vegetable soup with pasta* *½ cup white beans** 6 saltine crackers* ½ cup celery sticks Beverage: 1 cup fat-free milk **DINNER** Rigatoni with meat sauce: *1 cup rigatoni pasta (2 oz dry)* *2 ounces cooked ground beef (95% lean)* *2 tsp corn/canola oil (to cook beef)* *½ cup tomato sauce** *3 Tbsp grated parmesan cheese* Spinach salad: *1 cup raw spinach leaves* *½ cup tangerine sections* *½ ounce chopped walnuts* *4 tsp oil and vinegar dressing* Beverage: 1 cup water, coffee, or tea** **SNACKS** 1 cup nonfat fruit yogurt	**BREAKFAST** Cold cereal: *1 cup shredded wheat* *½ cup sliced banana* *½ cup fat-free milk* 1 slice whole wheat toast *2 tsp all-fruit preserves* Beverage: 1 cup fat-free chocolate milk **LUNCH** Turkey sandwich *1 whole wheat pita bread (2 oz)* *3 ounces roasted turkey, sliced* *2 slices tomato* *¼ cup shredded lettuce* *1 tsp mustard* *1 Tbsp mayonnaise* ½ cup grapes Beverage: 1 cup tomato juice* **DINNER** Steak and potatoes: *4 ounces broiled beef steak* *⅔ cup mashed potatoes made with milk and 2 tsp tub margarine* ½ cup cooked green beans *1 tsp tub margarine* *1 tsp honey* 1 ounce whole wheat roll *1 tsp tub margarine* Frozen yogurt and berries: *½ cup frozen yogurt (chocolate)* *¼ cup sliced strawberries* Beverage: 1 cup fat-free milk **SNACKS** 1 cup frozen yogurt (chocolate)	**BREAKFAST** French toast: *2 slices whole wheat bread* *3 Tbsp fat-free milk and ⅔ egg (in French toast)* *2 tsp tub margarine* *1 Tbsp pancake syrup* ½ large grapefruit Beverage: 1 cup fat-free milk **LUNCH** 3-bean vegetarian chili on baked potato: *¼ cup each cooked kidney beans,** *navy beans,** *and black beans** *½ cup tomato sauce** *¼ cup chopped onion* *2 Tbsp chopped jalapeno peppers* *1 tsp corn/canola oil (to cook onion and peppers)* *¼ cup cheese sauce* *1 large baked potato* ½ cup cantaloupe Beverage: 1 cup water, coffee, or tea** **DINNER** Hawaiian pizza *2 slices cheese pizza, thin crust* *1 ounce lean ham* *¼ cup pineapple* *¼ cup mushrooms* *1 tsp safflower oil (to cook mushrooms)* Green salad: *1 cup mixed salad greens* *4 tsp oil and vinegar dressing* Beverage: 1 cup fat-free milk **SNACKS** 3 Tbsp hummus 5 whole wheat crackers*	**BREAKFAST** Buckwheat pancakes with berries: *2 large (7") pancakes* *1 Tbsp pancake syrup* *¼ cup sliced strawberries* Beverage: 1 cup orange juice **LUNCH** New England clam chowder: *3 ounces canned clams* *½ small potato* *2 Tbsp chopped onion* *2 Tbsp chopped celery* *6 Tbsp evaporated milk* *¼ cup fat-free milk* *1 slice bacon* *1 Tbsp white flour* 10 whole wheat crackers* 1 medium orange Beverage: 1 cup fat-free milk **DINNER** Tofu-vegetable stir-fry: *4 ounces firm tofu* *½ cup chopped Chinese cabbage* *¼ cup sliced bamboo shoots* *2 Tbsp chopped sweet red peppers* *2 Tbsp chopped green peppers* *1 Tbsp corn/canola oil (to cook stir-fry)* 1 cup cooked brown rice (2 ounces raw) Honeydew yogurt cup: *¾ cup honeydew melon* *½ cup plain fat-free yogurt* Beverage: 1 cup water, coffee, or tea** **SNACKS** 1 large banana spread with 2 Tbsp peanut butter* 1 cup nonfat fruit yogurt

Notes:

*Foods that are reduced sodium, low sodium, or no-salt added products. These foods can also be prepared from scratch with no added salt. All other foods are regular commercial products, which contain variable levels of sodium. Average sodium level of the 7-day menu assumes that no salt is added in cooking or at the table.

**Unless indicated, all beverages are unsweetened and without added cream or whitener.

Italicized foods are part of the dish or food that precedes it.

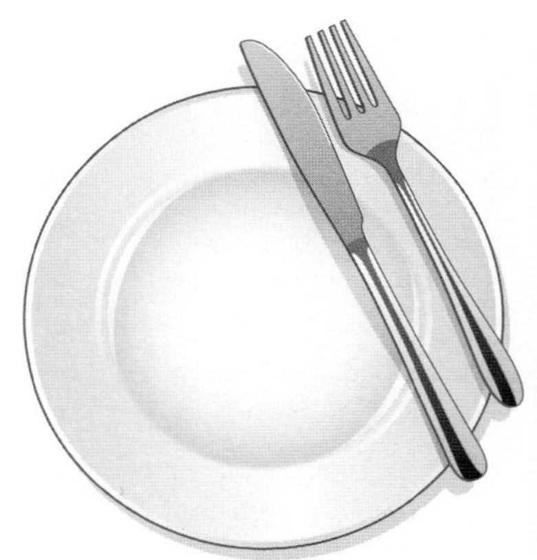

Average amounts for weekly menu:

Food group	Daily average over 1 week
GRAINS	6.2 oz eq
Whole grains	3.8
Refined grains	2.4
VEGETABLES	2.6 cups
Vegetable subgroups (amount per week)	
Dark green	1.6 cups per week
Red/Orange	5.6
Starchy	5.1
Beans and Peas	1.6
Other Vegetables	4.1
FRUITS	2.1 cups
DAIRY	3.1 cups
PROTEIN FOODS	5.7 oz eq
Seafood	8.8 oz per week
OILS	29 grams
CALORIES FROM ADDED FATS AND SUGARS	245 calories

Nutrient	Daily average over 1 week
Calories	1975
Protein	96 g
Protein	19% kcal
Carbohydrate	275 g
Carbohydrate	56% kcal
Total fat	59 g
Total fat	27% kcal
Saturated fat	13.2 g
Saturated fat	6.0% kcal
Monounsaturated fat	25 g
Polyunsaturated fat	16 g
Linoleic Acid	13 g
Alpha—linolenic Acid	1.8 g
Cholesterol	201 mg
Total dietary fiber	30 g
Potassium	4701 mg
Sodium	1810 mg
Calcium	1436 mg
Magnesium	468 mg
Copper	2.0 mg
Iron	18 mg
Phosphorus	1885 mg
Zinc	14 mg
Thiamin	1.6 mg
Riboflavin	2.5 mg
Niacin Equivalents	24 mg
Vitamin B6	2.4 mg
Vitamin B12	12.3 mcg
Vitamin C	146 mg
Vitamin E	11.8 mg (AT)
Vitamin D	9.1 mcg
Vitamin A	1090 mcg (RAE)
Dietary Folate Equivalents	530 mcg
Choline	386 mg

Student Workbook to Accompany

Alters & Schiff

Essential Concepts for Healthy Living

SEVENTH EDITION

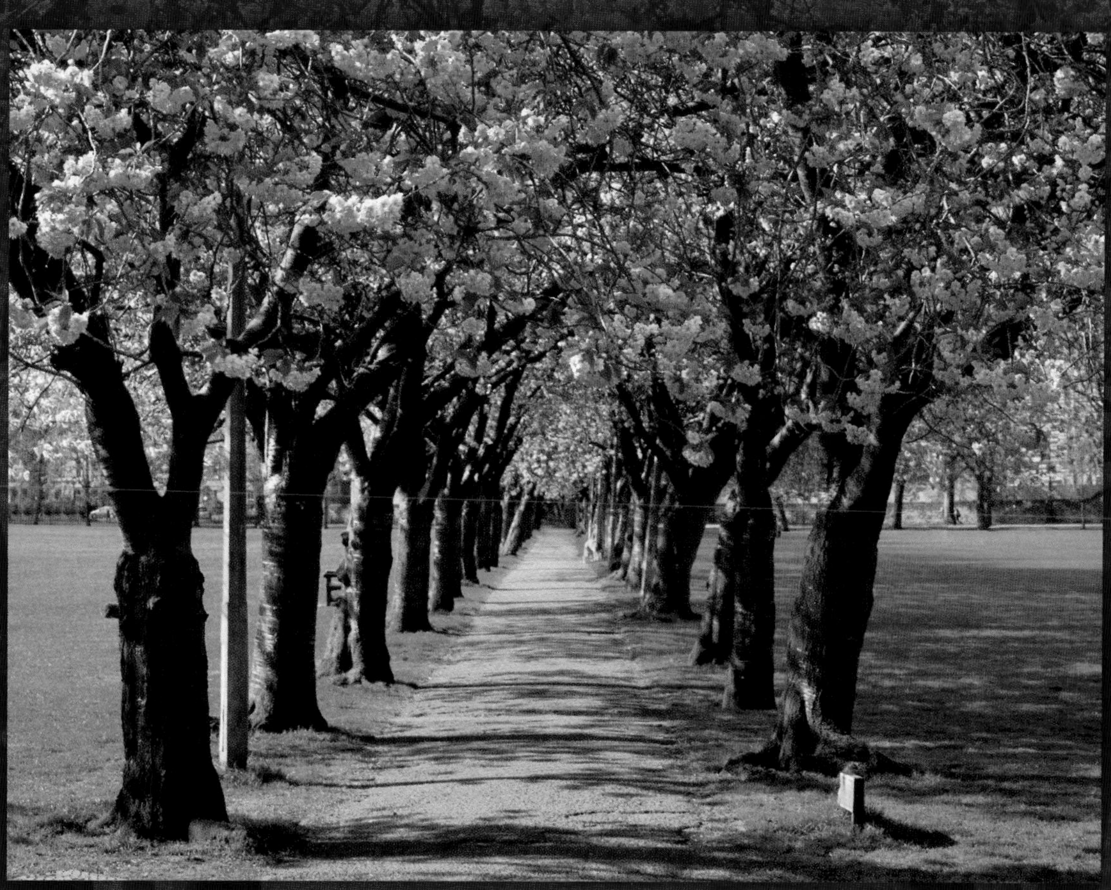

Jeff Housman

Mary Odum

CHAPTER 1

Student Workbook

SELF-ASSESSMENT 1

Healthstyle

This self-test, which is a modified version of one developed by the U.S. Public Health Service, assesses several health-related behaviors. Although these behaviors apply to most individuals, pregnant women, and people with chronic health concerns should follow the advice of their physicians. Answer each of the following questions by circling the number of the response that applies best to you. Add the number of points under each health-related behavior category to obtain a score for that category. Use the scoring guide at the end of the test to determine the level of risk you are incurring by your health-related behavior.

Tobacco, Alcohol, and Other Drugs

If you have never used tobacco products, enter a score of 10 for this section, and skip questions 1 and 2.

	Almost Always	Sometimes	Almost Never
1. I avoid using tobacco products.	2	1	0
2. I smoke only low-tar cigarettes.	2	1	0
		Smoking Score: ______	
3. I avoid drinking alcoholic beverages, or I drink no more than one or two drinks a day.	2	1	0
4. I avoid using alcohol or other drugs (especially illegal drugs) as a way of handling stressful situations or problems in my life.	2	1	0
5. I avoid driving while under the influence of alcohol and other drugs.	2	1	0
6. I am careful not to drink alcohol when taking certain pain medications or when pregnant.	2	1	0
7. I read and follow the label directions when using prescribed and over-the-counter drugs.	2	1	0
		Alcohol and Other Drugs Score: ______	

Eating Habits

	Almost Always	Sometimes	Almost Never
8. I eat a variety of foods each day, including fruits and vegetables, whole-grain products, lean meats, low-fat dairy products, seeds, nuts, and dry beans.	3	1	0
9. I limit the amount of animal fat in my food, which includes cream, butter, cheese, and fatty meats.	3	1	0
10. I limit the amount of salt that I eat, by avoiding salty foods and not using salt at the table.	2	1	0
11. I avoid eating too much sugar, by eating few sweet snacks and sugary soft drinks.	2	1	0
			Eating Habits Score: ______

Exercise/Fitness

	Almost Always	Sometimes	Almost Never
12. I maintain a body weight that is reasonable for my height.	3	1	0
13. I do vigorous exercise (for example, running, swimming, or brisk walking) for at least 30 minutes at least three times a week.	3	1	0
14. I do exercises to enhance my muscle tone and flexibility (for example, yoga or calisthenics) for 15 to 30 minutes at least three times a week.	2	1	0
15. I use part of my leisure time participating in individual, family, or team activities that increase my level of physical fitness (for example, gardening, bowling, or golf).	2	1	0
			Exercise/Fitness Score: ______

Stress Management

	Almost Always	Sometimes	Almost Never
16. I take time every day to relax.	2	1	0
17. I find it easy to express my feelings without harming others.	2	1	0
18. I recognize and prepare for events or situations that are likely to be stressful.	2	1	0
19. I have close friends, relatives, or others to whom I can talk about personal matters and contact for help when needed.	2	1	0
20. I participate in hobbies that I enjoy or group activities such as religious or community organizations.	2	1	0
			Stress Management Score: ______

Safety

	Almost Always	Sometimes	Almost Never
21. I wear a seat belt while riding in a motor vehicle.	2	1	0
22. I obey traffic rules and speed limits while driving.	2	1	0
23. I have a working smoke detector in my home.	2	1	0
24. I am careful when using potentially harmful products or substances, such as household cleaners, poisons, and electrical devices.	2	1	0
25. I avoid smoking in bed.	2	1	0
			Safety Score: ______

Student Workbook

What Your Scores Mean

Scores of 9 or 10 for each section: Excellent! Your responses show that you are aware of the importance of this area to your health, and that you are practicing good health-related habits. As long as you continue to do so, this area of health should not pose a risk.

Scores of 6 to 8 for each section: Your health practices in this area are good, but there is room for improvement. Look at the items that you answered with "Sometimes" or "Almost Never." What lifestyle changes can you make to improve your score and reduce your risk?

Scores of 3 to 5 for each section: Your health-related behaviors are risky. What lifestyle changes can you make to improve your score in this area of health and reduce your risk?

Scores of 0 to 2 for each section: You may be taking serious and unnecessary risks with your health and, possibly, the health of others. What lifestyle changes can you make to improve your score and reduce your risk?

Adapted from *Healthstyle: A Self-Test*, U.S. Department of Health and Human Services Public Health Service, DHHS Publication Number (PHS) 81-50155.

CHAPTER 1

SELF ASSESSMENT 2

Personal Health History

Being aware of your family's health history, especially which relatives had or have serious chronic diseases or inherited conditions, can help you and your physician assess your risk of such diseases or conditions. As a result of having this information, you can make choices concerning your lifestyle now that may reduce the likelihood of developing these health problems in the future.

To compile your personal health history and design a health history diagram, start with your own health and that of your brothers and sisters. Then indicate health conditions that affect your mother and father and their brothers and sisters. After completing health information for that generation, collect information about your grandparents' health. You may be aware of some family members' health problems, such as heart disease, obesity, drug addiction, or mental health conditions. In other instances, however, you will need to speak with your relatives to determine whether they have or had diseases or conditions such as prostate or breast cancer, diabetes, hypertension, liver disease, and so on. If you are adopted or cannot find information about individual family members, you may have to leave blanks.

A sample family health history diagram is shown in this assessment. Note that it has spaces for a person to fill in his or her personal health and the health of siblings, parents, aunts, uncles, and grandparents. Of course, your diagram will reflect your family's makeup. After developing your personal health history diagram, answer the following questions.

1. If a particular disease or condition occurs repeatedly in your family, it may be the result of inherited and/or lifestyle factors that are common within your family. Such repeated occurrences may indicate that your risk of the disease or condition is greater than average. Which serious health problems occur more than once in your family health history?

   ____

   ____

   ____

2. Which diseases or conditions in your family history do you think are related to lifestyle practices, such as food choices, lack of regular physical activity, or smoking?

   ____

   ____

   ____

3. Are you aware of actions you can take that may reduce your risk of developing the health problems that often affect or have affected members of your family? If so, list those actions.

____

____

____

4. The course of many diseases and conditions is influenced by lifestyle factors. Your physician can help you determine such factors. Therefore, consider discussing your family health history with your physician. Your physician can also provide advice concerning steps you can take to reduce your risk of developing the health problems that affect or have affected members of your family.

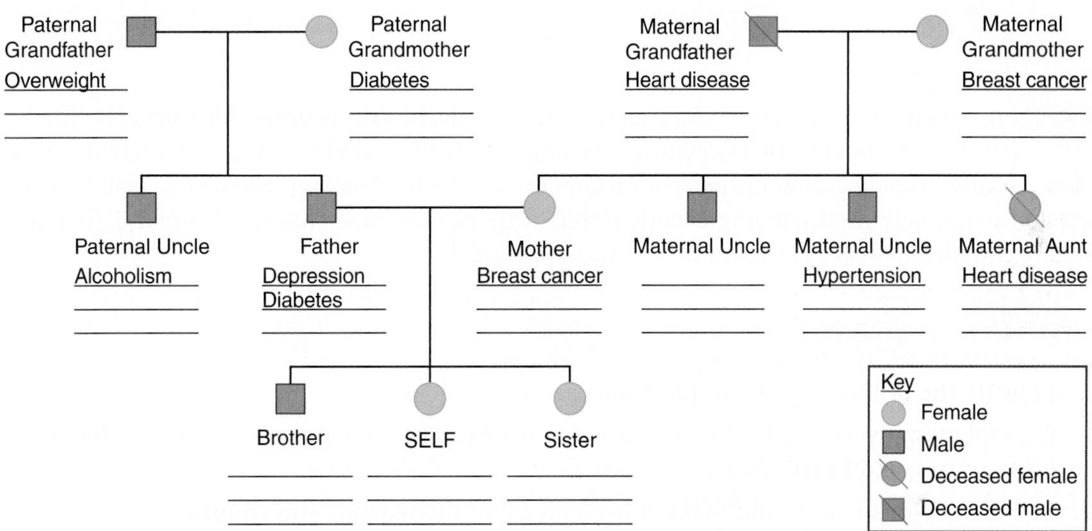

CHAPTER 1

CHANGING HEALTH HABITS

Model Activity for Better Health

This critical thinking feature describes a useful model of a decision-making process. The first part of the model involves deciding to change a health-related behavior; the second part describes implementing the behavioral change. To practice making responsible health-related decisions, complete the Changing Health Habits activities for each chapter. Chapter 1 (below) is already completed as an example of how to use this model.

Deciding to Change

1. **Identify the problem, goal, or question.**

   Example: I'm overweight. I know that being overweight increases my risk for diabetes, certain cancers, and heart disease.

2. **List the reasons you should make this change and the reasons you should not.** Assign each reason a point value from 1 to 5, with 5 being the highest (it has the most value to you) and 1 being the lowest (it has the least value to you).

Choices

Reasons to lose weight (pros):		Reasons not to lose weight (cons):	
Points	***Reasons***	***Points***	***Reasons***
3	Losing weight will reduce my risk of diabetes, certain cancers, and heart disease.	2	I'll have to spend money on new clothes.
5	Losing weight will improve the way my clothes fit.	2	I'll have to spend money to join a health club or weight loss group.
4	Losing weight will help me feel better about myself.	4	I'll have trouble keeping the weight off.
5	Losing weight will reduce my flab.	5	I can continue eating fatty and sugary foods
17	Total	13	Total

3. **Draw a conclusion.** Add the scores in each category. If the score of the positive reasons (pros) is greater than the score of the negative reasons (cons), you likely think that a change is in your best interest. Also, you are probably motivated to make the change and are likely to succeed. However, if your cons outweigh your pros, you likely think that changing is not in your best interest at this time. You may not be motivated to make the change now. Study your list of pros

and cons carefully, however, before making your final decision. You may decide to change even if your reasons not to change outrank your reasons to change.

Implementing the Change

1. **Set a target date to begin the new behavior or reach the goal.** Depending on the type of decision, a behavior change could involve setting a beginning date and a goal date. For example, you could decide to lose 10 pounds by May 31st, then begin changing your eating and physical activity patterns tomorrow.
2. **Identify and list the factors that will help you reach your goal and those that will stand in the way of reaching your goal.**

   Factors that help

   My roommate has also decided to lose weight.

   I just got a check for my birthday to buy a new outfit when I lose 10 pounds.

   My student fees include the use of the health facility.

   Factors that hinder

   My mother insists that I eat a lot of food when I visit.

   My roommate keeps lots of high-calorie snacks in the house.

   I'm so busy that finding a time to exercise is difficult.
3. **Prepare an action plan for making the change.** An action plan specifies how you will change your behavior to meet your goal.
   a. **Identify alternative methods for reaching your goal.**

      Example

      Alternative 1: Consume a 1,200-calorie diet that consists of eating only one meal a day and drinking a diet supplement for breakfast and lunch.

      Alternative 2: Consume a 1,200-calorie diet that permits three nutritious meals daily.

      Alternative 3: Consume a 1,200-calorie diet and increase exercise by 30 minutes a day.

      Alternative 4: Go to a weight loss clinic for help.

   b. **Gather information about each method.** Seek information that supports and criticizes each method. (People tend to gather data that only support what they think they want to do.) Ask yourself questions to guide your information gathering.

      Example: How long do people who reduce their caloric intake without exercising keep the weight off? By which method am I more likely to lose weight fastest? Is it better for my health to lose weight as quickly as possible, or does the length of time not matter? What changes will I have to make in my life if I decide to eat more nutritious foods and exercise? Are diet supplement drinks safe? Where can I find information about the caloric content of foods?

   c. **Choose the method that fits your situation best.**

      Example: After researching alternative methods, you decide to follow a 1,200-calorie-per-day, diet and increase the amount of exercise you engage in each day.

   d. **Consider the factors that can help or hinder your effort to change (see step 2).** What can you do that will take advantage of the helps and minimize the hindrances? For example, keep plenty of low-calorie snacks on hand to avoid being tempted by your roommate's supply of high-calorie munchies. Also, discuss the situation with your roommate to enlist his or her support in your effort.

4. **Change the lifestyle behavior that you have decided to improve by implementing the action plan you developed in step 3.**
5. **Chart your daily progress toward your goal.** Track your progress on a regular basis. Recording your weight once a week, for example, may be helpful. Are you losing weight?
6. **Evaluate how effective you were in reaching your goal.** Did your plan work? What can you learn from the experience?

   Example: You lost 5 pounds instead of 10 pounds. What seemed to keep you from reaching your goal? What can you do differently that might help you succeed? Do you need more time to lose weight, or do you need to reevaluate your decision?

CHAPTER 2

SELF-ASSESSMENT

The Self-Esteem Inventory

If the following statement describes how you usually feel, put a check in the column "Like Me." If the statement does not describe how you usually feel, put a check in the column "Unlike Me." There are no right or wrong answers. Read each statement quickly and answer the questions "off the top of your head."

Statement	Like Me	Unlike Me
1. I spend a lot of time daydreaming.	____	____
2. I'm pretty sure of myself.	____	____
3. I often wish I were someone else.	____	____
4. I'm easy to like.	____	____
5. My family and I have a lot of fun together.	____	____
6. I never worry about anything.	____	____
7. I find it very hard to talk in front of a group.	____	____
8. I wish I were younger.	____	____
9. There are lots of things about myself I'd change if I could.	____	____
10. I can make up my mind without too much trouble.	____	____
11. I'm a lot of fun to be with.	____	____
12. I get upset easily at home.	____	____
13. I always do the right thing.	____	____
14. I'm proud of my work.	____	____
15. Someone always has to tell me what to do.	____	____
16. It takes me a long time to get used to anything new.	____	____
17. I'm often sorry for the things I do.	____	____
18. I'm popular with people my own age.	____	____
19. My family usually considers my feelings.	____	____
20. I'm never unhappy.	____	____
21. I'm doing the best work that I can.	____	____
22. I give in very easily.	____	____
23. I can usually take care of myself.	____	____
24. I'm pretty happy.	____	____

Statement	Like Me	Unlike Me
25. I would rather associate with people younger than me.	_____	_____
26. My family expects too much of me.	_____	_____
27. I like everyone I know.	_____	_____
28. I like to be called on when I am in a group.	_____	_____
29. I understand myself.	_____	_____
30. It's pretty tough to be me.	_____	_____
31. Things are all mixed up in my life.	_____	_____
32. People usually follow my ideas.	_____	_____
33. No one pays much attention to me at home.	_____	_____
34. I never get scolded.	_____	_____
35. I'm not doing as well at work as I'd like to.	_____	_____
36. I can make up my mind and stick to it.	_____	_____
37. I really don't like being a man/woman.	_____	_____
38. I have a low opinion of myself.	_____	_____
39. I don't like to be with other people.	_____	_____
40. There are times when I'd like to leave home.	_____	_____
41. I'm never shy.	_____	_____
42. I often feel upset.	_____	_____
43. I often feel ashamed of myself.	_____	_____
44. I'm not as nice-looking as most people.	_____	_____
45. If I have something to say, I usually say it.	_____	_____
46. People pick on me very often.	_____	_____
47. My family understands me.	_____	_____
48. I always tell the truth.	_____	_____
49. My employer or supervisor makes me feel I'm not good enough.	_____	_____
50. I don't care what happens to me.	_____	_____
51. I'm a failure.	_____	_____
52. I get upset easily when I am scolded.	_____	_____
53. Most people are better liked than I am.	_____	_____
54. I usually feel as if my family is pushing me.	_____	_____
55. I always know what to say to people.	_____	_____
56. I often get discouraged.	_____	_____
57. Things usually don't bother me.	_____	_____
58. I can't be depended on.	_____	_____

Reproduced with permission from Ryden, Muriel B. (1978). An adult version of the Coopersmith Self-Esteem Inventory: Test-retest reliability and social desirability. *Psychological Reports, 43*:1189–1190.

Scoring the Self-Esteem Inventory

To determine your score, count the number of times your responses agree with the keyed responses below.

2. Like	22. Unlike	42. Unlike
3. Unlike	23. Like	43. Unlike
4. Like	24. Like	44. Unlike
5. Like	25. Unlike	45. Like
7. Unlike	26. Unlike	46. Unlike
8. Unlike	28. Like	47. Like
9. Unlike	29. Like	49. Unlike
10. Like	30. Unlike	50. Unlike
11. Like	31. Unlike	51. Unlike
12. Unlike	32. Like	52. Unlike
14. Like	33. Unlike	53. Unlike
15. Unlike	35. Unlike	54. Unlike
16. Unlike	36. Like	55. Like
17. Unlike	37. Unlike	56. Unlike
18. Like	38. Unlike	57. Like
19. Like	39. Unlike	58. Unlike
21. Like	40. Unlike	

The majority of the items measure self-esteem, but the eight items below that fall into the "Lie Scale" identify people who are trying to conceal their feelings about themselves. Count the number of times your responses to the questions listed agree with the responses shown below. If three or more responses agree, you may be trying to conceal feelings of low self-esteem.

1. Like	27. Like
6. Like	34. Like
13. Like	41. Like
20. Like	48. Like

How do you compare with other men and women taking this self-assessment? The average man obtains a score of 40; an average woman obtains a score of 39. Scores below 33 for men and 32 for women may indicate low self-esteem.

CHAPTER 2

CHANGING HEALTH HABITS

Are You Ready to Improve Your Psychological Health?

Do you need to change a behavior that relates to or affects your psychological health? For example, do you blame others for problems for which you should take responsibility? Do you eat too much fattening food or drink too much alcohol as a way of dealing with your problems? The "Deciding to Change" section of the worksheet can help you determine whether you are ready to alter your behavior to improve your psychological health. Use the "Implementing the Change" section of the worksheet if you decide to make the necessary changes.

Deciding to Change

1. Identify the problem, goal, or question.

   ____

   ____

2. List the reasons you should make this change and the reasons you should not. Assign each reason a point value from 1 to 5, with 5 being the highest (it has the most value to you) and 1 being the lowest (it has the least value to you).

Choices

Reasons to change thoughts or behaviors (pros):

Points	Reasons
____	______________
____	______________
____	______________
____ Total	

Reasons not to change thoughts or behaviors (cons):

Points	Reasons
____	______________
____	______________
____	______________
____ Total	

3. Draw a conclusion by adding the points in the pros section and then in the cons section. If the point total of the pros section is greater than the total of the cons section, you are probably ready to make a change that concerns your psychological health. If your cons outweigh your pros, you may not be motivated to make the change now. Study your list of pros and cons carefully, however, before making your final decision. You may decide to change even if your reasons not to change outrank your reasons to change.

Implementing the Change

1. Set a target date to begin the new behavior or reach the goal.

   ____

2. Identify and list the factors that will help you reach your goal and those that will stand in the way of reaching your goal.

   Factors that help: ______________________________

   ____

   ____

   ____

   Factors that hinder: ______________________________

   ____

   ____

   ____

3. Prepare an action plan for making the change.
   a. Identify alternative methods for reaching your goal.

   ____

   ____

   ____

   b. Gather information about each method.
   c. Choose the method that fits your situation best.
   d. Consider the factors that can help or hinder your effort to change (see step 2).

   Factors that help: ______________________________

   ____

   ____

   ____

   Factors that hinder: ______________________________

   ____

   ____

   ____

4. Change the lifestyle behavior that you have decided to improve by implementing the action plan that you developed in step 3.
5. Chart your daily progress toward your goal.
6. Evaluate how effective you were in reaching your goal.

   ____

   ____

   ____

   ____

   ____

   ____

CHAPTER 2

Student Workbook

SELF-ASSESSMENT 1

How Much Stress Have You Had Lately?

To estimate the amount of stress that you have endured recently, indicate the number of occasions (to a maximum of four) that you have experienced the following in the past year.

Event	Number of Occasions	Points	Total
1. Death of a spouse	___	87	___
2. Marriage	___	77	___
3. Death of a close relative	___	77	___
4. Divorce	___	76	___
5. Marital separation	___	74	___
6. Pregnancy, or fathered a pregnancy	___	64	___
7. Death of a close friend	___	68	___
8. Personal injury or illness	___	65	___
9. Loss of your job	___	62	___
10. Breakup of a marital engagement or a steady relationship	___	60	___
11. Sexual difficulties	___	58	___
12. Marital reconciliation	___	58	___
13. Major change in self-concept	___	57	___
14. Major change in health or behavior of a family member	___	56	___
15. Engagement to be married	___	54	___
16. Major change in financial status	___	53	___
17. Major change in the use of drugs (other than alcohol)	___	52	___
18. Mortgage or loan of less than $10,000	___	52	___
19. Entered college	___	50	___
20. A new family member	___	50	___
21. A conflict or change in values	___	50	___
22. Change to a different line of work	___	50	___
23. A major change in the number of arguments with spouse	___	50	___
24. Change to a new school		50	___

Event	Number of Occasions	Points	Total
25. A major change in amount of independence and responsibility	____	49	____
26. A major change in responsibilities at work	____	47	____
27. A major change in the use of alcohol	____	46	____
28. Revised personal habits	____	45	____
29. Being in trouble with school administration	____	44	____
30. A major change in social activities	____	43	____
31. Holding a job while attending school	____	43	____
32. Change of residence or living conditions	____	42	____
33. A major change in working hours or conditions	____	42	____
34. Trouble with in-laws	____	42	____
35. Your spouse beginning or stopping work outside the home	____	41	____
36. Change in dating habits	____	41	____
37. A change involving your major field of study	____	41	____
38. An outstanding personal achievement	____	40	____
39. Trouble with your boss	____	38	____
40. A major change in amount of participation in school activities	____	38	____
41. A major change in type and/or amount of recreation	____	37	____
42. A major change in religious activities	____	36	____
43. A major change in sleeping habits	____	34	____
44. A trip or vacation	____	33	____
45. A major change in eating habits	____	30	____
46. A major change in number of family get-togethers	____	26	____
47. Found guilty of minor violations of the law	____	22	____

Multiply the number of occasions times the point value for each event. Add the scores.

TOTAL POINTS ________

Your degree of stress is low if your score is lower than 347. If your score is higher than 1,435, you are under a high degree of stress.

Reproduced from Marx MB, Garrity TF, Bowers FR."The influence of recent life experiences on the health of college students." Reprinted from *Journal of Psychosomatic Research*, 19(1):87–98 with permission from Elsevier.

CHAPTER 2

SELF-ASSESSMENT 2

K6 Serious Psychological Distress Assessment

Answer the following questions by checking the statement that best applies.

During the past 30 days, how often did you feel?	All of the time 4	Most of the time 3	Some of the time 2	A little of the time 1	None of the time 0
So sad that nothing could cheer you up?					
Nervous?					
Restless or fidgety?					
Hopeless?					
That everything was an effort?					
Worthless?					
Total					

Scoring: To score the K6, add the points for each of the questions together. Scores can range from 0 to 24. A threshold of 13 or more points indicates a high degree of distress and possibility of serious mental illness.

National Center for Health Statistics (reviewed 2007). Serious psychological distress.

CHAPTER 3

CHANGING HEALTH HABITS

Taking Steps to Reduce Your Stress

Follow the steps of the decision-making and implementation model to identify and change a health-related habit that contributes to your level of stress. For example, do you work too many hours per week? Are you in a relationship that causes you continual stress? Are you trying to take care of your home and family with no help while going to school and working part-time?

Deciding to Change

1. Identify the problem, goal, or question.

   ____

   ____

2. List the reasons you should make this change and the reasons you should not. Assign each reason a point value from 1 to 5, with 5 being the highest (it has the most value to you) and 1 being the lowest (it has the least value to you).

Choices

Reasons to change behaviors (pros):

Points	***Reasons***
____	______________________
____	______________________
____	______________________
____	Total

Reasons not to change behaviors (cons):

Points	***Reasons***
____	______________________
____	______________________
____	______________________
____	Total

3. Draw a conclusion by adding the points in the pros section and then in the cons section. If the point total of the pros section is greater than the total of the cons section, you are probably ready to make a change in your life that reduces stress. If your cons outweigh your pros, you may not be motivated to make the change now. Study your list of pros and cons carefully, however, before making your final decision. You may decide to change even if your reasons not to change outrank your reasons to change.

Implementing the Change

1. Set a target date to begin the new behavior or reach the goal.

2. Identify and list the factors that will help you reach your goal and those that will stand in the way of reaching your goal.

   Factors that help:

   Factors that hinder:

3. Prepare an action plan for making the change.
   a. Identify alternative methods for reaching your goal.

   b. Gather information about each method.
   c. Choose the method that fits your particular situation best.
   d. Consider the factors that can help or hinder your effort to change (see step 2).

   Factors that help:

   Factors that hinder:

4. Change the lifestyle behavior that you have decided to improve by implementing the action plan you developed in step 3.
5. Chart your daily progress toward your goal.
6. Evaluate how effective you were in reaching your goal.

Student Workbook

CHAPTER 4

SELF-ASSESSMENT

Am I in an Abusive Intimate Relationship?

Read the following statements and indicate whether you agree or disagree with them. Draw a circle around your answer. Your responses can help you assess whether you are in an abusive intimate relationship.

1. My partner often embarrasses me in front of others.	Yes	No
2. My partner often criticizes my appearance, belittles my accomplishments, or makes fun of my ideas.	Yes	No
3. My partner frequently uses threats to make me to do what he/she wants.	Yes	No
4. My partner has told me that I'm worthless without him/her.	Yes	No
5. When my partner physically hurts me, he/she apologizes or says, "It was an accident," or "I didn't mean to hurt you."	Yes	No
6. My partner frequently has trouble controlling his/her anger.	Yes	No
7. My partner often makes me feel guilty when I want to spend time away from him/her.	Yes	No
8. My partner mistreats me when he/she gets drunk or high on drugs.	Yes	No
9. My partner usually blames me for his/her problems.	Yes	No
10. My partner pressures me for sex when I don't want it.	Yes	No
11. I often think about breaking up with my partner, but I don't because I'm afraid of what he/she might do to me or to himself/herself.	Yes	No
12. My friends and family members have told me that my partner is abusing me.	Yes	No
13. When I'm with others, I usually make excuses for my partner's abusive behavior.	Yes	No
14. I often sacrifice what I would like to do because I'm afraid of how my partner will respond if I don't follow his/her plans.	Yes	No
15. I often avoid saying or doing things that might anger my partner because I'm afraid that he/she will hurt me.	Yes	No

If you agreed with any of these statements, you may be in an abusive relationship. If you're not sure that your partner is abusive, seek counseling from a licensed professional therapist. If you are afraid of your partner, get help immediately. Contact your campus counseling center or a local domestic violence intervention center listed in your "Yellow Pages" phone book. The phone number for the National Domestic Violence Hotline is 1-800-799-7233.

CHAPTER 4

CHANGING HEALTH HABITS

Can You Reduce Your Risk of Violence?

Follow the steps of the decision-making and implementation model to identify and change a health-related habit that contributes to your risk of violence. For example, do you ignore basic security measures? Are you involved in an abusive relationship that you feel hopeless about improving or terminating? Does your work, family, and college schedule force you to be exposed to risky situations and places?

Deciding to Change

1. Identify the problem, goal, or question.

   ____

   ____

2. List the reasons you should make this change and the reasons you should not. Assign each reason a point value from 1 to 5, with 5 being the highest (it has the most value to you) and 1 being the lowest (it has the least value to you).

Choices

Reasons to change behaviors (pros):

Points	***Reasons***
____	____________________
____	____________________
____	____________________
____	Total

Reasons not to change behaviors (cons):

Points	***Reasons***
____	____________________
____	____________________
____	____________________
____	Total

3. Draw a conclusion by adding the points in the pros section and then in the cons section. If the point total of the pros section is greater than the total of the cons section, you are probably ready to make a change in your life that reduces your risk of violence. If your cons outweigh your pros, you may not be motivated to make the change now. Study your list of pros and cons carefully, however, before making your final decision. You may decide to change even if your reasons not to change outrank your reasons to change.

Implementing the Change

1. Set a target date to begin the new behavior or reach the goal.

2. Identify and list the factors that will help you reach your goal and those that will stand in the way of reaching your goal.

   Factors that help:

   Factors that hinder:

3. Prepare an action plan for making the change.

   a. Identify alternative methods for reaching your goal.

   b. Gather information about each method.

   c. Choose the method that fits your particular situation best.

   d. Consider the factors that can help or hinder your effort to change (see step 2).

   Factors that help:

   Factors that hinder:

4. Change the lifestyle behavior that you have decided to improve by implementing the action plan you developed in step 3.
5. Chart your daily progress toward your goal.
6. Evaluate how effective you were in reaching your goal.

CHAPTER 5

SELF-ASSESSMENT 1

Contraceptive Comfort and Confidence Scale

The following series of questions, which are adapted from the Contraceptive Comfort and Confidence Scale, is designed to help you assess whether the method of contraception that you are using or may be considering for future use is or will be effective for you.

With regard to the method of birth control you are currently using or are considering using, answer YES or NO to the following questions:

1. Have you had problems using this method before?
2. Are you afraid of using this method?
3. Would you really rather not use this method?
4. Will you have trouble remembering to use this method?
5. Have you ever become pregnant using this method? (Or, has your partner ever become pregnant using this method?)
6. Will you have trouble using this method correctly?
7. Do you still have unanswered questions about this method?
8. Does this method make menstrual periods longer or more painful?
9. Does this method cost more than you can afford?
10. Could this method cause you or your partner to have serious complications?
11. Are you opposed to this method because of religious beliefs?
12. Is your partner opposed to this method?
13. Are you using this method without your partner's knowledge?
14. Will using this method embarrass your partner?
15. Will using this method embarrass you?
16. Will you enjoy intercourse less because of this method?
17. Will your partner enjoy intercourse less because of this method?
18. If this method interrupts lovemaking, will you avoid using it?
19. Has a nurse or doctor ever told you (or your partner) not to use this method?
20. Is there anything about your personality that could lead you to use this method incorrectly?

21. Does this method leave you at risk of being exposed to HIV or other sexually transmissible infections?

Total number of YES answers: ____

Interpreting Your Score

Most individuals will have a few "yes" answers. Yes answers predict potential problems. If you have more than a few yes responses, you may want to talk to your physician, counselor, partner, or a friend. Talking it over can help you decide whether to use this method or how to use it so it will be effective. In general, the more yes answers you have, the less likely you are to use this method consistently and correctly.

In choosing a method of contraception, keep in mind that if you want a highly effective method of contraception and a method that is highly effective in preventing transmission of STIs, you may have to use two methods. Hence, any method of contraception (except abstinence, of course) should be combined with condom use for maximum protection against STIs.

Adapted from Hatcher, R. A., Stewart, F., Trussell, J., Kowal, D., Guest, F., Stewart, G. K., & Cates, W. (1990). *Contraceptive technology: 1990–1992* (15th ed., rev.) (p. 150). New York: Irvington.

CHAPTER 5

Student Workbook

SELF-ASSESSMENT 2

Attitudes Toward Timing of Parenthood Scale (ATOP)

Directions

Circle the response that most closely represents your feelings. The options are strongly agree (SA), agree (A), undecided (U), disagree (D), and strongly disagree (SD).

	SD	D	U	A	SA
1. The best time to begin having children is usually within the first two years of marriage.	1	2	3	4	5
2. It is important for a young couple to enjoy their social life first and to have children later in the marriage.	1	2	3	4	5
3. A marriage relationship is strengthened if children are born in the early years of marriage.	1	2	3	4	5
4. Women are generally happier if they have children early in the marriage.	1	2	3	4	5
5. Men are generally tied closer to the marriage when there are children in the home.	1	2	3	4	5
6. Most young married women lack self-fulfillment until they have a child.	1	2	3	4	5
7. Young couples who do not have children are usually unable to do so.	1	2	3	4	5
8. Married couples who have mature love for each other will be eager to have a child as soon as possible.	1	2	3	4	5
9. Couples who do not have children cannot share in the major interests of their friends who are parents, and are therefore left out of most social circles.	1	2	3	4	5
10. Children enjoy their parents more when the parents are nearer their own age; therefore, parents should have children while they are still young.	1	2	3	4	5
11. In general, research indicates that the majority of couples approaching parenthood for the first time have had little or no previous child care experience beyond sporadic babysitting, a course in child psychology, or occasional care of younger siblings. Considering your background preparation for parenthood, would you judge that you are well prepared for the parenting experience?	1	2	3	4	5

Items 1 through 10 are from the Attitudes Toward Timing of Parenthood Scale (Maxwell & Montgomery, 1969). Item 11 was an additional item constructed to determine perceived degree of preparation for parenthood.

Scoring: Response options that favor early parenthood receive the highest score (5 points), and those that favor delayed parenthood receive the lowest score (1 point). The range of possible scores is from 10 to 50. Item number 2 is reverse scored, so if you choose option 4, change it to 2 (or vice versa); if you chose option 5, change it to 1 (or vice versa). Then sum the value of the options you selected for all items to compute your total score.

Reliability and validity: No reliability information was provided. The scale's developers, Maxwell and Montgomery (1969), reported that in an item analysis, each of the original 10-scale items discriminated significantly between upper- and lower-quartile groups. In their study of 96 married women, consistent attitudes and behavior were found; those who waited longer before having their first child scored lower on the ATOP.

Interpreting your score: Maxwell and Montgomery (1969) found that the following factors related to lower scores (favoring delay of parenting): higher age of respondent, higher education level and socioeconomic status, and having fewer children. Studies in the decade following publication of this measure reveal that women in the late 1970s and early 1980s were more likely than Maxwell and Montgomery's original sample to favor delayed parenthood (Knaub, Eversol, & Voss, 1981, 1983). In the 1983 study of 213 female students at a large midwestern university (Knaub, Eversoll, & Voss, 1983), the mean total score (on items 1 through 10) on the ATOP was 21.

Researchers using this measure typically present the percentage of respondents who agree and disagree with each item. Following is a table that summarizes the responses of 213 female students at a large midwestern university (Knaub, Eversoll, & Voss, 1983) and 76 male students from colleges in four states (Eversoll, Voss, & Knaub, 1983). Percentages for the response options "strongly agree" and "agree" are combined, as are the percentages for "disagree" and "strongly disagree."

ATOP Items by Percent of Respondents Agreeing and Disagreeing (Refer to questions at the beginning of this assessment)

	Women			Men		
	Agree	Disagree	Undecided	Agree	Disagree	Undecided
Question 1	7.5	86.8	5.7	6.6	84.1	9.2
Question 2	78.8	10.8	11.3	76.0	11.8	13.2
Question 3	6.6	76.9	16.5	10.5	68.5	21.0
Question 4	5.2	72.7	22.1	5.3	58.0	36.5
Question 5	34.9	44.8	20.8	21.1	56.6	22.4
Question 6	8.9	81.7	9.4	7.9	72.4	19.7
Question 7	2.8	93.9	2.8	2.6	88.2	9.2
Question 8	4.3	84.4	11.3	9.2	81.6	9.2
Question 9	14.6	77.8	7.5	15.8	78.9	5.3
Question 10	15.6	71.2	13.2	19.8	64.5	15.8
Question 11	34.7	53.1	12.2			

Data from Eversoll, D. B., Voss, J. H., & Knaub, P. K. (1983). Attitudes of college females toward parenthood timing. *Journal of Home Economics*, 75:25–29.

Knaub, P. K., Eversoll, D. B., & Voss, J. H. (1981). Student attitudes toward parenthood: Implications for curricula in the 1980s. *Journal of Home Economics*, 73:34–37.

Knaub, P. K., Eversoll, D. B., & Voss, J. H. (1983). Is parenthood a desirable adult role? An assessment of attitudes held by contemporary women. *Sex Roles*, 9:355–362. Reprinted with kind permission from Springer Science and Business Media and Patricia K. Knaub.

Maxwell, J. W., & Montgomery, J. E. (1969). Societal pressure toward early parenthood. *Family Coordinator*, 18:340–344.

CHANGING HEALTH HABITS

Do You Want to Improve Your Reproductive Health?

Do you need to change a behavior that relates to or affects your reproductive health? For example, if you are sexually active, are you using contraception irregularly, risking pregnancy? Are you using a method that does not provide the level of protection you desire? The "Deciding to Change" section of the Changing Health Habits worksheet can help you determine whether you are ready to alter your behaviors to improve your reproductive health. Use the "Implementing the Change" section of the worksheet if you decide to make the necessary changes.

Deciding to Change

1. Identify the problem, goal, or question.

   ____

   ____

2. List the reasons you should make this change and the reasons you should not. Assign each reason a point value from 1 to 5, with 5 being the highest (it has the most value to you) and 1 being the lowest (it has the least value to you).

Choices

Reasons to change behaviors (pros):		Reasons not to change behaviors (cons):	
Points	***Reasons***	***Points***	***Reasons***
____	______________	____	______________
____	______________	____	______________
____	______________	____	______________
____	Total	____	Total

3. Draw a conclusion by adding the points in the pros section and then in the cons section. If the point total of the pros section is greater than the total of the cons section, you are probably ready to make a change in your life that improves your reproductive health. If your cons outweigh your pros, you may not be motivated to make the change now. Study your list of pros and cons carefully, however, before making your final decision. You may decide to change even if your reasons not to change outrank your reasons to change.

Implementing the Change

1. Set a target date to begin the new behavior or reach the goal.

2. Identify and list the factors that will help you reach your goal and those that will stand in the way of reaching your goal.

   Factors that help: ______

   Factors that hinder: ______

3. Prepare an action plan for making the change.

   a. Identify alternative methods for reaching your goal.

   b. Gather information about each method.

   c. Choose the method that fits your particular situation best.

   d. Consider the factors that can help or hinder your effort to change (see step 2).

   Factors that help: ______

   Factors that hinder: ______

4. Change the lifestyle behavior that you have decided to improve by implementing the action plan you developed in step 3.
5. Chart your daily progress toward your goal.
6. Evaluate how effective you were in reaching your goal.

CHAPTER 6

SELF-ASSESSMENT 1

Male Sexual Quotient Self-Assessment Questionnaire

This self-assessment addresses sexual function and satisfaction in men. It is designed to help men determine whether there are aspects of their sexual experience that could benefit from talking with their partner, consulting their physicians, and seeking treatment.

Answer this questionnaire honestly based on the last 6 months of your sex life, rating your answer as follows.

1 = Infrequently or rarely
2 = Sometimes
3 = Nearly 50% of the time
4 = Most of the time
5 = Always

1. Is your desire high enough to encourage you to initiate sexual intercourse? ____
2. Do you feel confident in your ability of seduction? ____
3. Do you feel that foreplay is enjoyable and satisfying for both you and your partner? ____
4. Is your own sexual performance affected by your partner's sexual satisfaction? ____
5. Can you maintain an erection sufficiently in order to complete sexual activity in a satisfactory way? ____
6. After sexual stimulation, is your erection hard enough to ensure satisfying intercourse? ____
7. Are you able to consistently obtain and maintain an erection whenever you have sexual activity? ____
8. Are you able to control ejaculation so that sexual activity lasts as long as you want? ____
9. Are you able to reach orgasm during sex? ____
10. Does your sexual performance encourage you to enjoy sex more frequently? ____

Male Sexual Quotient (MSQ) Scoring

Total maximum score: 50	
The MSQ equals total score multiplied by 2. Higher scores indicate greater sexual function and satisfaction with such function.	
82–100	Highly satisfied: I am very sexually satisfied and enjoy my sex life to the maximum.
62–80	Partially satisfied: I enjoy sex, but there is some room for improvement.
42–60	Average: I am concerned that my sexual enjoyment really could be better.
22–40	Dissatisfied: I feel that my sex life does not give me enough satisfaction.
0–20	Highly dissatisfied: I am very concerned that I don't get any satisfaction from my sex life.

Reproduced from Abdo, C. H. N. (2007). The Male Sexual Quotient: A brief, self-administered questionnaire to assess male sexual satisfaction. *Journal of Sexual Medicine, 4*:382–389. Reprinted with permission of Wiley-Blackwell.

CHAPTER 6

SELF-ASSESSMENT 2

The Love Attitudes Scale

Listed below are several statements that reflect different attitudes about love. For each statement, fill in the response that indicates how much you agree or disagree with the statement. The items refer to a specific love relationship. Whenever possible, answer the questions with your current partner in mind. If you are not currently in a love relationship, answer the questions with your most recent partner in mind. If you have never been in love, answer in terms of what you think your responses would most likely be.

For Each Statement

1 = strongly agree with the statement
2 = moderately agree with the statement
3 = neutral—neither agree nor disagree
4 = moderately disagree with the statement
5 = strongly disagree with the statement

1. My partner and I have the right physical "chemistry" between us. _____
2. I feel that my partner and I were meant for each other. _____
3. My partner and I really understand each other. _____
4. My partner fits my ideal standards of physical beauty/handsomeness. _____
5. I believe that what my partner doesn't know about me won't hurt him/her. _____
6. I have sometimes had to keep my partner from finding out about other lovers. _____
7. My partner would get upset if he/she knew of some of the things I've done with other people. _____
8. I enjoy playing the "game of love" with my partner and a number of other partners. _____
9. Our love is the best kind because it grew out of a long friendship. _____
10. Our friendship merged gradually into love over time. _____
11. Our love is really a deep friendship, not a mysterious, mystical emotion. _____
12. Our love relationship is the most satisfying because it developed from a good friendship. _____
13. A main consideration in choosing my partner was how he/she would reflect on my family. _____
14. An important factor in choosing my partner was whether or not he/she would be a good parent. _____
15. One consideration in choosing my partner was how he/she would reflect on my career. _____

16. Before getting very involved with my partner, I tried to figure out how compatible his/her hereditary background would be with mine in case we ever had children.	_____
17. When my partner doesn't pay attention to me, I feel sick all over.	_____
18. Since I've been in love with my partner I've had trouble concentrating on anything else.	_____
19. I cannot relax if I suspect that my partner is with someone else.	_____
20. If my partner ignores me for a while, I sometimes do stupid things to try to get his/her attention back.	_____
21. I would rather suffer myself than let my partner suffer.	_____
22. I cannot be happy unless I place my partner's happiness before my own.	_____
23. I am usually willing to sacrifice my own wishes to let my partner achieve his/hers.	_____
24. I would endure all things for the sake of my partner.	_____

Scoring

Add your scores for the following groups of questions: 1–4, 5–8, 9–12, 13–16, 17–20, and 21–24. Each of these six groupings of questions corresponds to one of Lee's six styles of loving. Your lowest group score means that you most closely align yourself with that style of loving. Table 6-1 in *Essential Concepts for Healthy Living*, Sixth Edition, lists meanings and characteristics for each of Lee's six styles of loving.

1–4 = Eros
5–8 = Ludus
9–12 = Storge
13–16 = Pragma
17–20 = Mania
21–24 = Agape

Modified from Hendrick, C., Hendrick, S. S., & Dicke, A. (1998). The love attitudes scale: Short form. *Journal of Social and Personal Relationships, 15*:147–159. Reprinted by permission of SAGE.

CHAPTER 6

CHANGING HEALTH HABITS

Would a Behavior Change Improve Your Relationship?

Do you need to change a behavior that relates to or affects your relationships? For example, are your communication patterns ineffective with those close to you, such as your lover, spouse, or parents? Are you having trouble communicating effectively with other persons, such as a friend or your boss? Do you want to change those patterns so that you will be more effective in maintaining successful relationships? The "Deciding to Change" section of the Changing Health Habits worksheet can help you determine whether you are ready to alter your behaviors to improve your communication skills. Use the "Implementing the Change" section of the worksheet if you decide to make the necessary changes.

Deciding to Change

1. Identify the problem, goal, or question.

    ____

    ____

2. List the reasons you should make this change and the reasons you should not. Assign each reason a point value from 1 to 5, with 5 being the highest (it has the most value to you) and 1 being the lowest (it has the least value to you).

Choices

Reasons to change behaviors (pros):

Points	*Reasons*
____	____________________
____	____________________
____	____________________
____	Total

Reasons not to change behaviors (cons):

Points	*Reasons*
____	____________________
____	____________________
____	____________________
____	Total

3. Draw a conclusion by adding the points in the pros section and then in the cons section. If the point total of the pros section is greater than the total of the cons section, you are probably ready to make a change in your life that improves your communications skills. If your cons outweigh your pros, you may not be motivated to make the change now. Study your list of pros and cons carefully, however, before making your final decision. You may decide to change even if your reasons not to change outrank your reasons to change.

Implementing the Change

1. Set a target date to begin the new behavior or reach the goal.

2. Identify and list the factors that will help you reach your goal and those that will stand in the way of reaching your goal.

   Factors that help:

   Factors that hinder:

3. Prepare an action plan for making the change.
   a. Identify alternative methods to reach your goal.

   b. Gather information about each method.
   c. Choose the method that fits your particular situation best.
   d. Consider the factors that can help or hinder your effort to change (see step 2).

   Factors that help:

   Factors that hinder:

4. Change the lifestyle behavior that you have decided to improve by implementing the action plan you developed in step 3.
5. Chart your daily progress toward your goal.
6. Evaluate how effective you were in reaching your goal.

CHAPTER 7

SELF-ASSESSMENT

Are You Dependent on Drugs?

Answer the following questions about your use and abuse of drugs.

	Yes	No
1. Have you used drugs other than those required for medical reasons?	____	____
2. Have you abused prescription drugs?	____	____
3. Do you abuse more than one drug at a time?	____	____
4. Can you get through the week without using drugs (other than those required for medical reasons)?*	____	____
5. Are you always able to stop using drugs when you want to?*	____	____
6. Do you abuse drugs on a continuous basis?	____	____
7. Do you try to limit your drug use to certain situations?*	____	____
8. Have you had "blackouts" or "flashbacks" as a result of drug use?	____	____
9. Do you ever feel bad about your drug abuse?	____	____
10. Does your spouse (or parents) ever complain about your involvement with drugs?	____	____
11. Do your friends or relatives know or suspect you abuse drugs?	____	____
12. Has drug abuse ever created problems between you and your spouse?	____	____
13. Has any family member ever sought help for problems related to your drug use?	____	____
14. Have you ever lost friends because of your use of drugs?	____	____
15. Have you ever neglected your family or missed work because of your use of drugs?	____	____
16. Have you ever been in trouble at work because of your use of drugs?	____	____
17. Have you ever lost a job because of drug abuse?	____	____
18. Have you gotten into fights while under the influence of drugs?	____	____
19. Have you ever been arrested because of unusual behavior while under the influence of drugs?	____	____
20. Have you ever been arrested while driving under the influence of drugs?	____	____
21. Have you engaged in illegal activities in order to obtain drugs?	____	____
22. Have you ever been arrested for possession of illegal drugs?	____	____

	Yes	No
23. Have you ever experienced withdrawal symptoms as a result of heavy drug intake?	____	____
24. Have you had medical problems as a result of your drug use (e.g., memory loss, hepatitis, convulsions, bleeding, etc.)?	____	____
25. Have you ever gone to anyone for help for a drug problem?	____	____
26. Have you ever been in a hospital for medical problems related to your drug use?	____	____
27. Have you ever been involved in a treatment program specifically related to drug use?	____	____
28. Have you ever been treated as an outpatient for problems related to drug abuse?	____	____

Scoring This Assessment

If you answered "yes" to 6 or more of these questions (including "no" answers to questions 4, 5, and 7), you may have a drug abuse problem.

*Items 4, 5, and 7 are scored in the "no" or false direction.

Reproduced with permission from Elsevier from Skinner, H. A. The Drug Screening Test. *Addictive Behaviors*, 7:363–371. Copyright Elsevier 1982.

Resources

If you are dependent on drugs, the following government agencies or private organizations may be able to provide you with help:

National Drug and Alcohol Treatment Referral Routing Service
1-800-662-HELP

Cocaine Anonymous World Services
21720 S. Wilmington Ave., Ste. 304
Long Beach, CA 90810
E-mail: cawso@ca.org
http://www.ca.org

Nar-Anon Family Groups
22527 Crenshaw Blvd., #200B
Torrance, CA 90505
(310) 534-8188
1-800-477-6291
http://nar-anon.org

Narcotics Anonymous World Services
P.O. Box 9999
Van Nuys, CA 91409
(818) 773-9999
E-mail: fsmail@na.org
http://www.na.org

National Council on Alcoholism and Drug Dependence
244 East 58th Street, 4th Floor
New York, NY 10022
Hope Line: 800-NCA-CALL (24-hour affiliate referral)
(212) 269-7797
http://www.ncadd.org

National Institute on Drug Abuse
National Institutes of Health
6001 Executive Blvd., Rm. 5213
Bethesda, MD 20892-9561
(301) 443-1124
E-mail: http://www.nida.nih.gov/nidahome.html
http://www.nida.nih.gov

CHAPTER 7

CHANGING HEALTH HABITS

Are You Using Drugs Inappropriately?

Student Workbook

Are you taking any drugs now, such as caffeine or much stronger drugs, that may be habit forming, may have negative health effects, and that were not prescribed by your healthcare practitioner? If you are using drugs inappropriately, follow the steps of the decision-making and implementation model to identify and change a drug-related habit.

Deciding to Change

1. Identify the problem, goal, or question.

____

____

2. List the reasons you should make this change and the reasons you should not. Assign each reason a point value from 1 to 5, with 5 being the highest (it has the most value to you) and 1 being the lowest (it has the least value to you).

Choices

Reasons to change behaviors (pros):

Points	*Reasons*
____	______________________
____	______________________
____	______________________
____	Total

Reasons not to change behaviors (cons):

Points	*Reasons*
____	______________________
____	______________________
____	______________________
____	Total

3. Draw a conclusion by adding the points in the pros section and then in the cons section. If the point total of the pros section is greater than the total of the cons section, you are probably ready to make a change in your life regarding a drug-related habit. If your cons outweigh your pros, you may not be motivated to make the change now. Study your list of pros and cons carefully, however, before making your final decision. You may decide to change even if your reasons not to change outrank your reasons to change.

Implementing the Change

1. Set a target date to begin the new behavior or reach the goal.

2. Identify and list the factors that will help you reach your goal and those that will stand in the way of reaching your goal.

   Factors that help:

   Factors that hinder:

3. Prepare an action plan for making the change.
   a. Identify alternative methods for reaching your goal.

   b. Gather information about each method.
   c. Choose the method that fits your particular situation best.
   d. Consider the factors that can help or hinder your effort to change (see step 2).

   Factors that help:

   Factors that hinder:

4. Change the lifestyle behavior that you have decided to improve by implementing the action plan you developed in step 3.
5. Chart your daily progress toward your goal.
6. Evaluate how effective you were in reaching your goal.

CHAPTER 8

Student Workbook

SELF-ASSESSMENT

Why Do You Smoke?

Directions

Answer the following questions by circling O (often), S (sometimes), or N (never).

	Often	Sometimes	Never
Group 1			
I smoke to keep from slowing down.	O	S	N
I reach for a cigarette when I need a lift.	O	S	N
When I'm tired, smoking perks me up.	O	S	N
Group 2			
I feel more comfortable with a cigarette in my hand.	O	S	N
I enjoy getting a cigarette out of the pack and lighting up.	O	S	N
I like to watch the smoke when I exhale.	O	S	N
Group 3			
Smoking cigarettes is pleasant and enjoyable.	O	S	N
Smoking makes good times better.	O	S	N
I want a cigarette most when I am comfortable and relaxed.	O	S	N
Group 4			
I light up a cigarette when something makes me angry.	O	S	N
Smoking relaxes me in a stressful situation.	O	S	N
When I'm depressed I reach for a cigarette to feel better.	O	S	N
Group 5			
When I run out of cigarettes, it's almost unbearable until I get more.	O	S	N
I am very aware of not smoking when I don't have a cigarette in my hand.	O	S	N
When I haven't smoked for a while I get a gnawing hunger for a cigarette.	O	S	N
Group 6			
I smoke cigarettes automatically without even being aware of it.	O	S	N
I light up a cigarette without realizing I have one burning in an ashtray.	O	S	N
I find a cigarette in my mouth and don't remember putting it there.	O	S	N

Interpretation: Look at each group separately. If you answer "often" or "sometimes" to the questions in a particular group, that signifies one reason you smoke.

Reasons:
Group 1: Smoking gives you more energy.
Group 2: You like to touch and handle cigarettes.
Group 3: Smoking is a pleasure.
Group 4: Smoking helps you relax when you're tense or upset.
Group 5: You crave cigarettes; you are addicted to smoking.
Group 6: Smoking is a habit.

Refer to the Managing Your Health essay "Tips for Quitters" in Chapter 8 for strategies to quit that address each of these reasons you smoke.

The National Cancer Institute. (1993). Learning why you smoke can teach you how to quit. Washington, DC: U.S. Department of Health and Human Services.

CHAPTER 8

CHANGING HEALTH HABITS

Student Workbook

Do You Want to Change a Smoking or Drinking Habit?

Follow the steps of the decision-making and implementation model to identify and change a health-related habit that concerns your drinking of alcoholic beverages or your use of tobacco. For example, are you a heavy smoker who would like to smoke less or stop smoking cigarettes completely? Do you have drinking habits that you would like to change, such as drinking a six-pack in front of the TV every night, drinking on an empty stomach, or drinking too much at parties and sporting events?

Deciding to Change

1. Identify the problem, goal, or question.

   ____

   ____

2. List the reasons you should make this change and the reasons you should not. Assign each reason a point value from 1 to 5, with 5 being the highest (it has the most value to you) and 1 being the lowest (it has the least value to you).

Choices

Reasons to change behaviors (pros):

Points	Reasons
____	____________________
____	____________________
____	____________________
____	Total

Reasons not to change behaviors (cons):

Points	Reasons
____	____________________
____	____________________
____	____________________
____	Total

3. Draw a conclusion by adding the points in the pros section and then in the cons section. If the point total of the pros section is greater than the total of the cons section, you are probably ready to make a change in your life regarding a smoking or drinking habit. If your cons outweigh your pros, you may not be motivated to make the change now. Study your list of pros and cons carefully, however, before making your final decision. You may decide to change even if your reasons not to change outrank your reasons to change.

Implementing the Change

1. Set a target date to begin the new behavior or reach the goal.

2. Identify and list the factors that will help you reach your goal and those that will stand in the way of reaching your goal.

   Factors that help:

   Factors that hinder:

3. Prepare an action plan for making the change.

   a. Identify alternative methods for reaching your goal.

   b. Gather information about each method.

   c. Choose the method that fits your particular situation best.

   d. Consider the factors that can help or hinder your effort to change (see step 2).

   Factors that help:

   Factors that hinder:

4. Change the lifestyle behavior that you have decided to improve by implementing the action plan you developed in step 3.
5. Chart your daily progress toward your goal.
6. Evaluate how effective you were in reaching your goal.

CHAPTER 9

SELF-ASSESSMENT 1

Assessing the Nutritional Quality of Your Diet

Measure or estimate the amounts of everything you eat and drink for 3 days. For each day, record this information on a daily food record-keeping form (see the next page). To determine the nutritional value of your food items, you can use the "SuperTracker" tools at http://www.choosemyplate.gov/

At the end of each day, add the amounts in each column and write the totals at the bottom of the form. Determine your average intake of calories and nutrients for that period. (Add the three daily totals for calories, then divide by 3. Do the same for each nutrient listed in the record-keeping form.) You can evaluate the nutritional quality of your diet by comparing your average intakes with the DRIs for those nutrients, which are shown in Appendix C.

1. Write a one-page description of the nutritional quality of your diet; in your summary, provide answers to the following questions:
   - **a.** Did your average intake of calories and nutrients meet at least 75% of the DRIs for your age and gender?
   - **b.** If your average intake of one or more nutrients did not meet 75% of the DRIs, which foods could you add to your diet to boost the amounts of the nutrient(s) you are lacking?
   - **c.** For each of the 3 days, what percentage of your calories were from protein, fat, and alcohol?
   - **d.** If the percentage of calories from fat exceeded 35%, which foods contributed to your high fat intake?

____

____

____

____

____

____

____

____

____

____

____

2. Do you need to make any changes to improve the nutritional quality of your diet? Would you like to eat more fruits or vegetables? Should you replace whole or reduced-fat (2%) milk with nonfat milk? Do you need more calcium or iron in your diet? Do you think you eat too much sugar, salt, or fat?

3. Use your responses to number 2 to complete the Changing Health Habits activity for this chapter.

Daily Food Record

Name ______________________

Date ________

Food Item	Amount Eaten	Calories	Prot. (g)	Fat* (g)	Vit. D (g)	Vit. C (mg)	Vit. E (mg)	Folate (μg)	Calcium (mg)	Iron (mg)
Totals										

*No DRI

Total calories from alcohol ____________

CHAPTER 9

SELF-ASSESSMENT 2

Diabetes Risk Test

American Diabetes Association.

ALERT!DA

ARE YOU AT RISK?

DIABETES RISK TEST

Calculate Your Chances for Type 2 or Pre-Diabetes

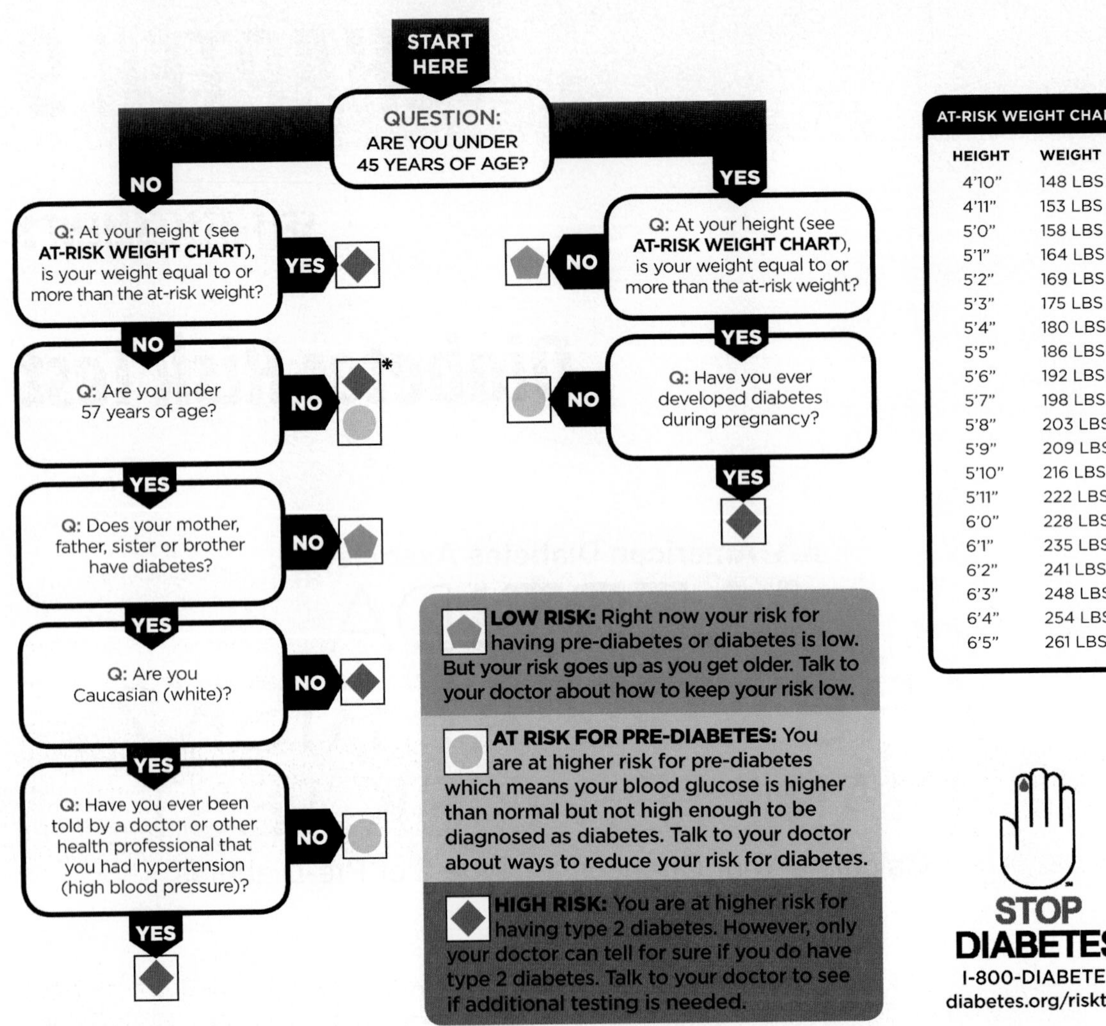
START HERE
QUESTION: ARE YOU UNDER 45 YEARS OF AGE?
NO
Q: At your height (see AT-RISK WEIGHT CHART), is your weight equal to or more than the at-risk weight?
YES
NO
Q: Are you under 57 years of age?
NO
*
YES
Q: Does your mother, father, sister or brother have diabetes?
NO
YES
Q: Are you Caucasian (white)?
NO
YES
Q: Have you ever been told by a doctor or other health professional that you had hypertension (high blood pressure)?
NO
YES
YES
Q: At your height (see AT-RISK WEIGHT CHART), is your weight equal to or more than the at-risk weight?
NO
YES
Q: Have you ever developed diabetes during pregnancy?
NO
YES
LOW RISK: Right now your risk for having pre-diabetes or diabetes is low. But your risk goes up as you get older. Talk to your doctor about how to keep your risk low.
AT RISK FOR PRE-DIABETES: You are at higher risk for pre-diabetes which means your blood glucose is higher than normal but not high enough to be diagnosed as diabetes. Talk to your doctor about ways to reduce your risk for diabetes.
HIGH RISK: You are at higher risk for having type 2 diabetes. However, only your doctor can tell for sure if you do have type 2 diabetes. Talk to your doctor to see if additional testing is needed.
STOP DIABETES.
1-800-DIABETES
diabetes.org/risktest

AT-RISK WEIGHT CHART

HEIGHT	WEIGHT
4'10"	148 LBS
4'11"	153 LBS
5'0"	158 LBS
5'1"	164 LBS
5'2"	169 LBS
5'3"	175 LBS
5'4"	180 LBS
5'5"	186 LBS
5'6"	192 LBS
5'7"	198 LBS
5'8"	203 LBS
5'9"	209 LBS
5'10"	216 LBS
5'11"	222 LBS
6'0"	228 LBS
6'1"	235 LBS
6'2"	241 LBS
6'3"	248 LBS
6'4"	254 LBS
6'5"	261 LBS

*Your risk for diabetes or pre-diabetes depends on additional risk factors including weight, physical activity and blood pressure.

CHAPTER 9

SELF-ASSESSMENT 3

Using MyPlate

To complete this self-assessment, you will need to access MyPlate via the Internet. When you open your Web browser, type http://www.choosemyplate.gov/myplate/index.aspx in the address window. This will take you to the U.S. Department of Agriculture's MyPlate page. Insert your age in the appropriate box. In the other boxes, select your sex, weight, height, and the activity level that approximates your physical activity habits, most days of the week. Fill in the same information below.

Age _____ Sex _____ Weight _____ Height _____

Physical Activity Level ____

Click on the Submit button. The next page provides a personalized plan that includes information about the number of calories you need to support your activity level as well as amounts of foods from each food group that you should eat daily. By following this food pattern, you are likely to obtain the nutrients you need each day and maintain your body weight.

Part I

Complete the following table with the information provided at your personal Daily Food Plan page. Note that vegetables are divided into subgroups, and amounts for weekly consumption are recommended for each subgroup. Daily amounts are suggested for the other food groups.

Food Group	Amount of Food
Grains *	____ ounces (refined grains)
	____ ounces (whole grains)
Vegetables (daily)	____ cups
Dark green (weekly)	____ cups
Red and orange (weekly)	____ cups
Beans and peas (weekly)	____ cups
Starchy (weekly)	____ cups
Other (weekly)	____ cups
Fruits	____ cups
Dairy	____ cups

Food Group	Amount of Food
Protein Foods	____ ounces
Oils (daily)	____ teaspoons

* At least half of your choices from the grains group should be whole grains.

Part II

Use the MyPlate Daily Food Record form to record everything you eat and drink for a day. You'll need to estimate the amounts of foods and beverages eaten and place that figure in the middle column. If you need to record information for more than one day, make copies of the form before you use it.

Name ______________________________

MyPlate Daily Food Record		
Food/Beverage Item Consumed	**Amount Consumed** (Ounces/Cups)	**MyPlate Plan Food Group**

Part III Self-Evaluation

1. According to your records, did you eat the recommended amounts of foods from each food group? _____ yes _____ no
   a. If you did not eat the recommended amounts, identify the food groups that had inadequate intakes.

   ____
   ____
   ____
   ____
   ____

2. Explain why this day's food intake was typical or unusual for you.

   ____
   ____
   ____
   ____
   ____

3. As a result of completing this activity, describe at least one step you can take to improve your daily food choices.

   ____
   ____
   ____
   ____
   ____

CHAPTER 9

CHANGING HEALTH HABITS

Are You Ready to Improve Your Diet?

After completing the summary for the nutritional assessment activity in self-assessments 1 and 3 of this chapter, do you think you need to improve the nutritional quality of your diet? The "Deciding to Change" section of the Changing Health Habits worksheet can help you determine whether you are ready to improve your diet and what the health benefits might be if you do so. If you decide to change some food-related habits, use the "Implementing the Change" section of the worksheet to help you make your dietary changes.

Deciding to Change

1. Identify the problem, goal, or question.

   ____

   ____

2. List the reasons you should make this change and the reasons you should not. Assign each reason a point value from 1 to 5, with 5 being the highest (it has the most value to you) and 1 being the lowest (it has the least value to you).

Choices

Reasons to change behaviors (pros):

Points	Reasons
____	____________________
____	____________________
____	____________________
____	Total

Reasons not to change behaviors (cons):

Points	Reasons
____	____________________
____	____________________
____	____________________
____	Total

3. Draw a conclusion by adding the points in the pros section and then in the cons section. If the point total of the pros section is greater than the total of the cons section, you are probably ready to make a change in your life that improves the nutritional qulaity of your diet. If your cons outweigh your pros, you may not be motivated to make the change now. Study your list of pros and cons carefully, however, before making your final decision. You may decide to change even if your reasons not to change outrank your reasons to change.

Implementing the Change

1. Set a target date to begin the new behavior or reach the goal.

2. Identify and list the factors that will help you reach your goal and those that will stand in the way of reaching your goal.

   Factors that help:

   Factors that hinder:

3. Prepare an action plan for making the change.
   a. Identify alternative methods for reaching your goal.

   b. Gather information about each method.
   c. Choose the method that fits your particular situation best.
   d. Consider the factors that can help or hinder your effort to change (see step 2).

   Factors that help:

   Factors that hinder:

4. Change the lifestyle behavior that you have decided to improve by implementing the action plan you developed in step 3.
5. Chart your daily progress toward your goal.
6. Evaluate how effective you were in reaching your goal.

Student Workbook

CHAPTER 10

SELF-ASSESSMENT

How Much Energy Do You Use Daily?

Use the following activity to estimate your daily caloric needs.

A. Estimating energy needs for basal metabolism:

1. Convert your body weight to kilograms. Since each pound equals about 2.2 kilograms, divide your weight in pounds by 2.2 to obtain your weight in kilograms.

   ____ weight in pounds ÷ 2.2 = ____ kilograms (kg)

2. To sustain its basal metabolic needs, the body needs about 1.0 calorie per kg of body weight per hour (men) or 0.9 calorie per kg of body weight per hour (women). To estimate the amount of calories you need for basal metabolism in an hour, multiply your body weight (kg) by 1.0 if you are male or 0.9 if you are female.

   ____ body weight (kg) × 1.0 or 0.9 = _____ calories per hour

3. To estimate the amount of calories you need for basal metabolism in a day, multiply the amount of calories you obtained in step 2 by 24 (hours in a day).

   ______ calories per hour × 24 hours = ______ calories per day (basal metabolism)

B. Estimating energy needs for physical activity:

4. To determine your energy needs for physical activity, you can keep records of every activity you perform during the day, and the time spent engaging in each activity. An easier, but less precise way to estimate your energy expenditures for physical activity is to use the following rule of thumb. To use this method, choose the category of physical activity in the table on the next page that best describes your usual physical activity level. For example, if you spend most of your day sitting while taking classes, studying, and watching TV, you probably have a very light level of activity. If you sit some of the time, but move around while working, you might rate your level of physical activity as light. If you are on your feet most of the time and engage in strenuous work such as lifting heavy objects, you are probably expending energy at the heavy level of intensity.

   My activity level is ____________________

5. Note the Activity Factor in the table below for your level of intensity and gender. For example, if you are male, and you consider your overall physical activity pattern to be in the moderate range, your Activity Factor is 1.7.

   The Activity Factor for my gender and level of physical activity intensity is ______

6. Multiply your basal metabolic energy needs (the number of calories per day estimated in step 3) by the Activity Factor (step 5).

   ___ calories for basal metabolism × ___ Activity Factor = _____calories for physical activity

7. To estimate the number of calories you expend each day for the thermic effect of food (TEF), multiply the number of calories determined in step 6 by 0.10.

   ______ calories × 0.10 = ____ calories for TEF

8. To estimate your total energy needs for a day, add the number of calories determined in steps 6 and 7.

   _________ calories for basal metabolism and physical activity

   \+ _________ calories for TEF

   = _________ total calories

   This is an estimation of the total number of calories you use each day. If you take in more calories than needed, they may be converted to body fat.

9. If you completed the assessment in Chapter 9, you were able to determine an average number of calories that you consumed during the three-day record-keeping period. Is your average caloric intake about the same, greater than, or less than the total number of calories that you need for a day?

   ____ about the same _____ greater than _____ less than

10. If you continue to consume this average amount of calories, explain what may happen to your body weight.

    ____

		Activity Factor	
Intensity	***Physical Activity***	***Men***	***Women***
Very light	Standing, sitting, driving, typing, sewing, cooking, playing cards or a musical instrument	1.3	1.3
Light	Walking on a level surface at 2.5 to 3.0 mph, carpentry, child care, golf, sailing, table tennis	1.6	1.5
Moderate	Walking 3.5 to 4.0 mph, gardening, carrying a load, cycling, skiing, tennis, dancing	1.7	1.6
Heavy	Walking uphill carrying a load; digging by hand; playing basketball, football, or soccer; climbing	2.1	1.9
Exceptionally heavy	Athletic training or participation in professional or world-class events	2.4	2.2

Data from *Recommended dietary allowances* (10th Ed.). Copyright © 1989 by the National Academy of Sciences. Courtesy of the National Academies Press, Washington, D.C.

CHAPTER 10

CHANGING HEALTH HABITS

Altering Caloric Intake and Physical Activity

Do you need to lose or gain weight? The "Deciding to Change" section of the Changing Health Habits worksheet can help you determine whether you are ready to alter your caloric intake and physical activity level to gain or lose weight. If you decide to change some of your eating and physical activity habits, use the "Implementing the Change" section of the worksheet to help you make the necessary lifestyle changes.

Deciding to Change

1. Identify the problem, goal, or question.

   ____

   ____

2. List the reasons you should make this change and the reasons you should not. Assign each reason a point value from 1 to 5, with 5 being the highest (it has the most value to you) and 1 being the lowest (it has the least value to you).

Choices

Reasons to change behaviors (pros):

Points	*Reasons*
____	______________________
____	______________________
____	______________________
____	Total

Reasons not to change behaviors (cons):

Points	*Reasons*
____	______________________
____	______________________
____	______________________
____	Total

3. Draw a conclusion by adding the points in the pros section and then in the cons section. If the point total of the pros section is greater than the total of the cons section, you are probably ready to make the lifestyle changes necessary to lose or gain weight. If your cons outweigh your pros, you may not be motivated to make the change now. Study your list of pros and cons carefully, however, before making your final decision. You may decide to change even if your reasons not to change outrank your reasons to change.

Implementing the Change

1. Set a target date to begin the new behavior or reach the goal.

   ____

2. Identify and list the factors that will help you reach your goal and those that will stand in the way of reaching your goal.

   Factors that help: ______________________________

   ____

   ____

   ____

   Factors that hinder: ______________________________

   ____

   ____

   ____

3. Prepare an action plan for making the change.

   a. Identify alternative methods for reaching your goal.

   ____

   ____

   ____

   b. Gather information about each method.

   c. Choose the method that fits your particular situation best.

   d. Consider the factors that can help or hinder your effort to change (see step 2).

   Factors that help: ______________________________

   ____

   ____

   ____

   Factors that hinder: ______________________________

   ____

   ____

   ____

4. Change the lifestyle behavior that you have decided to improve by implementing the action plan you developed in step 3.
5. Chart your daily progress toward your goal.
6. Evaluate how effective you were in reaching your goal.

   ____

   ____

   ____

   ____

   ____

   ____

CHAPTER 11

SELF-ASSESSMENT 1

Cardiorespiratory Fitness: The Rockport Fitness Walking Test™

This activity assesses cardiorespiratory (aerobic) fitness. To perform the test, you need a watch with a second hand to record your time, and you need to wear good walking shoes and loose clothes. You should have your physician's consent before undertaking this exercise test.

Instructions

1. Find a measured track or measure 1 mile using your car's odometer on a level uninterrupted road.
2. Warm up by walking slowly for 5 minutes.
3. Walk 1 mile as fast as you can, maintaining a steady pace. Note the time that you began walking.
4. When you complete the mile walk, record your time to the nearest second and keep walking at a slower pace. Count your pulse for 15 seconds and multiply by 4, then record this number. This gives you your heart rate per minute after your test walk.

   Heart rate at the end of a mile walk: ______ beats per minute

   Time to walk the mile: _____ minutes

5. Remember to stretch once you have cooled down.
6. To find your cardiorespiratory fitness level, refer to the appropriate Rockport Fitness Walking Test™ charts according to your age and sex. These show established fitness norms from the American Heart Association.

   Using your fitness level chart, find your time in minutes and your heart rate per minute. Follow these lines until they meet, and mark this point on your chart. This tells you how fit you are compared to other individuals of your sex and age category. Level 5 represents the highest fitness level.

   These charts are based on weights of 170 lb for men and 125 lb for women. If you weigh substantially less, your cardiovascular fitness will be slightly underestimated. Conversely, if you weigh substantially more, your cardiovascular fitness will be slightly overestimated.

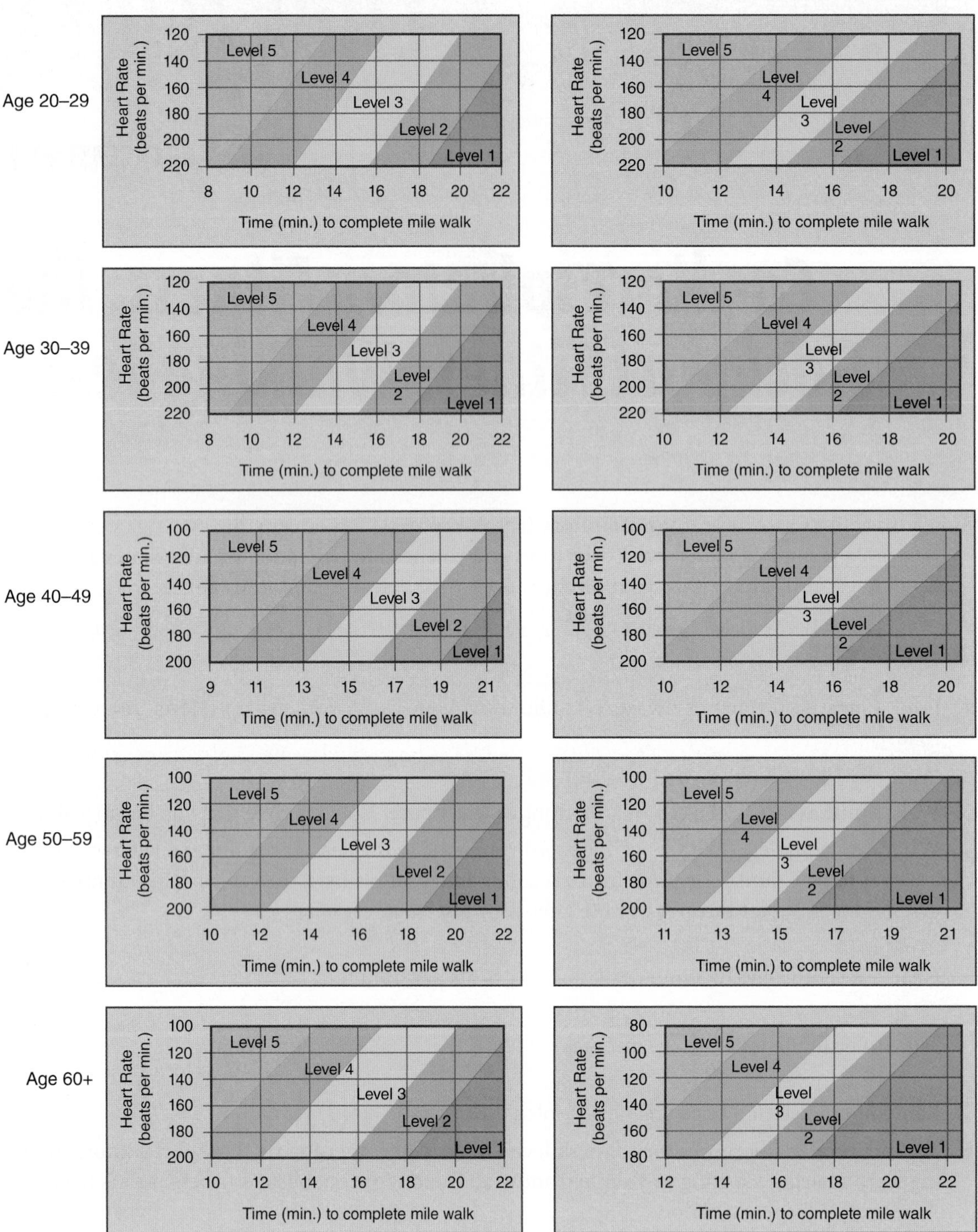
Men's Fitness Level Chart
Women's Fitness Level Chart
Age 20–29
Age 30–39
Age 40–49
Age 50–59
Age 60+
Heart Rate (beats per min.)
Level 5
Level 4
Level 3
Level 2
Level 1
Time (min.) to complete mile walk

SELF-ASSESSMENT 2

Push-Up Test for Muscular Endurance

The push-up test can help assess your muscular endurance. To take the test, follow these instructions.

Procedure

Men

- Assume the standard position for a push-up, with the body rigid and straight, toes tucked under, and hands about shoulder-width apart and straight under the shoulders.
- Lower the body until the elbows reach 90 degrees. Some prefer to place an object such as a paper cup beneath to touch.
- Return to the starting position with the arms fully extended.
- The most common error is not keeping the back straight and rigid throughout the entire push-up.
- Count the number of push-ups you can perform in one minute.
- See the accompanying table for your fitness level.

Women

Women tend to have less upper body strength and therefore should use the modified push-up position to assess their upper body endurance. The test is performed as follows:

- Directions are the same for women as for men, except that women should perform the test from the bent-knee position. Make sure that your hands are slightly ahead of your shoulders in the up position so that when you are in the down position, your hands are directly under the shoulders.
- Keep the back straight and rigid throughout the entire push-up.
- Count the number of push-ups you can perform in one minute.
- See the accompanying table to rate your muscular endurance.

Note: Women who wish to do full-body push-ups can rate their performances by using the table on the next page.

Muscular Endurance Ratings
1 Minute Push-Up

Males					
	Age				
%	20–29	30–39	40–49	50–59	
99	100	86	64	51	
95	62	52	40	39	Superior
90	57	46	36	30	
85	51	41	34	28	
80	47	39	30	25	Excellent
75	44	36	29	24	
70	41	34	26	21	
65	39	31	25	20	
60	37	30	24	19	Good
55	35	29	22	17	
50	33	27	21	15	
45	31	25	19	14	
40	29	24	18	13	Fair
35	27	21	16	11	
30	26	20	15	10	
25	24	19	13	9.5	
20	22	17	11	9	Poor
15	19	15	10	7	
10	18	13	9	6	
5	13	9	5	3	Very Poor
n	1,045	790	364	172	

Total n = 2,371

Note: Norms are based on worksite wellness program participants.

Reproduced with permission from The Cooper Institute®, Dallas, Texas from a book called "Physical Fitness Assessments and Norms for Adults and Law Enforcement". Available online at www.CooperInstitute.org

Muscular Endurance Ratings
1 Minute Modified Push-Up

Females

	Age				
%	20–29	30–39	40–49	50–59	
99	70	56	60	31	
95	45	39	33	28	Superior
90	42	36	28	25	
85	39	33	26	23	
80	36	31	24	21	Excellent
75	34	29	21	20	
70	32	28	20	19	
65	31	26	19	18	
60	30	24	18	17	Good
55	29	23	17	15	
50	26	21	15	13	
45	25	20	14	13	
40	23	19	13	12	Fair
35	22	17	11	10	
30	20	15	10	9	
25	19	14	9	8	
20	17	11	6	6	Poor
15	15	9	4	4	
10	12	8	2	1	
5	9	4	1	0	Very Poor
n	579	411	246	105	

Total n = 1,341

Note: Norms are based on worksite wellness program participants.

Reproduced with permission from The Cooper Institute®, Dallas, Texas from a book called "Physical Fitness Assessments and Norms for Adults and Law Enforcement". Available online at www.CooperInstitute.org

Muscular Endurance Ratings
1 Minute Full-Body Push-Up*

Females				
		Age		
%	20–29	30–39	40–49	Endurance Level
99	53	48	23	
95	42	39.5	20	Superior
90	37	33	18	
85	33	26	17	
80	28	23	15	Excellent
75	27	19	15	
70	24	18	14	
65	23	16	13	
60	21	15	13	Good
55	19	14	11	
50	18	14	11	
45	17	13	10	
40	15	11	9	Fair
35	14	10	8	
30	13	9	7	
25	11	9	7	
20	10	8	6	Poor
15	9	6.5	5	
10	8	6	4	
5	6	4	1	
1	3	1	0	Very Poor

* Full-body push-ups are generally used by law enforcement and public safety organizations. These norms are based on >1000 female U.S. Army soldiers who were tested in the 1990s by the U.S. Army.

Reproduced with permission from The Cooper Institute®, Dallas, Texas from a book called "Physical Fitness Assessments and Norms for Adults and Law Enforcement". Available online at www.CooperInstitute.org

SELF-ASSESSMENT 3

Sit-and-Reach Test for Flexibility Assessment

The sit-and-reach test can help assess your flexibility. Read the following precautions, and if they do not apply, take the test.

Precautions

If any of the following apply, seek medical advice before performing the test.

- You are presently suffering from acute back pain.
- You are currently receiving treatment for back pain.
- You have ever had a surgical operation on your back.
- A healthcare professional told you to never exercise your back.

Procedure

Warm up. Stop the test if pain occurs. Do not perform fast, jerky movements.

Step 1:

Sit on the floor with your legs straight and knees together. Your toes should point upward toward the ceiling and rest against the side of a box.

Step 2:

Place one hand over the other. The tips of your two middle fingers should be on top of each other.

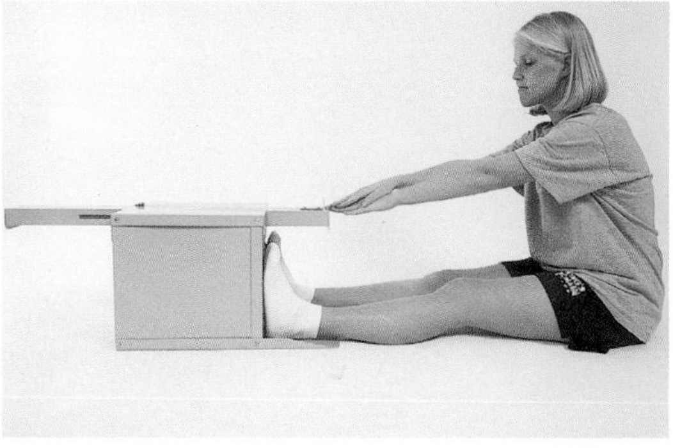

Step 3:

Slowly stretch forward without bouncing or jerking. Stop when tightness or discomfort occurs in the back or legs. Measure how far your hands reached on the top of the box.

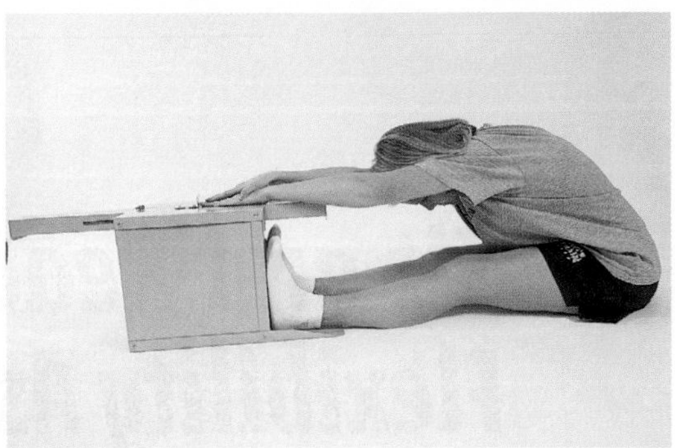

Step 4:

Repeat this test two more times and record scores.

First attempt ________ points

Second attempt ________ points

Third attempt ________ points

How to score (average of 3 attempts)	
Reached well past toes and side of box	1 point; excellent
Reached just to toes	2 points; good
Up to 4 inches from toes (did not reach side of box)	3 points; fair
More than 4 inches from toes (did not reach side of box)	4 points; poor
Reproduced from David Imrie. (1998). *Back power.* Toronto, Canada: Stoddart.	

Total points = _______ divided by 3 = ________ points, which is rated as _________.

SELF-ASSESSMENT 4

Check Your Physical Activity and Heart Disease IQ

Test your knowledge about the effects that physical activity can have on your heart. Mark each statement true or false. Answers are on the following page.

1. Regular physical activity can reduce your chances of getting heart disease.	T	F
2. Most people get enough physical activity from their normal daily routines.	T	F
3. You don't have to train like a marathon runner to become more physically fit.	T	F
4. Exercise programs do not require a lot of time to be very effective.	T	F
5. People who need to lose some weight are the only ones who will benefit from regular physical activity.	T	F
6. All exercises give you the same benefits.	T	F
7. The older you are, the less active you need to be.	T	F
8. It doesn't take a lot of money or expensive equipment to become physically fit.	T	F
9. There are many risks and injuries that can occur with exercise.	T	F
10. You should consult a doctor before starting a physical activity program.	T	F
11. People who have had a heart attack should not start any physical activity program.	T	F
12. To help stay physically active, include a variety of activities.	T	F

How well did you do?

Answers to the Check Your Physical Activity and Heart Disease IQ Quiz

1. *True.* Heart disease is almost twice as likely to develop in inactive people. Being physically inactive is a risk factor for heart disease, along with cigarette smoking, high blood pressure, high blood cholesterol, and being overweight. The more risk factors you have, the greater your chance for heart disease. Regular physical activity (even mild to moderate exercise) can reduce this risk.
2. *False.* Most Americans are very busy but not very active. Every American adult should make a habit of getting at least 30 minutes of low to moderate levels of physical activity daily. This includes walking, gardening, and walking up stairs. If you are inactive now, begin by doing a few minutes of activity each day. If you only do some activity every once in a while, try to work something into your routine everyday.
3. *True.* Low- to moderate-intensity activities, such as pleasure walking, stair climbing, yard work, housework, dancing, and home exercises can have both short- and long-term benefits. If you are inactive, the key is to get started. One great way is to take a walk for 10 to 15 minutes during your lunch break, or take your dog for a walk every day. At least 30 minutes of physical activity every day can help improve your heart health.
4. *True.* It takes only a few minutes a day to become more physically active. If you don't have 30 minutes in your schedule for an exercise break, try to find two 15-minute periods or even three 10-minute periods. These exercise breaks will soon become a habit you can't live without.
5. *False.* People who are physically active experience many positive benefits. Regular physical activity gives you more energy, reduces stress, and helps you to sleep better. It helps to lower high blood pressure and improves blood cholesterol levels. Physical activity helps to tone your muscles, burns off calories to help you lose extra pounds or stay at your desirable weight, and helps control your appetite. It can also increase muscle strength, help your heart and lungs work more efficiently, and let you enjoy your life more fully.
6. *False.* Low-intensity activities—if performed daily—can have some long-term health benefits and can lower your risk of heart disease. Regular, brisk, and sustained exercise for at least 30 minutes, three to four times a week, such as brisk walking, jogging, or swimming, is necessary to improve the efficiency of your heart and lungs and burn off extra calories. These activities are called aerobic—meaning the body uses oxygen to produce the energy needed for the activity. Other activities, depending on the type, may give you other benefits such as increased flexibility or muscle strength.
7. *False.* Although we tend to become less active with age, physical activity is still important. In fact, regular physical activity in older persons increases their capacity to do everyday activities. In general, middle-aged and older people benefit from regular physical activity just as young people do. What is important, at any age, is tailoring the activity program to your own fitness level.
8. *True.* Many activities require little or no equipment. For example, brisk walking only requires a comfortable pair of walking shoes. Many communities offer free or inexpensive recreation facilities and physical activity classes. Check your shopping malls, as many of them are open early and late for people who do not wish to walk alone, in the dark, or in bad weather.
9. *False.* Under normal conditions, exercise does not involve many risks and injuries. However, the most common risk in exercising is injury to the muscles and joints. Such injuries are usually caused by exercising too hard for too long, particularly if a person has been inactive. To avoid injuries, try to build up your level of activity gradually, listen to your body for warning pains, be aware of possible signs of heart problems (such as pain or pressure in the left or mid-chest

area, left neck, shoulder, or arm during or just after exercising, or sudden light-headedness, cold sweat, pallor, or fainting), and be prepared for special weather conditions.

10. *True*. You should ask your doctor before you start (or greatly increase) your physical activity **if** you have a medical condition such as high blood pressure, have pains or pressure in the chest and shoulder, feel dizzy or faint, get breathless after mild exertion, are middle-aged or older and have not been physically active, or plan a vigorous activity program. If none of these apply, start slow and get moving.
11. *False*. Regular physical activity can help reduce your risk of having another heart attack. People who include regular physical activity in their lives after a heart attack improve their chances of survival and can improve how they feel and look. If you have had a heart attack, consult your doctor to be sure you are following a safe and effective exercise program that will help prevent heart pain and further damage from overexertion.
12. *True*. Pick several different activities that you like doing. You will be more likely to stay with it. Plan short-term and long-term goals. Keep a record of your progress, and check it regularly to see the progress you have made. Get your family and friends to join in. They can help keep you going.

Reproduced from U.S. Department of Health and Human Services, National Institutes of Health, National Heart, Lung, and Blood Institute.

CHAPTER 11

CHANGING HEALTH HABITS

Do You Want to Be More Physically Active?

After completing the cardiorespiratory fitness assessment in the workbook, do you think you need to increase your physical activity level to become more fit? The "Deciding to Change" section of the Changing Health Habits worksheet can help you identify the health benefits of adding physical activity to your schedule and decide whether you are ready to do so. If you choose to increase your present level of physical activity, use the "Implementing the Change" section of the worksheet to help you.

Deciding to Change

1. Identify the problem, goal, or question.

   ____

   ____

2. List the reasons you should make this change and the reasons you should not. Assign each reason a point value from 1 to 5, with 5 being the highest (it has the most value to you) and 1 being the lowest (it has the least value to you).

Choices

Reasons to change behaviors (pros):		Reasons not to change behaviors (cons):	
Points	***Reasons***	***Points***	***Reasons***
___	____________	___	____________
___	____________	___	____________
___	____________	___	____________
___ Total		___ Total	

3. Draw a conclusion by adding the points in the pros section and then in the cons section. If the point total of the pros section is greater than the total of the cons section, you are probably ready to make a change that increases your level of physical activity. If your cons outweigh your pros, you may not be motivated to make the change now. Study your list of pros and cons carefully, however, before making your final decision. You may decide to change even if your reasons not to change outrank your reasons to change.

Implementing the Change

1. Set a target date to begin the new behavior or reach the goal.

2. Identify and list the factors that will help you reach your goal and those that will stand in the way of reaching your goal.

   Factors that help:

   Factors that hinder:

3. Prepare an action plan for making the change.
   a. Identify alternative methods for reaching your goal.

   b. Gather information about each method.
   c. Choose the method that fits your situation best.
   d. Consider the factors that can help or hinder your effort to change (see step 2).

   Factors that help:

   Factors that hinder:

4. Change the exercise-related behavior that you have decided to improve by implementing the action plan you developed in step 3.
5. Chart your daily progress toward your goal.
6. Evaluate how effective you were in reaching your goal.

Student Workbook

CHAPTER 12

Student Workbook

SELF-ASSESSMENT

What is Your Risk of Developing Heart Disease or Having a Heart Attack?

In general, the higher your LDL level and the more risk factors you have (other than LDL), the greater your chances of developing heart disease or having a heart attack. Some people are at high risk for a heart attack because they already have heart disease. Other people are at high risk for developing heart disease because they have diabetes (which is a strong risk factor) or a combination of risk factors for heart disease. Follow these steps to find out your risk for developing heart disease.

Step 1: Check the following table to see how many of the listed risk factors you have; these are the risk factors that affect your LDL goal.

Major Risk Factors That Affect Your LDL Goal
• Cigarette smoking
• High blood pressure (140/90 mmHg or higher or on blood pressure medication)
• Low HDL cholesterol (less than 40 mg/dl)*
• Family history of early heart disease (heart disease in father or brother before age 55; heart disease in mother or sister before age 65)
• Age (men 45 years or older; women 55 years or older)
* If your HDL cholesterol is 60 mg/dl or higher, subtract 1 from your total count.

Even though obesity and physical inactivity are not counted in this list, they are conditions that need to be corrected.

Step 2: How many major risk factors do you have? If you have two or more risk factors in the bulleted list above, use the risk scoring tables at the end of this assessment (which include your cholesterol levels) to find your risk score. Risk score refers to the chance of having a heart attack in the next 10 years, given as a percentage. My risk score is ________%.

Step 3: Use your medical history, number of risk factors, and risk score to find your risk of developing heart disease or having a heart attack in the following table.

If You Have	You Are in Category
Heart disease, diabetes, or risk score more than 20%*	I. High Risk
2 or more risk factors and risk score 10–20%	II. Next Highest Risk
2 or more risk factors and risk score less than 10%	III. Moderate Risk
0 or 1 risk factor	IV. Low-to-Moderate Risk
* Means that more than 20 of 100 people in this category will have a heart attack within 10 years.	

My risk category is ______________________.

Treating High Cholesterol

The main goal of cholesterol-lowering treatment is to lower your LDL level enough to reduce your risk of developing heart disease or having a heart attack. The higher your risk, the lower your LDL goal will be. To find your LDL goal, see the bulleted list that follows for your risk category. There are two main ways to lower your cholesterol:

1. Therapeutic lifestyle changes (TLC): Includes a cholesterol-lowering diet (called the TLC diet), physical activity, and weight management. TLC is for anyone whose LDL is above goal.
2. Drug treatment: If cholesterol-lowering drugs are needed, they are used together with TLC treatment to help lower your LDL.

If you are in . . .

- **Category I, Highest Risk**, your LDL goal is less than 100 mg/dl. You will need to begin the TLC diet to reduce your high risk even if your LDL is below 100 mg/dl. If your LDL is 100 or above, you will need to start drug treatment at the same time as the TLC diet. If your LDL is below 100 mg/dl, you may also need to start drug treatment together with the TLC diet if your doctor finds your risk is very high—for example, if you had a recent heart attack or have both heart disease and diabetes.
- **Category II, Next Highest Risk**, your LDL goal is less than 130 mg/dl. If your LDL is 130 mg/dl or above, you will need to begin treatment with the TLC diet. If your LDL is 130 mg/dl or more after 3 months on the TLC diet, you may need drug treatment along with the TLC diet. If your LDL is less than 130 mg/dl, you will need to follow the heart-healthy diet for all Americans, which allows a little more saturated fat and cholesterol than the TLC diet.
- **Category III, Moderate Risk**, your LDL goal is less than 130 mg/dl. If your LDL is 130 mg/dl or above, you will need to begin the TLC diet. If your LDL is 160 mg/dl or more after you have tried the TLC diet for 3 months, you may need drug treatment along with the TLC diet. If your LDL is less than 130 mg/dl, you will need to follow the heart-healthy diet for all Americans.
- **Category IV, Low-to-Moderate Risk**, your LDL goal is less than 160 mg/dl. If your LDL is 160 mg/dl or above, you will need to begin the TLC diet. If your LDL is still 160 mg/dl or more after 3 months on the TLC diet, you may need drug treatment along with the TLC diet to lower your LDL, especially if your LDL is 190 mg/dl or more. If your LDL is less than 160 mg/dl, you will need to follow the heart-healthy diet for all Americans.

To reduce your risk for heart disease or keep it low, it is very important to control any other risk factors you may have, such as high blood pressure and smoking.

Lowering Cholesterol with Therapeutic Lifestyle Changes

TLC is a set of things you can do to help lower your LDL cholesterol. The main parts of TLC are:

- *The TLC diet.* This is a low-saturated-fat, low-cholesterol eating plan that calls for less than 7% of calories from saturated fat and less than 200 mg of dietary cholesterol per day. The TLC diet recommends only enough calories to maintain a desirable weight and avoid weight gain. If your LDL is not lowered enough by reducing your saturated fat and cholesterol intakes, the amount of soluble fiber in your diet can be increased. Certain food products that contain plant stanols or plant sterols (for example, cholesterol-lowering margarines) can also be added to the TLC diet to boost its LDL-lowering power.
- *Weight management.* Losing weight if you are overweight can help lower LDL and is especially important for those with a cluster of risk factors that includes high triglyceride and/or low HDL levels and being overweight with a large waist measurement (more than 40 inches for men and more than 35 inches for women).
- *Physical activity.* Regular physical activity (30 minutes on most, if not all, days) is recommended for everyone. It can help raise HDL and lower LDL and is especially important for those with high triglyceride and/or low HDL levels who are overweight with a large waist measurement.

Foods low in saturated fat include fat-free or 1% dairy products, lean meats, fish, skinless poultry, whole-grain foods, and fruits and vegetables. Look for soft margarines (liquid or tub varieties) that are low in saturated fat and contain little or no trans fat (another type of dietary fat that can raise your cholesterol level). Limit foods high in cholesterol, such as liver and other organ meats, egg yolks, and full-fat dairy products.

Good sources of soluble fiber include oats, certain fruits (such as oranges and pears) and vegetables (such as brussels sprouts and carrots), and dried peas and beans.

Drug Treatment

Even if you begin drug treatment to lower your cholesterol, you will need to continue your treatment with lifestyle changes. This will keep the dose of medicine as low as possible, and lower your risk in other ways as well. There are several types of drugs available for cholesterol lowering, including statins, bile acid sequestrants, nicotinic acid, fibric acids, and cholesterol absorption inhibitors. Your doctor can help decide which type of drug is best for you. The statin drugs are very effective in lowering LDL levels and are safe for most people. Bile acid sequestrants also lower LDL and can be used alone or in combination with statin drugs. Nicotinic acid lowers LDL and triglycerides and raises HDL. Fibric acids lower LDL somewhat but are used mainly to treat high triglyceride and low HDL levels. Cholesterol absorption inhibitors lower LDL and can be used alone or in combination with statin drugs.

Note: Before beginning any diet and exercise regimen, you should speak with your physician to be sure it is right for you. Your physician will also advise you whether you should begin drug treatment to lower your cholesterol level.

Once your LDL goal has been reached, your doctor may prescribe treatment for high triglycerides and/or a low HDL level, if present. The treatment includes losing weight if needed, increasing physical activity, quitting smoking, and possibly taking a drug.

Resources

For more information about lowering cholesterol and lowering your risk for heart disease, write to the NHLBI Health Information Center, P.O. Box 30105, Bethesda, MD, 20824-0105 or call 301-592-8573.

Reproduced from National Heart, Lung, and Blood Institute. (2005). *High blood cholesterol: What you need to know*. Retrieved from http://www.nhlbi.nih.gov/health/public/heart/chol/hbc_what.htm.

Risk Scoring Tables: Estimate of Ten-Year Risk for Coronary Heart Disease

Men

(Framingham Point Scores)*

Age	Points
20–34	−9
35–39	−4
40–44	0
45–49	3
50–54	6
55–59	8
60–64	10
65–69	11
70–74	12
75–79	13

	Points				
Total Cholesterol	Age 20–39	Age 40–49	Age 50–59	Age 60–69	Age 70–79
<160	0	0	0	0	0
160–199	4	3	2	1	0
200–239	7	5	3	1	0
240–279	9	6	4	2	1
≥280	11	8	5	3	1

	Points				
	Age 20–39	Age 40–49	Age 50–59	Age 60–69	Age 70–79
Nonsmoker	0	0	0	0	0
Smoker	8	5	3	1	1

Women

(Framingham Point Scores)*

Age	Points
20–34	−7
35–39	−3
40–44	0
45–49	3
50–54	6
55–59	8
60–64	10
65–69	12
70–74	14
75–79	16

	Points				
Total Cholesterol	Age 20–39	Age 40–49	Age 50–59	Age 60–69	Age 70–79
<160	0	0	0	0	0
160–199	4	3	2	1	1
200–239	8	6	4	2	1
240–279	11	8	5	3	2
≥280	13	10	7	4	2

	Points				
	Age 20–39	Age 40–49	Age 50–59	Age 60–69	Age 70–79
Nonsmoker	0	0	0	0	0
Smoker	9	7	4	2	1

HDL (mg/dl)	Points
≥60	−1
50–59	0
40–49	1
<40	2

HDL (mg/dl)	Points
≥60	−1
50–59	0
40–49	1
<40	2

Systolic BP (mmHg)	If Untreated	If Treated
<120	0	0
120–129	0	1
130–139	1	2
140–159	1	2
≥160	2	5

Systolic BP (mmHg)	If Untreated	If Treated
<120	0	0
120–129	1	3
130–139	2	4
140–159	3	5
≥160	4	6

Point Total	10-Year Risk (%)
<0	<1
0	1
1	1
2	1
3	1
4	1
5	2
6	2
7	3
8	4
9	5
10	6
11	8
12	10
13	12
14	16
15	20
16	25
≥17	≥30

10-year risk ______%

Point Total	10-Year Risk (%)
<9	<1
9	1
10	1
11	1
12	1
13	2
14	2
15	3
16	4
17	5
18	6
19	8
20	11
21	14
22	17
23	22
24	27
≥25	≥30

10-year risk ______%

* Reproduced from The Framingham Heart Study is a long-term ongoing medical study conducted by the National Heart, Lung, and Blood Institute.

CHAPTER 12

CHANGING HEALTH HABITS

Reducing Your Risk of Cardiovascular Disease

In completing the "Applying What You Have Learned" questions for this chapter in the textbook, you analyzed your lifestyle to determine which modifiable risk factors are raising your probability of developing cardiovascular disease. Then you described how you could modify your behavior to lower your risk of developing cardiovascular disease. Pick one of these behaviors and take the following steps to facilitate change.

Deciding to Change

1. Identify the problem, goal, or question.

   ____

   ____

2. List the reasons you should make this change and the reasons you should not. Assign each reason a point value from 1 to 5, with 5 being the highest (it has the most value to you) and 1 being the lowest (it has the least value to you).

Choices

Reasons to change behaviors (pros):		Reasons not to change behaviors (cons):	
Points	***Reasons***	***Points***	***Reasons***
____	____________________	____	____________________
____	____________________	____	____________________
____	____________________	____	____________________
____	Total	____	Total

3. Draw a conclusion by adding the points in the pros section and then in the cons section. If the point total of the pros section is greater than the total of the cons section, you are probably ready to make a change in your life that reduces your risk of cardiovascular disease. If your cons outweigh your pros, you may not be motivated to make the change now. Study your list of pros and cons carefully, however, before making your final decision. You may decide to change even if your reasons not to change outrank your reasons to change.

Implementing the Change

1. Set a target date to begin the new behavior or reach the goal.

 ____

2. Identify and list the factors that will help you reach your goal and those that will stand in the way of reaching your goal.

 Factors that help: ______________________________

 ____

 ____

 ____

 Factors that hinder: ______________________________

 ____

 ____

 ____

3. Prepare an action plan for making the change.
   a. Identify alternative methods to reach your goal.

 ____

 ____

 ____

   b. Gather information about each method.
   c. Choose the method that fits your situation best.
   d. Consider the factors that can help or hinder your effort to change (see step 2).

 Factors that help: ______________________________

 ____

 ____

 ____

 Factors that hinder: ______________________________

 ____

 ____

 ____

4. Change the lifestyle behavior that you have decided to improve by implementing the action plan you developed in step 3.
5. Chart your daily progress toward your goal.
6. Evaluate how effective you were in reaching your goal.

 ____

 ____

 ____

 ____

 ____

 ____

SELF-ASSESSMENT

What Are Your Cancer Risks?

Breast or Ovarian Cancer

1. Are you female?	Yes	No
2. Do you have a family history of breast and/or ovarian cancer?	Yes	No
3. Are you over the age of 18?	Yes	No
4. Do you have at least one first-degree relative (mother, sister, or daughter) with breast or ovarian cancer?	Yes	No

If you answered yes to all of these questions, you may be at increased risk of developing breast or ovarian cancer.

Prostate Cancer

1. Are you male?	Yes	No
2. Are you African American?	Yes	No
3. Do you have a family history of prostate cancer?	Yes	No
4. Do you have one first-degree relative (father, brother, or son) with prostate cancer?	Yes	No
5. Was your relative diagnosed at a young age?	Yes	No

If you answered yes to most of these questions, or if you are an African American male, you may be at increased risk of developing prostate cancer.

Skin Cancer (Melanoma)

1. Do you have one or more first-degree relatives (parent, brother, sister, child) with a history of melanoma?	Yes	No
2. Do you experience severe blistering sunburns (especially at young ages)?	Yes	No
3. Do you sit in the sun with the purpose of getting tan, use tanning lamps, or tanning booths?	Yes	No
4. Do you have red or blond hair and fair skin that freckles or sunburns easily?	Yes	No

If you answered yes to any of these questions, you may be at increased risk of developing skin cancer (melanoma).

Liver Cancer

1. Have you been diagnosed with hepatitis B virus (HBV) or hepatitis C virus (HCV)?	Yes	No
2. Do you drink large amounts of alcohol?	Yes	No
3. Have you been diagnosed with cirrhosis of the liver (a progressive disorder that leads to scarring of the liver)?	Yes	No

If you answered yes to any of these questions, you may be at increased risk of developing liver cancer.

Gastrointestinal Cancer

1. Do you or one of your close relatives have a history of colorectal cancer, colon polyps, or other cancers (uterine, stomach, bile duct, urinary tract, or ovarian)?	Yes	No
2. Were you previously treated for colon cancer or polyps?	Yes	No
3. Do you have inflammatory bowel disease, such as ulcerative colitis or Crohn's disease?	Yes	No
4. Have you consumed foods that contain aflatoxins? Aflatoxins are a group of chemicals produced by a mold that can contaminate certain foods, such as peanuts, corn, grains, and seeds, and are carcinogens (cancer-causing agents) for liver cancer.	Yes	No

If you answered yes to one or more of these questions, you may be at increased risk of developing gastrointestinal cancer.

CHAPTER 13

CHANGING HEALTH HABITS

Modifying Behavior to Reduce Cancer Risk

Student Workbook

In completing the "Applying What You Have Learned" questions for this chapter in the textbook, you analyzed your lifestyle to determine which modifiable risk factors are raising your probability of developing cancer. Then you described how you could modify your behavior to lower your risk of developing cancer. Pick one of these behavior changes and follow the following steps to facilitate change.

Deciding to Change

1. Identify the problem, goal, or question.

   ____

   ____

2. List the reasons you should make this change and the reasons you should not. Assign each reason a point value from 1 to 5, with 5 being the highest (it has the most value to you) and 1 being the lowest (it has the least value to you).

Choices

Reasons to change behaviors (pros):

Points	***Reasons***
____	______________________
____	______________________
____	______________________
____	Total

Reasons not to change behaviors (cons):

Points	***Reasons***
____	______________________
____	______________________
____	______________________
____	Total

3. Draw a conclusion by adding the points in the pros section and then in the cons section. If the point total of the pros section is greater than the total of the cons section, you are probably ready to make a change that reduces your risk of cancer. If your cons outweigh your pros, you may not be motivated to make the change now. Study your list of pros and cons carefully, however, before making your final decision. You may decide to change even if your reasons not to change outrank your reasons to change.

Implementing the Change

1. Set a target date to begin the new behavior or reach the goal.

2. Identify and list the factors that will help you reach your goal and those that will stand in the way of reaching your goal.

   Factors that help:

   Factors that hinder:

3. Prepare an action plan for making the change.
   - **a.** Identify alternative methods for reaching your goal.
   - **b.** Gather information about each method.
   - **c.** Choose the method that fits your particular situation best.
   - **d.** Consider the factors that can help or hinder your effort to change (see step 2).

   Factors that help:

   Factors that hinder:

4. Change the lifestyle behavior that you have decided to improve by implementing the action plan you developed in step 3.
5. Chart your daily progress toward your goal.
6. Evaluate how effective you were in reaching your goal.

CHAPTER 14

SELF-ASSESSMENT

STI Attitude Scale

Directions

Please read each statement carefully: STIs are sexually transmitted infections, once called venereal diseases. Record your first reaction by circling the letter that best describes how much you agree or disagree with the idea.

Use this key:

SA = Strongly agree; A = Agree; U = Undecided;
D = Disagree; SD = Strongly disagree.

Remember: STIs means sexually transmitted infections, such as gonorrhea, syphilis, genital herpes, chlamydia, HPV, and AIDS.

1. How one uses his or her sexuality has nothing to do with STIs.
SA A U D SD

2. It is easy to use the prevention methods that reduce one's chances of getting an STI.
SA A U D SD

3. Responsible sex is one of the best ways of reducing the risk of STIs.
SA A U D SD

4. Getting early medical care is the main key to preventing harmful effects of STIs.
SA A U D SD

5. Choosing the right sex partner is important in reducing the risk of getting an STI.
SA A U D SD

6. A high rate of STIs should be a concern for all people.
SA A U D SD

7. People with an STI have a duty to get their sex partners to seek medical care.
SA A U D SD

8. The best way to get a sex partner to STI treatment is to take him or her to the doctor with you.
SA A U D SD

9. Changing one's sex habits is necessary once the presence of an STI is known.

SA A U D SD

10. I would dislike having to follow the medical steps for treating an STI.

SA A U D SD

11. If I were sexually active, I would feel uneasy doing things before and after sex to prevent getting an STI.

SA A U D SD

12. If I were sexually active, it would be insulting if a sex partner suggested we use a condom to avoid STIs.

SA A U D SD

13. I dislike talking about STIs with my peers.

SA A U D SD

14. I would be uncertain about going to the doctor unless I was sure I really had an STI.

SA A U D SD

15. I would feel that I should take my sex partner with me to a clinic if I thought I had an STI.

SA A U D SD

16. It would be embarrassing to discuss STIs with one's partner if one were sexually active.

SA A U D SD

17. If I were to have sex, the chance of getting an STI makes me uneasy about having sex with more than one person.

SA A U D SD

18. I like the idea of sexual abstinence (not having sex) as the best way of avoiding STIs.

SA A U D SD

19. If I had an STI, I would cooperate with public health persons to find the sources of the STI.

SA A U D SD

20. If I had an STI, I would avoid exposing others while I was being treated.

SA A U D SD

21. I would have regular STI checkups if I were having sex with more than one partner.

SA A U D SD

22. I intend to look for STI signs before deciding to have sex with anyone.

SA A U D SD

23. I will limit my sexual activity to just one partner because of the chances I might get an STI.

SA A U D SD

24. I will avoid sexual contact anytime I think there is even a slight chance of getting an STI.

SA A U D SD

25. The chance of getting an STI would not stop me from having sex.

SA A U D SD

26. If I had a chance, I would support community efforts toward controlling STIs.

SA A U D SD

27. I would be willing to work with others to make people aware of STI problems in my town.

SA A U D SD

Scoring Calculate total points for each subscale and total scale, using the point values below. For items 1, 10–14, 16, 25: Strongly agree = 5 points; Agree = 4 points; Undecided = 3 points; Disagree = 2 points; and Strongly disagree = 1 point.
For items 2–9, 15, 17–24, 26, 27: Strongly agree = 1 point; Agree = 2 points; Undecided = 3 points; Disagree = 4 points; and Strongly disagree = 5 points.

Total scale: items 1–27

Belief subscale: items 1–9

Feeling subscale: items 10–18

Intention to act subscale: items 19–27

Interpretation

High score predisposes one toward high-risk STI behavior. Low score predisposes one toward low-risk STI behavior.

Yarber, Torabi, and Veenker (1989) developed the STI Attitudes Scale by administering three experimental forms of 45 items each. Respondents were 2,980 students in six secondary school districts in the Midwest and East. Based on statistical analysis, the scale was reduced to the final 27 items. Reliability coefficients for the entire scale and the three subscales ranged from 0.48 to 0.73. The developers reported evidence of construct validity in that the scale was sensitive to positive attitude changes resulting from STI education.

CHAPTER 14

CHANGING HEALTH HABITS

Reducing Your Risk of Contracting an STI

In completing the "Applying What You Have Learned" questions for this chapter in the textbook, you analyzed your risk for contracting STIs. Then you determined what you could do to lower your risk of contracting a sexually transmitted infection. Pick one of these behavior changes and take the following steps to facilitate change.

Deciding to Change

1. Identify the problem, goal, or question.

 ____

 ____

2. List the reasons you should make this change and the reasons you should not. Assign each reason a point value from 1 to 5, with 5 being the highest (it has the most value to you) and 1 being the lowest (it has the least value to you).

Choices

Reasons to change behaviors (pros):		Reasons not to change behaviors (cons):	
Points	***Reasons***	***Points***	***Reasons***
____	____________	____	____________
____	____________	____	____________
____	____________	____	____________
____	Total	____	Total

3. Draw a conclusion by adding the points in the pros section and then in the cons section. If the point total of the pros section is greater than the total of the cons section, you are probably ready to make a change that reduces your risk of contracting an STI. If your cons outweigh your pros, you may not be motivated to make the change now. Study your list of pros and cons carefully, however, before making your final decision. You may decide to change even if your reasons not to change outrank your reasons to change.

Implementing the Change

1. Set a target date to begin the new behavior or reach the goal.

2. Identify and list the factors that will help you reach your goal and those that will stand in the way of reaching your goal.

   Factors that help:

   Factors that hinder:

3. Prepare an action plan for making the change.
   a. Identify alternative methods to reach your goal.

   b. Gather information about each method.
   c. Choose the method that fits your particular situation best.
   d. Consider the factors that can help or hinder your effort to change (see step 2).

   Factors that help:

   Factors that hinder:

4. Change the lifestyle behavior that you have decided to improve by implementing the action plan you developed in step 3.
5. Chart your daily progress toward your goal.
6. Evaluate how effective you were in reaching your goal.

Student Workbook

CHAPTER 15

SELF-ASSESSMENT

Preparing for Aging and Death

Answer the following questions. Depending on your situation, some of the questions may not apply.

1.	Are you doing anything to increase your chances of living a long and healthy life?	___ Yes	___ No
	If you answered yes, discuss the steps you are taking to live a long and healthy life.		
2.	How do you want to spend your retirement years? Are you doing anything to prepare for retirement?	___ Yes	___ No
	If you answered yes, what actions are you taking to prepare for retirement?		
3.	How do you feel about elderly people? Do you think they are "over the hill" and should be "put out to pasture?"	___ Yes	___ No
	Why do you feel this way about older adults?		
4.	Do you worry about growing old?	___ Yes	___ No
	If you do, what worries you about aging?		
5.	Have you prepared a will and a living will or durable power of attorney?	___ Yes	___ No
	If yes, have you informed your family about these documents?	___ Yes	___ No
	Have you selected a guardian for your children?	___ Yes	___ No
	Have you discussed guardianship with this individual?	___ Yes	___ No
6.	Have you thought about your funeral?	___ Yes	___ No
	If you have thought about your funeral, what kind of funeral would you want?		
	Do you want to be buried or cremated?		
	Have you discussed your wishes with your family?	___ Yes	___ No
	Have you made funeral prearrangements?	___ Yes	___ No
7.	Have you considered donating your body or your tissues or organs after your death?	___ Yes	___ No
	If you want to donate your body, tissues, or organs, have you made any preparations and informed relatives? Do you carry a card in your wallet that identifies you as a donor?	___ Yes	___ No
8.	If you were told that you have a terminal disease and have only 6 months to live, how would you spend these last months of your life?		
9.	Have you written your obituary?	___ Yes	___ No
	What would you like people to remember most about you?		

Examine your responses to these questions; there are no correct answers.

CHAPTER 15

CHANGING HEALTH HABITS

Can Changing a Health Habit Extend Your Life?

Do you have a habit, such as cigarette smoking, that increases your chances of dying prematurely? Which habit? The "Deciding to Change" section of the Changing Health Habits worksheet can help you determine whether you are ready to change this habit. If you decide to change, use the "Implementing the Change" section of the worksheet to help you make the necessary lifestyle changes.

Deciding to Change

1. Identify the problem, goal, or question.

   ____

   ____

2. List the reasons you should make this change and the reasons you should not. Assign each reason a point value from 1 to 5, with 5 being the highest (it has the most value to you) and 1 being the lowest (it has the least value to you).

Choices

Reasons to change behaviors (pros):

Points	*Reasons*
____	____________________
____	____________________
____	____________________
____	Total

Reasons not to change behaviors (cons):

Points	*Reasons*
____	____________________
____	____________________
____	____________________
____	Total

3. Draw a conclusion by adding the points in the pros section and then in the cons section. If the point total of the pros section is greater than the total of the cons section, you are probably ready to make the lifestyle changes necessary to change the unhealthy habit. If your cons outweigh your pros, you may not be motivated to make the change now. Study your list of pros and cons carefully, however, before making your final decision. You may decide to change even if your reasons not to change outrank your reasons to change.

Implementing the Change

1. Set a target date to begin the new behavior or reach the goal.

2. Identify and list the factors that will help you reach your goal and those that will stand in the way of reaching your goal.

   Factors that help:

   Factors that hinder:

3. Prepare an action plan for making the change.
   a. Identify alternative methods to reach your goal.

   b. Gather information about each method.
   c. Choose the method that fits your particular situation best.
   d. Consider the factors that can help or hinder your effort to change (see step 2).

   Factors that help:

   Factors that hinder:

4. Change the lifestyle behavior that you have decided to improve by implementing the action plan you developed in step 3.
5. Chart your daily progress toward your goal.
6. Evaluate how effective you were in reaching your goal.

Student Workbook

CHAPTER 16

SELF-ASSESSMENT 1

Poison Lookout Checklist

The home areas listed below are the most common sites of accidental poisonings. Follow this checklist to learn how to correct situations that may lead to poisonings. If you answer no to any questions, fix the situation quickly. Your goal is to have all your answers be yes.

The Kitchen

		Yes	No
1.	Do all harmful products in the cabinets have child-resistant caps? Products like furniture polishes, drain cleaners, and some oven cleaners should have safety packaging to keep little children from accidentally opening the packages.	___	___
2.	Are all potentially harmful products in their original containers? There are two dangers if products aren't stored in their original containers. Labels on the original containers often give first aid information if someone should swallow the product. And if products are stored in containers like drinking glasses or soda bottles, someone may think it is food and swallow it.	___	___
3.	Are harmful products stored away from food? If harmful products are placed next to food, someone may accidentally get a food and a poison mixed up and swallow the poison.	___	___
4.	Have all potentially harmful products been put up high and out of reach of children? The best way to prevent poisoning is making sure that it's impossible to find and get at the poisons. Locking all cabinets that hold dangerous products is the best poison prevention.	___	___

The Bathroom

		Yes	No
1.	Did you ever stop to think that medicines could poison if used improperly? Many children are poisoned each year by overdoses of aspirin. If aspirin can poison, just think of how many other poisons might be in your medicine cabinet.	___	___
2.	Do your aspirins and other potentially harmful products have child-resistant closures? Aspirins and most prescription drugs come with child-resistant caps. Check to see that yours have them, and that they are properly secured. Check your prescriptions before leaving the pharmacy to make sure the medicines are in child-resistant packaging. These caps have been shown to save the lives of children.	___	___

		Yes	No
3.	Have you thrown out all out-of-date prescriptions? As medicines get older, the chemicals inside them can change. So what was once a good medicine may now be a dangerous poison. Flush all old drugs down the toilet. Rinse the container well, then discard it.	___	___
4.	Are all medicines in their original containers with the original labels? Prescription medicines may or may not list ingredients. The prescription number on the label will, however, allow rapid identification by the pharmacist of the ingredients should they not be listed. Without the original label and container, you can't be sure of what you're taking. After all, aspirin looks a lot like poisonous roach tablets.	___	___
5.	If your vitamins or vitamin/mineral supplements contain iron, are they in child-resistant packaging? Most people think of vitamins and minerals as foods and, therefore, nontoxic, but a few iron pills can kill a child.	___	___

The Garage or Storage Area

Did you know that many things in your garage or storage area that can be swallowed are terrible poisons? Death may occur when people swallow such everyday substances as charcoal lighter, paint thinner and remover, antifreeze, and turpentine.

		Yes	No
1.	Do all these poisons have child-resistant caps?	___	___
2.	Are they stored in the original containers?	___	___
3.	Are the original labels on the containers?	___	___
4.	Have you made sure that no poisons are stored in drinking glasses or soda bottles?	___	___
5.	Are all these harmful products locked up and out of sight and reach?	___	___

When all your answers are yes, then continue this level of poison protection by making sure that whenever you buy potentially harmful products, they have child-resistant closures and are kept out of sight and reach. Post the number of the Poison Control Center near your telephone.

Courtesy of Consumer Product Safety Commission. CPSC Document 4383.

CHAPTER 16

SELF-ASSESSMENT 2

Checklist for the Prevention of Carbon Monoxide Poisoning

Carbon monoxide is often referred to as CO, which is its chemical symbol. Unlike many gases, CO is odorless, colorless, tasteless, and nonirritating. Red blood cells absorb CO over 200 times more readily than oxygen. As levels of CO in the air rise, this gas replaces oxygen in the bloodstream. As a result, body tissues are damaged and may die of a lack of oxygen. Knowing the major causes of carbon monoxide poisoning and using measures to eliminate them will prevent many needless tragedies.

The following questions relating to various areas in your environment will help you in dealing properly with the unseen, deadly hazard of carbon monoxide. The questions have been divided into sections that may directly apply to your particular situation. You can compare your answers with the correct explanation provided at the end of the list of questions.

Questions

Draw a circle around your answer.

The Home, Cabin, and Camper

Most questions will apply equally to homeowners, campers, and to those who rent. Renters, however, should refer any questions regarding maintenance to the management.

1.	Have you had the fireplace draft and the drafts of other fuel-burning appliances checked by an expert within the past year?	Yes	No
2.	Have all gas appliances been checked annually for proper operation?	Yes	No
3.	Are all combustion appliances properly vented?	Yes	No
4.	Has your chimney vent been checked for defects within the past year?	Yes	No
5.	Have you patched any vent pipe with tape, gum, or other substances?	Yes	No
6.	Are all horizontal vent pipes to fuel appliances perfectly level?	Yes	No
7.	Do you use your gas range or oven for heating?	Yes	No
8.	Does the cooling unit of your gas refrigerator give off an odor?	Yes	No
9.	Have you ever used a charcoal grill such as a barbecue grill for cooking within your home, cabin, or camper other than in a vented fireplace?	Yes	No
10.	Have you ever brought burning charcoal into your home, cabin, or camper for heating purposes?	Yes	No

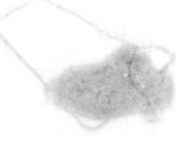

11.	Do you consider portable flameless chemical heaters (catalytic) safe for use in your cabin, camper, or home?	Yes	No
12.	Have you ever used a portable gas camp stove in your home, cabin, or camper for heating purposes?	Yes	No

The Auto

13.	Have you had a reliable mechanic check the exhaust system of your car within the past year?	Yes	No
14.	Do you ever run your auto engine in the garage while the garage door is shut?	Yes	No
15.	Do you leave the door closed between your attached garage and your house when you run your car engine?	Yes	No
16.	Do you keep your windows slightly open while driving in heavy traffic, although you have an air conditioner?	Yes	No
17.	While driving your station wagon, do you lower the tailgate to get a greater flow of air in the car?	Yes	No

Other

18.	When you are selecting gas equipment, do you buy only those items that carry the seal of a national testing agency, such as the American Gas Association or the Underwriters' Laboratory?	Yes	No
19.	Have you ever converted, or are you about to convert, a fuel burner from one fuel to another without having it done by an expert?	Yes	No
20.	As an overnight guest at motels or hotels that have heating units located in the room, do you read operating instructions or ask how such appliances operate?	Yes	No

Correct Answers

The Home, Cabin, and Camper

1. *Yes.* A yearly checkup of all fuel-burning venting systems in the home is desirable.
2. *Yes.* A yearly checkup of all combustion appliances is suggested. In many areas, upon request, the gas company will provide this service.
3. *Yes.* All gas appliances must have adequate ventilation so that CO will not accumulate.
4. *Yes.* Chimney vents often become blocked by debris, causing a buildup of CO. They should be checked annually.
5. *No.* Often a makeshift patch can lead to an accumulation of CO, and therefore should be avoided.
6. *No.* In-room vent pipes should be on a slight incline as they go toward the exterior. This will reduce leaking of toxic gases in case the joints or pipes are improperly fitted.
7. *No.* Using a gas range for heating can result in the accumulation of CO.
8. *No.* An unusual odor from a gas refrigerator often is the result of defects within the cooling unit. Odorless CO also may be given off.
9. *No.* The use of barbecue grills indoors will quickly result in dangerous levels of CO.
10. *No.* Burning charcoal—whether black, red, gray, or white—gives off CO.
11. *No.* Although catalytic heaters produce heat without flame, combustion is occurring that can cause the production of CO.

12. *No.* Using a gas camp stove for heating the home, cabin, or camper can result in the accumulation of CO.

The Auto

13. *Yes.* Small leaks in the exhaust system of a car can lead to an accumulation of CO in the interior.
14. *No.* CO can rapidly build up while your auto engine is operated in a closed garage. Never run your car in a garage unless the outside door is open to provide ventilation.
15. *Yes.* CO can easily escape from a garage through a connecting door that opens into the house, although the garage door is open. Doors connecting a garage and house should be kept closed when the auto is running.
16. *Yes.* Even with an air conditioner, CO can be drawn into a car while it is being driven slowly in heavy traffic. Therefore, windows should be slightly opened.
17. *No.* If the tailgate is open, be sure to open vents or windows to increase the flow of air in the car. If the tailgate window is open and the other windows or the vents are closed, CO from the exhaust will be drawn into the car.

Other

18. *Yes.* Buy only equipment carrying the seal of a national testing agency; otherwise, one may get poorly designed equipment, which may soon result in the production of CO.
19. *No.* An expert is needed to make proper modifications and to evaluate the venting capabilities of your appliance.
20. *Yes.* Even with adequately designed and properly installed heating equipment, the improper operation of this equipment can result in its malfunctioning and lead to the production of CO. Therefore, be sure you understand the correct way to operate any fuel-burning appliance before using it.

Courtesy of Centers for Disease Control and Prevention. HEW Pub. No.(CDC) 77 8335.

CHAPTER 16

CHANGING HEALTH HABITS

Can You Reduce Environmental Threats to Your Health?

In completing the "Applying What You Have Learned" questions for this chapter, you analyzed your interactions with the environment to develop a list of environmental threats to your health. Determine ways in which you could change your behavior to remove or reduce these environmental threats. Pick one of these behaviors and use the following steps to facilitate change.

Deciding to Change

1. Identify the problem, goal, or question.

   ____

   ____

2. List the reasons you should make this change and the reasons you should not. Assign each reason a point value from 1 to 5, with 5 being the highest (it has the most value to you) and 1 being the lowest (it has the least value to you).

Choices

Reasons to change behaviors (pros):		Reasons not to change behaviors (cons):	
Points	***Reasons***	***Points***	***Reasons***
____	__________________	____	__________________
____	__________________	____	__________________
____	__________________	____	__________________
____ Total		____ Total	

3. Draw a conclusion by adding the points in the pros section and then in the cons section. If the point total of the pros section is greater than the total of the cons section, you are probably ready to make a change in your life that reduces environmental risks to your health. If your cons outweigh your pros, you may not be motivated to make the change now. Study your list of pros and cons carefully, however, before making your final decision. You may decide to change even if your reasons not to change outrank your reasons to change.

Implementing the Change

1. Set a target date to begin the new behavior.

2. Identify and list the factors that will help you change this behavior and those that will stand in your way.

   Factors that help:

   Factors that hinder:

3. Prepare an action plan for making the change.

   a. Identify alternative methods for reaching your goal.

   b. Gather information about each method.

   c. Choose the method that fits your particular situation best.

   d. Consider the factors that can help or hinder your effort to change (see step 2).

   Factors that help:

   Factors that hinder:

4. Change the lifestyle behavior that you have decided to improve by implementing the action plan you developed in step 3.
5. Chart your daily progress toward your goal.
6. Evaluate how effective you were in reaching your goal.

Student Workbook

Glossary

abortion Removal of the embryo or fetus from the uterus before it is able to survive on its own.

absorption The passage of nutrients through the walls of the intestinal tract.

abstinence A method of birth control that involves refraining from vaginal intercourse.

abuse Taking advantage of a relationship to mistreat a person.

acid precipitation Rain, snow, or fog combined with sulfur dioxide from fossil fuel emissions.

acquired immune deficiency syndrome (AIDS) A set of certain diseases and conditions that results from infection by the human immunodeficiency virus (HIV).

acquired immunity Specific resistance to infection that is not inherited but develops during a person's lifetime.

acute A condition or illness that tends to develop quickly and resolve within a few days or weeks.

acute bronchitis A temporary inflammation of the mucous membranes.

adipose cells Cells that store fat.

aerobic Oxygen-requiring.

affect Observable expressions of mood.

affection Fondness.

ageism A bias against elderly people.

aging The sum of all changes that occur to an organism during its life.

Air Quality Index (AQI) A guide to air quality that uses levels of various pollutants to determine its values.

alcohol abuse Includes the symptoms of harmful use, but when drinking the abuser exhibits long-term social interaction problems and uses alcohol in physically dangerous situations.

alcohol dependence (alcoholism) A syndrome characterized by at least three of the following symptoms: a compulsion to drink, difficulty in controlling the amount of alcohol consumed, withdrawal symptoms when alcohol is not consumed, evidence of tolerance, progressive neglect of other interests because of drinking, and continuing to use alcohol despite its physical and psychological effects on the user.

Alzheimer's disease (AD) An incurable, progressive, degenerative disease that affects the functioning of the brain.

amino acids The chemical units that compose proteins.

amniocentesis A prenatal test performed generally between the 15th and 18th weeks of gestation, in which some of the amniotic fluid that surrounds the fetus is removed and studied to determine whether the fetus has a genetic abnormality.

anabolic steroids A group of drugs that can have muscle-building effects on the body.

analgesics (an-al-GEEZ-iks) Drugs that alleviate pain.

analogs Drugs that are chemically similar but have different effects on the body.

anecdotes Personal reports of individual experiences.

anesthetic Substance that interferes with normal sensations.

aneurysm (AN-you-rizm) A swollen, weakened blood vessel.

angina pectoris (an-JEYE-nah PECK-tor-iss) Chest pain caused by insufficient oxygen in a portion of the heart.

angioplasty (AN-jee-oh-PLAS-tee) The reconstruction of damaged blood vessels.

anorexia nervosa A severe psychological disturbance in which an individual refuses to eat enough food to maintain a healthy weight.

antibiotics (AN-tie-by-OT-iks) A group of chemicals that kill bacteria or inhibit their growth.

antibodies Proteins that interact in a lock-and-key fashion with antigens, interfering with the normal functioning of the antigen.

antigens (AN-tih-jenz) Proteins that are foreign or recognized as "nonself" by the body.

antioxidants Compounds that protect cells from free-radical damage.

appetite The psychological desire to eat foods that are appealing.

arrhythmias (uh-RITH-me-uhs) Abnormal heartbeats.

arteries Blood vessels that carry blood away from the heart.

arthritis A group of diseases characterized by inflammation of the joints.

asbestos (as-BES-tose) A fiber-like mineral found in rocks that, when inhaled, can cause lung cancer or other lung conditions.

asbestosis (AS-bes-TOE-sis) A condition in which scar tissue forms in the lungs as a response to irritation by asbestos.

assault The intentional use of force to injure another person physically.

asthma (AZ-mah) A common, chronic, childhood illness characterized by sensitive airways.

atherectomy (ATH-er-EK-toe-me) The removal of plaque from the interior of an artery.

atherosclerosis (ATH-er-oh-skle-ROW-sis) Disease of large and medium-sized arteries in which the inner lining has areas that are deteriorated, thickened, and inelastic.

atrial fibrillation (fih-brih-LAY-shun) A type of arrhythmia in which the upper chambers of the heart contract with no set pattern.

atrophy A condition in which muscles lose size and strength.

attachment The desire to spend time with someone to give and receive emotional support.

autoimmune diseases Diseases in which the body perceives its own cells as foreign, attacking them and causing localized and systemic (whole-body) reactions.

autonomy Sense of independence and self-control.

autopsy Various medical examinations and tests that usually determine the cause of death.

B cells Specialized white blood cells (lymphocytes) that function in antibody-mediated immunity and produce antibodies.

bacteria Unicellular, microscopic organisms with a simple cell structure; some are pathogenic to humans and produce infections such as strep throat, bacterial pneumonia, food poisoning, and infected cuts.

barrier methods Types of birth control that block the path that sperm must take to reach the ovum; these forms of contraception include male condoms, female condoms, diaphragms, and cervical caps.

basal (BAY-sl) cell carcinoma The most common cancer of the skin, which frequently develops on portions of the skin exposed to the sun.

benign (be-NINE) tumors Encapsulated masses of abnormal cells that remain in one location and do not invade surrounding tissues.

binge eating disorder A pattern of eating excessive amounts of food in response to distress such as anxiety or depression.

biopsy (BI-op-see) A small piece of tissue that is taken from a growth so that the cells can be studied and a diagnosis confirmed.

birth control (contraception) Methods to avoid pregnancy.

bisexual A person who engages in sexual activity with both sexes.

body mass index (BMI) A standard that correlates body weight with the risk of developing chronic health conditions associated with obesity.

Braxton-Hicks contractions False labor; preparatory contractions that are not a part of labor.

breech birth A delivery in which the baby presents feet or buttocks first instead of the usual head-first position.

bulimia nervosa An eating disorder characterized by a craving for food that is difficult to satisfy.

calorie A unit of energy.

cancer screening An examination to detect malignancies in a person who has no symptoms.

cancer staging A description of the extent of the growth and metastasis of a cancer to determine appropriate therapy and prognosis.

capillaries (KAP-ih-LAIR-eez) Microscopic blood vessels that permeate tissues, connecting small arteries to small veins.

carbohydrates A class of nutrients that includes sugars and starches.

carbon monoxide poisoning A toxic condition that affects red blood cells' ability to carry oxygen, caused by the inhalation of the gas carbon monoxide.

carcinogens (kar-SIN-oh-jenz) Cancer-causing substances.

carcinomas (KAR-si-NO-mahz) Cancers that arise from epithelial tissues.

cardiorespiratory fitness The ability to perform muscular work intensely and for long periods without becoming fatigued.

cardiovascular disease (CVD) Disorders of the heart and blood vessels.

caring The expression of concern for someone's -well-being.

carpal tunnel syndrome Numbness, pain, or pins-and-needles sensations in either of the hands that extends down the fingers, resulting from improper alignment of the wrist while engaging in repetitive-use activities.

cataracts A chronic condition in which the lens of the eye becomes cloudy and opaque, impairing vision.

celiac disease A condition characterized by hypersensitivity to gluten.

celibacy (sexual abstinence) Refrainment from sexual intercourse, usually by choice.

central nervous system (CNS) Of the two primary divisions of the nervous system, the one that consists of brain and spinal cord.

cerebral embolism A stroke caused by a floating blood clot that becomes lodged in a cerebral artery, blocking blood flow.

cerebral hemorrhage (HEM-ah-rij) A stroke caused by a burst artery that supplies the brain.

cerebral thrombosis A stroke caused by a stationary blood clot.

cervix The narrow neck of the uterus.

chain of infection The relationship among the factors important in the development of infectious diseases: the pathogen, transmission, and the host.

child physical abuse Physical violence against a child who is under 18 years of age.

child sexual abuse Sexual activity involving a child that takes place as a result of force or threat.

chlamydial (klah-MID-dee-ahl) infection An STI that results in gonorrhea-like symptoms.

cholesterol A type of lipid found only in animals.

MyPlate A practical guide for planning healthful diets.

chorionic villus sampling (CVS) A prenatal test performed generally between the 10th and 12th weeks of gestation, in which some of the fetal extraembryonic tissue is removed and analyzed to determine whether the fetus has a genetic abnormality.

chronic A condition or disease that often takes months or years to develop, progresses in severity, and can affect a person over a longer period.

chronic bronchitis A persistent inflammation and thickening of the lining of the bronchi.

chronic obstructive pulmonary disease (COPD) A syndrome that includes chronic bronchitis, asthma, and emphysema and that is characterized by extreme difficulty in breathing.

clitoris (KLIT-oh-ris) A female organ of sexual arousal. Located under a protective hood of tissue, the clitoris lies in front of the urethra.

cohabitation Unmarried persons living together.

coitus (KO-ih-tus) The act of a penis penetrating a vagina, often referred to as vaginal intercourse.

coitus interruptus (withdrawal) (KO-ih-tus in-ter-RUP-tus) A form of birth control in which the man removes his penis from his partner's vagina and genital area, interrupting intercourse before ejaculation.

colon Major segment of the large intestine.

colonoscopy (KO-lon-OS-ko-pee) A procedure in which a physician views the entire length of the colon using a flexible fiber-optic tube.

comatose Condition in which one is unresponsive to the environment and in a coma.

combined oral contraceptives "The pill" suppress ovulation through the combined actions of estrogen and progestin.

commitment The determination to maintain a relationship even when times are difficult.

communicable (ka-MYOO-ni-kah-bl) Transmissible from person to person.

community violence Violence between strangers or acquaintances that occurs in public settings.

compatible Capable of existing together in harmony.

compulsion The behavior that follows obsessive thoughts and reduces anxiety.

condom A sheath used to cover the penis during sexual intercourse to help prevent pregnancy or sexually transmitted infections.

constipation A condition characterized by having fewer than three bowel movements per week.

conventional medicine Form of medicine that relies on modern scientific principles, modern technolo-gies, and scientifically proven methods to prevent, diagnose, and treat health conditions.

coping strategies Behavioral responses and thought processes that people use to deal with stressors.

coronary arteries Blood vessels that arise from the base of the aorta and bring freshly oxygenated blood to the heart muscle.

coronary artery bypass graft (CABG) surgery A surgical procedure in which healthy blood vessels are used to redirect blood flow around blocked vessels of the heart.

coronary artery disease (CAD) A condition in which the coronary vessels are blocked partially or completely by fatty deposits, blood clots, or both. Also commonly called coronary heart disease (CHD).

coronary embolism (EM-bow-lizm) A floating blood clot that lodges in an artery that brings blood to the heart muscle, blocking blood flow.

coronary thrombosis (throm-BOW-sis) The development of a stationary blood clot that blocks blood flow in an artery that brings blood to the heart muscle.

corpus luteum (KOR-pus LOO-tea-um) The ruptured follicle left behind after ovulation.

cross-training Incorporating a variety of aerobic activities into a fitness program.

cunnilingus Use of the mouth and tongue to stimulate a woman's genitals.

cystic fibrosis (SIS-tik fie-BROH-sis) (CF) A common, lethal, inherited disease that affects the glands that secrete mucus and sweat, resulting in multiple disorders of the lungs and pancreas.

death The cessation of life, which occurs soon after a person's heart or lungs stop functioning.

defense mechanisms Ways of thinking and behaving that reduce or eliminate anxious and guilt feelings.

delusions Inaccurate and unreasonable beliefs that often result in decision-making errors.

dementia A brain disorder that seriously affects normal cognitive abilities.

detoxification The process of converting harmful substances into less dangerous compounds.

detraining A condition characterized by atrophied and weak muscles, which occurs when skeletal muscles are not used regularly.

diabetes mellitus ("diabetes") A group of chronic diseases characterized by the inability to metabolize carbohydrates properly.

diastolic (DIE-as-TOL-ik) pressure The lower number in the blood pressure reading, which is the pressure exerted by the blood on the artery walls when the left ventricle relaxes.

diet One's usual pattern of food choices.

dietary fiber Indigestible substances produced by plants.

Dietary Reference Intakes (DRIs) A set of standards for evaluating the nutritional quality of diets.

dietary supplement A product that is consumed to add nutrients, herbs, or other plant materials to a person's diet.

digestion The process of breaking down large food molecules into smaller molecules that the intestinal tract can absorb.

digital rectal exam A test in which a physician uses a gloved finger to feel the rectum or the prostate for abnormal growths.

disease A process that affects the proper functioning of the body and is usually accompanied by characteristic signs and symptoms.

distress Events or conditions that produce unwanted or negative outcomes.

diverticulosis An intestinal disorder that occurs when the colon lining forms small pouches that protrude through the outer wall of the colon.

douching (DOOSH-ing) The use of specially prepared solutions to cleanse the vagina; not an effective birth control method.

Down syndrome A genetic disease usually caused by the presence of three (rather than two) number 21 chromosomes; the child is usually intellectually disabled, with a short body and a broad, flat face.

drug abuse The intentional improper or nonmedical use of any drug.

drug dependence or addiction Occurs when users develop a habitual pattern of taking drugs that produces a compulsive need, which is both physical and psychological.

drug misuse The temporary and improper use of a legal drug.

drugs Nonfood chemicals that alter the way a person thinks, feels, functions, or behaves.

Duchenne/Becker muscular dystrophy (do-SHAYN BECK-er MUSS-ku-lar DIS-tro-fee) (DBMD) An inherited disease in which the muscles gradually weaken and degenerate. It usually strikes boys before the age of 6 years.

eating disorders Persistent, abnormal eating patterns that can threaten a person's health and well-being.

efficacy (EF-fih-ka-see) Regarding health education, the belief that one is capable of changing his or her behavior.

ejaculation The emission of semen from the penis during orgasm.

elder abuse Use of physical or sexual violence against an elderly person.

embolus (EM-bow-lus) A floating blood clot.

embryo The 3rd through 8th weeks of gestational development.

emergency contraception (EC) Birth control methods that help prevent pregnancy after sexual intercourse, rather than before or during sex.

emphysema (EM-fih-SEE-mah) A chronic condition in which the air sacs of the lungs lose their normal elasticity, impairing respiration.

endocrine system A group of glands that produce hormones.

endometrium (EN-doe-ME-tree-um) The inner lining of the uterus.

environmental health The effects of environmental factors on humans and the effects of humans on their environments.

environmental tobacco smoke (ETS) The smoke emitted from a lit cigarette, cigar, or pipe and the smoke exhaled by smokers.

epididymis (EP-ih-DID-ih-mis) A coiled tube that lies on the back of each testis and in which sperm mature.

episiotomy (uh-pee-zee-OT-uh-me) A cut in the tissue surrounding the vaginal opening to widen it during a vaginal delivery so that the surrounding skin and tissues will be less likely to tear.

erectile dysfunction (ED) A sexual dysfunction in which a man is unable to develop and/or sustain an erection firm enough for penetration of the vagina. Also called impotence.

ergogenic aids A variety of products that supposedly enhance physical development or performance.

estrogen (ES-tro-jen) A hormone secreted by ovarian follicles, the groups of cells within which ova mature. With progesterone, estrogen stimulates the continued development and thickening of the uterine lining.

euphoria (you-FOR-ee-a) An intense feeling of well-being commonly called a "high."

eustress (YOU-stress) Events or conditions that create positive effects, such as making one feel happy, challenged, or successful.

exercise Physical activity that is usually planned and performed to improve or maintain one's physical condition.

extrarelational sex Sexual relationships with individuals who are not one's spouse or primary sex partner.

fad diets Eating plans that are popular for a time, then quickly lose their widespread appeal.

family (domestic) violence Violence or abuse between family members, people who are involved in intimate relationships, or unrelated individuals who live together.

fecal occult (FEE-kle ok-KULT) blood test (FOBT) Home test that detects hidden blood in the stool.

fellatio Use of the mouth and tongue to stimulate a male's genitals.

fetal alcohol spectrum disorders (FASDs) A variety of incurable conditions and birth defects caused by alcohol exposure during prenatal development.

fetal alcohol syndrome (FAS) The most severe FASD. Children born with FAS may suffer intellectual disability and have characteristic facial anomalies, growth deficiency, and central nervous system abnormalities.

fetus The 9th through 38th weeks of gestational development.

fight-or-flight response The physical responses to stressful situations that enable the body to confront or leave dangerous situations.

flexibility The ability to move a muscle to any position in its normal range of motion.

follicles Masses of cells in the ovaries that contain immature ova (eggs) in various stages of development. Each follicle contains one ovum.

formaldehyde (form-AL-de-hide) A chemical used in the manufacture of certain building materials and furnishings; may cause health problems when released into indoor air.

fungi (FUN-jeye) Cellular organisms that cannot make their own food; some are pathogenic to humans and produce infections such as athlete's foot, ringworm, and yeast infections. *Fungus* is the singular term.

gender identity An individual's perception of himself or herself as male or female.

gender role Patterns of behavior, attitudes, and personality attributes that are traditionally considered in a particular culture to be feminine or masculine.

gender The classification of a person's sex based on many criteria, among them anatomic and chromosomal characteristics.

general adaptation syndrome (GAS) The three-stage manner in which the human body responds to stress: alarm, resistance, and exhaustion.

generalized anxiety disorder A condition characterized by uncontrollable chronic worrying and nervousness.

genes Segments of DNA.

genital herpes An STI caused by the herpes simplex virus that results in sores in the genital and anal areas.

genital warts An STI caused by the human papillomavirus that results in noncancerous skin tumors of the genital area.

genomics (Jee-nom-iks) The scientific study of an organism's entire set of genes.

gerontologists Scientists who study aging.

glaucoma (glaw-KO-mah) A chronic ailment that occurs when fluid pressure increases in the eye.

glucose The most important monosaccharide in the human body.

gonorrhea (GON-ah-REE-ah) An STI characterized by infection of the urethra in men and the cervix in women, usually resulting in a thick discharge from the penis or vagina.

good health The ability to function adequately and independently in a constantly changing environment.

grief The emotional state that nearly everyone experiences when they lose something or someone special.

hallucinations False sensory perceptions that have no apparent external cause.

harmful use Drinking alcoholic beverages while knowingly damaging one's physical and/or psychological health.

hazardous waste Toxic chemical refuse.

heart attack Myocardial infarction (MI); an area of heart muscle that dies because it does not receive enough oxygen as a result of insufficient blood supply.

heart failure Ineffective pumping of the heart, which results in the overfilling of the veins that bring blood to the heart.

heat cramps In a dehydrated and hot person, the signs and symptoms of heat cramps include muscular tightening and pain in the limbs or abdomen.

heat exhaustion A serious form of heat illness.

heatstroke A life-threatening form of heat illness.

hemorrhoids Painfully swollen veins in the rectal and anal areas.

hepatitis B virus (HBV) A serious infectious disease of the liver transmitted via blood or blood products.

heredity The transmission of biological information, coded within genes, from parents to offspring.

heterosexual A person who is sexually attracted to members of the opposite sex.

high-density lipoproteins (HDL) (LIP-oh-PRO-teenz or LIE-poe-PRO-teenz) "Good" cholesterol that carries cholesterol from the cells and to the liver for removal from the body.

holistic (hole-IS-tic) A characteristic involving all aspects of the person.

homophobia An intense fear of or hostility toward homosexuals.

homosexual A person who is sexually attracted to members of his or her own sex.

hormones Chemical messengers that convey information from a gland to other cells in the body.

hospice A form of health care specifically designed to give emotional support and pain relief to terminally ill people in the final stage of life.

host In reference to disease, an organism that supports the growth of a pathogen; the third, and last, link in the chain of infection.

human chorionic gonadotropin (hCG) In a pregnant woman, a hormone produced by embryonic tissues destined to become the placenta. Pregnancy tests rely on the detection of this hormone in the blood.

hunger The physiologic drive to seek and eat food.

hypertension Persistently high arterial blood pressure.

hyperthermia A condition that occurs when body temperature rises above the normal range.

hypertrophy A condition in which muscles become larger and stronger.

hypnotics Drugs that produce trancelike effects.

hypothermia Condition that occurs when the body's core temperature drops below 95°F.

immune system A collection of cells and organs of the body that recognizes and combats pathogens and other foreign substances with cells and proteins that are specific for particular invaders; The specific defenses of the body that include combating infectious agents. The immune system has two branches: antibody-mediated immunity and cell-mediated immunity.

immunity (im-MYOU-nih-tea) Resistance to disease.

immunotherapy Manipulation of the body's immune system to rid the body of cancer.

incest Sexual relations between family members who are not spouses.

infectious (in-FEK-shus) disease A disease caused by bacteria, rickettsias, viruses, fungi, protozoans, or parasitic worms.

infertility Inability to conceive a child after 1 year of unprotected sex.

inherited disease A genetic disease transmitted solely by gene transfer from parents to offspring.

institutional violence Violence that occurs mainly in institutional settings such as college campuses or workplaces.

integrative medicine System of medical care that emphasizes personalized health care and disease prevention.

interferons (IN-ter-FEAR-onz) Proteins produced by the body during a viral infection that protect uninfected cells from viral invasion.

intestinal ulcer A sore in the lining of the eso-phagus, stomach, or duodenum.

intimacy Disclosure of one's most personal thoughts and emotions to a trusted individual.

intoxication Impairment of the functioning of the central nervous system as a result of ingesting toxic substances such as alcohol. The state of being poisoned by a drug or other toxic substance.

intrauterine device (IUD) A small contraceptive device that either is covered with copper or contains a reservoir of progestin and is inserted into the uterus.

ischemia (is-KI-me-ah) Insufficient blood in part of the heart.

isometric A type of exercise in which the individual exerts muscular force against a fixed, immovable object.

isotonic A type of exercise in which the individual exerts muscular force against a movable but constant source of resistence.

joints The places where two or more bones come together.

labia majora (LAY-bee-ah mah-JOR-ah) Hairy, rounded, and thick folds of skin that lie adjacent to the labia minora and extend forward to unite at the mons pubis.

labia minora (LAY-bee-ah my NOR-ah) Two thin, hairless folds of skin that extend from over the clitoris to an area behind the vagina. The labia minor cover and protect the vaginal opening ad urethra.

labor (parturition) (PAR-too-RISH-un) The process of childbirth.

lead poisoning A toxic condition that affects the central nervous system, caused by the ingestion or inhalation of the metallic element lead.

leukemias (lew-KEY-me-ahz) Cancers of the blood and related cells.

leukocytes (LEWK-oh-sites) White blood cells; active in both specific and nonspecific defenses of the body.

life expectancy The average number of years that an individual of a particular age can expect to live.

life span The maximum number of years that members of a species can expect to live when conditions are optimal.

lifestyle A way of living including behaviors that promote or impair good health and longevity.

ligaments Tough bands of connective tissue that hold bones together at joints.

lipids A class of nutrients that includes triglycerides and cholesterol.

low-density lipoproteins (LDL) "Bad" cholesterol that carries cholesterol to the cells, including the cells that line the blood vessel walls.

lumpectomy (lum-PECK-toe-me) Surgical removal of a breast tumor, including a layer of surrounding tissue.

lymph (limf) Tissue fluid.

lymphomas (lim-FOE-mahz) Cancers of the lymphatic system.

macular degeneration A leading cause of vision loss for people age 60 years and older.

major depressive disorder A mood disorder characterized by persistent and profound sadness, hopelessness, helplessness, and feelings of worthlessness; lack of energy; loss of interest in usual activities; loss of the ability to concentrate; suicidal thoughts; and appetite and sleep disturbances.

malignant melanoma (MEL-ah-NO-mah) A deadly form of skin cancer that develops most often in persons who have been exposed to the sun in short, intense sessions, have had severe sunburn and extensive sun exposure in childhood, or have first-degree relatives who had the disease.

malignant (mah-LIG-nant) tumors Masses of cancer cells that invade body tissues and interfere with the normal functioning of tissues and organs.

malnutrition Overnutrition or undernutrition that results when diets supply improper amounts of nutrients.

medical abortion A method of drug-induced abortion performed within 9 weeks of the first day of the last period.

Medicare A federal health insurance program that provides benefits for people 65 years of age and older.

meditation An activity in which one relaxes by mentally focusing on a single word, object, or thought.

menarche (meh-NAR-key) The first menstruation.

menses (MEN-seez) The menstrual period; the sloughing of the endometrium.

menstrual (MEN-strool-al) cycle The monthly changes in the levels of the female sex hormones that orchestrate physiologic changes in the ovaries and uterus.

metabolic rate The amount of energy the body requires to fuel cellular activities during a specified time.

metabolism All chemical reactions that take place in the body.

metastasize (meh-TAS-tah-size) The ability of cancer cells to spread from where they develop to another part of the body.

minerals A class of inorganic nutrients that includes several elements, such as iron, calcium, and zinc.

mons pubis A mound of fatty tissue that lies over the pubic bone, cushioning it.

motivation The force or drive that leads people to take action.

mourning The culturally defined way in which survivors observe bereavement.

municipal solid waste Nonhazardous refuse generally collected from homes and offices.

muscular endurance A muscle's ability to contract repeatedly without becoming fatigued.

muscular strength The ability to apply maximum force against an object that is resisting this force.

mutation (mew-TAY-shun) In reference to human biology, a change in a gene or a chromosome; damaged genes.

myotonia An increase in muscle tension throughout the body during sexual arousal.

narcotics Drugs that induce euphoria and sleep as well as alter the perception of pain.

natural family planning (fertility awareness) Formerly called the rhythm method; a group of birth control techniques in which a couple abstains from sexual intercourse during the time of the month when a woman is most likely to conceive.

neurotransmitters Chemicals produced and released by nerves that convey information between most nerve cells.

nicotine An addictive psychoactive drug found in tobacco.

noncommunicable Not transmissible from person to person.

noninfectious (NON-in-FEK-shus) disease Illness caused by genetic abnormalities, by interactions between hereditary and environmental factors, or solely by environmental factors.

nonspecific immunity A variety of defense mechanisms that combat any type of damage to the body, including the invasion of infectious agents.

nutrient requirement The minimum amount of a nutrient that prevents that nutrient's deficiency disease.

nutrients Substances in food that are necessary for growth, repair, maintenance of tissues.

obesity A condition in which the body has an excessive and unhealthy amount of fat. Obese people have BMIs of 30 or more.

obsession A repetitive thought that produces anxious feelings.

oncogenes (ONG-ko-geenz) Tumor genes that manufacture altered proteins that speed cell growth and decrease the level of cell differentiation.

optimal wellness A sense that one is functioning at his or her best level.

orgasm The peak of sexual excitement.

osteoporosis An age-related condition in which bones lose density, becoming weak and breaking easily.

ovaries Internal organs of female sexual reproduction within which eggs (ova) develop.

overweight A condition in which the body has more fat, muscle, bone, and/or water than a person whose weight is normal. Overweight people have BMIs of between 25 and 30.

ovulation The maturation and release of an egg from an ovary, usually each month from puberty to menopause.

ozone holes Depleted areas of the ozone (O_3) layer in the upper atmosphere.

panic disorder Psychological condition that features panic attacks, unpredictable episodes of extreme anxiety, and loss of emotional control.

Papanicolaou (PAP-eh-nik-eh-LOUW) test (Pap test) A screening procedure for cervical cancer in which cells from the cervical canal are removed and then smeared on a glass slide for microscopic examination.

passive smoking The inhalation, by nonsmokers, of tobacco smoke in the air.

pathogen (PATH-oh-jen) A disease-causing agent of infection; the first link in the chain of infection.

pedophile (PE-doe-file) An individual who is sexually attracted to children.

penis A cylindrical external organ of sexual reproduction in males, which hangs in front of the scrotum.

periodontal (PER-ee-oh-DON-tal) disease A disorder of the tissues that support the teeth.

peripheral nervous system (PNS) Of the two primary divisions of the nervous system, the one that consists of nerves, which relay information to and from the CNS.

peripheral vascular disease Any blockage of vessels other than those to the heart.

persistent vegetative state Condition in which a person has a nonfunctioning cerebral cortex and is in an irreversible coma.

personality A set of distinct thoughts and behaviors that characterizes a person's response to situations.

pesticides Chemicals that kill plant and animal pests and that can cause poisoning when ingested.

phagocytosis (FAG-oh-sigh-TOE-sis) The process of white blood cells ingesting foreign cells and debris, such as the dirt or dead cells in a cut.

phobia An intense and irrational fear of an object or a situation.

physical activity Movement that occurs when skeletal muscles contract.

physiology The study of bodily functions.

phytochemicals A group of nonnutrients that are produced by plants and may have beneficial effects on the body.

placebo A sham treatment that has no known physical effects; an inactive substance.

placenta (plah-SEN-tah) A structure that develops after implantation of a fertilized ovum in the uterine wall and consists of maternal and fetal tissues that secrete hormones that help maintain the pregnancy.

plaques (plaks) Fatty deposits in artery walls.

polyabuse Abusing more than one drug at a time.

portal of entry Site on or in the body where pathogens enter.

pre-embryo The first 2 weeks of gestational development.

pregnancy The gestational process; the process of development of a new individual from fertilization until birth.

premature (rapid) ejaculation A common male sexual dysfunction in which a man consistently attains orgasm either before or shortly after intercourse and before he wishes it to occur.

premenstrual syndrome (PMS) Symptoms such as anxiety, mood swings, aches, and cramps that occur prior to the menses and that significantly interfere with daily life.

probiotics Live bacteria that may benefit health.

progesterone (pro-JES-te-rone) A hormone secreted by the corpus luteum. With estrogen, progesterone stimulates the continued development and thickening of the uterine lining.

progressive overload The training principle that placing increasing amounts of stress on the body causes adaptation that improves fitness.

prostate gland A single, walnut-sized gland that lies just below the bladder, surrounding the urethra. The prostate produces a milky alkaline fluid that is added to the ejaculate.

proteins A class of nutrients that are needed to build, maintain, and repair cells.

psychoactive Having mind-altering or mood-altering effects.

psychological adjustment Changing one's thoughts, attitudes, and behaviors to cope effectively with the demands of the environment.

psychological growth The process of learning from one's experiences.

psychology The study of the mental processes that influence human behavior.

psychoneuroimmunology (SIGH-ko-NEW-ro-im-mu-NOL-lo-gee) The study of the relationships between the nervous and immune systems.

puberty (PEW-ber-tea) A stage of sexual development during which the endocrine (hormone) and reproductive systems mature.

pubic louse A close relative of fleas that causes sexually transmitted infestation; also called crabs.

quackery The practice of medicine with-out having the proper training and credentials.

radical mastectomy Surgical removal of a breast, underlying muscle, and underarm fat and lymph nodes as a treatment for breast cancer.

radon gas A colorless, odorless, radioactive gas present in the rocks and soils in many areas in the United States that, when inhaled, can cause mutations in cells.

rape Sexual intercourse by force or with a person who is incapable of legal consent.

rectum The lower part of the large intestine.

respect The feeling that another has value and deserves attention.

risk factor A characteristic that increases an individual's chances of developing a health problem.

sarcomas (sar-KO-mahz) Cancers that arise from connective or muscle tissue.

satiety The feeling that enough food has been eaten to relieve hunger and turn off appetite.

scabies (SKAY-beez) An infestation of the pubic area in which a spider-like organism burrows into the skin and lays eggs there.

schizophrenia A form of psychosis.

scrotum (SKRO-tum) The sac of skin in which the testes are enclosed and hang outside the body.

sedatives Drugs that produce calming effects.

self-esteem The extent to which a person feels worthy and useful.

semen The ejaculate; the secretions of the accessory sex glands (called seminal fluid) and sperm.

seminal vesicles (SEM-ih-nal VES-ih-klz) Paired male sex organs located near the junction of the two vasa deferentia, which produce thick fructose-containing secretions that are added to the ejaculate.

senescence (seh-NES-ens) The stage of life that begins at age 65 years and ends with death.

set point A theoretical level of body fat that resists weight loss efforts.

sexism Discrimination and bias against one sex.

sexologists Scientists who study human sexuality.

sexual harassment Intentional use of annoying sexually related comments or behaviors to intimidate or coerce people into unwanted sexual activity.

sexual intercourse Penetration of the vagina by a penis.

sexual orientation The direction of a person's romantic thoughts, feelings, and attractions toward people of the same or different sex.

sexual reproduction The fertilization of an egg (*ovum*; plural, *ova*) by a sperm.

sexual stereotype The widespread association of certain perceptions with one gender.

sexual violence Gaining sexual activity through force or threat of force.

sexuality The aspect of personality that encompasses a person's sexual thoughts, feelings, attitudes, and actions.

sexually transmitted infection (STI) Infection spread from person to person by intimate sexual contact, primarily anal or vaginal intercourse and oral sex.

sick building syndrome A variety of vague health-related problems reported by many occupants of large buildings.

sigmoidoscopy (SIG-moid-OS-ko-pee) A procedure in which a physician views the lower portion of the colon via a flexible fiber-optic tube.

signs Observable and measurable features of an illness.

smog (smoke and fog) A haze in the atmosphere formed by various pollutants.

specific immunity Defense mechanism carried out by the immune system.

spermicides Chemicals that kill sperm.

sprain Generally refers to an injured ligament.

squamous (SKWAY-muss) cell carcinoma A common form of skin cancer that develops from exposure to noxious chemicals and high levels of x-rays, as well as from trauma.

stent A springlike mesh device that is implanted within an artery to cover compressed plaque, support the artery, and smooth the artery wall.

sterilization A permanent form of birth control that requires a surgical procedure.

strain Generally refers to an injured muscle or tendon.

stress A complex series of psychological and physical reactions that occur as one responds to a situation.

stressors Events that produce physical or psychological demands on an individual.

stroke A brain injury that occurs when arteries that supply the brain become blocked and prevent blood flow or become damaged and leak blood onto or into the brain.

sudden cardiac arrest Cessation of the heartbeat.

Suicide ideation Thinking about, considering, or planning for suicide.

surgical abortion Includes various methods of induced abortion in which the contents of the uterus are physically removed.

symptoms Subjective complaints of illness.

synergism (SIH-ner-jism) The multiplied effects produced by taking combinations of certain drugs.

syphilis (SIF-ih-lis) An STI that can progress from skin sores to more generalized symptoms (e.g., weight loss and muscle pain) to life-threatening, tissue-destroying skin abnormalities.

systolic (sis-TOL-ik) pressure The higher number in the blood pressure reading, which is the pressure exerted by the blood on the artery walls when the left ventricle contracts.

T cells specialized white blood cells (lymphocytes) that function in cell-mediated immunity; there are four types of T cells.

***T. vaginalis* infection** An STI caused by a protozoan, resulting in infection of the urethra in men and of the urethra and walls of the vagina in women.

targeted therapies Drugs or other substances that block the growth and spread of cancer by interfering with specific molecules involved in tumor growth and progression.

temperament The predictable way an individual responds to situations and others, such as being pleasant, outgoing, or shy.

temporomandibular (TEM-pe-row-man-DIB-you-ler) joint The place where the lower jaw bone (mandible) attaches to the temporal bone of the skull.

tendons Tough bands of tissue that connect many skeletal muscles to bones.

teratogens Various environmental influences such as drugs, alcohol, viruses, and dietary deficiencies that can damage the embryo or fetus early in pregnancy.

testes (TES-tease) The male reproductive organs that produce sperm (the male sex cells) and testosterone (a male sex hormone).

testicular (tes-TIK-you-lar) self-examination (TSE) A self-screening test that males can perform to detect cancer of the testicles.

testimonials Individual claims about the value of a product.

testosterone A male sex hormone (androgen) that plays a role in the development of functionally mature sperm and is responsible for the development and maintenance of male secondary sexual characteristics such as the deepening of the voice and the growth of facial hair.

thermic effect of food (TEF) The small amount of energy that the body uses to digest, absorb, and process the nutrients from foods.

thrombus (THROM-bus) A stationary blood clot.

tolerance A physiologic response in chronic users of drugs in which increased amounts of the drug are required to achieve effects previously produced by lower amounts.

total mastectomy (mas-TEK-toe-me) Surgical removal of a breast and involved lymph nodes for the treatment of breast cancer.

toxic chemicals Poisonous substances present in the home, workplace, or outdoor environments that affect human health.

toxicity (tok-SIH-si-tea) Poisonous quality.

transgender An umbrella term for various groups of people who do not conform to traditional gender roles.

transient ischemic (is-KI-mik) attacks (TIAs) Minor strokes that usually cause no permanent damage and have signs that last for only a short time.

transmission In reference to disease, the means by which a pathogen gets to a host; the second link in the chain of infection.

triglycerides The most prevalent form of lipids in foods; often called fat.

tubal ligation Female sterilization that is performed by cutting and tying off the uterine tubes so that the sperm and egg cannot unite.

tumor-suppressor genes Pieces of hereditary material that slow cell growth; anti-oncogenes.

urinary incontinence The inability to control the flow of urine from the bladder.

uterine tubes Passageways that extend from each ovary to the uterus.

uterus A hollow, muscular, pear-shaped organ that protects and nourishes the embryo/fetus during development.

vaccine A preparation of a killed or weakened pathogen or its antigenic parts to be administered to a person to induce immunity and thereby prevent infectious disease.

vagina A tube about 10 cm (approximately 4 in.) long that receives the penis during intercourse, allows the passage of the menstrual flow, and is a birth canal.

vaginismus A sexual dysfunction of women in which the lower portion of the vagina contracts involuntarily at the anticipation of penetration, preventing it.

value The belief that an idea, object, or action has worth.

vas deferens (VAS DEF-er-enz) A tube that links the epididymis and the urethra, the passageway through which sperm exit the body.

vasectomy Male sterilization that is performed by cutting and tying off the vas deferens to prevent sperm from becoming part of the ejaculate.

vasocongestion A condition in which the spongy tissue of the penis and clitoris expands with blood during sexual arousal.

veins Blood vessels that return blood to the heart.

violence Interpersonal uses of force that are not socially sanctioned.

virus Hereditary material surrounded by a coat of protein; some viruses are pathogenic to humans and produce infections such as the common cold, influenza, mumps, measles, chicken pox, hepatitis, and AIDS.

vitamins A class of organic nutrients that help regulate growth; release energy from carbohydrates, fats, and proteins; and maintain tissues.

vulva The collective term for the external female genitals. The vulva surrounds the vaginal opening.

withdrawal A temporary physical and psychological state that occurs when certain drugs are discontinued.

yeast infection A condition in which the fungus *Candida albicans* grows in the vagina or on the penis; also known as candidiasis or moniliasis.

Index

Note: Page numbers followed by *f*, or *t* indicate materials in figures, or tables respectively.

Welcome to ECONOMICS TODAY

UPDATED WITH

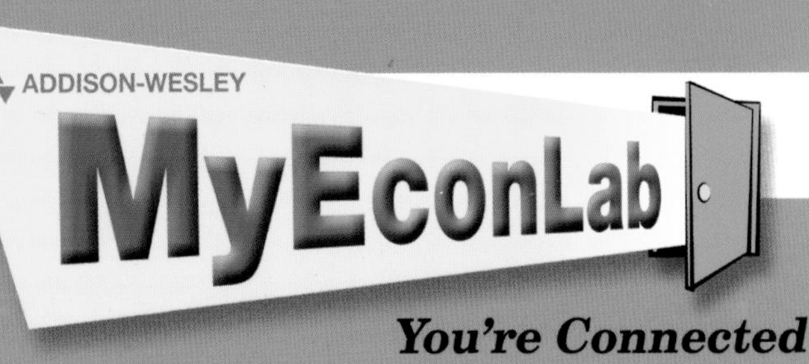

IMPORTANT

Your Student Access Code for MyEconLab

INSTRUCTIONS

1 Ask your instructor for your **MyEconLab Course ID** and record it here: ________________

2 Go to **http://www.myeconlab.com** and follow the instructions for getting started, installation, and registration for your course. You will need your **Course ID** and your **Student Access Code** only the first time you register for your course.

3 If you need help at any time during the registration process, please send an email to support@coursecompass.com or simply click on the Need Help? Icon.

Your unique **Student Access Code** is:

WSCDFR-AVOWS-ORIEL-BLUED-RETOT-AIDES

This Access Code can be used only once to register for your course. Your registration is not transferable. If you did not purchase a new textbook, your Access Code may not be valid.

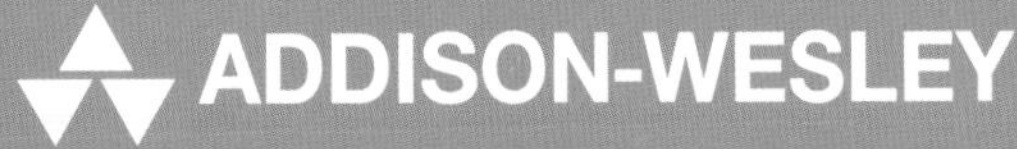

ECONOMICS TODAY

2001–2002 EDITION
MYECONLAB.COM UPDATE

Roger LeRoy Miller

The Addison-Wesley Series in Economics

Abel/Bernanke
Macroeconomics

Bade/Parkin
Foundations of Microeconomics

Bade/Parkin
Foundations of Macroeconomics

Bierman/Fernandez
Game Theory with Economic Applications

Binger/Hoffman
Microeconomics with Calculus

Boyer
Principles of Transportation Economics

Branson
Macroeconomic Theory and Policy

Bruce
Public Finance and the American Economy

Byrns/Stone
Economics

Carlton/Perloff
Modern Industrial Organization

Caves/Frankel/Jones
World Trade and Payments: An Introduction

Chapman
Environmental Economics: Theory, Application, and Policy

Cooter/Ulen
Law and Economics

Downs
An Economic Theory of Democracy

Eaton/Mishkin
Online Readings to Accompany The Economics of Money, Banking, and Financial Markets

Ehrenberg/Smith
Modern Labor Economics

Ekelund/Tollison
Economics: Private Markets and Public Choice

Fusfeld
The Age of the Economist

Gerber
International Economics

Ghiara
Learning Economics: A Practical Workbook

Gordon
Macroeconomics

Gregory
Essentials of Economics

Gregory/Stuart
Russian and Soviet Economic Performance and Structure

Hartwick/Olewiler
The Economics of Natural Resource Use

Hubbard
Money, the Financial System, and the Economy

Hughes/Cain
American Economic History

Husted/Melvin
International Economics

Jehle/Reny
Advanced Microeconomic Theory

Klein
Mathematical Methods for Economics

Krugman/Obstfeld
International Economics: Theory and Policy

Laidler
The Demand for Money: Theories, Evidence, and Problems

Leeds/von Allmen
The Economics of Sports

Lipsey/Courant/Ragan
Economics

McCarty
Dollars and Sense: An Introduction to Economics

Melvin
International Money and Finance

Miller
Economics Today

Miller/Benjamin/North
The Economics of Public Issues

Mills/Hamilton
Urban Economics

Mishkin
The Economics of Money, Banking, and Financial Markets

Parkin
Economics

Parkin/Bade
Economics in Action Software

Perloff
Microeconomics

Phelps
Health Economics

Riddell/Shackelford/Stamos/Schneider
Economics: A Tool for Critically Understanding Society

Ritter/Silber/Udell
Principles of Money, Banking, and Financial Markets

Rohlf
Introduction to Economic Reasoning

Ruffin/Gregory
Principles of Economics

Sargent
Rational Expectations and Inflation

Scherer
Industry Structure, Strategy, and Public Policy

Schotter
Microeconomics: A Modern Approach

Stock/Watson
Introduction to Econometrics

Studenmund
Using Econometrics: A Practical Guide

Tietenberg
Environmental and Natural Resource Economics

Tietenberg
Environmental Economics and Policy

Todaro/Smith
Economic Development

Waldman/Jensen
Industrial Organization: Theory and Practice

Williamson
Macroeconomics

ECONOMICS TODAY

2001–2002 Edition
MyEconLab.com Update

Roger LeRoy Miller

Institute for University Studies, Arlington, Texas

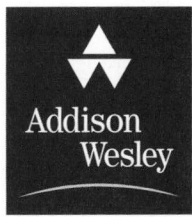

Boston San Francisco New York
London Toronto Sydney Tokyo Singapore Madrid
Mexico City Munich Paris Cape Town Hong Kong Montreal

Photo Credits

Pages 3 and 14, ©Grant LeDuc/Stock Boston; pages 26 and 43, ©Annie Griffiths Belt/CORBIS; pages 48 and 71, ©Keren Su/Stock Boston; pages 75 and 90, ©Tony Freeman/Photo Edit; pages 95 and 115, ©Bill Aron/Photo Edit; pages 120 and 135, ©CORBIS; pages 145 and 164, ©Miladinovic/Sygma CORBIS; pages 168 and 190, PN/The Slide file; page 170 left, Frank Siteman/The Picture Cube; page 170 right, Bernsau/The Image Works; pages 195 and 215, ©Bruce Forster/Tony Stone Images/Chicago Inc.; pages 225 and 241, ©Lee Snider/CORBIS; pages 246 and 265, ©Ilkka Uimonen/Sygma CORBIS; pages 269 and 292, ©Susan Van Etten; pages 298 and 314, ©Mark Richards/Photo Edit; pages 327 and 348, ©Grant LeDuc/Stock Boston; pages 353 and 378, ©Rob Crandall/Stock Boston; pages 383 and 398, ©Susan Van Etten; pages 402 and 419, ©AFP/CORBIS; pages 425 and 445, ©Tony Freeman/Photo Edit; pages 455 and 468, ©Susan Van Etten; pages 482 and 501, ©Susan Van Etten; pages 505 and 520, Stephen Ferry/Gamma Liaison; pages 531 and 555, *Chicago Tribune* photo by Bill Hogan; pages 560 and 582, ©Richard Hutchings/Photo Edit; pages 588 and 608, ©Martin Rogers/Tony Stone Images/Chicago Inc.; pages 612 and 634, permission granted by Lands' End.com; pages 638 and 656, ©Todd Gipstein/CORBIS; pages 665 and 684, ©Susan Van Etten; pages 689 and 707, ©Bettmann/CORBIS; pages 712 and 727, Copyright 2000–Wisconsin Department of Revenue–Lottery Division; pages 731 and 755, ©Ted Spiegel/CORBIS; pages 759 and 774, ©Jorie Butler Kent/Abercrombie & Kent; pages 783 and 800, ©Paul Conklin/Photo Edit; pages 805 and 827, ©Miladinovic/Sygma CORBIS.

Editor-in-Chief: Denise Clinton
Acquisitions Editor: Victoria Warneck
Developmental Editor: Rebecca Ferris
Web Project Manager: Karen Schmitt
Associate Editor: Roxanne Hoch
Managing Editor: James Rigney
Production Supervisor: Katherine Watson
Marketing Manager: Adrienne D'Ambrosio
Senior Media Producer: Melissa Honig
Design Manager: Regina Kolenda
Cover Designer: Regina Kolenda and Joyce Cosentino Wells
Senior Manufacturing Buyer: Hugh Crawford
Cover Collage Images: ©Digital Vision/PictureQuest; © Robert Cattan/Index Stock Imagery; ©PhotoDisc.
Compositor: Lynn Lowell
Art Studio: ElectraGraphics, Inc.
Printer and Binder: Quebecor World
Cover Printer: Coral Graphic Services, Inc.

ISBN 0-201-78615-X
12345678910—QWT—0605040302

To Bill Stryker,

It is rare to find one as
dedicated to superior effort
as you are. I thank you
for continuing always to
do the best work possible,
no matter what hurdles
are placed in front of you.

R. L. M.

Contents in Brief

CONTENTS IN DETAIL

Course Outline

MACROECONOMIC EMPHASIS

1. The Nature of Economics
2. Scarcity and the World of Trade-Offs
3. Demand and Supply
4. Extensions of Demand and Supply Analysis
5. The Public Sector and Public Choice
6. Your Future with Social Security
7. The Macroeconomy: Unemployment, Inflation, and Deflation
8. Measuring the Economy's Performance
9. Global Economic Growth and Development
10. Real GDP and the Price Level in the Long Run
11. Classical and Keynesian Macro Analyses
12. Consumption, Income, and the Multiplier
13. Fiscal Policy
14. Money and Banking Systems
15. Money Creation, Payment Systems, and Deposit Insurance
16. Electronic Banking
32. Comparative Advantage and the Open Economy
33. Exchange Rates and the Balance of Payments

MICROECONOMIC EMPHASIS

1. The Nature of Economics
2. Scarcity and the World of Trade-Offs
3. Demand and Supply
4. Extensions of Demand and Supply Analysis
6. Your Future with Social Security
19. Consumer Choice (Optional)
20. Demand and Supply Elasticity
21. The Global Financial Environment of Business (Optional)
22. The Firm: Cost and Output Determination
23. Perfect Competition
24. Monopoly
25. Monopolistic Competition, Oligopoly, and Strategic Behavior
26. Regulation and Antitrust Policy in a World of Multinational Firms
27. Labor Demand and Supply
28. Unions and Labor Market Monopoly Power
29. Rent, Interest, and Profits
30. Income, Poverty, and Health Care
31. Environmental Economics
32. Comparative Advantage and the Open Economy

BALANCED MICRO-MACRO

1. The Nature of Economics
2. Scarcity and the World of Trade-Offs
3. Demand and Supply
4. Extensions of Demand and Supply Analysis
6. Your Future with Social Security
20. Demand and Supply Elasticity
22. The Firm: Cost and Output Determination
23. Perfect Competition
24. Monopoly
27. Labor Demand and Supply
28. Unions and Labor Market Monopoly Power
7. The Macroeconomy: Unemployment, Inflation, and Deflation
10. Real GDP and the Price Level in the Long Run
11. Classical and Keynesian Macro Analyses
13. Fiscal Policy
14. Money and Banking Systems
15. Money Creation, Payment Systems, and Deposit Insurance
16. Electronic Banking

Acknowledgments

I am the most fortunate of economics textbook writers, for I receive the benefit of literally hundreds of suggestions from those of you who use *Economics Today*. I continue to be fully appreciative of the constructive criticisms that you offer. There are some professors who have been asked by my publisher to participate in a more detailed reviewing process of this edition. I list them below. I hope that each one of you so listed accepts my sincere appreciation for the fine work that you have done.

Bill Adamson, South Dakota State University
John Allen, Texas A&M University
John Baffoe-Bonnie, Pennsylvania State University
Kevin Baird, Montgomery County Community College
Daniel Benjamin, Clemson University
Abraham Bertisch, Nassau Community College
John Bethune, University of Tennessee
R. A. Blewett, St. Lawrence University
Melvin Borland, Western Kentucky University
James Carlson, Manatee Community College
Robert Carlsson, University of South Carolina
K. Merry Chambers, Central Piedmont Community College
Catherine Chambers, Central Missouri State University
Marc Chopin, Louisiana Tech University
Curtis Clarke, Mountain View College
Jerry Crawford, Arkansas State University
Andrew J. Dane, Angelo State University
Carl Enomoto, New Mexico State University
Abdollah Ferdowsi, Ferris State University
James Gale, Michigan Technical University
Neil Garston, California State University, Los Angeles
Paul Graf, Penn State University
William Henderson, Franklin University
Charles W. Hockert, Oklahoma City Community College
Yu Hsing, Southeastern Louisiana University
Scott Hunt, Columbus State Community College
Joseph W. Hunt Jr., Shippensburg University of Pennsylvania
John Ifediora, University of Wisconsin, Platteville
Allan Jenkins, University of Nebraska, Kearney
Alan Kessler, Providence College
Marie Kratochvil, Nassau Community College
James C. McBrearty, University of Arizona
Diego Méndez-Carbajo, Florida International University
Khan Mohabbat, Northern Illinois University
Zuohong Pan, Western Connecticut State University
Ginger Parker, Miami-Dade Community College
Bruce Pietrykowski, University of Michigan, Dearborn
Mannie Poen, Houston Community College
Robert Posatko, Shippensburg University of Pennsylvania
Jaishankar Raman, Valparaiso University
Richard Rawlins, Missouri Southern State College
Charles Roberts, Western Kentucky University
Larry Ross, University of Alaska, Anchorage
Stephen Rubb, Providence College
Henry Ryder, Gloucester County College
Swapan Sen, Christopher Newport University
Garvin Smith, Daytona Beach Community College
Alan Stafford, Niagara County College
Thomas Swanke, West Virginia State College
Lea Templer, College of the Canyons
David VanHoose, University of Alabama
Craig Walker, Delta State University
Mark Wohar, University of Nebraska, Omaha
Tim Wulf, Parkland College
Alex Yguado, Los Angeles Mission College

I also thank the reviewers of previous editions:

Esmond Adams
John Adams
John R. Aidem
Mohammed Akacem
M. C. Alderfer
Ann Al-Yasiri
Leslie J. Anderson
Fatima W. Antar
Aliakbar Ataiifar
Leonard Atencio
Glen W. Atkinson
Thomas R. Atkinson
James Q. Aylesworth
Charley Ballard
Maurice B. Ballabon
G. Jeffrey Barbour
Daniel Barszcz
Robin L. Bartlett
Kari Battaglia
Robert Becker
Charles Beem
Glen Beeson
Charles Berry
Scott Bloom
M. L. Bodnar
Mary Bone
Karl Bonnhi
Thomas W. Bonsor
John M. Booth
Wesley F. Booth
Thomas Borcherding
Tom Boston
Barry Boyer
Maryanna Boynton
Ronald Brandolini
Fenton L. Broadhead
Elba Brown
William Brown
Michael Bull
Maureen Burton
Conrad P. Caligaris
Kevin Carey
Dancy R. Carr
Doris Cash
Thomas H. Cate
Richard J. Cebula
Richard Chapman
Young Back Choi
Carol Cies
Joy L. Clark
Gary Clayton
Marsha Clayton
Warren L. Coats
Ed Coen
Pat Conroy
James Cox
Stephen R. Cox
Eleanor D. Craig
Joanna Cruse
John P. Cullity
Thomas Curtis
Mahmoud Davoudi
Edward Dennis
Carol Dimamro
William Dougherty
Barry Duman
Diane Dumont
Floyd Durham
G. B. Duwaji
James A. Dyal
Ishita Edwards
Robert P. Edwards
Alan E. Ellis
Mike Ellis
Steffany Ellis
Frank Emerson
Zaki Eusufzai
Sandy Evans
John L. Ewing-Smith
Frank Falero
Frank Fato
Grant Ferguson
David Fletcher
James Foley
John Foreman
Ralph G. Fowler
Arthur Friedberg
Peter Frost
E. Gabriel
Steve Gardner
Peter C. Garlick
Alexander Garvin
Joe Garwood
J. P. Gilbert
Otis Gilley
Frank Glesber
Jack Goddard
Allen C. Goodman
Richard J. Gosselin
Edward Greenberg
Gary Greene
Nicholas Grunt
William Gunther
Kwabena Gyimah-Brempong
Demos Hadjiyanis
Martin D. Haney
Mehdi Haririan
Ray Harvey
E. L. Hazlett
Sanford B. Helman
John Hensel
Robert Herman
Gus W. Herring
Charles Hill
John M. Hill
Morton Hirsch
Benjamin Hitchner
R. Bradley Hoppes
James Horner
Grover Howard
Nancy Howe-Ford
R. Jack Inch
Christopher Inya
Tomotaka Ishimine
E. E. Jarvis

Parvis Jenab
Mark Jensen
S. D. Jevremovic
J. Paul Jewell
Frederick Johnson
David Jones
Lamar B. Jones
Paul A. Joray
Daniel A. Joseph
Craig Justice
Septimus Kai Kai
Devajyoti Kataky
Timothy R. Keely
Ziad Keilany
Norman F. Keiser
Randall G. Kesselring
E. D. Key
M. Barbara Killen
Bruce Kimzey
Philip G. King
Terrence Kinal
E. R. Kittrell
David Klingman
Charles Knapp
Jerry Knarr
Faik Koray
Janet Koscianski
Peter Kressler
Michael Kupilik
Larry Landrum
Margaret Landman
Keith Langford
Anthony T. Lee
George Lieu
Stephen E. Lile
Lawrence W. Lovick
Akbar Marvasti
Warren T. Matthews
Robert McAuliffe
Howard J. McBride
Bruce McClung
John McDowell
E. S. McKuskey
James J. McLain
John L. Madden
Mary Lou Madden
Glen Marston
John M. Martin
Paul J. Mascotti
James D. Mason
Paul M. Mason
Tom Mathew
Warren Matthews
G. Hartley Mellish
Mike Melvin
Dan C. Messerschmidt
Michael Metzger
Herbert C. Milikien
Joel C. Millonzi
Glenn Milner
Thomas Molloy
Margaret D. Moore
William E. Morgan
Stephen Morrell
Irving Morrissett
James W. Moser
Martin F. Murray
George L. Nagy
Jerome Neadly
James E. Needham
Claron Nelson
Douglas Nettleton
Gerald T. O'Boyle
Lucian T. Orlowski
Diane S. Osborne
Jan Palmer
Gerald Parker
Randall E. Parker
Norm Paul
Raymond A. Pepin
Martin M. Perline
Timothy Perri
Jerry Petr
Maurice Pfannesteil
James Phillips
Raymond J. Phillips
I. James Pickl
Dennis Placone
William L. Polvent
Reneé Prim
Robert W. Pulsinelli
Rod D. Raehsler
Kambriz Raffiee
Sandra Rahman
John Rapp
Gautam Raychaudhuri
Ron Reddall
Mitchell Redlo
Charles Reichhelu
Robert S. Rippey
Ray C. Roberts
Richard Romano
Duane Rosa
Richard Rosenberg
Barbara Ross-Pfeiffer
Philip Rothman
John Roufagalas
Patricia Sanderson
Thomas N. Schaap
William A. Schaeffer
William Schaniel
David Schauer
A. C. Schlenker
Scott J. Schroeder
William Scott
Dan Segebarth
Augustus Shackelford
Richard Sherman Jr.
Liang-rong Shiau
David Shorow
Vishwa Shukla
R. J. Sidwell
David E. Sisk
Alden Smith
Howard F. Smith
Lynn A. Smith
Phil Smith
Steve Smith
William Doyle Smith
Lee Spector
George Spiva
Richard L. Sprinkle
Herbert F. Steeper
Columbus Stephens
William Stine
Allen D. Stone
Osman Suliman
J. M. Sullivan
Rebecca Summary
Joseph L. Swaffar
Frank D. Taylor
Daniel Teferra
Gary Theige
Robert P. Thomas
Deborah Thorsen
Richard Trieff
George Troxler
William T. Trulove
William N. Trumbull
Arianne K. Turner
Kay Unger
John Vahaly
Jim Van Beek
Lee J. Van Scyoc
Roy Van Til
Robert F. Wallace
Henry C. Wallich
Milledge Weathers
Robert G. Welch
Terence West
Wylie Whalthall
Everett E. White
Michael D. White
Mark A. Wilkening
Raburn M. Williams
James Willis
George Wilson
Travis Wilson
Ken Woodward
Peter R. Wyman
Whitney Yamamura
Donald Yankovic
Paul Young
Shik Young
Mohammed Zaheer
Ed Zajicek
Paul Zarembka
William J. Zimmer Jr.

This MyEconLab.com update required the labor of dozens of individuals and groups. Of course, I continue to be in debt to those who helped me on the original, underlying edition on which this version is based. In addition, the multimedia project manager, Karen Schmitt, made sure that all of the myriad elements of this extraordinary enterprise worked together. I thank her for the countless nights and weekends she devoted to this project. Melissa Honig helped with the technology every step of the way, as always. Rebecca Ferris, my ever-present developmental editor, conceptualized the project and stepped in on numerous occasions to make sure that the print and multimedia elements worked well together and came out on time. Victoria Warneck and Denise Clinton on the Addison-Wesley team supported this work from the very beginning. Others at Addison-Wesley who lent an invaluable hand included Katherine Watson, Production Supervisor, Scott Silva, Composition Manager, Lynn Lowell, Electronic Publisher, and Mansour Bethoney, Senior Web Designer.

The creators of the major animations, Ben Mallory, Matt Hampton, and Chris Bassolino of Fuse5, put in a lot more effort than planned, but came through with superb results. Dave VanHoose wrote the major scripts for all of the Economics in Motion features, while Debbie Mullen of the University of Colorado scripted the Graphs in Motion animations. All of the animations were scrutinized by our dedicated team of reviewers, including Paul Graf, Scott Hunt, Marie Kratochvil, Garvin Smith, Tim Wulf, and James Carlson.

I am also indebted to Steve Melzer of VidBoston and his top-notch crew, as well as Ken Kavanah of Newbury Sound and our voice talent, Ray Childs and Mary Ellen Whitaker, for their contributions. Thanks also to Henry Ryder and Debbie Mullin for their work preparing scripts for the glossary terms.

So, from the true bottom of my heart, I extend my appreciation to the above-mentioned individuals and companies. Putting together a regular book requires more effort than most imagine. Putting together a multimedia version extends the limits of such effort beyond reason. But the end result is, I am sure you will agree, worthy of a great team's travails.

I plan to add to this multimedia, interactive version of the *Economics Today* text. Please let me know what I can do to improve this project.

Roger LeRoy Miller

Preface

Economics Today has long led the field in offering students and instructors a dynamic, application-rich approach to learning and teaching economics. Often imitated but never duplicated, Miller remains on the cutting edge of economic teaching, defining what it means for a text to be user-friendly and student-oriented. With the introduction of the MyEconLab.com, powered by CourseCompass, it again zooms ahead of the pack.

The MyEconLab.com update presents an unprecedented wealth of specially designed multimedia resources, all available in an easy-to-use Web-based environment. It is contained within Addison-Wesley's premier Blackboard-based course management system, CourseCompass, allowing instructors to incorporate technology into the classroom with unprecedented ease.

Those of you who already teach from Miller's *Economics Today* will quickly notice the multimedia icons that have been inserted at strategic points throughout every textbook chapter. To view these new multimedia resources and see how effortlessly they will enhance your students' learning experience, please visit the MyEconLab.com Web site at **http://www.myeconlab.com**.

- **Flip and fumble no more.** Let's face it: Most introductory textbooks now come with a mind-boggling array of ancillary learning tools, both print and electronic. But do your students *use* those tools? Do they know what they are, or how they tie into their textbook? If not, how many take the time to find out? If your students are like most students, they will flip and fumble for a few minutes at most before giving up.

With MyEconLab.com, they don't need to search any further than the textbook page itself. The familiar design of their printed textbook — with the same layout, the same font, even the same page numbers—is a navigational tool that allows your students to painlessly access a wide array of video and audio clips, moving graphs, and full-scale animations of key concepts. All your students need to do is point and click. It's all at their fingertips!

NEW MULTIMEDIA ENHANCEMENTS

MyEconLab.com is tailored to match the *Economics Today* textbook; the Web site features an electronic version of the textbook that serves as a navigational tool for students to access animations, video clips, audio narration, and Internet activities. The goal of these multimedia features is to sharpen students' overall mastery of economics by reinforcing their command of economic theory and bolstering their ability to analyze graphs.

- **Seamless integration of the text and Web site.** Students experience multimedia content in the context of what they are learning in the textbook. Available in PDF format, the complete online textbook has the exact same layout as the printed version. Within each chapter PDF file, students can:
    - Preview the most critical concepts in an audio introduction by the author, Roger LeRoy Miller
    - Use the chapter outline to jump to a particular section
    - View animated graphs
    - Gauge their mastery of concepts in chapter quizzes
    - Link to Web sites cited in the Econ on the Net Internet Activities
    - View videos featuring the author, Roger LeRoy Miller, or

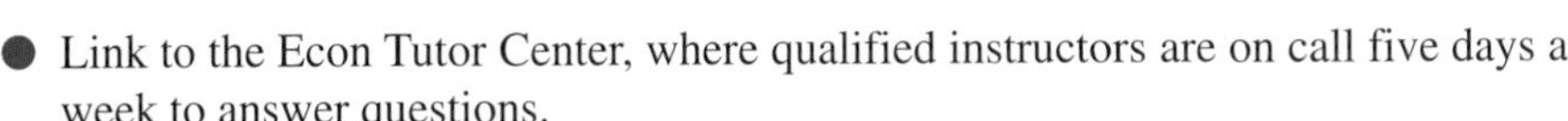

- Link to the Econ Tutor Center, where qualified instructors are on call five days a week to answer questions.

- **Media-rich learning resources.** The online version of the textbook includes a system of icons indicating the availability of innovative media tools:

In video clips, the author stresses the key points in every chapter and further clarifies concepts that students find most difficult to grasp.

To simplify the task of learning the vocabulary of economics, the key terms printed in bold type and defined in the text margin are available as audio clips. In addition to the definition, each clip includes an illuminating, relevant example or that extra word of explanation needed to cement students' understanding.

Each chapter also includes an upbeat audio introduction by the author during which he discusses the chapter topics and focuses student attention on the most critical concepts.

We have identified the ten key economic ideas in the textbook that are ideally suited to animated presentations. These *Economics in Motion* features are in-depth animations that guide students through these precise graphical presentations with detailed audio explanations. The step-by-step approach guides students through the action and makes clear the underlying economic theory. A Contents Guide in each animation allows students to focus in on the ideas that they are struggling with most.

Beginning students of economics are often apprehensive about working with graphs. Using the *Graphs in Motion* feature, with a click of the mouse curves shift, graphs come to life, and students' confidence builds. These animated graphs in every chapter foster graph-analyzing capabilities as points are plotted, curves are drawn, movement is simulated, and intersection points are called out.

EIA *Economics in Action*, the market-leading interactive tutorial software in principles of economics, is now available via the Web. Icons in the text indicate the availability of modules that aid students' mastery of concepts through review, demonstration, and interaction. In-depth tutorials guide students in their discovery of the relationship between economic theory and real-world applications, while the Draw Graph palette lets them test their graphing abilities.

Test Four ten-question quizzes per chapter with tutorial feedback allow students to gauge their understanding of the material.

SG One more tool to encourage students to succeed at economics is the Study Guide. Students can download a PDF version of the material from the print Study Guide for every chapter, all for no additional cost.

MyEconLab.com gives your students complimentary access to help from qualified economics instructors when you are not available. Five days a week, tutors answer questions via phone, fax, and e-mail.

THE COURSECOMPASS ADVANTAGE

MyEconLab.com is powered by CourseCompass. It allows you to easily build and manage online course materials that enhance your classroom teaching time. If you have an Internet connection and a Web browser, you can use CourseCompass. Because CourseCompass is nationally hosted, there is no need for anyone at your academic institution to have to set up and maintain CourseCompass.

Powered by the Blackboard online learning system, CourseCompass includes all the powerful Blackboard features for teaching and learning. Additionally, MyEconLab.com comes with preloaded, state-of-art course materials provided by Addison-Wesley. These course materials include a complete version of the textbook and study guide, extensive animations, video and audio clips, and more.

The advantages of CourseCompass include:

- **Flexibility**. CourseCompass lets you add files of any type to your course, from simple text documents to complex slide presentations and animations.
- **Automated grading**. CourseCompass grades student assessments as students complete them, and automatically posts scores to an online gradebook. As a result, you can spend more time teaching and less time grading.
- **Superior customer support.** CourseCompass provides customer support as well as an *Instructor Quick Start Guide* and comprehensive online Help system tailored to your needs. CourseCompass also includes a *Student Quick Start Guide* and online Help for students, so you can focus on teaching your course, not on teaching CourseCompass.

As an instructor, you will have a wealth of content and resources and powerful tools preloaded on to a customizable course that you download. In addition to the Multimedia Edition, you can:

- Access all of the supplementary items available with the text, including PowerPoint, Test Banks, and Instructor's Manual
- Set up a course calendar to post assignments and assess student performance with the gradebook
- Assign quizzes to students with time limits
- Add post-it notes to the online version of the text to point out particular items or to incorporate a favorite example
- Use communication tools such as e-mail and a course discussion board
- Direct students to submit documents electronically in the digital drop box.

And students can view announcements from the instructor, track their progress on testing features, or contribute to an online discussion board.

- **Value-added material.** For no additional cost, students who purchase the MyEconLab.com Update Edition receive access to the latest release of the Economics in Action software, an electronic version of the printed Study Guide, and access to the Addison-Wesley Tutor Center.

PEDAGOGY WITH PURPOSE

Economics Today, 2001–2002 Edtion, provides a fine-tuned teaching and learning system. This system is aimed at capturing student interest through the infusion of examples that capture the vitality of economics. Each of the following features has been carefully crafted to enhance the learning process:

- **Chapter-Opening Issues** Each chapter-opening issue whets student interest in core chapter concepts with compelling examples.

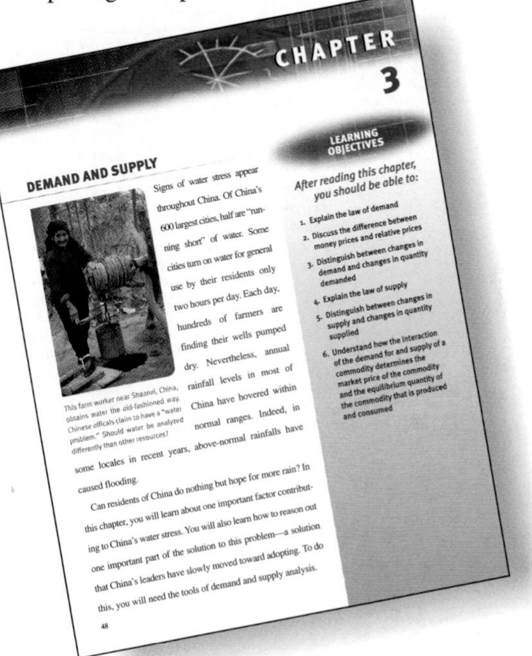

CHAPTER 3

DEMAND AND SUPPLY

This farm worker near Shaanxi, China, obtains water the old-fashioned way. Chinese officals claim to have a "water problem." Should water be analyzed differently than other resources?

Signs of water stress appear throughout China. Of China's 600 largest cities, half are "running short" of water. Some cities turn on water for general use by their residents only two hours per day. Each day, hundreds of farmers are finding their wells pumped dry. Nevertheless, annual rainfall levels in most of China have hovered within normal ranges. Indeed, in some locales in recent years, above-normal rainfalls have caused flooding.

Can residents of China do nothing but hope for more rain? In this chapter, you will learn about one important factor contributing to China's water stress. You will also learn how to reason out one important part of the solution to this problem—a solution that China's leaders have slowly moved toward adopting. To do this, you will need the tools of demand and supply analysis.

48

LEARNING OBJECTIVES

After reading this chapter, you should be able to:

1. Explain the law of demand
2. Discuss the difference between money prices and relative prices
3. Distinguish between changes in demand and changes in quantity demanded
4. Explain the law of supply
5. Distinguish between changes in supply and changes in quantity supplied
6. Understand how the interaction of the demand for and supply of a commodity determines the market price of the commodity and the equilibrium quantity of the commodity that is produced and consumed

- **Did You Know That . . . ?** Each chapter starts with a provocative question to engage students and to lead them into the content of the chapter.

Did You Know That... more than 75 million people currently own portable cellular phones? This is a huge jump from the mere 200,000 who owned them in 1985. Since 1992, two out of every three new telephone numbers have been assigned to cellular phones. There are several reasons for the growth of cellular phones, not the least being the dramatic reduction in both price and size due to improved and cheaper computer chips that go into making them. There is something else at work, though. It has to do with crime. In a recent survey, 46 percent of new cellular phone users said that personal safety was the main reason they bought a portable phone. In Florida, for example, most cellular phone companies allow users simply to dial *FHP to reach the Florida Highway Patrol. The rush to cellular phones is worldwide. Over the past decade, sales have grown by nearly 50 percent every year outside the United States.

We could attempt to explain the phenomenon by saying that more people like to use portable phones. But that explanation is neither satisfying nor entirely accurate. If we use the economist's primary set of tools, *demand and supply,* we will have a better understanding of the cellular phone explosion, as well as many other phenomena in our world. Demand and supply are two ways of categorizing the influences on the price of goods that you buy and the quantities available. As such, demand and supply form the basis of virtually all economic analysis of the world around us.

As you will see throughout this text, the operation of the forces of demand and supply take place in *markets.* A **market** is an abstract concept referring to all the arrangements individuals have for exchanging with one another. Goods and services are sold in markets, such as the automobile market, the health market, and the compact disc market. Workers offer their services in the labor market. Companies, or firms, buy workers' labor services in the labor market. Firms also buy other inputs in order to produce the goods and services that you buy as a consumer. Firms purchase machines, buildings, and land. These markets are in operation at all times. One of the most important activities in these markets is the setting of the prices of all of the inputs and outputs that are bought and sold in our complicated economy. To understand the determination of prices, you first need to look at the law of demand.

- **Learning Objectives** A clear statement of learning objectives on the first page of the chapter focuses students' studies.
- **Chapter Outline** The outline serves as a guide to the chapter coverage.
- **Graphs** Precise, four-color graphs clearly illustrate key concepts.
- **Key Terms** To simplify the task of learning the vocabulary of economics, key terms are printed in bold type and defined in the margin of the text the first time they appear.
- **Policy Examples** Students are exposed to important policy questions on both domestic and international fronts in over 40 policy examples.

POLICY EXAMPLE

Should Shortages in the Ticket Market Be Solved by Scalpers?

If you have ever tried to get tickets to a playoff game in sports, a popular Broadway play, or a superstar's rock concert, you know about "shortages." The standard ticket situation for a Super Bowl is shown in Figure 3-12. At the face-value price of Super Bowl tickets (P_1), the quantity demanded (Q_2) greatly exceeds the quantity supplied (Q_1). Because shortages last only so long as prices and quantities do not change, markets tend to exhibit a movement out of this disequilibrium toward equilibrium. Obviously, the quantity of Super Bowl tickets cannot change, but the price can go as high as P_2.

Enter the scalper. This colorful term is used because when you purchase a ticket that is being resold at a price that is higher than face value, the seller is skimming an extra profit off the top. If an event sells out, ticket prices by definition have been lower than market clearing prices. People without tickets may be willing to buy high-priced tickets because they place a greater value on the entertainment event than the face value of the ticket. Without scalpers, those individuals would not be able to attend the event. In the case of the Super Bowl, various forms of scalping occur nationwide. Tickets for a seat on the 50-yard line have been sold for more than $2,000 a piece. In front of every Super Bowl arena, you can find ticket scalpers hawking their wares.

In most states, scalping is illegal. In Pennsylvania, convicted scalpers are either fined $5,000 or sentenced to two years behind bars. For an economist, such legislation seems strange. As one New York ticket broker said, "I look at scalping like working as a stockbroker, buying low and selling high. If people are willing to pay me the money, what kind of problem is that?"

For Critical Analysis

What happens to ticket scalpers who are still holding tickets after an event has started?

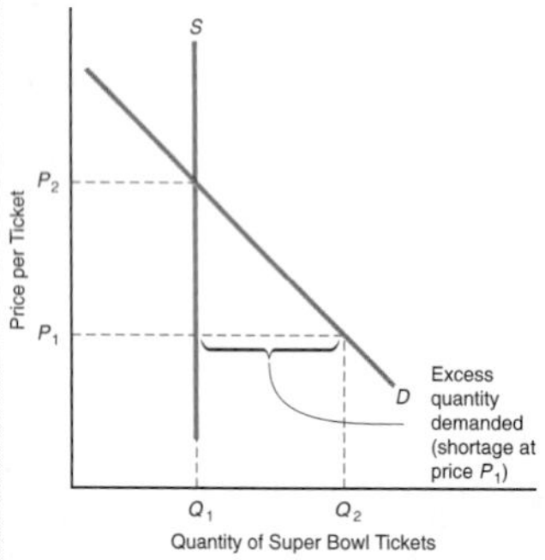

S
P_2
Price per Ticket
P_1
D
Excess quantity demanded (shortage at price P_1)
Q_1
Q_2
Quantity of Super Bowl Tickets

FIGURE 3-12
Shortages of Super Bowl Tickets
The quantity of tickets for any one Super Bowl is fixed at Q_1. At the price per ticket of P_1, the quantity demanded is Q_2, which is greater than Q_1. Consequently, there is an excess quantity demanded at the below-market-clearing price. Prices can go as high as P_2 in the scalpers' market.

- **International Examples** Over 30 international examples emphasize the interconnections of today's global economy.

INTERNATIONAL EXAMPLE

The High Relative Price of a U.S. Education

In 1993, about 40 percent of all college students classified as "international students"—students working toward degrees outside their home countries—were enrolled in U.S. colleges and universities. This figure has shrunk to just over 30 percent today, and it gradually continues to decline.

Have foreign students decided that the quality of American higher education is diminishing? Some may have made this judgment, but a more likely explanation for the falling U.S. share of international students is the higher relative price of a U.S. college education. Throughout the 1990s, tuition and other fees that U.S. colleges and universities charged for their services rose much faster than the average price of other goods and services. They also rose faster than tuition and fees at foreign universities. For instance, even before the sharp 1997–1998 economic contraction in Southeast Asia, increasing numbers of students from this region had begun studying at Australian universities. Colleges in Australia are not only closer to home but also less expensive.

For Critical Analysis

If the relative price of education at U.S. universities continues to increase, what other means could these universities use to try to regain their lost share of international students?

- **Examples** More than 50 thought-provoking and relevant examples highlight U.S. current events and demonstrate economic principles.

EXAMPLE

Garth Brooks, Used CDs, and the Law of Demand

A few years ago, country singer Garth Brooks tried to prevent his latest album from being sold to any chain or store that also sells used CDs. His argument was that the used-CD market deprived labels and artists of earnings. His announcement came after Wherehouse Entertainment, Inc., a 339-store retailer based in Torrance, California, started selling used CDs side by side with new releases, at half the price. Brooks, along with the distribution arms of Sony, Warner Music, Capitol-EMI, and MCA, was trying to quash the used-CD market. By so doing, it appears that none of these parties understands the law of demand.

Let's say the price of a new CD is $15. The existence of a secondary used-CD market means that to people who choose to resell their CDs for $5, the cost of a new CD is in fact only $10. Because we know that quantity demanded is inversely related to price, we know that more of a new CD will be sold at a price of $10 than of the same CD at a price of $15. Taking only this force into account, eliminating the used-CD market tends to reduce sales of new CDs.

But there is another force at work here, too. Used CDs are substitutes for new CDs. If used CDs are not available, some people who would have purchased them will instead purchase new CDs. If this second effect outweighs the incentive to buy less because of the higher effective price, then Brooks is behaving correctly in trying to suppress the used CD market.

For Critical Analysis

Can you apply this argument to the used-book market, in which both authors and publishers have long argued that used books are "killing them"?

- **For Critical Analysis** At the end of each example, students are asked to "think like economists" to answer the critical analysis questions. The answers to all questions are found in the Instructor's Manual.

- **Concepts in Brief** Following each major section, "Concepts in Brief" summarizes the main points of the section to reinforce learning and to encourage rereading of any difficult material.

- **FAQ** All-new sidebars encourage analysis by providing answers to frequently asked questions based on economic reasoning.

FAQ

Isn't postage a lot more expensive than it used to be?

No, in reality, the *relative price* of postage in the United States has fallen steadily over the years. The absolute dollar price of a first-class stamp rose from 3 cents in 1940 to 33 cents at the beginning of the twenty-first century. Nevertheless, the price of postage relative to the average of all other prices has declined since reaching a peak in 1975.

Click here to see how the U.S. Department of Agriculture seeks to estimate demand and supply conditions for major agricultural products.

- **Internet Resources** Margin notes link directly to interesting Web sites that illustrate chapter topics, giving students the opportunity to build their economic research skills by accessing the latest information on the national and global economy.

Market Equilibrium
Click here study market equilibrium in greater detail.

- **Economics in Action Icon** This marginal element directs students to "Economics in Action" modules corresponding to chapter content.

Netnomics The new "Netnomics" feature explores how innovations in information technology are changing economic theory and behavior.

NETNOMICS

Stealth Attacks by New Technologies

Successful new products often get off to a slow start. Eventually, however, consumers substitute away from the old products to the point at which demand for the old products effectively disappears. Consider handwritten versus printed manuscripts. For several years in the mid-fifteenth century, printed books were a rarity, and manuscript-copying monks and scribes continued to turn out the bulk of written forms of communication. By the 1470s, however, printed books were more common than handwritten manuscripts. By the end of the fifteenth century, manuscripts had become the rare commodity.

A more recent example involves train engines. Just before 1940, after the diesel-electric engine for train locomotives was invented, an executive of a steam-engine company declared, "They'll never replace the steam locomotive." In fact, it only took 20 years to prove the executive wrong. By 1960, steam engines were regarded as mechanical dinosaurs.

To generate the bulk of its profits, the U.S. Postal Service relies on revenues from first-class mail. To keep its first-class customers satisfied, it recently deployed a $5 billion automation system that reads nine addresses per second and paints envelopes with bar codes to speed sorting. Yet the postal service has lost about $4 billion in first-class mail business since 1994. Around that time, people began to compare the 25-cent cost of a one-minute phone call with the 32-cent cost of first-class postage. Then they began to substitute away from first-class letters to faxes. Other people got access to the Internet and began to send messages by electronic mail, at no additional charge. First-class mail increasingly looks like a steam-engine dinosaur.

Some observers of the software industry think the same sort of thing could happen to a powerhouse of the present: Microsoft Windows. Today the code for this program is on most personal computers on the planet. Competing operating system applications offered by Sun Microsystems's Java software and others currently run more slowly than Windows. But they consume many fewer lines of computer code and hence promise swift accessibility via the Internet. It is conceivable that someday people may log on to the Internet and pay by the minute to use such software to run their computers, thereby freeing up their hard drives for other uses. Thus today's dominant operating system may someday look a lot like a handwritten manuscript does to generations accustomed to reading printed books instead of handwritten manuscripts.

Issues and Applications Linked to the chapter-opening issue, the all-new "Issues and Applications" features are designed to encourage students to apply economic concepts to real-world situations. Each outlines the concepts being applied in the context of a particular issue and is followed by several critical thinking questions that may be used to prompt in-class discussion. Suggested answers to the critical thinking questions appear in the Instructor's Manual.

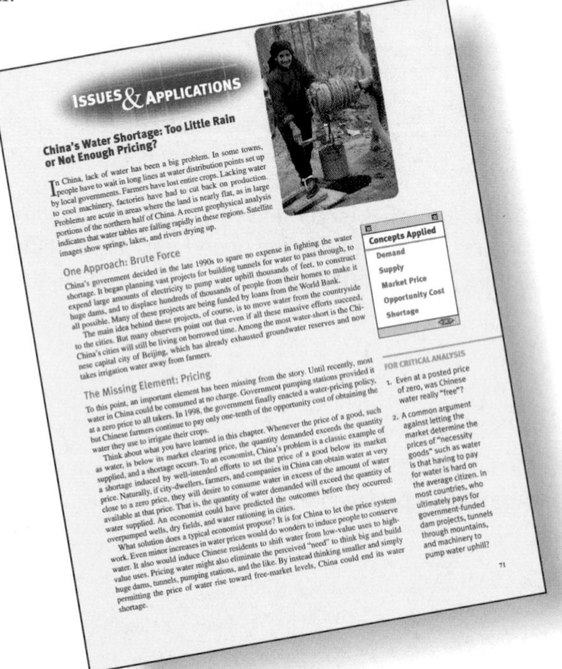

ISSUES & APPLICATIONS

China's Water Shortage: Too Little Rain or Not Enough Pricing?

In China, lack of water has been a big problem. In some towns, people have to wait in long lines at water distribution points set up by local governments. Farmers have lost entire crops. Lacking water to cool machinery, factories have had to cut back on production. Problems are acute in areas where the land is nearly flat, as in large portions of the northern half of China. A recent geophysical analysis indicates that water tables are falling rapidly in these regions. Satellite images show springs, lakes, and rivers drying up.

Concepts Applied
- Demand
- Supply
- Market Price
- Opportunity Cost
- Shortage

One Approach: Brute Force

China's government decided in the late 1990s to spare no expense in fighting the water shortage. It began planning vast projects for building tunnels for water to pass through, to expend large amounts of electricity to pump water uphill thousands of feet, to construct huge dams, and to displace hundreds of thousands of people from their homes to make it all possible. Many of these projects are being funded by loans from the World Bank.

The main idea behind these projects, of course, is to move water from the countryside to the cities. But many observers point out that even if all these massive efforts succeed, China's cities will still be living on borrowed time. Among the most water-short is the Chinese capital city of Beijing, which has already exhausted groundwater reserves and now takes irrigation water away from farmers.

The Missing Element: Pricing

To this point, an important element has been missing from the story. Until recently, most water in China could be consumed at no charge. Government pumping stations provided it at a zero price to all takers. In 1998, the government finally enacted a water-pricing policy, but Chinese farmers continue to pay only one-tenth of the opportunity cost of obtaining the water they use to irrigate their crops.

Think about what you have learned in this chapter. Whenever the price of a good, such as water, is below its market clearing price, the quantity demanded exceeds the quantity supplied, and a shortage occurs. To an economist, China's problem is a classic example of a shortage induced by well-intended efforts to set the price of a good below its market price. Naturally, if city-dwellers, farmers, and companies in China can obtain water at very close to a zero price, they will desire to consume water in excess of the amount of water available at that price. That is, the quantity of water demanded will exceed the quantity of water supplied. An economist could have predicted the outcomes before they occurred: overpumped wells, dry fields, and water rationing in cities.

What solution does a typical economist propose? It is for China to let the price system work. Even minor increases in water prices would do wonders to induce people to conserve water. It also would induce Chinese residents to shift water from low-value uses to high-value uses. Pricing water might also eliminate the perceived "need" to think big and build huge dams, tunnels, pumping stations, and the like. By instead thinking smaller and simply permitting the price of water rise toward free-market levels, China could end its water shortage.

FOR CRITICAL ANALYSIS

1. Even at a posted price of zero, was Chinese water really "free"?
2. A common argument against letting the market determine the prices of "necessity goods" such as water is that having to pay for water is hard on the average citizen. In most countries, who ultimately pays for government-funded dam projects, tunnels through mountains, and machinery to pump water uphill?

71

- **Summary Discussion of Learning Objectives** Every chapter ends with a concise, thorough summary of the important concepts organized around the learning objectives presented at the beginning of each chapter.
- **Key Terms** A list of key terms with page references is a handy study device.
- **Problems** A variety of problems support each chapter. Answers for all odd-numbered problems are provided at the back of the textbook.
- **Economics on the Net** Internet activities are designed to build student research skills and reinforce key concepts. The activities guide students to a Web site and provide a structured assignment for both individual and group work.

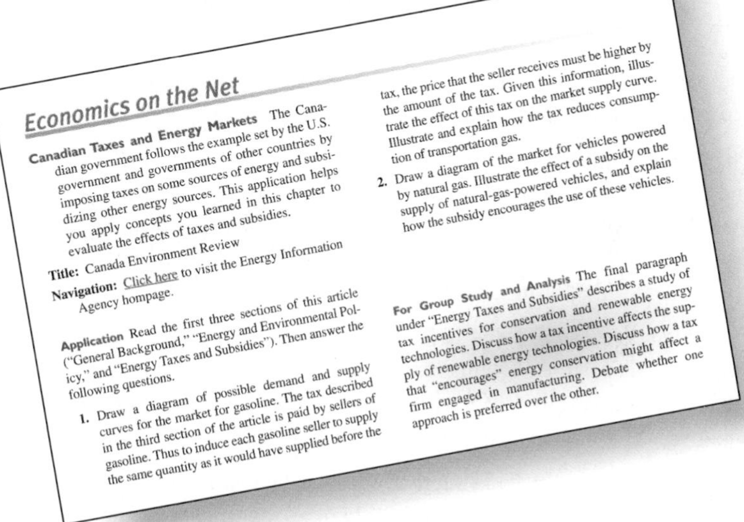

Economics on the Net

Canadian Taxes and Energy Markets The Canadian government follows the example set by the U.S. government and governments of other countries by imposing taxes on some sources of energy and subsidizing other energy sources. This application helps you apply concepts you learned in this chapter to evaluate the effects of taxes and subsidies.

Title: Canada Environment Review

Navigation: Click here to visit the Energy Information Agency hompage.

Application Read the first three sections of this article ("General Background," "Energy and Environmental Policy," and "Energy Taxes and Subsidies"). Then answer the following questions.

1. Draw a diagram of possible demand and supply curves for the market for gasoline. The tax described in the third section of the article is paid by sellers of gasoline. Thus to induce each gasoline seller to supply the same quantity as it would have supplied before the tax, the price that the seller receives must be higher by the amount of the tax. Given this information, illustrate the effect of this tax on the market supply curve. Illustrate and explain how the tax reduces consumption of transportation gas.
2. Draw a diagram of the market for vehicles powered by natural gas. Illustrate the effect of a subsidy on the supply of natural-gas-powered vehicles, and explain how the subsidy encourages the use of these vehicles.

For Group Study and Analysis The final paragraph under "Energy Taxes and Subsidies" describes a study of tax incentives for conservation and renewable energy technologies. Discuss how a tax incentive affects the supply of renewable energy technologies. Discuss how a tax that "encourages" energy conservation might affect a firm engaged in manufacturing. Debate whether one approach is preferred over the other.

- **Tying It All Together** This new feature captures the themes of each part in an extensive case application that demonstrates the relevance of concepts in a business decision-making context. Accompanying questions probe students to assess key issues and do additional research on the Internet. (The answers to all questions are found in the Instructor's Manual.)

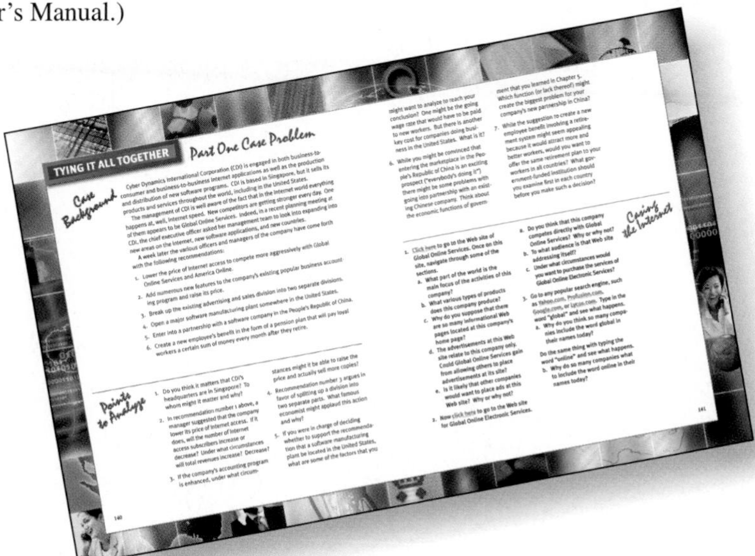

AN EXPANSIVE, INNOVATIVE TEACHING AND LEARNING PACKAGE

Economics Today is accompanied by a variety of technologically innovative and useful supplements for instructors and students.

TO THE INSTRUCTOR

The following supplementary materials are available to help busy instructors teach more effectively and to incorporate technological resources into their principles courses.

- **Instructor's Resource Disk (IRD) with PowerPoint Lecture Presentation** Fully compatible with the Windows NT, 95, and 98, and Macintosh computers, this CD-ROM provides numerous resources.
- The PowerPoint Lecture Presentation was developed by Jeff Caldwell, Steve Smith, and Mark Mitchell of Rose State College and revised by Andrew J. Dane of Angelo State University. With nearly 100 slides per chapter, the PowerPoint Lecture Presentation animates graphs from the text; outlines key terms, concepts, and figures; and provides direct links for in-class Internet activities.
- For added convenience, the IRD also includes Microsoft Word files for the entire content of the Instructor's Manual and Computerized Test Bank files. The easy-to-use testing software (**TestGen-EQ with QuizMaster-EQ** for Windows and Macintosh) is a valuable test preparation tool that allows professors to view, edit, and add questions.
- **Economics in Action** This interactive tutorial software has been developed by Michael Parkin and Robin Bade of the University of Western Ontario and adapted by David Van-Hoose of the University of Alabama for use with *Economics Today*. Available through **MyEconLab.com**, Economics in Action aids students' mastery of concepts through review, demonstration, and interaction. Step-by-step tutorials guide students in their discovery of the relationship between economic theory and real-world applications, while the Draw Graph palette tests their graphing abilities. Detailed, customizable quizzes help students prepare for exams by testing their grasp of concepts.

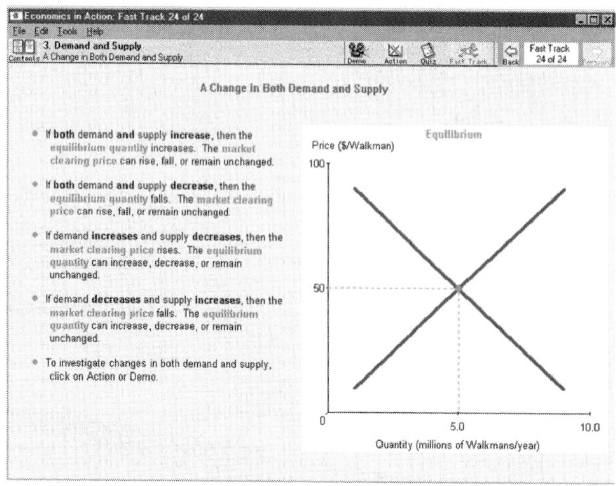

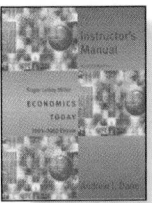

- **Instructor's Manual** Prepared by Andrew J. Dane of Angelo State University, the Instructor's Manual provides the following materials:
  - Chapter overviews, objectives, and outlines
  - Points to emphasize for those who wish to stress theory
  - Answers to "Issues and Applications" critical thinking questions
  - Further questions for class discussion
  - Answers to even-numbered end-of-chapter problems
  - Detailed step-by-step analysis of end-of-chapter problems
  - Suggested answers to "Tying It All Together" case questions
  - Annotated answers to selected student learning questions
  - Selected references

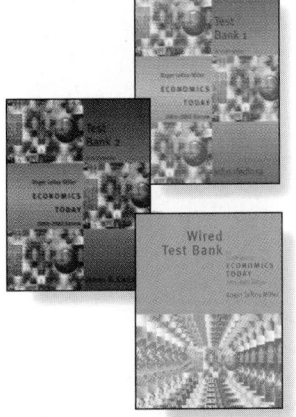

- **Test Bank 1** This Test Bank provides over 3,000 multiple-choice questions and more than 250 short-essay questions with answers. Revised by John Ifediora of the University of Wisconsin, the questions have been extensively classroom-tested for a number of years.
- **Test Bank 2** Revised by James R. Carlson of Manatee Community College, this test bank includes over 3,000 multiple-choice questions and more than 250 short-essay questions. These questions have been class-tested by many professors, including Clark G. Ross, coauthor of the National Competency Test for economics majors for the Educational Testing Service in Princeton, New Jersey.
- **Wired Test Bank** This all-new, innovative supplement is an indispensable aid for professors who are incorporating *Economics Today*'s many technology resources into their courses. It includes questions that allow you to test students on the "Economics in Action" modules, end-of-chapter "Economics on the Net" activities, and "Tying It All Together" cases' Internet feature.

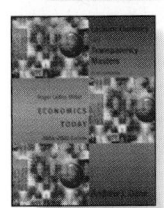

- **Lecture Outlines with Transparency Masters** Prepared by Andrew J. Dane of Angelo State University, this lecture system features more than 500 pages of lecture outlines and text illustrations, including numerous tables taken from the text. Its pages can be made into transparencies or handouts to assist student note taking.
- **Four-Color Overhead Transparencies** One hundred of the most important graphs from the textbook are reproduced as full-color transparency acetates. Many contain multiple overlays.

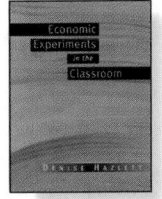

- **Economics Experiments in the Classroom** Developed by Denise Hazlett of Whitman College, these economics experiments involve students in actively testing economic theory. In addition to providing a variety of micro and macro experiments, this supplement offers step-by-step guidelines for successfully running experiments in the classroom.
- **Additional Homework Problems** For each text chapter, more than 20 additional problems are provided in two separate sets of homework assignments that are available for download from **www.myeconlab.com**. Each homework problem is accompanied by suggested answers.
- **Regional Case Studies for the East Coast, Texas, and California** Additional case studies, available at **www.myeconlab.com**, can be used for in-class team exercises or for additional homework assignments.

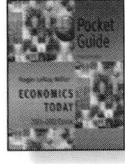

- **Pocket Guide to Economics Today for Printed and Electronic Supplements** The Pocket Guide is designed to coordinate the extensive teaching and learning package that accompanies *Economics Today*. For each chapter heading, the author has organized a list of print and electronic ancillaries with page references to help organize lectures, develop class assignments, and prepare examinations.

CHAPTER 1

THE NATURE OF ECONOMICS

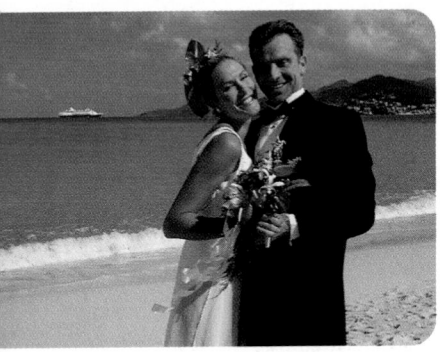

Men who are married earn, on average, higher incomes than those who are not married. Does this marriage premium mean that if you are single and decide to get married, you will automatically make a higher income?

In 1911, Edgar Watson Howe wrote, "Marriage is a good deal like a circus: There is not as much in it as is represented by the advertising." Nevertheless, for men (but not, apparently, for women), marriage has a concrete payoff: earnings 10 to 20 percent higher than those of unmarried men. Economists call this wage differential the "marriage premium."

One rationale for the marriage premium is that by settling down, men are able to be more successful in their careers. Another theory, however, is that the women do a good job of selecting their husbands. That is, women choose to marry men who are more successful than the men they choose not to marry.

Whether it is men deciding to marry for the good of their careers or women selecting a successful marriage partner, both make *choices.* A fundamental aspect of the science of economics is seeking to understand how people make choices.

LEARNING OBJECTIVES

After reading this chapter, you should be able to:

1. **Discuss the difference between microeconomics and macroeconomics**
2. **Evaluate the role that rational self-interest plays in economic analysis**
3. **Explain why the study of economics is a science**
4. **Distinguish between positive and normative economics**

Chapter Outline

- The Power of Economic Analysis
- Defining Economics
- Microeconomics Versus Macroeconomics
- The Economic Person: Rational Self-Interest
- Economics as a Science
- Positive Versus Normative Economics

Did You Know That... since 1989, the number of fax machines in U.S. offices and homes has increased by over 10,000 percent? During the same time period, the number of bike messengers in downtown New York City *decreased* by over 65 percent. The world around us is definitely changing. Much of that change is due to the dramatically falling cost of communications and information technology. Today the computers inside video games cost only about $100 yet have 50 times the processing power that a $10 million IBM mainframe had in 1975. Not surprisingly, American firms have been spending more on communications equipment and computers than on new construction and heavy machinery.

Cyberspace, the Internet, the World Wide Web—call it what you want, but your next home (if not your current one) will almost certainly have an address on it. The percentage of U.S. households that have at least one telephone is close to 100 percent, and those that have video game players is over 50 percent. Over half of homes have personal computers, and more than two-thirds of those machines are set up to receive and access information via phone lines. Your decisions about such things as when and what type of computer to buy, whether to accept a collect call from a friend traveling in Europe, and how much time you should invest in learning to use the latest Web browser involve an untold number of variables: where you live, the work your parents do, what your friends think, and so on. But as you will see, there are economic underpinnings for nearly all the decisions you make.

THE POWER OF ECONOMIC ANALYSIS

Knowing that an economic problem exists every time you make a decision is not enough. You also have to develop a framework that will allow you to analyze solutions to each economic problem—whether you are trying to decide how much to study, which courses to take, whether to finish school, or whether America should send troops abroad or raise tariffs. The framework that you will learn in this text is based on the *economic way of thinking.*

This framework gives you power—the power to reach informed conclusions about what is happening in the world. You can, of course, live your life without the power of economic analysis as part of your analytical framework. Indeed, most people do. But economists believe that economic analysis can help you make better decisions concerning your career, your education, financing your home, and other important matters. In the business world, the power of economic analysis can help you increase your competitive edge as an employee or as the owner of a business. As a voter, for the rest of your life you will be asked to make judgments about policies that are advocated by a particular political party. Many of these policies will deal with questions related to international economics, such as whether the U.S. government should encourage or discourage immigration, prevent foreigners from investing in domestic TV stations and newspapers, or restrict other countries from selling their goods here. Finally, just as taking an art, music, or literature appreciation class increases the pleasure you receive when you view paintings, listen to concerts, or read novels, taking an economics course will increase your understanding when watching the news on TV or reading the newspaper.

DEFINING ECONOMICS

What is economics exactly? Some cynics have defined *economics* as "common sense made difficult." But common sense, by definition, should be within everyone's grasp. You will encounter in the following pages numerous examples that show that economics is, in fact, pure and simple common sense.

Economics is part of the social sciences and as such seeks explanations of real events. All social sciences analyze human behavior, as opposed to the physical sciences, which generally analyze the behavior of electrons, atoms, and other nonhuman phenomena.

> Economics is the study of how people allocate their limited resources in an attempt to satisfy their unlimited wants. As such, economics is the study of how people make choices.

Economics 
The study of how people allocate their limited resources to satisfy their unlimited wants.

To understand this definition fully, two other words need explaining: *resources* and *wants.* **Resources** are things that have value and, more specifically, are used to produce things that satisfy people's wants. **Wants** are all of the things that people would consume if they had unlimited income.

Resources 
Things used to produce other things to satisfy people's wants.

Wants 
What people would buy if their incomes were unlimited.

Whenever an individual, a business, or a nation faces alternatives, a choice must be made, and economics helps us study how those choices are made. For example, you have to choose how to spend your limited income. You also have to choose how to spend your limited time. You may have to choose how much of your company's limited funds to spend on advertising and how much to spend on new-product research. In economics, we examine situations in which individuals choose how to do things, when to do things, and with whom to do them. Ultimately, the purpose of economics is to explain choices.

MICROECONOMICS VERSUS MACROECONOMICS 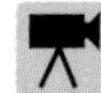

Economics is typically divided into two types of analysis: **microeconomics** and **macroeconomics.**

> Microeconomics is the part of economic analysis that studies decision making undertaken by individuals (or households) and by firms. It is like looking through a microscope to focus on the small parts of our economy.

> Macroeconomics is the part of economic analysis that studies the behavior of the economy as a whole. It deals with economywide phenomena such as changes in unemployment, the general price level, and national income.

Microeconomics 
The study of decision making undertaken by individuals (or households) and by firms.

Macroeconomics 
The study of the behavior of the economy as a whole, including such economywide phenomena as changes in unemployment, the general price level, and national income.

Microeconomic analysis, for example, is concerned with the effects of changes in the price of gasoline relative to that of other energy sources. It examines the effects of new taxes on a specific product or industry. If price controls were reinstituted in the United States, how individual firms and consumers would react to them would be in the realm of microeconomics. The raising of wages by an effective union strike would also be analyzed using the tools of microeconomics.

By contrast, issues such as the rate of inflation, the amount of economywide unemployment, and the yearly growth in the output of goods and services in the nation all fall into the realm of macroeconomic analysis. In other words, macroeconomics deals with **aggregates,** or totals—such as total output in an economy.

Aggregates 
Total amounts or quantities; aggregate demand, for example, is total planned expenditures throughout a nation.

Be aware, however, of the blending of microeconomics and macroeconomics in modern economic theory. Modern economists are increasingly using microeconomic analysis—the study of decision making by individuals and by firms—as the basis of macroeconomic analysis. They do this because even though in macroeconomic analysis aggregates are being examined, those aggregates are the result of choices made by individuals and firms.

THE ECONOMIC PERSON: RATIONAL SELF-INTEREST 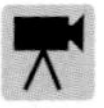

Economists assume that individuals act *as if* motivated by self-interest and respond predictably to opportunities for gain. This central insight of economics was first clearly articulated by Adam Smith in 1776. Smith wrote in his most famous book, *An Inquiry into the*

Click here to explore whether it is in a consumer's self-interest to shop on the Internet. Click on "To e-shoppers".

Nature and Causes of the Wealth of Nations, that "it is not from the benevolence of the butcher, the brewer, or the baker that we expect our dinner, but from their regard to their own interest." Otherwise stated, the typical person about whom economists make behavioral predictions is assumed to act as though motivated by self interest. Because monetary benefits and costs of actions are often the most easily measured, economists most often make behavioral predictions about individuals' responses to ways to increase their wealth, measured in money terms. Let's see if we can apply the theory of rational self-interest to explain an anomaly concerning the makeup of the U.S. population.

EXAMPLE

The Increasing Native American Population

Look at Figure 1-1. You see that the proportion of Native Americans increased quite dramatically from 1970 to 1990. Can we use Adam Smith's ideas to understand why so many Native Americans have decided to rejoin their tribes? Perhaps. Consider the benefits of being a member of the Mdewakanton *(bday-WAH-kan-toon),* a tribe of about 100 that runs a casino in which gamblers in a recent year wagered over $500 million. Each member of the tribe received over $400,000 from the casino's profits. There is now a clear economic reason for Native Americans to return home. Over 200 of the nation's 544 tribes have introduced gambling of some sort, and almost half of those have big-time casinos. Reservations are grossing almost $6 billion a year from gaming. Tribe members sometimes get direct payments and others get the benefits of better health care, subsidized mortgages, and jobs. Self-identified Native Americans increased in number by 150 percent between 1970 and 2000.

For Critical Analysis

What nonmonetary reasons are there for Native Americans to rejoin their tribes?

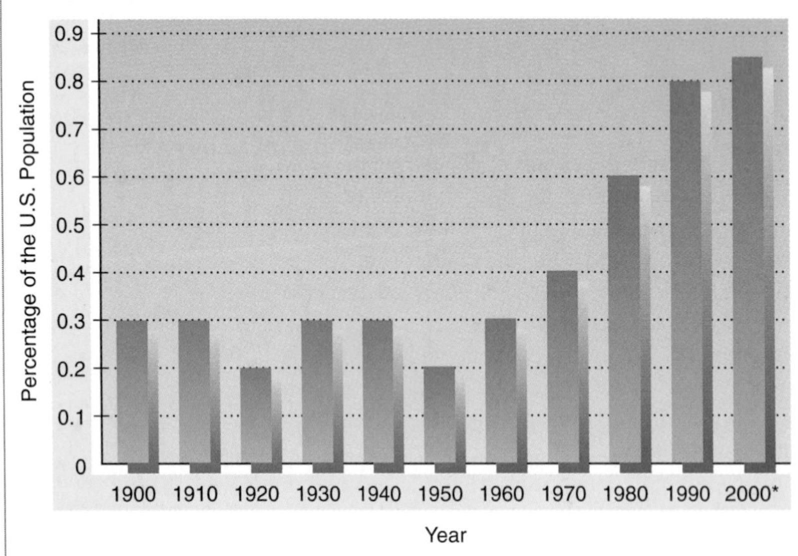

FIGURE 1-1

Native American Population of the United States

The percentage of the U.S. population identifying itself as Native American has increased substantially in recent decades. Is there an economic explanation for this demographic trend?

* Data for 2000 based on author's estimate

The Rationality Assumption

Rationality assumption

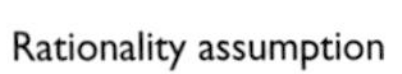
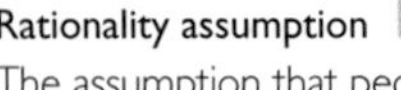

The assumption that people do not intentionally make decisions that would leave them worse off.

The **rationality assumption** of economics, simply stated, is as follows:

> We assume that individuals do not intentionally make decisions that would leave them worse off.

The distinction here is between what people may think—the realm of psychology and psychiatry and perhaps sociology—and what they do. Economics does *not* involve itself in analyzing individual or group thought processes. Economics looks at what people actually do in life with their limited resources. It does little good to criticize the rationality assumption by stating, "Nobody thinks that way" or "I never think that way" or "How unrealistic! That's as irrational as anyone can get!"

Take the example of driving. When you consider passing another car on a two-lane highway with oncoming traffic, you have to make very quick decisions: You must estimate the speed of the car that you are going to pass, the speed of the oncoming cars, the distance between your car and the oncoming cars, and your car's potential rate of acceleration. If we were to apply a model to your behavior, we would use the rules of calculus. In actual fact, you and most other drivers in such a situation do not actually think of using the rules of calculus, but to predict your behavior, we could make the prediction *as if* you understood the rules of calculus.

In any event, when you observe behavior around you, what may seem irrational often has its basis in the rationality assumption, as you can see by the following example.

EXAMPLE

When It May Be Rational *Not* to Learn New Technology

The standard young person's view of older people (particularly one's parents) is that they're reluctant to learn new things. The saying "You can't teach an old dog new tricks" seems to apply. Young people, in contrast, seem eager to learn about new technology—mastering computers and multimedia, playing interactive games, surfing the Internet. But there can be a rational reason for older people's reduced willingness to learn new technologies. If you are 20 years old and learn a new skill, you will be able to gain returns from your investment in learning over the course of many decades. If you are 60, however, and invest the same amount of time and effort learning the same skill, you will almost certainly not be able to reap those returns for as long a time period. Hence it can be perfectly rational for "old dogs" not to want to learn new tricks.

For Critical Analysis

Some older people do learn to use new technologies as they emerge. What might explain this behavior?

Responding to Incentives

If it can be assumed that individuals never intentionally make decisions that would leave them worse off, then almost by definition they will respond to different incentives. We define **incentives** as the potential rewards available if a particular activity is undertaken. Indeed, much of human behavior can be explained in terms of how individuals respond to changing incentives over time.

Incentives 
Rewards for engaging in a particular activity.

Schoolchildren are motivated to do better by a variety of incentive systems, ranging from gold stars and certificates of achievement when they are young to better grades with accompanying promises of a "better life" as they get older. There are, of course, negative incentives that affect our behavior, too. Children who disrupt the class are given after-school detention or sent to the vice principal for other punishment. Young people, like adults, respond to incentives.

For instance, consider the juvenile criminal justice system. Between the late 1970s and the mid-1990s, the number of arrests of adults for murder fell by 7 percent, but juvenile murder arrests increased by 177 percent. Arrests of juveniles for all violent crimes rose by 79 percent during the period, nearly three times the increase in adult arrests for these crimes.

Steven Levitt of the University of Chicago examined the incentives that juvenile criminals face. While the average number of adults incarcerated per violent crime rose by

60 percent over the same period, the corresponding ratio of juveniles imprisoned in youth detention centers *declined* by 20 percent. Levitt concluded that the probability of a juvenile offender's being jailed was less than half the probability of imprisonment that an adult faced.

Levitt also found changes in criminal behavior when youths face adult criminal justice at age 18. In states where incarceration rates for youths are high but those for adults are low, violent crimes committed by 18-year-olds rise by 23 percent. But crimes committed by 18-year-olds *fall* by 4 percent in states where incarceration rates for adults are relatively high.

Implicitly, all people, including juveniles contemplating crime, react to changing incentives after they have done some sort of rough comparison of the costs and benefits of various courses of action. In fact, making rational choices invariably involves balancing costs and benefits.

The linked concepts of incentives and costs and benefits can be used to explain much human behavior in the world around us. It can also explain how government policies can *induce* people to break the law.

INTERNATIONAL POLICY EXAMPLE

Chinese Smuggling

Recently, China's leaders announced the formation of a new antismuggling police force to try to stop the annual flow of tens of billions of dollars in illegal contraband.

One example of "illegal contraband" is cigarettes. Domestic taxes on cigarettes are so high that many Chinese cigarette manufacturers export half of their output, which they then smuggle back into China. Another example is diesel oil, the price of which the Chinese government sets at levels above prices elsewhere in the world. This gives consumers of diesel oil an incentive to smuggle foreign-produced diesel oil into the country.

Why does China need an antismuggling police force when it already has an army of border guards and customs inspectors? The answer is that the returns to smuggling are so high that many existing border guards and customs inspectors have become smugglers themselves. Thus the government feels that new police are needed in part to watch over the existing cadre of "law enforcers."

For Critical Analysis

What actions could the government take to end the incentives to smuggle cigarettes and diesel oil?

Defining Self-Interest

Self-interest does not always mean increasing one's wealth measured in dollars and cents. We assume that individuals seek many goals, not just increased wealth measured in monetary terms. Thus the self-interest part of our economic-person assumption includes goals relating to prestige, friendship, love, power, helping others, creating works of art, and many other matters. We can also think in terms of enlightened self-interest whereby individuals, in the pursuit of what makes them better off, also achieve the betterment of others around them. In brief, individuals are assumed to want the right to further their goals by making decisions about how things around them are used. The head of a charitable organization will usually not turn down an additional contribution because accepting it gains control over how that money is used, even if it is for other people's benefit.

Otherwise stated, charitable acts are not ruled out by self-interest. Giving gifts to relatives can be considered a form of charity that is nonetheless in the self-interest of the giver. But how efficient is such gift giving?

EXAMPLE

The Perceived Value of Gifts

Every holiday season, aunts, uncles, grandparents, mothers, and fathers give gifts to their college-aged loved ones. Joel Waldfogel, an economist at Yale University, surveyed several thousand college students after Christmas to find out the value of holiday gifts. He found that compact discs and outerwear (coats and jackets) had a perceived intrinsic value about equal to their actual cash equivalent. By the time he got down the list to socks, underwear, and cosmetics, the students' valuation was only about 85 percent of the cash value of the gift. He found out that aunts, uncles, and grandparents gave the "worst" gifts and friends, siblings, and parents gave the "best."

For Critical Analysis

What argument could you use against the idea of substituting cash or gift certificates for physical gifts?

CONCEPTS IN BRIEF

- Economics is a social science that involves the study of how individuals choose among alternatives to satisfy their wants, which are what people would buy if their incomes were unlimited.
- Microeconomics, the study of the decision-making processes of individuals (or households) and firms, and macroeconomics, the study of the performance of the economy as a whole, are the two main branches into which the study of economics is divided.
- In economics, we assume that people do not intentionally make decisions that will leave them worse off. This is known as the rationality assumption.
- Self-interest is not confined to material well-being but also involves any action that makes a person feel better off, such as having more friends, love, power, affection, or providing more help to others.

ECONOMICS AS A SCIENCE

Economics is a social science that employs the same kinds of methods used in other sciences, such as biology, physics, and chemistry. Like these other sciences, economics uses models, or theories. Economic **models,** or **theories,** are simplified representations of the real world that we use to help us understand, explain, and predict economic phenomena in the real world. There are, of course, differences between sciences. The social sciences—especially economics—make little use of laboratory methods in which changes in variables can be explained under controlled conditions. Rather, social scientists, and especially economists, usually have to examine what has already happened in the real world in order to test their models, or theories.

Models, or **theories**
Simplified representations of the real world used as the basis for predictions or explanations.

Models and Realism

At the outset it must be emphasized that no model in *any* science, and therefore no economic model, is complete in the sense that it captures *every* detail or interrelationship that exists. Indeed, a model, by definition, is an abstraction from reality. It is conceptually impossible to construct a perfectly complete realistic model. For example, in physics we cannot account for every molecule and its position and certainly not for every atom and subparticle. Not only is such a model impossibly expensive to build, but working with it would be impossibly complex.

The nature of scientific model building is such that the model should capture only the *essential* relationships that are sufficient to analyze the particular problem or answer the particular question with which we are concerned. *An economic model cannot be faulted as unrealistic simply because it does not represent every detail of the real world.* A map of a city that shows only major streets is not necessarily unrealistic if, in fact, all you need to know is how to pass through the city using major streets. As long as a model is realistic in terms of shedding light on the *central* issue at hand or forces at work, it may be useful.

A map is the quintessential model. It is always a simplified representation. It is always unrealistic. But it is also useful in making (refutable) predictions about the world. If the model—the map—predicts that when you take Campus Avenue to the north, you always run into the campus, that is a (refutable) prediction. If our goal is to explain observed behavior, the simplicity or complexity of the model we use is irrelevant. If a simple model can explain observed behavior in repeated settings just as well as a complex one, the simple model has some value and is probably easier to use.

Assumptions

Every model, or theory, must be based on a set of assumptions. Assumptions define the set of circumstances in which our model is most likely to be applicable. When scientists predicted that sailing ships would fall off the edge of the earth, they used the *assumption* that the earth was flat. Columbus did not accept the implications of such a model. He assumed that the world was round. The real-world test of his own model refuted the flat-earth model. Indirectly, then, it was a test of the assumption of the flat-earth model.

EXAMPLE

Getting Directions

Assumptions are a shorthand for reality. Imagine that you have decided to drive from your home in San Diego to downtown San Francisco. Because you have never driven this route, you decide to get directions from the local office of the American Automobile Association (AAA).

When you ask for directions, the travel planner could give you a set of detailed maps that shows each city through which you will travel—Oceanside, San Clemente, Irvine, Anaheim, Los Angeles, Bakersfield, Modesto, and so on—and then, opening each map, show you exactly how the freeway threads through each of these cities. You would get a nearly complete description of reality because the AAA travel planner will not have used many simplifying assumptions. It is more likely, however, that the travel planner will simply say, "Get on Interstate 5 going north. Stay on it for about 500 miles. Follow the signs for San Francisco. After crossing the toll bridge, take any exit marked 'Downtown.'" By omitting all of the trivial details, the travel planner has told you all that you really need and want to know. The models you will be using in this text are similar to the simplified directions on how to drive from San Diego to San Francisco—they focus on what is relevant to the problem at hand and omit what is not.

For Critical Analysis

In what way do small talk and gossip represent the use of simplifying assumptions?

Ceteris paribus [KAY-ter-us PEAR-uh-bus] assumption 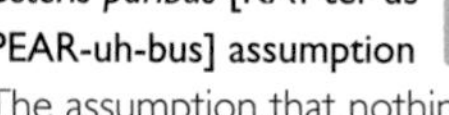
The assumption that nothing changes except the factor or factors being studied.

The *Ceteris Paribus* Assumption: All Other Things Being Equal. Everything in the world seems to relate in some way to everything else in the world. It would be impossible to isolate the effects of changes in one variable on another variable if we always had to worry about the many other variables that might also enter the analysis. As in other sciences, economics uses the ***ceteris paribus* assumption.** *Ceteris paribus* means "other things constant" or "other things equal."

Consider an example taken from economics. One of the most important determinants of how much of a particular product a family buys is how expensive that product is relative to other products. We know that in addition to relative prices, other factors influence decisions about making purchases. Some of them have to do with income, others with tastes, and yet others with custom and religious beliefs. Whatever these other factors are, we hold them constant when we look at the relationship between changes in prices and changes in how much of a given product people will purchase.

Deciding on the Usefulness of a Model

We generally do not attempt to determine the usefulness, or "goodness," of a model merely by evaluating how realistic its assumptions are. Rather, we consider a model good if it yields usable predictions and implications for the real world. In other words, can we use the model to predict what will happen in the world around us? Does the model provide useful implications of how things happen in our world?

Once we have determined that the model does predict real-world phenomena, the scientific approach to the analysis of the world around us requires that we consider evidence. Evidence is used to test the usefulness of a model. This is why we call economics an **empirical** science, *empirical* meaning that evidence (data) is looked at to see whether we are right. Economists are often engaged in empirically testing their models.

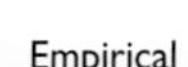 

Empirical
Relying on real-world data in evaluating the usefulness of a model.

Consider two competing models for the way students act when doing complicated probability problems to choose the best gambles. One model predicts that based on the assumption of rational self-interest, students who are paid more money for better performance will in fact perform better on average during the experiment. A competing model might be that students whose last names start with the letters *A* through *L* will do better than students with last names starting with *M* through *Z*, irrespective of how much they are paid. The model that consistently predicts more accurately is the model that we would normally choose. In this example, the "alphabet" model did not work well: The first letter of the last name of the students who actually did the experiment at UCLA was irrelevant in predicting how well they would perform the mathematical calculations necessary to choose the correct gambles. On average, students who received higher cash payments for better gambles did choose a higher percentage of better gambles. Thus the model based on rational self-interest predicted well.

FAQ: *Can economists rely on opinion polls to understand what motivates behavior?*

No, most economists are leery of trying to glean much from opinion polls. For instance, a psychology study once revolved around polls asking people at various income levels how "happy" they were, based on a scale of 1 to 10. The researchers who conducted the study received responses that appeared to indicate that many rich people were less happy, leading the researchers to conclude that wealth can be associated with lower satisfaction. Economics is a science of *revealed* preferences, however. We find out virtually no useful information by asking people to rate their happiness levels on an arbitrary scale. In response to this particular study, a typical economist would note that if "too much" wealth makes people unhappy, they can always give it away. No one forces them to keep it. The fact that we rarely observe people disposing of their wealth causes an economist to infer that higher wealth must be preferred to lower wealth.

Models of Behavior, Not Thought Processes

Take special note of the fact that economists' models do not relate to the way people *think;* they relate to the way people *act,* to what they do in life with their limited resources. Models tend to generalize human behavior. Normally, the economist does not attempt to predict how people will think about a particular topic, such as a higher price of oil products, accelerated inflation, or higher taxes. Rather, the task at hand is to predict how people will act, which may be quite different from what they *say* they will do (much to the consternation of poll takers and market researchers). The people involved in examining thought processes are psychologists and psychiatrists, not typically economists.

EXAMPLE

Incentives Work for Pigeons and Rats, Too

Researchers at Texas A&M University did a series of experiments with pigeons and rats. They allowed them to "purchase" food and drink by pushing various levers. The "price" was the number of times a lever had to be pushed. A piece of cheese required 10 pushes, a drop of root beer only one. The "incomes" that the animals were given equaled a certain number of total pushes per day. Once the income was used up, the levers did not work. The researchers discovered that holding income constant, when the price of cheese went down, the animals purchased more cheese. Similarly, they found that when the price of root beer was increased, the animals purchased less root beer. These are exactly the predictions that we make about human behavior.

For Critical Analysis

"People respond to incentives." Is this assumption also usable in the animal world?

POSITIVE VERSUS NORMATIVE ECONOMICS 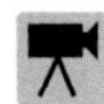

Economics uses *positive analysis,* a value-free approach to inquiry. No subjective or moral judgments enter into the analysis. Positive analysis relates to statements such as "If A, then B." For example, "If the price of gasoline goes up relative to all other prices, then the amount of it that people will buy will fall." That is a positive economic statement. It is a statement of *what is.* It is not a statement of anyone's value judgment or subjective feelings. For many problems analyzed in the hard sciences such as physics and chemistry, the analyses are considered to be virtually value-free. After all, how can someone's values enter into a theory of molecular behavior? But economists face a different problem. They deal with the behavior of individuals, not molecules. That makes it more difficult to stick to what we consider to be value-free or **positive economics** without reference to our feelings.

Positive economics 
Analysis that is strictly limited to making either purely descriptive statements or scientific predictions; for example, "If A, then B." A statement of *what is.*

When our values are interjected into the analysis, we enter the realm of **normative economics,** involving *normative analysis*. A positive economic statement is "If the price of gas rises, people will buy less." If we add to that analysis the statement "so we should not allow the price to go up," we have entered the realm of normative economics—we have expressed a value judgment. In fact, any time you see the word *should,* you will know that values are entering into the discussion. Just remember that positive statements are concerned with *what is,* whereas normative statements are concerned with *what ought to be.*

Normative economics 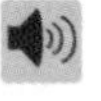
Analysis involving value judgments about economic policies; relates to whether things are good or bad. A statement of *what ought to be.*

Each of us has a desire for different things. That means that we have different values. When we express a value judgment, we are simply saying what we prefer, like, or desire. Because individual values are diverse, we expect—and indeed observe—people expressing widely varying value judgments about how the world ought to be.

A Warning: Recognize Normative Analysis

It is easy to define positive economics. It is quite another matter to catch all unlabeled normative statements in a textbook, even though an author goes over the manuscript many times before it is printed. Therefore, do not get the impression that a textbook author will be able to keep all personal values out of the book. They will slip through. In fact, the very choice of which topics to include in an introductory textbook involves normative economics. There is no value-free, or objective, way to decide which topics to use in a textbook. The author's values ultimately make a difference when choices have to be made. But from your own standpoint, you might want to be able to recognize when you are engaging in normative as opposed to positive economic analysis. Reading this text will help equip you for that task.

CONCEPTS IN BRIEF

- A model, or theory, uses assumptions and is by nature a simplification of the real world. The usefulness of a model can be evaluated by bringing empirical evidence to bear on its predictions.
- Models are not necessarily deficient simply because they are unrealistic and use simplifying assumptions, for every model in every science requires simplification compared to the real world.
- Most models use the *ceteris paribus* assumption, that all other things are held constant, or equal.
- Positive economics is value-free and relates to statements that can be refuted, such as "If A, then B." Normative economics involves people's values, and normative statements typically contain the word *should.*

NETNOMICS

Is It Irrational for People to Pay Amazon.com More for a Book They Can Buy for Less at Books.com?

To try to understand how consumers respond to changing incentives they face now that they can purchase goods and services on the Internet, Erik Brynjolfsson and Michael Smith of the Massachusetts Institute of Technology gathered more than 10,000 observations of the prices charged by traditional brick-and-mortar bookstores and Internet booksellers. What they found was what most economists would predict: The lower costs faced by Internet booksellers allowed them to charge about 8 percent less for a given book than traditional bookstores. Furthermore, the cost advantage of Internet booksellers allowed them to gain market share at the expense of traditional stores. (Indeed, some brick-and-mortar bookstores initially included in the study went out of business before the study ended.)

One finding seemed surprising, however. Amazon.com, which garnered an 80 percent share of all Internet-based book sales, charged an average of $1.60 more per book than Books.com, another Internet bookseller (now part of barnesandnoble.com). Yet Books.com could not seem to push its market share much above 2 percent during the period of the study. On the surface, this seemed to imply irrational consumers. After all, wouldn't everyone want to choose Books.com and save $1.60 per book?

As the authors point out, this would be true only if the *ceteris paribus* assumption had been satisfied. In their study, however, it was not. For one thing, Amazon.com spent a considerable amount on advertising and got a jump start on its Internet competitors. Indeed, even today, a great many Internet users have heard of Amazon.com but are unfamiliar with its competitors. This made Brynjolfsson and Smith wonder if perhaps people felt confident that Amazon.com really would deliver but might not have as much faith in less well-known Internet companies. Thus part of the $1.60 difference in the average price of a book might amount to a "trust premium." Furthermore, Brynjolfsson and Smith's study did not take into account differences in features of the two companies' Web sites. If people already knew how to use the Amazon.com Web site, then a legitimate question to ask is, would the average person consider $1.60 enough to compensate for having to learn how to order a book from another Web site?

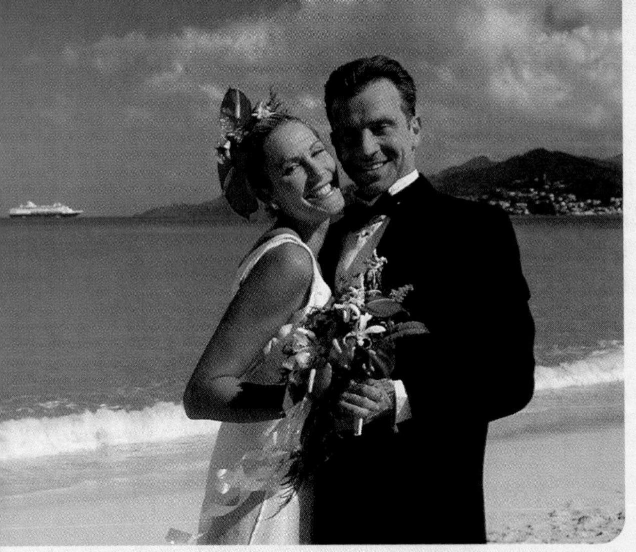

Issues & Applications

Marriage Isn't a Marxist Utopia, but It Can Pay Off

Concepts Applied

- Decision Making
- Rational Self-Interest
- Incentives

Karl Marx was a German economist who wrote a treatise called *Das Kapital* (Capital), in which he proposed that labor is the fundamental source of all value. With Friedrich Engels, he wrote an even more famous book, *The Communist Manifesto,* in which he promoted the virtues of state socialism. Economists largely have rejected his theory of value as overly narrow, and communism is on the decline worldwide. Nevertheless, Marx left a lasting legacy: the idea that people could achieve a perfect world, commonly called a *utopia.* The word was coined by Sir Thomas More in his book about a fictitious island by that name. More called his land Utopia (Greek for "no place") because he knew that a perfect world is impossible to achieve.

Nevertheless, on their wedding day, many women and men think they are entering a personal utopia: They convince themselves that they are embarking on the "perfect marriage." Jennifer Roback Morse of the Hoover Institution has written, "Utopianism in politics is destructive: Perfectionism in human relationships can be, too. The Marxist search for a perfect society has cost millions of lives. The American yearning for perfect marriages probably has ruined many lives."

Marriage as an Exercise in Self-Interest

A number of couples, however, remain married for decades even when they know that their marriages are imperfect. To outsiders looking at such a married couple and observing one spouse silently suffering for years while the other spouse continually behaves in some socially unacceptable manner, the rationality of the marriage can be hard to fathom. To an economist, this makes the institution of marriage an especially interesting case study of human choice.

Throughout history, literally billions of people have chosen to be married and to put up with the faults of their matrimonial partners. Why do they do this? One reason that economists have offered is that spouses show consideration for their marriage partners in the hope or expectation that the favor will be returned. This is self-interest at work. In addition, by entering into and staying faithful to a marriage, one spouse establishes a reputation with the other. By honoring their commitment to the marriage, they show more broadly that they are not afraid of commitments. This gives both a greater incentive to trust each other when they make joint financial decisions. By pooling their resources, both marriage partners can thereby make themselves better off than they would be alone. This is also an example of people responding in a self-interested way to incentives they face.

"Shotgun Weddings" and the Marriage Premium

Economists have evidence that there is something to this story. Recall from the opening to this chapter that most married men earn more than unmarried men. Donna Ginther of Washington University and Madeline Zavodny of the Federal Reserve Bank of Atlanta tried to evaluate whether this marriage premium is simply due to beneficial effects of marriage for men or instead results from careful spousal choices by women seeking committed husbands. To do this, they compared the wages of men married in so-called shotgun weddings—marriages followed within, say, seven months by the birth of a child—with the wages of men whose wives did not bear children until later on. After controlling for other factors, they found that men married in shotgun weddings typically did not earn a marriage premium. Presumably, many men in such situations are less committed to the marriage. Nevertheless, women expecting children may feel that their choices are constrained, so they are less likely to reject the marriage partner in a shotgun wedding. Thus it appears that in most instances, the marriage premium applies to the husbands of women who feel less constrained in choosing their mates.

FOR CRITICAL ANALYSIS

1. So far there is little evidence of a marriage premium for women. Can you think of any reasons why this is so?
2. What is the economic role of love in marriage?

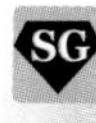

SUMMARY DISCUSSION OF LEARNING OBJECTIVES

1. **Microeconomics Versus Macroeconomics:** In general, economics is the study of how individuals make choices to satisfy wants. Economics is usually divided into microeconomics, which is the study of individual decision making by households and firms, and macroeconomics, which is the study of nationwide phenomena, such as inflation and unemployment.
2. **Self-Interest in Economic Analysis:** Rational self-interest is the assumption that individuals behave in a reasonable (rational) way in making choices to further their interests. That is, economists assume that individuals never intentionally make decisions that would leave them worse off. Instead, they are motivated primarily by their self-interest, keeping in mind that self-interest can relate to monetary and nonmonetary objectives, such as love, prestige, and helping others.
3. **Economics as a Science:** Like other scientists, economists use models, or theories, that are simplified representations of the real world to analyze and make predictions about the real world. Economic models are never completely realistic because by definition they are simplifications using assumptions that are not directly testable. Nevertheless, economists can subject the predictions of economic theories to empirical tests in which real-world data are used to decide whether or not to reject the predictions.
4. **The Difference Between Positive and Normative Economics:** Positive economics deals with *what is,* whereas normative economics deals with *what ought to be.* Positive economic statements are of the "if . . . then" variety; they are descriptive and predictive and are not related to what "should" happen. By contrast, whenever statements embodying values are made, we enter the realm of normative economics, or how individuals and groups think things ought to be.

Key Terms and Concepts

Problems

Answers to the odd-numbered problems appear at the back of the book.

1-1. Some people claim that the "economic way of thinking" does not apply to issues such as health care. Explain how economics does apply to this issue by developing a "model" of an individual's choice.

1-2. In a single sentence, contrast microeconomics and macroeconomics. Next, categorize the following issues as either a microeconomic issue, a macroeconomic issue, or not an economic issue.
- **a.** The national unemployment rate
- **b.** The decision of a worker to work overtime or not
- **c.** A family's choice of having a baby
- **d.** The rate of growth of the money supply
- **e.** The national government's budget deficit
- **f.** A student's allocation of study time across two subjects

1-3. One of your classmates, Sally, is a hardworking student, serious about her classes, and conscientious about her grades. Sally is also involved, however, in volunteer activities and an extracurricular sport. Is Sally displaying rational behavior? Based on what you read in this chapter, construct an argument supporting the conclusion that she is.

1-4. You have 10 hours in which to study for both a French test and an economics test. Construct a model to determine your allocation of study hours. Include as assumptions the points you "gain" from an hour of study time in each subject and your desired outcome on each test.

1-5. Use the model you constructed in Problem 1-4 to determine the allocation of study time across subjects.

1-6. Suppose you followed the model you constructed in Problem 1-4. Explain how you would "grade" the model.

1-7. Write a sentence contrasting positive and normative economic analysis.

1-8. Based on your answer to Problem 1-7, categorize the following conclusions as the result of positive analysis or normative analysis.
- **a.** Increasing the minimum wage will reduce minimum wage employment opportunities.
- **b.** Increasing the prospects of minimum wage employees is desirable, and raising the minimum wage is the best way to accomplish this.
- **c.** Everyone should enjoy open access to health care.
- **d.** Heath care subsidies will increase the demands for health care.

1-9. Consider the following statements, based on a positive economic analysis that assumes that all other things remain constant. List one other thing that might change and offset the outcome stated.
- **a.** Increased demand for laptop computers will drive up their price.
- **b.** Falling gasoline prices will result in additional vacation travel.
- **c.** A reduction of income tax rates will result in more people working.

1-10. Alan Greenspan, chairman of the U.S. Federal Reserve, referred to the high stock market prices of the late 1990s as a result of "irrational exuberance." Counter this statement by considering the rationality of stock market investors.

Economics on the Net

The Usefulness of Studying Economics This application helps you see how accomplished people benefited from their study of economics. It also explores ways in which these people feel others of all walks of life can gain from learning more about the economics field.

Navigation: Click here to visit the the Federal Reserve Bank of Minneapolis homepage. To access economics in *The Region* on Their Student Experiences and the Need for Economic Literacy, under Publications, click on *The Region*. Select the index of all issues and click on December 1998. Select the last article of the issue, Economics in *The Region* on Their Student Experiences and the Need for Economic Literacy.

Application Read the interviews of the six economists, and answer the following questions.

1. Based on your reading, what economists do you think other economists regard as influential? What educational institutions do you think are the most influential in economics?
2. Which economists do you think were attracted to microeconomics and which to macroeconomics?

For Group Study and Analysis Divide the class into three groups, and assign the groups the Blinder, Yellen, and Rivlin interviews. Have each group use the content of its assigned interview to develop a statement explaining why the study of economics is important, regardless of a student's chosen major.

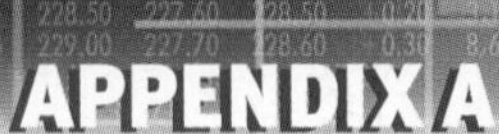

APPENDIX A

READING AND WORKING WITH GRAPHS

Independent variable 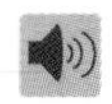
A variable whose value is determined independently of, or outside, the equation under study.

Dependent variable 
A variable whose value changes according to changes in the value of one or more independent variables.

TABLE A-1
Gas Mileage as a Function of Driving Speed

Miles per Hour	Miles per Gallon
45	25
50	24
55	23
60	21
65	19
70	16
75	13

Direct relationship 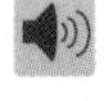
A relationship between two variables that is positive, meaning that an increase in one variable is associated with an increase in the other and a decrease in one variable is associated with a decrease in the other.

Inverse relationship 
A relationship between two variables that is negative, meaning that an increase in one variable is associated with a decrease in the other and a decrease in one variable is associated with an increase in the other.

A graph is a visual representation of the relationship between variables. In this appendix, we'll stick to just two variables: an **independent variable,** which can change in value freely, and a **dependent variable,** which changes only as a result of changes in the value of the independent variable. For example, if nothing else is changing in your life, your weight depends on the amount of food you eat. Food is the independent variable and weight the dependent variable.

A table is a list of numerical values showing the relationship between two (or more) variables. Any table can be converted into a graph, which is a visual representation of that list. Once you understand how a table can be converted to a graph, you will understand what graphs are and how to construct and use them.

Consider a practical example. A conservationist may try to convince you that driving at lower highway speeds will help you conserve gas. Table A-1 shows the relationship between speed—the independent variable—and the distance you can go on a gallon of gas at that speed—the dependent variable. This table does show a pattern of sorts. As the data in the first column get larger in value, the data in the second column get smaller.

Now let's take a look at the different ways in which variables can be related.

DIRECT AND INVERSE RELATIONSHIPS

Two variables can be related in different ways, some simple, others more complex. For example, a person's weight and height are often related. If we measured the height and weight of thousands of people, we would surely find that taller people tend to weigh more than shorter people. That is, we would discover that there is a **direct relationship** between height and weight. By this we simply mean that an *increase* in one variable is usually associated with an *increase* in the related variable. This can easily be seen in panel (a) of Figure A-1.

Let's look at another simple way in which two variables can be related. Much evidence indicates that as the price of a specific commodity rises, the amount purchased decreases—there is an **inverse relationship** between the variable's price per unit and quantity purchased. A table listing the data for this relationship would indicate that for higher and higher prices, smaller and smaller quantities would be purchased. We see this relationship in panel (b) of Figure A-1.

FIGURE A-1
Relationships

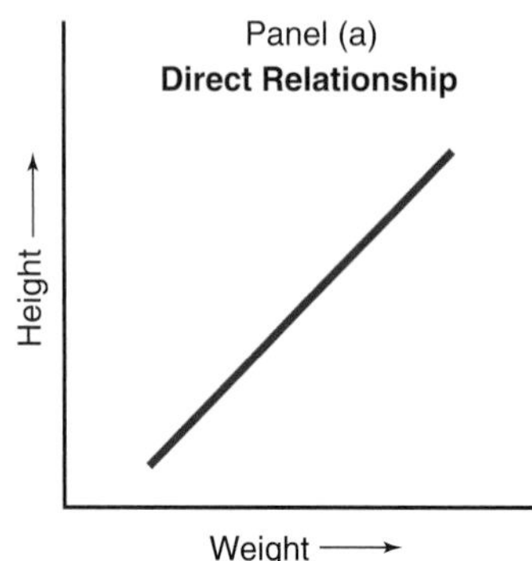

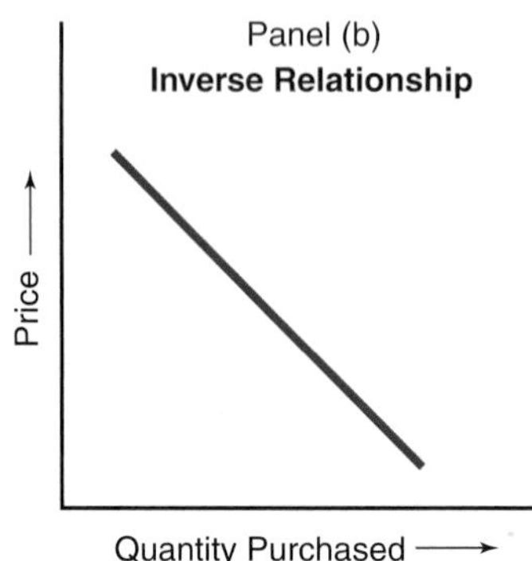

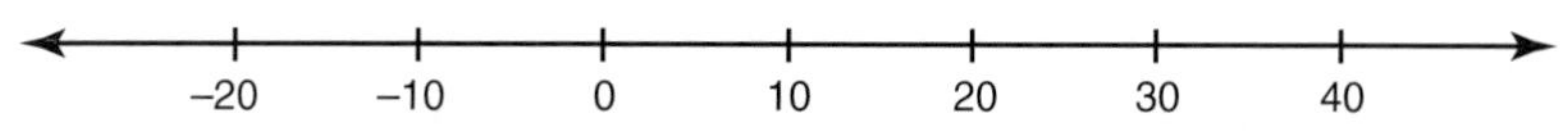

FIGURE A-2
Horizontal Number Line

CONSTRUCTING A GRAPH

Let us now examine how to construct a graph to illustrate a relationship between two variables.

A Number Line

The first step is to become familiar with what is called a **number line.** One is shown in Figure A-2. There are two things that you should know about it.

Number line 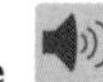
A line that can be divided into segments of equal length, each associated with a number.

1. The points on the line divide the line into equal segments.
2. The numbers associated with the points on the line increase in value from left to right; saying it the other way around, the numbers decrease in value from right to left. However you say it, what we're describing is formally called an *ordered set of points.*

On the number line, we have shown the line segments—that is, the distance from 0 to 10 or the distance between 30 and 40. They all appear to be equal and, indeed, are equal to $\frac{1}{2}$ inch. When we use a distance to represent a quantity, such as barrels of oil, graphically, we are *scaling* the number line. In the example shown, the distance between 0 and 10 might represent 10 barrels of oil, or the distance from 0 to 40 might represent 40 barrels. Of course, the scale may differ on different number lines. For example, a distance of 1 inch could represent 10 units on one number line but 5,000 units on another. Notice that on our number line, points to the left of 0 correspond to negative numbers and points to the right of 0 correspond to positive numbers.

Of course, we can also construct a vertical number line. Consider the one in Figure A-3. As we move up this vertical number line, the numbers increase in value; conversely, as we descend, they decrease in value. Below 0 the numbers are negative, and above 0 the numbers are positive. And as on the horizontal number line, all the line segments are equal. This line is divided into segments such that the distance between -2 and -1 is the same as the distance between 0 and 1.

FIGURE A-3
Vertical Number Line

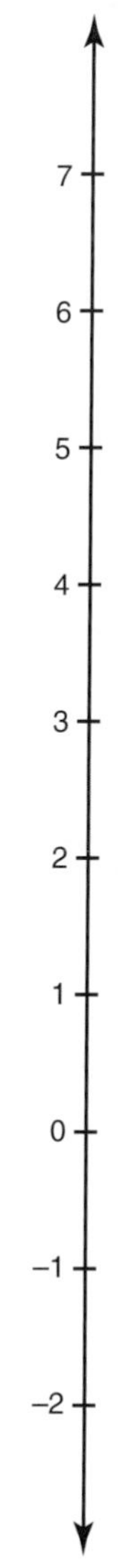

Combining Vertical and Horizontal Number Lines

By drawing the horizontal and vertical lines on the same sheet of paper, we are able to express the relationships between variables graphically. We do this in Figure A-4.

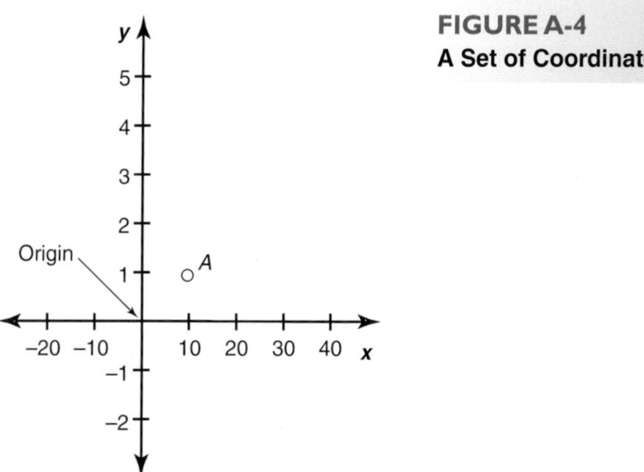

FIGURE A-4
A Set of Coordinate Axes

We draw them (1) so that they intersect at each other's 0 point and (2) so that they are perpendicular to each other. The result is a set of coordinate axes, where each line is called an *axis*. When we have two axes, they span a *plane*.

For one number line, you need only one number to specify any point on the line; equivalently, when you see a point on the line, you know that it represents one number or one value. With a coordinate value system, you need two numbers to specify a single point in the plane; when you see a single point on a graph, you know that it represents two numbers or two values.

y axis The vertical axis in a graph.

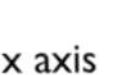

x axis The horizontal axis in a graph.

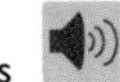

Origin The intersection of the *y* axis and the *x* axis in a graph.

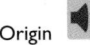

The basic things that you should know about a coordinate number system are that the vertical number line is referred to as the **y axis,** the horizontal number line is referred to as the ***x* axis,** and the point of intersection of the two lines is referred to as the **origin.**

Any point such as *A* in Figure A-4 represents two numbers—a value of *x* and a value of *y*. But we know more than that; we also know that point *A* represents a positive value of *y* because it is above the *x* axis, and we know that it represents a positive value of *x* because it is to the right of the *y* axis.

Point *A* represents a "paired observation" of the variables *x* and *y;* in particular, in Figure A-4, *A* represents an observation of the pair of values $x = 10$ and $y = 1$. Every point in the coordinate system corresponds to a paired observation of *x* and *y,* which can be simply written (x, y)—the *x* value is always specified first, then the *y* value. When we give the values associated with the position of point *A* in the coordinate number system, we are in effect giving the coordinates of that point. *A*'s coordinates are $x = 10$, $y = 1$, or (10, 1).

TABLE A-2
T-Shirts Purchased

(1) Price of T-Shirts	(2) Number of T-Shirts Purchased per Week
$10	20
9	30
8	40
7	50
6	60
5	70

GRAPHING NUMBERS IN A TABLE

Consider Table A-2. Column 1 shows different prices for T-shirts, and column 2 gives the number of T-shirts purchased per week at these prices. Notice the pattern of these numbers. As the price of T-shirts falls, the number of T-shirts purchased per week increases. Therefore, an inverse relationship exists between these two variables, and as soon as we represent it on a graph, you will be able to see the relationship. We can graph this relationship using a coordinate number system—a vertical and horizontal number line for each of these two variables. Such a graph is shown in panel (b) of Figure A-5.

FIGURE A-5
Graphing the Relationship Between T-Shirts Purchased and Price

Panel (a)

Price per T-Shirt	T-Shirts Purchased per Week	Point on Graph
$10	20	*I* (20, 10)
9	30	*J* (30, 9)
8	40	*K* (40, 8)
7	50	*L* (50, 7)
6	60	*M* (60, 6)
5	70	*N* (70, 5)

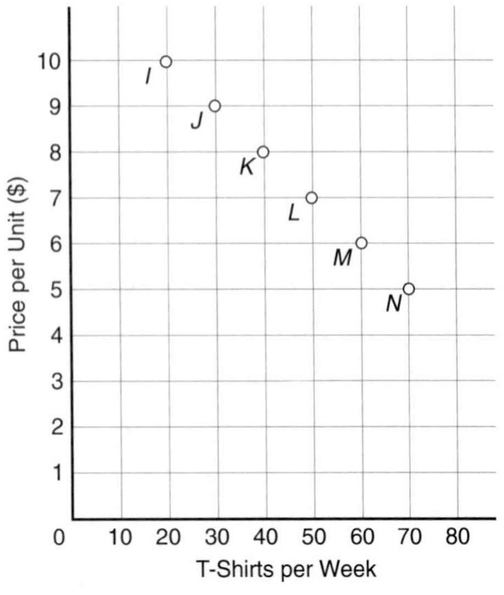

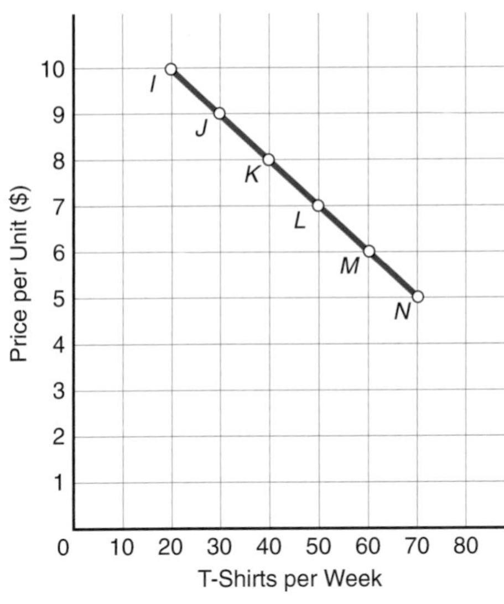

FIGURE A-6
Connecting the Observation Points

In economics, it is conventional to put dollar values on the *y* axis. We therefore construct a vertical number line for price and a horizontal number line, the *x* axis, for quantity of T-shirts purchased per week. The resulting coordinate system allows the plotting of each of the paired observation points; in panel (a), we repeat Table A-2, with a column added expressing these points in paired-data (*x*, *y*) form. For example, point *J* is the paired observation (30, 9). It indicates that when the price of a T-shirt is $9, 30 will be purchased per week.

If it were possible to sell parts of a T-shirt ($\frac{1}{2}$ or $\frac{1}{20}$ of a shirt), we would have observations at every possible price. That is, we would be able to connect our paired observations, represented as lettered points. Let's assume that we can make T-shirts perfectly divisible so that the linear relationship shown in Figure A-5 also holds for fractions of dollars and T-shirts. We would then have a line that connects these points, as shown in the graph in Figure A-6.

In short, we have now represented the data from the table in the form of a graph. Note that an inverse relationship between two variables shows up on a graph as a line or curve that slopes *downward* from left to right. (You might as well get used to the idea that economists call a straight line a "curve" even though it may not curve at all. Much of economists' data turn out to be curves, so they refer to everything represented graphically, even straight lines, as curves.)

THE SLOPE OF A LINE (A LINEAR CURVE)

An important property of a curve represented on a graph is its *slope*. Consider Figure A-7, which represents the quantities of shoes per week that a seller is willing to offer at different prices. Note that in panel (a) of Figure A-7, as in Figure A-5, we have expressed the coordinates of the points in parentheses in paired-data form.

Slope 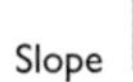
The change in the *y* value divided by the corresponding change in the *x* value of a curve; the "incline" of the curve.

The **slope** of a line is defined as the change in the *y* values divided by the corresponding change in the *x* values as we move along the line. Let's move from point *E* to point *D* in panel (b) of Figure A-7. As we move, we note that the change in the *y* values, which is the change in price, is +$20, because we have moved from a price of $20 to a price of $40 per pair. As we move from *E* to *D*, the change in the *x* values is +80; the number of pairs of shoes willingly offered per week rises from 80 to 160 pairs. The slope calculated as a change in the *y* values divided by the change in the *x* values is therefore

$$\frac{20}{80} = \frac{1}{4}$$

FIGURE A-7
A Positively Sloped Curve

Panel (a)

Price per Pair	Pairs of Shoes Offered per Week	Point on Graph
$100	400	*A* (400,100)
80	320	*B* (320, 80)
60	240	*C* (240, 60)
40	160	*D* (160, 40)
20	80	*E* (80, 20)

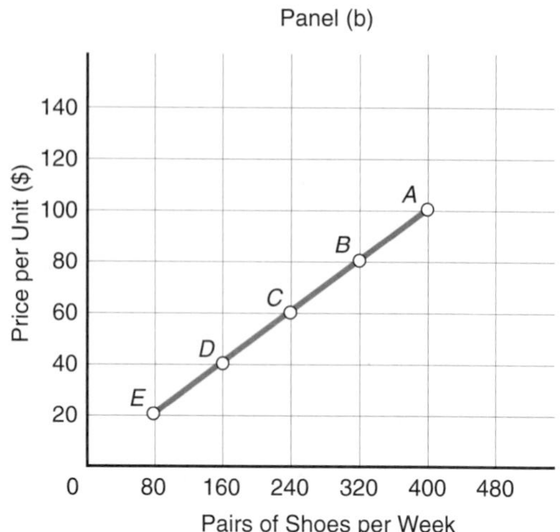

It may be helpful for you to think of slope as a "rise" (movement in the vertical direction) over a "run" (movement in the horizontal direction). We show this abstractly in Figure A-8. The slope is measured by the amount of rise divided by the amount of run. In the example in Figure A-8, and of course in Figure A-7, the amount of rise is positive and so is the amount of run. That's because it's a direct relationship. We show an inverse relationship in Figure A-9. The slope is still equal to the rise divided by the run, but in this case the rise and the run have opposite signs because the curve slopes downward. That means that the slope will have to be negative and that we are dealing with an inverse relationship.

Now let's calculate the slope for a different part of the curve in panel (b) of Figure A-7. We will find the slope as we move from point *B* to point *A*. Again, we note that the slope, or rise over run, from *B* to *A* equals

$$\frac{20}{80} = \frac{1}{4}$$

A specific property of a straight line is that its slope is the same between any two points; in other words, the slope is constant at all points on a straight line in a graph.

We conclude that for our example in Figure A-7, the relationship between the price of a pair of shoes and the number of pairs of shoes willingly offered per week is *linear,* which simply means "in a straight line," and our calculations indicate a constant slope. Moreover, we calculate a direct relationship between these two variables, which turns out to be an

FIGURE A-8 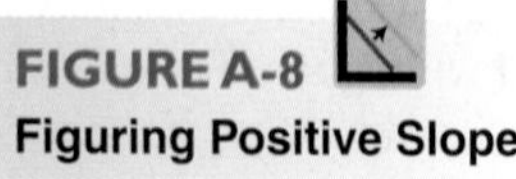
Figuring Positive Slope

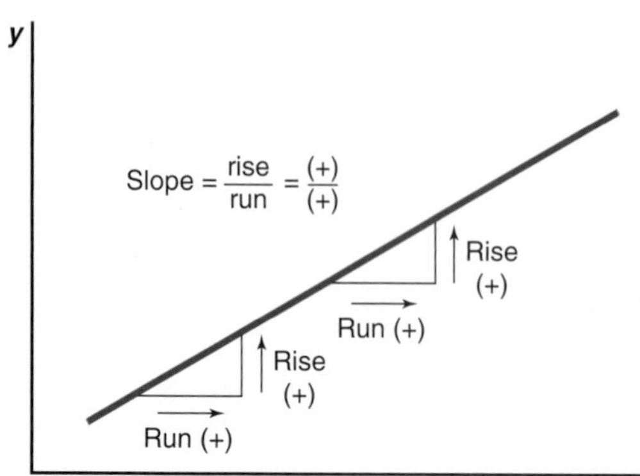

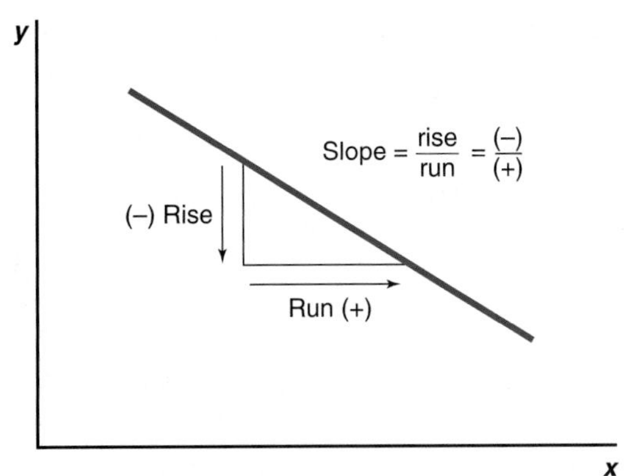

FIGURE A-9
Figuring Negative Slope

upward-sloping (from left to right) curve. Upward-sloping curves have positive slopes—in this case, it is $+\frac{1}{4}$.

We know that an inverse relationship between two variables shows up as a downward-sloping curve—rise over run will be a negative slope because the rise and run have opposite signs, as shown in Figure A-9. When we see a negative slope, we know that increases in one variable are associated with decreases in the other. Therefore, we say that downward-sloping curves have negative slopes. Can you verify that the slope of the graph representing the relationship between T-shirt prices and the quantity of T-shirts purchased per week in Figure A-6 is $-\frac{1}{10}$?

Slopes of Nonlinear Curves

The graph presented in Figure A-10 indicates a *nonlinear* relationship between two variables, total profits and output per unit of time. Inspection of this graph indicates that at first, increases in output lead to increases in total profits; that is, total profits rise as output increases. But beyond some output level, further increases in output cause decreases in total profits.

Can you see how this curve rises at first, reaches a peak at point *C,* and then falls? This curve relating total profits to output levels appears mountain-shaped.

Considering that this curve is nonlinear (it is obviously not a straight line), should we expect a constant slope when we compute changes in *y* divided by corresponding changes in *x* in moving from one point to another? A quick inspection, even without specific numbers, should lead us to conclude that the slopes of lines joining different points in this curve, such as between *A* and *B, B* and *C,* or *C* and *D,* will *not* be the same. The curve slopes upward (in a positive direction) for some values and downward (in a negative direction) for

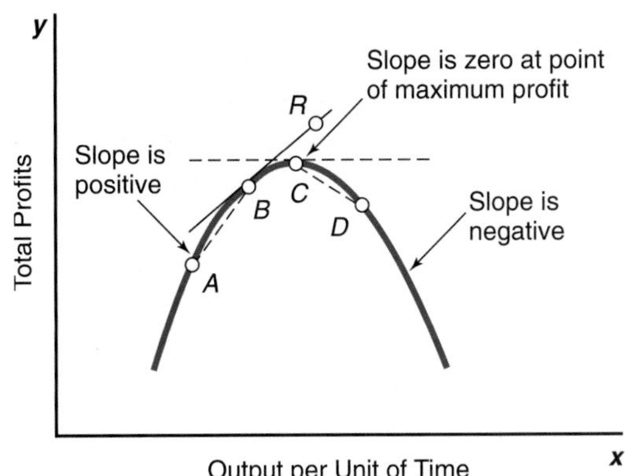

FIGURE A-10
The Slope of a Nonlinear Curve

other values. In fact, the slope of the line between any two points on this curve will be different from the slope of the line between any two other points. Each slope will be different as we move along the curve.

Instead of using a line between two points to discuss slope, mathematicians and economists prefer to discuss the slope *at a particular point.* The slope at a point on the curve, such as point B in the graph in Figure A-10, is the slope of a line *tangent* to that point. A tangent line is a straight line that touches a curve at only one point. For example, it might be helpful to think of the tangent at B as the straight line that just "kisses" the curve at point B.

To calculate the slope of a tangent line, you need to have some additional information besides the two values of the point of tangency. For example, in Figure A-10, if we knew that the point R also lay on the tangent line and we knew the two values of that point, we could calculate the slope of the tangent line. We could calculate rise over run between points B and R, and the result would be the slope of the line tangent to the one point B on the curve.

Appendix Summary

1. Direct relationships involve a dependent variable changing in the same direction as the change in the independent variable.
2. Inverse relationships involve the dependent variable changing in the opposite direction of the change in the independent variable.
3. When we draw a graph showing the relationship between two economic variables, we are holding all other things constant (the Latin term for which is *ceteris paribus*).
4. We obtain a set of coordinates by putting vertical and horizontal number lines together. The vertical line is called the y axis; the horizontal line, the x axis.
5. The slope of any linear (straight-line) curve is the change in the y values divided by the corresponding change in the x values as we move along the line. Otherwise stated, the slope is calculated as the amount of rise over the amount of run, where rise is movement in the vertical direction and run is movement in the horizontal direction.
6. The slope of a nonlinear curve changes; it is positive when the curve is rising and negative when the curve is falling. At a maximum or minimum point, the slope of the nonlinear curve is zero.

Key Terms and Concepts

Dependent variable (18)
Direct relationship (18)
Independent variable (18)
Inverse relationship (18)
Number line (19)
Origin (20)
Slope (21)
x axis (20)
y axis (20)

Problems Test

Answers to the odd-numbered problems appear at the back of the book.

A-1. Explain which is the independent variable and which is the dependent variable for the following examples.

a. Once you determine the price of a notebook at the college bookstore, you will decide how many notebooks to buy.

b. You will decide how many credit hours to register for this semester once the university tells you how many work-study hours you will be assigned.

c. You are anxious to receive your economics exam grade because you studied many hours in the weeks preceding the exam.

A-2. For the following items, state whether a direct or an inverse relationship is likely to exist.

a. The number of hours you study for an exam and your exam score
b. The price of pizza and the quantity purchased
c. The number of games the university basketball team won last year and the number of season tickets sold this year

A-3. Review Figure A-4, and then state whether the following paired observations are on, above, or below the x axis and on, to the left of, or to the right of the y axis.

a. $(-10, 4)$
b. $(20, -2)$
c. $(10, 0)$

A-4. State whether the following functions are linear or nonlinear.

a. $y = 5x$
b. $y = 5x^2$
c. $y = 3 + x$
d. $y = -3x$

A-5. Given the function $y = 5x$, complete the following schedule and plot the curve.

y	x
	−4
	−2
	0
	2
	4

A-6. Given the function $y = 5x^2$, complete the following schedule and plot the curve.

y	x
	−4
	−2
	0
	2
	4

A-7. Calculate the slope of the function you graphed in Problem A-5.

A-8. Indicate at each ordered pair whether the slope of the curve you plotted in Problem A-6 is positive, negative, or zero.

A-9. State whether the following functions imply a positive or negative relationship between x and y.

a. $y = 5\,x$
b. $y = 3 + x$
c. $y = -3\,x$

CHAPTER 2

SCARCITY AND THE WORLD OF TRADE-OFFS

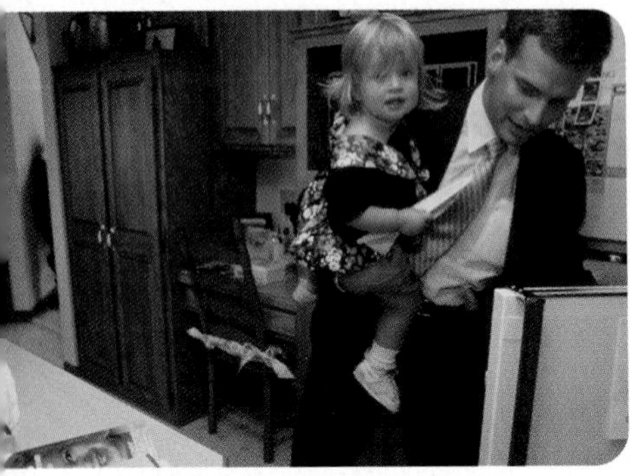

This harried father tries to balance the demands of work with those of child rearing. Why does it typically cost more for higher-income-earning parents to raise children than for those earning less income?

In Chapter 1, you learned that men and women can have good economic reasons to marry. Because children traditionally shared the family workload, couples have also had a strong incentive to have children. In most developed nations, however, this incentive for having children has largely disappeared. Even on today's "family farms," many tasks are now mechanized and even automated.

At the same time, the costs of raising children have increased. Of course, parents have always housed, fed, and clothed their children. In addition, they have sacrificed to provide "quality time" with their children. For many people today, the value of that time is greater than it was in years past. In this chapter you will learn how to put a value on time spent with children. This will help you understand why children are a more costly "commodity" than they used to be.

LEARNING OBJECTIVES

After reading this chapter, you should be able to:

1. Evaluate whether even affluent people face the problem of scarcity
2. Understand why economics considers individuals' "wants" but not their "needs"
3. Explain why the scarcity problem induces individuals to consider opportunity costs
4. Discuss why obtaining increasing increments of any particular good typically entails giving up more and more units of other goods
5. Explain why society faces a trade-off between consumption goods and capital goods
6. Distinguish between absolute and comparative advantage

Did You Know That... Chris Van Horn, president of CVK Group in Washington, D.C., grosses over $200,000 a year for having people wait in line? Adam Goldin loves working as a "line waiter" because he gets paid for "doing nothing." His job is to arrive early in the morning on Capitol Hill to hold places for lobbyists who must attend congressional hearings. Van Horn charges his more than 100 lobbyists and law firm clients $27 an hour and pays his part-time line waiters like Mr. Goldin $10 an hour. For example, when Congress was going to hold hearings for the proposed 1997 tax cut, $10-an-hour professional standees arrived to hold places for $300-an-hour lobbyists who would not show up until hours later. After all, lobbyists do not have an unlimited amount of time. Their time is scarce. It is worth more than what they are charged to "save" it.

Chapter Outline

SCARCITY

Whenever individuals or communities cannot obtain everything they desire simultaneously, choices occur. Choices occur because of *scarcity.* **Scarcity** is the most basic concept in all of economics. Scarcity means that we do not ever have enough of everything, including time, to satisfy our *every* desire. Scarcity exists because human wants always exceed what can be produced with the limited resources and time that nature makes available.

What Scarcity Is Not

Scarcity is not a shortage. After a hurricane hits and cuts off supplies to a community, TV newscasts often show people standing in line to get minimum amounts of cooking fuel and food. A news commentator might say that the line is caused by the "scarcity" of these products. But cooking fuel and food are always scarce—we cannot obtain all that we want at a zero price. Therefore, do not confuse the concept of scarcity, which is general and all-encompassing, with the concept of shortages as evidenced by people waiting in line to obtain a particular product.

Scarcity 
A situation in which the ingredients for producing the things that people desire are insufficient to satisfy all wants.

Scarcity is not the same thing as poverty. Scarcity occurs among the poor and among the rich. Even the richest person on earth faces scarcity because available time is limited. Low income levels do not create more scarcity. High income levels do not create less scarcity.

Scarcity is a fact of life, like gravity. And just as physicists did not invent gravity, economists did not invent scarcity—it existed well before the first economist ever lived. It exists even when we are not using all of our resources.

Scarcity and Resources 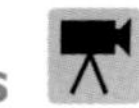

The scarcity concept arises from the fact that resources are insufficient to satisfy our every desire. Resources are the inputs used in the production of the things that we want. **Production** can be defined as virtually any activity that results in the conversion of resources into products that can be used in consumption. Production includes delivering things from one part of the country to another. It includes taking ice from an ice tray to put it in your soft-drink glass. The resources used in production are called *factors of production,* and some economists use the terms *resources* and *factors of production* interchangeably. The total quantity of all resources that an economy has at any one time determines what that economy can produce.

Production 
Any activity that results in the conversion of resources into products that can be used in consumption.

Land 
The natural resources that are available from nature. Land as a resource includes location, original fertility and mineral deposits, topography, climate, water, and vegetation.

Labor 
Productive contributions of humans who work, involving both mental and physical activities.

Physical capital 
All manufactured resources, including buildings, equipment, machines, and improvements to land that is used for production.

Human capital 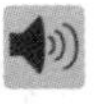
The accumulated training and education of workers.

Entrepreneurship 
The factor of production involving human resources that perform the functions of raising capital, organizing, managing, assembling other factors of production, and making basic business policy decisions. The entrepreneur is a risk taker.

Goods 
All things from which individuals derive satisfaction or happiness.

Economic goods 
Goods that are scarce, for which the quantity demanded exceeds the quantity supplied at a zero price.

Services 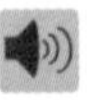
Mental or physical labor or help purchased by consumers. Examples are the assistance of doctors, lawyers, dentists, repair personnel, housecleaners, educators, retailers, and wholesalers; things purchased or used by consumers that do not have physical characteristics.

Factors of production can be classified in many ways. Here is one such classification:

1. Land. **Land** encompasses all the nonhuman gifts of nature, including timber, water, fish, minerals, and the original fertility of land. It is often called the *natural resource.*
2. Labor. **Labor** is the human resource, which includes all productive contributions made by individuals who work, such as steelworkers, ballet dancers, and professional baseball players.
3. Physical capital. **Physical capital** consists of the factories and equipment used in production. It also includes improvements to natural resources, such as irrigation ditches.
4. Human capital. **Human capital** is the economic characterization of the education and training of workers. How much the nation produces depends not only on how many hours people work but also on how productive they are, and that in turn depends in part on education and training. To become more educated, individuals have to devote time and resources, just as a business has to devote resources if it wants to increase its physical capital. Whenever a worker's skills increase, human capital has been improved.
5. Entrepreneurship. The factor of production known as **entrepreneurship** (actually a subdivision of labor) involves human resources that perform the functions of organizing, managing, and assembling the other factors of production to make business ventures. Entrepreneurship also encompasses taking risks that involve the possibility of losing large sums of wealth on new ventures. It includes new methods of doing common things and generally experimenting with any type of new thinking that could lead to making more money income. Without entrepreneurship, virtually no business organization could operate.

Goods Versus Economic Goods

Goods are defined as all things from which individuals derive satisfaction or happiness. Goods therefore include air to breathe and the beauty of a sunset as well as food, cars, and CD players.

Economic goods are a subset of all goods—they are goods derived from scarce resources about which we must constantly make decisions regarding their best use. By definition, the desired quantity of an economic good exceeds the amount that is directly available at a zero price. Virtually every example we use in economics concerns economic goods—cars, CD players, computers, socks, baseball bats, and corn. Weeds are a good example of *bads*—goods for which the desired quantity is much *less* than what nature provides at a zero price.

Sometimes you will see references to "goods and services." **Services** are tasks that are performed for someone else, such as laundry, cleaning, hospital care, restaurant meal preparation, car polishing, psychological counseling, and teaching. One way of looking at services is thinking of them as *intangible goods.*

WANTS AND NEEDS

Wants are not the same as needs. Indeed, from the economist's point of view, the term *needs* is objectively undefinable. When someone says, "I need some new clothes," there is no way to know whether that person is stating a vague wish, a want, or a lifesaving necessity. If the individual making the statement were dying of exposure in a northern country during the winter, we might argue that indeed the person does need clothes—perhaps not new ones, but at least some articles of warm clothing. Typically, however, the term *need* is used very casually in most conversations. What people mean, usually, is that they want something that they do not currently have.

Humans have unlimited wants. Just imagine if every single material want that you might have were satisfied. You can have all of the clothes, cars, houses, CDs, tickets to concerts, and other things that you want. Does that mean that nothing else could add to your total level of happiness? Probably not, because you might think of new goods and services that you could obtain, particularly as they came to market. You would also still be lacking in fulfilling all of your wants for compassion, friendship, love, affection, prestige, musical abilities, sports abilities, and so on.

In reality, every individual has competing wants but cannot satisfy all of them, given limited resources. This is the reality of scarcity. Each person must therefore make choices. Whenever a choice is made to do or buy something, something else that is also desired is not done or not purchased. In other words, in a world of scarcity, every want that ends up being satisfied causes one or more other wants to remain unsatisfied or to be forfeited.

CONCEPTS IN BRIEF

- Scarcity exists because human wants always exceed what can be produced with the limited resources and time that nature makes available.
- We use scarce resources, such as land, labor, physical and human capital, and entrepreneurship, to produce economic goods—goods that are desired but are not directly obtainable from nature to the extent demanded or desired at a zero price.
- Wants are unlimited; they include all material desires and all nonmaterial desires, such as love, affection, power, and prestige.
- The concept of need is difficult to define objectively for every person; consequently, we simply consider that every person's wants are unlimited. In a world of scarcity, satisfaction of one want necessarily means nonsatisfaction of one or more other wants.

SCARCITY, CHOICE, AND OPPORTUNITY COST

The natural fact of scarcity implies that we must make choices. One of the most important results of this fact is that every choice made (or not made, for that matter) means that some opportunity had to be sacrificed. Every choice involves giving up another opportunity to do or use something else.

Consider a practical example. Every choice you make to study one more hour of economics requires that you give up the opportunity to do any of the following activities: study more of another subject, listen to music, sleep, browse at a local store, read a novel, or work out at the gym. Many more opportunities are forgone also if you choose to study economics an additional hour.

Because there were so many alternatives from which to choose, how could you determine the value of what you gave up to engage in that extra hour of studying economics? First of all, no one else can tell you the answer because only you can *subjectively* put a value on the alternatives forgone. Only you know what is the value of another hour of sleep or of an hour looking for the latest CDs. That means that only you can determine the highest-valued, next-best alternative that you had to sacrifice in order to study economics one more hour. It is you who come up with the *subjective* estimate of the expected value of the next-best alternative.

Opportunity cost 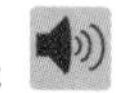
The highest-valued, next-best alternative that must be sacrificed to obtain something or to satisfy a want.

The value of the next-best alternative is called **opportunity cost.** The opportunity cost of any action is the value of what is given up—the next-highest-ranked alternative—because a choice was made. When you study one more hour, there may be many alternatives available for the use of that hour, but assume that you can do only one other thing in that hour—your next-highest-ranked alternative. What is important is the choice that you would have made if you hadn't studied one more hour. Your opportunity cost is the *next-highest-ranked* alternative, not *all* alternatives.

In economics, cost is always a forgone opportunity.

One way to think about opportunity cost is to understand that when you choose to do something, you lose. What you lose is being able to engage in your next-highest-valued alternative. The cost of your choice is what you lose, which is by definition your next-highest-valued alternative. This is your opportunity cost.

Let's consider a real-world example: the opportunity cost of a national monument.

POLICY EXAMPLE

The Trillion-Dollar Canyon

In September 1996, the U.S. government established the Grand Staircase/Escalante National Monument. If you visit the Monument's Web page (click here to visit the site), you will learn all about various activities available to visitors to the cliffs and canyons encompassed within the monument.

What the Web page does not tell you is that this 1.8 million-acre park in the southern Utah desert lies above the largest known reserve of coal in the United States: an underground bank of nearly 7 billion tons of coal with an estimated market value of about $1 trillion. That is the opportunity cost of this particular national monument.

For Critical Analysis

Recall that opportunity cost is the value of the next-best alternative. What does this tell us about the perceived social value of the Grand Staircase/Escalante National Monument?

THE WORLD OF TRADE-OFFS

Whenever you engage in any activity using any resource, even time, you are *trading off* the use of that resource for one or more alternative uses. The value of the trade-off is represented by the opportunity cost. The opportunity cost of studying economics has already been mentioned—it is the value of the next-best alternative. When you think of any alternative, you are thinking of trade-offs.

Let's consider a hypothetical example of a one-for-one trade-off between the results of spending time studying economics and accounting. For the sake of this argument, we will assume that additional time studying either economics or accounting will lead to a higher grade in the subject studied more. One of the best ways to examine this trade-off is with a graph. (If you would like a refresher on graphical techniques, study Appendix A at the end of Chapter 1 before going on.)

Graphical Analysis

In Figure 2-1, the expected grade in accounting is measured on the vertical axis of the graph, and the expected grade in economics is measured on the horizontal axis. We simplify the world and assume that you have a maximum of 10 hours per week to spend studying these two subjects and that if you spend all 10 hours on economics, you will get an A in the course. You will, however, fail accounting. Conversely, if you spend all of your 10 hours studying accounting, you will get an A in that subject, but you will flunk economics. Here the trade-off is a special case: one to one. A one-to-one trade-off means that the opportunity cost of receiving one grade higher in economics (for example, improving from a C to a B) is one grade lower in accounting (falling from a C to a D).

The Production Possibilities Curve (PPC)

The graph in Figure 2-1 illustrates the relationship between the possible results that can be produced in each of two activities, depending on how much time you choose to devote to each activity. This graph shows a representation of a **production possibilities curve (PPC).**

Consider that you are producing a grade in economics when you study economics and a grade in accounting when you study accounting. Then the graph in Figure 2-1 can be related to the production possibilities you face. The line that goes from A on one axis to A on the other axis therefore becomes a production possibilities curve. It is defined as the maximum quantity of one good or service that can be produced, given that a specific quantity of another is produced. It is a curve that shows the possibilities available for increasing the output of one good or service by reducing the amount of another. In the example in Figure 2-1, your time for studying was limited to 10 hours per week. The two possible outputs were grades in accounting and grades in economics. The particular production possibilities curve presented in Figure 2-1 is a graphical representation of the opportunity cost of studying one more hour in one subject. It is a *straight-line production possibilities curve,* which is a special case. (The more general case will be discussed next.) If you decide to be at point *x* in Figure 2-1, 5 hours of study time will be spent on accounting and 5 hours will be spent on economics. The expected grade in each course will be a C. If you are more interested in getting a B in economics, you will go to point *y* on the production possibilities curve, spending only 2.5 hours

Production possibilities curve (PPC)
A curve representing all possible combinations of total output that could be produced assuming (1) a fixed amount of productive resources of a given quality and (2) the efficient use of those resources.

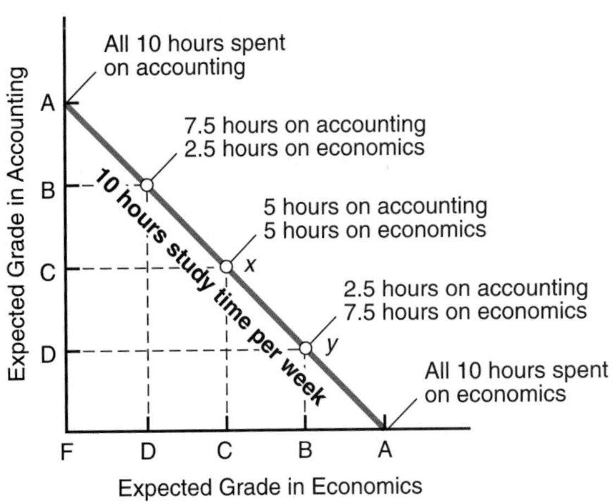

FIGURE 2-1
Production Possibilities Curve for Grades in Accounting and Economics (Trade-Offs)
We assume that only 10 hours can be spent per week on studying. If the student is at point *x*, equal time (5 hours a week) is spent on both courses and equal grades of C will be received. If a higher grade in economics is desired, the student may go to point *y*, thereby receiving a B in economics but a D in accounting. At point *y*, 2.5 hours are spent on accounting and 7.5 hours on economics.

on accounting but 7.5 hours on economics. Your expected grade in accounting will then drop from a C to a D.

Note that these trade-offs between expected grades in accounting and economics are the result of *holding constant* total study time as well as all other factors that might influence a student's ability to learn, such as computerized study aids. Quite clearly, if you wished to spend more total time studying, it would be possible to have higher grades in both economics and accounting. In that case, however, we would no longer be on the specific production possibilities curve illustrated in Figure 2-1. We would have to draw a new curve, farther to the right, to show the greater total study time and a different set of possible trade-offs.

CONCEPTS IN BRIEF

- Scarcity requires us to choose. Whenever we choose, we lose the next-highest-valued alternative.
- Cost is always a forgone opportunity.
- Another way to look at opportunity cost is the trade-off that occurs when one activity is undertaken rather than the next-best alternative activity.
- A production possibilities curve (PPC) graphically shows the trade-off that occurs when more of one output is obtained at the sacrifice of another. The PPC is a graphical representation of, among other things, opportunity cost.

THE CHOICES SOCIETY FACES

The straight-line production possibilities curve presented in Figure 2-1 can be generalized to demonstrate the related concepts of scarcity, choice, and trade-offs that our entire nation faces. As you will see, the production possibilities curve is a simple but powerful economic model because it can demonstrate these related concepts. The example we will use is the choice between the production of network computers and digital televisions (DTVs). We assume for the moment that these are the only two goods that can be produced in the nation. Panel (a) of Figure 2-2 gives the various combinations of computers and DTVs that are possible. If all resources are devoted to computer production, 25 million per year can be produced. If all resources are devoted to DTV production, 30 million per year can be produced. In between are various possible combinations. These combinations are plotted as points *A, B, C, D, E, F,* and *G* in panel (b) of Figure 2-2. If these points are connected with a smooth curve, the nation's production possibilities curve is shown, demonstrating the trade-off between the production of computers and DTVs. These trade-offs occur *on* the production possibilities curve.

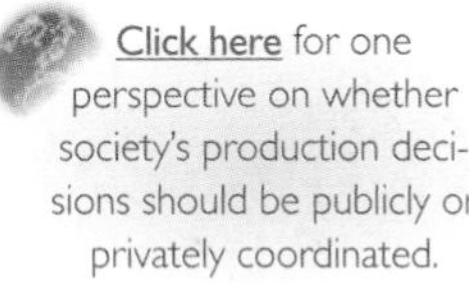

Click here for one perspective on whether society's production decisions should be publicly or privately coordinated.

Notice the major difference in the shape of the production possibilities curves in Figures 2-1 and 2-2. In Figure 2-1, there is a one-to-one trade-off between grades in economics and in accounting. In Figure 2-2, the trade-off between computer production and DTV production is not constant, and therefore the PPC is a *bowed* curve. To understand why the production possibilities curve for a society is typically bowed outward, you must understand the assumptions underlying the PPC.

Assumptions Underlying the Production Possibilities Curve

When we draw the curve that is shown in Figure 2-2, we make the following assumptions:

1. Resources are fully employed.
2. We are looking at production over a specific time period—for example, one year.

FIGURE 2-2

Society's Trade-Off Between Network Computers and Digital Televisions

The production of network computers and digital televisions are measured in millions of units per year. The various combinations are given in panel (a) and plotted in panel (b). Connecting the points *A*–*G* with a relatively smooth line gives the society's production possibilities curve for network computers and digital televisions. Point *R* lies outside the production possibilities curve and is therefore unattainable at the point in time for which the graph is drawn. Point *S* lies inside the production possibilities curve and therefore represents an inefficient use of available resources.

Panel (a)

Combination	Network Computers (millions per year)	Digital Televisions (millions per year)
A	25.00	0
B	24.00	5
C	22.50	10
D	20.00	15
E	16.50	20
F	11.25	25
G	0	30

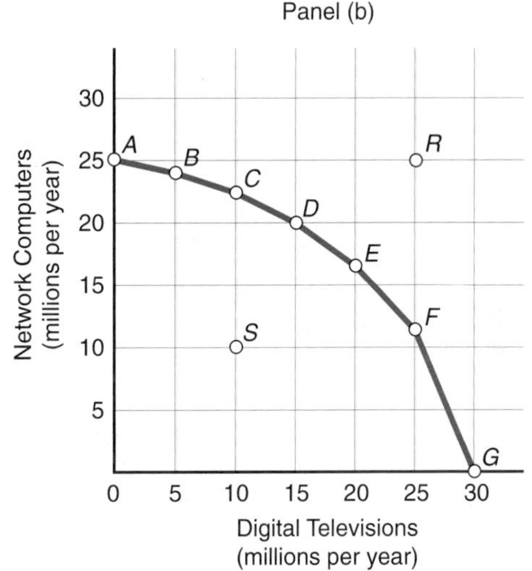

3. The resource inputs, in both quantity and quality, used to produce computers or digital televisions are fixed over this time period.
4. Technology does not change over this time period.

Technology is defined as society's pool of applied knowledge concerning how goods and services can be produced by managers, workers, engineers, scientists, and artisans, using land and capital. You can think of technology as the formula or recipe used to combine factors of production. (When better formulas are developed, more production can be obtained from the same amount of resources.) The level of technology sets the limit on the amount and types of goods and services that we can derive from any given amount of resources. The production possibilities curve is drawn under the assumption that we use the best technology that we currently have available and that this technology doesn't change over the time period under study.

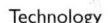

Technology 
Society's pool of applied knowledge concerning how goods and services can be produced.

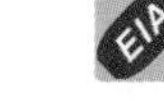

Production Possibilities Curve
Practice with the production possibilities curve.

Being off the Production Possibilities Curve

Look again at panel (b) of Figure 2-2. Point *R* lies *outside* the production possibilities curve and is *impossible* to achieve during the time period assumed. By definition, the production possibilities curve indicates the *maximum* quantity of one good given some quantity of the other.

It is possible, however, to be at point *S* in Figure 2-2. That point lies beneath the production possibilities curve. If the nation is at point *S*, it means that its resources are not being fully utilized. This occurs, for example, during periods of unemployment. Point *S* and all such points within the production possibilities curve are always attainable but usually not desirable.

Efficiency

The production possibilities curve can be used to define the notion of efficiency. Whenever the economy is operating on the PPC, at points such as *A, B, C,* or *D,* we say that its production is efficient. Points such as *S* in Figure 2-2, which lie beneath the production possibilities curve, are said to represent production situations that are not efficient.

Efficiency 
The case in which a given level of inputs is used to produce the maximum output possible. Alternatively, the situation in which a given output is produced at minimum cost.

Efficiency can mean many things to many people. Even within economics, there are different types of efficiency. Here we are discussing productive efficiency. An economy is productively efficient whenever it is producing the maximum output with given technology and resources.

A simple commonsense definition of efficiency is getting the most out of what we have as an economy. Clearly, we are not getting the most that we have if we are at point *S* in panel (b) of Figure 2-2. We can move from point *S* to, say, point *C,* thereby increasing the total quantity of network computers produced without any decrease in the total quantity of digital televisions produced. We can move from point *S* to point *E,* for example, and have both more computers and more DTVs. Point *S* is called an **inefficient point,** which is defined as any point below the production possibilities curve.

Inefficient point 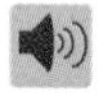
Any point below the production possibilities curve at which resources are being used inefficiently.

We can relate the concept of economic efficiency to how goods are distributed among different individuals and entities. In an efficient economy, people who value specific goods relatively the most end up with those goods. If you own a vintage electric Fender guitar but I value it more than you, I can buy it from you. Such trading benefits you and me mutually. In the process, the economy becomes more efficient. The maximum efficiency an economy can reach is when all such mutual benefits through trade have been exhausted.

The Law of Increasing Relative Cost

In the example in Figure 2-1, the trade-off between a grade in accounting and a grade in economics is one to one. The trade-off ratio was fixed. That is to say, the production possibilities curve was a straight line. The curve in Figure 2-2 is a more general case. We have re-created the curve in Figure 2-2 as Figure 2-3. Each combination, *A* through *G,* of network computers and digital televisions is represented on the production possibilities curve. Starting with the production of zero DTVs, the nation can produce 25 million units of computers with its available resources and technology. When we increase production of DTVs from zero to 5 million per year, the nation has to give up in computers that first vertical arrow, *Aa.* From panel (a) of Figure 2-2 you can see that this is 1 mil-

FIGURE 2-3 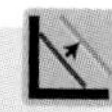
The Law of Increasing Relative Cost
Consider equal increments of digital television production, as measured on the horizontal axis. All of the horizontal arrows—*aB, bC,* and so on—are of equal length (5 million). The opportunity cost of going from 25 million DTVs per year to 30 million (*Ff*) is much greater than going from zero units to 5 million (*Aa*). The opportunity cost of each additional equal increase in DTV production rises.

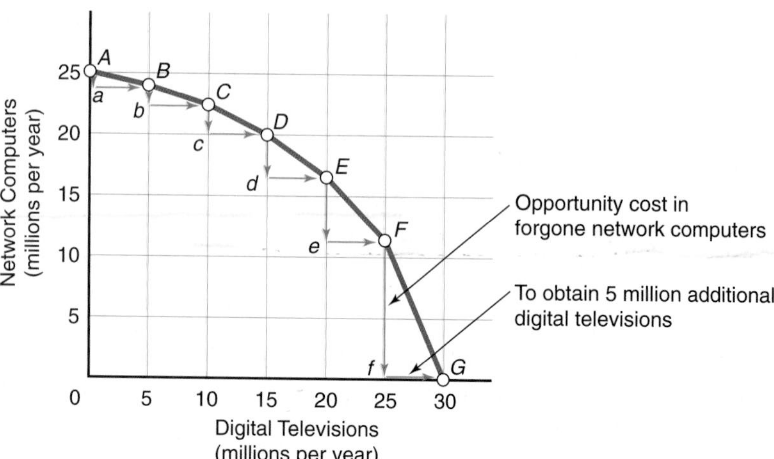

lion computers a year (25 million − 24 million). Again, if we increase production of DTVs by 5 million units per year, we go from *B* to *C*. In order to do so, the nation has to give up the vertical distance *Bb*, or 1.5 million computers a year. By the time we go from 25 million to 30 million digital televisions, to obtain that 5 million increase, we have to forgo the vertical distance *Ff*, or 11.25 million computers. In other words, we see an increase in the opportunity cost of the last 5 million digital televisions—11.25 million computers—compared to an equivalent increase in DTVs when we started with none being produced at all—1 million computers.

What we are observing is called the **law of increasing relative cost.** When society takes more resources and applies them to the production of any specific good, the opportunity cost increases for each additional unit produced. The reason that, as a nation, we face the law of increasing relative cost (which causes the production possibilities curve to bow outward) is that certain resources are better suited for producing some goods than they are for other goods. Resources are generally not *perfectly* adaptable for alternative uses. When increasing the output of a particular good, producers must use less suitable resources than those already used in order to produce the additional output. Hence the cost of producing the additional units increases. With respect to our hypothetical example here, at first the computer hardware specialists at computer firms would shift over to producing digital televisions. After a while, though, computer networking technicians, workers who normally build hard drives, and others would be asked to help design and manufacture television components. Clearly, they would be less effective in making televisions than the people who specialize in this task.

Law of increasing relative cost
The observation that the opportunity cost of additional units of a good generally increases as society attempts to produce more of that good. This accounts for the bowed-out shape of the production possibilities curve.

As a rule of thumb, *the more specialized the resources, the more bowed the production possibilities curve.* At the other extreme, if all resources are equally suitable for digital-television production or network computer production, the curves in Figures 2-2 and 2-3 would approach the straight line shown in our first example in Figure 2-1.

CONCEPTS IN BRIEF

- Trade-offs are represented graphically by a production possibilities curve showing the maximum quantity of one good or service that can be produced, given a specific quantity of another, from a given set of resources over a specified period of time—for example, one year.
- A PPC is drawn holding the quantity and quality of all resources fixed over the time period under study.
- Points outside the production possibilities curve are unattainable; points inside are attainable but represent an inefficient use or underuse of available resources.
- Because many resources are better suited for certain productive tasks than for others, society's production possibilities curve is bowed outward, following the law of increasing relative cost.

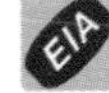

The Bowed-Out Curve
Practice with the concept of the law of increasing relative cost.

ECONOMIC GROWTH AND THE PRODUCTION POSSIBILITIES CURVE

Over any particular time period, a society cannot be outside the production possibilities curve. Over time, however, it is possible to have more of everything. This occurs through economic growth. (An important reason for economic growth, capital accumulation, is discussed next. A more complete discussion of why economic growth occurs is discussed in Chapter 9). Figure 2-4 shows the production possibilities curve for network computers and digital televisions shifting outward. The two additional curves shown represent new choices open to an economy that has experienced economic growth. Such economic growth

FIGURE 2-4

Economic Growth Allows for More of Everything

If the nation experiences economic growth, the production possibilities curve between network computers and digital televisions will move out, as is shown. This takes time, however, and it does not occur automatically. This means, therefore, that we can have more network computers and more DTVs only after a period of time during which we have experienced economic growth.

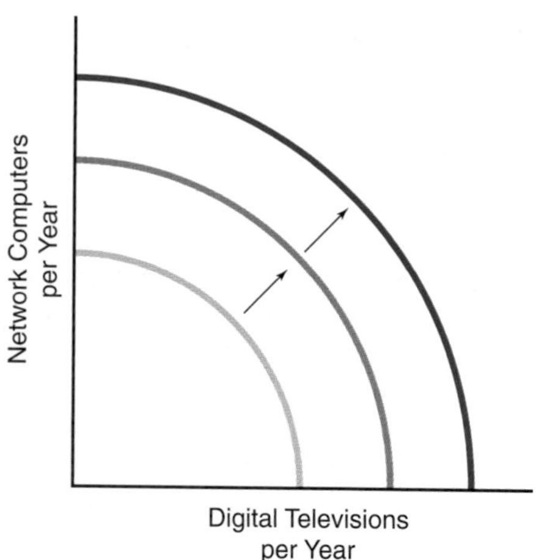

occurs because of many things, including increases in the number of workers and productive investment in equipment.

Scarcity still exists, however, no matter how much economic growth there is. At any point in time, we will always be on some production possibilities curve; thus we will always face trade-offs. The more we want of one thing, the less we can have of others.

If a nation experiences economic growth, the production possibilities curve between network computers and digital televisions will move outward, as shown in Figure 2-4. This takes time and does not occur automatically. One reason it will occur involves the choice about how much to consume today.

THE TRADE-OFF BETWEEN THE PRESENT AND THE FUTURE

Consumption
The use of goods and services for personal satisfaction.

The production possibilities curve and economic growth can be used to examine the trade-off between present **consumption** and future consumption. When we consume today, we are using up what we call consumption or consumer goods—food and clothes, for example. And we have already defined physical capital as the manufactured goods, such as machines and factories, used to make other goods and services.

Why We Make Capital Goods

Why would we be willing to use productive resources to make things—capital goods—that we cannot consume directly? For one thing, capital goods enable us to produce larger quantities of consumer goods or to produce them less expensively than we otherwise could. Before fish are "produced" for the market, equipment such as fishing boats, nets, and poles are produced first. Imagine how expensive it would be to obtain fish for market without using these capital goods. Catching fish with one's hands is not an easy task. The price per fish would be very high if capital goods weren't used.

Forgoing Current Consumption

Whenever we use productive resources to make capital goods, we are implicitly forgoing current consumption. We are waiting for some time in the future to consume the fruits that will be reaped from the use of capital goods. In effect, when we forgo current consumption to invest in capital goods, we are engaging in an economic activity that is forward-looking—we do not get instant utility or satisfaction from our activity. Indeed, if we were to produce only consumer goods now and no capital goods, our capacity to produce consumer goods in the future would suffer. Here we see a trade-off.

The Trade-Off Between Consumption Goods and Capital Goods

To have more consumer goods in the future, we must accept fewer consumer goods today. In other words, an opportunity cost is involved. Every time we make a choice for more goods today, we incur an opportunity cost of fewer goods tomorrow, and every time we make a choice of more goods in the future, we incur an opportunity cost of fewer goods today. With the resources that we don't use to produce consumer goods for today, we invest in capital goods that will produce more consumer goods for us later. The trade-off is shown in Figure 2-5. On the left in panel (a), you can see this trade-off depicted as a production possibilities curve between capital goods and consumption goods.

Assume that we are willing to give up $1 trillion worth of consumption today. We will be at point *A* in the left-hand diagram of panel (a). This will allow the economy to grow. We will have more future consumption because we invested in more capital goods today. In the right-hand diagram of panel (a), we see two goods represented, food and recreation. The production possibilities curve will move outward if we collectively decide to restrict consumption each year and invest in capital goods.

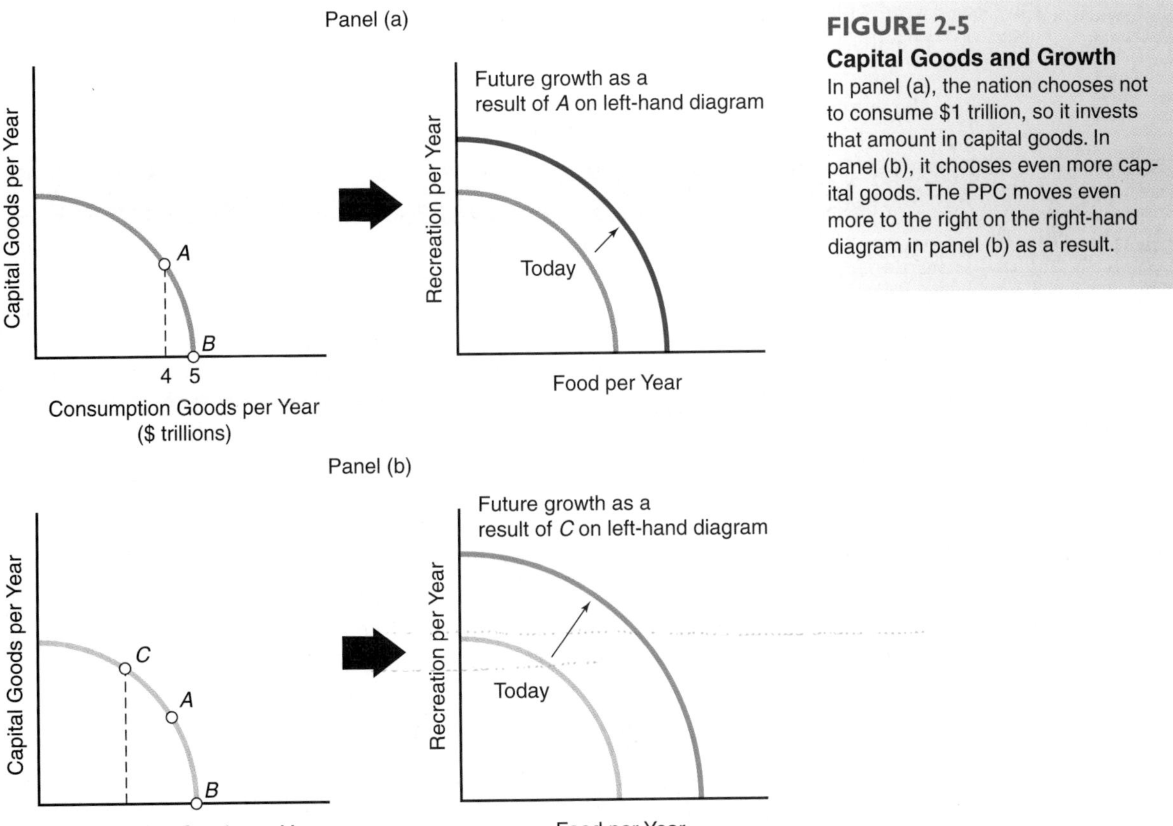

FIGURE 2-5
Capital Goods and Growth
In panel (a), the nation chooses not to consume $1 trillion, so it invests that amount in capital goods. In panel (b), it chooses even more capital goods. The PPC moves even more to the right on the right-hand diagram in panel (b) as a result.

In panel (b), we show the results of our willingness to forgo more current consumption. We move to point *C*, where we have many fewer consumer goods today but produce a lot more capital goods. This leads to more future growth in this simplified model, and thus the production possibilities curve in the right-hand side of panel (b) shifts outward more than it did in the right-hand side of panel (a).

In other words, the more we give up today, the more we can have tomorrow, provided, of course, that the capital goods are productive in future periods.

CONCEPTS IN BRIEF

- The use of capital requires using productive resources to produce capital goods that will later be used to produce consumer goods.
- A trade-off is involved between current consumption and capital goods or, alternatively, between current consumption and future consumption because the more we invest in capital goods today, the greater the amount of consumer goods we can produce in the future and the smaller the amount of consumer goods we can produce today.

SPECIALIZATION AND GREATER PRODUCTIVITY

Specialization The division of productive activities among persons and regions so that no one individual or one area is totally self-sufficient. An individual may specialize, for example, in law or medicine. A nation may specialize in the production of coffee, computers, or cameras.

Specialization involves working at a relatively well-defined, limited endeavor, such as accounting or teaching. It involves a division of labor among different individuals and regions. Most individuals do specialize. For example, you could change the oil in your car if you wanted to. Typically, though, you take your car to a garage and let the mechanic change the oil. You benefit by letting the garage mechanic specialize in changing the oil and in doing other repairs on your car. The specialist will get the job finished sooner than you could and has the proper equipment to make the job go more smoothly. Specialization usually leads to greater productivity, not only for each individual but also for the nation.

Specialization pays off for companies around the globe. This often has proved true in the automotive industry.

INTERNATIONAL POLICY EXAMPLE

Why the Light Turned Green Once the Trabi Was Parked

Among residents of eastern Germany, one of the best-recalled failures of communist rule was a little auto known as the "Trabi." Years after the reunification of Germany, people still joke about the car. For instance, "Why didn't the Trabi move when the light turned green? Because its tire got stuck on a piece of gum." Or "Why do deluxe Trabis have heated rear windows? To keep your hands warm as you push it." Another goes "How do you double a Trabi's value? Fill the gasoline tank."

Today the punch line is different, however. The company that once manufactured Trabis now has a booming business. The key to its success is that it no longer builds cars. Instead, it supplies auto parts to General Motors, Volkswagen, and DaimlerChrysler. What the company learned was that it was better off specializing in making auto parts—and leaving assembly of the parts to someone else.

For Critical Analysis

How do General Motors, Volkswagen, and DaimlerChrysler gain from specialization?

Absolute Advantage 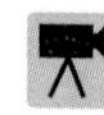

Specialization occurs because different individuals and different nations have different skills. Sometimes it seems that some individuals are better at doing everything than anyone else. A president of a large company might be able to type better than any of the typists, file better than any of the file clerks, and wash windows better than any of the window washers. The president has an **absolute advantage** in all of these endeavors—if he were to spend a given amount of time in one of these activities, he could produce more than anyone else in the company. The president does not, however, spend his time doing those other activities. Why not? Because he is being paid the most for undertaking the president's managerial duties. The president specializes in one particular task in spite of having an absolute advantage in all tasks. Indeed, absolute advantage is irrelevant in predicting how he uses his time; only *comparative advantage* matters.

Absolute advantage 
The ability to produce more units of a good or service using a given quantity of labor or resource inputs. Equivalently, the ability to produce the same quantity of a good or service using fewer units of labor or resource inputs.

Comparative Advantage

Comparative advantage is the ability to perform an activity at a lower opportunity cost. You have a comparative advantage in one activity whenever you have a lower opportunity cost of performing that activity. Comparative advantage is always a *relative* concept. You may be able to change the oil in your car; you might even be able to change it faster than the local mechanic. But if the opportunity cost you face by changing the oil exceeds the mechanic's opportunity cost, the mechanic has a comparative advantage in changing the oil. The mechanic faces a lower opportunity cost for that activity.

Comparative advantage 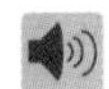
The ability to produce a good or service at a lower opportunity cost compared to other producers.

You may be convinced that everybody can do everything better than you. In this extreme situation, do you still have a comparative advantage? The answer is yes. What you need to do to discover your comparative advantage is to find a job in which your *disadvantage* relative to others is smaller. You do not have to be a mathematical genius to figure this out. The market tells you very clearly by offering you the highest income for the job for which you have a smaller disadvantage compared to others. Stated differently, to find your comparative advantage no matter how much better everybody else can do the jobs that you want to do, you simply find which job maximizes your income.

The coaches of sports teams are constantly faced with determining each player's comparative advantage. Babe Ruth was originally one of the best pitchers in professional baseball when he played for the Boston Red Sox. After he was traded to the New York Yankees, the owner and the coach decided to make him an outfielder, even though he was a better pitcher than anyone else on the team roster. They wanted "The Babe" to concentrate on his hitting. Good pitchers do not bring in as many fans as home-run kings. Babe Ruth's comparative advantage was clearly in hitting homers rather than practicing and developing his pitching game.

Scarcity, Self-Interest, and Specialization

In Chapter 1, you learned about the assumption of rational self-interest. To repeat, for the purposes of our analyses we assume that individuals are rational in that they will do what is in their own self-interest. They will not consciously carry out actions that will make them worse off. In this chapter, you learned that scarcity requires people to make choices. We assume that they make choices based on their self-interest. When they make these choices, they attempt to maximize benefits net of opportunity cost. In so doing, individuals choose their comparative advantage and end up specializing. Ultimately, when people specialize, they increase the money income they make and therefore become richer. When all individuals and businesses specialize simultaneously, the gains are seen in greater material well-being. With any given set of resources, specialization will result in higher output.

INTERNATIONAL EXAMPLE

Why Foreign Graduate Students Specialize When Studying in the United States

Specialization is evident in the fields of endeavor that foreign students choose when they come to the United States for graduate studies. Consider the following statistics: More than 60 percent of U.S. doctorates in engineering and 55 percent of those in mathematics, computer science, and the physical sciences are earned by foreign-born students. Yet foreign nationals are awarded relatively few advanced degrees in business, law, or medicine. The reason has nothing to do with intelligence or giftedness; it is simply that many more of the best American students choose schools in these professional fields rather than ones offering science and engineering programs.

Why does this specialization occur? For American students, the greatest returns for about the same effort come from business, law, and medicine. In contrast, foreign-born graduate students face fewer language and cultural obstacles (and hence better job prospects) if they choose technical subjects.

When students from foreign countries come to American graduate schools to obtain their Ph.D. degrees, more than 70 percent of them remain in the United States after graduation, thereby augmenting America's supply of engineers and scientists. Such specialization has helped the United States maintain its leadership in both the technoscientific and sociocultural areas.

For Critical Analysis

What type of capital do foreign-born students bring with them to the United States?

THE DIVISION OF LABOR

Division of labor 

The segregation of a resource into different specific tasks; for example, one automobile worker puts on bumpers, another doors, and so on.

In any firm that includes specialized human and nonhuman resources, there is a **division of labor** among those resources. The best-known example comes from Adam Smith, who in *The Wealth of Nations* illustrated the benefits of a division of labor in the making of pins, as depicted in the following example:

> One man draws out the wire, another straightens it, a third cuts it, a fourth points it, a fifth grinds it at the top for receiving the head; to make the head requires two or three distinct operations; to put it on is a peculiar business, to whiten the pins is another; it is even a trade by itself to put them into the paper.

Making pins this way allowed 10 workers without very much skill to make almost 48,000 pins "of a middling size" in a day. One worker, toiling alone, could have made perhaps 20 pins a day; therefore, 10 workers could have produced 200. Division of labor allowed for an increase in the daily output of the pin factory from 200 to 48,000! (Smith did not attribute all of the gain to the division of labor according to talent but credited also the use of machinery and the fact that less time was spent shifting from task to task.)

What we are discussing here involves a division of the resource called labor into different kinds of labor. The different kinds of labor are organized in such a way as to increase the amount of output possible from the fixed resources available. We can therefore talk about an organized division of labor within a firm leading to increased output.

COMPARATIVE ADVANTAGE AND TRADE AMONG NATIONS

Click here to find out about how much international trade takes place. Click on "Statistics" in the "A-Z list".

Though most of our analysis of absolute advantage, comparative advantage, and specialization has dealt with individuals, it is equally applicable to nations. First consider the United States. The Plains states have a comparative advantage in the production of grains and other agricultural goods. The states to the north and east tend to specialize in industrialized production, such as automobiles. Not surprisingly, grains are shipped from the Plains states to the northern states, and automobiles are shipped in the reverse direction. Such specialization and trade allow for higher incomes and standards of living. If both the Plains states and the northern states were politically defined as separate nations, the same analysis would still hold, but we would call it international trade. Indeed, Europe is comparable to the United States in area and population, but instead of one nation, Europe has 15. What in America we call *interstate* trade, in Europe they call *international* trade. There is no difference, however, in the economic results—both yield greater economic efficiency and higher average incomes.

Political problems that do not normally arise within a particular nation often do between nations. For example, if California avocado growers develop a cheaper method than growers in southern Florida to produce a tastier avocado, the Florida growers will lose out. They cannot do much about the situation except try to lower their own costs of production or improve their product. If avocado growers in Mexico, however, develop a cheaper method to produce better-tasting avocados, both California and Florida growers can (and likely will) try to raise political barriers that will prevent Mexican avocado growers from freely selling their product in America. U.S. avocado growers will use such arguments as "unfair" competition and loss of American jobs. In so doing, they are only partly right: Avocado-growing jobs may decline in America, but jobs will not necessarily decline overall. If the argument of U.S. avocado growers had any validity, every time a region in the United States developed a better way to produce a product manufactured somewhere else in the country, employment in America would decline. That has never happened and never will.

FAQ

Isn't too much international trade bad for the U.S. economy?

No, despite what you may read or hear, international trade is just like any other economic activity. Indeed, you can think of international trade as a production process that transforms goods that we sell to other countries (exports) into goods that we buy from other countries (imports). This process is a mutually beneficial exchange that takes place across political borders. Because international trade occurs only because it is in the interests of both buyers and sellers, people in both nations gain from trade.

When nations specialize where they have a comparative advantage and then trade with the rest of the world, the average standard of living in the world rises. In effect, international trade allows the world to move from inside the global production possibilities curve toward the curve itself, thereby improving worldwide economic efficiency.

CONCEPTS IN BRIEF

- With a given set of resources, specialization results in higher output; in other words, there are gains to specialization in terms of greater material well-being.
- Individuals and nations specialize in their areas of comparative advantage in order to reap the gains of specialization.
- Comparative advantages are found by determining which activities have the lowest opportunity cost—that is, which activities yield the highest return for the time and resources used.
- A division of labor occurs when different workers are assigned different tasks. Together, the workers produce a desired product.

NETNOMICS

Allocating Scarce Space on the Web

Nearly half of all users of the World Wide Web visit fewer than 10 Internet sites per month. Companies that want to sell their products on the Internet know this. They also know that when individuals access the Internet, their homepage is typically that of their Internet service provider (Netscape, Explorer) or a search engine such as Yahoo! Consequently, many companies advertise on those Web pages.

This is why each time you access the Net, you see advertising—banners, buttons, keywords, hot links, and other promotions. Some of the biggest advertisers on the Web are Microsoft, Toyota, General Motors, Disney, IBM, AT&T, and American Express. Internet-based companies such as Amazon.com also are major Web advertisers. It is estimated that by 2005, advertisers will be spending more than $25 billion a year on the Web.

The owner of any Web page that carries advertising faces an opportunity cost. For example, advertisers widely consider the opening page of the Yahoo! search engine "prime real estate" because so many people see it each day. But there is relatively little space on the screen. Thus when Yahoo! allocates space to promote its own services and products, it gives up space it could sell. But if it fills up too much of the screen with ads, some users will switch to a less cluttered search engine. That fact makes Web page design a crucial business concern.

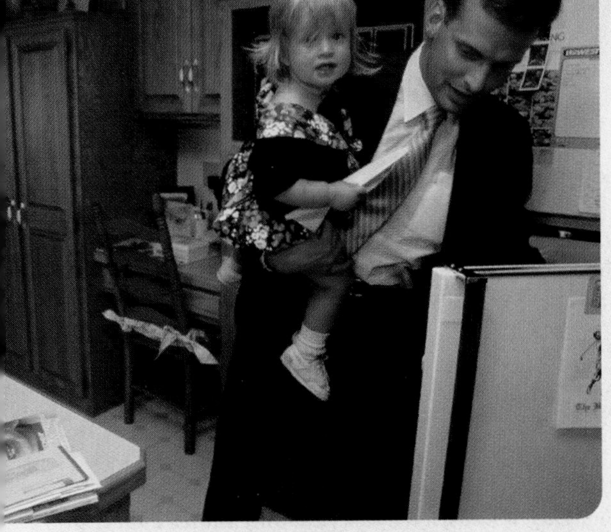

ISSUES & APPLICATIONS

The Costs of Raising a Child Are Not the Same for Everyone

The U.S. Department of Agriculture (USDA) has estimated the costs of raising a child. These include explicit expenses parents incur in providing the child with housing, food, clothing, day care, education, health care, and transportation. Panel (a) of Figure 2-6 shows the USDA's estimates of these expenses that typical American parents in upper-, middle-, and lower-income families with only one child born in 1997 will incur during each of the first 17 years of the child's life. (These estimates take into account projected inflation. Also, note that a wife often reduces or halts her income-earning activities before a child is born, so there is also an "age 0" in the chart.) As you might expect, higher-income parents incur greater direct expenses; they are more likely to buy high-tech toys and trendy clothing.

Concepts Applied

- Scarcity
- Choice
- Opportunity Cost

"Quality Time" with Kids Has a Market Value

Another key component of the cost of raising a child, however, is the wages that parents forgo when they spend time taking kids to school, the doctor, soccer games, and so on. In some families, one spouse stays home most of the time to provide these services. In others, both parents work but take turns allocating some of their time each day to these duties. No matter how they choose to balance the time, parents forgo wages they

FIGURE 2-6
The Full Cost of Raising a Child
As shown in panel (a), the dollar cost of raising a child increases with the child's age and is more for higher-income parents. The same is true of opportunity cost, as shown in panel (b). Panel (c) reveals that forgone wages (opportunity cost) make up the largest part of total child-rearing expenses.

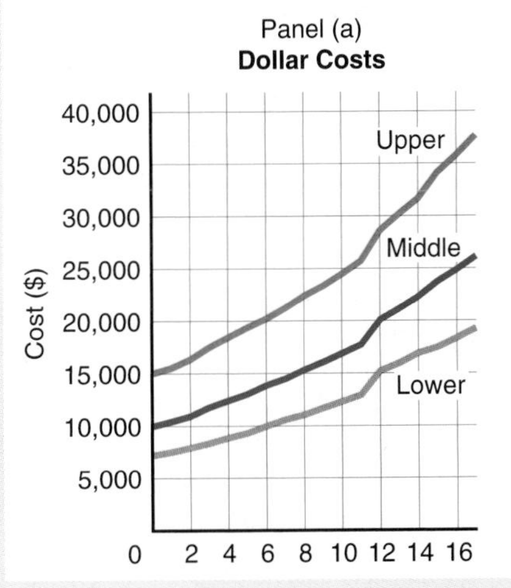

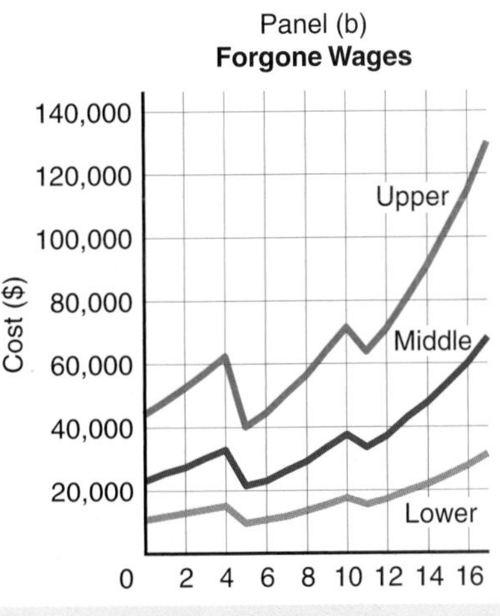

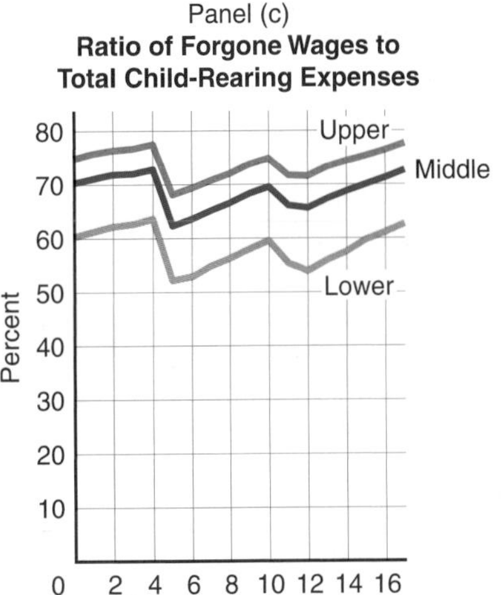

otherwise could have earned if they had allocated their time to income-generating activities.

Panel (b) shows the USDA's estimates of forgone wages for parents in a typical one-child family. Not surprisingly, the forgone wages are much higher for upper-income parents than for parents in middle- and lower-income families.

Forgone Wages and the Opportunity Cost of Raising a Child

The sum of explicit expenses and forgone wages constitutes the total opportunity cost of raising a child. Thus adding together the costs at each age in panels (a) and (b) would give the amounts that couples forgo by engaging in the activity of parenting rather than earning the highest possible wages and allocating their incomes to other activities. If you compare the dollar amounts in panels (a) and (b), however, it is clear that forgone wages are the key component of the total opportunity cost of child raising. Panel (c) verifies this fact. It shows the ratio of forgone wages to total child-raising expenses for each parental income category. Within each income group, and at each age of the child, forgone wages consistently exceed half the total opportunity cost of raising a child. For higher-income parents, forgone wages are consistently in excess of two-thirds of the total opportunity cost.

We can infer an important fact from Figure 2-6. When people acquire more training and education and move into higher-wage occupations, the opportunity cost of raising a child rises significantly. Other things being equal—for instance, if we assume that parents derive roughly the same satisfaction from raising children irrespective of their income—this is likely to induce higher-income people to have fewer children.

FOR CRITICAL ANALYSIS

1. Note in panel (b) that the forgone-wage component of the opportunity cost of child raising drops when a child reaches the age of 5 and then dips again slightly around age 11. What institutional factors do you suppose might account for this pattern?
2. In recent decades, population growth in lower-income countries has exceeded population growth in higher-income countries. Based on our discussion, can you provide a hypothesis explaining why?

SG

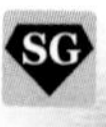

SUMMARY DISCUSSION OF LEARNING OBJECTIVES

1. **The Problem of Scarcity, Even for the Affluent:** Scarcity is very different from poverty. No one can obtain all one desires from nature without sacrifice. Thus even the richest people face scarcity, because they have to make choices among alternatives. Despite their high levels of income or wealth, affluent people, like everyone else, typically want more than they can have (in terms of goods, power, prestige, and so on).
2. **Why Economists Consider Individuals' Wants but Not Their "Needs":** Goods are all things from which individuals derive satisfaction. Economic goods are those for which the desired quantity exceeds that amount that is directly available from nature at a zero price. The goods that we want are not necessarily those that we need. To economists, the term *need* is undefinable, whereas humans have unlimited *wants,* which are defined as the goods and services on which we place a positive value.
3. **Why Scarcity Leads People to Evaluate Opportunity Costs:** We measure the opportunity cost of anything by the highest-valued alternative that one must give up to obtain it. The trade-offs that we face as individuals and as a society can be represented by a production possibilities curve (PPC), and moving from one point on a PPC to another entails incurring an opportunity cost. The reason is that along a PPC, all currently available resources and technology are being used, so obtaining more of one good requires shifting resources to production of that good and away from production of another. That is, there is an opportunity cost of allocating scarce resource toward producing one good instead of another good.

4. **Why Obtaining Increasing Increments of a Good Requires Giving Up More and More Units of Other Goods:** Typically, resources are specialized. Thus when society allocates additional resources to producing more and more of a single good, it must increasingly employ resources that would be better suited for producing other goods. As a result, the law of increasing relative cost holds. Each additional unit of a good can be obtained only by giving up more and more of other goods, which means that the production possibilities curve that society faces is bowed outward.
5. **The Trade-Off Between Consumption Goods and Capital Goods:** If we allocate more resources to producing capital goods today, then, other things being equal, the economy will grow by a larger amount. Thus the production possibilities curve will shift outward by a larger amount in the future, which means that we can have more consumption goods in the future. The trade-off, however, is that producing more capital goods today entails giving up consumption goods today.
6. **Absolute Advantage Versus Comparative Advantage:** A person has an absolute advantage if she can produce more of a specific good than someone else who uses the same amount of resources. This also means that she can produce the same amount of that good using fewer resources. Nevertheless, the individual may be better off producing a different good if she has a comparative advantage in producing the other good, meaning that she can produce the other good at lower opportunity cost than someone else. By specializing in producing the good for which she has a comparative advantage, she assures herself of reaping gains from specialization in the form of a higher income.

Key Terms and Concepts

Absolute advantage (39)
Comparative advantage (39)
Consumption (36)
Division of labor (40)
Economic goods (28)
Efficiency (34)
Entrepreneurship (28)
Goods (28)
Human capital (28)
Inefficient point (34)
Labor (28)
Land (28)
Law of increasing relative cost (35)
Opportunity cost (30)
Physical capital (28)
Production (27)
Production possibilities curve (PPC) (31)
Scarcity (27)
Services (28)
Specialization (38)
Technology (33)

Problems

Answers to the odd-numbered problems appear at the back of the book.

2-1. The following table illustrates the points a student can earn on examinations in economics and biology if the student uses all available hours for study.

Economics	Biology
100	40
90	50
80	60
70	70
60	80
50	90
40	100

Plot this student's production possibilities curve. Does the PPC illustrate increasing or decreasing opportunity costs?

2-2. Based on the information provided in Problem 2-1, what is the opportunity cost to this student of allocating sufficient additional study time on economics to move her grade up from a 90 to a 100?

2-3. Consider the following costs that a student incurs by attending a public university for one semester: $3,000 for tuition, $1,000 for room and board, $500 for books, $3,000 in wages lost that the student could have earned working, and 3 percent interest lost on the $4,500 paid for tuition, room and board, and books. Calculate the total opportunity cost that the student incurs by attending college for one semester.

2-4. Consider a change in the table in Problem 2-2. The student's set of opportunities is now as follows:

Economics	Biology
100	40
90	60
80	75
70	85
60	93
50	98
40	100

Plot this student's production possibilities curve. Does the PPC illustrate increasing or decreasing opportunity costs? What is the opportunity cost to this student for the additional amount of study time on economics required to move his grade from 60 to 70? From 90 to 100?

2-5. Construct a production possibilities curve for a nation facing increasing opportunity costs for producing food and video games. Show how the PPC changes given the following events.

a. A new and better fertilizer is invented.

b. There is a surge in labor, which can be employed in both the agricultural sector and the video game sector.

c. A new programming language is invented that is less costly to code and is more memory-efficient, enabling the use of smaller games cartridges.

d. A heat wave and drought results in a 10 percent decrease in usable farmland.

2-6. The president of a university announces to the local media that the university was able to construct its sports complex at a lower cost than it had previously projected. The president argues that the university can now purchase a yacht for the president at no additional cost. Explain why this statement is false by considering opportunity cost.

2-7. You can wash, fold, and iron a basket of laundry in two hours and prepare a meal in one hour. Your roommate can wash, fold, and iron a basket of laundry in three hours and prepare a meal in one hour. Who has the absolute advantage in laundry, and who has an absolute advantage in meal preparation? Who has the comparative advantage in laundry, and who has a comparative advantage in meal preparation?

2-8. Based on the information in Problem 2-7, should you and your roommate specialize in a particular task? Why? And if so, who should specialize in which task? Show how much labor time you save if you choose to "trade" an appropriate task with your roommate as opposed to doing it yourself.

2-9. On the one hand, Canada goes to considerable lengths to protect its television program and magazine producers from U.S. competitors. The United States, on the other hand, often seeks protection from food imports from Canada. Construct an argument showing that from an economywide viewpoint, these efforts are misguided.

2-10. Using only the concept of comparative advantage, evaluate this statement: "A professor with a Ph.D. in economics should never mow his or her own lawn, because this would fail to take into account the professor's comparative advantage."

2-11. Country A and country B produce the same consumption goods and capital goods and currently have *identical* production possibilities curves. They also have the same resources at present, and they have access to the same technology.

a. At present, does either country have a comparative advantage in producing capital goods? Consumption goods?

b. Currently, country A has chosen to produce more consumption goods, compared with country B. Other things being equal, which will experience the larger outward shift of its PPC during the next year?

c. Suppose that a year passes with no changes in technology or in factors other than the capital goods and consumption goods choices the countries initially made. Both countries' PPCs have shifted outward from their initial positions, but not in a parallel fashion. Country B's opportunity cost of producing consumption goods is now higher than in country A. Does either country have a comparative advantage in producing capital goods? Consumption goods?

Economics on the Net

Opportunity Cost and Labor Force Participation Many students choose to forgo full-time employment to concentrate on their studies, thereby incurring a sizable opportunity cost. This application explores the nature of this opportunity cost.

Title: College Enrollment and Work Activity of High School Graduates

Navigation: Click here to visit the Bureau of Labor Statistics (BLS) hompage. Select Topics A-Z, then click on Educational attainment, statistics. Finally, click on College Enrollment and Work Activity of High School Graduates.

Application Read the abbreviated report on college enrollment and work activity of high school graduates. Then answer the following questions.

1. Based on the article, explain who the BLS considers to be in the labor force and who it does not view as part of the labor force.
2. What is the difference in labor force participation rates between high school students entering four-year universities and those entering two-year universities? Using the concept of opportunity cost, explain the difference.
3. What is the difference in labor force participation rates between part-time college students and full-time college students? Using the concept of opportunity cost, explain the difference.

For Group Study and Analysis Read the last paragraph of the article, and then divide the class into two groups. The first group should explain, based on the concept of opportunity cost, the difference in labor force participation rates between youths not in school but with a high school diploma and youths not in school and without a high school diploma. The second half should explain, based on opportunity cost, the difference in labor force participation rates between men and women not in school but with a high school diploma and between men and women not in school and without a high school diploma.

CHAPTER 3

DEMAND AND SUPPLY

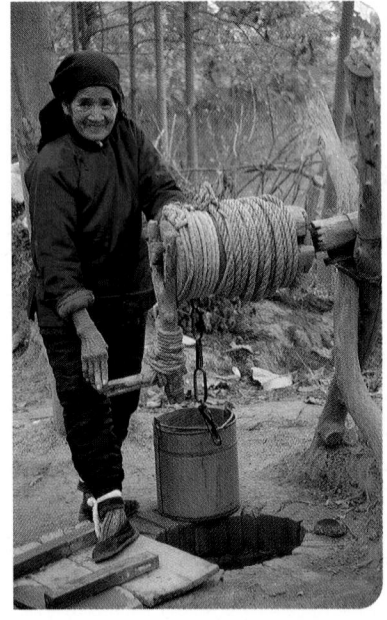
This farm worker near Shaanxi, China, obtains water the old-fashioned way. Chinese officals claim to have a "water problem." Should water be analyzed differently than other resources?

Signs of water stress appear throughout China. Of China's 600 largest cities, half are "running short" of water. Some cities turn on water for general use by their residents only two hours per day. Each day, hundreds of farmers are finding their wells pumped dry. Nevertheless, annual rainfall levels in most of China have hovered within normal ranges. Indeed, in some locales in recent years, above-normal rainfalls have caused flooding.

Can residents of China do nothing but hope for more rain? In this chapter, you will learn about one important factor contributing to China's water stress. You will also learn how to reason out one important part of the solution to this problem—a solution that China's leaders have slowly moved toward adopting. To do this, you will need the tools of demand and supply analysis.

LEARNING OBJECTIVES

After reading this chapter, you should be able to:

1. Explain the law of demand
2. Discuss the difference between money prices and relative prices
3. Distinguish between changes in demand and changes in quantity demanded
4. Explain the law of supply
5. Distinguish between changes in supply and changes in quantity supplied
6. Understand how the interaction of the demand for and supply of a commodity determines the market price of the commodity and the equilibrium quantity of the commodity that is produced and consumed

Chapter Outline

- The Law of Demand
- The Demand Schedule
- Shifts in Demand
- The Law of Supply
- The Supply Schedule
- Shifts in Supply
- Putting Demand and Supply Together

Did You Know That... more than 75 million people currently own portable cellular phones? This is a huge jump from the mere 200,000 who owned them in 1985. Since 1992, two out of every three new telephone numbers have been assigned to cellular phones. There are several reasons for the growth of cellular phones, not the least being the dramatic reduction in both price and size due to improved and cheaper computer chips that go into making them. There is something else at work, though. It has to do with crime. In a recent survey, 46 percent of new cellular phone users said that personal safety was the main reason they bought a portable phone. In Florida, for example, most cellular phone companies allow users simply to dial *FHP to reach the Florida Highway Patrol. The rush to cellular phones is worldwide. Over the past decade, sales have grown by nearly 50 percent every year outside the United States.

We could attempt to explain the phenomenon by saying that more people like to use portable phones. But that explanation is neither satisfying nor entirely accurate. If we use the economist's primary set of tools, *demand and supply,* we will have a better understanding of the cellular phone explosion, as well as many other phenomena in our world. Demand and supply are two ways of categorizing the influences on the price of goods that you buy and the quantities available. As such, demand and supply form the basis of virtually all economic analysis of the world around us.

As you will see throughout this text, the operation of the forces of demand and supply take place in *markets.* A **market** is an abstract concept referring to all the arrangements individuals have for exchanging with one another. Goods and services are sold in markets, such as the automobile market, the health market, and the compact disc market. Workers offer their services in the labor market. Companies, or firms, buy workers' labor services in the labor market. Firms also buy other inputs in order to produce the goods and services that you buy as a consumer. Firms purchase machines, buildings, and land. These markets are in operation at all times. One of the most important activities in these markets is the setting of the prices of all of the inputs and outputs that are bought and sold in our complicated economy. To understand the determination of prices, you first need to look at the law of demand.

Market 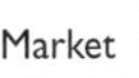 
All of the arrangements that individuals have for exchanging with one another. Thus we can speak of the labor market, the automobile market, and the credit market.

THE LAW OF DEMAND

Demand has a special meaning in economics. It refers to the quantities of specific goods or services that individuals, taken singly or as a group, will purchase at various possible prices, other things being constant. We can therefore talk about the demand for microprocessor chips, French fries, compact disc players, children, and criminal activities.

Demand 
A schedule of how much of a good or service people will purchase at any price during a specified time period, other things being constant.

Associated with the concept of demand is the **law of demand,** which can be stated as follows:

> When the price of a good goes up, people buy less of it, other things being equal.
> When the price of a good goes down, people buy more of it, other things being equal.

Law of demand 
The observation that there is a negative, or inverse, relationship between the price of any good or service and the quantity demanded, holding other factors constant.

The law of demand tells us that the quantity demanded of any commodity is inversely related to its price, other things being equal. In an inverse relationship, one variable moves up in value when the other moves down. The law of demand states that a change in price causes a change in the quantity demanded in the *opposite* direction.

Notice that we tacked on to the end of the law of demand the statement "other things being equal." We referred to this in Chapter 1 as the *ceteris paribus* assumption. It means, for example, that when we predict that people will buy fewer DVD (digital videodisk) players if their price goes up, we are holding constant the price of all other goods in the economy as well as people's incomes. Implicitly, therefore, if we are assuming that no other prices change when we examine the price behavior of DVD players, we are looking at the *relative* price of DVD players.

The law of demand is supported by millions of observations of people's behavior in the marketplace. Theoretically, it can be derived from an economic model based on rational behavior, as was discussed in Chapter 1. Basically, if nothing else changes and the price of a good falls, the lower price induces us to buy more over a certain period of time because we can enjoy additional net gains that were unavailable at the higher price. For the most part, if you examine your own behavior, you will see that it generally follows the law of demand.

Relative Prices Versus Money Prices 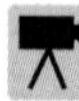

Relative price 
The price of one commodity divided by the price of another commodity; the number of units of one commodity that must be sacrificed to purchase one unit of another commodity.

Money price 
The price that we observe today, expressed in today's dollars. Also called the *absolute* or *nominal price*.

The **relative price** of any commodity is its price in terms of another commodity. The price that you pay in dollars and cents for any good or service at any point in time is called its **money price.** Consider an example that you might hear quite often around parents and grandparents. "When I bought my first new car, it cost only fifteen hundred dollars." The implication, of course, is that the price of cars today is outrageously high because the average new car might cost $25,000. But that is not an accurate comparison. What was the price of the average house during that same year? Perhaps it was only $12,000. By comparison, then, given that houses today average about $175,000, the price of a new car today doesn't sound so far out of line, does it?

The point is that money prices during different time periods don't tell you much. You have to find out relative prices. Consider an example of the price of CDs versus cassettes from last year and this year. In Table 3-1, we show the money price of CDs and cassettes for two years during which they have both gone up. That means that we have to pay out in today's dollars and cents more for CDs and more for cassettes. If we look, though, at the relative prices of CDs and cassettes, we find that last year, CDs were twice as expensive as cassettes, whereas this year they are only $1\frac{3}{4}$ times as expensive. Conversely, if we compare cassettes to CDs, last year they cost only half

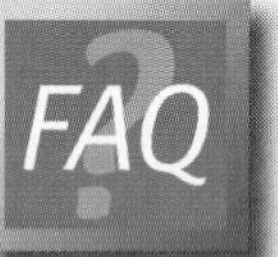

Isn't postage a lot more expensive than it used to be?

No, in reality, the *relative price* of postage in the United States has fallen steadily over the years. The absolute dollar price of a first-class stamp rose from 3 cents in 1940 to 33 cents at the beginning of the twenty-first century. Nevertheless, the price of postage relative to the average of all other prices has declined since reaching a peak in 1975.

TABLE 3-1
Money Price Versus Relative Price
The money price of both compact disks (CDs) and cassettes has risen. But the relative price of CDs has fallen (or conversely, the relative price of cassettes has risen).

	Money Price		Relative Price	
	Price Last Year	Price This Year	Price Last Year	Price This Year
CDs	$12	$14	$\frac{\$12}{\$6} = 2.0$	$\frac{\$14}{\$8} = 1.75$
Cassettes	$ 6	$ 8	$\frac{\$6}{\$12} = 0.5$	$\frac{\$8}{\$14} = 0.57$

as much as CDs, but today they cost about 57 percent as much. In the one-year period, though both prices have gone up in money terms, the relative price of CDs has fallen (and equivalently, the relative price of cassettes has risen).

INTERNATIONAL EXAMPLE

The High Relative Price of a U.S. Education

In 1993, about 40 percent of all college students classified as "international students"—students working toward degrees outside their home countries—were enrolled in U.S. colleges and universities. This figure has shrunk to just over 30 percent today, and it gradually continues to decline.

Have foreign students decided that the quality of American higher education is diminishing? Some may have made this judgment, but a more likely explanation for the falling U.S. share of international students is the higher relative price of a U.S. college education. Throughout the 1990s, tuition and other fees that U.S. colleges and universities charged for their services rose much faster than the average price of other goods and services. They also rose faster than tuition and fees at foreign universities. For instance, even before the sharp 1997–1998 economic contraction in Southeast Asia, increasing numbers of students from this region had begun studying at Australian universities. Colleges in Australia are not only closer to home but also less expensive.

For Critical Analysis

If the relative price of education at U.S. universities continues to increase, what other means could these universities use to try to regain their lost share of international students?

CONCEPTS IN BRIEF

- The law of demand posits an inverse relationship between the quantity demanded of a good and its price, other things being equal.
- The law of demand applies when other things, such as income and the prices of all other goods and services, are held constant.

THE DEMAND SCHEDULE

Let's take a hypothetical demand situation to see how the inverse relationship between the price and the quantity demanded looks (holding other things equal). We will consider the quantity of minidisks demanded *per year.* Without stating the *time dimension,* we could not make sense out of this demand relationship because the numbers would be different if we were talking about the quantity demanded per month or the quantity demanded per decade.

In addition to implicitly or explicitly stating a time dimension for a demand relationship, we are also implicitly referring to *constant-quality units* of the good or service in question. Prices are always expressed in constant-quality units in order to avoid the problem of comparing commodities that are in fact not truly comparable.

In panel (a) of Figure 3-1 on page 52, we see that if the price were $1 per minidisk, 50 disks would be bought each year by our representative individual, but if the price were $5 per disk, only 10 minidisks would be bought each year. This reflects the law of demand. Panel (a) is also called simply demand, or a *demand schedule,* because it gives a schedule of alternative quantities demanded per year at different possible prices.

FIGURE 3-1

The Individual Demand Schedule and the Individual Demand Curve

In panel (a), we show combinations *A* through *E* of the quantities of minidisks demanded, measured in constant-quality units at prices ranging from $5 down to $1 per disk. In panel (b), we plot combinations *A* through *E* on a grid. The result is the individual demand curve for minidisks.

Panel (a)

Combination	Price per Constant-Quality Minidisks	Quantity of Constant-Quality Minidisks per Year
A	$5	10
B	4	20
C	3	30
D	2	40
E	1	50

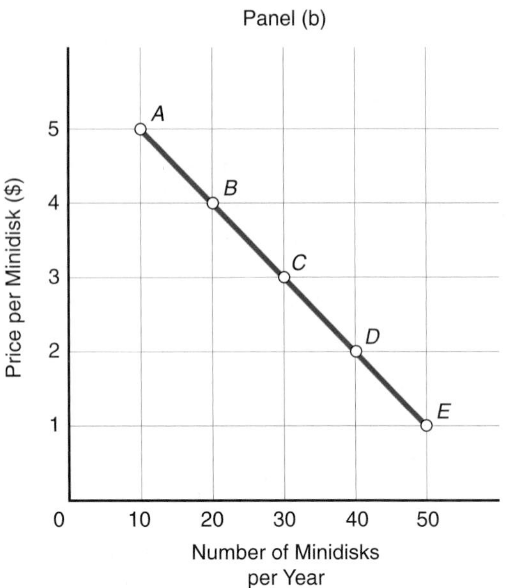

The Demand Curve

Demand curve A graphical representation of the demand schedule; a negatively sloped line showing the inverse relationship between the price and the quantity demanded (other things being equal).

Tables expressing relationships between two variables can be represented in graphical terms. To do this, we need only construct a graph that has the price per constant-quality minidisk on the vertical axis and the quantity measured in constant-quality minidisks per year on the horizontal axis. All we have to do is take combinations *A* through *E* from panel (a) of Figure 3-1 and plot those points in panel (b). Now we connect the points with a smooth line, and *voilà,* we have a **demand curve.*** It is downward-sloping (from left to right) to indicate the inverse relationship between the price of minidisks and the quantity demanded per year. Our presentation of demand schedules and curves applies equally well to all commodities, including toothpicks, hamburgers, textbooks, credit, and labor services. Remember, the demand curve is simply a graphical representation of the law of demand.

Individual Versus Market Demand Curves

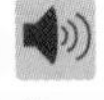

Market demand The demand of all consumers in the marketplace for a particular good or service. The summing at each price of the quantity demanded by each individual.

The demand schedule shown in panel (a) of Figure 3-1 and the resulting demand curve shown in panel (b) are both given for an individual. As we shall see, the determination of price in the marketplace depends on, among other things, the **market demand** for a particular commodity. The way in which we measure a market demand schedule and derive a market demand curve for minidisks or any other commodity is by summing (at each price) the individual demand for all buyers in the market. Suppose that the market demand for minidisks consists of only two buyers: buyer 1, for whom we've already shown the demand schedule, and buyer 2, whose demand schedule is displayed in column 3 of panel (a) of

*Even though we call them "curves," for the purposes of exposition we often draw straight lines. In many real-world situations, demand and supply curves will in fact be lines that do curve. To connect the points in panel (b) with a line, we assume that for all prices in between the ones shown, the quantities demanded will be found along that line.

FIGURE 3-2

The Horizontal Summation of Two Demand Schedules

Panel (a) shows how to sum the demand schedule for one buyer with that of another buyer. In column 2 is the quantity demanded by buyer 1, taken from panel (a) of Figure 3-1. Column 4 is the sum of columns 2 and 3. We plot the demand curve for buyer 1 in panel (b) and the demand curve for buyer 2 in panel (c). When we add those two demand curves horizontally, we get the market demand curve for two buyers, shown in panel (d).

Panel (a)

(1) Price per Minidisk	(2) Buyer 1's Quantity Demanded	(3) Buyer 2's Quantity Demanded	(4) = (2) + (3) Combined Quantity Demanded per Year
$5	10	10	20
4	20	20	40
3	30	40	70
2	40	50	90
1	50	60	110

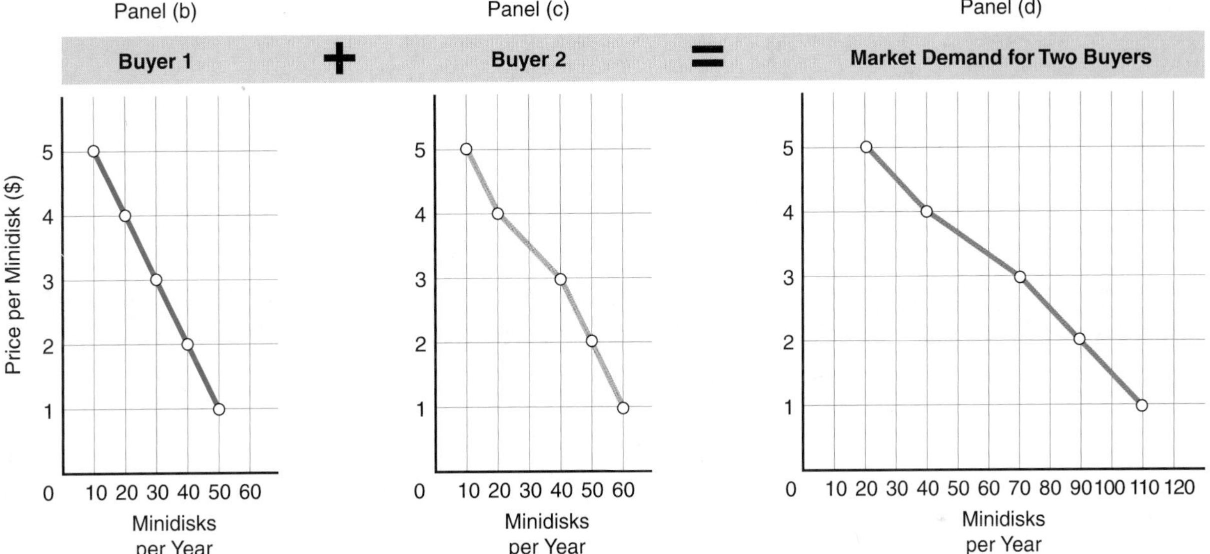

Figure 3-2. Column 1 shows the price, and column 2 shows the quantity demanded by buyer 1 at each price. These data are taken directly from Figure 3-1. In column 3, we show the quantity demanded by buyer 2. Column 4 shows the total quantity demanded at each price, which is obtained by simply adding columns 2 and 3. Graphically, in panel (d) of Figure 3-2, we add the demand curves of buyer 1 [panel (b)] and buyer 2 [panel (c)] to derive the market demand curve.

There are, of course, numerous potential consumers of minidisks. We'll simply assume that the summation of all of the consumers in the market results in a demand schedule, given in panel (a) of Figure 3-3 on page 54, and a demand curve, given in panel (b). The quantity demanded is now measured in millions of units per year. Remember, panel (b) in Figure 3-3 shows the market demand curve for the millions of users of minidisks. The "market" demand curve that we derived in Figure 3-2 was undertaken assuming that there were only two buyers in the entire market. That's why the "market" demand curve for two buyers in panel (d) of Figure 3-2 is not a smooth line, whereas the true market demand curve in panel (b) of Figure 3-3 is a smooth line with no kinks.

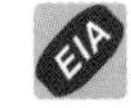

The Demand for Walkmans

Practice working with demand schedules.

Now consider some special aspects of the market demand curve for compact disks.

FIGURE 3-3

The Market Demand Schedule for Minidisks

In panel (a), we add up the existing demand schedules for minidisks. In panel (b), we plot the quantities from panel (a) on a grid; connecting them produces the market demand curve for minidisks.

Panel (a)

Price per Constant-Quality Minidisk	Total Quantity Demanded of Constant-Quality Minidisks per Year (millions)
$5	2
4	4
3	6
2	8
1	10

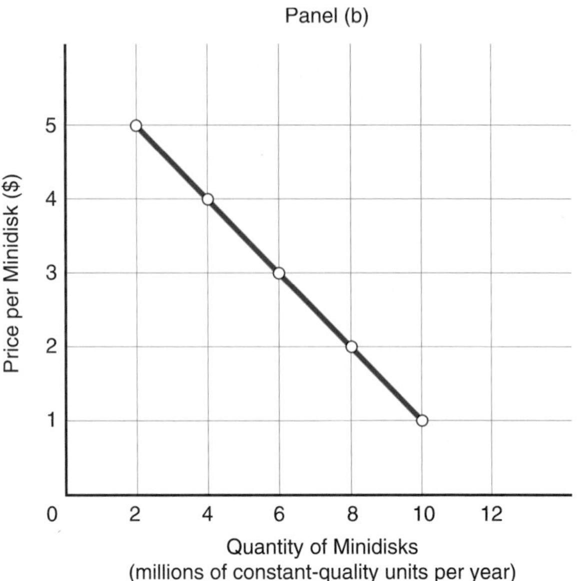

EXAMPLE

Garth Brooks, Used CDs, and the Law of Demand

A few years ago, country singer Garth Brooks tried to prevent his latest album from being sold to any chain or store that also sells used CDs. His argument was that the used-CD market deprived labels and artists of earnings. His announcement came after Wherehouse Entertainment, Inc., a 339-store retailer based in Torrance, California, started selling used CDs side by side with new releases, at half the price. Brooks, along with the distribution arms of Sony, Warner Music, Capitol-EMI, and MCA, was trying to quash the used-CD market. By so doing, it appears that none of these parties understands the law of demand.

Let's say the price of a new CD is $15. The existence of a secondary used-CD market means that to people who choose to resell their CDs for $5, the cost of a new CD is in fact only $10. Because we know that quantity demanded is inversely related to price, we know that more of a new CD will be sold at a price of $10 than of the same CD at a price of $15. Taking only this force into account, eliminating the used-CD market tends to reduce sales of new CDs.

But there is another force at work here, too. Used CDs are substitutes for new CDs. If used CDs are not available, some people who would have purchased them will instead purchase new CDs. If this second effect outweighs the incentive to buy less because of the higher effective price, then Brooks is behaving correctly in trying to suppress the used CD market.

For Critical Analysis

Can you apply this argument to the used-book market, in which both authors and publishers have long argued that used books are "killing them"?

CONCEPTS IN BRIEF

- We measure the demand schedule in terms of a time dimension and in constant-quality units.
- The market demand curve is derived by summing the quantity demanded by individuals at each price. Graphically, we add the individual demand curves horizontally to derive the total, or market, demand curve.

SHIFTS IN DEMAND

Assume that the federal government gives every student registered in a college, university, or technical school in the United States a minidisk player-recorder. The demand curve presented in panel (b) of Figure 3-3 would no longer be an accurate representation of total market demand for minidisks. What we have to do is shift the curve outward, or to the right, to represent the rise in demand. There will now be an increase in the number of minidisks demanded at *each and every possible price.* The demand curve shown in Figure 3-4 will shift from D_1 to D_2. Take any price, say, $3 per minidisk. Originally, before the federal government giveaway of player-recorders, the amount demanded at $3 was 6 million minidisks per year. After the government giveaway, however, the new amount demanded at $3 is 10 million minidisks per year. What we have seen is a shift in the demand for minidisks.

The shift can also go in the opposite direction. What if colleges uniformly outlawed the use of minidisk players by any of their students? Such a regulation would cause a shift inward—to the left—of the demand curve for minidisks. In Figure 3-4, the demand curve would shift to D_3; the amount demanded would now be less at each and every possible price.

The Other Determinants of Demand

The demand curve in panel (b) of Figure 3-3 is drawn with other things held constant, specifically all of the other factors that determine how much will be bought. There are many such determinants. The major other determinants are income; tastes and preferences; the prices of related goods; expectations regarding future prices, future incomes, and future product availability; and market size (number of buyers). Let's examine each determinant more closely.

Income. For most goods, an increase in income will lead to an increase in demand. The expression *increase in demand* always refers to a comparison between two different demand curves. Thus for most goods, an increase in income will lead to a rightward shift in the position of the demand curve from, say, D_1 to D_2 in Figure 3-4. You can avoid confusion about shifts in curves by always relating a rise in demand to a rightward shift in the

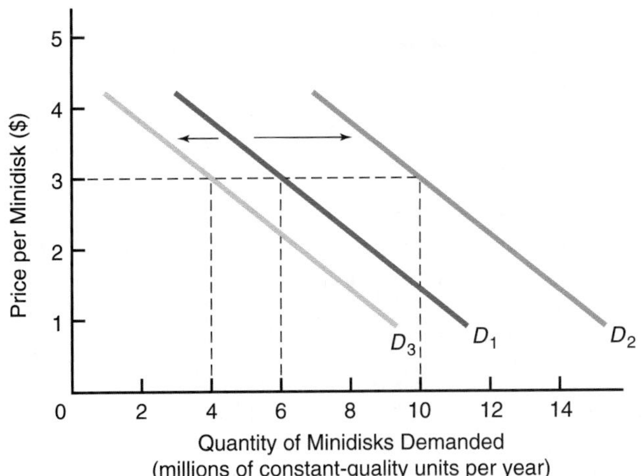

FIGURE 3-4 

A Shift in the Demand Curve

If some factor other than price changes, the only way we can show its effect is by moving the entire demand curve, say, from D_1 to D_2. We have assumed in our example that the move was precipitated by the government's giving a free minidisk player-recorder to every registered college student in America. That meant that at *all* prices, a larger number of minidisks would be demanded than before. Curve D_3 represents reduced demand compared to curve D_1, caused by a law prohibiting computers on campus.

Normal goods
Goods for which demand rises as income rises. Most goods are considered normal.

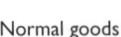

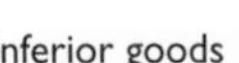
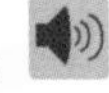
Inferior goods
Goods for which demand falls as income rises.

demand curve and a fall in demand to a leftward shift in the demand curve. Goods for which the demand rises when income rises are called **normal goods.** Most goods, such as shoes, computers, and CDs, are "normal goods." For some goods, however, demand *falls* as income rises. These are called **inferior goods.** Beans might be an example. As households get richer, they tend to spend less and less on beans and more and more on meat. (The terms *normal* and *inferior* are merely part of the economist's lexicon; no value judgments are associated with them.)

Remember, a shift to the left in the demand curve represents a fall in demand, and a shift to the right represents a rise, or increase, in demand.

EXAMPLE

Is Dental Care Becoming an Inferior Good?

A British health minister once claimed that the demand for health care is infinite because in the end everyone is in a losing battle against death. This is not so for American dentistry, however. As aggregate U.S. income levels have risen during the past 25 years, overall spending on dental care services has declined.

It isn't that fewer Americans are seeing dentists each year. They just do not require as many fillings or extractions. As incomes rose across the land, people purchased more expensive and effective toothpastes. More towns, cities, and counties began to fluoridate their water as the relative price of this anticavity agent declined, so changing relative prices have also played a role. And higher incomes of their residents have permitted more municipalities to purchase fluoridation systems.

At every age, the average American now has about two more teeth than 25 years ago. Unfortunately for dentists who specialize in treating decaying and diseased teeth, Americans' teeth are healthier than ever before.

For Critical Analysis

Many fledgling dentists have begun specializing in "cosmetic dentistry" desired by clients with healthy but less than beautiful teeth. Compared to traditional dental care services, is cosmetic dentistry more or less likely to be a normal good?

Tastes and Preferences. A change in consumer tastes in favor of a good can shift its demand curve outward to the right. When Frisbees® became the rage, the demand curve for them shifted outward to the right; when the rage died out, the demand curve shifted inward to the left. Fashions depend to a large extent on people's tastes and preferences. Economists have little to say about the determination of tastes; that is, they don't have any "good" theories of taste determination or why people buy one brand of product rather than others. Advertisers, however, have various theories that they use to try to make consumers prefer their products over those of competitors.

Prices of Related Goods: Substitutes and Complements. Demand schedules are always drawn with the prices of all other commodities held constant. That is to say, when deriving a given demand curve, we assume that only the price of the good under study changes. For example, when we draw the demand curve for butter, we assume that the price of margarine is held constant. When we draw the demand curve for stereo speakers, we assume that the price of stereo amplifiers is held constant. When we refer to *related goods,* we are talking about goods for which demand is interdependent. If a change in the price of one good shifts the demand for another good, those two goods are related. There are two types of related goods: *substitutes* and *complements.* We can define and distinguish between substitutes and complements in terms of how the change in price of one commodity affects the demand for its related commodity.

Butter and margarine are **substitutes.** Either can be consumed to satisfy the same basic want. Let's assume that both products originally cost $2 per pound. If the price of butter remains the same and the price of margarine falls from $2 per pound to $1 per pound, people will buy more margarine and less butter. The demand curve for butter will shift inward to the left. If, conversely, the price of margarine rises from $2 per pound to $3 per pound, people will buy more butter and less margarine. The demand curve for butter will shift outward to the right. In other words, an increase in the price of margarine will lead to an increase in the demand for butter, and an increase in the price of butter will lead to an increase in the demand for margarine. For substitutes, a price change in the substitute will cause a change in demand *in the same direction.*

Substitutes 

Two goods are substitutes when either one can be used for consumption to satisfy a similar want—for example, coffee and tea. The more you buy of one, the less you buy of the other. For substitutes, the change in the price of one causes a shift in demand for the other in the same direction as the price change.

For **complements,** goods typically consumed together, the situation is reversed. Consider stereo speakers and stereo amplifiers. We draw the demand curve for speakers with the price of amplifiers held constant. If the price per constant-quality unit of stereo amplifiers decreases from, say, $500 to $200, that will encourage more people to purchase component stereo systems. They will now buy more speakers, at any given speaker price, than before. The demand curve for speakers will shift outward to the right. If, by contrast, the price of amplifiers increases from $200 to $500, fewer people will purchase component stereo systems. The demand curve for speakers will shift inward to the left. To summarize, a decrease in the price of amplifiers leads to an increase in the demand for speakers. An increase in the price of amplifiers leads to a decrease in the demand for speakers. Thus for complements, a price change in a product will cause a change in demand *in the opposite direction.*

Complements 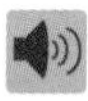

Two goods are complements if both are used together for consumption or enjoyment—for example, coffee and cream. The more you buy of one, the more you buy of the other. For complements, a change in the price of one causes an opposite shift in the demand for the other.

Are new learning technologies complements or substitutes for college instructors? Read on.

EXAMPLE

Getting Your Degree via the Internet

In this class and in others, you have most likely been exposed to such instructional technologies as films, videos, and interactive CD-ROM learning systems. The future for some of you, or at least the next few generations, may be quite different. All of the instructional technology that your professor provides may be packaged in the form of on-line courses. Many institutions of higher learning are now using the Internet to provide full instruction. It is called *distance learning* or *distributive learning.* And it is worldwide. For example, the University of Michigan, in conjunction with companies in Hong Kong, South Korea, and Europe, offers a global M.B.A. through the Internet. A professor teaches a course "live" via video and uses the software program Lotus Notes, which allows course information to be sent via the Internet. Students submit their homework assignments the same way. Duke University runs the Global Executive M.B.A. program, in which students "attend" CD-ROM video lectures, download additional video and audio materials, and receive interactive study aids, all via the Internet.

Virtually all major college publishers now have projects to develop distance learning via the Internet. In addition, a consortium of over 100 universities has put in place what is called Internet II. Internet II permits full-motion video and virtually instantaneous interactivity for participating universities. The age of fully interactive distance learning with full-motion video is not far off. Certainly, even better technology, as yet undeveloped, will speed up this process.

For Critical Analysis

What do you predict will happen to the demand curve for college professors in the future?

Expectations. Consumers' expectations regarding future prices, future incomes, and future availability may prompt them to buy more or less of a particular good without a change in its current money price. For example, consumers getting wind of a scheduled 100 percent price increase in minidisks next month may buy more of them today at today's prices. Today's demand curve for minidisks will shift from D_1 to D_2 in Figure 3-4. The opposite would occur if a decrease in the price of minidisks were scheduled for next month.

Expectations of a rise in income may cause consumers to want to purchase more of everything today at today's prices. Again, such a change in expectations of higher future income will cause a shift in the demand curve from D_1 to D_2 in Figure 3-4.

Finally, expectations that goods will not be available at any price will induce consumers to stock up now, increasing current demand.

Market Size (Number of Buyers). An increase in the number of buyers (holding per capita income constant) shifts the market demand curve outward. Conversely, a reduction in the number of buyers shifts the market demand curve inward.

Changes in Demand Versus Changes in Quantity Demanded 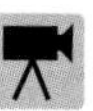

We have made repeated references to demand and to quantity demanded. It is important to realize that there is a difference between a *change in demand* and a *change in quantity demanded.*

Demand refers to a schedule of planned rates of purchase and depends on a great many nonprice determinants. Whenever there is a change in a nonprice determinant, there will be a change in demand—a shift in the entire demand curve to the right or to the left.

A quantity demanded is a specific quantity at a specific price, represented by a single point on a demand curve. When price changes, quantity demanded changes according to the law of demand, and there will be a movement from one point to another along the same demand curve. Look at Figure 3-5. At a price of \$3 per minidisk, 6 million disks per year are demanded. If the price falls to \$1, quantity demanded increases to 10 million per year. This movement occurs because the current market price for the product changes. In Figure 3-5, you can see the arrow pointing down the given demand curve *D*.

FIGURE 3-5
Movement Along a Given Demand Curve
A change in price changes the quantity of a good demanded. This can be represented as movement along a given demand schedule. If, in our example, the price of minidisks falls from \$3 to \$1 apiece, the quantity demanded will increase from 6 million to 10 million units per year.

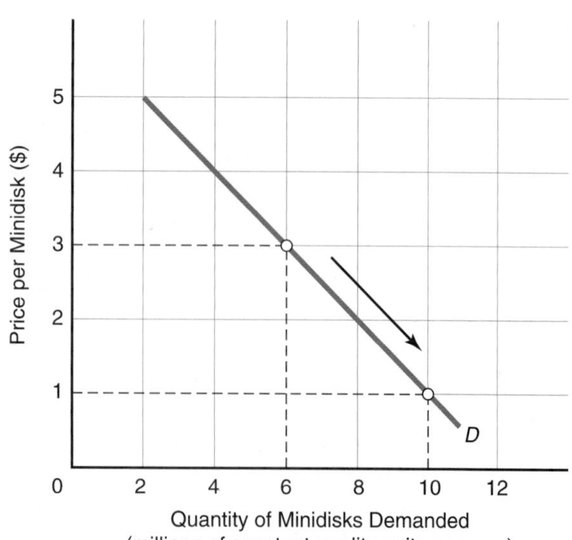

When you think of demand, think of the entire curve. Quantity demanded, in contrast, is represented by a single point on the demand curve.

A change or shift in demand causes the *entire* curve to move. The *only* thing that can cause the entire curve to move is a change in a determinant *other than its own price.*

In economic analysis, we cannot emphasize too much the following distinction that must constantly be made:

A change in a good's own price leads to a change in quantity demanded, for any given demand curve, other things held constant. This is a movement *on* the curve.

A change in any other determinant of demand leads to a change in demand. This causes a movement *of* the curve.

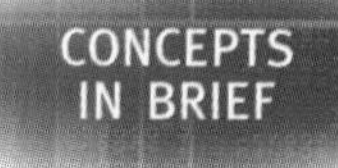

- Demand curves are drawn with determinants other than the price of the good held constant. These other determinants are (1) income; (2) tastes and preferences; (3) prices of related goods; (4) expectations about future prices, future incomes, and future availability of goods; and (5) market size (the number of buyers in the market). If any one of these determinants changes, the demand schedule will shift to the right or to the left.
- A change in demand comes about only because of a change in the other determinants of demand. This change in demand shifts the demand curve to the left or to the right.
- A change in the quantity demanded comes about when there is a change in the price of the good (other things held constant). Such a change in quantity demanded involves a movement along a given demand curve.

THE LAW OF SUPPLY

The other side of the basic model in economics involves the quantities of goods and services that firms will offer for sale to the market. The **supply** of any good or service is the amount that firms will produce and offer for sale under certain conditions during a specified time period. The relationship between price and quantity supplied, called the **law of supply,** can be summarized as follows:

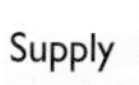 

Supply
A schedule showing the relationship between price and quantity supplied for a specified period of time, other things being equal.

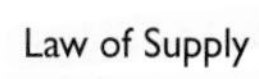 

Law of Supply
The observation that the higher the price of a good, the more of that good sellers will make available over a specified time period, other things being equal.

At higher prices, a larger quantity will generally be supplied than at lower prices, all other things held constant. At lower prices, a smaller quantity will generally be supplied than at higher prices, all other things held constant.

There is generally a direct relationship between quantity supplied and price. For supply, as the price rises, the quantity supplied rises; as price falls, the quantity supplied also falls. Producers are normally willing to produce and sell more of their product at a higher price than at a lower price, other things being constant. At $5 per minidisk, manufacturers would almost certainly be willing to supply a larger quantity than at $1 per unit, assuming, of course, that no other prices in the economy had changed.

As with the law of demand, millions of instances in the real world have given us confidence in the law of supply. On a theoretical level, the law of supply is based on a model in which producers and sellers seek to make the most gain possible from their a ctivities. For example, as a minidisk manufacturer attempts to produce more and more minidisks over the same time period, it will eventually have to hire more workers, pay overtime wages (which are higher), and overutilize its machines. Only if offered a higher price per minidisk will the minidisk manufacturer be willing to incur these higher costs. That is why the law of supply implies a direct relationship between price and quantity supplied.

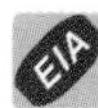

The Law of Supply
Gain more experience with the concept of the law of supply.

THE SUPPLY SCHEDULE

Just as we were able to construct a demand schedule, we can construct a *supply schedule*, which is a table relating prices to the quantity supplied at each price. A supply schedule can also be referred to simply as *supply*. It is a set of planned production rates that depends on the price of the product. We show the individual supply schedule for a hypothetical producer in panel (a) of Figure 3-6. At $1 per minidisk, for example, this producer will supply 20,000 minidisks per year; at $5, this producer will supply 55,000 minidisks per year.

The Supply Curve

Supply curve
The graphical representation of the supply schedule; a line (curve) showing the supply schedule, which generally slopes upward (has a positive slope), other things being equal.

We can convert the supply schedule in panel (a) of Figure 3-6 into a **supply curve,** just as we earlier created a demand curve in Figure 3-1. All we do is take the price-quantity combinations from panel (a) of Figure 3-6 and plot them in panel (b). We have labeled these combinations *F* through *J*. Connecting these points, we obtain an upward-sloping curve that shows the typically direct relationship between price and quantity supplied. Again, we have to remember that we are talking about quantity supplied *per year,* measured in constant-quality units.

The Market Supply Curve

Just as we had to sum the individual demand curves to get the market demand curve, we need to sum the individual producers' supply curves to get the market supply curve. Look at Figure 3-7, in which we horizontally sum two typical minidisk manufacturers' supply curves. Supplier 1's data are taken from Figure 3-6; supplier 2 is added. The numbers are presented in panel (a). The graphical representation of supplier 1 is in panel (b), of supplier 2 in panel (c), and of the summation in panel (d). The result, then, is the supply curve for minidisks for suppliers 1 and 2. We assume that there are more suppliers of minidisks, however. The total market supply schedule and total market demand curve for minidisks are represented in Figure 3-8, with the curve in panel (b) obtained by adding all of the supply

FIGURE 3-6
The Individual Producer's Supply Schedule and Supply Curve for Minidisks
Panel (a) shows that at higher prices, a hypothetical supplier will be willing to provide a greater quantity of minidisks. We plot the various price-quantity combinations in panel (a) on the grid in panel (b). When we connect these points, we find the individual supply curve for diskettes. It is positively sloped.

Panel (a)

Combination	Price per Constant-Quality Minidisk	Quantity of Minidisks Supplied (thousands of constant-quality units per year)
F	$5	55
G	4	40
H	3	35
I	2	25
J	1	20

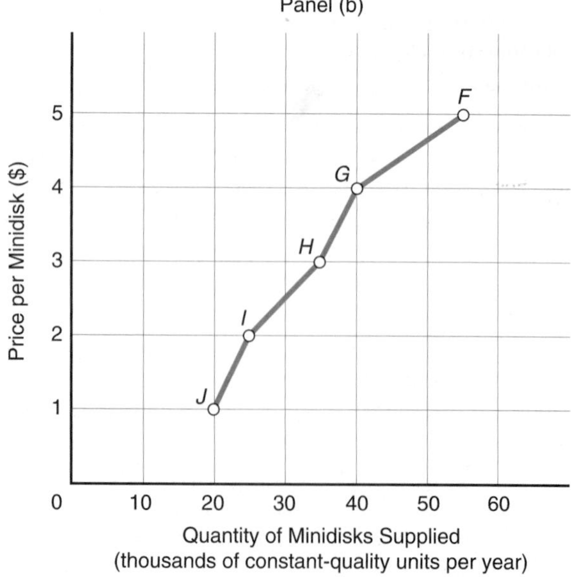

Panel (a)

(1) Price per Minidisk	(2) Supplier 1's Quantity Supplied (thousands)	(3) Supplier 2's Quantity Supplied (thousands)	(4) = (2) + (3) Combined Quantity Supplied per Year (thousands)
$5	55	35	90
4	40	30	70
3	35	20	55
2	25	15	40
1	20	10	30

FIGURE 3-7

Horizontal Summation of Supply Curves

In panel (a), we show the data for two individual suppliers of minidisks. Adding how much each is willing to supply at different prices, we come up with the combined quantities supplied in column 4. When we plot the values in columns 2 and 3 on grids in panels (b) and (c) and add them horizontally, we obtain the combined supply curve for the two suppliers in question, shown in panel (d).

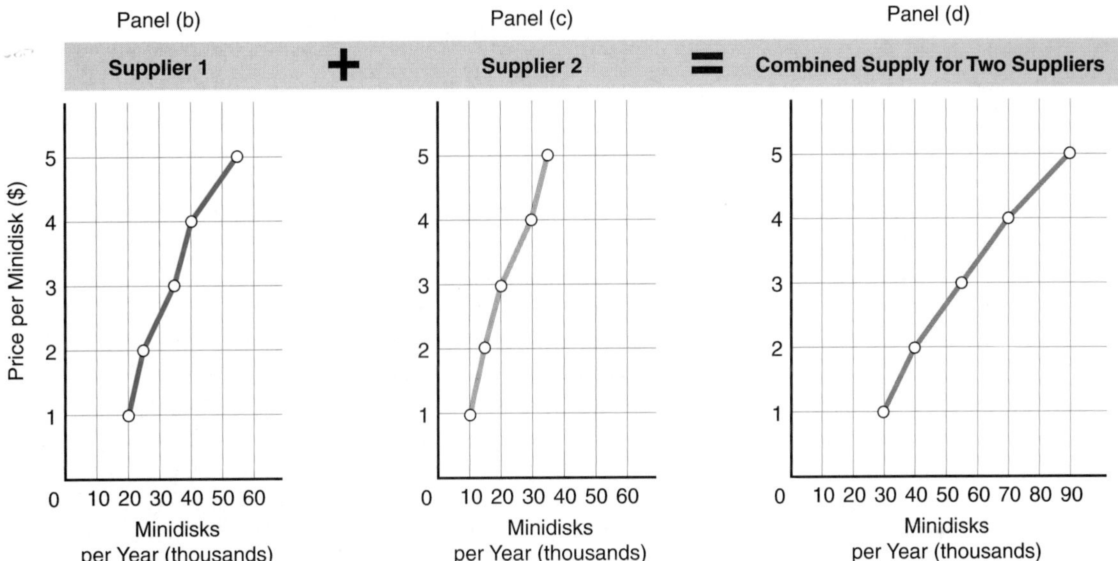

FIGURE 3-8

The Market Supply Schedule and the Market Supply Curve for Minidisks

In panel (a), we show the summation of all the individual producers' supply schedules; in panel (b), we graph the resulting supply curve. It represents the market supply curve for diskettes and is upward-sloping.

Panel (a)

Price per Constant-Quality Minidisk	Quantity of Minidisks Supplied (millions of constant-quality units per year)
$5	10
4	8
3	6
2	4
1	2

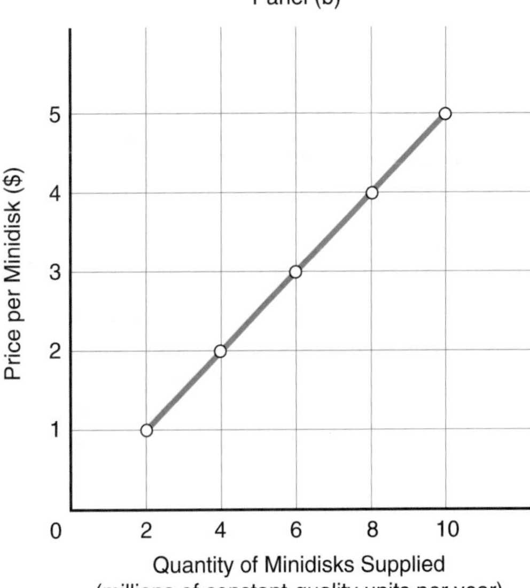

curves such as those shown in panels (b) and (c) of Figure 3-7. Notice the difference between the market supply curve with only two suppliers in Figure 3-7 and the one with a large number of suppliers—the entire true market—in panel (b) of Figure 3-8. We assume that the true total market supply curve is a straight line.

Notice what happens at the market level when price changes. If the price is \$3, the quantity supplied is 6 million. If the price goes up to \$4, the quantity supplied increases to 8 million per year. If the price falls to \$2, the quantity supplied decreases to 4 million per year. Changes in quantity supplied are represented by movements along the supply curve in panel (b) of Figure 3-8.

CONCEPTS IN BRIEF

- There is normally a direct, or positive, relationship between price and quantity of a good supplied, other things held constant.
- The supply curve normally shows a direct relationship between price and quantity supplied. The market supply curve is obtained by horizontally adding individual supply curves in the market.

SHIFTS IN SUPPLY

When we looked at demand, we found out that any change in anything relevant besides the price of the good or service caused the demand curve to shift inward or outward. The same is true for the supply curve. If something besides price changes and alters the willingness of suppliers to produce a good or service, then we will see the entire supply curve shift.

Consider an example. A new method of coating minidisks has been invented. It reduces the cost of production by 50 percent. In this situation, minidisk producers will supply more product at *all* prices because their cost of so doing has fallen dramatically. Competition among manufacturers to produce more at each and every price will shift the supply schedule outward to the right from S_1 to S_2 in Figure 3-9. At a price of \$3, the quantity supplied was originally 6 million per year, but now the quantity supplied (after the reduction in the costs of production) at \$3 a minidisk will be 9 million a year. (This is similar to what has happened to the supply curve of personal computers and fax machines in recent years as computer memory chip prices have fallen.)

Consider the opposite case. If the cost of making minidisks doubles, the supply curve in Figure 3-9 will shift from S_1 to S_3. At each and every price, the number of minidisks supplied will fall due to the increase in the price of raw materials.

FIGURE 3-9
A Shift in the Supply Schedule
If the cost of producing minidisks were to fall dramatically, the supply schedule would shift rightward from S_1 to S_2 such that at all prices, a larger quantity would be forthcoming from suppliers. Conversely, if the cost of production rose, the supply curve would shift leftward to S_3.

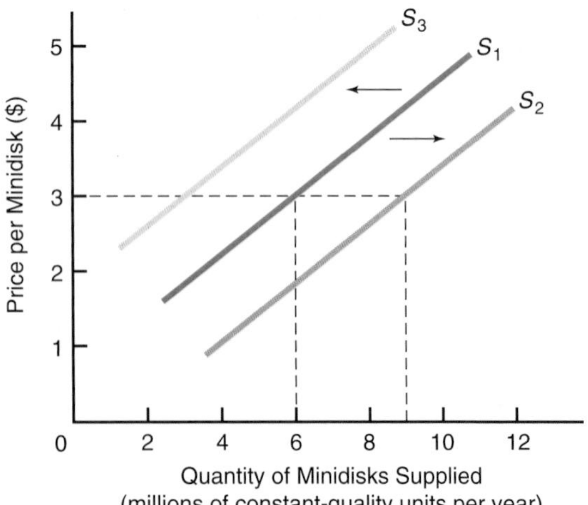

The Other Determinants of Supply

When supply curves are drawn, only the price of the good in question changes, and it is assumed that other things remain constant. The other things assumed constant are the costs of resources (inputs) used to produce the product, technology and productivity, taxes and subsidies, producers' price expectations, and the number of firms in the industry. These are the major nonprice determinants of supply. If *any* of them changes, there will be a shift in the supply curve.

Cost of Inputs Used to Produce the Product. If one or more input prices fall, the supply curve will shift outward to the right; that is, more will be supplied at each and every price. The opposite will be true if one or more inputs become more expensive. For example, when we draw the supply curve of new cars, we are holding the cost of steel (and other inputs) constant. When we draw the supply curve of blue jeans, we are holding the cost of cotton fabric fixed. Likewise, when we draw a supply curve for caviar, we are holding constant the cost of obtaining a fundamental input—a particular kind of fish.

INTERNATIONAL EXAMPLE

Caviar Poaching Is Making a Pricey Delicacy Even Pricier

You've probably heard that caviar is nothing but fish eggs. That is true, but the best caviar comes from a fish called the sturgeon, which thrives in the waters of the Volga River in Russia and the Caspian Sea. Caviar is a big but dwindling business. The reason is that in years past, poachers have removed so many sturgeon from their watery home that their population today is lower than in prior years.

The immediate effect? A leftward shift in the market supply curve. The market outcome? A big increase in the market price of caviar. In 1998, an ounce of prized caviar from a particular sturgeon, the beluga, sold for $55 in New York caviar boutiques. Since then, the market price has steadily risen, and within a few years it is expected to top $100 per ounce.

For Critical Analysis

The Russian government is trying to beef up its fisheries police force that patrols the Volga River, and nations bordering the Caspian Sea are working on a way to enforce the ban on poaching. If successful, how are these policies likely to affect the market price of caviar?

Technology and Productivity. Supply curves are drawn by assuming a given technology, or "state of the art." When the available production techniques change, the supply curve will shift. For example, when a better production technique for minidisks becomes available, the supply curve will shift to the right. A larger quantity will be forthcoming at each and every price because the cost of production is lower.

Taxes and Subsidies. Certain taxes, such as a per-unit tax, are effectively an addition to production costs and therefore reduce the supply. If the supply curve were S_1 in Figure 3-9, a per-unit tax increase would shift it to S_3. A **subsidy** would do the opposite; it would shift the curve to S_2. Every producer would get a "gift" from the government of a few cents for each unit produced.

Subsidy
A negative tax; a payment to a producer from the government, usually in the form of a cash grant.

Price Expectations. A change in the expectation of a future relative price of a product can affect a producer's current willingness to supply, just as price expectations affect a consumer's current willingness to purchase. For example, minidisk suppliers may withhold from the market part of their current supply if they anticipate higher prices in the future. The current amount supplied at each and every price will decrease.

Number of Firms in the Industry. In the short run, when firms can only change the number of employees they use, we hold the number of firms in the industry constant. In the long run, the number of firms (or the size of some existing firms) may change. If the number of firms increases, the supply curve will shift outward to the right. If the number of firms decreases, it will shift inward to the left.

Changes in Supply Versus Changes in Quantity Supplied 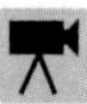

We cannot overstress the importance of distinguishing between a movement along the supply curve—which occurs only when the price changes for a given supply curve—and a shift in the supply curve—which occurs only with changes in other nonprice factors. A change in price always brings about a change in quantity supplied along a given supply curve. We move to a different coordinate on the existing supply curve. This is specifically called a *change in quantity supplied.* When price changes, quantity supplied changes, and there will be a movement from one point to another along the same supply curve.

When you think of *supply,* think of the entire curve. Quantity supplied is represented by a single point on the supply curve.

> A change or shift in supply causes the entire curve to move. The *only* thing that can cause the entire curve to move is a change in a determinant *other than price.*

Consequently,

> A change in the price leads to a change in the quantity supplied, other things being constant. This is a movement *on* the curve.
>
> A change in any other determinant of supply leads to a change in supply. This causes a movement *of* the curve.

CONCEPTS IN BRIEF

- If the price changes, we *move along* a curve—there is a change in quantity demanded or supplied. If some other determinant changes, we *shift* a curve—there is a change in demand or supply.
- The supply curve is drawn with other things held constant. If other determinants of supply change, the supply curve will shift. The other major determinants are (1) input costs, (2) technology and productivity, (3) taxes and subsidies, (4) expectations of future relative prices, and (5) the number of firms in the industry.

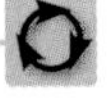

PUTTING DEMAND AND SUPPLY TOGETHER

In the sections on supply and demand, we tried to confine each discussion to supply or demand only. But you have probably already realized that we can't view the world just from the supply side or just from the demand side. There is an interaction between the two. In this section, we will discuss how they interact and how that interaction determines the prices that prevail in our economy. Understanding how demand and supply interact is essential to understanding how prices are determined in our economy and other economies in which the forces of supply and demand are allowed to work.

Let's first combine the demand and supply schedules and then combine the curves.

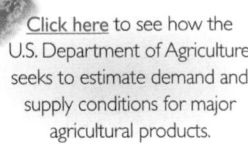

Click here to see how the U.S. Department of Agriculture seeks to estimate demand and supply conditions for major agricultural products.

Demand and Supply Schedules Combined

Let's place panel (a) from Figure 3-3 (the market demand schedule) and panel (a) from Figure 3-8 (the market supply schedule) together in panel (a) of Figure 3-10. Column 1 shows the price; column 2, the quantity supplied per year at any given price; and column 3,

FIGURE 3-10

Putting Demand and Supply Together

In panel (a), we see that at the price of $3, the quantity supplied and the quantity demanded are equal, resulting in neither an excess in the quantity demanded nor an excess in the quantity supplied. We call this price the equilibrium, or market clearing, price. In panel (b), the intersection of the supply and demand curves is at *E,* at a price of $3 and a quantity of 6 million per year. At point *E,* there is neither an excess in the quantity demanded nor an excess in the quantity supplied. At a price of $1, the quantity supplied will be only 2 million per year, but the quantity demanded will be 10 million. The difference is excess quantity demanded at a price of $1. The price will rise, so we will move from point *A* up the supply curve and point *B* up the demand curve to point *E.* At the other extreme, $5 elicits a quantity supplied of 10 million but a quantity demanded of only 2 million. The difference is excess quantity supplied at a price of $5. The price will fall, so we will move down the demand curve and the supply curve to the equilibrium price, $3 per minidisk.

Panel (a)

(1) Price per Constant-Quality Minidisk	(2) Quantity Supplied (minidisks per year)	(3) Quantity Demanded (minidisks per year)	(4) Difference (2) − (3) (minidisks per year)	(5) Condition
$5	10 million	2 million	8 million	Excess quantity supplied (surplus)
4	8 million	4 million	4 million	Excess quantity supplied (surplus)
3	6 million	6 million	0	Market clearing price—equilibrium (no surplus, no shortage)
2	4 million	8 million	–4 million	Excess quantity demanded (shortage)
1	2 million	10 million	–8 million	Excess quantity demanded (shortage)

Panel (b)

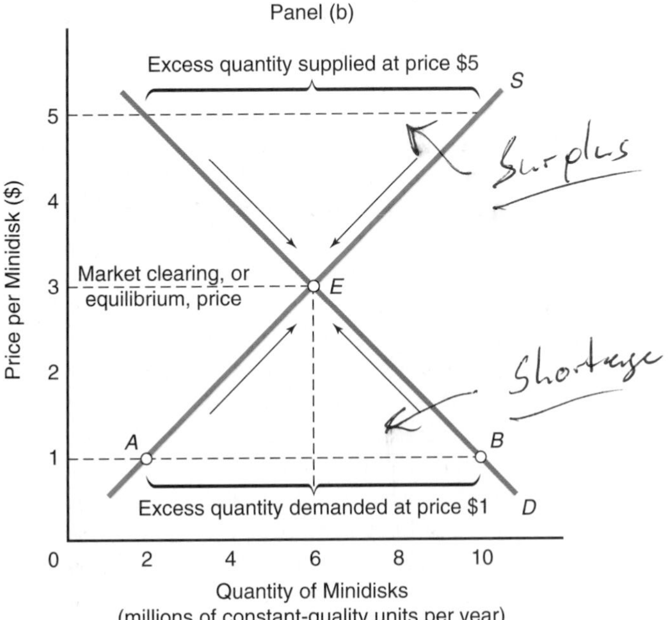

the quantity demanded. Column 4 is merely the difference between columns 2 and 3, or the difference between the quantity supplied and the quantity demanded. In column 5, we label those differences as either excess quantity supplied (called a *surplus,* which we shall discuss shortly) or excess quantity demanded (a commonly known as a *shortage,* discussed shortly). For example, at a price of $1, only 2 million minidisks would be supplied, but the quantity demanded would be 10 million. The difference would be -8 million, which we label excess quantity demanded (a shortage). At the other end of the scale, a price of $5 would elicit 10 million in quantity supplied, but quantity demanded would drop to 2 million, leaving a difference of +8 million units, which we call excess quantity supplied (a surplus).

Market clearing, or equilibrium, price 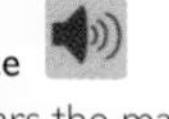
The price that clears the market, at which quantity demanded equals quantity supplied; the price where the demand curve intersects the supply curve.

Now, do you notice something special about the price of $3? At that price, both the quantity supplied and the quantity demanded per year are 6 million. The difference then is zero. There is neither excess quantity demanded (shortage) nor excess quantity supplied (surplus). Hence the price of $3 is very special. It is called the **market clearing price**—it clears the market of all excess supply or excess demand. There are no willing consumers who want to pay $3 per minidisk but are turned away by sellers, and there are no willing suppliers who want to sell minidisks at $3 who cannot sell all they want at that price. Another term for the market clearing price is the **equilibrium price,** the price at which there is no tendency for change. Consumers are able to get all they want at that price, and suppliers are able to sell the amount that they want at that price.

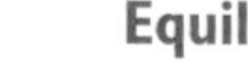

Equilibrium

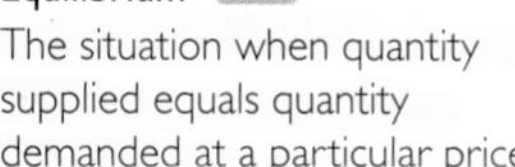

Equilibrium
The situation when quantity supplied equals quantity demanded at a particular price.

We can define **equilibrium** in general as a point at which quantity demanded equals quantity supplied at a particular price. There tends to be no movement away from this point unless demand or supply changes. Any movement away from this point will set into motion certain forces that will cause movement back to it. Therefore, equilibrium is a stable point. Any point that is not at equilibrium is unstable and cannot be maintained.

The equilibrium point occurs where the supply and demand curves intersect. The equilibrium price is given on the vertical axis directly to the left of where the supply and demand curves cross. The equilibrium quantity demanded and supplied is given on the horizontal axis directly underneath the intersection of the demand and supply curves. Equilibrium can change whenever there is a *shock.*

A shock to the supply-and-demand system can be represented by a shift in the supply curve, a shift in the demand curve, or a shift in both curves. Any shock to the system will result in a new set of supply-and-demand relationships and a new equilibrium; forces will come into play to move the system from the old price-quantity equilibrium (now a disequilibrium situation) to the new equilibrium, where the new demand and supply curves intersect.

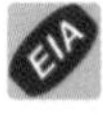

Putting Demand and Supply Together
Study market equilibrium in more detail.

Panel (b) in Figure 3-3 and panel (b) in Figure 3-8 are combined as panel (b) in Figure 3-10. The only difference now is that the horizontal axis measures both the quantity supplied and the quantity demanded per year. Everything else is the same. The demand curve is labeled *D,* the supply curve *S.* We have labeled the intersection of the supply curve with the demand curve as point *E,* for equilibrium. That corresponds to a market clearing price of $3, at which both the quantity supplied and the quantity demanded are 6 million units per year. There is neither excess quantity supplied nor excess quantity demanded. Point *E,* the equilibrium point, always occurs at the intersection of the supply and demand curves. This is the price toward which the market price will automatically tend to gravitate.

EXAMPLE

Why Babysitters Are Earning More

Though good data are hard to come by, parents today agree that the market price of babysitting is way up. Two factors have worked together to bring this about. To see how, take a look at Figure 3-11. There you see the original supply and demand curves for babysitting services in the early 1980s, labeled S_1 and D_1. The market price is P_1, and the equilibrium quantity is Q_1. Now let's think about two events that occurred in the 1990s and early 2000s.

First, there was a population shift. In 1980, there were about 39 million Americans aged 10 to 19, the typical age of babysitters. By the early 2000s, there were about 5 percent fewer people in this age group. Thus the number of suppliers of babysitting services declined at any given price; the market supply schedule shifted leftward, from S_1 to S_2.

At the same time, the number of children younger than 10 rose from 33 million in 1980 to nearly 40 million in the early 2000s. Furthermore, U.S. incomes rose, so more parents desired to eat out and be entertained without their children in tow. These two factors together increased the demand for babysitting services in the 2000s. That is, at any given price, the quantity of babysitting services demanded rose. The demand curve shifted from D_1 to D_2.

As you can see in Figure 3-11, the net effect of these two shifts is an unambiguous rise in the market price of babysitting services, from P_1 to P_2. The equilibrium quantity of babysitting services may increase or decrease. We have illustrated a situation in which it does not change. That is, it is entirely possible that parents in the 2000s are paying a lot more for exactly the same amount of babysitting services that parents purchased at a lower price in the 1980s.

For Critical Analysis

Suppose that in a few years, retiring baby boomers decide to earn extra income by offering to spend some of their time babysitting. What would happen to the equilibrium price of babysitting services? Why?

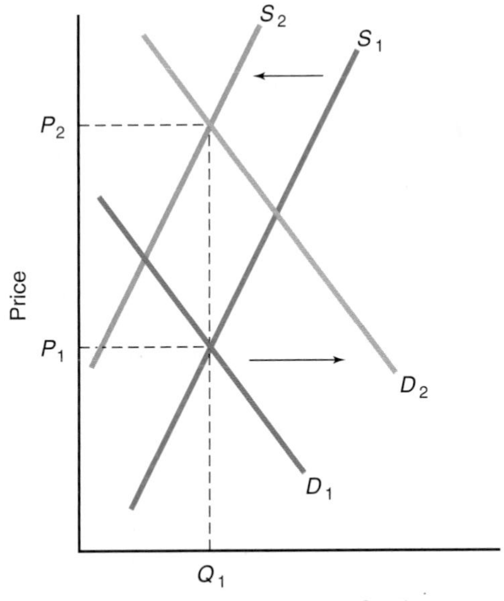

FIGURE 3-11

The Changing Price of Babysitting Services

Simultaneous shifts in the demand curve for babysitting services from D_1 to D_2 and in the supply curve for babysitting services from S_1 to S_2 will cause the equilibrium price of babysitting services to rise from P_1 to P_2. The equilibrium quantity may increase, decrease, or, as illustrated, remain unchanged.

Shortages

The demand and supply curves depicted in Figure 3-10 represent a situation of equilibrium. But a non-market-clearing, or disequilibrium, price will put into play forces that cause the price to change toward the market clearing price at which equilibrium will again be sustained. Look again at panel (b) in Figure 3-10 on page 65. Suppose that instead of being at the market clearing price of $3, for some reason the market price is $1. At this price, the quantity demanded exceeds the quantity supplied, the former being 10 million per year and the latter, 2 million per year. We have a situation of excess quantity demanded at the price of $1. This is usually called a **shortage.** Consumers of minidisks would find that they could not buy all that they wished at $1 apiece. But forces will cause the price to rise: Competing consumers will bid up the price, and suppliers will raise the price and increase output, whether explicitly or implicitly. (Remember, some buyers would pay $5 or more rather than do without minidisks. They do not want to be left out.) We would move from points *A* and *B* toward point *E.* The process would stop when the price again reached $3 per minidisk.

Shortage 
A situation in which quantity demanded is greater than quantity supplied at a price below the market clearing price.

At this point, it is important to recall a distinction made in Chapter 2:

Shortages and scarcity are not the same thing.

A shortage is a situation in which the quantity demanded exceeds the quantity supplied at a price *below* the market clearing price. Our definition of scarcity was much more general and all-encompassing: a situation in which the resources available for producing output are insufficient to satisfy all wants. Any choice necessarily costs an opportunity, and the opportunity is lost. Hence we will always live in a world of scarcity because we must constantly make choices, but we do not necessarily have to live in a world of shortages.

Surpluses

Now let's repeat the experiment with the market price at $5 rather than at the market clearing price of $3. Clearly, the quantity supplied will exceed the quantity demanded at that price. The result will be an excess quantity supplied at $5 per unit. This excess quantity supplied is often called a **surplus.** Given the curves in panel (b) in Figure 3-10, however, there will be forces pushing the price back down toward $3 per minidisk: Competing suppliers will attempt to reduce their inventories by cutting prices and reducing output, and consumers will offer to purchase more at lower prices. Suppliers will want to reduce inventories, which will be above their optimal level; that is, there will be an excess over what each seller believes to be the most profitable stock of minidisks. After all, inventories are costly to hold. But consumers may find out about such excess inventories and see the possibility of obtaining increased quantities of minidisks at a decreased price. It behooves consumers to attempt to obtain a good at a lower price, and they will therefore try to do so. If the two forces of supply and demand are unrestricted, they will bring the price back to $3 per minidisk.

Surplus 
A situation in which quantity supplied is greater than quantity demanded at a price above the market clearing price.

Shortages and surpluses are resolved in unfettered markets—markets in which price changes are free to occur. The forces that resolve them are those of competition: In the case of shortages, consumers competing for a limited quantity supplied drive up the price; in the case of surpluses, sellers compete for the limited quantity demanded, thus driving prices down to equilibrium. The equilibrium price is the only stable price, and all (unrestricted) market prices tend to gravitate toward it.

What happens when the price is set below the equilibrium price? Here come the scalpers.

POLICY EXAMPLE

Should Shortages in the Ticket Market Be Solved by Scalpers?

If you have ever tried to get tickets to a playoff game in sports, a popular Broadway play, or a superstar's rock concert, you know about "shortages." The standard ticket situation for a Super Bowl is shown in Figure 3-12. At the face-value price of Super Bowl tickets (P_1), the quantity demanded (Q_2) greatly exceeds the quantity supplied (Q_1). Because shortages last only so long as prices and quantities do not change, markets tend to exhibit a movement out of this disequilibrium toward equilibrium. Obviously, the quantity of Super Bowl tickets cannot change, but the price can go as high as P_2.

Enter the scalper. This colorful term is used because when you purchase a ticket that is being resold at a price that is higher than face value, the seller is skimming an extra profit off the top. If an event sells out, ticket prices by definition have been lower than market clearing prices. People without tickets may be willing to buy high-priced tickets because they place a greater value on the entertainment event than the face value of the ticket. Without scalpers, those individuals would not be able to attend the event. In the case of the Super Bowl, various forms of scalping occur nationwide. Tickets for a seat on the 50-yard line have been sold for more than $2,000 a piece. In front of every Super Bowl arena, you can find ticket scalpers hawking their wares.

In most states, scalping is illegal. In Pennsylvania, convicted scalpers are either fined $5,000 or sentenced to two years behind bars. For an economist, such legislation seems strange. As one New York ticket broker said, "I look at scalping like working as a stockbroker, buying low and selling high. If people are willing to pay me the money, what kind of problem is that?"

For Critical Analysis

What happens to ticket scalpers who are still holding tickets after an event has started?

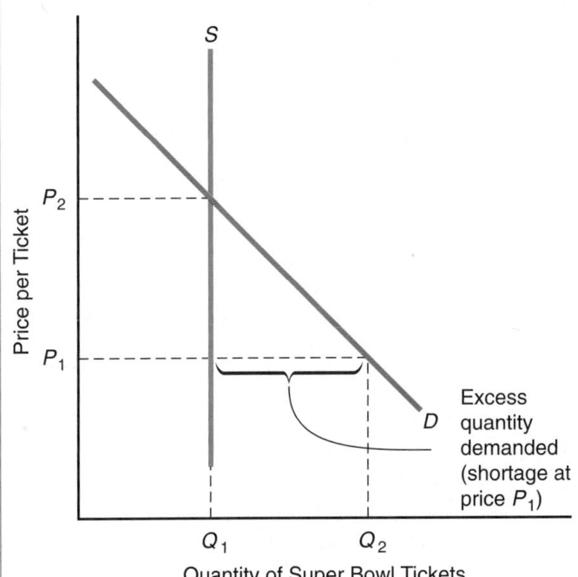

FIGURE 3-12

Shortages of Super Bowl Tickets

The quantity of tickets for any one Super Bowl is fixed at Q_1. At the price per ticket of P_1, the quantity demanded is Q_2, which is greater than Q_1. Consequently, there is an excess quantity demanded at the below-market-clearing price. Prices can go as high as P_2 in the scalpers' market.

CONCEPTS IN BRIEF

- The market clearing price occurs at the intersection of the market demand curve and the market supply curve. It is also called the equilibrium price, the price from which there is no tendency to change unless there is a change in demand or supply.
- Whenever the price is greater than the equilibrium price, there is an excess quantity supplied (a surplus).
- Whenever the price is less than the equilibrium price, there is an excess quantity demanded (a shortage).

NETNOMICS

Stealth Attacks by New Technologies

Successful new products often get off to a slow start. Eventually, however, consumers substitute away from the old products to the point at which demand for the old products effectively disappears. Consider handwritten versus printed manuscripts. For several years in the mid-fifteenth century, printed books were a rarity, and manuscript-copying monks and scribes continued to turn out the bulk of written forms of communication. By the 1470s, however, printed books were more common than handwritten manuscripts. By the end of the fifteenth century, manuscripts had become the rare commodity.

A more recent example involves train engines. Just before 1940, after the diesel-electric engine for train locomotives was invented, an executive of a steam-engine company declared, "They'll never replace the steam locomotive." In fact, it only took 20 years to prove the executive wrong. By 1960, steam engines were regarded as mechanical dinosaurs.

To generate the bulk of its profits, the U.S. Postal Service relies on revenues from first-class mail. To keep its first-class customers satisfied, it recently deployed a $5 billion automation system that reads nine addresses per second and paints envelopes with bar codes to speed sorting. Yet the postal service has lost about $4 billion in first-class mail business since 1994. Around that time, people began to compare the 25-cent cost of a one-minute phone call with the 32-cent cost of first-class postage. Then they began to substitute away from first-class letters to faxes. Other people got access to the Internet and began to send messages by electronic mail, at no additional charge. First-class mail increasingly looks like a steam-engine dinosaur.

Some observers of the software industry think the same sort of thing could happen to a powerhouse of the present: Microsoft Windows. Today the code for this program is on most personal computers on the planet. Competing operating system applications offered by Sun Microsystems's Java software and others currently run more slowly than Windows. But they consume many fewer lines of computer code and hence promise swift accessibility via the Internet. It is conceivable that someday people may log on to the Internet and pay by the minute to use such software to run their computers, thereby freeing up their hard drives for other uses. Thus today's dominant operating system may someday look a lot like a handwritten manuscript does to generations accustomed to reading printed books instead of handwritten manuscripts.

Issues & Applications

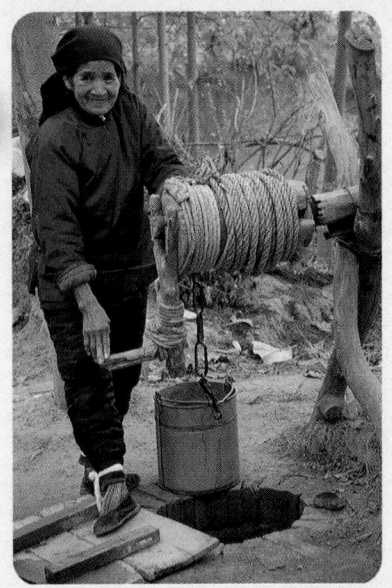

China's Water Shortage: Too Little Rain or Not Enough Pricing?

In China, lack of water has been a big problem. In some towns, people have to wait in long lines at water distribution points set up by local governments. Farmers have lost entire crops. Lacking water to cool machinery, factories have had to cut back on production. Problems are acute in areas where the land is nearly flat, as in large portions of the northern half of China. A recent geophysical analysis indicates that water tables are falling rapidly in these regions. Satellite images show springs, lakes, and rivers drying up.

One Approach: Brute Force

China's government decided in the late 1990s to spare no expense in fighting the water shortage. It began planning vast projects for building tunnels for water to pass through, to expend large amounts of electricity to pump water uphill thousands of feet, to construct huge dams, and to displace hundreds of thousands of people from their homes to make it all possible. Many of these projects are being funded by loans from the World Bank.

The main idea behind these projects, of course, is to move water from the countryside to the cities. But many observers point out that even if all these massive efforts succeed, China's cities will still be living on borrowed time. Among the most water-short is the Chinese capital city of Beijing, which has already exhausted groundwater reserves and now takes irrigation water away from farmers.

The Missing Element: Pricing

To this point, an important element has been missing from the story. Until recently, most water in China could be consumed at no charge. Government pumping stations provided it at a zero price to all takers. In 1998, the government finally enacted a water-pricing policy, but Chinese farmers continue to pay only one-tenth of the opportunity cost of obtaining the water they use to irrigate their crops.

Think about what you have learned in this chapter. Whenever the price of a good, such as water, is below its market clearing price, the quantity demanded exceeds the quantity supplied, and a shortage occurs. To an economist, China's problem is a classic example of a shortage induced by well-intended efforts to set the price of a good below its market price. Naturally, if city-dwellers, farmers, and companies in China can obtain water at very close to a zero price, they will desire to consume water in excess of the amount of water available at that price. That is, the quantity of water demanded will exceed the quantity of water supplied. An economist could have predicted the outcomes before they occurred: overpumped wells, dry fields, and water rationing in cities.

What solution does a typical economist propose? It is for China to let the price system work. Even minor increases in water prices would do wonders to induce people to conserve water. It also would induce Chinese residents to shift water from low-value uses to high-value uses. Pricing water might also eliminate the perceived "need" to think big and build huge dams, tunnels, pumping stations, and the like. By instead thinking smaller and simply permitting the price of water rise toward free-market levels, China could end its water shortage.

Concepts Applied

- Demand
- Supply
- Market Price
- Opportunity Cost
- Shortage

FOR CRITICAL ANALYSIS

1. Even at a posted price of zero, was Chinese water really "free"?
2. A common argument against letting the market determine the prices of "necessity goods" such as water is that having to pay for water is hard on the average citizen. In most countries, who ultimately pays for government-funded dam projects, tunnels through mountains, and machinery to pump water uphill?

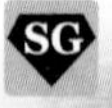
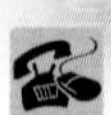

SUMMARY DISCUSSION OF LEARNING OBJECTIVES

1. **The Law of Demand:** According to the law of demand, other things being equal, individuals will purchase fewer units of a commodity at a higher price, and they will purchase more units of the commodity at a lower price.
2. **Relative Prices Versus Money Prices:** When determining the quantity of a commodity to purchase, people respond to changes in its relative price, the price of the commodities in terms of other commodities, rather than a change in the commodity's money price expressed in today's dollars. If the price of a CD rises by 50 percent next year while at the same time all other prices, including your wages, also increase by 50 percent, then the relative price of the CD has not changed. Thus in a world of generally rising prices, you have to compare the price of one good with the general level of prices of other goods in order to decide whether the relative price of that one good has gone up, gone down, or stayed the same.
3. **A Change in Quantity Demanded Versus a Change in Demand:** The demand schedule shows the relationship between various possible prices and respective quantities purchased per unit of time. Graphically, the demand schedule is a downward-sloping demand curve. A change in the price of the good generates a change in the quantity demanded, which is a movement along the demand curve. The determinants of the demand for a good other than the price of the good are (a) income, (b) tastes and preferences, (c) the prices of related goods, (d) expectations, and (e) market size (the number of buyers). Whenever any of these determinants of demand changes, there is a change in the demand for the good, and the demand curve shifts to a new position.
4. **The Law of Supply:** According to the law of supply, sellers will produce and offer for sale more units of a commodity at a higher price, and they will produce and offer for sale fewer units of the commodity at a lower price.
5. **A Change in Quantity Supplied Versus a Change in Supply:** The supply schedule shows the relationship between various possible prices and respective quantities produced and sold per unit of time. On a graph, the supply schedule is a supply curve that slopes upward. A change in the price of the good generates a change in the quantity supplied, which is a movement along the supply curve. The determinants of the supply of a good other than the price of the good are (a) input costs, (b) technology and productivity, (c) taxes and subsidies, (d) price expectations, and (e) the number of sellers. Whenever any of these determinants of supply changes, there is a change in the supply of the good, and the supply curve shifts to a new position
6. **Determining the Market Price and the Equilibrium Quantity:** The market price of a commodity and equilibrium quantity of the commodity that is produced and sold are determined by the intersection of the demand and supply curves. At this intersection point, the quantity demanded by buyers of the commodity just equals the quantity supplied by sellers. At the market price at this point of intersection, the plans of buyers and sellers mesh exactly. Hence there is neither an excess quantity of the commodity supplied (surplus) nor an excess quantity of the commodity demanded (shortage) at this equilibrium point.

Key Terms and Concepts

Complements (57)
Demand (49)
Demand curve (52)
Equilibrium (66)
Inferior goods (56)
Law of demand (49)
Law of supply (59)
Market (49)
Market clearing, or equilibrium, price (66)
Market demand (52)
Money price (50)
Normal goods (56)
Relative price (50)
Shortage (68)
Subsidy (63)
Substitutes (57)
Supply (59)
Supply curve (60)
Surplus (68)

Problems

Answers to the odd-numbered problems appear at the back of the book.

3-1. Suppose that in a recent market period, an industrywide survey determined the following relationship between the price of rock music CDs and the quantity supplied and quantity demanded.

Price	Quantity Demanded	Quantity Supplied
$9	100 million	40 million
$10	90 million	60 million
$11	80 million	80 million
$12	70 million	100 million
$13	60 million	120 million

Illustrate the supply and demand curves for rock CDs given the information in the table. What are the equilibrium price and quantity? If the industry price is $10, is there a shortage or surplus of CDs? How much is the shortage or surplus?

3-2. Suppose that a survey for a later market period indicates that the quantities supplied in the table in Problem 3-1 are unchanged. The quantity demanded, however, has increased by 30 million at each price. Construct the resulting demand curve in the illustration you made for Problem 3-1. Is this an increase or a decrease in demand? What are the new equilibrium quantity and the new market price? Give two examples that might cause such a change.

3-3. In the market for rock music CDs, explain whether the following event would cause an increase or a decrease in demand or an increase or a decrease in the quantity demanded. Also explain what happens to the equilibrium quantity and the market price.

a. The price of CD packaging material declines.
b. The price of CD players declines.
c. The price of cassette tapes increases dramatically.
d. A booming economy increases the income of the typical CD buyer.
e. Many rock fans suddenly develop a fondness for country music.

3-4. Give an example of a complement and a substitute in consumption for each of the following items.

a. Bacon
b. Tennis racquets
c. Coffee
d. Automobiles

3-5. At the end of the 1990s, the United States imposed high taxes on a number of European goods due to a trade dispute. One of these goods was Roquefort cheese. Show how this tax affects the market for Roquefort cheese, shifting the appropriate curve and indicating a new equilibrium quantity and market price.

3-6. Problem 3-5 described a tax imposed on Roquefort cheese. Illustrate the effect of the tax on Roquefort cheese on other types of blue cheese, shifting the appropriate curve and indicating a new equilibrium quantity and market price.

3-7. Consider the market for laptop computers. Explain whether the following events would cause an increase or a decrease in supply or an increase or a decrease in the quantity supplied. Illustrate each, and show what would happen to the equilibrium quantity and the market price.

a. The price of memory chips used in laptop computers declines.
b. The price of memory chips used in desktop personal computers declines.
c. The number of manufactures of laptop computers increases.
d. The price of computer peripherals, printers, fax-modems, and scanners decreases.

3-8. The United States offers significant subsidy payments to U.S. sugar growers. Describe the effects of the introduction of such subsidies on the market for sugar and the market for artificial sweeteners. Explain whether the demand curve or supply curve shifts in each market, and if so, in which direction. Also explain what happens to the equilibrium quantity and the market price in each market.

3-9. The supply curve for season tickets for basketball games for your school's team is vertical because there are a fixed number of seats in the school's gymnasium. Before preseason practice sessions begin, your school's administration commits itself to selling season tickets the day before the first basketball game at a predetermined price that it believes to be equal to the market price. The school will not change that price at any time prior to and including the day tickets go on sale. Illustrate, within a supply and demand framework, the effect of each of the following events on the market for season tickets on the day the school opens ticket sales, and indicate whether a surplus or a shortage would result.

a. The school's star player breaks a leg during preseason practice.

b. During preseason practice, a published newspaper poll of coaches of teams in your school's conference surprises everyone by indicating that your school's team is in the running to win the conference championship.

c. At a preseason practice session that is open to the public, the school president announces that all refreshments served during games will be free of charge throughout the season.

d. Most of your school's basketball fans enjoy an up-tempo, "run and gun" approach to basketball, but after the team's coach quits following the first preseason practice, the school's administration immediately hires a new coach who believes in a deliberate style of play that relies heavily on slow-tempo, four-corners offense.

3-10. Advances in computer technology allow individuals to purchase and download music from the Internet. Buyers may download single songs or complete tracks of songs that are also sold on CDs. Explain the impact of this technological advance on the market for CDs sold in retail stores.

Economics on the Net

Canadian Taxes and Energy Markets The Canadian government follows the example set by the U.S. government and governments of other countries by imposing taxes on some sources of energy and subsidizing other energy sources. This application helps you apply concepts you learned in this chapter to evaluate the effects of taxes and subsidies.

Title: Canada Environment Review

Navigation: Click here to visit the Energy Information Agency hompage.

Application Read the first three sections of this article ("General Background," "Energy and Environmental Policy," and "Energy Taxes and Subsidies"). Then answer the following questions.

1. Draw a diagram of possible demand and supply curves for the market for gasoline. The tax described in the third section of the article is paid by sellers of gasoline. Thus to induce each gasoline seller to supply the same quantity as it would have supplied before the tax, the price that the seller receives must be higher by the amount of the tax. Given this information, illustrate the effect of this tax on the market supply curve. Illustrate and explain how the tax reduces consumption of transportation gas.
2. Draw a diagram of the market for vehicles powered by natural gas. Illustrate the effect of a subsidy on the supply of natural-gas-powered vehicles, and explain how the subsidy encourages the use of these vehicles.

For Group Study and Analysis The final paragraph under "Energy Taxes and Subsidies" describes a study of tax incentives for conservation and renewable energy technologies. Discuss how a tax incentive affects the supply of renewable energy technologies. Discuss how a tax that "encourages" energy conservation might affect a firm engaged in manufacturing. Debate whether one approach is preferred over the other.

CHAPTER

4

EXTENSIONS OF DEMAND AND SUPPLY ANALYSIS

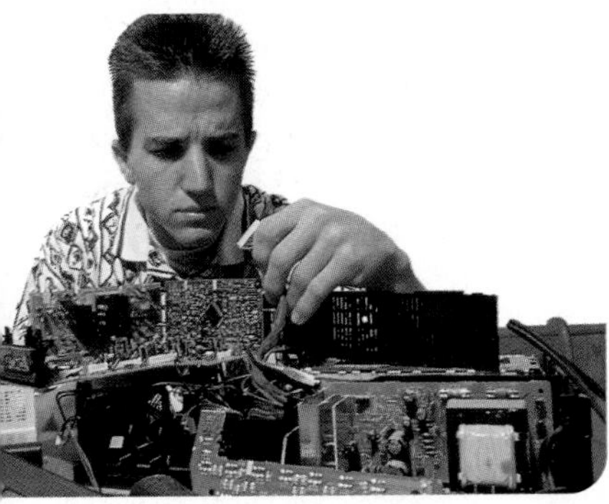

A basic principle in economics is that people respond to incentives. Why might this young person quit school to become a systems programmer?

A few years ago, after a top-flight college athlete turned professional following his sophomore season, a television news commentator called for a law prohibiting college stars from becoming pros "too soon." "He's too young to know what's in his own best interest," the commentator said, without noting that the athlete's salary would dwarf his own.

Other student stars, this time in the academic sphere, have also been responding to market incentives. In the face of soaring entry-level salaries, hordes of computer science students have been dropping their studies in favor of high-paying jobs. College deans and presidents have decried this trend, arguing that ultimately market salaries will fall. The students, they say, are grabbing near-term gains, but lacking degrees, they eventually face the prospect of lower future earnings. Do these academic naysayers have a point? To answer this question, you must learn more about how markets work.

LEARNING OBJECTIVES

After reading this chapter, you should be able to:

1. Discuss the essential features of the price system
2. Evaluate the effects on the market price and equilibrium quantity of changes in demand and supply
3. Understand the rationing function of prices
4. Explain the effects of price ceilings
5. Explain the effects of price floors
6. Describe various types of government-imposed quantity restrictions on markets

Chapter Outline

- The Price System
- Exchange and Markets
- Changes in Demand and Supply
- Price Flexibility and Adjustment Speed
- The Rationing Function of Prices
- The Policy of Government-Imposed Price Controls
- The Policy of Controlling Rents
- Price Floors in Agriculture
- Price Floors in the Labor Market
- Quantity Restrictions

Did You Know That... according to the U.S. Customs Service, the second most serious smuggling problem along the Mexican border, just behind drugs, involves the refrigerant Freon? Selling Freon is more profitable than dealing in cocaine, and illegal Freon smuggling is a bigger business than gunrunning. Freon is used in many air conditioners in cars and homes. Its use is already illegal in the United States, but residents of developing countries may legally use it until the year 2005. When an older U.S. air conditioner needs fixing, it is often cheaper to pay a relatively high price for illegally smuggled Freon than to modify the unit to use a replacement coolant. You can analyze illegal markets, such as the one for Freon, using the supply and demand analysis you learned in Chapter 3. Similarly, you can use this analysis to examine legal markets and the "shortage" of skilled information technology specialists, the "shortage" of apartments in certain cities, and many other phenomena. All of these examples are part of our economy, which we characterize as a *price system.*

THE PRICE SYSTEM

A **price system,** otherwise known as a *market system,* is one in which relative prices are constantly changing to reflect changes in supply and demand for different commodities. The prices of those commodities are the signals to everyone within the system as to what is relatively scarce and what is relatively abundant. Indeed, it is the *signaling* aspect of the price system that provides the information to buyers and sellers about what should be bought and what should be produced. In a price system, there is a clear-cut chain of events in which any changes in demand and supply cause changes in prices that in turn affect the opportunities that businesses and individuals have for profit and personal gain. Such changes influence our use of resources.

Price system 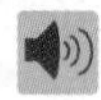
An economic system in which relative prices are constantly changing to reflect changes in supply and demand for different commodities. The prices of those commodities are signals to everyone within the system as to what is relatively scarce and what is relatively abundant.

EXCHANGE AND MARKETS

The price system features **voluntary exchange,** acts of trading between individuals that make both parties to the trade subjectively better off. The **terms of exchange**—the prices we pay for the desired items—are determined by the interaction of the forces underlying supply and demand. In our economy, the majority of exchanges take place voluntarily in markets. A market encompasses the exchange arrangements of both buyers and sellers that underlie the forces of supply and demand. Indeed, one definition of a market is a low-cost institution for facilitating exchange. A market increases incomes by helping resources move to their highest-valued uses by means of prices. Prices are the providers of information.

Voluntary exchange 
An act of trading, done on a voluntary basis, in which both parties to the trade are subjectively better off after the exchange.

Terms of exchange 
The terms under which trading takes place. Usually the terms of exchange are equal to the price at which a good is traded.

Transaction Costs

Individuals turn to markets because markets reduce the cost of exchanges. These costs are sometimes referred to as **transaction costs,** which are broadly defined as the costs associated with finding out exactly what is being transacted as well as the cost of enforcing contracts. If you were Robinson Crusoe and lived alone on an island, you would never incur a transaction cost. For everyone else, transaction costs are just as real as the costs of production. High-speed large-scale computers have allowed us to reduce transaction costs by increasing our ability to process information and keep records.

Consider some simple examples of transaction costs. The supermarket reduces transaction costs relative to your having to go to numerous specialty stores to obtain the items you desire. Organized stock exchanges, such as the New York Stock Exchange, have reduced transaction costs of buying and selling stocks and bonds. In general, the more organized the market, the lower the transaction costs. One group of individuals who constantly attempt to lower transaction costs are the much maligned middlemen.

Transaction costs 
All of the costs associated with exchanging, including the informational costs of finding out price and quality, service record, and durability of a product, plus the cost of contracting and enforcing that contract.

The Role of Middlemen

As long as there are costs to bringing together buyers and sellers, there will be an incentive for intermediaries, normally called middlemen, to lower those costs. This means that middlemen specialize in lowering transaction costs. Whenever producers do not sell their products directly to the final consumer, there are, by definition, one or more middlemen involved. Farmers typically sell their output to distributors, who are usually called wholesalers, who then sell those products to supermarkets.

Recently, technology has changed the way middlemen work.

EXAMPLE

Middlemen Flourish on the Internet

At one time, people speculated that the Internet would be bad news for middlemen. People would just click their mouse to head to a Web site where they could deal directly with a company. In fact, every day there are new companies establishing middleman sites all over the Web. For instance, one Web site, Kelley Blue Book (www.kbb.com), allows you to get exact dealer invoice prices and destination charges for automobiles so that you can learn what wholesale prices car dealers pay for the cars. You can even find out the prices of optional equipment.

To help consumers locate harder-to-find items, software companies have developed *intelligent shopping agents,* sometimes called "shopbots," which are programs that search the Web to find specific items. Even though human beings are not the middlemen in this instance, the software companies provide middleman services by offering to sell or lease these programs.

For Critical Analysis

Any of us connected to the Internet can find the same information that an Internet middleman (or shopbot, for that matter) can find. Why, then, would someone pay for the services of an Internet middleman?

CHANGES IN DEMAND AND SUPPLY

It is in markets that we see the results of changes in demand and supply. In certain situations, it is possible to predict what will happen to equilibrium price and equilibrium quantity when a change occurs in demand or supply. Specifically, whenever one curve is stable while the other curve shifts, we can tell what will happen to price and quantity. Consider the four possibilities in Figure 4-1 (p. 78). In panel (a), the supply curve remains stable but demand increases from D_1 to D_2. Note that the result is both an increase in the market clearing price from P_1 to P_2 and an increase in the equilibrium quantity from Q_1 to Q_2.

In panel (b), there is a decrease in demand from D_1 to D_3. This results in a decrease in both the relative price of the good and the equilibrium quantity. Panels (c) and (d) show the effects of a shift in the supply curve while the demand curve is stable. In panel (c), the supply

FIGURE 4-1

Shifts in Demand and in Supply: Determinate Results

In panel (a), the supply curve is stable at S. The demand curve shifts outward from D_1 to D_2. The equilibrium price and quantity rise from P_1, Q_1 to P_2, Q_2, respectively. In panel (b), again the supply curve remains stable at S. The demand curve, however, shifts inward to the left, showing a decrease in demand from D_1 to D_3. Both equilibrium price and equilibrium quantity fall. In panel (c), the demand curve now remains stable at D. The supply curve shifts from S_1 to S_2. The equilibrium price falls from P_1 to P_2. The equilibrium quantity increases, however, from Q_1 to Q_2. In panel (d), the demand curve is stable at D. Supply decreases as shown by a leftward shift of the supply curve from S_1 to S_3. The market clearing price increases from P_1 to P_3. The equilibrium quantity falls from Q_1 to Q_3.

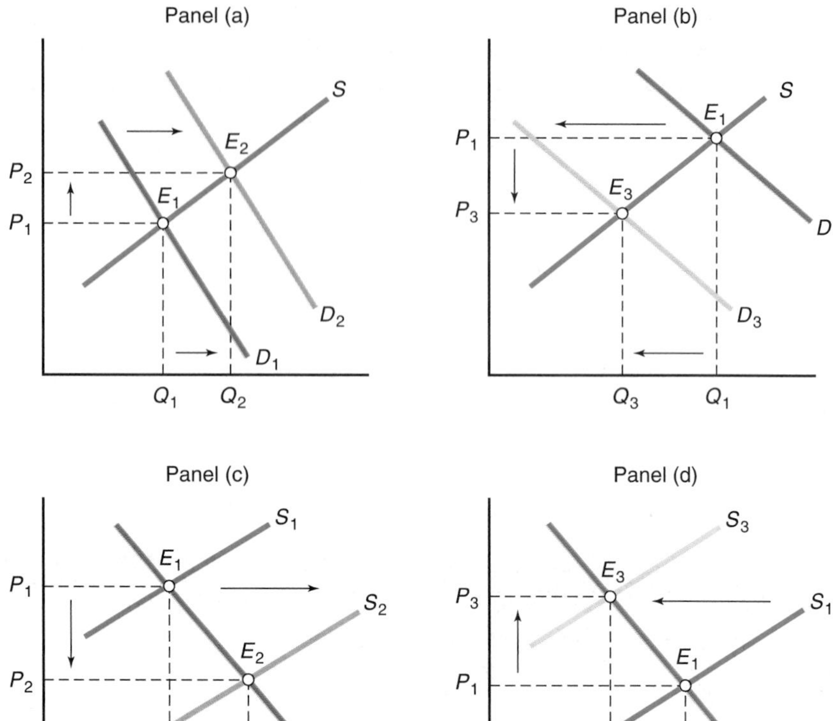

curve has shifted rightward. The relative price of the product falls; the equilibrium quantity increases. In panel (d), supply has shifted leftward—there has been a supply decrease. The product's relative price increases; the equilibrium quantity decreases.

EXAMPLE

The Upside of the Yo-Yo Cycle

Toymaking is a big business. It is also a volatile business. Consider the simple yo-yo. For years, kids couldn't get enough yo-yos, and the industry boomed. Then it fell on hard times—how could pieces of wood or plastic attached to a string compete with action figures and video games? But after years of dormant sales, yo-yos suddenly are hot again in places such as Australia, Japan, and the United Kingdom. Companies that manufacture yo-yos have found that they cannot keep up with this increasing worldwide demand at prevailing prices. Toy retailers can't keep yo-yos in stock. One San Francisco store maintains a yo-yo waiting list that runs to 200 names.

We can turn to demand and supply to see why this situation has arisen in the market for yo-yos. As you can see in Figure 4-2, when the demand schedule for yo-yos shifts rightward, the quantity of yo-yos demanded exceeds the quantity supplied, so at the initial market price, a shortage of yo-yos results. Adjustment to market equilibrium will entail a rise in the market price of yo-yos, which will raise the quantity of yo-yos supplied toward equality with the quantity demanded. Consistent

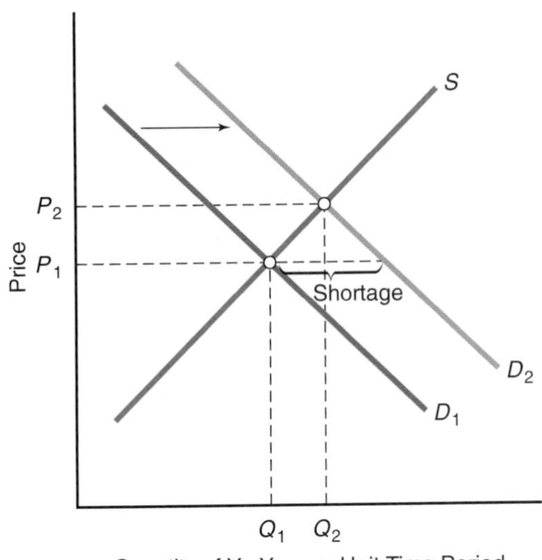

FIGURE 4-2

Responses to a Shift in Yo-Yo Demand

When demand shifts to D_2 but supply stays the same, there will be shortages at the prevailing price P. Eventually, price will rise to P_2 and equilibrium will occur at Q_2.

with this prediction, some yo-yo manufacturers report that their existing plants now run 24 hours a day, seven days a week. Many producers are opening new production lines. In the meantime, yo-yo prices have risen considerably at toy stores around the globe.

For Critical Analysis

The current yo-yo craze is unlikely to last. When it ends, what kinds of adjustments are likely to occur in the market for yo-yos?

When Both Demand and Supply Shift

The examples given in Figure 4-1 each showed a theoretically determinate outcome of a shift in either the demand curve holding the supply curve constant or the supply curve holding the demand curve constant. When both supply and demand curves change, the outcome is indeterminate for either equilibrium price or equilibrium quantity.

When both demand and supply increase, all we can be certain of is that equilibrium quantity will increase. We do not know what will happen to equilibrium price until we determine whether demand increased relative to supply (equilibrium price will rise) or supply increased relative to demand (equilibrium price will fall). The same analysis applies to decreases in both demand and supply, except that in this case equilibrium quantity falls.

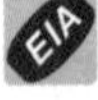

Predicting Changes in Price and Quantities

Improve your ability to reason through the effects of shifts in demand and supply.

We can be certain that when demand decreases and supply increases, the equilibrium price will fall, but we do not know what will happen to the equilibrium quantity unless we actually draw the new curves. If supply decreases and demand increases, we can be sure that equilibrium price will rise, but again we do not know what happens to equilibrium quantity without drawing the curves. In every situation in which both supply and demand change, you should always draw graphs to determine the resulting change in equilibrium price and quantity.

PRICE FLEXIBILITY AND ADJUSTMENT SPEED

We have used as an illustration for our analysis a market in which prices are quite flexible. Some markets are indeed like that. In others, however, price flexibility may take the form of indirect adjustments such as hidden payments or quality changes. For example, although the published price of bouquets of flowers may stay the same, the freshness of the flowers may change, meaning that the price per constant-quality unit changes. The published price of French bread might stay the same, but the quality could go up or down, thereby changing the price per constant-quality unit. There are many ways to change prices without actually changing the published price for a *nominal* unit of a product or service.

We must also consider the fact that markets do not return to equilibrium immediately. There must be an adjustment time. A shock to the economy in the form of an oil embargo, a drought, or a long strike will not be absorbed overnight. This means that even in unfettered market situations, in which there are no restrictions on changes in prices and quantities, temporary excess quantities supplied and excess quantities demanded may appear. Our analysis simply indicates what the market clearing price ultimately will be, given a demand curve and a supply curve. Nowhere in the analysis is there any indication of the speed with which a market will get to a new equilibrium if there has been a shock. The price may overshoot the equilibrium level. Remember this warning when we examine changes in demand and in supply due to changes in their nonprice determinants.

CONCEPTS IN BRIEF

- The terms of exchange in a voluntary exchange are determined by the interaction of the forces underlying demand and supply. These forces take place in markets, which tend to minimize transaction costs.
- When the demand curve shifts outward or inward with a stable supply curve, equilibrium price and quantity increase or decrease, respectively. When the supply curve shifts outward or inward given a stable demand curve, equilibrium price moves in the direction opposite of equilibrium quantity.
- When there is a shift in demand or supply, the new equilibrium price is not obtained instantaneously. Adjustment takes time.

THE RATIONING FUNCTION OF PRICES 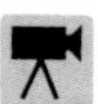

A shortage creates a situation that forces price to rise toward a market clearing, or equilibrium, level. A surplus brings into play forces that cause price to fall toward its market clearing level. The synchronization of decisions by buyers and sellers that creates a situation of equilibrium is called the *rationing function of prices.* Prices are indicators of relative scarcity. An equilibrium price clears the market. The plans of buyers and sellers, given the price, are not frustrated.* It is the free interaction of buyers and sellers that sets the price that eventually clears the market. Price, in effect, rations a commodity to demanders who are willing and able to pay the highest price. Whenever the rationing function of prices is frustrated by government-enforced price ceilings that set prices below the market clearing level, a prolonged shortage situation is not allowed to be corrected by the upward adjustment of the price.

---

*There is a difference between frustration and unhappiness. You may be unhappy because you can't buy a Rolls Royce, but if you had sufficient income, you would not be frustrated in your attempt to purchase one at the current market price. By contrast, you would be frustrated if you went to your local supermarket and could get only two cans of your favorite soft drink when you had wanted to purchase a dozen and had the necessary funds.

There are other ways to ration goods. *First come, first served* is one method. *Political power* is another. *Physical force* is yet another. Cultural, religious, and physical differences have been and are used as rationing devices throughout the world.

Consider first come, first served as a rationing device. In countries that do not allow prices to reflect true relative scarcity, first come, first served has become a way of life. We call this *rationing by queues,* where *queue* means "line," as in Britain. Whoever is willing to wait in line the longest obtains meat that is being sold at less than the market clearing price. All who wait in line are paying a higher *total* price than the money price paid for the meat. Personal time has an opportunity cost. To calculate the total price of the meat, we must add up the money price plus the opportunity cost of the time spent waiting.

Lotteries are another way to ration goods. You may have been involved in a rationing-by-lottery scheme during your first year in college when you were assigned a university-provided housing unit. Sometimes for popular classes, rationing by lottery is used to fill the available number of slots.

Rationing by *coupons* has also been used, particularly during wartime. In the United States during World War II, families were allotted coupons that allowed them to purchase specified quantities of rationed goods, such as meat and gasoline. To purchase such goods, you had to pay a specified price *and* give up a coupon.

Rationing by waiting may occur in situations in which entrepreneurs are free to change prices to equate quantity demanded with quantity supplied but choose not to do so. This results in queues of potential buyers. The most obvious conclusion seems to be that the price in the market is being held below equilibrium by some noncompetitive force. That is not true, however.

The reason is that queuing may also arise when the demand characteristics of a market are subject to large or unpredictable fluctuations, and the additional costs to firms (and ultimately to consumers) of constantly changing prices or of holding sufficient inventories or providing sufficient excess capacity to cover these peak demands are greater than the costs to consumers of waiting for the good. This is the usual case of waiting in line to purchase a fast-food lunch or to purchase a movie ticket a few minutes before the next show.

The Essential Role of Rationing

In a world of scarcity, there is, by definition, competition for what is scarce. After all, any resources that are not scarce can be had by everyone at a zero price in as large a quantity as everyone wants, such as air to burn in internal combustion engines. Once scarcity arises, there has to be some method to ration the available resources, goods, and services. The price system is one form of rationing; the others that we mentioned are alternatives. Economists cannot say which system of rationing is best. They can, however, say that rationing via the price system leads to the most efficient use of available resources. This means that generally in a price system, further trades could not occur without making somebody worse off. In other words, in a freely functioning price system, all of the gains from mutually beneficial trade will be exhausted.

CONCEPTS IN BRIEF

- Prices in a market economy perform a rationing function because they reflect relative scarcity, allowing the market to clear. Other ways to ration goods include first come, first served; political power; physical force; lotteries; and coupons.
- Even when businesspeople can change prices, some rationing by waiting will occur. Such queuing arises when there are large unexpected changes in demand coupled with high costs of satisfying those changes immediately.

THE POLICY OF GOVERNMENT-IMPOSED PRICE CONTROLS

Price controls 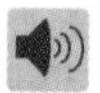
Government-mandated minimum or maximum prices that may be charged for goods and services.

The rationing function of prices is often not allowed to operate when governments impose price controls. **Price controls** typically involve setting a **price ceiling**—the maximum price that may be allowed in an exchange. The world has had a long history of price ceilings applied to some goods, wages, rents, and interest rates, among other things. Occasionally a government will set a **price floor**—a minimum price below which a good or service may not be sold. These have most often been applied to wages and agricultural products. Let's consider price controls in terms of price ceilings.

Price ceiling 
A legal maximum price that may be charged for a particular good or service.

Price Ceilings and Black Markets

Price floor 
A legal minimum price below which a good or service may not be sold. Legal minimum wages are an example.

As long as a price ceiling is below the market clearing price, imposing a price ceiling creates a shortage, as can be seen in Figure 4-3. At any price below the market clearing, or equilibrium, price of P_e, there will always be a larger quantity demanded than quantity supplied—a shortage, as you will recall from Chapter 3. Normally, whenever a shortage exists, there is a tendency for price and output to rise to equilibrium levels. This is exactly what we pointed out when discussing shortages in the labor market. But with a price ceiling, this tendency cannot be fully realized because everyone is forbidden to trade at the equilibrium price.

Nonprice rationing devices 
All methods used to ration scarce goods that are price-controlled. Whenever the price system is not allowed to work, nonprice rationing devices will evolve to ration the affected goods and services.

The result is fewer exchanges and **nonprice rationing devices.** In Figure 4-3, at an equilibrium price of P_e, the equilibrium quantity demanded and supplied (or traded) is Q_e. But at the price ceiling of P_1, the equilibrium quantity offered is only Q_s. What happens if there is a shortage? The most obvious nonprice rationing device to help clear the market is queuing, or long lines, which we have already discussed.

Black market 
A market in which goods are traded at prices above their legal maximum prices or in which illegal goods are sold.

Typically, an effective price ceiling leads to a **black market.** A black market is a market in which the price-controlled good is sold at an illegally high price through various methods. For example, if the price of gasoline is controlled at lower than the market clearing price, a gas station attendant may take a cash payment on the side in order to fill up a driver's car (as happened in the 1970s in the United States during price controls on gasoline). If the price of beef is controlled at below its market clearing price, the butcher may give special service to a customer who offers the butcher great seats at an upcoming foot-

FIGURE 4-3 

Black Markets

The demand curve is D. The supply curve is S. The equilibrium price is P_e. The government, however, steps in and imposes a maximum price of P_1. At that lower price, the quantity demanded will be Q_d, but the quantity supplied will only be Q_s. There is a "shortage." The implicit price (including time costs) tends to rise to P_2. If black markets arise, as they generally will, the equilibrium black market price will end up somewhere between P_1 and P_2.

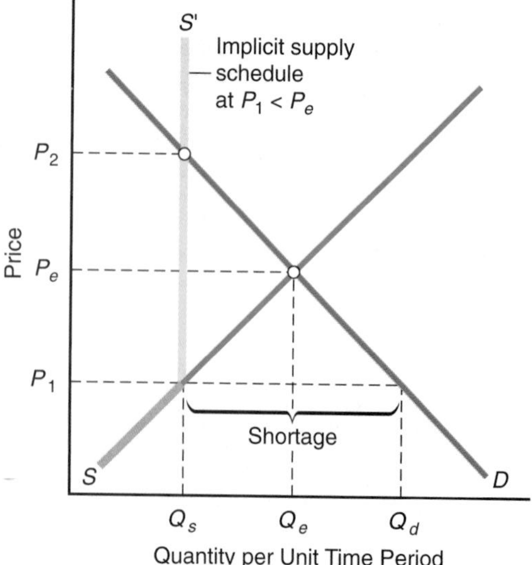

ball game. Indeed, the number of ways in which the true implicit price of a price-controlled good or service can be increased is infinite, limited only by the imagination. (Black markets also occur when goods are made illegal—their legal price is set at zero.)

Whenever a nation attempts to freeze all prices, a variety of problems arise. Many of them occurred a few years ago in one African country, Sierra Leone.

INTERNATIONAL EXAMPLE

Price Controls in Sierra Leone

Lisa Walker spent a year as a Peace Corps volunteer in Sierra Leone, West Africa, and she kept a diary of her experiences. One thing she wrote about was what happened when the government imposed price controls on many common items: "For the last five days," she wrote, "nobody has sold cigarettes, kerosene, Maggi [bouillon] cubes, or rice here . . . . This is the result of the government's new order. The government says that Maggi cubes have to be sold for 30 cents, but sellers bought them for 50 cents, so when military men enter the village to enforce the government price, those with Maggis hide them. Same story for cigarettes and kerosene. The rice supplies are now hidden because of government prices. Unless one is willing to pay an outrageous price, it is impossible to buy rice in the marketplace. The only way to get rice legally is to buy it from the government. This means standing in long lines for many hours to get a rationed amount. I don't know how Sierra Leoneans are managing or how long this artificial rice shortage will last."

For Critical Analysis

How would you graphically illustrate the market for rice in Sierra Leone in the presence of price controls?

CONCEPTS IN BRIEF

- Government policy can impose price controls in the form of price ceilings and price floors.
- An effective price ceiling is one that sets the legal price below the market clearing price and is enforced. Effective price ceilings lead to nonprice rationing devices and black markets.

THE POLICY OF CONTROLLING RENTS

Over 200 American cities and towns, including Berkeley and New York City, operate under some kind of rent control. **Rent control** is a system under which the local government tells building owners how much they can charge their tenants in rent. In the United States, rent controls date back to at least World War II. The objective of rent control is to keep rents below levels that would be observed in a freely competitive market.

Rent control The placement of price ceilings on rents in particular cities.

The Functions of Rental Prices

In any housing market, rental prices serve three functions: (1) to promote the efficient maintenance of existing housing and stimulate the construction of new housing, (2) to allocate existing scarce housing among competing claimants, and (3) to ration the use of existing housing by current demanders.

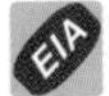

Competitive Housing Market Get practice examining the effects of rent controls.

Rent Controls and Construction. Rent controls have discouraged the construction of new rental units. Rents are the most important long-term determinant of profitability, and rent controls have artificially depressed them. Consider some examples. In a recent year in

Dallas, Texas, with a 16 percent rental vacancy rate but no rent control laws, 11,000 new rental housing units were built. In the same year in San Francisco, California, only 2,000 units were built. The major difference? San Francisco has only a 1.6 percent vacancy rate but stringent rent control laws. In New York City, until a change in the law in 1997, the only rental units being built were luxury units, which were exempt from controls.

Effects on the Existing Supply of Housing. When rental rates are held below equilibrium levels, property owners cannot recover the cost of maintenance, repairs, and capital improvements through higher rents. Hence they curtail these activities. In the extreme situation, taxes, utilities, and the expenses of basic repairs exceed rental receipts. The result is abandoned buildings. Numerous buildings have been abandoned in New York City. Some owners have resorted to arson, hoping to collect the insurance on their empty buildings before the city claims them for back taxes.

Rationing the Current Use of Housing. Rent controls also affect the current use of housing because they restrict tenant mobility. Consider the family whose children have gone off to college. That family might want to live in a smaller apartment. But in a rent-controlled environment, there can be a substantial cost to giving up a rent-controlled unit. In most rent-controlled cities, rents can be adjusted only when a tenant leaves. That means that a move from a long-occupied rent-controlled apartment to a smaller apartment can involve a hefty rent hike. This artificial preservation of the status quo became known in New York as "housing gridlock."

Attempts at Evading Rent Controls

The distortions produced by rent controls lead to efforts by both property owners and tenants to evade the rules. This leads to the growth of expensive government bureaucracies whose job it is to make sure that rent controls aren't evaded. In New York City, property owners have had an incentive to make life unpleasant for tenants to drive them out or to evict them on the slightest pretense as the only way to raise the rent. The city has responded by making evictions extremely costly for property owners. Eviction requires a tedious and expensive judicial proceeding. Tenants, for their part, routinely try to sublet all or part of their rent-controlled apartments at fees substantially above the rent they pay to the owner. Both the city and the property owners try to prohibit subletting and typically end up in the city's housing courts—an entire judicial system developed to deal with disputes involving rent-controlled apartments. The overflow and appeals from the city's housing courts is now clogging the rest of New York's judicial system.

Who Gains and Who Loses from Rent Controls?

The big losers from rent controls are clearly property owners. But there is another group of losers—low-income individuals, especially single mothers, trying to find their first apartment. Some observers now believe that rent controls have worsened the problem of homelessness in such cities as New York.

Typically, owners of rent-controlled apartments often charge "key money" before a new tenant is allowed to move in. This is a large up-front cash payment, usually illegal but demanded nonetheless—just one aspect of the black market in rent-controlled apartments. Poor individuals cannot afford a hefty key money payment, nor can they assure the owner that their rent will be on time or even paid each month. Because controlled rents are usually below market clearing levels, there is little incentive for apartment owners to take any risk on low-income-earning individuals as tenants. This is particularly true when a prospective tenant's chief source of income is a welfare check. Indeed, a large number of the litigants in the New York housing courts are welfare mothers who have missed their rent payments due to emergency expenses or delayed welfare checks. Often their appeals end in evictions and a new home in a temporary public shelter—or on the streets.

Who benefits from rent control? Ample evidence indicates that upper-income professionals benefit the most. These are the people who can use their mastery of the bureaucracy and their large network of friends and connections to exploit the rent control system. Consider that in New York, actresses Mia Farrow and Cicely Tyson live in rent-controlled apartments, paying well below market rates. So do State Senate Democratic leader Manfred Ohrenstein, the director of the Metropolitan Museum of Art, the chairman of Pathmark Stores, and writer Alistair Cooke.

INTERNATIONAL EXAMPLE

The End of Rent Controls in Egypt

Since Gamal Abdel Nasser's efforts to recast Egypt along socialist lines in the 1950s, farmland in this nation was subject to strict rent controls. Consequently, for more than 40 years, rents paid by tenant farmers—roughly 10 percent of the Egyptian populace—were frozen. Due to the considerable inflation that took place in Egypt during this period, the relative rental price of land was rapidly approaching zero. Tenants effectively took over lands they did not own, practically free of charge. A consequence was that the value of the land was very low to its owners, and this discouraged the adoption of modern cultivation techniques. Many tenant farmers in Egypt continued to plant only subsistence crops using their hands, hoes, and water buffaloes.

In 1992, Egypt adopted a law that reversed its rent controls. It phased in the law very gradually, however. Only recently has it permitted landowners to charge their tenants market prices. In some cases, landowners have evicted tenants to make way for more modern, less labor-intensive farming techniques. This has made the subject of rent control one of the most potent political issues in this Middle Eastern nation.

For Critical Analysis

What market-based policies might the Egyptian government adopt to reduce the impact of the removal of rent controls on tenant farmers?

CONCEPTS IN BRIEF

- Rental prices perform three functions: (1) allocating existing scarce housing among competing claimants, (2) promoting efficient maintenance of existing houses and stimulating new housing construction, and (3) rationing the use of existing houses by current demanders.
- Effective rent controls reduce or alter the three functions of rental prices. Construction of new rental units is discouraged. Rent controls decrease spending on maintenance of existing ones and also lead to "housing gridlock."
- There are numerous ways to evade rent controls; key money is one.

PRICE FLOORS IN AGRICULTURE

Another way that government can affect markets is by imposing price floors or price supports. In the United States, price supports are most often associated with agricultural products.

Price Supports

During the Great Depression, the federal government swung into action to help farmers. In 1933, it established a system of price supports for many agricultural products. Until recently, there were price supports for wheat, feed grains, cotton, rice, soybeans, sorghum, and

FIGURE 4-4
Agricultural Price Supports
Free market equilibrium occurs at *E*, with an equilibrium price of P_e and an equilibrium quantity of Q_e. When the government set a support price at P_s, the quantity demanded was Q_d, and the quantity supplied was Q_s. The difference was the surplus, which the government bought. Note that farmers' total income was from consumers $(P_s \times Q_d)$ plus taxpayers $[(Q_s - Q_d) \times P_s]$.

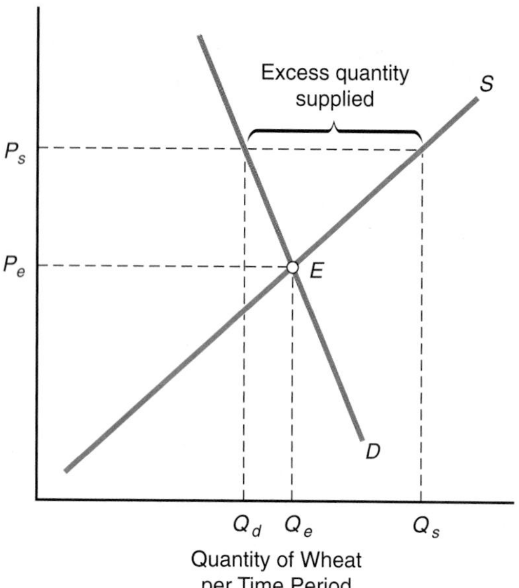

dairy products. The nature of the supports was quite simple: The government simply chose a *support price* for an agricultural product and then acted to ensure that the price of the product never fell below the support level. Figure 4-4 shows the market demand and supply of wheat. Without a price support program, competitive forces would yield an equilibrium price of P_e and an equilibrium quantity of Q_e. Clearly, if the government were to set the support price at P_e or below, the quantity of wheat demanded would equal the quantity of wheat supplied at point *E* because farmers can sell all they want at the market clearing price of P_e, above the price floor.

Until 1996, however, the government set the support price *above* P_e, at P_s. At a support price of P_s, the quantity demanded is only Q_d, but the quantity supplied is Q_s. The difference between them is called the *excess quantity supplied,* or *surplus.* As simple as this program seems, two questions arise: How did the government decide on the level of the support price P_s? And how did it prevent market forces from pushing the actual price down to P_e?

If production exceeded the amount consumers wanted to buy at the support price, what happened to the surplus? Quite simply, the government had to buy the surplus—the difference between Q_s and Q_d—if the price support program was to work. As a practical matter, the government acquired the quantity $Q_s - Q_d$ indirectly through a government agency. The government either stored the surplus or sold it to foreign countries at a greatly reduced price (or gave it away free of charge) under the Food for Peace program.

Who Benefited from Agricultural Price Supports?

Traditionally advocated as a way to guarantee a decent wage for low-income farmers, most of the benefits of agricultural price supports were skewed toward owners of very large farms. Price supports were made on a per-bushel basis, not on a per-farm basis. Thus traditionally, the larger the farm, the bigger the benefit from agricultural price supports. In addition, *all* of the benefits from price supports ultimately accrued to *landowners* on whose land price-supported crops could grow. Except for peanuts, tobacco, and sugar, the price support program was eliminated in 1996.

PRICE FLOORS IN THE LABOR MARKET  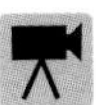

Minimum wage 
A wage floor, legislated by government, setting the lowest hourly rate that firms may legally pay workers.

The **minimum wage** is the lowest hourly wage rate that firms may legally pay their workers. Proponents want higher minimum wages to ensure low-income workers a "decent" standard of living. Opponents claim that higher minimum wages cause increased unemployment, particularly among unskilled minority teenagers.

The federal minimum wage started in 1938 at 25 cents an hour, about 40 percent of the average manufacturing wage at the time. Typically, its level has stayed at about 40 to 50 percent of average manufacturing wages. It was increased to $5.15 in 1995 and may be higher by the time you read this. Many states and cities have their own minimum wage laws that sometimes exceed the federal minimum.

What happens when the government passes a floor on wages? The effects can be seen in Figure 4-5. We start off in equilibrium with the equilibrium wage rate of W_e and the equilibrium quantity of labor demanded and supplied equal to Q_e. A minimum wage, W_m, higher than W_e, is imposed. At W_m, the quantity demanded for labor is reduced to Q_d, and some workers now become unemployed. Note that the reduction in employment from Q_e to Q_d, or the distance from *B* to *A*, is less than the excess quantity of labor supplied at wage rate W_m. This excess quantity supplied is the distance between *A* and *C*, or the distance between Q_d and Q_s. The reason the reduction in employment is smaller than the excess supply of labor at the minimum wage is that the latter also includes a second component that consists of the additional workers who would like to work more hours at the new, higher minimum wage. Some workers may become

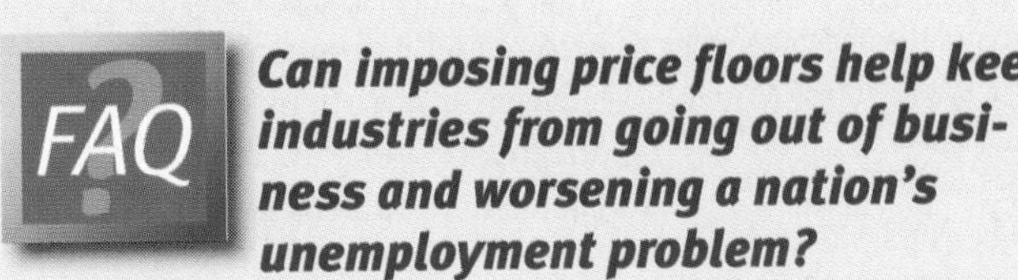

FAQ
Can imposing price floors help keep industries from going out of business and worsening a nation's unemployment problem?

Yes, certain price floor arrangements can induce companies to keep producing unsold output, at least for a while. The social cost of such a policy can be very high, however. China's government, for instance, recently became concerned when a number of industries were unable to sell all their output at government-mandated price floors. The industries were threatening to downsize and lay off millions of Chinese workers. The government began purchasing unsold goods and storing them in warehouses. Of course, China's taxpayers must foot the bill for all this overproduction.

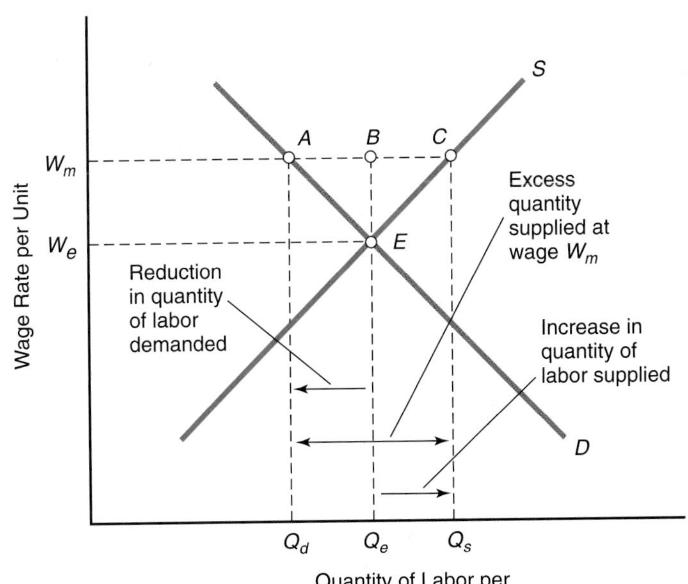

FIGURE 4-5

The Effect of Minimum Wages

The market clearing wage rate is W_e. The market clearing quantity of employment is Q_e, determined by the intersection of supply and demand at point *E*. A minimum wage equal to W_m is established. The quantity of labor demanded is reduced to Q_d; the reduction in employment from Q_e to Q_d is equal to the distance between *B* and *A*. That distance is smaller than the excess quantity of labor supplied at wage rate W_m. The distance between *B* and *C* is the increase in the quantity of labor supplied that results from the higher minimum wage rate.

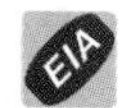
Click here to keep up to date on recent federal and state developments concerning minimum wages.

unemployed as a result of the minimum wage, but others will move to sectors where minimum wage laws do not apply; wages will be pushed down in these uncovered sectors.

In the long run (a time period that is long enough to allow for adjustment by workers and firms), some of the reduction in labor demanded will result from a reduction in the number of firms, and some will result from changes in the number of workers employed by each firm. Economists estimate that a 10 percent increase in the real minimum wage decreases total employment of those affected by 1 to 2 percent.*

QUANTITY RESTRICTIONS

EIA

A Market for Low-Skilled Labor
Gain further understanding of the effects of the minimum wage.

Governments can impose quantity restrictions on a market. The most obvious restriction is an outright ban on the ownership or trading of a good. It is presently illegal to buy and sell human organs. It is also currently illegal to buy and sell certain psychoactive drugs such as cocaine, heroin, and marijuana. In some states, it is illegal to start a new hospital without obtaining a license for a particular number of beds to be offered to patients. This licensing requirement effectively limits the quantity of hospital beds in some states. From 1933 to 1973, it was illegal for U.S. citizens to own gold except for manufacturing, medicinal, or jewelry purposes.

POLICY EXAMPLE

Should the Legal Quantity of Cigarettes Supplied Be Set at Zero?

Nicotine has been used as a psychoactive drug by the native peoples of the Americas for approximately 8,000 years. Five hundred years ago, Christopher Columbus introduced tobacco to the Europeans, who discovered that once they overcame the nausea and dizziness produced by chewing, snorting, or smoking the tobacco, they simply could not get along without it. Nicotine quickly joined alcohol and caffeine as one of the world's most popular psychoactive drugs.

In the century after Columbus returned from the Americas with tobacco, consumption of and addiction to nicotine spread rapidly around the world. There followed numerous efforts to quash what had become known as the "evil weed." In 1603, the Japanese prohibited the use of tobacco and repeatedly increased the penalties for violating the ban, which wasn't lifted until 1625. By the middle of the seventeenth century, similar bans on tobacco were in place in Bavaria, Saxony, Zurich, Turkey, and Russia, with punishments ranging from confiscation of property to execution. Even in the early twentieth century, several state governments in the United States attempted to ban the use of tobacco.

A proposed quantity restriction—outright prohibition—was in the news again a few years ago when the head of the Food and Drug Administration announced that his agency had concluded that nicotine is addictive. He even argued that it should be classified with marijuana, heroin, and cocaine.

What can we predict if tobacco were ever completely prohibited today? Because tobacco is legal, the supply of illegal tobacco is zero. If the use of tobacco were restricted, the supply of illegal tobacco would not remain zero for long. Even if U.S. tobacco growers were forced out of business, the production of tobacco in other countries would increase to meet the demand. Consequently, the supply curve of illegal tobacco products would shift outward to the right as more foreign sources determined they wanted to enter the illegal U.S. tobacco market. The demand curve for illegal tobacco products would emerge almost immediately after the quantity restriction. The price people pay to satisfy their nicotine addiction would go up.

For Critical Analysis

What other goods or services follow the same analysis as the one presented here?

*Because we are referring to a long-run analysis here, the reduction in labor demanded would be demonstrated by an eventual shift inward to the left of the short-run demand curve, *D*, in Figure 4-5.

Some of the most common quantity restrictions exist in the area of international trade. The U.S. government, as well as many foreign governments, imposes import quotas on a variety of goods. An **import quota** is a supply restriction that prohibits the importation of more than a specified quantity of a particular good in a one-year period. The United States has had import quotas on tobacco, sugar, and immigrant labor. For many years, there were import quotas on oil coming into the United States. There are also "voluntary" import quotas on certain goods. Japanese automakers have agreed since 1981 "voluntarily" to restrict the amount of Japanese cars they send to the United States.

Import quota 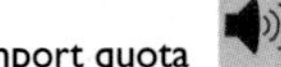
A physical supply restriction on imports of a particular good, such as sugar. Foreign exporters are unable to sell in the United States more than the quantity specified in the import quota.

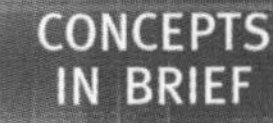

- With a price support system, the government sets a minimum price at which, say, qualifying farm products can be sold. Any farmers who cannot sell at that price can "sell" their surplus to the government. The only way a price support system can survive is for the government or some other entity to buy up the excess quantity supplied at the support price.
- When a floor is placed on wages at a rate that is above market equilibrium, the result is an excess quantity of labor supplied at that minimum wage.
- Quantity restrictions may take the form of import quotas, which are limits on the quantity of specific foreign goods that can be brought into the United States for resale purposes.

NETNOMICS

On-Line Ticket Scalpers Literally "Buy Out the House."

Recently, a large group of fans of a popular band from the 1970s, the Eagles, waited through the wee hours of the morning for the first tickets to go on sale for an upcoming concert at a Los Angeles arena. They had already waited so long that they were not overly concerned when the cashier opened the window to the ticket booth a couple of minutes late. They were a little more upset, however, when after making repeated attempts to place the ticket order of the first person in line, the cashier announced that only the highest-price seats to the show were still available—all the lower-priced seats had been completely sold out. It turned out that during the cashier's slight delay in opening the ticket booth, buyers on the Internet had, with a few clicks of a mouse, drained the pool of lower-priced tickets.

Although more people still buy tickets in person or over the phone, Internet buyers are purchasing tickets on-line in the largest permitted quantities. A number of buyers purchase additional lots using different names and credit cards. Once they have snapped up all the tickets they can, these on-line purchasers become scalpers, selling their tickets at on-line auctions. As noted in Chapter 3, scalping tickets is illegal in most states, but enforcement of these laws with respect to Internet sales is all but impossible. Auction sites such as eBay.com and Ubid.com provide forums that electronically bring together buyers and sellers of most anything, including tickets to entertainment and sporting events. For instance, when the movie *Star Wars: The Phantom Menace* was first released, tickets with a face value of $8.50 could be sold on eBay.com for as high as $40, a markup of 370 percent.

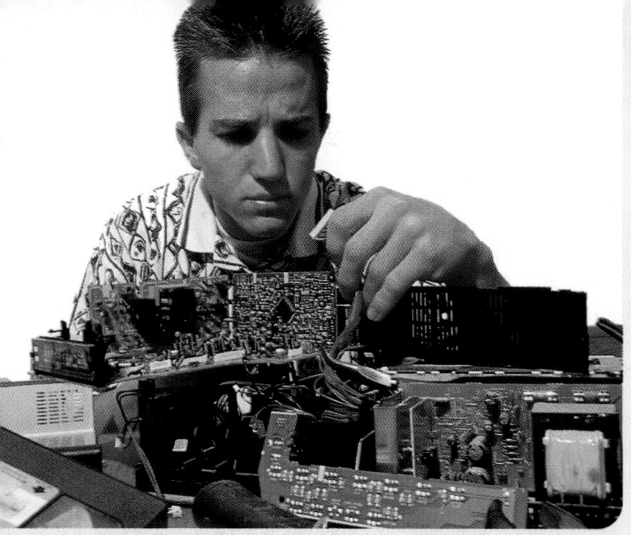

Issues & Applications

Computer Science Students Respond to Incentives, Just Like Everyone Else

The past several years have witnessed an upsurge of interest in computer courses. Across the nation, enrollments in computer courses rose by more than 40 percent in just four years.

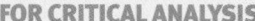

Concepts Applied

Shift in Supply

Shift in Demand

Equilibrium

A Shrinkage of Computer Science Students: Does It Compute?

At the same time, however, fewer students who begin training for graduate degrees in computer science are finishing their studies. This trend has filtered down to undergraduates as well. Increasingly, computer science majors are following the example set by college dropout Bill Gates, the Microsoft co-founder.

What is luring these students from their studies is high entry-level wages. The starting salary for a promising computer specialist without a college degree can be as high as $60,000. For students who already have undergraduate degrees and have completed some graduate-level training, far higher salaries beckon.

Will Dropping Out Pay Off in the End?

Computer science professors and college officials think many of these students are making a big mistake. They point, for instance, to the boom-and-bust cycles that have been so common in information technology (IT) professions. As shown in panel (a) of Figure 4-6, employment growth for computer programmers and systems analysts has seesawed from year to year before leveling off somewhat recently. Academics in computer science warn students that as so many of them leave their studies to enter the marketplace, a rise in the market supply of IT specialists will ultimately drive salaries below today's levels.

It is of course in the best interest of professors and university officials to try to stem the tide of student defectors from academia to the private marketplace. Could they have a point nonetheless? Take a look at panel (b) of Figure 4-6, in which the initial demand for and supply of IT specialists are D_1 and S_1, respectively. Now suppose that there is a big jump in the demand for people with training in this area, as shown by the shift from D_1 to D_2. The result is a rise in the equilibrium wage. This encourages more people who currently possess IT skills to provide their services, resulting in an increase in the quantity of employed IT specialists. Now consider what happens when additional people—such as today's undergraduate and graduate students who leave school early—expect to receive higher wages in the near future and enter this market. Recall that when the sellers of any service, including labor services, anticipate earning a higher price, the result is a rise in market supply. The supply schedule therefore shifts from S_1 to S_2 in panel (b), pushing the equilibrium wage back down somewhat.

Thus academic naysayers are correct that other things being equal, the entry of students without degrees into the market for IT specialists should ultimately tend to depress wages. Nevertheless, this argument is based on the *ceteris paribus* assumption (see Chapter 1) that the demand schedule will not shift any farther to the right. As more and more consumers move on-line, the demand for IT specialists may in fact continue to increase. If so, the academic field of computer science may continue to shrink.

FOR CRITICAL ANALYSIS

1. As noted, a key factor determining what happens to future earnings of IT specialists will be changes in the demand for their services. What other factors will matter?
2. If wages for IT specialists do eventually fall back to or below their previous levels, what is likely to happen to college enrollments?

FIGURE 4-6

The Market for Computer Science Specialists

Employment opportunities for computer science specialists have experienced booms and busts over the past decade, as seen in panel (a). Leaving school before getting a degree may still make sense nonetheless. As panel (b) shows, demand has increased sufficiently that even with an increase in supply, wage rates will remain higher than they are today for information technology workers.

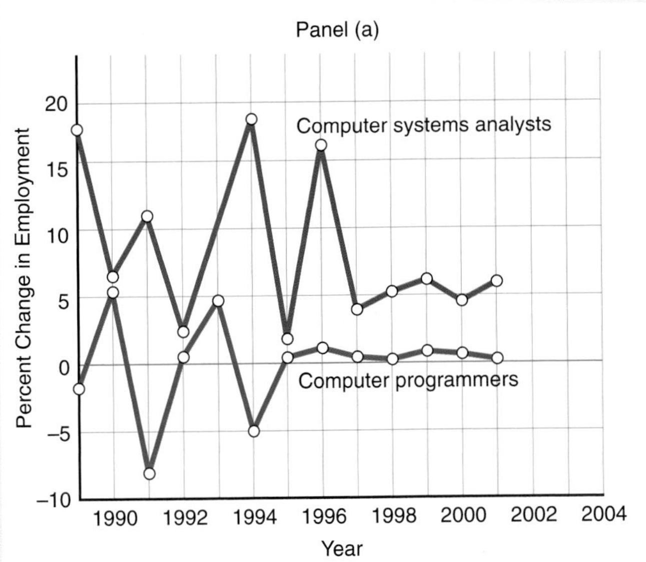

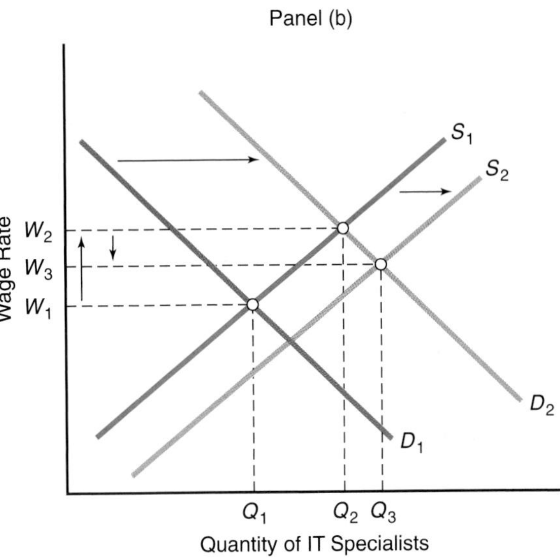

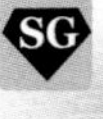

SUMMARY DISCUSSION OF LEARNING OBJECTIVES

1. **Essential Features of the Price System:** The price system, otherwise called the market system, allows prices to respond to changes in supply and demand for different commodities. Consumers' and business managers' decisions on resource use depend on what happens to prices. In the price system, exchange takes place in markets. The terms of exchange are communicated by prices in the marketplace, where individuals strive to minimize transaction costs, sometimes through the use of middlemen who bring buyers and sellers together.
2. **How Changes in Demand and Supply Affect the Market Price and Equilibrium Quantity:** With a stable supply curve, an increase in demand causes an increase in the market price and an increase in the equilibrium quantity, and a decrease in demand induces a fall in the market price and a decline in the equilibrium quantity. With a stable demand curve, an increase in supply causes a decrease in the market price and an increase in the equilibrium quantity, and a decrease in supply causes a rise in the market price and a decline in the equilibrium quantity. When both demand and supply shift at the same time, indeterminate results occur. We must know the direction and degree of each shift in order to predict the change in the market price and the equilibrium quantity.
3. **The Rationing Function of Prices:** In the market system, prices perform a rationing function—they ration scarce goods and services. Other ways of rationing include first come, first served; political power; physical force; lotteries; and coupons.
4. **The Effects of Price Ceilings:** Government-imposed price controls that require prices to be no

higher than a certain level are price ceilings. If a government sets a price ceiling below the market price, then at the ceiling price the quantity of the good demanded will exceed the quantity supplied. There will be a shortage of the good at the ceiling price. This can lead to nonprice rationing devices and black markets.

5. **The Effects of Price Floors:** Government-mandated price controls that require prices to be no lower than a certain level are price floors. If a government sets a price floor above the market price, then at the floor price the quantity of the good supplied will exceed the quantity demanded. There will be a surplus of the good at the floor price.
6. **Government-Imposed Restrictions on Market Quantities:** Quantity restrictions can take the form of outright government bans on the sale of certain goods, such as human organs or various psychoactive drugs. They can also arise from licensing requirements that limit the number of producers and thereby restrict the amount supplied of a good or service. Another example is an import quota, which limits the number of units of a foreign-produced good that can be legally sold domestically.

Key Terms and Concepts

Black market (82)
Import quota (89)
Minimum wage (87)
Nonprice rationing devices (82)
Price ceiling (82)
Price controls (82)
Price floor (82)
Price system (76)
Rent control (83)
Terms of exchange (76)
Transaction costs (77)
Voluntary exchange (76)

Problems Test

Answers to the odd-numbered problems appear at the back of the book.

4-1. Suppose that a rock band called the Raging Economists has released its first CD with Polyrock Records at a list price of $14.99. Explain how price serves as a purveyor of information to the band, the producer, and the consumer of rock CDs.

4-2. The pharmaceutical industry has benefited from advances in research and development that enable manufacturers to identify potential cures more quickly and therefore at lower cost. At the same time, our aging society has increased the demand for new drugs. Construct a supply and demand diagram of the market for pharmaceutical drugs. Illustrate the impact of these developments, and evaluate the effects on the market price and the equilibrium quantity.

4-3. The following table depicts the quantity demanded and quantity supplied of one-bedroom apartments in a small college town.

Monthly Rent	Quantity Demanded	Quantity Supplied
$400	3,000	1,600
$450	2,500	1,800
$500	2,000	2,000
$550	1,500	2,200
$600	1,000	2,400

What are the market price and equilibrium quantity of one-bedroom apartments in this town? Suppose that the mayor of this town decides to make housing more affordable for the local college students by imposing a rent control that holds the price of one-bedroom apartments to $450 a month. Explain the impact of this action on students desiring to live off campus and on owners of one-bedroom apartments. How many apartments are rented at the rate of $450 per month?

4-4. The United States provides considerable protection from foreign competition for its sugar industry. Suppose that one way it does this is by imposing a price floor that is above the market clearing price. Illustrate the U.S. sugar market with the price floor in place. Discuss the effects of the subsidy on conditions in the market for sugar in the United States.

4-5. The Canadian government and Canadian sugar industry have often complained that U.S. sugar manufacturers "dump" their sugar surpluses in the Canadian market. U.S. chocolate manufacturers and other U.S. businesses that use sugar as an input in their products have often complained that the high U.S. price of sugar hurts them in domestic and international markets. Explain how the imposition of a price floor for U.S. sugar, as described in Problem 4-4, affects these two markets. What are the changes in equilibrium quantities and market prices?

4-6. Suppose that the U.S. government places a ceiling on the price of Internet access. As a result, a black market for Internet providers arises, in which Internet service providers develop hidden means of connecting U.S. consumers. Illustrate the black market for Internet access, including the implicit supply schedule, the legal price, the black market supply and demand, and the black market equilibrium price and quantity. Also show why there is a shortage of Internet access at the legal price.

4-7. Airline routes are typically controlled by imposing a quota on the number of airline companies that may use the route and the number of flights on the route. Suppose that the following table illustrates the demand and supply schedules for seats on round-trip flights between Toronto and Chicago:

Price	Quantity Demanded	Quantity Supplied
$200	2,000	1,200
$300	1,800	1,400
$400	1,600	1,600
$500	1,400	1,800
$600	1,200	2,000

What are the market price and equilibrium quantity in this market? Now suppose that federal authorities limit the number of round-trip flights between the two cities to ensure that no more than 1,200 passengers can be flown. Explain the effects of this quota on the market price, quantity demanded, and quantity supplied.

4-8. The consequences of legalizing or decriminalizing illegal drugs have long been debated. Some individuals claim that legalization will lower the price of these drugs and therefore reduce related crime. Others claim that more people will use these drugs and the nation will face a health problem. Suppose that some of these drugs are legalized so that anyone may sell them and use them. Now consider the two claims—that price will fall and quantity will increase. Based on positive economic analysis, are these claims sound?

4-9. Look back at Figure 4-4. Suppose that the equilibrium price, P_e, is $1.00 per bushel of wheat and the support price is $1.25. In addition, suppose that the equilibrium quantity, Q_e, is 5 million bushels and the quantity supplied, Q_s, and quantity demanded, Q_d, with the price support are 8 million and 4 million, respectively. What was the total revenue of farmers before the price support program? What was the total revenue after the price support program? What is the cost of this program to taxpayers?

4-10. Using the information in Problem 4-9, calculate the total expenditures of wheat consumers before and after the price support program. Explain why these answers make sense.

Economics on the Net

The Floor on Milk Prices At various times the U.S. government has established price floors for milk. This application explains more about how governments implement floor prices and gives you an opportunity to apply what you have learned in this chapter to a real-world issue.

Title: Northeast Dairy Compact Commission

Navigation: Click here to visit the Web site of the Northeast Dairy Compact Commission.

Application Read the contents of the page, and answer the questions below.

1. Even though the federal government no longer formally sanctions the Northeast Dairy Compact, various states continue to coordinate their actions to regulate the price of milk. Based on the government-set price control concepts discussed in Chapter 4, explain the Northeast Dairy Compact that is in place in the Northeastern United States.

2. Draw a diagram illustrating the supply and demand of milk in the Northeast Dairy Compact and the supply and demand of milk outside of the Northeast Dairy Compact. Illustrate how the compact affects the quantities demanded and supplied for those participating in the compact. In addition, show how this affects the market for milk produced by those producers outside of the dairy compact.

3. In recent years, agricultural economists have found that Midwest dairy farmers are losing their dominance of milk production and sales. In light of your answer to question 2, explain how this occurred.

For Group Discussion and Analysis Discuss the impact of the Northeast Dairy Compact on farmers inside the compact and outside the compact. Discuss the impact of the Northeast Dairy Compact on consumers inside the compact and outside the compact. Debate the impact of eliminating the compact based on your earlier discussions. Identify in your debate arguments based on positive economic analysis and those based on normative arguments.

CHAPTER 5

THE PUBLIC SECTOR AND PUBLIC CHOICE

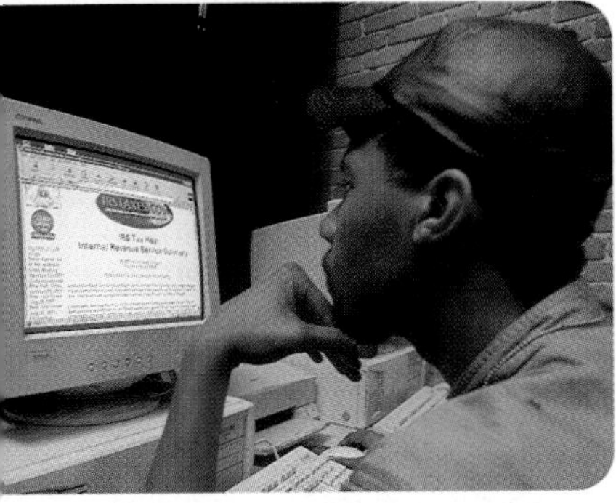

The average American reaches "tax freedom day" in early May. But the opportunity cost of filling out income tax forms is not considered in this calculation. On-line tax filing may reduce this cost but will never eliminate it.

In July 1776, John Adams wrote that Independence Day would be an occasion for "games, sports, guns, bells, bonfires, and illuminations, from one end of the continent to the other, from this time forevermore." For the average American, however, April 11 might also be a day to rejoice each year. This is touted as "tax freedom day"—the day when the average taxpayer has earned enough to pay all *federal* taxes for the current year. But don't overdo the celebrating. Almost another month's work will be required before the true tax freedom day arrives, on May 10. This is when the average American has earned enough to pay all federal, state, and local taxes *combined.* After nearly four and a half months of labor, U.S. taxpayers begin to earn income that they can keep for themselves.

Why does the U.S. government tax so much of its citizens' earnings for its own use? Before you can consider this question, you must learn some details about the public sector in America.

LEARNING OBJECTIVES

After reading this chapter, you should be able to:

1. **Explain how market failures such as externalities might justify economic functions of government**
2. **Distinguish between private goods and public goods and explain the nature of the free-rider problem**
3. **Describe political functions of government that entail its involvement in the economy**
4. **Distinguish between average tax rates and marginal tax rates**
5. **Explain the structure of the U.S. income tax system**
6. **Discuss the central elements of the theory of public choice**

Chapter Outline

Did You Know That... the U.S. government's total "take" from income taxes now exceeds $1 trillion each year? What is a trillion dollars? It is a million times a million. People earning an annual income of $200,000 or more typically pay just over 40 percent of these income taxes, and folks earning between $100,000 and $200,000 per year pay about 22 percent. Thus people earning more than $100,000 per year annually pay more than $620 billion in income taxes. People also pay miscellaneous other taxes, including sales and excise taxes. These also total to more than $1 trillion each year. So we cannot ignore the presence of government in our society. One of the reasons the government exists is to take care of what some people argue the price system does not do well.

WHAT A PRICE SYSTEM CAN AND CANNOT DO

Throughout the book so far, we have alluded to the benefits of a price system. High on the list is economic efficiency. In its most ideal form, a price system allows resources to move from lower-valued uses to higher-valued uses through voluntary exchange. The supreme point of economic efficiency occurs when all mutually advantageous trades have taken place. In a price system, consumers are sovereign; that is to say, they have the individual freedom to decide what they wish to purchase. Politicians and even business managers do not ultimately decide what is produced; consumers decide. Some proponents of the price system argue that this is its most important characteristic. A market organization of economic activity generally prevents one person from interfering with another in respect to most of his or her activities. Competition among sellers protects consumers from coercion by one seller, and sellers are protected from coercion by one consumer because other consumers are available.

Sometimes the price system does not generate these results, with too few or too many resources going to specific economic activities. Such situations are called **market failures.** Market failures prevent the price system from attaining economic efficiency and individual freedom, as well as other social goals. Market failures offer one of the strongest arguments in favor of certain economic functions of government, which we now examine.

Market failure 
A situation in which an unrestrained market economy leads to too few or too many resources going to a specific economic activity.

CORRECTING FOR EXTERNALITIES

In a pure market system, competition generates economic efficiency only when individuals know the true opportunity cost of their actions. In some circumstances, the price that someone actually pays for a resource, good, or service is higher or lower than the opportunity cost that all of society pays for that same resource, good, or service.

Consider a hypothetical world in which there is no government regulation against pollution. You are living in a town that until now has had clean air. A steel mill moves into town. It produces steel and has paid for the inputs—land, labor, capital, and entrepreneurship. The price it charges for the steel reflects, in this example, only the costs that the steel mill incurred. In the course of production, however, the mill gets one input—clean air—by simply taking it. This is indeed an input because in the making of steel, the furnaces emit smoke. The steel mill doesn't have to pay the cost of using the clean air; rather, it is the people in the community who pay that cost in the form of dirtier clothes, dirtier cars and houses, and more respiratory illnesses. The effect is similar to what would happen if the steel mill could take coal or oil or workers' services free. There has been an **externality,** an external cost. Some of the costs associated with the production of the steel have "spilled over" to affect **third parties,** parties other than the buyer and the seller of the steel.

Externality 
A consequence of an economic activity that spills over to affect third parties. Pollution is an externality.

Third parties 
Parties who are not directly involved in a given activity or transaction.

External Costs in Graphical Form

Look at panel (a) in Figure 5-1 on page 98. Here we show the demand curve for steel as D. The supply curve is S_1. The supply curve includes only the costs that the firms have to pay. The equilibrium, or market clearing, situation will occur at quantity Q_1. Let us take into account the fact that there are externalities—the external costs that you and your neighbors pay in the form of dirtier clothes, cars, and houses and increased respiratory disease due to the air pollution emitted from the steel mill; we also assume that all other suppliers of steel use clean air without having to pay for it. Let's include these external costs in our graph to find out what the full cost of steel production really is. This is equivalent to saying that the price of an input used in steel production increased. Recall from Chapter 3 that an increase in input prices shifts the supply curve. Thus in panel (a) of the figure, the supply curve shifts from S_1 to S_2; the external costs equal the vertical distance between A and E_1. If the external costs were somehow taken into account, the equilibrium quantity would fall to Q_2 and the price would rise to P_2. Equilibrium would shift from E to E_1. If the price does not account for external costs, third parties bear those costs—represented by the distance between A and E_1—in the form of dirtier clothes, houses, and cars and increased respiratory illnesses.

External Benefits in Graphical Form

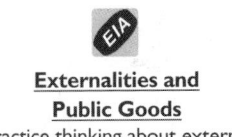

Externalities and Public Goods
Practice thinking about external costs and external benefits.

Externalities can also be positive. To demonstrate external benefits in graphical form, we will use the example of inoculations against communicable disease. In panel (b) of Figure 5-1, we show the demand curve as D_1 (without taking account of any external benefits) and the supply curve as S. The equilibrium price is P_1, and the equilibrium quantity is Q_1. We assume, however, that inoculations against communicable diseases generate external benefits to individuals who may not be inoculated but will benefit nevertheless because epidemics will not break out. If such external benefits were taken into account, the demand curve would shift from D_1 to D_2. The new equilibrium quantity would be Q_2, and the new equilibrium price would be P_2. With no corrective action, this society is not devoting enough resources to inoculations against communicable diseases.

When there are external costs, the market will tend to *overallocate* resources to the production of the good or service in question, for those goods or services will be deceptively low-priced. With the example of steel, too much will be produced because the steel mill owners and managers are not required to take account of the external cost that steel production is imposing on the rest of society. In essence, the full cost of production is unknown to the owners and managers, so the price they charge the public for steel is lower than it would be otherwise. And of course, the lower price means that buyers are willing and able to buy more. More steel is produced and consumed than is socially optimal.

When there are external benefits, the market *underallocates* resources to the production of that good or service because the good or service is relatively too expensive (because the demand is relatively too low). In a market system, too many of the goods that generate external costs are produced and too few of the goods that generate external benefits are produced.

How the Government Corrects Negative Externalities

The government can in theory correct externality situations in a variety of ways in all cases that warrant such action. In the case of negative externalities, at least two avenues are open to the government: special taxes and legislative regulation or prohibition.

FIGURE 5-1

External Costs and Benefits

In panel (a), we show a situation in which the production of steel generates external costs. If the steel mills ignore pollution, at equilibrium the quantity of steel will be Q_1. If the mills had to pay for the additional cost borne by nearby residents that is caused by the steel mill's production, the supply curve would shift the vertical distance A–E_1, to S_2. If consumers were forced to pay a price that reflected the spillover costs, the quantity demanded would fall to Q_2. In panel (b), we show the situation in which inoculations against communicable diseases generate external benefits to those individuals who may not be inoculated but who will benefit because epidemics will not occur. If each individual ignores the external benefit of inoculations, the market clearing quantity will be Q_1. If external benefits are taken into account by purchasers of inoculations, however, the demand curve would shift to D_2. The new equilibrium quantity would be Q_2 and the price would be higher, P_2.

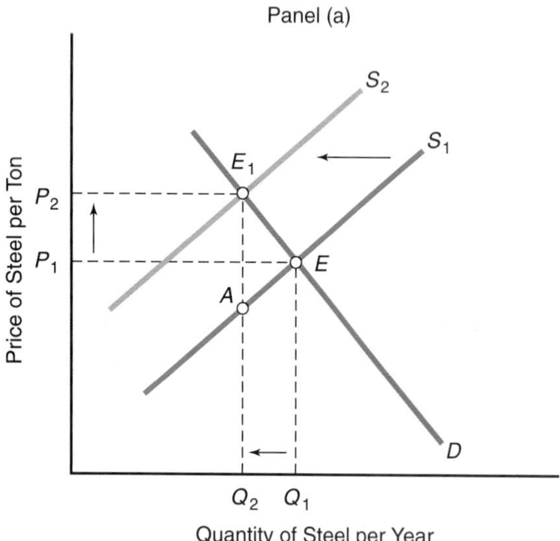

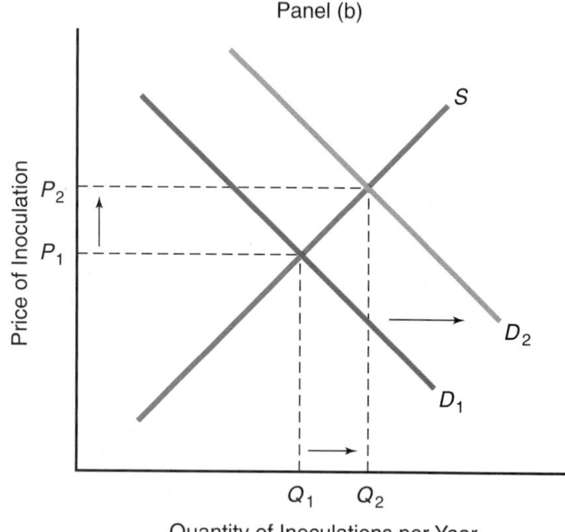

Special Taxes. In our example of the steel mill, the externality problem originates from the fact that the air as a waste disposal place is costless to the firm but not to society. The government could make the steel mill pay a tax for dumping its pollutants into the air. The government could attempt to tax the steel mill commensurate with the cost to third parties from smoke in the air. This, in effect, would be a pollution tax or an **effluent fee.** The ultimate effect would be to reduce the supply of steel and raise the price to consumers, ideally making the price equal to the full cost of production to society.

Effluent fee
A charge to a polluter that gives the right to discharge into the air or water a certain amount of pollution. Also called a *pollution tax*.

Regulation. To correct a negative externality arising from steel production, the government could specify a maximum allowable rate of pollution. This action would require that the steel mill install pollution abatement equipment at its facilities, that it reduce its rate of output, or some combination of the two. Note that the government's job would not be that simple, for it still would have to determine the level of pollution and then actually measure its output from steel production in order to enforce such regulation.

How the Government Corrects Positive Externalities

Click here to learn more about how the U.S. government uses regulations to try to protect the environment.

What can the government do when the production of one good spills *benefits* over to third parties? It has several policy options: financing the production of the good or producing the good itself, subsidies (negative taxes), and regulation.

Government Financing and Production. If the positive externalities seem extremely large, the government has the option of financing the desired additional production facilities so that the "right" amount of the good will be produced. Again consider inoculations against communicable diseases. The government could—and often does—finance campaigns to inoculate the population. It could (and does) even produce and operate centers for inoculation in which such inoculations would be given at no charge.

Subsidies. A subsidy is a negative tax; it is a payment made either to a business or to a consumer when the business produces or the consumer buys a good or a service. In the case of inoculations against communicable diseases, the government could subsidize everyone who obtains an inoculation by directly reimbursing those inoculated or by making payments to private firms that provide inoculations. If you are attending a state university, taxpayers are defraying part of the cost of providing your education; you are being subsidized by as much as 80 percent of the total cost. Subsidies reduce the net price to consumers, thereby causing a larger quantity to be demanded.

Regulation. In some cases involving positive externalities, the government can require by law that a certain action be undertaken by individuals in the society. For example, regulations require that all school-age children be inoculated before entering public and private schools. Some people believe that a basic school education itself generates positive externalities. Perhaps as a result of this belief, we have regulations—laws—that require all school-age children to be enrolled in a public or private school.

CONCEPTS IN BRIEF

- External costs lead to an overallocation of resources to the specific economic activity. Two possible ways of correcting these spillovers are taxation and regulation.
- External benefits result in an underallocation of resources to the specific activity. Three possible government corrections are financing the production of the activity, subsidizing private firms or consumers to engage in the activity, and regulation.

THE OTHER ECONOMIC FUNCTIONS OF GOVERNMENT

Besides correcting for externalities, the government performs many other economic functions that affect the way exchange is carried out. In contrast, the political functions of government have to do with deciding how income should be redistributed among households and selecting which goods and services have special merits and should therefore be treated differently. The economic and political functions of government can and do overlap.

Let's look at four more economic functions of government.

Providing a Legal System

The courts and the police may not at first seem like economic functions of government (although judges and police personnel must be paid). Their activities nonetheless have important consequences on economic activities in any country. You and I enter into contracts constantly, whether they be oral or written, expressed or implied. When we believe that we have been wronged, we seek redress of our grievances within our legal institutions. Moreover, consider the legal system that is necessary for the smooth functioning of our system. Our system has defined quite explicitly the legal status of businesses, the rights of private ownership, and a method for the enforcement of contracts. All relationships among consumers and businesses are governed by the legal rules of the game. We might consider the government in its judicial function, then, as the referee when there are disputes in the economic arena.

Property rights 
The rights of an owner to use and to exchange property.

Much of our legal system is involved with defining and protecting *property rights.* **Property rights** are the rights of an owner to use and to exchange his or her property. One might say that property rights are really the rules of our economic game. When property rights are well defined, owners of property have an incentive to use that property efficiently. Any mistakes in their decision about the use of property have negative consequences that the owners suffer. Furthermore, when property rights are well defined, owners of property have an incentive to maintain that property so that if those owners ever desire to sell it, it will fetch a better price.

Establishing and maintaining an independent constitutional judiciary, a familiar activity in the United States, is relatively new to Central and Eastern European countries.

INTERNATIONAL EXAMPLE

Post-Communist Rule of Law

Prior to the collapse of the Soviet empire, Central and Eastern European nations did not have an independent constitutional judiciary. Today that has changed. As a result, the institutional climate in these nations is more favorable for both domestic and foreign businesses.

The new constitutional frameworks in Central and Eastern European countries are based in large part on the U.S. Constitution. They emphasize the doctrines of separation of powers and checks and balances. They even give the courts the power of judicial review. (In the United States, this power allows the courts to declare laws unconstitutional.) A case in point is Hungary. There, legislators passed laws providing for restitution of nationalized land to pre-Communist owners. The court ruled that such laws were retroactive and thus invalid. The Hungarian court further stated that the only basis for returning land to former owners was through the transition to a market economy.

Bulgaria's constitutional court has consistently angered politicians. The court curbed government efforts to control radio and television. In Poland, the constitutional court voided a law passed by Parliament that would have lowered pensions of former state employees. This legal decision alone created a government obligation to pay almost $3 billion in compensation to almost 10 million Poles. This forced the government to sell bonds to pay for those pensions.

The trend toward highly independent court systems continues throughout Central and Eastern Europe.

For Critical Analysis

Why would an independent constitutional judiciary be important to someone who wished to invest in a new business in a Central or Eastern European country?

Promoting Competition

Antitrust legislation 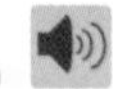
Laws that restrict the formation of monopolies and regulate certain anticompetitive business practices.

Monopoly 
A firm that has great control over the price of a good. In the extreme case, a monopoly is the only seller of a good or service.

Many people believe that the only way to attain economic efficiency is through competition. One of the roles of government is to serve as the protector of a competitive economic system. Congress and the various state governments have passed **antitrust legislation.** Such legislation makes illegal certain (but not all) economic activities that might restrain trade—that is, prevent free competition among actual and potential rival firms in the marketplace. The avowed aim of antitrust legislation is to reduce the power of **monopolies**—firms that have great control over the price of the goods they sell. A large number of antitrust laws have been passed that prohibit specific anticompetitive actions. Both the Antitrust Division of the Department of Justice and the Federal Trade Commission attempt to enforce these antitrust laws. Various state judicial agencies also expend efforts at maintaining competition.

Providing Public Goods 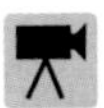

The goods used in our examples up to this point have been **private goods.** When I eat a cheeseburger, you cannot eat the same one. So you and I are rivals for that cheeseburger, just as much as rivals for the title of world champion are. When I use a CD-ROM player, you cannot use the same player. When I use the services of an auto mechanic, that person cannot work at the same time for you. That is the distinguishing feature of private goods—their use is exclusive to the people who purchase or rent them. The **principle of rival consumption** applies to all private goods by definition. Rival consumption is easy to understand. With private goods, either you use them or I use them.

Private goods 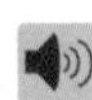
Goods that can be consumed by only one individual at a time. Private goods are subject to the principle of rival consumption.

Principle of rival consumption 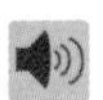
The recognition that individuals are rivals in consuming private goods because one person's consumption reduces the amount available for others to consume.

There is an entire class of goods that are not private goods. These are called **public goods.** The principle of rival consumption does not apply to them. That is, they can be consumed *jointly* by many individuals simultaneously. National defense, police protection, and the legal system, for example, are public goods. If you partake of them, you do not necessarily take away from anyone else's share of those goods.

Public goods 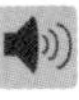
Goods to which the principle of rival consumption does not apply; they can be jointly consumed by many individuals simultaneously at no additional cost and with no reduction in quality or quantity.

Characteristics of Public Goods. Several distinguishing characteristics of public goods set them apart from all other goods.*

1. *Public goods are often indivisible.* You can't buy or sell $5 worth of our ability to annihilate the world with bombs. Public goods cannot usually be produced or sold very easily in small units.
2. *Public goods can be used by more and more people at no additional cost.* Once money has been spent on national defense, the defense protection you receive does not reduce the amount of protection bestowed on anyone else. The opportunity cost of your receiving national defense once it is in place is zero.
3. *Additional users of public goods do not deprive others of any of the services of the goods.* If you turn on your television set, your neighbors don't get weaker reception because of your action.
4. *It is difficult to design a collection system for a public good on the basis of how much individuals use it.* It is nearly impossible to determine how much any person uses or values national defense. No one can be denied the benefits of national defense for failing to pay for that public good. This is often called the **exclusion principle.**

Exclusion principle 
The principle that no one can be excluded from the benefits of a public good, even if that person hasn't paid for it.

One of the problems of public goods is that the private sector has a difficult, if not impossible, time providing them. There is little or no incentive for individuals in the private sector to offer public goods because it is so difficult to make a profit so doing. Consequently, true public goods must necessarily be provided by government.

INTERNATIONAL EXAMPLE

Is a Lighthouse a Public Good?

One of the most common examples of a public good is asserted to be a lighthouse. Arguably, it satisfies all the criteria listed in points 1 through 4. One historical example suggests, however, that a lighthouse was not a public good, in that a collection system was devised and enforced on the basis of how much individuals used it.

(cont.)

*Sometimes the distinction is made between pure public goods, which have all the characteristics we have described here, and quasi- or near-public goods, which do not. The major feature of near-public goods is that they are jointly consumed, even though nonpaying customers can be, and often are, excluded—for example, movies, football games, and concerts.

In the thirteenth century, the city of Aigues-Mortes, a French southern port, erected a tower, called the King's Tower, designed to assert the will and power of Louis IX (Saint Louis). The 105-foot tower served as a lighthouse for ships. More important, it served as a lookout so that ships sailing on the open sea, but in its view, did not escape paying for use of the lighthouse. Those payments were then used for the construction of the city walls.

For Critical Analysis

Explain how a lighthouse satisfies the characteristics of public goods described in points 1, 2, and 3.

Free-rider problem 

A problem that arises when individuals presume that others will pay for public goods so that, individually, they can escape paying for their portion without causing a reduction in production.

Free Riders. The nature of public goods leads to the **free-rider problem,** a situation in which some individuals take advantage of the fact that others will take on the burden of paying for public goods such as national defense. Free riders will argue that they receive no value from such government services as national defense and therefore really should not pay for it. Suppose that citizens were taxed directly in proportion to how much they tell an interviewer that they value national defense. Some people will probably tell interviewers that they are unwilling to pay for national defense because they don't want any of it—it is of no value to them. We may all want to be free riders if we believe that someone else will provide the commodity in question that we actually value.

The free-rider problem arises with respect to the international burden of defense and how it should be shared. A country may choose to belong to a multilateral defense organization, such as the North Atlantic Treaty Organization (NATO), but then consistently attempt to avoid contributing funds to the organization. The nation knows it would be defended by others in NATO if it were attacked but would rather not pay for such defense. In short, it seeks a "free ride."

Ensuring Economywide Stability

The government attempts to stabilize the economy by smoothing out the ups and downs in overall business activity. Our economy sometimes faces the problems of unemployment and rising prices. The government, especially the federal government, has made an attempt to solve these problems by trying to stabilize the economy. The notion that the federal government should undertake actions to stabilize business activity is a relatively new idea in the United States, encouraged by high unemployment rates during the Great Depression of the 1930s and subsequent theories about possible ways by which government could reduce unemployment. In 1946, the government passed the Employment Act, a landmark law concerning government responsibility for economic performance. It established three goals for government accountability: full employment, price stability, and economic growth. These goals have provided the justification for many government economic programs during the post–World War II period.

CONCEPTS IN BRIEF

- The economic activities of government include (1) correcting for externalities, (2) providing a judicial system, (3) promoting competition, (4) producing public goods, and (5) ensuring economywide stability.
- Public goods can be consumed jointly. The principle of rival consumption does not apply as it does with private goods.
- Public goods have the following characteristics: (1) They are indivisible; (2) once they are produced, there is no opportunity cost when additional consumers use them; (3) your use of a public good does not deprive others of its simultaneous use; and (4) consumers cannot conveniently be charged on the basis of use.

THE POLITICAL FUNCTIONS OF GOVERNMENT

At least two areas of government are in the realm of political, or normative, functions rather than that of the economic ones discussed in the first part of this chapter. These two areas are (1) the regulation and provision of merit and demerit goods and (2) income redistribution.

Merit good 
A good that has been deemed socially desirable through the political process. Museums are an example.

Merit and Demerit Goods

Certain goods are considered to have special merit. A **merit good** is defined as any good that the political process has deemed socially desirable. (Note that nothing inherent in any particular good makes it a merit good. The designation is entirely subjective.) Some examples of merit goods in our society are sports stadiums, museums, ballets, plays, and concerts. In these areas, the government's role is the provision of merit goods to the people in society who would not otherwise purchase them at market clearing prices or who would not purchase an amount of them judged to be sufficient. This provision may take the form of government production and distribution of merit goods. It can also take the form of reimbursement for payment on merit goods or subsidies to producers or consumers for part of the cost of merit goods. Governments do indeed subsidize such merit goods as professional sports, concerts, ballets, museums, and plays. In most cases, such merit goods would rarely be so numerous without subsidization.

Demerit good 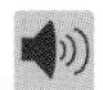
A good that has been deemed socially undesirable through the political process. Heroin is an example.

Demerit goods are the opposite of merit goods. They are goods that, through the political process, are deemed socially undesirable. Heroin, cigarettes, gambling, and cocaine are examples. The government exercises its role in the area of demerit goods by taxing, regulating, or prohibiting their manufacture, sale, and use. Governments justify the relatively high taxes on alcohol and tobacco by declaring them demerit goods. The best-known example of governmental exercise of power in this area is the stance against certain psychoactive drugs. Most psychoactives (except nicotine, caffeine, and alcohol) are either expressly prohibited, as is the case for heroin, cocaine, and opium, or heavily regulated, as in the case of prescription psychoactives.

FAQ

Do government-funded sports stadiums have a positive effect on local economies?

Probably not, even though in recent years many cities have decided that new football and baseball stadiums are merit goods worthy of public funding. Their rationale is that there is no collective mechanism besides government to ensure the construction of the stadiums that will draw big crowds. A local government, goes the argument, can regard a stadium as an investment because the crowds it draws benefit the local economy. Spending by the crowds can also generate tax revenues that help the government recoup its expenses. According to economist Andrew Zimbalist, however, "There has not been an independent study by an economist over the last 30 years that suggests you can anticipate a positive economic impact" from government investments in sports facilities.

Transfer payments 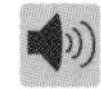
Money payments made by governments to individuals for which in return no services or goods are concurrently rendered. Examples are welfare, Social Security, and unemployment insurance benefits.

Income Redistribution

Another relatively recent political function of government has been the explicit redistribution of income. This redistribution uses two systems: the progressive income tax (described later in this chapter) and transfer payments. **Transfer payments** are payments made to individuals for which no services or goods are rendered in return. The three key money transfer payments in our system are welfare, Social Security, and unemployment insurance benefits. Income redistribution also includes a large amount of income **transfers in kind,** as opposed to money transfers. Some income transfers in kind are food stamps, Medicare and Medicaid, government health care services, and subsidized public housing.

Transfers in kind 
Payments that are in the form of actual goods and services, such as food stamps, subsidized public housing, and medical care, and for which in return no goods or services are rendered concurrently.

The government has also engaged in other activities as a form of redistribution of income. For example, the provision of public education is at least in part an attempt to redistribute income by making sure that the poor have access to education.

CONCEPTS IN BRIEF

- Political, or normative, activities of the government include the provision and regulation of merit and demerit goods and income redistribution.
- Merit and demerit goods do not have any inherent characteristics that qualify them as such; rather, collectively, through the political process, we make judgments about which goods and services are "good" for society and which are "bad."
- Income redistribution can be carried out by a system of progressive taxation, coupled with transfer payments, which can be made in money or in kind, such as food stamps and Medicare.

PAYING FOR THE PUBLIC SECTOR 

Jean-Baptiste Colbert, the seventeenth-century French finance minister, said the art of taxation was in "plucking the goose so as to obtain the largest amount of feathers with the least possible amount of hissing." In the United States, governments have designed a variety of methods of plucking the private-sector goose. To analyze any tax system, we must first understand the distinction between marginal tax rates and average tax rates.

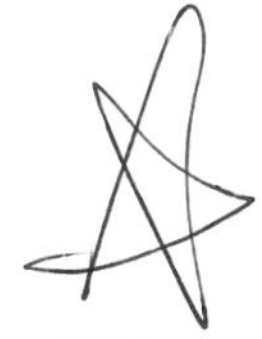

Marginal and Average Tax Rates

Marginal tax rate 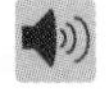
The change in the tax payment divided by the change in income, or the percentage of additional dollars that must be paid in taxes. The marginal tax rate is applied to the highest tax bracket of taxable income reached.

If somebody says, "I pay 28 percent in taxes," you cannot really tell what that person means unless you know if he or she is referring to average taxes paid or the tax rate on the last dollars earned. The latter concept refers to the **marginal tax rate.***

The marginal tax rate is expressed as follows:

$$\text{Marginal tax rate} = \frac{\text{change in taxes due}}{\text{change in taxable income}}$$

It is important to understand that the marginal tax rate applies only to the income in the highest **tax bracket** reached, where a tax bracket is defined as a specified level of taxable income to which a specific and unique marginal tax rate is applied.

Tax bracket 
A specified interval of income to which a specific and unique marginal tax rate is applied.

The marginal tax rate is not the same thing as the **average tax rate,** which is defined as follows:

$$\text{Average tax rate} = \frac{\text{total taxes due}}{\text{total taxable income}}$$

Average tax rate 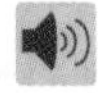
The total tax payment divided by total income. It is the proportion of total income paid in taxes.

Taxation Systems

No matter how governments raise revenues—from income taxes, sales taxes, or other taxes—all of those taxes fit into one of three types of taxation systems: proportional, progressive, and regressive, according to the relationship between the percentage of tax, or tax rate, paid and income. To determine whether a tax system is proportional, progressive, or regressive, we simply ask, What is the relationship between the average tax rate and the marginal tax rate?

*The word *marginal* means "incremental" (or "decremental") here.

Proportional Taxation. **Proportional taxation** means that regardless of an individual's income, taxes comprise exactly the same proportion. In terms of marginal versus average tax rates, in a proportional taxation system, the marginal tax rate is always equal to the average tax rate. If every dollar is taxed at 20 percent, then the average tax rate is 20 percent, as is the marginal tax rate.

A proportional tax system is also called a *flat-rate tax*. Taxpayers at all income levels end up paying the same *percentage* of their income in taxes. If the proportional tax rate were 20 percent, an individual with an income of $10,000 would pay $2,000 in taxes, while an individual making $100,000 would pay $20,000, the identical 20 percent rate being levied on both.

Proportional taxation 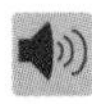
A tax system in which regardless of an individual's income, the tax bill comprises exactly the same proportion. Also called a *flat-rate tax*.

Progressive Taxation. Under **progressive taxation,** as a person's taxable income increases, the percentage of income paid in taxes increases. In terms of marginal versus average tax rates, in a progressive system, the marginal tax rate is above the average tax rate. If you are taxed 5 percent on the first $10,000 you make, 10 percent on the next $10,000 you make, and 30 percent on the last $10,000 you make, you face a progressive income tax system. Your marginal tax rate is always above your average tax rate.

Progressive taxation 
A tax system in which as income increases, a higher percentage of the additional income is taxed. The marginal tax rate exceeds the average tax rate as income rises.

Regressive Taxation. With **regressive taxation,** a smaller percentage of taxable income is taken in taxes as taxable income increases. The marginal rate is *below* the average rate. As income increases, the marginal tax rate falls, and so does the average tax rate. The U.S. Social Security tax is regressive. Once the legislative maximum taxable wage base is reached, no further Social Security taxes are paid. Consider a simplified hypothetical example: Every dollar up to $50,000 is taxed at 10 percent. After $50,000 there is no Social Security tax. Someone making $100,000 still pays only $5,000 in Social Security taxes. That person's average Social Security tax is 5 percent. The person making $50,000, by contrast, effectively pays 10 percent. The person making $1 million faces an average Social Security tax rate of only 0.5 percent in our simplified example.

Regressive taxation 
A tax system in which as more dollars are earned, the percentage of tax paid on them falls. The marginal tax rate is less than the average tax rate as income rises.

CONCEPTS IN BRIEF

- Marginal tax rates are applied to marginal tax brackets, defined as spreads of income over which the tax rate is constant.
- Tax systems can be proportional, progressive, or regressive, depending on whether the marginal tax rate is the same as, greater than, or less than the average tax rate as income rises.

THE MOST IMPORTANT FEDERAL TAXES

The federal government imposes income taxes on both individuals and corporations and collects Social Security taxes and a variety of other taxes.

The Federal Personal Income Tax

The most important tax in the U.S. economy is the federal personal income tax, which accounts for about 49 percent of all federal revenues. All American citizens, resident aliens, and most others who earn income in the United States are required to pay federal income taxes on all taxable income. The rates that are paid rise as income increases, as can be seen in Table 5-1. Marginal income tax rates at the federal level have varied from as

Click here to learn about what distinguishes recent so-called "flat-tax" proposals from a truly proportional income tax system. Next, click on "Flat Tax Proposals."

TABLE 5-1
Federal Marginal Income Tax Rates
These rates became effective in 2000. The highest rate includes a 10 percent surcharge on taxable income above $283,150.

Single Persons		Married Couples	
Marginal Tax Bracket	Marginal Tax Rate	Marginal Tax Bracket	Marginal Tax Rate
$0–$25,750	15%	$0–$43,050	15%
$25,751–$62,450	28%	$43,051–$104,050	28%
$62,451–$130,250	31%	$104,051–$158,550	31%
$130,251–$283,150	36%	$158,551–$283,150	36%
$283,151 and up	39.6%	$283,151 and up	39.6%

Source: U.S. Department of the Treasury.

low as 1 percent after the passage of the Sixteenth Amendment to as high as 94 percent (reached in 1944). There were 14 separate tax brackets prior to the Tax Reform Act of 1986, which reduced the number to three. Advocates of a more progressive income tax system in the United States argue that such a system redistributes income from the rich to the poor, taxes people according to their ability to pay, and taxes people according to the benefits they receive from government. Although there is much controversy over the redistributional nature of our progressive tax system, there is no strong evidence that in fact the tax system has ever done much income redistribution in this country. Currently, about 85 percent of all Americans, rich or poor, pay roughly the same proportion of their total income in federal taxes.

POLICY EXAMPLE

The Federal Income Tax, Then and Now

The United States first used an income tax during the Civil War. Congress ended the federal income tax in 1872. Adoption of the Sixteenth Amendment to the U.S. Constitution in 1913 brought back the income tax, however. Debate over the constitutional amendment was heated. One lawmaker argued passionately that ultimately "a hand from Washington will stretch out to every man's house." Many proponents of the amendment ridiculed him. After all, exempted from paying any taxes were single people with incomes below $3,000 (about $46,300 today) and married couples with incomes less than $4,000 (about $61,800 today). Thus initially, only U.S. citizens with relatively high incomes would be assessed income taxes of any significance.

Take a look at Table 5-2. It shows the tax rates imposed on various income brackets in 1913 and those same brackets expressed in 2000 dollars. A 1 percent tax rate would be in effect on incomes up to around $309,000. The highest rate, 7 percent, would apply to incomes over $7.7 million measured in 2000 dollars. Obviously, that is not the present situation—take a look at Table 5-1. Clearly, the federal income tax system as initiated in 1913 was a quite different animal from our current system. Looking back at Table 5-1, you can see that current tax rates are considerably higher than rates in 1913, and they affect virtually all Americans. A hand from Washington may not have stretched out to every house in 1913, but it certainly does today.

For Critical Analysis

The first income tax form was the size of a postcard. Why are tax forms so much thicker and more complicated today?

TABLE 5-2
1913 U. S. Income Tax Rates and Brackets

Tax Rate	Income Level in 1913	Equivalent Income Level in 2000 Dollars
1%	Up to $20,000	Up to $308,955
2%	$20,000–$50,000	$308,956–$772,388
3%	$50,000–$75,000	$772,389–$1,158,582
4%	$75,000–$100,000	$1,158,583–$1,544,776
5%	$100,000–$250,000	$1,544,777–$3,861,940
6%	$250,000–$500,000	$3,861,941–$7,723,881
7%	Over $500,000	Over $7,723,881

Source: U.S. Department of the Treasury.

The Treatment of Capital Gains

The difference between the buying and selling price of an asset, such as a share of stock or a plot of land, is called a **capital gain** if it is a profit and a **capital loss** if it is not. As of 2000, there were several capital gains tax rates.

Capital gain 
The positive difference between the purchase price and the sale price of an asset. If a share of stock is bought for $5 and then sold for $15, the capital gain is $10.

Capital loss 
The negative difference between the purchase price and the sale price of an asset.

Capital gains are not always real. If you pay $100,000 for a house in one year and sell it for 50 percent more 10 years later, your nominal capital gain is $50,000. But what if, during those 10 years, there has been inflation such that average prices also went up by 50 percent? Your *real* capital gain would be zero. But you still have to pay taxes on that $50,000. To counter this problem, many economists have argued that capital gains should be indexed to the rate of inflation. This is exactly what is done with the marginal tax brackets in the federal income tax code. Tax brackets for the purposes of calculating marginal tax rates each year are expanded at the rate of inflation, or the rate at which the average of all prices is rising. So if the rate of inflation is 10 percent, each tax bracket is moved up by 10 percent. The same concept could be applied to capital gains. So far, Congress has refused to enact such a measure.

The Corporate Income Tax 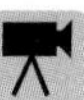

Corporate income taxes account for about 12 percent of all federal taxes collected and almost 8 percent of all state and local taxes collected. Corporations are generally taxed on the difference between their total revenues (or receipts) and their expenses. The federal corporate income tax structure is given in Table 5-3.

Double Taxation. Because individual stockholders must pay taxes on the dividends they receive, paid out of *after-tax* profits by the corporation, corporate profits are taxed twice.

TABLE 5-3
Federal Corporate Income Tax Schedule
The use rates were in effect through 2001.

Corporate Taxable Income	Corporate Tax Rate
$0–$50,000	15%
$50,001–$75,000	25%
$75,001–$10,000,000	34%
$10,000,000 and up	35%

Source: Internal Revenue Service.

If you receive $1,000 in dividends, you have to declare them as income, and you must pay taxes at your marginal tax rate. Before the corporation was able to pay you those dividends, it had to pay taxes on all its profits, including any that it put back into the company or did not distribute in the form of dividends. Eventually the new investment made possible by those **retained earnings**—profits not given out to stockholders—along with borrowed funds will be reflected in the increased value of the stock in that company. When you sell your stock in that company, you will have to pay taxes on the difference between what you paid for the stock and what you sold it for. In both cases, dividends and retained earnings (corporate profits) are taxed twice.

Retained earnings 
Earnings that a corporation saves, or retains, for investment in other productive activities; earnings that are not distributed to stockholders.

Who Really Pays the Corporate Income Tax? Corporations can exist only as long as consumers buy their products, employees make their goods, stockholders (owners) buy their shares, and bondholders buy their bonds. Corporations per se do not do anything. We must ask, then, who really pays the tax on corporate income. This is a question of **tax incidence.** (The question of tax incidence applies to all taxes, including sales taxes and Social Security taxes.) There remains considerable debate about the incidence of corporate taxation. Some economists say that corporations pass their tax burdens on to consumers by charging higher prices. Other economists believe that it is the stockholders who bear most of the tax. Still others believe that employees pay at least part of the tax by receiving lower wages than they would otherwise. Because the debate is not yet settled, we will not hazard a guess here as to what the correct conclusion may be. Suffice it to say that you should be cautious when you advocate increasing corporation income taxes. You may be the one who ultimately ends up paying the increase, at least in part, if you own shares in a corporation, buy its products, or work for it.

Tax incidence 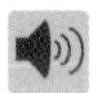
The distribution of tax burdens among various groups in society.

CONCEPTS IN BRIEF

- Because corporations must first pay an income tax on most earnings, the personal income tax shareholders pay on dividends received (or realized capital gains) constitutes double taxation.
- The corporate income tax is paid by one or more of the following groups: stockholder-owners, consumers of corporate-produced products, and employees in corporations.

Social Security and Unemployment Taxes

An increasing percentage of federal tax receipts is accounted for each year by taxes (other than income taxes) levied on payrolls. These taxes are for Social Security, retirement, survivors' disability, and old-age medical benefits (Medicare). As of 2000, the Social Security tax was imposed on earnings up to $72,600 at a rate of 6.2 percent on employers and 6.2 percent on employees. That is, the employer matches your "contribution" to Social Security. (The employer's contribution is really paid, at least in part, in the form of a reduced wage rate paid to employees.) A Medicare tax is imposed on all wage earnings at a combined rate of 2.9 percent. These taxes and the base on which they are levied are slated to rise in the next decade. Social Security taxes came into existence when the Federal Insurance Contributions Act (FICA) was passed in 1935. The future of Social Security is the subject of Chapter 6.

There is also a federal unemployment tax, which obviously has something to do with unemployment insurance. This tax rate is 0.8 percent on the first $7,000 of annual wages of each employee who earns more than $1,500. Only the employer makes the tax payment. This tax covers the costs of the unemployment insurance system and the costs of employment services. In addition to this federal tax, some states with an unemployment system impose an additional tax of up to about 3 percent, depending on the past record of the particular employer. An employer who frequently lays off workers will have a slightly higher state unemployment tax rate than an employer who never lays off workers.

SPENDING, GOVERNMENT SIZE, AND TAX RECEIPTS

The size of the public sector can be measured in many different ways. One way is to count the number of public employees. Another is to look at total government outlays. Government outlays include all government expenditures on employees, rent, electricity, and the like. In addition, total government outlays include transfer payments, such as welfare and Social Security. In Figure 5-2, you see that government outlays prior to World War I did not exceed 10 percent of annual national income. There was a spike during World War I, a general increase during the Great Depression, and then a huge spike during World War II. Contrary to previous postwar periods, after World War II government outlays as a percentage of total national income rose steadily before leveling off in the 1990s and 2000s.

Government Receipts

The main revenue raiser for all levels of government is taxes. We show in the two pie diagrams in Figure 5-3 on page 110 the percentage of receipts from various taxes obtained by the federal government and by state and local governments.

The Federal Government. The largest source of receipts for the federal government is the individual income tax. It accounts for 48.6 percent of all federal revenues. After that come social insurance taxes and contributions (Social Security), which account for 33.2 percent of total revenues. Next come corporate income taxes and then a number of other items, such as taxes on imported goods and excise taxes on such things as gasoline and alcoholic beverages.

State and Local Governments. As can be seen in Figure 5-3, there is quite a bit of difference in the origin of receipts for state and local governments and for the federal government. Personal and corporate income taxes account for only 20.4 percent of total state and

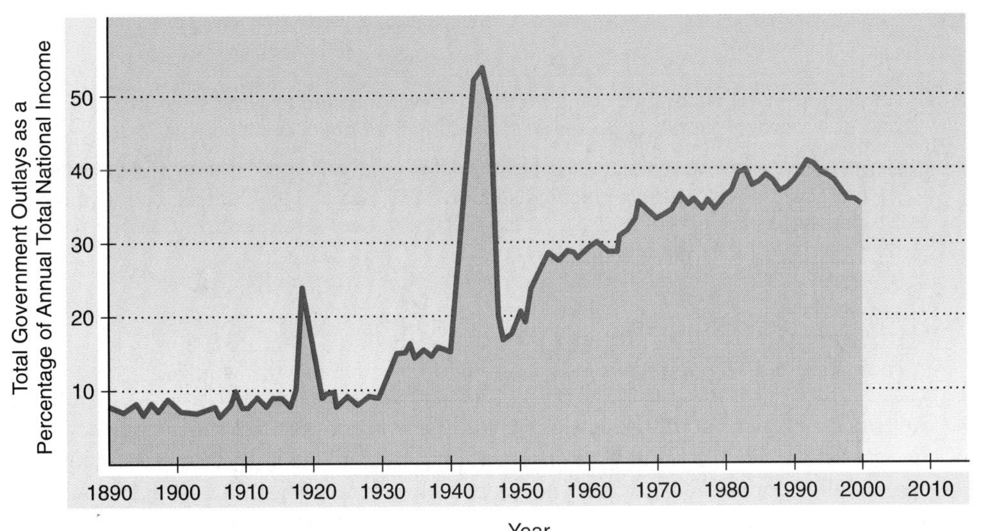

FIGURE 5-2
Total Government Outlays over Time
Here you see that total government outlays (federal, state, and local combined) remained small until the 1930s, except during World War I. Since World War II, government outlays have not fallen back to their historical average.

Sources: Facts and Figures on Government Finance and *Economic Indicators,* various issues.

FIGURE 5-3

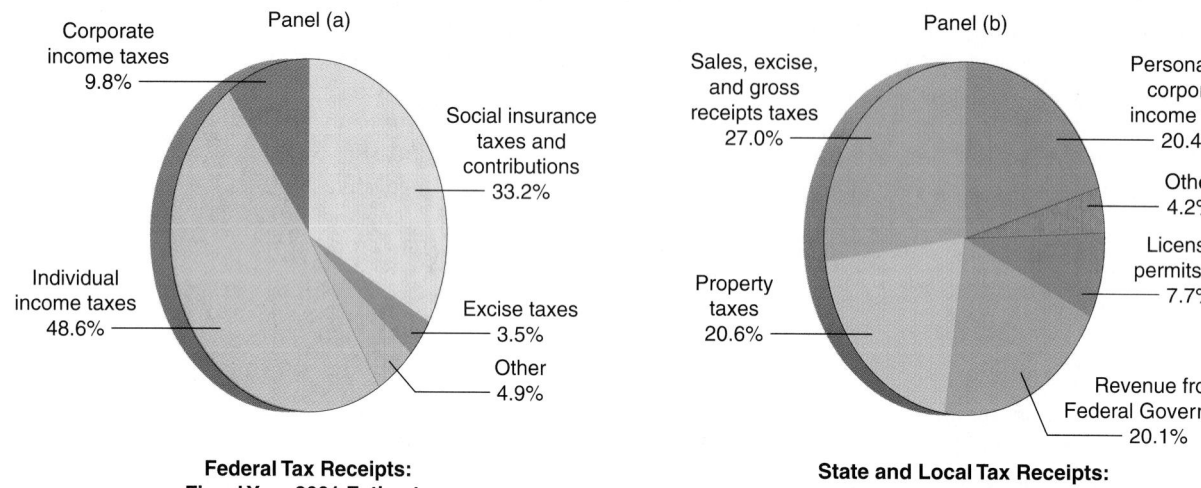

Sources of Government Tax Receipts

Over 82 percent of federal revenues come from income and Social Security taxes (a), whereas state government revenues are spread more evenly across sources (b), with less emphasis on taxes based on individual income.

Source: U.S. Department of Commerce, Bureau of Economic Analysis.

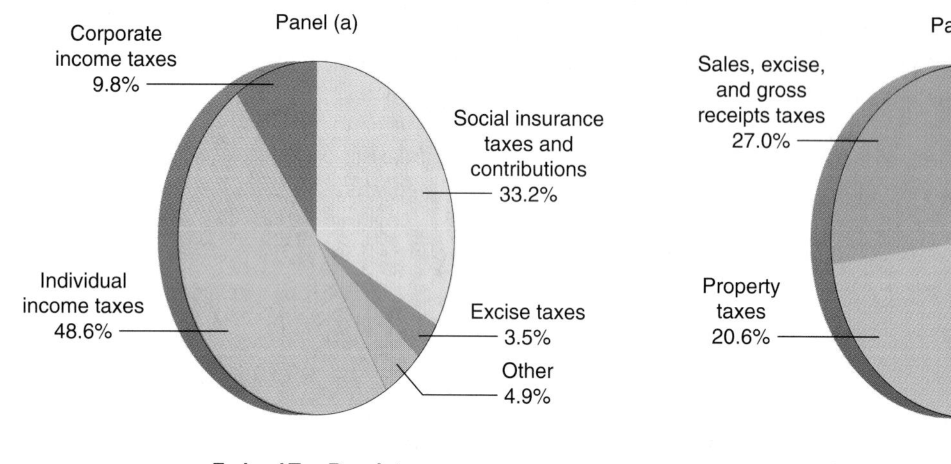

Click here to consider whether Internet sales should be taxed.

local revenues. There are even a number of states that collect no personal income tax. The largest sources of state and local receipts (other than from the federal government) are personal and corporate income taxes, sales taxes, and property taxes.

Comparing Federal with State and Local Spending. A typical federal government budget is given in panel (a) of Figure 5-4. The largest three categories are defense, income security, and Social Security, which together constitute 52.9 percent of the total federal budget.

The makeup of state and local expenditures is quite different. As panel (b) shows, education is the biggest category, accounting for 35.1 percent of all expenditures.

CONCEPTS IN BRIEF

- Total government outlays including transfers have continued to grow since World War II and now account for about 35 percent of yearly total national output.
- Government spending at the federal level is different from that at the state and local levels. At the federal level, defense, income security, and Social Security account for about 53 percent of the federal budget. At the state and local levels, education comprises 35 percent of all expenditures.

COLLECTIVE DECISION MAKING: THE THEORY OF PUBLIC CHOICE

Governments consist of individuals. No government actually thinks and acts; rather, government actions are the result of decision making by individuals in their roles as elected representatives, appointed officials, and salaried bureaucrats. Therefore, to understand how government works, we must examine the incentives for the people in government as well

FIGURE 5-4

Federal Government Spending Compared to State and Local Spending

The federal government's spending habits are quite different from those of the states and cities in panel (a), you can see that the categories of most importance in the federal budget are defense, income security, and Social Security, which make up 52.9 percent. In panel (b), the most important category at the state and local level is education, which makes up 35.1 percent. "Other" includes expenditures in such areas as waste treatment, garbage collection, mosquito abatement, and the judicial system.

Sources: Budget of the United States Government; Government Finances.

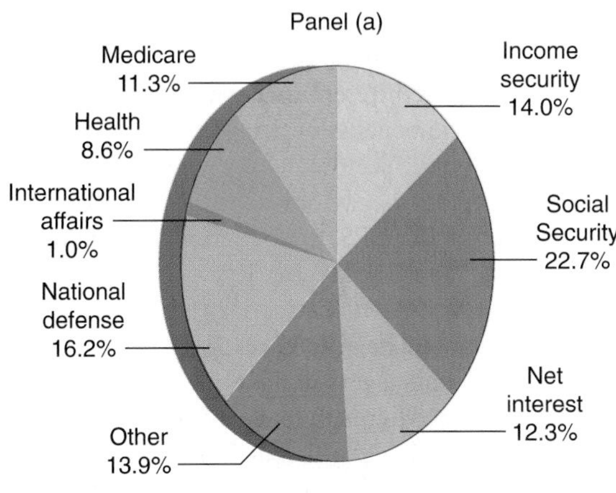

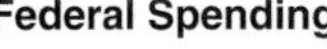

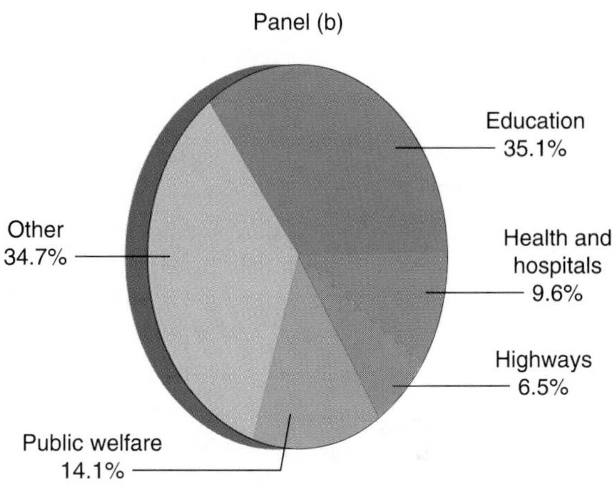

as those who would like to be in government—avowed or would-be candidates for elective or appointed positions—and special-interest lobbyists attempting to get government to do something. At issue is the analysis of **collective decision making.** Collective decision making involves the actions of voters, politicians, political parties, interest groups, and many other groups and individuals. The analysis of collective decision making is usually called the **theory of public choice.** It has been given this name because it involves hypotheses about how choices are made in the public sector, as opposed to the private sector. The foundation of public-choice theory is the assumption that individuals will act within the political process to maximize their *individual* (not collective) well-being. In that sense, the theory is similar to our analysis of the market economy, in which we also assume that individuals are motivated by self-interest.

Collective decision making 
How voters, politicians, and other interested parties act and how these actions influence nonmarket decisions.

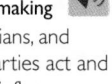

Theory of public choice
The study of collective decision making.

To understand public-choice theory, it is necessary to point out other similarities between the private market sector and the public, or government, sector; then we will look at the differences.

Similarities in Market and Public-Sector Decision Making

In addition to the similar assumption of self-interest being the motivating force in both sectors, there are other similarities.

Scarcity. At any given moment, the amount of resources is fixed. This means that for the private and the public sectors combined, there is a scarcity constraint. Everything that is spent by all levels of government, plus everything that is spent by the private sector, must add up to the total income available at any point in time. Hence every government action has an opportunity cost, just as in the market sector.

Competition. Although we typically think of competition as a private-market phenomenon, it is also present in collective action. Given the scarcity constraint government also faces, bureaucrats, appointed officials, and elected representatives will always be in competition for available government funds. Furthermore, the individuals within any government agency or institution will act as individuals do in the private sector: They will try to obtain higher wages, better working conditions, and higher job-level classifications. We assume that they will compete and act in their own, not society's, interest.

Similarity of Individuals. Contrary to popular belief, there are not two types of individuals, those who work in the private sector and those who work in the public sector; rather, individuals working in similar positions can be considered similar. The difference, as we shall see, is that the individuals in government face a different **incentive structure** than those in the private sector. For example, the costs and benefits of being efficient or inefficient differ when one goes from the private to the public sector.

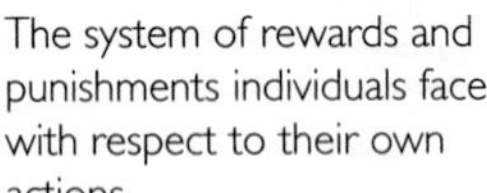
Incentive structure The system of rewards and punishments individuals face with respect to their own actions.

One approach to predicting government bureaucratic behavior is to ask what incentives bureaucrats face. Take the United States Postal Service (USPS) as an example. The bureaucrats running that government corporation are human beings with IQs not dissimilar to those possessed by workers in similar positions at Microsoft or American Airlines. Yet the USPS does not function like either of these companies. The difference can be explained, at least in part, in terms of the incentives provided for managers in the two types of institutions. When the bureaucratic managers and workers at Microsoft make incorrect decisions, work slowly, produce shoddy products, and are generally "inefficient," the profitability of the company declines. The owners—millions of shareholders—express their displeasure by selling some of their shares of company stock. The market value, as tracked on the stock exchange, falls. But what about the USPS? If a manager, a worker, or a bureaucrat in the USPS gives shoddy service, there is no straightforward mechanism by which the organization's owners—the taxpayers—can express their dissatisfaction. Despite the postal service's status as a "government corporation," taxpayers as shareholders do not really own shares of stock in the organization that they can sell.

The key, then, to understanding purported inefficiency in the government bureaucracy is not found in an examination of people and personalities but rather in an examination of incentives and institutional arrangements.

POLICY EXAMPLE

The U.S. Postal Service: Little Changed After More than Two Centuries

Like many private businesses, the federal government often desires to send urgent overnight mail. So to whom does it turn for delivery of the more than 8 million express letters and packages leaving federal offices for points around the nation and the world? Federal Express. Why not the U.S. Postal Service? The answer is that the USPS cannot legally reduce its prices to bid for competitive contracts. Even though the postal service now must make its own way without drawing on taxpayers, it still operates under a two-century-old mandate to serve every address, from backwoods farmhouses to crime-ridden urban apartments. It must do this while charging the same price to send a letter—whether regular first class or overnight delivery—from one point in New York City to another as it does from New York City to Anchorage, Alaska. This has made the postal service the provider of choice for transmitting items such as Pampers rebate coupons or proof-of-purchase seals from cereal boxes. But it has cost the USPS big revenues in the express-mail business. Its share of the overnight delivery pie is less than 10 percent. In recent years, supporters and critics of the postal service have both agreed that Congress must ultimately loosen the restraints that keep the USPS from competing with private firms in the marketplace. In the words of one member of Congress, if the postal service does not escape the bureaucratic shackles that bind it and compete in the private marketplace, it may "slowly strangle itself."

For Critical Analysis

If the U.S. Postal Service cannot reduce its prices, in what other ways can it try to compete for big overnight delivery contracts?

Differences Between Market and Collective Decision Making

There are probably more dissimilarities between the market sector and the public sector than there are similarities.

Government Goods at Zero Price. The majority of goods that governments produce are furnished to the ultimate consumers without direct money charge. **Government,** or **political, goods** can be either private or public goods. The fact that they are furnished to the ultimate consumer free of charge does *not* mean that the cost to society of those goods is zero, however; it only means that the price *charged* is zero. The full opportunity cost to society is the value of the resources used in the production of goods produced and provided by the government.

Government, or political, goods 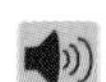
Goods (and services) provided by the public sector; they can be either private or public goods.

For example, none of us pays directly for each unit of consumption of defense or police protection. Rather, we pay for all these things indirectly through the taxes that support our governments—federal, state, and local. This special feature of government can be looked at in a different way. There is no longer a one-to-one relationship between consumption of a government-provided good and payment for that good. Consumers who pay taxes collectively pay for every political good, but the individual consumer may not be able to see the relationship between the taxes that he or she pays and the consumption of the good. Indeed, most taxpayers will find that their tax bill is the same whether or not they consume, or even like, government-provided goods.

Use of Force. All governments are able to engage in the legal use of force in their regulation of economic affairs. For example, governments can exercise the use of *expropriation,* which means that if you refuse to pay your taxes, your bank account and other assets may be seized by the Internal Revenue Service. In fact, you have no choice in the matter of paying taxes to governments. Collectively, we decide the total size of government through the political process, but individually, we cannot determine how much service we pay for just for ourselves during any one year.

Voting Versus Spending. In the private market sector, a dollar voting system is in effect. This dollar voting system is not equivalent to the voting system in the public sector. There are at least three differences:

1. In a political system, one person gets one vote, whereas in the market system, each dollar one spends counts separately.
2. The political system is run by **majority rule,** whereas the market system is run by **proportional rule.**
3. The spending of dollars can indicate intensity of want, whereas because of the all-or-nothing nature of political voting, a vote cannot.

Majority rule 
A collective decision-making system in which group decisions are made on the basis of more than 50 percent of the vote. In other words, whatever more than half of the electorate votes for, the entire electorate has to accept.

Proportional rule 
A decision-making system in which actions are based on the proportion of the "votes" cast and are in proportion to them. In a market system, if 10 percent of the "dollar votes" are cast for blue cars, 10 percent of the output will be blue cars.

Ultimately, the main distinction between political votes and dollar votes here is that political outcomes may differ from economic outcomes. Remember that economic efficiency is a situation in which, given the prevailing distribution of income, consumers get the economic goods they want. There is no corresponding situation using political voting. Thus we can never assume that a political voting process will lead to the same decisions that a dollar voting process will lead to in the marketplace.

Indeed, consider the dilemma every voter faces. Usually a voter is not asked to decide on a single issue (although this happens); rather, a voter is asked to choose among candidates who present a large number of issues and state a position on each of them. Just consider the average U.S. senator, who has to vote on several thousand different issues during a six-year term. When you vote for that senator, you are voting for a person who must make thousands of decisions during the next six years.

NETNOMICS

Protecting Private Property on the Internet: The Problem of Cyberpiracy

The U.S. Constitution grants Congress the power "to promote the Progress of Science and useful Arts, by securing for limited Times to Authors and Inventors the exclusive Rights to their respective Writings and Discoveries." Today, copyright laws are governed by the Copyright Act of 1976, as amended. This act has not been particularly effective, however, in preventing the theft of *intellectual property*. In contrast to physical property, intellectual property is any creation whose source is a person's mind or creativity.

Recent technological developments have greatly simplified the pirating of films, tapes, and CDs. Within days after the initial release of *Star Wars: The Phantom Menace*, people in China were selling tapes of the film that U.S. moviegoers had made by smuggling handheld videocassette recorders into theaters. The pirating of recorded music is also widespread. The International Federation of the Phonographic Industry (IFPI) estimates that one-fifth of all sales of recorded music are of pirated copies. The group estimates that one in three sales of CDs is pirated.

The IFPI's estimates are problematic, however. When estimating what legitimate CD sales would be in the absence of pirating, the IFPI assumes that pirated copies displace legitimate copies one for one, even though the pirated copies have much lower prices than legitimate copies. This assumption is a clear violation of the law of demand. In fact, there will be a larger quantity demanded at a lower price. Thus the lower-priced pirated copies of recorded music induce purchasers to buy more of them. If pirated copies did not exist, we could predict that legal sales of CDs would not simply replace them one for one.

This same analysis can apply to pirated copies of software. A person with a little computer background can develop relatively straightforward ways to transfer files from certain software programs for use by others who have not paid to use them. The Business Software Alliance estimates that a least half the global market for software is pirated products (remember the law of demand, however—this does not mean that if no pirating took place, legitimate sales of software would double).

There has been a significant change in pirating with the advent of the Internet: Not all pirates do so to profit. Some people, meaning to be kindhearted, offer downloadable copies of software and recorded music at no charge. Without ways to reduce this kind of unauthorized bootlegging, regardless of the motives of the bootleggers, people will reduce the time, effort, and creative energy they put into the development of software, recorded music, and other intellectual property.

This has led to calls from the film, recording, and software industries for stepped-up government efforts to protect their products under the copyright laws. Nonetheless, it is not clear how much the government can do when confronted with millions of Web sites to police. Many observers think that the solution will ultimately come from the private sector.

ISSUES & APPLICATIONS

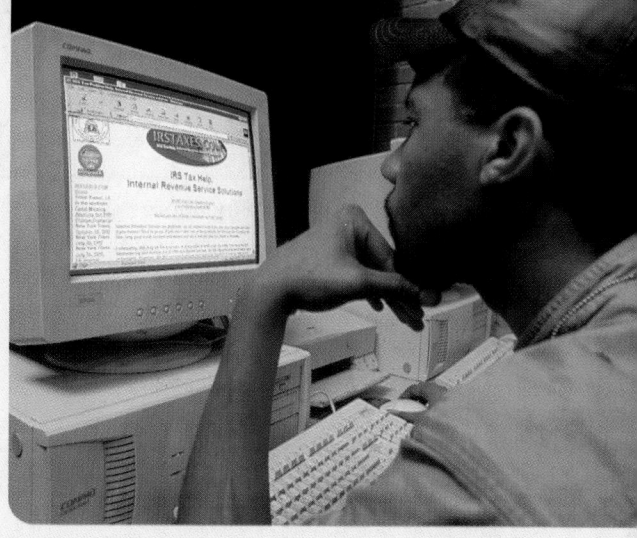

A Global Comparison of Income Tax Systems

Britain adopted the first national income tax in 1799 as a "temporary measure." Today residents of most developed nations pay income taxes every year. These nations typically strive to achieve progressivity of their tax structures.

Marginal Tax Rates in Other Nations

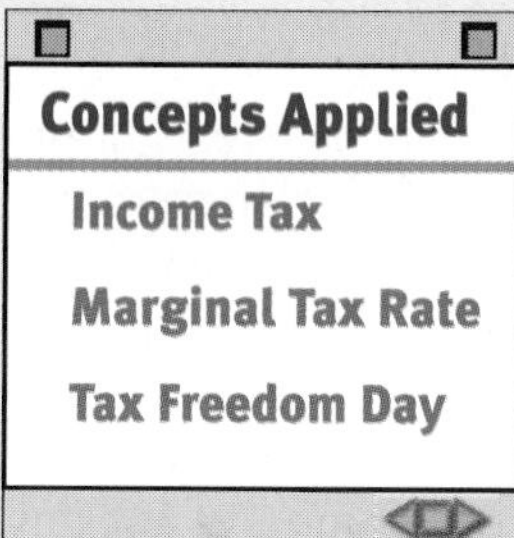

As you can see in panel (a) of Figure 5-5, Japan and several European nations have the highest marginal tax rates for the highest-income residents. By contrast, Hong Kong and Singapore stand out with much lower tax rates for the "rich." Residents with the lowest incomes also face lower marginal tax rates in these latter two nations.

FIGURE 5-5: Worldwide Income Tax Comparisons

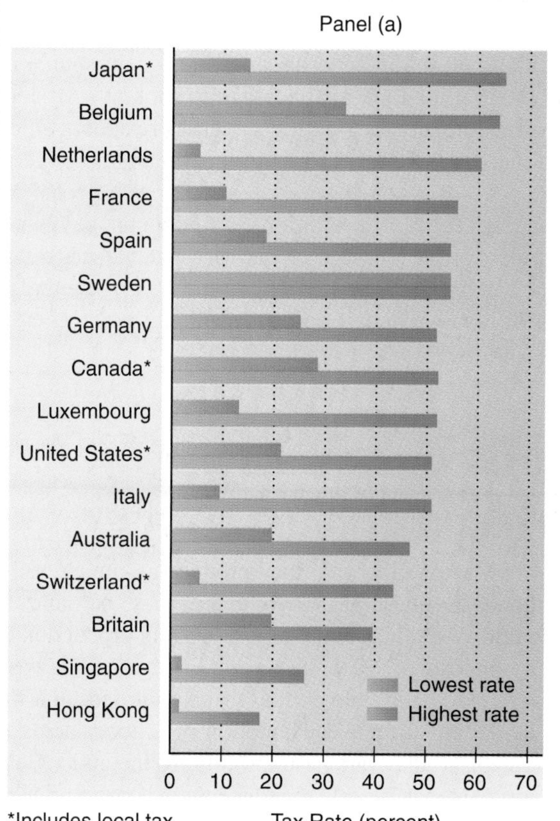

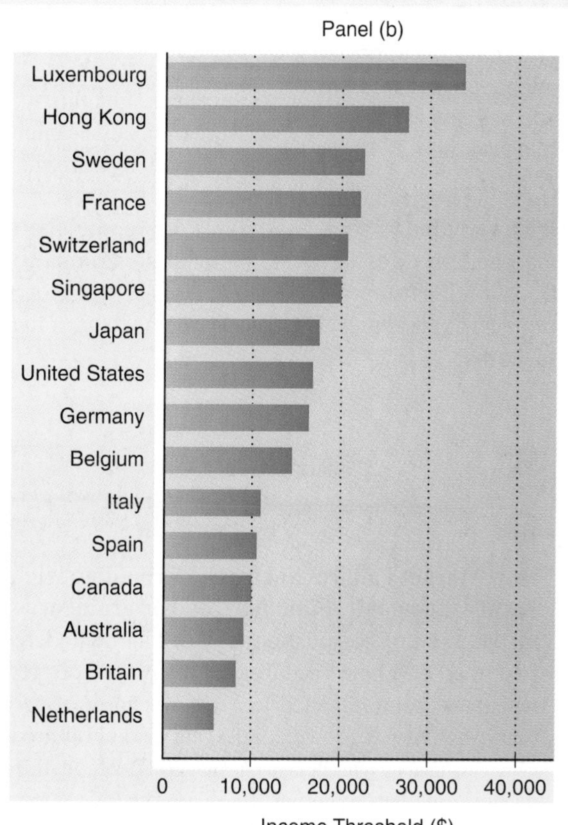

TABLE 5-4
Tax Freedom Day in Selected Nations
These figures exclude state, province, and local taxes.

Singapore	March 4	**Canada**	May 12
United States	April 11	**Germany**	May 23
Japan	April 12	**Italy**	June 2
Australia	April 25	**France**	June 12
Spain	May 5	**Netherlands**	June 12
Switzerland	May 6	**Belgium**	June 17
Britain	May 9	**Sweden**	July 3

Source: Organization for Economic Cooperation and Development.

Panel (b) of Figure 5-5 shows that some countries impose greater income tax burdens on lower-income residents than others do. A person can earn the equivalent of over $20,000 per year before owing any income taxes in Luxembourg, Hong Kong, Sweden, France, Switzerland, and Singapore. In contrast, in the United Kingdom and the Netherlands, a person earning less than the equivalent of $10,000 annually may owe income taxes to the government.

Tax Freedom Day—Anywhere Between March and July, Depending on Where You Live

Some governments rely more than others on the income tax as a significant source of tax revenues. For this reason, some international tax analysts like to look at a broader measure of tax assessments—the tax freedom day for a nation's average resident, which is the day each year when sufficient income has been earned to meet the nation's total tax bills.

Table 5-4 reports the "tax freedom day" for fourteen nations, based on tax payments to national governments. Based on this overall measure of tax assessments, residents of Sweden are the most tax-burdened people among developed nations: An average Swede begins to earn income on her or his own behalf only after the midpoint of each year!

FOR CRITICAL ANALYSIS

1. Some observers have attributed the strong employment and economic performance of Hong Kong and Singapore (despite the recession that affected Asian economies in 1997 and 1998) to the relatively small tax bite that they impose on income earners. Do you see any merit to this argument?
2. Does tax freedom day tell us anything about marginal tax rates? Does it tell us something about average tax rates?

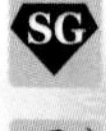

SUMMARY DISCUSSION OF LEARNING OBJECTIVES

1. **How Market Failures Such as Externalities Might Justify Economic Functions of Government:** A market failure is a situation in which an unhindered free market gives rise to too many or too few resources' being directed to a specific form of economic activity. A good example of a market failure is an externality, which is a spillover effect on third parties not directly involved in producing or purchasing a good or service. In the case of a negative externality, firms do not pay for the costs arising from spillover effects that their production of a good imposes on others, so they produce too much of the good in question. Government may be able to improve on the situation by restricting production or by imposing fees on producers. In the case of a positive externality, buyers fail to take into account the benefits that their consumption of a good yields to others, so they purchase too little of the good. Government may be able to induce more consumption of the good by regulating the market or subsidizing consumption. It can also provide a legal system to adjudicate disagreements about property rights, con-

duct antitrust policies to discourage monopoly and promote competition, provide public goods, and engage in policies designed to promote economic stability.

2. **Private Goods Versus Public Goods and the Free-Rider Problem:** Private goods are subject to the principle of rival consumption, meaning that one person's consumption of such a good reduces the amount available for another person to consume. This is not so for public goods, which can be consumed by many people simultaneously at no additional cost and with no reduction in quality or quantity of the good. Indeed, public goods are subject to the exclusion principle: No individual can be excluded from the benefits of a public good even if that person fails to help pay for it. This leads to the free-rider problem, which is that a person who thinks that others will pay for a public good will seek to avoid contributing to financing production of the good.
3. **Political Functions of Government That Lead to Its Involvement in the Economy:** Through the political process, people may decide that certain goods are merit goods, which they deem socially desirable, or demerit goods, which they feel are socially undesirable. They may call on government to promote the production of merit goods but to restrict or even ban the production and sale of demerit goods. In addition, the political process may determine that income redistribution is socially desirable, and governments may become involved in supervising transfer payments or in-kind transfers in the form of nonmoney payments.
4. **Average Tax Rates Versus Marginal Tax Rates:** The average tax rate is the ratio of total tax payments to total income. By contrast, the marginal tax rate is the change in tax payments induced by a change in total taxable income. Thus the marginal tax rate applies to the last dollar that a person earns.
5. **The U.S. Income Tax System:** The United States' income tax system assesses taxes against both personal and business incomes. It is designed to be a progressive tax system, in which the marginal tax rate increases as income rises, so that the marginal tax rate exceeds the average tax rate. This contrasts with a regressive tax system, in which higher-income people pay lower marginal tax rates, resulting in a marginal tax rate that is less than the average tax rate. The marginal tax rate equals the average tax rate only under proportional taxation, in which the marginal tax rate does not vary with income.
6. **Central Elements of the Theory of Public Choice:** The theory of public choice is the study of collective decision making, or the process through which voters, politicians, and other interested parties interact to influence nonmarket choices. Public choice theory emphasizes the incentive structures, or system of rewards or punishments, that affect the provision of government goods by the public sector of the economy. This theory points out that certain aspects of public-sector decision making, such as scarcity and competition, are similar to those that affect private-sector choices. Others, however, such as legal coercion and majority-rule decision making, differ from those involved in the market system.

Key Terms and Concepts

Problems

Answers to the odd-numbered problems appear at the back of the book.

5-1. Suppose that studies reveal that repeated application of a particular type of pesticide used on orange trees eventually causes harmful contamination of groundwater. The pesticide is produced by a large number of chemical manufacturers and is applied annually in orange groves throughout the world. Most orange growers regard the pesticide as a key input in their production of oranges.

a. Use a diagram of the market for the pesticides to illustrate the essential implications of a failure of pesticide manufacturers' costs to reflect the social costs associated with groundwater contamination.

b. Use your diagram from part (a) to explain a government policy that might be effective in achieving the socially optimal amount of pesticide production.

5-2. Now draw a diagram of the market for oranges. Explain how the government policy you discussed in part (b) of Problem 5-1 is likely to affect the market price and equilibrium quantity in the orange market. In what sense do consumers of oranges "pay" for dealing with the spillover costs of pesticide production?

5-3. The government of a major city in the United States has determined that mass transit, such as bus lines, helps alleviate traffic congestion, thereby benefiting both individual auto commuters and companies who desire to move workers, products, and factors of production speedily along streets and highways. Nevertheless, even though several private bus lines are in service, commuters in the city are failing to take the social benefits of the use of mass transit into account.

a. Use a diagram of the market for the bus service to illustrate the essential implications of a failure of commuters to take into account the social benefits associated with bus ridership.

b. Use your diagram from part (a) to explain a government policy that might be effective in achieving the socially optimal use of bus services.

5-4. Draw a diagram of the market for automobiles, which are a substitute means of transit. Explain how the government policy you discussed in part (b) of Problem 5-3 is likely to affect the market price and equilibrium quantity in the auto market. How are auto consumers affected by this policy to attain the spillover benefits of bus transit?

5-5. To promote increased use of port facilities in a major coastal city, a state government has decided to construct a state-of-the-art lighthouse at a projected cost of $10 million. The state proposes to pay half this cost and asks the city to raise the additional funds. Rather than raise its $5 million in funds via an increase in city taxes and fees, however, the city's government asks major businesses in and near the port area to contribute voluntarily to the project. Discuss key problems that the city is likely to face in raising the funds.

5-6. A senior citizen gets a part-time job at a fast-food restaurant. She earns $8 per hour for each hour she works, and she works exactly 25 hours per week. Thus her total pretax weekly income is $200. Her total income tax assessment each week is $40, but she has determined that she is assessed $3 in taxes for the final hour she works each week.

a. What is this individual's average tax rate each week?

b. What is the marginal tax rate for the last hour she works each week?

5-7. For purposes of assessing income taxes, there are three official income levels for workers in a small country: high, medium, and low. For the last hour on the job during a 40-hour workweek, a high-income worker pays a marginal income tax rate of 15 percent, a medium-income worker pays a marginal tax rate of 20 percent, and a low-income worker is assessed a 25 percent marginal income tax rate. Based only on this information, does this nation's income tax system appear to be progressive, proportional, or regressive?

5-8. Governments of country A and country B spend the same amount each year. In country A, the government allocates 25 percent of its spending to functions relating to dealing with market externalities and public goods, and it allocates the rest of its expenditures to funding the provision of merit goods and efforts to restrict the production of demerit goods. In country B, however, these relative spending allocations are reversed. Given this information, which country's government is more heavily involved in the economy through economic functions of government as opposed to political functions of government? Explain.

5-9. A government agency is contemplating launching an effort to expand the scope of its activities. One rationale for doing so is that another government agency could make the same effort and, if successful, receive larger budget allocations in future years. Another rationale for expanding the agency's activities is that this will make the jobs of its workers more interesting, which may help the agency attract better-qualified employees. Nevertheless, to broaden its legal mandate, the agency will have to convince more than half of the House of Representatives and the Senate to approve a formal proposal to expand its activities. In addition, to expand its activities, the agency must have the authority to force private companies it does not currently regulate to be officially licensed by agency personnel. Identify which aspects of this problem are similar to those faced by firms that operate in private markets and which aspects are specific to the public sector.

Economics on the Net

Putting Tax Dollars to Work In this application, you will learn about how the U.S. government allocates its expenditures. This will enable you to conduct your own evaluation of the current functions of the federal government within the U.S. economy.

Title: Historical Tables: Budget of the United States Government

Navigation: Click here to visit home page of the U.S. Government Printing Office. Select the most recent budget available, then click on Historical tables.

Application After the document downloads, examine Section 3, Federal Government Outlays by Function, and in particular Table 3.1, Outlays by Superfunction and Function. Then answer the following questions:

1. What government functions have been capturing growing shares of government spending in recent years? Which of these do you believe to be related to the problem of addressing externalities, providing public goods, or dealing with other market failures? Which appear to be related to political functions instead of economic functions?

2. Which government functions are receiving declining shares of total spending? Are any of these related to the problem of addressing externalities, providing public goods, or dealing with other market failures? Are any related to political functions instead of economic functions?

For Group Study and Analysis Assign groups to the following overall categories of government functions: national defense, health, income security, and Social Security. Have each group prepare a brief report concerning long-term and recent trends in government spending on each category. Each group should take a stand on whether specific spending on items in its category are likely to relate to resolving market failures, public funding of merit goods, regulating the sale of demerit goods, and so on.

CHAPTER 6

YOUR FUTURE WITH SOCIAL SECURITY

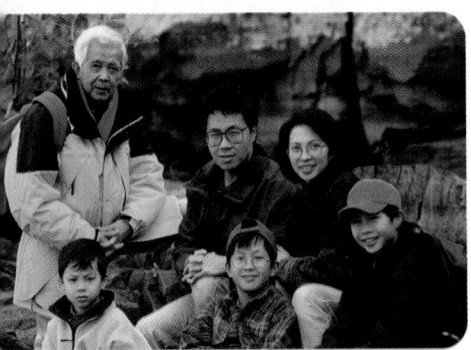

Of the three generations of this American family hiking in Vermont, the oldest will benefit the most from the Social Security system. Does that mean that the youngest may not benefit at all?

You've probably heard of chain letters. The basic notion is this: If you send, say, a dollar to each of several people on a list and then add your name to the list and mail it to your friends, you'll supposedly soon receive thousands of dollars from other people all over the world. There is a government program that has at times operated very much like a chain letter. The name of this program? Social Security.

The government retirement system that started 65 years ago was a good deal for your grandparents and probably will be a break-even proposition for your parents. But Social Security and a related program, Medicare, pose an enormous challenge for the economy.

Why have Social Security and Medicare become such problems? To find out, you need to learn more about how Social Security operates and what it will look like in your future.

LEARNING OBJECTIVES

After reading this chapter, you should be able to:

1. Identify the fundamental goals of Social Security and Medicare and the problems these programs pose for today's students
2. Analyze how Medicare affects the incentives to consume medical services
3. Explain why the Social Security Trust Fund is not a stock of savings we can draw on
4. Identify the key forces that caused the tremendous rise in Social Security spending
5. Explain how Social Security could be reformed

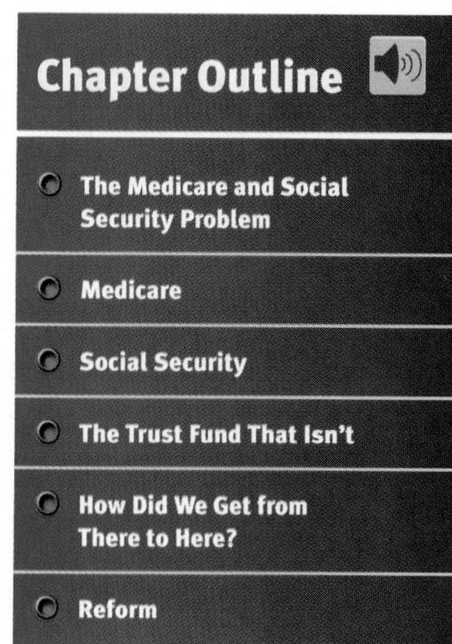

Did You Know That... America is getting old? The 78 million baby boomers born between 1946 and 1964 are entering middle age. Indeed, the future of America is now on display in Florida, where one person in five is over age 65. In 30 years, almost 20 percent of *all* Americans will be 65 or older.

Two principal forces are behind America's "senior boom." First, people are living longer. Average life expectancy in 1900 was 47. Today it is 77, and is likely to reach 80 within the next decade. Second, the birthrate is near record low levels. Today's mothers are having *half* the number of children that their mothers had. In short, the elderly are living longer, and the ranks of the young are growing too slowly to offset the added pressure of large numbers of retirees on the economy. Together, these forces are pushing the average age of the population higher and higher; in fact, the number of seniors is growing at *twice* the rate of the rest of the population. In 1970, the **median age** in the United States—the age that divides the older half of the population from the younger half—was 28; by 2000, the median age was over 35 and rising rapidly. Compounding these factors, the average age at retirement has been declining as well, from 65 in 1963 to 62 currently. Only 30 percent of the people age 55 and over hold jobs today, compared with 45 percent in 1930.

In this chapter, you will find out how the aging of America has caused an explosion of government spending, and you will learn about the potential impact of this increased spending on your future tax bills and retirement plans.

Median age 
The age that divides the older half of the population from the younger half.

THE MEDICARE AND SOCIAL SECURITY PROBLEM

Why should you be concerned with government programs designed to assist the elderly portion of the population? The main reason is that the elderly are expensive. In fact, people over 65 now consume over one-third of the federal government's budget. Social Security payments to retirees are the biggest item, now running over $300 billion a year. Medicare, the federal program that pays hospital and doctors' bills for the elderly, costs over $200 billion a year and is growing rapidly. Moreover, fully a third of the $150 billion-a-year budget for Medicaid, the government-sponsored program that helps pay medical bills for the poor of all ages, goes to people over the age of 65.

If current laws are maintained, the elderly will consume 40 percent of all federal spending within 10 years: Medicare's share of gross domestic product (GDP) will double, as will the number of "very old" people—those over 85, who are most in need of care. Within 25 years, probably *one-half* of the federal budget will go to caring for the elderly. In a nutshell, senior citizens are the beneficiaries of an expensive and rapidly growing share of all federal spending.

Click here for alternative perspectives on the problems of Social Security and Medicare.

Responsibility for paying the growing bills for Social Security and Medicare falls squarely on current and future workers, because both programs are financed by taxes on payrolls. Thirty years ago, these programs were adequately financed with a payroll levy of less than 10 percent of the typical worker's earnings. Today, the tax rate exceeds 15 percent of median wages, and it is expected to grow rapidly.

Consider what will happen if there is no change in the current structure of the Social Security system. By the year 2020, early baby boomers, born in the late 1940s and early 1950s, will have retired. Late baby boomers, born in the 1960s, will be nearing retirement. Both groups will leave today's college students, and their children, with a potentially staggering bill to pay. For Social Security and Medicare to be maintained, the payroll tax rate may have to rise to 25 percent of wages over the next 20 years. And a payroll tax rate of 40 percent is not unlikely by the middle of the twenty-first century.

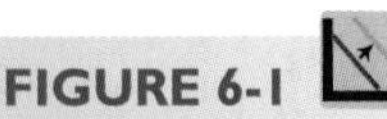

FIGURE 6-1

Workers Per Retiree

The average number of workers per Social Security retiree has declined dramatically since the program's inception.

Sources: Social Security Administration and author's estimates.

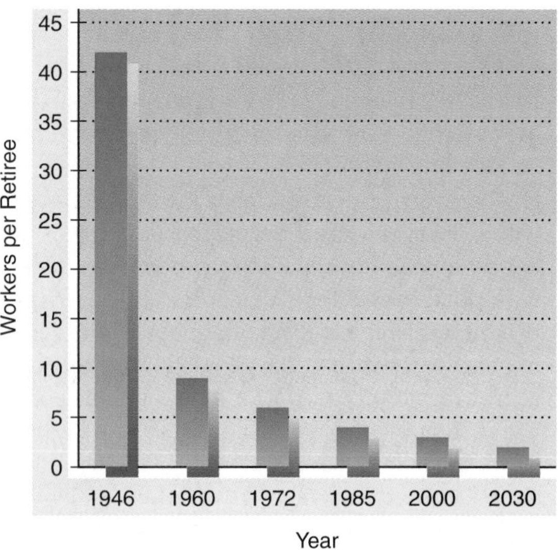

FAQ: *Why is the retirement age falling?*

Part of the exodus of the elderly from the workplace is due simply to their prosperity. Older people have higher disposable incomes than any other age group in the population, and they are using their wealth to consume more leisure. But early retirement is also being prompted by American businesses. Career advancement often slows after age 40; over 60 percent of American corporations offer early retirement plans, while only about 5 percent offer inducements to delay retirement. Even more important is the federal government's tax treatment of the elderly. Individuals age 70 and over, especially those in middle-income brackets, can be subject to a crushing array of taxes. They must pay taxes on up to 85 percent of their Social Security benefits, contribute payroll taxes if they keep working, and bear the loss of $1 in Social Security benefits for every $3 of wage income over about $10,000. Because these taxes can "piggyback" on each other, effective marginal tax rates can become astronomical for the elderly. In fact, for a fairly typical couple trying to supplement their retirement checks, income from work can be subject to a tax rate in excess of 80 percent, so little take-home pay remains after taxes. No wonder so many seniors are saying "no thanks" to seemingly attractive jobs.

One way to think about the future bill that could face today's college students and their successors in the absence of fundamental changes in Social Security is to consider the number of retirees each worker must support. In 1946, payroll taxes from 42 workers supported one Social Security recipient. By 1960, nine workers funded each retiree's Social Security benefits. Today, as shown in Figure 6-1, roughly three workers provide for each retiree's Social Security *and* Medicare benefits. Unless the current system is changed, by 2030 only two workers will be available to pay the Social Security and Medicare benefits due each recipient. In that event, a working couple would find itself responsible for supporting not only itself and its family but also someone outside the family who is receiving Social Security and Medicare benefits.

These figures illustrate why efforts to reform these programs have begun to dominate the nation's public agenda. Fortunately, the fact that Social Security and Medicare are your problems means that they are also your government's problems. What remains to be seen is how the government will ultimately resolve them.

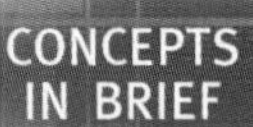

CONCEPTS IN BRIEF

- Social Security and Medicare payments are using up a large and growing portion of the federal budget.

- Because of a shrinking number of workers available to support each retiree, the expense for future workers to fund these programs will grow rapidly unless reforms are implemented.

MEDICARE 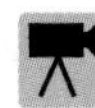

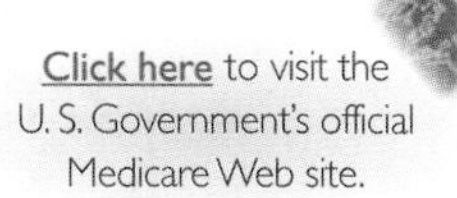
Click here to visit the U. S. Government's official Medicare Web site.

Not surprisingly, medical expenses are a major concern for many elderly Americans. Since 1965, that concern has been reflected in the existence of the Medicare program, which heavily subsidizes the medical expenses of persons over the age of 65. In return for paying a tax on their earnings while in the workforce (currently set at 2.9 percent of wages and salaries), retirees are ensured that the majority of their hospital and doctor's bills will be paid for with public monies.

The United States Compared to Other Nations

As we shall see, the design of the Medicare system encourages the consumption of medical services and drives up total spending on such services—spending that is paid for out of current taxes. Reflecting those facts, each person under the age of 65 in America currently pays an average of around $1,500 *per year* in federal taxes to subsidize medical care for the elderly. Some 30 percent of Medicare's budget goes to patients in their last year of life. Coronary bypass operations—costing over $30,000 apiece—are routinely performed on Americans in their sixties and even seventies. And for those over 65, Medicare picks up the tab. Even heart transplants are now performed on people in their sixties, paid for by Medicare for those over 65. Britain's National Health Service generally will not provide kidney dialysis for people over 55. Yet Medicare subsidizes dialysis for more than 200,000 people, whose average age is 63. The cost: more than $8 billion a year. Overall, the elderly receive Medicare benefits worth 5 to 20 times the payroll taxes (plus interest) they paid for this program.

The Simple Economics of Medicare

To understand how, in only 35 years, Medicare became the second-biggest domestic spending program in existence, a bit of economics is in order. Consider Figure 6-2 on page 124, which shows the demand and supply of medical care.

The initial equilibrium price is P_0, and equilibrium quantity is Q_0. Perhaps because the government believes that Q_0 is not enough medical care for these consumers, suppose that the government begins paying a subsidy that eventually is set at M for each unit of medical care consumed. This will simultaneously tend to raise the price per unit of care received by providers (doctors, hospitals, and so on) and lower the perceived price per unit that consumers see when they make decisions about how much medical care to consume. As presented in the figure, the price received by providers rises to P_s, while the price paid by demanders falls to P_d. As a result, demanders of medical care want to consume Q_m units, and suppliers are quite happy to provide it for them.

Medicare Incentives at Work

We can now understand the problems that plague the Medicare system today. First, one of the things that people observed during the 20 years after the founding of Medicare was a huge upsurge in physicians' incomes and medical school applications, the spread of private

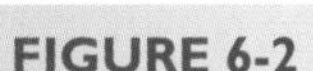
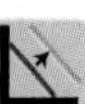

FIGURE 6-2

The Economic Effects of Medicare Subsidies

When the government pays a per-unit subsidy M for medical care, consumers pay the price P_d for the quantity of services Q_m. Providers receive the price P_s for supplying this quantity.

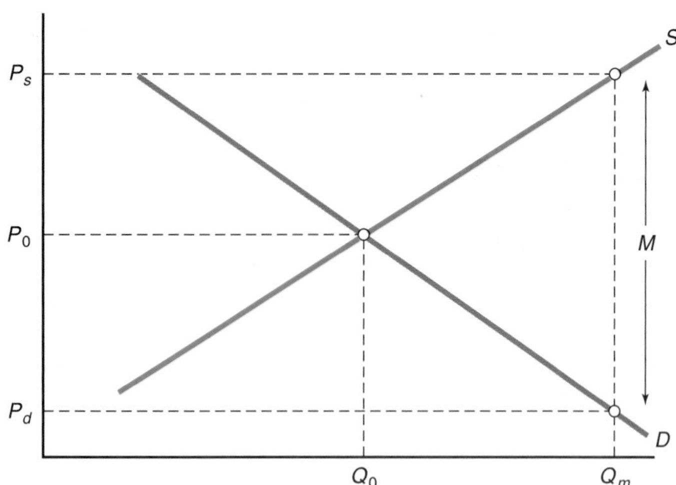

for-profit hospitals, and the rapid proliferation of new medical tests and procedures. All of this was being encouraged by the rise in the price of medical services from P_0 to P_s, which encouraged entry into this market.

Second, government expenditures on Medicare have routinely turned out to be far in excess of the expenditures forecast at the time the program was put in place or each time it was expanded. The reasons for this are easy to see. Bureaucratic planners often fail to recognize the incentive effects of government programs. On the demand side, they fail to account for the huge increase in consumption (from Q_0 to Q_m) that will result from a subsidy like Medicare. On the supply side, they fail to recognize that the larger amount of services can only be extracted from suppliers at a higher price, P_s. Consequently, original projected spending on Medicare was an area like $Q_0 \times (P_0 - P_d)$, because original plans for the program only allowed for consumption of Q_0 and assumed that the subsidy would have to be only $P_0 - P_d$ per unit. In fact, consumption rises to Q_m and marginal cost per unit of service rise to P_s, necessitating an increase in the per-unit subsidy to M. Hence actual expenditures turn out to be the far larger number $Q_m \times M$. The introduction of Medicare thus turned out to be more expensive than predicted, and every expansion of the program has followed the same pattern.

Third, total spending on medical services soars, consuming far more income than initially expected. Originally, total spending on medical services was $P_0 \times Q_0$. In the presence of Medicare, spending rises to $P_s \times Q_m$. This helps explain why current health care spending in the United States is 14 percent of GDP—the largest percentage spent anywhere in the world.

Finally, note that with the subsidy in place, consumers end up consuming many relatively low-value services that are nevertheless extremely costly to provide. For example, the value to consumers of the last few units of service consumed is only P_d per unit, but the cost of providing each of these units is P_s per unit. Hence the economic waste of having these last units provided—that is, the excess of cost over value received—is exactly equal to the subsidy per unit, M. This makes it clear why the United States spends so much money on high-cost procedures that have very low expected benefits for recipients: In America, the elderly are allowed to choose what they wish to consume at subsidized prices; in other countries, they often are not given the choice.

Spending and More Spending

Given these features of the Medicare system, it is little wonder that current health outlays per older person (over the age of 65) now average about $10,000 per year, a figure that has been rising at an inflation-adjusted rate of about 4 percent per year. At this sort of growth rate, real expenditures on each senior will average $25,000 per year by 2020. Moreover, the 65-and-older population will expand from 13 percent of the population today to 16.5 percent over that period. The combination of more elderly and more spending on each of them implies that medical spending is likely to rise to 20 percent of GDP over this period. As Victor Fuchs of Stanford University has observed, "Although people justifiably worry about Social Security, paying for old folks' health care is the real 800-pound gorilla facing the economy."

Public Versus Private Incentives

So far, the federal government's response to soaring Medicare costs has been to impose arbitrary reimbursement caps on specific procedures. Medicare's Prospective Payment System gives doctors and hospitals a flat fee for each of a wide variety of treatments and procedures. In principle, this should cap Medicare payments and give providers an incentive to cut costs by allowing them to pocket the difference. But as a practical matter, each of the caps is set in isolation from the others and without regard to the other incentives the caps give providers. Thus to avoid going over Medicare's reimbursement cap, hospitals often discharge patients too soon or in an unstable condition, making them more likely to end up back in the hospital or in a nursing home. For example, many hospitals fail to send elderly patients to rehabilitation centers after hip surgery. Six to 18 months later, the patients are back in the hospital with hip problems. Similarly, less than one-half of all Medicare heart patients receive anticlotting drugs after heart surgery, even though such drugs reduce the risk of a second heart attack by 50 percent. The result is elderly individuals who are sicker than they otherwise would be and Medicare costs that are actually higher *overall* because of the reimbursement caps on specific treatments and procedures.

Of course, even private health insurance companies and health maintenance organizations (HMOs)—organizations that are responsible for delivering, or arranging for the delivery of, and paying for their members' medical care—put limits on reimbursement levels. But they do so with a sharp eye to the reasonably predictable ways that physicians and patients are likely to respond to these caps. Hence insurers and HMOs go to great lengths to bundle services and reimbursement levels in ways that minimize the cost of achieving a given health outcome. Medicare administrators appear to pay far less attention to this issue.

CONCEPTS IN BRIEF

- Medicare subsidizes the consumption of medical care by the elderly, thus increasing the amount of such care consumed.
- Expenditures on programs such as Medicare almost invariably turn out to be more than forecasted because of a rise in consumption and a rise in the per-unit cost of providing the services.
- People tend to purchase large amounts of low-value, high-cost services in programs like Medicare because they do not directly bear the full cost of their decisions.
- Medicare managers do a poorer job of accounting for the incentive effects of their decisions than private sector managers because they have fewer incentives to do so.

SOCIAL SECURITY

The Social Security system was founded in 1935, as America was beginning to recover from the Great Depression. The financial resources of many people had been demolished during the previous six years: Jobs had been lost, stock prices had tumbled, and thousands of banks had failed, wiping out the accounts of their depositors. It was widely feared that recent retirees and workers soon to retire faced destitution. Moreover, many people argued that the elderly should be protected from any similar disasters in the future. Hence the decision was made to establish Social Security as a means of guaranteeing a minimum level of pension benefits to all persons. Today, many people regard Social Security as a kind of "social compact"—a national promise to successive generations that they will receive support in their old age.

Good Times for the First Retirees

The first Social Security taxes (called "contributions") were collected in 1937, but it was not until 1940 that retirement benefits were first paid. Ida May Fuller was the first person to receive a regular Social Security pension. She had paid a total of $25 in **Social Security contributions** before she retired. By the time she died in 1975 at age 100, she had received benefits totaling $23,000. Although Fuller did perhaps better than most, for the average retiree of 1940, the Social Security system was still more generous than any private investment plan anyone is likely to devise: After adjusting for inflation, the **rate of return** on their contributions was an astounding 135 percent. (Roughly speaking, every $100 of combined employer and employee contributions yielded $135 *per year* during each and every year of that person's retirement. This is also called the **inflation-adjusted return.**) Ever since then, however, the rate of return has decreased. Nonetheless, Social Security was an excellent deal for most retirees during the twentieth century. Figure 6-3 shows the rate of return for people retiring in different years.

Given that the inflation-adjusted long-term rate of return on the stock market is about 10 percent, it is clear that for retirees, Social Security was a good deal until at least 1970. In fact, because Social Security benefits are a lot less risky than stocks, Social Security actually remained a pretty good investment for many people until around 1990.

Social Security has managed to pay such high returns because at each point in time, current retirees are paid benefits out of the contributions of those who are currently working.

Social Security contributions
The mandatory taxes paid out of workers' wages and salaries. Although half are supposedly paid by employers, in fact the net wages of employees are lower by the full amount.

Rate of return
The interest rate necessary to make the present values of the costs and benefits of an action equal. For a situation in which a cost is incurred today and a benefit received one year from now, it is the percentage excess of the future benefit over the present cost.

Inflation-adjusted return
A rate of return that is measured in terms of real goods and services, that is, after the effects of inflation have been factored out.

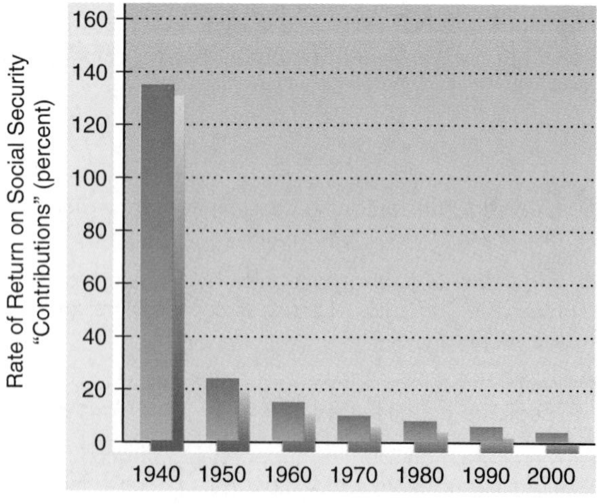

FIGURE 6-3
Private Rates of Return on Social Security Contributions, by Year of Retirement
The rate of return on Social Security contributions has steadily declined.
Sources: Social Security Administration and author's estimates.

(The contributions of today's retirees were long ago used to pay the benefits of previous retirees.) As long as Social Security was pulling in growing numbers of workers, either through a burgeoning workforce or by expanding its coverage of individuals in the workforce, the impressive rates of return during the early years of the program were possible. But as membership growth slowed as the post–World War II baby boom generation began to reach retirement age, the rate of return fell. Moreover, because the early participants received more than they contributed, it follows that later participants must receive less—and that ultimately means a *negative* rate of return. And for today's college students—indeed, for most people now under the age of 30 or so—that negative rate of return is what lies ahead, unless reforms are implemented.

Lesser Benefits for Some

Another aspect of today's low Social Security rate of return is worth noting. The system was originally designed to assist those most likely to be in need of assistance in their retirement years, and even today, low-income individuals do earn a higher rate of return on their contributions than higher-income people. But blacks do much worse than whites under the current system, because their life expectancy is significantly lower: Many collect nothing because they die before becoming eligible for their pensions. In addition, although women were generally net beneficiaries of the system in its early years, mainly through their spouses' contributions, that pattern has been changing as women entered the workforce in greater numbers: They are paying more in contributions but will receive proportionately less in benefits. In fact, families with two income earners now receive a substantially lower rate of return on their contributions than families with only one earner.

CONCEPTS IN BRIEF

- During the early years of the Social Security system, taxes were low and benefits were relatively robust, resulting in a high rate of return for retirees.
- As taxes have risen relative to benefits, the rate of return has fallen steadily.
- Blacks have often fared poorly under Social Security, as have two-earner families in recent years.

THE TRUST FUND THAT ISN'T 

During the early years of Social Security's existence, payroll taxes were collected, but no benefits were paid. The monies collected over this period were used to purchase bonds issued by the U.S. Treasury, and this accumulation of bonds was called the Social Security Trust Fund. (Medicare has a similar trust fund; because the basic principles apply to both funds, only Social Security's is discussed here in detail.) Even today, Social Security tax collections continue to exceed benefits, and so the trust fund has continued to grow. As the baby boomers move into retirement in a few years, benefit payments each year will exceed tax receipts, and the Social Security system will begin to sell the bonds in the trust fund to finance the difference. Eventually—current estimates are that in the absence of actions to alter the current system, it will be around the year 2030—all of the bonds in the trust fund will have been sold. Any further benefits will have to be explicitly financed out of current-day taxes.

Click here to learn more about Social Security. Next, click on "Understanding Social Security and Aging."

The Prefunding Myth

Many supporters of the current system argue that the "prefunding" of Social Security that has taken place so far is advantageous, because it has enabled the system to build up assets. This, these supporters contend, is much like a private pension fund that builds up assets for its members during their working years or the process by which individuals build up assets in their own individual retirement accounts to draw on during their retirement years. According to this line of reasoning, the Social Security Trust Fund represents net assets that society can use to finance future benefit payments. Nothing could be further from the truth.

The obligations of the Social Security system consist of the benefits that the system promises to pay. It is equally true that the financing for those obligations consists of the taxes on the public that will be levied over time. The question is this: Given the promised level of benefits, does it matter whether the taxes it will take to pay those benefits are levied before, during, or after the benefits are paid? The answer is no. A given stream of benefits can be paid for with smaller taxes now or larger taxes later, but the economic value of those taxes now or later must be exactly equivalent, given the stream of benefits that has been promised.

Congressional Meddling

Whenever current Social Security taxes exceed current benefits (as they have for the past 60 years), Congress has been unable to resist the temptation to spend the difference on other programs. For instance, in 1999, President Clinton and Congress quibbled over who should receive credit for the government budget surplus of nearly $123 billion. In fact, $124 billion of this "budget surplus" was the Social Security Trust Fund, which the president and Congress had borrowed to fund current spending. Thus the federal government actually operated at a *deficit* of about $1 billion that year.

But to maintain the fiction that the Social Security system is an insurance plan, Congress gives Social Security IOUs for the money that it spends. These IOUs are simply Treasury bonds, which of course are redeemable only for future taxes to be levied on the American people. Thus the "assets" owned by Social Security are nothing more than promises of the Treasury to make payments based on taxes collected from Americans.

Essentially, by borrowing from the Social Security Trust Fund and issuing IOUs, Congress transforms what looks like a prefunded system into a pay-as-you-go operation. After all, when it is time for the trust fund to redeem those IOUs, Congress must increase taxes, cut other spending, or borrow more money to raise the cash. But this would be true even if there were *no* Treasury bonds in the trust fund: All benefits must ultimately be paid for out of taxes. So although the design of the system's funding may originally have been well intentioned, the accounting fiction of the trust fund is nothing more than that: a fiction designed to disguise the true system.

POLICY EXAMPLE

Smoothing Taxes over Time

If the trust fund is a fiction, why would prefunding ever be the preferred means of financing the system? Tax smoothing is one possible explanation.

Whenever the government imposes taxes, the people who are expected to pay those taxes have a natural incentive to try to avoid or evade them. These efforts to avoid taxes (and the corresponding effort by the government to prevent such avoidance) use up ("waste") scarce resources. Moreover, as taxes rise relative to income in any given period, the efforts devoted to avoiding (and collecting) taxes tend to rise disproportionately, implying that so do the resources that are wasted in such activities.

Hence for any given level of taxes to be collected over time, the amount of resources that are wasted in avoiding and collecting those taxes can be minimized by following this rule: Keep the ratio of taxes to income constant over time; that is, smooth taxes over time. Suppose (as has been true) that Social Security benefits rise over time faster than income, implying that the ratio of benefits to income is expected to rise. Ideally, we want to keep the ratio of taxes to income constant, which implies that taxes will initially have to be high relative to benefits, eventually becoming low relative to the more rapidly growing benefits. The result is "prefunding" of benefits, much as we had during the early years of the Social Security system.

For Critical Analysis

What incentive does prefunding give to members of Congress who might be looking for additional funds to be used to pay for other programs?

CONCEPTS IN BRIEF

- Social Security is paid for out of taxes, regardless of when those taxes are imposed. Prefunding does not create any additional wealth that can be used to pay benefits.
- Congress has consistently reappropriated much or all of the excess of Social Security taxes over benefits that have been collected.

HOW DID WE GET FROM THERE TO HERE?

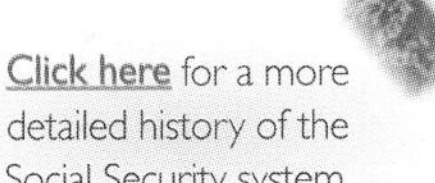
Click here for a more detailed history of the Social Security system.

If Social Security started as a system designed to relieve the misery of the destitute elderly in the aftermath of the Great Depression, it has certainly become something much different. There is no doubt that it has helped raise the standard of living of the 65-and-older age group to the highest of all the age groups. But it has also become the single largest drain on the U.S. taxpayer and the most important domestic policy problem facing politicians and public alike. What happened? There are many facets to the story, but we shall focus here on just two of them, both a mixture of economics and politics.

A Tale of Two Generations

The first of the forces that transformed Social Security is what we shall call the confluence of the generations. Until the 1960s, Social Security looked little different from when it had been founded three decades before. Tax collections still exceeded benefits, which had remained modest. And despite expansions of the system to cover industries and occupations not originally eligible, the political and economic scope of the system were relatively unobtrusive. Things began to change with the entry of the baby boom generation into the labor market: Taxes began flowing into the system at an unprecedented rate. And because the number of people then collecting benefits was small relative to the burgeoning labor force, and the boomers themselves were 40 years from collecting benefits themselves, the Social Security Trust Fund soon became a rich prize in the political arena.

In the early 1970s, the first members of the generation that had suffered through the Great Depression and then fought World War II began retiring. Most had private savings that were modest at best and strong memories of having endured much on behalf of their nation. Thus we had the confluence of a large source of cash (the taxes paid by the boomers) and a worthy cause on which to spend it (the retirement benefits of the generation that had fought to keep the world free in World War II). The result was enormous political pressure to expand Social Security benefits.

Inflation

At the same time, America was going through a period of inflation that was, by the standards of the day, quite significant, running as high as 4 percent per year. At the time, the dollar value of Social Security benefits was set by Congress and thus could be changed only by explicit congressional action. But a 4 percent rise in the price level in such circumstances meant a 4 percent decline in the real value of benefits that were fixed in dollar terms. This was not the sort of thing any member of Congress wanted to have happen to the deserving World War II generation who was collecting those benefits. And this was particularly true because the elderly were already well known for voting more regularly than any other age group. So Congress looked for a way to protect retirees from inflation, without at the same time having to vote on the level of Social Security benefits every year. With the aid of President Richard Nixon, who was himself facing reelection in 1972, Congress found what appeared to be the ideal answer: Benefits were indexed, or linked, to the Consumer Price Index (CPI), a measure of the dollar cost of consuming a fixed market basket of goods that we shall discuss in greater detail in Chapter 7. Once a year, the percentage increase in the CPI was computed, and nominal Social Security benefits were then automatically increased by the same percentage amount.

Bias in the CPI

There was one significant hitch in this process. The CPI is biased upward; that is, it tends to overstate the actual rate of inflation, by an amount estimated to be about 1.1 percent per year. Thus if the true inflation rate is 3 percent, the CPI will measure it at, say, 4.1 percent; if the true rate is 4.5 percent, the CPI will say 5.6 percent. What this meant was that every year, Social Security recipients were getting their benefits increased not just by enough to protect them from inflation but also by what amounted to an automatic raise in real benefits of about 1.1 percent per year. This may not sound like much, but over the next 30 years or so, the power of compounding translated this into a 50 percent increase in real benefits. Thus a simple device introduced to protect the elderly from the ravages of inflation became a powerful tool for increasing benefits well above the levels ever contemplated at the system's founding—and all without the necessity for any overt action by Congress.

CONCEPTS IN BRIEF

- The combination of a politically powerful older generation and a larger younger generation capable of paying payroll taxes into the system created the incentives for the huge increase in Social Security benefits over the past 30 years.
- The cost-of-living adjustment, calculated using the Consumer Price Index, was the means by which much of this increase in real benefits occurred because it did not compensate for the upward bias in the CPI.

REFORM

America now finds itself with a social compact—the Social Security system—that entails a flow of promised benefits that will exceed the inflow of taxes by about 2010. What, if anything, might be done about this? There have been several proposals, each of which will be discussed. But the point to keep in mind throughout is this: The entire burden of Social Security consists of the benefits that it promises to pay. Under the system currently in place, all of these benefits must be paid out of taxes levied on the American people. So unless we

Year	1935	1955	1975	2000
Payroll tax rate	2%	4%	11.7%	15.3%
Wage base to which tax is applied	$3,000	$4,200	$14,100	$72,600

Source: Social Security Administration and author's estimates.

TABLE 6-1
The Rise of Payroll Taxes
Both the payroll tax rate and the wage base are rising.

fundamentally alter the nature of the system, there are only four options—or combinations of these four options—for preserving the current social compact: (1) raise taxes, (2) reduce the number of people eligible for benefits, (3) cut the amount of benefits each person is eligible to receive, or (4) find a way to make the funding base of the system grow at a more robust rate.

Raising Taxes

The history of Social Security has been one of steadily increasing tax rates, applied to an ever-increasing wage base. Table 6-1 shows the tax rate (which includes Medicare taxes since 1965) for selected years, and the wage base to which that tax rate is applied.

The combination of a rising tax rate and a taxable base that in recent years has grown faster than the inflation rate means that payroll taxes are becoming an increasingly important source of revenue for the federal government. Indeed, as revealed in Figure 6-4, payroll taxes are now almost 40 times as important to the federal government as they were 65 years ago.

Given the steady rise in both the tax rate and the wage base to which it applies, it is perhaps not surprising that many of the proposals for "reforming" Social Security advocate more of the same: Raise the tax rate or increase the wage base. For example, one prominent proposal calls for increasing the payroll tax rate by 2.2 percentage points, lifting the overall rate to 17.5 percent. Such a move would generate additional tax collections of about $80 billion per year initially, an amount equivalent to a 10 percent increase in everyone's personal taxes. This is a huge tax hike, amounting to $880 per year for a worker earning $40,000; indeed, this would be the largest tax increase of any type in our nation's history. Even so, it will *at best* keep current taxes above current benefits until 2020, after which the system will again be in deficit. Although the long-run tax hike that it will take to keep

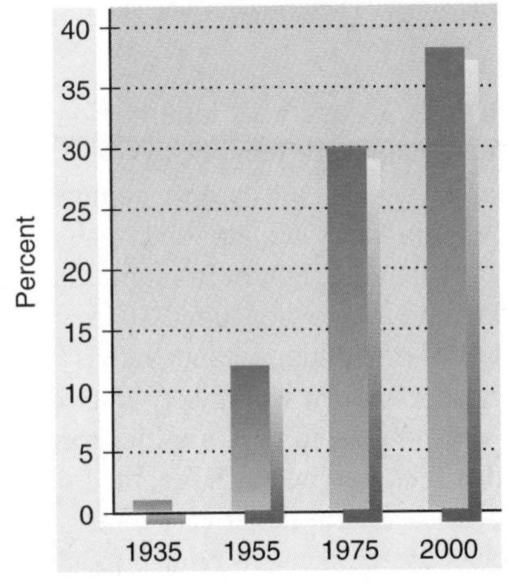

FIGURE 6-4
Payroll Taxes as a Share of Total Federal Tax Receipts, 1935–2000
Payroll taxes account for an increasing share of total federal tax revenues.
Sources: Social Security Administration, Council of Economic Advisers, and author's estimates.

Social Security solvent is subject to considerable uncertainty, best estimates now put that tax increase at around *seven* percentage points, not 2.2. Just to cover Social Security's projected deficits, the payroll tax will have to be increased to more than 22 percent.

Eliminating the Wage Cap

Another proposal is to eliminate the cap on the level of wages to which the payroll tax is applied. (This cap was lifted several years ago for the 2.9 percent Medicare component of payroll taxes.) All wage and salaries payments to workers would then be subject to the full brunt of payroll taxes. Although this proposal would not alter the tax obligations of workers earning less than $72,600 per year, it would result in a big hike in the marginal tax rate paid by millions of American workers. Indeed, the top rate paid would become 54.9 percent, the highest since the 1970s. Moreover, although this too would generate about $80 billion per year in additional tax revenues, it is not a long-term solution: Given projected benefit levels, the tax rate will eventually have to be increased. In fact, even the combination of eliminating the wage cap and a 2.2 percentage point tax increase is not enough to keep tax collections above benefit payments over the long run.

Cutting Benefits

The alternative to an increase in taxes is a cut in benefits. A small step in this direction has actually been taken, although not for the express purpose of reducing Social Security obligations. During the late 1990s, the Bureau of Labor Statistics revised the CPI to take better account of quality improvements in goods. One of the side effects of these revisions was to reduce slightly the upward bias in the CPI and thus reduce slightly the amount by which real benefits will be increased due to future cost-of-living adjustments.

No one has proposed cutting statutory benefits for existing retirees; future retirees are the target. One possibility is to raise the age of full eligibility. The eligibility age rose to 67 in 1999, but it could be increased further, perhaps to as high as 70. Another option is to cut benefits that are paid to nonworking spouses. A third proposal is to impose "means testing" on some or all Social Security benefits. As things stand now, all individuals covered by the system collect benefits when they retire, regardless of their assets or other sources of retirement income. Under a system of means testing, individuals with substantial alternative sources of retirement income would receive reduced Social Security benefits.

Immigration

Many experts believe that significant changes in America's immigration laws could offer the best hope for dealing with the tax burdens and workforce shrinkage of the future. About a million immigrants come to America each year, the largest number in our nation's history. Yet more than 90 percent of new immigrants are admitted on the basis of a selection system unchanged since 1952, under which the right of immigration is tied to family relationships. As a result, most people are admitted to the United States because they happen to be the spouses, children, or siblings of earlier immigrants, rather than because they have skills or training highly valued in the American workplace. Both Canada and Australia have modified their immigration laws to expand opportunities for immigrants who possess skills in short supply, with results that are generally regarded quite favorably in both nations. Unless Congress manages to overhaul America's immigration preference system, the taxes paid by new immigrants are unlikely to relieve much of the pressure building due to our aging population.

Investing in the Stock Market

Historically high returns were earned on most stock market investments during the 1990s. It is thus not surprising that some observers, including members of the Clinton administration, advocated that the Social Security system purchase stocks rather than Treasury bonds with the current excess of payroll taxes over current benefit payments. (Because this would necessitate that the Treasury borrow more from the public, this amounts to having the government borrow money from the public for the purpose of investing in the stock market.)

Although the added returns on stock investments could help stave off tax increases or benefit cuts, there are a few potential problems with this proposal. First, the rate of return on stocks during the 1990s was high by historical standards; we cannot expect such returns routinely in the future.

Second, the extra returns on stock market investments are not a sure thing; after all, during the early 1930s, the stock market dropped in value by nearly 90 percent. Despite the stock market's higher long-term returns, the inherent uncertainty of those returns is not entirely consistent with the function of Social Security as a source of *guaranteed* retirement income.

Finally, and most important, there is the issue of what stocks to invest in. There would surely be political pressure to invest in companies that happened to be politically popular and to refrain from investing in those that were unpopular, regardless of their returns. This sort of politically motivated investing would definitely reduce the expected returns from the government's stock portfolio—possibly even below the returns on Treasury bonds. This is exactly what has happened in Singapore: Workers there are required to pay 20 percent of their salary into the government-run Provident Fund, which has earned returns substantially below the market average.

INTERNATIONAL EXAMPLE

Privatizing Pensions in Chile

In 1981, Chile's state-run pension system was effectively bankrupt. So the government set up a mandatory system that was privately operated and funded. Workers were required to pay a minimum of 10 percent of their income each year into a private retirement account that the workers owned and controlled. To compensate workers for the public pensions they were giving up, the government issued "recognition bonds" that reflected the value of prior contributions to the old system. The government promised to redeem these bonds upon worker retirement, with the funding to come from a mixture of selling off state-owned enterprises and taxes on future workers and businesses.

The system is generally popular and well regarded by participants, perhaps in part because returns have averaged 13 percent per year. Annual retirement benefits are expected to be 50 percent to 70 percent above those payable under the old system. Nevertheless, the system is not flawless. Management charges on the retirement accounts have averaged nearly 3 percent per year, more than double the average charge on similar voluntary funds in the United States. Just as important, funds were initially restricted to investing only in Chile, a fact that depressed returns during the early years. Fund managers can now invest overseas, but 99 percent of fund assets remain invested in Chile, due to a peculiar incentive system imposed by the government. If a fund's return in any 12-month period is over two percentage points below the average for all funds, the firm managing that fund must make good the shortfall from its own capital. But there is no reward for outperforming the other funds. Not surprisingly, all of the funds have similar portfolios, and these portfolios are less risky—and yield lower average returns—than would be the case without this government-imposed reimbursement scheme.

For Critical Analysis

If the United States were to contemplate privatizing Social Security, what lessons might it learn from Chile's experience?

Growing the Economy

One way for the current Social Security problem to "go away" would be for the U.S. economy to grow at a faster pace. This would cause wages and salaries, which typically comprise more than 70 percent of total U.S. income, to increase, thereby expanding the tax base of the Social Security system. Additional funds would then flow into the Social Security system each year, thereby helping preserve the program's solvency.

As you learned in Chapter 2, expanding the economy's technological capabilities and producing more capital goods can help increase the nation's overall ability to produce and consume. Certainly, the U.S. economy has maintained steady growth in its productive capabilities. From the perspective of the Social Security system, however, the pace of growth has not been sufficient. As you will learn in Chapter 9, there are certain things that we could try to do to speed the pace of the nation's economic growth. Nevertheless, so far we have been unable to push the growth rate of national income much beyond 2 to 3 percent per year for more than a few years at a stretch. Saving the Social Security system without reforming it would require pushing long-term annual income growth up by at least 1 percentage point. In the absence of such a sustained increase in economic growth, the nation cannot postpone reforming its social compact.

CONCEPTS IN BRIEF

- One way or another, Social Security benefits will have to be cut, or taxes increased, or both.
- Although proposed tax increases will reduce the long-run Social Security deficit, no politicians have yet proposed raising them high enough to eliminate that deficit.
- Immigration would help the U.S. situation somewhat by increasing the workforce relative to the stock of retirees.
- Investing trust fund monies in the stock market might help, but there is a danger that political maneuvering with the funds would drastically reduce the returns.

ISSUES & APPLICATIONS

The Social Security Con Game

As we discussed in this chapter, Social Security offered retirees a rate of return in excess of 10 percent until around 1970. Given that the inflation-adjusted long-term rate of return on the stock market is about 10 percent, it is clear that for retirees, as noted, Social Security was an excellent deal for all beneficiaries until at least 1970 and for many until around 1990. But if investments on the stock market yielded only a 10 percent average real rate of return, how was Social Security able to offer such astonishingly high returns for so long? Moreover, why is it no longer able to do so?

Concepts Applied

Rate of Return

Inflation-adjusted Return

The answer is that Social Security has been operated exactly like a Ponzi scheme, named after Charles Ponzi, a con artist operating in Boston during the early 1920s. Ponzi offered potential investors returns much like those paid to early Social Security retirees and actually managed to pay them for a while, in the same manner Social Security paid them—out of the funds contributed by new entrants into the plan. Because nothing was actually being invested or even produced in the plan, Ponzi's scheme, to stay afloat, required increasing numbers of participants to make ever-larger contributions, used to pay off the promises made to earlier contributors. As soon as people realized what was going on, the scheme collapsed, and Ponzi was prosecuted for fraud and sent to jail—but not before 10,000 investors had been bilked.

Ponzi's Scheme

It is arguable that Social Security has operated in much the same manner since its inception, although its operation is legally sanctioned and it is not in danger of immediate collapse. At each point in time, current retirees are paid benefits out of the contributions of people who are currently working and paying in. (The contributions of today's retirees were long ago used to pay the benefits of previous retirees.) As membership growth slows, the rate of return falls. And as noted, because the early participants received more than they contributed, later participants must necessarily receive less—and that ultimately means a *negative* rate of return.

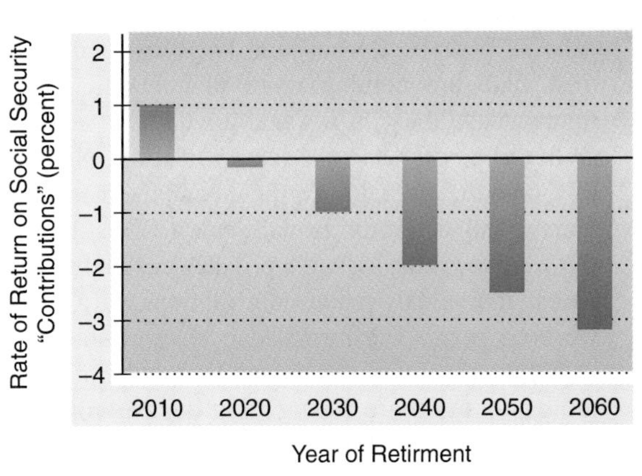

FIGURE 6-5

Projected Social Security Rates of Return for Future Retirees

While those who paid into Social Security in earlier years got a good deal, those who are now paying in and those who will pay in the future are facing low or negative rates of return.

Sources: Social Security Administration and author's estimates.

Parallels?

Indeed, as Figure 6-5 on the previous page shows, under any plausible assumptions about the future, unless the current Social Security system is changed, negative rates of returns will be the norm for retirees in the twenty-first century. In fact, for today's college students, who will begin retiring—if they can afford it—around 2040, in the absence of reform the situation looks particularly grim. As one economist has put it, "Today's students could get a better deal if they put their cash in a mattress—and then started smoking in bed." So unless you are not planning to retire, you'd better start saving now—or convincing your representatives in Congress to continue efforts to find a way to change the current system. Fortunately, there is every indication that the government is aware of the magnitude of the problem. It remains to be seen what proposed solution may ultimately be adopted.

FOR CRITICAL ANALYSIS

1. Based on what you have learned in this chapter, how might society find a way to avoid the negative projected rates of return displayed in Figure 6-5?
2. If the U.S. economy had grown at a much faster pace than it actually did between its inception and the present, would Social Security now look so much like a Ponzi scheme?

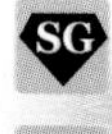

SUMMARY DISCUSSION OF LEARNING OBJECTIVES

1. **The Fundamental Problem That Social Security and Medicare Pose for Today's Students:** Both programs have promised (and paid) benefits far in excess of the amounts that can be sustained, given the taxes levied to finance the programs. In the future, taxes will have to be higher and benefits lower, and it is today's students who will suffer on both counts. In fact, the rate of return on both programs will almost surely be negative for anyone who is today under the age of 30. It is not surprising that Americans who are currently retired and those who are about to retire are very much in favor of keeping Social Security just the way it has always been. They have realized a very high rate of return on their "contributions" to the Social Security System.
2. **The Effect of Medicare on the Incentives to Consume Medical Services:** Medicare subsidizes the consumption of medical services by the elderly. As a result, the quantity consumed is higher, and so is the price per unit of those services. Thus Americans spend a larger proportion of GDP on medical care than any other nation in the world. Medicare also encourages people to consume medical services that are very low in value relative to the cost of providing them and places a substantial tax burden on other sectors of the economy. As Medicare has increasingly taken over the medical costs of the elderly, they have responded rationally by demanding more and better services. When the government foots the bill, decisions about what health services to purchase are not the same as in the private sector, where individuals pay the full opportunity cost of the products or services they use.
3. **The Myth That the Social Security Trust Fund Is a Stock of Savings:** Social Security benefits must be paid out of taxes. Because the Treasury bonds in the trust fund are nothing more than claims against future taxes, they do not add anything to society's ability to pay for Social Security benefits. Nonetheless, both the federal government and the media continue to talk about the Social Security Trust Fund as if it were the same as, say, a private pension fund into which individuals make contributions during their working years. The formal existence of something called a trust fund has allowed the government and the media to ignore the fact that our current Social Security system is a pay-as-you-go system.

4. **The Key Forces That Caused the Tremendous Rise in Social Security Spending:** The first force was the emergence of a politically powerful generation of elderly, who felt deserving of a retirement subsidized by younger persons. The second force was the entry of the huge baby boom generation into the workforce, which greatly increased the amount of money available to pay retirement benefits to the elderly. An important mechanism for creating higher real benefits has been the cost-of-living adjustment. Because of an upward bias in the index used to calculate this adjustment, real Social Security benefits have increased by 50 percent over the past several decades. This upward bias, however, is less today than in the past. The federal government has made some small corrections in how it calculates the price index in order to reduce the upward bias.

5. **How Social Security Could Be Reformed:** Because future benefits vastly exceed future scheduled taxes, some combination of higher taxes and lower benefits will have to be implemented. The situation could also be eased a bit if more immigration into the country were permitted. But an even better long-term reform would be to begin phasing out the current system and replacing it with one that is entirely privately run. Many possible replacement programs have been proposed by politicians and economists alike. Some have pointed to the apparent success of the privatization of the social security system in Chile. However, changing from a public system to a private system faces enormous political roadblocks in the United States.

Key Terms and Concepts

Inflation-adjusted return (126)

Median age (121)

Rate of return (126)

Social Security contributions (126)

Problems Test

Answers to the odd-numbered problems appear at the back of the book.

6-1. Suppose you invest $100 today and receive in return $150 exactly one year from now. What is the rate of return on this investment? (Hint: What is the percentage by which next year's benefit exceeds—or falls short of—this year's cost?)

6-2. Suppose you invest $100 today and receive in return $80 exactly one year from now. What is the rate of return on this investment? (Hint: What is the percentage by which next year's benefit exceeds—or falls short of—this year's cost?)

6-3. Suppose your employer is paying you a wage of $10 per hour, and you are working 40 hours per week. Now the government imposes a $2 per hour tax on your employment: $1 is collected from your employer and $1 is collected from you. The proceeds of the tax are used by the government to buy for you groceries that are valued by you at exactly $80 per week. You are eligible for the grocery program only as long as you continue to work. Once the plan is in place, what hourly wage will the employer pay you?

6-4. Suppose that the current price of a CD-ROM drive is $100 and that people are buying 1 million drives per year. In order to improve computer literacy, the government decides to begin subsidizing the purchase of new CD-ROM drives. The government believes that the appropriate price is $60 per drive, so the program offers to send people cash for the difference between $60 and whatever the people pay for each drive they buy.

a. If no one changes his or her drive-buying behavior, how much will this program cost the taxpayers?

b. Will the subsidy cause people to buy more, less, or the same number of drives? Explain.

c. Suppose people end up buying 1.5 million drives once the program is in place. If the market price of drives does not change, how much will this program cost the taxpayers?

d. Under the assumption that the program causes people to buy 1.5 million drives and also causes the market price of drives to rise to $120, how much will this program cost the taxpayers?

6-5. Scans of internal organs using magnetic resonance imaging (MRI) devices are often covered by subsidized health insurance programs such as Medicare. Consider the following table illustrating hypothetical quantities of individual MRI testing procedures demanded and supplied at various prices, and then answer the questions that follow.

Price	Quantity Demanded	Quantity Supplied
$100	100,000	40,000
$300	90,000	60,000
$500	80,000	80,000
$700	70,000	100,000
$900	60,000	120,000

a. In the absence of a government-subsidized health plan, what is the equilibrium price of a battery of MRI tests? What is the amount of society's total expense on MRI tests?

b. Suppose that the government establishes a health plan guaranteeing that all qualified participants can purchase MRI tests at an effective price (that is, out-of-pocket cost) to the individual of $100 per set of tests. How many batteries of MRI tests will people consume?

c. What is the per-unit cost incurred by producers to provide the amount of MRI tests demanded at the government-guaranteed price of $100? What is society's total expense on MRI tests?

d. Under the government's coverage of MRI tests, what is the per-unit subsidy it provides? What is the total subsidy that the government pays to support MRI testing at its guaranteed price?

6-6. Suppose that the following Social Security reform became law: All current Social Security recipients will continue to receive their benefits, but no increase will be made other than cost-of-living adjustments; Americans between age 40 and retirement not yet on Social Security can opt to continue with the current system; those who opt out can place what they would have "contributed" to Social Security into one or more government-approved mutual funds; and those under 40 must place their "contributions" into one or more government-approved mutual funds.

Now answer the following questions:

a. Who will be in favor of this reform and why?

b. Who will be against this reform and why?

c. What might happen to stock market indexes?

d. What additional risk is involved for those who end up in the private system?

e. What additional benefits are possible for the people in the private system?

f. Which firms in the mutual fund industry might not be approved by the federal government and why?

Economics on the Net

Social Security Privatization There are many proposals for reforming Social Security, but only one fundamentally alters the nature of the current system: privatization. The purpose of this exercise is to learn more about what would happen if Social Security were privatized.

Title: Social Security Privatization

Navigation: Click here to learn about Social Security Privatization. The entries you'll want to use are in the left-hand column.

Application For each of the entries noted, read the entry and answer the question.

1. Click on *African Americans and Social Security.* What are the likely consequences of Social Security privatization for African Americans? Why?

2. Click on *Women and Social Security.* What are the likely consequences of Social Security privatization for women? Why?

3. Click on *Low-Wage Workers and Social Security.* What are the likely consequences of Social Security privatization for low-wage workers? Why?

For Group Study and Analysis Taking into account the mix of gender, ethnic background, and other factors, is your group as a whole likely to be made better off or worse off if Social Security is privatized? Should your decision to support or oppose privatization be based solely on how it affects you personally? Or should your decision take into account how it might affect others in your group?

It will be worthwhile for those not nearing retirement age to examine what the "older" generation thinks about the idea of privatizing the Social Security system in the United States. So create two groups—one for and one against privatization. Each group will examine the following Web site and come up with arguments in favor or against the ideas expressed on it.

Click here to visit the Social Security Network homepage. Make sure that each side in this debate carefully reads the pages on the stance of the organization. Accept or rebut each statement, depending on the side to which you have been assigned. Be prepared to defend your reasons with more than just your feelings. At a minimum, be prepared to present arguments that are logical, if not entirely backed by facts.

TYING IT ALL TOGETHER

Part One Case Problem

Case Background

Cyber Dynamics International Corporation (CDI) is engaged in both business-to-consumer and business-to-business Internet applications as well as the production and distribution of new software programs. CDI is based in Singapore, but it sells its products and services throughout the world, including in the United States.

The management of CDI is well aware of the fact that in the Internet world everything happens at, well, Internet speed. New competitors are getting stronger every day. One of them appears to be Global Online Services. Indeed, in a recent planning meeting at CDI, the chief executive officer asked her management team to look into expanding into new areas on the Internet, new software applications, and new countries.

A week later the various officers and managers of the company have come forth with the following recommendations:

1. Lower the price of Internet access to compete more aggressively with Global Online Services and America Online.
2. Add numerous new features to the company's existing popular business accounting program and raise its price.
3. Break up the existing advertising and sales division into two separate divisions.
4. Open a major software manufacturing plant somewhere in the United States.
5. Enter into a partnership with a software company in the People's Republic of China.
6. Create a new employee's benefit in the form of a pension plan that will pay loyal workers a certain sum of money every month after they retire.

Points to Analyze

1. Do you think it matters that CDI's headquarters are in Singapore? To whom might it matter and why?
2. In recommendation number 1 above, a manager suggested that the company lower its price of Internet access. If it does, will the number of Internet access subscribers increase or decrease? Under what circumstances will total revenues increase? Decrease?
3. If the company's accounting program is enhanced, under what circumstances might it be able to raise the price and actually sell more copies?
4. Recommendation number 3 argues in favor of splitting up a division into two separate parts. What famous economist might applaud this action and why?
5. If you were in charge of deciding whether to support the recommendation that a software manufacturing plant be located in the United States, what are some of the factors that you

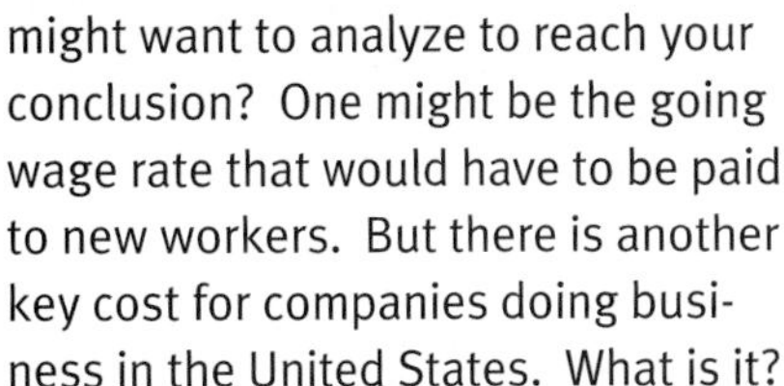

might want to analyze to reach your conclusion? One might be the going wage rate that would have to be paid to new workers. But there is another key cost for companies doing business in the United States. What is it?

6. While you might be convinced that entering the marketplace in the People's Republic of China is an exciting prospect ("everybody's doing it") there might be some problems with going into partnership with an existing Chinese company. Think about the economic functions of government that you learned in Chapter 5. Which function (or lack thereof) might create the biggest problem for your company's new partnership in China?

7. While the suggestion to create a new employee benefit involving a retirement system might seem appealing because it would attract more and better workers, would you want to offer the same retirement plan to your workers in all countries? What government-funded institution should you examine first in each country before you make such a decision?

Cruising the Internet

1. **Click here to go to the Web site of Global Online Services. Once on this site, navigate through some of the sections.**
   a. **What part of the world is the main focus of the activities of this company?**
   b. **What various types of products does this company produce?**
   c. **Why do you suppose that there are so many informational Web pages located at this company's home page?**
   d. **The advertisements at this Web site relate to this company only. Could Global Online Services gain from allowing others to place advertisements at its site?**
   e. **Is it likely that other companies would want to place ads at this Web site? Why or why not?**

2. **Now click here to go to the Web site for Global Online Electronic Services.**
   a. **Do you think that this company competes directly with Global Online Services? Why or why not?**
   b. **To what audience is that Web site addressing itself?**
   c. **Under what circumstances would you want to purchase the services of Global Online Electronic Services?**

3. **Go to any popular search engine, such as Yahoo.com, Profusion.com, Google.com, or Lycos.com. Type in the word "global" and see what happens.**
   a. **Why do you think so many companies include the word global in their names today?**

   Do the same thing with typing the word "online" and see what happens.

   b. **Why do so many companies what to include the word online in their names today?**

Part 2

Introduction to Macroeconomics and Economic Growth

CHAPTER 7

THE MACROECONOMY: UNEMPLOYMENT, INFLATION, AND DEFLATION

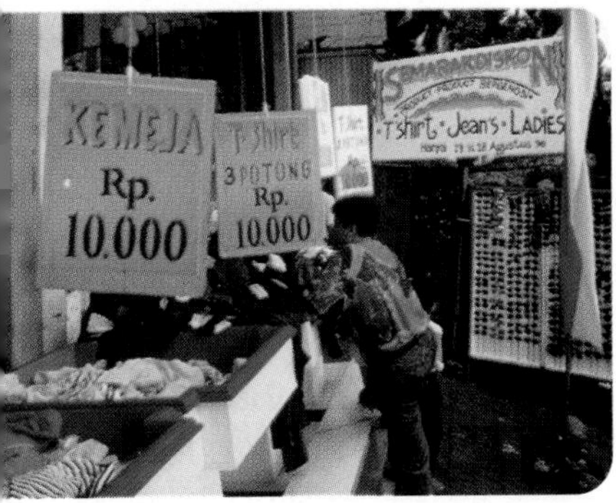

These signs in front of a shop in Bandung, the capital of West Java province in Indonesia, tell a tale of falling prices. Who is hurt by deflation?

For years, people have complained about rising prices for pretty much everything except electronics. Indeed, most Americans alive today have never experienced a time when the average of all prices did not go up, year in and year out. That has been true for people everywhere else in the world, too. So it came as a shock to learn that at the end of the 1990s, the average of all prices was no longer rising much in many parts of the world. Some countries, such as Japan, were even experiencing *falling* prices. Could falling prices cause serious problems in Asia? Could they spill over to Europe? Might there be repercussions in the United States? Before you can answer these questions, you need to learn more about unemployment, inflation, and deflation.

LEARNING OBJECTIVES

After reading this chapter, you should be able to:

1. Explain how the U.S. government calculates the official unemployment rate
2. Discuss the types of unemployment
3. Describe how price indexes are calculated and review the key types of price indexes
4. Distinguish between nominal and real interest rates
5. Evaluate who loses and who gains from inflation
6. Understand key features of business fluctuations

Chapter Outline

- Unemployment
- Inflation and Deflation
- Changing Inflation and Unemployment: Business Fluctuations

Did You Know That... although the United States is considered a highly advanced industrialized nation, less and less of its employment is involved in manufacturing? The same is true of Japan, Germany, France, Italy, and the United Kingdom, where the number of manufacturing workers has been dropping steadily since 1970, despite significant increases in total adult population. Yet the result has *not* been workers permanently out of jobs. Even so, work is a major policy issue facing many countries today. At the core of macroeconomics—the study of the performance and structure of the national economy—are the issues of employment and, more importantly, unemployment.

UNEMPLOYMENT

Unemployment The total number of adults (aged 16 years or older) who are willing and able to work and who are actively looking for work but have not found a job.

Unemployment is normally defined as adults actively looking for work, but without a job. Unemployment creates a cost to the entire economy in terms of lost output. One researcher estimated that at the beginning of the 1990s when unemployment was about 7 percent and factories were running at 80 percent of their capacity, the amount of output that the economy lost due to idle resources was almost 4 percent of the total production throughout the United States. (In other words, we were somewhere inside the production possibilities curve that we talked about in Chapter 2.) That was the equivalent of almost $275 billion of schools, houses, restaurant meals, cars, and movies that *could have been* produced. It is no wonder that policymakers closely watch the unemployment figures published by the Department of Labor's Bureau of Labor Statistics.

On a more personal level, the state of being unemployed often results in hardship and failed opportunities as well as a lack of self-respect. Psychological researchers believe that being fired creates at least as much stress as the death of a close friend. The numbers that we present about unemployment can never fully convey its true cost to this or any other nation.

Historical Unemployment Rates

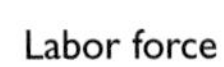

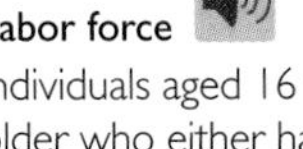

Labor force Individuals aged 16 years or older who either have jobs or are looking and available for jobs; the number of employed plus the number of unemployed.

The unemployment rate, defined as a proportion of the measured **labor force** that is unemployed, reached a low of 1.2 percent of the labor force at the end of World War II, after having reached 25 percent during the Great Depression in the 1930s. You can see in Figure 7-1 what happened to unemployment in the United States over the past century. The highest level ever was reached in the Great Depression, but unemployment was also very high during the Panic of 1893.

Employment, Unemployment, and the Labor Force

Figure 7-2 presents the population of individuals 16 years of age or older broken into three segments: (1) employed, (2) unemployed, and (3) not in the civilian labor force (a category that includes homemakers, full-time students, children, military personnel, persons in institutions, and retired persons). The employed and the unemployed, added together, make up the labor force. In 2000, the labor force amounted to 135.4 million + 5.8 million = 141.2 million Americans. To calculate the unemployment rate, we simply divide the number of unemployed by the number of people in the labor force and multiply by 100: 5.8 million/141.2 million × 100 = 4.1 percent.

FIGURE 7-1

More than a Century of Unemployment

Unemployment reached lows during World Wars I and II of less than 2 percent and highs during the Great Depression of more than 25 percent.

Source: U.S. Department of Labor, Bureau of Labor Statistics.

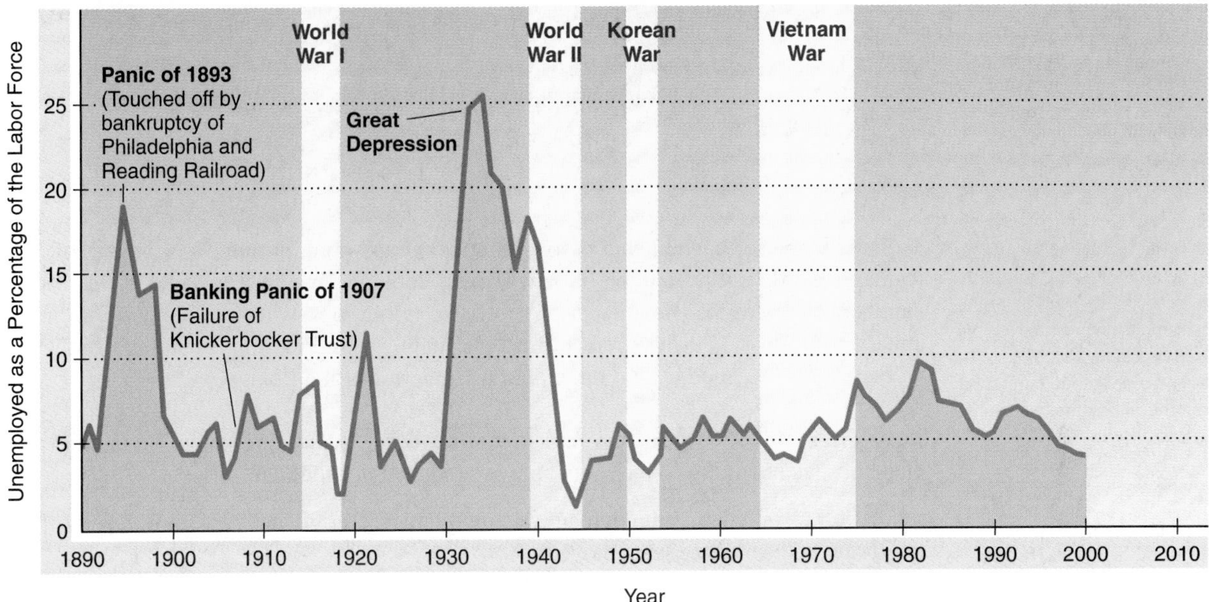

The Arithmetic Determination of Unemployment

Because there is a transition between employment and unemployment at any point in time—people are leaving jobs and others are finding jobs—there is a simple relationship between the employed and the unemployed, as can be seen in Figure 7-3 on page 148. People departing jobs are shown at the top of the diagram, and people taking new jobs are shown at the bottom. If job leavers and job finders are equal, the unemployment rate stays the same. If departures exceed new hires, the unemployment rate rises.

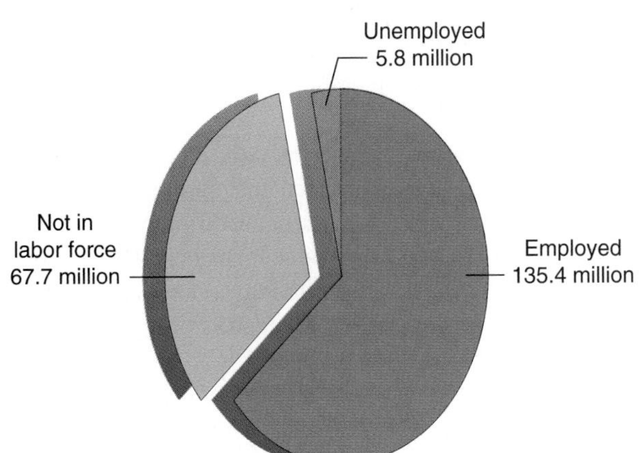

FIGURE 7-2

Adult Population

The population aged 16 and older can be broken down into three groups: people who are employed, those who are unemployed, and those not in the labor force.

Source: U.S. Department of Labor, Bureau of Labor Statistics.

FIGURE 7-3 

The Logic of the Unemployment Rate

Individuals who leave jobs but remain in the labor force are subtracted from the employed and added to the unemployed. When the unemployed find jobs, they are subtracted from the unemployed and added to the employed. In an unchanged labor force, if both flows are equal, the unemployment rate is stable. If more people leave jobs than find them, the unemployment rate increases, and vice versa.

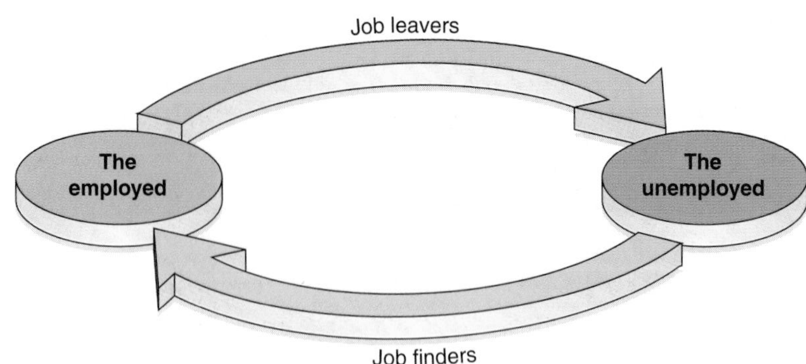

Stock 
The quantity of something, measured at a given point in time—for example, an inventory of goods or a bank account. Stocks are defined independently of time, although they are assessed at a point in time.

Flow 
A quantity measured per unit of time; something that occurs over time, such as the income you make per week or per year or the number of individuals who are fired every month.

Job loser 
An individual in the labor force whose employment was involuntarily terminated.

Reentrant 
An individual who used to work full time but left the labor force and has now reentered it looking for a job.

Job leaver 
An individual in the labor force who quits voluntarily.

New entrant 
An individual who has never held a full-time job lasting two weeks or longer but is now seeking employment.

Discouraged workers 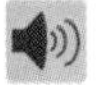
Individuals who have stopped looking for a job because they are convinced that they will not find a suitable one.

The number of unemployed is some number at any point in time. It is a **stock** of individuals who do not have a job but are actively looking for one. The same is true for the number of employed. The number of people departing jobs, whether voluntarily or involuntarily, is a **flow,** as is the number of people finding jobs. Picturing a bathtub like the one in Figure 7-4 is a good way of remembering how stocks and flows work.

Categories of Individuals Who Are Without Work. According to the Bureau of Labor Statistics, an unemployed individual may fall into any of four categories:

1. A **job loser,** whose employment was involuntarily terminated or who was laid off (40 to 60 percent of the unemployed)
2. A **reentrant,** having worked a full-time job before but having been out of the labor force (20 to 30 percent of the unemployed)
3. A **job leaver,** who voluntarily ended employment (less than 10 to around 15 percent of the unemployed)
4. A **new entrant,** who has never worked a full-time job for two weeks or longer (10 to 13 percent of the unemployed)

Duration of Unemployment. If you are out of a job for a week, your situation is typically much less serious than if you are out of a job for 14 weeks. An increase in the duration of unemployment can increase the unemployment rate because workers stay unemployed longer, thereby creating a greater number of them at any given time. The most recent information on duration of unemployment paints the following picture: 37.1 percent of those who become unemployed find a new job by the end of one month, an additional 31.8 percent find a job by the end of two months, and only 16.3 percent are still unemployed after six months. The average duration of unemployment for all unemployed has been 15.2 weeks over the past decade.

When overall business activity goes into a downturn, the duration of unemployment tends to rise, thereby causing much of the increase in the estimated unemployment rate. In a sense, then, it is the increase in the *duration* of unemployment during a downturn in national economic activity that generates the bad news that concerns policymakers in Washington, D.C. Furthermore, the individuals who stay unemployed longer than six months are the ones who create the pressure on Congress to "do something." What Congress does typically is extend and supplement unemployment benefits.

The Discouraged Worker Phenomenon. Critics of the published unemployment rate calculated by the federal government believe that it fails to reflect the true numbers of **discouraged workers** and "hidden unemployed." Though there is no exact definition or way

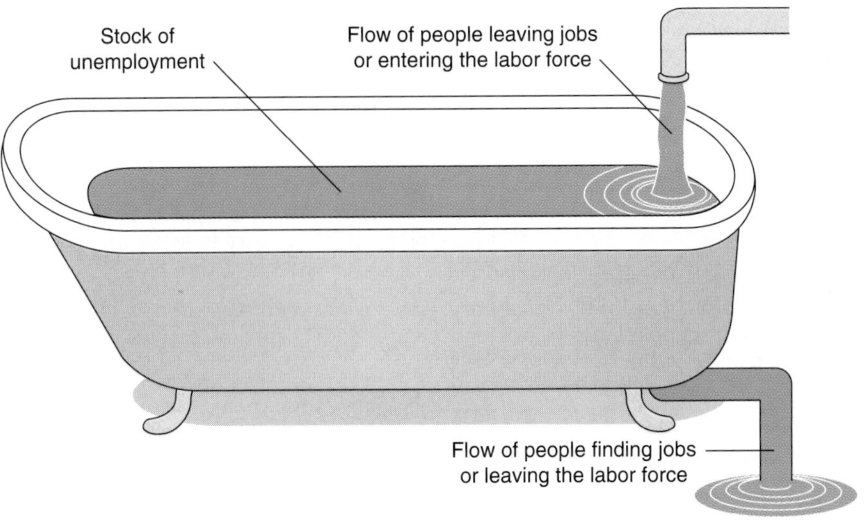

FIGURE 7-4
Visualizing Stocks and Flows
Unemployment at any point in time is some number that represents a stock, such as the amount of water in a bathtub. People who lose their jobs or enter the labor force constitute a new flow into the bathtub. Those who find jobs or leave the labor force can be thought of as the water that flows out by the drain.

to measure discouraged workers, the Department of Labor defines them as people who have dropped out of the labor force and are no longer looking for a job because they believe that the job market has little to offer them. To what extent do we want to include in the measured labor force individuals who voluntarily choose not to look for work or those who take only a few minutes a day to scan the want ads and then decide that there are no jobs?

Some economists argue that people who work part time but are willing to work full time should be classified as "semihidden" unemployed. Estimates range as high as 6 million workers at any one time. Offsetting this factor, though, is *overemployment.* An individual working 50 or 60 hours a week is still counted as only one full-time worker.

Labor Force Participation. The way in which we define unemployment and membership in the labor force will affect what is known as the **labor force participation rate.** It is defined as the proportion of working-age individuals who are employed or seeking employment.

Labor force participation rate 
The percentage of noninstitutionalized working-age individuals who are employed or seeking employment.

Figure 7-5 illustrates the labor force participation rates since 1950. The major change has been the increase in female labor force participation. If we take into account only

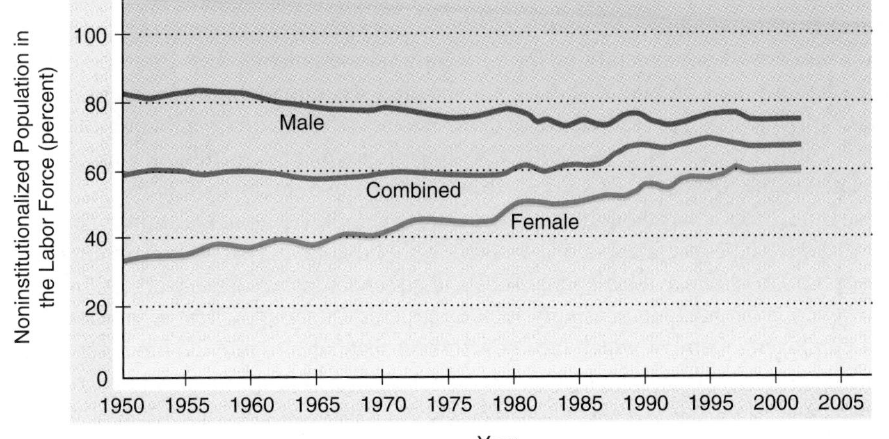

FIGURE 7-5
Labor Force Participation Rates by Sex
The combined labor force participation rate has increased in recent years. However, over the same period, the male participation rate has fallen, and the female rate has risen markedly.
Source: U.S. Department of Labor, Bureau of Labor Statistics, including projections.

married women aged 25 to 34, this increase is even more striking because it occurred over a shorter period of time. In 1960, about 29 percent of such women participated in the labor force outside of the home, compared with nearly 75 percent today.

CONCEPTS IN BRIEF

- Unemployed persons are adults who are willing and able to work and are actively looking for a job but have not found one. The unemployment rate is computed by dividing the number of unemployed by the total labor force, which is equal to those who are employed plus those who are unemployed.
- The unemployed are job losers, reentrants, job leavers, and new entrants to the labor force. The flow of people leaving jobs and people finding jobs determines the stock of unemployed as well as the stock of employed.
- The duration of unemployment affects the unemployment rate. The number of unemployed workers can remain the same, but if the duration of unemployment increases, the measured unemployment rate will go up.
- Whereas overall labor force participation has risen only a bit since World War II, there has been a major increase in female labor force participation, particularly among married women between the ages of 25 and 34.

The Major Types of Unemployment 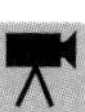

Unemployment has been categorized into four basic types: frictional, structural, cyclical, and seasonal.

Frictional Unemployment. Of the more than 135 million Americans in the labor force, more than 13 million will have either changed jobs or taken new jobs during the year; every single month, about one worker in 20 will have quit, been laid off (told to expect to be rehired later), or been permanently fired; another 6 percent will have gone to new jobs or returned to old ones. In the process, more than 20 million persons will have reported themselves unemployed at one time or another. What we call **frictional unemployment** is the continuous flow of individuals from job to job and in and out of employment. There will always be some frictional unemployment as resources are redirected in the market because transaction costs are never zero. To eliminate frictional unemployment, we would have to prevent workers from leaving their present jobs until they had already lined up other jobs at which they would start working immediately, and we would have to guarantee first-time job seekers a job *before* they started looking.

Frictional unemployment 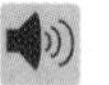
Unemployment due to the fact that workers must search for appropriate job offers. This takes time, and so they remain temporarily unemployed.

Structural Unemployment. Structural changes in our economy cause some workers to become unemployed permanently or for very long periods of time because they cannot find jobs that use their particular skills. This is called **structural unemployment.** Structural unemployment is not caused by general business fluctuations, although business fluctuations may affect it. And unlike frictional unemployment, structural unemployment is not related to the movement of workers from low-paying to high-paying jobs.

Structural unemployment 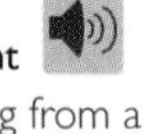
Unemployment resulting from a poor match of workers' abilities and skills with current requirements of employers.

At one time, economists thought about structural unemployment only from the perspective of workers. The concept applied to workers who did not have the ability, training, and skills necessary to obtain available jobs. Today, it still encompasses these workers. In addition, however, economists increasingly look at structural unemployment from the viewpoint of employers, many of which face government mandates to provide funds for social insurance programs for their employees, to announce plant closings months or even years in advance, and so on. There is now considerable evidence that government labor market policies influence how many positions businesses wish to fill, thereby affecting structural unemployment. In the United States, many businesses appear to have adjusted by hiring more "temporary workers" or establishing short-term contracts with "private consultants," which may have reduced the extent of U.S. structural unemployment in recent years. A similar adjustment to government labor market mandates may be taking place in Europe.

INTERNATIONAL EXAMPLE

Structural Unemployment in Europe Never Seems to Go Away

From 1980 to 2000, about 33 million jobs were created in the United States, mostly in the private sector. Yet in the European Union (EU), virtually no private-sector jobs were created during the same period. As U.S. unemployment dropped to a 30-year low of 4.1 percent, EU unemployment stayed well above 10 percent. Any modestly trained outside observer understands why the EU is in such trouble: high taxes paid by employers on all employees and rigid labor markets. Employers pay their governments an amount equal to 50 to 200 percent of employees' wages as "social charges." Moreover, government-mandated minimum wages often far exceed the value low-skilled workers might contribute to potential employers. Consequently, many low-skilled unemployed are unable to find jobs. Firing workers is legally difficult and always costly because obligatory severance pay is high. Even so, many fired European workers take their employers to court to try to regain their jobs or obtain even higher payments.

One result of this situation is that temporary employment is booming throughout Europe. One researcher estimated that 30 percent of the world's temporary labor market resides in France alone. Almost 90 percent of new hires in France, for example, are on short-term contracts.

Hardest hit is the portion of the labor force under age 25. In the EU, the average unemployment rate for that group is about 20 percent, and in France it exceeds 25 percent.

For Critical Analysis

If the reasons for the EU's high structural unemployment rate are so obvious, why aren't governments relaxing strict labor laws and reducing "social charges" levied on employers?

Cyclical Unemployment. **Cyclical unemployment** is related to business fluctuations. It is defined as unemployment associated with changes in business conditions—primarily recessions and depressions. The way to lessen cyclical unemployment would be to reduce the intensity, duration, and frequency of ups and downs of business activity. Economic policymakers attempt, through their policies, to reduce cyclical unemployment by keeping business activity on an even keel.

Cyclical unemployment
Unemployment resulting from business recessions that occur when aggregate (total) demand is insufficient to create full employment.

Seasonal Unemployment. **Seasonal unemployment** comes and goes with seasons of the year in which the demand for particular jobs rises and falls. In northern states, construction workers can often work only during the warmer months; they are seasonally unemployed during the winter. Summer resort workers can usually get jobs in resorts only during the summer season. They, too, become seasonally unemployed during the winter; the opposite is true for ski resort workers.

The unemployment rate that the Bureau of Labor Statistics releases each month is "seasonally adjusted." This means that the reported unemployment rate has been adjusted to remove the effects of variations in seasonal unemployment. Thus the unemployment rate that the media dutifully announce reflects only the sum of frictional unemployment, structural unemployment, and cyclical unemployment.

Seasonal unemployment
Unemployment resulting from the seasonal pattern of work in specific industries. It is usually due to seasonal fluctuations in demand or to changing weather conditions, rendering work difficult, if not impossible, as in the agriculture, construction, and tourist industries.

Full Employment

Does full employment mean that everybody has a job? Certainly not, for not everyone is looking for a job—full-time students and full-time homemakers, for example, are not. Is it possible for everyone who is looking for a job always to find one? No, because transaction costs in the labor market are not zero. Transaction costs include any activity whose goal is to enter into, carry out, or terminate contracts. In the labor market, these costs involve time spent looking for a job, being interviewed, negotiating the pay, and so on.

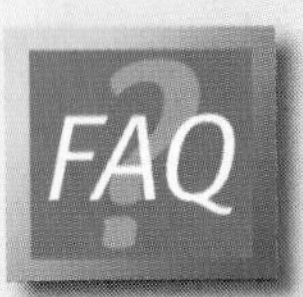

Isn't it true that much of today's employment consists of part-time jobs, contrary to the way it used to be?

That's the picture that seems to be written in the popular media, but it is inaccurate. Former Harvard Professor Lawrence Katz examined the data and discovered that despite minor ups and downs, there has not been a significant change in part-time employment in a decade and a half. Indeed, it is not much different from what it was 25 years ago. Moreover, surveys of part-time workers show that almost 80 percent of those interviewed say they do not want full-time jobs. These individuals include students, seniors, and parents with young children.

We will always have some frictional unemployment as individuals move in and out of the labor force, seek higher-paying jobs, and move to different parts of the country. **Full employment** is therefore a vague concept implying some sort of balance or equilibrium in an ever-shifting labor market. Of course, this general notion of full employment must somehow be put into numbers so that economists and others can determine whether the economy has reached the full-employment point.

Economists do this by estimating the **natural rate of unemployment,** the rate that is expected to prevail in the long run once all workers and employers have fully adjusted to any changes in the economy. If correctly estimated, the natural rate of unemployment should not reflect cyclical unemployment. When seasonally adjusted, the natural unemployment rate should take into account only frictional and structural unemployment.

Full employment 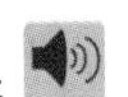
An arbitrary level of unemployment that corresponds to "normal" friction in the labor market. In 1986, a 6.5 percent rate of unemployment was considered full employment. Today, it is assumed to be 5 percent or possibly even less.

Natural rate of unemployment 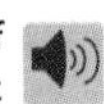
The rate of unemployment that is estimated to prevail in long-run macroeconomic equilibrium, when all workers and employers have fully adjusted to any changes in the economy.

A long-standing difficulty, however, has been a lack of agreement about how to estimate the natural unemployment rate. From the mid-1980s to the early 1990s, the President's Council of Economic Advisers (CEA) consistently estimated that the natural unemployment rate in the United States was about 6.5 percent. Even into the early 2000s, the approach to estimating the natural rate of unemployment that Federal Reserve staff economists have employed—which was intended to improve on the CEA's traditional method—yielded a natural rate just over 6 percent. Of course, when the measured unemployment rate fell below 5 percent in 1997 and hit 4.1 percent in 2000, economists began to rethink their approach to estimating the natural unemployment rate. This led some to alter their estimation methods to take into account such factors as greater rivalry among domestic businesses and increased international competition, which leads to an estimated natural rate of unemployment of roughly 5 percent. We shall return to the concept of the natural unemployment rate in Chapter 10.

Part of this reduction in the natural rate of unemployment in the United States may be due to a change in the age and sex composition of the labor force.

EXAMPLE

Why Is the Average Unemployment Rate Falling?

Of course, a booming economy for a decade has a lot to do with falling unemployment rates in the United States, which have become the envy of the world. But economists Robert Horn and Philip Heap of James Madison University believe that much of the change in the average unemployment rate has had to do with the change in the age and gender composition of the labor force. They point out that unemployment rates vary by age and to a lesser extent by gender. Thus any decreases in the relative importance of groups with historically high unemployment rates will reduce the overall unemployment rate. Specifically, they argue that the percentage of the labor force made up of teenage workers has dropped from 8.8 percent in 1970 to less than 6 percent today—thus reducing the overall unemployment rate. They further point out that the share of the labor force accounted for by women aged 25 to 44 rose from about 14 percent to almost 25 percent over the past three decades. This has tended also to reduce the unemployment rate, because women of this age bracket historically have lower unemployment rates than other groups. Their conclusion? If the age and gender composition of the labor force remains as it is today, the average rate of unemployment will also remain relatively low.

For Critical Analysis

Why do you think teenage unemployment rates are relatively high in general?

CONCEPTS IN BRIEF

- Frictional unemployment occurs because of transaction costs in the labor market. For example, workers do not have all the information necessary about vacancies. Structural unemployment occurs when the demand for a commodity permanently decreases so that workers find that the jobs that they are used to doing are no longer available.
- The level of frictional unemployment is used in part to determine our (somewhat arbitrary) definition of full employment.

INFLATION AND DEFLATION

During World War II, you could buy bread for 8 to 10 cents a loaf and have milk delivered fresh to your door for about 25 cents a half gallon. The average price of a new car was less than $700, and the average house cost less than $3,000. Today bread, milk, cars, and houses all cost more—a lot more. Prices are more than 10 times what they were in 1940. Clearly, this country has experienced quite a bit of *inflation* since then. We define **inflation** as an upward movement in the average level of prices. The opposite of inflation is **deflation,** defined as a downward movement in the average level of prices. Notice that these definitions depend on the *average* level of prices. This means that even during a period of inflation, some prices can be falling if other prices are rising at a faster rate. The prices of electronic equipment have dropped dramatically since the 1960s, even though there has been general inflation.

Inflation 
The situation in which the average of all prices of goods and services in an economy is rising.

Deflation 
The situation in which the average of all prices of goods and services in an economy is falling.

To discuss what has happened to prices here and in other countries, we have to know how to measure inflation.

Inflation and the Purchasing Power of Money

A rose is a rose is a rose, Gertrude Stein contended, but a dollar is not always a dollar. The value of a dollar does not stay constant when there is inflation. The value of money is usually talked about in terms of **purchasing power.** A dollar's purchasing power is the real goods and services that it can buy. Consequently, another way of defining inflation is as a decline in the purchasing power of money. The faster the rate of inflation, the greater the rate of decline in the purchasing power of money.

Purchasing power 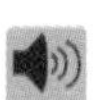
The value of money for buying goods and services. If your money income stays the same but the price of one good that you are buying goes up, your effective purchasing power falls, and vice versa.

One way to think about inflation and the purchasing power of money is to discuss dollar values in terms of *nominal* versus *real* values. The nominal value of anything is simply its price expressed in today's dollars. In contrast, the real value of anything is its value expressed in purchasing power, which varies with the overall price level. Let's say that you received a $100 bill from your grandparents this year. One year from now, the nominal value of that bill will still be $100. The real value will depend on what the purchasing power of money is after one year's worth of inflation. Obviously, if there has been a lot of inflation in one year, the real value of that $100 bill will have diminished.

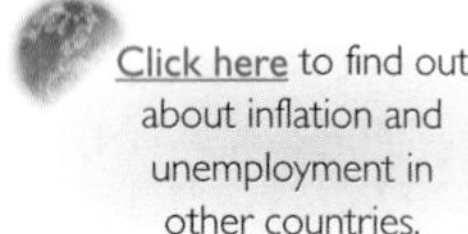

Click here to find out about inflation and unemployment in other countries.

Measuring the Rate of Inflation 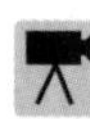

How can we measure the rate of inflation? This is a thorny problem for government statisticians. It is easy to determine how much the price of an individual commodity has risen: If last year a light bulb cost 50 cents and this year it costs 75 cents, there has been a 50 percent rise in the price of that light bulb over a one-year period. We can express the change in the individual light bulb price in one of several ways: The price has gone up 25 cents; the price is one and a half (1.5) times as high; the price has risen by 50 percent. An *index number* of this price rise is simply the second way (1.5) multiplied by 100, meaning that the index today would stand at 150. We multiply by 100 to eliminate decimals because it is easier to think in terms of percentage changes using integers. This is the standard convention adopted for convenience in dealing with index numbers or price levels.

Price index 
The cost of today's market basket of goods expressed as a percentage of the cost of the same market basket during a base year.

Base year 
The year that is chosen as the point of reference for comparison of prices in other years.

Computing a Price Index. The measurement problem becomes more complicated when it involves a large number of goods, especially if some prices have risen faster than others and some have even fallen. What we have to do is pick a representative bundle, a so-called market basket, of goods and compare the cost of that market basket of goods over time. When we do this, we obtain a **price index,** which is defined as the cost of a market basket of goods today, expressed as a percentage of the cost of that identical market basket of goods in some starting year, known as the **base year.**

$$\text{Price index} = \frac{\text{cost today of market basket}}{\text{cost of market basket in base year}} \times 100$$

In the base year, the price index will always be 100, because the year in the numerator and in the denominator of the fraction is the same; therefore, the fraction equals 1, and when we multiply it by 100, we get 100. A simple numerical example is given in Table 7-1. In the table, there are only two goods in the market basket—corn and computers. The *quantities* in the basket remain the same between the base year, 1992, and the current year, 2002; only the *prices* change. Such a *fixed-quantity* price index is the easiest to compute because the statistician need only look at prices of goods and services sold every year rather than actually observing how much of these goods and services consumers actually purchase each year.

Consumer Price Index (CPI) 
A statistical measure of a weighted average of prices of a specified set of goods and services purchased by wage earners in urban areas.

Producer Price Index (PPI) 
A statistical measure of a weighted average of prices of commodities that firms produce and sell.

GDP deflator 
A price index measuring the changes in prices of all new goods and services produced in the economy.

Real-World Price Indexes. Government statisticians calculate a number of price indexes. The most often quoted are the **Consumer Price Index (CPI),** the **Producer Price Index (PPI),** and the **GDP deflator.** The CPI attempts to measure changes only in the level of prices of goods and services purchased by wage earners. The PPI attempts to show what has happened to average price of goods and services produced and sold by a typical firm. There are also *wholesale price indexes* that track the price level for commodities that firms purchase from other firms. The GDP deflator attempts to show changes in the level of prices of all new goods and services produced in the economy. The most general indicator of inflation is the GDP deflator because it measures the changes in the prices of everything produced in the economy.

(1) Commodity Prices	(2) Market Basket Quantity	(3) 1992 Price per Unit	(4) Cost of Market Basket in 1992	(5) 2002 Price per Unit	(6) Cost of Market Basket at 200
Corn	100 bushels	$ 4	$ 400	$ 8	$ 800
Computers	2	500	1,000	425	850
Totals			$1,400		$1,650

$$\text{Price index} = \frac{\text{cost of market basket in 2002}}{\text{cost of market basket in base year 1992}} \times 100 = \frac{\$1{,}650}{\$1{,}400} \times 100 = 117.86$$

TABLE 7-1
Calculating a Price Index for a Two-Good Market Basket
In this simplified example, there are only two goods—corn and computers. The quantities and base-year prices are given in columns 2 and 3. The cost of the 1992 market basket, calculated in column 4, comes to $1,400. The 2002 prices are given in column 5. The cost of the market basket in 2002, calculated in column 6, is $1,650. The price index for 2002 compared with 1992 is 117.86.

The CPI. The Bureau of Labor Statistics (BLS) has the task of identifying a market basket of goods and services of the typical consumer. Today, the BLS uses as its base the time period 1982–1984. It intended to change the base to 1993–1995 but has yet to do so. It has, though, updated its market basket of goods to reflect consumer spending patterns for 1993–1995. All CPI numbers since February 1998 reflect the new expenditure weights.

Economists have known for years that the way the BLS measures changes in the Consumer Price Index is flawed. Specifically, the BLS has been unable to account for the way consumers substitute less expensive items for higher-priced items. The reason is that the CPI is a fixed-quantity price index, meaning that each month the BLS samples only prices, rather than relative quantities purchased by consumers. In addition, until recently, the BLS has been unable to take quality changes into account as they occur. Currently, though, the BLS is subtracting from certain list prices estimated effects of qualitative improvements and adding to other list prices for a deterioration in quality. A remaining flaw is that the CPI usually ignores successful new products until long after they have been introduced.

EXAMPLE

New Product Bias in the CPI: The Case of Cellular Phones

Any new product that is successful, by definition, makes the people who choose to purchase it better off. Successful new products should therefore reduce the cost of maintaining a given standard of living, and so successful new product introductions should reduce the CPI or at least lessen increases in it. Nevertheless, the government is often slow to recognize this fact when it calculates the CPI. Consider the research done by economist Jerry Hausman of MIT. He looked at cellular phones. Since the late 1980s, cell phone prices have dropped by 90 percent and quality has improved greatly. As of 1998, however, the price of cellular phones was still not included in the government's CPI calculations. Hausman estimated that Americans are $24 billion to $50 billion better off because cellular phones exist. That is about 0.5 percent of the nation's annual national output.

For Critical Analysis

"When people don't know about a new product, they don't miss it, and therefore they are not worse off." Analyze this statement.

The PPI. There are a number of Producer Price Indexes, including one for foodstuffs, another for intermediate goods (goods used in the production of other goods), and one for finished goods. Most of the producer prices included are in mining, manufacturing, and agriculture. The PPIs can be considered general-purpose indexes for nonretail markets.

Although in the long run the various PPIs and the CPI generally show the same rate of inflation, such is not the case in the short run. Most often the PPIs increase before the CPI because it takes time for producer price increases to show up in the prices that consumers pay for final products. Often changes in the PPIs are watched closely as a hint that inflation is going to increase or decrease.

The GDP Deflator. The broadest price index reported in the United States is the GDP deflator, where GDP stands for gross domestic product, or annual total national income. Unlike the CPI and the PPIs, the GDP deflator is not based on a fixed market basket of goods and services. The basket is allowed to change with people's consumption and investment patterns. In this sense, the changes in the GDP deflator reflect both price changes and the public's market responses to those price changes. Why? Because new expenditure patterns are allowed to show up in the GDP deflator as people respond to changing prices.

Historical Changes in the CPI. Until the mid-1990s, the Consumer Price Index showed a fairly dramatic trend upward since about World War II. Figure 7-6 shows the annual rate of change in the Consumer Price Index since 1860. Prior to World War II, there were numerous periods of deflation along with periods of inflation. Persistent year-in and year-out inflation seems to be a post–World War II phenomenon, at least in this country. As far back as before the American Revolution, prices used to rise during war periods but then would fall back to more normal levels afterward. This occurred after the Revolutionary War, the War of 1812, the Civil War, and to a lesser extent World War I. Consequently, the overall price level in 1940 wasn't much different from 150 years earlier.

POLICY EXAMPLE

The Labor Department Quietly Reduces Its Inflation Statistics

The Consumer Price Index has been inaccurate because it ignores many changes in quality, increased discount shopping at club warehouses, and other developments in the consumer market. The statisticians responsible for computing the CPI each month know this. As a result, they have made changes in the index. Without much fanfare, the Labor Department has modified the way it calculates the CPI. It altered its sampling procedure for food and nonfood items, and it made its treatment of rent, hospital prices, and generic drugs more accurate. After those adjustments, government-estimated inflation rates dropped by 0.2 to 0.3 percent. Further calculation changes in 1998 and 1999 reduced estimated inflation by another 0.75 percent.

For Critical Analysis

The government has not changed past published data on the CPI. Why is this fact important to a policymaker today?

CONCEPTS IN BRIEF

- Once we pick a market basket of goods, we can construct a price index that compares the cost of that market basket today with the cost of the same market basket in a base year.
- The Consumer Price Index (CPI) is the most often used price index in the United States. The Producer Price Index (PPI) is the second most mentioned.
- The GDP deflator measures what is happening to the average price level of *all* new, domestically produced final goods and services in our economy.

FIGURE 7-6

Inflation and Deflation in U.S. History

Since the Civil War, the United States has experienced alternating inflation and deflation. Here we show them as reflected by changes in the Consumer Price Index. Since World War II, the periods of inflation have not been followed by periods of deflation; that is, even during peacetime, the price index has continued to rise. The yellow areas represent wartime.

Source: U.S. Department of Labor, Bureau of Labor Statistics.

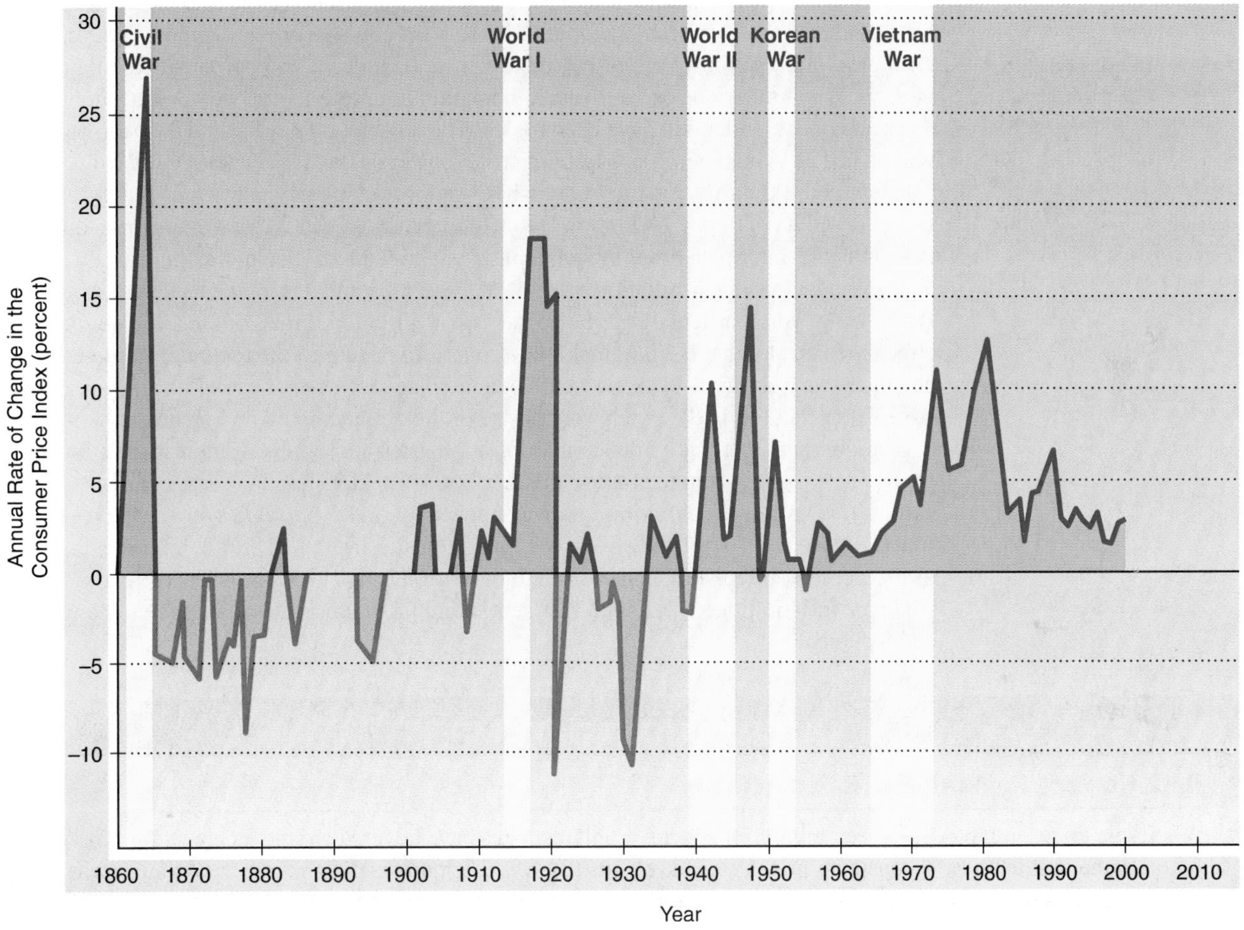

Anticipated Versus Unanticipated Inflation

To determine who is hurt by inflation and what the effects of inflation are in general, we have to distinguish between anticipated and unanticipated inflation. We will see that the effects on individuals and the economy are vastly different, depending on which type of inflation exists.

Anticipated inflation is the rate of inflation that the majority of individuals believe will occur. If the rate of inflation this year turns out to be 10 percent, and that's about what most people thought it was going to be, we are in a situation of fully anticipated inflation.

Unanticipated inflation is inflation that comes as a surprise to individuals in the economy. For example, if the inflation rate in a particular year turns out to be 10 percent when on average people thought it was going to be 5 percent, there will have been unanticipated inflation—inflation greater than anticipated.

Anticipated inflation 
The inflation rate that we believe will occur; when it does, we are in a situation of fully anticipated inflation.

Unanticipated inflation 
Inflation at a rate that comes as a surprise, either higher or lower than the rate anticipated.

Some of the problems caused by inflation arise when it is unanticipated, for when it is anticipated, many people are able to protect themselves from its ravages. Keeping the distinction between anticipated and unanticipated inflation in mind, we can easily see the relationship between inflation and interest rates.

Inflation and Interest Rates 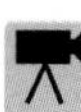

Nominal rate of interest The market rate of interest expressed in today's dollars.

Let's start in a hypothetical world in which there is no inflation and anticipated inflation is zero. In that world, you may be able to borrow money—to buy a computer or a car, for example—at a **nominal rate of interest** of, say, 10 percent. If you borrow the money to purchase a computer or a car and your anticipation of inflation turns out to be accurate, neither you nor the lender will have been fooled. The dollars you pay back in the years to come will be just as valuable in terms of purchasing power as the dollars that you borrowed.

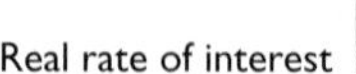 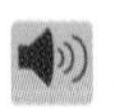

Real rate of interest The nominal rate of interest minus the anticipated rate of inflation.

What you ordinarily need to know when you borrow money is the *real rate of interest* that you will have to pay. The **real rate of interest** is defined as the nominal rate of interest minus the anticipated rate of inflation. If you are able to borrow money at 10 percent and you anticipated an inflation rate of 10 percent, your real rate of interest would be zero—lucky you, particularly if the actual rate of inflation turned out to be 10 percent. In effect, we can say that the nominal rate of interest is equal to the real rate of interest plus an *inflationary premium* to take account of anticipated inflation. That inflationary premium covers depreciation in the purchasing power of the dollars repaid by borrowers.*

There is fairly strong evidence that inflation rates and nominal interest rates move in parallel. Periods of rapid inflation create periods of high nominal interest rates. In the early 1970s, when the inflation rate was between 4 and 5 percent, average interest rates were around 8 to 10 percent. At the beginning of the 1980s, when the inflation rate was near 9 percent, interest rates had risen to between 12 and 14 percent. By the early 1990s, when the inflation rate was about 3 percent, nominal interest rates had fallen to between 4 and 8 percent.

INTERNATIONAL EXAMPLE

Deflation and Real Interest Rates in Japan

Wholesale prices in Japan have been falling for several years. In the past few years, consumer prices also have been falling, which means that Japan has been experiencing deflation. What does this have to do with real interest rates in Japan? Real interest rates are roughly equivalent to nominal, or market, rates minus the expected rate of inflation. Market interest rates are rarely negative. If the nominal interest rate a Japanese resident has to pay for a mortgage is 4 percent and the expected rate of *deflation* is 3 percent, then the expected real rate of interest is 7 percent, which is extremely high by historical standards. (In the United States, for example, real interest rates have hovered around 3 percent for most of its history.) The point is that in the United States, where we have learned to expect some inflation, we subtract that anticipated inflation from nominal interest rates to obtain real interest rates. In Japan, with expectations of deflation, the Japanese end up *adding* the expected deflationary rate to the nominal rate of interest to get real rates of interest.

For Critical Analysis

Why can't nominal interest rates be negative?

*Whenever there are relatively high rates of anticipated inflation, we must add an additional factor to the inflationary premium—the product of the real rate of interest times the anticipated rate of inflation. Usually this last term is omitted because the anticipated rate of inflation is not high enough to make much of a difference.

Does Inflation Necessarily Hurt Everyone?

Most people think that inflation is bad. After all, inflation means higher prices, and when we have to pay higher prices, are we not necessarily worse off? The truth is that inflation affects different people differently. Its effects also depend on whether it is anticipated or unanticipated.

Unanticipated Positive Inflation: Creditors Lose and Debtors Gain. In most situations, unanticipated inflation benefits borrowers because the nominal interest rate they are being charged does not fully compensate for the inflation that actually occurred. In other words, the lender did not anticipate inflation correctly. Whenever inflation rates are underestimated for the life of a loan, creditors lose and debtors gain. Periods of considerable unanticipated (higher than anticipated) inflation occurred in the late 1960s, the early 1970s, and the late 1970s. During those years, creditors lost and debtors gained.

Protecting Against Inflation. Banks attempt to protect themselves against inflation by raising nominal interest rates to reflect anticipated inflation. Adjustable-rate mortgages in fact do just that: The interest rate varies according to what happens to interest rates in the economy. Workers can protect themselves by **cost-of-living adjustments (COLAs),** which are automatic increases in wage rates to take account of increases in the price level.

Cost-of-living adjustments (COLAs) 
Clauses in contracts that allow for increases in specified nominal values to take account of changes in the cost of living.

To the extent that you hold non-interest-bearing cash, you will lose because of inflation. If you have put $100 in a mattress and the inflation rate is 10 percent for the year, you will have lost 10 percent of the purchasing power of that $100. If you have your funds in a non-interest-bearing checking account, you will suffer the same fate. Individuals attempt to reduce the cost of holding cash by putting it into interest-bearing accounts, a wide variety of which often pay nominal rates of interest that reflect anticipated inflation.

The Resource Cost of Inflation. Some economists believe that the main cost of unanticipated inflation is the opportunity cost of resources used to protect against inflation and the distortions introduced as firms attempt to plan for the long run. Individuals have to spend time and resources to figure out ways to cover themselves in case inflation is different from what it has been in the past. That may mean spending a longer time working out more complicated contracts for employment, for purchases of goods in the future, and for purchases of raw materials.

Inflation requires that price lists be changed. This is called the **repricing,** or **menu, cost of inflation.** The higher the rate of inflation, the higher the repricing cost of inflation.

Repricing, or **menu, cost of inflation** 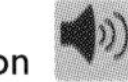
The cost associated with recalculating prices and printing new price lists when there is inflation.

Another major problem with inflation is that usually it does not proceed perfectly evenly. Consequently, the rate of inflation is not exactly what people anticipate. When this is so, the purchasing power of money changes in unanticipated ways. Because money is what we use as the measuring rod of the value of transactions we undertake, we have a more difficult time figuring out what we have really paid for things. As a result, resources tend to be misallocated in such situations because people have not really valued them accurately.

Think of any period during which you have to pay a higher price for something that was cheaper before. You are annoyed. But every time you pay a higher price, that represents the receipt of higher income for someone else. Therefore, it is impossible for all of us to be worse off because of rising prices. (Of course, we all become poorer if great variations in the rate of inflation cause us to incur the cost of resource misallocations.) There are numerous costs to inflation, but they aren't the ones commonly associated with inflation. One way to think of inflation is that it is simply a *change in the accounting system.* One year the price of fast-food hamburgers averages $1; 10 years later the price of fast-food hamburgers averages $2. Clearly, $1 doesn't mean the same thing 10 years later. If we changed the name of our unit of accounting each year so that one year we paid $1 for fast-food hamburgers and 10 years later we paid, say, 1 peso, this lesson would be driven home.

CONCEPTS IN BRIEF

- Whenever inflation is greater than anticipated, creditors lose and debtors gain. Whenever the rate of inflation is less than anticipated, creditors gain and debtors lose.
- Holders of cash lose during periods of inflation because the purchasing power of their cash depreciates at the rate of inflation.
- Households and businesses spend resources in attempting to protect themselves against unanticipated inflation, thus imposing a resource cost on the economy whenever there is unanticipated inflation.

Business fluctuations 
The ups and downs in overall business activity, as evidenced by changes in national income, employment, and the price level.

Expansion 
A business fluctuation in which overall business activity is rising at a more rapid rate than previously or at a more rapid rate than the overall historical trend for the nation.

Contraction 
A business fluctuation during which the pace of national economic activity is slowing down.

Recession 
A period of time during which the rate of growth of business activity is consistently less than its long-term trend or is negative.

Depression 
An extremely severe recession.

CHANGING INFLATION AND UNEMPLOYMENT: BUSINESS FLUCTUATIONS

Some years unemployment goes up, and some years it goes down. Some years there is a lot of inflation, and other years there isn't. We have fluctuations in all aspects of our macroeconomy. The ups and downs in economywide economic activity are sometimes called **business fluctuations.** When business fluctuations are positive, they are called **expansions** —speedups in the pace of national economic activity. The opposite of an expansion is a **contraction,** which is a slowdown in the pace of national economic activity. The top of an expansion is usually called its *peak,* and the bottom of a contraction is usually called its *trough.* Business fluctuations used to be called *business cycles,* but that term no longer seems appropriate because *cycle* implies regular or automatic recurrence, and we have never had automatic recurrent fluctuations in general business and economic activity. What we have had are contractions and expansions that vary greatly in length. For example, nine post–World War II expansions averaged 48 months, but three of those exceeded 55 months, and two lasted less than 25 months.

If the contractionary phase of business fluctuations becomes severe enough, we call it a **recession.** An extremely severe recession is called a **depression.** Typically, at the beginning of a recession, interest rates rise, and as the recession gets worse, they fall. At the same

FIGURE 7-7 
The Typical Course of Business Fluctuations
An idealized business cycle would go from peak to trough and back again in a regular cycle.

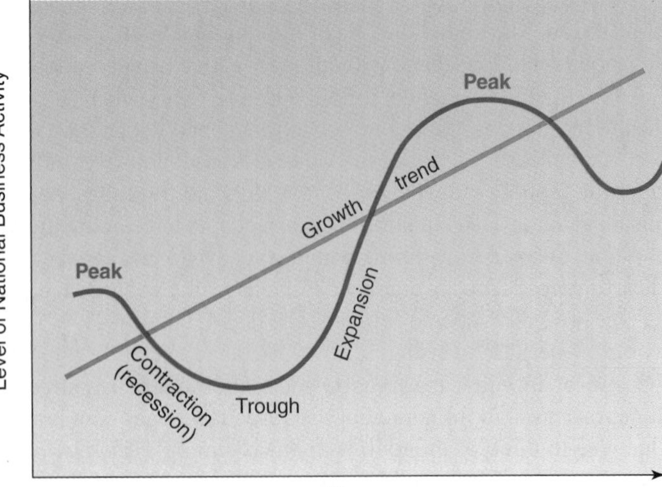

FIGURE 7-8

National Business Activity, 1880 to the Present

Variations around the trend of U.S. business activity have been frequent since 1880.

Sources: American Business Activity from 1790 to Today, 67th ed., AmeriTrust Co., January 1996, plus author's projections.

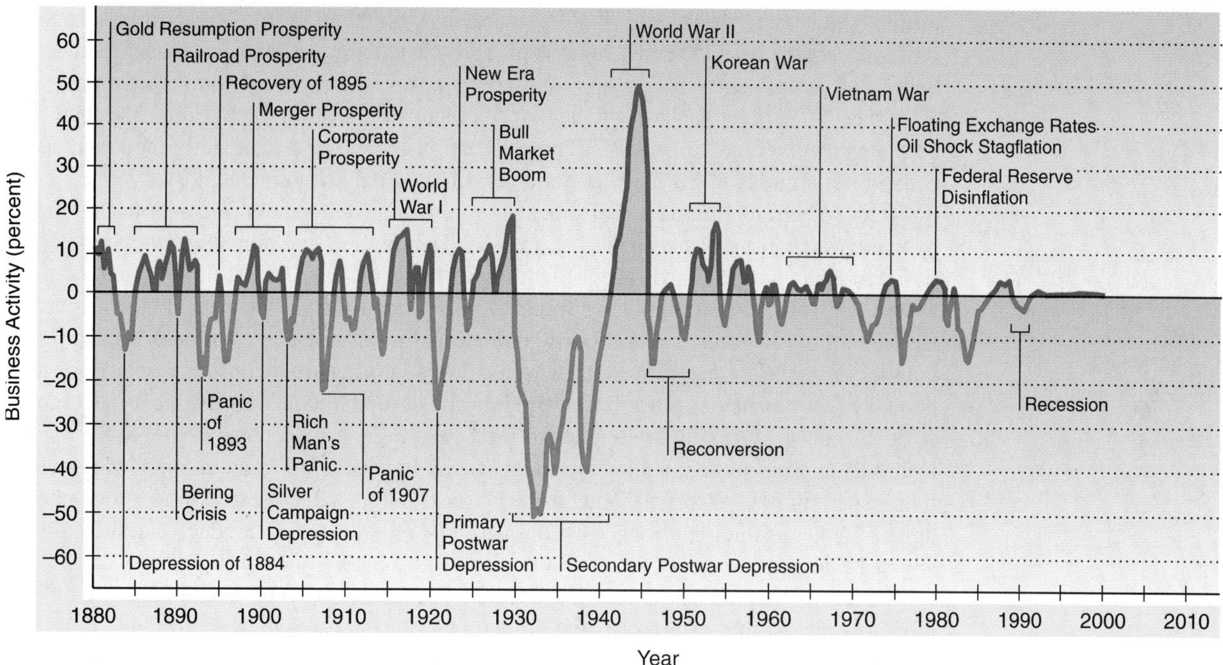

time, people's income starts to fall and the duration of unemployment increases so that the unemployment rate increases. In times of expansion, the opposite occurs.

In Figure 7-7, you see that typical business fluctuations occur around a growth trend in overall national business activity shown as a straight upward-sloping line. Starting out at a peak, the economy goes into a contraction (recession). Then an expansion starts that moves up to its peak, higher than the last one, and the sequence starts over again.

The official dating of business recessions is done by the National Bureau of Economic Research in New York City; Cambridge, Massachusetts; and Palo Alto, California.

Click here to learn about how economists formally determine when a recession is under way.

A Historical Picture of Business Activity in the United States

Figure 7-8 traces U.S. business activity from 1880 to the present. Note that the long-term trend line is shown as horizontal, so all changes in business activity focus around that trend line. Major changes in business activity in the United States occurred during the Great Depression and World War II. Note that none of the business fluctuations that you see in Figure 7-8 exactly mirror the idealized typical course of a business fluctuation shown in Figure 7-7.

Explaining Business Fluctuations: External Shocks

As you might imagine, because changes in national business activity affect everyone, economists for decades have attempted to understand and explain business fluctuations. For years, one of the most obvious explanations has been external events that tend to disrupt the economy. In many of the graphs in this chapter, you have seen that World War II was a critical point in this nation's economic history. A war is certainly an external shock—something that originates outside of our economy.

Other examples of external shocks, particularly for an agrarian nation, have to do with abrupt changes in the weather. Long-term drought tended to create downturns in national business activity when the majority of Americans worked on farms. Today, major droughts or floods usually affect specific regions of the U.S. economy. Even a hurricane or an earthquake that dramatically affects one area rarely causes a national economic downturn.

In the 1970s, due to actions on the part of certain countries in the Middle East, the United States received an "oil shock." The price of oil increased dramatically then, and some economists argue that this had a major effect on national economic activity.

To try to help identify external shocks that may induce business fluctuations and thereby make fluctuations easier to predict, the U.S. Department of Commerce tabulates a composite index (a weighted average) of **leading indicators.** These are factors that economists at the Commerce Department have found typically occur *before* changes in business activity. Economic downturns often follow reductions in the average workweek and a higher number of unemployment insurance claims, drops in orders that consumers place for new goods or that businesses place for new plants and equipment, an improvement in the ability of the sellers of inputs or supplies to meet new orders, a decrease in the prices of raw materials, a drop in the quantity of money in circulation, a fall in the number of new permits issued for new residential and business construction, a decline in average stock prices, or a drop in consumer confidence as revealed by a regular survey conducted at the University of Michigan.

Leading indicators 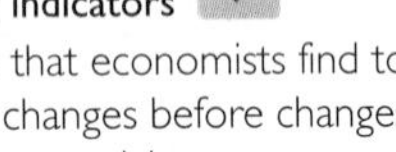
Factors that economists find to exhibit changes before changes in business activity.

The reason that the Commerce Department reports a composite index of leading indicators, however, is that external shocks sometimes cause these indicators to move in different directions. For instance, a fall in the average workweek and a rise in unemployment insurance claims may reflect a slight tapering off in the pace of a business expansion that businesspeople could regard as *good* news because it signals no inflationary pressures on the horizon—and hence little reason for the Federal Reserve to seek a rise in market interest rates. This could, for example, induce businesses to increase their orders for new plants and equipment, and it could encourage individuals to borrow to finance new home construction. It could even cause stock prices to rise.

Thus it is not enough for us to say simply that business downturns are caused by external shocks. In the first place, if that were the only determinant of recessions, there would be little reason to study macroeconomics. Second, we know that historically we have had business recessions in the absence of any external shocks. We therefore need a theory of why national economic activity changes. The remainder of the macro chapters in this book develop a series of models that will help you understand the ups and downs of our business fluctuations.

CONCEPTS IN BRIEF

- The ups and downs in economywide business activity are called business fluctuations, which consist of expansions and contractions in overall business activity.
- The lowest point of a contraction is called the trough; the highest point of an expansion is called the peak.
- A recession is a downturn in business activity for some length of time.
- One possible explanation for business fluctuations relates to external shocks, such as wars, dramatic increases in the prices of raw materials, and earthquakes, floods, and droughts.

NETNOMICS

Is Frictional Unemployment on Its Way Out?

Even in tight labor markets, frictional unemployment still exists because of the transaction costs required in changing jobs. The advent of the Internet, however, may be reducing frictional unemployment more than anticipated. Of course, some will always exist, but perhaps less than prior to the Internet.

The standard way of looking for another job is some combination of asking friends for contacts, looking at the "help wanted" ads, submitting résumés, using an employment agency, and even knocking on businesses' doors.

Now there's an Internet job market that is growing at lightning speed. Newspaper employment ads have started to instruct job seekers to send their résumés to a particular e-mail address. One reason is convenience, but an even more important reason is that electronic résumés allow prospective employers to scan for keywords and in that way rapidly locate qualified candidates for unfilled jobs. A big company like Intel, the chip maker for most of the world's computers, receives thousands of résumés electronically each year via the Internet. Those that it receives by conventional means it scans into a database using optical character recognition (OCR) technology. The company can then search both types electronically for key candidate qualifications.

Employment agencies on the Net are taking off. CareerPaths was cofounded by six major newspapers. It contains almost 500,000 job openings. Monster.com carries almost 300,000. CareerMosaic allows you to post your résumé, search for a job, and visit job fairs. Big-time power executives can go to Exec-U-Net and pay a fee to go job-searching on-line.

The Professional Job Network lets you select from over 1 million openings each month on-line, 24 hours a day. Some of these are jobs advertised in more than 1,000 newspapers and 500 trade journals; others are unadvertised opportunities with an additional 200,000 employers. There is also a listing from 200 professional job banks worldwide.

Job hunting will never be the same.

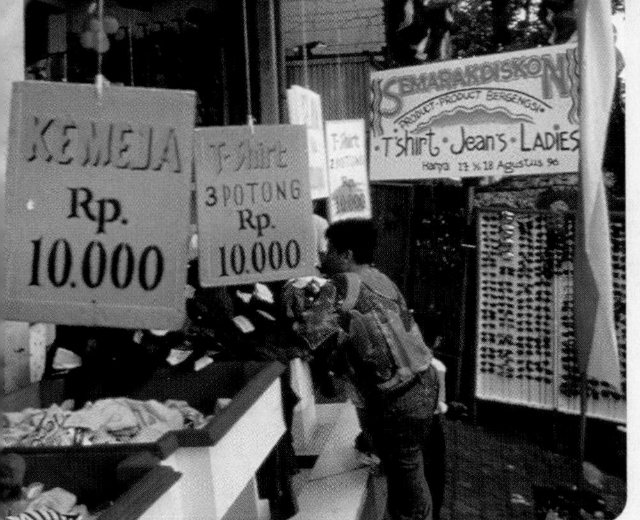

ISSUES & APPLICATIONS

Is the World Facing the Danger of Deflation?

In 1989, the number of newspaper articles around the world mentioning deflation was less than 50. Ten years later, more than 1,000 such articles appeared. What accounts for this new focus on falling prices?

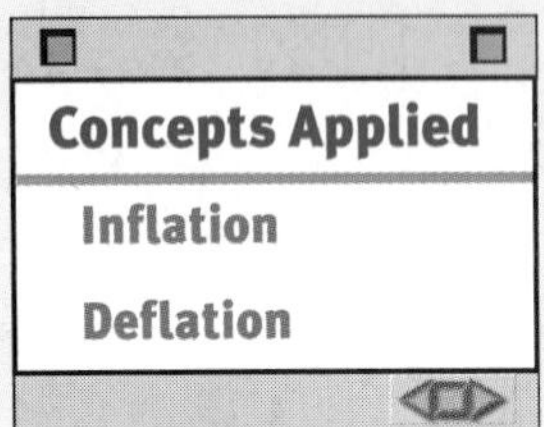

Concepts Applied

Inflation

Deflation

Inflation Trending Downward Worldwide

With a few exceptions, such as Russia, the rate of inflation in most of the world has declined. Indeed, by the year 2000, the rate of change of the Consumer Price Index in Europe was less than 1 percent. The rate of change of the Producer Price Index was negative. By 1999, Japan was already experiencing consistent deflation. The People's Republic of China had started to experience a similar deflation.

Causes for Concern

Commentators on the increase in deflation around the world contend that there are a number of causes for concern. First, they note that lower commodity prices cause real incomes in rich countries to go up but devastate producers in many economically troubled emerging economies.

They further argue that an even bigger risk is the failure of policymakers, workers, companies, and investors to adjust to the new reality. Nearly everyone in the post–World War II world has become used to high or even modest inflation and has no experience with deflation. The commentators point out that back in the nineteenth century, when deflation was a more common occurrence in the United States and elsewere, everyone was used to compensating for falling prices.

Few people alive today have had any such experience on any economywide level. Workers, particularly in unions, may need time to adapt to the notion of deflation. In the interim, they will demand higher nominal wage increases than are justified, because out of habit they will include an inflationary premium in their wage requests. Employers will resist, perhaps knowing better than employees that the inflationary premium should be zero or negative.

Deflation Versus Falling Relative Prices

Even during a period of low or nonexistent inflation, some prices rise and some prices fall. Some of the popular press has focused on price decreases in the goods sector, particularly in computers, telecommunications, and imported items. But at the same time, in the services sector, many prices have been rising—this is simple arithmetic, for if the Consumer Price Index is still going up, even at a relatively slow rate, some prices have to be rising. Remember that deflation is defined as a *consistent* decline in the average of *all* prices.

FOR CRITICAL ANALYSIS

1. When inflation occurs, most people complain about rising prices. If deflation occurs, why shouldn't everyone be happier?
2. How would you personally find it difficult to adjust to deflation?
3. How might you benefit from deflation?

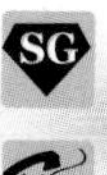

SUMMARY DISCUSSION OF LEARNING OBJECTIVES

1. **How the U.S. Government Calculates the Official Unemployment Rate:** The total number of workers who are officially unemployed are those people aged 16 or older who are willing and able to work and who are actively looking for work but have not found a job. To calculate the unemployment rate, the government determines what percentage this quantity is of the labor force, which consists of all people aged 16 years or older who either have jobs or are available for and actively seeking employment. Thus the official unemployment rate does not include discouraged workers who have stopped looking for work because they are convinced that they will not find suitable employment; these individuals are not included in the labor force.
2. **The Types of Unemployment:** Workers who are temporarily unemployed because they are searching for appropriate job offers are frictionally unemployed. The structurally unemployed lack the skills currently required by prospective employers. Unemployment resulting from business contractions are cyclically unemployed. And certain workers can find themselves seasonally unemployed because of the seasonal patterns of occupations within specific industries. The natural unemployment rate includes the portion of workers who are frictionally, structurally, and seasonally unemployed during a given interval. The overall rate of unemployment adds the portion of the labor force that is cyclically unemployed.
3. **How Price Indexes Are Calculated and Key Price Indexes:** To calculate any price index, economists multiply 100 times the ratio of the cost of a market basket of goods and services in the current year to the cost of the same market basket in a base year. The market basket used to compute the Consumer Price Index (CPI) is a weighted set of goods and services purchased by a typical consumer in urban areas. The Producer Price Index (PPI) is a weighted average of prices of goods sold by a typical firm. The GDP deflator measures changes in the overall level of prices of all goods produced in the economy during a given interval.
4. **Nominal Interest Rate Versus Real Interest Rate:** The nominal interest rate is the market rate of interest expressed in terms of current dollars. The real interest rate takes into account inflation that borrowers and lenders anticipate will erode the value of nominal interest payments during the period that a loan is repaid. Hence the real interest rate equals the nominal interest rate minus the expected inflation rate.
5. **Losers and Gainers from Inflation:** Creditors lose as a result of unanticipated inflation, or inflation that comes as a surprise after they have made a loan, because the real value of the interest payments they receive will turn out to be lower than they had expected. Borrowers gain when unanticipated inflation occurs, because the real value of their interest payments declines. Key costs of inflation are the expenses that individuals and businesses incur to protect themselves against inflation, costs of altering business plans because of unexpected changes in prices, and menu costs arising from expenses incurred in repricing goods and services.
6. **Key Features of Business Fluctuations:** Business fluctuations are increases and decreases in business activity. A positive fluctuation is an expansion, which is an upward movement in business activity from a trough, or low point, to a peak, or high point. A negative fluctuation is a contraction, which is a drop in the pace of business activity from a previous peak to a new trough.

Key Terms and Concepts

Anticipated inflation (157)
Base year (154)
Business fluctuations (160)
Consumer Price Index (CPI) (154)
Contraction (160)
Cost-of-living adjustments (COLAs) (159)
Cyclical unemployment (151)
Deflation (153)
Depression (160)
Discouraged workers (148)
Expansion (160)
Flow (148)
Frictional unemployment (150)
Full employment (152)

GDP deflator (154)
Inflation (153)
Job leaver (148)
Job loser (148)
Labor force (146)
Labor force participation rate (149)
Leading indicators (162)
Natural rate of unemployment (152)
New entrant (148)
Nominal rate of interest (158)
Price index (154)
Producer Price Index (PPI) (154)
Purchasing power (153)
Real rate of interest (158)
Recession (160)
Reentrant (148)
Repricing, or menu, cost of inflation (159)
Seasonal unemployment (151)
Stock (148)
Structural unemployment (150)
Unanticipated inflation (157)
Unemployment (146)

Problems

Answers to the odd-numbered problems appear at the back of the book.

7-1. Suppose that you receive two offers to begin employment after you complete your studies, which will be one year from now. You wish to take one of the two positions. You are indifferent between the jobs and their locations, however, and both job offers include the same benefits package. Job A will entail an annual salary of $24,000 beginning a year from now, and job B will pay an annual salary of $25,000. Neither salary will be adjusted until you complete a year of employment. After you study the regions where the firms are located, you determine that there is likely to be no inflation over the two years where employer A is located. By way of contrast, employer B is in an area where the annual inflation rate over the next two years is likely to be 5 percent. Which job should you accept?

7-2. Suppose that an elderly woman is retired, but she has become bored with retirement and is considering going back to work. She receives $3,000 in Social Security payments each month, and this is her only source of income. If she accepts other employment, her Social Security payment drops by $1 for every $2 in pretax earnings from that source of employment. She has been offered a job as an assistant manager of a fast-food restaurant at a pretax salary of $2,500 per month. Out of these earnings, she would have to pay a 7 percent Social Security tax and a 15 percent income tax. What would be her effective monthly earnings from working at the fast-food job, taking into account both the resulting change in her Social Security payment and the taxes that she would have to pay on her earned income?

7-3. During the course of a year, the labor force consists of the same 1,000 people. Of these, there are 20 who lack skills that employers desire and hence remain unemployed throughout the year. At the same time, every month during the year, 30 different people become unemployed and 30 other different people who were unemployed find jobs. There are no seasonal employment patterns.

a. What is the frictional unemployment rate?

b. What is the unemployment rate?

c. Suppose that a system of unemployment compensation is established. Each month, 30 new people (not including the 20 lacking required skills) continue to become unemployed, but each monthly group of newly unemployed now takes two months to find a job. After this change, what is the frictional unemployment rate?

d. After the change discussed in part (c), what is the unemployment rate?

7-4. Suppose that a nation has a labor force of 100 people. In January, Amy, Barbara, Carine, and Denise are unemployed; in February, those four find jobs, but Evan, Franceso, George, and Horatio become unemployed. Suppose further that every month, the previous four who were unemployed find jobs and four different people become unemployed. Throughout the year, however, the same three people—Ito, Jack, and Kelley—continually remain unemployed because they lack sufficient skills to obtain open jobs.

a. What is this nation's frictional unemployment rate?

b. What is its structural unemployment rate?

c. What is its unemployment rate?

7-5. In a country with a labor force of 200, a different group of 10 people becomes unemployed each month. Each group, however, becomes employed once again a month later. No others outside these groups are unemployed.

a. What is this country's unemployment rate?

b. What is the average duration of unemployment?

c. Suppose that institution of a system of unemployment compensation increases to two months the interval that it takes each group of job losers to become employed each month. Nevertheless, a different group of 10 people still becomes unemployed each month. Now what is the average duration of unemployment?

d. Following the change discussed in part (c), what is the country's unemployment rate?

7-6. A nation's frictional unemployment rate is 1 percent. Seasonal unemployment does not exist in this country. Its cyclical rate of unemployment is 3 percent, and its structural unemployment rate is 4 percent. What is this nation's overall rate of unemployment? What is its natural rate of unemployment?

7-7. In 1999, the cost of a market basket of goods was $2,000. In 2001, the cost of the same market basket of goods was $2,100. Use the price index formula to calculate the price index for 2001 if 1999 is the base year.

7-8. The real interest rate is 4 percent, and the nominal interest rate is 6 percent. What is the anticipated rate of inflation?

7-9. Suppose that in 2003 there is a sudden, unanticipated burst of inflation. Consider the situations faced by the following individuals. Who gains and who loses?

a. A homeowner whose wages will keep pace with inflation in 2003 but whose monthly mortgage interest payments to a savings bank will remain fixed

b. An apartment landlord who has guaranteed to his tenants that their monthly rent payments during 2003 will be the same as they were during 2002

c. A banker who made an auto loan that the auto buyer will repay at a fixed rate of interest during 2003

d. A retired individual who earns a pension with fixed monthly payments from her past employer during 2003

7-10. In January 2000, a nation's economic activity reached a peak, and a trough occurred in July 2000. The next peak occurs in August 2001, and another trough occurs in November 2002. Finally, there is another peak in October 2003. Identify the intervals of expansions and contractions (recessions).

Economics on the Net

Looking at the Unemployment and Inflation Data This chapter reviewed key concepts relating to unemployment and inflation. In this application, you get a chance to examine U.S. unemployment and inflation data on your own.

Title: Bureau of Labor Statistics: Most Requested Series

Navigation: Click here to visit the homepage of the Bureau of Labor Statistics. Click on Get Detailed Statistics, followed by Overall Most Requested BLS Series.

Application Perform the indicated operations, and answer the following questions:

1. Click checkmarks in the boxes for Civilian Labor Force, Employment, and Unemployment. Retreive the data. Can you identify periods of sharp cyclical swings? Do they show up in data for the labor force, employment, or unemployment?

2. Are cyclical factors important?

For Group Study and Analysis Divide the class into groups, and assign a price index to each group. Ask each group to take a look at the index for All Years and to identify periods during which their index accelerated or decelerated (or even fell). Do the indexes ever provide opposing implications about inflation and deflation?

CHAPTER 8

MEASURING THE ECONOMY'S PERFORMANCE

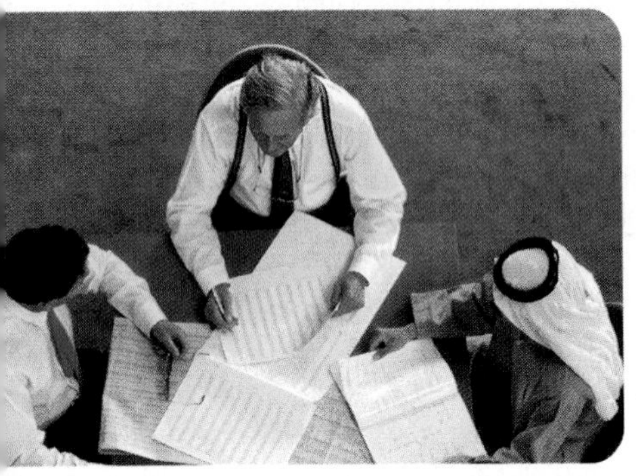

Mulitnational consulting firms often use large-scale economic models to predict economy wide chages. Why do such firms employ economists from all over the world??

If you watch the evening news, read newspapers and newsmagazines, or listen to news on the radio, you cannot miss hearing about the economy. One of the most eagerly awaited statistics, often touted in the media, concerns the federal government's quarterly estimate of how fast the economy is growing. Much is at stake here. Federal government policy aimed at stabilizing the economy hinges on these numbers. If the economy appears to be slowing down, that may indicate one policy; if the economy appears to be "overheating," that may lead to a different policy. A whole industry has developed to predict what will happen to the overall economy—and hence what the next policy change will be. How successful are those economic soothsayers? Before we can address this issue, you need to learn how the government derives its estimates of national economic performance.

LEARNING OBJECTIVES

After reading this chapter, you should be able to:

1. Describe the circular flow of income and output
2. Define gross domestic product (GDP)
3. Understand the limitations of using GDP as a measure of national welfare
4. Explain the expenditure approach to tabulating GDP
5. Explain the income approach to computing GDP
6. Distinguish between nominal GDP and real GDP

Did You Know That... whenever a single person who is currently paying a housekeeper marries that housekeeper, government statistics show that the economy's performance has declined? The reason for this seeming anomaly is that government statisticians do not yet consider unpaid housework as contributing to the total annual national income of the country (even though the same services would have to be purchased if not provided free of charge). In spite of such measurement problems, the statistics about the nation's economic performance are watched closely throughout the year by investors, bankers, businesspeople, and macroeconomic policymakers. After all, most people like to know where they stand financially at the end of each month or year. Why shouldn't we have similar information about the economy as a whole? The way we do this is by using what has become known as **national income accounting,** the main focus of this chapter.

But first we need to look at the flow of income within an economy, for it is the flow of goods and services from businesses to consumers and payments from consumers to businesses that constitutes economic activity.

Chapter Outline

THE SIMPLE CIRCULAR FLOW

The concept of a circular flow of income (ignoring taxes) involves two principles:

1. In every economic exchange, the seller receives exactly the same amount that the buyer spends.
2. Goods and services flow in one direction and money payments flow in the other.

In the simple economy shown in Figure 8-1 on page 170, there are only businesses and households. It is assumed that businesses sell their *entire* output *immediately* to households and that households spend their *entire* income *immediately* on consumer products. Households receive their income by selling the use of whatever factors of production they own, such as labor services.

National income accounting 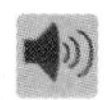
A measurement system used to estimate national income and its components; one approach to measuring an economy's aggregate performance.

Profits Explained

We have indicated in Figure 8-1 that profit is a cost of production. You might be under the impression that profits are not part of the cost of producing goods and services, but profits are indeed a part of this cost because entrepreneurs must be rewarded for providing their services or they won't provide them. Their reward, if any, is profit. The reward—the profit—is included in the cost of the factors of production. If there were no expectations of profit, entrepreneurs would not incur the risk associated with the organization of productive activities. That is why we consider profits a cost of doing business.

Total income 
The yearly amount earned by the nation's resources (factors of production). Total income therefore includes wages, rent, interest payments, and profits that are received, respectively, by workers, landowners, capital owners, and entrepreneurs.

Total Income or Total Output

The arrow that goes from businesses to households at the bottom of Figure 8-1 is labeled "Total income." What would be a good definition of **total income**? If you answered "the total of all individuals' income," you would be right. But all income is actually a payment for something, whether it be wages paid for labor services, rent paid for the use of land, interest paid for the use of capital, or profits paid to entrepreneurs. It is the amount paid to the resource suppliers. Therefore, total income is also defined as the annual *cost* of producing the entire output of **final goods and services.**

Final goods and services 
Goods and services that are at their final stage of production and will not be transformed into yet other goods or services. For example, wheat is not ordinarily considered a final good because it is usually used to make a final good, bread.

The arrow going from households to businesses at the top of the figure represents the dollar value of output in the economy. This is equal to the total monetary value of all final goods

FIGURE 8-1 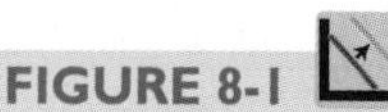

The Circular Flow of Income and Product

Businesses provide final goods and services to households (upper clockwise loop), who in turn pay for them with money (upper counterclockwise loop). Money flows in a counterclockwise direction and can be thought of as a circular flow. The dollar value of output is identical to total income because profits are defined as being equal to total business receipts minus business outlays for wages, rents, and interest.

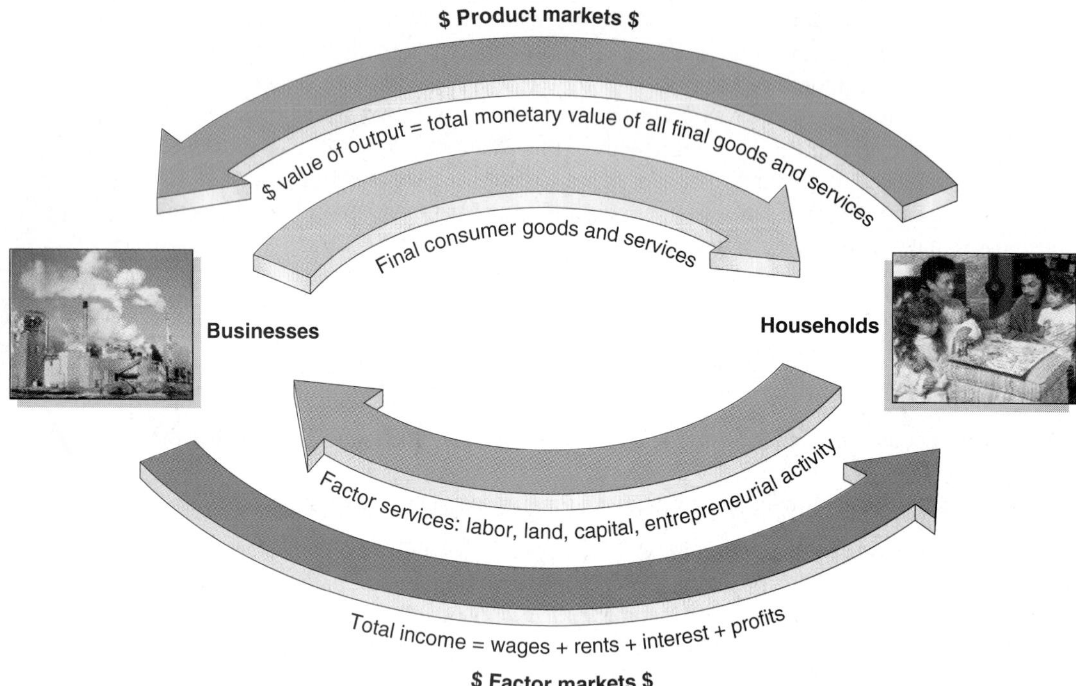

and services for this simple economy. In essence, it represents the total business receipts from the sale of all final goods and services produced by businesses and consumed by households. Business receipts are the opposite side of household expenditures. When households purchase goods and services with money, that money becomes a *business receipt.* Every transaction, therefore, simultaneously involves an expenditure as well as a receipt.

Product Markets. Transactions in which households buy goods take place in the product markets—that's where households are the buyers and businesses are the sellers of consumer goods. *Product market* transactions are represented in the upper loops in Figure 8-1. Note that consumer goods and services flow to household demanders, while money flows in the opposite direction to business suppliers.

Factor Markets. *Factor market* transactions are represented by the lower loops in Figure 8-1. In the factor market, households are the sellers; they sell resources such as labor, land, capital, and entrepreneurial ability. Businesses are the buyers in factor markets; business expenditures represent receipts or, more simply, income for households. Also, in the lower loops of Figure 8-1, factor services flow from households to businesses, while the money paid for these services flows in the opposite direction from businesses to households. Observe also the flow of money (counterclockwise) from households to businesses and back again from businesses to households: It is an endless circular flow.

Why the Dollar Value of Total Output Must Equal Total Income

Total income represents the income received by households in payment for the production of goods and services. Why must total income be identical to the dollar value of total output? First, as Figure 8-1 shows, spending by one group is income to another. Second, it is a matter of simple accounting and the economic definition of profit as a cost of production. Profit is defined as what is *left over* from total business receipts after all other costs—wages, rents, interest—have been paid. If the dollar value of total output is $1,000 and the total of wages, rent, and interest for producing that output is $900, profit is $100. Profit is always the *residual* item that makes total income equal to the dollar value of total output.

CONCEPTS IN BRIEF

- In the circular flow model of income and output, households sell factor services to businesses that pay for those factor services. The receipt of payments is total income. Businesses sell goods and services to households that pay for them.
- The dollar value of total output is equal to the total monetary value of all final goods and services produced.
- The dollar value of final output must always equal total income; the variable that makes this so is known as profit.

NATIONAL INCOME ACCOUNTING

We have already mentioned that policymakers need information about the state of the national economy. Historical statistical records on the performance of the national economy aid economists in testing their theories about how the economy really works. National income accounting is therefore important. Let's start with the most commonly presented statistic on the national economy.

Gross Domestic Product (GDP)

Gross domestic product (GDP) represents the total market value of the nation's annual final product, or output, produced per year by factors of production located within national borders. We therefore formally define GDP as the total market value of all final goods and services produced in an economy during a year. We are referring here to a *flow of production.* A nation produces at a certain rate, just as you receive income at a certain rate. Your income flow might be at a rate of $5,000 per year or $50,000 per year. Suppose you are told that someone earns $500. Would you consider this a good salary? There is no way to answer that question unless you know whether the person is earning $500 per month or per week or per day. Thus you have to specify a time period for all flows. Income received is a flow. You must contrast this with, for example, your total accumulated savings, which are a stock measured at a point in time, not over time. Implicit in just about everything we deal with in this chapter is a time period—usually one year. All the measures of domestic product and income are specified as *rates* measured in dollars per year.

Gross domestic product (GDP) 
The total market value of all final goods and services produced by factors of production located within a nation's borders.

Stress on Final Output

Intermediate goods 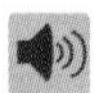
Goods used up entirely in the production of final goods.

Value added 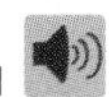
The dollar value of an industry's sales minus the value of intermediate goods (for example, raw materials and parts) used in production.

GDP does not count **intermediate goods** (goods used up entirely in the production of final goods) because to do so would be to count them twice. For example, even though grain that a farmer produces may be that farmer's final product, it is not the final product for the nation. It is sold to make bread. Bread is the final product.

We can use a numerical example to clarify this point further. Our example will involve determining the value added at each stage of production. **Value added** is the amount of dollar value contributed to a product at each stage of its production. In Table 8-1, we see the difference between total value of all sales and value added in the production of a donut. We also see that the sum of the values added is equal to the sale price to the final consumer. It is the 45 cents that is used to measure GDP, not the 96 cents. If we used the 96 cents, we would be double-counting from stages 2 through 5, for each intermediate good would be counted at least twice—once when it was produced and again when the good it was used in making was sold. Such double counting would grossly exaggerate GDP.

TABLE 8-1
Sales Value and Value Added at Each Stage of Donut Production

(1) Stage of Production	(2) Dollar Value of Sales	(3) Value Added
Stage 1: Fertilizer and seed	$.03	$.03
Stage 2: Growing	.06	.03
Stage 3: Milling	.12	.06
Stage 4: Baking	.30	.18
Stage 5: Retailing	.45	.15
Total dollar value of all sales	$.96	Total value added $.45

Stage 1: A farmer purchases 3 cents' worth of fertilizer and seed, which are used as factors of production in growing wheat.

Stage 2: The farmer grows the wheat, harvests it, and sells it to a miller for 6 cents. Thus we see that the farmer has added 3 cents' worth of value. Those 3 cents represent income paid to the farmer.

Stage 3: The miller purchases the wheat for 6 cents and adds 6 cents as the value added; that is, there is 6 cents for the miller as income. The miller sells the ground wheat flour to a donut-baking company.

Stage 4: The donut-baking company buys the flour for 12 cents and adds 18 cents as the value added. It then sells the donut to the final retailer.

Stage 5: The donut retailer sells fresh hot donuts at 45 cents apiece, thus creating an additional value of 15 cents.

We see that the total value of transactions involved in the production of one donut was 96 cents, but the total value added was 45 cents, which is exactly equal to the retail price. The total value added is equal to the sum of all income payments.

Exclusion of Financial Transactions, Transfer Payments, and Secondhand Goods 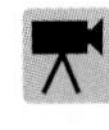

Remember that GDP is the measure of the value of all final goods and services produced in one year. Many more transactions occur that have nothing to do with final goods and services produced. There are financial transactions, transfers of the ownership of preexisting goods, and other transactions that should not and do not get included in our measure of GDP.

Financial Transactions. There are three general categories of purely financial transactions: (1) the buying and selling of securities, (2) government transfer payments, and (3) private transfer payments.

Securities. When you purchase a share of existing stock in Microsoft Corporation, someone else has sold it to you. In essence, there was merely a *transfer* of ownership rights. You paid $100 to obtain the stock certificate. Someone else received the $100 and gave up the stock certificate. No producing activity was consummated at that time. Hence the $100 transaction is not included when we measure gross domestic product.

Government Transfer Payments. Transfer payments are payments for which no productive services are concurrently provided in exchange. The most obvious government transfer payments are Social Security benefits, veterans' payments, and unemployment compensation. The recipients make no contribution to current production in return for such transfer payments (although they may have made contributions in the past to receive them). Government transfer payments are not included in GDP.

Click here for the most up-to-date U. S. economic data at the Web site of the Bureau of Economic Analysis.

Private Transfer Payments. Are you receiving money from your parents in order to live at school? Has a wealthy relative ever given you a gift of money? If so, you have been the recipient of a private transfer payment. This is merely a transfer of funds from one individual to another. As such, it does not constitute productive activity and is not included in gross domestic product.

Transfer of Secondhand Goods. If I sell you my two-year-old stereo, no current production is involved. I transfer to you the ownership of a sound system that was produced years ago; in exchange, you transfer to me $550. The original purchase price of the stereo was included in GDP in the year I purchased it. To include it again when I sell it to you would be counting the value of the stereo a second time.

Other Excluded Transactions. Many other transactions are not included in GDP for practical reasons:

- Household production—home cleaning, child care, and other tasks performed by people in their *own* households and for which they are not paid through the marketplace
- Otherwise legal underground transactions—those that are legal but not reported and hence not taxed, such as paying housekeepers in cash that is not declared as income
- Illegal underground activities—these include prostitution, illegal gambling, and the sale of illicit drugs

Many economists criticize measured GDP statistics because the underground economy is not included.

INTERNATIONAL EXAMPLE

The Underground Economy Is Alive and Thriving

To be sure, much of the underground economy has to do with illegal activities, particularly illegal drug sales. But in many countries outside the United States, the underground economy is a way of life for virtually all activities. This is true today in such countries as Russia, where even the use of money in many transactions has more or less disappeared. Professor Avi Shama of the University of Mexico believes that 90 percent of all private-sector production, sales, and profits are never reported to the tax authorities in Russia. But look at Figure 8-2. There you see the size of the underground economy in Europe, Canada, Australia, Japan, and the United States. Italy's underground economy is the most prominent. Why? Because the difference between an Italian worker's net take-home pay and his or her employer's cost for that worker—which includes taxes and other government-mandated employee costs—is 200 percent (the figure in the United States is 79 percent). It is not surprising that at least 25 percent of Italian economic activity takes place without the government's knowing it. But the Italian government does know what is happening. Consequently, Italian tax policemen stand outside of restaurants, beauty salons, and shops. They can ask for the legally required receipt. A customer without such a receipt can be fined on the spot.

For Critical Analysis

How can a country reduce the size of its underground economy?

FIGURE 8-2

The Size of the Underground Economy, by Country

These estimates indicate that Italy has the largest underground economy, relative to those of other nations.

Source: Friedrich Schneider, Linz University.

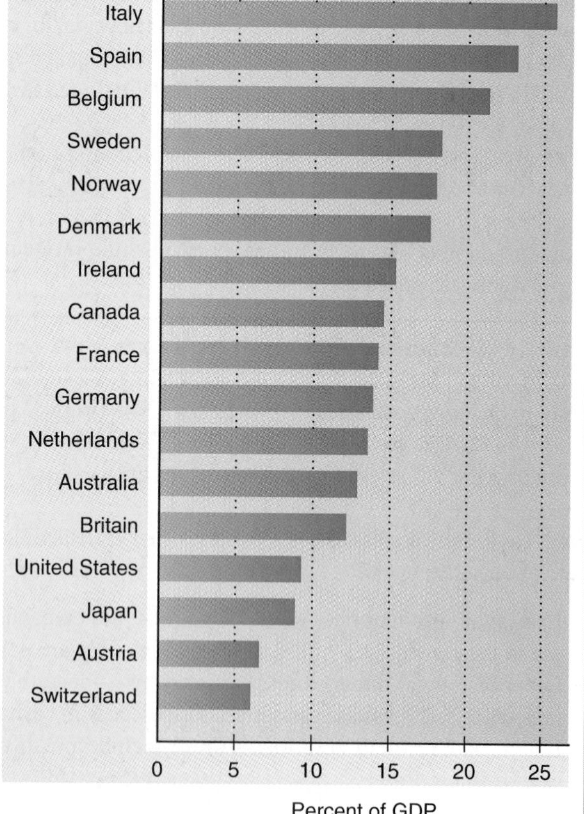

Recognizing GDP's Limitations

Like any statistical measure, gross domestic product is a concept that can be both well used and misused. Economists find it especially valuable as an overall indicator of a nation's economic performance. But it is important to realize that GDP has important weaknesses. Because it includes only the value of goods and services traded in markets, it excludes *nonmarket* production, such as the household services of homemakers discussed earlier. This can cause some problems in comparing the GDP of an industrialized country with the GDP of a highly agrarian nation in which nonmarket production is relatively more important. It also causes problems if nations have different definitions of legal versus illegal activities. For instance, a nation with legalized gambling will count the value of gambling services, which has a reported market value as a legal activity. But in a country in which gambling is illegal, individuals who provide such services will not report the market value of gambling activities, and so they will not be counted in that country's GDP. This can complicate comparing GDP in the nation where gambling is legal with GDP in the country that prohibits gambling.

Furthermore, although GDP is often used as a benchmark measure for standard-of-living calculations, it is not necessarily a good measure of the well-being of a nation. No measured figure of total national annual income can take account of changes in the degree of labor market discrimination, declines or improvements in personal safety, or the quantity or quality of leisure time. Measured GDP also says little about our environmental quality of life. As the now-defunct Soviet Union illustrated to the world, the large-scale production of such goods as minerals, electricity, and irrigation for farming can have negative effects on the environment: deforestation from strip mining, air and soil pollution from particulate emissions or nuclear accidents at power plants, and erosion of the natural balance between water and salt in bodies of water such as the Aral Sea. Hence it is important to recognize the following point:

GDP is a measure of production and an indicator of economic activity. It is not a measure of a nation's overall welfare.

Nonetheless, GDP is a relatively accurate and useful measure to map changes in the economy's domestic economic performance. Understanding GDP is thus important for recognizing changes in economic performance over time.

CONCEPTS IN BRIEF

- GDP is the total market value of final goods and services produced in an economy during a one-year period by factors of production within the nation's borders. It represents the dollar value of the flow of production over a one-year period.
- To avoid double counting, we look only at final goods and services produced or, alternatively, at value added.
- In measuring GDP, we must exclude (1) purely financial transactions, such as the buying and selling of securities; (2) government transfer payments and private transfer payments; and (3) the transfer of secondhand goods.
- Many other transactions are excluded from GDP, among them household services rendered by homemakers, underground economy transactions, and illegal economic activities.
- GDP is a useful measure for tracking changes in overall economic activity over time, but it is not a measure of the well-being of a nation's residents, because it fails to account for nonmarket transactions, the amount and quality of leisure time, environmental or safety issues, discrimination, and other factors that influence general welfare.

TWO MAIN METHODS OF MEASURING GDP 

If the definition of GDP is the total value of all final goods and services produced during a year, then to measure GDP we could add up the prices times the quantities of every individual commodity produced. But this would involve a monumental, if not impossible, task for government statisticians.

The circular flow diagram presented in Figure 8-1 gives us a shortcut method for calculating GDP. We can look at the *flow of expenditures,* which consists of consumption, investment, government purchases of goods and services, and net expenditures in the foreign sector (net exports). This is called the **expenditure approach** to measuring GDP, in which we add the dollar value of all final goods and services. We could also use the *flow of income,* looking at the income received by everybody producing goods and services. This is called the **income approach,** in which we add the income received by all factors of production.

Expenditure approach 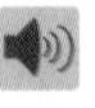
A way of computing national income by adding up the dollar value at current market prices of all final goods and services.

Income approach 
A way of measuring national income by adding up all components of national income, including wages, interest, rent, and profits.

Deriving GDP by the Expenditure Approach

To derive GDP using the expenditure approach, we must look at each of the separate components of expenditures and then add them together. These components are consumption expenditures, investment, government expenditures, and net exports.

Consumption Expenditures. How do we spend our income? As households or as individuals, we spend our income through consumption expenditure (C), which falls into three categories: **durable consumer goods, nondurable consumer goods,** and **services.** Durable goods are *arbitrarily* defined as items that last more than three years; they include automobiles, furniture, and household appliances. Nondurable goods are all the rest, such as food and gasoline. Services are intangible commodities: medical care, education, and so on.

Durable consumer goods 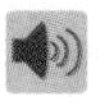
Consumer goods that have a life span of more than three years.

Nondurable consumer goods 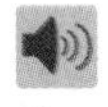
Consumer goods that are used up within three years.

Services 
Mental or physical labor or help purchased by consumers. Examples are the assistance of doctors, lawyers, dentists, repair personnel, housecleaners, educators, retailers, and wholesalers; things purchased or used by consumers that do not have physical characteristics.

Housing expenditures constitute a major proportion of anybody's annual expenditures. Rental payments on apartments are automatically included in consumption expenditure estimates. People who own their homes, however, do not make rental payments. Consequently, government statisticians estimate what is called the *implicit rental value* of owner-occupied homes. It is equal to the amount of rent you would have to pay if you did not own the home but were renting it from someone else.

Gross Private Domestic Investment. We now turn our attention to **gross private domestic investment** (I) undertaken by businesses. When economists refer to investment, they are referring to additions to productive capacity. **Investment** may be thought of as an activity that uses resources today in such a way that they allow for greater production in the future and hence greater consumption in the future. When a business buys new equipment or puts up a new factory, it is investing; it is increasing its capacity to produce in the future.

Gross private domestic investment 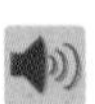
The creation of capital goods, such as factories and machines, that can yield production and hence consumption in the future. Also included in this definition are changes in business inventories and repairs made to machines or buildings.

Investment 
Any use of today's resources to expand tomorrow's production or consumption.

The layperson's notion of investment often relates to the purchase of stocks and bonds. For our purposes, such transactions simply represent the *transfer of ownership* of assets called stocks and bonds. Thus you must keep in mind the fact that in economics, investment refers *only* to *additions* to productive capacity, not to transfers of assets.

In our analysis, we will consider the basic components of investment. We have already mentioned the first one, which involves a firm's buying equipment or putting up a new factory. These are called **producer durables, or capital goods.** A producer durable, or a

Producer durables, or capital goods 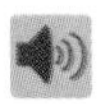
Durable goods having an expected service life of more than three years that are used by businesses to produce other goods and services.

capital good, is simply a good that is purchased not to be consumed in its current form but to be used to make other goods and services. The purchase of equipment and factories—capital goods—is called **fixed investment.**

Fixed investment 
Purchases by businesses of newly produced producer durables, or capital goods, such as production machinery and office equipment.

The other type of investment has to do with the change in inventories of raw materials and finished goods. Firms do not immediately sell off all their products to consumers. Some of this final product is usually held in inventory waiting to be sold. Firms hold inventories to meet future expected orders for their products. When a firm increases its inventories of finished products, it is engaging in **inventory investment.** Inventories consist of all finished goods on hand, goods in process, and raw materials.

Inventory investment 
Changes in the stocks of finished goods and goods in process, as well as changes in the raw materials that businesses keep on hand. Whenever inventories are decreasing, inventory investment is negative; whenever they are increasing, inventory investment is positive.

The reason that we can think of a change in inventories as being a type of investment is that an increase in such inventories provides for future increased consumption possibilities. When inventory investment is zero, the firm is neither adding to nor subtracting from the total stock of goods or raw materials on hand. Thus if the firm keeps the same amount of inventories throughout the year, inventory *investment* has been zero.

In estimating gross private domestic investment, government statisticians also add consumer expenditures on *new* residential structures because new housing represents an addition to our future productive capacity in the sense that a new house can generate housing services in the future.

POLICY EXAMPLE

Can the Government Catch Up with the Real-Life Economy?

For years, government statisticians have been classifying the industries in the United States according to the Standard Industrial Classification, or SIC. This system was developed in the 1930s. With so many complaints about how out outdated the SIC categories were, the government finally did start changing how it classifies industries. It has developed the North American Industry Classification System (NAICS). Three hundred new industries have been added, including satellite communications. It has also regrouped new and existing industries together. There is a grouping called "information," which includes publishing, software, broadcasting, telecommunications, and motion pictures. Unfortunately, the new NAICS data will not be fully integrated into federal statistics until around 2005.

For Critical Analysis

Does it matter whether we have accurate information on the growth or decline of industries that reflect the economy? Why or why not?

Government Expenditures. In addition to personal consumption expenditures, there are government purchases of goods and services (G). The government buys goods and services from private firms and pays wages and salaries to government employees. Generally, we value goods and services at the prices at which they are sold. But many government goods and services are not sold in the market. Therefore, we cannot use their market value when computing GDP. The value of these goods is considered equal to their *cost.* For example, the value of a newly built road is considered equal to its construction cost and is included in the GDP for the year it was built.

Net Exports (Foreign Expenditures). To get an accurate representation of gross domestic product, we must include the foreign sector. As Americans, we purchase foreign goods called *imports.* The goods that foreigners purchase from us are our *exports.* To get an idea of the *net* expenditures from the foreign sector, we subtract the value of imports from the value of exports to get net exports (X) for a year:

$$\text{Net exports } (X) = \text{total exports} - \text{total imports}$$

To understand why we subtract imports rather than ignoring them altogether, consider that we are using the expenditures approach. If we want to estimate *domestic* output, we have to subtract U.S. expenditures on the goods of other nations.

INTERNATIONAL EXAMPLE

What the GDP Figures in China Really Mean

For years, the Western world has been regaled by impressive figures on the growth in the Chinese economy. While the United States has been happy with growth rates of 3 and 4 percent per year, the Chinese economy has been growing at 7, 8, even 9 percent per year. But what do such statistics really mean? One Chinese economist in Beijing, Lu Feng, compared China's official production rate of meat, eggs, and fish products with what people actually consumed. He concluded that real output in these sectors had been exaggerated by over 40 percent. The reason is that local officials want to show good output performance, so they overstate agricultural output. The same problem plagues the industrial sector. The reality is that so long as China does not correct its reported output figures by doing many sampling surveys, it is bound to exaggerate its real GDP and thus its economic growth.

For Critical Analysis

Why do government statisticians in the United States not face a similar problem?

Mathematical Representation Using the Expenditure Approach

We have just defined the components of GDP using the expenditure approach. When we add them all together, we get a definition for GDP, which is as follows:

$$\text{GDP} = C + I + G + X$$

where

C = consumption expenditures

I = investment expenditures

G = government expenditures

X = net exports

The Historical Picture. To get an idea of the relationship among C, I, G, and X, look at Figure 8-3, which shows gross domestic product, personal consumption expenditures, government purchases, and gross private domestic investment plus net exports since 1929. When we add up the expenditures of the household, business, government, and foreign sectors, we get GDP.

Depreciation
Reduction in the value of capital goods over a one-year period due to physical wear and tear and also to obsolescence; also called *capital consumption allowance*.

Net domestic product (NDP)
GDP minus depreciation.

Depreciation and Net Domestic Product. We have used the terms *gross domestic product* and *gross private domestic investment* without really indicating what *gross* means. The dictionary defines it as "without deductions," the opposite of *net.* Deductions for what? you might ask. The deductions are for something we call **depreciation.** In the course of a year, machines and structures wear out or are used up in the production of domestic product. For example, houses deteriorate as they are occupied, and machines need repairs or they will fall apart and stop working. Most capital, or durable, goods depreciate. An estimate of this is subtracted from gross domestic product to arrive at a figure called **net domestic product (NDP),** which we define as follows:

FIGURE 8-3
GDP and Its Components
Here we see a display of gross domestic product, personal consumption expenditures, government purchases, and gross private domestic investment plus net exports for the years since 1929. Actually, during the Great Depression of the 1930s, gross private domestic investment *plus* net exports was negative because we were investing very little at that time.

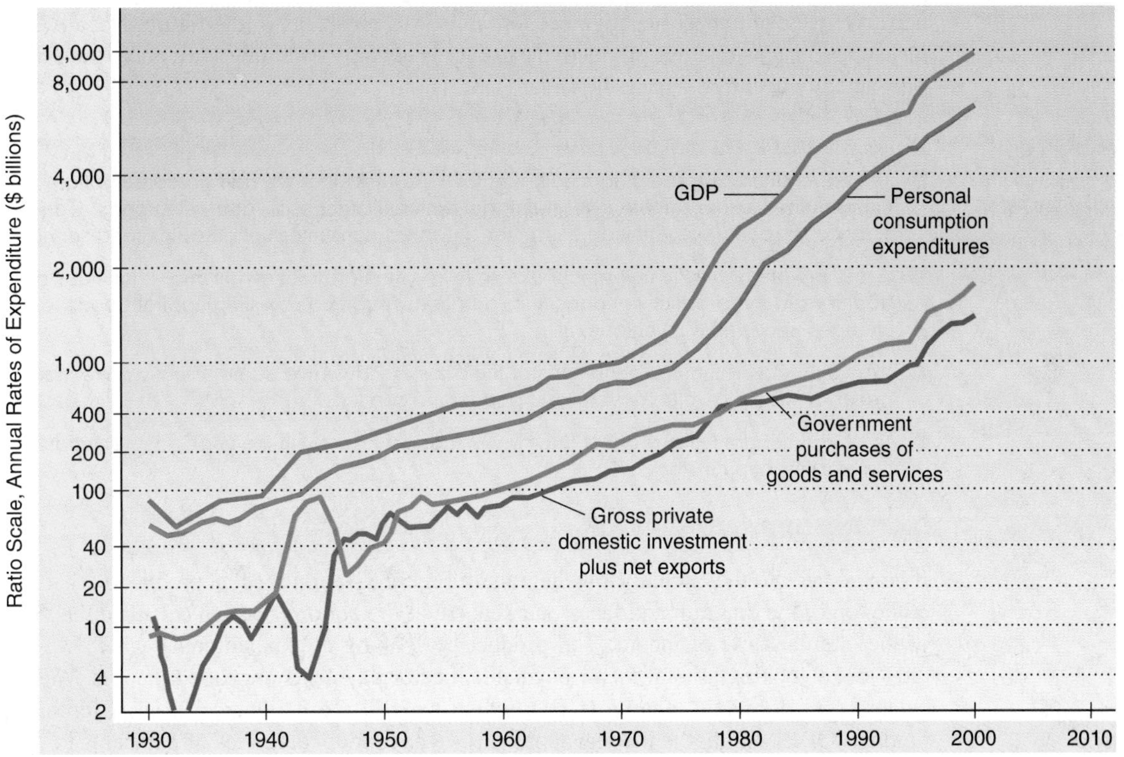

$$\text{NDP} = \text{GDP} - \text{depreciation}$$

Depreciation is also called **capital consumption allowance** because it is the amount of the capital stock that has been consumed over a one-year period. In essence, it equals the amount a business would have to put aside to repair and replace deteriorating machines. Because we know that

$$\text{GDP} = C + I + G + X$$

we know that the formula for NDP is

$$\text{NDP} = C + I + G + X - \text{depreciation}$$

Alternatively, because net $I = I -$ depreciation,

$$\text{NDP} = C + \text{net } I + G + X$$

Net investment measures *changes* in our capital stock over time and is positive nearly every year. Because depreciation does not vary greatly from year to year as a percentage of GDP, we get a similar picture of what is happening to our national economy by looking at either NDP or GDP data.

Capital consumption allowance 
Another name for depreciation, the amount that businesses would have to save in order to take care of the deterioration of machines and other equipment.

Net investment 
Gross private domestic investment minus an estimate of the wear and tear on the existing capital stock. Net investment therefore measures the change in capital stock over a one-year period.

Net investment is an important variable to observe over time nonetheless. If everything else remains the same in an economy, changes in net investment can have dramatic consequences for future economic growth (a topic we cover in more detail in Chapter 9). Positive net investment by definition expands the productive capacity of our economy. This means that there is increased capital, which will generate even more income in the future. When net investment is zero, we are investing just enough to take account of depreciation. Our economy's productive capacity remains unchanged. Finally, when net investment is negative, we can expect negative economic growth prospects in the future. Negative net investment means that our productive capacity is actually declining—we are disinvesting. This actually occurred during the Great Depression.

CONCEPTS IN BRIEF

- The expenditure approach to measuring GDP requires that we add up consumption expenditures, gross private investment, government purchases, and net exports. Consumption expenditures include consumer durables, consumer nondurables, and services.
- Gross private domestic investment *excludes* transfers of asset ownership. It includes only additions to the productive capacity of a nation, repairs on existing capital goods, and changes in business inventories.
- We value government expenditures at their cost because we do not usually have market prices at which to value government goods and services.
- To obtain net domestic product (NDP), we subtract from GDP the year's depreciation of the existing capital stock.

Deriving GDP by the Income Approach

If you go back to the circular flow diagram in Figure 8-1, you see that product markets are at the top of the diagram and factor markets are at the bottom. We can calculate the value of the circular flow of income and product by looking at expenditures—which we just did—or by looking at total factor payments. Factor payments are called income. We calculate **gross domestic income (GDI),** which we will see is identical to gross domestic product (GDP). Using the income approach, we have four categories of payments to individuals: wages, interest, rent, and profits.

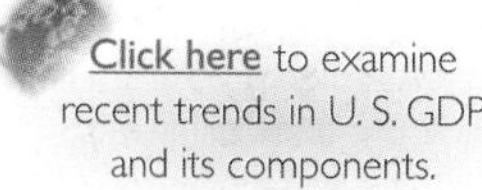

Gross domestic income (GDI)
The sum of all income—wages, interest, rent, and profits—paid to the four factors of production.

Click here to examine recent trends in U. S. GDP and its components.

1. *Wages.* The most important category is, of course, wages, including salaries and other forms of labor income, such as income in kind and incentive payments. We also count Social Security taxes (both the employees' and the employers' contributions).
2. *Interest.* Here interest payments do not equal the sum of all payments for the use of funds in a year. Instead, interest is expressed in *net* rather than in gross terms. The interest component of total income is only net interest received by households plus net interest paid to us by foreigners. Net interest received by households is the difference between the interest they receive (from savings accounts, certificates of deposit, and the like) and the interest they pay (to banks for mortgages, credit cards, and other loans).
3. *Rent.* Rent is all income earned by individuals for the use of their real (nonmonetary) assets, such as farms, houses, and stores. As stated previously, we have to include here the implicit rental value of owner-occupied houses. Also included in this category are royalties received from copyrights, patents, and assets such as oil wells.
4. *Profits.* Our last category includes total gross corporate profits plus *proprietors' income.* Proprietors' income is income earned from the operation of unincorporated businesses, which include sole proprietorships, partnerships, and producers' cooperatives. It is unincorporated business profit.

All of the payments listed are *actual* factor payments made to owners of the factors of production. When we add them together, though, we do not yet have gross domestic income. We have to take account of two other components: **indirect business taxes,** such as sales and business property taxes, and depreciation, which we have already discussed.

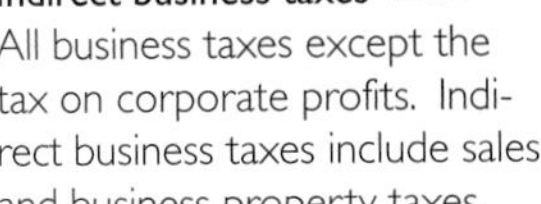

Indirect business taxes All business taxes except the tax on corporate profits. Indirect business taxes include sales and business property taxes.

Indirect Business Taxes. Indirect taxes are the (nonincome) taxes paid by consumers when they buy goods and services. When you buy a book, you pay the price of the book plus any state and local sales tax. The business is actually acting as the government's agent

FIGURE 8-4

Gross Domestic Product and Gross Domestic Income, 2000 (in billions of 2000 dollars per year)

By using the two different methods of computing the output of the economy, we come up with gross domestic product and gross domestic income, which are by definition equal. One approach focuses on expenditures, or the flow of product; the other approach concentrates on income, or the flow of costs.

Source: U.S. Department of Commerce. First quarter preliminary data annualized.

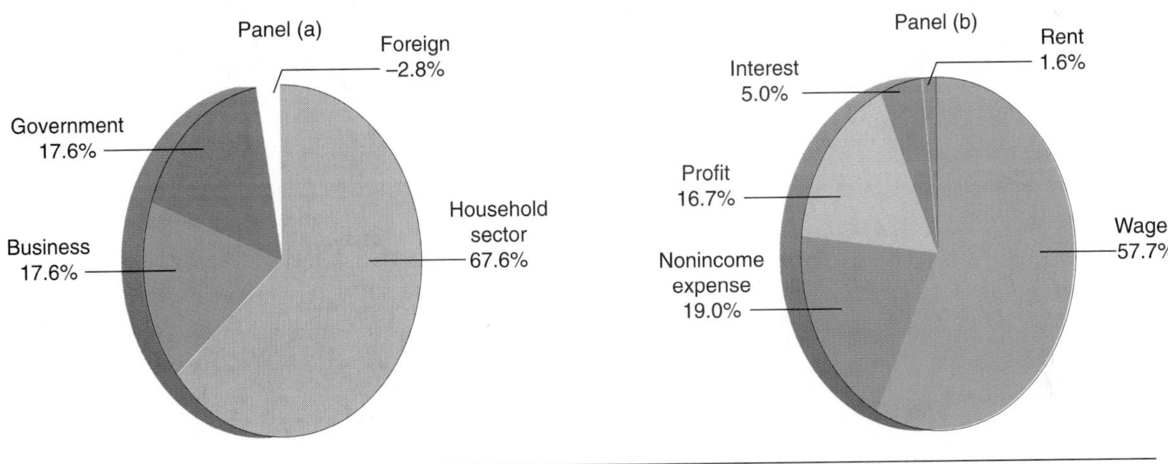

Expenditure Point of View—Product Flow Expenditures by Different Sectors:		Income Point of View—Cost Flow Domestic Income (at Factor Cost):	
Household sector		*Wages*	
Personal consumption expenses	$6,661.5	All wages, salaries, and supplemental employee compensation	$5,678.4
Government sector		*Rent*	
Purchase of goods and services	1,734.6	All rental income of individuals plus implicit rent on owner-occupied dwellings	155.4
Business sector		*Interest*	
Gross private domestic investment (including depreciation)	1,727.0	Net interest paid by business	490.2
Foreign sector		*Profit*	
Net exports of goods and services	−273.6	Proprietorial income	701.3
		Corporate profits before taxes deducted	952.0
		Nonincome expense items	
		Indirect business taxes and other adjustments	762.1
		Depreciation	1,215.4
		Statistical discrepancy	−105.3
Gross domestic product	$9,849.5	Gross domestic income	$9,849.5

in collecting the sales tax, which it in turn passes on to the government. Such taxes therefore represent a business expense and are included in gross domestic income.

Depreciation. Just as we had to deduct depreciation to get from GDP to NDP, so we must *add* depreciation to go from net domestic income to gross domestic income. Depreciation can be thought of as the portion of the current year's GDP that is used to replace physical capital consumed in the process of production. Because somebody has paid for the replacement, depreciation must be added as a component of gross domestic income.

Nonincome expense items
The total of indirect business taxes and depreciation.

The last two components of GDP—indirect business taxes and depreciation—are called **nonincome expense items.**

Figure 8-4 on the previous page shows a comparison between gross domestic product and gross domestic income for 2000. Whether you decide to use the expenditure approach or the income approach, you will come out with the same number. There are sometimes statistical discrepancies, but they are usually relatively small.

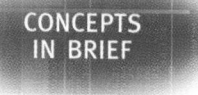

- To derive GDP using the income approach, we add up all factor payments, including wages, interest, rent, and profits.
- To get an accurate estimate of GDP with this method, we must also add indirect business taxes and depreciation to those total factor payments.

OTHER COMPONENTS OF NATIONAL INCOME ACCOUNTING

Gross domestic income or product does not really tell how much income people have access to for spending purposes. To get to those kinds of data, we must make some adjustments, which we now do.

National Income (NI)

We know that net domestic product (NDP) represents the total market value of goods and services available for both consumption, used in a broader sense here to mean "resource exhaustion," and net additions to the economy's stock of capital. NDP does not, however, represent the income available to individuals within that economy because it includes indirect business taxes, such as sales taxes. We therefore deduct these indirect business taxes from NDP to arrive at the figure for all factor income of resource owners. The result is what we define as **national income (NI)**—income *earned* by the factors of production.

National income (NI)
The total of all factor payments to resource owners. It can be obtained by subtracting indirect business taxes from NDP.

Personal Income (PI)

National income does not actually represent what is available to individuals to spend because some people obtain income for which they have provided no concurrent good or service and others earn income but do not receive it. In the former category are mainly recipients of transfer payments from the government, such as Social Security, welfare, and food stamps. These payments represent shifts of funds within the economy by way of the government, where no good or service is concurrently rendered in exchange. For the other category, income earned but not received, the most obvious examples are corporate retained earnings that are plowed back into the business, contributions to social insurance,

TABLE 8-2
Going from GDP to Disposable Income, 2000

	Billions of Dollars
Gross domestic product (GDP)	9,849.5
Minus depreciation	−1,215.4
Net domestic product (NDP)	8,634.1
Minus indirect business taxes and other adjustments	−762.1
National income (NI)	7,872.0
Minus corporate taxes, Social Security contributions, corporate retained earnings	−1,236.5
Plus government and business transfer payments	+1,606.8
Personal income (PI)	8,242.3
Minus personal income tax and nontax payments	−1,253.2
Disposable personal income (DPI)	6,989.1

Source: U.S. Department of Commerce.

and corporate income taxes. When transfer payments are added and when income earned but not received is subtracted, we end up with **personal income (PI)**—income *received* by the factors of production prior to the payment of personal income taxes.

Personal income (PI)
The amount of income that households actually receive before they pay personal income taxes.

Disposable Personal Income (DPI)

Everybody knows that you do not get to take home all your salary. To get **disposable personal income (DPI),** we subtract all personal income taxes from personal income. This is the income that individuals have left for consumption and saving.

Disposable personal income (DPI)
Personal income after personal income taxes have been paid.

Deriving the Components of GDP

Table 8-2 takes you through the steps necessary to derive the various components of GDP. It shows how you go from gross domestic product to net domestic product to national income to personal income and then to disposable personal income. On the endpapers of your book, you can see the historical record for GDP, NDP, NI, PI, and DPI for selected years since 1929.

We have completed our rundown of the different ways that GDP can be computed and of the different variants of national income and product. What we have not yet touched on is the difference between national income measured in this year's dollars and national income representing real goods and services.

CONCEPTS IN BRIEF

- To obtain national income, we subtract indirect business taxes from net domestic product. National income gives us a measure of all factor payments to resource owners.
- To obtain personal income, we must add government transfer payments, such as Social Security benefits and food stamps. We must subtract income earned but not received by factor owners, such as corporate retained earnings, Social Security contributions, and corporate income taxes.
- To obtain disposable personal income, we subtract all personal income taxes from personal income. Disposable personal income is income that individuals actually have for consumption or saving.

DISTINGUISHING BETWEEN NOMINAL AND REAL VALUES

Nominal values
The values of variables such as GDP and investment expressed in current dollars, also called *money values;* measurement in terms of the actual market prices at which goods are sold.

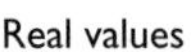

Real values
Measurement of economic values after adjustments have been made for changes in the average of prices between years.

So far we have shown how to measure *nominal* income and product. When we say "nominal," we are referring to income and product expressed in the current "face value" of today's dollar. Given the existence of inflation or deflation in the economy, we must also be able to distinguish between the **nominal values** that we will be looking at and the **real values** underlying them. Nominal values are expressed in current dollars. Real income involves our command over goods and services—purchasing power—and therefore depends on money income and a set of prices. Thus real income refers to nominal income corrected for changes in the weighted average of all prices. In other words, we must make an adjustment for changes in the price level. Consider an example. Nominal income *per person* in 1960 was only about $2,800 per year. In 2000, nominal income per person was close to $36,000. Were people really that bad off in 1960? No, for nominal income in 1960 is expressed in 1960 prices, not in the prices of today. In today's dollars, the per-person income of 1960 would be closer to $10,000, or about 28 percent of today's income per person. This is a meaningful comparison between income in 1960 and income today. Next we will show how we can translate nominal measures of income into real measures by using an appropriate price index, such as the CPI or the GDP deflator discussed in Chapter 7.

Correcting GDP for Price Changes

Constant dollars 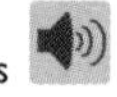
Dollars expressed in terms of real purchasing power using a particular year as the base or standard of comparison, in contrast to current dollars.

If a compact disk (CD) costs $15 this year, 10 CDs will have a market value of $150. If next year they cost $20 each, the same 10 CDs will have a market value of $200. In this case, there is no increase in the total quantity of CDs, but the market value will have increased by one-third. Apply this to every single good and service produced and sold in the United States and you realize that changes in GDP, measured in *current* dollars, may not be a very useful indication of economic activity. If we are really interested in variations in the *real* output of the economy, we must correct GDP (and just about everything else we look at) for changes in the average of overall prices from year to year. Basically, we need to generate an index that approximates the changes in average prices and then divide that estimate into the value of output in current dollars to adjust the value of output to what is called **constant dollars,** or dollars corrected for general price level changes. This price-corrected GDP is called *real GDP.*

EXAMPLE

Correcting GDP for Price Index Changes, 1990–2000

Let's take a numerical example to see how we can adjust GDP for changes in the price index. We must pick an appropriate price index in order to adjust for these price level changes. We mentioned the Consumer Price Index, the Producer Price Index, and the GDP deflator in Chapter 7. Let's use the GDP deflator to adjust our figures. Table 8-3 gives 13 years of GDP figures. Nominal GDP figures are shown in column 2. The price index (GDP deflator) is in column 3, with base year of 1996 when the GDP deflator equals 100. Column 4 shows real (inflation-adjusted) GDP in 1996 dollars.

The formula for real GDP is

$$\text{Real GDP} = \frac{\text{nominal GDP}}{\text{price level}} \times 100$$

The step-by-step derivation of real (constant-dollar) GDP is as follows: The base year is 1996, so the price index for that year must equal 100. In 1996, nominal GDP was $7,813.2 billion, and so too was real GDP expressed in 1996 dollars. In 1997, the price level increased to 101.7. Thus to correct 1997's nominal GDP for inflation, we divide the price index, 101.7, into the nominal GDP figure of $8,300.9 billion and

(1) Year	(2) Nominal GDP (billions of dollars per year)	(3) Price Level Index base year 1996 = 100)	(4) = [(2) ÷ (3)] × 100 Real GDP (billions of dollars per year (in constant 1996 dollars)
1990	5,803.2	86.8	6,683.5
1991	5,986.2	89.8	6,669.2
1992	6,318.9	91.7	6,891.1
1993	6,642.3	94.2	7,054.1
1994	7,054.3	96.1	7,337.8
1995	7,400.5	98.2	7,537.1
1996	7,813.2	100.0	7,813.2
1997	8,300.9	101.7	8,165.1
1998	8,759.9	102.9	8,516.3
1999	9,254.6	104.4	8,867.0
2000	9,849.5	106.4	9,256.2

Source: U.S. Department of Commerce, Bureau of Economic Analysis.

TABLE 8-3
Correcting GDP for Price Index Changes
To correct GDP for price index changes, we first have to pick a price index (the GDP deflator) with a specific year as its base. In our example, the base level is 1996 prices; the price index for that year is 100. To obtain 1996 constant-dollar GDP, we divide the price index into nominal GDP and multiply by 100. In other words, we divide column 3 into column 2 and multiply by 100. This gives us column 4, which is a measure of real GDP expressed in 1996 purchasing power.

then multiply it by 100. The result is $8,165.1 billion, which is 1997 GDP expressed in terms of the purchasing power of dollars in 1996. What about a situation when the price index is lower than in 1996? Look at 1990. Here the price index shown in column 3 is only 86.8. That means that in 1990, the average of all prices was about 87 percent of prices in 1996. To obtain 1990 GDP expressed in terms of 1996 purchasing power, we divide nominal GDP, $5,803.2 billion, by 86.8 and then multiply by 100. The result is a larger number—$6,683.5 billion. Column 4 in Table 8-3 is a better measure of how the economy has performed than column 2, which shows nominal GDP changes.

For Critical Analysis

A few years ago, the base year for the GDP deflator was 1992. What does a change in the base year for the price index affect?

Plotting Nominal and Real GDP

Nominal GDP and real GDP since 1970 are plotted in Figure 8-5 on page 186. Notice that there is quite a big gap between the two GDP figures, reflecting the amount of inflation that has occurred. Note, further, that the choice of a base year is arbitrary. We have chosen 1996 as the base year in our example. This happens to be the base year that is currently used by the government.

Per Capita GDP

Looking at changes in real gross domestic product may be deceiving, particularly if the population size has changed significantly. If real GDP over a 10-year period went up 100 percent, you might jump to the conclusion that the real income of a typical person in

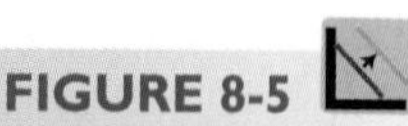

FIGURE 8-5

Nominal and Real GDP

Here we plot both nominal and real GDP. Real GDP is expressed in the purchasing power of 1996 dollars. The gap between the two represents price level changes.

Source: U.S. Department of Commerce.

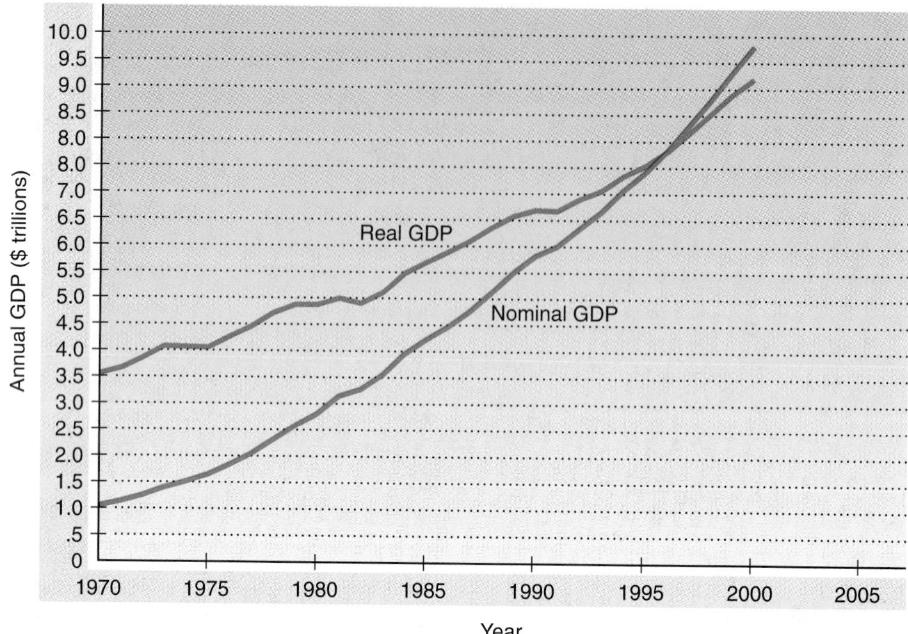

the economy had increased by that amount. But what if during the same period population increased by 200 percent? Then what would you say? Certainly, the amount of real GDP per person, or *per capita real GDP,* would have fallen, even though *total* real GDP had risen. What we must do to account not only for price changes but also for population changes is first deflate GDP and then divide by the total population, doing this for each year. If we were to look at certain less developed countries, we would find that in many cases, even though real GDP has risen over the past several decades, per capita real GDP has remained constant or fallen because the population has grown just as rapidly or more quickly.

The Chain-Weighted Measure of the Growth in Real GDP

In December 1995, the Commerce Department's Bureau of Economic Analysis (BEA) made a fundamental change in the way it computes real gross domestic product. Remember that real GDP consists of consumer spending, business investment, government expenditures on goods and services, and net foreign trade. To calculate real GDP, the BEA had used a weighted sum of 1,100 components of these four categories. Until 1996, these 1,100 components were fixed in weight, and their relative importance changed only periodically. For example, the last revision was made in 1987. Otherwise stated, the BEA had been using a *fixed-weight* measure of changes in real GDP.

Now the BEA changes the weights of the different components of real GDP to reflect changes in their relative prices and in their relative shares in the overall economy's output. The new measure is called *chain-weighted real GDP.* Rather than a specific number, an index is used. Thus to calculate a year's *change* in real GDP, it is necessary to compare one year's index with the previous year's index. The BEA publishes both the chain-weighted real GDP index and its dollar equivalent. You can find chain-weighted real GDP statistics on the endpapers of this book, which show our national income accounts.

CONCEPTS IN BRIEF

- To correct nominal GDP for price changes, we first use a base year for our price index and assign it the number 100. Then we construct an index based on how a weighted average of the price level has changed relative to that base year. For example, if in the next year a weighted average of the price level indicates that prices have increased by 10 percent, we would assign it the number 110. We then divide each year's price index, so constructed, into its respective nominal GDP figure (and multiply by 100).
- We can divide the population into real GDP to obtain per capita real GDP.

COMPARING GDP THROUGHOUT THE WORLD 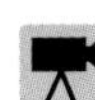

It is relatively easy to compare the standard of living of a family in Los Angeles with that of one living in Boston. Both families get paid in dollars and can buy the same goods and services at Kmart, McDonald's, and Costco. It is not so easy, however, to make a similar comparison between a family living in the United States and one in, say, India. The first problem concerns money. Indians get paid in rupees, their national currency, and buy goods and services with those rupees. But how do we compare the average standard of living measured in rupees with that measured in dollars?

Foreign Exchange Rates

In earlier chapters, you have encountered international examples that involved local currencies, but the dollar equivalent always has been given. The dollar equivalent is calculated by looking up the **foreign exchange rate** that is published daily in major newspapers throughout the world. If you know that you can exchange $1 for 5 francs, the exchange rate is 5 to 1 (or otherwise stated, a franc is worth 20 cents). So if French incomes per capita are, say, 100,000 francs, that translates at an exchange rate of 5 francs to $1, to $20,000. For years, statisticians calculated relative GDP by simply adding up each country's GDP in its local currency and dividing by each respective dollar exchange rate.

Foreign exchange rate
The price of one currency in terms of another.

True Purchasing Power

The problem with simply using foreign exchange rates to convert other countries' GDP and per capita GDP into dollars is that not all goods and services are bought and sold in a world market. Restaurant food, housecleaning services, and home repairs do not get exchanged across countries. In countries that have very low wages, those kinds of services are much cheaper than foreign exchange rate computations would imply. Government statistics claiming that per capita income in some poor country is only $300 a year seem shocking. But such a statistic does not tell you the true standard of living of people in that country. Only by looking at what is called **purchasing power parity** can you determine other countries' true standards of living compared to ours.

Purchasing power parity 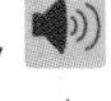
Adjustment in exchange rate conversions that takes into account differences in the true cost of living across countries.

INTERNATIONAL EXAMPLE

Purchasing Power Parity Comparisons of World Incomes

A few years ago, the International Monetary Fund accepted the purchasing power parity approach as the correct one. It started presenting international statistics on each country's GDP relative to every other's based on purchasing power parity. The results were surprising. As you can see from Table 8-4, India has a higher per capita GDP compared to what was measured at market foreign exchange rates.

For Critical Analysis

What percentage increase is there in per capita GDP in India when one switches from foreign exchange rates to purchasing power parity?

TABLE 8-4
Comparing GDP Internationally

Country	Annual GDP Based on Purchasing Power Parity (billions of U.S. dollars)	Per Capita GDP Based on Purchasing Power Parity (U.S. dollars)	Per Capita GDP Based on Foreign Exchange Rates (U.S. dollars)
United States	6,897.2	26,528	26,528
Japan	2,493.8	19,399	26,424
China	2,490.1	1,692	375
Germany	2,007.4	19,870	24,421
France	1,421.6	18,450	23,489
Russia	1,101.8	6,903	2,640
India	1,100.4	1,155	379
Italy	1,099.0	17,050	17,990
United Kingdom	1,088.0	16,352	16,804
Brazil	980.4	5,251	2,794

Sources: International Monetary Fund; World Bank; Organization for Economic Cooperation and Development.

CONCEPTS IN BRIEF

- The foreign exchange rate is the price of one currency in terms of another.
- Statisticians often calculate relative GDP by adding up each country's GDP in its local currency and dividing by the dollar exchange rate.
- Because not all goods and services are bought and sold in the world market, we must correct exchange rate conversions of other countries' GDP figures to take into account differences in the true cost of living across countries.

NETNOMICS

Has Real GDP Measurement Kept Pace with the Internet?

A key ingredient in the measurement of real GDP is of course the price index. Changes in the prices of things you buy eventually show up as changes in the measured price index. The price you pay for many items, however, consist really of two prices: the nominal price you pay in dollars plus the price of your time involved in the transaction, measured by its opportunity cost. If a good was sold at an artificially low price, thereby creating lines of people waiting to buy it, the measured price of the good would not reflect its true price.

Slowly but surely, the Internet is reducing the time spent engaging in many transactions. For example, people who trade stocks and bonds on-line do not have to spend any time dealing with securities brokers. Individuals who use the Internet for on-line banking spend considerably less time per transaction than they did only a few years ago. On-line purchasing of airline tickets also often saves time for each transaction.

There is a time saving on the seller's side also. But this time saving translates into lower costs for the sellers. These lower costs are generally picked up by government statisticians. In contrast, the other half of the equation—the consumer's reduced time spent per each transaction—is apparently not picked up by official government statistics.

The point is that in a world of increasing Internet use and consequent reductions in time spent per transaction, the level and rate of growth of real GDP may be greater than measured. Why? Because the price level may not be accurately reflecting the changes in true prices by including the opportunity cost of time.

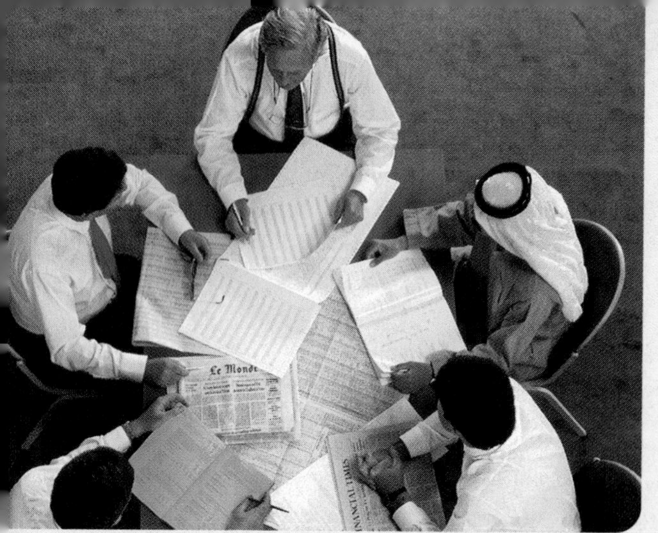

Issues & Applications

How Well Do Economists Predict GDP?

A joke among economists is that they have been able to forecast nine of the last seven recessions. Underlying this joke is a reality: The people who make their living forecasting changes in real GDP do not have a stellar track record. Actually, this assessment is a little too harsh. Forecasting economists have done a pretty good job predicting *long-run* trends in real GDP. Where they go wrong is in predicting downturns, otherwise known as recessions. In Table 8-5, you can see that forecasters missed four of the five past downturns in our economy since the 1960s. The best that can be said about typical economic forecasts of downturns is that they are usually late. In other words, downturns seemed to be recognized only after they have begun.

Concepts Applied

National Income Accounting

GDP

Real GDP

How the Forecasters Do It

Most forecasters use large-scale computer models to develop their estimates of changes in real GDP. These computer models attempt to make sense of how our multitrillion-dollar economy works. Sometimes these models involve hundreds of sectors. A sector, such as automobiles, may be shown to depend on a wide range of variables—interest rates, price changes, and so on. Some experts argue that even the largest-scale computer models of our economy can no longer handle its changing nature. Furthermore, the U.S. economy is increasingly part of an interconnected world. Little long-term research has been done to discover how changes in the rest of the world's economies ultimately affect the U.S. economy.

TABLE 8-5
Economic Forecasts: Missing the Mark
The forecasts given in the table are taken from *Business Week* surveys through the years. Only the recession that started at the beginning of 1980 was correctly anticipated by the economic forecasters surveyed. They missed the other four downturns completely.

Start of Recession	Date of Forecast	Forecasted Growth over the Next Year (%)	Actual Growth in Real GDP (%)
December 1969	December 1969	1.5	−.6
November 1973	December 1973	1.5	−1.8
January 1980	December 1979	−.7	−.3
July 1990	December 1989	2.1	−.1
July 1991	December 1990	2.2	.7

Source: Business Week, September 30, 1996, p. 92.

Other Difficulties in Predicting Downturns

The globalization of the American economy cannot be used as an excuse for missing the downturn that started in December 1969. The 1960s was a decade of sustained economic growth (similar to the 1990s). A year before the downturn started, economic forecasters as a group pegged the probability of recession in the coming year at less than 15 percent. Their excuse for missing this downturn was that they did not foresee federal government defense spending cuts and rising interest rates caused by contractionary government policies.

The forecasters' reasons for missing the 1973 downturn was that they could not predict the embargo imposed by oil-producing countries at that time. The recession of 1990 arrived without much warning at all. Indeed, virtually no economic model predicted that recession.

Economic forecasters defend themselves by stating that recessions that happen quickly are virtually impossible to predict. Those that commence slowly are countered by government policy and presumably do not actually occur. So, according to these forecasters, only when policymakers are caught by surprise do we have recessions.

FOR CRITICAL ANALYSIS

1. Explain how a business could be hurt by relying on an inaccurate forecast of changes in real GDP.
2. Computing power is relatively cheap and incredibly massive today compared to the 1960s. Nonetheless, large-scale computer economic models have done no better in predicting economic downturns? Why?

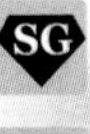

SUMMARY DISCUSSION OF LEARNING OBJECTIVES

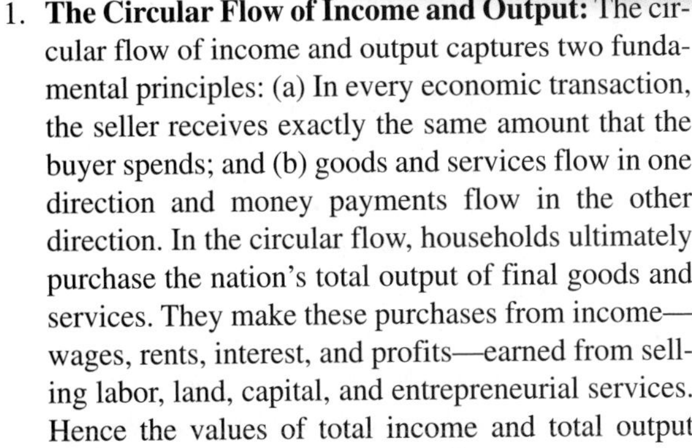

1. **The Circular Flow of Income and Output:** The circular flow of income and output captures two fundamental principles: (a) In every economic transaction, the seller receives exactly the same amount that the buyer spends; and (b) goods and services flow in one direction and money payments flow in the other direction. In the circular flow, households ultimately purchase the nation's total output of final goods and services. They make these purchases from income—wages, rents, interest, and profits—earned from selling labor, land, capital, and entrepreneurial services. Hence the values of total income and total output must be the same in the circular flow.
2. **Gross Domestic Product (GDP):** A nation's gross domestic product is the total market value of its final output of goods and services produced within a given year using factors of production located within the nation's borders. Because GDP measures a flow of production during a year, it is not a measure of a nation's wealth, which is a stock at a given point in time.
3. **The Limitations of Using GDP as a Measure of National Welfare:** Gross domestic product is a useful measure for tracking year-to-year changes in a nation's overall economic activity. Nevertheless, it excludes nonmarket transactions that may contribute to or detract from general welfare. It also fails to account for factors such as labor market discrimination, personal safety, environmental quality, and the amount of and quality of leisure time available to a nation's residents. Thus GDP is not a measure of national well-being.
4. **The Expenditure Approach to Tabulating GDP:** To calculate GDP using the expenditure approach, we sum consumption spending, investment expenditures, government spending, and net export expenditures. Thus we add the total amount spent on newly produced goods and services during the year to obtain the dollar value of the output produced and purchased during the year.
5. **The Income Approach to Computing GDP:** To tabulate GDP using the income approach, we first add total wages and salaries, rental income, interest income, profits, and nonincome expense items—indirect business taxes and depreciation—to obtain gross domestic income, which is equivalent to gross domestic product. Thus the total value of all income earnings (equivalent to total factor costs) equals GDP.

6. **Distinguishing Between Nominal GDP and Real GDP:** Nominal GDP is the value of newly produced output during the current year measured at current market prices. Real GDP adjusts the value of current output into constant dollars by correcting for changes in the overall level of prices from year to year. To calculate real GDP, we divide nominal GDP by the price level (the GDP deflator) and multiply by 100.

Key Terms and Concepts

Capital consumption allowance (179)
Constant dollars (184)
Depreciation (178)
Disposable personal income (DPI) (183)
Durable consumer goods (176)
Expenditure approach (176)
Final goods and services (169)
Fixed investment (177)
Foreign exchange rate (187)
Gross domestic income (GDI) (180)
Gross domestic product (GDP) (171)
Gross private domestic investment (176)
Income approach (176)
Indirect business taxes (181)
Intermediate goods (172)
Inventory investment (177)
Investment (176)
National income (NI) (182)
National income accounting (169)
Net domestic product (NDP) (178)
Net investment (179)
Nominal values (184)
Nondurable consumer goods (176)
Nonincome expense items (182)
Personal income (PI) (183)
Producer durables, or capital goods (176)
Purchasing power parity (187)
Real values (184)
Services (176)
Total income (169)
Value added (172)

Problems

Answers to the odd numbered problems appear at the back of the book.

8-1. Consider the following hypothetical data for the U.S. economy in 2005, where all amounts are in trillions of dollars.

Consumption	11.0
Indirect business taxes	.8
Depreciation	1.3
Government spending	1.8
Imports	1.7
Gross private domestic investment	2.0
Exports	1.5

a. Based on the data, what is GDP? NDP? NI?

b. Suppose that in 2006, exports fall to $1.3 trillion, imports rise to $1.85 trillion, and gross private domestic investment falls to $1.25 trillion. What will GDP be in 2006, assuming that other values do not change between 2005 and 2006?

c. Note that according to the fictitious data, depreciation (capital consumption allowance) exceeds gross private domestic investment in 2006. How would this affect future U.S. productivity, particularly if it were to continue beyond 2006?

8-2. Look back at Table 8-3, which explains how to calculate real GDP in terms of 1996 constant dollars. Change the base year to 1998. Recalculate the price index, and then recalculate real GDP—that is, express column 4 of Table 8-3 in terms of 1998 dollars instead of 1996 dollars.

8-3. Consider the following hypothetical data for the U.S. economy in 2005, and assume that there are no statistical discrepancies or other adjustments.

Profit	2.8
Indirect business taxes	.8
Rent	.7
Interest	.8
Wages	8.2

Depreciation	1.3
Consumption	11.0
Exports	1.5
Government and business transfer payments	2.0
Personal income taxes and nontax payments	1.7
Imports	1.7
Corporate taxes and retained earnings	.5
Social Security contributions	2.0
Government spending	1.8

a. What is gross domestic income? GDP?
b. What is gross private domestic investment?
c. What is personal income? Personal disposable income?

8-4. Which of the following are production activities that are included in GDP? Which are not?
a. Mr. King paints his own house.
b. Mr. King paints houses for a living.
c. Mrs. King earns income by taking baby photos in her home photography studio.
d. Mrs. King takes photos of planets and stars as part of her astronomy hobby.
e. E*Trade charges fees to process Internet orders for stock trades.
f. Mr. Ho purchases 300 shares of America Online stock via an Internet trade order.
g. Mrs. Ho receives a Social Security payment.
h. Ms. Chavez makes a $300 payment for an Internet-based course on stock trading.
i. Mr. Langham sells a used laptop computer to his neighbor.

8-5. Explain what happens to the official measure of GDP in each of the following situations.
a. A woman who makes a living charging for investment advice on her Internet Web site marries one of her clients, to whom she now provides advice at no charge.
b. A tennis player who recently had won two top professional tournaments earlier this year as an amateur turns professional and continues his streak by winning two more before the year is out.
c. A company that had been selling used firearms illegally finally gets around to obtaining an operating license and performing background checks as specified by law prior to each gun sale.

8-6. Which one of the following activities of a computer manufacturer during the current year are included in this year's measure of GDP?
a. The manufacturer purchases a chip in June, uses it as a component in a computer in August, and sells the computer to a customer in November.
b. A retail outlet of the company sells a computer manufactured during the current year.
c. A marketing arm of the company receives fee income during the current year when a buyer of a one of its computers elects to use the computer manufacturer as her Internet service provider.

8-7. Consider the following table for the economy of a nation whose residents produce five goods.

	1997		2002	
Good	Price	Quantity	Price	Quantity
Shampoo	$ 2	15	$ 4	20
DVD drives	200	10	250	10
Books	40	5	50	4
Milk	3	10	4	3
Candy	1	40	2	20

Assuming a 1997 baseyear:
a. What is nominal GDP for 1997 and 2002?
b. What is real GDP for 1997 and 2002?

8-8. In the table for Problem 8-7, if 1997 is the base year, what is the price index for 1997? For 2002? (Round decimal fractions to the nearest tenth.)

8-9. Suppose that early in a year, a hurricane hits a town in Florida and destroys a sizable amount of residential housing. A portion of this stock of housing, which had a market value of $100 million (not including the market value of the land), was uninsured. The owners of the houses spent a total of $5 million during the rest of the year to pay salvage companies to help them save remaining belongings. A small percentage of uninsured owners had sufficient resources to spend a total of $15 million during the year to pay construction companies to rebuild their homes. Some were able to devote their own time, the opportunity cost of which was valued at $3 million, to work on rebuilding their homes. The remaining people, however, chose to sell their land at its market value and abandon the remains of their houses. What was the combined effect of these transactions on GDP for this year? In what ways, if any, does the effect on GDP reflect a loss in welfare for these individuals?

8-10. Suppose that in 2004, geologists discover large reserves of oil under a barren tundra in Alaska. These reserves have a market value estimated at $50 billion at current oil prices. Oil companies spend $1 billion to hire workers and move and position equipment to begin exploratory pumping during that same year. In the process of loading some of the oil onto tankers at a port, one company accidentally creates a spill into a bay and ultimately pays more than $1 billion to other companies to clean it up. Nevertheless, the oil spill kills thousands of birds, seals, and other wildlife. What was the combined effect of these events on GDP for this year? In what ways, if any, does the effect on GDP reflect a loss in national welfare?

Economics on the Net

Tracking the Components of Gross Domestic Product One way to keep tabs on the components of GDP is via the FRED database at the Web site of the Federal Reserve Bank of St. Louis.

Title: Gross Domestic Product and Components

Navigation: Click here to visit the homepage of the Federal Reserve Bank of St. Louis. Click on FRED. Then click on Gross Domestic Product and Components.

Application

1. Click on Gross Domestic Product. Write down nominal GDP data for the past 10 quarters.
2. Back up to Real Gross Domestic Product in Fixed 1996 Dollars. Write down the amounts for the past 10 quarters. Use the formula on page 184 to calculate the price level for each quarter. Has the price level decreased or increased in recent quarters?

For Group Study and Analysis Divide the class into "consumption," "investment," "government sector," and "foreign sector" groups. Have each group evaluate the contribution of each category of spending to GDP and to its quarter-to-quarter volatility. Reconvene the class, and discuss the factors that appear to create the most variability in GDP.

CHAPTER 9

GLOBAL ECONOMIC GROWTH AND DEVELOPMENT

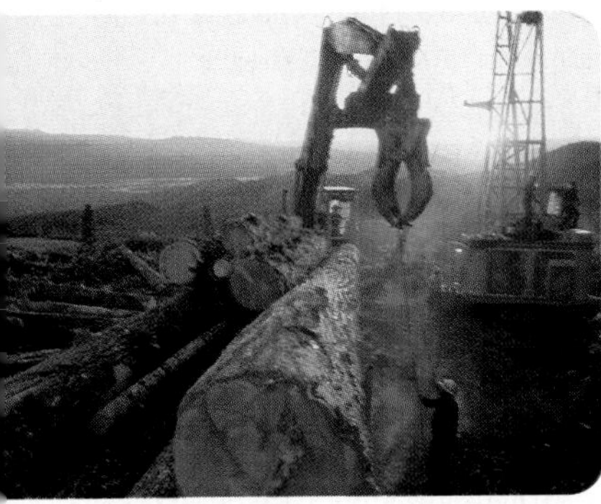

This type of logging operation at Mount Adams, Washington, may soon be a thing of the past. In today's modern facilities, newly felled trees slide onto platforms guided by computers. The logs then go into computer-automated sawing systems. How does such improved technology add to our economic growth?

In Portland, Oregon, a newly felled tree slides onto a platform. A spinning saw approaches the timber to start cutting 2-inch by 4-inch boards. Then it hesitates. Data received by a computer guiding the saw have indicated a rise in the market price of 4-inch by 4-inch boards. The computer has readjusted the saw's position to cut the timber into the larger boards. The saw begins to cut into the timber.

American companies have spent the past several years making huge investments in computers. As you will learn in this chapter, economists differ in their assessments of exactly how much computerization has contributed to growth of the American economy.

To understand why economists reach different conclusions about this issue, you need to know how to measure a nation's economic growth. You also need to understand the key determinants of economic growth. Both are central topics of this chapter.

LEARNING OBJECTIVES

After reading this chapter, you should be able to:

1. **Define economic growth**
2. **Recognize the importance of economic growth rates**
3. **Describe the fundamental determinants of economic growth**
4. **Explain why productivity increases are crucial for maintaining economic growth**
5. **Understand the basis of new growth theory**
6. **Discuss the fundamental factors that contribute to a nation's economic development**

Chapter Outline

Did You Know That... at the turn of the twentieth century, Argentina had the sixth highest per capita income in the world, whereas it is now around fortieth, somewhat below Iran? Consider also that 100 years ago, Hong Kong was basically a barren rock, whereas today its per capita income exceeds that of France and the United Kingdom. How can we explain such dramatic changes in relative living standards? From an arithmetic point of view, the answer is simple: Argentina experienced little and in some cases negative economic growth over the past century, whereas Hong Kong had significant economic growth. That answer, though, does not tell us why economic growth rates differed in these two countries. That is the task of this chapter. Should you care about the rate of economic growth in the United States? The answer is yes, if you care about your future standard of living and that of your children and grandchildren. You have already demonstrated that you care about your future standard of living; otherwise, you would not be bothering to obtain a higher education. Obviously, you want to make sure that you experience economic growth as an individual. Now it is time to consider the nation as a whole.

HOW DO WE DEFINE ECONOMIC GROWTH?

Remember from Chapter 2 that we can show economic growth graphically as an outward shift of a production possibilities curve, as is seen in Figure 9-1. If there is economic growth between 2000 and 2025, the production possibilities curve will shift outward toward the red curve. The distance that it shifts represents the amount of economic growth, defined as the increase in the productive capacity of a nation. Although it is possible to come up with a measure of a nation's increased productive capacity, it would not be easy. Therefore, we turn to a more readily obtainable definition of economic growth.

Most people have a general idea of what economic growth means. When a nation grows economically, its citizens must be better off in at least some ways, usually in terms of their material well-being. Typically, though, we do not measure the well-being of any nation solely in terms of its total output of real goods and services or in terms of real GDP without making some adjustments. After all, India has a GDP about three times as large as that of Switzerland. The population in India, though, is about 125 times greater than that of Switzerland. Consequently, we view India as a relatively poor country and Switzerland as a relatively rich country. That means that to measure how much a country is growing in terms of annual increases in real GDP, we have to adjust for population growth. Our formal definition becomes this: **Economic growth** occurs when there are increases in *per capita* real GDP; it is measured by the rate of change in per capita real GDP per year.

Economic growth 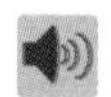
Increases in per capita real GDP measured by its rate of change per year.

FIGURE 9-1
Economic Growth
If there is growth between 2000 and 2025, the production possibilities curve for the entire economy will shift outward from the blue line labeled 2000 to the red line labeled 2025. The distance that it shifts represents an increase in the productive capacity of the nation.

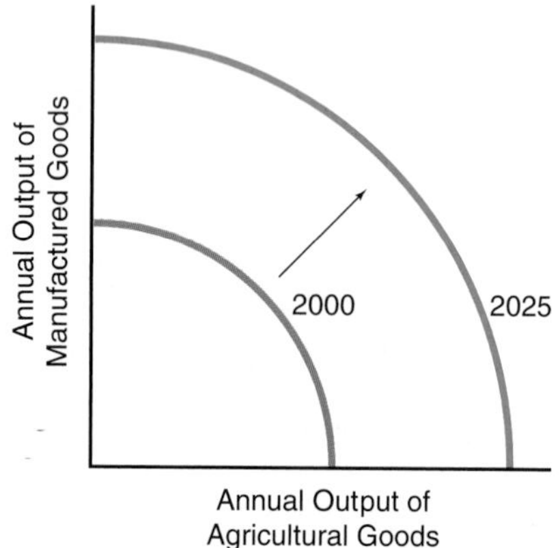

FIGURE 9-2
The Historical Record of U.S. Economic Growth
The graph traces per capita real GDP in the United States since 1900. Data are given in 1996 dollars.
Source: U.S. Department of Commerce.

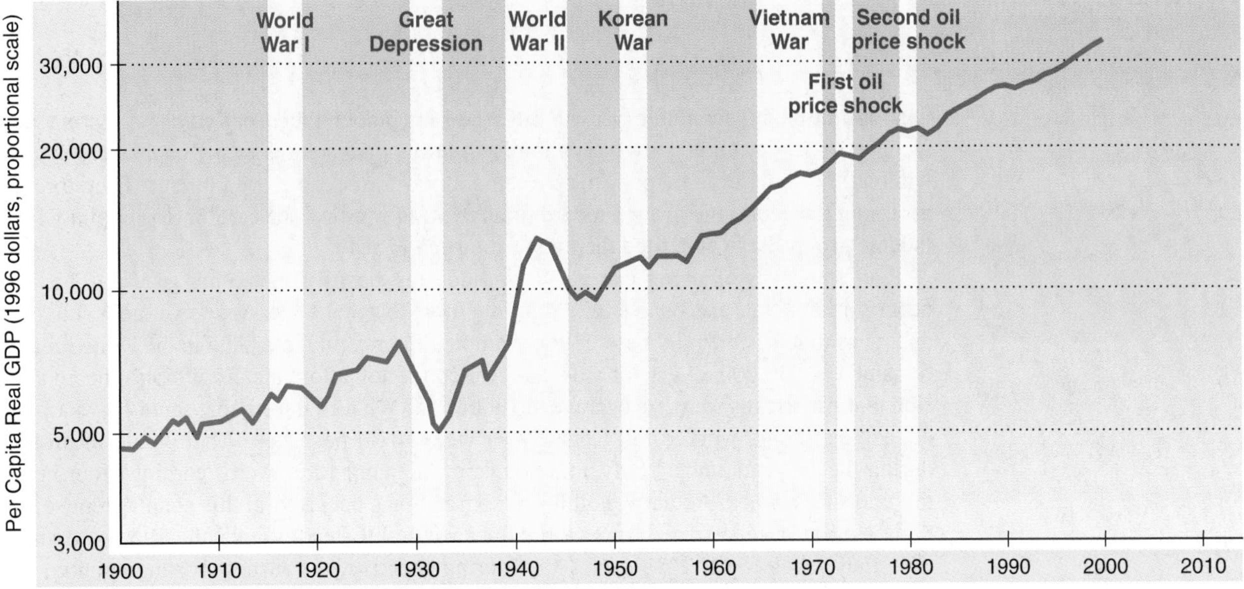

Figure 9-2 presents the historical record of real GDP per person in the United States.

INTERNATIONAL EXAMPLE

Growth Rates Around the World

Table 9-1 shows the annual average rate of growth of income per person in selected countries. Notice that the United States during the time period under study is positioned about midway in the pack. Even though we are one of the world's richest countries, our rate of economic growth through the 1990s was not particularly

TABLE 9-1
Per Capita Growth Rates in Various Countries

Country	Average Annual Rate of Growth of Income Per Capita, 1970–2000 (%)	Country	Average Annual Rate of Growth of Income Per Capita, 1970–2000 (%)
Switzerland	1.9	Italy	2.8
Sweden	2.0	United States	2.9
Germany	2.2	Spain	3.0
United Kingdom	2.3	Japan	3.9
Netherlands	2.4	Turkey	5.6
Canada	2.6	China	7.0
France	2.7		

Sources: World Bank; International Monetary Fund.

high. The reason that U.S. per capita income has remained higher than per capita incomes in most other nations is that the United States has been able to sustain growth over many decades. This is something that most other countries have so far been unable to accomplish.

For Critical Analysis

"The largest change is from zero to one." Does this statement have anything to do with relative growth rates in poorer versus richer countries?

Problems in Definition

Our definition of economic growth says nothing about the *distribution* of output and income. A nation might grow very rapidly in terms of increases in per capita real output, while at the same time its poor people remain poor or become even poorer. Therefore, in assessing the economic growth record of any nation, we must be careful to pinpoint which income groups have benefited the most from such growth.

Real standards of living can go up without any positive economic growth. This can occur if individuals are, on average, enjoying more leisure by working fewer hours but producing as much as they did before. For example, if per capita real GDP in the United States remained at $30,000 a year for a decade, we could not automatically jump to the conclusion that Americans were, on average, no better off. What if, during that same 10-year period, average hours worked fell from 37 per week to 33 per week? That would mean that during the 10 years under study, individuals in the labor force were "earning" four hours more leisure a week. Actually, nothing so extreme has occurred in this country, but something similar has. Average hours worked per week fell steadily until the 1960s, at which time they leveled off. That means that during much of the history of this country, the increase in per capita real GDP *understated* the actual economic growth that we were experiencing because we were enjoying more and more leisure as time passed.

Click here to get the latest figures and estimates on economic growth throughout the world.

Is Economic Growth Bad?

Some commentators on our current economic situation believe that the definition of economic growth ignores its negative effects. Some psychologists even contend that we are made worse off because of economic growth. They say that the more we grow, the more "needs" are created so that we feel worse off as we become richer. Our expectations are rising faster than reality, so we presumably always suffer from a sense of disappointment. Clearly, the economist's measurement of economic growth does not take into account the spiritual and cultural aspects of the good life. As with all activities, there are costs and benefits. You can see some of those listed in Table 9-2.

In any event, any measure of economic growth that we use will be imperfect. Nonetheless, the measures that we do have allow us to make comparisons across countries and over time and, if used judiciously, can enable us to gain important insights. Per capita real GDP,

TABLE 9-2
Costs and Benefits of Economic Growth

Benefits	Costs
Reduction in illiteracy	Environmental pollution
Reduction in poverty	Breakdown of the family
Improved health	Isolation and alienation
Longer lives	Urban congestion
Political stability	

used so often, is not always an accurate measure of economic well-being, but it is a serviceable measure of productive activity.

The Importance of Growth Rates 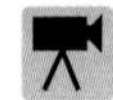

Notice back in Table 9-1 that the growth rates in real per capita income for most countries differ by very little—generally only a few percentage points. You might want to know why such small differences in growth rates are important. What would it matter if we grew at 3 percent rather than at 4 percent per year?

It matters a lot—not for next year or the year after but for the more distant future. The power of *compounding* is impressive. Let's see what happens with three different annual rates of growth: 3 percent, 4 percent, and 5 percent. We start with $1 trillion per year of gross domestic product of the United States at some time in the past. We then compound this $1 trillion, or allow it to grow, into the future at these three different growth rates. The difference is huge. In 50 years, $1 trillion per year becomes $4.38 trillion per year if compounded at 3 percent per year. Just one percentage point more in the growth rate, 4 percent, results in a real GDP of $7.11 trillion per year in 50 years, almost double the previous amount. Two percentage points difference in the growth rate—5 percent per year—results in a real GDP of $11.5 trillion per year in 50 years, or nearly three times as much. Obviously, there is a great difference in the results of economic growth for very small differences in annual growth rates. That is why nations are concerned if the growth rate falls even a little in absolute percentage terms.

Thus when we talk about growth rates, we are basically talking about compounding. In Table 9-3, we show how $1 compounded annually grows at different interest rates. We see in the 3 percent column that $1 in 50 years grows to $4.38. We merely multiplied $1 trillion times 4.38 to get the growth figure in our earlier example. In the 5 percent column, $1 grows to $11.50 after 50 years. Again, we multiplied $1 trillion times 11.50 to get the growth figure for 5 percent in the preceding example.

	Interest Rate						
Number of Years	3%	4%	5%	6%	8%	10%	20%
1	1.03	1.04	1.05	1.06	1.08	1.10	1.20
2	1.06	1.08	1.10	1.12	1.17	1.21	1.44
3	1.09	1.12	1.16	1.19	1.26	1.33	1.73
4	1.13	1.17	1.22	1.26	1.36	1.46	2.07
5	1.16	1.22	1.28	1.34	1.47	1.61	2.49
6	1.19	1.27	1.34	1.41	1.59	1.77	2.99
7	1.23	1.32	1.41	1.50	1.71	1.94	3.58
8	1.27	1.37	1.48	1.59	1.85	2.14	4.30
9	1.30	1.42	1.55	1.68	2.00	2.35	5.16
10	1.34	1.48	1.63	1.79	2.16	2.59	6.19
20	1.81	2.19	2.65	3.20	4.66	6.72	38.30
30	2.43	3.24	4.32	5.74	10.00	17.40	237.00
40	3.26	4.80	7.04	10.30	21.70	45.30	1,470.00
50	4.38	7.11	11.50	18.40	46.90	117.00	9,100.00

TABLE 9-3
One Dollar Compounded Annually at Different Interest Rates
Here we show the value of a dollar at the end of a specified period during which it has been compounded annually at a specified interest rate. For example, if you took $1 today and invested it at 5 percent per year, it would yield $1.05 at the end of one year. At the end of 10 years, it would equal $1.63, and at the end of 50 years, it would equal $11.50.

EXAMPLE

What If the United States Had Grown a Little Bit Less or More Each Year?

In 1870, the per-person real GDP expressed in 2000 dollars was $3,485. That figure had grown to $32,250 by the beginning of 2000. The average economic growth rate was therefore about 1.75 percent per year. What if the U.S. growth rate over the same century and a quarter had been simply 1 percent less—only 0.75 percent per year? Per capita real GDP in 2000 would have been only 30 percent of what it actually was. The United States would have ranked somewhere around thirty-fifth on the scale of per capita income throughout the world. We would have been poorer than Greece or Portugal.

Consider a rosier scenario: What if the U.S. economic rate of growth had been one point higher, or 2.75 percent per year? Today's per capita real GDP would be more than three times its actual value, or about $118,500!

For Critical Analysis

Can you relate this example to anything in your own life? (Hint: Use the compound interest rates in Table 9-3 to make various predictions about your future standard of living.)

CONCEPTS IN BRIEF

- Economic growth can be defined as the increase in real per capita output measured by its rate of change per year.
- The benefits of economic growth are reductions in illiteracy, poverty, and illness and increases in life spans and political stability. The costs of economic growth may include environmental pollution, alienation, and urban congestion.
- Small percentage-point differences in growth rates lead to large differences in real GDP over time. These differences can be seen by examining a compound interest table such as the one in Table 9-3.

PRODUCTIVITY INCREASES: THE HEART OF ECONOMIC GROWTH

Let's say that you are required to type 10 term papers and homework assignments a year. You have a computer; but you do not know how to touch-type. You end up spending an average of two hours per typing job. The next summer, you buy a touch-typing tutorial to use on your computer and spend a few minutes a day improving your typing speed. The following term, you spend only one hour per typing assignment, thereby saving 10 hours a semester. You have become more productive. This concept of productivity relates to your ability (and everyone else's) to produce the same output with fewer labor hours. Thus **labor productivity** is normally measured by dividing the total real domestic output (real GDP) by the number of workers or the number of labor hours. Labor productivity increases whenever average output produced per worker during a specified time period increases. Clearly, there is a relationship between economic growth and increases in labor productivity. If you divide all resources into just capital and labor, economic growth can be defined simply as the cumulative contribution to per capita GDP growth of three components: the rate of growth of capital, the rate of growth of labor, and the rate of growth of capital and labor productivity. If everything else remains constant, improvements in labor productivity ultimately lead to economic growth and higher living standards.

Labor productivity 
Total real domestic output (real GDP) divided by the number of workers (output per worker).

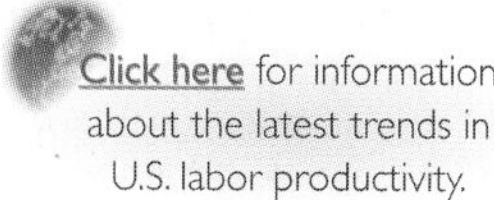
Click here for information about the latest trends in U.S. labor productivity.

Figure 9-3 traces measured U.S. productivity growth since 1970. Productivity in the manufacturing sector has grown at a steady pace. As we discuss later in this chapter, one

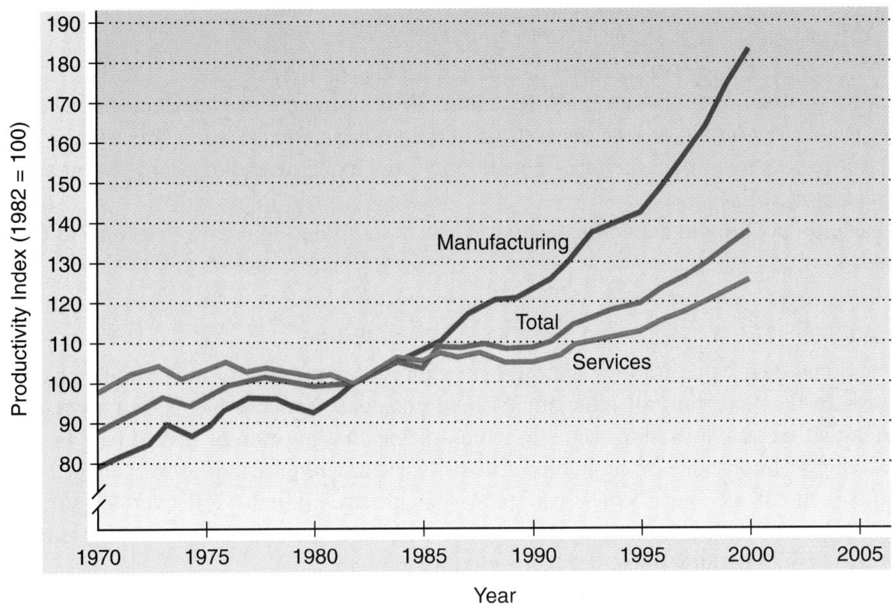

FIGURE 9-3
Nonfarm U.S. Productivity Growth
Whereas productivity in the services sector started increasing only in the early 1980s, productivity in the manufacturing sector has been increasing almost consistently since 1970.
Sources: U.S. Department of Commerce; U.S. Department of Labor, Bureau of Labor Statistics.

by-product of increased productivity in manufacturing has been a relative decline in employment in manufacturing industries. Greater productivity has led to reduced job growth in the manufacturing sector relative to other parts of the economy.

Growth of total productivity, however, has been slowed by stagnant growth in measured productivity in the service sector of the American economy.

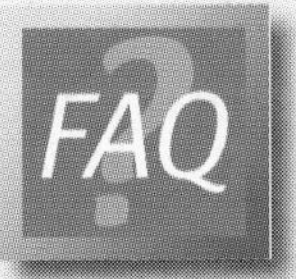

Isn't growth in a nation's manufacturing industries the key to growth in jobs and incomes?

No, this is not the case. In fact, information technology (IT) industries are now the biggest creators of jobs in the United States. Key IT employers produce such goods as software, computers, semiconductors, and telecommunications equipment. In recent years, more than one-third of all new American jobs have been in such industries.

EXAMPLE

The Productivity Paradox

In the course of a book review he wrote in 1987, Nobel economist Robert Solow made the offhand comment, "You can seen the computer age everywhere but in the productivity statistics." This comment summed up what has become known as the *productivity paradox*: the seeming lack of productivity gains from information technologies.

The service-sector productivity trend shown in Figure 9-3 illustrates the paradox. Widespread adoption of information technologies in service industries were supposed to allow these industries to reap big efficiency gains. Bar-coding of merchandise was supposed to allow salesclerks at retailers to do their work more efficiently. Financial electronic data interchange was supposed to provide big productivity enhancements in financial services. These productivity gains were slow to emerge—either that, or the data are wrong.

For Critical Analysis

Higher education is a good example of a service industry. College campuses are now full of computers. How would you propose to measure the effect of computers on productivity in higher education?

SAVING: A FUNDAMENTAL DETERMINANT OF ECONOMIC GROWTH

Economic growth does not occur in a vacuum. It is not some predetermined fate of a nation. Rather, economic growth depends on certain fundamental factors. One of the most important factors that affect the rate of economic growth and hence long-term living standards is the rate of saving.

A basic proposition in economics is that if you want more tomorrow, you have to take less today.

> To have more consumption in the future, you have to consume less today and save the difference between your consumption and your income.

On a national basis, this implies that higher saving rates eventually mean higher living standards in the long run, all other things held constant. Concern has been growing in America that we are not saving enough, which means that our rate of saving may be too low. Saving is important for economic growth because without saving, we cannot have investment. If all income is consumed each year, there is nothing left over for saving, which could be used by business for investment. If there is no investment in our capital stock, there could be little hope of much economic growth.

The relationship between the rate of savings and per capita real GDP is shown in Figure 9-4. Among the nations with the highest rates of saving are Japan and Germany.

INTERNATIONAL EXAMPLE

Japan and Germany Save and Invest More than the United States, but Does it Matter?

Japan and Germany have saving rates that are more than twice the U.S. rate. As a result, they have accumulated more capital. On a per capita basis, Japan has 22 percent more invested capital than the United States, and Germany has 13 percent more. Nevertheless, the United States creates more wealth per capita than Germany and Japan do. In 2000 dollars, the United States created an estimated $29,950 of new wealth per capita, compared with $23,600 for Japan and $24,750 for Germany.

At least part of the difference results from more efficient use of capital in the United States. Economists estimate that a unit of capital in Germany or Japan generates final output that is about a third lower than that in the United States. In other words, if a $1 million factory produces 1 million units of output per year in the United States, a comparable factory would produce about 670,000 units of output per year in Germany or Japan.

For Critical Analysis

"Americans overconsume, undersave, and underinvest." How do the figures presented here counter this statement?

CONCEPTS IN BRIEF

- Economic growth is numerically equal to the rate of growth of capital plus the rate of growth of labor plus the rate of growth in the productivity of capital and of labor. Improvements in labor productivity, all other things being equal, lead to greater economic growth and higher living standards.
- One fundamental determinant of the rate of growth is the rate of saving. To have more consumption in the future, we have to save rather than consume. In general, countries that have had higher rates of saving have had higher rates of growth in real GDP.

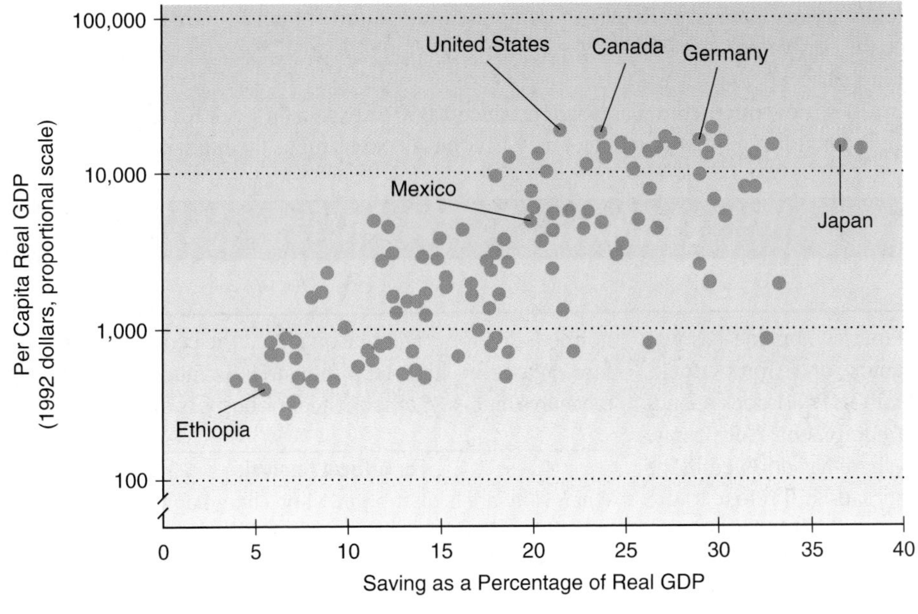

FIGURE 9-4

Relationship Between Rate of Saving and Per Capita Real GDP

This diagram shows the relationship between per capita real GDP and the rate of saving expressed as the average share of annual real GDP saved. The data cover several dozen nations since 1960. Centrally planned economies and major oil-producing countries are not shown.

Source: After Robert Summers and Alan Heston, "A New Set of International Comparisons of Real Product and Price Level," *Review of Income and Wealth,* March 1988.

NEW GROWTH THEORY AND THE DETERMINANTS OF GROWTH

New growth theory 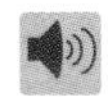
A theory of economic growth that examines the factors that determine why technology, research, innovation, and the like are undertaken and how they interact.

A simple arithmetic definition of economic growth has already been given. The growth rates of capital and labor plus the growth rate of their productivity constitute the rate of economic growth. Economists have had good data on the growth of the physical capital stock in the United States as well as on the labor force. But when you add those two growth rates together, you still do not get the total economic growth rate in the United States. The difference has to be due to improvements in productivity. Economists typically labeled this "improvements in technology," and that was that. More recently, proponents of what is now called the **new growth theory** argue that technology cannot simply be looked at as an outside factor without explanation. Technology must be understood in terms of what drives it. What are the forces that make productivity grow in America and elsewhere?

FAQ

Don't new technologies destroy jobs?

No, even though numerous "experts" in the media like to paint a gloomy picture of a future in which ordinary working people lose their livelihood to computers. Such claims have been popular since the weaving machine with a single operator replaced the work that 10 people did previously. But of course, the other nine were not unemployed forever. They and their offspring ultimately found new ways to earn a living. Theoretically, there is no limit on labor employment, which depends on the supply of and demand for labor. The demand for labor is not fixed. Workers released from industries that are more productive find work elsewhere, typically in other industries that can expand because of the freed-up resources made available by technological progress. In the end, technological change often *expands* employment opportunities for the nation's workforce.

Growth in Technology

Consider some startling statistics about the growth in technology. Microprocessor speeds may increase from 1,000 megahertz to 5,000 megahertz by the year 2011. By that same year, the size of the thinnest circuit line within a transistor will decrease by 77 percent. The typical memory capacity (RAM) of computers will jump from 128 megabytes, or about twice the equivalent text in the *Encyclopaedia Britannica,* to 128 gigabytes—a thousand-fold increase.

By 2005, new microchip plants will produce 1,000 transistors a week for every person on earth. Predictions are that computers may become as powerful as the human brain by 2020.

EXAMPLE

Our High-Tech Economy

Four decades ago, one in six American businesses was automotive-related. Today, autos and light trucks account for about 3.5 percent of GDP. So does spending on computers and related equipment. Yet despite the fact that high technology's share has doubled in the past decade, government statisticians still refuse to use chip inventories and personal computer sales as economic indicators. The reason is that the economic welfare created by high-tech industries is much harder to measure than, say, tons of steel or bushels of corn.

For Critical Analysis

When software is distributed at no charge on the Internet, does that contribute to the economy?

Technology: A Separate Factor of Production

We now recognize that technology must be viewed as a separate factor of production that is sensitive to rewards. Otherwise stated, one of the major foundations of new growth theory is this:

The greater the rewards, the more technological advances we will get.

Let's consider several aspects of technology here, the first one being research and development.

Research and Development

A certain amount of technological advance results from research and development (R&D) activities that have as their goal the development of specific new materials, new products, and new machines. How much spending a nation devotes to R&D can have an impact on its long-term economic growth. Part of how much a nation spends depends on what businesses decide is worth spending. That in turn depends on their expected rewards from successful R&D. If your company develops a new way to produce computer memory chips, how much will it be rewarded? The answer depends on whether others can freely copy the new technique.

Patent 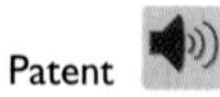
A government protection that gives an inventor the exclusive right to make, use, or sell an invention for a limited period of time (currently, 20 years).

Patents. To protect new techniques developed through R&D, we have a system of **patents,** protections whereby the federal government gives the patent holder the exclusive right to make, use, and sell an invention for a period of 20 years. One can argue that this special position given owners of patents increases expenditures on R&D and therefore adds to long-term economic growth.

Positive Externalities and R&D. As we discussed in Chapter 5, positive externalities are benefits from an activity that are not enjoyed by the instigator of the activity. In the case of R&D spending, a certain amount of the benefits go to other companies that do not have to pay for them. In particular, according to economists David Coe of the International Monetary Fund and Elhanan Helpman of Tel Aviv University, about a quarter of the global productivity gains of R&D investment in the top seven industrialized countries goes to foreigners. For every 1 percent rise in the stock of research and development in America alone, for example, productivity in the rest of the world increases by about 0.25 percent. One country's R&D expenditures benefit foreigners because foreigners are able to import goods from technologically advanced countries and then use them as inputs in making their own industries more efficient. In addition, countries that import high-tech goods are able to imitate the technology.

The Open Economy and Economic Growth

People who study economic growth today tend to emphasize the importance of the openness of the economy. Free trade encourages a more rapid spread of technology and industrial ideas. Moreover, open economies may experience higher rates of economic growth because their own industries have access to a bigger market. When trade barriers are erected in the form of tariffs and the like, domestic industries become isolated from global technological progress. This occurred for many years in former communist countries and in many developing countries in Latin America and elsewhere. Figure 9-5 shows the relationship between economic growth and the openness as measured by the level of protectionism of a given economy.

Innovation and Knowledge

We tend to think of technological progress as, say, the invention of the transistor. But invention means nothing by itself; **innovation** is required. Innovation involves the transformation of something new, such as an invention, into something that benefits the economy either by lowering production costs or providing new goods and services. Indeed, the new growth theorists believe that real wealth creation comes from innovation and that invention is but a facet of innovation.

Innovation 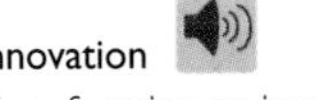
Transforming an invention into something that is useful to humans.

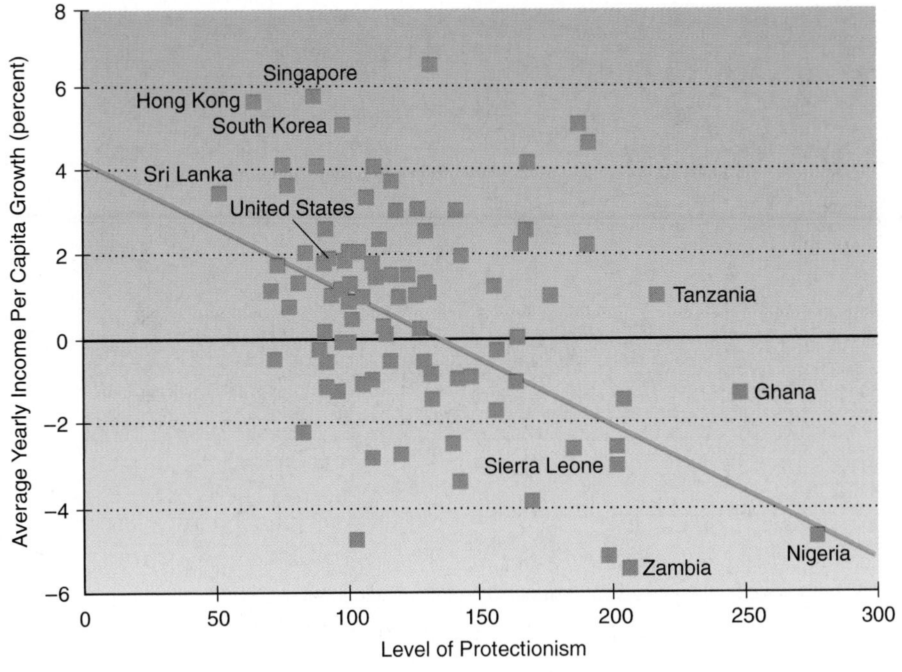

FIGURE 9-5
The Relationship Between Protectionism and Economic Growth
Closed economies are ones in which the government prevents imports from entering the country and sometimes exports from leaving the country. Such protectionism closes off the economy to new technologies. Here you see the relationship between the level of protectionism and economic growth rates measured on a per capita basis. The data seem to indicate that the more closed an economy, the lower its rate of growth, all other things held constant.
Source: Economic Review, Fourth Quarter 1993, p. 3.

Historically, technologies have moved relatively slowly from invention to innovation to widespread use, and the dispersion of new technology remains for the most part slow and uncertain. The inventor of the transistor thought it might be used to make better hearing aids. At the time it was invented, the *New York Times*'s sole reference to it was in a small weekly column called "News of Radio." When the laser was invented, no one really knew what it could be used for. It was initially used to help in navigation, measurement, and chemical research. Today, it is used in the reproduction of music, printing, surgery, and telecommunications. Tomorrow, who knows?

Figure 9-6 shows the process by which raw ideas turn into written ideas that are submitted for study in typical research and development laboratories. Businesses select a few of these for initial study and choose fewer still to evaluate in large research projects. Out of these full-scale research efforts, a few significant developments emerge and are launched as new products. If businesses are lucky, one or two of these product launches may ultimately pay off.

The Importance of Ideas and Knowledge

Economist Paul Romer has added at least one important factor that determines the rate of economic growth. He contends that production and manufacturing knowledge is just as important as the other determinants and perhaps even more so. He considers knowledge a factor of production that, like capital, has to be paid for by forgoing current consumption. Economies must therefore invest in knowledge just as they invest in machines. Because past investment in capital may make it more profitable to acquire more knowledge, there exists the possibility of an investment-knowledge cycle in which investment spurs knowl-

FIGURE 9-6

The Winnowing Process of Research and Development

Only a portion of new ideas are actually submitted for formal study, and just a fraction of these become subjects of research projects. Very few ideas actually lead to the development of new products.

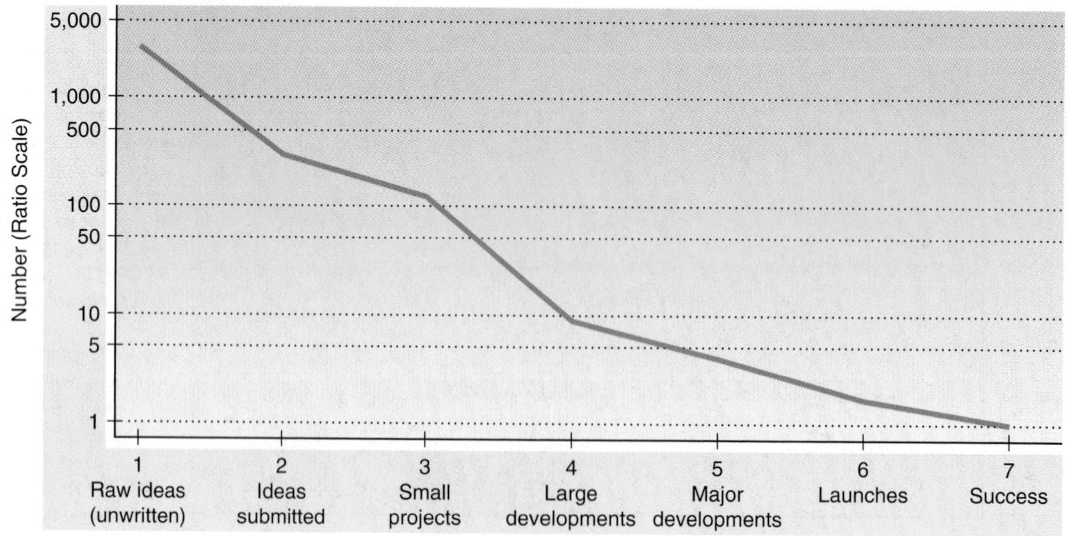

edge and knowledge spurs investment. A once-and-for-all increase in a country's rate of investment may permanently raise that country's growth rate. (According to traditional theory, a once-and-for-all increase in the rate of saving and therefore in the rate of investment simply leads to a new steady-state standard of living but not one that continues to increase.)

Another way of looking at knowledge is that it is a store of ideas. According to Romer, ideas are what drive economic growth. We have become, in fact, an idea economy. Consider Microsoft Corporation. A relatively small percentage of that company's labor force is involved in actually building products. Rather, a majority of Microsoft employees are attempting to discover new ideas that can be translated into computer code that can then be turned into products. The major conclusion that Romer and other new growth theorists draw is this:

Economic growth can continue as long as we keep coming up with new ideas.

EXAMPLE

Catch the Wave—It May Be the Shortest Yet

A major twentieth-century Austrian economist, Joseph Schumpeter, proposed the idea of "creative destruction." Schumpeter argued that a normal, healthy economy was not one that grew along a steady path. It was one that was constantly in a state of disruption because of a dizzying pace of technological innovations.

Inspired by the work of a Russian economist named Nikolai Kondratieff, Schumpeter concluded that industrial revolutions occur in cycles of about 50 to 60 years. Figure 9-7 illustrates the cycles that he had in mind, which are sometimes known as *Kondratieff waves*. In Schumpeter's view, each cycle is fueled by entirely different clusters of industries. Each cluster emerges following a period of fermentation of new technological discoveries and innovations. For instance, a first industrial wave was driven by new technologies for using water power, manufacturing textiles, and building with iron. A second wave developed from innovations in steam power, rail transportation, and the fabrication of steel. The adoption of technologies driven by electricity, chemicals, and the internal-combustion engine started a third wave. By the time Schumpeter died in 1950, a fourth industrial cycle, fueled by innovations in oil and natural gas, electronics, and air travel, had begun.

FIGURE 9-7

Waves of Industrial Revolution

Based on the ideas of Nikolai Kondratieff, the Austrian economist Joseph Schumpeter argued that industrial revolutions occur in waves. Schumpeter argued that four waves have taken place since the 1700s, and the advent of the new information technologies based on digital communications may represent the early years of a fifth wave.

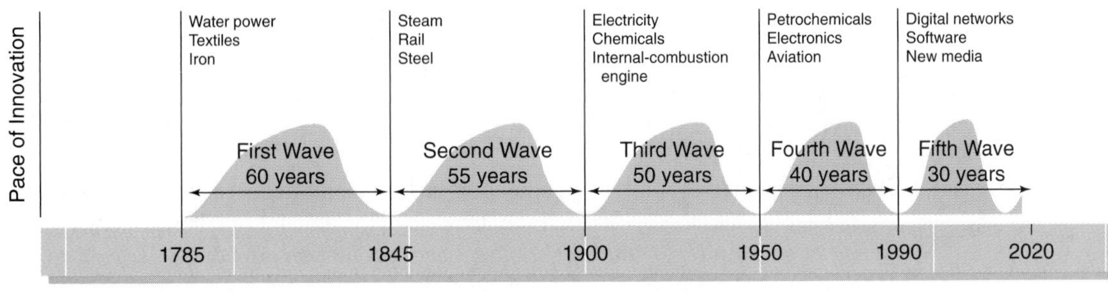

The figure depicts a fifth wave, driven by developments in digital networks, computer software, and new telecommunications technologies that may have begun in the early 1990s.

Economists who subscribe to Schumpeter's views argue that the tools of this new wave—computer analyzers, gene sequencers, Internet shopbots, patent searchers, text parsers, and the like—are getting better all the time. This, they argue, is likely to speed the pace of innovation. Thus the fifth wave could well be even shorter than the 40-year one that preceded it.

For Critical Analysis

New growth theorists like to stake a claim to developing a really "new" idea? Did Schumpeter beat them to the punch?

The Importance of Human Capital 

Knowledge, ideas, and productivity are all tied together. One of the threads is the quality of the labor force. Increases in the productivity of the labor force are a function of increases in human capital, the fourth factor of production discussed in Chapter 2. Recall that human capital is the knowledge and skills that people in the workforce acquire through education, on-the-job training, and self-teaching. To increase your own human capital, you have to invest by forgoing income-earning activities while you attend school. Society also has to invest in the form of libraries and teachers. According to the new growth theorists, human capital is at least as important as physical capital, particularly when trying to explain international differences in living standards.

It is therefore not surprising that one of the most effective ways that developing countries can become developed is by investing in secondary schooling.

One can argue that policy changes that increase human capital will lead to more technological improvements. One of the reasons why concerned citizens, policymakers, and politicians are looking for a change in America's schooling system is that our educational system seems to be falling behind that of other countries. This lag is greatest in science and mathematics—precisely the areas that are required for developing better technology.

CONCEPTS IN BRIEF

- New growth theory argues that the greater the rewards, the more rapid the pace of technology. And greater rewards spur research and development.
- The openness of a nation's economy seems to correlate with its rate of economic growth.
- Invention and innovation are not the same thing. Inventions are useless until innovation transforms them into things that people find valuable.
- According to the new growth economists, economic growth can continue as long as we keep coming up with new ideas.
- Increases in human capital can lead to greater rates of economic growth. These come about by increased education, on-the-job training, and self-teaching.

POPULATION AND IMMIGRATION AS THEY AFFECT ECONOMIC GROWTH

There are several ways to view population growth as it affects economic growth. On the one hand, population growth means an increase in the amount of labor, which is one component of economic growth. On the other hand, population growth can be seen as a drain on the economy because for any given amount of GDP, more population means lower per capita GDP. According to MIT economist Michael Kremer, the first view is historically correct. His conclusion is that population growth drives technological progress, which then increases economic growth. The theory is simple: If there are 50 percent more people in the United States, there will be 50 percent more geniuses. And with 50 percent more people, the rewards for creativity are commensurately greater. Otherwise stated, the larger the potential market, the greater the incentive to become ingenious.

Does the same argument apply to immigration? Yes, according to the late economist Julian Simon, who pointed out that "every time our system allows in one more immigrant, on average, the economic welfare of American citizens goes up. . . . Additional immigrants, both the legal and the illegal, raise the standard of living of U.S. natives and have little or no negative impact on any occupational or income class." He further argued that immigrants do not displace natives from jobs but rather create jobs through their purchases and by starting new businesses. Immigrants' earning and spending simply expand the economy.

Not all researchers agree with Simon, and few studies exist to test the theories advanced here. The area is currently the focus of much research.

PROPERTY RIGHTS AND ENTREPRENEURSHIP

If you were in a country where bank accounts and businesses were periodically expropriated by the government, how willing would you be to leave your money in a savings account or to invest in a business? Certainly you would be less willing than if such things never occurred. In general, the more certain private property rights are, the more capital accumulation there will be. People will be willing to invest their savings in endeavors that will increase their wealth in future years. They have property rights in their wealth that are sanctioned and enforced by the government. In fact, some economic historians have attempted to show that it was the development of well-defined private property rights that allowed Western Europe to increase its growth rate after many centuries of stagnation. The ability and certainty with which they can reap the gains from investing also determine the extent to which business owners in other countries will invest capital in developing countries. The threat of nationalization that hangs over some developing nations probably prevents the massive amount of foreign investment that might be necessary to allow these nations to develop more rapidly.

The property rights, or legal structure, in a nation are closely tied to the degree with which individuals use their own entrepreneurial skills. In Chapter 2, we identified entrepreneurship as the fifth factor of production. Entrepreneurs are the risk takers who seek out new ways to do things and create new products. To the extent that entrepreneurs are allowed to capture the rewards from their entrepreneurial activities, they will seek to engage in those activities. In countries where such rewards cannot be captured because of a lack of property rights, there will be less entrepreneurship. Typically, this results in fewer investments and a lower rate of growth.

CONCEPTS IN BRIEF

- While some economists argue that population growth stifles economic growth, others contend that the opposite is true. The latter economists consequently believe that immigration should be encouraged rather than discouraged.
- Well-defined and protected property rights are important for fostering entrepreneurship. In the absence of well-defined property rights, individuals have less incentive to take risks, and economic growth rates suffer.

ECONOMIC DEVELOPMENT

Development economics 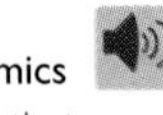
The study of factors that contribute to the economic development of a country.

How did developed countries travel paths of growth from extreme poverty to relative riches? That is the essential issue of **development economics,** which is the study of why some countries grow and develop and others do not and of policies that might help developing economies get richer. It is not enough simply to say that people in different countries are different and therefore that is why some countries are rich and some countries are poor. Economists do not deny that different cultures create different work ethics, but they are unwilling to accept such a pat and fatalistic answer.

Look at any world map. About four-fifths of the countries you will see on the map are considered relatively poor. The goal of economists who study development is to help the more than 4 billion today with low living standards join the 2 billion people who have at least moderately high living standards.

Putting World Poverty into Perspective

Most Americans cannot even begin to understand the reality of poverty in the world today. At least one-half, if not two-thirds, of the world's population lives at subsistence level, with just enough to eat for survival. Indeed, the World Bank estimates that nearly 30 percent of the world's people live on less than $1 per day. The official poverty line in the United States is set beyond the average income of at least half the human beings on the planet. This is not to say that we should ignore domestic problems with the poor and homeless simply because they are living better than many people elsewhere in the world. Rather, it is necessary for Americans to maintain an appropriate perspective on what are considered problems for this country relative to what are considered problems elsewhere.

The Relationship Between Population Growth and Economic Development

World population is growing at the rate of 2.8 people a second. That amounts to 242,000 a day or 88.3 million a year. Today, there are just over 6 billion people on earth. By 2030, according to the United Nations, there will be 8.5 billion. Panel (a) of Figure 9-8 shows which countries are growing the most. Panel (b) emphasizes an implication of panel (a), which is that virtually all the growth in population is occurring in developing nations. Some countries, such as Germany, are expected to lose population over the next several decades.

Ever since the Reverend Thomas Robert Malthus wrote *An Essay on the Principle of Population* in 1798, excessive population growth has been a concern. Modern-day Malthusians are able to generate just as much enthusiasm for the concept that population growth is bad. Over and over, media pundits and a number of scientists tell us that rapid population growth threatens economic development and the quality of life.

Nevertheless, Malthus's prediction that population would outstrip food supplies has never held true, according to economist Nicholas Eberstadt of the Harvard Center for Population Studies. As the world's population has grown, so has the world's food supply, measured by calories per person. Furthermore, the price of food, corrected for inflation, has been falling steadily for more than a century. That means that the supply of food has been expanding faster than the rise in demand caused by increased population.

Furthermore, economists have found that as nations become richer, average family size declines. Otherwise stated, the more economic development occurs, the slower the population growth rate becomes. Predictions of birthrates in developing countries have often turned out to be overstated if those countries experience rapid economic growth. This was

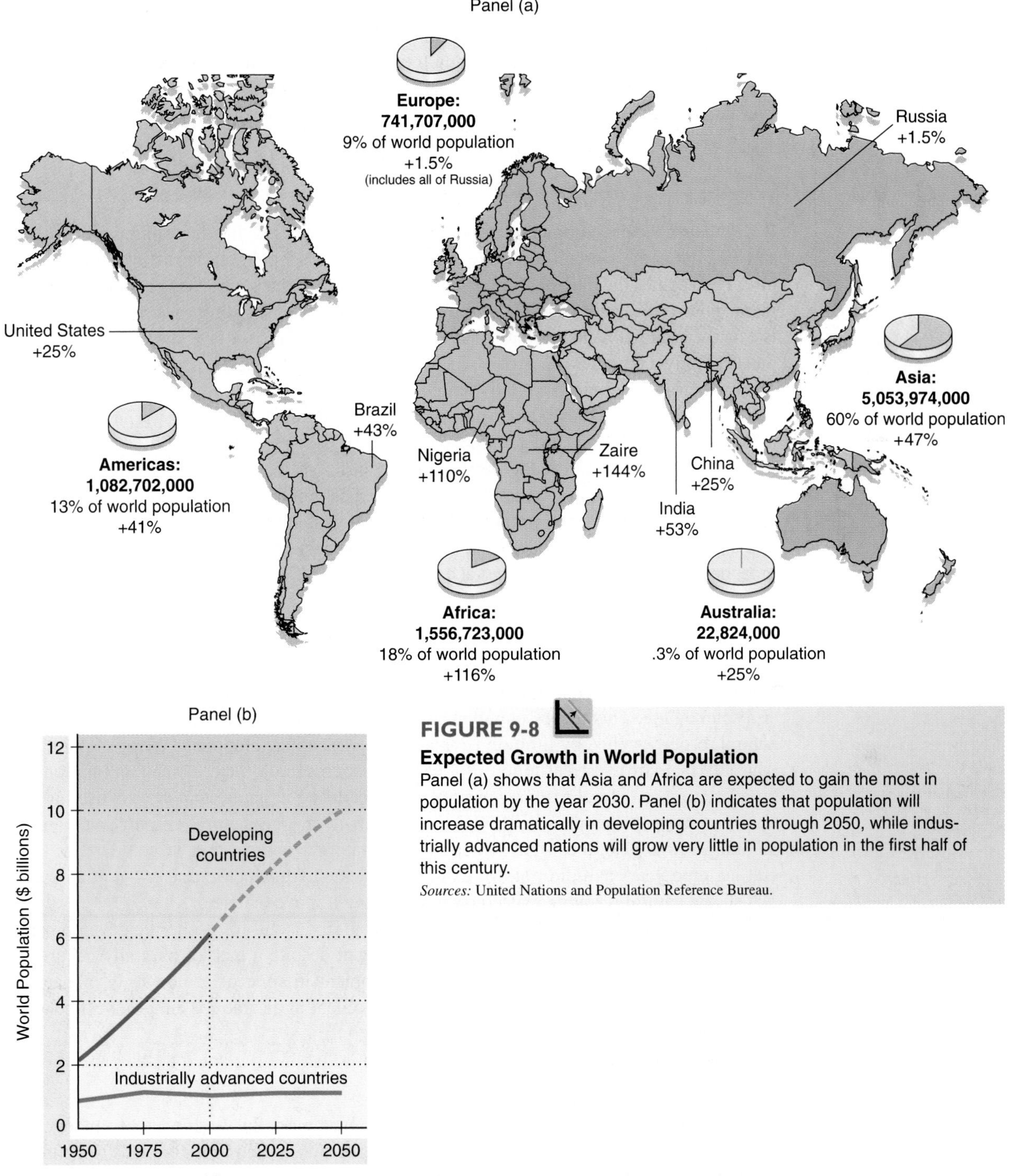

FIGURE 9-8

Expected Growth in World Population

Panel (a) shows that Asia and Africa are expected to gain the most in population by the year 2030. Panel (b) indicates that population will increase dramatically in developing countries through 2050, while industrially advanced nations will grow very little in population in the first half of this century.

Sources: United Nations and Population Reference Bureau.

the case in Hong Kong, Mexico, Taiwan, and Colombia. Recent research on population and economic development has revealed that social and economic modernization has been accompanied by what might be called a fertility revolution—the spread of deliberate family size limitation within marriage and a decline in childbearing. Modernization reduces infant mortality, which in turn reduces the incentive for couples to have many children to make sure that a certain number survive to adulthood. Modernization also lowers the demand for children for a variety of reasons, not the least being that couples in more developed countries do not need to rely on their children to take care of them in old age.

The Stages of Development: Agriculture to Industry to Services

If we analyze the development of modern rich nations, we find that they went through three stages. First is the agricultural stage, when most of the population is involved in agriculture. Then comes the manufacturing stage, when much of the population becomes involved in the industrialized sector of the economy. And finally there is a shift toward services. That is exactly what happened in the United States: The so-called tertiary, or service, sector of the economy continues to grow, whereas the manufacturing sector (and its share of employment) is declining in relative importance.

It is important to understand, however, the requirement for early specialization in a nation's comparative advantage (see Chapter 2). The doctrine of comparative advantage is particularly appropriate for the developing countries of the world. If trading is allowed among nations, a country is normally best off if it produces what it has a comparative advantage in producing and imports the rest (for more details, see Chapter 32). This means that many developing countries should continue to specialize in agricultural production or in labor-intensive manufactured goods.

Keys to Economic Development

Click here to contemplate whether there may be a relationship between inequality and a nation's growth, and to visit the home page of the World Bank's Thematic Group on Inequality, Poverty, and Socioeconomic Performance.

One theory of development states that for a country to develop, it must have a large natural resource base. This theory continues to assert that much of the world is running out of natural resources, thereby limiting economic growth and development. We must point out that only the narrowest definition of a natural resource could lead to such an opinion. In broader terms, a natural resource is something occurring in nature that we can use for our own purposes. As emphasized by the new growth theory, natural resources therefore include knowledge of the use of something. The natural resources that we could define several hundred years ago did not, for example, include hydroelectric power—no one knew that such a natural resource existed or how to bring it into existence.

Natural resources by themselves are not particularly useful for economic development, as demonstrated by Japan's extensive development despite a lack of naturally occurring crude oil and by Brazil's slow pace of development in spite of a vast array of natural resources. Resources must be transformed into something usable for either investment or consumption.

Economists have found that four factors seem to be highly related to the pace of economic development:

1. *An educated population.* Both theoretically and empirically, we know that a more educated workforce aids economic development because it allows individuals to build on the ideas of others. According to economists David Gould and Roy Ruffin, increasing the rate of enrollment in secondary schools by only 2 percentage points, from 8 percent to 10 percent, raises the average rate of economic growth by half a percent per year. Thus we must conclude that developing countries can advance more rapidly if they

invest more heavily in secondary education. Or stated in the negative, economic development cannot be sustained if a nation allows a sizable portion of its population to avoid education. After all, education allows young people who grew up poor to acquire skills that enable them to avoid poverty as adults.

2. *Establishing a system of property rights.* As noted, if you were in a country in which bank accounts and businesses were periodically expropriated by the government, you would be reluctant to leave your money in a savings account or to invest in a business. Expropriation of private property rarely takes place in developed countries. It has occurred in numerous developing countries, however. For example, private property was once nationalized in Chile and largely still is in Cuba. Economists have found that, other things being equal, the more certain private property rights are, the more private capital accumulation and economic growth there will be.
3. *Letting "creative destruction" run its course.* As discussed earlier, Harvard economist Joseph Schumpeter championed the concept of "creative destruction," through which new businesses ultimately create new jobs and economic growth after first destroying old jobs, old companies, and old industries. Such change is painful and costly, but it is necessary for economic advancement. Nowhere is this more important than in developing countries, where the principle is often ignored. Many developing nations have had a history of supporting current companies and industries by discouraging new technologies and new companies from entering the marketplace. The process of creative destruction has not been allowed to work its magic in these countries.
4. *Limiting protectionism.* Open economies experience faster economic development than economies closed to international trade. Trade encourages individuals and businesses to discover ways to specialize so that they can become more productive and earn higher incomes. Increased productivity and subsequent increases in economic growth are the results. Thus the less government protects the domestic economy by imposing trade barriers, the faster that economy will experience economic development. According to a study by economists Nouriel Roubini and Xavier Sala-i-Martin, when a country goes from being relatively open to relatively closed via government-enacted trade barriers, it will have a 2.5 percentage-point decrease in its annual rate of economic growth.

CONCEPTS IN BRIEF

- Although many people believe that population growth hinders economic development, there is little evidence to support that notion. What is clear is that economic development tends to lead to a reduction in the rate of population growth.
- Historically, there are three stages of economic development: the agricultural stage, the manufacturing stage, and the service-sector stage, when a large part of the workforce is employed in providing services.
- Although one theory of economic development holds that a sizable natural resource base is the key to a nation's development, this fails to account for the importance of the human element: The labor force must be capable of using a country's natural resources.
- Fundamental factors contributing to the pace of economic development are training and education, a well-defined system of property rights, allowing new generations of companies and industries to replace older generations, and promoting an open economy by allowing international trade.

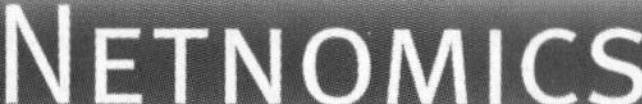

Direct Effects of Information Technology on Growth of Real Output: Computer Production

Some economists think that the solution to the "productivity paradox"—the seemingly slow response of productivity growth to computerization—is that we do a poor job of measuring the contribution of information technology to the economy's overall productivity. There is one growth effect of the computerization revolution that is relatively straightforward to measure, however. That is the direct impact of computer production on economic growth.

Fairly widespread use of the Internet for electronic mail began in 1993, and initial forays by companies into Internet commerce started shortly thereafter. As people started to learn about how much they could do on the Internet, they rapidly began to acquire computers. As you can see in the last line of Table 9-4, computer production then increased dramatically thereafter.

The Bureau of Economic Analysis (BEA), a unit of the Department of Commerce, has developed a way to track the effect of computers on the growth of aggregate real production in the U.S. economy. You can see how they do this in Table 9-4. The first line of the table shows annual growth rates for real GDP. The second line displays growth rates for real GDP *excluding* the production of computer components in all the various aspects of computing real GDP—for instance, in calculations of producers' durable equipment, personal consumption expenditures, and government spending.

The third line of the table gives the difference between the first and second lines. This difference is the BEA's estimate of the contribution of computer production to the growth of real GDP. As you can see, before Internet use became widespread in the mid-1990s, computers added no more than one- to two-tenths to the measured growth of real GDP. Now, however, computers have a direct growth effect—not taking into account indirect effects through changes in productivity of labor and capital—of close to one-half percentage point per year.

TABLE 9-4

Real GDP, Final Sales of Computers, and GDP less Final Sales of Computers: Percent Change from Preceding Year

	1989	1990	1991	1992	1993	1994	1995	1996	1997	1998	1999	2000*
Real GDP growth	3.5	1.8	−0.5	3.0	2.7	4.0	2.7	3.6	4.2	4.3	4.2	4.0
Real GDP growth less growth in final sales of computers	3.4	1.7	−0.6	2.9	2.5	3.9	2.3	3.2	3.9	3.9	3.8	3.5
Difference in growth rates	.1	.1	.1	.1	.2	.1	.4	.4	.3	.4	.4	.5
Growth in real final sales of computers, total	56.8	52.3	52.6	54.8	54.8	57.6	70.4	78.2	83.2	92.1	97.9	99.8

Sources: U.S. Department of Commerce, Bureau of Economic Analysis; author's estimates.

Issues & Applications

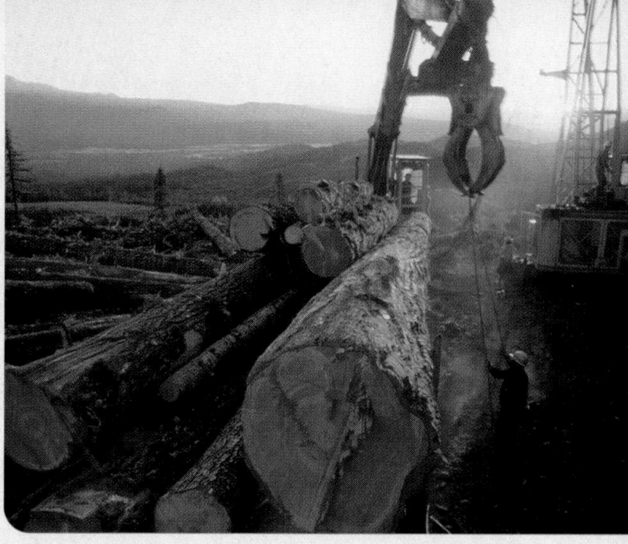

What Explains the Productivity Paradox?

For several years running, the acquisition of computers, telecommunications equipment, and other information technologies has been the main type of capital investment undertaken by U.S. businesses. Owners and managers anticipated big cost savings and revenue enhancements to result. Economists also anticipated higher productivity of labor and capital—and thus increased economic growth.

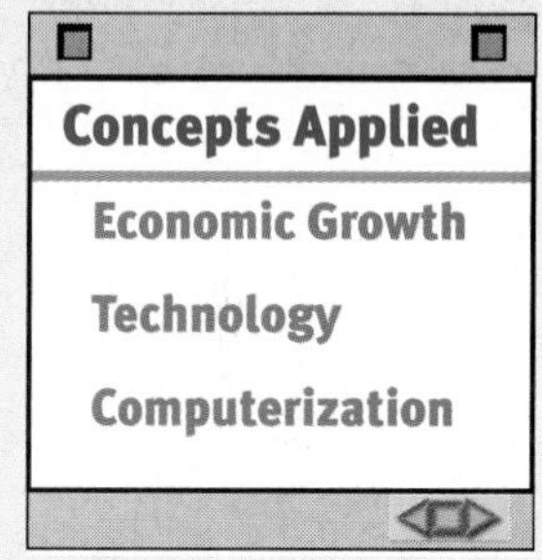

Looking at the Past

Take a look, however, at panel (a) of Figure 9-9 (p. 216). This chart traces movements in an overall index of the productivity of labor and capital since 1870. Two features of this chart are striking. One is the big upswing in the growth of overall productivity between the early 1930s and the mid-1970s. Another is the apparent lack of productivity growth since the late 1970s. This is the productivity paradox we noted earlier: So far, the widespread adoption of information technologies has not measurably increased productivity growth.

Accounting for the Productivity Paradox

What happened to the big productivity enhancements that the computer revolution was supposed to deliver? One possibility is that they are not there because computers have failed to provide the benefits that nearly everyone had expected. Some economists, for example, argue that in spite of all the recent investment in computers, they are still such a small portion of the aggregate capital stock that they are unlikely ever to be an important source of economic growth.

Another possibility is that other factors—perhaps weaker American public schools and diminished growth of human capital, as some analysts have argued—have tended to reduce overall productivity even as computers have added to it. Overall productivity therefore has remained flat.

A third possibility is that measures of overall productivity are wrong. Many economists have contended for years that current measures of the output of service industries understate the actual output rates of these industries, which include banks, insurance companies, brokerage firms, and other heavy users of new computer technologies. In spite of efforts to better measure service productivity in 1999, economists find that the U.S. banking industry is roughly half as productive as it was in the 1970s—yet no economist really believes this is so. As you can see in panel (b), the relative importance of service industries as employers has increased steadily since the 1960s. This means that the importance of productivity measurement difficulties in service industries are increasingly affecting aggregate productivity numbers. Look back at Figure 9-3. There you see that much slower measured growth of service productivity has pulled down the measure of total productivity in recent years.

There is a fourth possibility. Note in panel (a) of the figure that overall productivity in the U.S. economy remained relatively flat for some time after telephones, typewriters, electric lights, and automobiles came into use. Paul David of Stanford University suggests that we may have been witnessing a similar lag in the response of productivity to the inventions and innovations we have recently experienced. If he is right, U.S. productivity may jump to significantly higher levels in the future.

FIGURE 9-9

Productivity Growth and the Increasing Importance of Services

Panel (a) shows that following a period of heightened productivity growth from the 1930s through the early 1970s, overall productivity leveled off before increasing again in recent years. One possible explanation for the flattening of overall productivity growth is the upsurge in the production of services relative to total U.S. output depicted in panel (b). Measured service productivity growth has been weak relative to growth of manufacturing productivity.

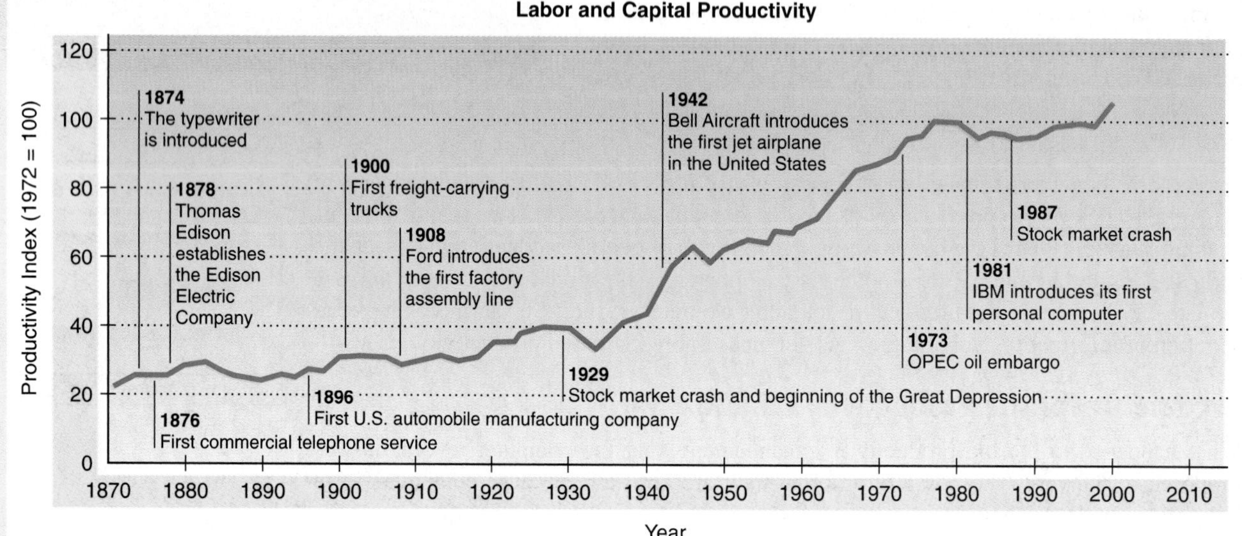

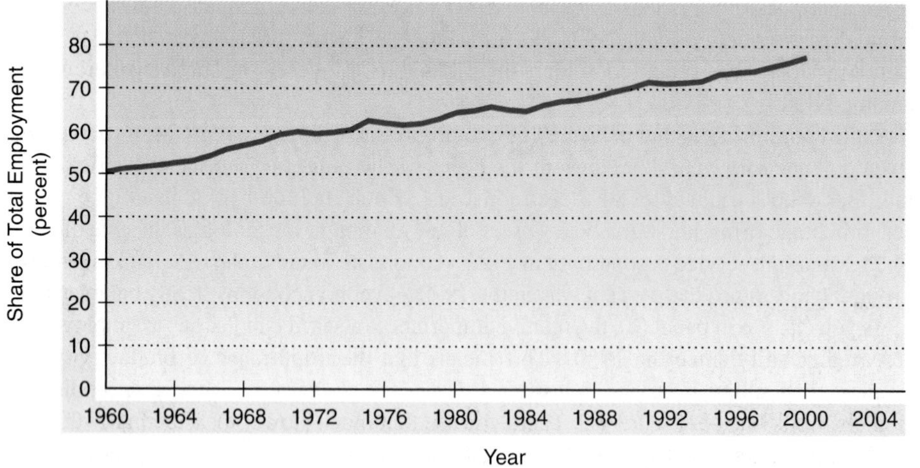

FOR CRITICAL ANALYSIS

1. What might account for a lagged response of productivity growth to new innovations?
2. A good example of a service industry is higher education. How would you propose to measure the output and productivity of higher education?

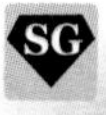

SUMMARY DISCUSSION OF LEARNING OBJECTIVES

1. **Economic growth:** The rate of economic growth is the annual rate of change in per capita real GDP. This measure of the growth of a nation's economy takes into account both its growth in overall production of goods and services and its population. It is an average measure that does not account for possible changes in the distribution of income or various welfare costs or benefits that may accompany growth of the economy.
2. **Why Economic Growth Rates Are Important:** Over long intervals, relatively small differences in the rate of economic growth can accumulate to produce large disparities in per capita incomes. The reason is that, like accumulations of interest, economic growth compounds over time. Thus a nation that experiences per capita income growth of 3 percent per year has a level of per capita income that is more than four times higher after 50 years, but a country with a per capita income growth rate of 4 percent per year ends up with a per capita income level more than seven times higher.
3. **The Key Determinants of Economic Growth:** The fundamental factors contributing to economic growth are growth in a nation's pool of labor, growth of its capital stock, and growth in the productivity of its capital and labor. A key determinant of capital accumulation is a nation's saving rate. Higher saving rates contribute to greater investment and hence increased capital accumulation and economic growth.
4. **Why Productivity Increases Are Crucial for Maintaining Economic Growth:** For a nation with a relatively stable population and a steady rate of capital accumulation, productivity growth emerges as the main factor influencing near-term changes in economic growth. Relatively slow measured growth of productivity in U.S. service industries during the past couple of decades appears to have contributed to relatively slow growth in overall U.S. productivity.
5. **New Growth Theory:** This is a relatively recent theory that examines why individuals and businesses conduct research into inventing and developing new technologies and how this process interacts with the rate of economic growth. This theory emphasizes how rewards to technological innovation contribute to higher economic growth rates. A key implication of the theory is that ideas and knowledge are crucial elements of the growth process.
6. **Fundamental Factors That Contribute to a Nation's Economic Development:** The key characteristics shared by nations that succeed in attaining higher levels of economic development are significant opportunities for their residents to obtain training and education, protection of property rights, policies that permit new companies and industries to replace older ones, and avoiding protectionist barriers that hinder international trade.

Key Terms and Concepts

Development economics (210)
Economic growth (196)
Innovation (205)
Labor productivity (200)
New growth theory (203)
Patent (204)

Problems 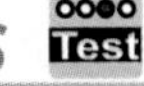

Answers to the odd-numbered problems appear at the back of the book.

9-1. The graph shows a production possibilities curve for 2003 and two potential production possibilities curves for 2004, denoted 2004_A and 2004_B.

a. Which of the labeled points corresponds to maximum feasible 2003 production that is more likely to be associated with the curve denoted 2004_A?

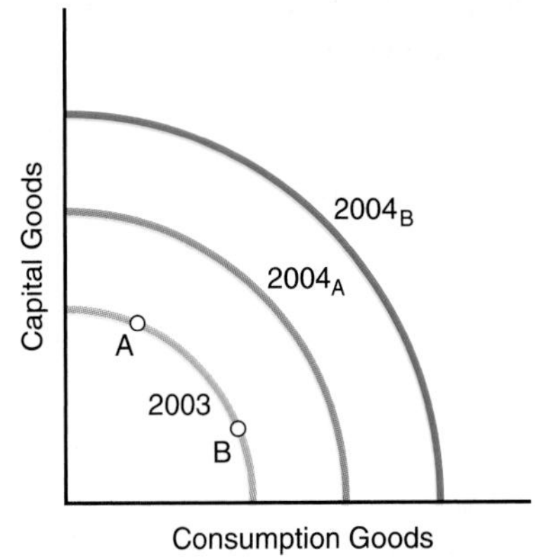

b. Which of the labeled points corresponds to maximum feasible 2003 production that is more likely to be associated with the curve denoted 2004_B?

9-2. Consider the following table displaying annual growth rates for nations X, Y, and Z, each of which entered 1999 with real per capita GDP equal to $20,000:

	Annual Growth Rate (%)			
Country	1999	2000	2001	2002
X	7	3	3	4
Y	4	5	7	9
Z	5	4	3	2

a. Which nation was most likely to have suffered a sizable 1999 earthquake that destroyed a significant portion of its stock of capital goods? What is this nation's per capita real GDP at the end of 2002, rounded to the nearest dollar?

b. Which nation was most likely to have adopted policies in 1999 that encouraged a gradual shift in production from capital goods to consumption goods? What is this nation's per capita real GDP at the end of 2002, rounded to the nearest dollar?

c. Which nation was most likely to have adopted policies in 1999 that encouraged a gradual shift in production from consumption goods to capital goods? What is this nation's per capita real GDP at the end of 2002, rounded to the nearest dollar?

9-3. Per capita real GDP in country F grows at a rate of 3 percent and in country G at a rate of 6 percent. Both begin with equal levels of per capita real GDP. Use Table 9-3 to determine how much higher per capita real GDP will be in country G after 20 years. How much higher will real GDP be in country G after 40 years?

9-4. Per capita real GDP in country L is three times as high as in country M. The economic growth rate in country M, however, is 8 percent, while country L's economy grows at a rate of 5 percent. Use Table 9-3 to determine approximately how many years it will be before per capita real GDP in country M surpasses per capita real GDP in country L?

9-5. Per capita real GDP in country S is only half as great as per capita real GDP in country T. Country T's rate of economic growth is 4 percent. The government of country S, however, enacts policies that achieve a growth rate of 20 percent. Use Table 9-3 to determine how long country S must maintain this growth rate before its per capita real GDP surpasses that of country T.

9-6. In 2001, a nation's population was 10 million. Its nominal GDP was $40 billion, and its price index was 100. In 2002, its population had increased to 12 million. Its nominal GDP had risen to $57.6 billion, and its price index had increased to 120. What was this nation's economic growth rate during the year?

9-7. Between the start of 2001 and the start of 2002, a country's economic growth rate was 4 percent. Its population did not change during the year, nor did its price level. What was the rate of increase of the country's nominal GDP during this one-year interval?

9-8. A nation's government determines that a 5 percent increase in its human capital generates a 3 percent increase in per capita real GDP in the same year. Initially, per capital real GDP in this nation was $10,000. The government launches an "education initiative" that causes its human capital level to rise by 5 percent per year for three years. Other things being equal, what is per capita real GDP in this nation three years hence, rounded to the nearest hundred dollars?

Economics on the Net

Multifactor Productivity and Its Growth Growth in productivity is a key factor determining a nation's overall economic growth. This application helps you perform your own evaluation of the factors contributing to U.S. growth.

Title: Bureau of Labor Statistics: Multifactor Productivity Trends

Navigation: Click here to visit the multifactor productivity homepage of the Bureau of Labor Statistics.

Application Read the summary and answer following questions.

1. What does multifactor productivity measure? Based on your reading of this chapter, how does multifactor productivity relate to the determination of economic growth?
2. Click on Manufacturing Industries: Multifactor Productivity Trends. According to these data, which industries have exhibited the greatest productivity growth in recent years? Which industries have shown the least productivity growth?

For Group Study and Analysis Divide the class into three groups to examine multifactor productivity data for the private business sector, the private nonfarm business sector, and the manufacturing sector. (Be sure to tell the groups to read the Sources and Footnotes discussion following the multifactor productivity tables so that they will know how the sectors are defined.) Have each group identify periods when multifactor productivity growth was particularly fast or slow. Then compare notes. Does it appear to make a big difference which sector one looks at when evaluating periods of largest and smallest growth in multifactor productivity?

TYING IT ALL TOGETHER

Part 2 Case Problem

Case Background

Web Capital, Inc., is an Internet service provider (ISP). Its owners and managers have launched an effort to develop a worldwide clientele. Currently, Web Capital's managers are focusing their attention on the People's Republic of China.

Evaluating the Chinese Environment As early as 1981, reformers within the Chinese government had pushed for expanding the nation's telecommunications network as part of an overall effort to modernize the national economy. Nevertheless, during the following decade, the nation's investment in its information technology infrastructure was meager by the standards of developing nations. Furthermore, the nation experienced rising inflation that by 1994 was in excess of 24 percent per year. The central government began to worry that it had no effective means for controlling an overheating economy that it perceived as prone to rapid booms followed by hard-to-predict busts.

By late 1994, both reformers and hard-liners in the Chinese leadership had reached a consensus that creation of a modern information technology infrastructure was a desirable objective. In 1998, China launched a major effort to develop an Internet of its own, and it sought to link businesses and, ultimately, consumers within a centralized telecommunications network. Current estimates indicate that as many as 75 million Chinese people could have access to Web-connected computers by 2003.

The Management Issue at Web Capital Web Capital is exploring the potential for the company to negotiate a contract to become one of two or three primary providers of Internet service for this emerging Chinese network.

Following a meeting with top government telecommunications officials, a review committee comprised of mid-level managers identified the following key factors that senior officers should contemplate before making a final decision about whether the company should enter into the contract:

1. In the current working draft of the contract, the Chinese government requires Web Capital to commit to a specific, sizable investment measured in current-year quantities of yuan, the Chinese currency. It cannot invest more or less.
2. Initially, the contract grants Web Capital the right to market its services to up to 2 million households in a specific geographic region. How quickly the potential for new ISP subscribers in this region might grow during the following years will largely depend on the economy's growth.
3. Actual company sales of Internet access services will depend on a number of factors, including the hours of employment and the average hourly wages earned by Chinese households during the term of the contract.
4. There is some evidence that structural, seasonal, and frictional unemployment have trended downward throughout China in recent years.
5. There is considerable evidence that per capita income growth in China is far from equally spread across Chinese households.

Points to Analyze

1. What are the near-term risks that Web Capital is likely to face if it makes a significant investment in China?
2. Looking into the longer term, are there reasons to be optimistic about China's overall growth and, by implication, growth in the market for ISP services in China? Are there reasons to be pessimistic? Be as specific as you can.
3. Web Capital has determined that successful market penetration in China will require a minimal real capital investment that is very close to the amount the contract specifies. Although China's annual inflation rate has been below 3 percent since 1997, the average rate of increase in consumer prices was 16 percent per year between 1993 and 1996, and inflation has picked up in recent quarters. Given the current terms of the contract, is this a legitimate area of concern for Web Capital's management?
4. In what ways does the recent experience with high growth rates in per capita incomes make the terms of the contract look more advantageous for Web Capital? In what ways do the terms look less advantageous? Why?
5. Based on experiences in North America, Europe, and South America, Web Capital has learned that high- and middle-income individuals are most likely to be willing to include ISP fees in their monthly household budgets. Should this raise any management concerns with respect to a potential investment in China?

Casing the Internet

1. **Is there really evidence of a boom-and-bust cycle in China? To investigate this issue, click here to go to the International Monetary Fund's home page. Then click on "Publications." In the right-hand column, click on "World Economic Outlook." At this site, you can download the final file of this report.**
   a. **Look at Table 6, titled "Developing Countries—by Country: Real GDP." Has China's economy experienced a recession during the past decade?**
   b. **Now examine Table 12, titled "Developing Countries—by Country: Consumer Prices." Has China's inflation rate been volatile during the past decade?**
   c. **Based on your answers to parts (a) and (b), has nominal GDP been volatile during the past decade?**
2. **The World Bank has funded projects intended to support increased economic growth in rural parts of China. You can read about one of these projects by clicking here.**
   a. **Based on this article, in what ways might World Bank loans assist in improving China's economic growth?**
   b. **Can you see any way that World Bank loans to China could, under some circumstances, actually hinder China's growth prospects?**

Part 3

National Income Determination and Fiscal Policy

CHAPTER

10

REAL GDP AND THE PRICE LEVEL IN THE LONG RUN

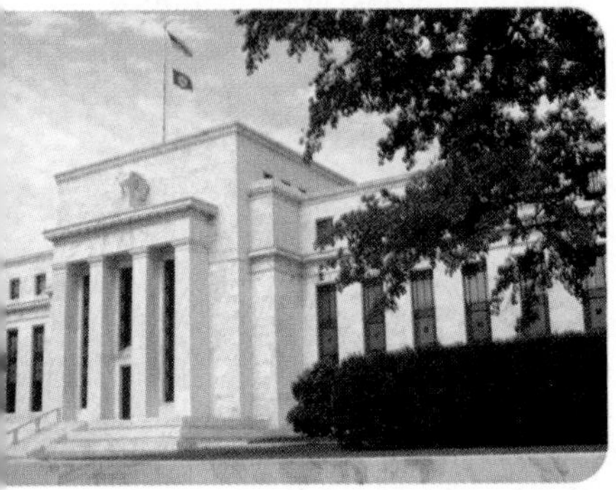

What goes on inside the Federal Reserve building is a mystery to many. But the policymakers inside can and do influence various aspects of our economy. Why should the Fed be concerned about such things as the long-run equilibrium price level?

In January 1989, a *New York Times* feature article focused on a "new theory" that Federal Reserve economists had developed, known as the P^* model. The theory's aim was to identify a price level consistent with the economy's long-run growth path. The idea was that if the Fed could identify this price level, called P^*, it could adjust the quantity of money in circulation appropriately to achieve long-run price stability and essentially eliminate inflation. Other economists chuckled when they read about this so-called new theory because they knew something the article's author apparently didn't—that the thinking behind the P^* model had been around for a long, long time. Nevertheless, research to identify P^* continues. By the time you complete your study of this chapter, you will understand the basis of the P^* model. It will also be clear why economists today remain interested in its implications.

LEARNING OBJECTIVES

After reading this chapter, you should be able to:

1. **Understand the concept of long-run aggregate supply**
2. **Describe the effect of economic growth on the long-run aggregate supply curve**
3. **Explain why the aggregate demand curve slopes downward and list key factors that cause this curve to shift**
4. **Discuss the meaning of long-run equilibrium for the economy as a whole**
5. **Evaluate why economic growth can cause deflation**
6. **Evaluate likely reasons for persistent inflation in recent decades**

Chapter Outline

Did You Know That... the children's classic *The Wonderful Wizard of Oz,* written in 1900 by L. Frank Baum, was also an allegory about how a nation should achieve long-run price stability? According to economist Hugh Rockoff of Rutgers University, Baum's book was intended to support the populist political movement that arose in the 1890s. The economic issue of central concern to the populists was widespread *deflation*. The U.S. price level had generally declined since the end of the Civil War, and from time to time unexpected drops in prices greatly disrupted the lives of farmers, shopkeepers, and workers in the Midwest and West. According to Rockoff, the small-minded Munchkins that Dorothy meets after a tornado transports her to the Land of Oz probably symbolize inhabitants of eastern states whom Baum perceived as insensitive to the plight of informally educated but commonsensical western farmers (symbolized by the Scarecrow) and urban workers in danger of losing their hearts and souls (symbolized by the Tin Man). The city inhabited by the Wizard of Oz, the Emerald City (symbolic of Washington, D.C.) is green—the color of money. The same is true of the Wizard's home, the Emerald Palace (representing the White House). Before Dorothy and her friends enter the Emerald City, however, they must put on green-colored glasses held together with gold buckles, symbolizing the U.S. government's forcing westerners to use money supported only by gold. The populists believed that the way to halt the nation's persistent and variable deflation was to expand the quantity of money in circulation by basing money's value on silver as well as gold. For this reason, in Baum's book the slippers that help Dorothy get back to Kansas are made of silver (the writers of the 1939 movie version of the book changed these to ruby slippers). Rockoff speculates that the Cowardly Lion represents William Jennings Bryan, the "roaring orator" and presidential candidate who decried gold but then retreated—in a way that Baum evidently found cowardly—for political reasons. Oz, of course, is the abbreviation for ounces, in which gold is measured, and the yellow brick road is paved with bars of gold.

Why did the United States experience persistent deflation during the latter part of the nineteenth century? Did the populists and their literary supporter, L. Frank Baum, have a legitimate point in arguing that the United States ought to expand the quantity of money in circulation to halt deflation? To answer these questions, you must learn about the factors that influence the long-run stability of the price level.

OUTPUT GROWTH AND THE LONG-RUN AGGREGATE SUPPLY CURVE

In Chapter 2, we showed the derivation of the production possibilities curve. At any point in time, the economy can be inside or on the PPC but never outside it. Along the PPC, a country's resources are fully employed in the production of goods and services, and the sum total of all goods and services produced is the nation's real output, or real GDP. Economists refer to the total of all planned production for the entire economy as the **aggregate supply** of real output.

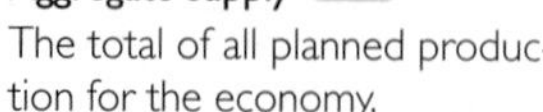

Aggregate supply The total of all planned production for the economy.

The Long-Run Aggregate Supply Curve 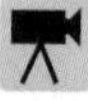

Put yourself in a world in which nothing has been changing, year in and year out. The price level has not changed. Technology has not changed. The prices of inputs that firms must purchase have not changed. Labor productivity has not changed. All resources are fully employed, so the economy operates on its production possibilities curve, such as the one

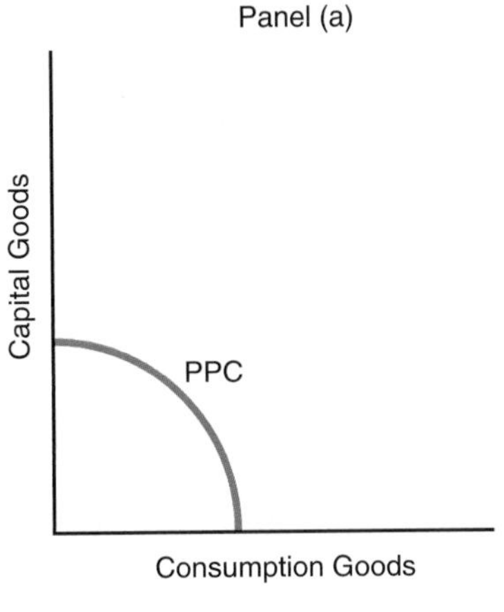

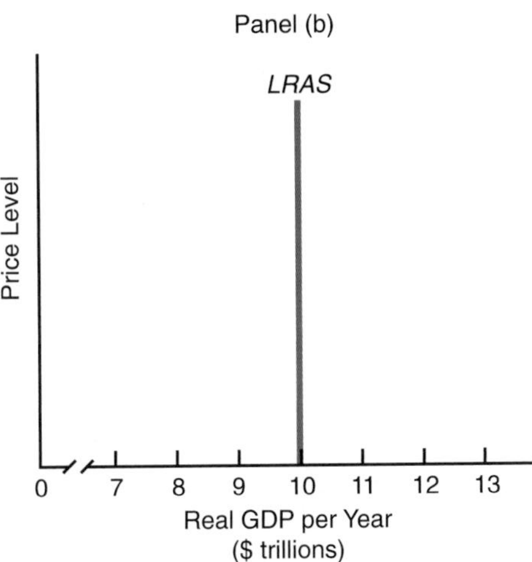

FIGURE 10-1

The Production Possibilities and the Economy's Long-Run Aggregate Supply Curve

At a point in time, a nation's base of resources and its technological capabilities define the position of its production possibilities curve, as shown in panel (a). This defines the real GDP that the nation can produce when resources are fully employed, which determines the position of the long-run aggregate supply curve (*LRAS*) displayed in panel (b). Because people have complete information and input prices adjust fully to changes in output prices in the long run, the *LRAS* is vertical.

depicted in panel (a) of Figure 10-1. This is a world that is fully adjusted and in which people have all the information they are ever going to get about that world. The **long-run aggregate supply curve** (*LRAS*) in this world is some amount of output of real goods and services—say, $10 trillion of real GDP. We can show long-run aggregate supply simply by a vertical line at $10 trillion of real GDP. This is what you see in panel (b) of the figure. That curve, labeled *LRAS*, is a vertical line determined by technology and **endowments,** or resources that exist in our economy. It is the full-information and full-adjustment level of real output of goods and services. It is the level of real output that will continue being produced year after year, forever, if nothing changes.

Long-run aggregate supply curve 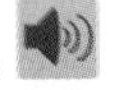
A vertical line representing real output of goods and services after full adjustment has occurred. Can also be viewed as representing the real output of the economy under conditions of full employment—the full-employment level of real GDP.

Endowments 
The various resources in an economy, including both physical resources and such human resources as ingenuity and management skills.

Another way of viewing the *LRAS* is to think of it as the full-employment level of real GDP. When the economy reaches full employment along its production possibilities curve, no further adjustments will occur unless a change occurs in the other variables that we are assuming constant and stable. Some economists like to think of the *LRAS* as occurring at the level of real GDP consistent with the natural rate of unemployment, the unemployment rate that occurs in an economy with full adjustment in the long run. As we discussed in Chapter 7, many economists like to think of the natural rate of unemployment as consisting of frictional and structural unemployment.

To understand why the long-run aggregate supply curve is vertical, think about the long run, which is a sufficiently long period that all factors of production and prices, including wages and other input prices, can change. A change in the level of prices of goods and services has no effect on real output (real GDP per year) in the long run, because higher output prices will be accompanied by comparable changes in input prices. Suppliers will therefore have no incentive to increase or decrease output. Remember that in the long run, everybody has full information, and there is full adjustment to price level changes.

Click here to find out how fast one key input price—wages—are adjusting. Next click on "Employment Cost Index."

Economic Growth and Long-Run Aggregate Supply

In Chapter 9, you learned about the factors that determine growth in per capita output: the annual growth rate of labor, the rate of year-to-year capital accumulation, and the rate of growth of the productivity of labor and capital. As time goes by, population gradually

FIGURE 10-2

The Long-Run Aggregate Supply Curve and Shifts in It

In panel (a), we repeat a diagram that we used in Chapter 2 to show the meaning of economic growth. Over time, the production possibilities curve shifts outward. In panel (b), we demonstrate the same principle by showing the long-run aggregate supply curve as initially a vertical line at *LRAS* at $10 trillion of real GDP per year. As our endowments increase, the *LRAS* moves outward to $LRAS_{2004}$.

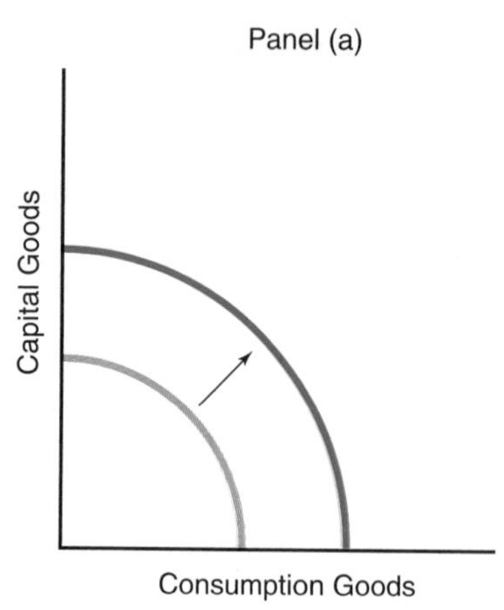

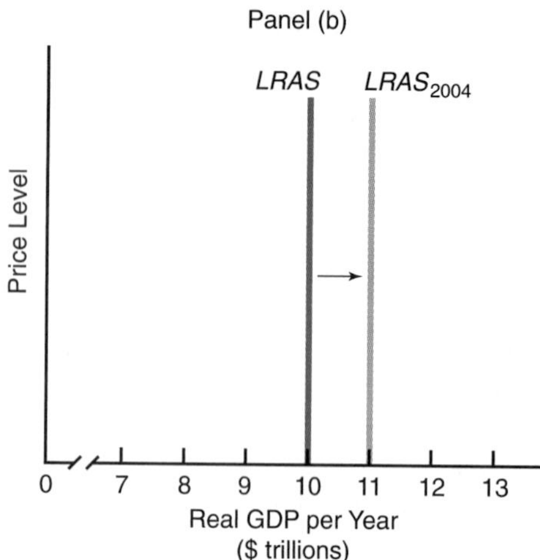

increases, and labor force participation rates change. The capital stock typically grows as businesses add such capital equipment as new information technology hardware. Furthermore, technology improves. Thus the economy's production possibilities increase, and the production possibilities curve shifts outward, as shown in panel (a) of Figure 10-2.

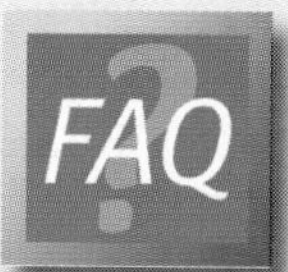

Does the government include business software when tracking investment and growth?

Yes, but it only began doing so in late 1999. Now the Bureau of Economic Analysis (BEA), a unit of the U.S. Department of Commerce, treats business software purchases as a type of capital accumulation. Estimates are that this change will add 0.15 to 0.30 percentage point to estimates of GDP growth in the 1990s and 2000s. Furthermore, the BEA's revisions have for some periods boosted measured private-sector capital accumulation by as much as a third. This isn't surprising, perhaps, given that in recent years about half the approximately $8,000 in annual per-employee capital spending by businesses was allocated to expenditures on information technology—much of which went to purchases of new and updated software.

The result is economic growth: Aggregate real GDP and real GDP per capita increase. This means that at least in a growing economy such as ours, *LRAS* will shift outward to the right, as in panel (b). We have drawn *LRAS* for the year 2004 to the right of our original *LRAS* of $10 trillion of real GDP. The number we have attached to $LRAS_{2004}$ is $11 trillion of real GDP, but that is only a guess. The point is that it is to the right of today's *LRAS* curve.

We may conclude that in a growing economy, the *LRAS* shifts ever farther to the right over time. If it were the case that the pace at which *LRAS* shifts rightward were constant, real GDP would increase at a steady annual rate. As shown in Figure 10-3, this means that real GDP would increase along a long-run, or *trend*, path that is an upward-sloping line. Thus if the *LRAS* shifts rightward from $10 trillion to $11 trillion between now and 2004 and then increases at a steady pace of $500 billion per year every year thereafter, in 2006 long-run real GDP will equal $12 trillion, in 2008 it will equal $13 trillion, and so on.

CONCEPTS IN BRIEF

- The long-run aggregate supply curve, *LRAS,* is a vertical line determined by amounts of available resources such as labor and capital and by technology and resource productivity. The position of the *LRAS* gives the full-information and full-adjustment level of real output of goods and services.

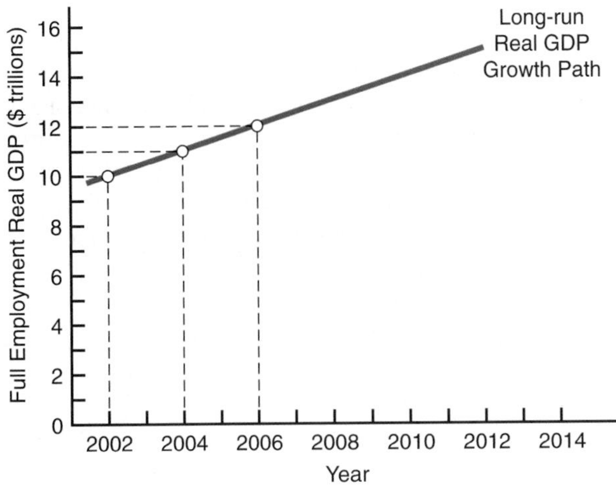

FIGURE 10-3
A Sample Long-Run Growth Path for Real GDP
Year-to-year shifts in the long-run aggregate supply curve yield a long-run trend path for real GDP growth. In this example, real GDP grows by a steady amount of $500 billion each year.

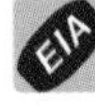

Long-Run Aggregate Supply
Practice with the long-run aggregate supply.

- The natural rate of unemployment occurs at the long-run level of real GDP given by the position of the *LRAS*.
- If labor or capital increases from year to year or if the productivity of either of these resources rises from one year to the next, the *LRAS* shifts rightward. In a growing economy, therefore, real GDP gradually rises over time.

SPENDING AND TOTAL EXPENDITURES

In equilibrium, individuals, businesses, and governments purchase all the goods and services produced, valued in trillions of real dollars. As explained in Chapters 7 and 8, GDP is the dollar value of total expenditures on domestically produced final goods and services. Because all expenditures are made by individuals, firms, or governments, the total value of these expenditures must be what each of these market participants decides it shall be. The decisions of individuals, managers of firms, and government officials determine the annual dollar value of total expenditures. You can certainly see this in your role as an individual. You decide what the total dollar amount of your expenditures will be in a year. You decide how much you want to spend and how much you want to save. Thus if we want to know what determines the total value of GDP, the answer would be clear: the spending decisions of individuals like you; firms; and local, state, and national governments. In an open economy, we must also include foreign individuals, firms, and governments (foreigners, for short) that decide to spend their money income in the United States.

Simply stating that the dollar value of total expenditures in this country depends on what individuals, firms, governments, and foreigners decide to do really doesn't tell us much, though. Two important issues remain:

1. What determines the total amount that individuals, firms, governments, and foreigners want to spend?
2. What determines the equilibrium price level and the rate of inflation (or deflation)?

The *LRAS* tells us only about the economy's long-run, or trend, real GDP. To answer these additional questions, we must consider another important concept. This is **aggregate demand,** which is the total of all planned real expenditures in the economy.

Aggregate demand 
The total of all planned expenditures for the entire economy.

AGGREGATE DEMAND

Aggregate demand curve
A curve showing planned purchase rates for all final goods and services in the economy at various price levels, all other things held constant.

The **aggregate demand curve,** *AD,* gives the various quantities of all final commodities demanded at various price levels, all other things held constant. Recall the components of GDP that you studied in Chapter 8: consumption spending, investment expenditures, government purchases, and net foreign demand for domestic production. They are all components of aggregate demand. Throughout this chapter and the next, whenever you see the aggregate demand curve, realize that it is a shorthand way of talking about the components of GDP that are measured by government statisticians when they calculate total economic activity each year. In Chapter 12, you will look more closely at the relationship between these components and in particular how consumption spending depends on income.

The Aggregate Demand Curve

The aggregate demand curve gives the total amount of *real* domestic output that will be purchased at each price level. This consists of the output of final goods and services in the economy—everything produced for final use by households, businesses, the government, and foreign residents. It includes stereos, socks, shoes, medical and legal services, computers, and millions of other goods and services that people buy each year. A graphical representation of the aggregate demand curve is seen in Figure 10-4. On the horizontal axis is measured real gross domestic output, or real GDP. For our measure of the price level, we use the GDP price deflator on the vertical axis. The aggregate demand curve is labeled *AD.* If the GDP deflator is 100, aggregate quantity demanded is \$10 trillion per year (point *A*). At price level 120, it is \$9 trillion per year (point *B*). At price level 140, it is \$8 trillion per year (point *C*). The higher the price level, the lower the total real output demanded by the economy, everything else remaining constant, as shown by the arrow along *AD* in Figure 10-4. Conversely, the lower the price level, the higher the total real output demanded by the economy, everything else staying constant.

Let's take the year 2000. Looking at U.S. Department of Commerce preliminary statistics reveals the following information:

FIGURE 10-4 

The Aggregate Demand Curve
Because of the real-balance, interest rate, and open economy effects, the aggregate demand curve, *AD,* slopes downward. If the price level is 100, we will be at point *A* with \$10 trillion of real GDP demanded per year. As the price level increases to 120 and 140, we will move up the aggregate demand curve to points *B* and *C.*

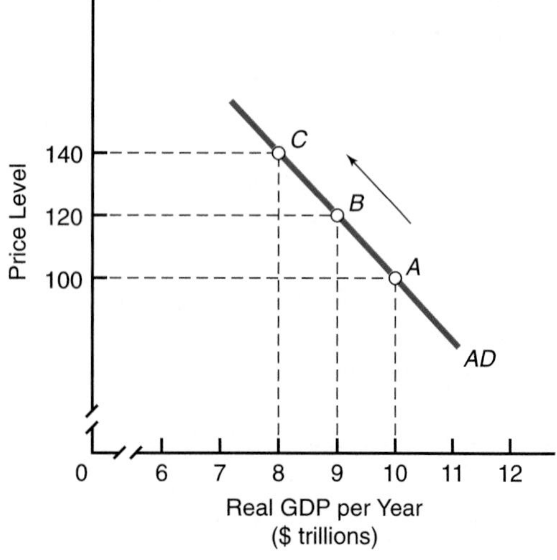

- GDP was $9,849.5 billion.
- The price level as measured by GDP deflator was 106.41 (base year is 1996, for which the index equals 100).
- Real GDP (output) was $9,256.2 billion in 1996 dollars.

What can we say about 2000? Given the dollar cost of buying goods and services and all of the other factors that go into spending decisions by individuals, firms, governments, and foreigners, the total amount of real domestic output demanded by firms, individuals, governments, and foreigners was $9,256.2 billion in 2000 (in terms of 1996 dollars).

What Happens When the Price Level Rises? 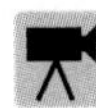

What if the price level in the economy rose to 160 tomorrow? What would happen to the amount of real goods and services that individuals, firms, governments, and foreigners wish to purchase in the United States? We know from Chapter 3 that when the price of one good or service rises, the quantity of it demanded will fall. But here we are talking about the *price level*—the average price of *all* goods and services in the economy. The answer is still that the total quantities of real goods and services demanded would fall, but the reasons are different. When the price of one good or service goes up, the consumer substitutes other goods and services. For the entire economy, when the price level goes up, the consumer doesn't simply substitute one good for another, for now we are dealing with the demand for *all* goods and services in the nation. There are *economywide* reasons that cause the aggregate demand curve to slope downward. They involve at least three distinct forces: the *real-balance effect,* the *interest rate effect,* and the *open economy effect.*

The Real-Balance Effect. A rise in the price level will have an effect on spending. Individuals, firms, governments, and foreigners carry out transactions using money, a portion of which consists of currency and coins that you have in your pocket (or stashed away) right now. Because people use money to purchase goods and services, the amount of money that people have influences the amount of goods and services they want to buy. For example, if you found a $10 bill on the sidewalk, the amount of money you had would rise. Given your now greater level of money balances—currency in this case—you would almost surely increase your spending on goods and services. Similarly, if while on a trip downtown you had your pocket picked, there would be an effect on your desired spending. For example, if your wallet had $30 in it when it was stolen, the reduction in your cash balances—in this case currency—would no doubt cause you to reduce your planned expenditures. You would ultimately buy fewer goods and services. This response is sometimes called the **real-balance effect** (or *wealth effect*) because it relates to the real value of your cash balances. While your *nominal* cash balances may remain the same, any change in the price level will cause a change in the *real* value of those cash balances—hence the real-balance effect on the quantity of aggregate goods and services demanded.

Real-balance effect 
The change in expenditures resulting from the real value of money balances when the price level changes, all other things held constant. Also called the *wealth effect.*

When you think of the real-balance effect, just think of what happens to your real wealth if you have, say, a $100 bill hidden under your mattress. If the price level increases by 10 percent, the purchasing power of that $100 bill drops by 10 percent, so you have become less wealthy. That will reduce your spending on all goods and services by some small amount.

The Interest Rate Effect. There is a more subtle but equally important effect on your desire to spend. As the price level rises, interest rates increase. This raises borrowing costs for consumers and businesses. They will borrow less and consequently spend less. The fact that a higher price level pushes up interest rates and thereby reduces borrowing and spending is known as the **interest rate effect.**

Interest rate effect 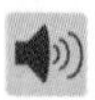
One of the reasons that the aggregate demand curve slopes downward is that higher price levels increase the interest rate, which in turn causes businesses and consumers to reduce desired spending due to the higher price of borrowing.

Higher interest rates make it more costly for people to buy houses and cars. Higher interest rates also make it less profitable for firms to install new equipment and to erect new office buildings. Whether we are talking about individuals or firms, the effect of a rise in the price level will cause higher interest rates, which in turn reduces the amount of goods and services that people are willing to purchase. Therefore, an increase in the price level will tend to reduce the aggregate quantity of goods and services demanded. (The opposite occurs if the price level declines.)

The Open Economy Effect: The Substitution of Foreign Goods. Recall from Chapter 8 that GDP includes net exports—the difference between exports and imports. In an open economy, we buy imports from other countries and ultimately pay for them through the foreign exchange market. The same is true for foreigners who purchase our goods (exports). Given any set of exchange rates between the U.S. dollar and other currencies, an increase in the price level in the United States makes American goods more expensive relative to foreign goods. Foreigners have downward-sloping demand curves for American goods. When the relative price of American goods goes up, foreigners buy fewer American goods and more of their own. At home, relatively cheaper prices for foreign goods cause Americans to want to buy more foreign goods instead of American goods. The result is a fall in exports and a rise in imports when the domestic price level rises. That means that a price level increase tends to reduce net exports, thereby reducing the amount of real goods and services purchased in the United States. This is known as the **open economy effect.**

Open economy effect 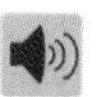
One of the reasons that the aggregate demand curve slopes downward is that higher price levels result in foreigners' desiring to buy fewer American-made goods while Americans now desire more foreign-made goods, thereby reducing net exports. This is equivalent to a reduction in the amount of real goods and services purchased in the United States.

What Happens When the Price Level Falls?

What about the reverse? Suppose now that the GDP deflator falls to 100 from an initial level of 120. You should be able to trace the three effects on desired purchases of goods and services. Specifically, how do the real-balance, interest rate, and open economy effects cause people to want to buy more? You should come to the conclusion that the lower the price level, the greater the quantity of output of goods and services demanded.

The aggregate demand curve, *AD,* shows the quantity of aggregate output that will be demanded at alternative price levels. It is downward-sloping, just like the demand curve for individual goods. The higher the price level, the lower the quantity of aggregate output demanded, and vice versa.

Demand for All Goods and Services Versus Demand for a Single Good or Serivce

Even though the aggregate demand curve, *AD,* in Figure 10-4 on page 230 looks similar to the one for individual demand, *D,* for a single good or service that you encountered in Chapters 3 and 4, the two are not the same. When we derive the aggregate demand curve, we are looking at the entire economic system. The aggregate demand curve, *AD,* differs from an individual demand curve, *D,* because we are looking at the *entire* circular flow of income and product when we construct *AD.*

SHIFTS IN THE AGGREGATE DEMAND CURVE 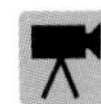

In Chapter 3, you learned that any time a nonprice determinant of demand changed, the demand curve shifted inward to the left or outward to the right. The same analysis holds for the aggregate demand curve, except we are now talking about the non-price-level determinants of aggregate demand. So when we ask the question, "What determines the position of the aggregate demand curve?" the fundamental proposition is as follows:

> Any non-price-level change that increases aggregate spending (on domestic goods) shifts *AD* to the right. Any non-price-level change that decreases aggregate spending (on domestic goods) shifts *AD* to the left.

The list of potential determinants of the position of the aggregate demand curve is long. Some of the most important "curve shifters" for aggregate demand are presented in Table 10-1.

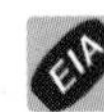

Aggregate Demand and Supply
Gain further understanding of the effects of aggregate demand and aggregate supply.

TABLE 10-1
Determinants of Aggregate Demand
Aggregate demand consists of the demand for domestically produced consumption goods, investment goods, government purchases, and net exports. Consequently, any change in the demand for any one of these components of real GDP will cause a change in aggregate demand. Some possibilities are listed here.

Changes That Cause an Increase in Aggregate Demand	Changes That Cause a Decrease in Aggregate Demand
A drop in the foreign exchange value of the dollar	A rise in the foreign exchange value of the dollar
Increased security about jobs and future income	Decreased security about jobs and future income
Improvements in economic conditions in other countries	Declines in economic conditions in other countries
A reduction in real interest rates (nominal interest rates corrected for inflation) not due to price level changes	A rise in real interest rates (nominal interest rates corrected for inflation) not due to price level changes
Tax decreases	Tax increases
An increase in the amount of money in circulation	A decrease in the amount of money in circulation

CONCEPTS IN BRIEF

- Aggregate demand is the total of all planned expenditures in the economy, and aggregate supply is the total of all planned production in the economy. The aggregate demand curve shows the various quantities of all commodities demanded at various price levels; it is downward-sloping.
- There are three reasons why the aggregate demand curve is downward-sloping: the real-balance effect, the interest rate effect, and the open economy effect.
- The real-balance effect occurs because price level changes alter the real value of cash balances, thereby causing people to desire to spend more or less, depending on whether the price level decreases or increases.
- The interest rate effect is caused via interest rate changes that mimic price level changes. At higher interest rates, people desire to buy fewer houses and cars, and vice versa.
- The open economy effect occurs because of a shift toward foreign goods when the domestic price level increases and a shift away from foreign goods when the domestic price level decreases.

FIGURE 10-5 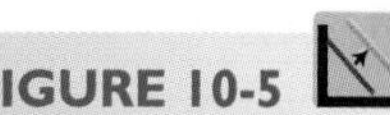

Long-Run Economywide Equilibrium

For the economy as a whole, long-run equilibrium occurs at the price level where the aggregate demand curve crosses the long-run aggregate supply curve. At this long-run equilibrium price level, which is 120 in the diagram, total planned real expenditures equal total planned production at full employment, which in our example is a real GDP of $10 trillion.

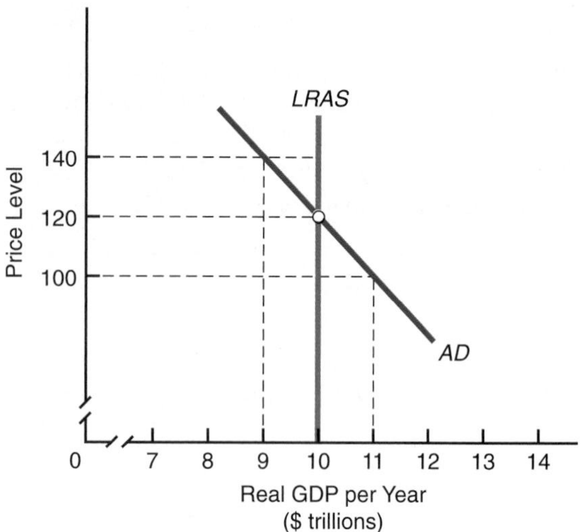

LONG-RUN EQUILIBRIUM AND THE PRICE LEVEL

As noted in Chapter 3, equilibrium occurs where the demand and supply curves intersect. The same is true for the economy as a whole, as shown in Figure 10-5: The equilibrium price level occurs at the point where the aggregate demand curve *(AD)* crosses the long-run aggregate supply curve *(LRAS)*. At this equilibrium price level of 120, the total of all planned real expenditures for the entire economy is equal to total planned production along the economy's trend growth path for real GDP. Thus the equilibrium depicted in Figure 10-5 is the economy's *long-run equilibrium*.

Note that if the price level were to increase to 140, total planned production would exceed total planned real expenditures. Inventories of unsold goods would begin to accumulate, and firms would stand ready to offer services that people would not wish to purchase. As a result, the price level would tend to fall. If the price level were 100, then total planned real expenditures by individuals, businesses, and the government would exceed total planned production by firms, and the price level would move toward 120.

THE EFFECTS OF ECONOMIC GROWTH ON THE PRICE LEVEL

We now have a basic theory of how real output and the price level are determined in the long run when all of a nation's resources can change over time and all input prices can adjust fully to changes in the overall level of prices of goods and services that firms produce. Let's begin by evaluating the effects of economic growth on the nation's price level.

Take a look at panel (a) of Figure 10-6, which shows what happens, other things being equal, when the *LRAS* shifts rightward over time. If the economy were to grow steadily during, say, a 10-year interval, the long-run aggregate supply schedule would shift to the right, from $LRAS_1$ to $LRAS_2$. In the example illustrated in the figure, this results in a downward movement along the aggregate demand schedule. The equilibrium price level falls, from 120 to 60. Thus if all factors that affect total planned real expenditures are unchanged, so that the aggregate demand curve does not noticeably move during the 10-year period of real GDP growth, the growing economy in the example would experience deflation. This is

FIGURE 10-6

Secular Deflation Versus Long-Run Price Stability in a Growing Economy

Panel (a) illustrates what happens when economic growth occurs without a corresponding increase in aggregate demand. The result is a decline in the price level over time, known as *secular deflation.* Panel (b) shows that in principle, secular deflation can be avoided if the aggregate demand curve shifts rightward at the same pace that the long-run aggregate supply curve shifts to the right.

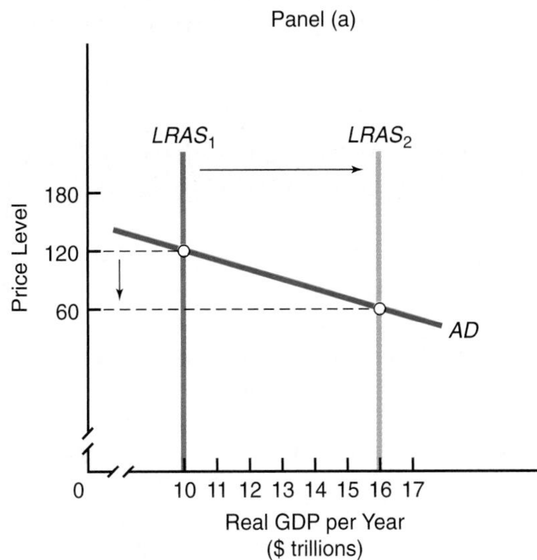

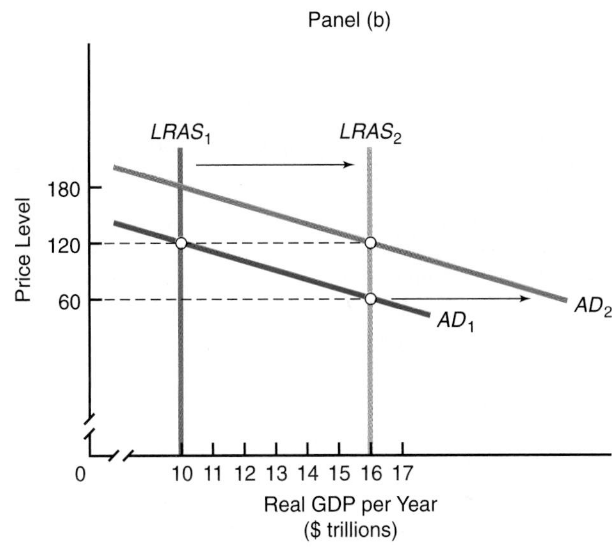

known as **secular deflation,** or a persistently declining price level resulting from economic growth in the presence of relatively unchanged aggregate demand.

L. Frank Baum and his contemporaries experienced secular deflation during the three decades preceding publication of *The Wonderful Wizard of Oz*. For instance, compared with 1872 levels, by 1894 the price of bricks had fallen by 50 percent, the price of sugar by 67 percent, the price of wheat by 69 percent, the price of nails by 70 percent, and the price of copper by nearly 75 percent. Baum and other populists at the turn of the twentieth century offered a proposal for ending deflation and achieving long-run price stability: They wanted the government to expand the quantity of money in circulation by issuing new money backed by silver. As we discussed earlier, an increase in the quantity of money in circulation raises total planned real expenditures at any given price level and thereby causes the aggregate demand curve to shift to the right. Although economic historians have been divided about how effectively silver-backed money would have maintained long-run price stability, it is clear from panel (b) of Figure 10-6 that the increase in the quantity of money surely would have pushed the price level back upward. As you can see in panel (b), in principle just the right increase in aggregate demand could indeed stabilize the equilibrium price level at its initial value of 120.

In fact, in 1890 Congress passed the Treasury Note Act, otherwise known as the Silver Purchase Act, which required the U.S. Treasury to purchase silver and issue currency known as silver certificates. This effort to expand the quantity of money barely got off the ground, however, before stock market panics hit in the spring and summer of 1893. People began to hoard gold, and the price of silver fell. To limit the government's losses on its silver holdings, Congress, at the urging of President Grover Cleveland, repealed the Silver

Secular deflation 
A persistent decline in prices resulting from economic growth in the presence of stable aggregate demand.

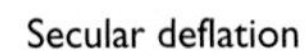
Click here to learn about how the price level has changed during recent years. Next click on "Gross Domestic Product and Components" (for GDP deflators) or "Consumer Price Indexes."

Purchase Act. William Jennings Bryan sought the Democratic presidential nomination to oppose Republican William McKinley in 1896, and in an emotional speech, he decried the repeal of the Silver Purchase Act, saying, "You shall not press down upon the brow of labor this crown of thorns, you shall not crucify mankind upon a cross of gold." Although Bryan's speechmaking abilities made him a public sensation, he nonetheless lost the election, which sounded the death knell of the populist effort to increase the quantity of money in circulation via silver certificates. According to Rutgers economist Hugh Rockoff, Baum represented the twin enemies of silver, Presidents Cleveland (of New York) and McKinley (of Ohio), as the Wicked Witch of the East and the Wicked Witch of the West.

INTERNATIONAL EXAMPLE

Corporations Adjust to Potential and True Deflation

For decades, conventional wisdom among corporate financial officers was that they can lower their companies' costs by financing purchases of capital by borrowing—taking out loans from banks, selling commercial paper, issuing new bonds, and the like. The reason is that debt has traditionally been less expensive to a firm than the issuing of new shares. Corporate managers could count on inflation to erode the value of the firm's debts even as the selling price of the company's output increased.

In a deflationary environment, however, these dynamics are reversed. Deflation *increases* the real value of outstanding debts. At the same time, companies find that to repay their loans, they must dip into profits that are declining because of falling output prices. In 1997 and 1998, companies based in Southeast Asia learned this lesson with a vengeance. From Russia to Thailand to Indonesia, companies faced lower selling prices and mounting real values of indebtedness. Of course, they were hit by a double whammy: The relative values of local currencies also fell during 1997 and 1998, and many debts of these companies were denominated in dollars. Thus companies found themselves having to give up more of their profits denominated in domestic currencies to obtain the dollars they required to make their debt payments.

Closer to home, however, even some U.S. corporate managers are getting nervous. A few have openly called for changing their long-term fundraising philosophies now in anticipation of future deflation, even though the overall rate of inflation remains positive. For some industries, however, the deflationary future has already arrived. Companies specializing in manufacturing, chemicals, oil, and natural gas products already are seeing their selling prices decline year in and year out. Corporate treasurers in these industries are now talking about a "new balance sheet paradigm" in which companies will rely much more heavily on issuing stock instead of borrowing.

For Critical Analysis

In what ways might deflation affect the average individual's financial well-being?

CAUSES OF INFLATION

Of course, so far during your lifetime, deflation has not been a problem in the United States. Figure 10-7 shows annual U.S. inflation rates for the past few decades. Clearly, inflation rates have been variable. The other obvious fact, however, is that inflation rates have consistently been *positive*. The price level in the United States has *risen* almost every year. For today's United States, secular deflation has not been a big political issue. If anything, it is a secular *inflation* that has plagued the nation.

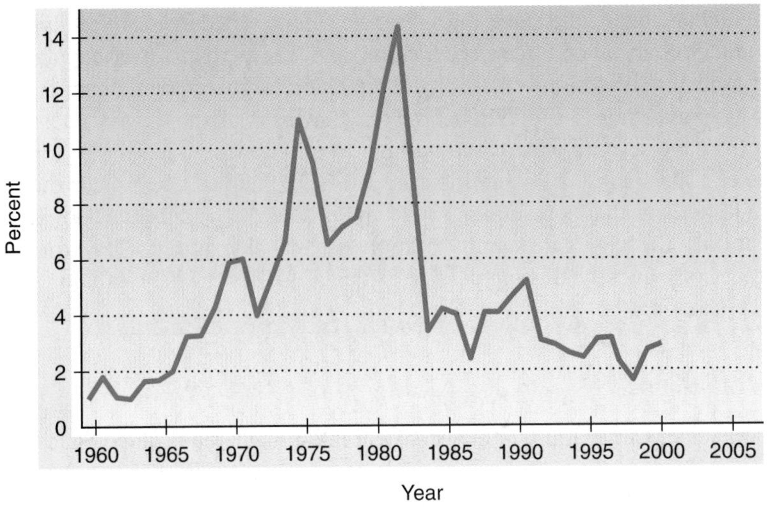

FIGURE 10-7

Inflation Rates in the United States

U.S. inflation rates rose considerably during the 1970s but declined to lower levels since the 1980s. Nevertheless, the United States has experienced inflation every year since 1959.

Sources: Economic Report of the President; Economic Indicators, various issues.

Supply-Side Inflation?

What causes such persistent inflation? The classical model provides two possible explanations for inflation. One potential rationale is depicted in panel (a) of Figure 10-8. This panel shows a rise in the price level caused by a *decline in long-run aggregate supply.* Hence one possible reason for persistent inflation would be continual reductions in the production of real output.

FIGURE 10-8

Explaining Persistent Inflation

As shown in panel (a), it is possible for a decline in long-run aggregate supply to cause a rise in the price level. Long-run aggregate supply *increases,* however, in a growing economy, so this cannot explain the observation of persistent U.S. inflation. Panel (b) provides the true explanation of persistent inflation, which is that increases in aggregate demand push up the long-run equilibrium price level. Thus it is possible to explain persistent inflation in a growing economy if the aggregate demand curve shifts rightward at a faster pace than the long-run aggregate supply curve.

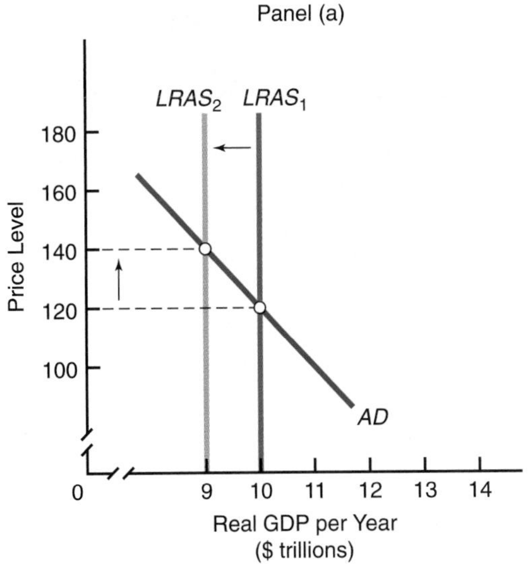

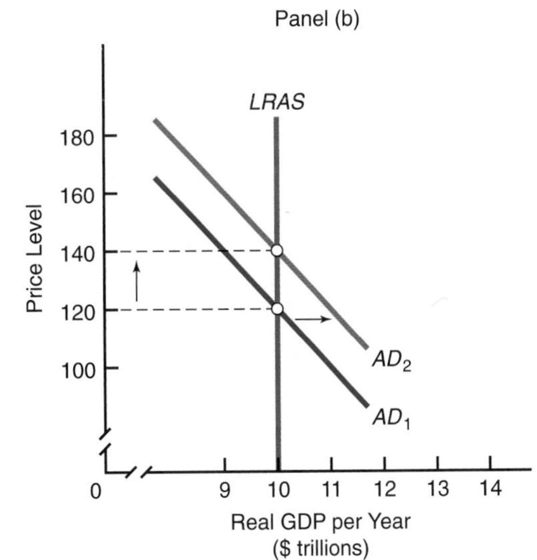

Recall now the factors that would cause the aggregate supply schedule to shift leftward. One might be reductions in labor force participation, induced perhaps by a population decline, higher marginal tax rates on wages, or the provision of government benefits that give households incentives not to supply labor services to firms. Although tax rates and government benefits have definitely increased during recent decades, so has the U.S. population. Nevertheless, the significant overall rise in real GDP that has taken place during the past few decades tells us that population growth and productivity gains have dominated other factors. In fact, the aggregate supply schedule has actually shifted *rightward,* not leftward, over time. Consequently, this supply-side explanation for persistent inflation *cannot* be the true explanation.

Demand-Side Inflation

This leaves only one other explanation for the persistent inflation that the United States has experienced in recent decades. This explanation is depicted in panel (b) of Figure 10-8. If aggregate demand increases for a given level of long-run aggregate supply, the price level must increase. The reason is that at an initial price level such as 120, people desire to purchase more goods and services than firms are willing and able to produce given currently available resources and technology. As a result, the rise in aggregate demand leads only to a general rise in the price level, such as the increase to a value of 140 depicted in the figure.

From a long-run perspective, we are left with only one possibility: Persistent inflation in a growing economy is possible only if the aggregate demand curve shifts rightward over time at a faster pace than rightward progression of the long-run aggregate supply curve. Thus in contrast to the experience of people who lived in the latter portion of the nineteenth century, in which aggregate demand grew too slowly relative to aggregate supply to maintain price stability, your grandparents, parents, and you have lived in times during which

FIGURE 10-9

Economic Growth and Inflation in the United States, 1970 to the Present

This figure shows the points where aggregate demand and aggregate supply have intersected each year from 1970 to the present. The United States has experienced economic growth over this period, but not without inflation.

Sources: Economic Report of the President; Economic Indicators, various issues.

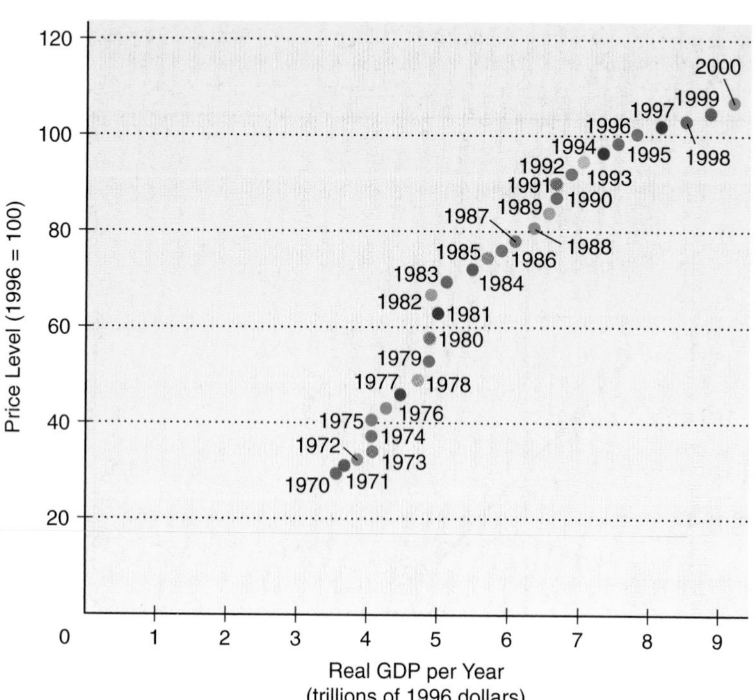

aggregate demand grew too *speedily.* The result has been a continual upward drift in the price level, or long-term inflation.

Take a look at Figure 10-9, which shows that real output has grown in most years since 1970. Apparently, however, the U.S. economy has been unable to experience economic growth without higher prices every single year.

POLICY EXAMPLE

Is There a Simple Explanation for the Price Level's Upward Drift?

As you will learn in more detail in Chapter 17, a group of economists known as *monetarists* have been given this name because they believe that changes in the quantity of money in circulation are the predominant cause of changes in the position of the aggregate demand curve. Consequently, they also believe that changes in the quantity of money are the fundamental determinant of movements in the price level.

Take a look at panel (a) of Figure 10-10. There you can see that two key measures of the price level—the GDP deflator and the Consumer Price Index (CPI)—have persistently drifted upward over recent decades, though at a somewhat reduced pace in recent years. Now look at panel (b) of the figure. This panel plots the Federal Reserve's primary measure of the total quantity of money in circulation, M2, which among other things includes the total amount of currency and coins, checking accounts, and savings accounts in the United States. As you can see, the amount of money circulating in the U.S. economy has also drifted persistently upward in recent decades, although its pace of growth has also tapered off in recent years. To monetarists, the correspondence of these trends is not coincidence. Money growth, they conclude, is the predominant factor explaining the rate of inflation.

For Critical Analysis

If the monetarists are correct, what U.S. policymaker is most responsible for attaining, or failing to attain, stability of the long-run equilibrium price level?

FIGURE 10-10

The GDP Deflator and Consumer Price Index and the Quantity of Money in Circulation

Panel (a) shows that both the GDP deflator and the CPI have risen during recent decades. As indicated in panel (b), so has the quantity of money in circulation.

Sources: Economic Report of the President; Economic Indicators, various issues.

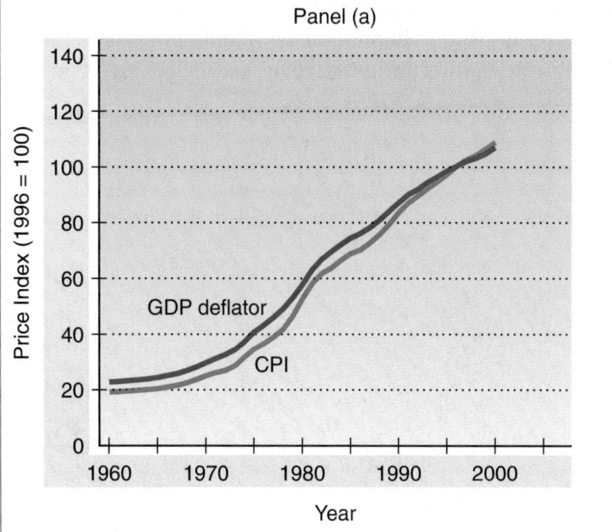

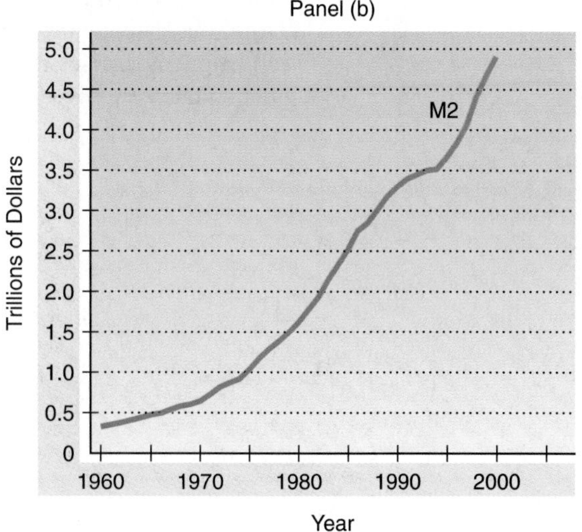

CONCEPTS IN BRIEF

- When the economy is in long-run equilibrium, the price level adjusts to equate total planned real expenditures by individuals, businesses, and the government with total planned production by firms.
- Economic growth causes the long-run aggregate supply schedule to shift rightward over time. If the position of the aggregate demand curve does not change, therefore, the long-run equilibrium price level tends to decline, and there is secular deflation.
- Because the U.S. economy has generally grown in recent decades, the persistent inflation during those years has been caused by the aggregate demand curve shifting rightward at a faster pace than the long-run aggregate supply curve.

NETNOMICS

The "New" Economy, the Long-Run Aggregate Supply Curve, and Inflation

Call it what you may, the Internet economy, the new economy, the network economy, or even the information economy. The most promising technologies today are chiefly due to communications among computers—connections rather than computations. We are currently enhancing and extending the relationships between all businesses and all people.

Sometimes it may seem that economists do not seem to agree about much. Nevertheless, one thing they do agree about is a likely high rate of growth in the portion of GDP marketed and sold on the Internet. The value of electronic-commerce transactions, including those among businesses, grew from almost zero in 1996 to $43 billion, or 0.5 percent of U.S. GDP, in 1998. Current forecasts call for commerce over the Internet to more than double every year and reach as much as $1.3 trillion by 2003, which likely would be more than 10 percent of GDP.

Furthermore, the growth of the Internet has allowed for the creation of more entrepreneurial talent among people whose creative lives have become enmeshed in the Web. Recall from Chapter 2 that entrepreneurship is an important factor of production. If in fact the new economy creates more entrepreneurship, then the long-run aggregate supply curve *(LRAS)* may be moving out to the right faster than previously thought possible. This could well help temper rises in the long-run equilibrium price level and help keep a lid on the inflation rate.

ISSUES & APPLICATIONS

What Is P^*, and Why Should We Care?

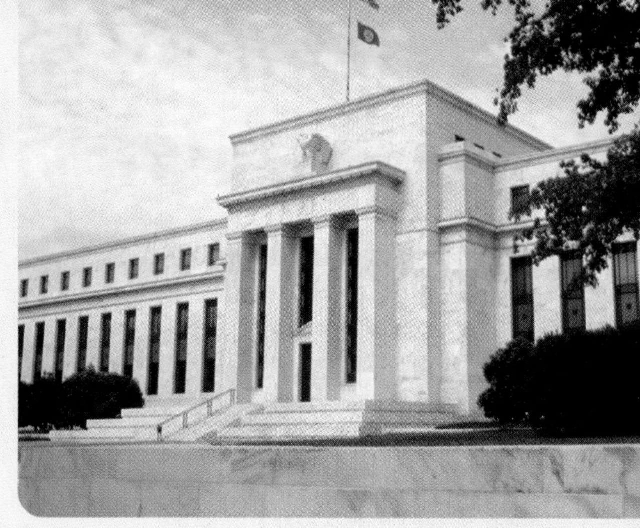

In 1991, the *American Economic Review* published a study by Federal Reserve economists Jeffrey Hallman, Richard Porter, and David Small. This study proposed the so-called P^* model. This was a theory of what the price level ought to be in long-run equilibrium for the U.S. economy. By the time of its formal publication, however, many economists were already well aware of the study, because the *New York Times* and the *Washington Post* had previously published feature articles about the study's "new theory" and its implications for Federal Reserve policymaking.

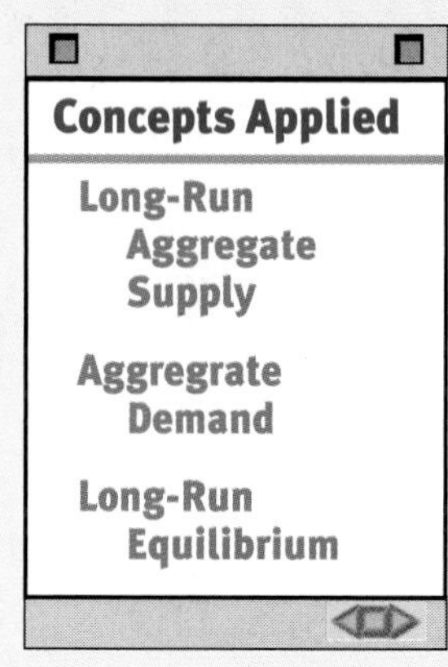

Concepts Applied

Long-Run Aggregate Supply

Aggregrate Demand

Long-Run Equilibrium

There Is Nothing Novel About the Theory of P^*

After the newspaper stories appeared, a few economists poked some good-natured fun at the three Fed economists. On bulletin boards around the country, a mock front-page story purported to be from a well-known "tabloid" (actually computer-generated) appeared. Above second-level headlines shouting that "Elvis Found Alive" and "Boy Shaves Head to Rent as Advertising Space" was a giant headline saying "Three Fed Economists Think of P^* *at the Same Time*!!!" Below the headline was a *New York Times* photo of the three economists that had been spliced into the mock front page.

The reason this was a joke among economists was that the theory of P^* was news to no one with an even rudimentary background in macroeconomics. Indeed, it should not be news to you now that you have nearly completed your study of this chapter. The reason is that P^* is nothing other than the equilibrium price level that emerges in the economy's long-run equilibrium. Poorly informed news reporters had not realized this fact, even though the economists who did the study had probably done their best to make this fact clear in interviews—or perhaps news editors realized that a headline about a new application of an old theory might not attract their readers' attention.

What Is New Is the Fed's Interest

What Hallman, Porter, and Small had successfully accomplished, however, was to refocus economists' attention on thinking about what the price level ought to be in long-run equilibrium. Prior to their study, most economists concentrated on trying to understand short-term movements in the price level. The study highlighted how it might be possible to estimate the price level that ought to emerge in the absence of variations in short-term factors that can often cause the price level to deviate from its long-run equilibrium value. (This is a key subject of Chapter 11.) More important, the Federal Reserve itself seemed narrowly focused on short-term factors as well. Evidence for this was the phenomenon of *base drift,* which is a tendency for the quantity of money in circulation to vary over time without necessarily returning to a level consistent with a single long-run average growth rate.

To see how base drift occurs, consider point *A* in Figure 10-11, where we assume that in the fourth quarter of a given year, Fed announces a desired growth rate for the quantity of money in circulation of no less than 4 percent and no greater than 8 percent. The midrange of these two growth rates is its announced *target* growth rate of 6 percent. During the weeks that follow, however, the Fed permits money growth to drift toward the upper part of its target growth range. Then, at the time indicated by point *B,* Fed officials reaffirm their commitment to the same target growth rate and range of permitted deviations from this target. The

FIGURE 10-11
Base Drift
If the Federal Reserve permits the quantity of money in circulation to drift toward the upper part of its target growth range during one year and then resets its target growth ranges at the beginning of a second year, the result is base drift. This can cause the price level to fail to settle at a single long-run average level.

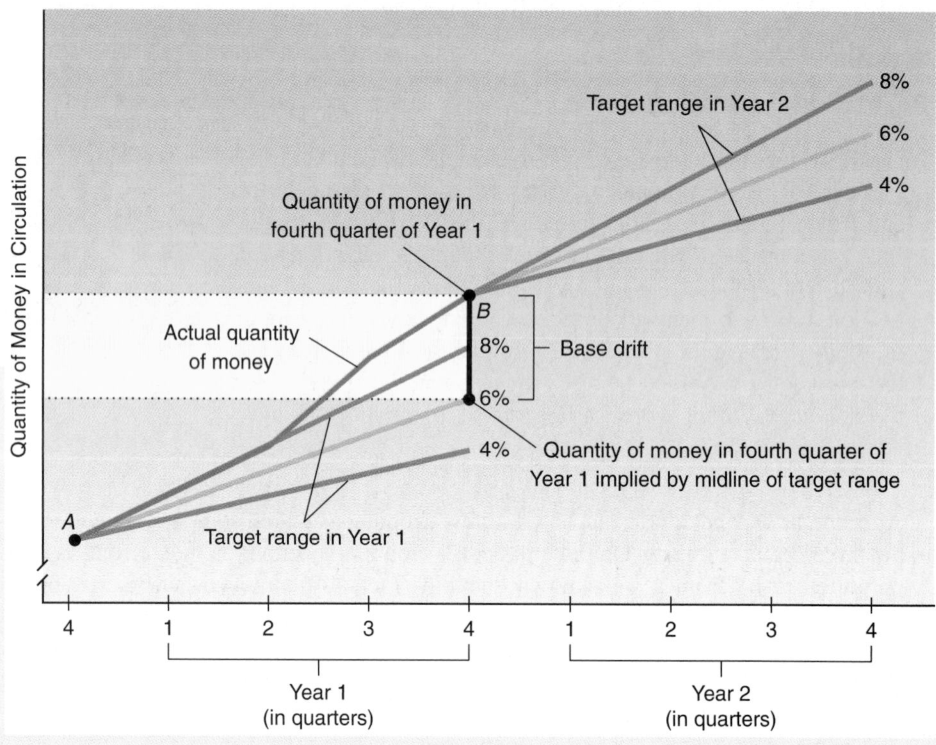

FOR CRITICAL ANALYSIS

1. Why is a stable price level desirable?
2. How might random meanderings of the price level affect creditors and debtors, and under what circumstances might one of these groups be pleased with upward drift of the price level?

result, however, is *upward drift* of the quantity of money. As a result, there is no stable rate of money growth, and the Fed contributes to intermittent outward shifts of the aggregate demand curve.

A result of base drift is that the price level never settles down to a long-run average level. Instead, the price level meanders with no clear long-run trend. Consistent with the general upward drift in the quantity of money in circulation, the general pattern of price level drift has been upward.

Since the Hallman-Porter-Small study, economists have endeavored to determine the best way to estimate the long-run equilibrium price level. The hope is that if a foolproof way of estimating this price level can be determined, it might serve as a guide for monetary policy. This would allow the Fed to ignore short-run movements in the price level and aim directly at a long-run objective of price stability.

SG

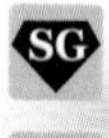

SUMMARY DISCUSSION OF LEARNING OBJECTIVES

1. **Long-Run Aggregate Supply:** The long-run aggregate supply curve is vertical at the amount of real GDP that firms plan to produce when they have full information and when complete adjustment of input prices to any changes in output prices has taken place. This is the full-employment level of real output, or the output level at which the natural rate of unemployment—the sum of frictional and structural unemployment as a percentage of the labor force—arises.

2. **Economic Growth and the Long-Run Aggregate Supply Curve:** Economic growth is an expansion of a country's production possibilities. Thus the production possibilities curve shifts rightward when the economy grows, and so does the nation's long-run aggregate supply curve. In a growing economy, the changes in full-employment output defined by the shifting long-run aggregate supply curve define the nation's long-run, or trend, growth path.
3. **Why the Aggregate Demand Curve Slopes Downward and Factors That Cause It to Shift:** A rise in the price level reduces the real value of cash balances in the hands of the public, which induces people to cut back on spending. This is the real-balance effect. In addition, higher interest rates typically accompany increases in the price level, and this interest rate effect induces people to cut back on borrowing and, consequently, spending. Finally, a rise in the price level at home causes domestic goods to be relatively more expensive relative to foreign goods, so that there is a fall in exports and a rise in imports, both of which cause domestic planned expenditures to fall. These three factors together account for the downward slope of the aggregate demand curve. A shift in the aggregate demand curve results from a change in total planned real expenditures at any given price level and may be caused by a number of factors, including changes in security about jobs and future income, tax changes, variations in the quantity of money in circulation, changes in real interest rates, movements in exchange rates, and changes in economic conditions in other countries.
4. **Long-Run Equilibrium for the Economy:** In a long-run economywide equilibrium, the price level adjusts until total planned real expenditures equal total planned production. Thus the long-run equilibrium price level is determined at the point where the aggregate demand curve intersects the long-run aggregate supply curve. If the price level is below its long-run equilibrium value, total planned real expenditures exceed total planned production, and the level of prices of goods and services tends to rise back toward the long-run equilibrium price level. By contrast, if the price level is above its long-run equilibrium value, total planned production is greater than total planned real expenditures, and the price level declines in the direction of the long-run equilibrium price level.
5. **Why Economic Growth Can Cause Deflation:** If the aggregate demand curve is relatively stable during a period of economic growth, the long-run aggregate supply curve shifts rightward along the aggregate demand curve. The long-run equilibrium price level falls, so there is deflation. Historically, economic growth has in this way generated secular deflation, or relatively long periods of decline prices.
6. **Likely Reasons for Recent Persistent Inflation:** One event that can induce inflation is a decline in long-run aggregate supply, because this causes the long-run aggregate supply curve to shift leftward along the aggregate demand curve. In a growing economy, however, the long-run aggregate supply curve generally shifts rightward. This indicates that a much more likely cause of persistent inflation is a pace of aggregate demand growth that exceeds the pace at which long-run aggregate supply increases.

Key Terms and Concepts

Aggregate demand (229)	Endowments (227)	Open economy effect (232)
Aggregate demand curve (230)	Interest rate effect (232)	Real-balance effect (231)
Aggregate supply (226)	Long-run aggregate supply curve (227)	Secular deflation (235)

Problems Test

Answers to the odd-numbered problems appear at the back of the book.

10-1. Many economists view the natural rate of unemployment as arising when the economy is producing a level of real GDP consistent with the position of its long-run aggregate supply curve. How can there be positive unemployment in this situation?

10-2. Suppose that the long-run aggregate supply curve is positioned at a real GDP level of $12 trillion, and the long-run equilibrium price level (in index number form) is 120. What is the full-employment level of *nominal* GDP?

10-3. Continuing from Problem 10-2, suppose that the full-employment level of *nominal* GDP in the following year rises to $16.8 trillion. The long-run equilibrium price level, however, remains unchanged. By how much (in real dollars) has the long-run aggregate supply curve shifted to the right in the following year?

10-4. The position of a nation's long-run aggregate supply curve has not changed, but its long-run equilibrium price level has increased. Which of the following factors might account for this event?

a. A rise in the value of the domestic currency relative to other world currencies

b. An increase in the quantity of money in circulation

c. An increase in the real interest rate

d. A decrease in taxes

e. A rise in real incomes of countries that are key trading partners of this nation

f. Increased long-run economic growth

10-5. Suppose that there is a sudden rise in the price level. What happens to economywide spending on purchases of goods and services? Why?

10-6. Suppose that the economy is a long-run situation with complete information and speedy adjustment of input prices to changes in the prices of goods and services. If there is a sudden rise in the price level, what happens to economywide production of goods and services?

10-7. Consider the accompanying diagram when answering the questions that follow.

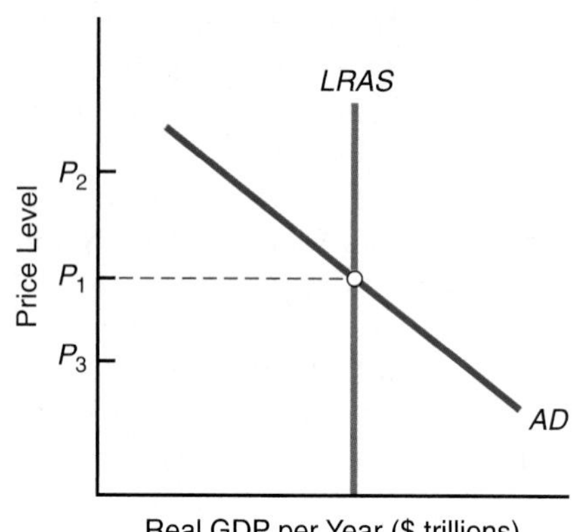

a. Suppose that the current price level is P_2. Explain why the price level will decline toward P_1.

b. Suppose that the current price level is P_3. Explain why the price level will rise toward P_1.

10-8. A country's long-run equilibrium price level has increased, but the position of its aggregate demand schedule has not changed. What has happened? What specific factors might have accounted for this event?

10-9. Most economists argue that the main reason that price level nonstationarity is undesirable is that it is often unpredictable. Explain the rationale behind this argument.

10-10. Is predictable deflation necessarily undesirable? Support your position.

Economics on the Net

Wages, Productivity, and Aggregate Supply How much firms pay their employees and the productivity of those employees influence firms' total planned production, so changes in these factors affect the position of the aggregate supply curve. This application gives you the opportunity to examine recent trends in measures of the overall wages and productivity of workers.

Title: Bureau of Labor Statistics: Economy at a Glance

Navigation: Click here to visit the Bureau of Labor Statistics web site. Then click on Economy at a Glance, then on U.S. Economy at a Glance.

Application Perform the indicated operations, and answer the following questions.

1. Click on the graph box next to Employee Cost Index. What are the recent trends in wages and salaries and

in benefits? In the long run, how should these trends be related to movements in the overall price level?

2. Back up to U.S. Economy at a Glance, and now click on the graph box next to Productivity. How has labor productivity behaved recently? What does this imply for the long-run aggregate supply curve?

3. Back up to U.S. Economy at a Glance, and now click on the graph box next to "Change in Payroll Employment." Does it appear that the U.S. economy is currently in a long-run growth equilibrium?

For Group Study and Analysis

1. Divide the class into aggregate demand and long-run aggregate supply groups. Have each group search the Internet for data on factors that influence their assigned curve. For which factors do data appear to be most readily available? For which factors are data more sparse or more subject to measurement problems?

2. Click on "EAG Home." The opening page of Economy at a Glance displays a map of the United States. Assign regions of the nation to different groups, and have each group develop a short report about current and future prospects for economic growth within its assigned region. In what ways are there similarities across regions? In what ways are there regional differences?

CHAPTER

11

CLASSICAL AND KEYNESIAN MACRO ANALYSES

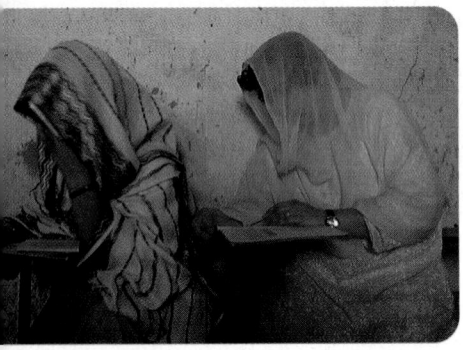

These veiled Afghan women are attending a clandestine school. Afghanistan's Taliban government bars women from working or acquiring a formal education. What is the cost to Afghan society of such restrictions?

In the United States, there are over 135 million people in the measured labor force. Approximately 54 percent are males, and the remaining 46 percent are females. Try to imagine what would happen if Congress passed a law forbidding all females from working outside the home. The active labor force would fall sharply. To be sure, the economy would be much worse off, not to speak of the female members of the labor force. This hypothetical scenario actually happened a few years ago when the Muslim clerics who ruled Afghanistan issued a decree forbidding women to work. To analyze what happened to the labor market and the economy in Afghanistan, you need to understand where the labor market fits into the classical and Keynesian views of macroeconomics.

LEARNING OBJECTIVES

After reading this chapter, you should be able to:

1. Discuss the central assumptions of the classical model
2. Describe the short-run determination of equilibrium real GDP and the price level in the classical model
3. Explain circumstances under which the short-run aggregate supply curve may be either horizontal or upward-sloping
4. Understand what factors cause shifts in the short-run and long-run aggregate supply curves
5. Evaluate the effects of aggregate demand and supply shocks on equilibrium real output in the short run
6. Determine the causes of short-run variations in the inflation rate

Did You Know That... in spite of continuing general inflation, magazine publishers tend to keep the same magazine prices for more than a year? According to one study by economist Stephen G. Cecchetti, the typical magazine publisher lets inflation eat away at a fourth of the magazine's price before a new price is printed on the magazine. This common example of "sticky" prices gives just a hint that our economy may not instantaneously adapt itself to changes in macroeconomic variables such as an increase in the overall price level. Economists want to know what causes fluctuations in employment, output, and the price level. The fact that magazine prices are sticky is just one empirical observation that would lead researchers to develop macroeconomic models that somehow reflect the less flexible nature of certain prices. Such was not the case with the classical economists, who had a different view of how the macroeconomy operated. We will start this chapter with a look at the classical model of the economy and then examine a model developed in the twentieth century.

Chapter Outline 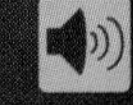

THE CLASSICAL MODEL

The classical model, which traces its origins to the 1770s, was the first systematic attempt to explain the determinants of the price level and the national levels of output, income, employment, consumption, saving, and investment. The term *classical model* was coined by John Maynard Keynes (pronounced "kainz"), a Cambridge University economist, who used the term to refer to the way in which earlier economists had analyzed economic aggregates. Classical economists—Adam Smith, J. B. Say, David Ricardo, John Stuart Mill, Thomas Malthus, A. C. Pigou, and others—wrote from the 1770s to the 1930s. They assumed, among other things, that all wages and prices were flexible and that competitive markets existed throughout the economy.

Say's Law 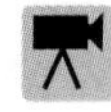

Every time you produce something for which you receive income, you generate the income necessary to make expenditures on other goods and services. That means that an economy producing $10 trillion of GDP (final goods and services) simultaneously produces the income with which these goods and services can be purchased. As an accounting identity, *actual* aggregate output always equals *actual* aggregate income. Classical economists took this accounting identity one step further by arguing that total national supply creates its own national demand. They asserted what has become known as **Say's law:**

> Supply creates its own demand; hence it follows that *desired* expenditures will equal *actual* expenditures.

Say's law 
A dictum of economist J. B. Say that supply creates its own demand; producing goods and services generates the means and the willingness to purchase other goods and services.

What does Say's law really mean? It states that the very process of producing specific goods (supply) is proof that other goods are desired (demand). People produce more goods than they want for their own use only if they seek to trade them for other goods. Someone offers to supply something only because he or she has a demand for something else. The implication of this, according to Say, is that no general glut, or overproduction, is possible in a market economy. From this reasoning, it seems to follow that full employment of labor and other resources would be the normal state of affairs in such an economy.

Say acknowledged that an oversupply of some goods might occur in particular markets. He argued that such surpluses would simply cause prices to fall, thereby decreasing production as the economy adjusted. The opposite would occur in markets in which shortages temporarily appeared.

All this seems reasonable enough in a simple barter economy in which households produce most of the goods they want and trade for the rest. This is shown in Figure 11-1, where there is a simple circular flow. But what about a more sophisticated economy in which people work for others and there is no barter but rather the use of money? Can these complications create the possibility of unemployment? And does the fact that laborers receive money income, some of which can be saved, lead to unemployment? No, said the classical economists to these last two questions. They based their reasoning on a number of key assumptions.

Assumptions of the Classical Model

The classical model makes four major assumptions:

1. *Pure competition exists.* No single buyer or seller of a commodity or an input can affect its price.
2. *Wages and prices are flexible.* The assumption of pure competition leads to the notion that prices, wages, interest rates, and the like are free to move to whatever level supply and demand dictate (as the economy adjusts). Although no *individual* buyer can set a price, the community of buyers or sellers can cause prices to rise or to fall to an equilibrium level.
3. *People are motivated by self-interest.* Businesses want to maximize their profits, and households want to maximize their economic well-being.
4. *People cannot be fooled by money illusion.* Buyers and sellers react to changes in relative prices. That is to say, they do not suffer from **money illusion.** For example, a worker will not be fooled into thinking that he or she is better off by a doubling of wages if the price level has also doubled during the same time period.

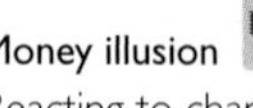

Money illusion

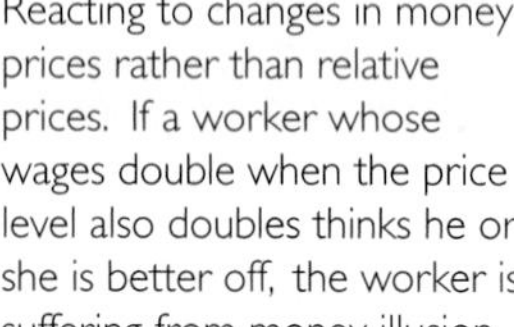

Reacting to changes in money prices rather than relative prices. If a worker whose wages double when the price level also doubles thinks he or she is better off, the worker is suffering from money illusion.

The classical economists concluded, after taking account of the four major assumptions, that the role of government in the economy should be minimal. If all prices and wages are flexible, any problems in the macroeconomy will be temporary. The market will come to the rescue and correct itself.

FIGURE 11-1
Say's Law and the Circular Flow
Here we show the circular flow of income and output. The very act of supplying a certain level of goods and services necessarily equals the level of goods and services demanded, in Say's simplified world.

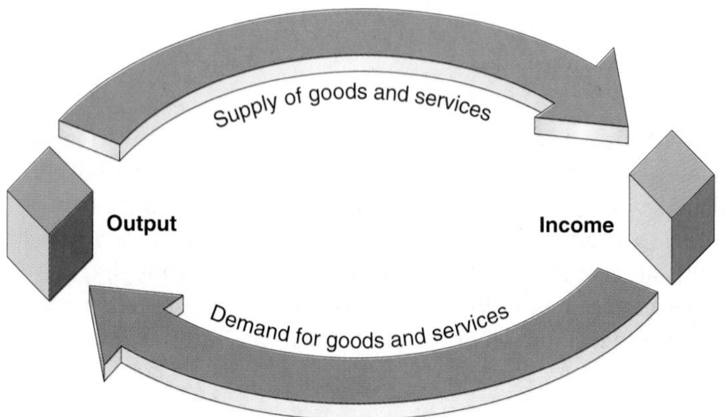

Equilibrium in the Credit Market

When income is saved, it is not reflected in product demand. It is a type of *leakage* from the circular flow of income and output because saving withdraws funds from the income stream. Therefore, consumption expenditures *can* fall short of total current output. In such a situation, it does not appear that supply necessarily creates its own demand.

The classical economists did not believe that the complicating factor of saving in the circular flow model of income and output was a problem. They contended that each dollar saved would be invested by businesses so that the leakage of saving would be matched by the injection of business investment. *Investment* here refers only to additions to the nation's capital stock. The classical economists believed that businesses as a group would intend to invest as much as households wanted to save.

Equilibrium between the saving plans of consumers and the investment plans of businesses comes about, in the classical economists' world, through the working of the credit market. In the credit market, the *price* of credit is the interest rate. At equilibrium, the price of credit—the interest rate—ensures that the amount of credit demanded equals the amount of credit supplied. Planned investment just equals planned saving, so there is no reason to be concerned about the leakage of saving. This is illustrated graphically in Figure 11-2.

Click here to track U.S. interest rates.

In the figure, the vertical axis measures the rate of interest in percentage terms; on the horizontal axis are the amounts of desired saving and desired investment per unit time period. The desired saving curve is really a supply curve of saving. It shows that people wish to save more at higher interest rates than at lower interest rates.

By contrast, the higher the rate of interest, the more expensive it is to invest and the lower the level of desired investment. Thus the desired investment curve slopes downward. In this simplified model, the equilibrium rate of interest is 10 percent, and the equilibrium quantity of saving and investment is $700 billion per year.

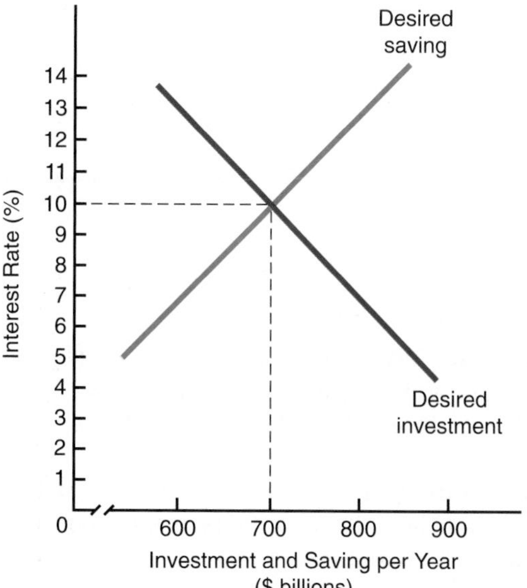

FIGURE 11-2
Equating Desired Saving and Investment in the Classical Model
The schedule showing planned investment is labeled "Desired investment." The supply of resources used for investment occurs when individuals do not consume but save instead. The desired saving curve is shown as an upward-sloping supply curve of saving. The equilibrating force here is, of course, the interest rate. At higher interest rates, people desire to save more. But at higher interest rates, businesses wish to engage in less investment because it is more expensive to invest. In this model, at an interest rate of 10 percent, the planned investment just equals planned saving, which is $700 billion per year.

POLICY EXAMPLE

Personal Saving Rates Are Nearly Zero

At various times in the past few years, the measured personal saving rate has fallen to 1 percent. Imagine what this means in terms of Figure 11-2. Because desired saving and investment are equal in equilibrium, it would seem that investment should be very low also. That hasn't happened, though. Nonetheless, government economists express concern. They argue that U.S. consumers have been borrowing heavily against future income gains.

But perhaps American consumers aren't so spending-crazy after all. Many Americans made large gains in the stock market and other personal investments in the latter part of the 1990s. Not surprisingly, they spent some of those gains. Because capital gains are excluded from U.S. government figures on disposable income, statistically the U.S. personal saving rate looks extemely low, but it really isn't.

In addition, we have not had to worry about funds for investment. For years, foreigners have poured hundreds of billions of dollars into the United States. Also, businesses have retained earnings and reinvested them—to the tune of over $1 trillion per year recently. Finally, governments at the state and federal levels have been running surpluses. Figure 11-3 shows the *gross* saving rate for the past decade. It includes personal, business, and government saving as a percentage of GDP. It has actually gone up since 1992, not down.

For Critical Analysis

Why should government policymakers care how much individuals spend or save?

FIGURE 11-3
Gross Saving and Personal Saving Rates in the United States, 1990–Present

As the U.S. personal saving rate has fallen, the gross saving rate has increased.
Source: U.S. Department of Commerce.

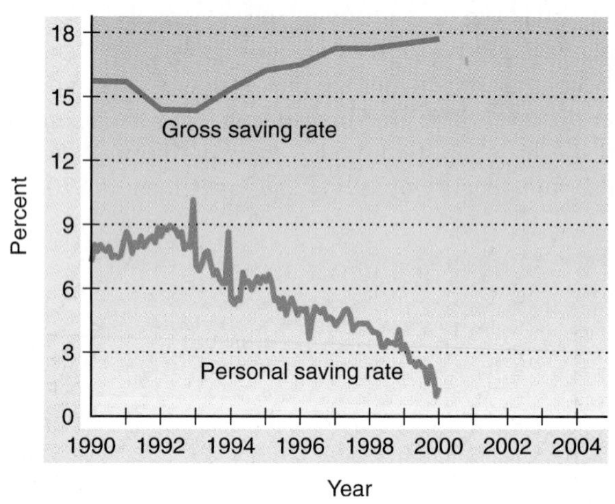

Equilibrium in the Labor Market

Click here to find out the latest U.S. saving rate. Select "Personal saving as a percentage of disposable personal income."

Now consider the labor market. If an excess quantity of labor is supplied at a particular wage level, the wage level must be above equilibrium. By accepting lower wages, unemployed workers will quickly be put back to work. We show equilibrium in the labor market in Figure 11-4.

Assume that full-employment equilibrium exists at $12 per hour and 135 million workers employed. If the wage rate were $14 an hour, there would be unemployment—145 million workers would want to work, but businesses would want to hire only 125 million. In the classical model, this unemployment is eliminated rather rapidly by wage rates dropping back to $12 per hour.

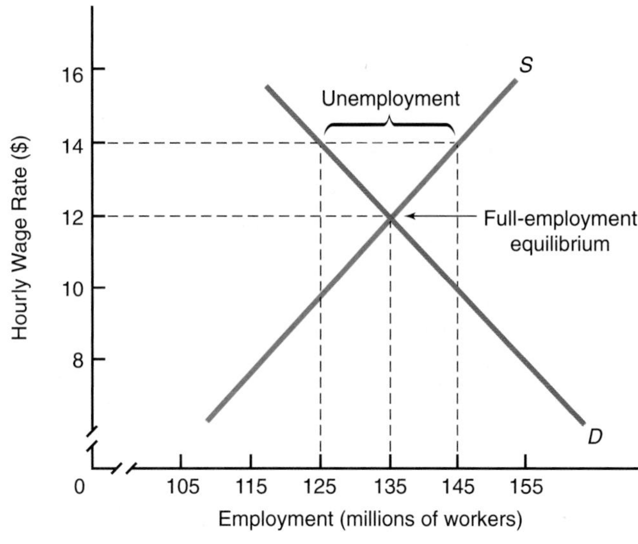

FIGURE 11-4
Equilibrium in the Labor Market
The demand for labor is downward sloping; at higher wage rates, firms will employ fewer workers. The supply of labor is upward sloping; at higher wage rates, more workers will work longer and more people will be willing to work. The equilibrium wage rate is $12 with an equilibrium employment per year of 135 million workers.

The Relationship Between Employment and Real GDP. Employment is not to be regarded simply as some isolated figure that government statisticians estimate. Rather, the level of employment in an economy determines its real GDP (output), other things held constant. A hypothetical relationship between input (number of employees) and output (rate of real GDP per year) is shown in Table 11-1. We have highlighted the row that has 135 million workers per year as the labor input. That might be considered a hypothetical level of full employment, and it is related to a rate of real GDP of $10 trillion per year.

Classical Theory, Vertical Aggregate Supply, and the Price Level

In the classical model, long-term unemployment is impossible. Say's law, coupled with flexible interest rates, prices, and wages, would always tend to keep workers fully employed so that the aggregate supply curve, as shown in Figure 11-5 on page 252, is vertical at Y_0. We have labeled the supply curve *LRAS,* consistent with the long-run aggregate supply curve introduced in Chapter 10. It was defined there as the quantity of output that would be produced in an economy with full information and full adjustment of wages and prices year in and year out. In the classical model, this happens to be the *only* aggregate supply curve that exists. *LRAS* is therefore at the full (natural) rate of unemployment. The classical economists made little distinction between the long run and the short run. Prices adjust so fast that the economy is essentially always on or quickly moving toward *LRAS.*

TABLE 11-1
The Relationship Between Employment and Real GDP

Labor Input per Year (millions of workers)	Real GDP per Year ($ trillions)
98	7
104	8
120	9
135	10
145	11
160	12

FIGURE 11-5

Classical Theory and Increases in Aggregate Demand

The classical theorists believed that Say's law, flexible interest rates, prices, and wages would always lead to full employment at Y_0 along the vertical aggregate supply curve, *LRAS*. With aggregate demand, AD_1, the price level is 100. An increase in aggregate demand shifts AD_1 to AD_2. At price level 100, the quantity of real GDP per year demanded is *A* on AD_2, or Y_1. But this is greater than at full employment. Prices rise, and the economy quickly moves from E_1 to E_2 at the higher price level of 110. It will be at Point *A* for only a very brief interval.

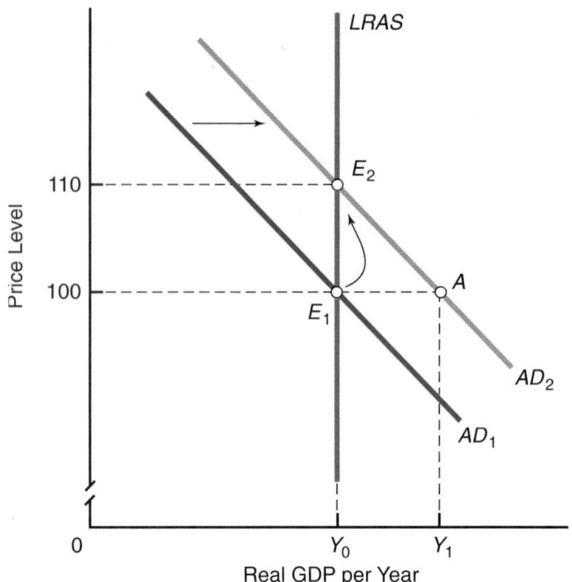

Furthermore, because the labor market adjusts rapidly, Y_0 is always at, or soon to be at, full employment. Full employment does not mean zero unemployment because there is always some frictional and structural unemployment (discussed in Chapter 7), even in the classical world. This is the natural rate of unemployment.

Effect of an Increase in Aggregate Demand in the Classical Model. In this model, any change in aggregate demand will quickly cause a change in the price level. Consider starting at E_1, at price level 100. If aggregate demand shifts to AD_2, the economy will tend toward point *A,* but because this is beyond full employment, prices will rise, and the economy will find itself back on the vertical *LRAS* at point E_2 at a higher price level, 110. The price level will increase as a result of the increase in *AD* because employers will end up bidding up wages for now more relatively scarce workers. In addition, factories will be bidding up the price of other inputs.

The level of real GDP per year clearly does not depend on the level of aggregate demand. Hence we say that in the classical model, the equilibrium level of real GDP per year is completely *supply determined.* Changes in aggregate demand affect only the price level, not the output of real goods and services.

Effect of a Decrease in Aggregate Demand in the Classical Model. The effect of a decrease in aggregate demand in the classical model is the converse of the analysis just presented for an increase in aggregate demand. You can simply reverse AD_2 and AD_1 in Figure 11-5. To help you see how this analysis works, consider the flowchart in Figure 11-6.

FIGURE 11-6

Effect of a Decrease in Aggregate Demand in the Classical Model

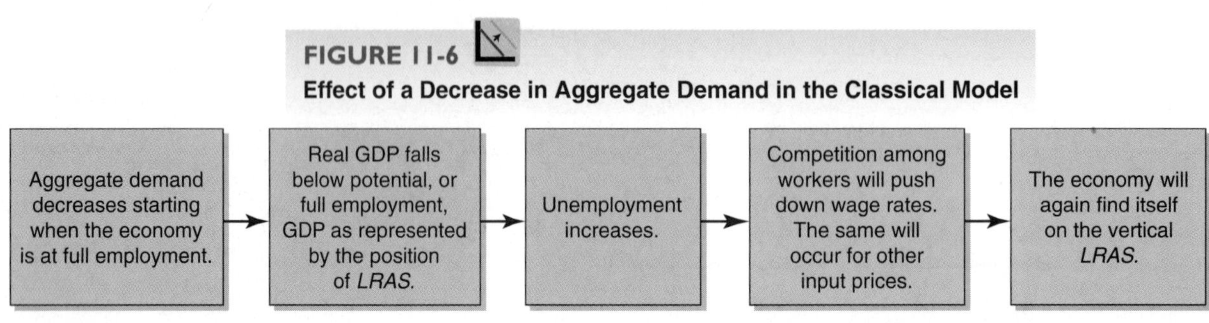

CONCEPTS IN BRIEF

- Say's law states that supply creates its own demand and therefore *desired* expenditures will equal *actual* expenditures.
- The classical model assumes that (1) pure competition exists, (2) wages and prices are completely flexible, (3) individuals are motivated by self-interest, and (4) they cannot be fooled by money illusion.
- When saving is introduced into the model, equilibrium occurs in the credit market through changes in the interest rate such that desired saving equals desired investment at the equilibrium rate of interest.
- In the labor market, full employment occurs at a wage rate at which quantity demanded equals quantity supplied. That particular level of employment is associated with a full-employment value of real GDP per year.
- In the classical model, because the *LRAS* is vertical, the equilibrium level of real GDP is supply determined. Any changes in aggregate demand simply change the price level.

KEYNESIAN ECONOMICS AND THE KEYNESIAN SHORT-RUN AGGREGATE SUPPLY CURVE 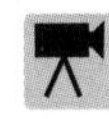

The classical economists' world was one of fully utilized resources. There would be no unused capacity and no unemployment. But then post–World War I Europe entered a period of long-term economic decline that could not be explained by the classical model. John Maynard Keynes developed an explanation that has since become known as the Keynesian model. Keynes and his followers argued that prices, especially the price of labor (wages), were inflexible downward due to the existence of unions and of long-term contracts between businesses and workers. That meant that prices were "sticky." Keynes argued that in such a world, which has large amounts of excess capacity and unemployment, an increase in aggregate demand will not raise the price level, and a decrease in aggregate demand will not cause firms to lower prices. This situation is depicted in Figure 11-7. For simplicity, Figure 11-7 does not show the point where the economy reaches capacity, and that is why *SRAS* never starts to slope upward. Moreover, we don't show *LRAS* in Figure 11-7 either. It would be a vertical line at the level of real GDP per year that is consistent with full employment. The short-run aggregate supply curve is labeled as the horizontal line *SRAS.* If we start out in equilibrium with aggregate demand at AD_1, the equilibrium level of real GDP per year will be Y_1 and the equilibrium price level will be P_0. If there is a rise in aggregate demand, so that the aggregate demand curve

Price Level
P_0
SRAS
AD_3
AD_1
AD_2
Y_3 Y_1 Y_2
Real GDP per Year

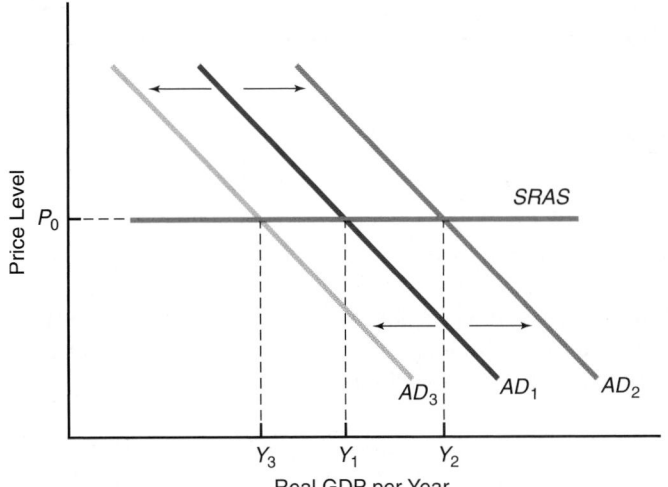

FIGURE 11-7
Demand-Determined Equilibrium Output at Less than Full Employment
Keynes assumed that prices will not fall when aggregate demand falls and that there is excess capacity so that prices will not rise when aggregate demand increases. Thus the short-run aggregate supply curve is simply a horizontal line at the given price level, P_0, represented by *SRAS.* An aggregate demand shock that increases aggregate demand to AD_2 will increase the equilibrium level of real output per year to Y_2. An aggregate demand shock that decreases aggregate demand to AD_3 will decrease the equilibrium level of real output to Y_3. The equilibrium price level will not change.

FIGURE 11-8
Real GDP and the Price Level, 1934–1940
In a depressed economy, increased aggregate spending can increase output without raising prices. This is what Keynes believed, and the data for the United States' recovery from the later years of the Great Depression seem to bear this out. In such circumstances, the level of real output is demand determined.

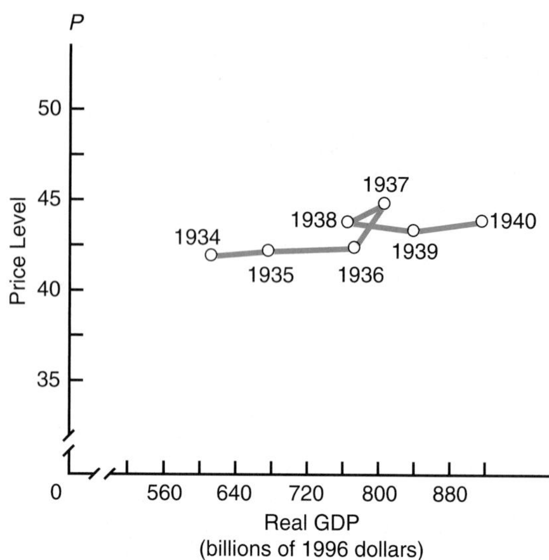

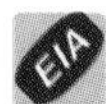

Aggregate Demand
Practice with the aggregate demand curve.

shifts outward to the right to AD_2, the equilibrium price level will not change; only the equilibrium level of real GDP per year will increase, to Y_2. Conversely, if there is a fall in demand that shifts the aggregate demand curve to AD_3, the equilibrium price level will again remain at P_0, but the equilibrium level of real GDP per year will fall to Y_3.

Under such circumstances, the equilibrium level of real GDP per year is completely *demand determined.*

Keynesian short-run aggregate supply curve 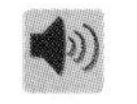
The horizontal portion of the aggregate supply curve in which there is unemployment and unused capacity in the economy.

The horizontal short-run aggregate supply curve represented in Figure 11-7 is often called the **Keynesian short-run aggregate supply curve.** According to Keynes, unions and long-term contracts are real-world factors that explain the inflexibility of *nominal* wage rates. Such stickiness of wages makes *involuntary* unemployment of labor a distinct possibility. The classical assumption of everlasting full employment no longer holds.

A pretty good example of a horizontal short-run aggregate supply curve can be seen by examining data from the aftermath of the Great Depression of the 1930s. Look at Figure 11-8, where you see real GDP in billions of 1996 dollars on the horizontal axis and the price level index on the vertical axis. From the early days of recovery from the Great Depression to the outbreak of World War II, real GDP increased without much rise in the price level. During this period, the economy experienced neither supply constraints nor any dramatic changes in the price level. The most simplified Keynesian model in which prices do not change is essentially an immediate post-Depression model that fits the data very well during this period.

OUTPUT DETERMINATION USING AGGREGATE DEMAND AND AGGREGATE SUPPLY: FIXED VERSUS CHANGING PRICE LEVELS IN THE SHORT RUN

The underlying assumption of the simplified Keynesian model is that the relevant range of the short-run aggregate supply schedule (*SRAS*) is horizontal, as depicted in panel (a) of Figure 11-9. There you will see that short-run aggregate supply is fixed at price level 120. If aggregate demand is AD_1, then the equilibrium level of real GDP is \$9 trillion per year. If aggregate demand increases to AD_2, then the equilibrium level of real GDP increases to \$10 trillion per year.

As discussed in Chapter 10, the price level has clearly drifted upward during recent decades. Hence the assumption of totally sticky prices is an oversimplification. Modern

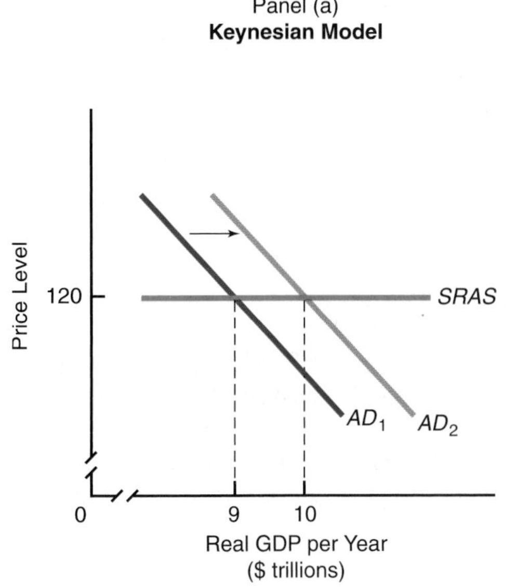

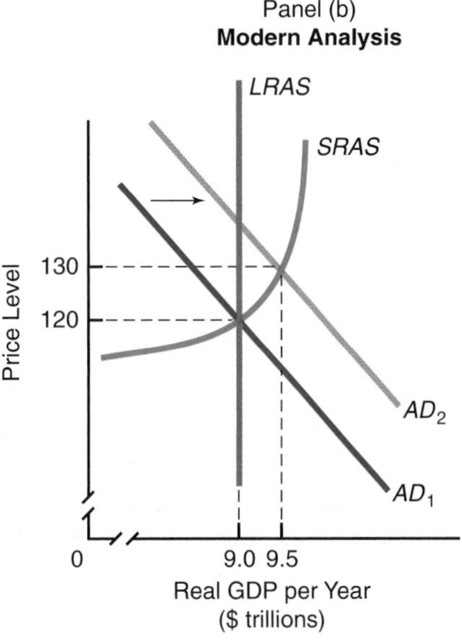

FIGURE 11-9

Income Determination with Fixed Versus Flexible Prices

In panel (a), the price level index is fixed at 120. An increase in aggregate demand from AD_1 to AD_2 moves the equilibrium level of real GDP from $9 trillion per year to $10 trillion per year. In panel (b), *SRAS* is upward-sloping. The same shift in aggregate demand yields an equilibrium level of real GDP of only $9.5 trillion per year and a higher price level index at 130.

Keynesian analysis recognizes that *some*—but not complete—price adjustment takes place in the short run. Panel (b) of Figure 11-9 displays a more general **short-run aggregate supply curve** (*SRAS*). This curve represents the relationship between the price level and real output of goods and services in the economy with incomplete price adjustment and in the absence of complete information in the short run. Allowing for partial price adjustment implies that *SRAS* slopes upward, and its slope is steeper after it crosses long-run aggregate supply, *LRAS*. This is because higher and higher prices of output are required to induce firms to raise their output to levels temporarily exceed full-employment output. With gradual price adjustment in the short run, if aggregate demand is AD_1, then the equilibrium level of real GDP in panel (b) is also $9 trillion per year, also at a price level of 120. A similar increase in aggregate demand to AD_2 as occurred in panel (a) produces a different equilibrium, however. Equilibrium real GDP increases to $9.5 trillion per year, which is less than in panel (a) because part of the increase in *nominal* GDP has occurred through an increase in the price level to 130.

Short-run aggregate supply curve 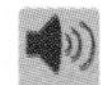
The relationship between aggregate supply and the price level in the short run, all other things held constant. If prices adjust gradually in the short run, the curve is positively sloped.

In the modern Keynesian short run, when the price level rises gradually, output can be expanded beyond the level consistent with its long-run growth path, discussed in Chapter 10, for a variety of reasons:

1. In the short run, most labor contracts implicitly or explicitly call for flexibility in hours of work at the given wage rate. Therefore, firms can use existing workers more intensively in a variety of ways: They can get them to work harder. They can get them to work more hours per day. And they can get them to work more days per week. Workers can also be switched from *uncounted* production, such as maintenance, to *counted* production, which generates counted output. The distinction between counted and uncounted is simply what is measured in the marketplace, particularly by government statisticians and accountants. If a worker cleans a machine, there is no measured output. But if that worker is put on the production line and helps increase the number of units produced each day, measured output will go up. That worker's production has then been counted.
2. Existing capital equipment can be used more intensively. Machines can be worked more hours per day. Some can be made to work at a faster speed. Maintenance can be delayed.

3. Finally, and just as important, if wage rates are held constant, a higher price level means that profits go up, which induces firms to hire more workers. The duration of unemployment falls, and thus the unemployment rate falls. And people who were previously not in the labor force (homemakers and younger or older workers) can be induced to enter.

All these adjustments cause national output to rise as the price level increases.

SHIFTS IN THE AGGREGATE SUPPLY CURVE

Just as there were non-price-level factors that could cause a shift in the aggregate demand curve, there are non-price-level factors that can cause a shift in the aggregate supply curve. The analysis here is not quite so simple as the analysis for the non-price-level determinants for aggregate demand, for here we are dealing with both the short run and the long run—*SRAS* and *LRAS*. Still, anything other than the price level that affects output production will shift aggregate supply curves.

Shifts in Both Short- and Long-Run Aggregate Supply

There is a core class of events that causes a shift in both the short-run aggregate supply curve and the long-run aggregate supply curve. These include any change in our endowments of the factors of production.* Any change in a factor influencing economic growth—labor, capital, or technology—will shift *SRAS and LRAS*. Look at Figure 11-10. Initially, the two curves are $SRAS_1$ and $LRAS_1$. Now consider a big oil discovery in Tennessee in an area where no one thought oil existed. This shifts $LRAS_1$ to $LRAS_2$ at $10.5 trillion of real GDP. $SRAS_1$ also shifts outward horizontally to $SRAS_2$.

FIGURE 11-10
Shifts in Both Short- and Long-Run Aggregate Supply
Initially, the two supply curves are $SRAS_1$ and $LRAS_1$. Now consider a big oil find in Tennessee in an area where no one thought oil existed. This shifts $LRAS_1$ to $LRAS_2$ at $10.5 trillion of real GDP. $SRAS_1$ also shifts outward horizontally to $SRAS_2$.

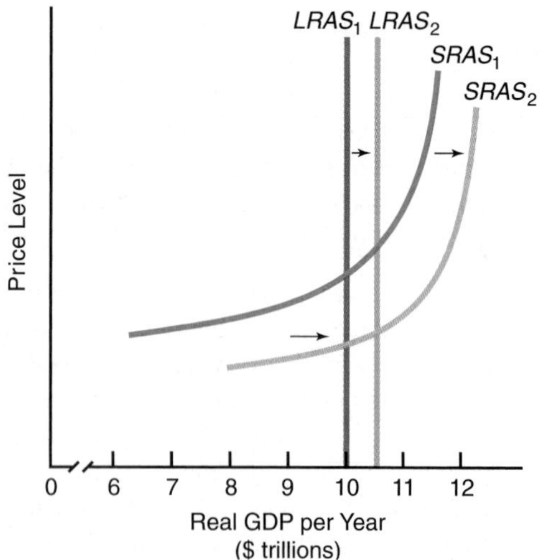

*There is a complication here. A big enough increase in natural resources not only shifts aggregate supply outward but also affects aggregate demand. Aggregate demand is a function of people's wealth, among other things. A big oil discovery in America will make enough people richer that desired total spending will increase. For the sake of simplicity, we ignore this complication.

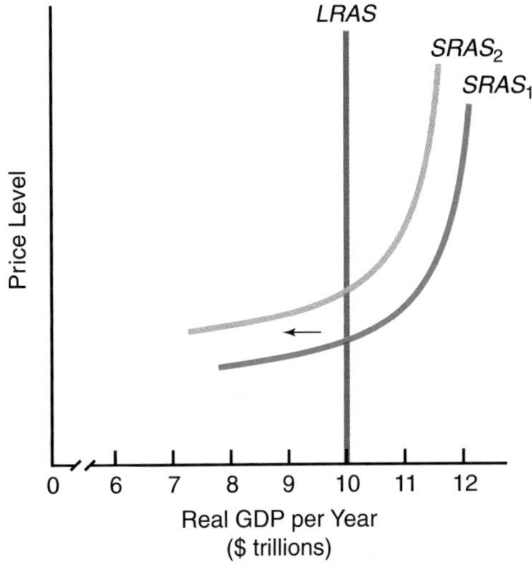

FIGURE 11-11
Shifts in *SRAS* Only
A temporary increase in an input price will shift the short-run aggregate supply curve from $SRAS_1$ to $SRAS_2$.

Shifts in *SRAS* Only

Some events, particularly those that are short-lived, will temporarily shift *SRAS* but not *LRAS*. One of the most obvious is a change in input prices, particularly those caused by external events that are not expected to last forever. Consider the possibility of an announced 90-day embargo of oil from the Middle East to the United States. Oil is an important input in many production activities. The 90-day oil embargo will cause at least a temporary increase in the price of this input. You can see what happens in Figure 11-11. *LRAS* remains fixed, but $SRAS_1$ shifts to $SRAS_2$, reflecting the increase in input prices—the higher price of oil. This is because the rise in the costs of production at each level of real GDP per year requires a higher price level to cover those increased costs.

We summarize the possible determinants of aggregate supply in Table 11-2. These determinants will cause a shift in either the short-run or the long-run aggregate supply curve, or both, depending on whether they are temporary or permanent.

TABLE 11-2
Determinants of Aggregate Supply
The determinants listed here can affect short-run or long-run aggregate supply (or both), depending on whether they are temporary or permanent.

Changes That Cause an Increase in Aggregate Supply	Changes That Cause a Decrease in Aggregate Supply
Discoveries of new raw materials	Depletion of raw materials
Increased competition	Decreased competition
A reduction in international trade barriers	An increase in international trade barriers
Fewer regulatory impediments to business	More regulatory impediments to business
An increase in labor supplied	A decrease in labor supplied
Increased training and education	Decreased training and education
A decrease in marginal tax rates	An increase in marginal tax rates
A reduction in input prices	An increase in input prices

CONCEPTS IN BRIEF

- If we assume that we are operating on a horizontal short-run aggregate supply curve, the equilibrium level of real GDP per year is completely demand determined.

- The horizontal short-run aggregate supply curve has been called the Keynesian short-run aggregate supply curve because Keynes believed that many prices, especially wages, would not be reduced even when aggregate demand decreased.
- The modern Keynesian theory short-run aggregate supply curve, *SRAS,* shows the relationship between the price level and the real output of goods and services in the economy without full adjustment or full information. It is upward sloping because it allows only for partial price adjustment in the short run.
- Output can be expanded in the short run because firms can use existing workers and capital equipment more intensively. Also, in the short run, when input prices are fixed, a higher price level means higher profits, which induces firms to hire more workers.
- Any change in factors influencing long-run output growth, such as labor, capital, or technology, will shift both *SRAS* and *LRAS*. A temporary shift in input prices, however, will shift only *SRAS*.

CONSEQUENCES OF CHANGES IN AGGREGATE SHORT-RUN DEMAND

We now have a basic model to apply when evaluating short-run adjustments of the equilibrium price level and the equilibrium real GDP when there are shocks to the economy. Whenever there is a shift in our economy's curves, the equilibrium price level or real GDP level (or both) may change. These shifts are called **aggregate demand shocks** on the demand side and **aggregate supply shocks** on the supply side.

Aggregate demand shock 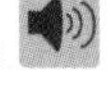
Any shock that causes the aggregate demand curve to shift inward or outward.

Aggregate supply shock 
Any shock that causes the aggregate supply curve to shift inward or outward.

Effects When Aggregate Demand Falls While Aggregate Supply Is Stable

Now we can show what happens in the short run when aggregate supply remains stable but aggregate demand falls. The short-run outcome may be the possible cause of a recession and can under certain circumstances explain a rise in the unemployment rate.

FIGURE 11-12
The Short-Run Effects of Stable Aggregate Supply and a Decrease in Aggregate Demand: The Recessionary Gap
If the economy is at equilibrium at E_1, with price level 120 and real GDP per year of $10 trillion, a shift inward of the aggregate demand curve to AD_2 will lead to a new short-run equilibrium at E_2. The equilibrium price level will fall to 115, and the short-run equilibrium level of real GDP per year will fall to $9.8 trillion. There will be a recessionary gap.

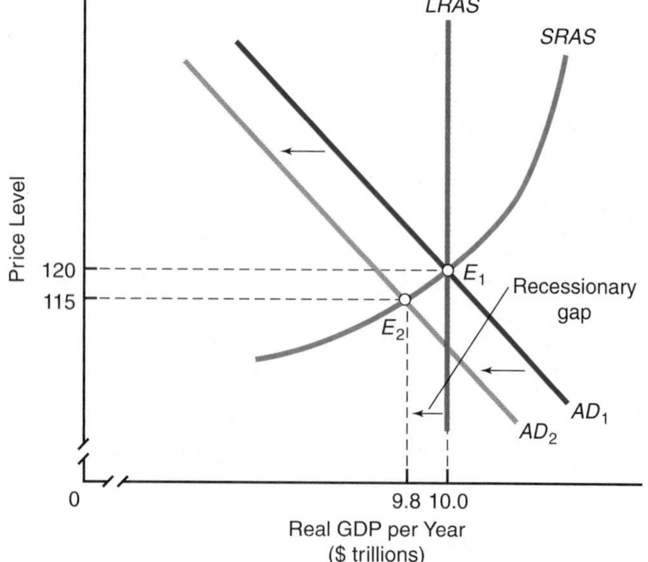

In Figure 11-12, you see that with AD_1, both long-run and short-run equilibrium are at \$10 trillion of real GDP per year (because *SRAS* and *LRAS* also intersect AD_1 at that level of real GDP). The long-run equilibrium price level is 120. A reduction in aggregate demand shifts the aggregate demand curve to AD_2. The new intersection with *SRAS* is at \$9.8 trillion per year, which is below the economy's long-run aggregate supply. The difference between \$10 trillion and \$9.8 trillion is called the **recessionary gap,** which is defined as the difference between the short-run equilibrium level of real GDP and how much the economy could be producing if it were operating at full employment on its *LRAS*.

In effect, at E_2, the economy is in short-run equilibrium at less than full employment. With too many unemployed inputs, input prices will begin to fall. Eventually, *SRAS* will have to shift down. Where will it intersect AD_2?

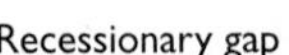

Recessionary gap 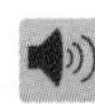
The gap that exists whenever the equilibrium level of real national income per year is less than the full-employment level as shown by the position of the long-run aggregate supply curve.

Inflationary gap 
The gap that exists whenever the equilibrium level of real national income per year is greater than the full-employment level as shown by the position of the long-run aggregate supply curve.

The Short-Run Effects When Aggregate Demand Increases

We can reverse the situation and have aggregate demand increase to AD_2, as is shown in Figure 11-13. The initial equilibrium conditions are exactly the same as in Figure 11-12. The move to AD_2 increases the short-run equilibrium from E_1 to E_2 such that the economy is operating at \$10.2 trillion of real GDP per year, which exceeds *LRAS*. This is a condition of an overheated economy, typically called an **inflationary gap.**

At B_2 in Figure 11-13, the economy is at a short-run equilibrium that is beyond full employment. In the short run, more can be squeezed out of the economy than what occurs in the long run, full-information, full-adjustment situation. Firms would be operating beyond long-run capacity. Inputs would be working too hard. Input prices would begin to rise. That would eventually cause *SRAS* to shift upward. At what point on AD_2 in Figure 11-13 would the new *SRAS* stop shifting?

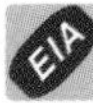

Short-Run Macroeconomic Equilibrium
Practice Thinking about how real GDP and the price level are determined in the short run.

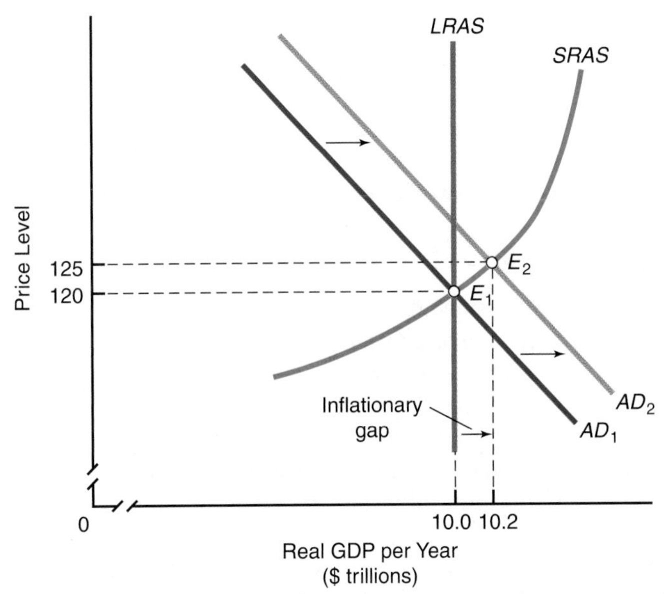

FIGURE 11-13
The Effects of Stable Aggregate Supply with an Increase in Aggregate Demand: The Inflationary Gap
The economy is at equilibrium at E_1. An increase in aggregate demand of AD_2 leads to a new short-run equilibrium at E_2 with the price level rising from 120 to 125 and the equilibrium level of real GDP per year rising from \$10 trillion to \$10.2 trillion. The difference, \$200 billion, is called the inflationary gap.

EXAMPLE

Effects on the Domestic Economy of a Short-Lived Foreign War

One way we can show what happens to the equilibrium price level and the equilibrium real GDP level with an aggregate demand shock is to consider a short-lived war (we actually had one in the Persian Gulf from August 1990 to early 1991). In Figure 11-14 you see the equilibrium price level of 110 and the equilibrium real GDP level of $10 trillion at the long-run aggregate supply curve. The quick war shifts aggregate demand from AD_{prewar} to $AD_{\text{quick war}}$. Equilibrium moves from E_1 to E_2, and the price level moves from 110 to 115. The short-run equilibrium real GDP increases to $10.2 trillion per year. The government's spending for the short-lived war caused *AD* to shift outward to the right. Also notice that the quick war temporarily pushed the economy above its long-run aggregate supply curve.

For Critical Analysis

What would happen if the short-lived war became permanent? How would you show it in Figure 11-14?

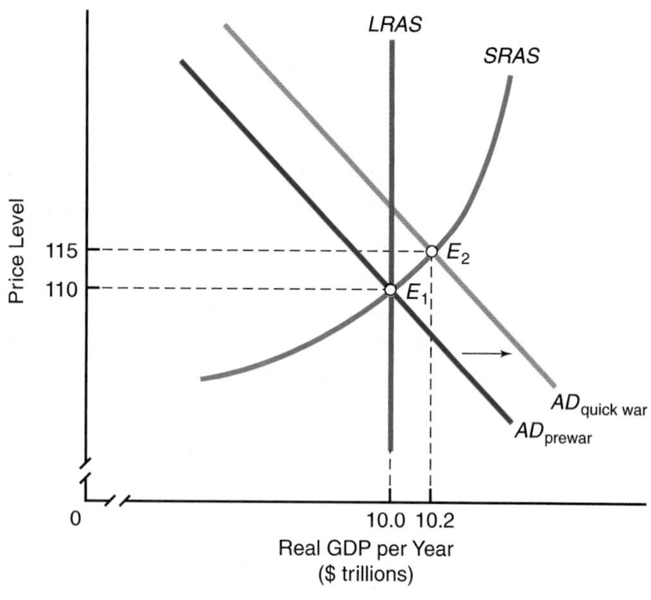

FIGURE 11-14
The Short-Run Effects of a War
A quick war will shift aggregate demand to $AD_{\text{quick war}}$. Equilibrium will move from E_1 to E_2 temporarily.

EXPLAINING SHORT-RUN VARIATIONS IN INFLATION: DEMAND-PULL OR COST-PUSH?

In Chapter 10, we noted that in a growing economy, the explanation for persistent inflation is that aggregate demand rises over time at a faster pace than the full-employment output level. Short-run variations in inflation, however, can arise as a result of both demand *and* supply factors. Figure 11-13 presents a demand-side theory explaining a short-run jump in inflation, sometimes called *demand-pull inflation.* Whenever the general level of prices rises in the short run because of increases in aggregate demand, we say that the economy is experiencing **demand-pull inflation**—inflation caused by increases in aggregate demand.

Demand-pull inflation
Inflation caused by increases in aggregate demand not matched by increases in aggregate supply.

An alternative explanation for near-term increases in the price level comes from the supply side. Look at Figure 11-15. The initial equilibrium conditions are the same as in

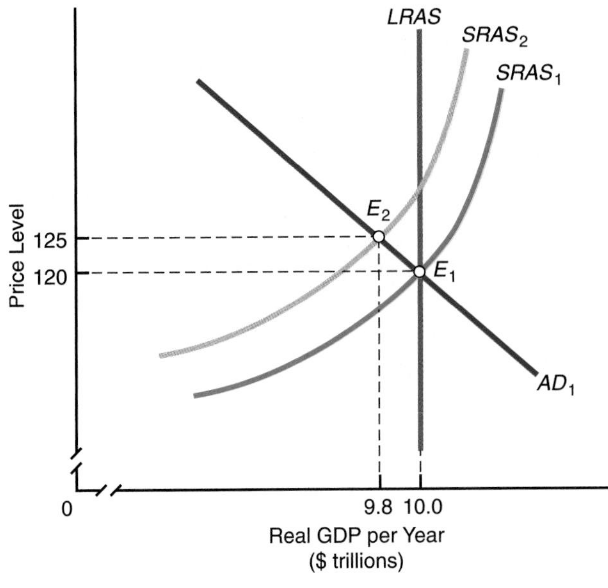

FIGURE 11-15
The Short-Run Effects of Stable Aggregate Demand and a Decrease in Aggregate Supply: Supply-Side Inflation
If aggregate demand remains stable but $SRAS_1$ shifts to $SRAS_2$, equilibrium changes from E_1 to E_2. The price level rises from 120 to 125. If there are continual decreases in aggregate supply of this nature, the situation is called cost-push inflation.

Figures 11-13 and 11-14. Now, however, there is a decrease in the aggregate supply curve, from $SRAS_1$ to $SRAS_2$. Equilibrium shifts from E_1 to E_2. The price level has increased from 120 to 125, too, while the equilibrium level of real GDP per year decreased from $10 trillion to $9.8 trillion. If there are continual decreases in aggregate supply, the situation is called **cost-push inflation.**

Cost-push inflation
Inflation caused by a continually decreasing short-run aggregate supply curve.

As the example of cost-push inflation shows, if the economy is initially in equilibrium on its *LRAS,* a decrease in *SRAS* will lead to a rise in the price level. Thus any abrupt change in one of the factors that determine aggregate supply will alter the equilibrium level of real GDP and the equilibrium price level. If the economy is for some reason operating to the left of its *LRAS,* an increase in *SRAS* will lead to a simultaneous *increase* in the equilibrium level of real GDP per year and a *decrease* in the price level. You should be able to show this in a graph similar to Figure 11-15.

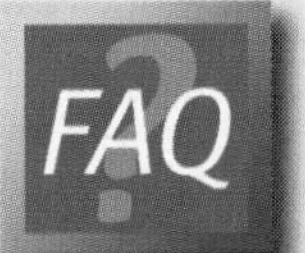

My parents talk about paying only a quarter for a gallon of gas. Why was gas so cheap then?

You have to distinguish between the real and nominal price of a gallon of gas. Even if the nominal price of a gallon of gas in 1999 was around a dollar, or four times what it was in the 1950s, it still was actually cheaper in *real* terms. The price level had increased more than four times since then. At the beginning of the twenty-first, century, the real price of gas was probably the lowest it had ever been in the history of civilization.

EXAMPLE

The Oil Price Shock of the 1970s

One of the best examples of an aggregate supply shock occurred in the 1970s. Several times, the supply of crude oil to the United States was restricted. These restrictions were the result of actions taken by the Organization of Petroleum Exporting Countries (OPEC). The oil embargo had an almost immediate impact on the price of oil and petroleum products, mainly gasoline and heating oil. Higher oil prices raised the cost of production in many U.S. industries that relied on petroleum. The result was a shift in the aggregate supply curve as shown in Figure 11-16. The equilibrium shifted from E_1—\$3 trillion of real GDP per year and a price level of 115—to E_2—equilibrium real GDP of \$2.8 trillion and a price level of 120.

For Critical Analysis

If the price of oil had remained permanently high, what would have happened to *LRAS* in Figure 11-16?

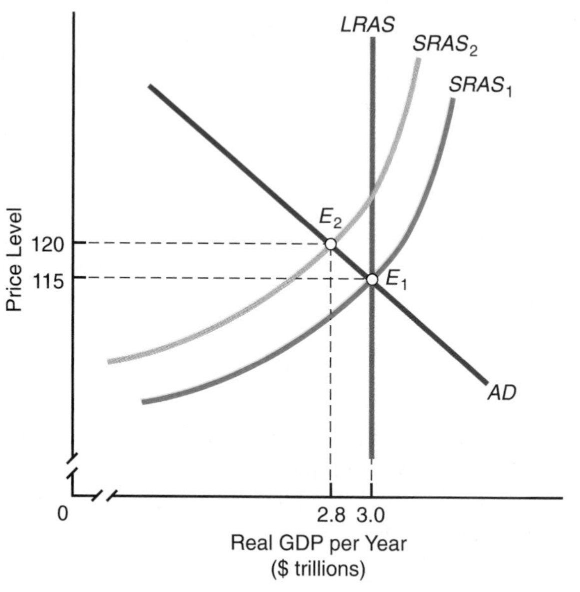

FIGURE 11-16
The Effects of Oil Price Shocks on the Economy
In the 1970s, the supply of crude oil to the United States was restricted. Higher oil prices raised the cost of production. $SRAS_1$ shifted to $SRAS_2$ and equilibrium went from E_1 to E_2 with a higher price level and a lower equilibrium real GDP per year.

AGGREGATE DEMAND AND SUPPLY IN AN OPEN ECONOMY

In many of the international examples in the preceding chapters, we had to translate foreign currencies into dollars when the open economy was discussed. We used the exchange rate, or the price of the dollar relative to other currencies. In Chapter 10, you also discovered that the open economy effect was one of the reasons why the aggregate demand curve slopes downward. When the domestic price level rises, Americans want to buy cheaper-priced foreign goods. The opposite occurs when the American domestic price level falls. Currently, the foreign sector of the American economy constitutes over 12 percent of all economic activities.

How a Stronger Dollar Affects Aggregate Supply

Assume that the dollar becomes stronger in international foreign exchange markets. If last week the dollar could buy 1 euro but this week it now buys 1.25 euros, it has become stronger. To the extent that American companies import raw and partially processed goods from abroad, a stronger dollar can lead to lower input prices. This will lead to a shift outward to the right in the short-run aggregate supply curve as shown in panel (a) of Figure 11-17. In that simplified model, equilibrium GDP would rise and the price level would fall. The result might involve increased employment and lower inflation.

FIGURE 11-17
The Effects of a Stronger Dollar
When the dollar increases in value in the international currency market, lower prices for imported inputs result, causing a shift outward to the right in the short-run aggregate supply schedule from $SRAS_1$ to $SRAS_2$ in panel (a). If nothing else changes, equilibrium shifts from E_1 to E_2 at a lower price level and a higher equilibrium real GDP per year. A stronger dollar can also affect the aggregate demand curve because it will lead to fewer net exports and cause AD_1 to fall to AD_2 in panel (b). Equilibrium would move from E_1 to E_2, a lower price level, and a lower equilibrium real GDP per year.

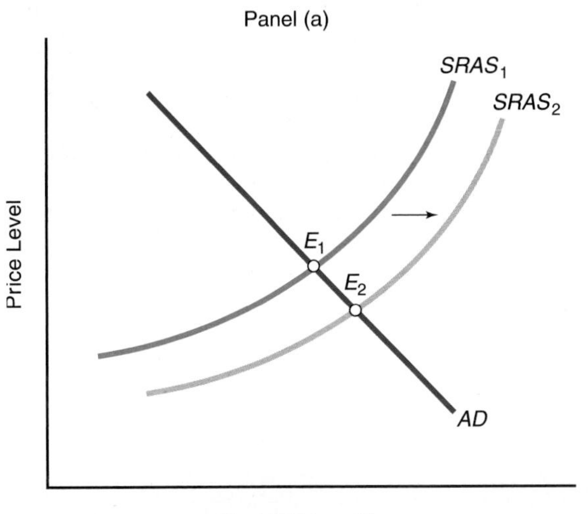

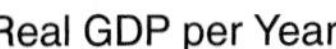

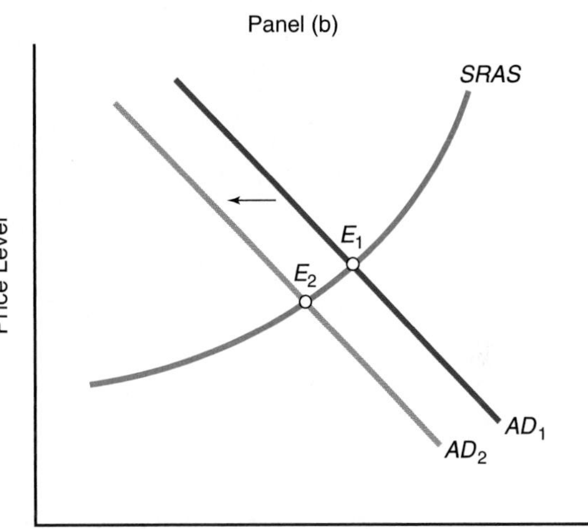

How a Stronger Dollar Affects Aggregate Demand

There is another effect of a stronger dollar that we must consider. Foreigners will find that American goods are now more expensive, expressed in their own currency. After all, a $10 compact disk before the stronger dollar cost a French person 10 euros when the exchange rate was 1 to 1. After the dollar became stronger and the exchange rate increased to 1.25 to 1, that same $10 CD would cost 12.5 euros. Conversely, Americans will find that the stronger dollar makes imported goods cheaper. The result for Americans is fewer exports and more imports, or lower net exports (exports minus imports). If net exports fall, employment in export industries will fall: This is represented in panel (b) of Figure 11-17. After the dollar becomes stronger, the aggregate demand curve shifts inward from AD_1 to AD_2. The result is a tendency for equilibrium real GDP and the price level to fall and for unemployment to rise.

Click here to track how the dollar's value is changing relative to other currencies.

The Net Effect

We have learned, then, that a stronger dollar *simultaneously* leads to an increase in *SRAS* and a decrease in *AD*. Remember from Chapter 4 that in such situations, the effect on real output depends on which curve shifts more. If the aggregate demand curve shifts more than the short-run aggregate supply curve, equilibrium real GDP will fall. Conversely, if the aggregate supply curve shifts more than the aggregate demand curve, equilibrium real GDP will rise.

You should be able to redo this entire analysis for a weaker dollar.

CONCEPTS IN BRIEF

- Short-run equilibrium occurs at the intersection of the aggregate demand curve, *AD*, and the short-run aggregate supply curve, *SRAS*. Long-run equilibrium occurs at the intersection of *AD* and the long-run aggregate supply curve, *LRAS*. Any unanticipated shifts in aggregate demand or supply are called aggregate demand shocks or aggregate supply shocks.
- When aggregate demand shifts while aggregate supply is stable, a recessionary gap can occur, defined as the difference between the equilibrium level of real GDP and how much the economy could be producing if it were operating on its *LRAS*. The reverse situation leads to an inflationary gap.
- With stable aggregate supply, an abrupt shift in *AD* may lead to what is called demand-pull inflation. With a stable aggregate demand, an abrupt shift inward in *SRAS* may lead to what is called cost-push inflation.
- A change in the international value of the dollar can affect both the *SRAS* and aggregate demand. A stronger dollar will reduce the cost of imported inputs, thereby causing the *SRAS* to shift outward to the right, leading to a lower price level and a higher equilibrium real GDP per year, given no change in aggregate demand. In contrast, a stronger dollar will lead to lower net exports, causing the aggregate demand curve to shift inward, leading to a lower price level and a lower equilibrium real GDP per year. The net effect depends on which shift is more important. The opposite analysis applies to a weakening dollar in international currency markets.

NETNOMICS

Are New Information Technologies Making the Short-Run Aggregate Supply Schedule Less Steeply Sloped?

Evidence has been increasing that the short-run aggregate supply curve (*SRAS*) has become less steeply sloped since the early 1990s. Some economists credit widespread deregulation in the 1970s and 1980s with laying the foundation for a more shallowly sloped *SRAS* curve. The increase in domestic and international rivalry among sellers of goods and services, they argue, has made consumers much more sensitive to price differences across products. In equilibrium, therefore, the general level of prices exhibits less change, relative to years past, in response to a given change in output—hence a less steeply sloped *SRAS* curve.

Now continuing developments in information technologies promise to take this trend a step further. For the first time ever, information technologies are the biggest job creators. Depending on whose statistics you look at, such industries are producing between 25 and 40 percent of all new jobs. An information economy is fundamentally different from an industrial economy. Software and databases, for example, can be scaled up to gigantic capacity at little cost. Indeed, because of the ease of communicating data over the Internet, they have unlimited capacity at the very beginning. In other words, capacity as previously defined may be an outdated concept.

Hence beyond the point at which the *SRAS* curve crosses the *LRAS* curve, there will likely be less of a tendency for the *SRAS* curve to bend upward as the United States becomes more of an information economy. Perhaps today's and especially tomorrow's *SRAS* will have to be represented by a curve that is more nearly horizontal.

ISSUES & APPLICATIONS

Banning Women from the Labor Force: Its Effect on Afghanistan's Economy

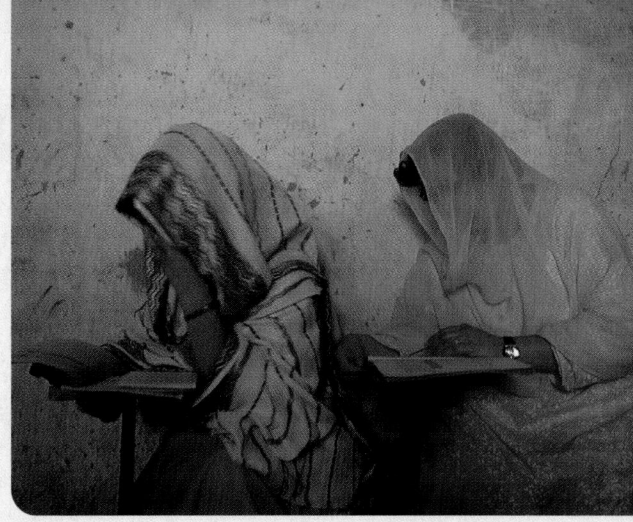

Afghanistan suffered through 18 years of war until the mid-1990s, when the Taliban militia took over and proclaimed a Muslim fundamentalist state. As part of the Muslim principles as interpreted by the ruling clerics, women's activities were severely restricted. Women and girls were forbidden to go to offices and schools. The restriction on gainful employment for women was particularly painful to those who were sole supporters of their families. After 18 years of war, there were many fewer men around to support families.

Concepts Applied

- Labor Force
- Supply and Demand of Labor
- Relationship Between Employment and Real GDP

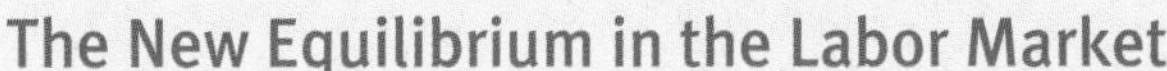

The New Equilibrium in the Labor Market

Let's re-create Figure 11-4 for the Afghan labor market as Figure 11-18. In panel (a) you see the demand curve for labor, *D*, intersecting the former supply curve, *S*, at E_0. Employment in Afghanistan was in equilibrium at 6.6 million workers. The equilibrium wage rate was estimated to be 7,150 afghani, the national currency. (Of course, we are ignoring a very large nonmarket economy in Afghanistan.)

It was estimated that women made up 10 percent of the labor force. So after the ban, the supply curve shifted to S_1 such that total employment was reduced to 5.9 million

FIGURE 11-18

The Effects of Curtailing Female Employment in Afghanistan

Panel (a) shows that forbidding women and girls to be gainfully employed reduces the supply of labor, thereby causing a reduction in equilibrium employment and an increase in the market wage rate. As shown in panel (b), this reduction in productive labor caused the short-run aggregate supply curve to shift upward, causing an increase in the equilibrium price level and a reduction in equilibrium real GDP.

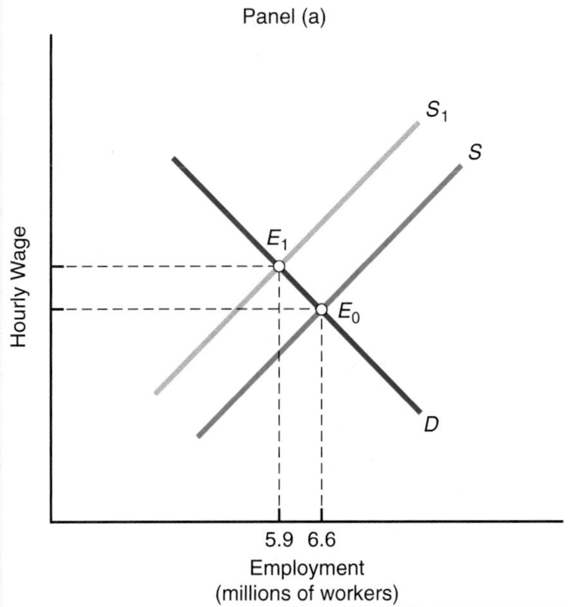

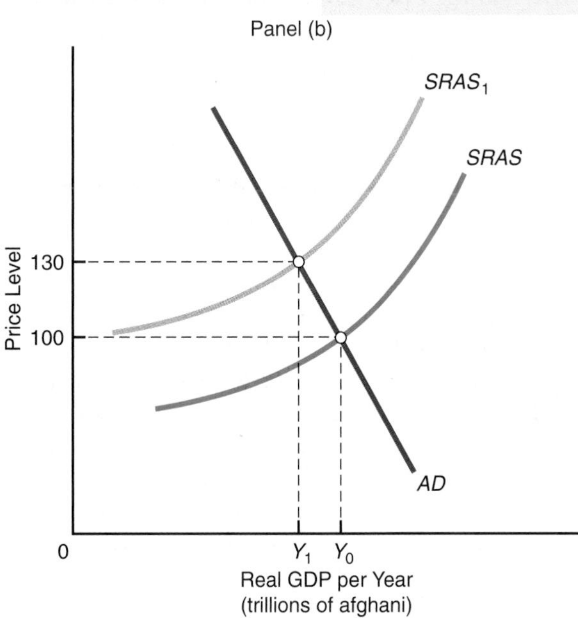

workers. The wage rate of those who continued to work—males—obviously had to go up. Those continuing to work were better off. But the economy as a whole had to have suffered from the ban on female work. Remember the relationship between employment and real GDP in Table 11-1. The smaller the labor input per year, the smaller the resulting real GDP per year.

The Reduction in Equilibrium Real GDP

Look at panel (b). The aggregate demand curve is labeled *AD*. The original short-run aggregate supply curve is labeled *SRAS*. After the ban on female work, Afghanistan had in essence lost a significant part of its productive inputs. The price of the remaining labor input did, of course, rise. The short-run aggregate supply curve shifted upward to $SRAS_1$. Equilibrium real GDP fell from Y_0 to Y_1. The price level rose from 100 to 130.

FOR CRITICAL ANALYSIS

1. How would the analysis change, if at all, if we used a traditional Keynesian horizontal *SRAS* curve?
2. What would happen to the measured unemployment rate in Afghanistan after the ban on female work?

SG

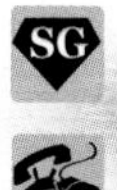

SUMMARY DISCUSSION OF LEARNING OBJECTIVES

1. **Central Assumptions of the Classical Model:** There are four fundamental assumptions of the classical model: (a) Pure competition prevails, so that no individual buyer or seller of a good or service or of a factor of production can affect its price; (b) wages and prices are completely flexible; (c) people are motivated by self-interest; and (d) buyers and sellers do not experience money illusion, meaning that they respond only to changes in relative prices.
2. **Short-Run Determination of Equilibrium Real GDP and the Price Level in the Classical Model:** Under the four assumptions of the classical model, the short-run aggregate supply curve is vertical at the full-employment output level and thus corresponds to the long-run aggregate supply curve. So even in the short run, real GDP cannot increase in the absence of changes in factors, such as labor, capital, and technology, which induce longer-term economic growth. Given the current position of the classical aggregate supply curve, short-run movements in the equilibrium price level are generated by variations in aggregate demand.
3. **Circumstances Under Which the Short-Run Aggregate Supply Curve May Be Horizontal or Upward-Sloping:** If output prices and wages and other input prices are "sticky," perhaps because of the unions or labor contracts, the short-run aggregate supply schedule can be horizontal over much of its range. This is the Keynesian short-run aggregate supply curve. More generally, however, to the extent that there is gradual but incomplete adjustment of prices in the short run, the short-run aggregate supply curve slopes upward.
4. **Factors That Induce Shifts in the Short-Run and Long-Run Aggregate Supply Curves:** The long-run aggregate supply curve shifts in response to changes in the availability of labor or capital or to changes in technology and productivity, and changes in these factors also cause the short-run aggregate supply curve to shift. Because output prices may adjust only partially to changing input prices in the short run, however, a widespread change in the prices of factors of production, such as an economy-wide change in wages, can cause a shift in the short-run aggregate supply curve without affecting the long-run aggregate supply curve.
5. **Effects of Aggregate Demand and Supply Shocks on Equilibrium Real Output in the Short Run:** An aggregate demand shock that causes the aggregate demand curve to shift leftward pushes equilibrium real output below the full-employment output level in the short run, so that there is a recessionary gap. An aggregate demand shock that induces a rightward shift in the aggregate demand curve results in an inflationary gap in which the short-run equilibrium level of real GDP exceeds the full-employment GDP level.
6. **Causes of Short-Run Variations in the Inflation Rate:** In the short run, an upward movement in the

price level can occur in the form of demand-pull inflation when the aggregate demand curve shifts rightward along an upward-sloping short-run aggregate supply curve. Cost-push inflation can arise in the short run when the short-run aggregate supply curve shifts leftward along the aggregate demand curve.

Key Terms and Concepts

Aggregate demand shock (258)
Aggregate supply shock (258)
Cost-push inflation (261)
Demand-pull inflation (260)
Inflationary gap (259)
Keynesian short-run aggregate supply curve (254)
Money illusion (248)
Recessionary gap (259)
Say's law (247)
Short-run aggregate supply curve (255)

Problems

Answers to the odd-numbered problems appear at the back of the book.

11-1. Consider a country whose economic structure matches the assumptions of the classical model. After reading a recent best-seller documenting a growing population of low-income elderly people who were ill-prepared for retirement, most residents of this country decide to increase their saving at any given interest rate. Explain whether or how this could affect the following:

a. The current equilibrium interest rate
b. Current equilibrium national output
c. Current equilibrium employment
d. Current equilibrium investment
e. Future equilibrium national output

11-2. "There is *absolutely no distinction* between the classical model and the model of long-run equilibrium discussed in Chapter 10." Is this statement true or false? Support your answer.

11-3. A nation in which the classical model applies experiences a decline in the quantity of money in circulation. Use an appropriate aggregate demand and aggregate supply diagram to explain what happens to equilibrium output and to the equilibrium price level.

11-4. The classical model is appropriate for a country that has suddenly experienced an influx of immigrants who possess a wide variety of employable skills and who have reputations for saving relatively large portions of their incomes, as compared with native-born residents, at any given interest rate. Evaluate the effects of this event on the following:

a. Current equilibrium employment
b. Current equilibrium national output
c. The current equilibrium interest rate
d. Current equilibrium investment
e. Future equilibrium national output

11-5. Suppose that the Keynesian short-run aggregate supply curve is applicable for a nation's economy. Use appropriate diagrams to assist in answering the following questions:

a. What are two factors that can cause the nation's real GDP to increase in the short run?
b. What are two factors that can cause the nation's real GDP to increase in the long run?

11-6. What determines how steeply the short-run aggregate supply curve is sloped?

11-7. At a point along the short-run aggregate supply curve that is to the right of the point where it crosses the long-run aggregate supply curve, what must be true of the unemployment rate relative to the natural rate of unemployment? Why?

11-8. The stock market crashes in an economy with an upward-sloping short-run aggregate supply curve, and consumer and business confidence plummets. What are the short-run effects on equilibrium real GDP and the equilibrium price level?

11-9. Consider an open economy in which the aggregate supply curve slopes upward in the short run and businesses buy a large portion of their nonhuman factors of production from abroad. In contrast, consumers import few foreign-made goods, and foreign residents purchase few domestically produced goods. What is the most likely short-run effect on this nation's economy if the value of its currency weakens sharply and for a prolonged period in foreign exchange markets?

11-10. Consider an open economy in which the aggregate supply curve slopes upward in the short run. Firms in this nation do not import raw materials or any other productive inputs from abroad, but foreign residents purchase many of the nation's export goods. What is the most likely short-run effect on this nation's economy if there is a significant downturn in economic activity in other nations around the world?

Economics on the Net

Money, the Price Level, and Real GDP The classical and Keynesian theories have differing predictions about how changes in the quantity of money in circulation should affect the equilibrium price level and equilibrium real GDP. Here you get a chance to take your own look at the data on growth in the money supply, the price level, and real GDP in the United States.

Title: Federal Reserve Bank of St. Louis Monetary Trends

Navigation: Click here to visit the Federal Reserve Bank of St. Louis. Click on Gross Domestic Product and M2.

Application Read the article; then answer the questions that follow.

1. Classical theory indicates that, *ceteris paribus*, changes in the price level should be closely related to changes in aggregate demand induced by variations in the quantity of money. Take a look at the charts showing "Gross Domestic Product Price Index" and "M2." Are annual percentage changes in these variables closely related?

2. Keynesian theory predicts that, *ceteris paribus*, changes in GDP and the quantity of money should be directly related. Take a look at the charts showing "Real Gross Domestic Product" and "M2." Are annual percentage changes in these variables closely related?

For Group Study and Analysis Both classical and Keynesian theories of relationships among real GDP, the price level, and the quantity of money hinge on specific assumptions. Have class groups search through the FRED database to evaluate factors that provide support for either theory's predictions. Which approach appears to receive greater support from recent data? Does this necessarily imply that this is the "true theory"? Why or why not?

CHAPTER 12

CONSUMPTION, INCOME, AND THE MULTIPLIER

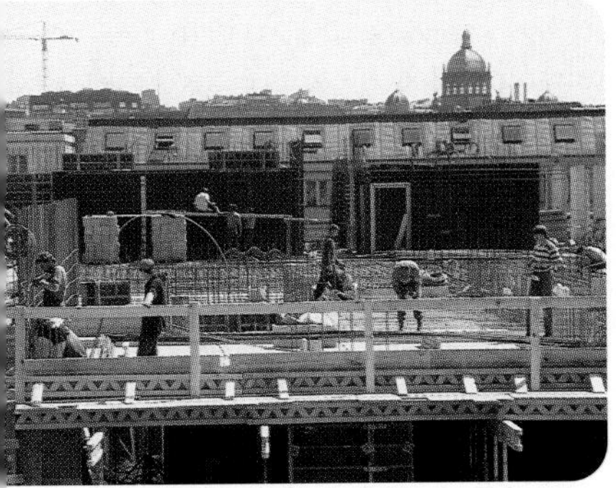

Some countries are allocating a much larger percentage of GDP to net investment. The Czech Republic is one of them. Should the U.S. be worried about being "overtaken" by those countries that are investing so much?

During the 1990s and the early 2000s, the United States allocated about 17 percent of its GDP to net investment. This compares with an average of more than 20 percent in Western Europe and approximately 30 percent in Japan. Some commentators in the media have speculated that the lower measured investment rate in the United States will ultimately threaten the nation's long-term growth. A few go even further, arguing that because a relatively low investment rate depresses total spending, it serves as a drag on *current* U.S. output. How do changes in net investment spending affect economic activity? Is the U.S. investment rate really lagging so far behind the rest of the world? Studying this chapter will help you contemplate these and other questions about how total expenditures affect equilibrium U.S. national income.

LEARNING OBJECTIVES

After reading this chapter, you should be able to:

1. Distinguish between saving and savings and explain how saving and consumption are related
2. Explain the key determinants of consumption and saving in the Keynesian model
3. Identify the primary determinants of planned investment
4. Describe how equilibrium national income is established in the Keynesian model
5. Evaluate why autonomous changes in total planned expenditures have a multiplier effect on equilibrium national income
6. Understand the relationship between total planned expenditures and the aggregate demand curve

Chapter Outline

Did You Know That... personal consumption expenditures in the United States have averaged about two-thirds of gross domestic product for decades? Each year, Americans purchase millions of television sets, millions of pairs of shoes, millions of compact disks, and billions of stress-reducing pills, among other products and services. We are a nation of spenders, and our personal consumption expenditures keep the American economic machine moving day in and day out. As it turns out, John Maynard Keynes focused much of his research on what determines how much you and I decide to spend each year. Remember that total planned expenditures consist of consumption expenditures, plus expenditures for investment purposes, what the government spends, and what foreigners spend on domestically produced output, less what U.S. residents spend on foreign goods and services. Keynes focused on the relationship between how much people earn and their willingness to engage in personal consumption expenditures. In this chapter, you will learn about that relationship as well as the influence of investment, government, and the foreign sector on the economy's equilibrium level of real GDP—the values of both income and output in the circular flow—per year.

SOME SIMPLIFYING ASSUMPTIONS IN A KEYNESIAN MODEL

Continuing in the Keynesian tradition, we will assume that the short-run aggregate supply curve within the current range of real GDP is horizontal. That is to say, we assume that it is similar to Figure 11-7 on page 253, meaning that the equilibrium level of real GDP is demand determined. That is why Keynes wished to examine the elements of desired aggregate expenditures. Because of the Keynesian assumption of inflexible prices, inflation is not a concern. Hence real values are identical to nominal values.

To simplify the income determination model that follows, a number of assumptions are made:

1. Businesses pay no indirect taxes (for example, sales taxes).
2. Businesses distribute all of their profits to shareholders.
3. There is no depreciation (capital consumption allowance), so gross private domestic investment equals net investment.
4. The economy is closed—that is, there is no foreign trade.

Given all these simplifying assumptions, real disposable income will be equal to real national income minus taxes.*

Another Look at Definitions and Relationships

You can do only two things with a dollar of disposable income: consume it or save it. If you consume it, it is gone forever. If you save the entire dollar, however, you will be able to

*Strictly speaking, we are referring here to net taxes—the difference between taxes paid and transfer payments received. If taxes are $1 trillion but individuals receive transfer payments—Social Security, unemployment benefits, and so forth—of $300 billion, net taxes are equal to $700 billion.

consume it (and perhaps more if it earns interest) at some future time. That is the distinction between **consumption** and **saving.** Consumption is the act of using income for the purchase of consumption goods. **Consumption goods** are goods purchased by households for immediate satisfaction. Consumption goods are such things as food, clothing, and movies. By definition, whatever you do not consume you save and can consume at some time in the future.

Consumption 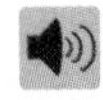
Spending on new goods and services out of a household's current income. Whatever is not consumed is saved. Consumption includes such things as buying food and going to a concert.

Stocks and Flows: The Difference Between Saving and Savings. It is important to distinguish between *saving* and *savings. Saving* is an action that occurs at a particular rate—for example, $10 a week or $520 a year. This rate is a flow. It is expressed per unit of time, usually a year. Implicitly, then, when we talk about saving, we talk about a *flow* or rate of saving. *Savings,* by contrast, is a *stock* concept, measured at a certain point or instant in time. Your current *savings* are the result of past *saving.* You may presently have *savings* of $2,000 that are the result of four years' *saving* at a rate of $500 per year. Consumption is also a flow concept. You consume from after-tax income at a certain rate per week, per month, or per year.

Saving 
The act of not consuming all of one's current income. Whatever is not consumed out of spendable income is, by definition, saved. *Saving* is an action measured over time (a flow), whereas *savings* are a stock, an accumulation resulting from the act of saving in the past.

Relating Income to Saving and Consumption. Obviously, a dollar of take-home income can be either consumed or not consumed. Realizing this, we can see the relationship among saving, consumption, and disposable income:

$$\text{Consumption} + \text{saving} \equiv \text{disposable income}$$

Consumption goods 
Goods bought by households to use up, such as food, clothing, and movies.

This is called an *accounting identity.* It has to hold true at every moment in time. From it we can derive the definition of saving:

$$\text{Saving} \equiv \text{disposable income} - \text{consumption}$$

Recall that disposable income is what you actually have left to spend after you pay taxes.

Investment 
Spending by businesses on things such as machines and buildings, which can be used to produce goods and services in the future. The investment part of total output is the portion that will be used in the process of producing goods in the future.

Investment

Investment is also a flow concept. As noted earlier, *investment* as used in economics differs from the common use of the term. In common speech, it is often used to describe putting money into the stock market or real estate. In economic analysis, investment is defined as expenditures by firms on new machines and buildings—**capital goods**—that are expected to yield a future stream of income. This is called *fixed investment.* We also include changes in business inventories in our definition. This we call *inventory investment.*

Capital goods 
Producer durables; nonconsumable goods that firms use to make other goods.

CONCEPTS IN BRIEF

- If we assume that we are operating on a horizontal short-run aggregate supply curve, the equilibrium level of real GDP per year is completely demand determined.
- *Saving* is a flow, something that occurs over time. It equals disposable income minus consumption. *Savings* are a stock. They are the accumulation resulting from saving.
- Investment is also a flow. It includes expenditures on new machines, buildings, and equipment and changes in business inventories.

DETERMINANTS OF PLANNED CONSUMPTION AND PLANNED SAVING

In the classical model, the supply of saving was determined by the rate of interest: The higher the rate of interest, the more people wanted to save and therefore the less people wanted to consume. According to Keynes, the interest rate is not the most important determinant of an individual's saving and consumption decisions.

> Keynes argued that saving and consumption decisions depend primarily on an individual's current real disposable income.

Consumption function 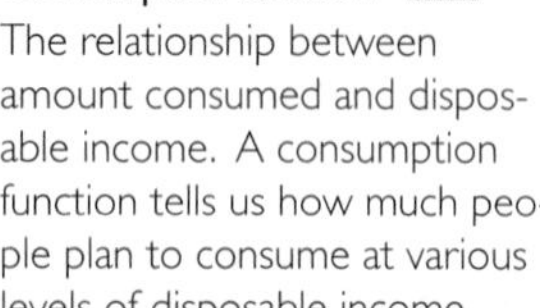
The relationship between amount consumed and disposable income. A consumption function tells us how much people plan to consume at various levels of disposable income.

Dissaving 
Negative saving; a situation in which spending exceeds income. Dissaving can occur when a household is able to borrow or use up existing assets.

The relationship between planned consumption expenditures of households and their current level of real disposable income has been called the **consumption function.** It shows how much all households plan to consume per year at each level of real disposable income per year. The first two columns of Table 12-1 illustrate a consumption function for a hypothetical household.

We see from Table 12-1 that as real disposable income rises, planned consumption also rises, but by a smaller amount, as Keynes suggested. Planned saving also increases with disposable income. Notice, however, that below an income of $10,000, the planned saving of this hypothetical family is actually negative. The further that income drops below that level, the more the family engages in **dissaving,** either by going into debt or by using up some of its existing wealth.

TABLE 12-1
Real Consumption and Saving Schedules: A Hypothetical Case

Column 1 presents real disposable income from zero up to $20,000 per year; column 2 indicates planned consumption per year; column 3 presents planned saving per year. At levels of disposable income below $10,000, planned saving is negative. In column 4, we see the average propensity to consume, which is merely planned consumption divided by disposable income. Column 5 lists average propensity to save, which is planned saving divided by disposable income. Column 6 is the marginal propensity to consume, which shows the proportion of *additional* income that will be consumed. Finally, column 7 shows the proportion of *additional* income that will be saved, or the marginal propensity to save.

Combination	(1) Real Disposable Income per Year (Y_d)	(2) Planned Real Consumption per Year (C)	(3) Planned Real Saving Per Year ($S \equiv Y_d - C$) (1) − (2)	(4) Average Propensity to Consume (APC $\equiv C/Y_d$) (2) ÷ (1)	(5) Average Propensity to Save (APS $\equiv S/Y_d$) (3) ÷ (1)	(6) Marginal Propensity to Consume (MPC $\equiv \Delta C/\Delta Y_d$)	(7) Marginal Propensity to Save (MPS $\equiv \Delta S/\Delta Y_d$)
A	$ 0	$ 2,000	$−2,000	—	—	—	—
B	2,000	3,600	−1,600	1.8	−.8	.8	.2
C	4,000	5,200	−1,200	1.3	−.3	.8	.2
D	6,000	6,800	− 800	1.133	−.133	.8	.2
E	8,000	8,400	− 400	1.05	−.05	.8	.2
F	10,000	10,000	0	1.0	.0	.8	.2
G	12,000	11,600	400	.967	.033	.8	.2
H	14,000	13,200	800	.943	.057	.8	.2
I	16,000	14,800	1,200	.925	.075	.8	.2
J	18,000	16,400	1,600	.911	.089	.8	.2
K	20,000	18,000	2,000	.9	.1	.8	.2

Graphing the Numbers

We now graph the consumption and saving relationships presented in Table 12-1. In the upper part of Figure 12-1, the vertical axis measures the level of planned real consumption per year, and the horizontal axis measures the level of real disposable income per year. In the lower part of the figure, the horizontal axis is again real disposable income per year, but now the vertical axis is planned real saving per year. All of these are on a dollars-per-year basis, which emphasizes the point that we are measuring flows, not stocks.

As you can see, we have taken income-consumption and income-saving combinations *A* through *K* and plotted them. In the upper part of Figure 12-1, the result is called the *consumption function.* In the lower part, the result is called the *saving function.* Mathematically, the saving function is the *complement* of the consumption function because consumption plus saving always equals disposable income. What is not consumed is, by definition, saved. The difference between actual disposable income and the planned rate of consumption per year *must* be the planned rate of saving per year.

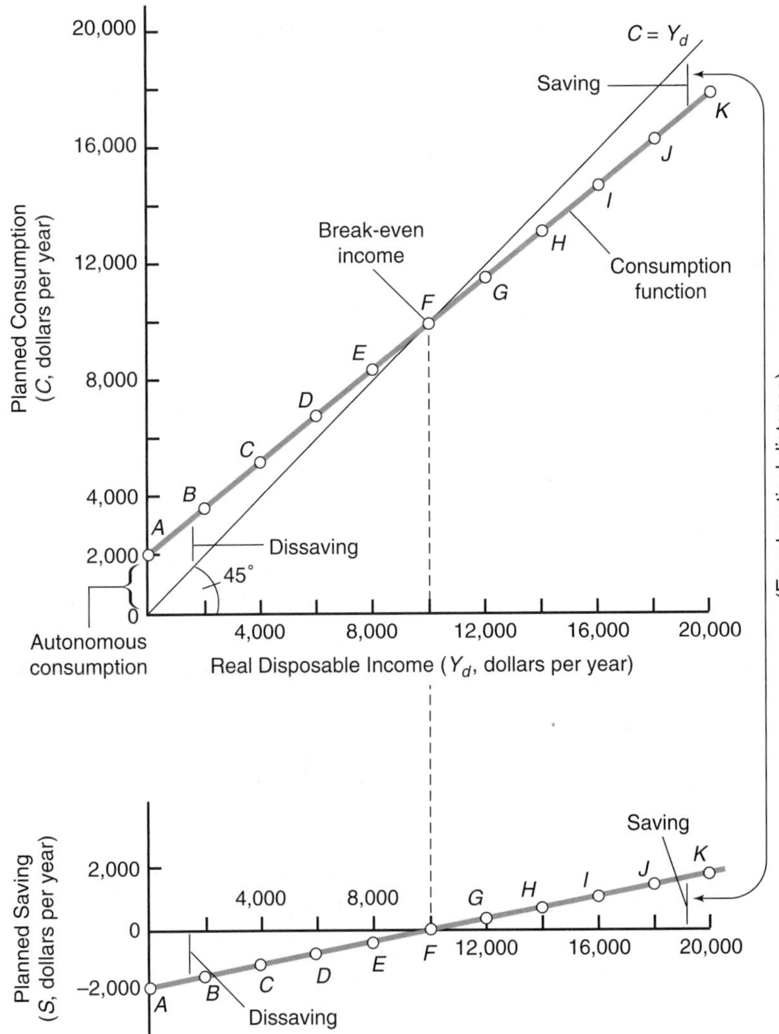

FIGURE 12-1

The Consumption and Saving Functions

If we plot the combinations of real disposable income and planned real consumption from columns 1 and 2 in Table 12-1, we get the consumption function. At every point on the 45-degree line, a vertical line drawn to the income axis is the same distance from the origin as a horizontal line drawn to the consumption axis. Where the consumption function crosses the 45-degree line at *F*, we know that planned real consumption equals real disposable income and there is zero saving. The vertical distance between the 45-degree line and the consumption function measures the rate of real saving or dissaving at any given income level. If we plot the relationship between column 1, real disposable income, and column 3, planned real saving, from Table 12-1, we arrive at the saving function shown in the lower part of this diagram. It is the complement of the consumption function presented above it.

45-degree reference line 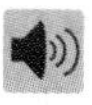
The line along which planned real expenditures equal real national income per year.

How can we find the rate of saving or dissaving in the upper part of Figure 12-1? We draw a line that is equidistant from both the horizontal and the vertical axes. This line is 45 degrees from either axis and is often called the **45-degree reference line.** At every point on the 45-degree reference line, a vertical line drawn to the income axis is the same distance from the origin as a horizontal line drawn to the consumption axis. Thus at point *F*, where the consumption function intersects the 45-degree line, real disposable income equals planned real consumption. Point *F* is sometimes called the *break-even income point* because there is neither positive nor negative real saving. This can be seen in the lower part of Figure 12-1 as well. The planned annual rate of real saving at a real disposable income level of $10,000 is indeed zero.

Dissaving and Autonomous Consumption

To the left of point *F* in either part of Figure 12-1, this hypothetical family engages in dissaving, either by going into debt or by consuming existing assets, including savings. The rate of real saving or dissaving in the upper part of the figure can be found by measuring the vertical distance between the 45-degree line and the consumption function. This simply tells us that if our hypothetical family starts above $10,000 of real disposable income per year and then temporarily finds its real disposable income below $10,000, it will not cut back its real consumption by the full amount of the reduction. It will instead go into debt or consume existing assets in some way to compensate for part of the loss.

Autonomous consumption 
The part of consumption that is independent of (does not depend on) the level of disposable income. Changes in autonomous consumption shift the consumption function.

Now look at the point on the diagram where real disposable income is zero but planned consumption per year is $2,000. This amount of real planned consumption, which does not depend at all on actual real disposable income, is called **autonomous consumption.** The autonomous consumption of $2,000 is *independent* of the level of disposable income. That means that no matter how low the level of real income of our hypothetical family falls, the family will always attempt to consume at least $2,000 per year. (We are, of course, assuming here that the family's real disposable income does not equal zero year in and year out. There is certainly a limit to how long our hypothetical family could finance autonomous consumption without any income.) That $2,000 of yearly consumption is determined by things other than the level of income. We don't need to specify what determines autonomous consumption; we merely state that it exists and that in our example it is $2,000 per year. Just remember that the word *autonomous* means "existing independently." In our model, autonomous consumption exists independently of the hypothetical family's level of real disposable income. (Later we will review some of the non-real-disposable-income determinants of consumption.) There are many possible types of autonomous expenditures. Hypothetically, we can consider that investment is autonomous—independent of income. We can assume that government expenditures are autonomous. We will do just that at various times in our discussions to simplify our analysis of income determination.

Average propensity to consume (APC) 
Consumption divided by disposable income; for any given level of income, the proportion of total disposable income that is consumed.

Average Propensity to Consume and to Save

Let's now go back to Table 12-1, and this time let's look at columns 4 and 5: **average propensity to consume (APC)** and **average propensity to save (APS).** They are defined as follows:

Average propensity to save (APS) 
Saving divided by disposable income; for any given level of income, the proportion of total disposable income that is saved.

$$\text{APC} \equiv \frac{\text{consumption}}{\text{real disposable income}}$$

$$\text{APS} \equiv \frac{\text{savings}}{\text{real disposable income}}$$

Notice from column 4 in Table 12-1 that for this hypothetical family, the average propensity to consume decreases as real disposable income increases. This decrease simply means that the fraction of the family's real disposable income going to consumption falls as income rises. The same fact can be found in column 5. The average propensity to save (APS), which at first is negative, finally hits zero at an income level of $10,000 and then becomes positive. In this example, the APS reaches a value of 0.1 at income level $20,000. This means that the household saves 10 percent of a $20,000 income.

It's quite easy for you to figure out your own average propensity to consume or to save. Just divide your total real disposable income for the year into what you consumed and what you saved. The result will be your personal APC and APS, respectively, at your current level of income. This gives the proportions of total income that are consumed and saved.

Marginal Propensity to Consume and to Save 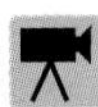

Now we go to the last two columns in Table 12-1: **marginal propensity to consume (MPC)** and **marginal propensity to save (MPS).** The term *marginal* refers to a small incremental or decremental change (represented by the Greek letter delta, Δ, in Table 12-1). The marginal propensity to consume, then, is defined as

$$\text{MPC} \equiv \frac{\text{change in consumption}}{\text{change in real disposable income}}$$

The marginal propensity to save is defined similarly as

$$\text{MPS} \equiv \frac{\text{change in saving}}{\text{change in real disposable income}}$$

Marginal propensity to consume (MPC) 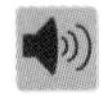
The ratio of the change in consumption to the change in disposable income. A marginal propensity to consume of 0.8 tells us that an additional $100 in take-home pay will lead to an additional $80 consumed.

Marginal propensity to save (MPS) 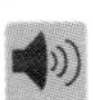
The ratio of the change in saving to the change in disposable income. A marginal propensity to save of 0.2 indicates that out of an additional $100 in take-home pay, $20 will be saved. Whatever is not saved is consumed. The marginal propensity to save plus the marginal propensity to consume must always equal 1, by definition.

What do MPC and MPS tell you? They tell you what percentage of a given increase or decrease in income will go toward consumption and saving, respectively. The emphasis here is on the word *change*. The marginal propensity to consume indicates how much you will change your planned consumption if there is a change in your real disposable income. If your marginal propensity to consume is 0.8, that does not mean that you consume 80 percent of *all* disposable income. The percentage of your real disposable income that you consume is given by the average propensity to consume, or APC. As Table 12-1 indicates, the APC is not equal to 0.8. In contrast, an MPC of 0.8 means that you will consume 80 percent of any *increase* in your disposable income. Hence the MPC cannot be less than zero or greater than one. We assume that individuals increase their planned consumption by more than zero and less than 100 percent of any increase in real disposable income that they receive.

Consider a simple example in which we show the difference between the average propensity to consume and the marginal propensity to consume. Assume that your consumption behavior is exactly the same as our hypothetical family's behavior depicted in Table 12-1. You have an annual real disposable income of $18,000. Your planned consumption rate, then, from column 2 of Table 12-1 is $16,400. So your average propensity to consume is $16,400/$18,000 = 0.911. Now suppose that at the end of the year your boss gives you an after-tax bonus of $2,000. What would you do with that additional $2,000 in real disposable income? According to the table, you would consume $1,600 of it and save $400. In that case, your *marginal* propensity to consume would be $1,600/$2,000 = 0.8, and your marginal propensity to save would be $400/$2,000 = 0.2. What would happen to your *average* propensity to consume? To find out, we add $1,600 to $16,400 of planned consumption, which gives us a new consumption rate of $18,000. The average propensity to consume is then $18,000 divided by the new higher salary of $20,000. Your APC drops from 0.911 to 0.9. By contrast, your MPC remains, in our simplified example, 0.8 all the time. Look at column 6 in Table 12-1. The MPC is 0.8 at every level of income. (Therefore, the MPS is always equal to 0.2 at every level of income.) Underlying the constancy of MPC is the assumption that the amount that you are willing to consume out of additional income will remain the same in percentage terms no matter what level of real disposable income is your starting point.

Some Relationships

Consumption plus saving must equal income. Both your total real disposable income and the change in total real disposable income are either consumed or saved. The proportions of either measure must equal 1, or 100 percent. This allows us to make the following statements:

$$\text{APC} + \text{APS} = 1 \ (= 100 \text{ percent of total income})$$

$$\text{MPC} + \text{MPS} = 1 \ (= 100 \text{ percent of the } \textit{change} \text{ in income})$$

The average propensities as well as the marginal propensities to consume and save must total 1, or 100 percent. Check the two statements by adding the figures in columns 4 and 5 for each level of real disposable income in Table 12-1. Do the same for columns 6 and 7.

Causes of Shifts in the Consumption Function

Wealth 
The stock of assets owned by a person, household, firm, or nation. For a household, wealth can consist of a house, cars, personal belongings, stocks, bonds, bank accounts, and cash.

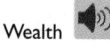

A change in any other relevant economic variable besides real disposable income will cause the consumption function to shift. There is a virtually unlimited number of such nonincome determinants of the position of the consumption function. When population increases or decreases, for example, the consumption function will shift up or down, respectively. Real household **wealth** is also a determinant of the position of the consumption function. An increase in real wealth of the average household will cause the consumption function to shift upward. A decrease in real wealth will cause it to shift downward. So far we have been talking about the consumption function of an individual or a household. Now let's move on to the national economy. We'll consider the consumption function for the entire nation.

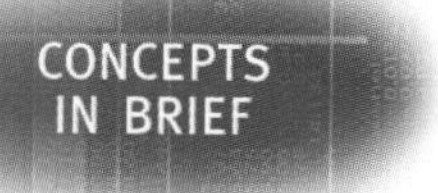

- The consumption function shows the relationship between planned rates of consumption and real disposable income per year. The saving function is the complement of the consumption function because saving plus consumption must equal real disposable income.
- The average propensity to consume (APC) is equal to consumption divided by real disposable income. The average propensity to save (APS) is equal to saving divided by real disposable income.
- The marginal propensity to consume (MPC) is equal to the change in planned consumption divided by the change in real disposable income. The marginal propensity to save (MPS) is equal to the change in planned saving divided by the change in real disposable income.
- Any change in real disposable income will cause the planned rate of consumption to change; this is represented by a movement along the consumption function. Any change in a nonincome determinant of consumption will shift the consumption function.

DETERMINANTS OF INVESTMENT 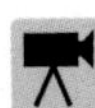

Investment, you will remember, consists of expenditures on new buildings and equipment and changes in business inventories. Real gross private domestic investment in the United States has been extremely volatile over the years relative to real consumption. If we were to look at net private domestic investment (investment after depreciation has been deducted), we would see that in the depths of the Great Depression and at the peak of the World War II effort, the figure was negative. In other words, we were eating away at our capital stock—we weren't even maintaining it by completely replacing depreciated equipment.

If we compare real investment expenditures historically with real consumption expenditures, we find that the latter are less variable over time than the former. Why is this so? One possible reason is that the real investment decisions of businesspeople are based on highly variable, subjective estimates of how the economic future looks.

The Planned Investment Function

Consider that at all times, businesses perceive an array of investment opportunities. These investment opportunities have rates of return ranging from zero to very high, with the number (or dollar value) of all such projects inversely related to the rate of return. Because a project is profitable only if its rate of return exceeds the opportunity cost of the investment—the rate of interest—it follows that as the interest rate falls, planned investment spending increases, and vice versa. Even if firms use retained earnings (internal financing) to fund an investment, the higher the market rate of interest, the greater the *opportunity cost* of using those retained earnings. Thus it does not matter in our analysis whether the firm must seek financing from external sources or can obtain such financing by using retained earnings. Just consider that as the interest rate falls, more investment opportunities will be profitable, and planned investment will be higher.

It should be no surprise, therefore, that the investment function is represented as an inverse relationship between the rate of interest and the value of planned investment. A hypothetical investment schedule is given in panel (a) of Figure 12-2 and plotted in panel (b). We see from this schedule that if, for example, the rate of interest is 7 percent, the dollar value of planned investment will be $1.1 trillion per year. Notice, by the way, that planned investment is also given on a per-year basis, showing that it represents a flow, not a stock. (The stock counterpart of investment is the stock of capital in the economy measured in dollars at a point in time.)

What Causes the Investment Function to Shift?

Because planned investment is assumed to be a function of the rate of interest, any non-interest-rate variable that changes can have the potential of shifting the investment function. Expectations of businesspeople is one of those variables. If higher future sales are expected, more machines and bigger plants will be planned for the future. More investment will be undertaken because of the expectation of higher future profits. In this case, the investment schedule, *I*, would shift outward to the right, meaning that more investment would be desired at all rates of interest. Any change in productive technology can potentially shift the investment function. A positive change in productive technology would stimulate demand for additional capital goods and shift the *I* outward to the right. Changes in business taxes can also shift the investment schedule. If they increase, we predict a leftward shift in the planned investment function because higher taxes imply a lower (after-tax) rate of return.

Click here to see how U.S. real private investment has varied in recent years.

FIGURE 12-2
Planned Investment
In the hypothetical planned investment schedule in panel (a), the rate of planned investment is inversely related to the rate of interest. If we plot the data pairs from panel (a), we obtain the investment function, *I*, in panel (b). It is negatively sloped.

Panel (a)

Rate of Interest (percent per year)	Planned Investment per Year ($ trillions)
12	0.6
11	0.7
10	0.8
9	0.9
8	1.0
7	1.1
6	1.2
5	1.3
4	1.4
3	1.5

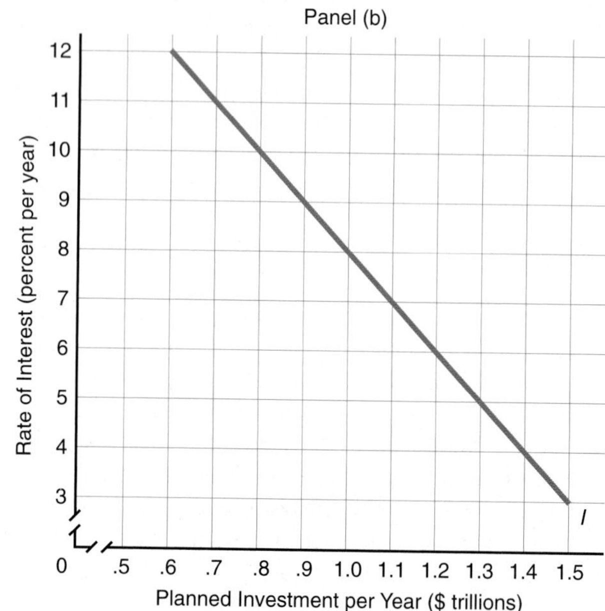

CONCEPTS IN BRIEF

- The planned investment schedule shows the relationship between investment and the rate of interest; it slopes downward.
- The non-interest-rate determinants of planned investment are expectations, innovation and technological changes, and business taxes.
- Any change in the non-interest-rate determinants of planned investment will cause the planned investment function to shift so that at each and every rate of interest a different amount of planned investment will be obtained.

CONSUMPTION AS A FUNCTION OF REAL NATIONAL INCOME

We are interested in determining the equilibrium level of real national income per year. But when we examined the consumption function earlier in this chapter, it related planned consumption expenditures to the level of real disposable income per year. We have already shown where adjustments must be made to GDP in order to get real disposable income (see Table 8-2 in Chapter 8). Real disposable income turns out to be less than real national income because net taxes (taxes minus government transfer payments) are usually about 11 to 18 percent of national income. A representative average is about 15 percent, so disposable income, on average, has in recent years been around 85 percent of national income.

If we are willing to assume that real disposable income, Y_d, differs from real national income by an amount *T* every year, we can relatively easily substitute real national income for real disposable income in the consumption function.

We can now plot any consumption function on a diagram in which the horizontal axis is no longer real disposable income but rather real national income, as in Figure 12-3. Notice that there is an autonomous part of consumption that is so labeled. The difference between this graph and the graphs presented earlier in this chapter is the change in the horizontal axis from real disposable income to real national income per year. For the rest of this chapter, assume that this calculation has been made, and the result is that the MPC out of real national income equals 0.8, suggesting that 20 percent of changes in real national income are either saved or paid in taxes: In other words, of an additional \$100 earned, an additional \$80 will be consumed.

The 45-Degree Reference Line

Like the earlier graphs, Figure 12-3 shows a 45-degree reference line. The 45-degree line bisects the quadrant into two equal spaces. Thus along the 45-degree reference line, planned consumption expenditures, *C,* equal real national income per year, *Y.* One can see, then, that at any point where the consumption function intersects the 45-degree reference line, planned consumption expenditures will be exactly equal to real national income per year, or $C = Y$. Note that in this graph, because we are looking only at planned consumption on the vertical axis, the 45-degree reference line is where planned consumption, *C,* is always equal to real national income per year, *Y.* Later, when we add investment, government spending, and net exports to the graph, the 45-degree reference line with respect to *all* planned expenditures will be labeled as such on the vertical axis. In any event, consumption and real national income are equal at \$7.5 trillion per year. That is where the consumption curve, *C,* intersects the 45-degree reference line. At that income level, all income is consumed.

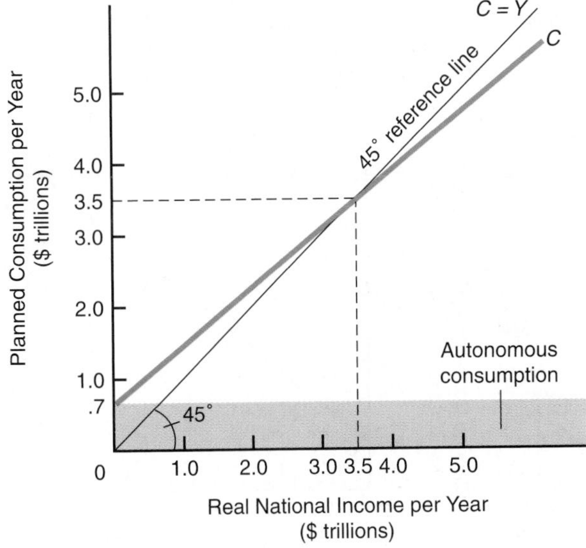

FIGURE 12-3
Consumption as a Function of Real National Income
This consumption function shows the rate of planned expenditures for each level of real national income per year. In this example, there is an autonomous component in consumption equal to \$0.7 trillion (\$700 billion). Along the 45-degree reference line, planned consumption expenditures per year, *C,* are identical to real national income per year, *Y.* The consumption curve intersects the 45-degree reference line at a value of \$3.5 trillion per year.

Adding the Investment Function

Another component of private aggregate demand is, of course, investment spending, *I*. We have already looked at the planned investment function, which related investment to the rate of interest. You see that as the downward-sloping curve in panel (a) of Figure 12-4. Recall from Figure 11-2 that the equilibrium rate of interest is determined at the intersection of the desired savings schedule, which is labeled *S* and is upward-sloping. The equilibrium rate of interest is 7 percent, and the equilibrium rate of investment is $1.1 trillion per year. The $1.1 trillion of real investment per year is *autonomous* with respect to real national income—that is, it is independent of real national income. In other words, given that we have a determinant investment level of $1.1 trillion at a 7 percent rate of interest, we can treat this level of investment as constant, regardless of the level of national income. This is shown in panel (b) of Figure 12-4. The vertical distance of investment spending is $1.1 trillion. Businesses plan on investing a particular amount—$1.1 trillion per year—and will do so no matter what the level of real national income.

How do we add this amount of investment spending to our consumption function? We simply add a line above the *C* line that we drew in Figure 12-3 that is higher by the vertical distance equal to $1.1 trillion of autonomous investment spending. This is shown by the arrow in panel (c) of Figure 12-4. Our new line, now labeled $C + I$, is called the *consumption plus investment line.* In our simple economy without government expenditures and net exports, the $C + I$ curve represents total planned expenditures as they relate to different levels of real national income per year. Because the 45-degree reference line shows all the points where planned expenditures (now $C + I$) equal real national income, we label it $C + I = Y$. Equilibrium *Y* equals $9 trillion per year. Equilibrium occurs when total planned expenditures equal total planned production (given that any amount of production in this model in the short run can occur without a change in the price level).

FIGURE 12-4

Combining Consumption and Investment

In panel (a), we show the determination of real investment in trillions of dollars per year. It occurs where the investment schedule intersects the saving schedule at an interest rate of 7 percent and is equal to $1.1 trillion per year. In panel (b), investment is a constant $1.1 trillion per year. When we add this amount to the consumption line, we obtain in panel (c) the *C* + *I* line, which is vertically higher than the *C* line by exactly $1.1 trillion. Real national income is equal to *C* + *I* at $9 trillion per year where total planned expenditure, *C* + *I*, is equal to actual real national income, for this is where the *C* + *I* line intersects the 45-degree reference line, on which *C* + *I* is equal to *Y* at every point.

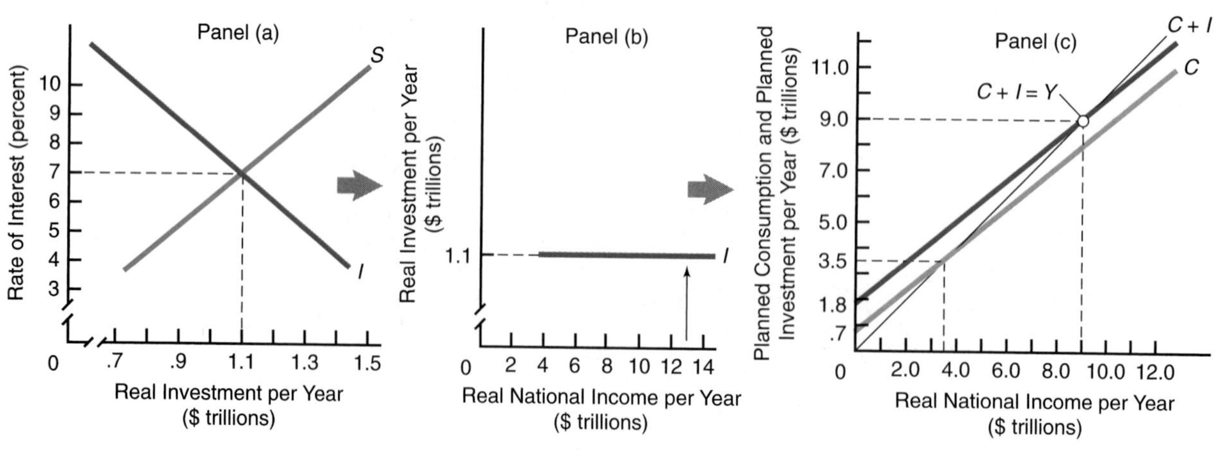

SAVING AND INVESTMENT: PLANNED VERSUS ACTUAL

Figure 12-5 shows the planned investment curve as a horizontal line at $1.1 trillion per year. Investment is completely autonomous in this simplified model—it does not depend on the level of income.

The planned saving curve is represented by *S*. Because in our model whatever is not consumed is, by definition, saved, the planned saving schedule is the complement of the planned consumption schedule, represented by the *C* line in Figure 12-3. For better exposition, we look at only a part of the saving and investment schedules—real national incomes between $7 and $11 trillion per year.

Why does equilibrium have to occur at the intersection of the planned saving and planned investment schedules? If we are at *E* in Figure 12-5, planned saving equals planned investment. All anticipations are validated by reality. There is no tendency for businesses to alter the rate of production or the level of employment because they are neither increasing nor decreasing their inventories in an unplanned way.

If we are producing at a real national income level of $11 trillion instead of $9 trillion, planned investment, as usual, is $1.1 trillion per year, but it is exceeded by planned saving, which is $1.5 trillion per year. This means that consumers will purchase less of total output than businesses had anticipated. Unplanned business inventories will now rise at the rate of $400 billion per year, bringing actual investment into line with actual saving because the $400 billion increase in inventories is included in actual investment. But this rate of output cannot continue for long. Businesses will respond to this unplanned increase in inventories by cutting back production and employment, and we will move toward a lower level of real national income.

Conversely, if the real national income is $7 trillion per year, planned investment continues annually at $1.1 trillion; but at that output rate, planned saving is only $700 billion. This means that households and businesses are purchasing more of real national income than businesses had planned. Businesses will find that they must draw down their inventories below the planned level by $400 billion (business inventories will fall now at the unplanned rate of $400 billion per year), bringing actual investment into equality with

FIGURE 12-5

Planned and Actual Rates of Saving and Investment

Only at the equilibrium level of real national income of $9 trillion per year will planned saving equal actual saving, planned investment equal actual investment, and hence planned saving equal planned investment.

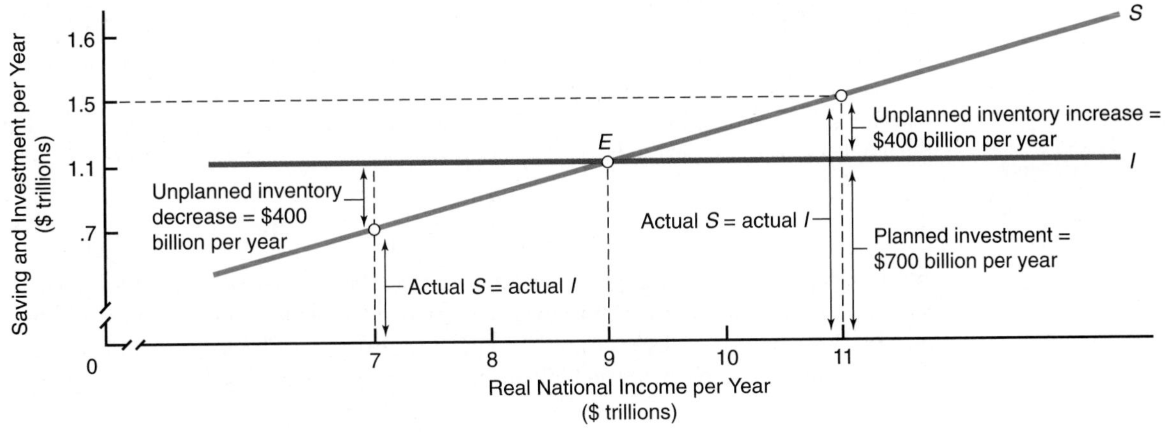

actual saving because the $400 billion decline in inventories is included in actual investment (thereby decreasing it). But this situation cannot last forever either. In their attempt to increase inventories to the desired previous level, businesses will increase output and employment, and real national income will rise toward its equilibrium value of $9 trillion per year. Figure 12-5 demonstrates the necessary equality between actual saving and actual investment. Inventories adjust so that saving and investment, after the fact, are *always* equal in this simplified model. (Remember that changes in inventories count as part of investment.)

Every time the saving rate planned by households differs from the investment rate planned by businesses, there will be a shrinkage or an expansion in the circular flow of income and output (introduced in Chapter 8) in the form of unplanned inventory changes. Real national income and employment will change until unplanned inventory changes are again zero—that is, until we have attained the equilibrium level of real national income.

CONCEPTS IN BRIEF

- We assume that the consumption function has an autonomous part that is independent of the level of real national income per year. It is labeled "autonomous consumption."
- For simplicity, we assume that investment is autonomous with respect to real national income and therefore unaffected by the level of real national income per year.
- The equilibrium level of real national income can be found where planned saving equals planned investment.
- Whenever planned saving exceeds planned investment, there will be unplanned inventory accumulation, and national income will fall as producers reduce output. Whenever planned saving is less than planned investment, there will be unplanned inventory depletion, and national income will rise as producers increase output.

KEYNESIAN EQUILIBRIUM WITH GOVERNMENT AND THE FOREIGN SECTOR ADDED

Government

We have to add government spending, *G*, to our macroeconomic model. We assume that the level of resource-using government purchases of goods and services (federal, state, and local), *not* including transfer payments, is determined by the political process. In other words, *G* will be considered autonomous, just like investment (and a certain component of consumption). In the United States, resource-using government expenditures are around 25 percent of real national income. The other side of the coin, of course, is that there are taxes, which are used to pay for much of government spending. We will simplify our model greatly by assuming that there is a constant **lump-sum tax** of $1.5 trillion a year to finance $1.5 trillion of government spending. This lump-sum tax will reduce disposable income and consumption by the same amount. We show this in Table 12-2 (column 2), where we give the numbers for a complete model.

Lump-sum tax
A tax that does not depend on income or the circumstances of the taxpayer. An example is a $1,000 tax that every family must pay, irrespective of its economic situation.

The Foreign Sector

Not a week goes by without a commentary in the media about the problem of our foreign trade deficit. For many years, we have been buying merchandise and services from foreign residents—imports—the value of which exceeds the value of the exports we have been selling to them. The difference between exports and imports is *net exports,* which we label *X* in our graphs.

TABLE 12-2

The Determination of Equilibrium Real National Income with Net Exports

Figures are trillions of dollars.

(1) Real National Income	(2) Taxes	(3) Real Disposable Income	(4) Planned Consumption	(5) Planned Saving	(6) Planned Investment	(7) Government Spending	(8) Net Exports (exports − imports)	(9) Total Planned Expenditures (4) + (6) + (7) + (8)	(10) Unplanned Inventory Changes	(11) Direction of Change in Real National Income
4.0	1.5	2.5	2.7	−.2	1.1	1.5	−.1	5.2	−1.2	Increase
5.0	1.5	3.5	3.5	0	1.1	1.5	−.1	6.0	−1.0	Increase
6.0	1.5	4.5	4.3	.2	1.1	1.5	−.1	6.8	−.8	Increase
7.0	1.5	5.5	5.1	.4	1.1	1.5	−.1	7.6	−.6	Increase
8.0	1.5	6.5	5.9	.6	1.1	1.5	−.1	8.4	−.4	Increase
9.0	1.5	7.5	6.7	.8	1.1	1.5	−.1	9.2	−.2	Increase
10.0	1.5	8.5	7.5	1.0	1.1	1.5	−.1	10.0	0	Neither (equilibrium)
11.0	1.5	9.5	8.3	1.2	1.1	1.5	−.1	10.8	+.2	Decrease
12.0	1.5	10.5	9.1	1.4	1.1	1.5	−.1	11.6	+.4	Decrease

The level of exports depends on international economic conditions, especially in the countries that buy our products. Imports depend on economic conditions here at home. For simplicity, let us assume that imports exceed exports (net exports, X, is negative) and furthermore that the level of net exports is autonomous—independent of national income. Assume a level of X of −$100 billion per year, as shown in column 8 of Table 12-2.

Click here to find out how the North American Free Trade Agreement has affected U.S. imports and exports.

Determining the Equilibrium Level of Real National Income per Year

We are now in a position to determine the equilibrium level of real national income per year under the continuing assumptions that the price level is unchanging; that investment, government, and the foreign sector are autonomous; and that planned consumption expenditures are determined by the level of real national income. As can be seen in Table 12-2, total planned expenditures of $10 trillion per year equal real national income of $10 trillion per year, and this is where we reach equilibrium.

Remember that equilibrium *always* occurs when total planned expenditures equal total production (given that any amount of production in this model in the short run can occur without a change in the price level).

Now look at Figure 12-6, which shows the equilibrium level of real national income. There are two curves, one showing the consumption function, which is the exact duplicate of the one shown in Figure 12-3, and the other being the $C + I + G + X$ curve, which intersects the 45-degree reference line (representing equilibrium) at $10 trillion per year.

Whenever total planned expenditures differ from real national income, there are unplanned inventory changes. When total planned expenditures are greater than real

FIGURE 12-6

The Equilibrium Level of Real National Income

The consumption function, with no government and thus no taxes, is shown as *C*. When we add autonomous investment, government, taxes, and net exports, we obtain $C + I + G + X$. We move from E_1 to E_2. The equilibrium level of real national income is \$10 trillion per year.

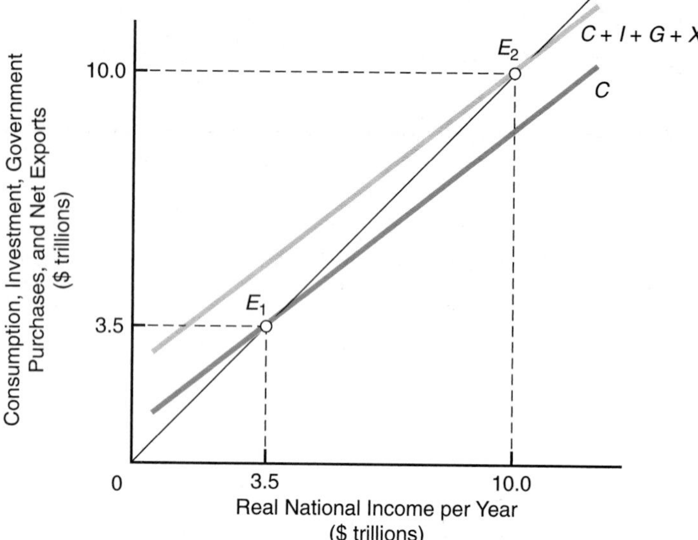

national income, inventory levels drop in an unplanned manner. To get them back up, firms seek to expand their production, which increases real national income. Real national income rises toward its equilibrium level. Whenever total planned expenditures are less than real national income, the opposite occurs. There are unplanned inventory increases, causing firms to cut back on their production. The result is a drop in real national income toward the equilibrium level.

CONCEPTS IN BRIEF

- When we add autonomous investment, *I*, and autonomous government spending, *G*, to the consumption function, we obtain the $C + I + G$ curve, which represents total planned expenditures for a closed economy. In an open economy, we add the foreign sector, which consists of exports minus imports, or net exports, *X*. Total planned expenditures are thus represented by the $C + I + G + X$ curve.
- The equilibrium level of real national income can be found by locating the intersection of the total planned expenditures curve with the 45-degree reference line. At that level of real national income per year, planned consumption plus planned investment plus government expenditures plus net exports will equal real national income.
- Whenever total planned expenditures exceed real national income, there will be unplanned decreases in inventories; the size of the circular flow of income will increase, and a higher level of equilibrium real national income will prevail. Whenever planned expenditures are less than real national income, there will be unplanned increases in inventories; the size of the circular flow will shrink, and a lower equilibrium level of real national income will prevail.

THE MULTIPLIER

Look again at panel (c) of Figure 12-4. Assume for the moment that the only expenditures included in real national income are consumption expenditures. Where would the equilibrium level of income be in this case? It would be where the consumption function (*C*) intersects the 45-degree reference line, which is at \$3.5 trillion per year. Now we add the autonomous amount of planned investment, \$1.1 trillion, and then determine what the new equilibrium level of income will be. It turns out to be \$9 trillion per year. Adding \$1.1 trillion per year of investment spending increased the equilibrium level of income by *five* times that amount, or by \$5.5 trillion per year.

What is operating here is the multiplier effect of changes in autonomous spending. The **multiplier** is the number by which a permanent change in autonomous investment or autonomous consumption is multiplied to get the change in the equilibrium level of real national income. Any permanent increases in autonomous investment or in any autonomous component of consumption will cause an even larger increase in real national income. Any permanent decreases in autonomous spending will cause even larger decreases in the equilibrium level of real national income per year. To understand why this multiple expansion (or contraction) in the equilibrium level of real national income occurs, let's look at a simple numerical example.

Multiplier 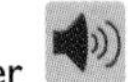
The ratio of the change in the equilibrium level of real national income to the change in autonomous expenditures; the number by which a change in autonomous investment or autonomous consumption, for example, is multiplied to get the change in the equilibrium level of real national income.

We'll use the same figures we used for the marginal propensity to consume and to save. MPC will equal 0.8, or $\frac{4}{5}$, and MPS will equal 0.2, or $\frac{1}{5}$. Now let's run an experiment and say that businesses decide to increase planned investment permanently by \$100 billion a year. We see in Table 12-3 that during what we'll call the first round in column 1, investment is increased by \$100 billion; this also means an increase in real national income of \$100 billion, because the spending by one group represents income for another, shown in column 2. Column 3 gives the resultant increase in consumption by households that received this additional \$100 billion in real income. This is found by multiplying the MPC by the increase in real income. Because the MPC equals 0.8, consumption expenditures during the first round will increase by \$80 billion.

TABLE 12-3

The Multiplier Process

We trace the effects of a permanent \$100 billion increase in autonomous investment spending on the equilibrium level of real national income. If we assume a marginal propensity to consume of 0.8, such an increase will eventually elicit a \$500 billion increase in the equilibrium level of real national income per year.

Assumption: MPC = 0.8, or $\frac{4}{5}$

(1) Round	(2) Annual Increase in Real National Income (\$ billions per year)	(3) Annual Increase in Planned Consumption (\$ billions per year)	(4) Annual Increase in Planned Saving (\$ billions per year)
1 (\$100 billion per year increase in *I*)	100.00	80.000	20.000
2	80.00	64.000	16.000
3	64.00	51.200	12.800
4	51.20	40.960	10.240
5	40.96	32.768	8.192
.	.	.	.
.	.	.	.
.	.	.	.
All later rounds	163.84	131.072	32.768
Totals ($C + I + G$)	500.00	400.000	100.000

But that's not the end of the story. This additional household consumption is also spending, and it will provide \$80 billion of additional real income for other individuals. Thus during the second round, we see an increase in real income of \$80 billion. Now, out of this increased real income, what will be the resultant increase in consumption expenditures? It will be 0.8 times \$80 billion, or \$64 billion. We continue these induced expenditure rounds and find that because of an initial increase in autonomous investment expenditures of \$100 billion, the equilibrium level of real national income will eventually increase by \$500 billion. A permanent \$100 billion increase in autonomous investment spending has induced an additional \$400 billion increase in consumption spending, for a total increase in real national income of \$500 billion. In other words, the equilibrium level of real national income will change by an amount equal to five times the change in investment.

The Multiplier Formula 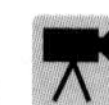

It turns out that the autonomous spending multiplier is equal to the reciprocal of the marginal propensity to save. In our example, the MPC was $\frac{4}{5}$; therefore, because MPC + MPS = 1, the MPS was equal to $\frac{1}{5}$. The reciprocal is 5. That was our multiplier. A \$100 billion increase in planned investment led to a \$500 billion increase in the equilibrium level of real income. Our multiplier will always be the following:

$$\text{Multiplier} \equiv \frac{1}{1 - \text{MPC}} \equiv \frac{1}{\text{MPS}}$$

You can always figure out the multiplier if you know either the MPC or the MPS. Let's consider some examples. If MPS = $\frac{1}{4}$,

$$\text{Multiplier} = \frac{1}{\frac{1}{4}} = 4$$

Repeating again that MPC + MPS = 1, then MPS = 1 − MPC. Hence we can always figure out the multiplier if we are given the marginal propensity to consume. In this example, if the marginal propensity to consume were given as $\frac{3}{4}$,

$$\text{Multiplier} = \frac{1}{1 - \frac{3}{4}} = \frac{1}{\frac{1}{4}} = 4$$

By taking a few numerical examples, you can demonstrate to yourself an important property of the multiplier:

The smaller the marginal propensity to save, the larger the multiplier.

Otherwise stated:

The larger the marginal propensity to consume, the larger the multiplier.

Demonstrate this to yourself by computing the multiplier when the marginal propensities to save equal $\frac{3}{4}$, $\frac{1}{2}$, and $\frac{1}{4}$. What happens to the multiplier as the MPS gets smaller?

When you have the multiplier, the following formula will then give you the change in the equilibrium level of real national income due to a permanent change in autonomous spending:

$$\text{Multiplier} \times \text{change in autonomous spending} = \text{change in equilibrium level of real national income}$$

The multiplier, as we have mentioned, works for a permanent increase or permanent decrease in autonomous spending. In our earlier example, if the autonomous component of consumption had fallen by \$100 billion, the reduction in the equilibrium level of real national income per year would have been \$500 billion per year.

Significance of the Multiplier

Depending on the size of the multiplier, it is possible that a relatively small change in planned investment or autonomous consumption can trigger a much larger change in the equilibrium level of real national income per year. In essence, the multiplier magnifies the fluctuations in the equilibrium level of real national income initiated by changes in autonomous spending.

As was just stated, the larger the marginal propensity to consume, the larger the multiplier. If the marginal propensity to consume is $\frac{1}{2}$, the multiplier is 2. In that case, a $1 billion decrease in (autonomous) investment will elicit a $2 billion decrease in the equilibrium level of real national income per year. Conversely, if the marginal propensity to consume is $\frac{9}{10}$, the multiplier will be 10. That same $1 billion decrease in planned investment expenditures with a multiplier of 10 will lead to a $10 billion decrease in the equilibrium level of real national income per year.

EXAMPLE

Changes in Investment and the Great Depression

Changes in autonomous spending lead to shifts in the total expenditures ($C + I + G + X$) curve and, as you have seen, cause a multiplier effect on the equilibrium level of real GDP per year. A classic example apparently occurred during the Great Depression. Indeed, some economists believe that it was an autonomous downward shift (collapse) in the investment function that provoked the Great Depression. Look at panel (a) of Figure 12-7. There you see the net investment (gross investment minus depreciation) in the United States from 1929 to 1941 (expressed in 1992 dollars). Clearly, during business contractions, decision makers in the

FIGURE 12-7

Net Private Domestic Investment and Real GDP During the Great Depression

In panel (a), you see how net private investment expressed in billions of 1992 dollars became negative starting in 1931 and stayed negative for several years. It became positive in 1936 and 1937, only to become negative again in 1938. Look at panel (b). There you see how changes in GDP seem to mirror changes in net private domestic investment.

Source: U.S. Bureau of the Census.

Panel (a)

Year	Net Private Domestic Investment (billions of 1992 dollars)
1929	85.96
1930	24.48
1931	–26.89
1932	–83.34
1933	–80.20
1934	–43.51
1935	– 6.13
1936	18.39
1937	54.20
1938	– 9.54
1939	24.27
1940	66.89
1941	107.71

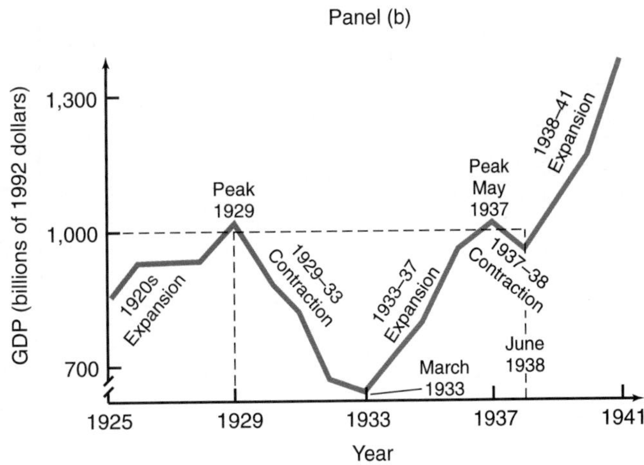

business world can and do decide to postpone long-range investment plans for buildings and equipment. This causes the business recovery to be weak unless those business plans are revised. If you examine real GDP in panel (b) of Figure 12-7, you see that the contraction that started in 1929 reached its trough in 1933. The expansion was relatively strong for the following four years, and then there was another contraction from 1937 to 1938. Some researchers argue that even though the 1937–1938 contraction initially was more severe than the one that started in 1929, it was short-lived because long-range investment plans were revised upward by the end of 1938.

For Critical Analysis

Why might businesses have revised their investment plans upward in 1938?

THE MULTIPLIER EFFECT WHEN THE PRICE LEVEL CAN CHANGE

Clearly, the multiplier effect on the equilibrium overall level of *real* national income will not be as great if part of the increase in *nominal* national income occurs because of increases in the price level. We show this in Figure 12-8. The intersection of AD_1 and *SRAS* is at a price level of 120 with equilibrium real national income of $10 trillion per year. An increase in autonomous spending shifts the aggregate demand curve outward to the right to AD_2. If price level remained at 120, the short-run equilibrium level of real GDP would increase to $10.5 trillion per year because, for the $100 billion increase in autonomous spending, the multiplier would be 5, as it was in Table 12-3. But the price level does not stay fixed because ordinarily the *SRAS* curve is positively sloped. In this diagram, the new short-run equilibrium level of real national income is hypothetically $10.3 trillion of real national income per year. Instead of the multiplier being 5, the multiplier with respect to equilibrium changes in the output of real goods and services—real national income—is only 3. The multiplier is smaller because part of the additional income is used to pay higher prices; not all is spent on increased output, as is the case when the price level is fixed.

If the economy is at an equilibrium level of real national income that is greater than *LRAS*, the implications for the multiplier are even more severe. Look again at Figure 12-8. The *SRAS* curve starts to slope upward more dramatically after $10 trillion of real national income per year. Therefore, any increase in aggregate demand will lead to a proportionally

FIGURE 12-8

Multiplier Effect on Equilibrium of Real National Income

A $100 billion increase in autonomous spending (investment, government, or net exports), which moves AD_1 to AD_2, will yield a full multiplier effect only if prices are constant. If the price index increases from 120 to 125, the multiplier effect is less, and the equilibrium level of real national income goes up only to, say, $10.3 trillion per year instead of $10.5 trillion per year.

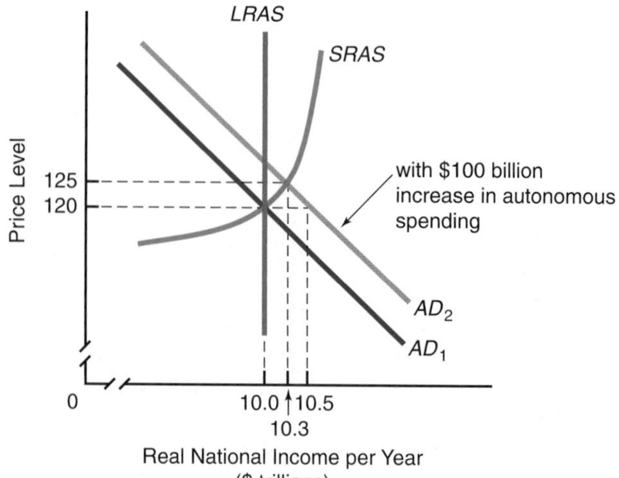

greater increase in the price level and a smaller increase in the equilibrium level of real national income per year. The multiplier effect of any increase in autonomous spending will be relatively small because most of the changes will be in the price level. Moreover, any increase in the short-run equilibrium level of real national income will tend to be temporary because the economy is temporarily above *LRAS*—the strain on its productive capacity will raise prices.

THE RELATIONSHIP BETWEEN AGGREGATE DEMAND AND THE *C* + *I* + *G* + *X* CURVE

There is clearly a relationship between the aggregate demand curves that you studied in Chapters 10 and 11 and the $C + I + G + X$ curve developed in this chapter. After all, aggregate demand consists of consumption, investment, and government purchases, plus the foreign sector of our economy. There is a major difference, however, between the aggregate demand curve, *AD*, and the $C + I + G + X$ curve: The latter is drawn with the price level held constant, whereas the former is drawn, by definition, with the price level changing. In other words, the $C + I + G + X$ curve shown in Figure 12-6 is drawn with the price level fixed. To derive the aggregate demand curve, we must now allow the price level to change. Look at the upper part of Figure 12-9. Here we show the $C + I + G + X$

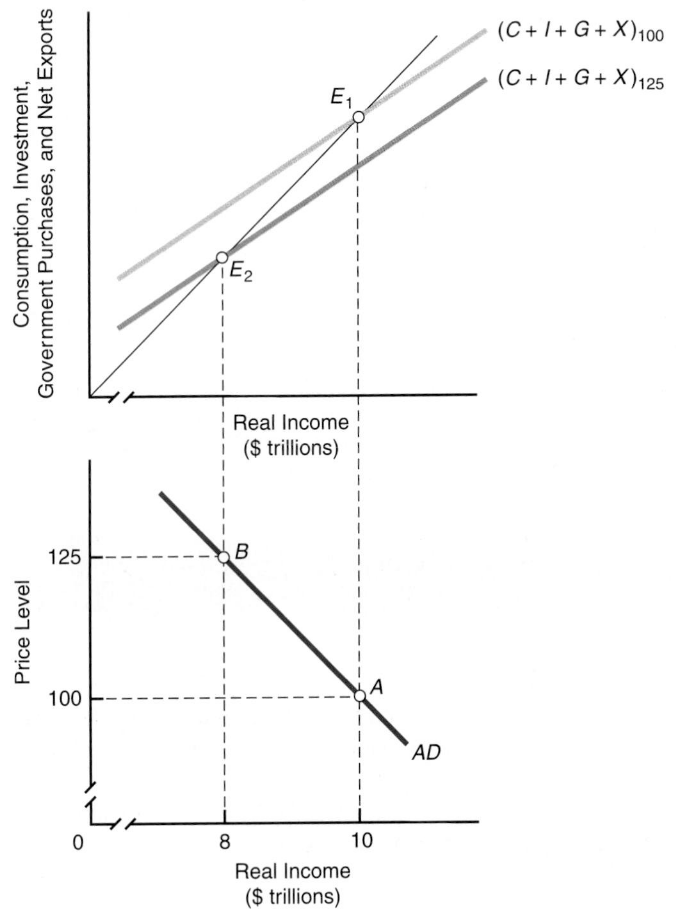

FIGURE 12-9

The Relationship Between *AD* and the *C* + *I* + *G* + *X* Curve

In the upper graph, the $C + I + G + X$ curve at a price level equal to 100 intersects the 45-degree reference line at E_1, or \$10 trillion of real income per year. That gives us point *A* (price level = 100; real income = \$10 trillion) in the lower graph. When the price level increases to 125, the $C + I + G + X$ curve shifts downward, and the new equilibrium level of real income is at E_2 at \$8 trillion per year. This gives us point *B* in the lower graph. Connecting points *A* and *B*, we obtain the aggregate demand curve.

curve at a price level equal to 100 and equilibrium at $10 trillion of income per year. This gives us point *A* in the lower graph, for it shows what real income would be at a price level of 100.

Now let's assume that in the upper graph, the price level increases to 125. What are the effects?

1. A higher price level can decrease the purchasing power of any cash that people hold (the real-balance effect). This is a decrease in real wealth, and it causes consumption expenditures, *C*, to fall, thereby putting downward pressure on the $C + I + G + X$ curve.
2. Because individuals attempt to borrow more to replenish their real cash balances, interest rates will rise, which will make it more costly for people to buy houses and cars (the interest rate effect). Higher interest rates make it more costly, for example, to install new equipment and to erect new buildings. Therefore, the rise in the price level indirectly causes a reduction in the quantity of aggregate goods and services demanded.
3. In an open economy, our higher price level causes the foreign demand for our goods to fall (the open economy effect). Simultaneously, it increases our demand for others' goods. If the foreign exchange price of the dollar stays constant for a while, there will be an increase in imports and a decrease in exports, thereby reducing the size of *X*, again putting downward pressure on the $C + I + G + X$ curve.

The result is that a new $C + I + G + X$ curve at a price level equal to 125 generates an equilibrium at E_2 at $8 trillion of real income per year. This gives us point *B* in the lower part of Figure 12-9. When we connect points *A* and *B*, we obtain the aggregate demand curve, *AD*.

CONCEPTS IN BRIEF

- Any change in autonomous spending shifts the expenditure curve and causes a multiplier effect on the equilibrium level of real national income per year.
- The multiplier is equal to the reciprocal of the marginal propensity to save.
- The smaller the marginal propensity to save, the larger the multiplier. Otherwise stated, the larger the marginal propensity to consume, the larger the multiplier.
- The $C + I + G + X$ curve is drawn with the price level held constant, whereas the *AD* curve allows the price level to change. Each different price level generates a new $C + I + G + X$ curve.

NETNOMICS

The Internet Is Making Investment a Fuzzier Concept

Before 1999, the government had treated spending on the software used to post Web pages, download programs, or transmit Internet orders the same as electricity that powered computers and equipment that linked people to the Internet: as a once-and-for-all cost of production. Of course, unlike electricity, software can last for a long time. This is why the government now counts business software expenditures as investment spending, classifying these expenditures as equivalent to spending on the computers and high-speed communications equipment that are the nuts and bolts of the Internet.

Many economists had pushed for this change for years, but now some are having second thoughts. Currently, most businesses purchase new or updated software for on-site installation on the hard drives of office computers. Sun Microsystems and other companies, however, are championing a new approach to computer software distribution that would fundamentally change how businesses use software. In this proposed model for computer operations, businesses would no longer store software on hard drives. Instead, companies would pay monthly or annual fees to software providers in exchange for real-time access to computer operating systems, word processing software, and computer spreadsheet programs directly from the Internet. The Internet-based providers of these new "software services" would automatically update the software as often as new versions became available.

Currently, fees that companies pay for services rendered are costs of doing business and are not counted as investment. Even though there is no *functional* distinction between software stored on a hard drive for months or years and software accessed in real time on the Internet for a fee, the new approach to measuring investment makes a distinction: Spending on software that businesses purchase and store on hard drives is investment, but fees paid for real-time computer operations using software downloaded from the Internet are a short-term cost of doing business. It remains to be seen how government statisticians will deal with this new wrinkle.

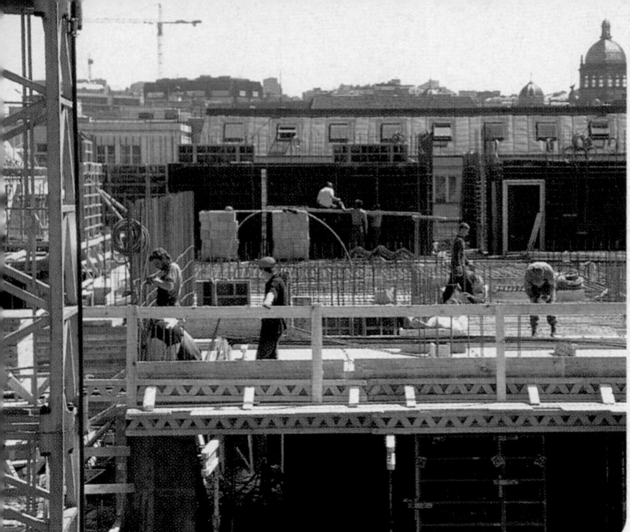

Issues & Applications

Is the U.S. Rate of Net Investment Understated?

Concepts Applied

- Investment
- Total Planned Expenditures
- National Income

As tabulated in the national income accounts, net investment includes spending only on physical capital—plants and equipment, infrastructure, and housing—and adjustments in inventories of produced goods. Using this measure of net investment, the portion of real GDP that U.S. residents allocate to net investment tends to lag behind much of the rest of the developed world. Some observers have interpreted this lower rate of investment as a factor that tends to depress total planned expenditures and hence equilibrium U.S. national income. After all, they point out, any reduction in investment cuts into total planned spending and thereby pulls down equilibrium real income via the multiplier. These observers also worry about a longer-term effect of lower U.S. investment: a fall-off in capital accumulation and reduced growth.

A Measurement Problem?

Other economists are less concerned because they think that the current measure of net investment, which has remained more or less unchanged since national income accounting was developed more than 60 years ago, fails to capture the true meaning of the term. Recall that much investment is spending on capital, resources that may be used to produce output in the future. There are several types of expenditures that appear to fit economists' definition of investment but are not counted as investment:

Education: Spending on education yields returns over long periods of time, but only expenditures on schools and educational equipment are currently included in the official definition of investment spending. In recent years, the United States has allocated nearly 7 percent of its GDP to education. In Japan, this figure is less than 4 percent, and in most other countries it rarely exceeds 5.5 percent.

Research and development: As you learned in Chapter 9, some theories of economic growth view research and development as a fundamental aspect of the growth process. Nevertheless, in the national income accounts, government R&D expenses are counted as government consumption. Business R&D expenses are treated solely as a cost of production, so they are excluded from tabulations of private business investment. The United States spends close to 3 percent of its GDP on research and development, while in many other developed countries such expenses rarely top 2 percent of GDP.

Consumer durables: Only household spending on housing is counted as investment in the national income accounts. Yet U.S. households spend about 6 percent of GDP on durable goods such as automobiles, personal computers, and other relatively long-lived gadgets that yield service flows for years. The comparable figure in other industrialized countries is about 5 percent. All this spending shows up as consumption spending in the official statistics.

U.S. Investment Spending May Be a Bargain

Another neglected factor in comparing the U.S. investment rate with the rate of investment in other countries is that U.S. investment goods are less expensive. That is, a given dollar of spending on factories or computers provides more units of these goods in the United States relative to other countries.

What happens when all factors—relative differences in the prices of investment goods and spending on education, research and development, and consumer durables—are taken into account? The answer is a dramatic change in the international comparison: The adjusted measure of the U.S. investment rate exceeds 35 percent of GDP per year, while the average rate (adjusted in the same way) for other industrialized is about 30 percent. It is possible, therefore, that the United States actually leads the way in investment as broadly defined by economists.

FOR CRITICAL ANALYSIS

1. Some economists argue that military expenditures protect a nation's capital stock from seizure from other powers and thereby ensure returns on other forms of investment, so military spending should somehow count as "investment." What are pros and cons of this proposal?
2. Why is "investment" difficult to define?

SG

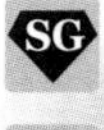

SUMMARY DISCUSSION OF LEARNING OBJECTIVES

1. **The Difference Between Saving and Savings and the Relationship Between Saving and Consumption:** Saving is a flow over time, whereas savings is a stock of resources at a point in time. Thus, the portion of your disposable income you do not consume during a week, a month, or a year is an addition to your stock of savings. By definition, saving during a year plus consumption during that year must equal total disposable (after-tax) income earned that year.
2. **Key Determinants of Consumption and Saving in the Keynesian Model:** In the classical model, the interest rate is the fundamental determinant of saving, but in the Keynesian model, the primary determinant is disposable income. The reason is that as real disposable income increases, so do real consumption expenditures. Because consumption and saving equal disposable income, this means that saving must also vary with changes in disposable income. Of course, factors other than disposable income can affect consumption and saving. The portion of consumption that is not related to disposable income is called autonomous consumption. The ratio of saving to disposable income is the average propensity to save (APS), and the ratio of consumption to disposable income is the average propensity to consume (APC). A change in saving divided by the corresponding change in disposable income is the marginal propensity to save (MPS), and a change in consumption divided by the corresponding change in disposable income is the marginal propensity to consume (MPC).
3. **The Primary Determinants of Planned Investment:** An increase in the interest rate raises the opportunity cost of retaining earnings for investment, so planned investment varies inversely with the interest rate. Hence the investment schedule slopes downward. Other factors that influence planned investment, such as business expectations, productive technology, or business taxes, can cause the investment schedule to shift. In the basic Keynesian model, changes in real national income do not affect planned investment, meaning that investment is autonomous with respect to national income.
4. **How Equilibrium National Income Is Established in the Keynesian Model:** In equilibrium, total planned consumption, investment, government, and net export expenditures equal total national income,

so that $C + I + G + X = Y$. This occurs at the point where the $C + I + G + X$ curve crosses the 45-degree reference line. In a world without government spending and taxes, equilibrium also occurs when planned saving is equal to planned investment. Furthermore, at the equilibrium level of national income, there is no tendency for business inventories to expand or contract.

5. **Why Autonomous Changes in Total Planned Expenditures Have a Multiplier Effect on Equilibrium National Income:** Any increase in autonomous expenditures, such as an increase in investment caused by a rise in business confidence, causes a direct rise in national income. This income increase in turn stimulates increased consumption, and the amount of this increase is the marginal propensity to consume multiplied by the rise in disposable income that results. As consumption increases, however, so does income, which induces a further increase in consumption spending. The ultimate expansion of income is equal to the multiplier, 1/(1 − MPC), times the increase in autonomous expenditures.
6. **The Relationship Between Total Planned Expenditures and the Aggregate Demand Curve:** An increase in the price level decreases the purchasing power of money holdings, which induces households and businesses to cut back on expenditures. In addition, as individuals and firms seek to borrow to replenish their cash balances, the interest rate tends to rise, which increases borrowing costs and further discourages spending. Furthermore, a higher price level reduces exports as foreign residents cut back on purchases of domestically produced goods. These effects combined shift the C + I + G + X curve downward following a rise in the price level, so that equilibrium real national income falls. This yields the downward-sloping aggregate demand curve.

Key Terms and Concepts

Autonomous consumption (274)
Average propensity to consume (APC) (274)
Average propensity to save (APS) (274)
Capital goods (271)
Consumption (271)
Consumption function (272)
Consumption goods (271)
Dissaving (272)
45-degree reference line (274)
Investment (271)
Lump-sum tax (282)
Marginal propensity to consume (MPC) (275)
Marginal propensity to save (MPS) (275)
Multiplier (285)
Saving (271)
Wealth (276)

Problems

Answers to the odd-numbered problems appear at the back of the book.

12-1. Complete the accompanying table.
  a. Complete the table.
  b. Add two columns to the right of the table. Calculate the average propensity to save and the average propensity to consume at each level of disposable income. (Round to the nearest hundredth.)
  c. Determine the marginal propensity to save and the marginal propensity to consume.

Disposable Income	Saving	Consumption
$ 200	−$ 40	____
400	0	____
600	40	____
800	80	____
1,000	120	____
1,200	160	____

12-2. Classify each of the following as either a stock or a flow.

a. Myung Park earns $850 per week.
b. America Online purchases $100 million in new computer equipment this month.
c. Sally Schmidt has $1,000 in a savings account at a credit union.
d. XYZ, Inc., produces 200 units of output per week.
e. Giorgio Giannelli owns three private jets.
f. DaimlerChrysler's inventories decline by 750 autos per month.
g. Russia owes $25 billion to the International Monetary Fund.

12-3. An Internet service provider (ISP) is contemplating an investment of $50,000 in new comptuer servers and related hardware. The ISP projects an annual rate of return on this investment of 6 percent.

a. The current market interest rate is 5 percent per year. Will the ISP undertake the investment?
b. Suddenly there is an economic downturn. Although the market interest rate does not change, the ISP anticipates will reduce the projected rate of return on the investment to 4 percent per year. Will the ISP now undertake the investment?

12-4. Consider the table when answering the following questions. For this hypothetical economy, the marginal propensity to save is constant at all levels of income, and investment spending is autonomous. There is no government.

Real National Income	Consumption	Saving	Investment
$ 2,000	$2,200	$____	$400
4,000	4,000	____	____
6,000	____	____	____
8,000	____	____	____
10,000	____	____	____
12,000	____	____	____

a. Complete the table. What is the marginal propensity to save? What is the marginal propensity to consume?
b. Draw a graph of the consumption function. Then add the investment function to obtain $C + I$.
c. Under the graph of $C + I$, draw another graph showing the saving and investment curves. Note that the $C + I$ curve crosses the 45-degree reference line in the upper graph at the same level of real national income where the saving and investment curves cross in the lower graph. (If not, redraw your graphs.) What is this level of real national income?
d. What is the numerical value of the multiplier?
e. What is the equilibrium level of real national income without investment? What is the multiplier effect from the inclusion of investment?
f. What is the average propensity to consume at the equilibrium level of real national income?
g. If autonomous investment declines from $400 to $200, what happens to equilibrium real national income?

12-5. Consider the table when answering the following questions. For this hypothetical economy, the marginal propensity to consume is constant at all levels of income, and investment spending is autonomous. The equilibrium level of real national income is equal to $8,000. There is no government.

Real National Income	Consumption	Saving	Investment
$ 2,000	$ 2,000	____	____
4,000	3,600	____	____
6,000	5,200	____	____
8,000	6,800	____	____
10,000	8,400	____	____
12,000	10,000	____	____

a. Complete the table. What is the marginal propensity to consume? What is the marginal propensity to save?
b. Draw a graph of the consumption function. Then add the investment function to obtain $C + I$.
c. Under the graph of $C + I$, draw another graph showing the saving and investment curves. Does the $C + I$ curve cross the 45-degree reference line in the upper graph at the same level of real national income where the saving

and investment curves cross in the lower graph, at the equilibrium real national income level of \$8,000? (If not, redraw your graphs.)

d. What is the average propensity to save at the equilibrium level of real national income?

e. If autonomous consumption were to rise by \$100, what would happen to equilibrium real national income?

12-6. Calculate the multiplier for the following cases.

a. MPS $= .25$

b. MPC $= \frac{5}{6}$

c. MPS $= .125$

d. MPC $= \frac{6}{7}$

e. $C = \$200 + .85Y$

Economics on the Net

The Relationship Between Consumption and Real GDP According to the basic consumption function we considered in this Chapter, comsumption rises at a fixed rate when both disposable income and real GDP increase. Your task here is to evaluate how reasonable this assumption is and to determine the relative extent to which variations in consumption appear to be related to variations in real GDP.

Title: Gross Domestic Product and Components

Navigation: Click here to visit the Federal Reserve Bank of St. Louis' web page on Gross Domestic Product and Components.

Application

1. Click on Personal Consumption Expenditures. Write down consumption expenditures for the past eight quarters. Now back up to Gross Domestic Product and Components, click on Gross Domestic Product, and write down GDP for the past eight quarters. Use these data to calculate implied values for the marginal propensity to consume, assuming that taxes do not vary with income. Is there any problem with this assumption?

2. Back up to Gross Domestic Product and Components. Now click on Gross Domestic Product in Chained (1996) Dollars. Scan through the data since the mid-1960s. In what years did the largest variations in GDP take place? What component or components of GDP appear to have accounted for these large movements?

For Group Study and Analysis Assign groups to use the FRED database to try to determine the best measure of aggregate U.S. disposable income for the past eight quarters. Reconvene the class, and discuss each group's approach to this issue.

THE KEYNESIAN CROSS AND THE MULTIPLIER

We can see the multiplier effect more clearly if we look at Figure B-1, in which we see only a small section of the graphs that we used in Chapter 12. We start with an equilibrium level of real national income of \$9.5 trillion per year. This equilibrium occurs with total planned expenditures represented by $C + I + G + X$. The $C + I + G + X$ curve intersects the 45-degree reference line at \$6.5 trillion per year. Now we increase investment, *I*, by \$100 billion. This increase in investment shifts the entire $C + I + G + X$ curve vertically to $C + I' + G + X$. The vertical shift represents that \$100 billion increase in autonomous investment. With the higher level of planned expenditures per year, we are no longer in equilibrium at *E*. Inventories are falling. Production will increase. Eventually, planned production will catch up with total planned expenditures. The new equilibrium level of real national income is established at *E'* at the intersection of the new $C + I' + G + X$ curve and the 45-degree reference line, along which $C + I + G + X = Y$ (total planned expenditures equal real national income). The new equilibrium level of real national income is \$10 trillion per year. Thus the increase in equilibrium real national income is equal to five times the permanent increase in planned investment spending.

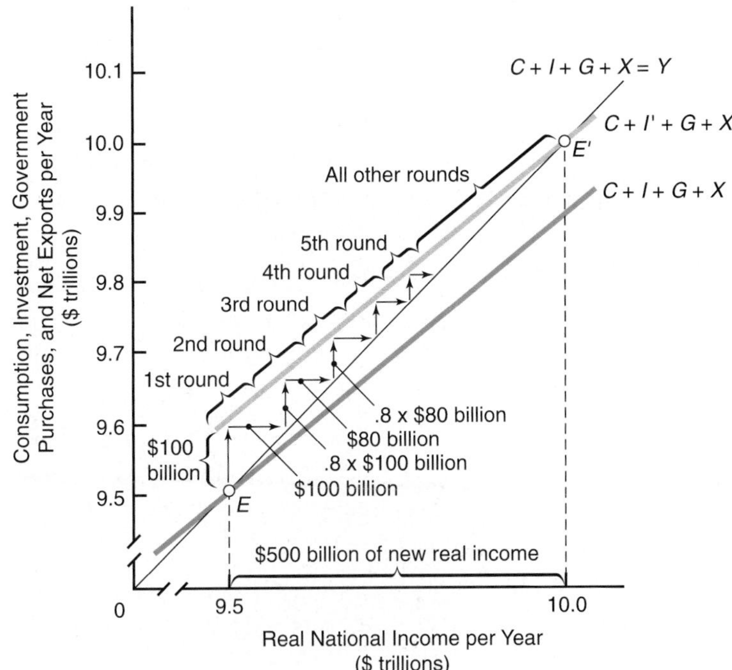

FIGURE B-1

Graphing the Multiplier

We can translate Table 12-3 in Chapter 12 into graphic form by looking at each successive round of additional spending induced by an autonomous increase in planned investment of \$100 billion. The total planned expenditures curve shifts from $C + I + G + X$, with its associated equilibrium level of real national income of \$9.5 trillion, to a new curve labeled $C + I' + G + X$. The new equilibrium level of real national income is \$10 trillion. Equilibrium is again established.

CHAPTER 13

FISCAL POLICY

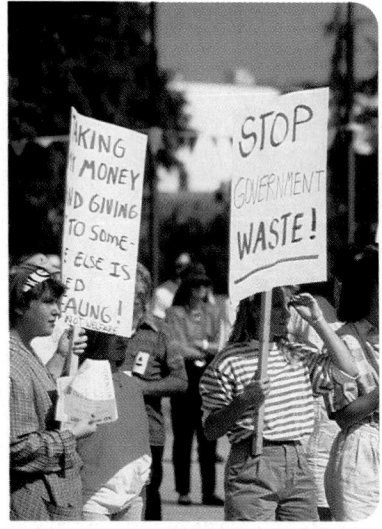

After years of running deficits, the federal government started running surpluses at the end of the 1990s. How would this group of protesters suggest that the surpluses be eliminated?

In recent years, politicians across America have squabbled about whether the nation should "protect" current and expected future federal budget surpluses—government tax receipts in excess of government expenditures—and use them to pay off the government's debts. Others advocate spending the surpluses (in which case, of course, there would no longer be surpluses) on "crucial government programs." Still others argue that surpluses should be "returned to the American people" via tax cuts (in which case there would also no longer be surpluses). What kinds of budgetary policies, known as *fiscal policies,* should the government pursue? To contemplate this question, you must learn more about how changes in government spending and taxes affect the economy. Those effects are the subject of this chapter.

LEARNING OBJECTIVES

After reading this chapter, you should be able to:

1. **Use traditional Keynesian analysis to evaluate the effects of discretionary fiscal policies**
2. **Discuss ways in which indirect crowding out and direct expenditure offsets can reduce the effectiveness of fiscal policy actions**
3. **Explain why the Ricardian equivalence theorem calls into question the usefulness of tax changes**
4. **List and define fiscal policy time lags and explain why they complicate efforts to engage in fiscal "fine tuning"**
5. **Describe how certain aspects of fiscal policy function as automatic stabilizers for the economy**
6. **Distinguish between government deficits and the public debt**

Did You Know That... the first type of income tax was probably established in the 1200s and 1300s during times of war in the Italian city-states? America's first income tax, enacted in 1861 to help pay for the Civil War, was 3 percent on incomes over $800 a year. Not until the Sixteenth Amendment to the Constitution was ratified in 1913 did most Americans come to know of the federal income tax, and even then very few had to pay it. Today, federal income taxes are taken for granted. More important for this chapter, the federal tax system is now viewed as being capable of affecting the equilibrium level of real GDP. On the spending side of the budget, changes in the federal government's expenditures are also viewed as potentially capable of changing the equilibrium level of real GDP.

Chapter Outline

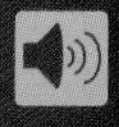

DISCRETIONARY FISCAL POLICY

Deliberate, discretionary changes in government expenditures or taxes (or both) to achieve certain national economic goals is the realm of **fiscal policy.** Some national goals are high employment (low unemployment), price stability, economic growth, and improvement in the nation's international payments balance. Fiscal policy can be thought of as a deliberate attempt to cause the economy to move to full employment and price stability more quickly than it otherwise might.

Fiscal policy 

The discretionary changing of government expenditures or taxes to achieve national economic goals, such as high employment with price stability.

Fiscal policy has typically been associated with the economic theories of John Maynard Keynes and what is now called *traditional* Keynesian analysis. Recall from Chapter 11 that Keynes's explanation of the Great Depression was that there was insufficient aggregate demand. Because he believed that wages and prices were "sticky downward," he argued that the classical economists' picture of an economy moving automatically and quickly toward full employment was inaccurate. To Keynes and his followers, government had to step in to increase aggregate demand. In other words, expansionary fiscal policy initiated by the federal government was the way to ward off recessions and depressions.

Traditional Keynesian economics dominated academic discussion and government policymaking in the 1960s and 1970s. Perhaps the best-known policy action based on traditional Keynesian theory was the Kennedy-Johnson tax cut of 1964. When John F. Kennedy took office in 1961 promising to "get the country moving again," his advisers recommended a tax cut. The tax cut was not implemented until after Kennedy's death, but in 1964, federal taxes were slashed by $11 billion; within a year, the unemployment rate had fallen from 5.2 percent to 4.5 percent.

As you will see in Chapter 18, modern-day variants of Keynesian analysis are now taking center stage in policymaking discussions.

Changes in Government Spending

In Chapter 11, we looked at the recessionary gap and the inflationary gap (see Figures 11-12 and 11-13). The recessionary gap was defined as the amount by which the current level of real GDP fell short of the economy's potential production if it were operating on its *LRAS*. The inflationary gap was defined as the amount by which the equilibrium level of real GDP exceeds the long-run equilibrium level as given by *LRAS*. Let us examine fiscal policy first in the context of a recessionary gap.

When There Is a Recessionary Gap. The government, along with firms, individuals, and foreigners, is one of the spending agents in the economy. When the government decides to spend more, all other things held constant, the dollar value of total spending must rise.

FIGURE 13-1
Expansionary and Contractionary Fiscal Policy: Changes in *G*
If there is a recessionary gap and short-run equilibrium is at E_1 in panel (a), fiscal policy can presumably increase aggregate demand to AD_2. The new equilibrium is at E_2 at higher real GDP per year and a higher price level. In panel (b), the economy is at short-run equilibrium at E_1, which is at a higher real income than the *LRAS*. To reduce this inflationary gap, fiscal policy can be used to decrease aggregate demand from AD_1 to AD_2. Eventually, equilibrium will fall to E_2, which is on the *LRAS*.

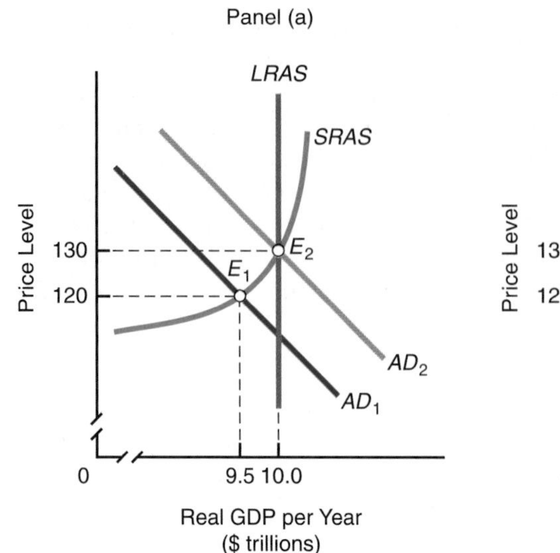

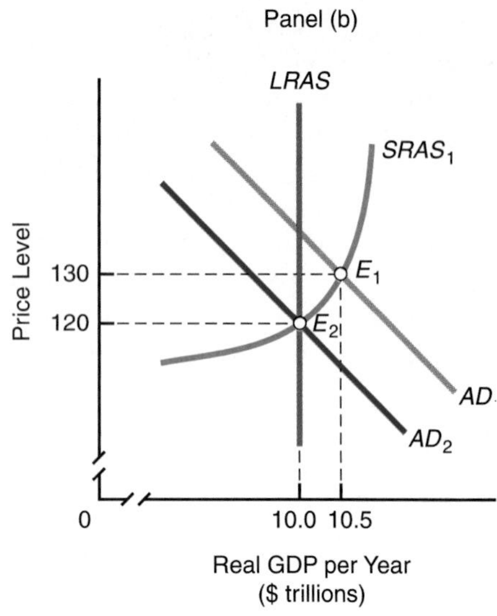

Look at panel (a) of Figure 13-1. We start at short-run equilibrium with AD_1 intersecting *SRAS* at \$9.5 trillion of real GDP per year. There is a recessionary gap of \$500 billion of real GDP per year—the difference between *LRAS* (the economy's long-run potential) and the short-run equilibrium level of real GDP per year. When the government decides to spend more (expansionary fiscal policy), the aggregate demand curve shifts to the right to AD_2. Here we assume that the government knows exactly how much more to spend so that AD_2 intersects *SRAS* at \$10 trillion, or at *LRAS*. Because of the upward-sloping *SRAS,* the price level rises from 120 to 130 as real GDP goes to \$10 trillion per year.

Click here to find out the fractions of GDP allocated to government spending and taxes in the most recent period.

When There Is an Inflationary Gap. The entire process shown in panel (a) of Figure 13-1 can be reversed, as shown in panel (b). An inflationary gap occurs at the intersection of $SRAS_1$ and AD_1, at point E_1. The economy cannot be sustained at \$10.5 trillion indefinitely, because this exceeds long-run aggregate supply, which is in real terms \$10 trillion. If the government recognizes this and reduces its spending (pursues a contractionary fiscal policy), this action reduces aggregate demand from AD_1 to AD_2. Equilibrium will fall to E_2, where real GDP per year is \$10 trillion, which is on the *LRAS.* The price level will fall from 130 to 120.

Changes in Taxes

The spending decisions of firms, individuals, and foreigners depend on the taxes levied on them. Individuals in their role as consumers look to their disposable (after-tax) income when determining their desired rates of consumption. Firms look at their after-tax profits when deciding on the levels of investment to undertake. Foreigners look at the tax-inclusive

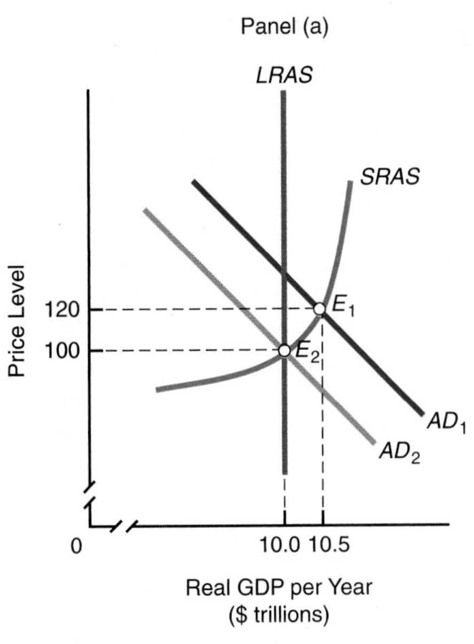

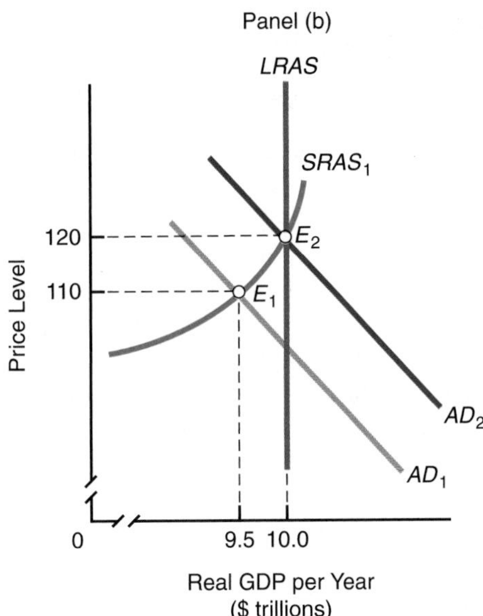

FIGURE 13-2

Contractionary and Expansionary Fiscal Policy: Changes in *T*

In panel (a), the economy is initially at E_1, which exceeds *LRAS*. Contractionary fiscal policy can move aggregate demand to AD_2 so that the new equilibrium is at E_2 at a lower price level and now at *LRAS*. In panel (b), with a recessionary gap (in this case of $500 billion), taxes are cut. AD_1 moves to AD_2. The economy moves from E_1 to E_2, and real GDP is now at $10 trillion per year, the *LRAS* level.

cost of goods when deciding whether to buy in the United States or elsewhere. Therefore, holding all other things constant, a rise in taxes causes a reduction in aggregate demand because it reduces consumption, investment, or net exports. What actually happens depends, of course, on the parties on whom the taxes are levied.

When the Current Short-Run Equilibrium Is Greater than *LRAS*. Assume that aggregate demand is AD_1 in panel (a) of Figure 13-2. It intersects *SRAS* at E_1, which is at a level greater than *LRAS*. In this situation, an increase in taxes shifts the aggregate demand curve inward to the left. For argument's sake, assume that it intersects *SRAS* at E_2, or exactly where *LRAS* intersects AD_2. In this situation, the equilibrium level of real GDP falls from $10.5 trillion per year to $10 trillion per year. The price level falls from 120 to 100.

When the Current Short-Run Equilibrium Is Less than *LRAS*. Look at panel (b) in Figure 13-2. AD_1 intersects *SRAS* at E_1, with real GDP at $9.5 trillion, less than the *LRAS* of $10 trillion. In this situation, a decrease in taxes shifts the aggregate demand curve outward to the right. At AD_2, equilibrium is established at E_2, with the price level at 120 and equilibrium real GDP at $10 trillion per year.

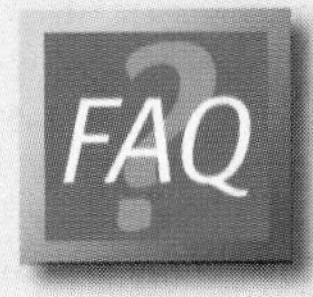

Don't cuts in income tax rates necessarily reduce the government's tax revenues by exactly the same percentage of income?

No, because cuts in income tax rates cause equilibrium national income to rise. Certainly, one effect of a cut in tax rates is a reduction in tax collections at the *current* level of national income. To jump to the conclusion implied by the question, however, assumes that the economy is static and unchanging in response to reduced tax rates. Lower income tax rates generate higher consumption, which pushes up equilibrium national income. This tends to push the government's tax receipts back up, because more income is taxed at the new lower rates. In theory, it is even possible that this "dynamic effect" of income tax rate cuts could lead to *higher* net tax revenues following cuts in income tax rates.

POLICY EXAMPLE

Did the New Deal Really Provide a Stimulus?

Many researchers have pointed out that Franklin Roosevelt's New Deal was influenced by Keynes's view that government had to increase "effective" aggregate demand. To be sure, the New Deal included what appeared on the surface to be large federal government expenditures and numerous government jobs programs. We have to look at the total picture, however. During the Great Depression, taxes were raised repeatedly. The Revenue Act of 1932, for example, passed during the depths of the Depression, brought the largest percentage increase in federal taxes in the history of the United States in peacetime—it almost doubled total federal tax revenues. Federal government deficits during the Depression years were small. In fact, in 1937 the total government budget—for federal, state, and local levels—was in surplus by $300 million. For many years during the period, at the same time that the federal government was increasing expenditures, local and state governments were decreasing them. If we measure the total of federal, state, and local fiscal policies, we find that they were truly expansive only in 1931 and 1936 compared to what the government was doing prior to the Great Depression. These two years were expansive only because of large payments to veterans, passed by Congress in both years over the vigorous opposition of the president.

For Critical Analysis

What other aspects of the New Deal might be studied to see if they had expansionary effects on the national economy?

CONCEPTS IN BRIEF

- Fiscal policy is defined as the discretionary change in government expenditures or taxes to achieve such national goals as high employment or reduced inflation.
- If there is a recessionary gap and the economy is operating at less than long-run average supply *(LRAS)*, an increase in government spending can shift the aggregate demand curve to the right and perhaps lead to a higher equilibrium level of real GDP per year.
- If there is an inflationary gap, a decrease in government spending can shift the aggregate demand curve to the left, reducing the equilibrium level of real GDP per year to be consistent with *LRAS*.
- Changes in taxes can have similar effects on the equilibrium rate of real GDP and the price level. A decrease in taxes can lead to an increase in real GDP. In contrast, if there is an inflationary gap, an increase in taxes can decrease equilibrium real GDP.

POSSIBLE OFFSETS TO FISCAL POLICY

Fiscal policy does not operate in a vacuum. Important questions have to be answered: If government expenditures increase, how are those expenditures financed, and by whom? If taxes are increased, what does the government do with the taxes? What will happen if individuals worry about increases in *future* taxes because there is more government spending today with no increased taxes? All of these questions involve *offsets* to the effects of fiscal policy. We will look at each of them and others in detail.

Indirect Crowding Out 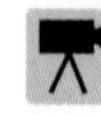

Let's take the first example of fiscal policy in this chapter, an increase in government expenditures. If government expenditures rise and taxes are held constant, something has to give. Our government does not simply take goods and services when it wants them. It has to pay for them. When it pays for them and does not simultaneously collect the same amount in taxes, it must borrow. That means that an increase in government spending without raising taxes creates additional government borrowing from the private sector (or from foreigners).

Induced Interest Rate Changes. Holding everything else constant, if the government attempts to borrow more from the private sector to pay for its increased budget deficit, it is not going to have an easy time selling its bonds. If the bond market is in equilibrium, when the government tries to sell more bonds, it is going to have to offer a better deal in order to get rid of them. A better deal means offering a higher interest rate. This is the interest rate effect of expansionary fiscal policy financed by borrowing from the public. In this sense, when the federal government finances increased spending by additional borrowing, it will push interest rates up. When interest rates go up, it is more expensive for firms to finance new construction, equipment, and inventories. It is also more expensive for individuals to finance their cars and homes. Thus a rise in government spending, holding taxes constant (in short, deficit spending), tends to crowd out private spending, dampening the positive effect of increased government spending on aggregate demand. This is called the **crowding-out effect.** In the extreme case, the crowding out may be complete, with the increased government spending having no net effect on aggregate demand. The final result is simply more government spending and less private investment and consumption. Figure 13-3 shows how the crowding-out effect occurs.

Crowding-out effect
The tendency of expansionary fiscal policy to cause a decrease in planned investment or planned consumption in the private sector; this decrease normally results from the rise in interest rates.

The Firm's Investment Decision. To understand the interest rate effect better, consider a firm that is contemplating borrowing $100,000 to expand its business. Suppose that the interest rate is 7 percent. The interest payments on the debt will be 7 percent times $100,000, or $7,000 per year ($583 per month). A rise in the interest rate to 10 percent will push the payments to 10 percent of $100,000, or $10,000 per year ($833 per month). The extra $250 per month in interest expenses will discourage some firms from making the investment. Consumers face similar decisions when they purchase houses and cars. An increase in the interest rate causes their monthly payments to go up, thereby discouraging some of them from purchasing cars and houses.

Graphical Analysis. You see in Figure 13-4 that the initial equilibrium, E_1, is below *LRAS*. But suppose that government expansionary fiscal policy in the form of increased government spending (without increasing current taxes) shifts aggregate demand from AD_1 to AD_2. In the absence of the crowding-out effect, the real output of goods and

FIGURE 13-3
The Crowding-Out Effect, Step-by-Step

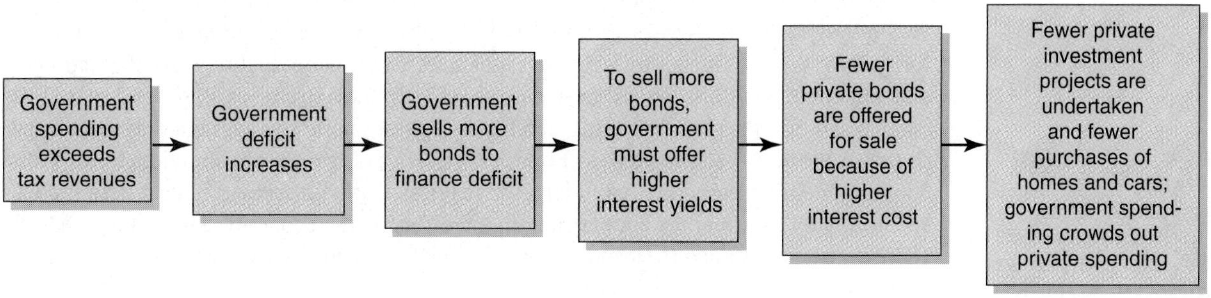

Government spending exceeds tax revenues → Government deficit increases → Government sells more bonds to finance deficit → To sell more bonds, government must offer higher interest yields → Fewer private bonds are offered for sale because of higher interest cost → Fewer private investment projects are undertaken and fewer purchases of homes and cars; government spending crowds out private spending

FIGURE 13-4

The Crowding-Out Effect

Expansionary fiscal policy that causes deficit financing initially shifts AD_1 to AD_2. Equilibrium initially moves toward E_2. But expansionary fiscal policy pushes up interest rates, which reduces interest-sensitive spending. This effect causes the aggregate demand curve to shift inward to AD_3, and the new short-run equilibrium is at E_3.

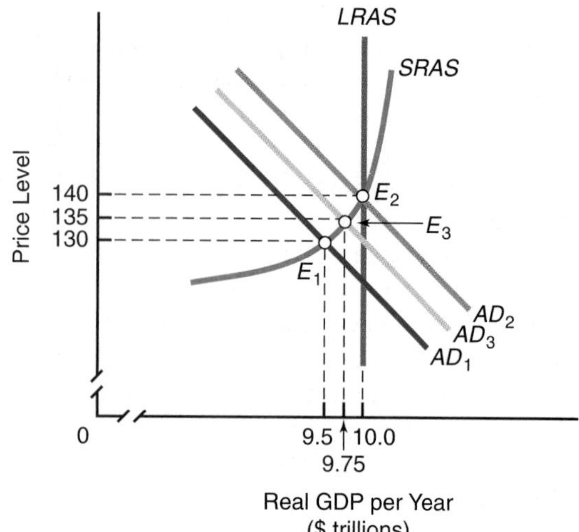

services would increase to $10 trillion per year, and the price level would rise to 140 (point E_2). With the (partial) crowding-out effect, however, as investment and consumption decline, partly offsetting the rise in government spending, the aggregate demand curve shifts inward to the left to AD_3. The new equilibrium is now at E_3, with real GDP of $9.75 trillion per year at a price level of 135. In other words, crowding out dilutes the effect of expansionary fiscal policy, and a recessionary gap remains.

Planning for the Future: The Ricardian Equivalence Theorem

Economists have implicitly assumed that people look at changes in taxes or changes in government spending only in the present. What if people actually think about the size of *future* tax payments? Does this have an effect on how they react to an increase in government spending with no tax increases? Some economists believe that the answer is yes. What if people's horizons extend beyond this year? Don't we then have to take into account the effects of today's government policies on the future?

Consider an example. The government wants to reduce taxes by $100 billion today. Assume that government spending remains constant. Assume further that the government initially has a balanced budget. Thus the only way for the government to pay for this $100 billion tax cut is to borrow $100 billion today. The public will owe $100 billion plus interest later. Realizing that a $100 billion tax cut today is mathematically equivalent to $100 billion plus interest later, people may wish to save the tax cut to meet future tax liabilities—payment of interest and repayment of debt.

Consequently, a tax cut may not affect total planned expenditures. A reduction in taxes without a reduction in government spending, according to the new classical economists, will therefore not necessarily have a large impact on aggregate demand.

Similarly, increased government spending without an increase in taxes will not necessarily have a large impact on aggregate demand. In terms of Figure 13-4, the aggregate demand curve will shift inward from AD_1 to AD_3. In the extreme case, if consumers fully compensate for a higher future tax liability by saving more, the aggregate demand curve shifts all the way back to AD_1 in Figure 13-4. This is the case of individuals fully discounting their increased tax liabilities. The result is that an increased budget deficit created entirely by a current tax cut has literally no effect on the economy. This is known as the **Ricardian equivalence theorem,** after the nineteenth-century economist David Ricardo, who first developed the argument publicly.

Ricardian equivalence theorem The proposition that an increase in the government budget deficit has no effect on aggregate demand.

For economists who believe in the Ricardian equivalence theorem, it does not matter how government expenditures are financed—by taxes or by issuing debt. Is the Ricardian equivalence theorem correct? Research so far has not provided much compelling evidence either way.

Direct Expenditure Offsets

Government has a distinct comparative advantage over the private sector in certain activities such as diplomacy and national defense. Otherwise stated, certain resource-using activities in which the government engages do not compete with the private sector. In contrast, some of what government does competes directly with the private sector, such as education. When government competes with the private sector, **direct expenditure offsets** to fiscal policy may occur. For example, if the government starts providing milk at no charge to students who are already purchasing milk, there is a direct expenditure offset. Households spend less directly on milk, but government spends more.

Direct expenditure offsets 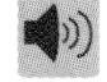
Actions on the part of the private sector in spending income that offset government fiscal policy actions. Any increase in government spending in an area that competes with the private sector will have some direct expenditure offset.

The normal way to analyze the impact of an increase in government spending on aggregate demand is implicitly to assume that government spending is *not* a substitute for private spending. This is clearly the case for a cruise missile. Whenever government spending is a substitute for private spending, however, a rise in government spending causes a direct reduction in private spending to offset it.

The Extreme Case. In the extreme case, the direct expenditure offset is dollar for dollar, so we merely end up with a relabeling of spending from private to public. Assume that you have decided to spend $100 on groceries. Upon your arrival at the checkout counter, you are met by a U.S. Department of Agriculture official. She announces that she will pay for your groceries—but only the ones in the cart. Here increased government spending is $100. You leave the store in bliss. But just as you are deciding how to spend the $100, an Internal Revenue Service agent meets you. He announces that as a result of the current budgetary crisis, your taxes are going to rise by $100. You have to pay right now. Increases in taxes have now been $100. We have a balanced-budget increase in government spending. In this scenario, there would be no change in total spending. We simply end up with higher government spending, which directly offsets exactly the same amount of consumption. Aggregate demand and GDP are unchanged. Otherwise stated, if there is a full direct expenditure offset, the government spending multiplier is zero.

The Less Extreme Case. Much government spending has a private-sector substitute. When government expenditures increase, there is a tendency for private spending to decline somewhat (but not in proportion), thereby mitigating the upward impact on total aggregate demand. To the extent that there are some direct expenditure offsets to expansionary fiscal policy, predicted changes in aggregate demand will be lessened. Consequently, real output and the price level will be less affected.

POLICY EXAMPLE

Crowding-Out Effects During World War II

Most American history books point to World War II as a clear-cut example of beneficial expansionary fiscal policy in action. The U.S. economy was pulled out of the Great Depression by enormous governmental outlays for the war effort—or so the story goes. The actual situation was a little more complex, though. The U.S. economy's growth rate from 1933 to 1941 was already higher than that of any other recorded peacetime period of the same length. Moreover, the increase in military expenditures during World War II was not matched by a similar increase in total output. In fact, it looks as if the crowding-out effect was relatively large, at least much greater than the history books indicate. This can be readily observed in terms of what happened to per capita personal consumption expenditures. They dropped by 3.5 percent in real terms from 1941 and 1942 and did not rebound to 1941 levels until after 1944. In other words, the average American saw no real increase in living standards during the war, in spite of massive military expenditures.

For Critical Analysis

Given the information presented here, what could you say about the government's spending multiplier during World War II?

The Supply-Side Effects of Changes in Taxes

We have talked about changing taxes and changing government spending, the traditional tools of fiscal policy. We have not really talked about the possibility of changing marginal tax rates. Recall from Chapter 5 that the marginal tax rate is the rate applied to the last bracket of taxable income. In our federal tax system, higher marginal tax rates are applied as income rises. In that sense, the United States has a progressive federal individual income tax system. Expansionary fiscal policy might involve reducing marginal tax rates. Advocates of such changes argue that lower tax rates will lead to an increase in productivity because individuals will work harder and longer, save more, and invest more and that increased productivity will lead to more economic growth, which will lead to higher real GDP. The government, by applying lower marginal tax rates, will not necessarily lose tax revenues, for the lower marginal tax rates will be applied to a growing tax base because of economic growth—after all, tax revenues are the product of a tax rate times a tax base.

This relationship is sometimes called the Laffer curve, named after economist Arthur Laffer, who developed it in front of some journalists and politicians in 1974. It is reproduced in Figure 13-5. On the vertical axis are tax revenues, and on the horizontal axis is the marginal tax rate. As you can see, total tax revenues rise and then eventually fall as tax rates increase after some unspecified tax-revenue-maximizing rate.

People who support the notion that reducing taxes does not necessarily lead to reduced tax revenues are called supply-side economists. **Supply-side economics** involves changing the tax structure to create incentives to increase productivity. Due to a shift in the aggregate

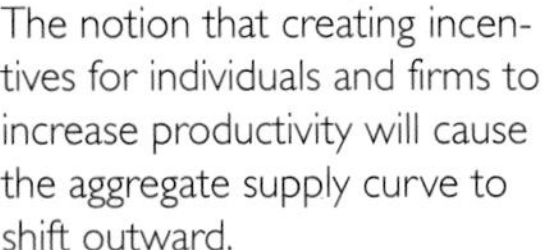

The notion that creating incentives for individuals and firms to increase productivity will cause the aggregate supply curve to shift outward.

FIGURE 13-5

Laffer Curve

The Laffer Curve indicates that tax revenues initially rise with a higher tax rate. Eventually, however, tax revenues decline as the tax rate increases.

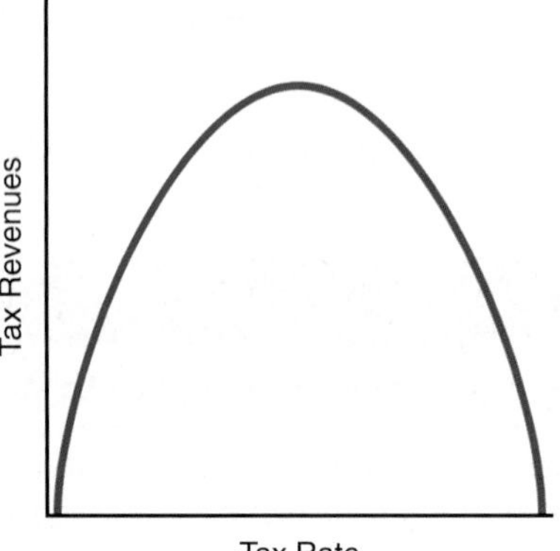

supply curve to the right, there can be greater output without upward pressure on the price level.

Consider the supply-side effects of changes in marginal tax rates on labor. An increase in tax rates reduces the opportunity cost of leisure, thereby inducing individuals (at least on the margin) to reduce their work effort and to consume more leisure. But an increase in tax rates will also reduce spendable income, thereby shifting the demand curve for leisure inward to the left. Here a reduction in real spendable income shifts the demand curve for all goods and services, including leisure, inward to the left. The outcome of these two effects on the choice of leisure (and thus work) depends on which of them is stronger. Supply-side economists argue that in the 1970s and 1980s, the first effect dominated: Increases in marginal tax rates caused workers to work less, and decreases in marginal tax rates caused workers to work more.

INTERNATIONAL EXAMPLE

Islam and Supply-Side Economics

Supply-side economics has a long history, dating back to at least the fourteenth century. The greatest of medieval Islamic historians, Abu Zayd Abd-ar-Rahman Ibn Khaldun (1332–1406), included an Islamic view of supply-side economics in his monumental book *The Muqaddimah* (1377). He pointed out that "when tax assessments . . . upon the subjects are low, the latter have the energy and desire to do things. Cultural enterprises grow and increase . . . . [Therefore] the number of individual imposts [taxes] and assessments mounts." If taxes are increased both in size and rates, "the result is that the interest of subjects in cultural enterprises disappears, because when they compare expenditures and taxes with their income and gain and see little profit they make, they lose all hope." Ibn Khaldun concluded that "at the beginning of a dynasty, taxation yields a large revenue from small assessments. At the end of a dynasty, taxation yields a small revenue from large assessments."

For Critical Analysis

How do this Islamic scholar's economic theories apply to the modern world?

CONCEPTS IN BRIEF

- Indirect crowding out occurs because of an interest rate effect in which the government's efforts to finance its deficit spending cause interest rates to rise, thereby crowding out private investment and spending, particularly on cars and houses. This is called the crowding-out effect.
- Direct expenditure offsets occur when government spending competes with the private sector and is increased. A direct crowding-out effect may occur.
- Many new classical economists believe in the Ricardian equivalence theorem, which holds that an increase in the government budget deficit has no effect on aggregate demand because individuals correctly perceive their increased future taxes and therefore save more today to pay for them.
- Changes in marginal tax rates may cause supply-side effects if a reduction in marginal tax rates induces enough additional work, saving, and investing. Government tax receipts can actually increase. This is called supply-side economics.

DISCRETIONARY FISCAL POLICY IN PRACTICE: COPING WITH TIME LAGS

We can discuss fiscal policy in a relatively precise way. We draw graphs with aggregate demand and supply curves to show what we are doing. We could even in principle estimate the offsets that we just discussed. However, even if we were able to measure all of these offsets exactly, would-be fiscal policymakers still face a problem: The conduct of fiscal policy involves a variety of time lags.

Recognition time lag 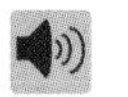
The time required to gather information about the current state of the economy.

Policymakers must be concerned with time lags. Quite apart from the fact that it is difficult to measure economic variables, it takes time to collect and assimilate such data. Thus policymakers must contend with the **recognition time lag,** the months that may elapse before economic problems can be identified.*

Action time lag 
The time between recognizing an economic problem and implementing policy to solve it. The action time lag is quite long for fiscal policy, which requires congressional approval.

After an economic problem is recognized, a solution must be formulated; thus there will be an **action time lag,** the period between the recognition of a problem and the implementation of policy to solve it. For fiscal policy, the action time lag is particularly long. Such policy must be approved by Congress and is subject to political wrangling and infighting. The action time lag can easily last a year or two. Then it takes time to put the policy into effect. After Congress enacts fiscal policy legislation, it takes time to decide such matters as who gets new federal construction contracts.

Effect time lag 
The time that elapses between the onset of policy and the results of that policy.

Finally, there is the **effect time lag:** After fiscal policy is enacted, it takes time for it to affect the economy. To demonstrate the effects, economists need only shift curves on a chalkboard, but in real time, multiplier effects take quite a while to work their way through the economy.

Because the various fiscal policy time lags are long, a policy designed to combat a recession might not produce results until the economy is already out of recession and perhaps experiencing inflation, in which case the fiscal policy would worsen the situation. Or a fiscal policy designed to eliminate inflation might not produce effects until the economy is in a recession; in that case, too, fiscal policy would make the economic problem worse rather than better.

Furthermore, because fiscal policy time lags tend to be *variable* (by anywhere from one to three years), policymakers have a difficult time fine-tuning the economy. Clearly, fiscal policy is more an art than a science.

INTERNATIONAL POLICY EXAMPLE

Keynesian Fiscal Policy Loses Its Luster

Some analysts argue that John Maynard Keynes was the most influential economist of the twentieth century, for he supposedly armed policymakers with fiscal weapons that allowed them to fight recession. Yet at the beginning of the twenty-first century, influential policymakers throughout the world are ignoring the concept of government spending as a way out of recessions.

Even though European governments have long favored welfare spending, the 11 that joined together to use the common currency called the euro also agreed to some specific anti-government-spending stipulations. These countries, including France and Germany, are committed to keeping public deficits at 3 percent or less of gross domestic product. Whenever a country's public deficit exceeds this figure, the offending government can be fined up to 0.5 percent of its GDP. Deficit spending—a favorite Keynesian fiscal policy action—is tightly constrained in these countries.

In 1999, Brazil's president, Fernando Enrique Cardoso, stated that in the face of the then current recession, "we will need to put in place as rapidly as possible a fiscal austerity plan so that interest rates can fall and

*Final annual data for GDP, after various revisions, are not forthcoming for three to six months after the year's end.

Brazil can begin to grow again." He publicly announced that the country's government sector should shrink by 3 percent the following year even when his government economists predicted a probable 4 percent decrease in real GDP.

The International Monetary Fund did a study on fiscal policy a few years ago. It examined attempts by governments to reduce public spending and public debt. It looked at 62 attempts over two and a half decades. Its conclusion was that in the 14 cases for which the governments had aggressively reduced government spending, as in Denmark and Ireland, those economies had the fastest growth rates. The IMF contended that there may have been a "virtuous circle between economic growth and debt-reduction programs."

For Critical Analysis

How might Keynes have responded to this increase in anti-Keynesianism?

AUTOMATIC STABILIZERS

Not all changes in taxes (or in tax rates) or in government spending (including government transfers) constitute discretionary fiscal policy. There are several types of automatic (or nondiscretionary) fiscal policies. Such policies do not require new legislation on the part of Congress. Specific automatic fiscal policies—called **automatic,** or **built-in, stabilizers**—include the tax system itself and the government transfer system; the latter includes unemployment compensation and welfare spending.

Automatic, or built-in, stabilizers 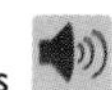
Special provisions of certain federal programs that cause changes in desired aggregate expenditures without the action of Congress and the president. Examples are the federal tax system and unemployment compensation.

The Tax System as an Automatic Stabilizer

You know that if you work less, you are paid less, and therefore you pay fewer taxes. The amount of taxes that our government collects falls automatically during a recession. Basically, incomes and profits fall when business activity slows down, and the government's take drops too. Some economists consider this an automatic tax cut, which therefore stimulates aggregate demand. It reduces the extent of any negative economic fluctuation.

The progressive nature of both the federal personal and corporate income tax systems magnifies any automatic stabilization effect that might exist. If your hours of work are reduced because of a recession, you still pay federal personal income taxes. But because of our progressive system, you may drop into a lower tax bracket, thereby paying a lower marginal tax rate. As a result, your disposable income falls by a smaller percentage than your before-tax income falls.

Unemployment Compensation and Welfare Payments

Like our tax system unemployment compensation payments stabilize aggregate demand. Throughout the business cycle, unemployment compensation reduces *changes* in people's disposable income. When business activity drops, most laid-off workers automatically become eligible for unemployment compensation from their state governments. Their disposable income therefore remains positive, although certainly it is less than when they were employed. During boom periods there is less unemployment, and consequently fewer unemployment payments are made to the labor force. Less purchasing power is being added to the economy because fewer unemployment checks are paid out. Historically, the relationship between the unemployment rate and unemployment compensation payments has been strongly positive.

FIGURE 13-6
Automatic Stabilizers
Here we assume that as real national income rises, tax revenues rise and government transfers fall, other things remaining constant. Thus as the economy expands from Y_f to Y_1, a budget surplus automatically arises; as the economy contracts from Y_f to Y_2, a budget deficit automatically arises. Such automatic changes tend to drive the economy back toward its full-employment real national income.

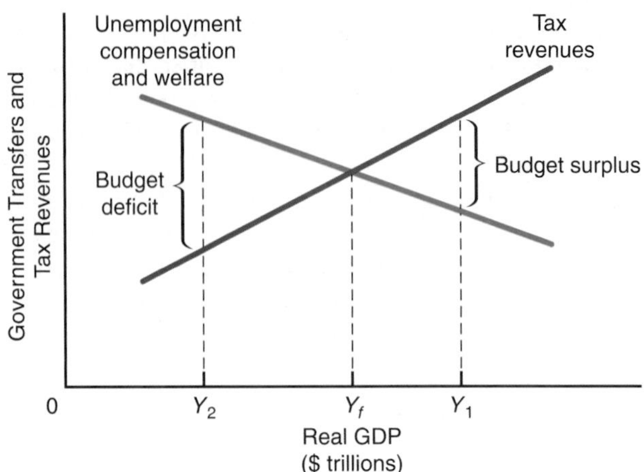

Welfare payments act similarly as an automatic stabilizer. When a recession occurs, more people become eligible for welfare payments. Therefore, those people do not experience so dramatic a drop in disposable income as they would have otherwise.

Stabilizing Impact

The key stabilizing impact of our tax system, unemployment compensation, and welfare payments is their ability to mitigate undesirable changes in disposable income, consumption, and the equilibrium level of national income. If disposable income is prevented from falling as much as it would during a recession, the downturn will be moderated. In contrast, if disposable income is prevented from rising as rapidly as it would during a boom, the boom is less likely to get out of hand. The progressive income tax and unemployment compensation thus provide automatic stabilization to the economy. We present the argument graphically in Figure 13-6.

WHAT DO WE REALLY KNOW ABOUT FISCAL POLICY?

There are two ways of looking at fiscal policy, one that prevails during normal times and the other during abnormal times.

Fiscal Policy During Normal Times

Click here to learn about the current outlook for the budget of the U. S. government.

During normal times (without "excessive" unemployment, inflation, or problems in the national economy), we know that due to the recognition time lag and the modest size of any fiscal policy action that Congress will actually take, discretionary fiscal policy is probably not very effective. Congress ends up doing too little too late to help in a minor recession. Moreover, fiscal policy that generates repeated tax changes (as it has done) creates uncertainty, which may do more harm than good. To the extent that fiscal policy has any effect during normal times, it probably achieves this by way of automatic stabilizers rather than by way of discretionary policy.

Fiscal Policy During Abnormal Times

During abnormal times, fiscal policy may be effective. Consider some classic examples: the Great Depression and war periods.

The Great Depression. When there is a catastrophic drop in real GDP, as there was during the Great Depression, fiscal policy may be able to stimulate aggregate demand. Because so many people are income-constrained during such periods, government spending is a way to get income into their hands.

Wartime. Wars are in fact reserved for governments. War expenditures are not good substitutes for private expenditures—they have little or no direct expenditure offsets. Consequently, war spending as part of expansionary fiscal policy usually has noteworthy effects, such as occurred while we were waging World War II, during which real GDP increased dramatically.

The "Soothing" Effect of Keynesian Fiscal Policy

One view of traditional Keynesian fiscal policy does not relate to its being used on a regular basis. As you have learned in this chapter, there are many problems associated with attempting to use fiscal policy. But if we should encounter a severe downturn, fiscal policy is available. Knowing this may reassure consumers and investors. After all, the ability of the federal government to prevent another Great Depression—given what we know about how to use fiscal policy today—may take some of the large risk out of consumers' and investors' calculations. This may induce more buoyant and stable expectations of the future, thereby smoothing investment spending.

DEFICIT FINANCING AND THE PUBLIC DEBT

Discretionary fiscal policy has mostly resulted in the government's purposely spending more than it receives. This is often called *deficit financing* and creates a federal budget deficit. Sometimes it has even been called *Keynesian deficit financing,* for many economists consider increased government spending (without raising taxes) stimulative. Indeed, you have been reading about using discretionary fiscal policy to close a recessionary gap.

Flows Versus Stocks: Deficits and Debts

Each year that the government spends more than it collects in revenues, it runs a deficit. This is a flow, something that happens on a yearly basis or over time. The accumulation of deficits results in an increasing government debt. The debt is a stock, which is an accumulation of years' deficits.

For decades, federal budget deficits were common and indeed almost expected. That changed in 1998, when the federal government ran its first official surplus since 1969. Yet even though the government may not be running a budget deficit, the United States still has the stock of accumulated deficits: its net public debt.

The Federal Public Debt

All federal public debt, taken together, is called the **gross public debt.** Many government agencies own government securities. This interagency borrowing really has no effect on anything—it's like taking one IOU out of your left pocket and putting it into your right pocket. Therefore, when we subtract out the portion of the gross public debt held by government agencies, we arrive at the **net public debt.** The net public debt is currently about $2.6 trillion. You can see in Figure 13-7 on page 312 what has happened to the net U.S.

Gross Public Debt 
All federal government debt irrespective of who owns it.

Net Public Debt 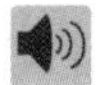
Gross public debt minus all government interagency borrowing.

FIGURE 13-7

Net U.S. Public Debt as a Percentage of GDP

During World War II, the net public debt grew dramatically. It fell until the 1970s, rose again until the early 1990s, and has been declining ever since.

Source: U.S. Department of the Treasury.

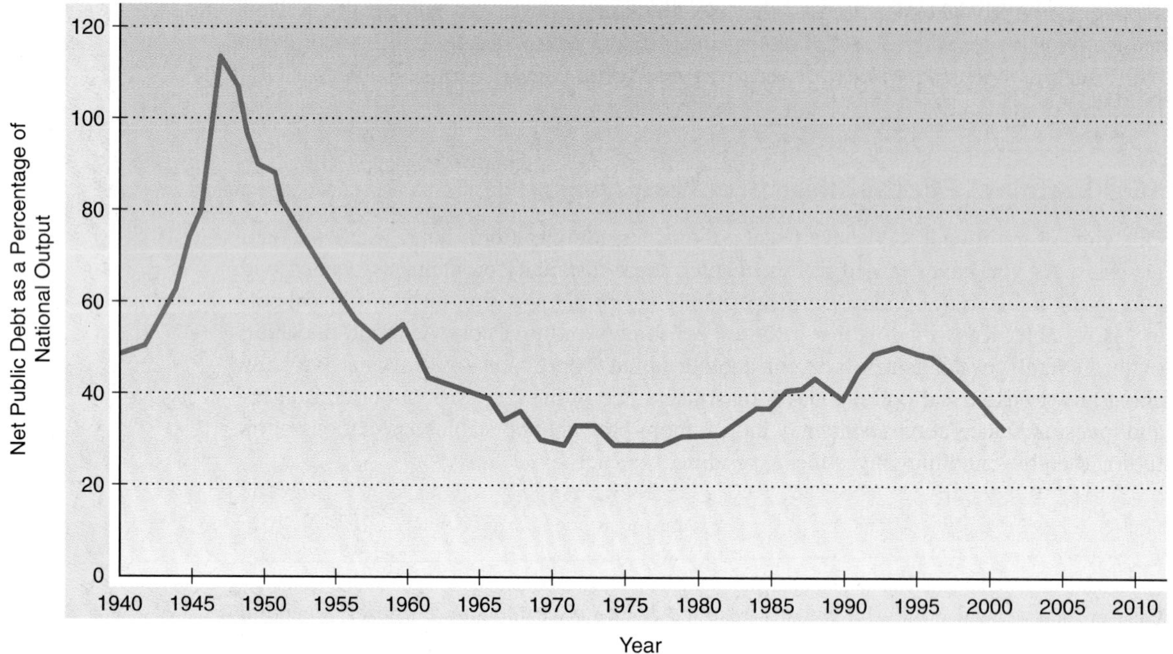

public debt expressed as a percentage of GDP. It reached its peak right after World War II, fell until the 1970s, rose again until the early 1990s, and has been declining ever since.

CONCEPTS IN BRIEF

- Time lags of various sorts reduce the effectiveness of fiscal policy. These include the recognition time lag, the action time lag, and the effect time lag.
- Two automatic, or built-in, stabilizers are the tax system, unemployment compensation, and welfare payments.
- Built-in stabilizers tend automatically to moderate changes in disposable income resulting from changes in overall business activity.
- Though discretionary fiscal policy may not necessarily be a useful policy tool in normal times because of crowding out and time lags, it may work well during abnormal times, such as depressions and wartime. In addition, the existence of fiscal policy may have a soothing effect on consumers and investors.
- If the federal government's spending flow exceeds the taxes that it collects, the government runs a deficit. The gross public debt is the total accumulation of past years' deficits. The net public debt subtracts off the part of the gross public debt held by agencies of the government.

NETNOMICS

Deficit Financing: A Thing of the Past?

Governments throughout the world have often resorted to deficit financing when they have expanded government spending faster than tax collections. Most governments in Europe, for example, since World War II have gradually added more welfare programs. In addition, European governments have frequently argued that they can "create jobs" by expanding public-sector employment. Recently, for example, the French prime minister said that he would create 350,000 new jobs by hiring young people to engage in worthwhile public jobs. Such "job creation" requires funding nonetheless. The French government, like virtually all European governments, has been unable to match government spending with government revenues. It has consistently issued government securities to pay for increased government spending—debt financing.

Enter the Internet, and over goes the apple cart. Today, information about all aspects of governmental activities—spending, revenues, and the like—is available to everyone in the world on a second's notice via the Internet. Even more important, dealers in government securities can obtain this information at the speed of light. Because capital flows worldwide depend on perceived real rates of return—that is, rates of return corrected for inflation in whatever currency the securities are denominated—the owners of government securities anywhere in the world (pension plans, mutual funds, speculators, and the like) can instantaneously pull their capital out of a country when they get a sense that things aren't right. If the French government announces a new jobs program that must be financed by the sale of additional French government securities, the French government could be punished. How? By a quick net outflow of capital from France, thereby increasing its domestic interest rates.

The Internet helps spread information about government actions, the possibility of their positive or negative effects, and the economic growth outlook as a result. It also allows capital to be moved in and out of countries with the click of a mouse. Consequently, no government has the ability to engage in serious deficit financing anymore without being instantly punished.

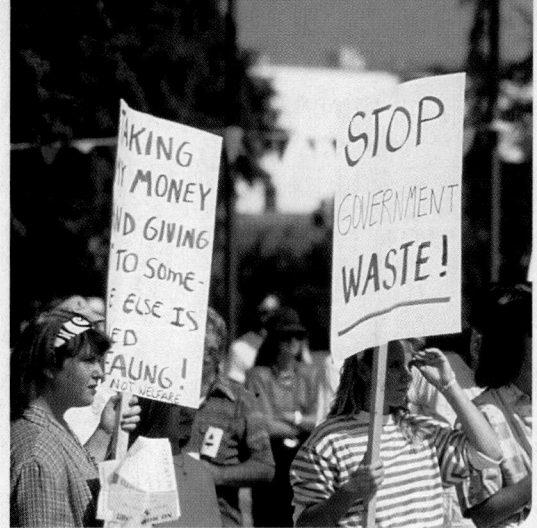

ISSUES & APPLICATIONS

Will the Government Allow the U.S. Economy to Drown in Black Ink?

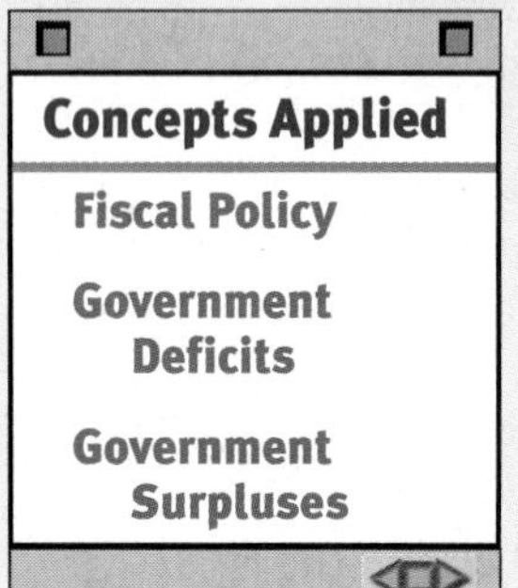

During the 1970s, 1980s, and early 1990s, many economists strenuously argued that the federal government should end its deficit spending. Indeed, at one point in the 1990s, close to two-thirds of both houses of the U.S. Congress was swayed by arguments that the sea of red ink generated by spending on government consumption was crowding out private investment and slowing economic growth. The Senate, however, came up one vote short of passing a balanced-budget amendment to the U.S. Constitution.

Of course, many on the other side of the debate viewed private investment and government investment as equally productive and were unconcerned about any crowding-out effect. Ultimately, therefore, the *macroeconomic* argument about government deficits hinged on the amount of government spending on long-term capital investment and on the relative efficiency of government versus private investment.

A New Debate . . .

The terms of the debate have shifted as the government has taken in more taxes than it spends. Some forecasts indicate that in the absence of big tax cuts or increases in the rate of government expenditures, there may be federal budget surpluses for years into the future. During the latter years of the Clinton presidency, the U.S. Treasury used annual surpluses to pay off some of the government's accumulated debt from years past. The rosiest forecasts indicated the possibility of completely paying off the debt by 2015.

Nevertheless, a number of economists—many of whom had argued previously against large government deficits—now argue against running big federal surpluses. Their concern, once again, is the possibility of ill effects on economic growth.

. . . Or Just a Return to an Old Argument?

To understand why some might contend that budget surpluses can harm economic growth, note that when the government runs a surplus (meaning that it does not spend any excess of tax revenues over planned government expenditures), it adds to the total flow of saving in the economy. That is, the government becomes a net saver. So far, the government has saved by repurchasing some of its debt. In principle, it could save by buying privately placed debt, such as corporate bonds or stock.

If the government adds to national saving, then a likely result is an interest rate decline that stimulates private investment. Other things being equal, increased private investment tends to spur greater capital accumulation and push up the rate of economic growth. So why do some economists now grumble that government surpluses may *hinder* growth? Their argument hinges on the fact that when the government runs a surplus, it effectively saves *on behalf* of private individuals. It extracts taxes in excess of the amount required to cover the government's own expenses and then channels unspent taxes to financial markets. What critics of government surpluses question is the government's capability to channel this "forced saving" to the most productive uses. They worry that "too much" government saving may be directed to activities with low rates of return. If so, they argue, persistent government surpluses will lead to lower rates of economic growth than the nation could otherwise achieve.

This, of course, is the flip side of the argument against government deficits. In the case of deficits, a key issue is whether government investment is as productive as private investment. Likewise, in the case of surpluses, a fundamental issue is whether government saving is allocated as efficiently as private saving.

FOR CRITICAL ANALYSIS

1. How might we judge whether government saving is more or less efficient than private saving?
2. Some critics argue that attaining high rates of return on saving entails taking risks that are inappropriate for government institutions to take. Explain why you agree or disagree.

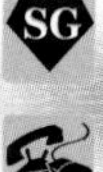

SUMMARY DISCUSSION OF LEARNING OBJECTIVES

1. **The Effects of Discretionary Fiscal Policies Using Traditional Keynesian Analysis:** Within the Keynesian short-run framework of analysis, a deliberate increase in government spending or reduction in taxes can raise aggregate demand. Thus, these fiscal policy actions can shift the aggregate demand curve outward along the short-run aggregate supply curve and thereby close a recessionary gap in which current real GDP is less than the long-run level of real GDP. Likewise, an intentional reduction in government spending or tax increase will reduce aggregate demand. These fiscal policy actions thereby shift the aggregate demand curve inward along the short-run aggregate supply curve and close an inflationary gap in which current real GDP exceeds the long-run level of real GDP.

2. **How Indirect Crowding Out and Direct Expenditure Offsets Can Reduce the Effectiveness of Fiscal Policy Actions:** Indirect crowding out occurs when the government engages in expansionary fiscal policy actions by running deficits, which it must finance by issuing bonds that compete with private bonds and thereby drive up market interest rates. This reduces, or crowds out, interest-sensitive private spending, thereby reducing the net effect of the fiscal expansion on aggregate demand. As a result, the aggregate demand curve shifts by a smaller amount than it would have in the absence of the crowding out effect, and fiscal policy has a somewhat lessened net effect on equilibrium national income. Increased government spending may also substitute directly for private expenditures, and the resulting decline in private spending directly offsets the increase in total planned expenditures that the government had intended to bring about. This also mutes the net change in aggregate demand brought about by a fiscal policy action.

3. **The Ricardian Equivalence Theorem:** According to this proposition, when the government cuts taxes and borrows to finance the tax reduction, people realize that eventually the government will have to repay the loan. Thus they anticipate that in the future there will have to be a tax increase. This induces them to save the proceeds of the tax cut to meet their future tax liabilities. Consequently, a tax cut fails to induce an increase in aggregate consumption spending. On net, therefore, a tax cut has no effect on total planned expenditures and aggregate demand if the Ricardian equivalence theorem is valid.

4. **Fiscal Policy Time Lags and the Effectiveness of Fiscal "Fine Tuning":** Efforts to engage in fiscal policy actions intended to bring about carefully planned changes in aggregate demand are often complicated by policy time lags. One of these is the recognition time lag, which is the time required to collect information about the economy's current situation. Another is the action time lag, the period between recognition of a problem and implementation of a policy intended to address it. Finally, there is the effect time lag, which is the interval that passes between policy implementation and the policy's effects on the economy. For fiscal policy, all of these lags can be very lengthy and variable, often lasting anywhere from one to three years. Hence, fiscal "fine tuning" may be a misnomer.
5. **Automatic Stabilizers:** In our tax system, income taxes diminish automatically when economic activity drops, and unemployment compensation and welfare payments increase. Thus, when there is a decline in national income, the automatic reduction in income tax collections and increases in unemployment compensation and welfare payments tends to mute the reduction in total planned expenditures that otherwise would have resulted. The existence of these government programs thereby tends to stabilize the economy automatically in the face of variations in autonomous expenditures that induce fluctuations in economic activity.
6. **Government Deficits Versus the Public Debt:** When governments run budget deficits, government spending during a given time interval exceeds tax collections during that period. Thus deficits are a flow over time. Governments finance deficits by issuing bonds, so deficit spending year after year leads to an accumulated public debt, which is a stock at a given point in time. The entire outstanding debt of the federal government is the gross public debt. Some of this debt is held by public agencies. When we subtract out their holdings of government debt, we tabulate the net public debt. The net public debt increased from the end of the 1960s until 1998, when the federal government officially began to operate with budget surpluses again. Since 1998 the net public debt has declined somewhat.

Key Terms and Concepts

Action time lag (308)
Automatic, or built-in, stabilizers (309)
Crowding-out effect (303)
Direct expenditure offsets (305)
Effect time lag (308)
Fiscal policy (299)
Gross public debt (311)
Net public debt (311)
Recognition time lag (308)
Ricardian equivalence theorem (304)
Supply-side economics (306)

Problems

Answers to the odd-numbered problems appear at the back of the book.

13-1. Suppose that Congress and the president decide that economic performance is weakening and that the government should "do something" about the situation. They make no tax changes but do enact new laws increasing government spending on a variety of programs.

a. Prior to congressional and presidential action, careful studies by government economists indicated that the direct multiplier effect of a rise in government expenditures on equilibrium national income is equal to 6. Within the 12 months after the increase in government spending, however, it has become clear that the actual ultimate multiplier effect on real GDP will be unlikely to exceed half of that amount. What factors might account for this?

b. Another year and a half elapses following passage of the government-spending boost. The government has undertaken no additional policy actions, nor have there been any other events of significance. Nevertheless, by the end of the second year, real national income has returned to its original level, and the price level has increased sharply. Provide a possible explanation for this outcome.

13-2. Suppose that Congress enacts a significant tax cut with the expectation that this action will stimulate aggregate demand and push up real GDP in the short run. In fact, however, neither real national income nor the price level changes significantly following the tax cut. What might account for this outcome?

13-3. Explain how time lags in discretionary fiscal policymaking could thwart the efforts of Congress and the president to stabilize real national income in the face of an economic downturn. Is it possible that these time lags could actually cause discretionary fiscal policy to *destabilize* real national income?

13-4. Under what circumstance might a tax reduction be associated with a long-run increase in real national income and a long-run reduction in the price level?

13-5. Which of the following is an example of a discretionary fiscal policy action?

a. A recession occurs, and government-funded unemployment compensation payments are paid out to laid-off workers as a result.

b. Congress votes to fund a new jobs program designed to put unemployed workers to work.

c. The Federal Reserve decides to reduce the quantity of money in circulation in an effort to slow inflation.

d. Under powers authorized by an act of Congress, the president decides to authorize an emergency release of funds for spending programs intended to head off economic crises.

13-6. Which of the following is an example of an automatic fiscal stabilizer?

a. The Federal Reserve arranges to make loans to banks automatically whenever an economic downturn begins.

b. As the economy heats up, the resulting increase in equilibrium income immediately results in higher income tax payments, which dampens consumption spending somewhat.

c. As the economy starts to recover from a recession and more people go back to work, government-funded unemployment compensation payments begin to decline.

d. To stem an overheated economy, the president, using special powers granted by Congress, authorizes emergency impoundment of funds that Congress had previously authorized for spending on government programs.

13-7. There is an inflationary gap. Discuss one discretionary fiscal policy action that might eliminate it.

13-8. There is a recessionary gap. Discuss one discretionary fiscal policy action that might eliminate it.

13-9. If the Ricardian equivalence theorem is not relevant, then a cut in the income tax rate should affect both the level of equilibrium real income and its stability. Explain why.

13-10. Suppose that Congress enacts a lump-sum tax cut of $750 billion. The marginal propensity to consume is equal to .75. If Ricardian equivalence holds true, what is the effect on equilibrium real income? On saving?

Economics on the Net

Federal Government Spending and Taxation A quick way to keep up with the federal government's spending and taxation is by examining federal budget data at the White House Internet address.

Title: Historical Tables: Budget of the United States Government

Navigation: Click here to visit the Office of Management and Budget. Select the most recent budget. Then click on Historical Tables.

Application After the document downloads, perform the indicated operations and answer the questions.

1. Go to section 2, titled "Composition of Federal Government Receipts." Take a look at Table 2.2, "Percentage Composition of Receipts by Source." Before World War II, what was the key source of revenues of the federal government? What has been the key revenue source since World War II?

2. Now scan down the document to Table 2.3 "Receipts by Source as Percentages of GDP." Have any government revenue sources declined as a percentage of GDP? Which ones have noticeably risen in recent years?

3. In the Table of Contents in the left-hand margin of the Historical Tables, click on Table 7.1: Federal Debt at the End of the Year, 1940-2006. In light of the discussion in this chapter, which column shows the net public debt? What is the conceptual difference between the gross public debt and the net public debt? Last year, what was the dollar difference between these two amounts?

4. Table 7.1 includes estimates of the gross and net public debt through 2006. Suppose that these estimates turn out to be accurate. Calculate how much the net public debt should decline on average each year from 1997 to 2006. If the government managed to reduce its indebtedness by this amount every year indefinitely, how many years would it take to completely pay off the debt?

For Group Study and Analysis Split into four groups, and have each group examine section 3, "Federal Government Outlays by Function," and in particular Table 3.1, "Outlays by Superfunction and Function." Assign groups to the following functions: national defense, health, income security, and Social Security. Have each group prepare a brief report concerning long-term and recent trends in government spending on each function. Which functions are capturing growing shares of government spending in recent years? Which are receiving declining shares of total spending?

APPENDIX C

FISCAL POLICY: A KEYNESIAN PERSPECTIVE

The traditional Keynesian approach to fiscal policy differs in three ways from that presented in Chapter 13. First, it emphasizes the underpinnings of the components of aggregate demand. Second, it assumes that government expenditures are not substitutes for private expenditures and that current taxes are the only taxes taken into account by consumers and firms. Third, the traditional Keynesian approach focuses on the short run and so assumes that as a first approximation, the price level is constant.

CHANGES IN GOVERNMENT SPENDING

Figure C-1 measures real national income along the horizontal axis and total planned expenditures (aggregate demand) along the vertical axis. The components of aggregate demand are consumption (C), investment (I), government spending (G), and net exports (X). The height of the schedule labeled $C + I + G + X$ shows total planned expenditures (aggregate demand) as a function of income. This schedule slopes upward because consumption depends positively on income. Everywhere along the 45-degree reference line, planned spending equals income. At the point Y^*, where the $C + I + G + X$ line intersects the 45-degree line, planned spending is consistent with real national income. At any income less than Y^*, spending exceeds income, and so income and thus spending will tend to rise. At any level of income greater than Y^*, planned spending is less than income, and so income and thus spending will tend to decline. Given the determinants of C, I, G, and X, total spending (aggregate demand) will be Y^*.

The Keynesian approach assumes that changes in government spending cause no direct offsets in either consumption or investment spending because G is not a substitute for C, I, or X. Hence a rise in government spending from G to G' causes the $C + I + G + X$ line to shift upward by the full amount of the rise in government spending, yielding the line $C + I + G' + X$. The rise in government spending causes income to rise, which in turn causes consumption spending to rise, which further increases income. Ultimately, aggregate demand rises to Y^{**}, where spending again equals income. A key conclusion of the Keynesian analysis is that total spending rises by *more* than the original rise in government spending because consumption spending depends positively on income.

FIGURE C-1
The Impact of Higher Government Spending on Aggregate Demand
Government spending increases, causing $C + I + G + X$ to move to $C + I + G' + X$. Equilibrium increases to Y^{**}.

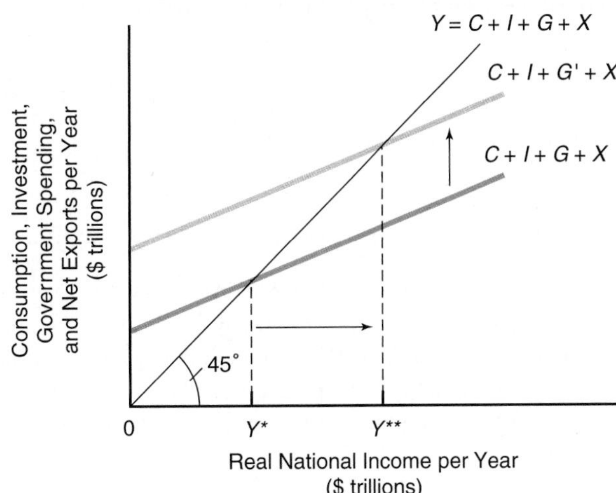

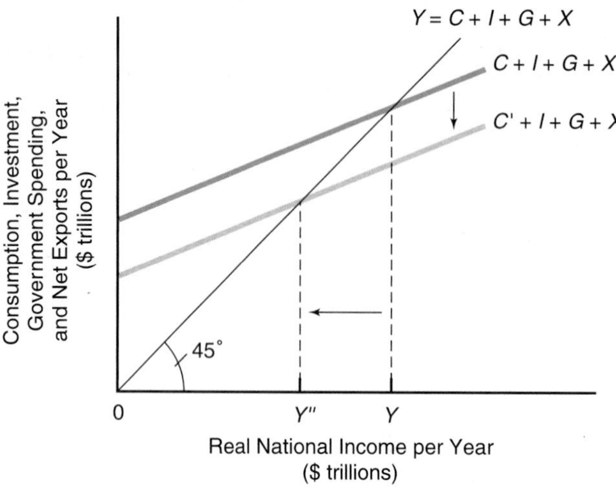

FIGURE C-2
The Impact of Higher Taxes on Aggregate Demand
Higher taxes cause consumption to fall to C'. Equilibrium decreases to Y''.

CHANGES IN TAXES

According to the Keynesian approach, changes in current taxes affect aggregate demand by changing the amount of disposable (after-tax) income available to consumers. A rise in taxes reduces disposable income and thus reduces consumption; conversely, a tax cut raises disposable income and thus causes a rise in consumption spending. The effects of a tax increase are shown in Figure C-2. Higher taxes cause consumption spending to decline from C to C', causing total spending to shift downward to $C' + I + G + X$. In general, the decline in consumption will be less than the increase in taxes because people will also reduce their saving to help pay the higher taxes.

THE BALANCED-BUDGET MULTIPLIER

One interesting implication of the Keynesian approach concerns the impact of a balanced-budget change in government spending. Suppose that the government increases spending by $1 billion and pays for it by raising current taxes by $1 billion. Such a policy is called a *balanced-budget increase in spending.* Because the higher spending tends to push aggregate demand *up* by *more* than $1 billion while the higher taxes tend to push aggregate demand *down* by *less* than $1 billion, a most remarkable thing happens: A balanced-budget increase in G causes total spending to rise by *exactly* the amount of the rise in G—in this case, $1 billion. We say that the *balanced-budget multiplier* is equal to 1. Similarly, a balanced-budget reduction in spending will cause total spending to fall by exactly the amount of the spending cut.

THE FIXED PRICE LEVEL ASSUMPTION

The final key feature of the Keynesian approach is that it typically assumes that as a first approximation, the price level is fixed. Recall that nominal income equals the price level multiplied by real output. If the price level is fixed, an increase in government spending that causes nominal income to rise will show up exclusively as a rise in *real* output. This will in turn be accompanied by a decline in the unemployment rate because the additional output can be produced only if additional factors of production, such as labor, are utilized.

Problems

Answers to the odd-numbered problems appear at the back of the book.

C-1. Assume that equilibrium income is \$10.20 trillion and full-employment equilibrium is \$10.55 trillion. The marginal propensity to save is $\frac{1}{7}$. Answer the questions using the data in the following graph.

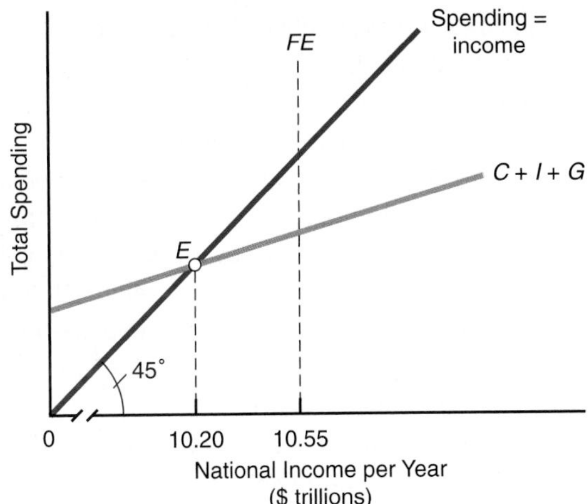

a. What is the marginal propensity to consume?
b. By how much must new investment or government spending increase to bring the economy up to full employment?
c. By how much must government cut personal taxes to stimulate the economy to the full-employment equilibrium?

C-2. Assume that MPC $= \frac{4}{5}$; then answer the following questions.

a. If government expenditures rise by \$2 billion, by how much will the aggregate expenditure curve shift upward? By how much will equilibrium income change?
b. If taxes increase by \$2 billion, by how much will the aggregate expenditure curve shift downward? By how much will equilibrium income change?

C-3. Assume that MPC $= \frac{4}{5}$; then answer the following questions.

a. If government expenditures rise by \$1 billion, by how much will the aggregate expenditure curve shift upward?
b. If taxes rise by \$1 billion, by how much will the aggregate expenditure curve shift downward?
c. If both taxes and government expenditures rise by \$1 billion, by how much will the aggregate expenditure curve shift? What will happen to the equilibrium level of income?
d. How does our conclusion in the second part of (c) change if MPC $= \frac{3}{4}$? If MPC $= \frac{1}{2}$?

TYING IT ALL TOGETHER

Part 3 Case Problem

Case Background

The year is 2013. It wasn't supposed to turn out this way. After successive years of federal surpluses that have paid down much of the U.S. government's debt and added to the Social Security trust fund, the nation is now mired in a severe recession.

The Current Situation Before leaving the Oval Office for the East Wing meeting, the president clicks the mouse on his computer and sees that this year real investment spending has declined by 3.6 percent, and export spending is down by 5 percent. Inflation is quite low, at an annual rate of 0.5 percent, which is near its average for the preceding three years. Nominal government spending actually fell by 2 percent last year and was down by an annualized rate of 3 percent in the most recent quarter.

The Fed's primary measure of the quantity of money in circulation has declined at an average rate of 1 percent during the past year. A broader measure of money has barely changed. Market interest rates have declined, however, by an average of about 1 percentage point, during the past 12 months. The value of the dollar relative to the currencies of the euro and the yen has risen by 12 percent during the same period.

Labor productivity is stagnant. Claims for unemployment compensation are up by 3.2 percent from last year. This understates the scope of the unemployment problem, however, because such a large portion of the labor force, relative to 10 years earlier, is now composed of temporary workers and consultants who are struggling to find steady employment. The overall unemployment rate last month was 7.5 percent, and the CEA estimates that it may increase to as much as 7.8 percent next month. Even so, information technology companies complain that they cannot find enough well-trained workers for many of the jobs that they would like to fill because job seekers lack the requisite technical training.

Trying to Reach a Consensus The president convenes the meeting, and key cabinet officials and the Fed chair each suggest a course of action.

- *Secretary of the Treasury:* In keeping with the president's commitment to paying off the national debt, the Treasury proposes no fundamental change in the stance of fiscal policy. The Treasury secretary does propose, however, selling dollars in foreign exchange markets in an effort to drive down the dollar's value.

- *Secretary of State:* The secretary of state proposes quick passage of legislation lowering barriers to entry by the most highly qualified immigrants in an effort to boost U.S. labor productivity.

- *Secretary of Labor:* The secretary recommends holding fast to the president's budgetary promises but cutting back on spending in some areas so that available public funds may be redirected toward job training programs targeted at preparing young people for high-tech jobs.

- *Federal Reserve Chair:* The Fed chair argues that its number one job is to contain inflation, and she notes that the Fed has done its job well for the past 3 1/2 years.

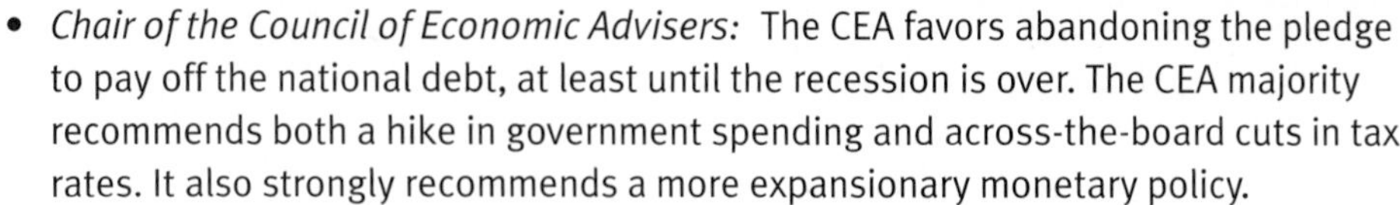

- *Chair of the Council of Economic Advisers:* The CEA favors abandoning the pledge to pay off the national debt, at least until the recession is over. The CEA majority recommends both a hike in government spending and across-the-board cuts in tax rates. It also strongly recommends a more expansionary monetary policy.

Points to Analyze

1. Which viewpoints are consistent with potential short-run efforts to stem the downturn in U.S. business activity? Which are directed at longer-term solutions?
2. Which perspective is most consistent with Keynesian economic analysis?
3. Which perspective is most consistent with classical economic analysis?
4. If the president takes the politically easy way out in light of the Fed chair's stance, how might this action help raise equilibrium real GDP?
5. If you were the president, what broad economic plan would you pull together from these suggestions? Why?

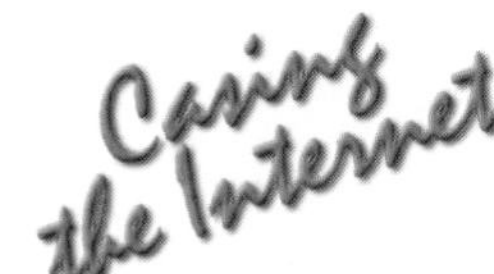

1. **Click here to go the homepage of the Bureau of Economic Analysis. Click on "GDP and related data." Next to "GDP and other major NIPA series," click on "PDF" to download the latest data from the national income product accounts.**
   a. **Look at Table 1. Exports and imports made up what percentages of GDP in 1960? In 1980? In the most recent full year for which data are available? By these measures, does the United States appear to be a more open economy than in years past?**
   b. **In Table 1, what was government spending as a percentage of GDP in 1960? In 1980? In the most recent full year for which data are available? Is the government consuming a larger or smaller share of U.S. GDP than in earlier years?**
2. **Click here to visit the homepage of the International Monetary Fund. Click on "Publications" and then on "World Economic Outlook" (most recent issue). Download the file which contains the statistical appendix.**
   a. **Look at Table 3, "Advanced Economies: Components of Real GDP." Across countries, which component of GDP tends to grow at the most stable pace over time?**
   b. **Again looking across countries, which component of GDP tends to exhibit the greatest stability over time?**

Part 4
Money, Monetary Policy, and Stabilization

CHAPTER

14

MONEY AND BANKING SYSTEMS

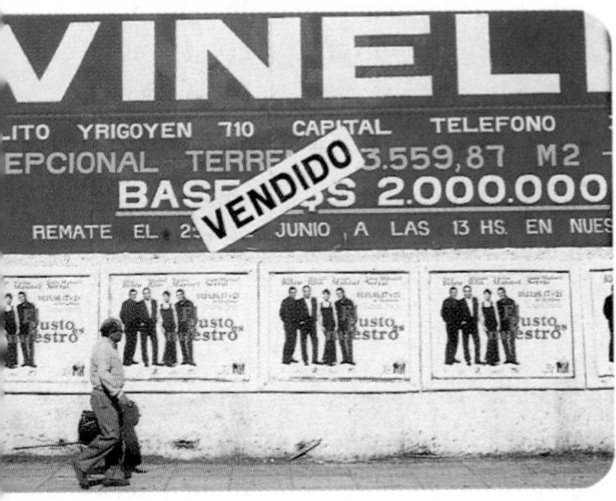

This advertising billboard in Buenos Aires, Argentina, may someday be displaying prices in dollars instead of the local currency. If Argentina used dollars instead of pesos, would Argentineans necessarily be better off?

A couple of years ago, Argentina's government made a startling announcement. It was, it said, thinking about scrapping the nation's currency, the peso. Furthermore, it might not even replace the peso with a new national money. Instead, the government might declare U.S. dollars to be the legal money of Argentina. Since then, a few other Latin American nations have contemplated the same plan. A similar idea has even emerged in Canada, where some economists floated a plan for dropping the Canadian dollar in favor of the dollar issued by their big neighbor to the south. Why would these countries think about giving up their own national currencies and using U.S. dollars instead? Before you can consider this question, you must learn about the functions of money. You must also understand how economists measure the total quantity of money in circulation. These are key topics in this chapter.

LEARNING OBJECTIVES

After reading this chapter, you should be able to:

1. Define the fundamental functions of money
2. Identify key properties that any good that functions as money must possess
3. Explain official definitions of the quantity of money in circulation
4. Understand why financial intermediaries such as banks exist
5. Describe the basic structure of the Federal Reserve System
6. Discuss the major functions of the Federal Reserve

Chapter Outline

Did You Know That... the typical dollar bill changes hands 50 times a year? Paper bills and coins are not the only things we use as money, however. As you will see in this chapter, *money* is a much broader concept.

Money has been important to society for thousands of years. In 300 B.C., Aristotle claimed that everything had to "be accessed in money, for this enables men always to exchange their services, and so makes society possible." Money is indeed a part of our everyday existence. Nevertheless, we have to be careful when we talk about money. Often a person may say, "I wish I had more money," instead of "I wish I had a higher income," thereby confusing the concepts of money and income. Economists use the term ***money*** to mean anything that people generally accept in exchange for goods and services. Table 14-1 provides a list of some items that various civilizations have used as money. The best way to understand how these items served this purpose is to examine the functions of money.

THE FUNCTIONS OF MONEY 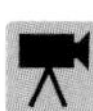

Money traditionally has four functions. The one that most people are familiar with is money's function as a *medium of exchange.* Money also serves as a *unit of accounting,* a *store of value* or *purchasing power,* and a *standard of deferred payment.* Anything that serves these four functions is money. Anything that could serve these four functions could be considered money.

Money
Any medium that is universally accepted in an economy both by sellers of goods and services as payment for those goods and services and by creditors as payment for debts.

Medium of exchange 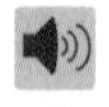
Any asset that sellers will accept as payment.

Barter 
The direct exchange of goods and services for other goods and services without the use of money.

Money as a Medium of Exchange

When we say that money serves as a **medium of exchange,** what we mean is that sellers will accept it as payment in market transactions. Without some generally accepted medium of exchange, we would have to resort to *barter.* In fact, before money was used, transactions took place by means of barter. **Barter** is simply a direct exchange—people do not use money as an intermediate item in conducting exchanges. In a barter economy, the shoemaker who wants to obtain a dozen water glasses must seek out a glassmaker who at exactly the same time is interested in obtaining a pair of shoes. For this to occur, there has to be a *double coincidence of wants* for each specific item to be exchanged. If there isn't, the shoemaker must go through several trades in order to obtain the desired dozen glasses—perhaps first trading shoes for jewelry, then jewelry for some pots and pans, and then the pots and pans for the desired glasses.

Money facilitates exchange by reducing the transaction costs associated with means-of-payment uncertainty—that is, with regard to goods that the partners in any exchange are willing to accept, the existence of money means that individuals no longer have to hold a diverse collection of goods as an exchange inventory. As a medium of exchange, money allows individuals to specialize in any area in which they have a comparative advantage and to receive money payments for their labor. Money payments can then be exchanged for the fruits of other people's labor. The use of money as a medium of exchange permits more specialization and the inherent economic efficiencies that come with it (and hence greater economic growth). Money is even more important when used for large amounts of trade.

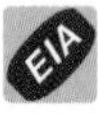

The Functions of Money
Gain further understanding of the concept of money.

TABLE 14-1

Types of Money

This is a partial list of things that have been used as money. Native Americans used *wampum,* beads made from shells. Fijians used whale teeth. The early colonists in North America used tobacco. And cigarettes were used in prisoner-of-war camps during World War II and in post–World War II Germany.

Iron	Boar tusk	Playing cards
Copper	Red woodpecker scalps	Leather
Brass	Feathers	Gold
Wine	Glass	Silver
Corn	Polished beads (wampum)	Knives
Salt	Rum	Pots
Horses	Molasses	Boats
Sheep	Tobacco	Pitch
Goats	Agricultural implements	Rice
Tortoise shells	Round stones with centers removed	Cows
Porpoise teeth	Crystal salt bars	Paper
Whale teeth	Snail shells	Cigarettes

Source: Roger LeRoy Miller and David D. VanHoose, *Money, Banking, and Financial Markets with Their Inter-national and Cyber Nexus* (Cincinnati: Southwestern, 2001), p. 6.

Money as a Unit of Accounting

Unit of accounting 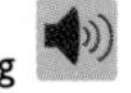
A measure by which prices are expressed; the common denominator of the price system; a central property of money.

A **unit of accounting** is a way of placing a specific price on economic goods and services. It is the common denominator, the commonly recognized measure of value. The dollar is the monetary unit in the United States. It is the yardstick that allows individuals easily to compare the relative value of goods and services. Accountants at the U.S. Department of Commerce use dollar prices to measure national income and domestic product, a business uses dollar prices to calculate profits and losses, and a typical household budgets regularly anticipated expenses using dollar prices as its unit of accounting.

Another way of describing money as a unit of accounting is to say that it serves as a *standard of value* that allows economic actors to compare the relative worth of various goods and services. This allows for comparison shopping, for example.

FAQ: Must debts be specified in terms of the local currency?

Not all countries, or the firms and individuals in those countries, will specify that debts owed must be paid in their own national monetary unit. For example, individuals, private corporations, and governments in other countries incur debts in terms of the U.S. dollar, even though the dollar is neither the medium of exchange nor the monetary unit in those countries. In the late 1990s, this became a significant problem for firms in Thailand, Malaysia, Indonesia, and South Korea when the values of the currencies in which they earned revenues—the Thai baht, the Malaysian ringgit, the Indonesian rupiah, and the South Korean won—all declined significantly in value relative to their dollar-denominated debts.

Money as a Store of Value

One of the most important functions of money is that it serves as a **store of value** or purchasing power. The money you have today can be set aside to purchase things later on. In the meantime, money retains its nominal value, which you can apply to those future purchases. If you have $1,000 in your checking account, you can choose to spend it today on goods and services, spend it tomorrow, or spend it a month from now. In this way, money provides a way to transfer value (wealth) into the future.

Store of value 
The ability to hold value over time; a necessary property of money.

Money as a Standard of Deferred Payment

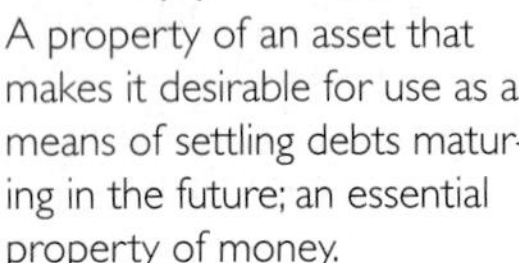

Standard of deferred payment
A property of an asset that makes it desirable for use as a means of settling debts maturing in the future; an essential property of money.

The fourth function of the monetary unit is as a **standard of deferred payment.** This function involves the use of money both as a medium of exchange and as a unit of accounting. Debts are typically stated in terms of a unit of accounting; they are paid with a monetary medium of exchange. That is to say, a debt is specified in a dollar amount and paid in currency (or by check). A corporate bond, for example, has a face value—the dollar value stated on it, which is to be paid upon maturity. The periodic interest payments on that corporate bond are specified and paid in dollars, and when the bond comes due (at maturity), the corporation pays the face value in dollars to the holder of the bond.

LIQUIDITY

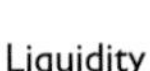

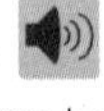

Liquidity
The degree to which an asset can be acquired or disposed of without much danger of any intervening loss in *nominal* value and with small transaction costs. Money is the most liquid asset.

Money is an asset—something of value—that accounts for part of personal wealth. Wealth in the form of money can be exchanged later for other assets, goods, or services. Although it is not the only form of wealth that can be exchanged for goods and services, it is the most widely and most readily accepted one. This attribute of money is called **liquidity.** We say that an asset is *liquid* when it can easily be acquired or disposed of without high transaction costs and with relative certainty as to its value. Money is by definition the most liquid asset. Compare it, for example, with a share of stock listed on the New York Stock Exchange. To sell that stock, you usually call a stockbroker, who will place the sell order for you. This generally must be done during normal business hours. You have to pay a commission to the broker. Moreover, there is a distinct probability that you will get more or less for the stock than you originally paid for it. This is not the case with money. People can easily convert money to other asset forms. Therefore, most individuals hold at least a part of their wealth in the form of the most liquid of assets, money. You can see how assets rank in liquidity relative to one another in Figure 14-1.

When we hold money, however, we pay a price for this advantage of liquidity. Because cash in your pocket and many checking account balances do not earn interest, that price is the interest yield that could have been obtained had the asset been held in another form—for example, in the form of stocks and bonds.

The cost of holding money (its opportunity cost) is measured by the alternative interest yield obtainable by holding some other asset.

MONETARY STANDARDS, OR WHAT BACKS MONEY 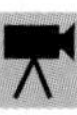

In the past, many different monetary standards have existed. For example, commodity money, which is a physical good that may be valued for other uses it provides, has been used (see Table 14-1). The main forms of commodity money were gold and silver. Today,

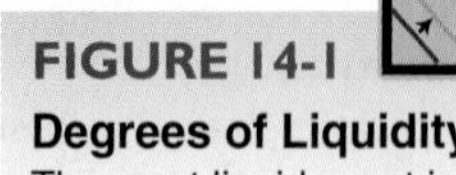

FIGURE 14-1
Degrees of Liquidity
The most liquid asset is cash. Liquidity decreases as you move from right to left.

Antique furniture | Commercial office buildings | Old Masters paintings | Houses | Cars | Stocks and Bonds | Certificates of deposit | Transactions accounts | Cash

Low Liquidity ← → **High Liquidity**

though, most people throughout the world accept coins, paper currency, and balances in **transactions accounts** (checking accounts with banks and other financial institutions; also called checkable deposits) in exchange for items sold, including labor services. The question remains, why are we willing to accept as payment something that has no intrinsic value? After all, you could not sell checks to anybody for use as a raw material in manufacturing. The reason is that payments in the modern world arise from a **fiduciary monetary system.** This means that the value of the payments rests on the public's confidence that such payments can be exchanged for goods and services. *Fiduciary* comes from the Latin *fiducia,* which means "trust" or "confidence." In our fiduciary monetary system, money, in the form of currency or transactions accounts, is not convertible to a fixed quantity of gold, silver, or some other precious commodity. The bills are just pieces of paper. Coins have a value stamped on them that today is much greater than the market value of the metal in them. Nevertheless, currency and transactions accounts are money because of their acceptability and predictability of value.

Transactions accounts 
Checking account balances in commercial banks and other types of financial institutions, such as credit unions and mutual savings banks; any accounts in financial institutions on which you can easily write checks without many restrictions.

Fiduciary monetary system 
A system in which currency is issued by the government and its value is based uniquely on the public's faith that the currency represents command over goods and services.

INTERNATIONAL EXAMPLE

Is Gold Worth Its Weight?

For centuries, gold has been precious because it has been scarce. Today, however, this glittering metal may be overabundant, especially for international agencies, governments, and central banks. Gold accounts for more than a third of the official international reserves of a number of developed nations. Combined gold holdings of the International Monetary Fund (IMF) and the world's central banks exceed 30,000 tons, or the equivalent of about a dozen years of global mining output. All this gold is very expensive to move around. For this reason, it typically just sits unused, in sturdy vaults surrounded by armed guards. This is an expensive use for a metal. Moreover, over the past 25 years, gold has turned out to be a poor store of value. Returns on relatively low-risk bonds have been much higher than the rate of return from holding gold. Switzerland, for instance, determined that the cost of interest forgone by holding gold rather than U.S. Treasury bonds is about $400 a year per Swiss household.

Recently, the Swiss government began selling off half its 2,600 tons of gold reserves, third-largest in the world behind the United States and the European Monetary Union. More recently, the IMF has auctioned off some of its gold holdings to finance debt relief for poor countries. The European System of Central Banks, which began the new century with 30 percent of its reserves in the form of gold, decided to reduce this fraction to 15 percent.

Official gold sales until late 1999 contributed to a decline in the world price of gold, thereby worsening the return to holding gold. This led companies operating gold mines in United States to lobby their representatives and senators, who successfully pushed through a law threatening a reduction of U.S. funding of the IMF unless it agreed to scale back gold sales it had planned for the early 2000s. It did so, and central banks also agreed to stop selling gold.

For Critical Analysis

It appears that today central banks' portfolios are weighted too heavily in favor of gold. Under what circumstances might central banks again determine that huge stocks of gold are worth holding?

Acceptability

Transactions accounts and currency are money because they are accepted in exchange for goods and services. They are accepted because people have confidence that these items can later be exchanged for other goods and services. This confidence is based on the knowledge that such exchanges have occurred in the past without problems. Even during a period of inflation, we might still be inclined to accept money in exchange for goods and services because it is so useful. Barter is a costly and time-consuming alternative.

Realize always that money is socially defined. Acceptability is not something that you can necessarily predict. For example, the U.S. government has tried to circulate types of money, such as the $2 bill, that were socially unacceptable. How many $2 bills have you seen lately? The answer is probably none. No one wanted to make room for $2 bills in register tills or billfolds.

Predictability of Value

The purchasing power of the dollar (its real value) varies inversely with the price level. The more rapid the rate of increase of some price level index, such as the Consumer Price Index, the more rapid the decrease in the real value, or purchasing power, of a dollar. Money still retains its usefulness even if its purchasing power is declining year in and year out, as in periods of inflation, if it still retains the characteristic of predictability of value. If you anticipate that the inflation rate is going to be around 10 percent during the next year, you know that any dollar you receive a year from now will have a purchasing power equal to 10 percent less than that same dollar today. Thus you will not necessarily refuse to accept money in exchange simply because you know that its value will decline by the rate of inflation during next year. You may, however, wish to be compensated for that expected decline in money's real value.

CONCEPTS IN BRIEF

- Money is defined by its functions, which are as a medium of exchange, a unit of accounting or standard of value, a store of value or purchasing power, and a standard of deferred payment.
- Because money is a highly liquid asset, it can be disposed of with low transaction costs and with relative certainty as to its value.
- Today's nations have fiduciary monetary systems—national currencies are not convertible into a fixed quantity of a commodity such as gold or silver.
- Money is accepted in exchange for goods and services because people have confidence that it can later be exchanged for other goods and services. Another reason for this is that it has predictable value.

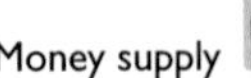
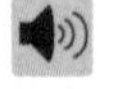

Money supply The amount of money in circulation.

Transactions approach A method of measuring the money supply by looking at money as a medium of exchange.

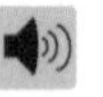

Liquidity approach A method of measuring the money supply by looking at money as a temporary store of value.

The Money Supply
Practice thinking about how to measure the money supply.

DEFINING MONEY

Money is important. Changes in the total **money supply**—the amount of money in circulation—and changes in the rate at which the money supply increases or decreases affect important economic variables (at least in the short run), such as the rate of inflation, interest rates, employment, and the equilibrium level of real national income. Although there is widespread agreement among economists that money is indeed important, they have struggled to reach agreement about defining and measuring it. There are two basic approaches: the **transactions approach,** which stresses the role of money as a medium of exchange, and the **liquidity approach,** which stresses the role of money as a temporary store of value.

The Transactions Approach to Measuring Money: M1

Using the transactions approach to measuring money, the money supply consists of currency, checkable deposits, and traveler's checks.

FIGURE 14-2

Composition of the U.S. M1 and M2 Money Supply, 2000

Panel (a) shows the M1 money supply, of which the greatest component is checkable deposits (over 65 percent). M2 consists of M1 plus three other components, the most important of which is small time deposits at all depository institutions (over 50 percent).

Sources: Federal Reserve Bulletin, Economic Indicators, various issues.

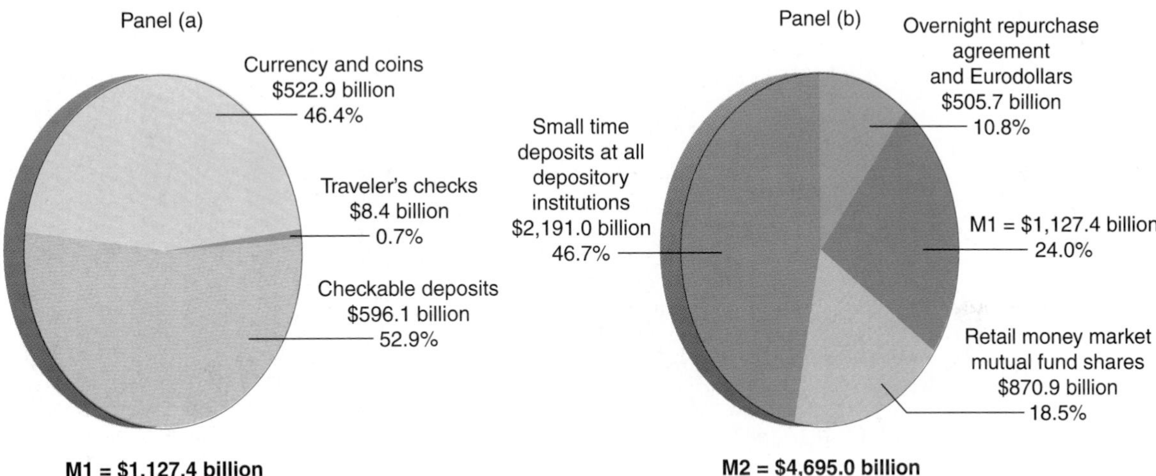

The official designation of the money supply, including currency, checkable deposits, and traveler's checks not issued by banks, is **M1.** The various elements of M1 for a typical year are presented in panel (a) of Figure 14-2.

M1 

The money supply, taken as the total value of currency plus checkable deposits plus traveler's checks not issued by banks.

Currency. In the United States, currency includes coins minted by the U.S. Treasury and paper currency in the form of Federal Reserve notes issued by the Federal Reserve banks (to be discussed shortly). In other nations, currency also consists of coins and paper bills. The typical resident of another nation uses currency denominated in local money terms, but in many countries the U.S. dollar is the preferred currency for many transactions. For this reason, the bulk of U.S. currency "in circulation" actually does not circulate within the borders of the United States. Figure 14-3 on page 334 displays the estimated value of U.S. currency in circulation elsewhere in the world. In any given year, at least two-thirds of the dollars in existence circulate outside the United States!

Checkable Deposits 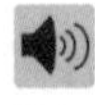

Any deposits in a thrift institution or a commercial bank on which a check may be written.

Checkable Deposits. Most major transactions today are done with checks. The convenience and safety of using checks and debit cards has made checkable deposit accounts the most important component of the money supply. For example, it is estimated that in 2000, currency transactions accounted for only 0.5 percent of the dollar amount of all transactions. The rest, excluding barter, involved checks. Checks are a way of transferring the ownership of deposits in financial institutions. They are normally acceptable as a medium of exchange. The financial institutions that offer checkable deposits are numerous and include commercial banks and virtually all **thrift institutions**—savings banks, savings and loan associations (S&Ls), and credit unions.

Thrift institutions 

Financial institutions that receive most of their funds from the savings of the public; they include mutual savings banks, savings and loan associations, and credit unions.

Traveler's Checks. **Traveler's checks** are paid for by the purchaser at the time of transfer. The total quantity of traveler's checks outstanding issued by institutions other than

Traveler's checks 

Financial instruments purchased from a bank or a nonbanking organization and signed during purchase that can be used as cash upon a second signature by the purchaser.

FIGURE 14-3
The Value of American Currency in Circulation Outside the United States
The amount of U.S. dollars circulating beyond American borders has grown steadily in recent years.
Source: Board of Governors of the Federal Reserve System.

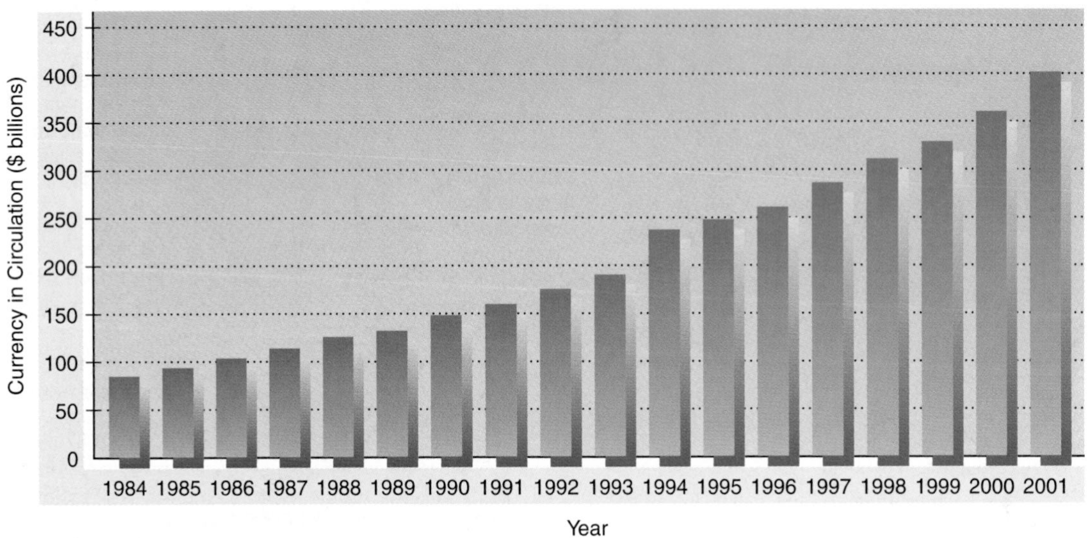

FAQ: Why aren't credit cards part of the money supply?

Even though a large percentage of U.S. transactions are accomplished using plastic credit cards, the credit card itself cannot be considered money. Remember the functions of money: a unit of accounting, a store of value, a standard of deferred payment—a credit card is none of these things. The use of your credit card in fact constitutes a *loan* to you by the issuer of the card, be it a bank, a retail store, a gas company, or American Express. The proceeds of the loan are paid to the business that sold you something. You must pay back the loan to the issuer of the credit card, either in full when you get your statement or with interest over time. Thus credit cards *defer* rather than complete transactions that ultimately involve the use of money.

banks is part of the M1 money supply.* American Express, Citibank, Cook's, and other institutions issue traveler's checks.

The Liquidity Approach to Measuring Money: M2

The liquidity approach to defining and measuring the U.S. money supply involves taking into account not only the most liquid assets that people use as money, which are already included in the definition of M1, but also other assets that are highly liquid—that is, that can be converted into money quickly without loss of nominal dollar value and without much cost. Any (non-M1) assets that come under this definition have been called **near moneys.** Thus the liquidity approach to the definition of the money supply views money as a temporary store of value and so includes all of M1 *plus* all near moneys. Panel (b) of Figure 14-2 shows the components of **M2**—money as a temporary store of value. We examine each of these components in turn.

Near moneys
Assets that are almost money. They have a high degree of liquidity; they can be easily converted into money without loss in value. Time deposits and short-term U.S. government securities are examples.

*Banks place the funds that are to be used to redeem traveler's checks in a special deposit account, and they are therefore already counted as checkable accounts. Nonbank issuers, however, do not place these funds in checkable accounts. Improvements in data collection have made it possible to estimate the total amount of nonbank traveler's checks, and since June 1981 they have been included in M1.

Savings Deposits. Total **savings deposits** in all **depository institutions** (such as commercial banks, savings banks, savings and loan associations, and credit unions) are part of the M2 money supply. A savings deposit has no set maturity.

Small-Denomination Time Deposits. A basic distinction has always been made between a checkable deposit, which is a checking account, and a **time deposit,** which theoretically requires notice of withdrawal and on which the financial institution pays the depositor interest. The name indicates that there is an agreed period during which the funds must be left in the financial institution. If the deposit holder withdraws funds before the end of that period, the institution issuing the deposit may apply a penalty. Time deposits include savings certificates and small **certificates of deposit (CDs).** The owner of a savings certificate is given a receipt indicating the amount deposited, the interest rate to be paid, and the maturity date. A CD is an actual certificate that indicates the date of issue, its maturity date, and other relevant contractual matters.

The distinction between checkable deposits and time deposits has blurred over time, but it is still used in the official definition of the money supply. To be included in the M2 definition of the money supply, however, time deposits must be less than $100,000—hence the name *small-denomination time deposits.* A variety of small-denomination time deposits are available from depository institutions, ranging in maturities from one month to 10 years.

Money Market Deposit Accounts (MMDAs). Since 1982, banks and thrift institutions have offered **money market deposit accounts (MMDAs),** which usually require a minimum balance and set limits on the number of monthly transactions (deposits and withdrawals by check).

Overnight Repurchase Agreements at Commercial Banks (REPOs, or RPs). A **repurchase agreement (REPO,** or **RP)** is made by a bank to sell Treasury or federal agency securities to its customers, coupled with an agreement to repurchase them at a price that includes accumulated interest. REPOs fill a gap in that depository institutions are not yet allowed to offer to businesses interest-bearing commercial checking accounts. Therefore, REPOs can be thought of as a financial innovation that bypasses regulations because businesses can deposit their excess cash in REPOs instead of leaving it in non-interest-bearing commercial checking accounts.

Overnight Eurodollars. **Eurodollar deposits** are dollar-denominated deposits in foreign commercial banks and in foreign branches of U.S. banks. *Dollar-denominated* simply means that although the deposit might be held at, say, a Caribbean commercial bank, its value is stated in terms of U.S. dollars rather than in terms of the local currency. The term *Eurodollar* is not completely accurate because banks outside continental Europe participate in the Eurodollar market and also because banks in some countries issue deposits denominated in German marks, Swiss francs, British pounds sterling, and Dutch guilders. This has led to wide use of the broader term *Eurocurrency deposits,* even though this is also not fully accurate given that banks in some countries also issue deposits denominated in non-European currencies such as the Japanese yen. (Note that Eurodollars and other Eurocurrencies are not the same as the *euro,* the monetary unit used by 11 European nations.)

M2  
M1 plus (1) savings and small-denomination time deposits at all depository institutions, (2) overnight repurchase agreements at commercial banks, (3) overnight Eurodollars held by U.S. residents other than banks at Caribbean branches of member banks, (4) balances in retail money market mutual funds, and (5) money market deposit accounts (MMDAs).

Savings deposits 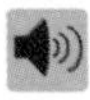
Interest-earning funds that can be withdrawn at any time without payment of a penalty.

Depository institutions 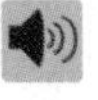
Financial institutions that accept deposits from savers and lend those deposits out at interest.

Time deposit 
A deposit in a financial institution that requires notice of intent to withdraw or must be left for an agreed period. Withdrawal of funds prior to the end of the agreed period may result in a penalty.

Certificate of deposit (CD) 
A time deposit with a fixed maturity date offered by banks and other financial institutions.

Money market deposit accounts (MMDAs) 
Accounts issued by banks yielding a market rate of interest with a minimum balance requirement and a limit on transactions. They have no minimum maturity.

Repurchase agreement (REPO, or RP) 
An agreement made by a bank to sell Treasury or federal agency securities to its customers, coupled with an agreement to repurchase them at a price that includes accumulated interest.

Eurodollar deposits 
Deposits denominated in U.S. dollars but held in banks outside the United States, often in overseas branches of U.S. banks.

Money market mutual funds Funds of investment companies that obtain funds from the public that are held in common and used to acquire short-maturity credit instruments, such as certificates of deposit and securities sold by the U.S. government.

Money Market Mutual Fund Balances. Many individuals keep part of their assets in the form of shares in **money market mutual funds.** These retail mutual funds invest only in short-term credit instruments. The majority of these money market funds allow check-writing privileges, provided that the size of the check exceeds some minimum amount, usually $250. All money market mutual fund balances except those held by large institutions (which typically use them more like large time deposits) are included in M2.

M2 and Other Money Supply Definitions. When all of these assets are added together, the result is M2. The composition of M2 is given in panel (b) of Figure 14-2.

Economists and researchers have come up with even broader definitions of money than M2.* More assets are simply added to the definition. Just remember that there is no best definition of the money supply. For different purposes and under varying institutional circumstances, different definitions are appropriate. The definition that seems to correlate best with economic activity on an economywide basis for most countries is probably M2.

CONCEPTS IN BRIEF

- The money supply can be defined in a variety of ways, depending on whether we use the transactions approach or the liquidity approach. Using the transactions approach, the money supply consists of currency, checkable deposits, and traveler's checks. This is called M1.
- Checkable deposits (transactions accounts) are any deposits in financial institutions on which the deposit owner can write checks.
- Credit cards are not part of the money supply, for they simply defer transactions that ultimately involve the use of money.
- When we add savings deposits, small-denomination time deposits (certificates of deposit), money market deposit accounts, overnight REPOs, overnight Eurodollars, and retail money market mutual fund balances to M1, we obtain the measure known as M2, which comes close to reflecting economywide economic activity.

Click here to find out about the latest trends in the monetary aggregates.

FINANCIAL INTERMEDIATION AND BANKS

Central bank A banker's bank, usually an official institution that also serves as a country's treasury's bank. Central banks normally regulate commercial banks.

Most nations, including the United States, have a banking system that consists of two types of institutions. One type consists of private banking institutions. These include commercial banks, which are privately owned profit-seeking institutions, and savings institutions, such as savings banks, savings and loan associations, and credit unions. Savings institutions may be profit-seeking institutions, or they may be *mutual* institutions that are owned by their depositors. The other type of institution is a **central bank,** which typically serves as a banker's bank and as a bank for the national treasury or finance ministry.

Direct Versus Indirect Financing

When individuals choose to hold some of their savings in new bonds issued by a corporation, their purchases of the bonds are in effect direct loans to the business. This is an example of *direct finance,* in which people lend funds directly to a business. Business financing

*They include M3, which is equal to M2 plus large-denomination time deposits and REPOs (in amounts over $100,000) issued by commercial banks and thrift institutions, Eurodollars held by U.S residents and foreign branches of U.S. banks worldwide and all banking offices in the United Kingdom and Canada, and balances in both taxable and tax-exempt institution-only money market mutual funds. An even broader definition is called L, for *liquidity.* It is defined as M3 plus nonbank public holdings of U.S. savings bonds, Treasury bills, and other short-term securities.

is not always so direct. Individuals might choose instead to hold a time deposit at a bank. The bank may then lend to the same company. In this way, the same people can provide *indirect finance* to a business. The bank makes this possible by *intermediating* the financing of the company.

Financial intermediation 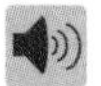
The process by which financial institutions accept savings from businesses, households, and governments and lend the savings to other businesses, households, and governments.

Financial Intermediation

Banks and other financial institutions are all in the same business—transferring funds from savers to investors. This process is known as **financial intermediation,** and its participants, such as banks and savings institutions, are **financial intermediaries.** The process of financial intermediation is illustrated in Figure 14-4.

Financial intermediaries 
Institutions that transfer funds between ultimate lenders (savers) and ultimate borrowers.

Asymmetric Information, Adverse Selection, and Moral Hazard. Why might people wish to direct their funds through a bank instead of lending them directly to a business? One important reason is **asymmetric information,** the fact that the business may have better knowledge of its own current and future prospects than potential lenders do. For instance, the business may know that it intends to use borrowed funds for projects with a high risk of failure that would make repaying the loan difficult. This potential for those who wish to borrow funds to use in unworthy projects is known as **adverse selection.** Alternatively, a business that had intended to undertake low-risk projects may change management after receiving a loan, and the new managers may use borrowed funds in riskier ways. The possibility that a borrower might engage in behavior that increases risk after borrowing funds is called **moral hazard.**

Asymmetric information 
Possession of information by one party in a financial transaction but not by the other party.

Adverse selection 
The likelihood that individuals who seek to borrow money may use the funds that they receive for unworthy, high-risk projects.

Moral hazard 
The possibility that a borrower might engage in riskier behavior after a loan has been obtained.

To minimize the possibility that a business might fail to repay on a loan, people thinking about lending funds directly to the business must study the business carefully before making the loan, and they must continue to monitor its performance afterward. Alternatively, they can choose to avoid the trouble by holding deposits with financial intermediaries,

FIGURE 14-4
The Process of Financial Intermediation
The process of financial intermediation is depicted here. Note that ultimate lenders and ultimate borrowers are the same economic units—households, businesses, and governments—but not necessarily the same individuals. Whereas individual households can be net lenders or borrowers, households as an economic unit are net lenders. Specific businesses or governments similarly can be net lenders or borrowers; as economic units, both are net borrowers.

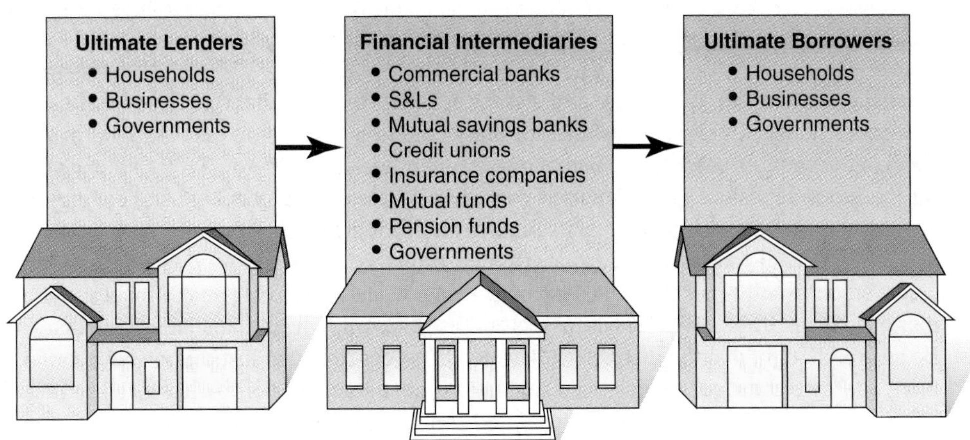

which then specialize in evaluating the creditworthiness of business borrowers and in keeping tabs on their progress until loans are repaid. Thus asymmetric information helps explain why people use financial intermediaries. Moral hazard can be involved when billions of dollars are lent to foreign governments. This is exactly what happened in Russia.

INTERNATIONAL EXAMPLE

Russia and Moral Hazard

Whenever funds are borrowed from a lender, the potential for moral hazard exists. On an international level, this is exactly what happened with the International Monetary Fund (which is financed in large part by U.S. taxpayers). Soon after the Soviet Union collapsed at the end of 1989, the largest new republic, Russia, asked Western nations to help it out. The IMF did just that with a $15 billion "bailout" loan. In order to get the loan, the Russian government agreed to undertake extensive market reforms, cut back on its military spending, and do whatever was necessary to change its economy and make sure it could pay back the money borrowed. Lo and behold, as soon as the billions were lent to Russia, government officials changed their behavior. Moral hazard slipped in as the Russian government suddenly found new uses for the funds that had more to do with encouraging people to vote for current leaders than to enact true reforms. The loan became more risky as a result. Not surprisingly, a few years later, the Russian government asked for even more funds from the IMF. But of course the inevitable was to happen again—no matter what the Russian government agreed to do to get the additional IMF loans, it started to renege as soon as the funds were received.

For Critical Analysis

Once the IMF makes a loan to a country "in trouble," what, if anything, can be done to reduce the moral hazard problem?

Larger Scale and Lower Management Costs. Another important reason that financial intermediaries exist is that they make it possible for many people to pool their funds, thereby increasing the size, or *scale,* of the total amount of savings managed by an intermediary. This centralization of management reduces fund management costs and risks below the levels savers would incur if all were to manage their savings alone. *Pension fund companies,* which are institutions that specialize in managing funds that individuals save for retirement, owe their existence largely to their abilities to provide such cost savings to individual savers. Likewise, *investment companies,* which are institutions that manage portfolios of financial instruments called mutual funds on behalf of shareholders, also exist largely because of cost savings from their greater scale of operations.

Liabilities 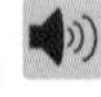
Amounts owed; the legal claims against a business or household by nonowners.

Assets 
Amounts owned; all items to which a business or household holds legal claim.

Financial Institution Liabilities and Assets. Every financial intermediary has its own sources of funds, which are **liabilities** of that institution. When you deposit $100 in your checking account in a bank, the bank creates a liability—it owes you $100—in exchange for the funds deposited. A commercial bank gets its funds from checking and savings accounts; an insurance company gets its funds from insurance policy premiums.

Each financial intermediary has a different primary use of its **assets.** For example, a credit union usually makes small consumer loans, whereas a savings bank makes mainly mortgage loans. Table 14-2 lists the assets and liabilities of typical financial intermediaries. Be aware, though, that the distinction between different financial institutions is becoming more and more blurred. As laws and regulations change, there will be less need to make any distinction. All may ultimately be treated simply as financial intermediaries.

TABLE 14-2
Financial Intermediaries and Their Assets and Liabilities

Financial Intermediary	Assets	Liabilities
Commercial banks	Car loans and other consumer debt, business loans, government securities, home mortgages	Transactions accounts, savings deposits, various other time deposits, money market deposit accounts
Savings and loan associations	Home mortgages, some consumer and business debt	Savings and loan shares, transactions accounts, various time deposits, money market deposit accounts
Mutual savings banks	Home mortgages, some consumer and business debt	Transactions accounts, savings accounts, various time deposits, money market deposit accounts
Credit unions	Consumer debt, long-term mortgage loans	Credit union shares, transactions accounts
Insurance companies	Mortgages, stocks, bonds, real estate	Insurance contracts, annuities, pension plans
Pension and retirement funds	Stocks, bonds, mortgages, time deposits	Pension plans
Money market mutual funds	Short-term credit instruments such as large-bank CDs, Treasury bills, and high-grade commercial paper	Fund shares with limited checking privileges

Financial Intermediation Across National Boundaries

Some countries' governments restrict the financial intermediation process to within their national boundaries. They do so by imposing legal restraints called **capital controls** that bar certain flows of funds across their borders. Nevertheless, today many nations have reduced or even eliminated capital controls. This permits their residents to strive for **international financial diversification** by engaging in the direct or indirect financing of companies located in various nations.

Capital controls 
Legal restrictions on the ability of a nation's residents to hold and trade assets denominated in foreign currencies.

Because business conditions may be good in one country, as they were in the United States in the late 1990s, at the same time that they are poor in another, such as Japan in the late 1990s, people can limit their overall lending risks through international financial diversification. One way to do this is to hold a portion of one's savings with an investment company that offers a **world index fund.** This is carefully designed set of globally issued bonds yielding returns that historically tend to move in offsetting directions. By holding world index funds, individuals can earn the average return on bonds from a number of nations while keeping overall risk of loss to a minimum.

International financial diversification 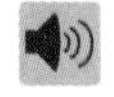
Financing investment projects in more than one country.

World index fund 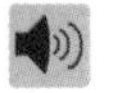
A portfolio of bonds issued in various nations whose yields generally move in offsetting directions, thereby reducing the overall risk of losses.

Holding shares in a world index fund is an example of indirect finance across national borders through financial intermediaries. Banks located in various countries take part in the process of international financial intermediation by using some of the funds of depositors in their home nations to finance loans to companies based in other nations. Today, bank financing of U.S. business activities increasingly stems from loans by non-U.S. banks.

TABLE 14-3
The World's Largest Banks
There usually are few U.S. banks among the world's top ten.

Bank	Country	Assets ($ Billions)
Fuji Industrial Bank	Japan	1,380
Asahi Sanwa Bank	Japan	1,044
Sumitomo Bank	Japan	1,002
Deutsche Bank	Germany	765
Bank of Tokyo-Mitsubishi	Japan	721
Citigroup Inc.	United States	717
BNP Paribas Group	France	702
Bank of America Corp.	United States	633
UBS AG	Switzerland	615
HSBC Holdings PLC	United Kingdom	569

Source: American Banker, March 31, 2000.

Indeed, as Table 14-3 indicates, the world's largest banks are not based in the United States. Today, most of the largest banking institutions, sometimes called *megabanks,* are based in Europe and Japan. These megabanks typically take in deposits and lend throughout the world. Although they report their profits and pay taxes in their home nations, these megabanks are in all other ways international banking institutions.

BANKING STRUCTURES THROUGHOUT THE WORLD

Multinational businesses have relationships with megabanks based in many nations. Individuals and companies increasingly retain the services of banks based outside their home countries. The business of banking varies from nation to nation, however. Each country has its own distinctive banking history, and this fact helps explain unique features of the world's banking systems. Countries' banking systems differ in a number of ways. In some nations, banks are the crucial component of the financial intermediation process, but in others, banking is only part of a varied financial system. In addition, some countries have only a few large banks, while others, such as the United States, have relatively large numbers of banks of various sizes. The legal environments regulating bank dealings with individual and business customers also differ considerably across nations.

A World of National Banking Structures

Click here to learn more about worldwide banking developments. Select "Annual Report."

The extent to which banks are the predominant means by which businesses finance their operations is a key way that national banking systems differ. For instance, in Britain, nearly 70 percent of funds raised by businesses typically stem from bank borrowings, and the proportions for Germany and Japan are on the order of 50 percent and 65 percent, respectively. By way of contrast, U.S. businesses normally raise less than 30 percent of their funds through bank loans.

The relative sizes of banks also differ from one country to another. The five largest banks in Belgium, Denmark, France, Italy, Luxembourg, Portugal, Spain, and the United Kingdom have over 30 percent of the deposits of their nations' residents. In Greece and the Netherlands, this figure is over 80 percent. In contrast, the top five U.S. banks account for less than 15 percent of the deposit holdings of U.S. residents. In Germany, Japan, and Britain, about two-thirds of total bank assets are held by the largest 10 banks. In the United States, this figure is less than one-third.

Traditionally, another feature that has distinguished national banking systems has been the extent to which they have permitted **universal banking.** Under this form of banking, there are few, if any, limits on the ability of banks to offer a full range of financial services and to own shares of corporate stock. In Germany, Britain, and other European nations, banks have had the right to sell insurance and to own stock for many years. Japanese banks face greater restrictions on their activities than European banks, but many Japanese banks have long had the authority to buy stocks. Until very recently, U.S. banks could not hold *any* shares of stock, even for brief periods and were subject to limitations on their ability to offer insurance policies to their customers. This state of affairs changed, however, with passage of the Gramm-Leach-Bliley Act of 1999. This legislation authorized U.S. commercial banks to market insurance and to own stock. Consequently, national differences in banking powers are much narrower than they were just a few years ago.

Universal banking 
Environment in which banks face few or no restrictions on their power to offer a full range of financial services and to own shares of stock in corporations.

Central Banks and Their Roles

The first central bank, which began operations in 1668, was Sweden's Sveriges Riksbank (called the Risens Standers Bank until 1867). In 1694, the British Parliament established the most historically famous of central banks, the Bank of England. It authorized the Bank of England to issue currency notes redeemable in silver, and initially the Bank of England's notes circulated alongside currency notes issued by the government and private finance companies. Until 1800, the Riksbank and the Bank of England were the only central banks. The number of central banks worldwide remained less than 10 as late as 1873. The number expanded considerably toward the end of the nineteenth century and again during the second half of the twentieth century, as shown in Figure 14-5.

FIGURE 14-5
The Number of Central Banking Institutions, 1670 to the Present
The twentieth century witnessed considerable growth in the number of central banks.

Source: Data from Forrest Capie, Charles Goodhart, and Norbert Schnadt, "The Development of Central Banking," in Forrest Capie et al., *The Future of Central Banking: The Tercentenary Symposium of the Bank of England* (Cambridge: Cambridge University Press, 1994.)

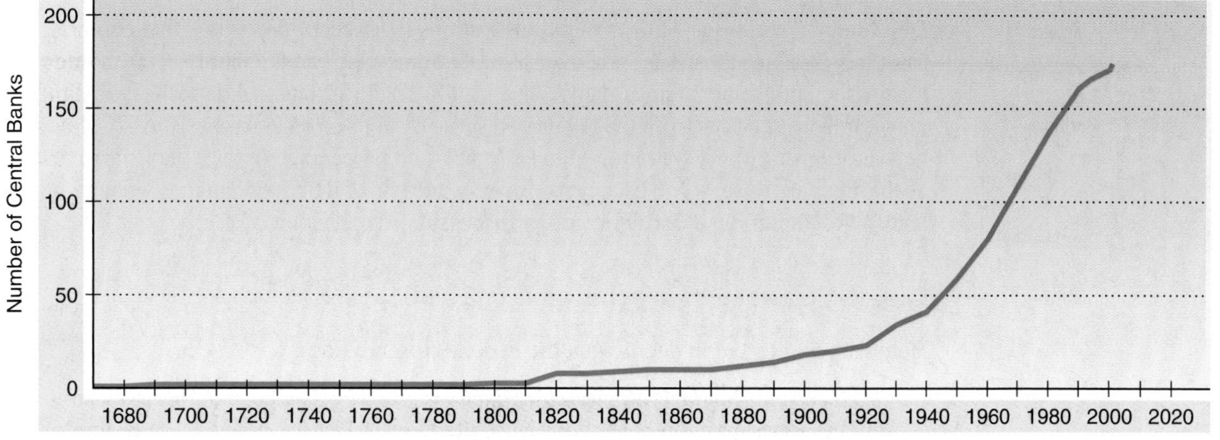

The duties of central banks fall into three broad categories:

1. Central banks perform banking functions for their nations' governments.
2. Central banks provide financial services for private banks.
3. Central banks conduct their nations' monetary policies.

The third is the area of central banking that receives most media attention, even though most central banks devote the bulk of their resources to the other two tasks.

THE FEDERAL RESERVE SYSTEM

The Federal Reserve System, also known simply as **the Fed,** is the most important regulatory agency in the United States' monetary system and is usually considered the monetary authority. The Fed was established by the Federal Reserve Act, signed on December 23, 1913, by President Woodrow Wilson. The act was the outgrowth of recommendations from the National Monetary Commission, which had been authorized by the Aldridge-Vreeland Act of 1908. Basically, the commission had attempted to find a way to counter the periodic financial panics that had occurred in our country. Based on the commission's recommendations, which were developed after considerable study of the Bank of England and other central banks, Congress established the Federal Reserve System to aid and supervise banks and also to provide banking services for the U.S. Treasury.

The Fed 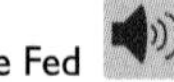 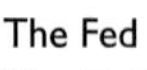
The Federal Reserve System; the central bank of the United States.

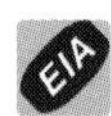

The Federal Reserve System
Reinforce your understanding of the Federal Reserve's structure and functions.

Organization of the Federal Reserve System

Figure 14-6 shows how the Federal Reserve System is organized. It is managed by the Board of Governors, composed of seven full-time members appointed by the U.S. president with the approval of the Senate. The 12 Federal Reserve district banks have a total of 25 branches. The boundaries of the 12 Federal Reserve districts and the cities in which Federal Reserve banks are located are shown in Figure 14-7. The Federal Open Market Committee (FOMC) determines the future growth of the money supply and other important variables. This committee is composed of the members of the Board of Governors, the president of the New York Federal Reserve Bank, and presidents of four other Reserve banks, rotated periodically.

Depository Institutions

Depository institutions—all financial institutions that accept deposits—that comprise our monetary system consist of just over 8,500 commercial banks, about 1,100 savings and loan associations and savings banks, and 12,000 credit unions. All depository institutions may purchase services from the Federal Reserve System on an equal basis. Also, almost all depository institutions are required to keep a certain percentage of their deposits in reserve at the Federal Reserve district banks or as vault cash. This percentage depends on the bank's volume of business. (For further discussion, see Chapter 15.)

Functions of the Federal Reserve System

Here we will present in detail what the Federal Reserve does.

1. *The Fed supplies the economy with fiduciary currency.* The Federal Reserve banks supply the economy with paper currency called Federal Reserve notes. For example, dur-

FIGURE 14-6
Organization of the Federal Reserve System
The 12 Federal Reserve district banks are headed by 12 separate presidents. The main authority of the Fed resides with the Board of Governors of the Federal Reserve System, whose seven members are appointed for 14-year terms by the president of the United States and confirmed by the Senate. Open market operations are carried out through the Federal Open Market Committee (FOMC), consisting of the seven members of the Board of Governors plus five presidents of the district banks (always including the president of the New York bank, with the others rotating).
Source: Board of Governors of the Federal Reserve System, *The Federal Reserve System: Purposes and Functions,* 7th ed. (Washington, D.C., 1984), p. 5.

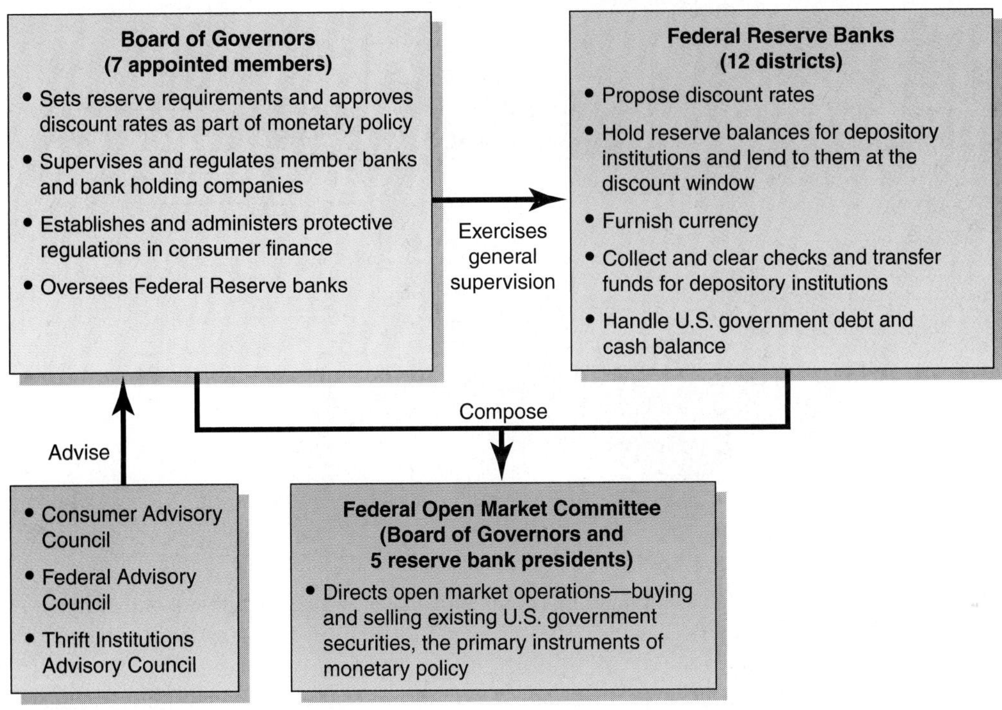

ing holiday seasons, when there is an abnormally large number of currency transactions, more paper currency is desired. Commercial banks find this out as deposit holders withdraw large amounts of cash from their accounts. Commercial banks turn to the Federal Reserve banks to replenish vault cash. Hence the Federal Reserve banks must have on hand a sufficient amount of cash to accommodate the demands for paper currency at different times of the year. Note that even though all Federal Reserve notes are printed at the Bureau of Printing and Engraving in Washington, D.C., each note is assigned a code indicating from which of the 12 Federal Reserve banks it "originated." Moreover, each of these notes is an obligation (liability) of the Federal Reserve System, *not* the U.S. Treasury.

2. *The Fed provides a system for check collection and clearing.* The Federal Reserve System has established a clearing mechanism for checks. Suppose that John Smith in Chicago writes a check to Jill Jones, who lives in San Francisco. When Jill receives the check in the mail, she deposits it at her commercial bank. Her bank then deposits the check in the Federal Reserve Bank of San Francisco. In turn, the Federal Reserve Bank of San Francisco sends the check to the Federal Reserve Bank of Chicago. The Chicago Fed

FIGURE 14-7
The Federal Reserve System
The Federal Reserve System is divided into 12 districts, each served by one of the Federal Reserve district banks, located in the cities indicated. The Board of Governors meets in Washington, D.C.

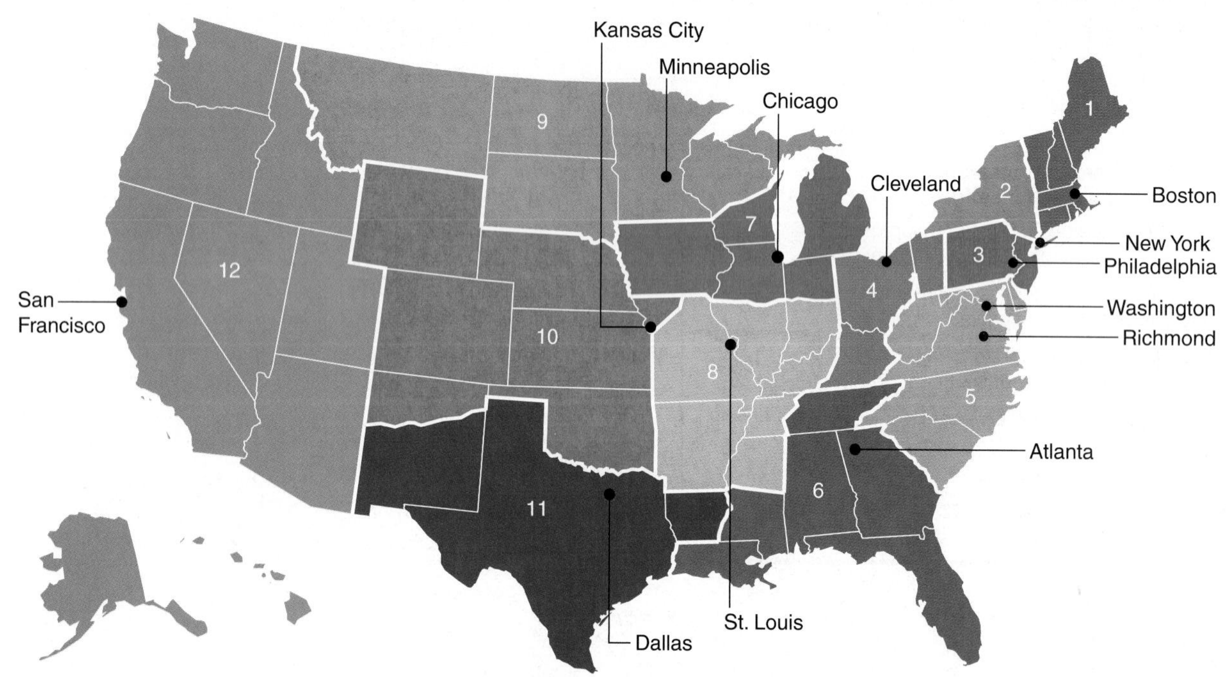

then sends the check to John Smith's commercial bank, where the amount of the check is deducted from John's account. The schematic diagram in Figure 14-8 illustrates this check-clearing process.

The Fed's check collection and clearing operations compete with private clearinghouses. Since the Fed began charging for these services, a considerable volume of this business has shifted back to the private sector. At present, the Federal Reserve processes about one-third of all checks in the United States.

3. *The Fed holds depository institutions' reserves.* The 12 Federal Reserve district banks hold the reserves (other than vault cash) of depository institutions. As you will see in Chapter 15, depository institutions are required by law to keep a certain percentage of their deposits as reserves. Even if they weren't required to do so by law, they would still wish to keep some reserves. Depository institutions act just like other businesses. A firm would not try to operate with a zero balance in its checking account. It would keep a positive balance on hand from which it could draw for expected and unexpected transactions. So, too, would a depository institution desire to have reserves in its banker's bank (the Federal Reserve) on which it could draw funds needed for expected and unexpected transactions.
4. *The Fed acts as the government's fiscal agent.* The Federal Reserve is the banker and fiscal agent for the federal government. The government, as we are all aware, collects large sums of money through taxation. The government also spends and distributes equally large sums. Consequently, the U.S. Treasury has a checking account with the Federal Reserve. Thus the Fed acts as the government's banker, along with commer-

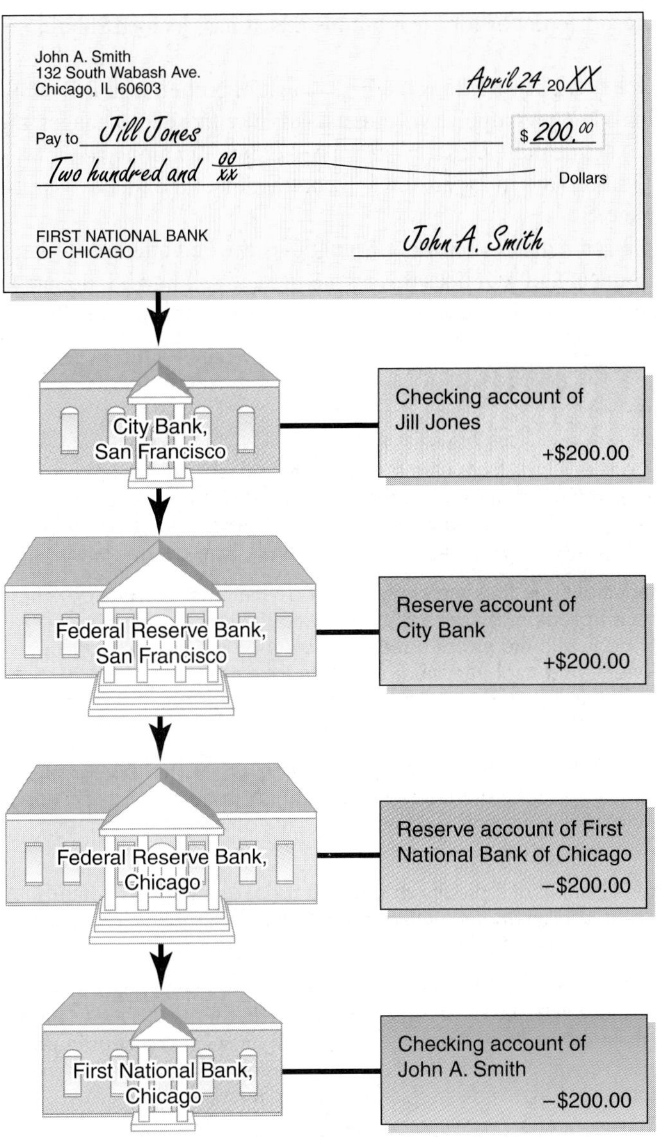

FIGURE 14-8 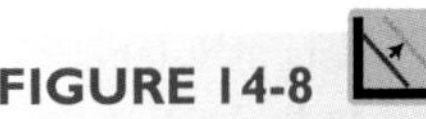

How a Check Clears

The check-clearing process for an out-of-town check normally involves four steps, including two with Federal Reserve district banks.

cial banks that hold government deposits. The Fed also helps the government collect certain tax revenues and aids in the purchase and sale of government securities.

5. *The Fed supervises depository institutions.* The Fed (along with the comptroller of the currency, the Federal Deposit Insurance Corporation, the Office of Thrift Supervision in the Treasury Department, and the National Credit Union Administration) is a supervisor and regulator of depository institutions. The Fed and other regulators periodically and without warning examine depository institutions to see what kinds of loans have been made, what has been used to back the loans, and who has received them. Whenever such an examination indicates that a bank is not conforming to current banking rules and standards, the Fed can exert pressure on the bank to alter its banking practices.
6. *The Fed acts as the "lender of last resort."* As a central bank, the Fed stands ready to assist, temporarily, any part of the banking system that is in trouble. In this sense, it

acts as a lender of last resort to depository institutions that it has decided should not fail.

7. *The Fed regulates the money supply.* Perhaps the Fed's most important task is its ability to regulate the nation's money supply. To understand how the Fed manages the money supply, we must examine more closely its reserve-holding function and the way in which depository institutions aid in expansion and contraction of the money supply. We will do this in Chapter 15.
8. *The Fed intervenes in foreign currency markets.* Sometimes the Fed attempts to keep the value of the dollar from changing. It does this by buying and selling U.S. dollars in foreign exchange markets. You will read more about this important topic in Chapter 33.

CONCEPTS IN BRIEF

- Financial intermediaries transfer funds from ultimate lenders (savers) to ultimate borrowers. This process of financial intermediation is undertaken by depository institutions such as commercial banks, savings and loan associations, savings banks, and credit unions, as well as by insurance companies, mutual funds, pension funds, and governments.
- Financial intermediaries specialize in tackling problems of asymmetric information. They address the adverse selection problem by carefully reviewing the creditworthiness of loan applicants, and they deal with the moral hazard problem by monitoring borrowers after they receive loans. Many financial intermediaries also take advantage of cost reductions arising from the centralized management of funds pooled from the savings of many individuals.
- In the absence of capital controls that inhibit flows of funds across national borders, many financial intermediaries also take advantage of overall risk reductions made possible by international financial diversification. This has led to the development of megabanks, which operate in many countries.
- A central bank is a banker's bank that typically acts as the fiscal agent for its nation's government as well. The central bank in the United States is the Federal Reserve System, which was established on December 13, 1913.
- There are 12 Federal Reserve district banks, with 25 branches. The Federal Reserve is managed by the Board of Governors in Washington, D.C. The Fed interacts with virtually all depository institutions in the United States, most of which must keep a certain percentage of deposits on reserve with the Fed. The Fed serves as chief regulatory agency for all depository institutions that have Federal Reserve System membership.
- The functions of the Federal Reserve System are to supply fiduciary currency, provide for check collection and clearing, hold depository institution reserves, act as the government's fiscal agent, supervise depository institutions, act as lender of last resort, regulate the supply of money, and intervene in foreign currency markets.

NETNOMICS

Electronic Check Processing

The typical U.S. resident writes nearly three times as many checks as a typical resident of Canada, France, or the United Kingdom. In 2000, the Federal Reserve banks and private clearinghouses processed over 70 billion checks. For a 365-day year, which contains 31,536,000 seconds, this implies that on an average day, these institutions processed well over 2,000 checks per second!

Most of the Federal Reserve's annual $2 billion budget, 25,000 employees (only about 1,600 of whom have job functions related to monetary policy), and small air force of 47 jets and cargo planes are devoted to check-clearing services. To clear checks, the Fed uses automated clearing mechanisms. Since the 1970s, checks have been encrypted with magnetic ink that machines can read directly, which permits automatic sorting, computer crediting, and machine-assisted distribution of checks.

At the time of its introduction, this magnetic encryption system increased the cost efficiency of check collection considerably. Today, however, the technology that the Fed and private clearinghouses use to clear checks looks increasingly antiquated. Current estimates are that alternative electronic payment technologies cost between one-third and one-half as much to use. In an effort to make the check-clearing process more efficient, therefore, the Fed is moving toward full implementation of *electronic check processing* (ECP). Once ECP is in place—which will require large initial setup costs for new hardware and software—magnetic encryption information will be fully scannable for processing by electronic transfer systems already in place. Under ECP, therefore, once a check is turned in to a bank, clearinghouses will essentially convert it to an electronic impulse.

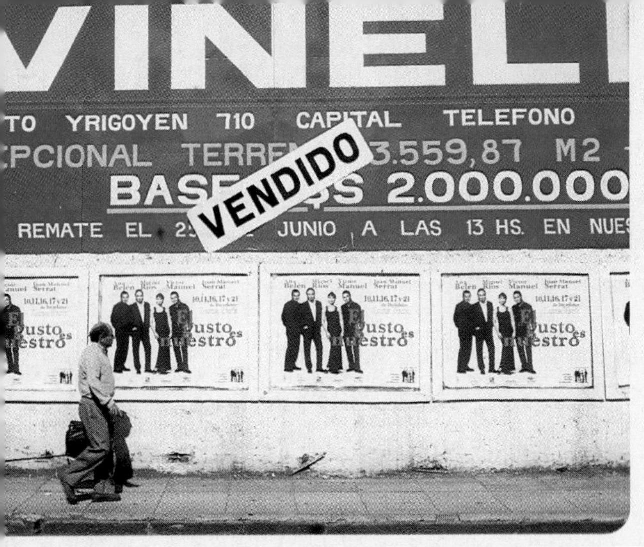

Issues & Applications

The Dollarization Movement: Is the Fed Destined to Be a Multinational Central Bank?

In 1998, Brazil faced an economic crisis, and Brazilian interest rates shot up considerably. So did interest rates in Argentina, Brazil's main international trading partner. This spillover from Brazil's crisis induced Argentina to contemplate a radical change in its monetary arrangements.

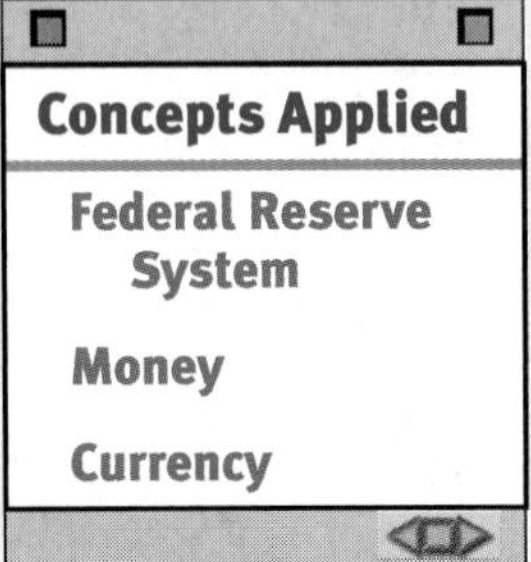

The Prospect of Latin American Dollarization

The change that Argentina's leaders considered was *dollarization.* This would entail abandoning Argentina's peso in favor of the U.S. dollar as a medium of exchange, unit of accounting, store of value, and standard of deferred payment. To implement dollarization, Argentina would have to import sufficient U.S. currency for people to use in hand-to-hand transactions. It also would have to convert all Argentine financial accounts and contracts to dollars at the prevailing fixed rate of exchange. Such a conversion would not be too difficult for Argentina, however, because it already has a *currency board* system, in which Argentina issues pesos on a one-to-one basis with the number of U.S. dollars it has on reserve. Thus Argentina's monetary system is already closely linked to that of the United States.

Since Argentina's leaders floated the dollarization proposal, several Latin American nations have revealed that they have been considering the same idea. Dollarization of part of Latin America would have both costs and benefits for the United States. It would simplify efforts by U.S. companies to do business with Latin America, which accounts for about a fifth of U.S. trade. Greater use of the dollar outside the United States could also create a financial windfall for the U.S. government, because Argentina would purchase dollars, giving the U.S. government interest-bearing securities in exchange. The U.S. government would earn the interest on those securities, but as usual, it would not pay interest on its currency. The worldwide return of about $15 billion per year that the U.S. government earns overseas on use of the dollar would undoubtedly increase.

Nevertheless, Federal Reserve and U.S. Treasury officials have expressed concerns about dollarization. Fed policy actions consistent with stabilizing the U.S. economy could have negative consequences outside the United States, fostering resentment and encouraging policymakers in dollarized countries to deflect blame onto U.S. policymakers. This could give governments of dollarized countries political cover for dodging tough decisions regarding appropriate economic policies.

A North American Monetary Union?

So far, Latin American nations, except for Ecuador, have not pursued the dollarization idea any further. Nevertheless, it has now moved north of U.S. borders. Recently, a Toronto-based think tank released a study proposing "North American currency integration" by establishing the U.S. dollar as the single circulating currency in Canada. The authors of the Canadian proposal were not quite as willing as Latin Americans to contemplate unilateral dollarization, however. Their proposal called for the Federal Reserve's Board of Governors to have one Canadian member.

So far the United States has expressed little interest in sharing control of its central bank, but many Canadians seem to be coming around to the idea. After watching the value of the Canadian dollar fall from about 0.90 Canadian dollar per U.S. dollar in 1991 to about 0.65 Canadian dollar per U.S. dollar today, more than a third of Canadians surveyed in public opinion polls indicated support for abolishing the Canadian currency altogether. Three-fourths of Canadians polled said they expected to see a common dollar for the United States and Canada by 2020.

FOR CRITICAL ANALYSIS

1. What would Argentina and Canada give up by dollarizing their economies?
2. Do you see any merit to the arguments by critics of dollarization proposals, who argue that unilateral dollarization in Latin America and Canada would lead to "taxation without representation"?

SG

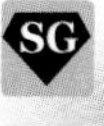

SUMMARY DISCUSSION OF LEARNING OBJECTIVES

1. **The Key Functions of Money:** Money has four functions. It is a medium of exchange, which means that people use money to make payments for goods, services, and financial assets. It is also is a unit of accounting, meaning that prices are quoted in terms of money values. In addition, money is a store of value, so that people can hold money for future use in exchange. Furthermore, money is a standard of deferred payment, so that the lenders make loans and buyers repay those loans with money.
2. **Important Properties of Goods That Serve as Money:** A good will successfully function as money only if people are widely willing to accept the good in exchange for other goods and services. People must have confidence that others will be willing to trade their goods and services for the good used as money. In addition, while people may continue to use money even if inflation erodes its real purchasing power, they will do so only if the value of money is relatively predictable.
3. **Official Definitions of the Quantity of Money in Circulation:** The narrow definition of the quantity of money in circulation, called M1, focuses on money's role as a medium of exchange. It includes only currency, checkable deposits, and traveler's checks. A broader definition, called M2, stresses money's role as a temporary store of value. M2 is equal to M1 plus near-money assets such as savings deposits, small-denomination time deposits, money market deposit accounts, overnight repurchase agreements and Eurodollars, and noninstitutional holdings of money market mutual fund balances.
4. **Why Financial Intermediaries Such as Banks Exist:** Financial intermediaries help reduce problems stemming from the existence of asymmetric information in financial transactions. Asymmetric information can lead to adverse selection, in which uncreditworthy individuals and firms seek loans, and moral hazard problems, in which an individual or business that has been granted credit begins to engage in riskier practices. Financial intermediaries may also permit savers to benefit from economies of scale, which is the ability to reduce the costs and risks of managing funds by pooling funds and spreading costs and risks across many savers.
5. **The Basic Structure of the Federal Reserve System:** The central bank of the United States is the Federal Reserve System, which consists of 12 district banks with 25 branches. The governing body of the Federal Reserve System is the Board of Governors, which is based in Washington, D.C. Decisions about the quantity of money in circulation are made

by the Federal Open Market Committee, which is composed of the Board of Governors and five Federal Reserve bank presidents.

6. **Major Functions of the Federal Reserve:** The main functions of the Federal Reserve System are supplying the economy with fiduciary currency, providing a system for check collection and clearing, holding depository institutions' reserves, acting as the government's fiscal agent, supervising banks, acting as a lender of last resort, regulating the money supply, and intervening in foreign exchange markets.

Key Terms and Concepts

Adverse selection (337)
Assets (338)
Asymmetric information (337)
Barter (328)
Capital controls (339)
Central bank (336)
Certificate of deposit (CDs) (335)
Checkable deposits (333)
Depository institutions (335)
Eurodollar deposits (335)
The Fed (342)
Fiduciary monetary system (331)
Financial intermediaries (337)
Financial intermediation (337)
International financial diversification (339)
Liabilities (338)
Liquidity (330)
Liquidity approach (332)
M1 (333)
M2 (335)
Medium of exchange (328)
Money (328)
Money market deposit account (MMDAs) (335)
Money market mutual funds (336)
Money supply (332)
Moral hazard (337)
Near moneys (334)
Repurchase agreement (REPO, or RP) (335)
Savings deposits (335)
Standard of deferred payment (330)
Store of value (329)
Thrift institutions (333)
Time deposit (335)
Transactions accounts (331)
Transactions approach (332)
Traveler's checks (333)
Unit of accounting (329)
Universal banking (341)
World index fund (339)

Problems

Answers to the odd-numbered problems appear at the back of the book.

14-1. On the island of Yap, natives until 1946 used large doughnut-shaped stones as financial assets. Although prices of goods and services were not quoted in terms of the stones, the stones were often used in exchange for particularly large purchases, such as payments for livestock. To make the transaction, several individuals would place a large stick through a stone's center and carry it to its new owner. A stone was difficult for any one person to steal, so an owner typically would lean it against the side of his or her home as a sign to others of accumulated purchasing power that would hold value for later use in exchange. Loans would often be repaid using the stones. In what ways did these stones function as money?

14-2. During the late 1970s, prices quoted in terms of the Israeli currency, the shekel, rose so fast that grocery stores listed their prices in terms of the U.S. dollar and provided customers with dollar-shekel conversion tables that they updated daily. Although people continued to buy goods and services and make loans using shekels, many Israeli citizens converted shekels to dollars to avoid a reduction in their wealth due to inflation. In what way did the U.S. dollar function as money in Israel during this period?

14-3. During the 1945–1946 Hungarian hyperinflation, when the rate of inflation reached 41.9 *quadrillion* percent per month, the Hungarian government discovered that the real value of its tax receipts was falling dramatically. To keep real tax income more stable, it created a good called a "tax pengö," in which all bank deposits were denominated for purposes of taxation. Nevertheless, payments for goods and services were made only in terms of the real Hungarian currency, whose value tended to fall rapidly even though the value of a tax pengö remained stable. Prices were quoted only in terms of the regular currency also. Lenders, however, began denominating loan payments in terms of tax pengös. In what ways did the tax pengö function as money in Hungary in 1945 and 1946?

14-4. Considering the following data (expressed in billions of U.S. dollars), calculate M1 and M2.

Currency	450
Savings deposits and money market deposit accounts	1,400
Small-denomination time deposits	1,000
Traveler's checks	10
Overnight repurchase agreements	100
Total money market mutual funds	500
Institution-only money market mutual funds	200
Overnight Eurodollars	50
Demand deposits	450
Other checkable deposits	490

14-5. Identify whether the following item is counted in M1, M2, or neither:

a. A $1,000 balance in a checking account at a mutual savings bank

b. A $100,000 certificate of deposit issued by a New York bank

c. A $10,000 time deposit an elderly widow holds at her credit union

d. A Eurodollar deposit that matures in three months

e. A $50,000 money market deposit account balance

14-6. In the early 1990s, many pension funds and mutual funds began offering U.S. savers special portfolios composed only of financial instruments issued by companies and governments located in other nations. In 1997 and 1998, many of those savers who held these portfolios earned very low, and sometimes negative, returns. By way of contrast, most people who allocated 100 percent of their savings only to U.S. financial instruments earned higher returns. Does this experience mean that international financial diversification is a mistake? Explain your reasoning.

14-7. A few years ago, a Florida county commissioner and her husband, a Washington lobbyist, were indicted for securities laws violations. Allegedly, they sought to improve the terms under which the county could issue new municipal bonds. Suppose this information had not come to light and had made the municipal bonds more risky than they otherwise might have seemed to potential buyers. Would this have been an example of adverse selection or of moral hazard? Explain your reasoning.

14-8. In what sense is currency a liability of the Federal Reserve System?

14-9. In what respects is the Fed like a private banking institution? In what respects is it more like a government agency?

14-10. Take a look at the map of the locations of the Federal Reserve districts and their headquarters in Figure 14-7. Today, the U.S. population is centered just west of the Mississippi River—that is, about half of the population is either to the west or the east of a line running roughly just west of this river. Can you reconcile the current locations of Fed districts and banks with this fact? Why do you suppose the Fed has its current geographic structure?

Economics on the Net

What's Happened to the Money Supply? Deposits at banks and other financial institutions comprise a portion of the U.S. money supply. This application gives you the chance to see how changes in these deposits influence the Fed's measures of money.

Title: FRED (Federal Reserve Economic Data)

Navigation: Click here to visit the Web page of the Federal Reserve Bank of St. Louis.

Application

1. Under Daily/Weekly U.S. Financial Data, select the data series for demand deposits (either seasonally adjusted or not). Scan through the data. Do you notice any recent trend? (Hint: Compare the growth in the figures before 1993 with their growth after 1993.) In addition, take a look at the data series for currency and for other checkable deposits. Do you observe similar recent trends in these series?

2. Now take a look at the M1 series (again, either seasonally adjusted or not). Does it show any recent trend (pre-1993 versus post-1993)?

For Group Study and Analysis FRED contains considerable financial data series. Assign individual members or groups of the class the task of examining data on assets included in M1, M2, and M3. Have each student or group look for big swings in the data. Then ask the groups to report to the class as a whole. When did clear changes occur in various categories of the monetary aggregates? Were there times that people appeared to shift funds from one aggregate to another? Are there any other noticeable patterns that may have had something to do with economic events during various periods?

CHAPTER 15

MONEY CREATION, PAYMENT SYSTEMS, AND DEPOSIT INSURANCE

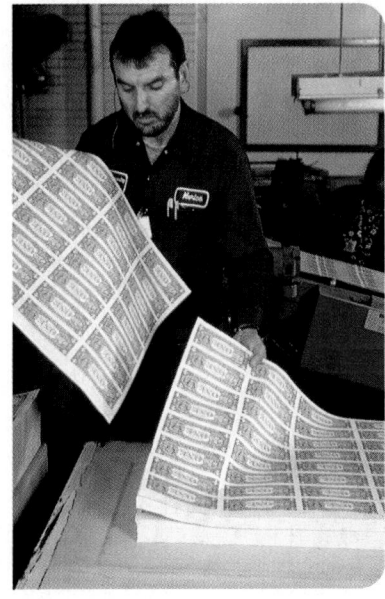

Federal Reserve notes are part of the money supply. But they constitute only a small part of the legal reserves that depository institutions keep. In what form are most legal reserves held?

In the early 1990s, banks and other depository institutions held about $30 billion in funds on deposit with Federal Reserve Banks — funds known as *depository institution reserves.* Today, that amount has declined to about $9 billion. In the late 1990s, Federal Reserve Board Chair Alan Greenspan expressed his concern that this development "could adversely affect the ability of the Federal Reserve to gauge the supply of reserves consistent with the Federal Open Market Committee's intended policy stance." Translated, this means that the Fed is worried that the big decline in depository institution reserves at Federal Reserve banks may make it hard for the Fed to control the money supply. Why have banks cut back so much on their reserves on deposit with Federal Reserve banks? What does this have to do with the money supply? In this chapter, you will learn about the concepts you must understand in order to answer these questions.

LEARNING OBJECTIVES

After reading this chapter, you should be able to:

1. Describe how the Federal Reserve assesses reserve requirements on banks and other depository institutions
2. Understand why the money supply is unaffected when someone deposits in a depository institution a check drawn on another depository institution
3. Explain why the money supply changes when someone deposits in a depository institution a check drawn on the Federal Reserve System
4. Determine the maximum potential extent to which the money supply will change following a Federal Reserve purchase or sale of government securities
5. Describe the structure of the U.S. payment system and the associated risks it poses for individual depository institutions and the banking system as a whole
6. Explain the essential features of federal deposit insurance

Chapter Outline

Did You Know That... virtually overnight, Nick Leeson, a 27-year-old manager in the Singapore branch of Barings Bank, was able to inflict losses of several billion dollars on the institution? Barings was founded in 1762. In 1803, it helped the United States purchase the Louisiana Territory from France. It provided credit to the British government during the Napoleonic Wars (1803–1815). When Barings collapsed in the mid-1990s—as a result of Leeson's actions—it was bought by former competitors, thereby ending the life of one of the longest-running financial institutions in the world. Could the collapse of such an important bank lead to serious problems in the world's banking sector? A lot depends on whether the losses suffered by Barings's depositors would cause other banks to shrink. That in turn depends on the relationship between deposits in different banks.

If you were to attend a luncheon of local bankers and ask the question, "Do you as bankers create money?" you would get a uniformly negative response. Bankers are certain that they do not create money. Indeed, *by itself* no individual bank can create money. But through actions initiated by a central bank such as the Federal Reserve, depository institutions *together* do create money; they determine the total deposits outstanding. In this chapter, we will examine the money multiplier process, which explains how an injection of new money into the banking system leads to an eventual multiple expansion in the total money supply. We will also take a look at our payment system and how it creates risks for depository institutions, including the potential for widespread bank failures. Then we shall examine federal deposit insurance and its role in provoking the 1980s crisis in the savings and loan industry.

LINKS BETWEEN CHANGES IN THE MONEY SUPPLY AND OTHER ECONOMIC VARIABLES

How fast the money supply grows or does not grow is important because no matter what model of the economy is used, theories link the money supply growth rate to economic growth or to business fluctuations. There is in fact a long-standing relationship between changes in the money supply and changes in GDP. Some economists use this historical evidence to argue that money is an important determinant of the level of economic activity in the economy.

Another key economic variable in our economy is the price level. As you learned in Chapter 10, both the quantity of money and the price level have risen since the 1950s, and at least one theory attributes changes in the rate of inflation to changes in the growth rate of money in circulation. Figure 15-1 shows the relationship between the rate of growth of the money supply and the inflation rate. There seems to be a loose, long-run, direct relationship between changes in the money supply and changes in the rate of inflation. Increases in the money supply growth rate seem to lead to increases in the inflation rate, after a time lag.

THE ORIGINS OF FRACTIONAL RESERVE BANKING

As early as 1000 B.C., uncoined gold and silver were being used as money in Mesopotamia. Goldsmiths weighed and assessed the purity of those metals; later they started issuing paper notes indicating that the bearers held gold or silver of given weights and purity on deposit with the goldsmith. These notes could be transferred in exchange for goods and became the first paper currency. The gold and silver on deposit with the goldsmiths were

FIGURE 15-1

Money Supply Growth Versus the Inflation Rate

These time-series curves indicate a loose correspondence between money supply growth and the inflation rate. Actually, closer inspection reveals a direct relationship between changes in the growth rate of money and changes in the inflation rate *in a later period.* This relationship seemed to hold well into the 1990s, when it became less strong.

Sources: Economic Report of the President; Federal Reserve Bulletin; Economic Indicators, various issues.

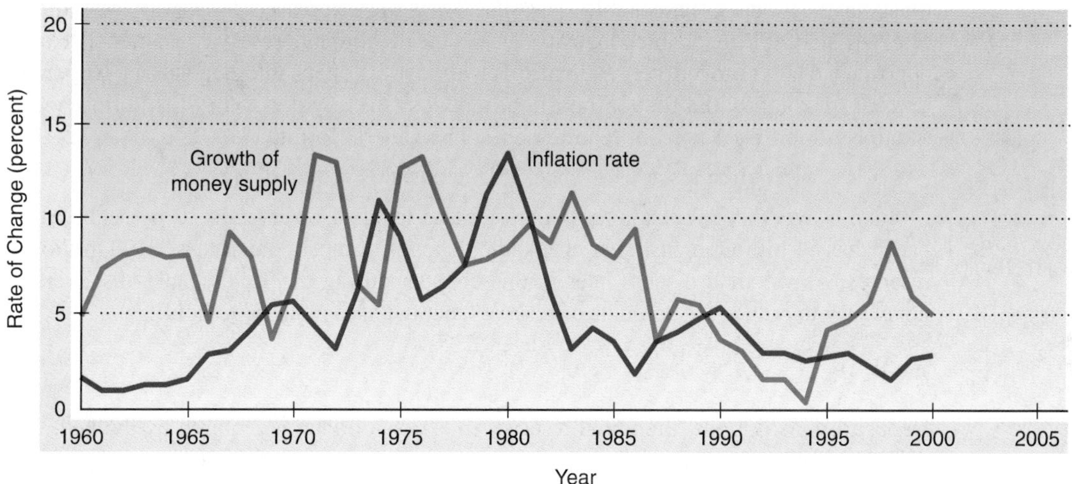

the first bank deposits. Eventually, goldsmiths realized that the amount of gold and silver on deposit always exceeded the average amount of gold and silver withdrawn at any given time—often by a predictable ratio. These goldsmiths started making loans by issuing to borrowers paper notes that exceeded in value the amount of gold and silver they actually kept on hand. They charged interest on these loans. This constituted the earliest form of what is now called **fractional reserve banking.** We know that goldsmiths operated this way in Delphi, Didyma, and Olympia in Greece as early as the seventh century B.C. In Athens, fractional reserve banking was well developed by the sixth century B.C.

Fractional reserve banking 
A system in which depository institutions hold reserves that are less than the amount of total deposits.

DEPOSITORY INSTITUTION RESERVES 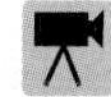

In a fractional reserve banking system, banks do not keep sufficient reserves on hand to cover 100 percent of their depositors' accounts. And the reserves that are held by depository institutions in the United States are not kept in gold and silver, as they were with the early goldsmiths, but rather in the form of deposits on reserve with Federal Reserve district banks and in vault cash. Depository institutions are required by the Fed to maintain a specified percentage of their customer deposits as **reserves.** There are three distinguishable types of reserves: legal, required, and excess.

Reserves 
In the U.S. Federal Reserve System, deposits held by Federal Reserve district banks for depository institutions, plus depository institutions' vault cash.

Legal Reserves

For depository institutions, **legal reserves** constitute anything that the law permits them to claim as reserves. Today, that consists only of deposits held at the Federal Reserve district bank plus vault cash. Government securities, for example, are not legal reserves, even

Legal reserves 
Reserves that depository institutions are allowed by law to claim as reserves—for example, deposits held at Federal Reserve district banks and vault cash.

though the owners and managers of the depository institutions may consider them such because they can easily be turned into cash, should the need arise, to meet unusually large net withdrawals by customers. Economists refer to all legal reserves that banks hold with the Federal Reserve or keep in their vaults as their *total reserves.*

Required Reserves

Required reserves 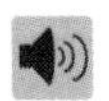
The value of reserves that a depository institution must hold in the form of vault cash or deposits with the Fed.

Required reserve ratio 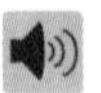
The percentage of total deposits that the Fed requires depository institutions to hold in the form of vault cash or deposits with the Fed.

Required reserves are the minimum amount of legal reserves that a depository institution must have to "back" checkable deposits. They are expressed as a ratio of required reserves to total checkable deposits (banks need hold no reserves on noncheckable deposits). The **required reserve ratio** for almost all checkable deposits is 10 percent (except for roughly the first \$50 million in deposits at any depository institution, which is subject to only a 3 percent requirement). The general formula is

$$\text{Required reserves} = \text{checkable deposits} \times \text{required reserve ratio}$$

Take a hypothetical example. If the required level of reserves is 10 percent and the bank* has \$1 billion in customer checkable deposits, it must hold at least \$100 million as reserves. As we shall discuss later in this chapter, during the 1990s banks discovered a novel way to reduce the amounts of reserves that they are required to hold.

Excess Reserves

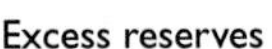
Excess reserves 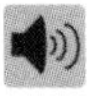
The difference between legal reserves and required reserves.

Depository institutions often hold reserves in excess of what is required by the Fed. This difference between actual (legal) reserves and required reserves is called **excess reserves.** (Excess reserves can be negative, but they rarely are. Negative excess reserves indicate that depository institutions do not have sufficient reserves to meet their required reserves. When this happens, they borrow from other depository institutions or from a Federal Reserve district bank, sell assets such as securities, or call in loans.) Excess reserves are an important potential determinant of the rate of growth of the money supply, for as we shall see, it is only to the extent that depository institutions have excess reserves that they can make new loans. Because reserves produce no income, profit-seeking financial institutions have an incentive to minimize excess reserves, disposing of them either to purchase income-producing securities or to make loans with which they earn income through interest payments received. In equation form, we can define excess reserves in this way:

$$\text{Excess reserves} = \text{legal reserves} - \text{required reserves}$$

In the analysis that follows, we examine the relationship between the level of reserves and the size of the money supply. This analysis implies that factors influencing the level of the reserves of the banking system as a whole will ultimately affect the size of the money supply, other things held constant. We show first that when someone deposits in one depository institution a check that is written on another depository institution, the two depository institutions involved are individually affected, but the overall money supply does not change. Then we show that when someone deposits in a depository institution a check that is written on the Fed, a multiple expansion in the money supply results.

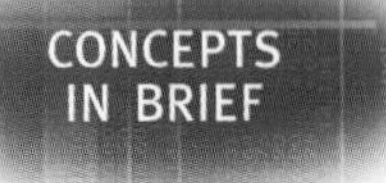

- Ours is a fractional reserve banking system in which depository institutions must hold only a percentage of their deposits as reserves, either on deposit with a Federal Reserve district bank or as vault cash.

*The term *bank* will be used interchangeably with the term *depository institution* in this chapter because distinctions among financial institutions are becoming less and less meaningful.

- Required reserves are usually expressed as a ratio, in percentage terms, of required reserves to total deposits.

THE RELATIONSHIP BETWEEN RESERVES AND TOTAL DEPOSITS

To show the relationship between reserves and depository institution deposits, we first analyze a single bank (existing alongside many others). A single bank is able to make new loans to its customers only to the extent that it has reserves above the level legally required to cover the new deposits. When an individual bank has no excess reserves, it cannot make loans.

How a Single Bank Reacts to an Increase in Reserves

To examine the **balance sheet** of a single bank after its reserves are increased, let's make the following assumptions:

Balance sheet 
A statement of the assets and liabilities of any business entity, including financial institutions and the Federal Reserve System. Assets are what is owned; liabilities are what is owed.

1. The required reserve ratio is 10 percent for all checkable deposits.
2. Checkable deposits are the bank's only liabilities; reserves at a Federal Reserve district bank and loans are the bank's only assets. Loans are promises made by customers to repay some amount in the future; that is, they are IOUs and as such are assets to the bank.
3. An individual bank can lend as much as it is legally allowed.
4. Every time a loan is made to an individual (consumer or business), all the proceeds from the loan are put into a checkable deposit account; no cash (currency or coins) is withdrawn.
5. Depository institutions seek to keep zero excess reserves because reserves do not earn interest. (Depository institutions are run to make profits; we assume that all depository institutions wish to convert excess reserves that do not pay interest into interest-bearing loans.)
6. Depository institutions have zero **net worth.** (In reality, all depository institutions are required to have some positive owners' equity, or capital, which is another name for net worth. It is usually a small percentage of the institutions' total assets.)

Net worth 
The difference between assets and liabilities.

Look at the simplified initial position of Typical Bank in Balance Sheet 15-1. Liabilities consist of $1 million in checkable deposits. Assets consist of $100,000 in reserves and $900,000 in loans to customers. Total assets of $1 million equal total liabilities of $1 million. With a 10 percent reserve requirement and $1 million in checkable deposits, the bank has required reserves of $100,000 and therefore no excess reserves.

Balance Sheet 15-1
Typical Bank

ASSETS			LIABILITIES	
Total reserves		$100,000	Checkable deposits	$1,000,000
Required reserves	$100,000			
Excess reserves	0			
Loans		900,000		
Total		$1,000,000	Total	$1,000,000

Assume that a depositor deposits in Typical Bank a $100,000 check drawn on another depository institution. Checkable deposits in Typical Bank immediately increase by $100,000, bringing the total to $1.1 million. Once the check clears, total reserves of Typical Bank increase to $200,000. A $1.1 million total in checkable deposits means that required reserves will have to be 10 percent of $1.1 million, or $110,000. Typical Bank now has excess reserves equal to $200,000 minus $110,000, or $90,000. This is shown in Balance Sheet 15-2.

Balance Sheet 15-2
Typical Bank

ASSETS			LIABILITIES	
Total reserves		$200,000	Checkable deposits	$1,100,000
Required reserves	$110,000			
Excess reserves	90,000			
Loans		900,000		
Total		$1,100,000	Total	$1,100,000

Effect on Typical Bank's Balance Sheet. Look at excess reserves in Balance Sheet 15-2. Excess reserves were zero before the $100,000 deposit, and now they are $90,000—that's $90,000 worth of assets not earning any income. By assumption, Typical Bank will now lend out this entire $90,000 in excess reserves in order to obtain interest income. Loans will increase to $990,000. The borrowers who receive the new loans will not leave them on deposit in Typical Bank. After all, they borrow money to spend it. As they spend it by writing checks that are deposited in other banks, actual reserves will fall to $110,000 (as required), and excess reserves will again become zero, as indicated in Balance Sheet 15-3.

Balance Sheet 15-3
Typical Bank

ASSETS			LIABILITIES	
Total reserves		$110,000	Checkable deposits	$1,100,000
Required reserves	$110,000			
Excess reserves	0			
Loans		990,000		
Total		$1,100,000	Total	$1,100,000

In this example, a person deposited a $100,000 check drawn on another bank. That $100,000 became part of the reserves of Typical Bank. Because that deposit immediately created excess reserves in Typical Bank, further loans were possible for Typical Bank. The excess reserves were lent out to earn interest. A bank will not lend more than its excess reserves because, by law, it must hold a certain amount of required reserves.

Effect on the Money Supply. A look at the balance sheets for Typical Bank might give the impression that the money supply increased because of the new customer's $100,000 deposit. Remember, though, that the deposit was a check written on *another* bank. Therefore, the other bank suffered a *decline* in its checkable deposits and its reserves. While total assets and liabilities in Typical Bank have increased by $100,000, they have *decreased* in the other bank by $100,000. The total amount of money and credit in the economy is unaffected by the transfer of funds from one depository institution to another.

The thing to remember is that new reserves are not created when checks written on one bank are deposited in another bank. The Federal Reserve System can, however, create new reserves; that is the subject of the next section.

THE FED'S DIRECT EFFECT ON THE OVERALL LEVEL OF RESERVES

Now we shall examine the Fed's direct effect on the level of reserves, showing how a change in the level of reserves causes a multiple change in the total money supply. Consider the Federal Open Market Committee (FOMC), whose decisions essentially determine the level of reserves in the monetary system.

Federal Open Market Committee

Open market operations are the purchase and sale of existing U.S. government securities in the open market (the private secondary U.S. securities market in which people exchange government securities that have not yet matured) by the FOMC in order to change the money supply. If the FOMC decides that the Fed should buy or sell bonds, it instructs the New York Federal Reserve Bank trading desk to do so.*

Open market operations The purchase and sale of existing U.S. government securities (such as bonds) in the open private market by the Federal Reserve System.

A Sample Transaction

Assume that the trading desk at the New York Fed has determined that in order to comply with the latest directive from the FOMC, it must purchase $100,000 worth of U.S. government securities.† The Fed pays for these securities by writing a check on itself for $100,000. This check is given to the bond dealer in exchange for the $100,000 worth of bonds. The bond dealer deposits the $100,000 check in its checkable account at a bank, which then sends the $100,000 check back to the Federal Reserve. When the Fed receives the check, it adds $100,000 to the reserve account of the bank that sent it the check. The Fed has created $100,000 of reserves. The Fed can create reserves because it has the ability to add to the reserve accounts of depository institutions whenever it buys U.S. securities. When the Fed buys a U.S. government security in the open market, it initially expands total reserves by the amount of the purchase.

Using Balance Sheets. Consider the balance sheets of the Fed and of the depository institution receiving the check. Balance Sheet 15-4 on page 360 shows the results for the Fed after the bond purchase and for the bank after the bond dealer deposits the $100,000 check.‡ The Fed' balance sheet (which here reflects only account changes) shows that after the purchase, the Fed's assets have increased by $100,000 in the form of U.S. government securities. Liabilities have also increased by $100,000 in the form of an increase in the reserve account of the bank. The balance sheet for the bank shows an increase in assets of

*Actually, the Fed usually deals in Treasury bills that have a maturity date of one year or less.

†In practice, the trading desk is never given a specific dollar amount to purchase or to sell. The account manager uses personal discretion in determining what amount should be purchased or sold in order to satisfy the FOMC's latest directive.

‡Strictly speaking, the balance sheets that we are showing should be called the *consolidated balance sheets* for the 12 Federal Reserve district banks. We will simply refer to these banks as the Fed, however.

$100,000 in the form of reserves with its Federal Reserve district bank. The bank also has an increase in its liabilities in the form of a $100,000 deposit in the checkable account of the bond dealer; this is an immediate $100,000 increase in the money supply.

Balance Sheet 15-4
Balance Sheets for the Fed and the Bank When a U.S. Government Security is Purchased by the Fed, Showing Changes Only in Assets and Liabilities

The Fed		Bank	
ASSETS	LIABILITIES	ASSETS	LIABILITIES
+$100,000 U.S. government securities	+$100,000 depository institution's reserves	+$100,000 reserves	+$100,000 checkable deposit owned by bond dealer

Sale of a $100,000 U.S. Government Security by the Fed

The process is reversed when the account manager at the New York Fed trading desk sells a U.S. government security from the Fed's portfolio.

Sale of a Security by the Fed. When the individual or institution buying the security from the Fed writes a check for $100,000 and the check clears, the Fed reduces the reserves and deposits of the bank on which the check was written. The $100,000 sale of the U.S. government security leads to a reduction in reserves in the banking system and a reduction in checkable deposits. Hence the money supply declines.

Using Balance Sheets Again. Balance Sheet 15-5 shows the results for the sale of a U.S. government security by the Fed. When the $100,000 clears, the Fed reduces by $100,000 the reserve account of the bank on which the check is written. The Fed's assets are also reduced by $100,000 because it no longer owns the U.S. government security. The bank's checkable deposit liabilities are reduced by $100,000 when that amount is deducted from the account of the bond purchaser, and the money supply is thereby reduced by that amount. The bank's assets are also reduced by $100,000, because the Fed has reduced its total reserves by that amount.

Balance Sheet 15-5
Balance Sheets After the Fed Has Sold $100,000 of U.S. Government Securities, Showing Changes Only in Assets and Liabilities

The Fed		Bank	
ASSETS	LIABILITIES	ASSETS	LIABILITIES
−$100,000 U.S. government securities	−$100,000 depository institution's reserves	−$100,000 reserves	−$100,000 checkable deposit balances

CONCEPTS IN BRIEF

- If a check is written on one depository institution and deposited in another, there is no change in total deposits or in the total money supply. No additional reserves in the banking system have been created.
- The Federal Reserve, through its Federal Open Market Committee (FOMC), can directly increase depository institutions' reserves and the money supply by purchasing U.S. government securities from bond dealers in the open market; it can decrease depository institutions' reserves and the money supply by selling U.S. government securities to bond dealers in the open market.

MONEY EXPANSION BY THE BANKING SYSTEM

Consider now the entire banking system. For practical purposes, we can look at all depository institutions taken as a whole. To understand how money is created, we must understand how depository institutions respond to Fed actions that increase reserves in the entire system.

Fed Purchases of U.S. Government Securities

Assume that the Fed purchases a $100,000 U.S. government security from a bond dealer. The bond dealer deposits the $100,000 check in Bank 1, which prior to this transaction is in the position depicted in Balance Sheet 15-6. The check, however, is not written on another depository institution; rather, it is written on the Fed itself.

Balance Sheet 15-6
Bank 1

ASSETS			LIABILITIES	
Total reserves		$100,000	Checkable deposits	$1,000,000
Required reserves	$100,000			
Excess reserves	0			
Loans		900,000		
Total		$1,000,000	Total	$1,000,000

Now look at the balance sheet for Bank 1 shown in Balance Sheet 15-7. Reserves have been increased by $100,000 to $200,000, and checkable deposits have also been increased by $100,000. Because required reserves on $1.1 million of checkable deposits are only $110,000, the depository institution has $90,000 in excess reserves.

Balance Sheet 15-7
Bank 1

ASSETS			LIABILITIES	
Total reserves		$200,000	Checkable deposits	$1,100,000
Required reserves	$110,000			
Excess reserves	90,000			
Loans		900,000		
Total		$1,100,000	Total	$1,100,000

Effect on the Money Supply. The purchase of a $100,000 U.S. government security by the Federal Reserve from the public (a bond dealer, for example) increases the money supply immediately by $100,000 because checkable deposits held by the public—the bond dealers are members of the public—are part of the money supply, and no other bank has lost deposits.

The process of money creation does not stop here. Look again at Balance Sheet 15-7. Bank 1 has excess reserves of $90,000. No other depository institution (or combination of depository institutions) has negative excess reserves of $90,000 as a result of the Fed's bond purchase. (Remember, the Fed simply created the reserves to pay for the bond purchase.)

Bank 1 will not wish to hold non-interest-bearing excess reserves. Assume that it will expand its loans by $90,000. This is shown in Balance Sheet 15-8.

Balance Sheet 15-8
Bank 1

ASSETS			LIABILITIES	
Total reserves		$110,000	Checkable deposits	$1,100,000
Required reserves	$110,000			
Excess reserves	0			
Loans		990,000		
Total		$1,100,000	Total	$1,100,000

The individual or business that has received the $90,000 loan will spend these funds, which will then be deposited in other banks. For the sake of simplicity, concentrate only on the balance sheet *changes* resulting from this new deposit, as shown in Balance Sheet 15-9. For Bank 2, the $90,000 deposit, after the check has cleared, becomes an increase in reserves as well as an increase in checkable deposits and hence the money supply. Because the reserve requirement is 10 percent, required reserves increase $9,000, so Bank 2 will have excess reserves of $81,000. But of course, excess reserves are not income producing, so by assumption Bank 2 will reduce them to zero by making a loan of $81,000 (which will earn interest income). This is shown in Balance Sheet 15-10.

Balance Sheet 15-9
Bank 2 (Changes Only)

ASSETS			LIABILITIES	
Total reserves		+$90,000	New checkable deposits	+$90,000
Required reserves	+$9,000			
Excess reserves	+81,000			
Total		+$90,000	Total	+$90,000

Balance Sheet 15-10
Bank 2 (Changes Only)

ASSETS			LIABILITIES	
Total reserves		+$9,000	Checkable deposits	+$90,000
Required reserves	+$9,000			
Excess reserves	+0			
Loans		+81,000		
Total		+$90,000	Total	+$90,000

Remember that in this example, the original $100,000 deposit was a check issued by a Federal Reserve bank to the bond dealer. That $100,000 constituted an immediate increase in the money supply of $100,000 when deposited in the bond dealer's checkable account. The deposit creation process (in addition to the original $100,000) occurs because of the fractional reserve banking system, coupled with the desire of depository institutions to maintain a minimum level of excess reserves. Under fractional reserve banking, banks must only hold a portion of new deposits as reserves, and in their quest to earn profits they seek to transform excess reserves into holdings of loans and securities.

Continuation of the Deposit Creation Process. Look at Bank 3's simplified account in Balance Sheet 15-11, where again only *changes* in the assets and liabilities are shown. Assume that the firm borrowing from Bank 2 writes a check for $81,000 that is deposited in Bank 3; checkable deposits and the money supply increase by $81,000. Legal reserves of Bank 3 rise by that amount when the check clears.

Balance Sheet 15-11
Bank 3 (Changes Only)

ASSETS			LIABILITIES	
Total reserves		+$81,000	New checkable deposits	+$81,000
Required reserves	+$8,100			
Excess reserves	+72,900			
Total		+$81,000	Total	+$81,000

Because the reserve requirement is 10 percent, required reserves rise by $8,100, and excess reserves therefore increase by $72,900. We assume that Bank 3 will want to lend all of those non-interest-earning assets (excess reserves). When it does, loans (and newly created checkable deposits) will increase by $72,900. This bank's legal reserves will fall to $8,100, and excess reserves become zero as checks are written on the new deposit. This is shown in Balance Sheet 15-12 on page 364.

Balance Sheet 15-12
Bank 3 (Changes Only)

ASSETS			LIABILITIES	
Total reserves		+$8,100	Checkable deposits	+$81,000
Required reserves	+$8,100			
Excess reserves	0			
Loans		+72,900		
Total		+$81,000	Total	+$81,000

Progression to Other Banks. This process continues to Banks 4, 5, 6, and so forth. Each bank obtains smaller and smaller increases in deposits because 10 percent of each deposit must be held in required reserves; therefore, each succeeding depository institution makes correspondingly smaller loans. Table 15-1 shows the new deposits, possible loans, and required reserves for the remaining depository institutions in the system.

Effect on Total Deposits. In this example, deposits (and the money supply) increased initially by the $100,000 that the Fed paid the bond dealer in exchange for a bond. Deposits (and the money supply) were further increased by a $90,000 deposit in Bank 2, and they were again increased by an $81,000 deposit in Bank 3. Eventually, total deposits and the money supply will increase by $1 million, as shown in Table 15-1. The $1 million consists of the original $100,000 created by the Fed, plus an extra $900,000 generated by deposit-creating bank loans. The money multiplier process is portrayed graphically in Figure 15-2 on page 364.

Increase in Total Banking System Reserves

Even with fractional reserve banking, if there are zero excess reserves, deposits cannot expand unless total banking system reserves are increased. The original new deposit in Bank 1, in our example, was in the form of a check written on a Federal Reserve district bank. It therefore represented new reserves to the banking system. Had that check been written on Bank 3, by contrast, nothing would have happened to the total amount of checkable deposits; there would have been no change in the total money supply. To repeat: Checks written on banks within the system, without any expansion of overall reserves within the banking system, represent transfers of reserves and deposits among depository

TABLE 15-1

Maximum Money Creation with 10 Percent Required Reserves

This table shows the maximum new loans plus investments that banks can make, given the Fed's deposit of a $100,000 check in Bank 1. The required reserve ratio is 10 percent. We assume that all excess reserves in each bank are used for new loans or investments.

Bank	New Deposits	New Required Reserves	Maximum New Loans
1	$100,000 (from Fed)	$10,000	$90,000
2	90,000	9,000	81,000
3	81,000	8,100	72,900
4	72,900	7,290	65,610
.	.	.	.
.	.	.	.
.	.	.	.
All other banks	656,100	65,610	590,490
Totals	$1,000,000	$100,000	$900,000

FIGURE 15-2

The Multiple Expansion in the Money Supply Due to $100,000 in New Reserves When the Required Reserve Ratio Is 10 Percent

The banks are all aligned in decreasing order of new deposits created. Bank 1 receives the $100,000 in new reserves and lends out $90,000. Bank 2 receives the $90,000 and lends out $81,000. The process continues through banks 3 to 19 and then the rest of the banking system. Ultimately, assuming no leakages, the $100,000 of new reserves results in an increase in the money supply of $1 million, or 10 times the new reserves, because the required reserve ratio is 10 percent.

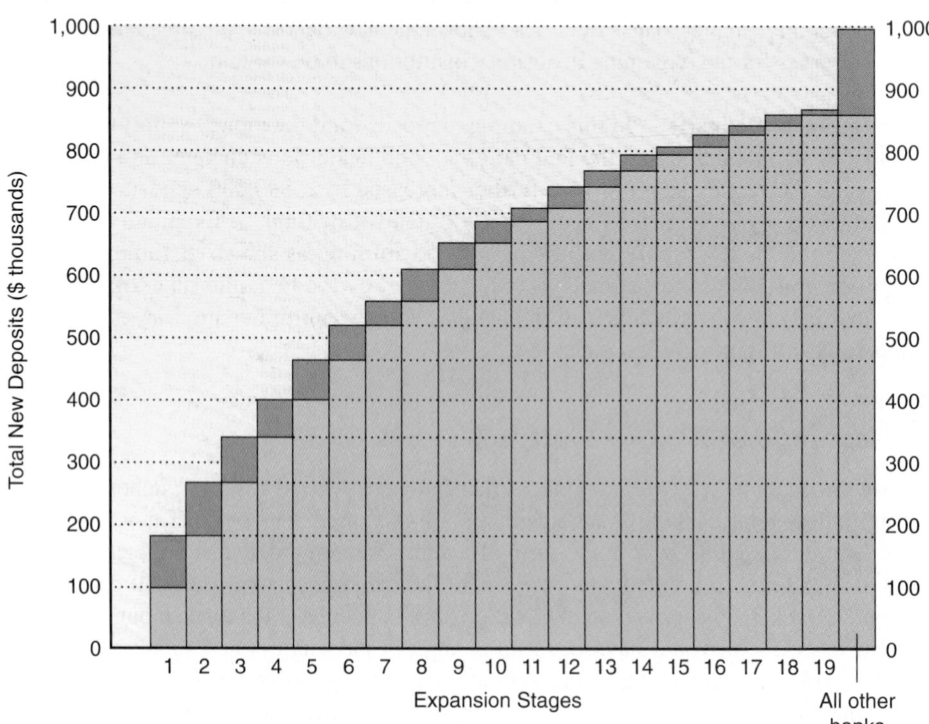

institutions that do not affect the money supply. Only when additional new reserves and deposits are created by the Federal Reserve System does the money supply increase.

You should be able to work through the foregoing example to show the reverse process when there is a decrease in reserves because the Fed sells a $100,000 U.S. government security. The result is a multiple contraction of deposits and therefore of the total money supply in circulation.

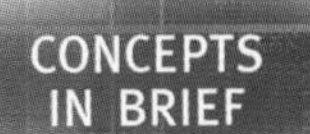

- When the Fed increases reserves through a purchase of U.S. government securities, the result is a multiple expansion of deposits and therefore of the supply of money.
- When the Fed reduces the banking system's reserves by selling U.S. government securities, the result is a multiple contraction of deposits and therefore of the money supply.

THE MONEY MULTIPLIER

In the example just given, a $100,000 increase in excess reserves generated by the Fed's purchase of a security yielded a $1 million increase in total deposits; deposits increased by a multiple of 10 times the initial $100,000 increase in overall reserves. Conversely, a $100,000 decrease in excess reserves generated by the Fed's sale of a security will yield a $1 million decrease in total deposits; they will decrease by a multiple of 10 times. The initial $100,000 decrease in overall reserves.

We can now make a generalization about the extent to which the money supply will change when the banking system's reserves are increased or decreased. The **money multiplier** gives the change in the money supply due to a change in reserves. If we assume that no excess reserves are kept and that all loan proceeds are deposited in depository institutions in the system, the following equation applies:

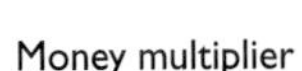 

The reciprocal of the required reserve ratio, assuming no leakages into currency and no excess reserves. It is equal to 1 divided by the required reserve ratio.

$$\text{Potential money multiplier} = \frac{1}{\text{required reserve ratio}}$$

That is, the maximum possible value of the money multiplier is equal to 1 divided by the required reserve ratio for checkable deposits. The *actual* change in the money supply—currency plus checkable account balances—will be equal to the following:

Actual change in money supply = actual money multiplier × change in total reserves

Now we examine why there is a difference between the potential money multiplier—1 divided by the required reserve ratio—and the actual multiplier.

Forces That Reduce the Money Multiplier

We made a number of simplifying assumptions to come up with the potential money multiplier. In the real world, the actual money multiplier is considerably smaller. Several factors account for this.

Depository Institution Reserves
Get additional experience thinking about how a change in overall depository institution reserves the total quantity of deposits in the banking system.

Leakages. The entire loan (check) from one bank is not always deposited in another bank. At least two leakages can occur:

- *Currency drains.* When deposits increase, the public may want to hold more currency. Currency that is kept in a person's wallet remains outside the banking system and cannot be held by banks as reserves from which to make loans. The greater the amount of cash leakage, the smaller the actual money multiplier.

- *Excess reserves.* Depository institutions may wish to maintain excess reserves greater than zero. For example, they may wish to keep them because they want to be able to make speedy loans when good deals arise unexpectedly. To the extent that they want to keep positive excess reserves, the money multiplier will be smaller. The greater the excess reserves that banks maintain, the smaller the actual money multiplier.

Empirically, the currency drain is more significant than the effect of desired positive excess reserves.

Real-World Money Multipliers. The maximum potential money multiplier is the reciprocal of the required reserve ratio. The maximum is never attained for the money supply as a whole because of currency drains and excess reserves. Also, each definition of the money supply, M1 or M2, will yield different results for money multipliers. For several decades, the M1 multiplier has varied between 2.5 and 3.0. The M2 multiplier, however, has shown a trend upward, ranging from 6.5 at the beginning of the 1960s to over 12 in the 2000s.

Ways in Which the Federal Reserve Changes the Money Supply

As we have just seen, the Fed can change the money supply by directly changing reserves available to the banking system. It does this by engaging in open market operations. To repeat: The purchase of a U.S. government security by the Fed results in an increase in reserves and leads to a multiple expansion in the money supply. A sale of a U.S. government security by the Fed results in a decrease in reserves and leads to a multiple contraction in the money supply.

The Fed changes the money supply in two other ways, both of which will have multiplier effects similar to those outlined earlier in this chapter.

Discount rate
The interest rate that the Federal Reserve charges for reserves that it lends to depository institutions. It is sometimes referred to as the *rediscount rate* or, in Canada and England, as the *bank rate*.

Borrowed Reserves and the Discount Rate. If a depository institution wants to increase its loans but has no excess reserves, it can borrow reserves. One place it can borrow reserves is from the Fed itself. The depository institution goes to the Federal Reserve and asks for a loan of a certain amount of reserves. The Fed charges these institutions for any reserves that it lends them. The interest rate that the Fed charges is the **discount rate.** When newspapers report that the Fed has decreased the discount rate from 5 to 4 percent, you know that the Fed has decreased its charge for lending reserves to depository institutions. Borrowing from the Fed increases reserves and thereby enhances the ability of the depository institution to engage in deposit creation, thus increasing the money supply.

Often the Federal Reserve System makes changes in the discount rate not necessarily to encourage or discourage depository institutions from borrowing from the Fed but rather as a signal to the banking system and financial markets that there has been a change in the Fed's monetary policy. We discuss monetary policy in more detail in Chapter 17.

Federal funds market 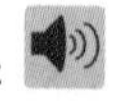
A private market (made up mostly of banks) in which banks can borrow reserves from other banks that want to lend them. Federal funds are usually lent for overnight use.

Depository institutions actually do not often go to the Fed to borrow reserves because the Fed will not lend them all they want. In fact, the Fed can even refuse to lend reserves when the depository institutions need the reserves to make their reserve accounts meet legal requirements. Since the early 1990s, the Fed has been much more restrictive in lending to depository institutions than it was in the 1970s and 1980s. There are, however, alternative sources for the banks to tap when they want to expand their reserves or when they need reserves to meet a requirement. The primary source is the **federal funds market.** The federal funds market is an interbank market in reserves, with one bank borrowing the excess reserves of another. The generic term *federal funds market* refers to the borrowing or lending reserve funds that are usually repaid within the same 24-hour period.

Depository institutions that borrow in the federal funds market pay an interest rate called the **federal funds rate.** Because the federal funds rate is a ready measure of the price that banks must pay to raise funds, the Federal Reserve often uses it as a yardstick by which to measure the effects of its policies. Consequently, the federal funds rate is a closely watched indicator of the Fed's anticipated intentions.

Federal funds rate 
The interest rate that depository institutions pay to borrow reserves in the interbank federal funds market.

Reserve Requirement Changes. In principle, another method by which the Fed can alter the money supply is by changing the reserve requirements it imposes on all depository institutions. Earlier we assumed that reserve requirements were fixed. Actually, these requirements are set by the Fed within limits established by Congress. The Fed can vary reserve requirements within these broad limits.

What would a change in reserve requirements from 10 to 20 percent do (if there were no excess reserves and if we ignore currency leakages)? We already discovered that the maximum money multiplier was the reciprocal of the required reserve ratio. If the required reserve ratio is 10 percent, then the maximum money multiplier is the reciprocal of $\frac{1}{10}$ or 10 (assuming no leakages). If, for some reason, the Fed decided to increase reserve requirements to 20 percent, the maximum money multiplier would equal the reciprocal of $\frac{1}{5}$, or 5. The maximum money multiplier is therefore inversely related to the required reserve ratio. If the Fed decides to increase reserve requirements, there will be a decrease in the maximum money multiplier. With any given level of legal reserves already in existence, the money supply will therefore contract.

In practice, open market operations allow the Federal Reserve to control the money supply much more precisely than changes in reserve requirements do, and they also allow the Fed to reverse itself quickly. In contrast, a small change in reserve requirements could, at least initially, result in a very large change in the money supply. Reserve requirement changes also impose costs on banks by restricting the portion of funds that they can lend, thereby inducing them to find legal ways to evade reserve requirements. That is why the Federal Reserve does not change reserve requirements very often.

CONCEPTS IN BRIEF

- The maximum potential money multiplier is equal to the reciprocal of the required reserve ratio.
- The actual multiplier is smaller than the maximum money multiplier because of currency drains and excess reserves voluntarily held by banks.
- The Fed can change the money supply in three ways: It can change reserves and hence the money supply through open market operations in which it buys and sells existing U.S. government securities (open market operations are the primary form of monetary policy), it can encourage change in reserves by changing the discount rate, and it can change the amount of deposits created from reserves by changing reserve requirements.

PAYMENT SYSTEMS, THEIR RISKS, AND DEPOSIT INSURANCE

The word *bank* derives from the Italian merchant's bench, or *banco,* across which bankers and borrowers exchanged funds in medieval Europe. In today's electronic trading environments, however, the word has become truly antiquated. Increased electronic trading has also complicated the lives of central bank policymakers, including those at the Fed.

Financial Trading Systems

Financial trading system 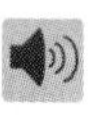
A mechanism linking buyers and sellers of stocks and bonds.

Key terms in the vocabulary of bankers and other financial market traders are acronyms such as MATIF and CORES, which refer to automated **financial trading systems.** These are mechanisms linking buyers and sellers of government securities and corporate bonds and stocks. MATIF, the Marché à Terme International de France, is located in Paris, and CORES, the Computer-Assisted Order Routing and Execution System, is a trading system based in Tokyo. Most developed nations have similar systems. These and other trading systems in locales such as Germany, Singapore, Switzerland, and the United Kingdom permit traders to place orders for purchases and sales of securities via computers.

For some time now, the U.S. Chicago Mercantile Exchange (CME) has operated a system known as Globex. People make trades on Globex via computer terminals. A trader uses Globex software programs to access data on market prices of financial contracts. The trader then can interact with the system to initiate and complete financial transactions.

Automated trading permits people to engage in financial transactions at any time of the day or night. For example, a trader who logs on to the Globex system at 10 P.M. Central Time may see a profit opportunity and initiate a transaction on the system. If the trader can transact business at 10 P.M., however, there is no reason to confine trading only to an exchange open during the day. It is also possible, after all, to trade electronically via an exchange in Tokyo, where 10 P.M. in the middle portion of the United States is late morning in Australia, Hong Kong, Japan, and Singapore.

Payment Systems and Payment Intermediaries

Payment system 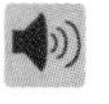
An institutional structure by which consumers, businesses, governments, and financial institutions exchange payments.

Payment intermediary 
An institution that facilitates the transfer of funds between buyer and seller during the course of any purchase of goods, services, or financial assets.

Financial trading systems allow people to conduct financial transactions. Actual transferals of *funds,* however, take place on **payment systems,** which are institutional structures through which people, businesses, governments, and financial institutions transmit payments of funds for goods, services, or financial assets. In most nations, people continue to use coins and currency to conduct transactions. For instance, U.S. residents use coin and currency to make over three-fourths of their exchanges. When a person buys something using coins and currency, the exchange is final at the moment that it occurs. By way of contrast, check transactions are final only after banks transfer funds from the account of the purchaser to the seller. Hence using checks requires people to rely on banks as **payment intermediaries,** or go-betweens in clearing payments that arise from exchanges of goods, services, or financial assets. Not all countries use checks as much as we do in the United States, though.

INTERNATIONAL EXAMPLE

Other Countries Are Not So Fond of Checks

Table 15-2 shows that U.S. residents use paper-based, *nonelectronic* (check) transactions much more than people in other countries. A typical U.S. resident makes over 200 check transactions a year. This is at least three times more—and in comparison with a few nations as much as 100 times more—than the numbers of check transactions made by people outside the United States. Other forms of noncash, nonelectronic payments conducted via payment intermediaries include credit card, money order, and paper-based *giro* transactions, which are payment order transmittals between banks and other financial institutions. Nonelectronic giro systems are common in both Europe and Asia and link a number of payment intermediaries besides banks, such as post offices.

For Critical Analysis

Why do Americans still write so many checks when credit cards are so easy to use?

TABLE 15-2
Annual Noncash Transactions per Person in Selected Countries
In comparison with Italy and the United States, other developed nations use more electronic means of payment.

Country	Number of Transactions per Person: Paper-Based	Electronic	Electronic Share of All Transactions
Switzerland	2	65	97%
Netherlands	19	128	87%
Belgium	16	85	84%
Denmark	24	100	81%
Japan	9	31	78%
Germany	36	103	74%
Sweden	24	68	74%
Finland	40	81	67%
United Kingdom	57	58	50%
France	86	71	45%
Canada	76	53	41%
Norway	58	40	41%
Italy	23	6	20%
United States	234	59	20%

Source: Data from David Humphrey, Lawrence Pulley, and Jukka Vesala, "Cash, Paper, and Electronic Payments: A Cross-Country Analysis," *Journal of Money, Credit, and Banking,* 28 (November 1996, p. 2), pp. 914–939.

Electronic Payment Systems: The Electronic Giro. Table 15-2 indicates that people in other nations use electronic means of payment to a greater extent than U.S. and Italian residents. For instance, many Europeans commonly use *electronic giro* systems, in which banks, post offices, and other payment intermediaries transfer funds over the telephone lines or other electronic pathways.

The closest U.S. counterpart to the electronic giro system is the **automated clearing house (ACH),** which is a computer-based clearing and settlement facility for the transmittal of funds via electronic messages instead of checks. Typical ACH transfers are automatic payroll deposits, in which businesses make wage and salary payments directly into employees' deposit accounts within one or two business days. The U.S. government distributes Social Security benefits via ACH direct-deposit mechanisms and disperses an increasing percentage of welfare and food stamp payments using an *electronic benefits transfer (EBT)* system. The EBT system functions much like an ACH, but to a welfare and food stamp recipient it works much like an ATM, because EBT machines disperse welfare funds or food stamps just as an ATM machine disperses cash.

Automated clearinghouse (ACH) 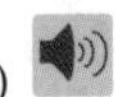
A computer-based clearing and settlement facility that replaces check transactions by interchanging credits and debits electronically.

Point-of-sale (POS) network 
System in which consumer payments for retail purchases are made by means of direct deductions from their deposit accounts at depository institutions.

POS and ATM Networks. Since the 1970s, technology has permitted the development of **point-of-sale (POS) networks,** which are systems allowing consumers to make immediate payments via direct deductions from their deposit accounts at depository institutions. POS networks have not caught on very quickly in the United States, perhaps because U.S. residents so commonly use **automated teller machine (ATM) networks.** These are systems linking more than 90,000 depository institution computer terminals activated by magnetically encoded bank cards. An average U.S. ATM machine is used

Automated teller machine (ATM) network 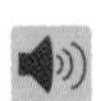
A system of linked depository institution computer terminals that are activated by magnetically encoded bank cards.

for about 100,000 transactions each year, most of which are cash withdrawals. Such ready access to cash helps reduce the extent to which U.S. residents might use POS networks.

Payment Systems
Visit for an over of the various issues associated with payment systems.

By contrast, in places such as the Scandinavian countries, POS networks have caught on quickly, leaving ATM networks much less developed. Current trends toward higher U.S. consumer use of on-line banking via the Internet could lead to greater worldwide interest in POS networks in the future. At present, however, even though a growing number of U.S. retailers make POS systems available to their customers, consumer-oriented electronic payment systems process a negligible percentage of the value of U.S. electronic payments. This may be because the U.S. check-clearing system remains relatively more cost-efficient. Nonetheless, as discussed in greater detail in Chapter 16, most economists believe that ultimately POS networks will become more widespread in the United States.

Large-Value Payment Systems

Large-value wire transfer system 
A payment system that permits the electronic transmission of large dollar sums.

Although U.S. consumers have been slow to adopt electronic payment systems for retail transactions, over 80 percent of the total *dollar value* of annual U.S. payments take place via **large-value wire transfer systems.** These are payment systems that banks, other financial institutions, and multinational corporations uses to transmit sizable payment transactions. Large-value wire transfer systems are also commonplace in other developed nations and handle the bulk of the value of total payments in those countries. Table 15-3 lists the world's major large-value payment systems and provides data on annual transactions and flows of funds on these systems. The largest of these outside the United States is the Bank of Japan's BOJ-NET system. Japan has another private system, and Germany and the United Kingdom both have major large-value payment systems.

TABLE 15-3
Transactions and Payment Flows in Major National Payment Systems
The world's major large-value payment systems are in Europe, Japan, and the United States.

Country and Payment System	Transactions (millions)	Value ($ trillions)
Germany		
ELS	13.5	22.4
EAF	22.5	107.0
Japan		
FEYCS	11.2	81.6
BOJ-NET	5.3	329.2
United Kingdom		
CHAPS	18.0	68.8
United States		
Fedwire	98.1	328.7
CHIPS	59.1	350.4

Source: Bank for International Settlements, 2000.

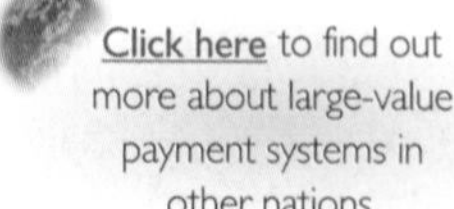
Click here to find out more about large-value payment systems in other nations.

Fedwire. In the United States, there are two key large-value wire transfer systems. One is **Fedwire,** which is owned and operated by the Federal Reserve System. All financial institutions that must hold reserves at Federal Reserve banks may transmit payments using Fedwire. They pay fees to the Fed to use the system. Financial institutions commonly use Fedwire to make *book-entry securities transactions,* which are electronic payments for U.S. Treasury securities, and to process interbank payments, such as payments for federal funds market loans. The average Fedwire payment is more than $3 million, and the average daily payment volume on the Fedwire system now is well over $1 trillion.

Fedwire 
A large-value wire transfer system operated by the Federal Reserve that is open to all depository institutions that legally must maintain required reserves with the Fed.

CHIPS. The other major U.S. large-value wire transfer system is the **Clearing House Interbank Payments System (CHIPS).** This is a privately owned system managed by the New York Clearing House Association, which has about 100 member banks. These banks use CHIPS primarily to transfer funds for foreign exchange and Eurocurrency transactions. The average value of a CHIPS transaction is about $6 million, and the average daily payment flow on the CHIPS system now also exceeds $1 trillion.

Clearing House Interbank Payment System (CHIPS) 
A large-value wire transfer system linking about 100 banks that permits them to transmit large sums of money related primarily to foreign exchange and Eurodollar transactions.

Payment System Risks

Even before the advent of electronic trading, there was some element of risk inherent in any financial transaction. For instance, when a nineteenth-century frontier store accepted coins from a fur trader, there was a remote possibility that the customer's payment might be counterfeit. A Wal-Mart store faces the same risk today every time its clerks accept a cash payment from a customer. Nonetheless, Wal-Mart and other retailers commonly accept currency and coin payments, because the risk of loss is normally limited to a relatively small payment value. The risk of loss for every multimillion-dollar transfer on a large-value wire transfer system, however, is much greater.

Click here to learn more about the Clearing House Interbank Payment System.

Three types of risk naturally arise in any payment system: *liquidity risk, credit risk,* and *systemic risk.*

Liquidity Risk. You probably know a few people who are not very punctual in keeping scheduled appointments. Some almost seem to be intent on being late for meetings and other engagements. Likewise, people sometimes fail to make payments at promised times, which creates a risk of loss for payment recipients. This risk often is an opportunity cost, because the recipient could have used the funds for other purposes. **Liquidity risk** is the risk that such losses may arise from late receipt of payments.

Liquidity risk 
The risk of loss that may occur if a payment is not received when due.

Before the advent of electronic payment systems, banks and other payment intermediaries had to depend on courier or postal services for hand delivery of paper orders for payment and of currency and coins. Unanticipated delays in these services exposed them to significant liquidity risks. The development of electronic payment systems stems largely from a desire by banks and other payment intermediaries to speed up the process of transferring payments in an effort to reduce these risks. Using large-value wire transfer systems, for instance, banks can initiate payment orders in minutes, and actual transfers take place nearly instantaneously.

Credit Risk. In any exchange, often one person transfers funds before the other party reciprocates with the transfer of a good, service, or financial asset. When this happens, the individual who transfers the funds essentially extends credit to the other party in the transaction. Hence the person who transfers funds first takes on **credit risk,** which is the possibility that the other party in the exchange may ultimately fail to honor the terms of the exchange. Payment intermediaries have developed intricate systems of rules intended to reduce exposure to credit risks. These rules lay out the responsibilities of both parties. They clearly spell out penalties that are assessed if someone fails to settle transactions on a timely basis.

Credit risk 
The risk of loss that might occur if one party to an exchange fails to honor the terms under which the exchange was to take place.

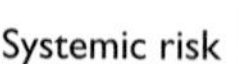
Systemic risk 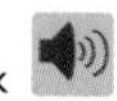
The risk that some payment intermediaries may not be able to meet the terms of their credit agreements because of failures by other institutions to settle other transactions.

Systemic Risk. Liquidity and credit risks are payment system risks that payment intermediaries assume on an individual basis. Because the payment intermediaries that participate in large-value wire transfer systems are all interconnected, however, they share some payment system risks. Payment flows among these intermediaries are interdependent, and that gives rise to **systemic risk**—the risk that some payment intermediaries may not be able to honor financial commitments because of payment settlement breakdowns in otherwise unrelated transactions.

INTERNATIONAL EXAMPLE

Another Risk in the Payment System: Some Customers May Be Crooks!

With the assistance of officials of the Bank of New York, federal investigators spent months tracking wire transfers made by the bank on behalf of Russian clients. The Bank of New York had spent years trying to build customer relationships with these companies because it anticipated big boosts in its profitability when the Russian economy would finally burst into bloom following big privatization efforts. Toward this end, the bank had employed a couple of vice presidents who were originally from Russia and who were well connected with emerging private companies there.

In the summer of 1999, however, the bank's efforts garnered little but unfavorable publicity. It turned out that the vice presidents it had hired may have been well connected with another big Russian private-sector institution: the Russian mafia. Billions of dollars of illegal transactions related to organized crime took place via a complex series of globe-spanning transactions involving Russian clients of the Bank of New York and other international clearing banks. A number of the transactions originated from the Russian central bank, and as much as $2 billion (or perhaps even more—we may never know the actual amounts) transferred from the central bank's accounts were funds that it had received via loans from the International Monetary Fund. Thus funds provided by taxpayers in the United States and other nations that contribute to the IMF may have been "laundered" for ultimate use by criminal elements in Russian society.

Officials at the Bank of New York were asked why they had not done more to monitor the billions of dollars that the bank had transferred on behalf of Russian companies. They replied that these transfers were only a drop in the bucket compared with all the funds they transmit each year. They also pointed out that all they can do is report suspicious activities to federal authorities and cooperate with government investigations, as they had done in this case. For its part, the IMF said that it traditionally relies on governments that borrow its funds to put them to use as promised. It rarely follows up to make sure that this actually happens.

For Critical Analysis

Which of the various parties involved in all these Russian-related wire transfers—clearing banks such as the Bank of New York, Russian companies, the Russian mafia, the Russian government, the people of Russia, and U.S. and other IMF-supporting taxpayers—incurred the largest payment system risks?

Federal Deposit Insurance 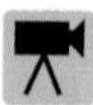

Federal Deposit Insurance Corporation (FDIC) 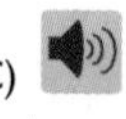
A government agency that insures the deposits held in banks and most other depository institutions; all U.S. banks are insured this way.

Central banks and governments worry about systemic risk in banking because systemic breakdowns can cause widespread bank failures. When businesses fail, they create hardships for creditors, owners, and customers. But when a depository institution fails, an even greater hardship results because many individuals and businesses depend on the safety and security of banks. Figure 15-3 indicates that during the 1920s, an average of about 600 banks failed each year. In the 1930s, during the Great Depression, that average soared to 2,000 failures each year.

In 1933, at the height of such bank failures, the **Federal Deposit Insurance Corporation (FDIC)** was founded to insure the funds of depositors and remove the reason for

FIGURE 15-3
Bank Failures
During the Great Depression, a tremendous number of banks failed. Federal deposit insurance was created in 1933. Thereafter, bank failures were few until around 1984. Failures peaked at over 200 in 1989 and are now fewer than a dozen per year.
Source: Federal Deposit Insurance Corporation.

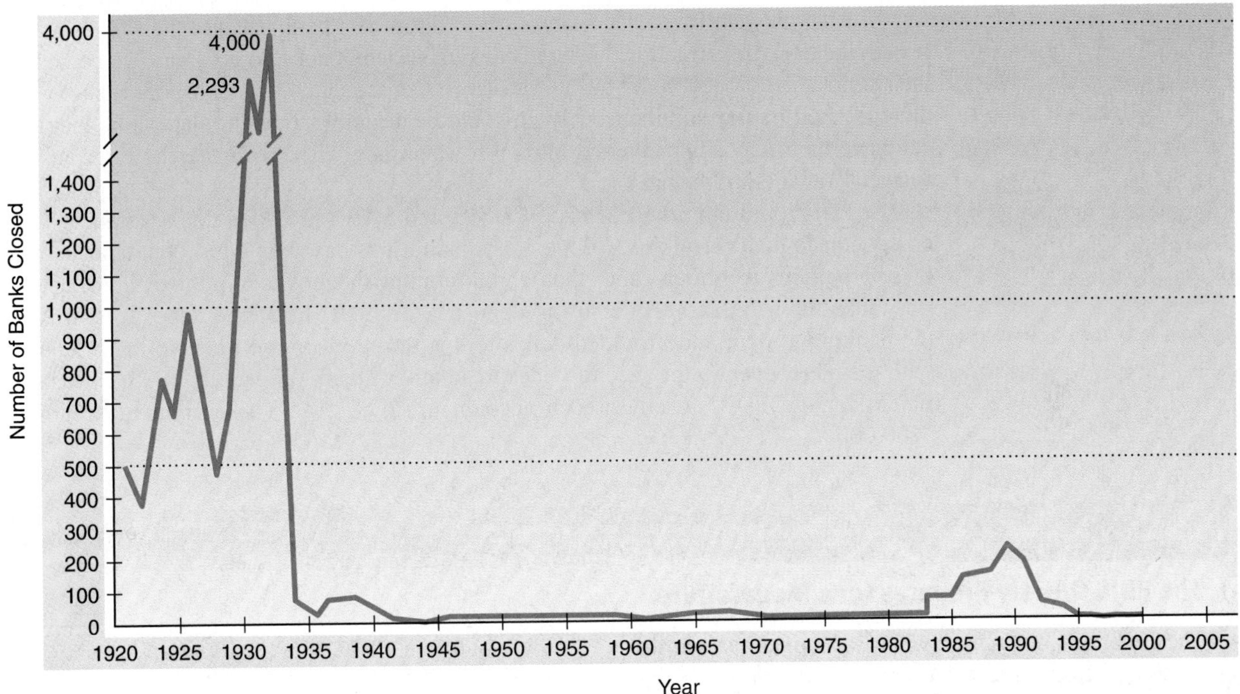

ruinous runs on banks. In 1934, the Federal Savings and Loan Insurance Corporation (FSLIC) was installed to insure deposits in savings and loan associations and mutual savings banks. In 1971, the National Credit Union Share Insurance Fund (NCUSIF) was created to insure deposits in credit unions. In 1989, the FSLIC was dissolved and the Savings Association Insurance Fund (SAIF) was established to protect the deposits of those institutions.

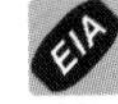

Federal Deposit Insurance
Gain further understanding of deposit insurance.

As can be seen in Figure 15-3, a tremendous drop in bank failure rates occurred after passage of the early federal legislation. The long period from 1935 until the 1980s was relatively quiet. From World War II to 1984, fewer than nine banks failed per year. From 1985 until the beginning of 1993, however, 1,065 commercial banks failed—an annual average of nearly 120 bank failures per year, more than 10 times the average for the preceding years! We will examine the reasons shortly. But first we need to understand how deposit insurance works.

The Rationale for Deposit Insurance

The FDIC, FSLIC, and NCUSIF were established to mitigate the primary cause of bank failures, **bank runs**—the simultaneous rush of depositors to convert their demand deposits or time deposits into currency.

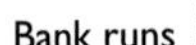

Bank runs
Attempts by many of a bank's depositors to convert checkable and time deposits into currency out of fear for the bank's solvency.

Consider the following scenario. A bank begins to look shaky; its assets may not seem sufficient to cover its liabilities. If the bank has no deposit insurance, depositors in this bank (and any banks associated with it) will all want to withdraw their money from the bank at the same time. Their concern is that this shaky bank will not have enough money to return their deposits to them in the form of currency. Indeed, this is what happens in a bank failure when insurance doesn't exist. Just as with the failure of a regular business, the creditors of the bank may not all get paid, or if they do, they will get paid less than 100 percent of what they are owed. Depositors are creditors of a bank because their funds are on loan to the bank. In a fractional reserve banking system, banks do not hold 100 percent of their depositors' money in the form of reserves. Consequently, all depositors cannot withdraw all their money simultaneously. It would be desirable to assure depositors that they can have their deposits converted into cash when they wish, no matter how serious the financial situation of the bank.

Click here to keep up with the latest issues in deposit insurance and banking issues.

The FDIC (and later the FSLIC, NCUSIF, and SAIF) provided this assurance. They charged insurance premiums to depository institutions based on their total deposits, and these premiums went into funds that would reimburse depositors in the event of depository institution failures. By insuring deposits, the FDIC bolstered depositors' trust in the banking system and provided depositors with the incentive to leave their deposits with the bank, even in the face of widespread talk of bank failures. In 1933, it was sufficient for the FDIC to cover each account up to $2,500. The current maximum is $100,000.

POLICY EXAMPLE

The FDIC Quietly Prepares for a Megafailure

The 1990s and 2000s have witnessed numerous record-breaking bank mergers. The days of $100 billion-asset banks seem to be here to stay. What might happen if one of these megabanks were to fail? The FDIC is quietly preparing for such a possibility. It has formed what has become known as the Mega-Merger Committee, which is trying to answer the following questions:

- When should the government pledge to refund uninsured deposits in order to avoid system-wide chaos?
- Who would manage such a failed megabank's loans and securities until it could be auctioned off?
- How much new staff would the downsized FDIC need to hire in case of a megafailure?
- How could the FDIC hire such a staff on short notice?
- Would the FDIC have to send its employees to other countries to monitor the failed bank's foreign branches?

It would not be easy for the FDIC to sell a $100 billion-asset bank. Consequently, the Mega-Merger Committee has determined that it would break a failed megabank into smaller pieces. The FDIC could, for example, break the bank up along geographic lines or along business lines.

For Critical Analysis

Would U.S. banking authorities have the legal ability to shut down a failed megabank's foreign branches?

How Deposit Insurance Causes Increased Risk Taking by Bank Managers

Until very recently, all insured depository institutions paid the same small fee for coverage. (In 1996, the fee was reduced to zero for most banks.) The fee that they paid was completely unrelated to how risky their assets were. A depository institution that made loans to companies such as General Motors and Microsoft Corporation paid the same deposit insurance premium as another depository institution that made loans (at higher interest rates) to the governments of developing countries that were teetering on the brink of financial collapse. Although deposit insurance premiums for a while were adjusted somewhat in response to the riskiness of a depository institution's assets, they never reflected all of the relative risk. This can be considered a flaw in the deposit insurance scheme.

Because bank managers do not have to pay higher insurance premiums when they make riskier loans, they have an incentive to invest in more assets of higher yield, and therefore higher risk, than they would if there were no deposit insurance. The insurance premium rate is artificially low, permitting institution managers to obtain deposits at less than full cost (because depositors will accept a lower interest payment on insured deposits). Consequently, depository institution managers can increase their profits using lower-cost insured deposits to purchase higher-yield, higher-risk assets. The gains to risk taking accrue to the managers and stockholders of the depository institutions; the losses go to the deposit insurer (and, as we will see, ultimately to taxpayers).

To combat the inherent flaws in the financial industry and in the deposit insurance system, a vast regulatory apparatus was installed. The FDIC was given regulatory powers to offset the risk-taking temptations to depository institution managers; those powers included the ability to require higher capital investment; the ability to regulate, examine, and supervise bank affairs; and the ability to enforce its decisions. Still higher capital requirements were imposed in the early 1990s and then adjusted somewhat beginning in 2000, but the basic flaws in the system remain.

Deposit Insurance, Adverse Selection, and Moral Hazard

As a deposit insurer, the FDIC effectively acts as a government-run insurance company. This means that the FDIC's operations expose the federal government to the same kinds of asymmetric information problems that other financial intermediaries face.

Adverse Selection in Deposit Insurance. One of these problems, as discussed in Chapter 14, is *adverse selection,* which arises when there is asymmetric information before a transaction takes place. Adverse selection is often a problem when insurance is involved because people or firms that are relatively poor risks are sometimes able to disguise that fact from insurers. It is instructive to examine the way this works with the deposit insurance provided by the FDIC. Deposit insurance shields depositors from the potential adverse effects of risky decisions and so makes depositors willing to accept riskier investment strategies by their banks. Clearly, this encourages more high-flying, risk-loving entrepreneurs to become managers of banks. Moreover, because depositors have so little incentive to monitor the activities of insured banks, it is also likely that the insurance actually encourages outright crooks—embezzlers and con artists—to enter the industry. The consequences for the FDIC—and for the taxpayer—are larger losses.

Moral Hazard in Deposit Insurance and the U.S. Savings and Loan Debacle. As you learned in Chapter 14, *moral hazard* arises as the result of information asymmetry after a transaction has occurred. Moral hazard is also an important phenomenon in the presence of insurance contracts, such as the deposit insurance provided by the FDIC. Insured depositors know that they will not suffer losses if their bank fails. Hence they have little incentive to monitor their bank's investment activities or to punish their bank by withdrawing their funds if the bank assumes too much risk. This means that insured banks have incentives to take on more risks than they otherwise would—and with those risks come higher losses for the FDIC and for taxpayers.

For a variety of reasons, by the mid-1980s, the savings and loan (S&L) industry in the United States was facing disaster. What was occurring at that time was a perfect example of the perverse incentives that occur when government-provided deposit insurance exists. S&L institution managers undertook riskier actions than they otherwise would have because of the existence of deposit insurance. Moreover, because of the existence of deposit insurance, depositors in savings and loan associations had little incentive to investigate the financial dealings and stability of those institutions. After all, deposits were guaranteed by an agency of the federal government, so why worry? Hence there was little incentive for households and firms to monitor savings and loan institutions or even to diversify their deposits across institutions. From an S&L manager's point of view, as long as deposit insurance protected depositors, the manager could feel confident to "go for the gold." One result was an increase in the amount of high-risk, high-yielding assets purchased by many savings and loan associations.

The first year of the S&L crisis, 135 institutions failed. Over the next two years, another 600 went bankrupt. By the end of the crisis, 1,500 thrift institutions had gone under. Politicians chose to solve the crisis by passing the Financial Institutions Reform, Recovery and Enforcement Act (FIRREA), popularly known as the Thrift Bailout Act of 1989. The estimated cost to American taxpayers was about $200 billion. Congress followed up in 1991 by passing the FDIC Improvement Act (FDICIA). This law toughened regulatory standards and required the FDIC to close weak depository institutions promptly, rather than letting their managers continue to roll the dice with taxpayers' dollars at stake.

POLICY EXAMPLE

Letting the Market Do the Regulators' Work

Some observers contend that there should be less regulation of banks. They argue that markets could do the regulators' work. Indeed, two top Federal Reserve officials have argued just that. The first one was Federal Reserve Bank of Richmond President J. Alfred Broaddus, Jr. The other was Federal Reserve Governor Laurence H. Meyer, who presented a detailed approach to how such a system would work.

Meyer argued that "large, internationally active banks" should be required to issue a minimum amount of "subordinated debt"—such as bonds that are redeemed only after bank depositors and other claimants are repaid following a default—to investors. Such debt would provide an extra cushion of protection for taxpayers. In addition, however, the market price that investors would pay for such subordinated bank debt would depend on how investors evaluate the management strategy of each particular bank. Any subordinated debt holder could lose everything if the bank failed. Thus owners of such debt have an incentive to monitor closely any issuer's activities. This is exactly the type of monitoring that the FDIC currently does on behalf of the insurance funds.

The risk premium a bank's subordinated debt carried would give a signal to the FDIC. Indeed, the FDIC could use the observed risk premiums as a simple way to determine how much an insured bank should be charged in premiums. Imagine a situation in which a certain bank's subordinated debt could be sold only at a very high interest rate. This would be an early warning to regulators that this bank was encountering financial trouble.

For Critical Analysis

Why is it more important to worry about "large internationally active banks" than small banks?

CONCEPTS IN BRIEF

- Banks and other financial institutions function as payment intermediaries, transferring funds used to pay for goods, services, or finanicial assets between the payers and receivers of the funds.
- In most countries, people use nonelectronic payment mechanisms, such as currency, checks, and paper-based giro systems, for the largest portion of their daily payment transactions. The bulk of the total *value* of payments, however, is processed on large-value payment systems. In the United States, Fedwire and the Clearing House Interbank Payment System (CHIPS) are the two key large-value payment systems.
- Their role as payment intermediaries exposes banks to liquidity, credit, and systemic risks. The last of these risks exposes the entire banking system to the threat of bank runs.
- To limit the fallout from systemic failures and bank runs, Congress created the Federal Deposit Insurance Corporation (FDIC) in 1933. Since the advent of federal deposit insurance, there have been no true bank runs at federally insured banks.
- Because of the way deposit insurance is set up in the United States, it encourages bank managers to invest in riskier assets to make higher rates of return.

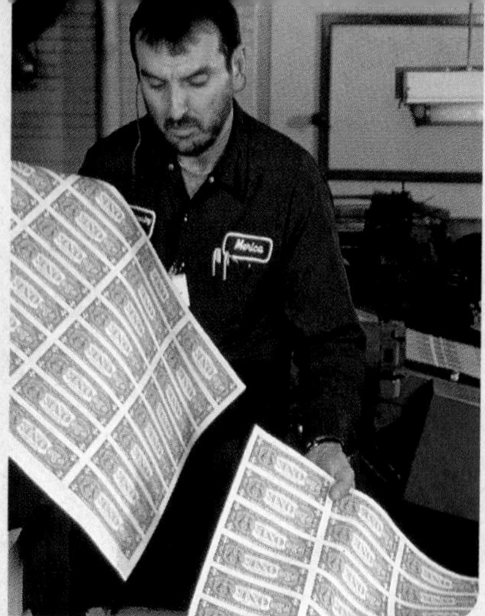

ISSUES & APPLICATIONS

Are Reserve Requirements on the Way Out or In?

To many economists, reserve requirements are an outdated relic. They argue that reserve requirements might prove useful as a stabilizing tool if central banks really sought to achieve targets for the quantity of money in circulation, but they note that most central banks today pay little attention to variations in money growth. Hence, they contend, reserve requirements around the world should be reduced or even eliminated.

Concepts Applied

Reserve Requirements

Money Creation

Table 15-4 shows that banks in many industrialized countries face lower required reserve ratios than they did a decade ago. Relative to the required reserve ratios of other nations in the table, the official 10 percent ratio for transactions deposits in the United States stands out. This is misleading, however, because the *effective* U.S. required reserve ratio has been much lower than this since the mid-1990s.

The Great Reserve-Requirement Loophole: Sweep Accounts

A key simplifying assumption in our example of the money creation process was that checkable deposits were the only bank liability system that changes when total reserves change. Of course, banks also issue savings and time deposits. In addition, they offer *automatic transfer accounts.* In these accounts, which banks have offered since the 1970s, funds are automatically transferred from savings deposits to checkable deposits whenever the account holder writes a check that would otherwise cause the balance of checkable deposits to become negative. Automatic transfer accounts thereby protected individuals and businesses from overdrawing their checking accounts.

TABLE 15-4
Required Reserve Ratios in Selected Nations
Several nations have reduced their required reserve ratios in recent years.

Required Reserve Ratio	1989	2000
Checkable Deposits		
Canada	10.0%	0%
European Monetary Union*	—	2.0%
Japan	1.75%	1.2%
New Zealand	0%	0%
United Kingdom	.45%	.35%
United States	12.0%	10.0%
Noncheckable Deposits		
Canada	3.0%	0%
European Monetary Union*	—	2.0%
Japan	2.5%	1.3%
New Zealand	0%	0%
United Kingdom	.45%	.35%
United States	3.0%	0%

*The European Monetary Union was formed in 1999.
Sources: Gordon Sellon Jr. and Stuart Weiner, "Monetary Policy Without Reserve Requirements: Analytical Issues," Federal Reserve Bank of Kansas City *Economic Review,* 81 (Fourth Quarter 1996), pp. 5–24; Bank for International Settlements.

FIGURE 15-4

Sweep Accounts and Reserves of U.S. Depository Institutions at Federal Reserve Banks

Panel (a) depicts the growth of sweep accounts, which shift funds from transactions deposits subject to reserve requirements to savings deposits with no legal required reserve ratios. Panel (b) shows that the effect of the existence of sweep accounts has been a steady decline in reserve balances that depository institutions hold with Federal Reserve Banks.

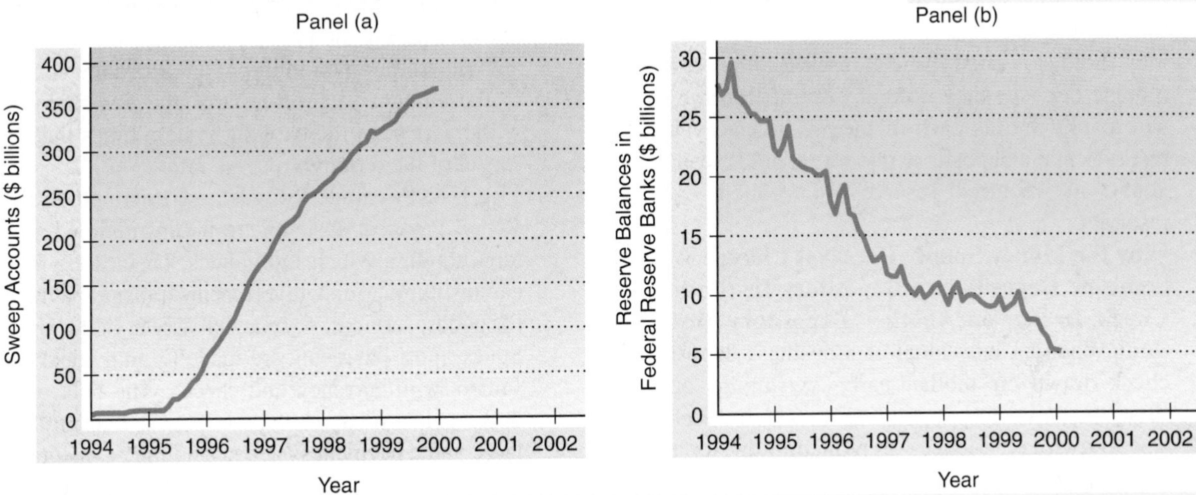

Beginning in 1993, several U.S. banks discovered a way to use automatic transfer accounts to reduce their required reserves. This permitted the banks to shift funds *out of* their customers' checkable deposit accounts, which are subject to reserve requirements, and *into* the customers' savings deposits—mainly money market deposit accounts—which are *not* subject to reserve requirements. Automatic transfer accounts with provisions permitting banks to shift funds from checkable deposits to savings deposits to avoid reserve requirements are called **sweep accounts.** Banks gave the accounts this name because they effectively used them to "sweep" funds from one deposit to another.

As panel (a) of Figure 15-4 shows, total funds in U.S. sweep accounts (and hence total funds exempt from the 10 percent required reserve ratio) have increased dramatically since June 1995. Panel (b) indicates that the result has been a significant decline in the reserves that U.S. banks hold at Federal Reserve banks.

Sweep account 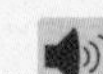
A depository institution account that entails regular shifts of funds from transaction deposits that are subject to reserve requirements to savings deposits that are exempt from reserve requirements.

Reserve Requirements on an Upswing in Europe

Even as the United States has joined the movement toward significant reductions in effective reserve requirements, however, European central bank officials successfully imposed *higher* reserve requirements on many banks in European Union countries. When the European Monetary Union began in 1999, the European System of Central Banks established a 2 percent reserve requirement ratio that applies to nearly all bank deposits, including saving and time deposits as well as checkable deposits. Their rationale for this proposal is simple: If European banks have to hold more reserves with central banks, then the central banks can earn interest on the funds, which is a steady source of income to fund their operations. This justification for higher reserve requirements relies on their usefulness as a tax on banks and their customers. It has nothing to do with issues of monetary, financial, or economic stability.

FOR CRITICAL ANALYSIS

1. What incentive do banks have to establish sweep accounts, and how might bank customers benefit from sweep accounts?
2. What actions, short of forbidding sweep accounts, can the Federal Reserve take to keep reserve changes caused by the growth of sweep accounts from affecting the money supply?

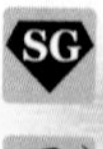

SUMMARY DISCUSSION OF LEARNING OBJECTIVES

1. **How the Federal Reserve Assesses Reserve Requirements:** The Federal Reserve establishes a required reserve ratio, which is currently 10 percent of nearly all checkable deposits at depository institutions. Legal reserves that depository institutions may hold to satisfy their reserve requirements include deposits they hold at Federal Reserve district banks and as cash in their vaults. Any legal reserves that a depository institution holds over and above its required reserves are called excess reserves.
2. **Why the Money Supply Does Not Change When Someone Deposits in a Depository Institution a Check Drawn on Another Depository Institution:** When an individual or a business deposits a check drawn on another party, two things occur. First, the depository institution on which the check was drawn experiences a reduction in its total deposits when the check clears. Second, the depository institution that receives the deposit experiences an equal-sized increase in its total deposits. For the banking system as a whole, therefore, total deposits remain unchanged. Thus the money supply is unaffected by the transaction.
3. **Why the Money Supply Does Change When Someone Deposits in a Depository Institution a Check Drawn on the Federal Reserve System:** When an individual or a business (typically a bond dealer) deposits a check drawn on the Federal Reserve System, the depository institution that receives the deposit experiences an equal-sized increase in its total deposits. Consequently, there is an immediate increase in total deposits in the banking system as a whole, and the money supply increases by the amount of the initial deposit. Furthermore, the depository institution that receives this deposit can lend any reserves in excess of requires reserves, which will generate a rise in deposits at another bank. This process continues as each bank receiving a deposit has additional funds over and above required reserves that it can lend.
4. **The Maximum Potential Change in the Money Supply Following a Federal Reserve Purchase or Sale of U.S. Government Securities:** When the Federal Reserve buys or sells securities, the maximum potential change in the money supply occurs when there are no leakages of currency or excess reserves during the process of money creation. The amount of the maximum potential change is equal to the amount of reserves that the Fed injects or withdraws from the banking system times the reciprocal of the required reserve ratio.
5. **The U.S. Payment System and Payment System Risks:** Payment systems are the institutional structures through which individuals, businesses, financial institutions, and governments transmit payments for goods, services, or financial assets. In the United States, most payments are made by individual consumers with currency and checks. The bulk of the dollar value of payments, however, is transmitted in large-value payment systems handling payments that average millions of dollars each. Any payment system exposes its users to liquidity, credit, and systemic risks. Systemic risk exposes more than one financial institution to the potential for failure, which can give rise to bank runs.
6. **Features of Federal Deposit Insurance:** To help prevent runs on banks, the U.S. government in 1933 established the Federal Deposit Insurance Corporation (FDIC). This government agency provides deposit insurance by charging depository institutions premiums based on the value of their deposits, and it places these funds in accounts for use in closing failed banks and reimbursing their depositors. One difficulty associated with providing deposit insurance is the problem of adverse selection, because the availability of deposit insurance can potentially attract risk-taking individuals into the banking business. Another difficulty is the moral hazard problem. This problem arises when deposit insurance premiums fail to reflect the full extent of the risks taken on by depository institution managers and when depositors who know they are insured have little incentive to monitor the performance of the institutions that hold their deposit funds.

Key Terms and Concepts

Automated clearing house (ACH) (369)

Automated teller machine (ATM) networks (369)

Balance sheet (357)

Bank runs (373)

Clearing House Interbank Payments System (CHIPS) (371)

Credit risk (371)

Discount rate (366)

Excess reserves (356)

Federal Deposit Insurance Corporation (FDIC) (372)

Federal funds market (366)

Federal funds rate (367)

Fedwire (371)

Financial trading systems (368)

Fractional reserve banking (355)

Large-value wire transfer systems (370)

Legal reserves (355)

Liquidity risk (371)

Money multiplier (365)

Net worth (357)

Open market operations (359)

Payment intermediaries (368)

Payment systems (368)

Point-of-sale (POS) networks (369)

Required reserve ratio (356)

Required reserves (356)

Reserves (355)

Sweep accounts (379)

Systemic risk (372)

Problems Test

Answers to the odd-numbered problems appear at the back of the book.

15-1. A bank's only liabilities are $15 million in checkable deposits. The bank currently meets its reserve requirement, and it holds no excess reserves. The required reserve ratio is 10 percent. Assuming that its only assets are legal reserves, loans, and securities, what is the value of loans and securities held by the bank?

15-2. Draw an empty bank balance sheet, with the heading "Assets" on the left-hand side and the heading "Liabilities" on the right-hand side. Then place the following items on the proper side of the balance sheet:

a. Loans to a private company

b. Borrowings from a Federal Reserve district bank

c. Deposits with a Federal Reserve district bank

d. U.S. Treasury bills

e. Vault cash

f. Loans to other banks in the federal funds market

g. Checkable deposits

15-3. Suppose that the total liabilities of a depository institution are checkable deposits equal to $2 billion. It has $1.65 billion in loans and securities, and the required reserve ratio is .15. Does this institution hold any excess reserves? If so, how much?

15-4. A bank has $120 million in total assets, which are composed of legal reserves, loans, and securities. Its only liabilities are $120 million in checkable deposits. The bank exactly satisfies its reserve requirement, and its total legal reserves equal $6 million. What is the required reserve ratio?

15-5. The Federal Reserve purchases $1 million in U.S. Treasury bonds from a bond dealer, and the dealer's bank credits the dealer's account. The required reserve ratio is .15, and the bank typically lends any excess reserves immediately. Assuming that no currency leakage occurs, how much will the bank be able to lend to its customers following the Fed's purchase?

15-6. A depository institution holds $150 million in required reserves and $10 million in excess reserves. Its remaining assets include $440 million in loans and $150 million in securities. If the institution's only liabilities are checkable deposits, what is the required reserve ratio?

15-7. Suppose that the value of the maximum potential money multiplier is equal to 4. What is the required reserve ratio?

15-8. Why is it that you cannot induce any net multiple deposit expansion in the banking system by buying a U.S. government security, yet the Federal Reserve can do so?

15-9. Consider a world in which there is no currency and depository institutions issue only checkable deposits and desire to hold no excess reserves. The required reserve ratio is 20 percent. The central bank sells $1 billion in government securities. What happens to the money supply?

15-10. Assume a 1 percent required reserve ratio, zero excess reserves, and no currency leakages. What is the maximum potential money multiplier? How will total deposits in the banking system change if the Federal Reserve purchases $5 million in U.S. government securities?

Economics on the Net

Statistics on Payment Systems in the Group of Ten Countries Every nation's overall payment system is different. This application gives you the opportunity to evaluate just how different national payment systems can be.

Title: Bank for International Settlements

Navigation: Click here to visit the Bank for International Settlements. Scan down the list and click Statistics on Payment Systems in the Group of Ten Countries (most recent year). Download the entire PDF file, which contains tables displaying payment system data for G-10 countries listed in alphabetical order; then answer the application questions.

Application You can use the data in this report to make a number of cross-country comparisons. Here let's focus on comparing the relative use of checks and automated teller machines (ATMs) in Belgium and the United States.

1. Look at Table 1 ("Basic Statistical Data") for Belgium (the first country in the report) and the United States (the last country in the report). On a separate sheet of paper, write down each nation's population in the latest available year and the average exchange rate for the Belgian franc, or BEF (given in francs per dollar), for that year. Next scroll to Table 13 ("Indicators of Use of Various Cashless Payment Instruments: Values of Transactions") for each country. What was the *dollar value* of total checks (spelled *cheques* in the tables) issued in each nation during this year? (Use the average BEF exchange rate for the year to convert the Belgian value of checks issued into dollars.) What was the average *per capita dollar value* of checks issued in each nation? (Divide each nation's dollar value of checks issued by its population.) Based on your per capita figures, in which of the two nations are checks a more important means of payment for the average resident?
2. Now consider Table 6 ("Cash Dispensers, ATMs, and EFTPOS Terminals") for each nation. For the most recent year, what was the total *dollar value* of all transactions on ATMs in each country? What was the average *per capita dollar value* of ATM transactions in each nation? Based on your per capita figures, in which of the two nations are ATM transactions a more common means of transferring funds?

For Group Study and Analysis Assign each student or group to repeat the exercise for other countries included in this report.

CHAPTER 16

ELECTRONIC BANKING

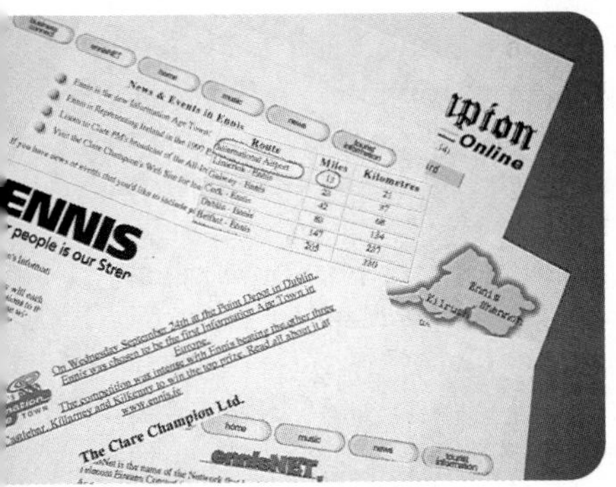

The village of Ennis, Ireland, became Europe's first Internet-age town. All 6,000 Ennis households are now equipped with voice mail, Internet access, and "smart cards." Many more electronic commerce solutions are in the works. Will wider use of digital cash eliminate our banking system?

Recently, the village of Ennis, in County Clare, became Ireland's "Information Age Town." About 6,000 Ennis households were equipped with voice mail, personal computers, and Internet access. They also received *smart cards,* which can store data, process computer messages, and communicate with cell phones, screen phones, personal computers, parking meters, and vending machines. Department stores, supermarkets, gas stations, taxicabs, and pubs were also equipped with smart-card devices. Participating banks deployed card-accessible, cash-loading stations in parking lots, shopping centers, schools, and bank branches. All this was designed to find out what aspects of "smart-card technology" would and would not work in an ordinary community.

Why are so many banks and companies around the world striving to decide how much, and how quickly, they should invest in the kinds of technologies available to residents of Ennis? What is the expected payoff? To help you to contemplate these questions, let's look at the various forms of electronic payment, including smart cards, and their uses in the emerging world of *e-money* (electronic money) and *cyberbanking*.

LEARNING OBJECTIVES

After reading this chapter, you should be able to:

1. **Distinguish among the functions of stored-value cards, debit cards, and smart cards**
2. **Explain the importance of digital certification for the ultimate acceptability of digital cash**
3. **Explain the security features of digital cash versus physical cash**
4. **Understand how on-line banking has developed and why regulators have given it special attention**
5. **Consider how the widespread adoption of digital cash may affect the money multiplier and the money supply**

Chapter Outline

- Current Electronic Means of Payment
- The Precursor to E-Money: Stored-Value Cards
- From Stored-Value Cards to Debit Cards
- Smart Cards and Digital Cash
- Cyberpayment Intermediaries
- On-Line Banking
- Regulating E-Money and Internet Banking
- Digital Cash and the Money Multiplier

Did You Know That... the Treasury Department estimates that the total annual cost of handling physical cash throughout the United States is approximately $60 billion? This includes all the costs of replacing worn-out currency, printing hard-to-counterfeit currency and minting new coins, and transporting boxes and bags full of currency and coins between banks and retailers. It also includes the cost of sorting and counting billions of coins every day. Since the nation's founding, the Treasury has searched for ways to reduce the costs of producing and handling money. After all, society could direct funds not spent on shuffling cash to a number of alternative uses.

Today, the use of **digital cash,** which consists of funds contained on the computer software stored on microchips and other computer devices, promises to drastically reduce the nation's costs of transferring funds. The reason is that people can store and instantaneously transmit digital cash along preexisting electronic networks. People can keep digital cash on diskettes, compact disks, and hard drives. They can send digital cash payments along telephone lines, between cell phones, or over fiber-optic cables. Certainly, digital cash is in its early stages of experimentation and adoption. Nevertheless, the use of digital cash promises to change the nature of money. It is also beginning to transform the world of banking.

In this chapter, you will find out about the new world of smart cards and digital cash, efforts by bank regulators to try to keep up with the explosion in cyberbanking, and ways in which the use of digital cash may affect the money supply.

Digital cash 
Funds contained on computer software, in the form of secure programs stored on microchips and other computer devices.

CURRENT ELECTRONIC MEANS OF PAYMENT

The idea of electronic payments is not new. Most Americans use paper checks to pay for groceries and other items. The checks we write have magnetic ink encryptions that special machines use to sort and distribute checks automatically. Increasingly, the information on paper checks is transformed into digital information to permit computers to credit and debit accounts electronically. This large-scale automation of check sorting, accounting, and distribution has kept the per-check cost of clearing checks very low. Today, banking institutions clear millions of checks each day—a total of more than 70 billion per year. It was not always this way, however. Fifty years ago, checking accounts were offered primarily to higher-income and upper-middle-income individuals, and bank employees cleared checks by hand using paper accounting ledgers. Because checking accounts were so expensive to maintain, most other people made their purchases using cash or money orders.

Today, most U.S. consumers have experience using automated teller machine (ATM) networks. As noted in Chapter 15, many consumers regularly use ATM networks to make deposits, withdraw cash from their accounts, transfer funds among accounts, and pay bills. Even though all these ATM functions are commonplace today, three decades ago about all an ATM machine could do was dispense cash. Furthermore, banks had to work hard to convince many skeptical customers to trust ATMs to handle even this simple function.

Without knowing it, many of us have used the services of automated clearing house (ACH) systems, as also noted in Chapter 15. Banks began to put ACH payment-clearing and settlement systems into place back in the days when the only computers were mainframes. Anyone who has received a direct deposit, such as an automatic payroll deposit, has taken advantage of the services of an ACH. So has a person who has arranged for a regular monthly insurance or mortgage payment to be debited automatically from a checking account. This is yet another example of an electronic means of payment that did not exist all that long ago. Nevertheless, many of us commonly use them today.

Clearly, various forms of electronic payments have been with us for some time. What is new and different is the potential to replace *physical* cash—coins and paper currency—with *virtual* cash in the form of electronic impulses. This is the unique promise of digital cash.

THE PRECURSOR TO E-MONEY: STORED-VALUE CARDS

According to the Bank for International Settlements, an international institution operated by major central banks, U.S. residents make more than 300 billion cash transactions (or nearly 1,100 per person) every year. Of these, 270 billion are in amounts of less than $2. It is easy to see why people use paper currency and coins to purchase a soft drink, a candy bar, or a magazine. Why would they use e-money, however, instead of currency and coins?

To understand why people might use e-money instead of physical cash, let's begin by thinking about the simplest kind of e-money system, one that uses **stored-value cards.** These are plastic cards embossed with magnetic stripes containing magnetically encoded data. Using a stored-value card, a person purchases specific goods and services offered by the card issuer. For example, a number of college and university libraries have copy machines that students operate by inserting a stored-value card. Each time a student makes copies, the copy machine deducts the per-copy fee. When the balance on the student's card runs low in the middle of copying a news article, the student can replenish the balance by placing the card in a separate machine and inserting physical cash. The machine stores the value of the cash on the card. Then the student can go back to a copy machine, reinsert the card, and finish copying the article.

Stored-value card 
A card bearing magnetic stripes that hold magnetically encoded data, providing access to stored funds.

Some stored-value cards are disposable. The cardholder throws away the card after spending the value stored on it. But many banks and other issuers prefer reusable stored-value cards. Bearers of these cards may use them to purchase goods and services offered by any participating merchant.

FROM STORED-VALUE CARDS TO DEBIT CARDS

Plastic cards used in *open* funds transfer systems are called **debit cards.** These cards essentially adapt the technology of stored-value cards to permit authorization of direct funds transfers. People can use them to authorize transfers of funds from their accounts to those of merchants.

Debit card 
A plastic card that allows the bearer to transfer funds to a merchant's account, provided that the bearer authorizes the transfer by providing personal identification.

Debit Cards as Electronic Checking

Figure 16-1 on page 386 illustrates a sample transaction flow in a debit card system. A card issuer, Bank A, provides cards to its customers, who use their cards to make purchases from retailers. The retailers' electronic cash registers record the value of the purchases and the routing numbers of the issuing banks. The retailers then submit the recorded data to their own bank, Bank B. This bank then forwards claims for funds to the system operator. The operator transmits these claims to each issuing bank, including Bank A. Once Bank A honors its obligations to Bank B by debiting your checking account, the latter bank credits the deposit accounts of the retailers.

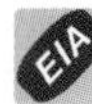

Electronic Banking and Payments
Learn more about stored-value, debit, and smart cards.

Note that Figure 16-1 could just as easily show the workings of a system of paper checks. Instead of using debit cards to buy goods and services, bank customers could use checks to make their purchases. Then the retailers could send the checks on to their own banks. The banks could then submit them to a clearinghouse, which could then process the

FIGURE 16-1
A Debit Card System
Holders of cards issued by Bank A can automatically authorize payments directly to retailers, who in turn transmit claims to Bank B. This bank then transmits payment claims to the operator of the system, which then transmits the claims to Bank A.

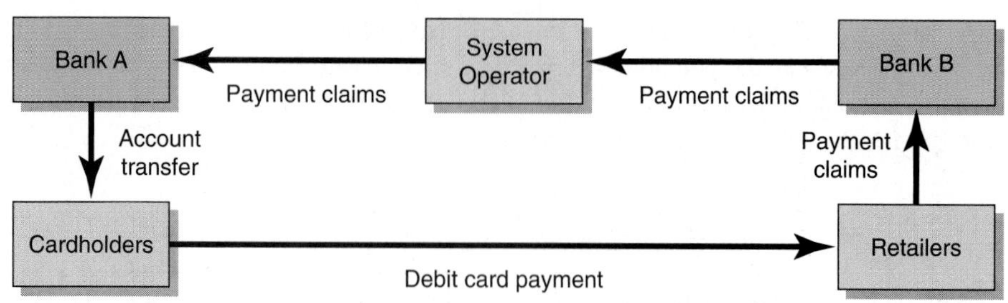

interbank payments required for the retailers to receive final payment of funds. Thus a fully electronic debit card system effectively amounts to electronic checking. As with check clearing, behind-the-scenes interbank clearing must take place to finalize a transaction.

The Trouble and Expense of Debit Cards

The security features of debit card systems make them somewhat cumbersome. When a cardholder presents a typical debit card to a retailer, the retailer's electronic cash register routes a request for authorization to the issuing bank. The bank's computer checks the cardholder's account number against a file of lost or stolen cards. It also verifies that funds are available in the customer's account. Then the bank sends confirmation of payment authorization.

This authorization system helps reduce the chance that someone who stole the card can use it. The thief would have to steal the customer's authorization codes as well as the card. Thus the authorization procedure enhances the security of the system for the legitimate cardholder. In addition, the system guarantees that the retailer will receive final payment. Nevertheless, the telecommunication costs of standard on-line authorizations range from 8 cents to 15 cents per transaction. This is typically much higher than the per-transaction cost of paper currency and coins. In addition, retailers such as fast-food restaurants are not enthused about the slow speed of this kind of authorization system. After all, employees awaiting payment authorizations for customers they have already served cannot start serving customers who are waiting in line.

For these reasons, debit cards represent a purely technical innovation in retail payments. Unless debit card systems become speedier and more cost-effective, they are unlikely to alter fundamentally the nature of retail payments.

SMART CARDS AND DIGITAL CASH 

Smart card 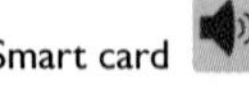
A card containing a microprocessor that permits storage of funds via security programming, can communicate with other computers, and does not require on-line authorization for funds transfers.

A more dramatic innovation has been the development of **smart cards;** plastic cards containing minute computer microchips that can hold far more information than a magnetic stripe. Thanks to microchip technology, a smart card can do much more than maintain a running cash balance in its memory or authorize the transfer of funds.

Smart Cards

A smart card carries and processes security programming. This capability of smart cards gives them a technical advantage over stored-value cards. Magnetic stripe cards fail to communicate a transaction correctly about 250 times in every million transactions. Smart cards fail to communicate properly less than 100 times per million transactions. Furthermore, smart cards are no more expensive to produce than standard stored-value cards or debit cards. Many smart cards are designed to be disposable.

The microprocessors on smart cards can also authenticate the validity of transactions. Retailers can program electronic cash registers to confirm the authenticity of the smart card by examining a unique "digital signature" stored on its microchip. The digital signature is created by software called a *cryptographic algorithm.* This is a secure program loaded onto the microchip of the card. The digital signature guarantees to the retailer's electronic cash register that the information on the smart card's chip is genuine. Figure 16-2 shows how digital encryption helps guarantee the security of electronic payments.

In a smart-card-based system for e-money transfers, the user of a smart card can remain anonymous. There is also no need for on-line authorization using expensive telecommunication services. Each time a cardholder uses a smart card, the amount of a purchase is deducted automatically and credited to a retailer. The retailer can in turn store its electronic cash receipts in specially adapted point-of-sale terminals and transfer accumulated balances to its bank at the end of the day via telephone links. This permits payments to be completed within seconds. Effectively, smart cards can do anything that paper currency and coins can do.

The Convenience of Digital Cash

What does a smart card have that paper currency and coins do not? The answer is potentially greater convenience. Smart cards' microchips can communicate with any computing device equipped with the appropriate software. ATMs and retailers' electronic cash registers are examples, but so are desktop and laptop computers.

People cannot use paper currency and coins, checks, or stored-value cards to complete transactions over the Internet. Instead, they usually provide credit card numbers and finalize payments to credit card issuers when they pay their monthly bills. Using smart cards or other microchip-bearing devices, however, they can send cash directly across cyberspace and finalize a transaction instantly, just as they could by handing over physical cash in person.

FIGURE 16-2

Digital Encryption and Electronic Payment Security

An electronic payment instruction starts out in a form readable by a human being, called "plaintext." When this instruction is entered into a computer, it is secured, or encrypted, using an "encryption key," which is a software code. In computer-readable form, the payment instruction is called "ciphertext," which the computer transmits to another location. A computer at the other location uses another software code, called a "decryption key," to read the data and turn it back into a plaintext form that a human operator can read.

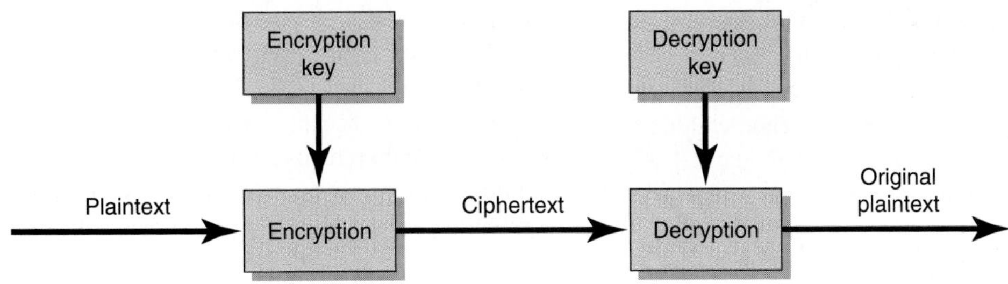

For instance, it is now technologically feasible for someone to use smart card technology to make a digital cash purchase of a service from an Internet-based retailer. Suppose that a student who likes classical music wishes to hear the latest rendition of a Mozart concerto by a favorite set of performers. The student can do this by using a smart-card-reading device connected to her personal computer—hardware manufacturers began introducing these devices at retail prices between $80 and $140 in the late 1990s—or she can load digital cash onto a program located on the hard drive of the computer. As long as the performer's recording company also has the necessary software, the student can enter a designated location on the recording company's Web site, point, click, and download the music as a digital file. The student's computer automatically sends digital cash as payment for this service. Then the student can listen to the latest concerto recording on her computer's speakers.

CYBERPAYMENT INTERMEDIARIES

Of course, the fact that people have the ability to adopt a technology does not mean that they actually will. After all, the basic technology for stored-value cards has been available since the 1970s. Only recently, however, have people made widespread use of stored-value cards to purchase such items as telephone calls and gasoline.

The Shaky Start of On-line Payments

Some initial experiments with on-line payments did not encourage consumers to adopt the new technology. Consider the 1996 experience of a woman in California who thought she had arranged to use financial software to pay her electric bill on the Internet. In fact, what she did when she clicked her computer's mouse was send a pay order to the software company's computers in Illinois. The company automatically wired instructions to a Utah location, where a clerk printed a paper check and sent it by surface mail to the San Francisco power company that provided the woman's electricity. The utility customer learned of this tangled payment chain after power to her home was shut off. The power company had rejected the check after it arrived from Utah because it was missing a payment stub.

Naturally, customers have been unwilling to adopt cyberpayment technologies until they are convinced that their payments are secure from transmission errors, fraud, and theft. They also want to know that technologies such as smart cards will be accepted by many other consumers and merchants before going to the trouble of learning to use them. At the same time, retailers do not want to install systems for

FAQ

Are smart cards too hard for the average person to use?

No, because even children can use them. A big fear of banks and companies interested in introducing smart cards and digital cash systems has been the supposedly unsophisticated U.S. consumer. Since the late 1990s, however, elementary school children in Westport, Connecticut, have been using smart cards to buy lunch at the school cafeteria. Each child has an account set up by the school. At the end of each month, parents receive a statement of purchases. Whenever funds are low, a computer generates a letter sent automatically to the parent. Each cafeteria cash register is equipped with a computer, software, printer, external floppy drive, scanner, and digital camera. Each pupil's photo is stored on a host computer for verification purposes. So even though fraud is not completely impossible, the probability of fraudulent card use has been significantly diminished. Today, most Westport schoolchildren—kids as young as 5 years old—use smart cards every day. Clearly, it doesn't take grown-up smarts to use smart cards.

reading smart cards and processing digital cash payments until more customers are willing to use them.

Convincing People That Digital Cash Is "Real Money"

As you learned in Chapter 15, banks have traditionally served as payment intermediaries. Today, many banks have memberships in such credit card industry groups as Visa International, MasterCard, and American Express. As a result, many banks are indirectly members of the Global Chipcard Alliance, an industry trade group that has promoted the standardization of smart card technology. An example is so-called smart card dial tones, which are sophisticated computer programs that allow any smart card to be accepted by any card-reading terminal.

Such standardization is necessary before widespread—indeed, worldwide—adoption of smart cards will be feasible. Today, U.S. videotapes cannot work on European videocassette players. In future years, will U.S. residents who travel to Europe find that their smart cards do not work in European equipment or with European software? Will they find that their smart cards will not function in on-line systems installed in Japan, China, or South Africa? Closer to home, will a New Orleans resident discover that his smart card doesn't work in Des Moines?

At present, every smart card system has a digital cash **certificate authority.** This is a designated payment intermediary that administers and regulates the terms under which people legitimately engage in e-money transactions. A certificate authority's key job is to approve and implement standards for digital signatures of smart cards, thereby enabling smartcard systems to connect all users. Because the security of their funds and the unrestricted ability to spend them when they wish are so important to people, a lot of effort is currently being devoted to standardizing the functions and interactions among certificate authorities. Once this is accomplished, smart cards should work in most locales.

Certificate authority 
A group charged with supervising the terms governing how buyers and sellers can legitimately make digital cash transfers.

Nearly all economists agree that there is likely to be an incentive for people to shift a portion of their paper-based transactions to exchanges using digital cash. No one can say for sure, however, if people will make this shift quickly or only gradually, perhaps over a period spanning a decade or more. In addition, it is impossible to estimate exactly what portion of retail transactions will ultimately be settled using digital cash. One thing is certain, however: Worldwide distribution of funds transfer cards such as debit cards and smart cards is growing rapidly. In 1989, there was one such card for every 100 people in the world. Today, the ratio is closer to one card for every eight people in the world.

CONCEPTS IN BRIEF

- Stored-value cards are capable of storing computer-accessible data. They do not process data, so they are most often used in closed systems operated by a single business.
- Debit cards permit transfers of funds among accounts. They essentially perform the same functions as checks, but without paper.
- Smart cards contain microprocessors that can tabulate data, process security programs, and communicate directly with other computers. Smart cards or any other computing device can store and transmit digital cash, which consists of funds in the form of secure software programs.
- Digital cash transactions between different cyberpayment systems can be accomplished only if digital signatures used in one system can be recognized by the other system. This has induced software companies and payment intermediaries to develop digital certification techniques in an effort to make digital cash more widely acceptable.

ON-LINE BANKING

Banks were initially hesitant to jump into cyberspace. But they now recognize that they have an interest in seeing smart cards catch on. The reason is that widespread smart card adoption holds the promise of significant profits. Funds stored on customers' bank-issued smart cards are still, technically speaking, on deposit with their banks. Thus just as with traditional checking accounts, banks can earn profits by lending out unused balances of excess reserves on cards to other customers.

Banks also see the promise of fees that they will be able to charge retailers who accept the cards. They also anticipate getting to keep any spare change that customers leave on a card if they decide to throw it away. For instance, suppose that a bank finds that during a given week, a "typical" customer using a disposable smart card has 21 cents in "spare change" left on the card that the customer does not think worth the effort to spend before throwing away the card. If 10,000 customers are "typical," then each week a bank will get to keep a total amount of $2,100. Over the course of a year, this "spare change" will accumulate to $109,200!

Before most people become comfortable about sending digital cash to retailers across cyberspace, they must be sure that they can have secure on-line dealings with their own banks. This process is further along than the development of digital cash.

The Development of On-Line Banking

On-line banking began through the efforts of home financial management software developers, such as Quicken. These businesses wanted to include attractive features to induce people to buy their software, so they started offering to help software users consolidate bills and initiate payments over the Internet. Bill payments are typically issued from bank accounts, so ultimately the financial software companies formed alliances with banks.

Soon banks realized that they might be able to earn fee income by providing these kinds of services themselves. By 2000, nearly 1,000 U.S. banks offered on-line banking services via the Internet. A survey indicated that about a third of the more than 8,000 U.S. banks were implementing on-line banking and that more than another third were in the planning stages for offering such services.

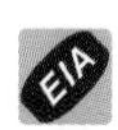

The Emergence of Online Banking
Learn more about developments in online banking.

Most on-line bank customers use three kinds of services. One of the most popular is still bill consolidation and payment. Another is transferring funds among accounts. This on-line service eliminates the need to make trips to a bank branch or ATM. The third is applying for loans, which many banks now permit customers to do over the Internet. Customers typically have to appear in person to finalize the terms of a loan. Nonetheless, they can save some time and effort by starting the process at home.

The Chicken-or-Egg Problem of On-Line Banking

There are two important banking activities generally not available on-line: depositing and withdrawing funds. This, of course, is where smart cards can come into the picture. With smart cards, people could transfer funds on the Internet, thereby effectively transforming their personal computers into home ATMs. This, in turn, would give them more incentive to bank from home via the Internet. Yet many observers believe that on-line banking is the way to introduce people to e-money and to induce them to think about using smart cards.

This raises the potential for a chicken-or-egg problem to develop. Bank customers may wait for widespread acceptability of smart cards before exploring home banking options. At the same time, banks may wait for more customers to choose on-line banking before making big investments in smart card technology.

Nevertheless, many bankers have decided that there are two very good reasons to promote on-line banking irrespective of smart cards. One is that once in place, on-line banking is less expensive for the bank. Banks require fewer employees to maintain automated systems, so on-line banking saves banks from incurring significant expenses associated with large systems of branch offices. The potential cost savings of on-line banking are hard to quantify. This has not stopped some banks from seeking to convert customers to Internet-based banking services, however. A number of banks have adopted explicit targets for portions of their customers that they wish to entice into on-line banking within the next few years. Many are aiming to convince more than half their customers to bank on-line by before 2010.

Click here to find out about the latest on-line banking options. Select your state to find an online bank.

Competitive Pressures for On-Line Banking

Another key rationale that bankers have for developing on-line services is the threat of competition. Many banks worry that if they do not figure out how to provide services on-line, someone else will—and steal away many of their best customers.

Since the late 1990s, several banks have operated exclusively on the Internet. These "virtual banks" have no physical branch offices. Because few people are equipped to send virtual banks funds via smart card technologies, the virtual banks have accepted deposits through physical delivery systems, such as the U.S. Postal Service or Federal Express. This saves the expense of maintaining a costly branch network with buildings and tellers, which sharply reduced the costs that virtual banks incur relative to traditional banks. These Internet-only banks pass on part of the cost savings to customers in the form of lower banking fees and lower interest rates on loans. Some even offer free checking with very low minimum deposits, such as $100, and no-fee money market accounts with average monthly balances of $2,500 or more.

Virtual banks have not been the only on-line competition faced by traditional banks. Today, there are several Internet loan brokers, such as QuickenMortgage, E-Loan, GetSmart, Lending Tree, and Microsoft's HomeAdviser. Each of these broker systems uses software that matches consumers with appropriate loans. The consumer supplies information to the program. The program then searches among available loan products for the best fit. The loans are available from lenders with whom the broker has a contractual relationship.

Internet loan brokers' biggest forays into banks' turf have been in the credit card and mortgage markets. In the credit card business, Internet brokers have been especially successful in providing credit card debt consolidation services. They do not always compete with banks; often they act as marketers for traditional credit-card-issuing banks. Credit card issuers pay the brokers fees to match with new customers. This saves the issuers from having to create lists of potential prospects and to develop and mail card offers.

In the mortgage market, however, the competition is more direct. When mortgage rates fell in the late 1990s, people who wished to refinance flooded the telephone lines of traditional banking institutions. Many experienced busy signals, long waits on hold, and slow responses from loan officers. This induced them to turn to the Internet. One Internet broker reported that visitors to its Web site increased from about 35,000 per month to over

500,000 per month. Some real estate experts estimate that within a few years, at least 10 percent of U.S. mortgage loan refinancings will be initiated through the Internet.

REGULATING E-MONEY AND INTERNET BANKING

Electronic banking technologies make some people nervous. Some people hesitate to adopt digital cash for the same kinds of reasons that have slowed adoption of other new technologies: Until they have time to evaluate what's new, people often begin by assuming the worst.

The Security of Digital Cash

As we all know, from time to time airplanes crash. In the years following the introduction of commercial air passenger service, many people refused to fly. Over time, however, it became clear that flying was often much more convenient than other forms of transportation. Air travel eventually turned out to be safer, too, as reflected by lower average injury and death rates compared to other forms of transportation.

It remains to be seen whether people will find digital cash more convenient than other means of payment. A big issue in the minds of most potential users of smart cards or online banking services is the security of the e-money payments they make. For bank regulators, the security of digital cash is one of two key issues raised by electronic banking. The other concerns the potential for an upsurge of fraudulent banking practices.

Potential Security Concerns

Just because smart cards can be equipped with authentication software does not mean they are 100 percent secure. Criminals can be ingenious. There are a number of ways that one could imagine them stealing or otherwise interfering with digital cash. To thwart such efforts, banks and crime enforcement officials must anticipate them and develop ways to hinder potential criminals.

Digital Counterfeiting. One possible way that a crook could pilfer digital money is old-fashioned but potentially lucrative: counterfeiting. The most obvious way to counterfeit would be to produce smart cards that look, feel, and function just like legitimate smart cards.

Issuers of smart cards have already undertaken a number of defensive measures aimed at preventing such counterfeiting efforts from succeeding. One is to make counterfeit smart cards easier to recognize. Smart card issuers typically place holographic images on their own legitimate cards, just as credit card issuers do. Issuers also place special features in the computer code on smart card microprocessor that complicate efforts to access data stored in memory. They place these features in a portion of the microprocessor's memory that can be changed only by altering its internal functions. Issuers also equip smart cards with physical barriers intended to inhibit optical or electrical analysis of the microprocessor's memory. Most smart card chips are also coated with several layers of wiring, making it difficult to remove the chip without damaging it beyond repair.

Stealing Digital Cash Off-Line and On-Line. One of the most common types of bank robbery today entails driving a pickup truck through the front window of a bank branch or supermarket containing an automated teller machine. Two or three people quickly lift the ATM into the bed of the truck, drive to their hideout, and remove the cash from the machine. An *off-line theft* of digital cash is only slightly more sophisticated. Thieves break into a merchant's establishment, physically remove electronic devices used to store value from customers' smart cards, and download these funds onto their own cards. The threat of this kind of off-line theft is likely to be a bigger problem for small retailers that do not wish to incur the expense required to process all smart card transactions immediately.

More sophisticated thieves might attempt to engage in *on-line thefts.* They could try to intercept payment messages as they are transmitted from smart cards and other electronic funds storage devices to host computers. For instance, thieves might learn the times of day that a large upscale department store transmits its receipts to a central computer. Then they could attempt to tap into the store's transmission line and steal the funds. These kinds of on-line theft are most likely to be "inside jobs," in which employees pilfer their own companies' funds using their knowledge of internal systems for transmitting digital cash.

Making E-Money "Catch a Cold." A key feature of digital cash is its dependence on smoothly functioning microprocessors and software. This exposes electronic money to special security dangers, such as computer viruses that could damage the input-output mechanisms of smart card microprocessors.

Malfunctioning Money. Paper currency can wear out. Magnetic-ink-scanning devices can misread checks. But people can still exchange physical units of money during electricity outages. Power failures or other equipment breakdowns can bring e-money transactions to a grinding halt.

The widespread use of digital cash could also contribute to a problem that is already well known to today's law enforcement officials. Many people already try to move funds from place to place to avoid reporting the funds to tax authorities or to hide illegalities associated with the funds. These activities could become even more common in a world of digital cash.

Click here to learn about the U.S. government's efforts to prevent money laundering.

POLICY EXAMPLE

E-Cash and Money Laundering

Tax evaders, drug traffickers, and others seek to "launder" money every day. That is, they try moving funds around the world without their actions being traced. Estimates are that about $500 billion is "laundered" worldwide every year. Congress has passed several laws aimed at minimizing money laundering, including the Money Laundering Control Act of 1986 and the Money Laundering Suppression Act of 1994.

A U.S. Treasury Department division, the Financial Crimes Enforcement Network (FinCEN), seeks to fight money laundering. Every year, FinCEN receives 11 million reports covering everything from casino earnings to foreign bank accounts maintained by U.S. citizens. Money launderers today invest in bars, restaurants, travel agencies, jewelry stores, and construction companies—virtually any business through which they can channel cash earned illegally.

The Financial Action Taskforce, a group of 26 countries fighting money laundering, believes that the speed, security, and anonymity of new Internet payment systems will lead to massive additional money laundering. Drug traffickers in particular will no longer need to smuggle currency across borders—they will be able to move funds through the Internet. Technology will permit anonymous transactions outside the regulated banking sector. Consequently, all restrictions on the banking system to make money laundering riskier and costlier will be for naught. Even when digital cash enters the banking system, it will have already bounced among numerous intermediaries, making the funds hard to trace. By definition, e-cash will be heavily encrypted. Thus law enforcement authorities will not be able to reconstruct transactions, nor will private providers of e-cash. DigiCash, a major European electronic money provider, indicates that it cannot track how its customers spend their money.

For Critical Analysis

Imagine yourself as a FinCEN employee trying to hinder money-laundering activities, and you know that banks that transfer cash into digital money systems have a limit of a few hundred dollars per transfer. How might money launderers overcome this constraint?

CONCEPTS IN BRIEF

- Key factors spurring on-line banking have been banks' interest in earning fee income and their concerns about competition from other banks and nonbanking firms that offer financial services over the Internet.
- In some respects, the potential security problems of digital cash, such as counterfeiting and outright theft, are simply high-tech versions of security concerns people already experience when they use physical currency and coins.
- In other ways, however, digital cash has its own special security difficulties. Unlike physical money, digital cash can potentially be infected by computer viruses. In addition, during periods of hardware breakdowns or power failures, digital cash transactions may be hindered or halted. On-line banking and the provision of digital cash also expose bank customers to new types of fraudulent practices on the part of unscrupulous virtual banks.

DIGITAL CASH AND THE MONEY MULTIPLIER 

How is digital cash likely to affect the process by which the amount of money in circulation is determined? To address this question, the first thing to do is to recognize that the broad adoption of smart cards and other mechanisms for using digital cash will undoubtedly require redefining measures of the money supply. Because digital cash will function as a medium of exchange, it will ultimately be included in the M1 definition of money. In turn, M1 is included within the broader money measures, so M2 and M3 will also include digital cash. Thus the money multiplier will link changes in reserves in the banking system to measures of money that include digital cash.

Immediate Effects of Digital Cash on the Money Supply Process

To envision the most likely immediate effect of digital cash on the deposit expansion process, suppose that the Fed in a cybereconomy of the not-so-distant future buys \$1 million in government securities. Naturally, transactions deposits initially increase by \$1 million. The recipient of these funds, however, allocates a portion of the \$1 million to both government-issued currency *and* digital cash. The recipient's bank can lend out the remaining deposits less an amount that it must hold to meet its reserve requirement. This generates a deposit at another institution, and the depositor will allocate some of these funds to government currency *and* to digital cash. Thus allocations of funds to digital cash holdings constitute "leakages" from transactions deposits at each stage of the deposit expansion process.

Funds held as digital cash are included in our revised definition of the money supply, however. At every stage of the deposit expansion process, therefore, new digital cash is "created" and included in M1 and other money measures. When the Fed injects more reserves into the banking system, a multiple increase in deposits results, and this causes an increase in digital cash holdings as individuals shift a desired portion of funds from deposit accounts to smart cards and other digital cash storage devices. Unlike government currency holdings, which together with reserves are constrained by the government and the Federal Reserve, privately issued digital cash will vary directly with the extent of transactions deposit expansion. On balance, therefore, the overall quantity of money *increases* with the addition of digital cash. Consequently, the multiplier linking this measure of money to bank reserves must also rise in value. The immediate effect of digital cash, therefore, is likely to be a rise in the value of the money multiplier.

Indirect Effects of Digital Cash on the Money Supply Process

Our reasoning indicates that, other things being equal, the near-term effect of a widespread adoption of digital cash will be an increase in the quantity of money and a rise in the value of the money multiplier. Over time, however, we would not expect that other things will remain equal. For this reason, the money multiplier implications of digital cash will not be so clear-cut in the more distant future.

Substitution of Private Digital Cash for Government Currency. For instance, if many people begin to prefer digital cash to government-provided currency as a means of payment, digital cash could begin to displace government currency. This would have the direct effect of decreasing the government currency component of M1 and other money measures. Although this also would reduce the extent of currency drains—as you learned in Chapter 15, other things being equal, currency drains tend to raise the size of the money multiplier somewhat—the direct effect would dominate. Thus declining use of government-provided currency as people switch to increased use of digital cash will tend to reduce the money multiplier and the money supply.

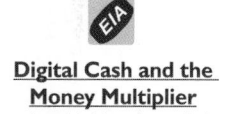

Digital Cash and the Money Multiplier
Practice thinking through how digital cash may affect the money supply process.

On-line Banking and the Money Supply Process. What if on-line banking permits people to make payments directly from their checking accounts without the need to write checks? Will this affect the money supply process?

By transferring transactions deposit funds electronically from their accounts via debit cards, automated bill payments, or Internet-based on-line payment mechanisms, people simply avoid writing paper checks. The money multiplier implications of the transactions are the same as those that arise if paper checks change hands, however, provided that the funds are redeposited in another depository institution. So if normal redepositing occurs, all that changes is the nature of the transactions that lie behind the normal deposit expansion process. Even if many of these are electronic, effects on balance sheets are unchanged. Thus on-line transmission of checking funds by itself has no fundamental effect on the money supply process.

This is true, however, only if all transactions deposits from which people can transmit funds on-line are maintained at depository institutions and are subject to reserve requirements. If other, nondepository institutions find ways to issue transactions deposits via on-line mechanisms such as the Internet, these deposits will also function as money, yet they will not be subject to reserve requirements. In that event, the money multiplier will rise, potentially by a sizable amount. At present, any such activities are illegal, because only government-regulated banking institutions have the legal authority to issue transactions deposits accessible either by check or via the Internet. If nonbanking institutions find a way to get around this restriction, however, the money multiplier could increase dramatically.

CONCEPTS IN BRIEF

- If digital cash is included in M1 and other money measures, widespread adoption of digital cash will have the immediate effect of raising the money multiplier and the amount of money in circulation.
- An offsetting effect that can take place over the longer term is the gradual displacement of government-provided currency by digital cash, which would tend to reduce the money multiplier and money supply somewhat.
- On-line banking services involving transactions deposits will not fundamentally affect the money multiplier. Nevertheless, if nonbanking institutions find ways to offer such deposits while avoiding reserve requirements, the money multiplier could increase significantly.

NETNOMICS

What Will Digital Cash Replace?

If people start to use smart cards, personal computers, and cellular phones to store and transmit digital cash, presumably they will have less desire to use other forms of money. To understand why, consider Table 16-1, which lists the key characteristics of checks, government-issued currency, and digital cash.

In comparing currency with checks, it is clear that people must trade off features that each offers. Checks promise greater security, because if a thief steals a woman's handbag containing cash and checks, she can contact her depository institution to halt payment on all checks in the handbag. Currency payments are final, however, so the thief can spend all the cash he has taken from her. She can send checks through the mail, but using currency requires face-to-face contact. In addition, currency transactions are anonymous, which may be desirable under some circumstances. Nevertheless, not everyone will accept a check in payment for a transaction, and a check payment is not final until the check clears. Check transactions are also more expensive. After evaluating these features of currency and checks, people typically choose to hold both payment instruments.

People will likewise compare the features that digital cash offers with the features currently offered by government-provided currency and checking accounts available from depository institutions. As Table 16-1 indicates, the acceptability of digital cash is uncertain at present. Nonetheless, we are contemplating an environment with wide acceptability, and in such an

TABLE 16-1
Features of Alternative Forms of Money
Digital cash tends to overshadow government-issued currency.

Feature	Checks	Currency	Digital Cash
Security	High	Low	High(?)
Per-Transfer Cost	High	Medium	Low
Payment Final, Face-to-face	No	Yes	Yes
Payment Final, Non-Face-to-Face	No	No	Yes
Anonymity	No	Yes	Yes
Acceptability	Restricted	Wide	Uncertain at present

Source: Aleksander Berentsen, "Monetary Policy Implications of Digital Money," *Kyklos,* 51 (1998), p. 92.

environment, digital cash would be nearly as acceptable as government-provided currency. Digital cash held on smart cards without special security features such as personal identification numbers will be as susceptible to theft as government currency. Some digital cash, however, may be held on devices, such as laptop computers or even wristwatches (Swiss watch manufacturers have already developed watches with microchips for storing digital cash), requiring an access code before a microchip containing digital cash can be accessed. Overall, therefore, digital cash is likely to be somewhat more secure than government-provided currency, though not as secure as check transactions.

Digital cash transactions are likely to be less costly to undertake, because people will not have to go to depository institution branches or automated teller machines to obtain digital cash (although they will be able to do this if they wish). They will also be able to access digital cash at home on their personal computers. In addition, they will be able to send digital cash from remote locations using the Internet, and digital cash transactions will be instantaneously final. Unlike transactions using currency, therefore, digital cash transactions need not be conducted face to face. Like currency transactions, however, most digital cash transfers will be anonymous.

In most respects, therefore, digital cash looks like a better means of payment than government-provided currency. Certainly, for some time to come, a number of items—canned beverages and candy in vending machines, for example—will be easiest to purchase using government-provided currency. Many economists, however, believe that widespread adoption of privately issued digital cash will ultimately tend to crowd out government-provided currency. On many college campuses, vending machines already accept stored-value cards. Eventually, vending machines on street corners are likely to have smart card readers.

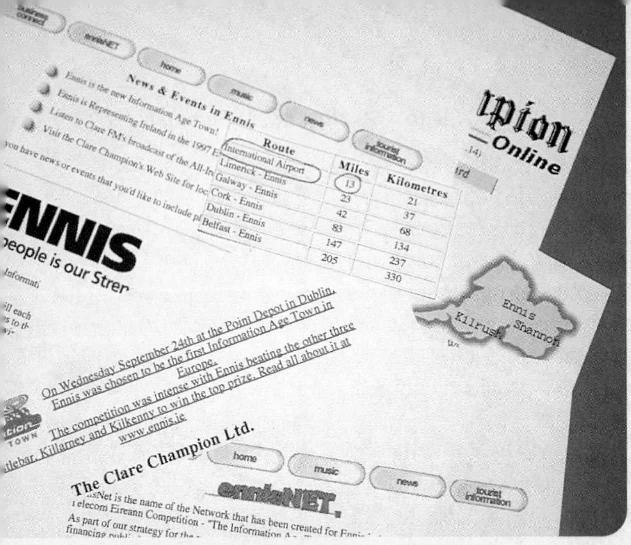

ISSUES & APPLICATIONS

Investing in Digital Cash Systems

Security and standardization are not the only issues that payment intermediaries such as banks must confront when trying to develop e-money systems. Companies invested millions of dollars in Ennis, Ireland, to make cyberpayments a reality for a few thousand households. How much would it cost for the United States to permit widespread use of digital cash?

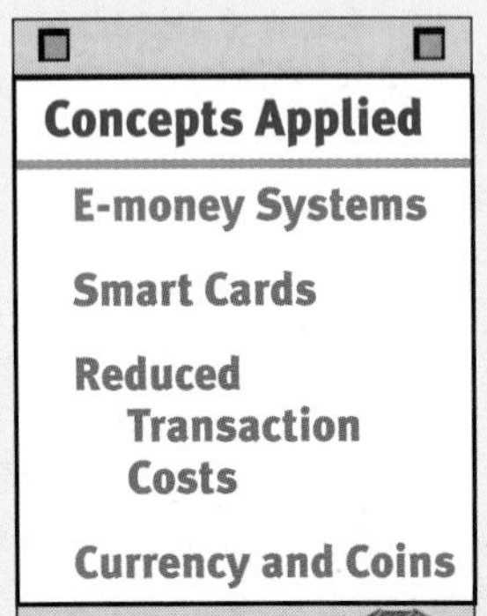
Concepts Applied

- E-money Systems
- Smart Cards
- Reduced Transaction Costs
- Currency and Coins

The High Cost of Setting Up Digital Cash Systems

The initial setup costs of e-money systems will likely be very high. Banks will have to provide smart cards to their customers at an estimated cost of $2 to $10 apiece. If 100 million U.S. residents use smart cards, this implies a total investment of between $200 million and $1 billion. Some banks have already begun to work to reduce the initial costs of distributing smart cards by turning credit cards into smart cards. Beginning in 1998, for instance, First USA began issuing credit cards with both stripes and microchips with limited e-money capabilities. Other banks and American Express since have followed the same strategy.

In addition, banks will have to replace the nation's 150,000 automated teller machines with new ATMs that can communicate with smart cards. Depending on the level of sophistication, the purchase price of a typical ATM ranges from $7,000 to $50,000. Thus the aggregate investment that banks will have to undertake solely to make their ATMs part of a digital cash network is somewhere between $1 billion and $7.5 billion.

Although large retailers have sophisticated electronic cash registers, most do not. Current estimates are that to function in a fully digital cash environment, retailers will have to purchase a total of 25 to 35 million new cash registers. The prices of these machines range from $500 to $2,000 apiece. This implies a likely total investment expense for retailers of between $10 billion and $15 billion.

Balancing Costs Against Benefits

Banks and retailers will be willing to undertake capital investments totaling somewhere between $12 billion and $23 billion if e-money systems for digital cash exchange generate cost savings at least as large. As noted at the beginning of the chapter, the U.S. Treasury has estimated that the total cost of handling paper currency and coins amounts to about $60 billion per year. Thus if the use of digital cash becomes sufficiently widespread to reduce this cost by only 10 percent, the cost savings will be $6 billion per year, which will justify the aggregate investment by banks and retailers within a two- to six-year horizon.

The wide ranges in these rough estimates illustrate the degree of uncertainty surrounding the speed at which e-money trading will catch on in the United States. Nevertheless, nearly all economists agree that there is likely to be an incentive for people to shift at least a portion of their paper-based transactions to exchanges using digital cash.

FOR CRITICAL ANALYSIS

1. When must a bank make the decision to invest in electronic banking?
2. Why do U.S. citizens persist in using currency and coins so much?

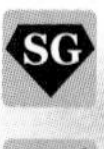

SUMMARY DISCUSSION OF LEARNING OBJECTIVES

1. **The Distinction Between Stored-Value Cards, Debit Cards, and Smart Cards:** Consumers can use stored-value cards to maintain balances of electronic money that they can use to purchase specific goods or service. Stored-value cards are most often used in closed systems operated by a single business or institution, but in an open, on-line system, they can function as debit cards. Debit cards permit individuals to authorize direct transfers of funds from their bank accounts to retailers, effectively transforming paper-based checking accounts into electronic checking deposits. Smart cards contain computer microchips that permit them to communicate directly with other computers to process software containing programs that store and transmit digital cash. In contrast to stored-value cards, transferring funds with smart cards can be done anonymously.
2. **Digital Certification and the Acceptability of Digital Cash:** Widespread use of digital cash via smart cards and other cybertechnologies will arise only if people have confidence that digital cash payments will be widely accepted by others. For this reason, banks and other payment intermediaries are working to establish digital certification authorities. These groups will develop standards for digital certification, or official recognition that digital cash payments are genuine. This will permit people to transmit digital cash between different payment systems and across national boundaries.
3. **The Security of Digital Cash:** Counterfeiting and theft are potential problems with digital cash, just as they are with physical currency and coins. Special security problems of digital cash are the threat of infection by computer viruses and the potential for monetary breakdowns caused by power outages or hardware malfunctions.
4. **On-Line Banking and Its Regulation:** Banks first offered on-line banking services in conjunction with marketers of home financial software packages. Today, they seek to earn fee income from offering bill consolidation services, providing the capability to transfer funds among accounts via home computers, and processing loan applications. Some observers argue that unique security concerns and an increased potential for bank fraud justify special care in regulating virtual banks that specialize in on-line banking. A few recent cases of on-line banking fraud have heightened the concerns of regulators.
5. **Digital Cash and the Money Supply:** If the use of digital cash becomes sufficiently widespread that digital cash is included in M1 and other money measures, the immediate effect is likely to be a rise in the money multiplier and an increase in the quantity of money in circulation. Over the longer term, if digital cash begins to displace government-provided currency, there may be an offsetting effect as the amount of government-provided currency in circulation declines. If nonbanking institutions find ways to get around current prohibitions on their ability to issue on-line transactions deposits not subject to reserve requirements, the money multiplier could rise dramatically in the future.

Key Terms and Concepts

Certificate authority (389)
Debit card (385)
Digital cash (384)
Smart card (386)
Stored-value card (385)

Problems

Answers to the odd-numbered problems appear at the back of the book.

16-1. A bank is contemplating issuing smart cards to its 10,000 household customers this year. Producing and distributing the smart cards will cost $2.50 per card. The bank has estimated that the cards will bring in $50 in additional revenues per customer during the year. It will have to pay five people to supervise an existing system for processing transfers and payments generated by the cards, and the average salary of each employee is

$75,000. If there are no other costs or benefits for the bank, and if it only cares about being sure that it will at least break even on smart cards during the current year, should it issue the cards?

16-2. After the bank discussed in Problem 16-1 has made a tentative decision, the head of its legal department convinces the bank's overall management team that it should install devices that provide both audio and video assistance for disabled customers who use smart cards. The cost of installing these devices is $80,000. Should the bank change its original decision?

16-3. As discussed in Chapter 5, an *externality* is a consequence of production or consumption activities in a market that spills over to affect third parties. Some economists argue that payment systems are subject to positive externalities called *network externalities.* Essentially, their argument is that a person who is not currently using a means of payment is more likely to switch to using it if others already use it. Could the existence of network externalities help explain why the average American does not yet carry a smart card?

16-4. In Chapter 15, you learned that there are also some potential *negative* externalities that can arise in payment systems. Based on this chapter's overview of smart cards and on-line banking, can you think of any potential negative externalities associated with digital cash and on-line banking?

16-5. Suppose that FinCEN discovers that individuals and companies seeking to avoid paying taxes on legitimately earned income laundered $100 million in funds using on-line transfers of digital cash during the latest year. FinCEN determines that it can capture one-half of all launderers and force them to pay taxes and penalties. The average rate of taxes and penalties that the government assesses against apprehended money launderers is 50 percent of the laundered funds. Suppose that FinCEN's records indicate that the agency spends $20 million each year investigating these laundering activities and bringing the perpetrators to justice. Ignoring all other factors except recovered taxes and penalties and enforcement costs (that is, abstracting from the issue of whether FinCEN should try to stop all money laundering because it is morally wrong), were FinCEN's activities justified during this year?

16-6. Some bankers have become concerned that their biggest competition for customers of on-line financial services might come from software companies and Internet service providers. What competitive advantages might the latter firms have over banks in providing on-line financial services? What advantages might banks have in providing such services?

16-7. In terms of the effects on the money multiplier and the money supply, if all transactions deposits are issued by banks that must meet legal reserve requirements, does it matter if their customers make payments from transactions account deposits using paper checks, debit cards, or on-line transfers directly from their checking accounts via the Internet?

16-8. Does your answer to Problem 16-7 change if nonbanking institutions not subject to reserve requirements also offer transfers from transactions deposits using paper checks, debit cards, or on-line transactions?

16-9. Suppose that the Federal Reserve is authorized by Congress to subject any firm that issues transactions-deposit-type liabilities over the Internet to reserve requirements. At the same time, Congress decides to follow the free banking laws of the nineteenth century by allowing any firm to offer such accounts, as long as it submits to the Fed's reserve requirements and meets other minimal standards to operate as a bank. The Fed immediately imposes the same required reserve ratio on firms that enter the on-line banking business that it imposes on traditional banks. What is the implication for the money multiplier?

16-10. Imagine a future world in which both banks and other nonbanking firms find a way to offer transactions deposits on-line while evading all reserve requirements. In this world, nearly all funds are digital cash in bank computer files and on consumers' personal computing equipment and smart cards. What is the potential money multiplier in such a world? What factors are likely to constrain the money multiplier to a lower value?

Economics on the Net

Digital Cash Versus E-Checks In this chapter, we focused on the potential for smart card technology to allow people to purchase goods and services over the Internet and other electronic delivery systems without the need to provide identification codes. The same technology, however, may permit people to write electronic checks that they could also use in this manner.

Title: What Is eCheck?

Navigation: Click here to go to the eCheck homepage. Select Overview, then click on *What Is eCheck?*

Application Read the explanation of eCheck, and then answer the following questions.

1. People are likely to use digital cash in place of government-issued currency and coins. Would people be more likely to use e-checks in place of traditional paper checks?
2. Based on the discussion in the article, who are likely to be the main providers of e-check technology? In light of the answer to this question, do e-checks pose the same fundamental questions for monetary policy that arise from the use of digital cash?

For Group Study and Analysis The article indicates that consumer acceptance of e-check technology could set the stage for more widespread consumer use of other electronic delivery systems. As a group, review the arguments in favor of this view. Identify some arguments that run counter to this perspective. Does the banking industry have a vested interest in e-checks' catching on?

CHAPTER

17

DOMESTIC AND INTERNATIONAL MONETARY POLICY

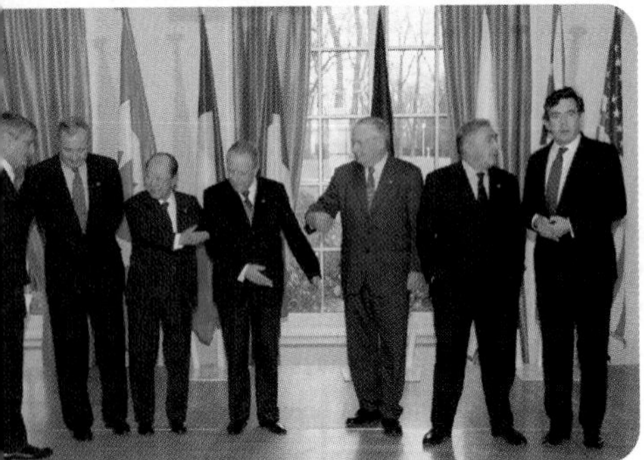

The so-called Group of Seven, or G-7, meets informally and attempts to coordinate monetary and fiscal policies among their governments. Do their decisions have the force of law in these countries?

Security is tight. The heads of the departments of treasury or finance of some of the most powerful economies throughout the world are meeting again. These are usually called the meetings of the Group of Seven (G-7) large industrials world economies. It used to be the G-5, sometimes it's the G-8 if Russia is included, and sometimes it's referred to as the G-10 if other nations are asked to send their ministers of finance. The goal is always the same—to coordinate macroeconomic policies and, more specifically, monetary policies. Can monetary policy be coordinated throughout the world? This is a complex question. Before you can attempt to understand it, though, you must learn about the ins and outs of monetary policy at home.

LEARNING OBJECTIVES

After reading this chapter, you should be able to:

1. Identify the key factors that influence the quantity of money that people desire to hold
2. Describe how the Federal Reserve's tools of monetary policy influence market interest rates
3. Evaluate how expansionary and contractionary monetary policy actions affect equilibrium real GDP and the price level in the short run
4. Understand the equation of exchange and its importance in the crude quantity theory of money and prices
5. Distinguish between the Keynesian and monetarist views on the transmission mechanism of monetary policy
6. Explain why the Federal Reserve cannot stabilize both the money supply and the interest rate simultaneously

Did You Know That... you can now purchase the securities of the United States government in amounts as low as $1,000? The program is called Treasury Direct. Through Treasury Direct, you can buy Treasury bills, which have maturities of 3, 6, or 12 months; Treasury notes, with maturities of 1 to 10 years; and Treasury bonds, with maturities of 10 years or more. All you have to do is open an account with Treasury Direct and then call (800)-943-6864 to buy government securities. Or alternatively, you can do it all via the Bureau of Public Debt's Web site at http://www.publicdebt.treas.gov/sec/sec.htm by clicking on "Treasury Direct." What all this means is that you don't need to be a superrich person who flies off to the Federal Reserve to buy U.S. Treasury securities. As you'll see in this chapter, when the Federal Reserve itself buys and sells U.S. Treasury securities (it usually deals in Treasury bills on a daily basis), it is engaging in monetary policy.

Monetary policy is the Fed's changing of the supply of money or the rate at which it grows in order to achieve national economic goals. When you were introduced to aggregate demand in Chapter 10, you discovered that the position of the aggregate demand curve is determined by the willingness of firms, individuals, governments, and foreigners to purchase domestically produced goods and services. Monetary policy works in a variety of ways to change this willingness, both directly and indirectly.

Think about monetary policy in an intuitive way: An increase in the money supply adds to the amount of money that firms and individuals have on hand and so increases the amount that they wish to spend. The result is an increase in aggregate demand. A decrease in the money supply reduces the amount of money that people have on hand to spend and so decreases aggregate demand.

Chapter Outline 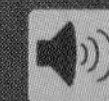

WHAT'S SO SPECIAL ABOUT MONEY?

By definition, monetary policy has to do, in the main, with money. But what is so special about money? Money is the product of a "social contract" in which we all agree to do two things:

1. Express all prices in terms of a common unit of account, which in the United States we call the dollar
2. Use a specific medium of exchange for market transactions

These two features of money distinguish it from all other goods in the economy. As a practical matter, money is involved on one side of every nonbarter transaction in the economy—and trillions of them occur every year. What this means is that something that changes the amount of money in circulation will have some effect on many transactions and thus on elements of GDP. If something affects the number of snowmobiles in existence, probably only the snowmobile market will be altered. But something that affects the amount of money in existence is going to affect *all* markets.

Holding Money

All of us engage in a flow of transactions. We buy and sell things all of our lives. But because we use money—dollars—as our medium of exchange, all *flows* of nonbarter transactions involve a *stock* of money. We can restate this as follows:

To use money, one must hold money.

Given that everybody must hold money, we can now talk about the *demand* to hold it. People do not demand to hold money just to look at pictures of past leaders. They hold it to be able to use it to buy goods and services.

The Demand for Money: What People Wish to Hold 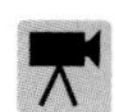

People have a certain motivation that causes them to want to hold money balances. Individuals and firms could try to have zero non-interest-bearing money balances. But life is inconvenient without a ready supply of money balances. There is a demand for money by the public, motivated by several factors.

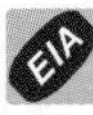

The Demand for Money
Get more exposure to the concept of the demand for money.

The Transactions Demand. The main reason why people hold money is that money can be used to purchase goods and services. People are paid at specific intervals (once a week, once a month, and so on), but they wish to make purchases more or less continuously. To free themselves from making expenditures on goods and services only on payday, people find it beneficial to hold money. The benefit they receive is convenience: They willingly forgo interest earnings in order to avoid the inconvenience and expense of cashing in such nonmoney assets as bonds every time they wish to make a purchase. Thus people hold money to make regular, *expected* expenditures under the **transactions demand.** As national income rises, people will want to hold more money because they will be making more transactions.

Transactions demand 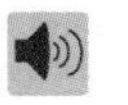
Holding money as a medium of exchange to make payments. The level varies directly with nominal national income.

The Precautionary Demand. The transactions demand involves money held to make *expected* expenditures. People also hold money for the **precautionary demand** to make *unexpected* purchases or to meet emergencies. When people hold money for the precautionary demand, they incur a cost in forgone interest earnings that they balance against the benefit that having cash on hand provides. The higher the rate of interest, the lower the money balances people wish to hold for the precautionary demand.

Precautionary demand 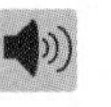
Holding money to meet unplanned expenditures and emergencies.

The Asset Demand. Remember that one of the functions of money is a store of value. People can hold money balances as a store of value, or they can hold bonds or stocks or other interest-earning assets. The desire to hold money as a store of value leads to the **asset demand** for money. People choose to hold money rather than other assets for two reasons: its liquidity and the lack of risk. Moreover, if deflation is expected, money balances can yield an extra return by rising in real value as prices fall.

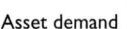

Asset demand 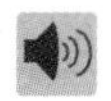
Holding money as a store of value instead of other assets such as certificates of deposit, corporate bonds, and stocks.

The disadvantage of holding money balances as an asset, of course, is the interest earnings forgone. Each individual or business decides how much money to hold as an asset by looking at the opportunity cost of holding money. The higher the interest rate—which is the opportunity cost of holding money—the lower the money balances people will want to hold as assets. Conversely, the lower the interest rate offered on alternative assets, the higher the money balances people will want to hold as assets.

The Demand for Money Curve

Assume that the amount of money demanded for transactions purposes is fixed, given a certain level of income. That leaves the precautionary and asset demands for money, both determined by the opportunity cost of holding money. If we assume that the interest rate represents the cost of holding money balances, we can graph the relationship between the interest rate and the quantity of money demanded. In Figure 17-1, the demand for money curve shows a familiar downward slope. The horizontal axis measures the quantity of

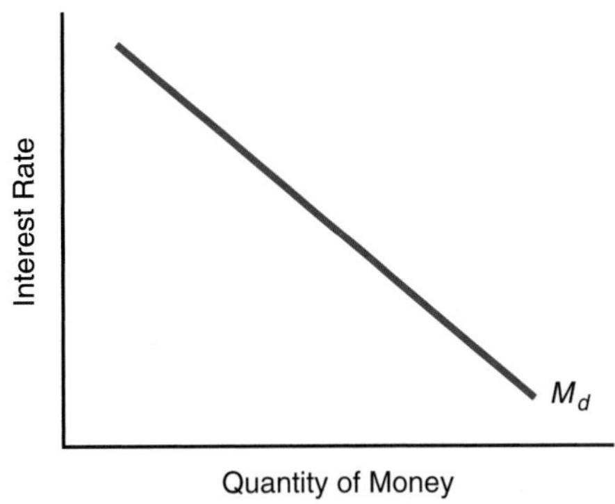

FIGURE 17-1

The Demand for Money Curve

If we use the interest rate as a proxy for the opportunity cost of holding money balances, the demand for money curve, M_d, is downward sloping, similar to other demand curves.

money demanded, and the vertical axis is the interest rate. In this sense, the interest rate is the price of holding money. At a higher price, a lower quantity of money is demanded, and vice versa.

Imagine two scenarios. In the first one, you can earn 20 percent a year if you put your cash into purchases of U.S. government securities. In the other scenario, you can earn 1 percent if you put your cash into purchases of U.S. government securities. If you have $1,000 average cash balances in a non-interest-bearing checking account, in the second scenario over a one-year period, your opportunity cost would be 1 percent of $1,000, or $10. In the first scenario, your opportunity cost would be 20 percent of $1,000, or $200. Under which scenario would you hold more cash instead of securities?

CONCEPTS IN BRIEF

- To use money, people must hold money. Therefore, they have a demand for money balances.
- The determinants of the demand for money balances are the transactions demand, the precautionary demand, and the asset demand.
- Because holding money carries with it an opportunity cost—the interest income forgone—the demand for money curve showing the relationship between money balances and the interest rate slopes downward.

THE TOOLS OF MONETARY POLICY

The Fed seeks to alter consumption, investment, and aggregate demand as a whole by altering the rate of growth of the money supply. The Fed has three tools at its disposal as part of its policymaking action: open market operations, discount rate changes, and reserve requirement changes.

Open Market Operations

The Fed changes the amount of reserves in the system by its purchases and sales of government bonds issued by the U.S. Treasury. To understand how the Fed does this, you must first start out in an equilibrium in which everybody, including the holders of bonds, is satisfied with the current situation. There is some equilibrium level of interest rate (and bond prices). Now if the Fed wants to conduct open market operations, it must somehow induce individuals, businesses, and foreigners to hold more or fewer U.S. Treasury bonds. The inducement must be in the form of making people better off. So if the Fed wants to buy bonds, it is going

Click here to learn about the Federal Reserve's current policy stance regarding openmarket operations. Select the "Minutes" for the most recent month.

FIGURE 17-2

Determining the Price of Bonds

In panel (a), the Fed offers more bonds for sale. The price drops from P_1 to P_2. In panel (b), the Fed purchases bonds. This is the equivalent of a reduction in the supply of bonds available for private investors to hold. The price of bonds must rise from P_1 to P_3 to clear the market.

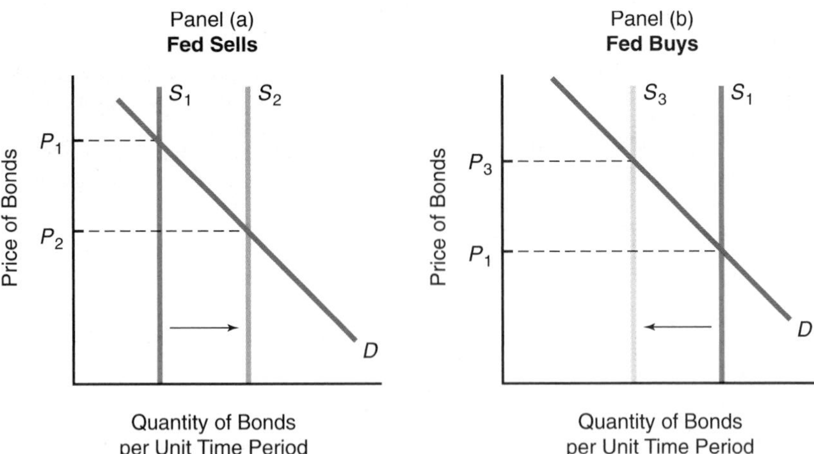

to have to offer to buy them at a higher price than exists in the marketplace. If the Fed wants to sell bonds, it is going to have to offer them at a lower price than exists in the marketplace. Thus an open market operation must cause a change in the price of bonds.

Graphing the Sale of Bonds. The Fed sells some of the bonds in its portfolio. This is shown in panel (a) of Figure 17-2. Notice that the supply of bonds is shown here as a vertical line with respect to price. The demand for bonds is downward-sloping. If the Fed offers more bonds for sale, it shifts the supply curve from S_1 to S_2. It cannot induce people to buy the extra bonds at the original price of P_1, so it must lower the price to P_2.

The Fed's Purchase of Bonds. The opposite occurs when the Fed purchases bonds. In panel (b) of Figure 17-2, the original supply curve is S_1. The new supply curve of outstanding bonds will end up being S_3 because of the Fed's purchases of bonds. You can view this purchase of bonds as a reduction in the stock of bonds available for private investors to hold. To get people to give up these bonds, the Fed must offer them a more attractive price. The price will rise from P_1 to P_3.

Relationship Between the Price of Existing Bonds and the Rate of Interest. There is an inverse relationship between the price of existing bonds and the rate of interest. Assume that the average yield on bonds is 5 percent. You decide to purchase a bond. A local corporation agrees to sell you a bond that will pay you $50 a year forever. What is the price you are willing to pay for the bond? It is $1,000. Why? Because $50 divided by $1,000 equals 5 percent, which is as good as the best return you can earn elsewhere. You purchase the bond. The next year something happens in the economy, and you can now obtain bonds that have effective yields of 10 percent. (In other words, the prevailing interest rate in the economy is now 10 percent.) What has happened to the market price of the existing bond that you own, the one you purchased the year before? It will have fallen. If you try to sell it for $1,000, you will discover that no investors will buy it from you. Why should they when they can obtain the same $50-a-year yield from someone else by paying only $500? Indeed, unless you offer your bond for sale at a price of $500, no buyers will be forthcoming. Hence an increase in the prevailing interest rate in the economy has caused the market value of your existing bond to fall.

The important point to be understood is this:

The market price of existing bonds (and all fixed-income assets) is inversely related to the rate of interest prevailing in the economy.

Changes in the Discount Rate

When the Fed was founded in 1913, the most important tool in its monetary policy kit was changes in the discount rate, discussed in Chapter 15. The Fed originally relied on the discount rate to carry out monetary policy because it had no power over reserve requirements. More important, its initial portfolio of government bonds was practically nonexistent and hence insufficient to conduct open market operations. As the Fed has come increasingly to rely on open market operations, it has used the discount rate less frequently as a tool of monetary policy—especially since the end of World War II.

Recall that the discount rate is the interest rate the Fed charges depository institutions when they borrow reserves directly from the Fed. An increase in the discount rate increases the cost of funds for depository institutions that seek loans from the Fed. That means that the price of one of their major lending inputs—the cost of money—has just gone up. Depository institutions pass at least part of this increased cost on to their borrowing customers by raising the interest rates they charge on loans.

Conversely, a reduction in the discount rate lowers depository institutions' cost of funds. It enables them to lower the rates they charge their customers for borrowing.

Changes in Reserve Requirements

Although the Fed rarely uses changes in reserve requirements as a form of monetary policy, most recently it did so in 1992, when it decreased reserve requirements on checkable deposits to 10 percent. In any event, here is how changes in reserve requirements affect the economy.

If the Fed increases reserve requirements, this makes it more expensive for banks to meet their reserve requirements. They must replenish their reserves by reducing their lending. They induce potential borrowers not to borrow so much by raising the interest rates they charge on the loans they offer.

Conversely, when the Fed decreases reserve requirements, as it did in 1992, some depository institutions attempt to lend their excess reserves out. To induce customers to borrow more, depository institutions cut interest rates.

CONCEPTS IN BRIEF

- Monetary policy consists of open market operations, discount rate changes, and reserve requirement changes undertaken by the Fed.
- When the Fed sells bonds, it must offer them at a lower price. When the Fed buys bonds, it must pay a higher price.
- There is an inverse relationship between the prevailing rate of interest in the economy and the market price of existing bonds.

EFFECTS OF AN INCREASE IN THE MONEY SUPPLY

To understand how monetary policy works in its simplest form, we are going to run an experiment in which you increase the money supply in a very direct way. Assume that the government has given you hundreds of millions of dollars in just-printed bills that you load into a helicopter. You then fly around the country, dropping the money out of the window. People pick it up and put it in their billfolds. Some deposit the money in their checking accounts. The first thing that happens is that they have too much money—not in the sense that they want to throw it away but rather in relation to other things that they own. There are a variety of ways to dispose of this "new" money.

Direct Effect

The simplest thing that people can do when they have excess money balances is to go out and spend it on goods and services. Here we have a direct impact on aggregate demand. Aggregate demand rises because with an increase in the money supply at any given price level, people now want to purchase more output of real goods and services.

Indirect Effect

Not everybody will necessarily spend the newfound money on real output. Some people may wish to deposit some or all of this excess cash in banks. The recipient banks now discover that they have higher reserves than they need to hold. As you learned in Chapter 15, one thing that banks can do to get interest-earning assets is to lend out the excess reserves. But banks cannot induce people to borrow more money than they were borrowing before unless the banks lower the interest rate that they charge on loans. This lower interest rate encourages people to take out those loans. Businesses will therefore engage in new investment with the money loaned. Individuals will engage in more consumption of such durable goods as housing, autos, and home entertainment centers. Either way, the increased loans have created a rise in aggregate demand. More people will be involved in more spending, even those who did not pick up any of the money that was originally dropped out of your helicopter.

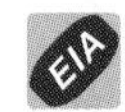

Monetary Policy
Get more experience thinking about how monetary policy affects the price level and real output in the short run and in the long run.

Graphing the Effects of an Expansionary Monetary Policy

Look at Figure 17-3. We start out in a situation in which the economy is operating at less than full employment. You see a recessionary gap in the figure, which is measured as the difference between *LRAS* and the current equilibrium. Short-run equilibrium is at E_1, with a price level of 120 and real GDP of $9.5 trillion. The long-run aggregate supply curve is

FIGURE 17-3
Expansionary Monetary Policy with Underutilized Resources
If we start out with equilibrium at E_1, expansionary monetary policy will shift AD_1 to AD_2. The new equilibrium will be at E_2.

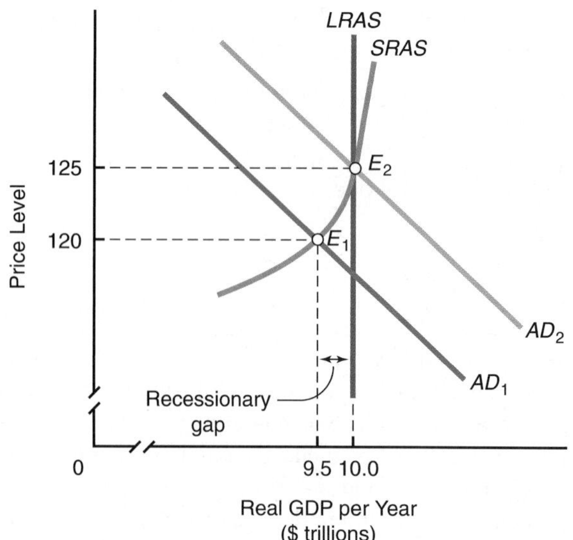

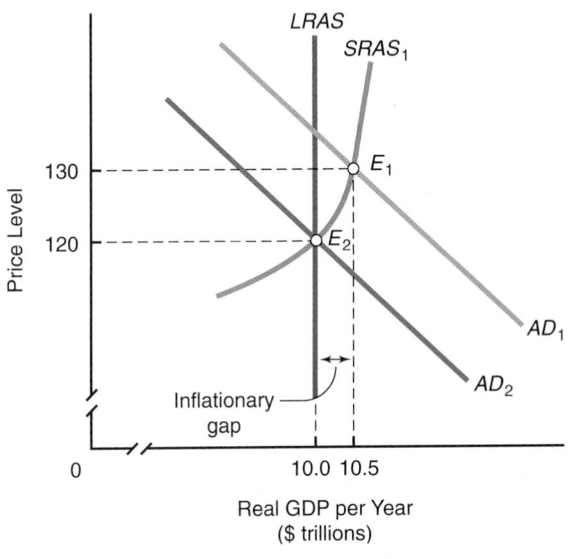

FIGURE 17-4
Contractionary Monetary Policy with Overutilized Resources
If we begin at an equilibrium at point E_1, contractionary monetary policy will shift the aggregate demand curve from AD_1 to AD_2. The new equilibrium will be at point E_2.

at \$10 trillion. Assume now that the money supply is increased by the Fed. Because of the direct and indirect effects of this increase in the money supply, aggregate demand shifts outward to the right to AD_2. The new equilibrium is at an output rate of \$10 trillion of real GDP per year and a price level of 125. Here expansionary monetary policy can move the economy toward its *LRAS* sooner than otherwise.

Graphing the Effects of Contractionary Monetary Policy

Assume that there is an inflationary gap as shown in Figure 17-4. There you see that the short-run average supply curve, $SRAS_1$, intersects aggregate demand, AD_1, at E_1. This is to the right of the *LRAS* of real GDP per year of \$10 trillion. Contractionary monetary policy can eliminate this inflationary gap. Because of both the direct and indirect effects of monetary policy, the aggregate demand curve shifts inward from AD_1 to AD_2. Equilibrium is now at E_2, which is at a lower price level, 120. Equilibrium real GDP has now fallen from \$10.5 trillion to \$10 trillion.

Note that contractionary monetary policy involves a reduction in the money supply, with a consequent decline in the price level (deflation). In the real world, contractionary monetary policy normally involves reducing the *rate of growth* of the money supply, thereby reducing the rate of increase in the price level (inflation). Similarly, real-world expansionary monetary policy typically involves increasing the rate of growth of the money supply.

CONCEPTS IN BRIEF

- The direct effect of an increase in the money supply arises because people desire to spend more on real goods and services when they have excess money balances.
- The indirect effect of an increase in the money supply works through a lowering of the interest rates, which encourages businesses to make new investments with the money loaned to them. Individuals will also engage in more consumption (on consumer durables) because of lower interest rates.

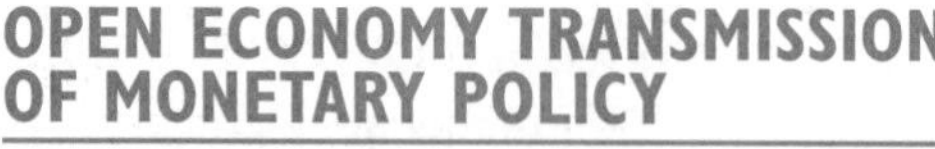

OPEN ECONOMY TRANSMISSION OF MONETARY POLICY

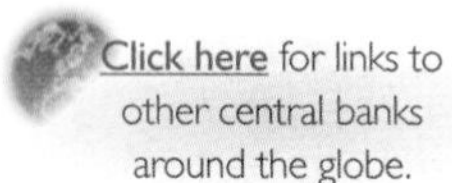

Click here for links to other central banks around the globe.

So far we have discussed monetary policy in a closed economy. When we move to an open economy, in which there is international trade and the international purchase and sale of all assets including dollars and other currencies, monetary policy becomes more complex. Consider first the effect on exports of any type of monetary policy.

The Net Export Effect

When we examined fiscal policy, we pointed out that deficit financing can lead to higher interest rates. Higher (real, after-tax) interest rates do something in the foreign sector—they attract foreign financial investment. More people want to purchase U.S. government securities, for example. But to purchase U.S. assets, people first have to obtain U.S. dollars. This means that the demand for dollars goes up in foreign exchange markets. The international price of the dollar therefore rises. This is called an *appreciation* of the dollar, and it tends to reduce net exports because it makes our exports more expensive in terms of foreign currency and imports cheaper in terms of dollars. Foreigners demand fewer of our goods and services, and we demand more of theirs. In this way, expansionary fiscal policy that creates deficit spending financed by U.S. government borrowing can lead to a reduction in net exports.

But what about expansionary monetary policy? If expansionary monetary policy reduces real, after-tax U.S. interest rates, there will be a positive net export effect because foreigners will want fewer U.S. financial instruments, demanding fewer dollars and thereby causing the international price of the dollar to fall. This makes our exports cheaper for the rest of the world, which then demands a larger quantity of our exports. It also means that foreign goods and services are more expensive in the United States, so we therefore demand fewer imports. We come up with two conclusions:

1. Expansionary fiscal policy may cause interest rates to rise and thereby attract international flows of financial capital. The resulting appreciation of the dollar causes net exports to decline, which reduces the effectiveness of fiscal policy to some extent.
2. Expansionary monetary policy may cause interest rates to fall. Such a fall will induce international outflows of financial capital, thereby lowering the value of the dollar and making American goods more attractive. The net export effect of expansionary monetary policy will be in the same direction as the monetary policy effect, thereby enhancing the effect of such policy.

Contractionary Monetary Policy

Now assume that the economy is experiencing inflation and the Federal Reserve wants to pursue a contractionary monetary policy. In so doing, it may cause interest rates to rise. Rising interest rates will cause financial capital to flow into the United States. The demand for dollars will increase, and their international price will go up. Foreign goods will now look cheaper to Americans, and imports will rise. Foreigners will not want our exports as much, and exports will fall. The result will be a reduction in our international trade balance, that is, a decline in net exports. Again, the international consequences reinforce the domestic consequences of monetary policy.

Globalization of International Money Markets

On a broader level, the Fed's ability to control the rate of growth of the money supply may be hampered as U.S. money markets become less isolated. With the push of a computer button, billions of dollars can change hands halfway around the world. In the world dollar market, the Fed finds an increasing number of dollars coming from *private* institutions. If the Fed reduces the growth of the money supply, individuals and firms in the United States can increasingly obtain dollars from other sources. People in the United States who want more liquidity can obtain their dollars from foreign residents. Indeed, it is possible that as world markets become increasingly integrated, U.S. residents may someday conduct transactions in *foreign* currencies.

CONCEPTS IN BRIEF

- Monetary policy in an open economy has repercussions for net exports.
- If expansionary monetary policy reduces U.S. interest rates, there is a positive net export effect because foreigners will demand fewer U.S. financial instruments, thereby demanding fewer dollars and hence causing the international price of the dollar to fall. This makes our exports cheaper for the rest of the world.
- When contractionary monetary policy causes interest rates to rise, foreign residents will want more U.S. financial instruments. The resulting increase in the demand for dollars will raise the dollar's value in foreign exchange markets, leading to a decline in net exports.

MONETARY POLICY AND INFLATION

Most theories of inflation relate to the short run. The price index in the short run can fluctuate because of events such as oil price shocks, labor union strikes, or discoveries of large amounts of new natural resources. In the long run, however, empirical studies show a relatively stable relationship between excessive growth in the money supply and inflation.

Simple supply and demand can explain why the price level rises when the money supply is increased. Suppose that a major oil discovery is made, and the supply of oil increases dramatically relative to the demand for oil. The relative price of oil will fall; now it will take more units of oil to exchange for specific quantities of non-oil products. Similarly, if the supply of money rises relative to the demand for money, it will take more units of money to purchase specific quantities of goods and services. That is merely another way of stating that the price level has increased or that the purchasing power of money has fallen. In fact, the classical economists referred to inflation as a situation in which more money is chasing the same quantity of goods and services.

The Equation of Exchange and the Quantity Theory 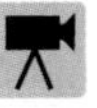

Equation of exchange 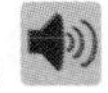
The formula indicating that the number of monetary units times the number of times each unit is spent on final goods and services is identical to the price level times output (or nominal national income).

A simple way to show the relationship between changes in the quantity of money in circulation and the price level is through the **equation of exchange,** developed by Irving Fisher:

$$M_sV \equiv PY$$

where

M_s = actual money balances held by the nonbanking public
V = **income velocity of money,** or the number of times, on average, each monetary unit is spent on final goods and services
P = price level or price index
Y = real national output (real GDP)

Income velocity of money 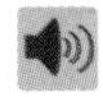
The number of times per year a dollar is spent on final goods and services; equal to GDP divided by the money supply.

Consider a numerical example involving a one-commodity economy. Assume that in this economy, the total money supply, M_s, is \$5 trillion; the quantity of output, Y, is \$10 trillion (in base-year dollars); and the price level, P, is 1.5 (150 in index number terms). Using the equation of exchange,

$$M_sV \equiv PY$$
$$\$5 \text{ trillion} \times V \equiv 1.5 \times \$10 \text{ trillion}$$
$$\$5 \text{ trillion} \times V \equiv \$15 \text{ trillion}$$
$$V \equiv 3$$

Thus each dollar is spent an average of three times a year.

The Equation of Exchange as an Identity. The equation of exchange must always be true—it is an *accounting identity.* The equation of exchange states that the total amount of money spent on final output, M_sV, is equal to the total amount of money *received* for final output, PY. Thus a given flow of money can be seen from either the buyers' side or the producers' side. The value of goods purchased is equal to the value of goods sold.

If Y represents real national output and P is the price level, PY equals the dollar value of national output, or *nominal* national income. Thus

$$M_sV \equiv PY \equiv \text{nominal national income}$$

The Crude Quantity Theory of Money and Prices. If we now make some assumptions about different variables in the equation of exchange, we come up with the simplified theory of why prices change, called the **crude quantity theory of money and prices.** If we assume that the velocity of money, V, is constant and that real national output, Y, is basically stable, the simple equation of exchange tells us that a change in the money supply can lead only to a proportionate change in the price level. Continue with our numerical example. Y is 50 units of the good. V equals 5. If the money supply increases to 200, the only thing that can happen is that the price index, P, has to go up from 10 to 20. Otherwise the equation is no longer in balance.

Crude quantity theory of money and prices 
The belief that changes in the money supply lead to proportional changes in the price level.

INTERNATIONAL EXAMPLE

Hyperinflation in Belarus: The "Bunny" Breeds Rapidly!

In Belarus, formerly part of the Soviet Union, the national currency is called the *zaichik*, or little hare. People in that country count their currency in "bunnies." The government there is fond of letting the bunnies breed rapidly, that is, printing more and more of them. Not long ago, the government announced that it would issue more bunnies to pay for the fall harvest. Not surprisingly, Belarus's domestic currency dropped in value. In one five-month period, it lost half of its purchasing power. In one week alone, it lost more than 10 percent. Foreign investors simply disappeared.

Officially, there is no inflation in Belarus. The government has instituted price controls while increasing the rate of growth of the money supply. The only country that Belarus has much trade with now is Russia, and most of that trade is through barter.

For Critical Analysis

How might price controls work in a situation in which the money supply is growing rapidly?

Empirical Verification. There is considerable evidence of the empirical validity of the relationship between monetary growth and high rates of inflation. Figure 17-5 tracks the

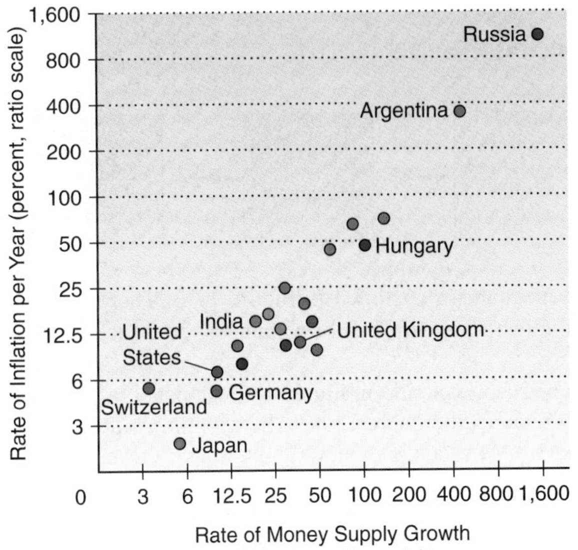

FIGURE 17-5

The Relationship Between Money Supply Growth Rates and Rates of Inflation

If we plot rates of inflation and rates of monetary growth for different countries, we come up with a scatter diagram that reveals an obvious direct relationship. If you were to draw a line through the "average" of the points in this figure, it would be upward-sloping, showing that an increase in the rate of growth of the money supply leads to an increase in the rate of inflation.

Source: International Monetary Fund. Data are for latest available periods.

correspondence between money supply growth and the rates of inflation in various countries around the world.

CONCEPTS IN BRIEF

- The equation of exchange states that the expenditures by some people will equal income receipts by others, or $M_sV \equiv PY$ (money supply times velocity equals nominal national income).
- Viewed as an accounting identity, the equation of exchange is always true, because the amount of money spent on final output must equal the total amount of money received for final output.
- The crude quantity theory of money and prices states that a change in the money supply will bring about an equiproportional change in the price level.

MONETARY POLICY IN ACTION: THE TRANSMISSION MECHANISM

At the start of this chapter, we talked about the direct and indirect effects of monetary policy. The direct effect is simply that an increase in the money supply causes people to have excess money balances. To get rid of these excess money balances, people increase their expenditures. The indirect effect occurs because some people have decided to purchase interest-bearing assets with their excess money balances. This causes the price of such assets—bonds—to go up. Because of the inverse relationship between the price of existing bonds and the interest rate, the interest rate in the economy falls. This lower interest rate induces people and businesses to spend more than they otherwise would have spent.

The Keynesian Transmission Mechanism

One school of economists believes that the indirect effect of monetary policy is the more important. This group, typically called Keynesian because of its belief in Keynes's work, asserts that the main effect of monetary policy occurs through changes in the interest rate.

FIGURE 17-6
The Keynesian Money Transmission Mechanism

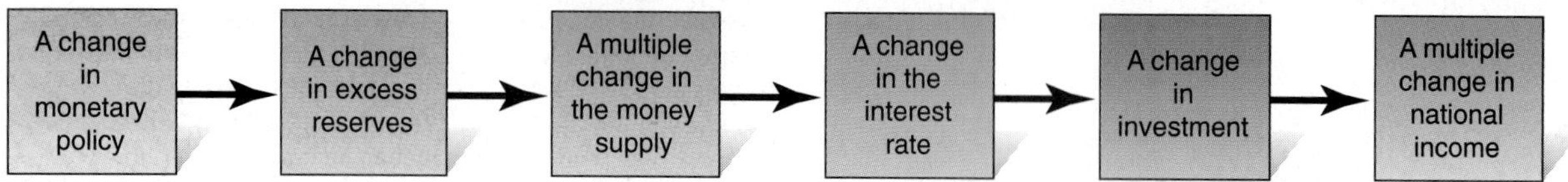

The Keynesian money transmission mechanism is shown in Figure 17-6. There you see that the money supply changes the interest rate, which in turn changes the desired rate of investment.

This transmission mechanism can be seen explicitly in Figure 17-7. In panel (a), you see that an increase in the money supply reduces the interest rate. The economywide demand curve for money is labeled M_d in panel (a). At first, the money supply is at M_s, a vertical line determined by our central bank, the Federal Reserve System. The equilibrium interest rate is r_1. This occurs where the money supply curve intersects the money demand curve. Now assume that the Fed increases the money supply, say, via open market operations. This will shift the money supply curve outward to the right to M_s'. People find themselves with too much cash (liquidity). They buy bonds. When they buy bonds, they bid up the prices of bonds, thereby lowering the interest rate. The interest rate falls to r_2, where the new money supply curve M_s' intersects the money demand curve M_d. This reduction in the interest rate

FIGURE 17-7
Adding Monetary Policy to the Keynesian Model
In panel (a), we show a demand for money function, M_d. It slopes downward to show that at lower rates of interest, a larger quantity of money will be demanded. The money supply is given initially as M_s, so the equilibrium rate of interest will be r_1. At this rate of interest, we see from the planned investment schedule given in panel (b) that the quantity of planned investment demanded per year will be I_1. After the shift in the money supply to M_s', the resulting increase in investment from I_1 to I_2 shifts the aggregate demand curve in panel (c) outward from AD_1 to AD_2. Equilibrium moves from E_1 to E_2, at \$10 trillion real GDP per year.

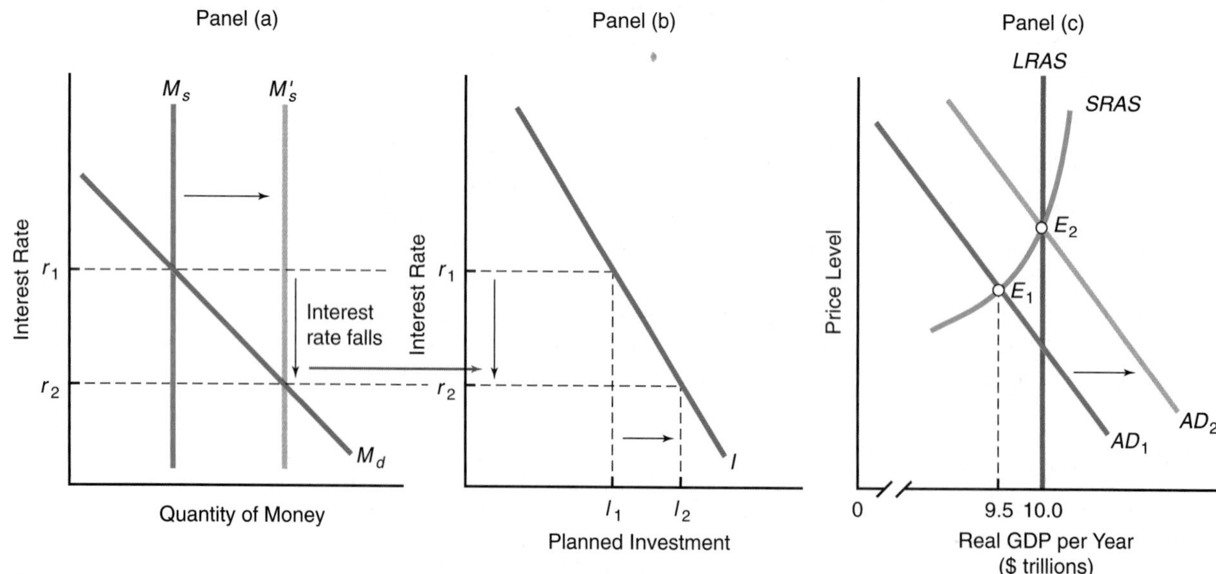

from r_1 to r_2 has an effect on planned investment, as can be seen in panel (b). Planned investment per year increases from I_1 to I_2. An increase in investment will increase aggregate demand, as shown in panel (c). Aggregate demand increases from AD_1 to AD_2. Equilibrium in the economy increases from real GDP per year of $9.5 trillion, which is not on the *LRAS,* to equilibrium real GDP per year of $10 trillion, which is on the *LRAS.*

The Monetarists' Transmission Mechanism

Monetarists, economists who believe in a modern quantity theory of money and prices, contend that monetary policy works its way more directly into the economy. They believe that changes in the money supply lead to changes in nominal GDP in the same direction. An increase in the money supply because of expansionary open market operations (purchases of bonds) by the Fed leads the public to have larger money holdings than desired. This excess quantity of money supplied induces the public to buy more of everything, especially more durable goods such as cars, stereos, and houses. If the economy is starting out at its long-run equilibrium rate of output, there can only be a short-run increase in real GDP. Ultimately, though, the public cannot buy more of everything; it simply bids up prices so that the price level rises.

Monetarists 

Macroeconomists who believe that inflation is always caused by excessive monetary growth and that changes in the money supply affect aggregate demand both directly and indirectly.

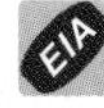

Monetary Policy and Interest Rates

Get additional practice thinking through the monetary policy transmission mechanism.

Monetarists' Criticism of Monetary Policy 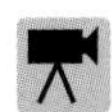

The monetarists' belief that monetary policy works through changes in desired spending does not mean that they consider such policy an appropriate government stabilization tool. According to the monetarists, although monetary policy can affect real GDP (and employment) in the short run, the length of time required before money supply changes take effect is so long and variable that such policy is difficult to conduct. For example, an expansionary monetary policy to counteract a recessionary gap may not take effect for a year and a half, by which time inflation may be a problem. At that point, the expansionary monetary policy will end up making the then current inflation worse. Monetarists therefore see discretionary monetary policy as a *destabilizing* force in the economy.

According to the monetarists, policymakers should consequently follow a **monetary rule:** Increase the money supply *smoothly* at a rate consistent with the economy's long-run potential growth rate. *Smoothly* is an important word here. Increasing the money supply at 20 percent per year half the time and decreasing it at 17 percent per year the other half of the time would average out to about a 3 percent increase, but the results would be disastrous, say the monetarists. Instead of permitting the Fed to use its discretion in setting monetary policy, monetarists would force it to follow a rule such as "Increase the money supply smoothly at 3.5 percent per year" or "Abolish the Fed and replace it with a computer program allowing for a steady rise in the money supply."

Monetary rule 

A monetary policy that incorporates a rule specifying the annual rate of growth of some monetary aggregate.

FED TARGET CHOICE: INTEREST RATES OR MONEY SUPPLY?

It is not possible to stabilize the money supply and interest rates simultaneously. The Federal Reserve has often sought to achieve an *interest rate target*. There is a fundamental tension between targeting interest rates and controlling the money supply, however. Interest rate targets force the Fed to abandon control over the money supply; money stock growth targets force the Fed to allow interest rates to fluctuate.

Figure 17-8 on page 416 shows the relationship between the total demand for money and the supply of money. Note that in the short run (in the sense that nominal national

FIGURE 17-8
Choosing a Monetary Policy Target
The Fed, in the short run, can select an interest rate or a money supply target but not both. It cannot, for example, choose r_e and M_S'; if it selects r_e, it must accept M_S; if it selects M_S', it must allow the interest rate to fall to r_1. The Fed can obtain point *A* or *B*. It cannot get to point *C* or *D*. It must therefore choose one target or the other.

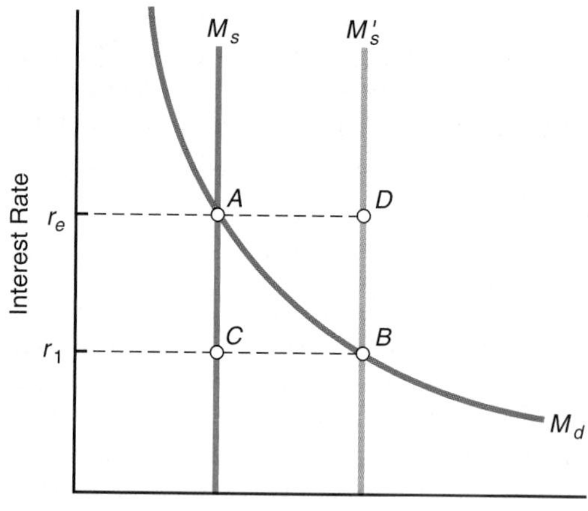

income is fixed), the demand for money is constant; short-run money supply changes leave the demand for money curve unaltered. In the short run, the Fed can choose either a particular interest rate (r_e or r_1) or a particular money supply (M_s or M_s').

If the Fed wants interest rate r_e, it must select money supply M_s; if it desires a lower interest rate in the short run, it must increase the money supply. Thus by targeting an interest rate, the Fed must relinquish control of the money supply. Conversely, if the Fed wants to target the money supply at, say, M_s', it must allow the interest rate to fall to r_1.

But which should the Fed target, interest rates or monetary aggregates? (And which interest rate or which money stock?) It is generally agreed that the answer depends on the source of instability in the economy. If the source of instability is variations in private or public spending, monetary aggregate (money supply) targets should be set and pursued, because with a fixed interest rate, spending variations cause maximum volatility of real national income. However, if the source of instability is an unstable demand for (or perhaps supply of) money, interest rate targets are preferred, because the Fed's effort to keep the interest rate stable automatically offsets the effect of the money demand (or supply) change.

Click here to find out about the Fed's latest monetary policy actions.

One perennial critic of the Federal Reserve, Milton Friedman, argues that no matter what, "the idea that a central bank can target interest rates is utterly false. Interest rates are partly a real magnitude, partly a nominal magnitude. The Federal Reserve cannot target real interest rates and has done great damage by trying to do so." Here Friedman is referring to the concept of the nominal rate of interest being comprised of the real interest rate plus the future expected inflation rate.

Consider the case in which the Fed wants to maintain the present level of interest rates. If actual market interest rates in the future rise persistently above the present (desired) rates, the Fed will be continuously forced to increase the money supply. The initial increase in the money supply will only temporarily lower interest rates. The increased money stock will eventually induce inflation, and inflationary premiums will be included in nominal interest rates. To pursue its low-interest-rate policy, the Fed must *again* increase the money stock because interest rates are still rising. Note that to attempt to maintain an interest rate target (stable interest rates), the Fed must abandon an independent money stock target.

CONCEPTS IN BRIEF

- In the Keynesian model, monetary transmission operates through a change in interest rates, which changes investment, causing a multiple change in the equilibrium level of national income.
- Monetarists believe that changes in the money supply lead to changes in nominal GDP in the same direction. The effect is both direct and indirect, however, as individuals spend their excess money balances on cars, stereos, houses, and other items.
- Monetarists argue in favor of a monetary rule—increasing the money supply smoothly at a rate consistent with the economy's long-run potential growth rate. Monetarists do not believe in discretionary monetary (or fiscal) policy.
- The Fed can choose to stabilize interest rates or to change the money supply but not both.

THE WAY FED POLICY IS CURRENTLY ANNOUNCED

No matter what the Fed is actually targeting, it only announces an interest rate target. You should not be fooled, however. When the chair of the Fed states that the Fed is lowering "the" interest rate from, say, 5.75 percent to 5.25 percent, he really means something else. In the first place, the interest rate referred to is the federal funds rate, or the rate at which banks can borrow excess reserves from other banks. In the second place, even if the Fed talks about changing interest rates, it can do so only by actively entering the market for federal government securities (usually Treasury bills). So if the Fed wants to lower "the" interest rate, it essentially must engage in expansionary open market operations. That is to say, it must buy more Treasury securities than it sells, thereby increasing the money supply. This tends to lower the rate of interest. Conversely, when the Fed wants to increase "the" rate of interest, it engages in contractionary open market operations, thereby decreasing the money supply (or the rate of growth of the money supply).

What is the correct interest rate policy for the Fed to pursue? This is a question being answered by some young people across the country today.

POLICY EXAMPLE

Predict Monetary Policy Correctly and Win a $10,000 Scholarship

Every year since 1995, there has been a "Fed Challenge." This is a contest sponsored by the Federal Reserve Board and Citibank (now a division of Citigroup). More than 200 high schools throughout the country participate. Each school has a five-member team. Each team recommends whether the Fed ought to raise interest rates, keep them the same, or reduce them.

The vice-chair of the Federal Reserve Board and two colleagues judge the national finals at the beginning of May each year. The finalists give presentations of their models reflecting what they think should happen at meetings of the Federal Reserve's Open Market Committee. The winning team members each get a $10,000 scholarship, and their school receives a $50,000 grant to establish an "economics laboratory."

For Critical Analysis

What criteria do you think the judges should use to determine which team has presented the best monetary policy recommendations?

NETNOMICS

Will Digital Cash Weaken Monetary Policy?

In Chapter 16 you learned about digital cash, or e-money. In this chapter, you learned that monetary policy usually works through a process that involves changes in the money supply, which then affect interest rates and nationwide economic activity.

Whether money takes the form of coins, paper, or deposits makes little difference to officials who are charged with conducting monetary policy, as long as it does not interfere with their ability to control the total *quantity* of money in circulation. It is this issue that makes policymakers nervous about digital cash.

If the Federal Reserve and other central banks desire to control, or at least influence, the quantity of money in circulation, it is helpful for them to have direct or indirect oversight over the process by which money is placed into circulation.

It is conceivable that traditional banking institutions, such as commercial banks, savings institutions, and credit unions, may not be the only ones that choose to issue digital cash. To a central bank such as the Federal Reserve, this is the *fundamental* monetary policy issue posed by the development of e-money. Like banks and their customers, the Federal Reserve does not particularly care what form money takes. Nevertheless, it does have some reason to be concerned about who has the power to issue money.

In principle, anyone can issue digital cash accounts. Even if the government were to decide that only traditional banking institutions that fall under the Federal Reserve's regulatory umbrella can issue smart cards, what is to stop other firms from setting up e-money accounts over the Internet? That is, what is to stop firms that technically are not banks from issuing Internet-based digital checking accounts that effectively function as money? Presumably, one answer is that Congress could pass laws prohibiting such accounts, and the Federal Reserve and other bank regulators would have to police the Internet to ensure that only traditional banks issue such accounts.

Another possible answer, however, is that ultimately nothing may be able to stop a host of firms from pecking away at legal loopholes and eventually finding a way to enter the banking business by issuing e-money accounts. Balances stored in these digital cash accounts would be as much a part of the nation's quantity of circulating money as government currency and checkable deposits at traditional banks. As a result, the Fed's central-banking task of measuring and regulating this quantity would become much more complicated.

This is one way in which the new electronic banking systems have the potential to alter profoundly monetary affairs in the United States and worldwide. This potential development, more than any other, may be the *truly* fundamental change brought about by the use of digital cash.

ISSUES & APPLICATIONS

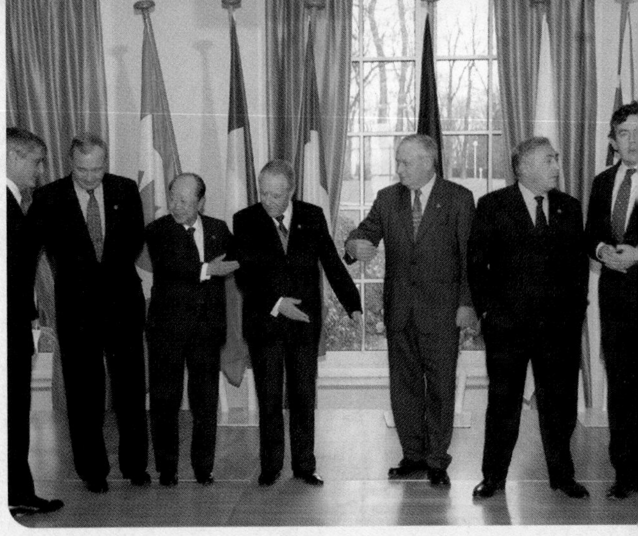

Can Monetary Policy Be Coordinated Worldwide?

For years now, high-level officials, usually from the departments of treasury or finance or the central banks of major industrialized nations, have been meeting on an irregular basis. Every time they do so, the world waits with bated breath to see what has been decided on a global level. Will the G-7 (representatives from the Group of Seven industrialized nations) decide to lower interest rates? Will they decide to increase interest rates? Will they decide to prop up the dollar or some other currency? Will they decide to stop the dollar from increasing in foreign exchange value?

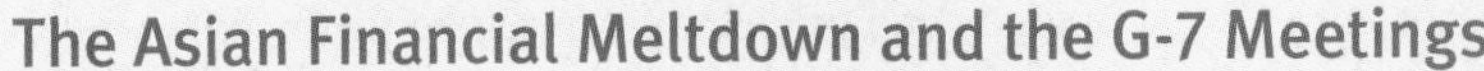

The Asian Financial Meltdown and the G-7 Meetings

A few years ago, many Asian nations experienced a sort of financial meltdown. These economies saw their stock markets drop precipitously, along with the value of their domestic currencies in foreign currency markets. This was referred to at the time as the Asian disease or the Asian contagion, out of fear that other nations, including the United States, would catch it.

While it was happening, then U.S. President Clinton called for a global meeting to deal with the crisis. This caused a major rally in the U.S. stock market. Some analysts argue that this reaction was entirely rational. It is a variant on what military historians call the "mask of command": If one can give the impression that everything is under control, it may be possible to restore confidence and prevent panic from spreading.

Concepts Applied

- Monetary Policy
- Coordination
- Contractionary Policies
- Expansionary Policies
- interest Rate Changes

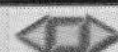

A Dose of Reality

The Asian contagion was contained—but not by the G-7. The reality is that every country acts in its own best interest, not the world's. So no matter how often top officials from the G-7 meet, they are all beholden to their own constituents. Thus ideas that sound promising at a G-7 meeting may fall on deaf ears back home.

Furthermore, the Fed is not the world's central bank. Important as it is as an engine of economic policymaking, its impact beyond U.S. borders should not be overstated. The Fed can change the rate of growth of the money supply in the United States. But it cannot change the rate of growth of the money supply in Japan or Europe, and if Japan or Europe is having economic problems, a slight change in monetary policy in the United States is not going to make much difference anyway.

Even in a country that does business in dollars and whose currency is pegged to the dollar, the Fed's actions have little impact. If investors in Argentina, for example, believe, for whatever reason, that their loans will not be paid back in that country, they will simply move their capital somewhere else.

So What About a Global Central Bank?

Some observers have argued that to regulate the world's economies, or at least the world's currencies and rates of inflation, a global central bank should be created. Realistically, this would require a single global currency. The countries in Europe that are switching to a single currency, the euro, and a single central bank, the European Central Bank, took decades to do so. For the rest of the world to follow suit on a global scale is highly—nay, completely—improbable.

FOR CRITICAL ANALYSIS

1. If meetings of the G-7 cannot make much of a difference, why does the press pay so much attention to them?
2. Why shouldn't the world just adopt the U.S. dollar as its only currency and let the Fed run monetary policy?

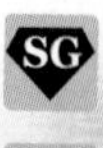

SUMMARY DISCUSSION OF LEARNING OBJECTIVES

1. **Key Factors that Influence the Quantity of Money That People Desire to Hold**: People generally make more transactions when real national income rises, and they require more money to make these transactions. Consequently, they desire to hold more money when real national income increases. People also hold money as a precaution against unexpected expenditures they may wish to make, and the interest rate is the opportunity cost of holding money for this purpose. In addition, money is a store of value that people may hold alongside bonds, stocks, and other interest-earning assets, and the opportunity cost of holding money as an asset is again the interest rate. Thus the quantity of money demanded declines as the market interest rate increases.
2. **How the Federal Reserve's Monetary Policy Tools Influence Market Interest Rates:** An open market purchase of government securities, a reduction in the discount rate, or a decrease in the required reserve ratio are all ways that the Federal Reserve can bring about an increase in total reserves in the banking system and an increase in the money supply. The rise in reserve levels that banks have available to lend leads them to bid down interest rates on loans. Thus market interest rates tend to fall in response to any of these changes in the Fed's tools of monetary policy.
3. **How Expansionary and Contractionary Monetary Policies Affect Equilibrium Real GDP and the Price Level in the Short Run:** By pushing up the money supply and inducing a fall in market interest rates, an expansionary monetary policy action causes total planned expenditures to rise at any given price level. Hence the aggregate demand curve shifts rightward, which can eliminate a short-run recessionary gap in real GDP. In contrast, a contractionary monetary policy action reduces the money supply and causes an increase in market interest rates, thereby generating a fall in total planned expenditures at any given price level. This results in a leftward shift in the aggregate demand curve, which can eliminate a short-run inflationary gap in real GDP.
4. **The Equation of Exchange and the Crude Quantity Theory of Money and Prices:** The equation of exchange is a truism that states that the quantity of money in circulation times the average number of times a unit of money is used in exchange—the income velocity of money—must equal nominal national income, or the price level times real national output. According to the crude quantity theory of money and prices, we can regard the income velocity of money as constant and real GDP as relatively stable. Thus a rise in the quantity of money must lead to a proportionate increase in the price level.
5. **Keynesian and Monetarist Views on the Transmission Mechanism of Monetary Policy:** The Keynesian approach to the monetary policy transmission mechanism operates through effects of monetary policy actions on market interest rates, which bring about changes in desired investment and thereby affect equilibrium real national income via the Keynesian multiplier effect. By contrast, monetarists propose a transmission mechanism in which money supply changes influence total desired expenditures on goods and services.
6. **Why the Federal Reserve Cannot Stabilize the Money Supply and the Interest Rate Simultaneously:** To target a market interest rate, the Federal Reserve must be willing to adjust the money supply as necessary when there are variations in the demand for money. Hence stabilizing the interest rate typically requires variations in the money supply. To target the money supply, however, the Federal Reserve must be willing to let the market interest rate vary whenever the demand for money rises or falls. Consequently, stabilizing the money supply usually entails some degree of interest rate volatility.

Key Terms and Concepts

Asset demand (404)
Crude quantity theory of money and prices (412)
Equation of exchange (411)
Income velocity of money (411)
Monetarists (415)
Monetary rule (415)
Precautionary demand (404)
Transactions demand (404)

Problems

Answers to the odd-numbered problems appear at the back of the book.

17-1. Let's denote the price of a nonmaturing bond (called a consol) as P_b. The equation that indicates this price is = I/r, where I is the annual net income the bond generates and r is the market nominal interest rate.

a. Suppose that a bond promises the holder $500 per year forever. If the market nominal interest rate is 5 percent, what is the bond's current price?

b. What happens to the bond's price if the market interest rate rises to 10 percent?

17-2. Based on Problem 17-1, imagine that initially the market interest rate is 5 percent and at this interest rate you have decided to hold half of your financial wealth as bonds and half as holdings of non-interest-bearing money. You notice that the market interest rate is starting to rise, however, and you become convinced that it will ultimately rise to 10 percent.

a. In what direction do you expect the value of your bond holdings to go when the interest rate increases?

b. If you wish to prevent the value of your financial wealth from declining in the future, how should you adjust the way you split your wealth between bonds and money? What does this imply about the demand for money?

17-3. You learned in Chapter 11 that if there is an inflationary gap in the short run, then in the long run a new equilibrium arises when input prices and expectations adjust upward, causing the aggregate supply curve to shift upward and to the left and pushing equilibrium real GDP back to its long-run potential value. In this chapter, however, you learned that the Federal Reserve can eliminate an inflationary gap in the short run by undertaking a policy action that reduces aggregate demand.

a. Outline one monetary policy action that could eliminate an inflationary gap in the short run.

b. In what way might society gain if the Fed implements the policy you have proposed instead of simply permitting long-run adjustments to take place?

17-4. In addition, you learned in Chapter 11 that if there is a recessionary gap in the short run, then in the long run a new equilibrium arises when input prices and expectations adjust downward, causing the aggregate supply curve to shift downward and to the right and pushing equilibrium real GDP back to its long-run potential value. In this chapter, however, you learned that the Federal Reserve can eliminate a recessionary gap in the short run by undertaking a policy action that raises aggregate demand.

a. Outline a monetary policy action that could eliminate a contractionary gap in the short run but uses a different tool of monetary policy than the one you considered in Problem 17-3.

b. In what way might society gain if the Fed implements the policy you have proposed instead of simply permitting long-run adjustments to take place?

17-5. Explain why the net export effect of a contractionary monetary policy reinforces the usual impact that monetary policy has on equilibrium real GDP in the short run.

17-6. Use a chart to illustrate how the Fed can reduce inflationary pressures by conducting open market sales of U.S. government securities.

17-7. Suppose that the quantity of money in circulation is fixed but the income velocity of money doubles. If real GDP remains at its long-run potential level, what happens to the equilibrium price level?

17-8. Suppose that following the events described in Problem 17-7, the Federal Reserve implements policies that cut the money supply in half. How does the price level now compare with its value before the income velocity of money and the money supply both changed?

17-9. Consider the following data: The money supply is equal to $1 trillion, the price level equals 2, and real output of goods and services is $5 quadrillion in base-year dollars. What is the income velocity of money for this economy?

17-10. Suppose that the Federal Reserve wishes to keep the nominal interest rate at a target level of

6 percent. Draw a money supply and demand diagram in which the current equilibrium interest rate is 6 percent. Explain a specific policy action that the Fed, using one of its three tools of monetary policy, could take to keep the interest rate at its target level if the demand for money suddenly declines.

Economics on the Net

The Fed's Policy Report to Congress Congress requires the Fed to make periodic reports on the scope of its recent policymaking activities. In this application, you will study recent reports to learn about what factors affect Fed decisions.

Title: Monetary Policy Report to the Congress

Navigation: Click here to start at the homepage of the Federal Reserve's Monetary Policy Report to the Congress (formerly called the Humphrey-Hawkins Report). Then click on Report for the most recent date. Finally, click on Monetary Policy and the Economic Outlook.

Application: Read the report; then answer the following questions:

1. According to the report, what economic events played the most important role in shaping recent monetary policy actions?
2. Based on the report, what are the Fed's current monetary policy goals?

For Group Study and Analysis Divide the class into "domestic" and "foreign" groups. Have each group read the past four Humphrey-Hawkins reports and then explain to the class how domestic and foreign factors, respectively, appear to have influenced recent Fed monetary policy decisions. Which of the two types of factors seem to have mattered most during the past year?

MONETARY POLICY: A KEYNESIAN PERSEPCTIVE

According to the traditional Keynesian approach to monetary policy, changes in the money supply can affect the level of aggregate demand only through their effect on interest rates. Moreover, interest rate changes act on aggregate demand solely by changing the level of investment spending. Finally, the traditional Keynesian approach argues that there exist plausible circumstances under which monetary policy may have little or no effect on interest rates and thus on aggregate demand.

Figure D-1 measures real national income along the horizontal axis and total planned expenditures (aggregate demand) along the vertical axis. The components of aggregate demand are consumption (C), investment (I), government spending (G), and net exports (X). The height of the schedule labeled $C + I + G + X$ shows total planned expenditures (aggregate demand) as a function of income. This schedule slopes upward because consumption depends positively on income. Everywhere along the line labeled $Y = C + I + G + X$, planned spending equals income. At point Y^*, where the $C + I + G + X$ line intersects this 45-degree reference line, planned spending is consistent with income. At any income less than Y^*, spending exceeds income, so income and thus spending will tend to rise. At any level of income greater than Y^*, planned spending is less than income, so income and thus spending will tend to decline. Given the determinants of C, I, G, and X, total spending (aggregate demand) will be Y^*.

INCREASING THE MONEY SUPPLY

According to the Keynesian approach, an increase in the money supply pushes interest rates down. This reduces the cost of borrowing and thus induces firms to increase the level of investment spending from I to I'. As a result, the $C + I + G + X$ line shifts upward in Figure D-1 by the full amount of the rise in investment spending, thus yielding the line $C + I' + G + X$. The rise in investment spending causes income to rise, which in turn causes consumption spending to rise, which further increases income. Ultimately, aggregate demand rises to Y^{**}, where spending again equals income. A key conclusion of the

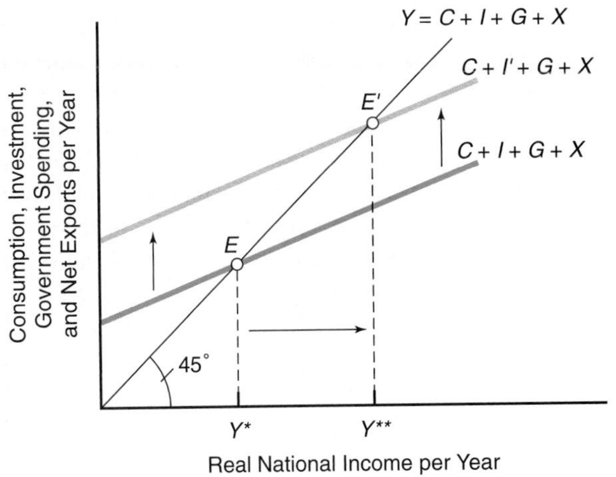

FIGURE D-1
An Increase in the Money Supply
An increase in the money supply increases income by lowering interest rates and thus increasing investment from I to I'.

Keynesian analysis is that total spending rises by *more* than the original rise in investment spending because consumption spending depends positively on income.

DECREASING THE MONEY SUPPLY

Not surprisingly, contractionary monetary policy works in exactly the reverse manner. A reduction in the money supply pushes interest rates up, which increases the cost of borrowing. Firms respond by reducing their investment spending, and this starts income downward. Consumers react to the lower income by scaling back on their consumption spending, which further depresses income. Thus the ultimate decline in income is larger than the initial drop in investment spending. Indeed, because the change in income is a multiple of the change in investment, Keynesians note that changes in investment spending (similar to changes in government spending) have a *multiplier* effect on the economy.

ARGUMENTS AGAINST MONETARY POLICY

It might be thought that this multiplier effect would make monetary policy a potent tool in the Keynesian arsenal, particularly when it comes to getting the economy out of a recession. In fact, however, many traditional Keynesians argue that monetary policy is likely to be relatively ineffective as a recession fighter. According to their line of reasoning, although monetary policy has the potential to reduce interest rates, changes in the money supply have little actual impact on interest rates. Instead, during recessions, people try to build up as much as they can in liquid assets to protect themselves from risks of unemployment and other losses of income. When the monetary authorities increase the money supply, individuals are willing to allow most of it to accumulate in their bank accounts. This desire for increased liquidity thus prevents interest rates from falling very much, which in turn means that there will be virtually no change in investment spending and thus little change in aggregate demand.

Problem

The answer to this problem appears at the back of the book.

D-1. Assume that the following conditions exist:

a. All banks are fully loaned up—there are no excess reserves, and desired excess reserves are always zero.
b. The money multiplier is 3.
c. The planned investment schedule is such that at a 7 percent rate of interest, investment is $200 billion; at 6 percent, investment is $225 billion.
d. The investment multiplier is 3.
e. The initial equilibrium level of national income is $2 trillion.
f. The equilibrium rate of interest is 7 percent.

Now the Fed engages in expansionary monetary policy. It buys $1 billion worth of bonds, which increases the money supply, which in turn lowers the market rate of interest by 1 percent. Indicate by how much the money supply increased, and then trace out the numerical consequences of the associated reduction in interest rates on all the other variables mentioned.

CHAPTER

18

STABILIZATION IN AN INTEGRATED WORLD ECONOMY

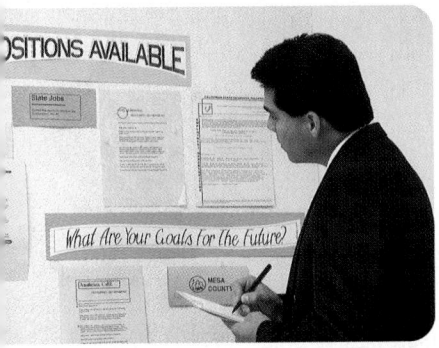

At the start of the 2000s, unemployment had dropped to around 4 percent, but the rate of inflation had not budged for several years. So where did economists get the idea that low unemployment can cause higher rates of inflation?

At one time, it was a concept of central importance to economic policymakers. Many economists devoted their careers to trying to understand it. The concept is something known as the *Phillips curve*—a potential policy trade-off between the inflation rate and the unemployment rate arising from a proposed inverse relationship between the two. Today, however, a number of economists regard the idea of a Phillips curve as an anachronism. After all, in recent years inflation and unemployment have been *positively* related. As the unemployment rate declined from the 1990s into the early 2000s, so did the inflation rate. Why did anyone ever suggest that an inverse relationship between the inflation rate and the unemployment was the norm? Why do some economists continue to believe that it is, in spite of the experience of the past decade? You will learn the answers to these questions in this chapter.

LEARNING OBJECTIVES

After reading this chapter, you should be able to:

1. **Explain why the actual unemployment rate might depart from the natural rate of unemployment**
2. **Describe why economic theory implies that there may be an inverse relationship between the inflation rate and the unemployment rate, reflected by the Phillips curve**
3. **Evaluate how expectations affect the relationship between the actual inflation rate and the unemployment rate**
4. **Understand the fundamental hypotheses of the new classical theory and their implications for economic policymaking**
5. **Identify the central features and predictions of real business cycle theory**
6. **Distinguish among alternative new Keynesian theories of business fluctuations**

Chapter Outline

- Active Versus Passive Policymaking
- The Natural Rate of Unemployment
- Rational Expectations and the New Classical Model
- Real Business Cycle Theory
- New Keynesian Economics
- Macroeconomic Models and Their Implications for Stabilization Policy

Did You Know That... since November 1948, Congress has passed at least a dozen bills aimed at fighting recession with fiscal policy? In the mid-1990s, in one 17-month period, the Fed increased short-term interest rates seven times and cut them once. And over a longer period, the Fed has even changed its basic operating targets.

ACTIVE VERSUS PASSIVE POLICYMAKING

All of these actions constitute part of what is called **active (discretionary) policymaking.** At the other extreme is **passive (nondiscretionary) policymaking,** in which there is no deliberate stabilization policy at all. You have already been introduced to one nondiscretionary policymaking idea in Chapter 17—the *monetary rule,* by which the money supply is allowed to increase at a fixed rate per year. In the fiscal arena, passive (nondiscretionary) policy might be simply to balance the federal budget over the business cycle. Recall from Chapter 13 that there are lags between the time when the national economy enters a recession or a boom and the time when that fact becomes known and acted on by the economy. Proponents of passive policy argue strongly that such time lags often render short-term stabilization policy ineffective or, worse, procyclical.

Active (discretionary) policymaking 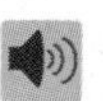
All actions on the part of monetary and fiscal policymakers that are undertaken in response to or in anticipation of some change in the overall economy.

Passive (nondiscretionary) policymaking 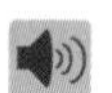
Policymaking that is carried out in response to a rule. It is therefore not in response to an actual or potential change in overall economic activity.

To take a stand on this debate concerning active versus passive policymaking, you first need to know what the potential trade-offs are that policymakers believe they face. Then you need to see what the data actually show. The most important policy trade-off appears to be between price stability and unemployment. Before exploring that, however, we need first to look at the economy's natural, or long-run, rate of unemployment.

THE NATURAL RATE OF UNEMPLOYMENT 

Recall from Chapter 7 that there are different types of unemployment: frictional, cyclical, structural, and seasonal. Frictional unemployment arises because individuals take the time to search for the best job opportunities. Except when the economy is in a recession or a depression, much unemployment is of this type.

Note that we did not say that frictional unemployment was the *sole* form of unemployment during normal times. *Structural unemployment* is caused by a variety of "rigidities" throughout the economy. Structural unemployment results from factors such as these:

1. Union activity that sets wages above the equilibrium level and also restricts the mobility of labor
2. Government-imposed licensing arrangements that restrict entry into specific occupations or professions
3. Government-imposed minimum wage laws and other laws that require all workers to be paid union wage rates on government contract jobs
4. Welfare and unemployment insurance benefits that reduce incentives to work
5. A mismatch of worker training and skills with available jobs

In each case, these factors reduce individuals' abilities or incentives to choose employment rather than unemployment.

Consider the effect of unemployment insurance benefits on the probability of an unemployed person's finding a job. When unemployment benefits run out, according to economists Lawrence Katz and Bruce Meyer, the probability of an unemployed person's finding a job doubles. The conclusion is that unemployed workers are more serious about finding a job when they are no longer receiving such benefits.

Frictional unemployment and structural unemployment both exist even when the economy is in long-run equilibrium—they are a natural consequence of costly information (the need to conduct a job search) and the existence of rigidities such as those noted. Because these two types of unemployment are a natural consequence of imperfect and costly information and rigidities, they are related to what economists call the natural rate of unemployment. As we discussed in Chapter 7, this is defined as the rate of unemployment that would exist in the long run after everyone in the economy fully adjusted to any changes that have occurred. Recall that national output tends to return to the level implied by the long-run aggregate supply curve (*LRAS*). Thus whatever rate of unemployment the economy tends to return to can be called the natural rate of unemployment.

EXAMPLE

The U.S. Natural Rate of Unemployment

At the end of World War II, the unemployment rate was below 4 percent. By the early 1990s, it was above 6 per cent. These two endpoints for half a cycle of unemployment rates prove nothing by themselves. But look at Figure 18-1. There you see not only what has happened to the unemployment rate over that same time period but an estimate of the natural rate of unemployment. The solid line labeled "Natural rate of unemployment" is esti-

FIGURE 18-1

Estimated U.S. Natural Rate of Unemployment

As you can see in this figure, the actual rate of unemployment has varied widely in the United States in recent decades. If we estimate the natural rate of unemployment by averaging unemployment rates from five years earlier to five years later at each point in time, we get the heavy solid line so labeled. It rose from the 1950s until the mid-1980s and seems to be gradually descending since then.

Sources: Economic Report of the President; Economic Indicators, various issues.

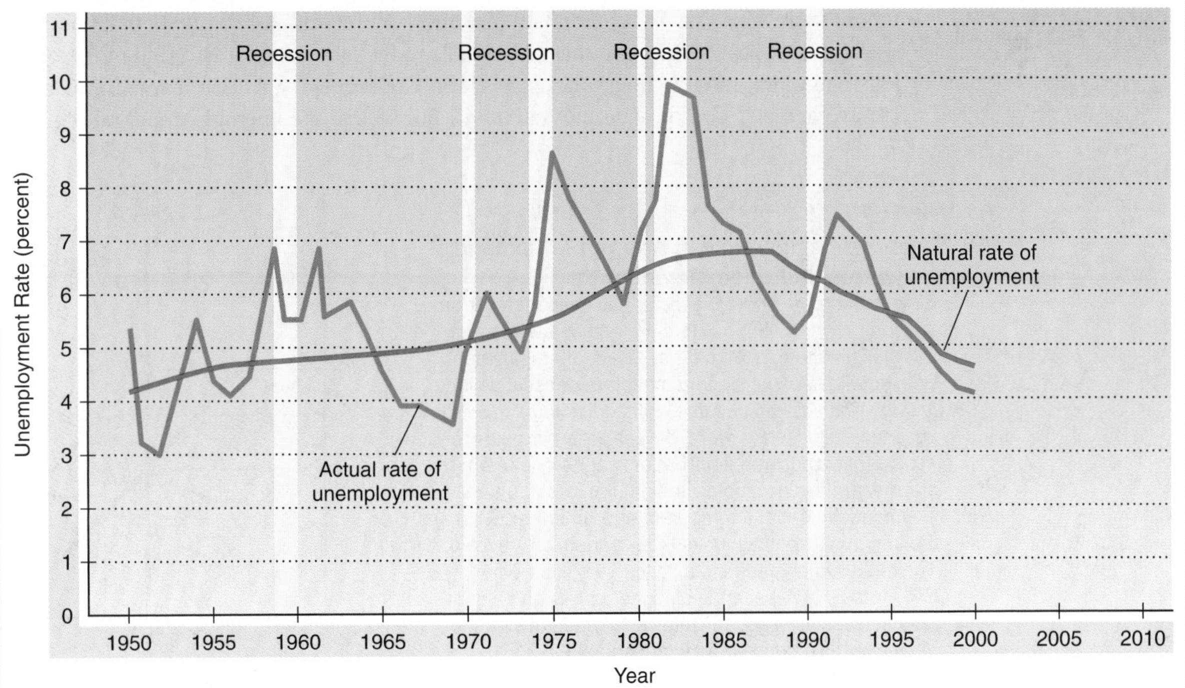

mated by averaging unemployment rates from five years earlier to five years later at each point in time. This computation reveals that until about 1983, the natural rate of unemployment was rising. But since then, a downward trend appears to have taken hold.

For Critical Analysis

Of the various factors that create structural unemployment, which ones do you think explained the gradual trend upward in the natural rate of unemployment from the late 1940s until the 1990s in the United States?

Departures from the Natural Rate of Unemployment

Even though the unemployment rate has a strong tendency to stay at and return to the natural rate, it is possible for fiscal and monetary policy to move the actual unemployment rate away from the natural rate, at least in the short run. Deviations of the actual unemployment rate from the natural rate are called *cyclical unemployment* because they are observed over the course of nationwide business fluctuations. During recessions, the overall unemployment rate exceeds the natural rate; cyclical unemployment is positive. During periods of economic booms, the overall unemployment rate can go below the natural rate; at such times, cyclical unemployment is in essence negative.

To see how departures from the natural rate of unemployment can occur, let's consider two examples. Referring to Figure 18-2, we begin in equilibrium at point E, with the associated price level P_1 and real GDP per year of level Y_1.

The Impact of Expansionary Policy. Now imagine that the government decides to use fiscal or monetary policy to stimulate the economy. Further suppose, for reasons that will soon become clear, that this policy surprises decision makers throughout the economy in the sense that they did not anticipate that the policy would occur. The aggregate demand curve shifts from AD_1 to AD_2 in Figure 18-2, so both the price level and real GDP rise to P_2 and Y_2, respectively. In the labor market, individuals would find that conditions had improved markedly relative to what they expected. Firms seeking to expand output will want to hire more workers. To accomplish this, they will recruit more actively and possibly ask workers to work overtime, so that individuals in the labor market will find more job openings and more possible hours they can work. Consequently, as you learned in Chapter 7, the average duration of unemployment will fall so that the unemployment rate falls. This

FIGURE 18-2
Impact of an Increase in Aggregate Demand on Output and Unemployment
If the economy is operating at E_1, it is in both short-run and long-run equilibrium. Here the actual rate of unemployment is equal to the natural rate of unemployment. Subsequent to expansionary monetary or fiscal policy, the aggregate demand curve shifts outward to AD_2. The price level rises to P_2; real GDP per year increases to Y_2. The new short-run equilibrium is at E_2. The unemployment rate is now below the natural rate of unemployment. We are at a temporary equilibrium at E_2. In the long run, expectations of input owners are revised. The short-run aggregate supply curve shifts from $SRAS_1$ to $SRAS_2$ because of higher prices and higher resource costs. Real GDP returns to the $LRAS$ level of Y_1 per year. The price level increases to P_3.

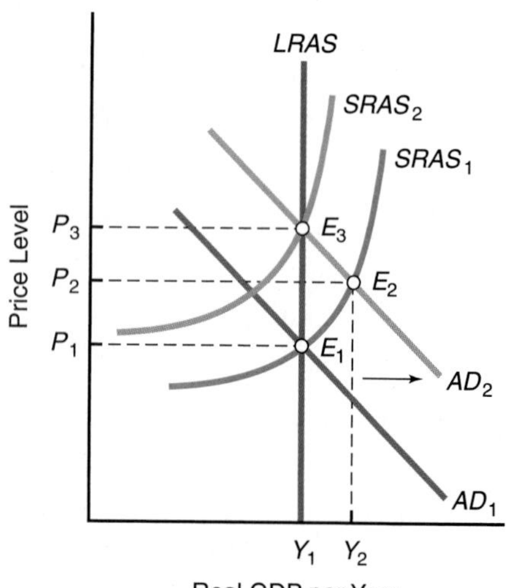

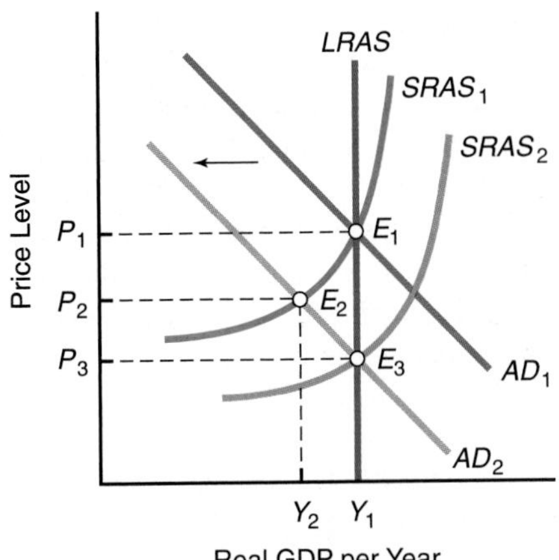

FIGURE 18-3
Impact of a Decline in Aggregate Demand on Output and Unemployment
Starting from equilibrium at E_1, a decline in aggregate demand to AD_2 leads to a lower price level, P_2, and real GDP declines to Y_2. The unemployment rate will rise above the natural rate of unemployment. Equilibrium at E_2 is temporary, however. At the lower price level, the expectations of input owners will be revised. $SRAS_1$ will shift to $SRAS_2$. The new equilibrium will be at E_3, with real GDP equal to Y_1 and a price level of P_3.

unexpected increase in aggregate demand simultaneously causes the price level to rise to P_2 and the unemployment rate to fall. The *SRAS* curve will not stay at $SRAS_1$, however. A change in the expectations of input owners, such as workers and owners of capital and raw materials, will be revised. The short-run aggregate supply curve shifts to $SRAS_2$ as input prices rise. We find ourselves at a new equilibrium at E_3, which is on the *LRAS*. Long-run real GDP per year is Y_1 again, but at a higher price level, P_3.

The Consequences of Contractionary Policy. Instead of expansionary policy, the government could have decided to engage in contractionary (or deflationary) policy. As shown in Figure 18-3, the sequence of events would have been in the opposite direction of those in Figure 18-2. Again, beginning from an initial equilibrium E_1, an unanticipated reduction in aggregate demand puts downward pressure on both prices and real GDP; the price level falls to P_2, and real GDP declines to Y_2. Fewer firms will be hiring, and those that are hiring will offer fewer overtime possibilities. Individuals looking for jobs will find that it takes longer than predicted. As a result, unemployed individuals will remain unemployed longer. The average duration of unemployment will rise, and so will the rate of unemployment. The unexpected decrease in aggregate demand simultaneously causes the price level to fall to P_2 and the unemployment rate to rise. This is a short-run situation only at E_2. $SRAS_1$ will shift to $SRAS_2$ with a change in the expectations of input owners about future prices, and input prices fall. The new equilibrium will be at E_3, which is on the long-run aggregate supply curve, *LRAS*. The price level will have fallen to P_3.

The Phillips Curve: A Trade-Off?

Let's recap what we have just observed. An *unexpected* increase in aggregate demand causes the price level to rise and the unemployment rate to fall. Conversely, an *unexpected* decrease in aggregate demand causes the price level to fall and the unemployment rate to rise. Moreover, although not shown explicitly in either diagram, two additional points are true:

1. The greater the unexpected increase in aggregate demand, the greater the amount of inflation that results, and the lower the unemployment rate.
2. The greater the unexpected decrease in aggregate demand, the greater the deflation that results, and the higher the unemployment rate.

The Negative Relationship Between Inflation and Unemployment. Figure 18-4 summarizes these findings. The inflation rate (*not* the price level) is measured along the vertical axis, and the unemployment rate is measured along the horizontal axis. Point *A* shows an initial starting point, with the unemployment rate at the natural rate, *U**. Note that as a matter of convenience, we are starting from an equilibrium in which the price level is stable (the inflation rate is zero). Unexpected increases in aggregate demand cause the price level to rise—the inflation rate becomes positive—and cause the unemployment rate to fall. Thus the economy moves up to the left from *A* to *B*. Conversely, unexpected decreases in aggregate demand cause the price level to fall and the unemployment rate to rise above the natural rate—the economy moves from point *A* to point *C*. If we look at both increases and decreases in aggregate demand, we see that high inflation rates tend to be associated with low unemployment rates (as at *B*) and that low (or negative) inflation rates tend to be accompanied by high unemployment rates (as at *C*).

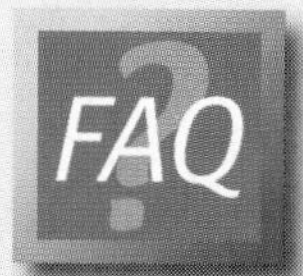

Americans say they are working more hours than ever before. Is that true?

Well, it seems to be true if you ask American workers. Survey after survey shows that full-time workers say they are working more than they were in the 1960s. A more telling examination of 10,000 workers' diaries collected by Professor John Robinson of the University of Maryland tells another story, however. It turns out that Americans today have an average of 40 hours of leisure a week, which is five hours more than their counterparts enjoyed in the 1960s. It is true that Americans still work more hours each year than virtually all Europeans, but they are not working more than previous generations of Americans.

Phillips curve 
A curve showing the relationship between unemployment and changes in wages or prices. It was long thought to reflect a trade-off between unemployment and inflation.

Is There a Trade-Off? The apparent negative relationship between the inflation rate and the unemployment rate shown in Figure 18-4 has come to be called the **Phillips curve,** after A. W. Phillips, who discovered that a similar relationship existed historically in Great Britain. Although Phillips presented his findings only as an empirical regularity, economists quickly came to view the relationship as representing a *trade-off* between inflation and unemployment. In particular, policymakers believed that they could *choose* alternative combinations of unemployment and inflation (or worse, that the trade-off was inevitable because you could not get more of one without giving up the other). Thus it seemed that a government that disliked unemployment could select a point like *B* in Figure 18-4, with a positive inflation rate but a relatively low unemployment rate. Conversely, a government that feared inflation could choose a stable price level at *A*, but only at the expense of a higher associated unemployment rate. Indeed, the Phillips curve seemed to suggest that it was possible for policymakers to fine-tune the economy by selecting the

FIGURE 18-4

The Phillips Curve

Unanticipated changes in aggregate demand produce a negative relationship between the inflation rate and unemployment. *U* * is the natural rate of unemployment.

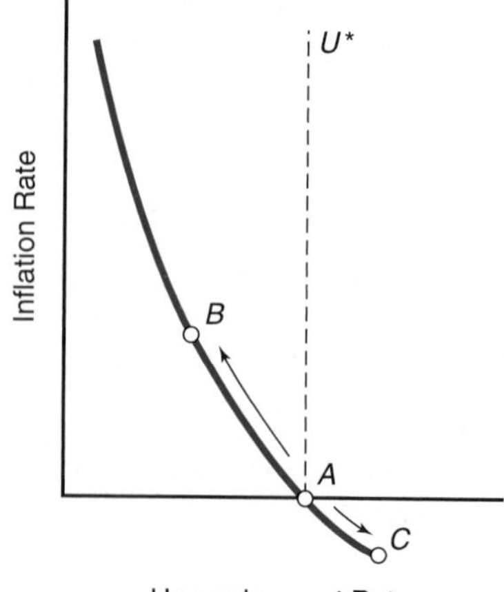

policies that would produce the exact mix of unemployment and inflation that suited current government objectives. As it turned out, matters are not so simple.

The NAIRU. If we accept that a trade-off exists between the rate of inflation and the rate of unemployment, then the notion of "noninflationary" rates of unemployment seems appropriate. In fact, some economists have proposed what they call the **nonaccelerating inflation rate of unemployment (NAIRU).** The NAIRU is therefore the rate of unemployment that corresponds to a stable rate of inflation. When the unemployment rate is less than the NAIRU, the rate of inflation tends to increase. When the unemployment rate is more than the NAIRU, the rate of inflation tends to decrease. When the rate of unemployment is equal to the NAIRU, inflation continues at an unchanged rate. If the Phillips curve trade-off exists and if the NAIRU can be estimated, that estimate will define the short-run trade-off between the rate of unemployment and the rate of inflation. Economists who have estimated the NAIRU for the world's 24 richest industrial countries claim that it has been steadily rising since the 1960s. Critics of the NAIRU concept argue that inflationary expectations must be taken into account.

Nonaccelerating inflation rate of unemployment (NAIRU)
The rate of unemployment below which the rate of inflation tends to rise and above which the rate of inflation tends to fall.

The Importance of Expectations

The reduction in unemployment that takes place as the economy moves from *A* to *B* in Figure 18-4 occurs because the wage offers encountered by unemployed workers are unexpectedly high. As far as the workers are concerned, these higher *nominal* wages appear, at least initially, to be increases in *real* wages; it is this fact that induces them to reduce their duration of search. This is a sensible way for the workers to view the world if aggregate demand fluctuates up and down at random, with no systematic or predictable variation one way or another. But if policymakers attempt to exploit the apparent trade-off in the Phillips curve, according to some macroeconomists, aggregate demand will no longer move up and down in an *unpredictable* way.

The Effects of an Unanticipated Policy. Consider Figure 18-5, for example. If the Federal Reserve attempts to reduce the unemployment rate to U_1, it must increase the money

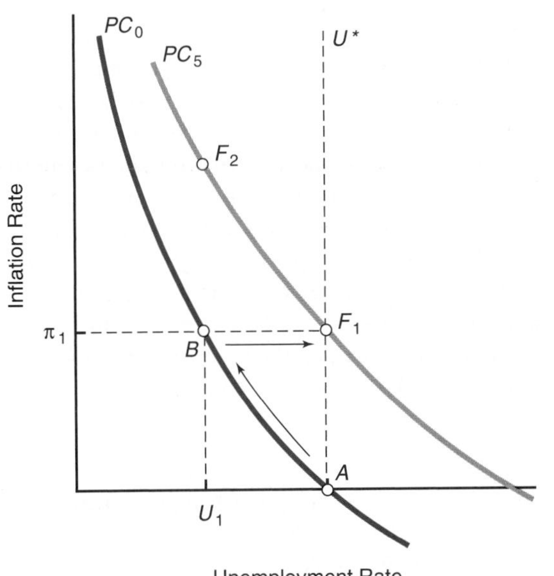

FIGURE 18-5
A Shift in the Phillips Curve
When there is a change in the expected inflation rate, the Phillips curve (*PC*) shifts to incorporate the new expectations. PC_0 shows expectations of zero inflation; PC_5 reflects an expected inflation rate of 5 percent.

supply enough to produce an inflation rate of π_1. If this is an unexpected one-shot affair in which the money supply is first increased and then held constant, the inflation rate will temporarily rise to π_1 and the unemployment rate will temporarily fall to U_1; but as soon as the money supply stops growing, the inflation rate will return to zero and unemployment will return to U^*, its natural rate. Thus an unexpected one-shot increase in the money supply will move the economy from point *A* to point *B*, and the economy will move of its own accord back to *A*.

If the authorities wish to prevent the unemployment rate from returning to U^*, some macroeconomists argue that the Federal Reserve must keep the money supply growing fast enough to keep the inflation rate up at π_1. But if the Fed does this, all of the economic participants in the economy—workers and job seekers included—will come to *expect* that inflation rate to continue. This, in turn, will change their expectations about wages. For example, suppose that π_1 equals 5 percent per year. When the expected inflation rate was zero, a 5 percent rise in nominal wages meant a 5 percent expected rise in real wages, and this was sufficient to induce some individuals to take jobs rather than remain unemployed. It was this perception of a rise in real wages that reduced search duration and caused the unemployment rate to drop from U^* to U_1. But if the expected inflation rate becomes 5 percent, a 5 percent rise in nominal wages means *no* rise in *real* wages. Once workers come to expect the higher inflation rate, rising nominal wages will no longer be sufficient to entice them out of unemployment. As a result, as the *expected* inflation rate moves up from 0 percent to 5 percent, the unemployment rate will move up also.

Click here to try using the Phillips curve as a guide for policymaking in the United Kingdom.

The Role of Expected Inflation. In terms of Figure 18-5, as authorities initially increase aggregate demand, the economy moves from point *A* to point *B*. If the authorities continue the stimulus in an effort to keep the unemployment rate down, workers' expectations will adjust, causing the unemployment rate to rise. In this second stage, the economy moves from *B* to point F_1: The unemployment rate returns to the natural rate, U^*, but the inflation rate is now π_1 instead of zero. Once the adjustment of expectations has taken place, any further changes in policy will have to take place along a curve such as PC_5, say, a movement from F_1 to F_2. This new schedule is also a Phillips curve, differing from the first, PC_0, in that the actual inflation rate consistent with any given unemployment rate is higher because the expected inflation rate is higher.

Not surprisingly, when economic policymakers found that economic participants engaged in such adjustment behavior, they were both surprised and dismayed. If decision makers can adjust their expectations to conform with fiscal and monetary policies, then policymakers cannot choose a permanently lower unemployment rate of U_1, even if they are willing to tolerate an inflation rate of π_1. Instead, the policymakers would end up with an unchanged unemployment rate in the long run, at the expense of a permanently higher inflation rate.

Initially, however, there did seem to be a small consolation, for it appeared that in the short run—before expectations adjusted—the unemployment rate could be *temporarily* reduced from U^* to U_1, even though eventually it would return to the natural rate. If an important national election were approaching, it might be possible to stimulate the economy long enough to get the unemployment rate low enough to assure reelection. However, policymakers came to learn that not even this was likely to be a sure thing.

The U.S. Experience with the Phillips Curve

In separate articles in 1968, Milton Friedman and E. S. Phelps published pioneering studies suggesting that the apparent trade-off suggested by the Phillips curve could not be exploited by policymakers. Friedman and Phelps both argued that any attempt to reduce

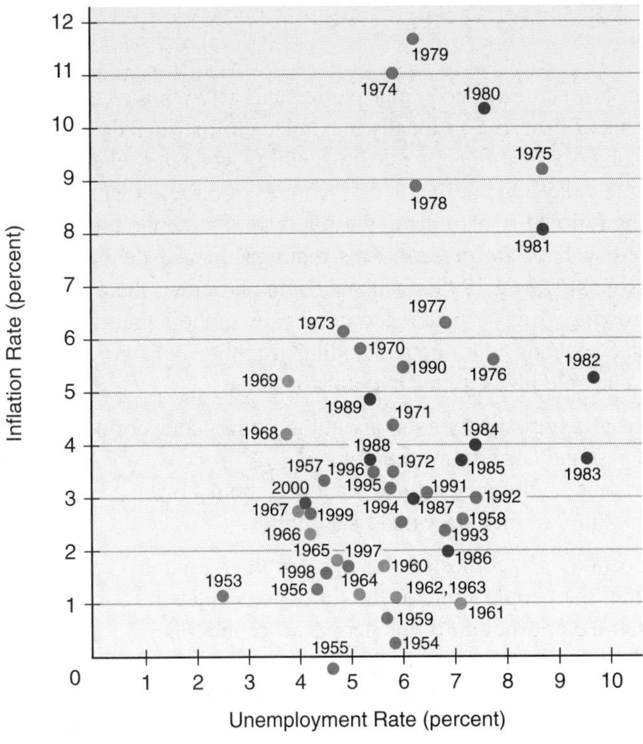

FIGURE 18-6

The Phillips Curve: Theory Versus Data

If you plot points representing the rate of inflation and the rate of unemployment for the United States from 1953 to the present, there does not appear to be any Phillips curve trade-off between the two variables.

Sources: Economic Report of the President; Economic Indicators, various issues.

unemployment by inflating the economy would soon be thwarted by economic participants' incorporating the new higher inflation rate into their expectations. The Friedman-Phelps research thus implies that for any given unemployment rate, *any* inflation rate is possible, depending on the actions of policymakers. As reflected in Figure 18-6, the propositions of Friedman and Phelps were to prove remarkably accurate.

When we examine the data for unemployment and inflation in the United States over the past half century, we see virtually no clear relationship between them. Although there seemed to have been a Phillips curve trade-off between unemployment and inflation from the mid-1950s to the mid-1960s, apparently once people in the economy realized what was happening, they started revising their forecasts accordingly. So once policymakers attempted to exploit the Phillips curve, the presumed trade-off between unemployment and inflation disappeared.

CONCEPTS IN BRIEF

- The natural rate of unemployment is the rate that exists in long-run equilibrium, when workers' expectations are consistent with actual conditions.
- Departures from the natural rate of unemployment can occur when individuals encounter unanticipated changes in fiscal or monetary policy. An unexpected rise in aggregate demand will reduce unemployment below the natural rate, whereas an unanticipated decrease in aggregate demand will push unemployment above the natural rate.
- The Phillips curve exhibits a negative relationship between the inflation rate and the unemployment rate that can be observed when there are *unanticipated* changes in aggregate demand.
- It was originally believed that the Phillips curve represented a trade-off between inflation and unemployment. In fact, no trade-off exists because workers' expectations adjust to any systematic attempts to reduce unemployment below the natural rate.

RATIONAL EXPECTATIONS AND THE NEW CLASSICAL MODEL

You already know that economists assume that economic participants act *as though* they were rational and calculating. We think of firms that rationally maximize profits when they choose today's rate of output and consumers who rationally maximize utility when they choose how much of what goods to consume today. One of the pivotal features of current macro policy research is the assumption that rationality also applies to the way that economic participants think about the future as well as the present. This relationship was developed by Robert Lucas, who won the Nobel Prize in 1995 for his work. In particular, there is widespread agreement among a growing group of macroeconomics researchers that the **rational expectations hypothesis** extends our understanding of the behavior of the macroeconomy. There are two key elements to this hypothesis:

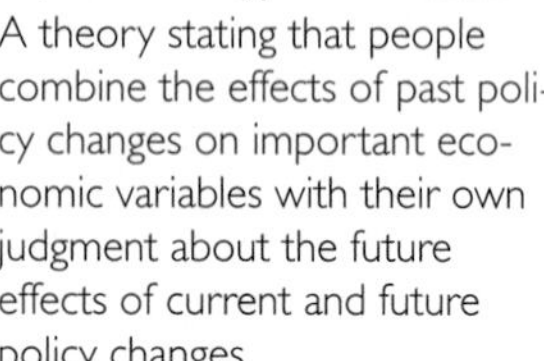

Rational expectations hypothesis
A theory stating that people combine the effects of past policy changes on important economic variables with their own judgment about the future effects of current and future policy changes.

1. Individuals base their forecasts (or expectations) about the future values of economic variables on all available past and current information.
2. These expectations incorporate individuals' understanding about how the economy operates, including the operation of monetary and fiscal policy.

In essence, the rational expectations hypothesis holds that Abraham Lincoln was correct when he said, "You may fool all the people some of the time; you can even fool some of the people all of the time; but you can't fool *all* of the people *all* of the time."

If we further assume that there is pure competition in all markets and that all prices and wages are flexible, we obtain the **new classical model** (referred to in Chapter 13 when discussing the Ricardian equivalence theorem). To see how rational expectations operate within the context of this model, let's take a simple example of the economy's response to a change in monetary policy.

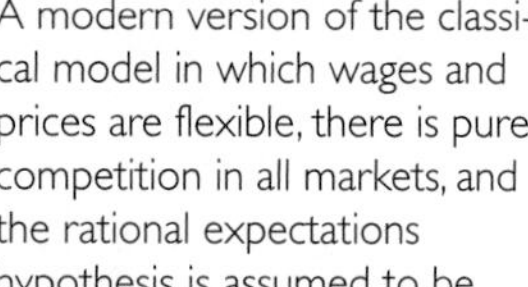

New classical model
A modern version of the classical model in which wages and prices are flexible, there is pure competition in all markets, and the rational expectations hypothesis is assumed to be working.

The New Classical Model

Consider Figure 18-7, which shows the long-run aggregate supply curve (*LRAS*) for the economy, as well as the initial aggregate demand curve (AD_1) and the short-run aggregate supply curve ($SRAS_1$). The money supply is initially given by $M = M_1$, and the price level and real GDP are shown by P_1 and Y_1, respectively. Thus point *A* represents the initial equilibrium.

FIGURE 18-7
Response to an Unanticipated Rise in Aggregate Demand
Unanticipated changes in aggregate demand have real effects. In this case, the rise in demand causes real output to rise from Y_1 to Y_2.

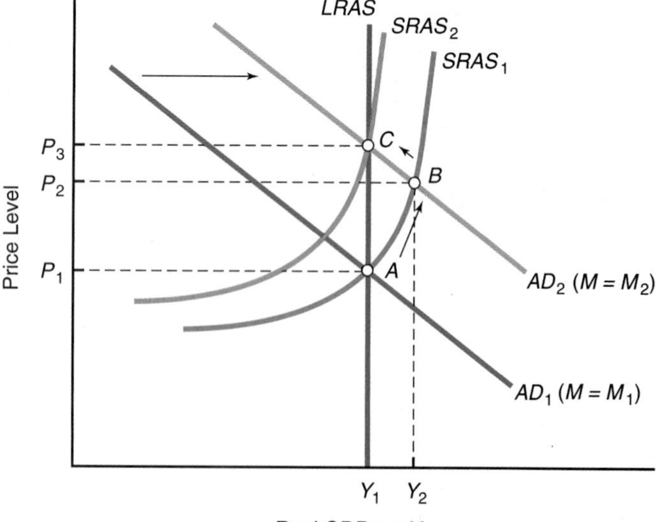

Suppose now that the money supply is unexpectedly increased to M_2, thereby causing the aggregate demand curve to shift outward to AD_2. Given the location of the short-run aggregate supply curve, this increase in aggregate demand will cause output and the price level to rise to Y_2 and P_2, respectively. The new short-run equilibrium is at *B*. Because output is *above* the long-run equilibrium level of Y_1, unemployment must be below long-run levels (the natural rate), and so workers will soon respond to the higher price level by demanding higher nominal wages. This will cause the short-run aggregate supply curve to shift upward vertically, moving the economy to the new long-run equilibrium at *C*. The price level thus continues its rise to P_3, even as real GDP declines back down to Y_1 (and unemployment returns to the natural rate). So as we have seen before, even though an increase in the money supply can raise output and lower unemployment in the short run, it has no effect on either variable in the long run.

The Response to Anticipated Policy. Now let's look at this disturbance with the perspective given by the rational expectations hypothesis, as it is embedded in the new classical model. Suppose that workers (and other input owners) know ahead of time that this increase in the money supply is about to take place. Assume also that they know when it is going to occur and understand that its ultimate effect will be to push the price level from P_1 to P_3. Will workers wait until after the price level has increased to insist that their nominal wages go up? The rational expectations hypothesis says that they will not. Instead, they will go to employers and insist on nominal wages that move upward in step with the higher prices. From the workers' perspective, this is the only way to protect their real wages from declining due to the anticipated increase in the money supply.

The Policy Irrelevance Proposition. As long as economic participants behave in this manner, when we draw the *SRAS* curve, we must be explicit about the nature of their expectations. This we have done in Figure 18-8. In the initial equilibrium, the short-run

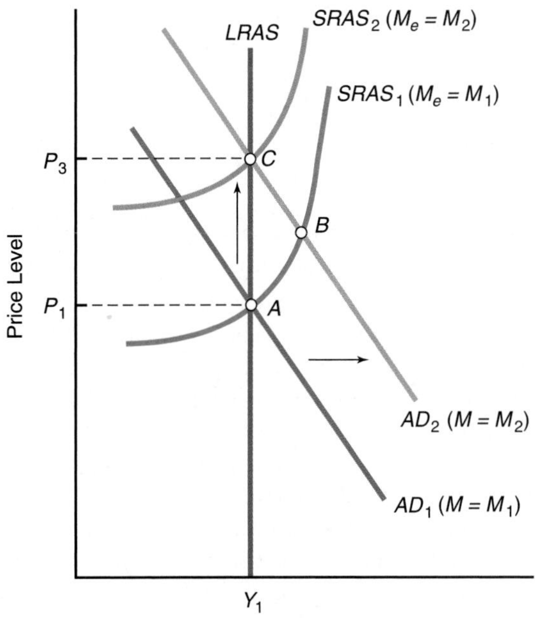

FIGURE 18-8
Effects of an Anticipated Rise in Aggregate Demand
When policy is fully anticipated, a rise in the money supply causes a rise in the price level from P_1 to P_3, with no change in real output.

aggregate supply curve is labeled to show that the expected money supply (M_e) and the actual money supply (M_1) are equal ($M_e = M_1$). Similarly, when the money supply changes in a way that is anticipated by economic participants, the aggregate supply curve shifts to reflect this expected change in the money supply. The new short-run aggregate supply curve is labeled ($M_e = M_2$) to reveal this. According to the rational expectations hypothesis, the short-run aggregate supply will shift upward *simultaneously* with the rise in aggregate demand. As a result, the economy will move directly from point *A* to point *C* in Figure 18-8 without passing through *B:* The *only* response to the rise in the money supply is a rise in the price level from P_1 to P_3; neither output nor unemployment changes at all. This conclusion—that fully anticipated monetary policy is irrelevant in determining the levels of real variables—is called the **policy irrelevance proposition:**

Policy irrelevance proposition 
The new classical and rational expectations conclusion that policy actions have no real effects in the short run if the policy actions are anticipated and none in the long run even if the policy actions are unanticipated.

> Under the assumption of rational expectations on the part of decision makers in the economy, anticipated monetary policy cannot alter either the rate of unemployment or the level of real GDP. Regardless of the nature of the anticipated policy, the unemployment rate will equal the natural rate, and real GDP will be determined solely by the economy's long-run aggregate supply curve.

What Must People Know? There are two important matters to keep in mind when considering this proposition. First, our discussion has assumed that economic participants know in advance exactly what the change in monetary policy is going to be and precisely when it is going to occur. In fact, the Federal Reserve does not announce exactly what the future course of monetary policy (down to the last dollar) is going to be. Instead, the Fed tries to keep most of its plans secret, announcing only in general terms what policy actions are intended for the future. It is tempting to conclude that because the Fed's intended policies are not freely available, they are not available at all. But such a conclusion would be wrong. Economic participants have great incentives to learn how to predict the future behavior of the monetary authorities, just as businesses try to forecast consumer behavior and college students do their best to forecast what their next economics exam will look like. Even if the economic participants are not perfect at forecasting the course of policy, they are likely to come a lot closer than they would in total ignorance. The policy irrelevance proposition really assumes only that *people don't persistently make the same mistakes in forecasting the future.*

What Happens If People Don't Know Everything? This brings us to our second point. Once we accept the fact that people are not perfect in their ability to predict the future, the possibility emerges that some policy actions will have systematic effects that look much like the movements *A* to *B* to *C* in Figure 18-7. For example, just as other economic participants sometimes make mistakes, it is likely that the Federal Reserve sometimes make mistakes—meaning that the money supply may change in ways that even the Fed does not predict. And even if the Fed always accomplished every policy action it intended, there is no guarantee that other economic participants would fully forecast those actions. What happens if the Fed makes a mistake or if firms and workers misjudge the future course of policy? Matters will look much as they do in panel (a) of Figure 18-9, which shows the effects of an unanticipated increase in the money supply. Economic participants expect the money supply to be M_1, but the actual money supply turns out to be M_2. Because $M_2 > M_1$, aggregate demand shifts relative to aggregate supply. The result is a rise in real output (real GDP) in the short run from Y_1 to Y_2; corresponding to this rise in real output will be an increase in employment and hence a fall in the unemployment rate. So even under the

FIGURE 18-9
Effects of an Unanticipated Rise in Aggregate Demand
Even with rational expectations, an unanticipated change in demand can affect output in the short run.

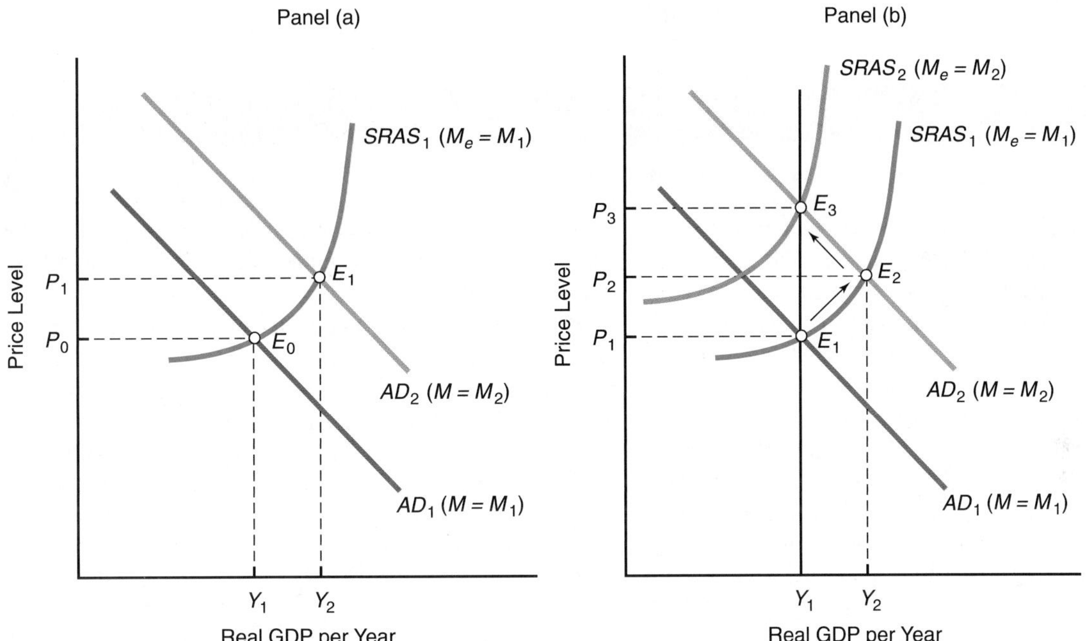

rational expectations hypothesis, monetary policy *can* have an effect on real variables in the short run, but only if the policy is unsystematic and therefore unanticipated.

In the long run, this effect on real variables will disappear because people will figure out that the Fed either accidentally increased the money supply or intentionally increased it in a way that somehow fooled individuals. Either way, people's expectations will soon be revised so that the short-run aggregate supply curve will shift upward. As shown in panel (b) of Figure 18-9, real GDP will return to long-run levels, meaning that so will the employment and unemployment rates.

The Policy Dilemma

Perhaps the most striking and disturbing feature of the new classical model is that it seems to suggest that only mistakes can have real effects. If the Federal Reserve always does what it intends to do and if other economic participants always correctly anticipate the Fed's actions, monetary policy will affect only the price level and nominal input prices. It appears that only if the Fed makes a mistake in executing monetary policy or people err in anticipating that policy will changes in the money supply cause fluctuations in real output and employment. If this reasoning is correct, the Fed is effectively precluded from using monetary policy in any rational way to lower the unemployment rate or to raise the level of real GDP. This is because fully anticipated changes in the money supply will lead to exactly offsetting changes in prices and hence no real effects. Many economists were disturbed at the prospect that if the economy happened to enter a recessionary period, policymakers would be powerless to push real GDP and unemployment back to long-run levels. As a result, they asked, in light of the rational expectations hypothesis, is it *ever* possible for systematic policy to have predictable real effects on the economy? The answer has led to even more developments in the way we think about macroeconomics.

INTERNATIONAL POLICY EXAMPLE

The New Policy Rulebook in a Globalized Economy

Economic events in other countries, such as the financial crises in Eastern Europe and in Asia during the 1990s, have apparently forced the Federal Reserve to take a more global view. This is particularly relevant in how is sets interest rate policies for the United States.

When the economies of Asia suffered severe economic crises, the value of their domestic curriencies fell in international markets. This allowed U.S. companies to buy comodities from these countries at much lower prices in terms of U.S. dollars. These falling commodity prices apparently helped reduce any threat of inflation in the United States during this period. Some observers argue that is why we saw robust economic growth without inflation as well as a surging stock market. Policymakers at the Fed realized that they could continue to increase the money supply at a historically rapid pace without fear of immediate inflation.

At the start of the Asian financial crisis, the U.S. stock market began to falter. The Fed immediately announced several interest rate cuts. Fed policymakers later stated that they wanted to cut rates to avert a credit crunch that could have triggered a global recession.

Clearly, the Fed is taking international developments into account more than ever before when deciding what policy to make for the United States.

For Critical Analysis

In what ways can global events affect the U.S. economy?

CONCEPTS IN BRIEF

- The rational expectations hypothesis assumes that individuals' forecasts incorporate all available information, including an understanding of government policy and its effects on the economy.
- The new classical economics assumes that the rational expectations hypothesis is valid and also that there is pure competition and that all prices and wages are flexible.
- The policy irrelevance proposition says that under the assumptions of the new classical model, fully anticipated monetary policy cannot alter either the rate of unemployment or the level of real GDP.
- The new classical model implies that policies can alter real economic variables only if the policies are unsystematic and therefore unanticipated; otherwise people learn and defeat the desired policy goals.

REAL BUSINESS CYCLE THEORY

The modern extension of new classical theory involves reexamining the first principles that assume fully flexible prices.

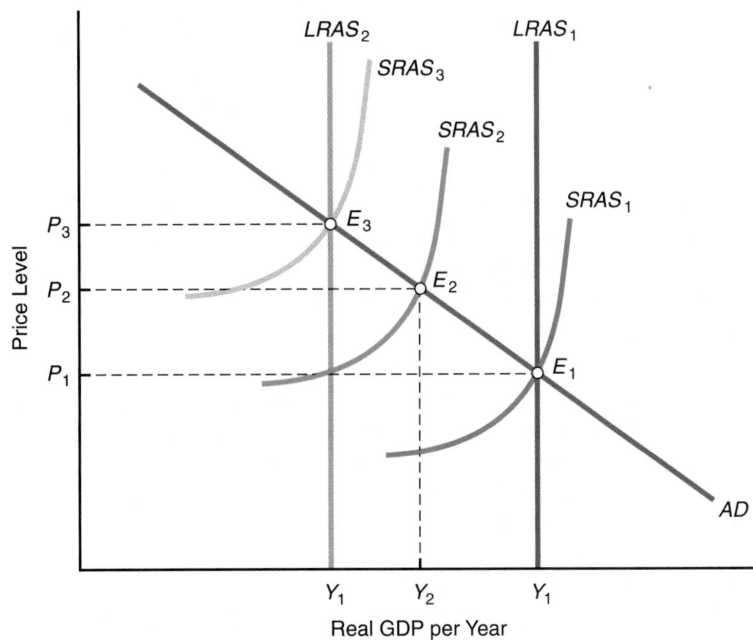

FIGURE 18-10
Effects of a Reduction in the Supply of Resources
The position of the *LRAS* depends on our endowments of all types of resources. Hence a reduction in the supply of one of those resources, such as oil, causes a reduction—an inward shift—in the aggregate supply curve. In addition, there is a rise in the equilibrium price level and a fall in the equilibrium rate of real GDP per year (output).

The Distinction Between Real and Monetary Shocks

The research of the new business cycle theorists differs importantly from that of new classical theorists in that business cycle theorists seek to determine whether real, as opposed to purely monetary, forces might help explain aggregate economic fluctuations. An important stimulus for the development of **real business cycle theory,** as it has come to be known, was the economic turmoil of the 1970s. During that decade, world economies were staggered by two major disruptions to the supply of oil. The first occurred in 1973, the second in 1979. In both episodes, members of the Organization of Petroleum Exporting Countries (OPEC) reduced the amount of oil they were willing to supply and raised the price at which they offered it for sale. Each time, the price level rose sharply in the United States, and real GDP declined. Thus each episode produced a period of "stagflation"—real economic stagnation combined with high inflation. Figure 18-10 illustrates the pattern of events.

Real business cycle theory 
An extension and modification of the theories of the new classical economists of the 1970s and 1980s, in which money is neutral and only real, supply-side factors matter in influencing labor employment and real output.

We begin at point E_1 with the economy in both short- and long-run equilibrium, with the associated supply curves, $SRAS_1$ and $LRAS_1$. Initially, the level of real GDP is Y_1, and the price level is P_1. Because the economy is in long-run equilibrium, the unemployment rate must be at the natural rate.

A reduction in the supply of oil, as occurred in 1973 and 1979, causes the *SRAS* curve to shift to the left to $SRAS_2$ because fewer goods will be available for sale due to the reduced supplies. If the reduction in oil supplies is (or is believed to be) permanent, the *LRAS* shifts to the left also. This assumption is reflected in Figure 18-10, where $LRAS_2$ shows the new long-run aggregate supply curve associated with the lowered output of oil.

In the short run, two adjustments begin to occur simultaneously. First, the prices of oil and petroleum-based products begin to rise, so that the overall price level rises to P_2. Second, the higher costs of production occasioned by the rise in oil prices induce firms to cut back production, so total output falls to Y_2 in the short run. The new temporary short-run equilibrium occurs at E_2, with a higher price level (P_2) and a lower level of real GDP (Y_2).

Impact on the Labor Market

If we were to focus on the labor market while this adjustment from E_1 to E_2 was taking place, we would find two developments occurring. The rise in the price level pushes the real wage rate downward, even as the scaled-back production plans of firms induce them to reduce the amount of labor inputs they are using. So not only does the real wage rate fall, but the level of employment declines as well. On both counts, workers are made worse off due to the reduction in the supply of oil.

Now this is not the full story, because owners of non-oil inputs (such as labor) who are willing to put up with reduced real payments in the short run simply will not tolerate them in the long run. Thus, for example, some workers who were willing to continue working at lower wages in the short run will eventually decide to retire, switch from full-time work to part-time employment, or drop out of the labor force altogether. In effect, there is a reduction in the supply of non-oil inputs, reflected in an upward shift in the *SRAS* from $SRAS_2$ to $SRAS_3$. This puts additional upward pressure on the price level and exerts a downward force on real GDP. The final long-run equilibrium thus occurs at point E_3, with the price level at P_3 and real GDP at Y_3. (In principle, because the oil supply shock has had no direct effect on labor markets, the natural rate of unemployment does not change when equilibrium moves from E_1 to E_3.)

Generalizing the Theory

Naturally, the focus of real business cycle theory goes well beyond the simple "oil shock" that we have discussed here, for it encompasses all types of real disturbances, including technological changes and shifts in the composition of the labor force. Moreover, a complete treatment of real shocks to the economy is typically much more complex than we have allowed for in our discussion. For example, an oil shock such as is shown in Figure 18-10 would likely also have effects on the real wealth of Americans, causing a reduction in aggregate demand as well as aggregate supply. Nevertheless, our simple example still manages to capture the flavor of the theory.

It is clear that real business cycle theory has improved our understanding of the economy's behavior, but economists agree that it alone is incapable of explaining all of the facets of business cycles that we observe. For example, it is difficult to imagine a real disturbance that could possibly account for the Great Depression in this country, when real income fell more than 30 percent and the unemployment rate rose to 25 percent. Moreover, real business cycle theory continues to assume that prices are perfectly flexible and so fails to explain a great deal of the apparent rigidity of prices throughout the economy.

New Keynesian economics
A macroeconomic approach that emphasizes that the prices of some goods and services adjust sluggishly in response to changing market conditions. Thus an unexpected decrease in the price level results in some firms with higher-than-desired prices. A consequence is a reduction in sales for those firms.

NEW KEYNESIAN ECONOMICS

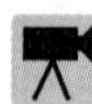

Although the new classical and real business cycle theories both embody pure competition and flexible prices, a body of research called the **new Keynesian economics** drops both of these assumptions. The new Keynesian economists do not believe that market clearing models of the economy can explain business cycles. Consequently, they argue that macroeconomic models must contain the "sticky" wages and prices assumption that Keynes outlined in his major work (see Chapter 11). Thus the new Keynesian research has as its goal a refinement of the theory of aggregate supply that explains how wages and prices behave in the short run. There are several such theories. The first one relates to the cost of changing prices.

Small Menu Cost Theory

If prices do not respond to demand changes, two conditions must be true: Someone must be consciously deciding not to change prices, and that decision must be in the decision maker's self-interest. One combination of facts that is consistent with this scenario is the **small menu cost theory,** which supposes that much of the economy is characterized by imperfect competition and that it is costly for firms to change their prices in response to changes in demand. The costs associated with changing prices are called *menu costs,* and they include the costs of renegotiating contracts, printing price lists (such as menus), and informing customers of price changes. (But see *Netnomics* on page 444.)

Small menu cost theory
A hypothesis that it is costly for firms to change prices in response to demand changes because of the cost of renegotiating contracts, printing price lists, and so on.

Many such costs may not be very large in magnitude; that is why they are called *small menu costs.* Some of the costs of changing prices, however, such as those incurred in bringing together business managers from points around the nation or the world for meetings on price changes or renegotiating deals with customers, may be significant.

Firms in different industries have different cost structures. Such differences explain diverse small menu costs. Therefore, the extent to which firms hold their prices constant in the face of changes in demand for their products will vary across industries. Not all prices will be rigid. Nonetheless, new Keynesian theorists argue that many—even most—firms' prices are sticky for relatively long time intervals. As a result, the aggregate level of prices could be very nearly rigid because of small menu costs.

Although most economists agree that such costs exist, there is considerably less agreement on whether they are sufficient to explain the extent of price rigidity that is observed.

Efficiency Wage Theory

An alternative approach within the new Keynesian framework is called the **efficiency wage theory.** It proposes that worker productivity actually *depends on* the wages that workers are paid, rather than being independent of wages, as is assumed in other theories. According to this theory, higher real wages encourage workers to work harder, improve their efficiency, increase morale, and raise their loyalty to the firm. Across the board, then, higher wages tend to increase workers' productivity, which in turn discourages firms from cutting real wages because of the damaging effect that such an action would have on productivity and profitability. Under highly competitive conditions, there will generally be an optimal wage—called the *efficiency wage*—that the firm should continue paying, even in the face of large fluctuations in the demand for its output.

Efficiency wage theory
The hypothesis that the productivity of workers depends on the level of the real wage rate.

The efficiency wage theory model is a rather simple idea, but it is somewhat revolutionary. All of the models of the labor market adopted by traditional classical, traditional Keynesian, monetarist, new classical, and new Keynesian theorists alike do not consider such real-wage effects on worker productivity.

There are significant, valid elements in the efficiency wage theory, but its importance in understanding national business fluctuations remains uncertain. For example, although the theory explains rigid real wages, it does not explain rigid prices. Moreover, the theory ignores the fact that firms can (and apparently do) rely on a host of incentives other than wages to encourage their workers to be loyal, efficient, and productive.

EXAMPLE

Are the Secretaries of Investment Bankers Overpaid?

Numerous studies have been done to show that secretaries for investment bankers earn considerably more than their counterparts in other sectors of the economy. These studies have taken account of age, education, and length of time on the job. Even when the salary data are corrected for these factors, secretarial pay in the investment banking sector is still much higher than in other sectors. Economist F. R. Mehta of Purdue University suggests that the efficiency wage theory may explain this wage disparity. He argues that in high-productivity industries, managers' time is more valuable. Thus it is more costly for such managers to spend time monitoring employees. To reduce the time highly productive managers (such as investment bankers) spend supervising secretaries, secretaries need additional incentives to keep them working harder and more efficiently. One such incentive is a relatively high rate of pay, one that may seem at an above-market rate. It is therefore rational for highly productive managers as investment bankers to "overpay" their secretaries and others who work under their guidance.

For Critical Analysis

Can you think of other reasons why more profitable firms might pay their secretaries and other workers more than the going wage rate?

Effect of Aggregate Demand Changes on Output and Employment in the Long Run

Some new Keynesian economists argue that a reduction in aggregate demand that causes a recession may affect output and employment even in the long run. They point out that workers who are fired or laid off may lose job skills during their period of unemployment. Consequently, they will have a more difficult time finding new employment later. Furthermore, those who remain unemployed over long periods of time may change their attitudes toward work. They may even have a reduced desire to find employment later on. For these reasons and others, a recession could permanently raise the amount of frictional unemployment.

As yet, little research has been done to quantify this theory.

MACROECONOMIC MODELS AND THEIR IMPLICATIONS FOR STABILIZATION POLICY

Although it is impossible to compare accurately and completely every single detail of the various macroeconomic approaches we have examined, it is useful to summarize and contrast some of their key aspects. Table 18-1 presents features of our five key models: traditional classical, traditional Keynesian, new (modern) classical, new (modern) Keynesian, and modern monetarist. Realize when examining the table that we are painting with a broad brush.

TABLE 18-1
A Comparison of Macroeconomic Models

	Macroeconomic Model				
Issue	Traditional Classical	Traditional Keynesian	New Classical	New Keynesian	Modern Monetarist
Stability of capitalism	Yes	No	Yes	Yes, but can be enhanced by policy	Yes
Price-wage flexibility	Yes	No	Yes	Yes, but imperfect	Yes, but some restraints
Belief in natural rate of employment hypothesis	Yes	No	Yes	Yes	Yes
Factors sensitive to interest rate	Saving, consumption, investment	Demand for money	Saving, consumption, investment	Saving, consumption, investment	Saving, consumption, investment
View of the velocity of money	Stable	Unstable	No consensus	No consensus	Stable
Effect of changes in money supply on economy	Changes aggregate demand	Changes interest rates, which change investment and real output	No effect on real variables if anticipated	Changes aggregate demand	Directly changes aggregate demand
Effects of fiscal policy on the economy	Not applicable	Multiplier changes in aggregate demand and output	Generally ineffective*	Changes aggregate demand	Ineffective unless money supply changes also
Causes of inflation	Excess money growth	Excess real aggregate demand	Excess money growth	Excess money growth	Excess money growth
Stabilization policy	Unnecessary	Fiscal policy necessary and effective; monetary policy ineffective	Too difficult to conduct	Both fiscal and monetary policy may be useful	Too difficult to conduct

*Some fiscal policies affect relative prices (interest rates) and so many have real effects on economy.

CONCEPTS IN BRIEF

- Real business cycle theory holds that even if all prices and wages are perfectly flexible, shocks to the economy (such as technological change and changes in the supply of factors of production) can cause national business fluctuations.
- The new Keynesian economics explains why various features of the economy, such as small menu costs and wage rates that affect productivity, make it possible for monetary shocks to cause real effects.
- Although there remain significant differences between the classical and Keynesian branches of macroeconomics, the rivalry between them is an important source of innovation that helps improve our understanding of the economy.

NETNOMICS

New Keynesian Economics, Sticky Prices, and the Internet

You have read about new Keynesian economics in this chapter. You discovered that new Keynesian economists support the supposition that prices are "sticky." One resulting model is the small menu cost theory. It supposes that much of the economy is characterized by imperfect competition because it is costly for firms to change their prices and respond to changes in demand. Today, many economists believe that the Internet will reduce such supposed price stickiness.

Prices change only when the cost of *not* changing them is greater than the expense of adjusting them. We know that there is virtually no stickiness in prices in financial markets—stocks, bonds, foreign currencies, and so on—because the cost of such price stickiness can be dramatic. The same is true for anyone selling perishable goods. If prices are not reduced downward to eliminate excess quantities supplied, financial losses can be quite great. The existence of the Internet will not change these markets much. Before the Internet, we saw quick movements in prices in response to changing supply and demand in these markets.

Not so elsewhere. Electronic price tags are relatively costless to change. Thus anything that is sold over the Internet can have its price changed instantaneously at the click of a mouse. A travel agency, for example, selling holiday excursions can alter its vacation package prices digitally without any reprinting. Notice also that comparison shopping has become a major activity on the Internet. Any retailer who does not change prices downward in response to an excess quantity supplied will be driven out of the marketplace very quickly. Comparison shopping on the Internet for hotel rooms, airline tickets, CDs, books, and other commodities should cause prices to be far less sticky than just a few years ago. Thus in a sense, the Internet is making competition more intense. Prices will adjust more quickly, thereby undermining macro models that rely on the assumption of price stickiness.

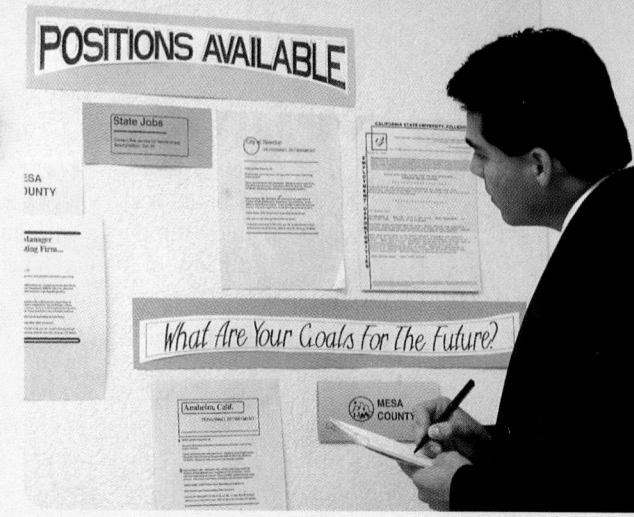

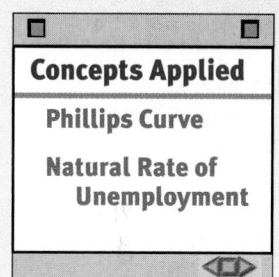

ISSUES & APPLICATIONS

What Happened to the Phillips Curve?

In the 1990s, Dana Mead, the chief executive officer of Tenneco, Inc., quipped, "NAIRU is to economics what the Nehru jacket is to fashion: outdated." (See page 431.) Figure 18-11 provides a rationale for this view. Since 1991, the relationship between inflation and unemployment rates has been shallow and upward-sloping. Through the 1990s, reductions in the unemployment rate were accompanied—to the experts' surprise—by lower, rather than higher, inflation.

Concepts Applied

- Phillips Curve
- Natural Rate of Unemployment

Good News and Bad News

This change in the relationship between inflation and unemployment sparked considerable optimism. Many commentators contended that the Internet and other information technologies had transformed the economic landscape. These new sources of economic growth, they claimed, had become self-perpetuating. America had crossed into the territory of a "new economy," and inflation would become a distant memory.

For the Federal Reserve, however, the inverted slope of the Phillips curve posed problems. Fed economists' forecasts of future inflation have been based on Phillips curve models of the inflation process. Starting in the 1990s, the Fed's inflation-forecasting models indicated that inflation was "too low" relative to actual unemployment rates—or, alternatively stated, unemployment was "too low" relative to observed rates of inflation. The Fed's forecasting models consistently indicated that the natural rate of unemployment was close to 6 percent but, as Figure 18-11 indicates, the unemployment rate was consistently 1 to $1\frac{1}{2}$ percent below this level.

Attempting an Explanation

Economists have struggled to explain the shifting inflation-unemployment relationship. Two theories have emerged. One focuses on greater competition in markets for goods and

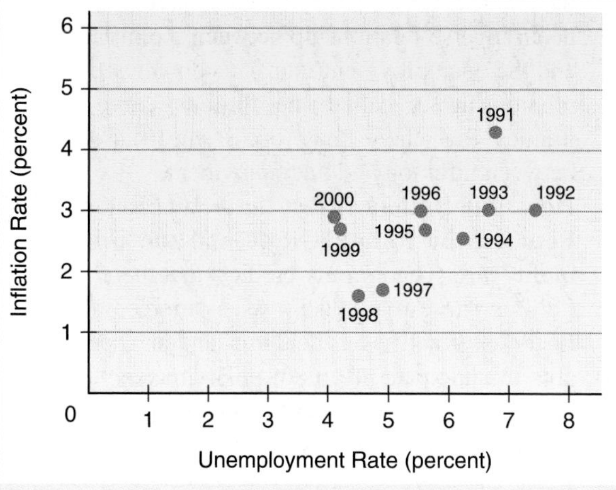

FIGURE 18-11
Inflation and Unemployment Rates Since 1991
During the 1990s, in an apparent contradiction to the standard theory of the short-run Phillips curve, there was an *upward*-sloping relationship between inflation and unemployment rates in the United States.
Sources: Economic Report of the President; Economic Indicators various issues.

FOR CRITICAL ANALYSIS

1. Can the unemployment rate ever be "too low"?
2. If the age distribution hypothesis concerning the behavior of unemployment rates is correct, when might we expect an upturn in the natural unemployment rate as a result of the "baby boomlet" of the early and mid-1990s, other things being equal?

services following widespread deregulation of many industries, reduced barriers to international trade, and the growth of Internet commerce. This hypothesis proposes that firms in most industries found that the demand for their products was more price-sensitive than it had been before. This left less scope for price changes, which automatically tended to restrain price increases in the face of rising demand. At any given unemployment rate, therefore, increased competition across the economy tends to restrain inflation even as the unemployment rate falls, making the short-run Phillips curve more shallow. In addition, greater competition for goods and services can theoretically reduce the natural rate of unemployment. Both these effects are consistent with the declines in inflation and unemployment depicted in Figure 18-11.

Another theory focuses on the age distribution of the U.S. population. A large fraction of the current population consists of the baby boom generation born between the late 1940s and the late 1950s. This large group reached working age (16) in the 1960s and 1970s. In contrast, fewer people were born between the early 1970s and the early 1980s. These people reached their working years in the late 1980s and 1990s. Unemployment rates for teenagers are always higher than for other groups in the labor force, because most teenagers have only the most rudimentary of skills to offer prospective employers. If we combine this fact with the timing at which different generations reached its teens, we can develop a very simple explanation for why unemployment was higher from the mid-1960s and to the late 1970s: There were a lot of teenagers around, and many of them were unemployed. This factor pushed up the unemployment rate during those years. As the rate of population growth declined, fewer teens were in the labor force, and the unemployment rate naturally fell.

Studies indicate that these two theories can account for 1 to $1\frac{1}{2}$ percentage points of the observed reduction in the U.S. unemployment rate, thereby potentially explaining why unemployment has been "so low" since the early 1990s.

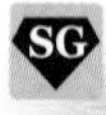

SUMMARY DISCUSSION OF LEARNING OBJECTIVES

1. **Why the Actual Unemployment Rate Might Depart from the Natural Rate of Unemployment:** According to the basic theory of aggregate demand and short- and long-run aggregate supply, an unexpected increase in aggregate demand can cause real GDP to rise in the short run, which results in a reduction in the unemployment rate. Consequently, for a time the actual unemployment rate can fall below the natural rate of unemployment. Likewise, an unanticipated reduction in aggregate demand can push down real GDP in the short run, thereby causing the actual unemployment rate to rise above the natural unemployment rate.
2. **The Phillips Curve:** An unexpected increase in aggregate demand that causes a drop in the unemployment rate also induces a rise in the equilibrium price level and, consequently, inflation. Thus the basic aggregate demand-aggregate supply model indicates that, other things being equal, there should be an inverse relationship between the inflation rate and the unemployment rate. This downward-sloping relationship is called the Phillips curve, and it implies that there may be a short-run trade-off between inflation and unemployment.
3. **How Expectations Affect the Actual Relationship Between the Inflation Rate and the Unemployment Rate:** Theory only predicts that there will be a Phillips curve relationship when another important factor, expectations, is held unchanged. If people are able to anticipate efforts of policymakers to exploit the Phillips curve trade-off by engaging in inflationary policies to push down the unemployment rate,

then basic theory also suggests that input prices such as nominal wages will adjust more rapidly to an increase in the price level. As a result, the Phillips curve will shift outward, and the economy will adjust more speedily toward the natural rate of unemployment. When plotted on a chart, therefore, the actual relationship between the inflation rate and the unemployment rate will not be a smooth, downward-sloping Phillips curve.

4. **The New Classical Theory and Its Implications for Economic Policymaking:** A key innovation of the new classical approach was the rational expectations hypothesis. According to this hypothesis, people form expectations of future economic variables such as inflation using all available past and current information and based on their understanding of the how the economy functions. A fundamental implication of the new classical theory is that only unanticipated policy actions can induce even short-run changes in real GDP. If people completely anticipate the actions of policymakers, wages and other input prices adjust immediately, so that real GDP remains unaffected. Thus a key implication of new classical theory is the policy irrelevance proposition, which states that the unemployment rate is unaffected by fully anticipated policy actions.
5. **Central Features and Predictions of Real Business Cycle Theory:** The key emphasis of real business cycle theory is on the importance of technological changes and labor market shocks such as variations in the composition of the labor force as factors that can induce business fluctuations. Therefore, this theory focuses on how shifts in aggregate supply curves can cause real GDP to vary over time.
6. **Alternative New Keynesian Views of Business Fluctuations:** New Keynesian approaches to understanding the sources of business fluctuations highlight wage and price stickiness. Small-menu cost theory proposes that imperfectly competitive firms that face costs of adjusting their prices may be slow to change prices in the face of variations in demand, so that real GDP may exhibit greater short-run variability than it otherwise would. Another new Keynesian approach, efficiency wage theory, proposes that worker productivity depends on the real wages that workers earn, which dissuades firms from reducing real wages and thereby leads to widespread wage stickiness. Finally, some new Keynesian theorists propose that short-term downturns in economic activity can affect the natural unemployment rate because people who lose their jobs in the short run also lose the opportunities to develop skills while unemployed or may change their attitudes toward work.

Key Terms and Concepts

Active (discretionary) policymaking (426)

Efficiency wage theory (441)

New classical model (434)

New Keynesian economics (440)

Nonaccelerating inflation rate of unemployment (NAIRU) (431)

Passive (nondiscretionary) policymaking (426)

Phillips curve (430)

Policy irrelevance proposition (436)

Rational expectations hypothesis (434)

Real business cycle theory (439)

Small menu cost theory (441)

Problems

Answers to the odd-numbered problems appear at the back of the book.

18-1. Suppose that the government were to alter the computation of the unemployment rate by including people in the military as part of the labor force.

a. How would this affect the actual unemployment rate?

b. How would such a change affect estimates of the natural rate of unemployment?

c. If this computational change were made, would it in any way affect the logic of the short-run and long-run Phillips curve analysis and its implications for policymaking? Why might the government wish to make such a change?

18-2. When Alan Greenspan was nominated for his third term as chair of the Federal Reserve's Board of Governors, a few senators held up his nomination. One of them acted as spokesperson in explaining their joint action to hinder his approval, saying, "Every time growth starts to go up, they [the Federal Reserve] push on the brakes, robbing working families and businesses of the benefits of faster growth." Evaluate this statement in the context of short-run and long-run perspectives on the Phillips curve.

18-3. Economists have not reached agreement on how lengthy the time horizon for "the long run" is in the context of analysis of the Phillips curve. Would you anticipate that this period is likely to have been shortened or extended by the advent of more sophisticated computer and communications technology? Explain your reasoning.

18-4. The natural rate of unemployment depends on factors that affect the behavior of both workers and firms. Make lists of possible factors affecting both workers and firms that you believe are likely to influence the natural rate of unemployment.

18-5. People called "Fed watchers" earn their living by trying to forecast what policies the Federal Reserve will implement within the next few weeks and months. Suppose that Fed watchers discover that the current group of Fed officials is following very systematic and predictable policies intended to reduce the unemployment rate, and they sell this information to firms, unions, and others in the private sector. If the new classical theory is correct, are the Fed's policies likely to have their intended effects on the unemployment rate?

18-6. Evaluate the following statement: "In an important sense, the term *policy irrelevance proposition* is misleading because even in the new classical model, economic policy actions can have significant effects on real GDP and the unemployment rate."

18-7. Real business cycle theory attributes even short-run increases in real GDP largely to changes in aggregate supply. Rightward shifts in aggregate supply tend to push down the equilibrium price level. How, then, could a real business cycle theorist explain the low but persistent inflation that the United States has experienced in recent years?

18-8. Does the Federal Reserve have any role in real business cycle theory? If so, what is it?

18-9. Use an aggregate demand and aggregate supply diagram to illustrate why the existence of widespread stickiness in prices established by businesses throughout the economy would be extremely important to predicting the potential effects of policy actions on real GDP.

18-10. Economists have also established that higher productivity due to technological improvements tends to push up real wages. Now suppose that the economy experiences a host of technological improvements. If the efficiency wage theory is correct, meaning that worker productivity responds positively to higher real wages, will this effect tend to add to or subtract from the economic growth initially induced by the improvements in technology?

Economics on the Net

The Inflation-Unemployment Relationship

According to the basic aggregate demand and aggregate supply model, the unemployment rate should be inversely related to changes in the inflation rate, other things being equal. This application allows you to take a direct look at unemployment and inflation data to judge for yourself whether or not the two variables appear to be related.

Title: Bureau of Labor Statistics: Economy at a Glance

Navigation: Click here to visit the Bureau of Labor Statistics Economy at a Glance homepage.

Application Perform the indicated operations, and then answer the following questions.

1. Click on the graph box next to Consumer Price Index. Take a look at the solid line showing inflation. How much has inflation varied in recent years? Compare this with previous years, especially the mid-1970s to mid-1980s.

2. Back up to Economy at a Glance, and now click on the graph box next to Unemployment Rate. During what recent years was the unemployment rate approaching and at its peak value? Do you note any appearance of an inverse relationship between the unemployment rate and the inflation rate?

For Group Study and Analysis Divide the class into groups, and have each group search through the Economy at a Glance site to develop an explanation for the key factors accounting for the recent behavior of the unemployment rate. Have each group report on its explanation. Is there any one factor that best explains the recent behavior of the unemployment rate?

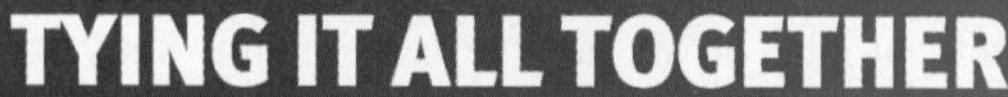

TYING IT ALL TOGETHER

Part 4 Case Problem

Case Background

The year is 2029. A special Federal Reserve task force is gathered around the huge mahogany table in the Federal Reserve Board's headquarters meeting room in its building on Constitution Avenue in Washington, D.C. The mission of the task force is to chart the Federal Reserve System's long-term future. At the moment, that future is not bright.

More than a Decade of Change The senior economist whom the task force has charged with researching the current situation summarizes the findings of the Board's economic staff. Estimates indicate that 75 percent of all Americans conduct their financial affairs on-line directly from home. Roughly 95 percent use smart cards to make cash purchases on-line, either from their homes or using kiosks in a wide variety of locations. Only in pockets of rural America is physical cash still the predominant means of payment.

Furthermore, there are now literally tens of thousands of issuers of digital cash accounts that people access using the FinNet, the nationwide on-line financial services network. Any business can issue what once were called transactions deposits (some old-fashioned economists at the Fed still use this term, but *smart accounts* is the more common name for these accounts). The many firms that offer smart accounts settle their payments obligations using private payment intermediaries based on the FinNet. Smart cards and debit cards became indistinguishable a decade ago. Retailers commonly add surcharges to the purchase prices of goods and services when people use paper checks, so even the stodgiest of retired baby boomers have given up on using checks.

These changes have already had significant effects on the Federal Reserve. Its retail product office in Atlanta, which once processed many millions of checks each day, is now a cavernous shell with a handful of employees. The wholesale product office in New York continues to serve as a central conduit for trillions of dollars of daily "interbank" payments, but it now specializes in providing these clearing services on-line in competition with a dozen private providers.

Sharpening the Fed's Mission The Fed has already undergone some major downsizing. Employment at the Fed has shrunk by 70 percent since the turn of the century, and half of current employees do work related to payment clearing, compared to about 80 percent 20 years ago. Many of these work as financial "cyberpolice," seeking to protect the FinNet from hackers, scam artists, and money launderers. Fed examiners also audit the virtual accounting ledgers of the conglomerates that provide financial services, a task assigned to it since the Gramm-Leach-Bliley Act was passed at the end of the last century.

Nevertheless, concludes the senior economist in her briefing of the Fed's task force, it may be time to contemplate additional steps. She proposes that the task force consider the following possibilities for a new Fed of the mid-twenty-first century:

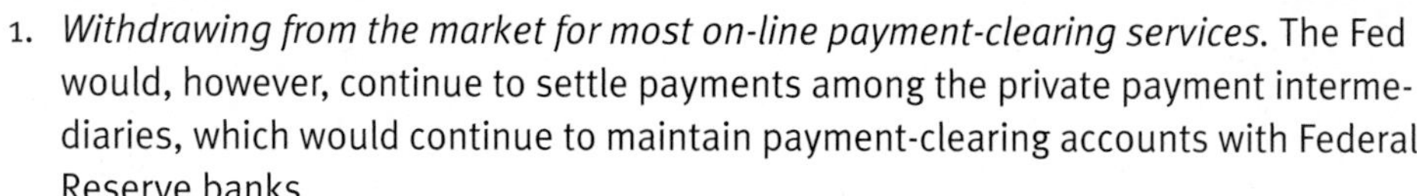

1. *Withdrawing from the market for most on-line payment-clearing services.* The Fed would, however, continue to settle payments among the private payment intermediaries, which would continue to maintain payment-clearing accounts with Federal Reserve banks.

2. *Continuing to supervise the activities of financial services conglomerates.* The Fed has long-standing expertise in this area. Other agencies of the U.S. government would be hard-pressed to duplicate this function.

3. *Ceding the Fed's current cyberpolicing role to the Treasury's Secret Service and to the Federal Bureau of Investigation.* This would eliminate wasteful duplication within the government that has attracted the ire of several powerful members of the Senate and House of Representatives, who also complain that the Fed has sometimes come close to violations of Net privacy laws enacted early in the century.

Points to Analyze

1. In what ways is this Fed of the not-so-distant future much different from today's Federal Reserve System?
2. In what ways is this Fed of the not-so-distant future very much like today's Federal Reserve System?
3. Should this future Fed, or other government agencies, act as a cyberpolice force? Why or why not?
4. Should this future Fed—or, for that matter, today's Fed—"worry" about volatility of interest rates? Why?

Casing the Internet

1. **Click here to go to the electronic banking Web page of the Office of the Comptroller of the Currency. Click on "Internet Banking in the U.S." to download a summary of recent trends.**
   a. **What progress are Internet banks making in the marketplace?**
   b. **How promising does the future appear to be for Internet banking?**
2. **Click here to learn about efforts to develop different forms of electronic payments by eCash Technologies, Inc.**
   a. **How is this company revamping familiar means of payment?**
   b. **Click on "PayAnyone." Do you think e-mail payments are likely to make people more comfortable using digital cash?**
3. **Click here and get up to date on the most recent developments in smart card technology at the home page of the Smart Card Industry Association.**
   a. **Explore this Web site. In the above scenario, digital cash and smart cards are commonplace. Nevertheless, smart cards have not yet caught on in the United States. Based on what you have learned in this text and your review of the information available at this Web site, why do you think that people are not yet rushing to use smart cards?**
   b. **Should the U.S. government use taxpayer funds to promote the use of smart cards in the interest of "the greater good"? Take a stand, and support your answer.**

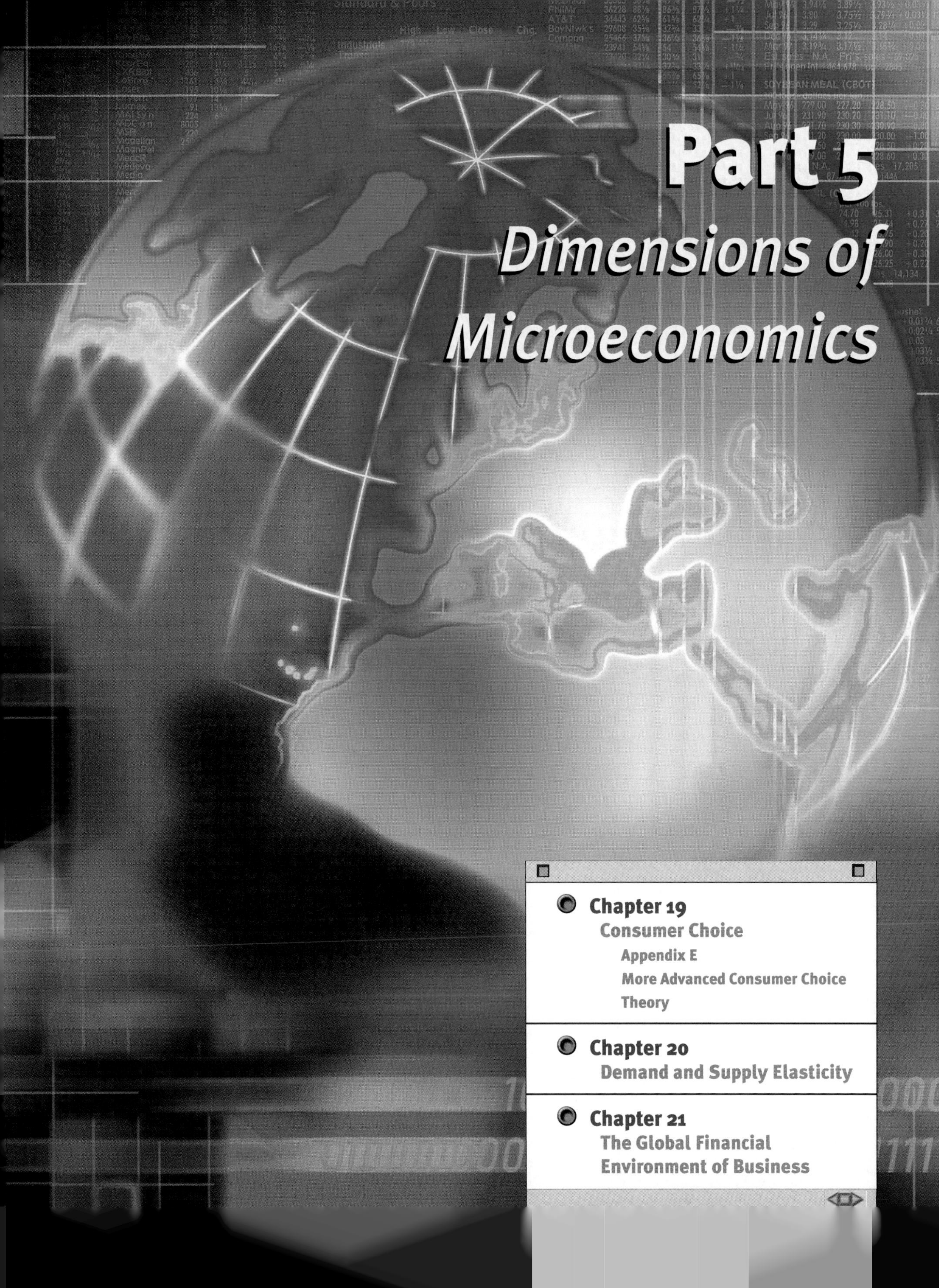

Part 5
Dimensions of Microeconomics

CHAPTER 19

CONSUMER CHOICE

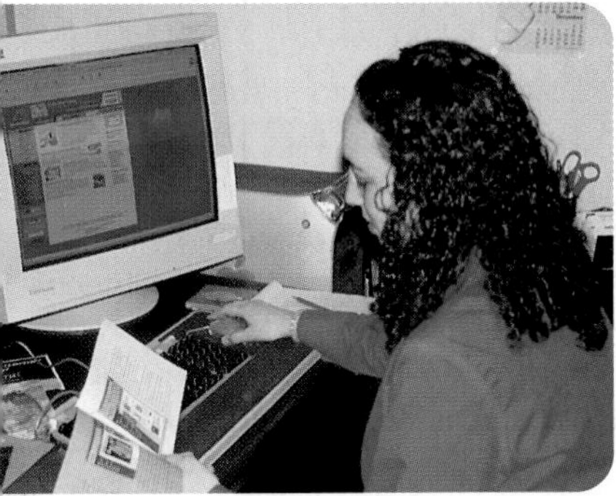

Internet access is offered by over 6,000 Internet service providers (ISPs) in the United States. What determines whether someone uses a high-priced service such as America Online at $21.95 per month or a lower-priced service such as VirtuallyFreeInternet.com at $15 per month?

Once you pay a connection fee to an Internet service provider such as America Online, you are "in." You incur no explicit fees for the time that you actually spend browsing the Internet. The only cost you incur is the opportunity cost of your time. Undoubtedly, the sweeping growth of the Internet owes much to this fact. A number of economists believe that the failure to price Internet use could also pose big problems for the system in the future. They claim that a very low price of Internet use induces people to spend too much time surfing the Web, thereby contributing to Internet congestion problems. To understand and evaluate this argument, you will need to understand the theory of consumer choice. This theory, it turns out, tells us how to value the last minute of time that a person spends on the Internet each day. It also permits us to speculate about whether the price of Internet usage is too low.

LEARNING OBJECTIVES

After reading this chapter, you should be able to:

1. Distinguish between total utility and marginal utility
2. Discuss why marginal utility at first rises but ultimately tends to decline as a person consumes more of a good or service
3. Explain why an individual's optimal choice of how much to consume of each good or service entails equalizing the marginal utility per dollar spent across all goods and services
4. Describe the substitution effect of a price change on quantity demanded of a good or service
5. Understand how the real-income effect of a price change affects the quantity demanded of a good or service
6. Evaluate why the price of diamonds is so much higher than the price of water even though people cannot survive long without water

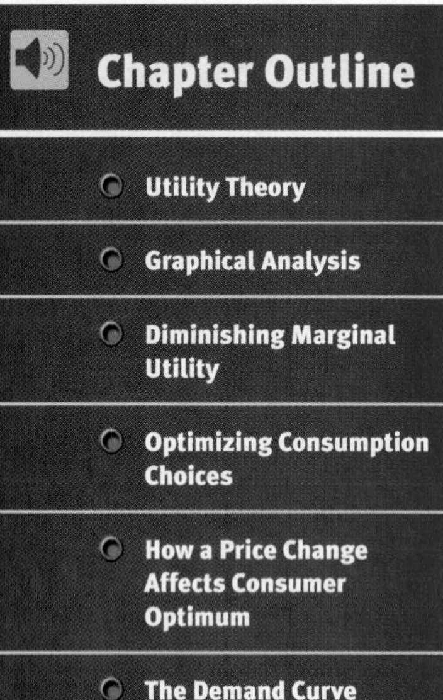

Did You Know That... more than 100 million people in the United States now have access to the Internet? Many of these people have decided to buy computers and to pay for regular access to the Internet at home. A significant portion of them own no computers, however. They choose to browse the Web at local schools or public libraries. What determines how much people spend on computers, Internet access, and other family budget items? One explanation is simply tastes—the values that family members place on different items on which they can spend their income. Different individuals have different preferences for how to allocate their limited incomes. Although there is no real theory of what determines people's tastes, we can examine some of the behavior that underlies how consumers react to changes in the prices of the goods and services that they purchase. Recall from Chapter 3 that people generally purchase less at higher prices than at lower prices. This is called the law of demand.

Understanding the derivation of the law of demand is useful because it allows us to arrange the relevant variables, such as price, income, and tastes, in such a way as to make better sense of the world and even perhaps generate predictions about it. One way of deriving the law of demand involves an analysis of the logic of consumer choice in a world of limited resources. In this chapter, therefore, we discuss what is called *utility analysis.*

UTILITY THEORY

Utility 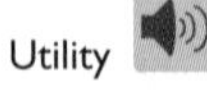
The want-satisfying power of a good or service.

When you buy something, you do so because of the satisfaction you expect to receive from having and using that good. For everything that you like to have, the more you have of it, the higher the level of satisfaction you receive. Another term that can be used for satisfaction is **utility,** or want-satisfying power. This property is common to all goods that are desired. The concept of utility is purely subjective, however. There is no way that you or I can measure the amount of utility that a consumer might be able to obtain from a particular good, for utility does not imply "useful" or "utilitarian" or "practical." For this reason, there can be no accurate scientific assessment of the utility that someone might receive by consuming a frozen dinner or a movie relative to the utility that another person might receive from that same good or service.

The utility that individuals receive from consuming a good depends on their tastes and preferences. These tastes and preferences are normally assumed to be given and stable for a given individual. An individual's tastes determine how much utility that individual derives from consuming a good, and this in turn determines how that individual allocates his or her income. People spend a greater proportion of their incomes on goods they like. But we cannot explain why tastes are different between individuals. For example, we cannot explain why some people like yogurt but others do not.

Utility analysis 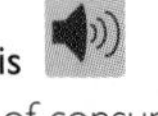
The analysis of consumer decision making based on utility maximization.

We can analyze in terms of utility the way consumers decide what to buy, just as physicists have analyzed some of their problems in terms of what they call force. No physicist has ever seen a unit of force, and no economist has ever seen a unit of utility. In both cases, however, these concepts have proved useful for analysis.

Throughout this chapter, we will be discussing **utility analysis,** which is the analysis of consumer decision making based on utility maximization.

Utility and Utils

Economists once believed that utility could be measured. In fact, there is a philosophical school of thought based on utility theory called *utilitarianism,* developed by the English philosopher Jeremy Bentham (1748–1832). Bentham held that society should seek the greatest happiness for the greatest number. He sought to apply an arithmetic formula for measuring happiness. He and his followers developed the notion of measurable utility and invented the **util** to measure it. For the moment, we will also assume that we can measure satisfaction using this representative unit. Our assumption will allow us to quantify the way we examine consumer behavior.* Thus the first chocolate bar that you eat might yield you 4 utils of satisfaction; the first peanut cluster, 6 utils; and so on. Today, no one really believes that we can actually measure utils, but the ideas forthcoming from such analysis will prove useful in our understanding of the way in which consumers choose among alternatives.

Util 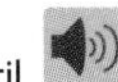
A representative unit by which utility is measured.

Total and Marginal Utility

Consider the satisfaction, or utility, that you receive each time that you rent and watch a video on your VCR. To make the example straightforward, let's say that there are hundreds of videos to choose from each year and that each of them is of the same quality. Let's say that you normally rent one video per week. You could, of course, rent two, or three, or four per week. Presumably, each time you rent another video per week, you will get additional satisfaction, or utility. The question, though, that we must ask is, given that you are already renting one per week, will the next one rented that week give you the same amount of additional utility?

That additional, or incremental, utility is called **marginal utility,** where *marginal,* as before, means "incremental" or "additional." (Marginal changes also refer to decreases, in which cases we talk about *decremental* changes.) The concept of marginality is important in economics because we make decisions at the margin. At any particular point, we compare additional (marginal) benefits with additional (marginal) costs.

Marginal utility
The change in total utility due to a one-unit change in the quantity of a good or service consumed.

Applying Marginal Analysis to Utility

The specific example presented in Figure 19-1 (p. 458) will clarify the distinction between total utility and marginal utility. The table in panel (a) shows the total utility and the marginal utility of watching videos each week. Marginal utility is the difference between total utility derived from one level of consumption and total utility derived from another level of consumption within a given time interval. A simple formula for marginal utility is this:

$$\text{Marginal utility} = \frac{\text{change in total utility}}{\text{change in number of units consumed}}$$

In our example, when a person has already watched two videos in one week and then watches another, total utility increases from 16 utils to 19. Therefore, the marginal utility (of watching one more video after already having watched two in one week) is equal to 3 utils.

---

*What follows is typically called *cardinal utility analysis* because it requires cardinal measurement. Numbers such as 1, 2, and 3 are cardinals. We know that 2 is exactly twice as many as 1 and that 3 is exactly three times as many as 1. You will see in Appendix E at the end of this chapter a type of consumer behavior analysis that requires only *ordinal* (ranked or ordered) measurement of utility. *First, second,* and *third* are ordinal numbers; nothing can be said about their exact size relationships; we can only talk about their importance relative to each other. Temperature, for example, is an ordinal ranking. One hundred degrees Celsius is not twice as warm as 50 degrees Celsius. All we can say is that 100 degrees Celsius is warmer than 50 degrees Celsius.

FIGURE 19-1

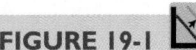

Total and Marginal Utility of Watching Videos

If we were able to assign specific values to the utility derived from watching videos each week, we could obtain a marginal utility schedule similar in pattern to the one shown in panel (a). In column 1 is the number of videos watched per week; in column 2, the total utility derived from each quantity; and in column 3, the marginal utility derived from each additional quantity, which is defined as the change in total utility due to a change of one unit of watching videos per week. Total utility from panel (a) is plotted in panel (b). Marginal utility is plotted in panel (c), where you see that it reaches zero where total utility hits its maximum at between 4 and 5 units.

Panel (a)

(1) Number of Videos Watched per Week	(2) Total Utility (utils per week)	(3) Marginal Utility (utils per week)
0	0	
		10 (10 – 0)
1	10	
		6 (16 – 10)
2	16	
		3 (19 – 16)
3	19	
		1 (20 – 19)
4	20	
		0 (20 – 20)
5	20	
		–2 (18 – 20)
6	18	

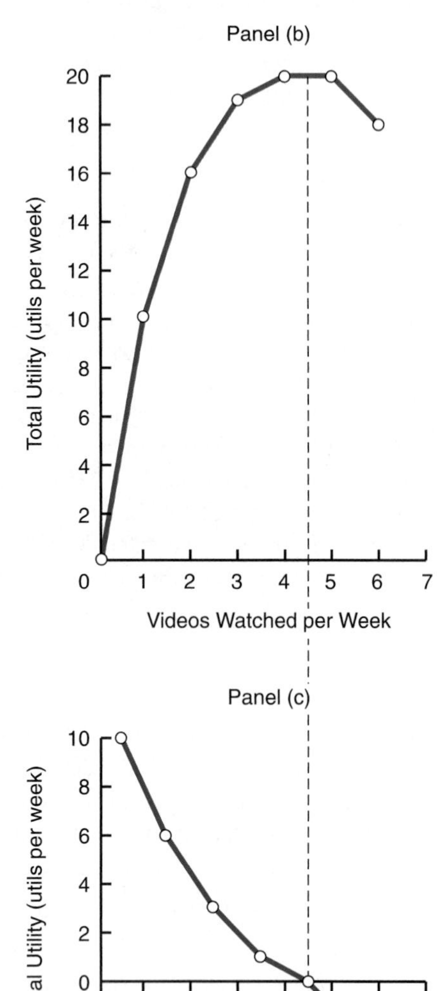

GRAPHICAL ANALYSIS

We can transfer the information in panel (a) onto a graph, as we do in panels (b) and (c) of Figure 19-1. Total utility, which is represented in column 2 of panel (a), is transferred to panel (b).

Total utility continues to rise until four videos are watched per week. This measure of utility remains at 20 utils through the fifth video, and at the sixth video per week it falls to 18 utils; we assume that at some quantity consumed per unit time period, boredom sets in. This is shown in panel (b).

Marginal Utility

If you look carefully at panels (b) and (c) of Figure 19-1, the notion of marginal utility becomes very clear. In economics, the term *marginal* always refers to a change in the total. The marginal utility of watching three videos per week instead of two videos per week is the increment in total utility and is equal to 3 utils per week. All of the points in panel (c) are taken from column 3 of the table in panel (a). Notice that marginal utility falls throughout the graph. A special point occurs after four videos are watched per week because the total utility curve in panel (b) is unchanged after the consumption of the fourth video. That means that the consumer receives no additional (marginal) utility from watching the fifth video. This is shown in panel (c) as *zero* marginal utility. After that point, marginal utility becomes negative.

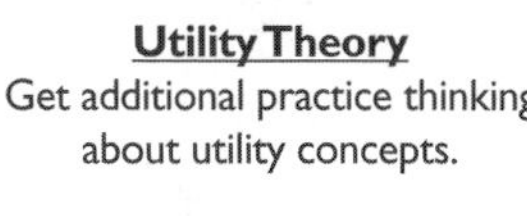

Utility Theory
Get additional practice thinking about utility concepts.

In our example, when marginal utility becomes negative, it means that the consumer is fed up with watching videos and would require some form of compensation to watch any more. When marginal utility is negative, an additional unit consumed actually lowers total utility by becoming a nuisance. Rarely does a consumer face a situation of negative marginal utility. Whenever this point is reached, goods become in effect "bads." A rational consumer will stop consuming at the point at which marginal utility becomes negative, even if the good is available at a price of zero.

CONCEPTS IN BRIEF

- Utility is defined as want-satisfying power; it is a power common to all desired goods and services.
- We arbitrarily measure utility in units called utils.
- It is important to distinguish between total utility and marginal utility. Total utility is the total satisfaction derived from the consumption of a given quantity of a good or service. Marginal utility is the *change* in total utility due to a one-unit change in the consumption of the good or service.

DIMINISHING MARGINAL UTILITY

Notice that in panel (c) of Figure 19-1, marginal utility is continuously declining. This property has been named the principle of **diminishing marginal utility.** There is no way that we can prove diminishing marginal utility; nonetheless, economists and others have for years believed strongly in the notion. Diminishing marginal utility has even been called a law. This supposed law concerns a psychological, or subjective, utility that you receive as you consume more and more of a particular good. Stated formally, the law is as follows:

Diminishing marginal utility
The principle that as more of any good or service is consumed, its extra benefit declines. Otherwise stated, increases in total utility from the consumption of a good or service become smaller and smaller as more is consumed during a given time period.

As an individual consumes more of a particular commodity, the total level of utility, or satisfaction, derived from that consumption usually increases. Eventually, however, the *rate* at which it increases diminishes as more is consumed.

Click here to see how diminishing marginal utility can complicate the task that wine tasters face when comparing different wines.

Take a hungry individual at a dinner table. The first serving is greatly appreciated, and the individual derives a substantial amount of utility from it. The second serving does not have quite as much pleasurable impact as the first one, and the third serving is likely to be even less satisfying. This individual experiences diminishing marginal utility of food until he or she stops eating, and this is true for most people. All-you-can-eat restaurants count on this fact; a second helping of ribs may provide some marginal utility, but the third helping would have only a little or even negative marginal utility. The fall in the marginal utility of other goods is even more dramatic.

Consider for a moment the opposite possibility—increasing marginal utility. Under such a situation, the marginal utility after consuming, say, one hamburger would increase. The second hamburger would be more valuable to you, and the third would be even more valuable yet. If increasing marginal utility existed, each of us would consume only one good or service! Rather than observing that "variety is the spice of life," we would see that monotony in consumption was preferred. We do not observe this, and therefore we have great confidence in the concept of diminishing marginal utility.

Consider an example. Your birthday is on December 25. Suppose that you derive utility from listening to new CDs each month. Even if you receive exactly the same number of CDs as presents on December 25 that you would have if your birthday were six months later, your total level of utility from these presents will be lower. Why? Because of diminishing marginal utility. Let's say that your relatives and friends all give you CDs as birthday and Christmas presents. The total utility you receive from, say, 20 CDs on December 25 is less than if you received 10 on December 25 and 10 on an alternative birthdate several months later.

EXAMPLE

Newspaper Vending Machines Versus Candy Vending Machines

Have you ever noticed that newspaper vending machines nearly everywhere in the United States allow you to put in the correct change, lift up the door, and take as many newspapers as you want? Contrast this type of vending machine with candy machines. They are completely locked at all times. You must designate the candy that you wish, normally by using some type of keypad. The candy then drops down to a place where you reach to retrieve it but from which you cannot grab any other candy.

The difference between these two types of vending machines is explained by diminishing marginal utility. Newspaper companies dispense newspapers from coin-operated boxes that allow dishonest people to take more copies than they pay for. What would a dishonest person do with more than one copy of a newspaper, however? The marginal utility of a second newspaper is normally zero. The benefit of storing excessive newspapers is usually nil because yesterday's news has no value. But the same analysis does not hold for candy. The marginal utility of a second candy bar is certainly less than the first, but it is normally not zero. Moreover, one can store candy for relatively long periods of time at relatively low cost. Consequently, food vending machine companies have to worry about dishonest users of their machines and must make their machines much more theftproof than newspaper companies do.

For Critical Analysis

Can you think of a circumstance under which a substantial number of newspaper purchasers might be inclined to take more than one newspaper out of a vending machine?

OPTIMIZING CONSUMPTION CHOICES 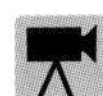

Every consumer has a limited income. Choices must be made. When a consumer has made all of his or her choices about what to buy and in what quantities, and when the total level of satisfaction, or utility, from that set of choices is as great as it can be, we say that the consumer has *optimized.* When the consumer has attained an optimum consumption set of goods and services, we say that he or she has reached **consumer optimum.***

Consumer optimum 
A choice of a set of goods and services that maximizes the level of satisfaction for each consumer, subject to limited income.

Consider a simple two-good example. The consumer has to choose between spending income on the rental of videos at $5 each and on purchasing deluxe hamburgers at $3 each. Let's say that when the consumer has spent all income on videos and hamburgers, the last dollar spent on hamburgers yields 3 utils of utility but the last dollar spent on video rentals yields 10 utils. Wouldn't this consumer increase total utility if some dollars were taken away from hamburger consumption and allocated to video rentals? The answer is yes. Given diminishing marginal utility, more dollars spent on video rentals will reduce marginal utility per last dollar spent, whereas fewer dollars spent on hamburger consumption will increase marginal utility per last dollar spent. The optimum—where total utility is maximized—might occur when the satisfaction per last dollar spent on both hamburgers and video rentals per week is equal for the two goods. Thus the amount of goods consumed depends on the prices of the goods, the income of the consumers, and the marginal utility derived from each good.

Table 19-1 presents information on utility derived from consuming various quantities of videos and hamburgers. Columns 4 and 8 show the marginal utility per dollar spent on videos and hamburgers, respectively. If the prices of both goods are zero, individuals will consume each as long as their respective marginal utility is positive (at least five units of

TABLE 19-1
Total and Marginal Utility from Consuming Videos and Hamburgers on an Income of $26

(1) Videos per Period	(2) Total Utility of Videos per Period (utils)	(3) Marginal Utility (utils) MU_v	(4) Marginal Utility per Dollar Spent (MU_v/P_v) (price = $5)	(5) Hamburgers per Period	(6) Total Utility of Hamburgers per Period (utils)	(7) Marginal Utility (utils) MU_h	(8) Marginal Utility per Dollar Spent (MU_h/P_h) (price = $3)
0	0.0	—	—	0	0	—	—
1	50.0	50.0	10.0	1	25	25	8.3
2	95.0	45.0	9.0	2	47	22	7.3
3	135.0	40.0	8.0	3	65	18	6.0
4	171.5	36.5	7.3	4	80	15	5.0
5	200.0	28.5	5.7	5	89	9	3.0

*Optimization typically refers to individual decision-making processes. When we deal with many individuals interacting in the marketplace, we talk in terms of an equilibrium in the marketplace. Generally speaking, equilibrium is a property of markets rather than of individual decision making.

each and probably much more). It is also true that a consumer with infinite income will continue consuming goods until the marginal utility of each is equal to zero. When the price is zero or the consumer's income is infinite, there is no effective constraint on consumption.

Consumer optimum is attained when the marginal utility of the last dollar spent on each good yields the same utility and income is completely exhausted. The individual's income is $26. From columns 4 and 8 of Table 19-1, equal marginal utilities per dollar spent occur at the consumption level of four videos and two hamburgers (the marginal utility per dollar spent equals 7.3). Notice that the marginal utility per dollar spent for both goods is also (approximately) equal at the consumption level of three videos and one hamburger, but here total income is not completely exhausted. Likewise, the marginal utility per dollar spent is (approximately) equal at five videos and three hamburgers, but the expenditures necessary for that level of consumption ($28) exceed the individual's income.

Table 19-2 shows the steps taken to arrive at consumer optimum. The first video would yield a marginal utility per dollar of 10 (50 units of utility divided by $5 per video), while the first hamburger would yield a marginal utility of only 8.3 per dollar (25 units of utility divided by $3 per hamburger). Because it yields the higher marginal utility per dollar, the video is purchased. This leaves $21 of income. The second video yields a higher marginal utility per dollar (9, versus 8.3 for hamburgers), so it is also purchased, leaving an unspent income of $16. At the third purchase, the first hamburger now yields a higher marginal utility per dollar than the next video (8.3 versus 8), so the first hamburger is purchased. This leaves income of $13 to spend. The process continues until all income is exhausted and the marginal utility per dollar spent is equal for both goods.

To restate, consumer optimum requires the following:

> A consumer's money income should be allocated so that the last dollar spent on each good purchased yields the same amount of marginal utility (when all income is spent).

TABLE 19-2

Steps to Consumer Optimum

In each purchase situation described here, the consumer always purchases the good with the higher marginal utility per dollar spent (*MU/P*). For example, at the time of the third purchase, the marginal utility per last dollar spent on videos is 8, but it is 8.3 for hamburgers, and $16 of income remains, so the next purchase will be a hamburger. Here $P_v = \$5$, $P_h = \$3$, MU_v is the marginal utility of video consumption, and MU_h is the marginal utility of hamburger consumption.

	Choices					
	Videos		Hamburgers			
Purchase	Unit	(MU_v/P_v)	Unit	$(MU_h/(P_h)$	Buying Decision	Remaining Income
1	First	10.0	First	8.3	First video	$26 – $5 = $21
2	Second	9.0	First	8.3	Second video	$21 – $5 = $16
3	Third	8.0	First	8.3	First hamburger	$16 – $3 = $13
4	Third	8.0	Second	7.3	Third video	$13 – $5 = $ 8
5	Fourth	7.3	Second	7.3	Fourth video and second hamburger	$ 8 – $5 = $ 3 $ 3 – $3 = $ 0

A Little Math

We can state the rule of consumer optimum in algebraic terms by examining the ratio of marginal utilities and prices of individual products. This is sometimes called the *rule of equal marginal utilities per dollar spent* on a basket of goods. The rule simply states that a consumer maximizes personal satisfaction when allocating money income in such a way that the last dollars spent on good A, good B, good C, and so on, yield equal amounts of marginal utility. Marginal utility (*MU*) from good A is indicated by "*MU* of good A." For good B, it is "*MU* of good B." Our algebraic formulation of this rule, therefore, becomes

$$\frac{MU \text{ of good A}}{\text{Price of good A}} = \frac{MU \text{ of good B}}{\text{price of good B}} = \cdots = \frac{MU \text{ of good Z}}{\text{price of good Z}}$$

The letters A, B, . . . , Z indicate the various goods and services that the consumer might purchase.

We know, then, that the marginal utility of good A divided by the price of good A must equal the marginal utility of any other good divided by its price in order for the consumer to maximize utility. Note, though, that the application of the rule of equal marginal utility per dollar spent is not an explicit or conscious act on the part of consumers. Rather, this is a model of consumer optimum.

HOW A PRICE CHANGE AFFECTS CONSUMER OPTIMUM

Consumption decisions are summarized in the law of demand, which states that the amount purchased is inversely related to price. We can now see why by using the law of diminishing marginal utility.

When a consumer has optimally allocated all her income to purchases, the marginal utility per dollar spent at current prices of goods and services is the same for each good or service she buys. No consumer will, when optimizing, buy 10 units of a good per unit time period when the marginal utility per dollar spent on the tenth unit of that good is less than the marginal utility per dollar spent on some other item.

If we start out at a consumer optimum and then observe a good's price decrease, we can predict that consumers will respond to the price decrease by consuming more of that good. This is because before the price change, the marginal utility per dollar spent on each good or service consumed was the same. Now, when a specific good's price is lower, it is possible to consume more of that good while continuing to equalize the marginal utility per dollar spent on that good with the marginal utility per dollar spent on other goods and services. If the law of diminishing marginal utility holds, then the purchase and consumption of additional units of the lower-priced good will cause the marginal utility from consuming the good to fall. Eventually it will fall to the point at which the marginal utility per dollar spent on the good is once again equalized with the marginal utility per dollar spent on other goods and services. At this point, the consumer will stop buying additional units of the lower-priced good.

A hypothetical demand curve for video rentals per week for a typical consumer is presented in Figure 19-2. At a rental price of \$5 per video, the marginal utility of the last video rented per week is MU_1. At a rental price of \$4 per video per week, the marginal utility is represented by MU_2. Because of the law of diminishing marginal utility—with the consumption of more videos, the marginal utility of the last unit of these additional videos is lower—MU_2 must be less than MU_1. What has happened is that at a lower price, the number of video rentals per week increased from two to three; marginal utility must

FIGURE 19-2
Video Rental Prices and Marginal Utility
The rate of video rentals per week will increase as long as the marginal utility per last video rental per week exceeds the cost of that rental. A reduction in price from $5 to $4 per video rental causes consumers to increase consumption until marginal utility falls from MU_1 to MU_2 (because of the law of diminishing marginal utility).

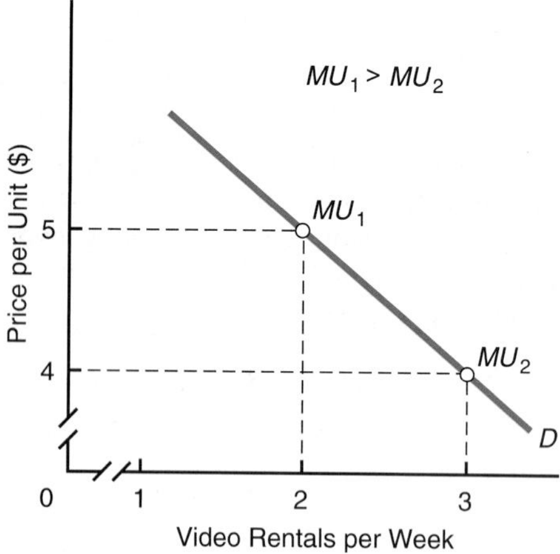

have fallen. At a higher consumption rate, the marginal utility falls in response to the rise in video consumption so that the marginal utility per dollar spent is equalized across purchases.

The Substitution Effect 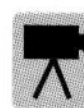

Substitution effect 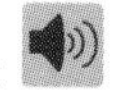
The tendency of people to substitute cheaper commodities for more expensive commodities.

Principle of substitution 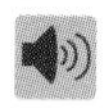
The principle that consumers and producers shift away from goods and resources that become priced relatively higher in favor of goods and resources that are now priced relatively lower.

What is happening as the price of video rental falls is that consumers are substituting the now relatively cheaper video rentals for other goods and services, such as restaurant meals and live concerts. We call this the **substitution effect** of a change in price of a good because it occurs when consumers substitute relatively cheaper goods for relatively more expensive ones.

We assume that people desire a variety of goods and pursue a variety of goals. That means that few, if any, goods are irreplaceable in meeting demand. We are generally able to substitute one product for another to satisfy demand. This is commonly referred to as the **principle of substitution.**

Let's assume now that there are several goods, not exactly the same, and perhaps even very different from one another, but all serving basically the same purpose. If the relative price of one particular good falls, we will most likely substitute in favor of the lower-priced good and against the other similar goods that we might have been purchasing. Conversely, if the price of that good rises relative to the price of the other similar goods, we will substitute in favor of them and not buy as much of the now higher-priced good. An example is the growth in purchases of personal computers since the late 1980s. As the relative price of computers has plummeted, people have substituted away from other, now relatively more expensive goods in favor of purchasing additional computers to use in their homes.

If the price of some item that you purchase goes down while your money income and all other prices stay the same, your ability to

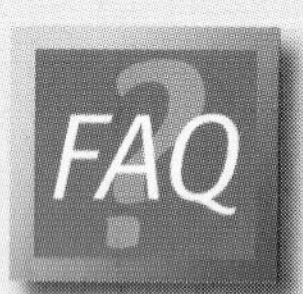

Is there a racial "digital divide" in home computer use and Internet access?

Yes. A study by Donna Hoffman and Thomas Novak of Vanderbilt University found that more than 40 percent of all white Americans now own a personal computer, whereas only about 25 percent of African Americans and Hispanic Americans have a computer at home. A key factor explaining different rates of computer ownership was income differences among the groups. There are smaller differences among Internet access rates for these groups, however. The reason is that many people who do not own personal computers can still get connected to the Internet at work or school.

purchase goods goes up. That is to say that your effective **purchasing power** is increased, even though your money income has stayed the same. If you purchase 20 gallons of gas a week at $1.60 per gallon, your total outlay for gas is $32. If the price goes down by 50 percent, to 80 cents a gallon, you would have to spend only $16 a week to purchase the same number of gallons of gas. If your money income and the prices of other goods remain the same, it would be possible for you to continue purchasing 20 gallons of gas a week *and* to purchase more of other goods. You will feel richer and will indeed probably purchase more of a number of goods, including perhaps even more gasoline.

Purchasing power 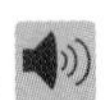
The value of money for buying goods and services. If your money income stays the same but the price of one good that you are buying goes up, your effective purchasing power falls, and vice versa.

The converse will also be true. When the price of one good you are purchasing goes up, without any other change in prices or income, the purchasing power of your income will drop. You will have to reduce your purchases of either the now higher-priced good or other goods (or a combination).

In general, this **real-income effect** is usually quite small. After all, unless we consider broad categories, such as housing or food, a change in the price of one particular item that we purchase will have a relatively small effect on our total purchasing power. Thus we expect the substitution effect usually to be more important than the real-income effect in causing us to purchase more of goods that have become cheaper and less of goods that have become more expensive.

Real-income effect 
The change in people's purchasing power that occurs when, other things being constant, the price of one good that they purchase changes. When that price goes up, real income, or purchasing power, falls, and when that price goes down, real income increases.

THE DEMAND CURVE REVISITED

Linking the "law" of diminishing marginal utility and the rule of equal marginal utilities per dollar gives us a negative relationship between the quantity demanded of a good or service and its price. As the relative price of video rentals goes up, for example, the quantity demanded will fall; and as the relative price of video rentals goes down, the quantity demanded will rise. Figure 19-2 shows this demand curve for video rentals. As the price of video rentals falls, the consumer can maximize total utility only by renting more videos, and vice versa. In other words, the relationship between price and quantity desired is simply a downward-sloping demand curve. Note, though, that this downward-sloping demand curve (the law of demand) is derived under the assumption of constant tastes and incomes. You must remember that we are keeping these important determining variables constant when we look at the relationship between price and quantity demanded.

Marginal Utility, Total Utility, and the Diamond-Water Paradox

Even though water is essential to life and diamonds are not, water is cheap and diamonds are dear. The economist Adam Smith in 1776 called this the "diamond-water paradox." The paradox is easily understood when we make the distinction between total utility and marginal utility. The total utility of water greatly exceeds the total utility derived from diamonds. What determines the price, though, is what happens on the margin. We have relatively few diamonds, so the marginal utility of the last diamond consumed is relatively high. The opposite is true for water. Total utility does not determine what people are willing to pay for a unit of a particular commodity; marginal utility does. Look at the situation graphically in Figure 19-3 on page 466. We show the demand curve for diamonds, labeled D_{diamonds}. The demand curve for water is labeled D_{water}. We plot quantity in terms of kilograms per unit time period on the horizontal axis. On the vertical axis we plot price in dollars per kilogram. We use kilograms as our common unit of measurement for water and for diamonds. We could just as well have used gallons, acre-feet, or liters.

FIGURE 19-3

The Diamond-Water Paradox

We pick kilograms as a common unit of measurement for both water and diamonds. To demonstrate that the demand and supply of water is immense, we have put a break in the horizontal quantity axis. Although the demand for water is much greater than the demand for diamonds, the marginal valuation of water is given by the marginal value placed on the last unit of water consumed. To find that, we must know the supply of water, which is given as S_1. At that supply, the price of water is P_{water}. But the supply for diamonds is given by S_2. At that supply, the price of diamonds is $P_{diamonds}$. The total valuation that consumers place on water is tremendous relative to the total valuation consumers place on diamonds. What is important for price determination, however, is the marginal valuation, or the marginal utility received.

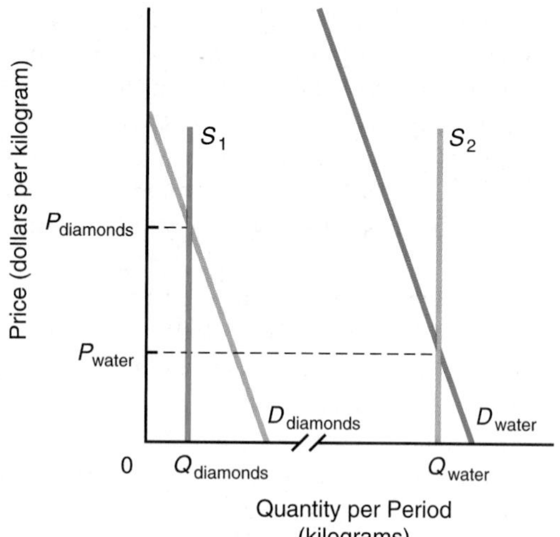

Notice that the demand for water is many, many times the demand for diamonds (even though we really don't show this in the diagram). We draw the supply curve of water as S_1 at a quantity of Q_{water}. The supply curve for diamonds is given as S_2 at quantity $Q_{diamonds}$. At the intersection of the supply curve of water with the demand curve of water, the price per kilogram is P_{water}. The intersection of the supply curve of diamonds with the demand curve of diamonds is at $P_{diamonds}$. Notice that $P_{diamonds}$ exceeds P_{water}. Diamonds sell at a higher price than water.

INTERNATIONAL EXAMPLE

Water in Saudi Arabia

The diamond-water paradox deals with the situation in which water, although necessary for life, may be much cheaper than some luxury item. In Saudi Arabia, as you might expect, the contrary can be true. A liter of water costs five times as much as a liter of gasoline, whereas a pair of custom-made British wool dress pants costs only $20. These relative prices are quite different from what we are used to seeing in America. Water costs next to nothing, a liter of gas about 40 cents, and custom-made wool pants at least $200. To understand what has happened in Saudi Arabia, simply substitute gasoline for water and water for diamonds in Figure 19-3.

For Critical Analysis

List some of the effects on human behavior that such a high relative price of water would cause.

CONCEPTS IN BRIEF

- The law of diminishing marginal utility tells us that each successive marginal unit of a good consumed adds less extra utility.
- Each consumer with a limited income must make a choice about the basket of commodities to purchase; economic theory assumes that the consumer chooses the basket of commodities that yields optimum consumption. The consumer maximizes total utility by equating the marginal utility of the last dollar spent on one good with the marginal utility per last dollar spent on all other goods. That is the state of consumer optimum.
- To remain in consumer optimum, a price decrease requires an increase in consumption; a price increase requires a decrease in consumption.

- Each change in price has a substitution effect and a real-income effect. When price falls, the consumer substitutes in favor of the relatively cheaper good. When price falls, the consumer's real purchasing power increases, causing the consumer to purchase more of most goods. The opposite would occur when price increases. Assuming that the law of diminishing marginal utility holds, the demand curve must slope downward.

NETNOMICS

The Meat and Potatoes of On-Line Shopping

In their quest to avoid time-consuming phone calls to travel agents or trips to shopping malls, millions of American consumers now routinely order airline tickets, books, and videos over the Internet. Nevertheless, even though the typical household goes to the grocery store two to three times per week, grocery shopping over the Internet has been slow to take off. Sales of groceries are small potatoes in comparison with the Internet sales of products offered by companies such as Amazon.com or Ticketmaster.

Consider the experience of NetGrocer Inc., a New York company that had worked out special promotional arrangements with America Online and Yahoo! Within a year after setting up a Web site modeled on that of Amazon.com—but designed for placing orders for items such as canned goods, toilet paper, and toothpaste instead of books—NetGrocer had laid off more than half of its staff and fired its chief executive officer. The company's problem was simple, provided that you think like an economist who understands consumer choice. The big advantage of Internet shopping is that it can save an individual the time and trouble of shopping in person. That is, Internet shopping reduces the opportunity cost of shopping, which reduces the *total* price that a person must pay for an airline ticket, a book, or a basket of groceries.

Like other Internet-grocery startups, NetGrocer shipped only dry goods and bottled beverages. It did not ship perishable goods that must be refrigerated, such as milk, butter, and eggs. Consequently, people who made Web purchases from NetGrocer still had to shop at their local grocery store. As long as shoppers had to go to the store anyway, few could see a big cost advantage in buying their nonrefrigerated grocery items over the Net.

Thus the grocery business has been a tough market for new Internet companies to crack. Indeed, some observers of the industry think that the biggest opportunities to earn profits by selling groceries on the Internet are available to existing grocers. Many of these companies already have chains of grocery stores spread across large regions. To start competing via the Internet, all these companies have to do is post Web pages, lease delivery trucks, and hire clerks to stock orders and drivers to make home deliveries. Indeed, a number of existing grocers are entering the Internet-shopping business, which some in the industry project could ultimately account for between 5 and 10 percent of total grocery sales within the next five years.

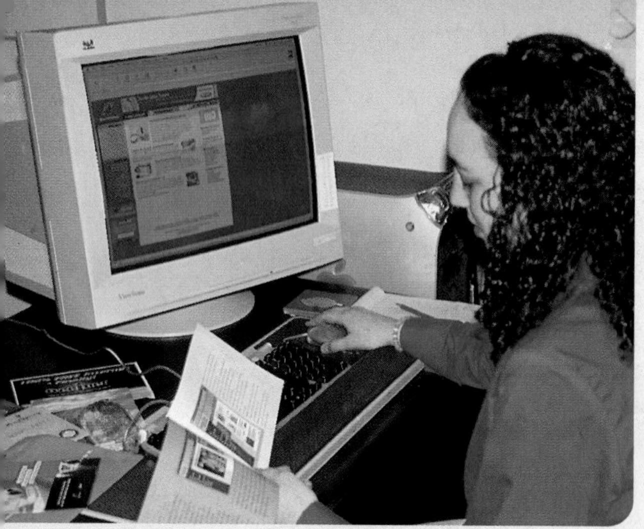

ISSUES & APPLICATIONS

Should You Be Charged to Use the Internet?

Many Internet users continue to experience intermittent problems with delays in data transmission. System failures occur from time to time. A few years ago, Internet traffic in Scandanavia became so congested that network administrators temporarily shut down all Internet transmissions throughout much of northern Europe. It turned out that a single user had tried to download a huge multimedia file and had overloaded the system. Network administrators were able to restore access to other users once they located and disconnected the computer belonging to the individual who had tried to download the file. He said that he didn't mean to cause a problem; he was just bored and was spending some free time "playing around" on the Internet.

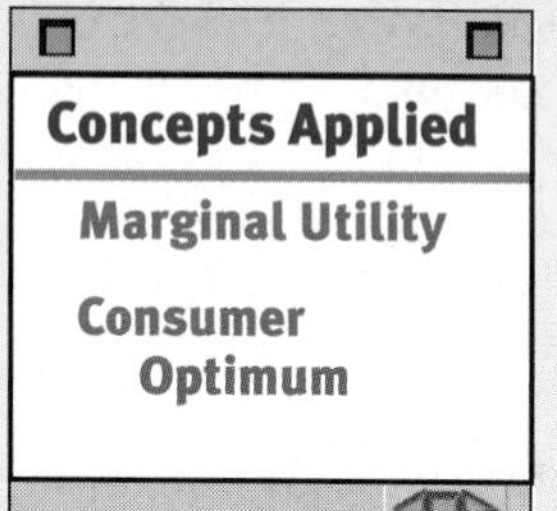

Consumer Choice with a Nearly Zero Price of Usage

Some economists believe that the Internet congestion problem will get worse before it gets better. The problem, they argue, is that for many users, the price of using the Internet is much too low. Recall that as a result of the choices a consumer makes, for the last dollar spent on each good or service, the ratio of marginal utility to price will be the same.

For example, suppose that for a typical individual, a consumer optimum is attained when the ratio of marginal utility to price for each good or service consumed is a relatively small positive number, such as 1 unit of utility per dollar spent. Now suppose that another good that a typical individual consumes is Internet access time, which has an explicit price very close to zero. At a consumer optimum in which the marginal utility per dollar is not a huge number (such as 1), this will require spending sufficient time on the Internet to push the marginal utility of surfing the Net very close to zero as well. Compared to the units of utility from consuming other goods, how could a consumer derive such little additional utility from an hour's worth of time on the Internet? The law of diminishing marginal utility tells us that utility ultimately declines with greater consumption of a good. Thus pushing the marginal utility from surfing the Net close to zero likely entails spending *many* hours surfing the Web. Because spending time on the Internet is such a low-cost activity, the individual ends up spending a large number of hours on the Internet, thereby contributing to the potential for Internet congestion.

Good News for the Internet: People Value Their Time

The *effective* price of Internet usage is probably much higher than "nearly zero," however. Most people place a value on their time that is well above zero. After all, an hour spent surfing the Net could otherwise be allocated to earning income at a market wage. Even for a person possessing very few skills, this opportunity cost of time is likely to be at least a couple of dollars per hour. For the average person, the effective price of using the Internet—inclusive of both explicit and implicit costs—is probably several dollars per hour. In the context of our numerical example, suppose that this effective price is $10 per hour. At this price, attaining a ratio of 1 unit of utility per dollar spent on the last hour of Internet access entails a marginal utility of 10 units per hour. The law of diminishing marginal utility thereby implies that a person who places a relatively high value on his time will likely spend much less time surfing the Net.

Explicit pricing of Internet usage would undoubtedly reduce Internet congestion problems. Nonetheless, a big check on "overuse" of the Net is that many people value their time at more than $0 per hour.

FOR CRITICAL ANALYSIS

1. How could time-based fees for Internet usage be assessed?
2. Who could assess fees for using the Internet? What might they do with the funds?

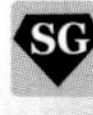

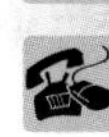

SUMMARY DISCUSSION OF LEARNING OBJECTIVES

1. **Total Utility Versus Marginal Utility:** Total utility is the total satisfaction that an individual derives from consuming a given amount of a good or service during a given period. By way of contrast, marginal utility is the additional satisfaction that a person gains by consuming an additional unit of the good or service.
2. **The Law of Diminishing Marginal Utility:** For at least the first unit of consumption of a good or service, a person's marginal utility increases with increased consumption. Eventually, however, the rate at which an individual's utility rises with greater consumption tends to fall. Thus marginal utility ultimately declines as the person consumes more and more of the good or service.
3. **The Consumer Optimum:** An individual optimally allocates available income to consumption of all goods and services when the marginal utility per dollar spent on the last unit consumed of each good is equalized. Thus a consumer optimum occurs when the ratio of the marginal utility derived from consuming a good or service to the price of that good or service is equal across all goods and services that the person consumes and when the person spends all available income.
4. **The Substitution Effect of a Price Change:** One effect of a change in the price of a good or service is that the price change induces people to substitute among goods. For example, if the price of a good rises, the individual will tend to consume some other good that has become relatively less expensive as a result. In addition, the individual will tend to reduce consumption of the good whose price increased.
5. **The Real-Income Effect of a Price Change:** Another effect of a price change is that it affects the purchasing power of an individual's available income. For instance, if there is an increase in the price of a good, a person must reduce purchases of either the now higher-priced good or other goods (or a combination of both of these responses). Normally, we anticipate that the real-income effect is smaller than the substitution effect, so that when the price of a good or service increases, people will purchase more of goods or services that have lower relative prices as a result.
6. **Why the Price of Diamonds Exceeds the Price of Water Even Though People Cannot Long Survive Without Water:** The reason for this price difference is that marginal utility, not total utility, determines how much people are willing to pay for any particular good. Because there are relatively few diamonds, the number of diamonds consumed by a typical individual is relatively small, which means that the marginal utility derived from consuming a diamond is relatively high. By contrast, water is abundant, so people consume relatively large volumes of water, and the marginal utility for the last unit of water consumed is relatively low. It follows that at a consumer optimum, in which the marginal utility per dollar spent is equalized for diamonds and water, people are willing to pay a much higher price for diamonds.

Key Terms and Concepts

Consumer optimum (461)
Diminishing marginal utility (459)
Marginal utility (457)
Principle of substitution (464)
Purchasing power (465)
Real-income effect (465)
Substitution effect (464)
Util (457)
Utility (456)
Utility analysis (456)

Problems

Answers to the odd-numbered problems appear at the back of the book.

19-1. The campus pizzeria sells a single pizza for $12. If you order a second pizza, however, its price is only $5. Explain how this relates to marginal utility.

19-2. As an individual consumes more units of an item, the person eventually experiences diminishing marginal utility. This means that in order to increase marginal utility, the person must often consume less of an item. This seems paradoxical. Explain the logic of this using the example in Problem 19-1.

19-3. Complete the missing cells in the table.

Number of Cheese-burgers	Total Utility of Cheese-burgers	Marginal Utility of Cheese-burgers	Bags of French Fries	Total Utility of French Fries	Marginal Utility of French Fries
0	0	—	0	0	—
1	20	—	1	—	8
2	36	—	2	—	6
3	—	12	3	—	4
4	—	8	4	20	—
5	—	4	5	20	—

19-4. If the price of a cheeseburger is $2 and the price of a bag of french fries is $1 and you have $6 to spend (and you spend all of it), what is the utility-maximizing combination of cheeseburgers and french fries?

19-5. Suppose that you observe that total utility rises as more of an item is consumed. What can you say for certain about marginal utility? Can you say for sure that it is rising or falling or that it is positive or negative?

19-6. After monitoring your daily consumption patterns, you determine that your daily consumption of soft drinks is 3 and your daily consumption of tacos is 4 when the prices per unit are 50 cents and $1, respectively. Explain what happens to your consumption bundle, the marginal utility of soft drinks, and the marginal utility of tacos when the price of soft drinks rises to 75 cents.

19-7. At a consumer optimum, for all goods purchased, marginal utility per dollar spent is equalized. A high school student is deciding between attending Western State University and Eastern State University. The student cannot attend both universities simultaneously. Both are fine universities, but the reputation of Western is slightly higher, as is the tuition. Use the rule of consumer optimum to explain how the student will go about deciding which university to attend.

19-8. Suppose that 5 apples and 6 bananas generate a total utility of 50 for you. In addition, 4 apples and 8 bananas generate a total utility of 50. Given this information, what can you say about the marginal utility of apples relative to the marginal utility of bananas?

19-9. Return to Problem 19-4. Suppose that the price of cheeseburgers falls to $1. Determine the new utility-maximizing combination of cheeseburgers and french fries. Use this new combination of goods to explain the income and substitution effects.

19-10. Using your answers to Problems 19-4 and 19-9, illustrate a simple demand curve for cheeseburgers.

Economics on the Net

Book Prices and Consumer Optimum This application helps you see how a consumer optimum can be attained when one engages in Internet shopping.

Title: Amazon.com Web Site

Navigation: Click here to start at Amazon.com's homepage. Click on the Books tab.

Application

1. On the right-hand side of the page, find the list of the top books in the Amazon.com 100 section. Click on the number 1 book. Record the price of the book. Then, locate the Search window. Type in Roger LeRoy Miller. Scroll down until you find your class text listed. Record the price.
2. Suppose you are an individual who has purchased both the number 1 book and your class text through Amazon.com. Describe how economic analysis would explain this choice.
3. Using the prices you recorded for the two books, write an equation that relates the prices and your marginal utilities of the two books. Use this equation to explain verbally how you might quantify the magnitude of your marginal utility for the number 1 book relative to your marginal utility for your class text.

For Group Study and Analysis Discuss what changes might occur if the price of the number 1 book were lowered but the student remains enrolled in this course. Discuss what changes might take place regarding the consumer optimum if the student was not enrolled in this course.

APPENDIX E

MORE ADVANCED CONSUMER CHOICE THEORY

It is possible to analyze consumer choice verbally, as we did for the most part in Chapter 19. The theory of diminishing marginal utility can be fairly well accepted on intuitive grounds and by introspection. If we want to be more formal and perhaps more elegant in our theorizing, however, we can translate our discussion into a graphical analysis with what we call *indifference curves* and the *budget constraint.* Here we discuss these terms and their relationship and demonstrate consumer equilibrium in geometric form.

ON BEING INDIFFERENT

What does it mean to be indifferent? It usually means that you don't care one way or the other about something—you are equally disposed to either of two alternatives. With this interpretation in mind, we will turn to two choices, video rentals and restaurant meals. In panel (a) of Figure E-1, we show several combinations of video rentals and restaurant meals per week that a representative consumer considers equally satisfactory. That is to say, for each combination, *A, B, C,* and *D,* this consumer will have exactly the same level of total utility.

The simple numerical example that we have used happens to concern video rentals and restaurant meals per week. This example is used to illustrate general features of indifference curves and related analytical tools that are necessary for deriving the demand curve. Obviously, we could have used any two commodities. Just remember that we are using a *specific* example to illustrate a *general* analysis.

We can plot these combinations graphically in panel (b) of Figure E-1, with restaurant meals per week on the horizontal axis and video rentals per week on the vertical axis. These are our consumer's indifference combinations—the consumer finds each combination as acceptable as the others. When we connect these combinations with a smooth curve, we obtain

FIGURE E-1

Combinations That Yield Equal Levels of Satisfaction

A, B, C, and *D* represent combinations of video rentals and restaurant meals per week that give an equal level of satisfaction to this consumer. In other words, the consumer is indifferent among these four combinations.

Panel (a)

Combination	Video Rentals per Week	Restaurant Meals per Week
A	1	7
B	2	4
C	3	2
D	4	1

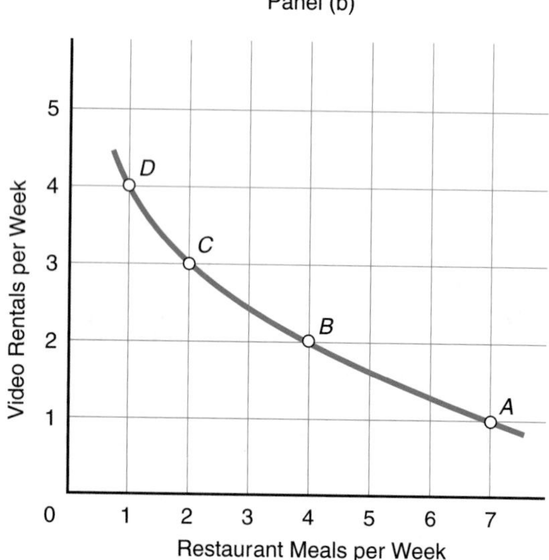

what is called the consumer's **indifference curve.** Along the indifference curve, every combination of the two goods in question yields the same level of satisfaction. Every point along the indifference curve is equally desirable to the consumer. For example, four video rentals per week and one restaurant meal per week will give our representative consumer exactly the same total satisfaction as two video rentals per week and four restaurant meals per week.

Indifference curve 
A curve composed of a set of consumption alternatives, each of which yields the same total amount of satisfaction.

PROPERTIES OF INDIFFERENCE CURVES

Indifference curves have special properties relating to their slope and shape.

Downward Slope

The indifference curve shown in panel (b) of Figure E-1 slopes downward; that is, it has a negative slope. Now consider Figure E-2. Here we show two points, *A* and *B*. Point *A* represents four video rentals per week and two restaurant meals per week. Point *B* represents five video rentals per week and six restaurant meals per week. Clearly, *B* is always preferred to *A* because *B* represents more of everything. If *B* is always preferred to *A*, it is impossible for points *A* and *B* to be on the same indifference curve because the definition of the indifference curve is a set of combinations of two goods that are preferred equally.

Curvature

The indifference curve that we have drawn in panel (b) of Figure E-1 is special. Notice that it is curved. Why didn't we just draw a straight line, as we have usually done for a demand curve? To find out why we don't posit straight-line indifference curves, consider the implications. We show such a straight-line indifference curve in Figure E-3 (p. 474). Start at point *A*. The consumer has no restaurant meals and five video rentals per week. Now the consumer wishes to go to point *B*. He or she is willing to give up only one video rental in order to get one restaurant meal. Now let's assume that the consumer is at point *C*, consuming one video rental and four restaurant meals per week. If the consumer wants to go to point *D*, he or she is again willing to give up one video rental in order to get one more restaurant meal per week.

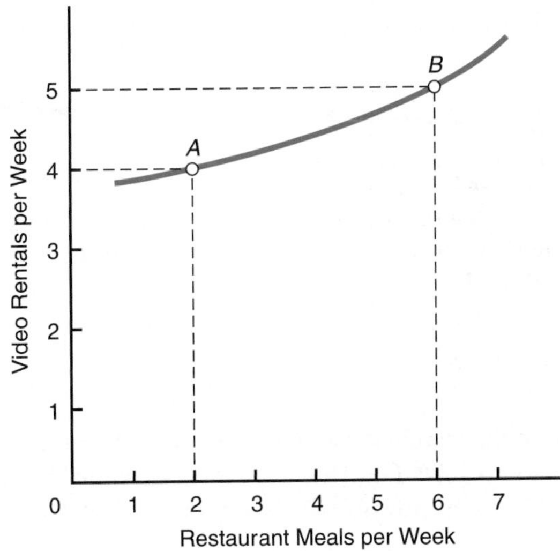

FIGURE E-2
Indifference Curves: Impossibility of an Upward Slope
Point *B* represents a consumption of more video rentals per week and more restaurant meals per week than point *A*. *B* is always preferred to *A*. Therefore, *A* and *B* cannot be on the same indifference curve, which is positively sloped, because an indifference curve shows *equally preferred* combinations of the two goods.

FIGURE E-3

Implications of a Straight-Line Indifference Curve

If the indifference curve is a straight line, the consumer will be willing to give up the same number of video rentals (one for one in this simple example) to get one more restaurant meal per week, whether the consumer has no restaurant meals or a lot of restaurant meals per week. For example, the consumer at point *A* has five video rentals and no restaurant meals per week. He or she is willing to give up one video rental in order to get one restaurant meal per week. At point *C,* however, the consumer has only one video rental and four restaurant meals per week. Because of the straight-line indifference curve, this consumer is willing to give up the last video rental in order to get one more restaurant meal per week, even though he or she already has four.

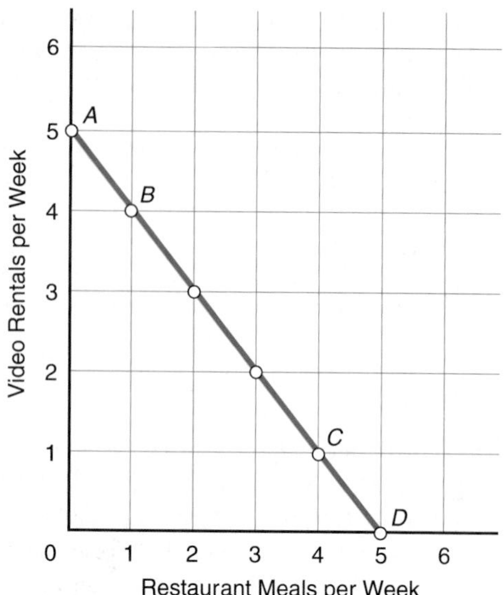

In other words, no matter how many videos the consumer rents, he or she is willing to give up one video rental to get one restaurant meal per week—which does not seem plausible. Doesn't it make sense to hypothesize that the more videos the consumer rents per week, the less he or she will value an *additional* video rental? Presumably, when the consumer has five video rentals and no restaurant meals per week, he or she should be willing to give up more than one video rental in order to get one restaurant meal. Therefore, a straight-line indifference curve as shown in Figure E-3 no longer seems plausible.

In mathematical jargon, an indifference curve is convex with respect to the origin. Let's look at this in panel (a) of Figure E-1 on page 472. Starting with combination *A,* the consumer has one video rental but seven restaurant meals per week. To remain indifferent, the consumer would have to be willing to give up three restaurant meals to obtain one more video rental (as shown in combination *B*). However, to go from combination *C* to combination *D,* notice that the consumer would have to be willing to give up only one restaurant meal for an additional video rental per week. The quantity of the substitute considered acceptable changes as the rate of consumption of the original item changes.

Consequently, the indifference curve in panel (b) of Figure E-1 will be convex when viewed from the origin.

THE MARGINAL RATE OF SUBSTITUTION

Instead of using marginal utility, we can talk in terms of the *marginal rate of substitution* between restaurant meals and video rentals per week. We can formally define the consumer's marginal rate of substitution as follows:

> The marginal rate of substitution is equal to the change in the quantity of one good that just offsets a one-unit change in the consumption of another good, such that total satisfaction remains constant.

We can see numerically what happens to the marginal rate of substitution in our example if we rearrange panel (a) of Figure E-1 into Table E-1. Here we show restaurant meals in the second column and video rentals in the third. Now we ask the question, what change

(1) Combination	(2) Restaurant Meals Per Week	(3) Video Rentals Per Week	(4) Marginal Rate of Substitution of Restaurant Meals for Video Rentals
A	7	1	
			3:1
B	4	2	
			2:1
C	2	3	
			1:1
D	1	4	

TABLE E-1

Calculating the Marginal Rate of Substitution

As we move from combination *A* to combination *B*, we are still on the same indifference curve. To stay on that curve, the number of restaurant meals decreases by three and the number of video rentals increases by one. The marginal rate of substitution is 3:1. A three-unit decrease in restaurant meals requires an increase in one video rental to leave the consumer's total utility unaltered.

in the consumption of video rentals per week will just compensate for a three-unit change in the consumption of restaurant meals per week and leave the consumer's total utility constant? The movement from *A* to *B* increases video rental consumption by one. Here the marginal rate of substitution is 3:1—a three-unit decrease in restaurant meals requires an increase of one video rental to leave the consumer's total utility unaltered. Thus the consumer values the three restaurant meals as the equivalent of one video rental. We do this for the rest of the table and find that as restaurant meals decrease further, the marginal rate of substitution goes from 3:1 to 2:1 to 1:1. The marginal rate of substitution of restaurant meals for video rentals per week falls as the consumer obtains more video rentals. That is, the consumer values successive units of video rentals less and less in terms of restaurant meals. The first video rental is valued at three restaurant meals; the last (fourth) video rental is valued at only one restaurant meal. The fact that the marginal rate of substitution falls is sometimes called the *law of substitution.*

In geometric language, the slope of the consumer's indifference curve (actually, the negative of the slope) measures the consumer's marginal rate of substitution. Notice that this marginal rate of substitution is purely subjective or psychological.

THE INDIFFERENCE MAP

Let's now consider the possibility of having both more video rentals *and* more restaurant meals per week. When we do this, we can no longer stay on the same indifference curve that we drew in Figure E-1. That indifference curve was drawn for equally satisfying combinations of video rentals and restaurant meals per week. If the individual can now obtain more of both, a new indifference curve will have to be drawn, above and to the right of the one shown in panel (b) of Figure E-1. Alternatively, if the individual faces the possibility of having less of both video rentals and restaurant meals per week, an indifference curve will have to be drawn below and to the left of the one in panel (b) of Figure E-1. We can map out a whole set of indifference curves corresponding to these possibilities.

Figure E-4 on page 476 shows three possible indifference curves. Indifference curves that are higher than others necessarily imply that for every given quantity of one good, more of the other good can be obtained on a higher indifference curve. Looked at another way, if one goes from curve I_1 to I_2, it is possible to consume the same number of restaurant meals *and* be able to rent more videos per week. This is shown as a movement from point *A* to point *B* in Figure E-4. We could do it the other way. When we move from a lower to a higher indifference

FIGURE E-4

A Set of Indifference Curves

An infinite number of indifference curves can be drawn. We show three possible ones. Realize that a higher indifference curve represents the possibility of higher rates of consumption of both goods. Hence a higher indifference curve is preferred to a lower one because more is preferred to less. Look at points *A* and *B*. Point *B* represents more video rentals than point *A;* therefore, bundles on indifference curve I_2 have to be preferred over bundles on I_1 because the number of restaurant meals per week is the same at points *A* and *B*.

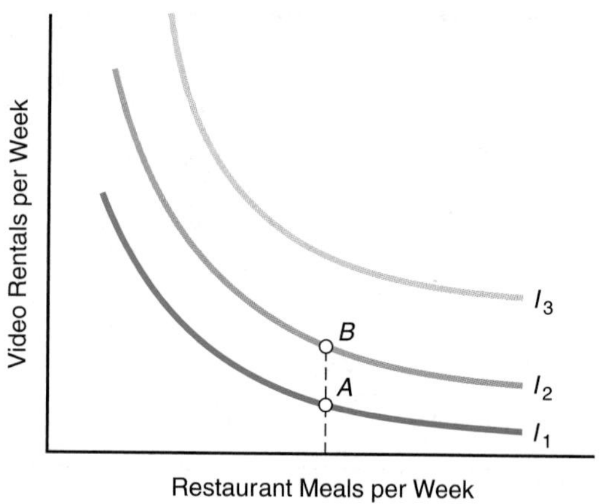

curve, it is possible to rent the same number of videos *and* to consume more restaurant meals per week. Thus the higher a consumer is on the indifference map, the greater that consumer's total level of satisfaction.

THE BUDGET CONSTRAINT

Budget constraint 
All of the possible combinations of goods that can be purchased (at fixed prices) with a specific budget.

Our problem here is to find out how to maximize consumer satisfaction. To do so, we must consult not only our *preferences*—given by indifference curves—but also our *market opportunities*—given by our available income and prices, called our **budget constraint.** We might want more of everything, but for any given budget constraint, we have to make choices, or trade-offs, among possible goods. Everyone has a budget constraint; that is, everyone faces a limited consumption potential. How do we show this graphically? We must find the prices of the goods in question and determine the maximum consumption of each allowed by our budget. For example, let's assume that videos rent for \$10 apiece and restaurant meals cost \$20. Let's also assume that our representative consumer has a total budget of \$60 per week. What is the maximum number of videos the consumer can rent? Six. And the maximum number of restaurant meals per week he or she can consume? Three. So now, as shown in Figure E-5, we have two points on our budget line, which is sometimes called the *consumption possibilities curve.* These anchor points of the budget line are obtained by dividing money income by the price of each product. The first point is at *b* on the vertical axis; the second, at *b′* on the horizontal axis. The budget line is linear because prices are given.

Any combination along line *bb′* is possible; in fact, any combination in the colored area is possible. We will assume, however, that the individual consumer completely uses up the available budget, and we will consider as possible only those points along *bb′*.

Slope of the Budget Constraint

The budget constraint is a line that slopes downward from left to right. The slope of that line has a special meaning. Look carefully at the budget line in Figure E-5. Remember from our discussion of graphs in Appendix A that we measure a negative slope by the ratio of the fall in *Y* over the run in *X*. In this case, *Y* is video rentals per week and *X* is restaurant meals per week. In Figure E-5, the fall in *Y* is − 2 video rentals per week (a drop from 4 to 2) for

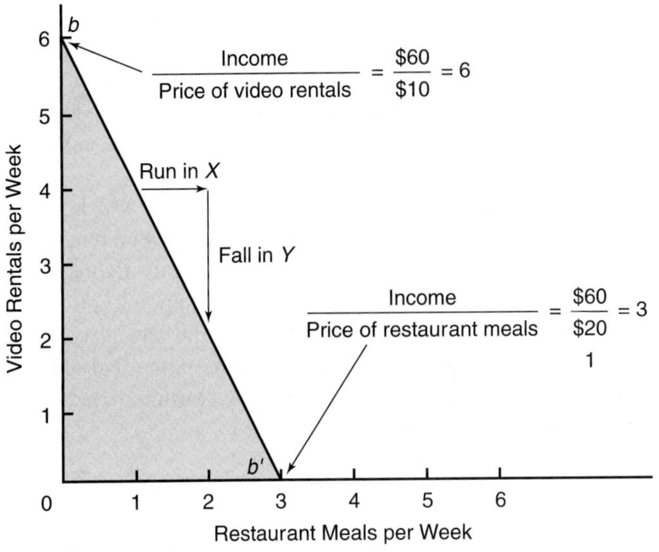

FIGURE E-5
The Budget Constraint
The line *bb′* represents this individual's budget constraint. Assuming that video rentals cost $10 each, restaurant meals cost $20 each, and the individual has a budget of $60 per week, a maximum of six video rentals or three restaurant meals can be bought each week. These two extreme points are connected to form the budget constraint. All combinations within the colored area and on the budget constraint line are feasible.

a run in *X* of one restaurant meal per week (an increase from 1 to 2); therefore, the slope of the budget constraint is $-2/1$, or -2. This slope of the budget constraint represents the rate of exchange between video rentals and restaurant meals.

Now we are ready to determine how the consumer achieves the optimum consumption rate.

CONSUMER OPTIMUM REVISITED

Consumers will try to attain the highest level of total utility possible, given their budget constraints. How can this be shown graphically? We draw a set of indifference curves similar to those in Figure E-4, and we bring in reality—the budget constraint *bb′*. Both are drawn in Figure E-6. Because a higher level of total satisfaction is represented by a higher indifference curve, we know that the consumer will strive to be on the highest indifference

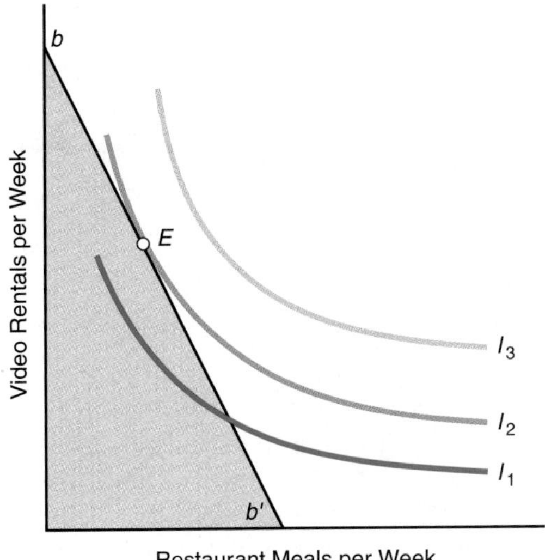

FIGURE E-6
Consumer Optimum
A consumer reaches an optimum when he or she ends up on the highest indifference curve possible, given a limited budget. This occurs at the tangency between an indifference curve and the budget constraint. In this diagram, the tangency is at *E*.

curve possible. However, the consumer cannot get to indifference curve I_3 because the budget will be exhausted before any combination of video rentals and restaurant meals represented on indifference curve I_3 is attained. This consumer can maximize total utility, subject to the budget constraint, only by being at point E on indifference curve I_2 because here the consumer's income is just being exhausted. Mathematically, point E is called the *tangency point* of the curve I_2 to the straight line bb'.

Click here for a numerical example illustrating the consumer optimum.

Consumer optimum is achieved when the marginal rate of substitution (which is subjective) is just equal to the feasible, or realistic, rate of exchange between video rentals and restaurant meals. This realistic rate is the ratio of the two prices of the goods involved. It is represented by the absolute value of the slope of the budget constraint. At point E, the point of tangency between indifference curve I_2 and budget constraint bb', the rate at which the consumer wishes to substitute video rentals for restaurant meals (the numerical value of slope of the indifference curve) is just equal to the rate at which the consumer *can* substitute video rentals for restaurant meals (the slope of the budget line).

EFFECTS OF CHANGES IN INCOME

A change in income will shift the budget constraint bb' in Figure E-6. Consider only increases in income and no changes in price. The budget constraint will shift outward. Each new budget line will be parallel to the original one because we are not allowing a change in the relative prices of video rentals and restaurant meals. We would now like to find out how an individual consumer responds to successive increases in income when relative prices remain constant. We do this in Figure E-7. We start out with an income that is represented by a budget line bb'. Consumer optimum is at point E, where the consumer attains the highest indifference curve I_1, given the budget constraint bb'. Now we let income increase. This is shown by a shift outward in the budget line to cc'. The consumer attains a new optimum at point E'. That is where a higher indifference curve, I_2, is reached. Again, the consumer's income is increased so that the new budget line is dd'. The new optimum now moves to E''. This is where indifference curve I_3 is reached. If we connect the three consumer optimum points, E, E', and E'', we have what is called an income-consumption curve. The **income-consumption curve** shows the optimum consumption points that

Income-consumption curve The set of optimum consumption points that would occur if income were increased, relative prices remaining constant.

FIGURE E-7

Income-Consumption Curve

We start off with income sufficient to yield budget constraint bb'. The highest attainable indifference curve is I_1, which is just tangent to bb' at E. Next we increase income. The budget line moves outward to cc', which is parallel to bb'. The new highest indifference curve is I_2, which is just tangent to cc' at E'. We increase income again, which is represented by a shift in the budget line to dd'. The new tangency point of the highest indifference curve, I_3, with dd', is at point E''. When we connect these three points, we obtain the income-consumption curve.

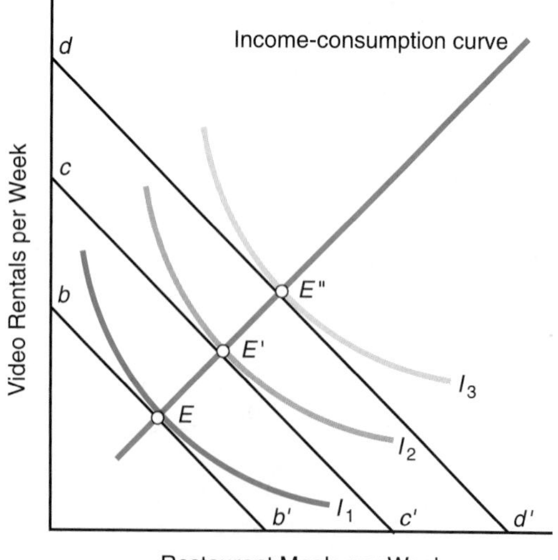

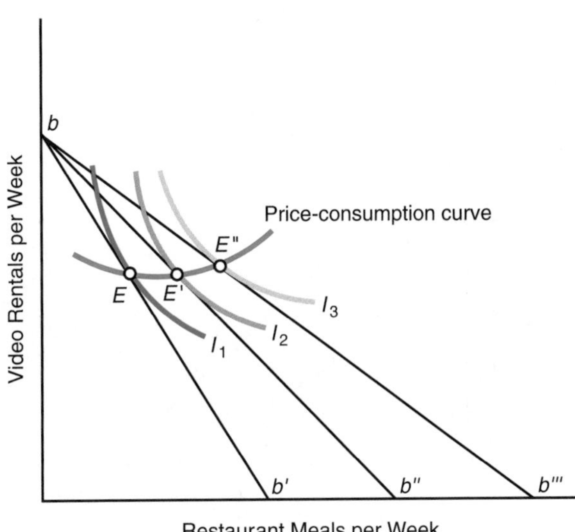

FIGURE E-8

Price-Consumption Curve

As we lower the price of restaurant meals, income measured in terms of restaurant meals per week increases. We show this by rotating the budget constraint from *bb'* to *bb''* and finally to *bb'''*. We then find the highest indifference curve that is attainable for each successive budget constraint. For budget constraint *bb'*, the highest indifference curve is I_1, which is tangent to *bb'* at point *E*. We do this for the next two budget constraints. When we connect the optimum points, *E*, *E'*, and *E''*, we derive the price-consumption curve, which shows the combinations of the two commodities that a consumer will purchase when money income and the price of one commodity remain constant while the other commodity's price changes.

would occur if income for that consumer were increased continuously, holding the prices of video rentals and restaurant meals constant.

THE PRICE-CONSUMPTION CURVE

In Figure E-8, we hold money income and the price of video rentals constant while we lower the price of restaurant meals. As we keep lowering the price of restaurant meals, the quantity of meals that could be purchased if all income were spent on restaurant meals increases; thus the extreme points for the budget constraint keep moving outward to the right as the price of restaurant meals falls. In other words, the budget line rotates outward from *bb'* to *bb''* and *bb'''*. Each time the price of restaurant meals falls, a new budget line is formed. There has to be a new optimum point. We find it by locating on each new budget line the highest attainable indifference curve. This is shown at points *E*, *E'*, and *E''*. We see that as price decreases for restaurant meals, the consumer purchases more restaurant meals per week. We call the line connecting points *E*, *E'*, and *E''* the **price-consumption curve.** It connects the tangency points of the budget constraints and indifference curves, thus showing the amounts of two goods that a consumer will buy when money income and the price of one commodity are held constant while the price of the remaining good changes.

Price-consumption curve
The set of consumer optimum combinations of two goods that the consumer would choose as the price of one good changes, while money income and the price of the other good remain constant.

DERIVING THE DEMAND CURVE

We are now in a position to derive the demand curve using indifference curve analysis. In panel (a) of Figure E-9 on page 480, we show what happens when the price of restaurant meals decreases, holding both the price of video rentals and income constant. If the price of restaurant meals decreases, the budget line rotates from *bb'* to *bb''*. The two optimum points are given by the tangency at the highest indifference curve that just touches those two budget lines. This is at *E* and *E'*. But those two points give us two price-quantity pairs. At point *E*, the price of restaurant meals is \$20; the quantity demanded is 2. Thus we have one point that we can transfer to panel (b) of Figure E-9. At point *E'*, we have another price-quantity pair. The price has fallen to \$10; the quantity demanded has increased to 5. We therefore transfer this other point to panel (b). When we connect these two points (and all the others in between), we derive the demand curve for restaurant meals; it slopes downward.

FIGURE E-9

Deriving the Demand Curve

In panel (a), we show the effects of a decrease in the price of restaurant meals from $20 to $10. At $20, the highest indifference curve touches the budget line *bb′* at point *E*. The quantity of restaurant meals consumed is two. We transfer this combination—price, $20; quantity demanded, 2—down to panel (b). Next we decrease the price of restaurant meals to $10. This generates a new budget line, or constraint, which is *bb″*. Consumer optimum is now at *E′*. The optimum quantity of restaurant meals demanded at a price of $10 is five. We transfer this point—price, $10; quantity demanded, 5—down to panel (b). When we connect these two points, we have a demand curve, *D*, for restaurant meals.

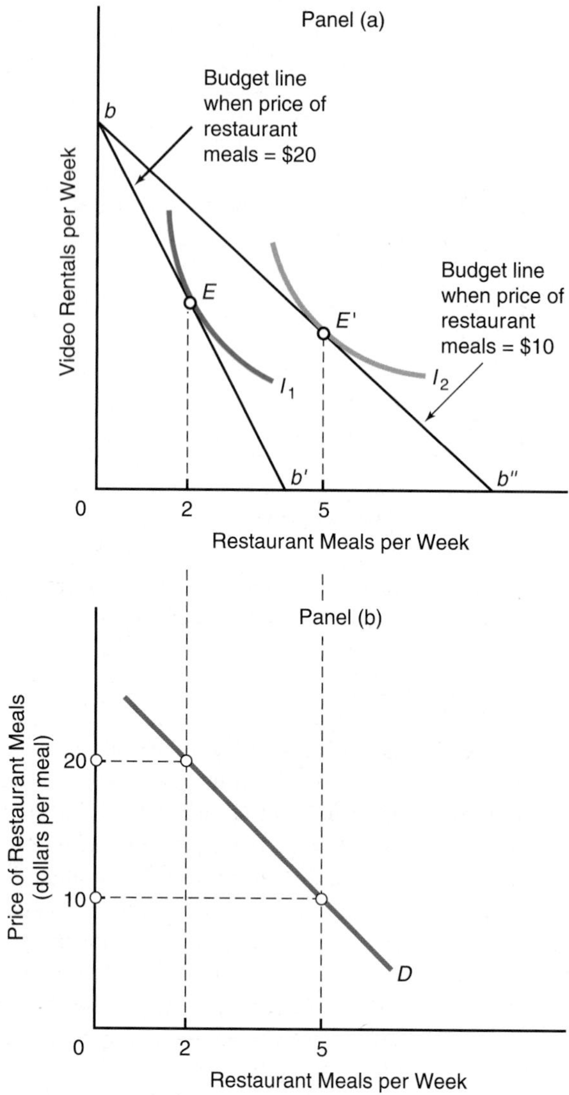

Appendix Summary

1. Along an indifference curve, the consumer experiences equal levels of satisfaction. That is to say, along any indifference curve, every combination of the two goods in question yields exactly the same level of satisfaction.
2. Indifference curves usually slope downward and are usually convex to the origin.
3. To measure the marginal rate of substitution, we find out how much of one good has to be given up in order to allow the consumer to consume one more unit of the other good while still remaining on the same indifference curve. The marginal rate of substitution falls as one moves down an indifference curve.
4. Indifference curves represent preferences. A budget constraint represents opportunities—how much can be purchased with a given level of income. Consumer optimum is obtained when the highest indifference curve is just tangent to the budget constraint line; at that point, the consumer reaches the highest feasible indifference curve.
5. When income increases, the budget constraint shifts outward to the right, parallel to the previous budget constraint line.

6. As income increases, the consumer optimum moves up to higher and higher indifference curves. When we connect those points with a line, we derive the income-consumption curve.
7. As the price of one good decreases, the budget line rotates. When we connect the tangency points of the highest indifference curves to these new budget lines, we derive the price-consumption curve.

Problems

Answers to the odd-numbered problems appear at the back of the book.

E-1. Consider the indifference curve illustrated in Figure E-1. Explain, in economic terms, why the curve is convex to the origin.

E-2. Your classmate tells you that he is indifferent between three soft drinks and two hamburgers or two soft drinks and three hamburgers. He is also indifferent between two soft drinks and three hamburgers and one soft drink and four hamburgers. However, he prefers three soft drinks and two hamburgers to one soft drink and four hamburgers. Illustrate your friend's preferences as described. How many indifference curves are in your illustration? Explain why he can have these preferences.

E-3. The following table represents Sue's preferences for bottled water and soft drinks, which yield the same level of utility.

Combination of Bottled Water and Soft Drinks	Bottled Water per Month	Soft Drinks per Month
A	5	11
B	10	7
C	15	4
D	20	2
E	25	1

Calculate Sue's marginal rate of substitution of soft drinks for bottled water. Relate the marginal rate of substitution to marginal utility.

E-4. Using the information provided in Problem E-3, illustrate Sue's indifference curve, with water on the horizontal axis and soft drinks on the vertical axis.

E-5. Sue's monthly budget for bottled water and soft drinks is $23. Bottled water costs $1 per bottle, and soft drinks cost $2 per bottle. Calculate the slope of Sue's budget constraint. Given this information and the information provided in Problem E-3, find the combination of goods that satisfies Sue's utility maximization problem in light of her budget constraint.

E-6. Using the indifference curve diagram you constructed in Problem E-4, add in Sue's budget constraint given the information in Problem E-5. Illustrate the utility-maximizing combination of bottled water and soft drinks.

E-7. Using the information provided in Problem E-5, suppose now that the price of a soft drink falls to $1. Now Sue's constant-utility preferences are as follows:

Combination of Bottled Water and Soft Drinks	Bottled Water per Month	Soft Drinks per Month
A	5	22
B	10	14
C	15	8
D	20	4
E	25	2

Calculate the slope of Sue's new budget constraint. Next, find the combination of goods that satisfies Sue's utility maximization problem in light of her budget constraint.

E-8. Illustrate Sue's new budget constraint and indifference curve in the diagram you constructed for Problem E-6. Illustrate also the utility-maximizing combination of goods. Finally, draw the price-consumption curve.

E-9. Given your answers to Problems E-5 and E-7, are Sue's preferences for soft drinks consistent with the law of demand?

E-10. Using your answer to Problem E-8, draw Sue's demand curve for soft drinks.

CHAPTER

20

DEMAND AND SUPPLY ELASTICITY

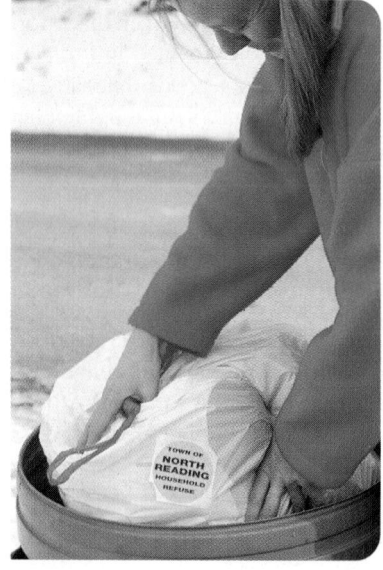

This resident of North Reading, Massachusetts, must place a "paid for" sticker on each trash bag that is to be picked up. Can charging explicit prices for hauling away trash reduce the flow of garbage? Can people vary the amount of garbage they generate?

For some American cities, the crisis began in the 1980s. It spread to other municipalities during the 1990s, and today most villages, towns, counties, and cities throughout the nation are affected. The affliction they share is an overabundance of trash. Even though landfill prices have declined in many areas, municipalities foresee a time when local landfills will be full, requiring big expenses to transport trash to more remote areas. Municipal sanitation department managers everywhere are searching for places to send future trash and affordable ways to get it there. Some municipalities, however, have discovered that charging explicit prices to haul away trash can help stem the flow of garbage. Experiments are under way to determine how high prices must go to induce people to cut back significantly on how much they throw away. To understand how successful a trash-pricing policy may turn out to be, you must learn more about how people respond to changing prices.

LEARNING OBJECTIVES

After reading this chapter, you should be able to:

1. **Express and calculate price elasticity of demand**
2. **Understand the relationship between the price elasticity of demand and total revenues**
3. **Discuss the factors that determine the price elasticity of demand**
4. **Describe the cross price elasticity of demand and how it may be used to indicate whether two goods are substitutes or complements**
5. **Explain the income elasticity of demand**
6. **Classify supply elasticities and explain how the length of time for adjustment affects the price elasticity of supply**

Did You Know That... the government predicted it would raise $6 million per year in new revenues from a new 10 percent luxury tax on private airplane and yacht sales a few years ago, but it actually collected only $53,000? How can that be? The answer lies in understanding the relationship between the quantities that people demand at lower prices relative to the quantities that people demand at higher prices. The year during which the 10 percent luxury tax was imposed also saw expensive new yacht sales fall to almost nothing. Clearly, even rich people respond to rising prices, which in this case were caused by the new tax.

The government isn't alone in having to worry about how individuals respond to rising prices; it is perhaps even more important that businesses take into account consumer response to changing prices. If McDonald's lowers its prices by 10 percent, will fast-food consumers respond by buying so many more Big Macs that the company's revenues will rise? At the other end of the spectrum, can Rolls Royce dealers "get away" with a 2 percent increase in prices? Otherwise stated, will Rolls Royce purchasers respond so little to the relatively small increase in price that the total revenues received for Rolls Royce sales will not fall and may actually rise? The only way to answer these questions is to know how responsive people in the real world will be to changes in prices. Economists have a special name for price responsiveness—*elasticity*, which is the subject of this chapter.

Chapter Outline

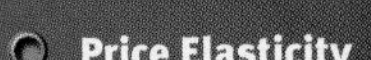

- Price Elasticity
- Price Elasticity Ranges
- Elasticity and Total Revenues
- Determinants of the Price Elasticity of Demand
- Cross Price Elasticity of Demand
- Income Elasticity of Demand
- Elasticity of Supply

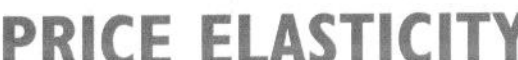

PRICE ELASTICITY

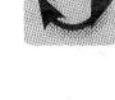

To begin to understand what elasticity is all about, just keep in mind that it means "responsiveness." Here we are concerned with the price elasticity of demand. We wish to know the extent to which a change in the price of, say, petroleum products will cause the quantity demanded to change, other things held constant. We want to determine the percentage change in quantity demanded in response to a percentage change in price.

Price Elasticity of Demand

We will formally define the **price elasticity of demand,** which we will label E_p, as follows:

$$E_p = \frac{\text{percentage change in quantity demanded}}{\text{percentage change in price}}$$

Price elasticity of demand (E_p) 
The responsiveness of the quantity demanded of a commodity to changes in its price; defined as the percentage change in quantity demanded divided by the percentage change in price.

What will price elasticity of demand tell us? It will tell us the relative amount by which the quantity demanded will change in response to a change in the price of a particular good.

Consider an example in which a 10 percent rise in the price of oil leads to a reduction in quantity demanded of only 1 percent. Putting these numbers into the formula, we find that the price elasticity of demand for oil in this case equals the percentage change in quantity demanded divided by the percentage change in price, or

$$E_p = \frac{-1\%}{+10\%} = -.1$$

An elasticity of $-.1$ means that a 1 percent *increase* in the price would lead to a mere .1 percent *decrease* in the quantity demanded. If you were now told, in contrast, that the price elasticity of demand for oil was -1, you would know that a 1 percent increase in the price of oil would lead to a 1 percent decrease in the quantity demanded.

Relative Quantities Only. Notice that in our elasticity formula, we talk about *percentage* changes in quantity demanded divided by *percentage* changes in price. We are therefore

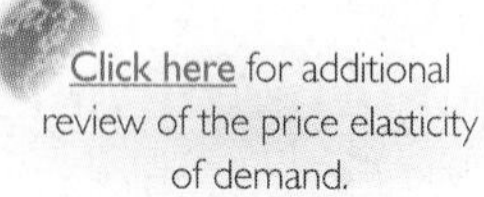
Click here for additional review of the price elasticity of demand.

not interested in the absolute changes, only in relative amounts. This means that it doesn't matter if we measure price changes in terms of cents, dollars, or hundreds of dollars. It also doesn't matter whether we measure quantity changes in ounces, grams, or pounds. The percentage change will be independent of the units chosen.

Always Negative. The law of demand states that quantity demanded is *inversely* related to the relative price. An *increase* in the price of a good leads to a *decrease* in the quantity demanded. If a *decrease* in the relative price of a good should occur, the quantity demanded would *increase* by a certain percentage. The point is that price elasticity of demand will always be negative. By convention, however, *we will ignore the minus sign in our discussion from this point on.*

Basically, the greater the *absolute* price elasticity of demand (disregarding sign), the greater the demand responsiveness to relative price changes—a small change in price has a great impact on quantity demanded. The smaller the absolute price elasticity of demand, the smaller the demand responsiveness to relative price changes—a large change in price has little effect on quantity demanded.

EXAMPLE

To Cut Teen Drug Use, Make the Price of a "High" Higher

Recently, John Tauras of the University of Illinois at Chicago and Michael Grossman of the City University of New York conducted a study of teen use of cocaine. They found that compared with adults, youthful drug abusers are three times more sensitive to price changes. Whereas adult cocaine demand is inelastic, teen cocaine demand is nearly unit-elastic over the range of market prices tabulated by the Drug Enforcement Administration. In other words, a 33 percent increase in the market price of cocaine likely would reduce the teen purchases and consumption of cocaine by a third. Undoubtedly, some teens would substitute other drugs. Nonetheless, cocaine and a derivative drug, crack cocaine, are considered addictive substances. Inducing teens to reduce cocaine use might therefore take a significant bite out of the nation's longer-term problems with drug abuse. An implication of this study is that legal crackdowns on cocaine dealers that restrict the supply of the drug and push up its price might be an appropriate strategy in the war against drugs.

For Critical Analysis

If teen price elasticity of demand for cocaine equals 1, what will happen to drug dealers' revenues from sales to teens if cocaine prices rise?

CONCEPTS IN BRIEF

- Elasticity is a measure of the price responsiveness of the quantity demanded and quantity supplied.
- The price elasticity of demand is equal to the percentage change in quantity demanded divided by the percentage change in price.
- Price elasticity of demand is calculated in terms of percentage changes in quantity demanded and in price. Thus it is expressed as a unitless, dimensionless number.
- The law of demand states that quantity demanded and price are inversely related. Therefore, the price elasticity of demand is always negative, because an increase in price will lead to a decrease in quantity demanded and a decrease in price will lead to an increase in quantity demanded. By convention, we ignore the negative sign in discussions of the price elasticity of demand.

Calculating Elasticity

To calculate the price elasticity of demand, we have to compute percentage changes in quantity demanded and in relative price. To obtain the percentage change in quantity demanded, we divide the change in the quantity demanded by the original quantity demanded:

$$\frac{\text{Change in quantity demand}}{\text{Original quantity demand}}$$

To find the percentage change in price, we divide the change in price by the original price:

$$\frac{\text{Change in price}}{\text{Original price}}$$

There is an arithmetic problem, though, when we calculate percentage changes in this manner. The percentage change, say, from 2 to 3—50 percent—is not the same as the percentage change from 3 to 2—$33\frac{1}{3}$ percent. In other words, it makes a difference where you start. One way out of this dilemma is simply to use average values.

To compute the price elasticity of demand, we need to deal with the average change in quantity demanded caused by the average change in price. That means that we take the average of the two prices and the two quantities over the range we are considering and compare the change with these averages. For relatively small changes in price, the formula for computing the price elasticity of demand then becomes

$$E_p = \frac{\text{change in quantity}}{\text{sum of quantities/2}} \div \frac{\text{change in price}}{\text{sum of prices/2}}$$

We can rewrite this more simply if we do two things: (1) We can let Q_1 and Q_2 equal the two different quantities demanded before and after the price change and let P_1 and P_2 equal the two different prices. (2) Because we will be dividing a percentage by a percentage, we simply use the ratio, or the decimal form, of the percentages. Therefore,

$$E_p = \frac{\Delta Q}{(Q_1 + Q_2)/2} \div \frac{\Delta P}{(P_1 + P_2)/2}$$

where the Greek letter Δ stands for "change in."

INTERNATIONAL EXAMPLE

The Price Elasticity of Demand for Newspapers

Newspaper owners are always seeking to increase their paper's circulation, not because they want the revenue generated from the sales of the paper, but because the larger the circulation, the more the newspaper can charge for its advertising space. The source of most of a paper's revenues—and profits—comes from its advertisers.

One newspaper owner, Rupert Murdoch, ran an experiment to see how high he could boost sales of a particular newspaper by lowering its price. For one day, he lowered the price of the British daily paper *Today* from 25 pence to 10 pence. According to London's *Financial Times,* sales of *Today* almost doubled that day, increasing the circulation from 590,000 to 1,050,000 copies. We can estimate the price elasticity of demand for *Today* by using the formula presented earlier (under the assumption, of course, that all other things were held constant):

$$E_p = \frac{\Delta Q}{(Q_1 + Q_2)/2} \div \frac{\Delta P}{(P_1 + P_2)/2}$$

$$= \frac{1{,}050{,}000 - 590{,}000}{(590{,}000 + 1{,}050{,}000)/2} \div \frac{25 \text{ pence} - 10 \text{ pence}}{(10 \text{ pence} + 25 \text{ pence})/2}$$

$$= \frac{460{,}000}{820{,}000} \div \frac{15 \text{ pence}}{17.5 \text{ pence}} = .66$$

The price elasticity of demand of .66 means that a 1 percent decrease in price will lead to a .66 percent increase in quantity demanded.

For Critical Analysis

Would the estimated price elasticity of the *Today* newspaper have been different if we had *not* used the average-values formula? How?

PRICE ELASTICITY RANGES

We have names for the varying ranges of price elasticities, depending on whether a 1 percent change in price elicits more or less than a 1 percent change in the quantity demanded.

- We say that a good has an **elastic demand** whenever the price elasticity of demand is greater than 1. A 1 percent change in price causes a greater than 1 percent change in the quantity demanded.
- In a situation of **unit elasticity of demand,** a 1 percent change in price causes exactly a 1 percent change in the quantity demanded.
- In a situation of **inelastic demand,** a 1 percent change in price causes a change of less than 1 percent in the quantity demanded.

When we say that a commodity's demand is elastic, we are indicating that consumers are relatively responsive to changes in price. When we say that a commodity's demand is inelastic, we are indicating that its consumers are relatively unresponsive to price changes. When economists say that demand is inelastic, it does not mean that quantity demanded is totally unresponsive to price changes. Remember, the law of demand suggests that there will be some responsiveness in quantity demanded to a price change. The question is how much. That's what elasticity attempts to determine.

Elastic demand 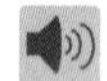
A demand relationship in which a given percentage change in price will result in a larger percentage change in quantity demanded. Total expenditures and price changes are inversely related in the elastic region of the demand curve.

Unit elasticity of demand 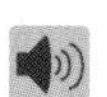
A demand relationship in which the quantity demanded changes exactly in proportion to the change in price. Total expenditures are invariant to price changes in the unit-elastic region of the demand curve.

Inelastic demand 
A demand relationship in which a given percentage change in price will result in a less than proportionate percentage change in the quantity demanded. Total expenditures and price are directly related in the inelastic region of the demand curve.

Extreme Elasticities

There are two extremes in price elasticities of demand. One extreme represents total unresponsiveness of quantity demanded to price changes, which is referred to as **perfectly inelastic demand,** or zero elasticity. The other represents total responsiveness, which is referred to as infinitely or **perfectly elastic demand.**

We show perfect inelasticity in panel (a) of Figure 20-1. Notice that the quantity demanded per year is 8 million units, no matter what the price. Hence for any percentage price change, the quantity demanded will remain the same, and thus the change in the quantity demanded will be zero. Look back at our formula for computing elasticity. If the change in the quantity demanded is zero, the numerator is also zero, and a nonzero number divided into zero results in an answer of zero too. This is true at any point along the demand curve. Hence there is perfect inelasticity. At the opposite extreme is the situation depicted in panel (b) of Figure 20-1. Here we show that at a price of 30 cents, an unlimited quantity will be demanded. At a price that is only slightly above 30 cents, no quantity will be demanded. There is complete, or infinite, responsiveness at each point along this curve, and hence we call the demand schedule in panel (b) infinitely elastic.

Perfectly inelastic demand 
A demand that exhibits zero responsiveness to price changes; no matter what the price is, the quantity demanded remains the same.

Perfectly elastic demand 
A demand that has the characteristic that even the slightest increase in price will lead to zero quantity demanded.

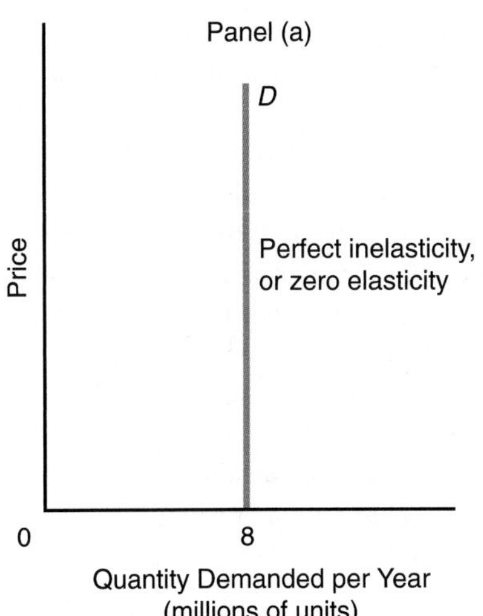

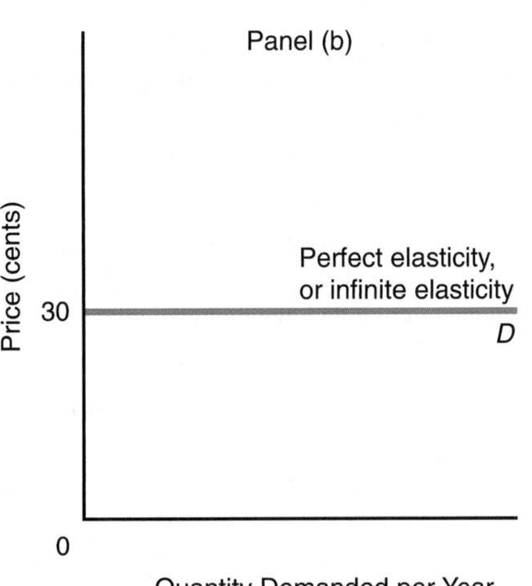

FIGURE 20-1

Extreme Price Elasticities

In panel (a), we show complete price unresponsiveness. The demand curve is vertical at the quantity of 8 million units per year. This means that the price elasticity of demand is zero. In panel (b), we show complete price responsiveness. At a price of 30 cents, in this example, consumers will demand an unlimited quantity of the particular good in question. This is a case of infinite price elasticity of demand.

POLICY EXAMPLE

Who Pays Higher Cigarette Taxes?

In recent years, Congress and state legislatures have steadily pushed up taxes on cigarettes, which are assessed as a flat amount per physical unit of sales (that is, per standard pack of cigarettes). These taxes are paid by sellers of cigarettes from the revenues they earn from their total sales. Thus to receive the same effective price for selling a given quantity, a cigarette seller must charge an actual price that is higher by exactly the amount of the tax. As shown in panel (a) of Figure 20-2, this means that imposing a cigarette tax shifts the supply

FIGURE 20-2

Price Elasticity and a Cigarette Tax

Placing a per-pack tax on cigarettes causes the supply curve to shift upward by the amount of the tax, as illustrated in panel (a), in order for sellers to earn the same effective price for any given quantity of cigarettes they sell. If the demand for cigarettes were perfectly inelastic, as depicted in panel (b), imposing the tax causes the market price of cigarettes to rise by the amount of the tax, so that cigarette consumers would effectively pay all the tax. Conversely, if the demand for cigarettes were perfectly elastic, as shown in panel (c), the market price would not change, and sellers would pay all the tax. The quantity demanded would fall to Q_2.

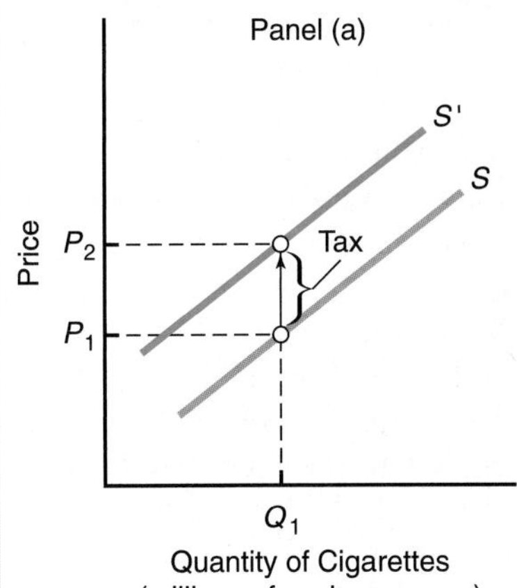

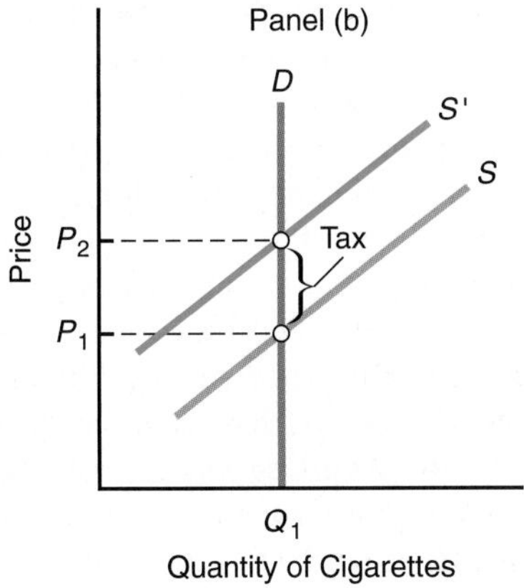

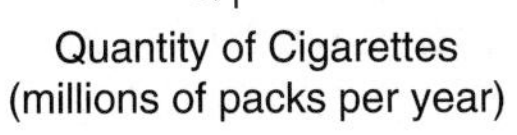

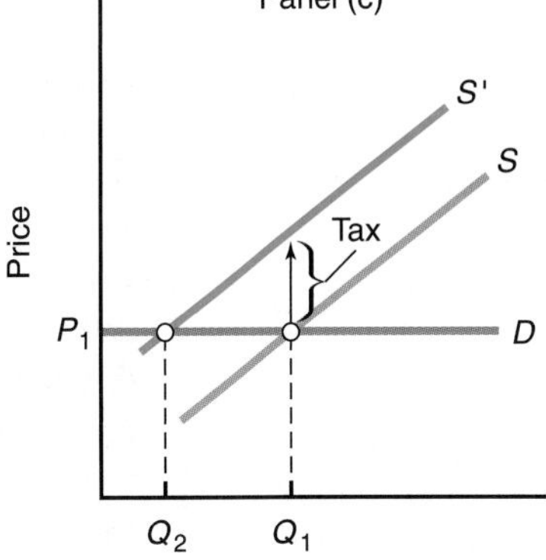

curve upward by the amount of the tax. At any given quantity of cigarettes sold, sellers supply the same quantity of cigarettes, but at a price that is higher by the amount of the tax that they will have to pass along to the government.

Who *truly* pays the tax depends on the price elasticity of demand, however. Take a look at panel (b) of Figure 20-2, which illustrates what happens to the market price in the case of perfectly inelastic demand for cigarettes. In this instance, the market price rises by the full amount that the supply curve shifts upward. This amount, of course, is the amount of the tax. Consequently, if cigarette consumers have a perfectly inelastic demand for cigarettes, they effectively pay the entire tax in the form of higher prices. Panel (c) illustrates the opposite case, in which the demand for cigarettes is perfectly elastic. In this situation, the market price is unresponsive to a tax-induced shift in the supply curve, so sellers must pay all the tax.

Realistically, many cigarette smokers are "addicted" and have a very low price elasticity of demand for cigarettes. Most studies indicate that these people are also often of lower socioeconimic status. But some consumers are "recreational smokers" who cut back on their consumption when they face higher prices. These people tend to fall into higher-income categories. Thus as the federal and state governments continue to ratchet up cigarette taxes, the burden of those taxes, in the form of higher prices for consumers, increasingly tends to fall on lower-income smokers.

For Critical Analysis

Do cigarette taxes appear to be progressive or regressive?

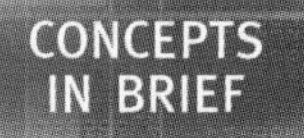

- One extreme elasticity occurs when a demand curve is vertical. It has zero price elasticity of demand; it is completely inelastic.
- Another extreme elasticity occurs when a demand curve is horizontal. It has completely elastic demand; its price elasticity of demand is infinite.

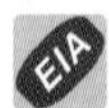

Who Pays the Sales Tax?
Gain further understanding of how the price elasticity of demand influences the burden of taxation.

ELASTICITY AND TOTAL REVENUES

Suppose that you are in charge of the pricing decision for a cellular telephone service company. How would you know when it is best to raise or not to raise prices? The answer depends in part on the effect of your pricing decision on total revenues, or the total receipts of your company. (The rest of the equation is, of course, your cost structure, a subject we examine in Chapter 22.) It is commonly thought that the way to increase total receipts is to increase price per unit. But is this always the case? Is it possible that a rise in price per unit could lead to a decrease in total revenues? The answers to these questions depend on the price elasticity of demand.

Let's look at Figure 20-3. In panel (a), column 1 shows the price of cellular telephone service in dollars per minute, and column 2 represents billions of minutes per year. In column 3, we multiply column 1 times column 2 to derive total revenue because total revenue is always equal to the number of units (quantity) sold times the price per unit, and in column 4, we calculate values of elasticity. Notice what happens to total revenues throughout the schedule. They rise steadily as the price rises from 10 cents to 50 cents per minute; but when the price rises further to 60 cents per minute, total revenues remain constant at $3 billion. At prices per minute higher than 60 cents, total revenues fall as price increases. Indeed, if prices are above 60 cents per minute, total revenues can be increased only by *cutting* prices, not by raising them.

FIGURE 20-3

The Relationship Between Price Elasticity of Demand and Total Revenues for Cellular Phone Service

In panel (a), we show the elastic, unit-elastic, and inelastic sections of the demand schedule according to whether a reduction in price increases total revenues, causes them to remain constant, or causes them to decrease, respectively. In panel (b), we show these regions graphically on the demand curve. In panel (c), we show them on the total revenue curve.

Panel (a)

(1) Price, P, per Minute of cellular phone service	(2) Quantity Demanded, D (billions of minutes)	(3) Total Revenue ($ billions) = (1) X (2)	(4) Elasticity, $E_p = \dfrac{\text{Change in } Q}{(Q_1 + Q_2)/2} \div \dfrac{\text{Change in } P}{(P_1 + P_2)/2}$	
$1.10	0	0		
			21.000	Elastic
1.00	1	1.0		
			6.330	Elastic
.90	2	1.8		
			3.400	Elastic
.80	3	2.4		
			2.143	Elastic
.70	4	2.8		
			1.144	Elastic
.60	5	3.0		
			1.000	Unit-elastic
.50	6	3.0		
			.692	Inelastic
.40	7	2.8		
			.467	Inelastic
.30	8	2.4		
			.294	Inelastic
.20	9	1.8		
			.158	Inelastic
.10	10	1.0		

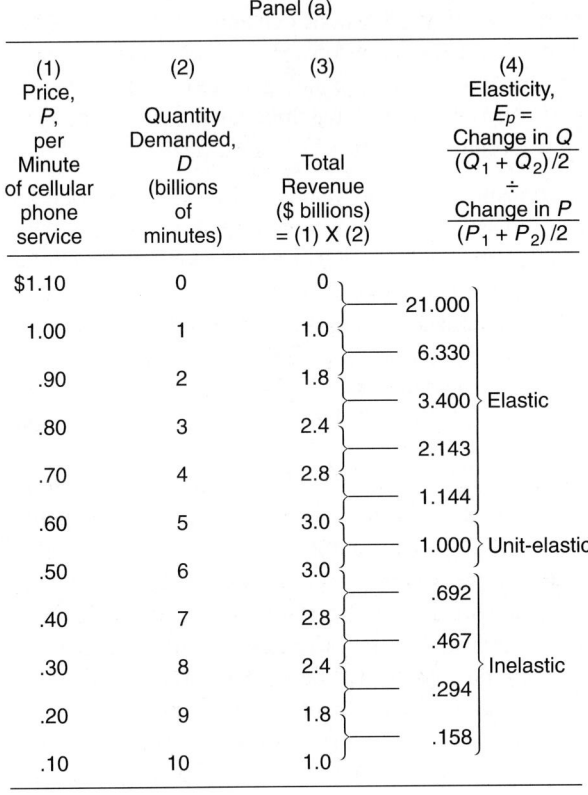

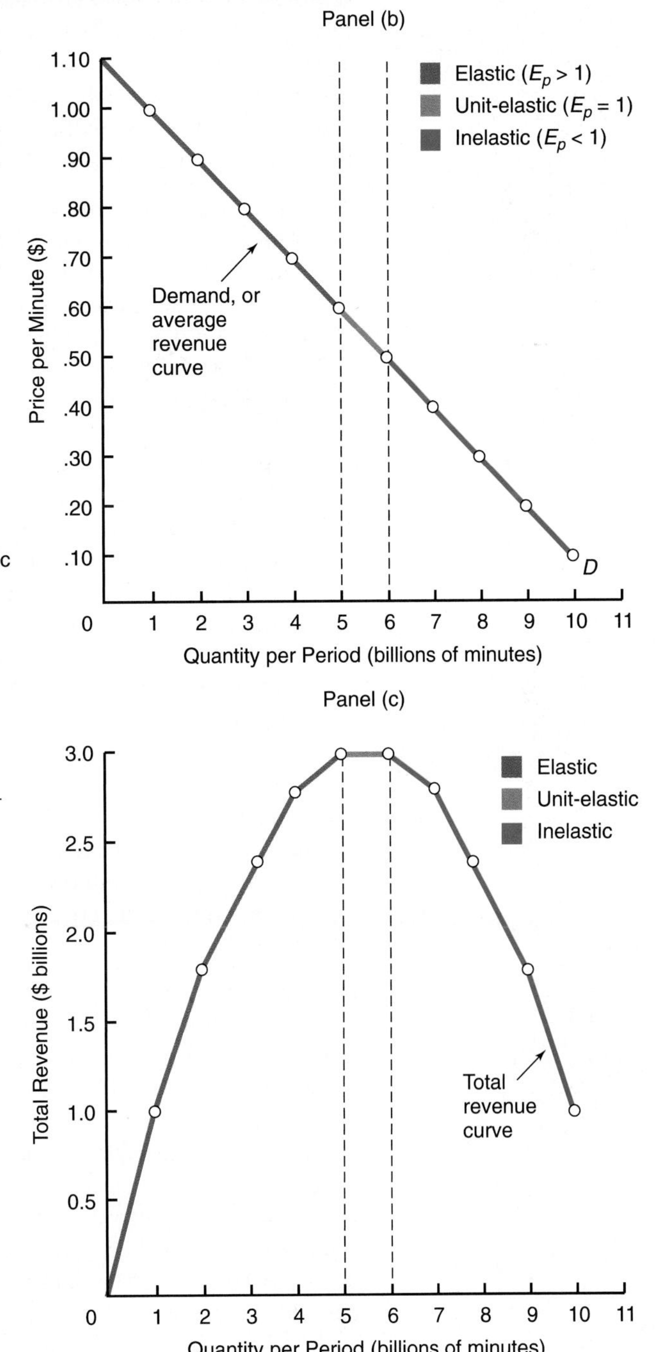

Labeling Elasticity

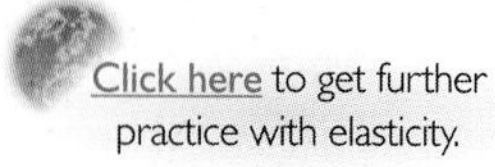
Click here to get further practice with elasticity.

The relationship between price and quantity on the demand schedule is given in columns 1 and 2 of panel (a) in Figure 20-3. In panel (b), the demand curve, *D,* representing that schedule is drawn. In panel (c), the total revenue curve representing the data in column 3 is drawn. Notice first the level of these curves at small quantities. The demand curve is at a maximum height, but total revenue is zero, which makes sense according to this demand schedule—at a price of $1.10 and above, no units will be purchased, and therefore total revenue will be zero. As price is lowered, we travel down the demand curve, and total revenues increase until price is 60 cents per minute, remain constant from 60 cents to 50 cents per minute, and then fall at lower unit prices. Corresponding to those three sections, demand is elastic, unit-elastic, and inelastic. Hence we have three relationships among the three types of price elasticity and total revenues.

- *Elastic demand.* A negative relationship exists between small changes in price and changes in total revenues. That is to say, if price is lowered, total revenues will rise when the firm faces demand that is elastic, and if it raises price, total revenues will fall. Consider another example. If the price of Diet Coke were raised by 25 percent and the price of all other soft drinks remained constant, the quantity demanded of Diet Coke would probably fall dramatically. The decrease in quantity demanded due to the increase in the price of Diet Coke would lead in this example to a reduction in the total revenues of the Coca-Cola Company. Therefore, if demand is elastic, price and total revenues will move in *opposite* directions.
- *Unit-elastic demand.* Changes in price do not change total revenues. When the firm is facing demand that is unit-elastic, if it increases price, total revenues will not change; if it decreases price, total revenues will not change either.
- *Inelastic demand.* A positive relationship exists between changes in price and total revenues. When the firm is facing demand that is inelastic, if it raises price, total revenues will go up; if it lowers price, total revenues will fall. Consider another example. You have just invented a cure for the common cold that has been approved by the Food and Drug Administration for sale to the public. You are not sure what price you should charge, so you start out with a price of $1 per pill. You sell 20 million pills at that price over a year. The next year, you decide to raise the price by 25 percent, to $1.25. The number of pills you sell drops to 18 million per year. The price increase of 25 percent has led to a 10 percent decrease in quantity demanded. Your total revenues, however, will rise to $22.5 million because of the price increase. We therefore conclude that if demand is inelastic, price and total revenues move in the *same* direction.

The elastic, unit-elastic, and inelastic areas of the demand curve are shown in Figure 20-3. For prices from $1.10 per minute of cellular phone time to 60 cents per minute, as price decreases, total revenues rise from zero to $3 billion. Demand is price-elastic. When price changes from 60 cents to 50 cents, however, total revenues remain constant at $3 billion; demand is unit-elastic. Finally, when price falls from 50 cents to 10 cents, total revenues decrease from $3 billion to $1 billion; demand is inelastic. In panels (b) and (c) of Figure 20-3, we have labeled the sections of the demand curve accordingly, and we have also shown how total revenues first rise, then remain constant, and finally fall.

The relationship between price elasticity of demand and total revenues brings together some important microeconomic concepts. Total revenues, as we have noted, are the product of price per unit times number of units sold. The law of demand states that along a given demand curve, price and quantity changes will move in opposite directions: One increases as the other decreases. Consequently, what happens to the product of price times quantity

TABLE 20-1
Relationship Between Price Elasticity of Demand and Total Revenues

Price Elasticity of Demand		Effect of Price Change on Total Revenues (TR)	
		Price Decrease	Price Increase
Inelastic	($E_p < 1$)	TR ↓	TR ↑
Unit-elastic	($E_p = 1$)	No change in TR	No change in TR
Elastic	($E_p > 1$)	TR ↑	TR ↓

depends on which of the opposing changes exerts a greater force on total revenues. But this is just what price elasticity of demand is designed to measure—responsiveness of quantity demanded to a change in price. The relationship between price elasticity of demand and total revenues is summarized in Table 20-1.

INTERNATIONAL EXAMPLE

A Pricing Decision at Disneyland Paris

Several years after it opened with great fanfare, the $4 billion investment in Disneyland Paris (formerly called EuroDisney) was in trouble. In an attempt to improve profits (actually, decrease losses), Disney management decided to lower prices. Entrance fees during peak periods (April 1 to October 1) dropped from 250 francs (about $50) to 195 francs (about $40). Was this 22 percent reduction in ticket prices a good management strategy for Disney officials? That depends in part on what happened to total revenues. As it turned out, park attendance increased by 700,000 visitors, and total revenues increased by more than 22 percent. This indicates that the demand for Disneyland Paris was elastic in the price range of $40 to $50.

For Critical Analysis

What other factors may have affected attendance at Disneyland Paris?

CONCEPTS IN BRIEF

- Price elasticity of demand is related to total revenues (and total consumer expenditures).
- When demand is *elastic,* the change in price elicits a change in total revenues (and total consumer expenditures) in the direction opposite that of the price change.
- When demand is *unit-elastic,* a change in price elicits no change in total revenues (or in total consumer expenditures).
- When demand is *inelastic,* a change in price elicits a change in total revenues (and in consumer expenditures) in the same direction as the price change.

DETERMINANTS OF THE PRICE ELASTICITY OF DEMAND 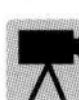

We have learned how to calculate the price elasticity of demand. We know that theoretically it ranges numerically from zero, completely inelastic, to infinity, completely elastic. What we would like to do now is come up with a list of the determinants of the price elasticity of demand. The price elasticity of demand for a particular commodity at any price depends, at a minimum, on the following:

- The existence, number, and quality of substitutes
- The percentage of a consumer's total budget devoted to purchases of that commodity
- The length of time allowed for adjustment to changes in the price of the commodity

Existence of Substitutes

The closer the substitutes for a particular commodity and the more substitutes there are, the greater will be its price elasticity of demand. At the limit, if there is a perfect substitute, the elasticity of demand for the commodity will be infinity. Thus even the slightest increase in the commodity's price will cause an enormous reduction in the quantity demanded: Quantity demanded will fall to zero. We are really talking about two goods that the consumer believes are exactly alike and equally desirable, like dollar bills whose only difference is serial numbers. When we talk about less extreme examples, we can speak only in terms of the number and the similarity of substitutes that are available. Thus we will find that the more narrowly we define a good, the closer and greater will be the number of substitutes available. For example, the demand for a Diet Coke may be highly elastic because consumers can switch to Diet Pepsi. The demand for diet drinks in general, however, is relatively less elastic because there are fewer substitutes.

Share of Budget

We know that the greater the percentage of a total budget spent on the commodity, the greater the person's price elasticity of demand for that commodity. The demand for pepper is thought to be very inelastic merely because individuals spend so little on it relative to their total budgets. In contrast, the demand for things such as transportation and housing is thought to be far more elastic because they occupy a large part of people's budgets—changes in their prices cannot be ignored so easily without sacrificing a lot of other alternative goods that could be purchased.

Consider a numerical example. A household earns $40,000 a year. It purchases $4 of pepper per year and $4,000 of transportation services. Now consider the spending power of this family when the price of pepper and the price of transportation both double. If the household buys the same amount of pepper, it will now spend $8. It will thus have to reduce other expenditures by $4. This $4 represents only .01 percent of the entire household budget. By contrast, a doubling of transportation costs requires that the family spend $8,000, or $4,000 more on transportation, if it is to purchase the same quantity. That increased expenditure on transportation of $4,000 represents 10 percent of total expenditures that must be switched from other purchases. We would therefore predict that the household will react differently to the doubling of prices for pepper than it will for transportation. It will buy almost the same amount of pepper but will buy significantly less transportation.

Time for Adjustment

When the price of a commodity changes and that price change persists, more people will learn about it. Further, consumers will be better able to revise their consumption patterns the longer the time period they have to do so. And in fact, the longer the time they do take, the less costly it will be for them to engage in this revision of consumption patterns. Consider a price decrease. The longer the price decrease persists, the greater will be the number of new uses that consumers will discover for the particular commodity, and the greater will be the number of new users of that particular commodity.

It is possible to make a very strong statement about the relationship between the price elasticity of demand and the time allowed for adjustment:

> The longer any price change persists, the greater the elasticity of demand, other things held constant. Elasticity of demand is greater in the long run than in the short run.

Let's take an example. Suppose that the price of electricity goes up 50 percent. How do you adjust in the short run? You can turn the lights off more often, you can stop using the stereo as much as you do, and so on. Otherwise it's very difficult to cut back on your consumption of electricity. In the long run, though, you can devise methods to reduce your consumption. Instead of using electric heaters, the next time you have a house built you will install gas heaters. Instead of using an electric stove, the next time you move you will have a gas stove installed. You will purchase fluorescent bulbs because they use less electricity. The more time you have to think about it, the more ways you will find to cut your electricity consumption. We would expect, therefore, that the short-run demand curve for electricity would be relatively less elastic (in the price range around P_e), as demonstrated by D_1 in Figure 20-4. However, the long-run demand curve may exhibit much more elasticity (in the neighborhood of P_e), as demonstrated by D_3. Indeed, we can think of an entire family of demand curves such as those depicted in the figure. The short-run demand curve is for the period when there is no time for adjustment. As more time is allowed, the demand curve goes first to D_2 and then all the way to D_3. Thus in the neighborhood of P_e, elasticity differs for each of these curves. It is greater for the less steep curves (but slope alone does not measure elasticity for the entire curve).

How to Define the Short Run and the Long Run. We've mentioned the short run and the long run. Is the short run one week, two weeks, one month, two months? Is the long run three years, four years, five years? The answer is that there is no single answer. What we mean by the long run is the period of time necessary for consumers to make a full adjustment to a given price change, all other things held constant. In the case of the demand for electricity, the long run will be however long it takes consumers to switch over to cheaper sources of heating, to buy houses that are more energy-efficient, to purchase

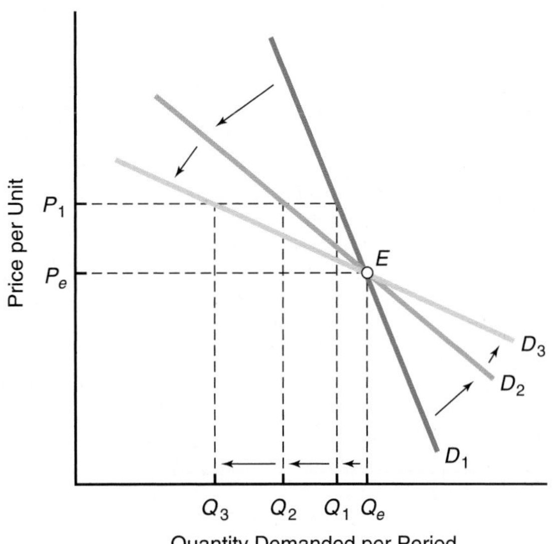

FIGURE 20-4

Short-Run and Long-Run Price Elasticity of Demand

Consider an equilibrium situation in which the market price is P_e and the quantity demanded is Q_e. Then there is a price increase to P_1. In the short run, as evidenced by the demand curve D_1, we move from equilibrium quantity demanded, Q_e, to Q_1. After more time is allowed for adjustment, the demand curve rotates at original price P_e to D_2. Quantity demanded falls again, now to Q_2. After even more time is allowed for adjustment, the demand curve rotates at price P_e to D_3. At the higher price P_1, in the long run, the quantity demanded falls all the way to Q_3.

appliances that are more energy-efficient, and so on. The long-run elasticity of demand for electricity therefore relates to a period of at least several years. The short run—by default—is any period less than the long run.

EXAMPLE

What Do Real-World Price Elasticities of Demand Look Like?

In Table 20-2, we present demand elasticities for selected goods. None of them is zero, and the largest is 3.8—a far cry from infinity. Remember that even though we are leaving off the negative sign, there is an inverse relationship between price and quantity demanded, and the minus sign is understood. Also remember that these elasticities represent averages over given price ranges. Choosing different price ranges would yield different elasticity estimates for these goods.

Economists have consistently found that estimated price elasticities of demand are greater in the long run than in the short run, as seen in Table 20-2. There you see, for example, in the far-right column that the long-run price elasticity of demand for tires and related items is 1.2, whereas the estimate for the short run is .8. Throughout the table, you see that all estimates of long-run price elasticities of demand exceed their short-run counterparts.

For Critical Analysis

Explain the intuitive reasoning behind the difference between long-run and short-run price elasticity of demand.

TABLE 20-2

Demand Elasticity for Selected Goods

Here are estimated demand elasticities for selected goods. All of them are negative, although we omit the minus sign. We have given some estimates of the long-run price elasticities of demand. The long run is associated with the time necessary for consumers to adjust fully to any given price change.

	Estimated Elasticity	
Category	Short Run	Long Run
Lamb	2.7	—
Bread	.2	—
Tires and related items	.8	1.2
Auto repair and related services	1.4	2.4
Radio and television repair	.5	3.8
Legitimate theater and opera	.2	.3
Motion pictures	.9	3.7
Foreign travel by U.S. residents	.1	1.8
Taxicabs	.6	—
Local public transportation	.6	1.2
Intercity bus	.6	2.2
Electricity	.1	1.8
Jewelry and watches	.4	.6

CROSS PRICE ELASTICITY OF DEMAND 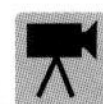

In Chapter 3, we discussed the effect of a change in the price of one good on the demand for a related good. We defined substitutes and complements in terms of whether a reduction in the price of one caused a decrease or an increase, respectively, in the demand for the other. If the price of compact disks is held constant, the amount of CDs demanded (at any price) will certainly be influenced by the price of a close substitute such as audiocassettes. If the price of stereo speakers is held constant, the amount of stereo speakers demanded (at any price) will certainly be affected by changes in the price of stereo amplifiers.

What we now need to do is come up with a numerical measure of the price responsiveness of demand to the prices of related goods. This is called the **cross price elasticity of demand (E_{xy}),** which is defined as the percentage change in the demand for one good (a shift in the demand curve) divided by the percentage change in the price of the related good. In equation form, the cross price elasticity of demand for good X with good Y is

Cross price elasticity of demand (E_{xy}) 
The percentage change in the demand for one good (holding its price constant) divided by the percentage change in the price of a related good.

$$E_{xy} = \frac{\text{percentage change in demand for good X}}{\text{percentage change in price of good Y}}$$

Alternatively, the cross price elasticity of demand for good Y with good X would use the percentage change in the demand for good Y as the numerator and the percentage change in the price of good X as the denominator.

When two goods are substitutes, the cross price elasticity of demand will be positive. For example, when the price of margarine goes up, the demand for butter will rise too as consumers shift away from the now relatively more expensive margarine to butter. A producer of margarine could benefit from a numerical estimate of the cross price elasticity of demand between butter and margarine. For example, if the price of butter went up by 10 percent and the margarine producer knew that the cross price elasticity of demand was 1, the margarine producer could estimate that the demand for margarine would also go up by 10 percent at any given price. Plans for increasing margarine production could then be made.

FAQ

Are people substituting away from public libraries to the Internet as their main source of information?

Yes. Although careful studies have not yet been done, there is considerable anecdotal evidence that the relatively inexpensive accessibility of the Internet together with the availability of Internet search engines has reduced the price of on-line information services. This has induced a decline in the demand for traditional public library services. No one has yet explicitly computed the cross price elasticity of demand for traditional library services. One key indicator that extensive substitution is taking place, however, is that libraries are hiring fewer librarians. Today, they mainly wish to hire people skilled in information technologies—people who can assist visitors who mainly desire to use the libraries' computers to search the Internet.

When two related goods are complements, the cross price elasticity of demand will be negative (and we will not disregard the minus sign). For example, when the price of stereo amplifiers goes up, the demand for stereo speakers will fall. This is because as prices of amplifiers increase, the quantity of amplifiers demanded will naturally decrease. Because amplifiers and stereo speakers are often used together, the demand for speakers is likely to fall. Any manufacturer of stereo speakers must take this into account in making production plans.

If goods are completely unrelated, their cross price elasticity of demand will be zero.

INCOME ELASTICITY OF DEMAND

In Chapter 3, we discussed the determinants of demand. One of those determinants was income. Briefly, we can apply our understanding of elasticity to the relationship between changes in income and changes in demand. We measure the responsiveness of quantity demanded to income changes by the **income elasticity of demand (E_i):**

Income elasticity of demand (E_i)
The percentage change in demand for any good, holding its price constant, divided by the percentage change in income; the responsiveness of demand to changes in income, holding the good's relative price constant.

$$E_i = \frac{\text{percentage change in demand}}{\text{percentage change in income}}$$

holding relative price constant.

Income elasticity of demand refers to a *horizontal shift* in the demand curve in response to changes in income, whereas price elasticity of demand refers to a *movement along* the curve in response to price changes. Thus income elasticity of demand is calculated at a given price, and price elasticity of demand is calculated at a given income.

A simple example will demonstrate how income elasticity of demand can be computed. Table 20-3 gives the relevant data. The product in question is compact disks. We assume that the price of CDs remains constant relative to other prices. In period 1, six CDs per month are purchased. Income per month is \$400. In period 2, monthly income increases to \$600, and the quantity of CDs demanded per month is increased to eight. We can apply the following calculation:

$$E_i = \frac{(8-6)/6}{(600-400)/400} = \frac{1/3}{1/2} = \frac{2}{3} = .667$$

Hence measured income elasticity of demand for CDs for the individual represented in this example is .667. Note that this holds only for the move from six CDs to eight CDs purchased per month. If the situation were reversed, with income decreasing from \$600 to \$400 per month and CDs purchased dropping from eight to six CDs per month, the calculation becomes

$$E_i = \frac{(6-8)/8}{(400-600)/600} = \frac{-2/8}{-1/3} = \frac{-1/4}{-1/3} = \frac{3}{4} = .75$$

In this case, the measured income elasticity of demand is equal to .75.

To get the same income elasticity of demand over the same range of values regardless of direction of change (increase or decrease), we can use the same formula that we used in computing the price elasticity of demand. When doing so, we have

Elasticities and Applications
Review additional elasticity concepts and choose the type of elasticity you wish to study.

$$E_i = \frac{\text{change in quantity}}{\text{sum of quantities}/2} \div \frac{\text{change in income}}{\text{sum of incomes}/2}$$

You have just been introduced to three types of elasticities. All three elasticities are important in influencing the quantity demanded for most goods. Reasonably accurate estimates of these can go a long way toward making accurate forecasts of demand for goods or services.

TABLE 20-3
How Income Affects Quantity of CDs Demanded

Period	Number of CDs Demanded per Month	Income per Month
1	6	\$400
2	8	600

CONCEPTS IN BRIEF

- Some determinants of price elasticity of demand are (1) the existence, number, and quality of substitutes; (2) the share of the total budget spent on the good in question; and (3) the length of time allowed for adjustment to a change in prices.
- Cross price elasticity of demand measures one good's demand responsiveness to another's price changes. For substitutes, it is positive; for complements, it is negative.
- Income elasticity of demand tells you by what percentage demand will change for a particular percentage change in income.

ELASTICITY OF SUPPLY

The **price elasticity of supply (E_s)** is defined similarly to the price elasticity of demand. Supply elasticities are generally positive; this is because at higher prices, larger quantities will generally be forthcoming from suppliers. The definition of the price elasticity of supply is as follows:

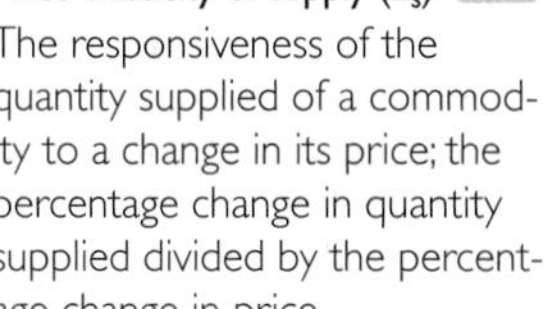

Price elasticity of supply (E_s) The responsiveness of the quantity supplied of a commodity to a change in its price; the percentage change in quantity supplied divided by the percentage change in price.

$$E_s = \frac{\text{percentage change in quantity supplied}}{\text{percentage change in price}}$$

Classifying Supply Elasticities

Just as with demand, there are different ranges of supply elasticities. They are similar in definition to the ranges of demand elasticities.

If a 1 percent increase in price elicits a greater than 1 percent increase in the quantity supplied, we say that at the particular price in question on the supply schedule, *supply is elastic.* The most extreme elastic supply is called **perfectly elastic supply**—the slightest reduction in price will cause quantity supplied to fall to zero.

Perfectly elastic supply A supply characterized by a reduction in quantity supplied to zero when there is the slightest decrease in price.

If, conversely, a 1 percent increase in price elicits a less than 1 percent increase in the quantity supplied, we refer to that as an *inelastic supply.* The most extreme inelastic supply is called **perfectly inelastic supply**—no matter what the price, the quantity supplied remains the same.

Perfectly inelastic supply A supply for which quantity supplied remains constant, no matter what happens to price.

If the percentage change in the quantity supplied is just equal to the percentage change in the price, we call this *unit-elastic supply.*

We show in Figure 20-5 two supply schedules, S and S'. You can tell at a glance, without reading the labels, which one is infinitely elastic and which one is perfectly inelastic.

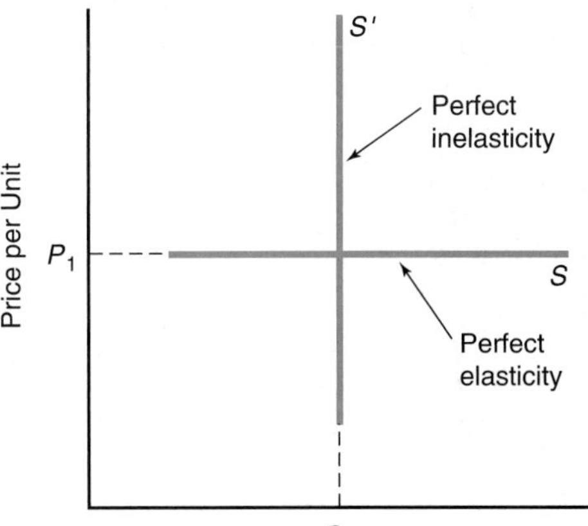

FIGURE 20-5
The Extremes in Supply Curves
Here we have drawn two extremes of supply schedules; S is a perfectly elastic supply curve; S' is a perfectly inelastic one. In the former, an unlimited quantity will be supplied at price P_1. In the latter, no matter what the price, the quantity supplied will be Q_1. An example of S' might be the supply curve for fresh fish on the morning the boats come in.

As you might expect, most supply schedules exhibit elasticities that are somewhere between zero and infinity.

Price Elasticity of Supply and Length of Time for Adjustment

We pointed out earlier that the longer the time period allowed for adjustment, the greater the price elasticity of demand. It turns out that the same proposition applies to supply. The longer the time for adjustment, the more elastic the supply curve. Consider why this is true:

1. The longer the time allowed for adjustment, the more resources can flow into (or out of) an industry through expansion (or contraction) of existing firms.
2. The longer the time allowed for adjustment, the more firms are able to figure out ways to increase (or decrease) production in an industry.

We therefore talk about short-run and long-run price elasticities of supply. The short run is defined as the time period during which full adjustment has not yet taken place. The long run is the time period during which firms have been able to adjust fully to the change in price.

Consider an increase in the price of housing. In the immediate run, when there is no time allowed for any adjustment, the amount of housing offered for rent or for sale is perfectly inelastic. However, as more time is allowed for adjustment, current owners of the housing stock can find ways to increase the amount of housing they will offer for rent from given buildings. The owner of a large house can decide, for example, to have two children move into one room so that a "new" extra bedroom can be rented out. This can also be done by the owner of a large house who decides to move into an apartment and rent each floor of the house to a separate family. Thus the quantity of housing supplied will increase. With more time, landlords will find it profitable to build new rental units.

We can show a whole set of supply curves similar to the ones we generated for demand. As Figure 20-6 shows, when nothing can be done in the immediate run, the supply curve is vertical, S_1. As more time is allowed for adjustment, the supply curve rotates to S_2 and then to S_3, becoming more elastic as it rotates.

FIGURE 20-6

Short-Run and Long-Run Price Elasticity of Supply

Consider a situation in which the price is P_e and the quantity supplied is Q_e. In the immediate run, we hypothesize a vertical supply curve, S_1. With the price increase to P_1, therefore, there will be no change in the short run in quantity supplied; it will remain at Q_e. Given some time for adjustment, the supply curve will rotate to S_2. The new amount supplied will increase to Q_1. The long-run supply curve is shown by S_3. The amount supplied again increases to Q_2.

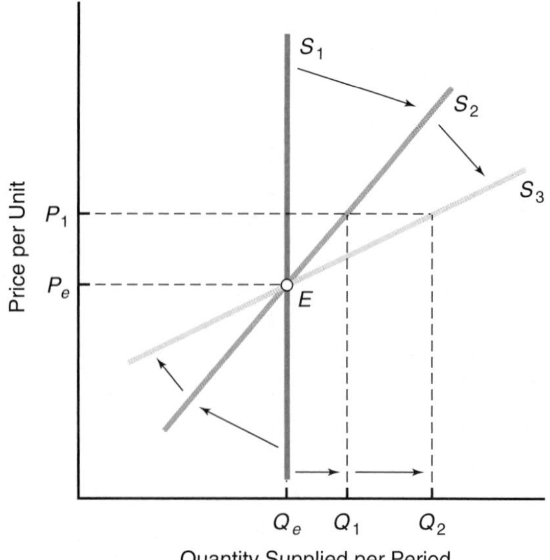

INTERNATIONAL EXAMPLE

French Truffle Production Takes a Nosedive

Some of the best truffles in the world come from the seven *départements* (counties) in the middle of France that make up the Périgord region. Black truffles are often called "black diamonds" because they are so expensive and also because they have a faceted skin. Their official name is *Tuber melanosporum.* Ranging in size from that of a hazelnut to that of a baseball, truffles are sliced fine and used in cooking as a pungent addition to many refined dishes. Their prices range from $250 to $500 a pound wholesale to as much as $1,000 a pound retail. Yet things are not well in the French truffle industry. The Chinese have started exporting their version of truffles, considered inferior by the French but popular nonetheless in the open market. By 1996, the average price for French-grown truffles had dropped by 30 percent. Many French farmers, fed up with lower prices, simply gave up on truffles. French production subsequently decreased by 25 percent. Hence the estimated short-run price elasticity of supply of French truffles was .83. (Why?)

For Critical Analysis

There is a company in the United States that will sell you trees inoculated with the truffle organism so that you can "grow your own." How will this affect the price of truffles and thus French production?

CONCEPTS IN BRIEF

- Price elasticity of supply is calculated by dividing the percentage change in quantity supplied by the percentage change in price.
- Usually, price elasticities of supply are positive—higher prices yield larger quantities supplied.
- Long-run supply curves are more elastic than short-run supply curves because the longer the time allowed, the more resources can flow into or out of an industry when price changes.

NETNOMICS

How Clever Internet Companies Infer Their Customers' Price Elasticity of Demand

As you learned in this chapter, a company that wishes to increase its revenues should raise the price it charges customers with an inelastic demand for the goods it sells. By contrast, a firm can bring about an increase in its revenues by reducing the price it charges customers whose demand is elastic.

Increasingly, companies are using the Internet to try to have it both ways. One California software firm has developed a program that allows Internet sellers to track the shopping patterns of customers who visit their Web sites. The software studies a Web surfer's "clickstream"—the manner in which the customer navigates through the site. For example, if the customer quickly zeroes in on a specific item and makes little effort to shop around for better prices, the software program tags the customer as one whose demand for that item is likely to be relatively inelastic. The program then automatically quotes a relatively high price. If another Web surfer who visits the site behaves like a price-sensitive shopper—perhaps by comparing many different products without jumping to buy—the program concludes that the customer's demand is more likely to be relatively elastic. It then automatically quotes a lower price to this customer.

Thus new technologies are making it easier for Net-based firms to increase their revenues, and thus their profits, by charging higher prices to customers whose price elasticity of demand is less than 1 and lower prices to customers whose price elasticity of demand is greater than 1. (Charging different prices for the same product, as you will learn in Chapter 27, is known as *price discrimination.*) Of course, this is an old idea extended to a high-tech age. After all, makers of breakfast cereals, disposable diapers, and other retail products have done the same sort of thing for years by offering rebates to people who save boxtops or proof-of-purchase seals. These rebates effectively amount to lower prices for penny-pinchers, whose demand is relatively elastic. Busy people with less elastic demands end up paying the full, undiscounted, and effectively higher retail price.

What remains to be seen is whether Internet customers will respond to the new pricing strategies of Internet sellers. Will spendthrifts with a low price elasticity of demand try to masquerade as skinflints with a high price elasticity of demand by displaying artificially cautious clickstreams? Probably not. People with a low price elasticity of demand are typically in a hurry to get what they want. They will not wish to waste precious time trying to fool Internet sellers' pricing programs.

ISSUES & APPLICATIONS

Discovering the Value of Garbage

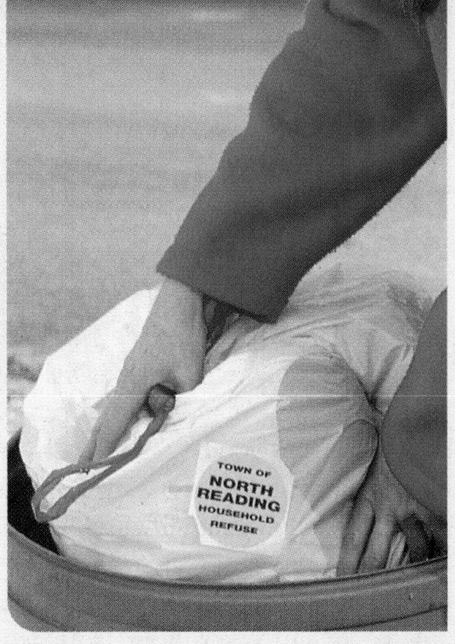

Each day, a massive volume of garbage flows away from the driveways and doorsteps of American homes. It has to go somewhere. Although some trash is incinerated, today most goes into landfills. Increasing land values, however, have put landfill space at a premium for municipalities that collect and dump their residents' trash.

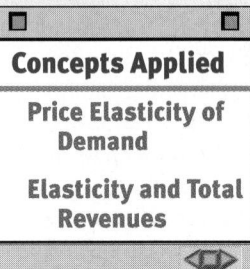

Trying to Make the Market Work

The town of Charlottesville, Virginia, recently experimented with charging a per-unit price for trash collection. Previously, like most municipalities, Charlottesville had financed its trash collection from property taxes. Of course, this meant that the effective price to a household of putting each additional bag of trash out for curbside collection was zero. Once they had paid their taxes, Charlottesville residents could set out as many bags of garbage as they wished on trash pickup day.

In light of the high cost of finding a place to put all the town's trash, Charlottesville decided to try to let market forces work by charging a fee of 80 cents per 32-gallon bag or can of residential garbage collected at the curb. Just as predicted by the law of demand, the amount of trash that Charlottesville's residents wished to dump declined following the imposition of this fee. The percentage reduction in quantity of trash collection services demanded was 37 percent, which translated into about 1,500 fewer tons of trash for the town to handle each year. Thus charging a fee to haul trash from people's homes significantly reduced the volume of trash collected in Charlottesville by over one-third. Because the initial explicit price of dumping trash was zero, the change in price to 80 cents per bag occurred along the inelastic range of the demand curve for trash collection services. Thus raising the per-bag collection fee increased the town's revenues from trash collection—from zero to positive revenues.

Some Unintended Consequences

What did Charlottesville residents do with all the garbage they withheld from collection following the imposition of the per-bag fee? Residents found that they could recycle about a third of it, and they were able to compost roughly another third of the garbage. Unfortunately, some residents apparently illegally engaged in "midnight dumping": To avoid paying the fee, they dumped trash along roadsides and in vacant lots. Trying to increase enforcement of antilittering laws was a costly activity for the town. So was the cost of administering the pricing program. Printing tags for all the trash bags the town collected and keeping track of residents' payments turned out to be a high-cost activity also.

On net, it turned out that the costs of enforcing and administering the pricing program were so high that trash collection revenues failed to cover the costs of the program. Thus Charlottesville suffered an economic loss on its trash collection business. In light of Charlottesville's experience, other municipalities are currently contemplating ways to implement similar pricing programs while containing administrative costs.

FOR CRITICAL ANALYSIS

1. If the demand for trash collection services is inelastic over a relatively large range of prices above 80 cents per bag, how might Charlottesville try to push up its trash collection revenues to earn a profit from hauling trash?
2. Critics of city trash collection pricing programs contend that they are unlikely to be profitable whenever governments administer the programs and argue that trash collection should be done by private firms. Do you agree with this perspective? Why or why not?

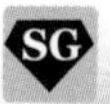

SUMMARY DISCUSSION OF LEARNING OBJECTIVES

1. **Expressing and Calculating the Price Elasticity of Demand:** The price elasticity of demand is the responsiveness of the quantity demanded of a good to a change in the price of the good. It is the percentage change in quantity demanded divided by the percentage change in price. To calculate the price elasticity of demand for relatively small changes in price, the percentage change in quantity demanded is equal to the change in the quantity resulting from a price change divided by the average of the initial and final quantities, and the percentage change in price is equal to the price change divided by the average of the initial and final prices.
2. **The Relationship Between the Price Elasticity of Demand and Total Revenues:** Demand is elastic when the price elasticity of demand exceeds 1, and over the elastic range of a demand curve, an increase in price reduces total revenues. Demand is inelastic when the price elasticity of demand is less than 1, and over this range of a demand curve, an increase in price raises total revenues. Finally, demand is unit-elastic when the price elasticity of demand equals 1, and over this range of a demand curve, an increase in price does not affect total revenues.
3. **Factors That Determine the Price Elasticity of Demand:** Three factors affect the price elasticity of demand. If there are more close substitutes for a good, the price elasticity of demand increases. The price elasticity of demand for a good also tends to be higher when a larger portion of a person's budget is spent on the good. In addition, if people have a longer period of time to adjust to a price change and change their consumption patterns, the price elasticity of demand tends to be higher.
4. **The Cross Price Elasticity of Demand and Using It to Determine Whether Two Goods Are Substitutes or Complements:** The cross price elasticity of demand for a good is the percentage change in the demand for that good divided by the percentage change in the price of a related good. If two goods are substitutes in consumption, a percentage increase in the price of one of the goods induces a percentage increase in the demand for the other good, so that the cross price elasticity of demand is positive. By contrast, if two goods are complements in consumption, a percentage increase in the price of one of the goods brings about a percentage decrease in the demand for the other good, so that the cross price elasticity of demand is negative.
5. **The Income Elasticity of Demand:** The income elasticity of demand for any good is the responsiveness of the demand for the good to a change in income, holding the good's relative price unchanged. It is equal to the percentage change in demand for the good divided by the percentage change in income.
6. **Classifying Supply Elasticities and How the Length of Time for Adjustment Affects the Price Elasticity of Supply:** The price elasticity of supply is equal to the percentage change in quantity supplied divided by the percentage change in price. If the price elasticity of supply is greater than 1, supply is elastic, and if the price elasticity of supply is less than 1, supply is inelastic. Supply is unit-elastic if the price elasticity of supply equals 1. Supply is more likely to be elastic when sellers have more time to adjust to price changes. One reason for this is that the more time sellers have to adjust, the more resources can flow into (or out of) an industry via expansion (or contraction) of firms. Another reason is that the longer the time allowed for adjustment, the more firms are able to find ways to increase (or decrease) production in response to a price increase (or decrease).

Key Terms and Concepts

Cross price elasticity of demand (E_{xy}) (495)

Elastic demand (486)

Income elasticity of demand (E_i) (496)

Inelastic demand (486)

Perfectly elastic demand (497)

Perfectly elastic supply (486)

Perfectly inelastic demand (486)

Perfectly inelastic supply (497)

Price elasticity of demand (E_p) (483)

Price elasticity of supply (E_s) (497)

Unit elasticity of demand (486)

Problems

Answers to the odd-numbered problems appear at the back of the book.

20-1. A student organization finds that when it prices shirts emblazoned with the college logo at $10, the organization sells 150 per week. When the price is reduced to $9, the organization sells 200 per week. Based on this information, calculate the price elasticity of demand for logo-emblazoned shirts.

20-2. Table 20-2 indicates that the price elasticity of demand for motion picture tickets is 0.9. If a theater raises the price of a movie ticket from $5 to $6, by what percentage should it expect the quantity of tickets sold to change?

20-3. When Joe's Campus Grill priced its famous hamburgers at $1, it sold 200 a week. When the price was $2, Joe's sold only 100 a week. Based on this information, calculate the price elasticity of demand for Joe's hamburgers.

20-4. Using the information in Problem 20-3, calculate the price elasticity of demand. Is demand elastic, unit-elastic, or inelastic?

20-5. It is difficult, if not impossible, to find commodities with perfectly elastic or perfectly inelastic demand. We can, however, find commodities that lie near these extremes. Characterize the following goods as being near perfectly elastic or near perfectly inelastic.

a. Corn grown and harvested by a small farmer in Iowa
b. Heroin for a drug addict
c. The services of the only dentist in town
d. The required text for the only section of a required economics course

20-6. A craftsman who makes guitars by hand finds that when he prices his guitars at $800, his annual revenue is $64,000. When he prices his guitars at $700, his annual revenue is $63,000. Over this range of guitar prices, does the craftsman face elastic, unit-elastic, or inelastic demand?

20-7. Suppose that over a range of prices, the price elasticity of demand varies from 15.0 to 2.5. Over another range of prices, price elasticity of demand varies from 1.5 to .75. What can you say about total revenue and the total revenue curve over these two ranges of the demand curve as price falls?

20-8. Based on the information provided alone, characterize the following goods as being more elastic or more inelastic.

a. A 45-cent box of kosher salt that you buy once a year
b. A type of high-powered ski boat that you can rent from any one of a number of rental agencies
c. A specific brand of bottled water
d. Automobile insurance in a state that requires autos to be insured but has few insurance companies
e. A 75-cent guitar pick for the lead guitarist of a major rock band

20-9. The value of cross price elasticity of demand between goods X and Y is 1.25, while the cross price elasticity of demand between goods X and Z is 2.0. Characterize X and Y, X and Z, and Y and Z as substitutes or complements.

20-10. Suppose that the cross price elasticity of demand between eggs and bacon is $-.5$. What would you expect to happen to the sales of bacon if the price of eggs rises by 10 percent?

20-11. Assume that the income elasticity of demand for hot dogs is -1.25 and that the income elasticity of demand for lobster is 1.25. Explain why the measure for hot dogs is negative while that for lobster is positive. Based on this information alone, are these normal or inferior goods? (Hint: You may want to refer to the discussion of normal and inferior goods in Chapter 3.)

20-12. The price elasticity of supply of a basic commodity that a nation produces domestically and that it also imports is 2. What would you expect to happen to the volume of imports if the price of this commodity rises by 10 percent?

Economics on the Net

Cigarettes, Elasticity, and Government Policy In recent years, state and federal governments have focused considerable attention on cigarettes. This application helps you understand the role that elasticity plays in this issue.

Title: Measures to Reduce the Demand for Tobacco

Navigation: Click here to go directly to the Web page provided by UICC GLOBALink: The International Tobacco Control Network.

Application Read the article and answer the following questions.

1. In general, is the elasticity of demand for cigarettes elastic, unit-elastic, or inelastic? Explain why.
2. Would a tax hike on cigarettes have much of an impact on cigarette smoking?
3. Based on the forecasts provided in the article, is cigarette consumption perfectly elastic?

For Group Study and Analysis Explore the impact of the government subsidies to tobacco growers and of taxes on the consumption of cigarettes. Illustrate the effects of these two programs in a supply and demand diagram for cigarettes. Discuss the logic of the government's approaches to cigarette consumption. Attempt to reach a consensus on the "right" approach for the government to take.

CHAPTER

21

THE GLOBAL FINANCIAL ENVIRONMENT OF BUSINESS

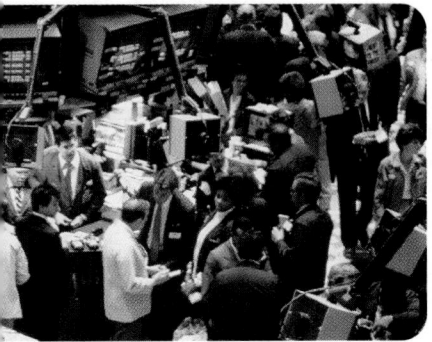

This scene from the floor of a stock exchange used to be of little interest to most Americans. Today, in contrast, at least 40 percent of American families own stocks. How might changes in the stock market affect consumer spending?

Someone in your family probably owns stock in at least one American corporation. And you undoubtedly know plenty of other people who own corporate stock. Stock ownership has become much more widespread in America over the past half century. In 1952, for example, only 4 percent of Americans owned stock. But the proportion has risen more than 10-fold. The economic consequences of this wider ownership of American corporations are considerable. For example, upturns and downturns in the stock market now have a much stronger impact on consumer spending than they used to. But the fact that all parts of the income distribution now have a stake in Wall Street also has political implications, ranging from opposition to particular tax policies to support for certain types of foreign policy. Before you can grasp the full importance of America's love affair with the stock market, however, you need to know more about the global financial environment of business.

LEARNING OBJECTIVES

After reading this chapter, you should be able to:

1. **Distinguish among the main organizational forms of business and explain the chief advantages and disadvantages of each**
2. **Explain the three main sources of corporate funds**
3. **Discuss the difference between stocks and bonds**
4. **Evaluate the economic impact of on-line trading of stocks and bonds**
5. **Explain the global nature of capital markets**
6. **Understand the problems of corporate control**

Chapter Outline

- The Legal Organization of Firms
- Methods of Corporate Financing
- The Markets for Stocks and Bonds
- Global Capital Markets
- Electronic Securities Trading
- Problems in Corporate Governance

Did You Know That... at the start of the twenty-first century, nearly one-half of all retail purchases of corporate stock in the United States were made over the Internet? Moreover, corporate bonds and many other financial assets could also be purchased over the Internet with just the click of a mouse. In fact, some corporations seeking **financial capital** had begun to make initial public offerings (IPOs)—their initial start-up sales of stocks—over the Internet. Just five years before, none of this was possible. As it is doing to so much of life, the Internet is changing the nature of global financial markets.

You were introduced to the term *physical capital* as one of the five factors of production. In that context, capital consists of the goods that do not directly satisfy human wants but are used to make other goods. *Financial capital* is the money that is made available to purchase capital goods.

Different types of businesses are able to raise financial capital in different ways. And because of the Internet, raising capital is becoming easier and less costly. The first step in understanding the firm's financial environment is to understand the way firms are organized.

THE LEGAL ORGANIZATION OF FIRMS

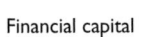

Financial capital 
Money used to purchase capital goods such as buildings and equipment.

We all know that firms differ from one another. Some sell frozen yogurt, others make automobiles; some advertise, some do not; some have annual sales of a few thousand dollars, others have sales in the billions of dollars. The list of differences is probably endless. Yet for all this diversity, the basic organization of *all* firms can be thought of in terms of a few simple structures, the most important of which are the proprietorship, the partnership, and the corporation.

Proprietorships

Proprietorship 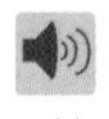
A business owned by one individual who makes the business decisions, receives all the profits, and is legally responsible for all the debts of the firm.

The most common form of business organization is the **proprietorship;** as shown in Table 21-1, more than 73 percent of all firms in the United States are proprietorships. Each is owned by a single individual who makes the business decisions, receives all the profits, and is legally responsible for all the debts of the firm. Although proprietorships are numerous, they are generally rather small businesses, with annual sales typically under $50,000. For this reason, even though there are more than 10 million proprietorships in the United States, they account for only about 5 percent of all business revenues.

TABLE 21-1
Forms of Business Organization

Type of Firm	Percentage of U.S. Firms	Average Size (annual sales in dollars)	Percentage of Total Business Revenues
Proprietorship	73.1	49,000	5.1
Partnership	7.0	540,000	5.5
Corporation	19.9	3,122,000	89.4

Sources: U.S. Bureau of the Census; *2000 Statistical Abstract.*

Advantages of Proprietorships. Proprietorships offer several advantages as a form of business organization. First, they are *easy to form and to dissolve.* In the simplest case, all one must do to start a business is to start working; to dissolve the firm, one simply stops working. Second, *all decision-making power resides with the sole proprietor.* No partners, shareholders, or board of directors need be consulted. The third advantage is that its *profit is taxed only once.* All profit is treated by law as the net income of the proprietor and as such is subject only to personal income taxation.

Disadvantages of Proprietorships. The most important disadvantage of a proprietorship is that the proprietor faces **unlimited liability** *for the debts of the firm.* This means that the owner is personally responsible for all of the firm's debts. The second disadvantage is that it has *limited ability to raise funds,* to expand the business or even simply to help it survive bad times. Because of this, many lenders are reluctant to lend large sums to a proprietorship. The third disadvantage of proprietorships is that they normally *end with the death of the proprietor,* which creates added uncertainty for prospective lenders or employees.

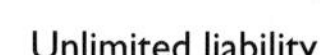

A legal concept whereby the personal assets of the owner of a firm can be seized to pay off the firm's debts.

Partnerships

The second important form of business organization is the **partnership.** As shown in Table 21-1, partnerships are far less numerous than proprietorships but tend to be significantly larger, with average sales about 10 times greater. A partnership differs from a proprietorship chiefly in that there are two or more co-owners, called partners. They share the responsibilities of operating the firm and its profits, and they are *each* legally responsible for *all* of the debts incurred by the firm. In this sense, a partnership may be viewed as a proprietorship with more than one owner.

Partnership 
A business owned by two or more joint owners, or partners, who share the responsibilities and the profits of the firm and are individually liable for all of the debts of the partnership.

Advantages of Partnerships. The first advantage of a partnership is that it is *easy to form.* In fact, it is almost as easy as forming a proprietorship. Second, partnerships, like proprietorships, often help *reduce the costs of monitoring job performance.* This is particularly true when interpersonal skills are important for successful performance and in lines of business where, even after the fact, it is difficult to measure performance objectively. Thus attorneys and physicians often organize themselves as partnerships. A third advantage of the partnership is that it *permits more effective specialization* in occupations in which, for legal or other reasons, the multiple talents required for success are unlikely to be uniform across individuals. Finally, the income of the partnership is treated as personal income and thus is *subject only to personal taxation.*

Disadvantages of Partnerships. Partnerships also have their disadvantages. First, the *partners each have unlimited liability.* Thus the personal assets of *each* partner are at risk due to debts incurred on behalf of the partnership by *any* of the partners. Second, *decision making is generally more costly* in a partnership than in a proprietorship; there are more people involved in making decisions, and they may have differences of opinion that must be resolved before action is possible. Finally, *dissolution of the partnership is generally necessary* when a partner dies or voluntarily withdraws or when one or more partners wish to remove someone from the partnership. This creates potential uncertainty for creditors and employees.

Corporations

Corporation 
A legal entity that may conduct business in its own name just as an individual does; the owners of a corporation, called shareholders, own shares of the firm's profits and enjoy the protection of limited liability.

A **corporation** is a legal entity that may conduct business in its own name just as an individual does. The owners of a corporation are called *shareholders* because they own shares of the profits earned by the firm. By law, shareholders enjoy **limited liability,** so that if the corporation incurs debts that it cannot pay, the shareholders' personal property is shielded from claims by the firm's creditors. As shown in Table 21-1, corporations are far less numerous than proprietorships, but because of their large size, they are responsible for about 90 percent of all business revenues in the United States.

Limited liability 
A legal concept whereby the responsibility, or liability, of the owners of a corporation is limited to the value of the shares in the firm that they own.

Advantages of Corporations. Perhaps the greatest advantage of corporations is that their owners (the shareholders) enjoy *limited liability.* The liability of shareholders is limited to the value of their shares. The second advantage arises because legally, the corporation *continues to exist* even if one or more owners cease to be owners. A third advantage of the corporation stems from the first two: Corporations are well positioned to *raise large sums of financial capital.* People are able to buy ownership shares or lend money to the corporation knowing that their liability is limited to the amount of money they invest and confident that the corporation's existence does not depend on the life of any one of the firm's owners.

Disadvantages of Corporations. The chief disadvantage of the corporation is that corporate income is subject to *double taxation.* The profits of the corporation are subject first to corporate taxation. Then, if any of the after-tax profits are distributed to shareholders as **dividends,** such payments are treated as personal income to the shareholders and subject to personal taxation. Owners of corporations pay about twice as much in taxes on corporate income as they do on other forms of income.

Dividends 
Portion of a corporation's profits paid to its owners (shareholders).

A second disadvantage of the corporation is that corporations are potentially subject to problems associated with the *separation of ownership and control.* The owners and managers of a corporation are typically different persons and may have different incentives. The problems that can result are discussed later in the chapter.

CONCEPTS IN BRIEF

- Proprietorships are the most common form of business organization, comprising 73 percent of all firms. Each is owned by a single individual who makes all business decisions, receives all the profits, and has unlimited liability for the firm's debts.
- Partnerships are much like proprietorships, except that two or more individuals, or partners, share the decisions and the profits of the firm. In addition, each partner has unlimited liability for the debts of the firm.
- Corporations are responsible for the largest share of business revenues. The owners, called shareholders, share in the firm's profits but normally have little responsibility for the firm's day-to-day operations. They enjoy limited liability for the debts of the firm.

METHODS OF CORPORATE FINANCING

When the Dutch East India Company was founded in 1602, it raised financial capital by selling shares of its expected future profits to investors. The investors thus became the owners of the company, and their ownership shares eventually became known as "shares of stock," or simply *stocks.* The company also issued notes of indebtedness, which involved borrowing money in return for interest on the funds, plus eventual repayment of the principal amount borrowed. In modern parlance, these notes of indebtedness are called *bonds*. As the company prospered over time, some of its revenues were used to pay lenders the interest and principal owed them; of the profits that remained, some were paid to shareholders in the form of dividends, and some were retained by the company for reinvestment in further enterprises. The methods of financing used by the Dutch East India Company four centuries ago—stocks, bonds, and reinvestment—remain the principal methods of financing for today's corporations.

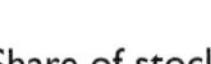

Share of stock
A legal claim to a share of a corporation's future profits; if it is *common stock*, it incorporates certain voting rights regarding major policy decisions of the corporation; if it is *preferred stock*, its owners are accorded preferential treatment in the payment of dividends.

A **share of stock** in a corporation is simply a legal claim to a share of the corporation's future profits. If there are 100,000 shares of stock in a company and you own 1,000 of them, you own the right to 1 percent of that company's future profits. If the stock you own is *common stock,* you also have the right to vote on major policy decisions affecting the company, such as the selection of the corporation's board of directors. Your 1,000 shares would entitle you to cast 1 percent of the votes on such issues. If the stock you own is *preferred stock,* you also own a share of the future profits of the corporation, but you do *not* have regular voting rights. You do, however, get something in return for giving up your voting rights: preferential treatment in the payment of dividends. Specifically, the owners of preferred stock generally must receive at least a certain amount of dividends in each period before the owners of common stock can receive *any* dividends.

Bond
A legal claim against a firm, usually entitling the owner of the bond to receive a fixed annual coupon payment, plus a lump-sum payment at the bond's maturity date. Bonds are issued in return for funds lent to the firm.

A **bond** is a legal claim against a firm, entitling the owner of the bond to receive a fixed annual *coupon* payment, plus a lump-sum payment at the maturity date of the bond.* Bonds are issued in return for funds lent to the firm; the coupon payments represent interest on the amount borrowed by the firm, and the lump-sum payment at maturity of the bond generally equals the amount originally borrowed by the firm. Bonds are *not* claims on the future profits of the firm; legally, bondholders must be paid whether the firm prospers or not. To help ensure this, bondholders generally receive their coupon payments each year, along with any principal that is due, before *any* shareholders can receive dividend payments.

Reinvestment
Profits (or depreciation reserves) used to purchase new capital equipment.

Reinvestment takes place when the firm uses some of its profits to purchase new capital equipment rather than paying the money out as dividends to shareholders. Although sales of stock are an important source of financing for new firms, reinvestment and borrowing are the primary means of financing for existing firms. Indeed, reinvestment by established firms is such an important source of financing that it dominates the other two sources of corporate finance, amounting to roughly 75 percent of new financial capital for corporations in recent years. Also, small businesses, which are the source of much current growth, often cannot rely on the stock market to raise investment funds.

THE MARKETS FOR STOCKS AND BONDS

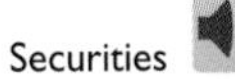

Securities
Stocks and bonds.

Economists often refer to the "market for wheat" or the "market for labor," but these are concepts rather than actual places. For **securities** (stocks and bonds), however, there really are markets—centralized, physical locations where exchange takes place. The most prestigious of these are the New York Stock Exchange (NYSE) and the New York Bond Exchange, both located in New York City. Numerous other stock and bond markets, or exchanges, exist throughout the United States and in various financial capitals of the world, such as London and Tokyo. Although the exact process by which exchanges are conducted

---

*Coupon payments on bonds get their name from the fact that bonds once had coupons attached to them when they were issued. Each year, the owner would clip a coupon off the bond and send it to the issuing firm in return for that year's interest on the bond.

in these markets varies slightly from one to another, the process used on the NYSE is representative of the principles involved.*

FAQ: What is the Dow Jones Industrial Average?

The Dow Jones Industrial Average—"the Dow" for short—is an index that measures the average price of the stocks of 30 major American corporations, including McDonald's (fast food), Hewlett-Packard (computers and printers), and Wal-Mart (retail sales). The Dow was set up in 1896 (with just 12 stocks) by publisher Charles Dow and has been expanded and revised ever since by the editors of the *Wall Street Journal*. In principle, changes in the Dow mirror changes in the average price of the thousands of American stocks. But in reality, the Dow reflects only the average price of the specific stocks that comprise it: A $1 per share change in the price of a component stock causes a 4-point change in the Dow. Because the Dow comprises so few stocks, many observers think its usefulness as a measure of the overall stock market is limited. Still, it remains the most widely watched stock index in the world, and when it broke 10,000 for the first time in 1999, every major newspaper and newscast in America covered the story.

More than 2,500 stocks are traded on the NYSE, which is sometimes called the "Big Board." Leading brokerage firms—about 600 of them—own seats on the NYSE. These seats, which are actually rights to buy and sell stocks on the floor of the Big Board, are themselves regularly exchanged. In recent years, their value has fluctuated between $350,000 and $2 million each. These prices reflect the fact that stock trades on the NYSE are ultimately handled by the firms owning these seats, and the firms earn commissions on each trade.

The Theory of Efficient Markets 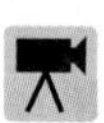

At any point in time, there are tens of thousands, even millions of persons looking for any bit of information that will enable them to forecast correctly the future prices of stocks. Responding to any information that seems useful, these people try to buy low and sell high. The result is that all publicly available information that might be used to forecast stock prices gets taken into account by those with access to the information and the knowledge and ability to learn from it, leaving no forecastable profit opportunities. And because so many people are involved in this process, it occurs quite swiftly. Indeed, there is some evidence that *all* information entering the market is fully incorporated into stock prices within less than a minute of its arrival. One view is that any information about specific stocks will prove to have little value by the time it reaches you.

Random walk theory 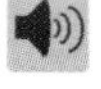
The theory that there are no predictable trends in securities prices that can be used to "get rich quick."

Consequently, stock prices tend to follow a *random walk,* which is to say that the best forecast of tomorrow's price is today's price. This is called the **random walk theory.** Although large values of the random component of stock price changes are less likely than small values, nothing else about the magnitude or direction of a stock price change can be predicted. Indeed, the random component of stock prices exhibits behavior much like what would occur if you rolled two dice and subtracted 7 from the resulting total. On average, the dice will show a total of 7, so after you subtract 7, the average result will be zero. It is true that rolling a 12 or a 2 (resulting in a total of +5 or −5) is less likely than rolling an 8 or a 6 (yielding a total of +1 or −1). Nevertheless, positive and negative totals are equally likely, and the expected total is zero.

Inside Information

Inside information 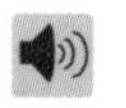
Information that is not available to the general public about what is happening in a corporation.

Isn't there any way to "beat the market"? The answer is yes—but normally only if you have **inside information** that is not available to the public. Suppose that your best friend is in charge of new product development at the country's largest software firm, Microsoft Corporation.

*A number of stocks and bonds are traded in so-called over-the-counter (OTC) markets, which, although not physically centralized, otherwise operate in much the same way as the NYSE and so are not treated separately in this text.

Your friend tells you that the company's smartest programmer has just come up with major new software that millions of computer users will want to buy. No one but your friend and the programmer—and now you—is aware of this. You could indeed make money using this information by purchasing shares of Microsoft and then selling them (at a higher price) as soon as the new product is publicly announced. There is one problem: Stock trading based on inside information such as this is illegal, punishable by substantial fines and even imprisonment. So unless you happen to have a stronger than average desire for a long vacation in a federal prison, you might be better off investing in Microsoft after the new program is publicly announced.

Click here to explore how the U.S. Securities and Exchange Commission seeks to prevent the use of inside information.

EXAMPLE

How to Read the Financial Press: Stock Prices

Table 21-2, reproduced from the *Wall Street Journal,* contains information about the stocks of four companies. Across the top of the financial page are a series of column headings. Under the heading "Stock" we find the name of the company—in the second row, for example, is Eastman Kodak, the photographic materials firm. The two columns to the left of the company's name show the highest and lowest prices at which

TABLE 21-2
Reading Stock Quotes

52 Weeks											
Hi	Low	Stock	Sym	Div.	Yld %	PE	Vol 100s	Hi	Lo	Close	Net Chg
$69\frac{9}{16}$	$40\frac{3}{16}$	Eastman Chm	EMN	1.76	3.4	21	2838	52	51	51	$+\frac{3}{4}$
$88\frac{15}{16}$	$60\frac{13}{16}$	EKodak	EK	1.76	2.4	18	17286	74	$72\frac{3}{8}$	73	$-2\frac{9}{16}$
$92\frac{7}{16}$	57	Eaton	ETN	1.76	2.1	19	4198	$89\frac{1}{8}$	84	85	$-4\frac{9}{16}$
$29\frac{5}{8}$	$17\frac{5}{8}$	Eaton/Vance	EV	.30	1.0	na	710	$30\frac{5}{8}$	$29\frac{9}{16}$	30	$+\frac{7}{16}$

The summary of stock market information presented on the financial pages of many newspapers reveals the following:

52 Weeks Hi/Lo: The highest and lowest prices, in dollars per share, of the stock during the previous 52 weeks

Stock: The name of the company (frequently abbreviated)

Sym: Highly abbreviated name of the company, as it appears on the stock exchange ticker tape

Div: Dividend paid, in dollars per share

Yld %: Yield in percent per year; the dividend divided by the price of the stock

PE: Price-earnings ratio; the price of the stock divided by the earnings (profits) per share of the company

Vol 100s: Number of shares traded during the day, in hundreds of shares

Hi: Highest price at which the stock traded that day

Lo: Lowest price at which the stock traded that day

Close: Last price at which the stock traded that day

Net Chg: Net change in the stock's price from the previous day's closing price

shares of that company's stock traded during the past 52 weeks. These prices are typically quoted in dollars and fractions of dollars.

Immediately to the right of the company's name you will find the company's *symbol* on the NYSE. This symbol (omitted by some newspapers) is simply the unique identifier used by the exchange when it reports information about the stock. For example, the designation EK is used by the exchange as the unique identifier for the firm Eastman Kodak.

The last four columns of information for each firm summarize the behavior of the firm's stock price on the latest trading day. On this particular day, the highest price at which Kodak stock traded was $74.50, the lowest price was $72.375, and the last (or closing) price at which it traded was $73.00 per share. The *net change* in the price of Kodak stock was −$2.5625, which means that it *closed* the day at a price about $2.56 per share below the price at which it closed the day before.

The dividend column, headed "Div," shows the annual dividend (in dollars and cents) that the company has paid over the preceding year on each share of its stock. In Kodak's case, this amounts to $1.76 a share. If the dividend is divided by the closing price of the stock ($1.76 ÷ $73.00), the result is 2.4 percent, which is shown in the yield percentage ("Yld %") column for Kodak. In a sense, the company is paying interest on the stock at a rate of about 2.4 percent. At first glance, this seems like an absurdly low amount; after all, at the time this issue of the *Wall Street Journal* was printed, ordinary checking accounts were paying about this much. The reason people tolerate this seemingly low yield on Kodak (or any other stock) is that they expect that the price of the stock will rise over time, yielding capital gains.

The column heading "PE" stands for *price-earnings ratio.* To obtain the entries for this column, the firm's total earnings (profits) for the year are divided by the number of the firm's shares in existence to give the earnings per share. When the price of the stock is divided by the earnings per share, the result is the price-earnings ratio.

The column to the right of the PE ratio shows the total *volume* of the shares of the stock traded that day, measured in hundreds of shares.

For Critical Analysis

Is there necessarily any relationship between the net change in a stock's price and how many shares have been sold on a particular day?

CONCEPTS IN BRIEF

- Many economists believe that asset markets, especially the stock market, are efficient, meaning that one cannot make a higher than normal rate of return without having inside information (information that the general public does not possess).
- Stock prices normally follow a random walk, meaning that you cannot predict changes in future stock prices based on information about stock price behavior in the past.

GLOBAL CAPITAL MARKETS

Financial institutions in the United States are tied to the rest of the world via their lending capacities. In addition, integration of all financial markets is increasing. Indeed, recent changes in world finance have been nothing short of remarkable. Distinctions among financial institutions and between financial institutions and nonfinancial institutions have blurred. As the legal barriers that have preserved such distinctions are dismantled, multinational corporations offering a wide array of financial services are becoming dominant worldwide.

The globalization of financial markets is not entirely new. U.S. banks developed worldwide branch networks in the 1960s and 1970s for loans, check clearing, and foreign exchange (currency) trading. Also in the 1970s, firms dealing in U.S. securities expanded their operations in London (on the Eurobond market) and then into other financial centers, including Tokyo. Similarly, foreign firms invaded U.S. shores: first the banks, then securities firms. The "big four" Japanese securities firms now have offices in New York and London.

Money and capital markets today are truly international. Markets for U.S. government securities, interbank lending and borrowing, foreign exchange trading, and common stocks are now trading continuously, in vast quantities, around the clock and around the world.

Trading for U.S. government securities has been described as "the world's fastest-growing 24-hour market." This market was made possible by (1) sophisticated communications and computer technology, (2) deregulation of financial markets in foreign countries to permit such trading, (3) U.S. legislation in 1984 to enable foreign investors to buy U.S. government securities tax-free, and (4) huge annual U.S. government budget deficits, which have poured a steady stream of tradable debt into the world markets.

Foreign exchange—the buying and selling of foreign currencies—became a 24-hour, worldwide market in the 1970s. Instruments tied to government bonds, foreign exchange, stock market indexes, and commodities (grains, metals, oil) are now traded increasingly in financial futures markets in all the world's major centers of commerce. Most financial firms are coming to the conclusion that to survive as a force in any one of the world's leading financial markets, a firm must have a significant presence in all of them. As we enter the twenty-first century, between 30 and 50 financial institutions are at the centers of world finance—New York, London, Tokyo, and Frankfurt—and they are competing in all those markets to do business with the world's major corporations and portfolio managers. Today, major corporate borrowers throughout the world can choose to borrow from a wide variety of lenders, also located throughout the world. Moreover, as discussed in the next section, on-line securities trading is transforming finanical markets into a unified whole.

EXAMPLE

Going Global Without Knowing It

Although it seems much easier to buy and sell stocks of American companies than stocks of foreign companies, it is in fact quite easy to invest globally, even without realizing it. Consider recent retirees Mary Jo and George Paoni, residents of Illinois. Part of their savings are in a money market fund with ties to J. P. Morgan, the investment banker. Morgan has in turn engaged in $1 billion in high-risk trades in the baht, the national currency of Thailand. The Paonis' money market fund also had assets tied up with Bangkok Land, a real estate development company. Bangkok Land currently owns a modern—and largely worthless—ghost town near Bangkok airport that was supposed to be a city of 700,000. Mrs. Paoni's stake in the Illinois State Pension Fund turns out to have connections even more farflung. For example, the pension fund owns a piece of Aracruz Cellulose S.A., a Brazilian pulp and paper company hit by a sharp drop in commodity prices in the late 1990s. The drop in pulp prices from $850 a ton to $420 a ton drove the value of the pension fund's investment in the same direction. The fund also indirectly owns a stake in the Russian department store GUM (doing as poorly as the Russian economy) and in Peregrine Investments, a Hong Kong investment bank. Peregrine collapsed in 1998 with more than 2,000 creditors owed more than $4 billion. Although Mrs. Paoni's retirement check is as yet in no danger, the Illinois Pension Fund's investment in Peregrine is currently worthless.

For Critical Analysis

Should pension funds be limited by law in the nature of the investments they are allowed to make?

CONCEPTS IN BRIEF

- Financial markets throughout the world have become increasingly integrated, leading to a global financial market. Interbank lending and borrowing, foreign exchange trading, and stock sales now occur virtually 24 hours a day throughout the world.
- Many U.S. government or government-guaranteed securities trade 24 hours a day.

ELECTRONIC SECURITIES TRADING

On-line trading of shares of corporate stock is transforming the market for these securities. It all began in the mid-1990s with the establishment of just a few Internet addresses, such as www.etrade.com, www.schwab.com, and www.lombard.com. These Web sites offered something never before available: the capability to buy shares of stock on-line.

Benefits of On-Line Trading

What these Internet sites also offered were low brokerage fees. To buy 100 shares of stock in AOL–Time Warner from a traditional brokerage firm entailed fees in the neighborhood of $100; on-line brokers typically charged about $10 to make the same transaction. The result was predictable: On-line securities trading took off. By 2000, more than 2 million on-line trading accounts had been established. Total on-line stock trading had grown to about $200 billion. Observers expect that by 2003, the number of on-line stock-trading accounts will increase to as many as 11 million, with at least $700 billion traded via those accounts.

These estimates could prove to be low. They take into account only "hard-wired" trading via desktop and laptop computers. Recently, some high-tech firms have begun to introduce on-line securities trading systems that use cellular telephones, two-way pagers, and handheld computers connected to wireless modems. Today, there are more than 200 million mobile telephone subscribers, and that figure is expected to exceed 500 million worldwide by 2003. Thus there is a significant potential for even more growth in on-line securities trading.

Trading Speed

On-line trading does not just entail lower explicit expenses. It is faster, too. Anyone can reach Internet-based brokerage accounts from any computer with a secure Web browser. Today, literally at one's fingertips are hundreds of sites offering investment research sources and trading capabilities—all of which help make the Web a logical fit with the fast-paced, high-tech world of Wall Street.

To connect to an on-line trading site, an Internet trader punches in an ID and account password. Typically, she then has access to a package of services that might otherwise be quite costly if purchased separately. These include portfolio-tracking software and databases containing information about the market capitalization and earnings growth of listed companies. After conducting market research, an Internet trader can scan her portfolio of holdings, search for key information on companies whose stock she owns, and send an order to buy or sell more stock.

Moreover, she can do all this in a few minutes. That saves time, and time is valuable. Any time that she spends trading securities is time that she could have allocated to other endeavors. Thus the speed of on-line trading reduces the opportunity cost of trading.

EXAMPLE

Funding a Start-Up Company on the Internet

Getting a business off the ground requires more than lots of hard work. It requires raising hard cash. Many small businesses have trouble raising seed money to get started. But those that succeed in raising the initial funds can seek out venture capital firms for additional financing. Eventually they can "go public" by floating a stock issue.

Today, a business can to go public on the Net—it can sell shares of stock to the public directly. Spring Street Brewing Company made history in 1995 when it became the first company to conduct an initial public offering (IPO) over the Internet. It made history again in March 1996 when the Securities and Exchange Commission (SEC) allowed Spring Street to trade its shares via its Web site without registering as a broker-dealer. The SEC only required Spring Street to use an independent agent, such as a bank or an escrow agent, to process the funds it raised on the Net.

The SEC estimates that going public via the traditional, non-Internet route takes about 900 hours of work. Most of this time is devoted to preparing a prospectus prior to the sale of stock. Companies also have to hire specialized lawyers and use an underwriter, who normally charges a fee equal to about 10 percent of the value of the IPO. The cyber-based alternative is to buy a computer program called CapScape. This program automates the process of compiling the offer documents, permitting a company to sell shares directly to investors over the Internet.

Who will ultimately benefit from Internet IPOs? Small businesses.

For Critical Analysis

Who stands to lose if Internet IPOs become commonplace?

Can Brokerage Firms Keep Up?

Internet trading benefits the brokerage firms that offer it. Most Wall Street discount brokers now accept on-line orders. Internet-based brokerage firms can get by with less printed marketing material to send to clients, smaller customer service staffs, and fewer physical branches.

On July 16, 1996, U.S. stock prices suddenly dropped. Home computer screens flickered as stock prices then recovered somewhat while thousands of people followed the events on-line. For many brand-new Internet brokers, that day turned out to be a supreme test of the capacities of their systems.

Some brokerage firms almost failed the test, however. People across the nation reacted to the sudden fluctuation in stock prices by turning on their home computers to conduct a speedy on-line reshuffling of their portfolios. Many, however, discovered after a few clicks of their mouse buttons that they were frozen out of their Internet trading accounts. One New Jersey trader, for instance, indicated that found himself "stuck in Never-Never Land" for two hours that day. During that time, he was unable to log on to his account, check his account status, obtain stock price quotes, or even check the values of market indexes such as the Dow Jones Industrial Average. He was finally able to get connected later in the day, but even then the system reported incorrect stock prices. Ultimately, his on-line broker sent him a negotiated payment to try to compensate for its inability to handle the unexpectedly large volume of Internet traffic it experienced that day.

Nowadays, Internet brokers are much better equipped to handle huge trading volumes. Nevertheless, the July 1996 experience showed that Internet traders cannot rule out the possibility of a new kind of stock market crash: the crash of an on-line system along with the market itself. When Internet traders crowd on-line at once, computer systems can fail to handle the overflow. As a result, active traders who like the minute-to-minute control offered by on-line trading might actually find themselves completely frozen out of the market.

A Lower Return to "Day Trading"?

Click here to see one way that day traders keep up with scheduled initial public offerings and news of mergers and acquisitions.

Not everyone possesses the savvy to be a successful stock trader. The average customer of a traditional stockbroker makes just four or five transactions a year. By contrast, the typical Internet trader makes more than 20 transactions per year, and some, known as "day traders," spend significant portions of each day buying and selling stocks on-line in pursuit of quick profits.

Unfortunately for some of these day traders, researchers Terrance Odean and Brad Barber of the University of California, Davis, have found evidence that people who engage in more stock purchases and sales tend to earn lower overall returns on their portfolios. One possible reason for this is that many people who trade less often may think more carefully about the trades they make. Some people who trade more frequently may be more inclined to act on impulse. Such hasty decision making can result in lower earnings.

According to some observers—particularly traditional brokers facing growing competition from on-line brokers—the spontaneity of Internet trading could actually make some people worse off. Many of us know otherwise reasonable people who sometimes act as impulsive consumers, wasting hard-earned income on goods or services they realize later they did not really desire. Likewise, some Internet stock traders can end up losing hard-earned savings by impulsively buying stocks that perform worse than they expected.

Currently, around one person in 10 who trade stocks does so on-line. Furthermore, the $1.5 trillion in retail on-line trading predicted for 2003 would account for less than 10 percent of the total volume of securities trading likely to take place. This indicates that people have not given up on traditional stockbrokers. So in fact, a two-tiered stock market seems to be emerging. One group of savers will trade on their own accounts on-line. The other will continue to rely on brokers, both to offer advice and to execute transactions.

Policy Issues of Globalized On-Line Trading

For the myriad financial firms setting up shop on the Internet, the promise of avoiding the costs of physical offices has been perceived as a key advantage. Nevertheless, the on-line broker E*Trade ran into a snag in the late 1990s when it attempted to offer its services in Australia, Canada, New Zealand, and the United Kingdom. It found that securities regulators required the company to open bricks-and-mortar offices in those countries before having the legal right to do any business there. The United Kingdom's Securities and Investments Board (SIB) even threatened to require E*Trade to locate some of its computers within Britain as well. The SIB was unconvinced by E*Trade's argument that cyberspace is both everywhere and anywhere. The British agency noted that the United Kingdom has laws forbidding solicitation by unauthorized foreign securities firms. It ruled that merely setting up a Web site constitutes solicitation. It held that whenever a British-based computer was used to make offers to buy or sell securities over the Internet, those offers were legally made in Britain. The SIB therefore concluded that anyone establishing financial trading Web sites must comply with Britain's laws or else face penalties of prison or a fine.

Should national securities trading regulators cooperate by enforcing the rules of all other nations? For instance, should the U.S. Securities and Exchange Commission compel companies such as E*Trade to abide by the rules of the British SIB and all other national regulators? Alternatively, should all countries follow the example set by the European Union and automatically authorize companies in other nations to sell their services across borders under the rules of the nations in which the companies themselves are based? For example, should the SIB concentrate only on regulating British Internet trading firms, thereby risking a flight of business away from the United Kingdom? These are the kinds of questions that public policymakers are struggling to answer as Internet trading continues to spread.

CONCEPTS IN BRIEF

- On-line securities trading has grown rapidly in recent years, largely because on-line brokers' fees are much lower than those of full-service brokers and because people can execute on-line trades more quickly.
- On-line brokerage firms have struggled to keep up with the growing volumes of Internet stock trading, particularly during periods of rapid stock price swings that have generated big increases in trading activity. This has exposed some on-line traders to problems when on-line systems have crashed.
- In principle, on-line trading can span national borders, but securities regulators have offered different legal interpretations about the extent to which on-line brokers are subject to national regulations.

PROBLEMS IN CORPORATE GOVERNANCE

Many corporations issue stock to raise financial capital that they will use to fund expansion or modernization. The decision to raise capital in this way is ordinarily made not by the owners of the corporation—the holders of its stock—but by the company's managers. This **separation of ownership and control** in corporations leads to incentive problems. Managers may not act in the best interest of shareholders. Further incentive problems arise when corporations borrow money in financial markets. These corporate governance problems have to do with information that is not the same for everyone.

Separation of ownership and control 
The situation that exists in corporations in which the owners (shareholders) are not the people who control the operation of the corporation (managers). The goals of these two groups are often different.

Asymmetric Information: The Perils of Adverse Selection and Moral Hazard

If you invest in a corporation, you give purchasing power to the managers of that corporation. Those managers have much more information about what is happening to the corporation and its future than you do. As you learned in Chapter 14 the inequality of knowledge between the two parties is called *asymmetric information.* If asymmetric information exists before a transaction takes place, we have a circumstance of *adverse selection.* In financial markets, adverse selection occurs because borrowers who are the worst credit risks (and thus likely to yield the most adverse outcomes) are the ones most likely to seek, and perhaps to receive, loans.

Consider two firms seeking to borrow funds by selling bonds. Suppose that one of the firms, the Dynamic Corporation, is pursuing a project with a small chance of yielding large profits and a large chance of bankruptcy. The other firm, the Reliable Company, intends to invest in a project that is guaranteed to yield the competitive rate of return, thereby ensuring repayment of its debts. Because Dynamic knows the chance is high that it will go bankrupt and never have to pay its debts, it can offer a high interest rate on the bonds it issues. Unless prospective bond purchasers can distinguish perfectly between the two firms' projects, they will select the high-yielding bonds offered by Dynamic and refuse to buy the low-yielding bonds offered by Reliable. Firms like Reliable will be unable to get funding, yet lenders will lose money on firms like Dynamic. Adverse selection thus makes investors less likely to lend to anyone and more inclined to charge higher interest rates when they do lend.

Moral hazard occurs as a result of asymmetric information *after* a transaction has occurred. To continue with our example of the Dynamic Corporation, once the firm has sold the bonds, it must choose among alternative strategies in executing its project. Lenders face the hazard that Dynamic may choose strategies contrary to the lenders' well-being and thus "immoral" from their perspective. Because bondholders are entitled to a fixed amount regardless of the firm's profits, Dynamic has an incentive to select strategies offering a small chance of high profits, thereby enabling the owners to keep the largest amount after paying bondholders. Such strategies are also the riskiest—ones that make it more likely that lenders will not be repaid—so the presence of moral hazard makes lenders less likely to lend to anyone and more inclined to charge higher interest rates when they do lend.

The Principal-Agent Problem 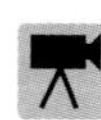

Principal-agent problem 
The conflict of interest that occurs when agents—managers of firms—pursue their own objectives to the detriment of the goals of the firms' principals, or owners.

A type of moral hazard problem that occurs within firms is called the **principal-agent problem.** The shareholders who own a firm are referred to as *principals,* and the managers who operate the firm are the *agents* of the owners. When the managers do not own all of a firm (as is usually the case), a separation of ownership and control exists, and if the stockholders have less information about the firm's opportunities and risks than the managers do (as is also usually the case), the managers may act in their own self-interest rather than in the interest of the shareholders.

Consider, for example, the choice between two investment projects, one of which involves an enormous amount of work but also promises high profits, while the other requires little effort and promises small returns. Because the managers must do all the work while the shareholders receive all the profits, the managers' incentives are different from those of the shareholders. In this case, the presence of moral hazard will induce the managers to choose the "good life," the easy but low-yielding project—an outcome that fails to maximize the economic value of the firm.

Solving Principal-Agent and Moral Hazard Problems

Collateral 
An asset pledged to guarantee the repayment of a loan.

Incentive-compatible contract
A loan contract under which a significant amount of the borrower's assets are at risk, providing an incentive for the borrower to look after the lender's interests.

The dangers associated with asymmetric information are well known to participants in financial markets, who regularly undertake vigorous steps to minimize its costly consequences. For example, research companies such as Standard & Poor's gather financial data and other information about corporations and sell the information to their subscribers. When even this is insufficient to eliminate the dangers of adverse selection, lenders often require that borrowers post **collateral**—assets that the borrower will forfeit in the event that repayment of a debt is not made. A variant of this strategy, designed to reduce moral hazard problems, is called the **incentive-compatible contract:** Lenders make sure that borrowers have a large amount of their own assets at risk so that the incentives of the borrower are compatible with the interests of the lender. Although measures such as these cannot eliminate the losses caused by asymmetric information, they reduce them below what would otherwise be the case.

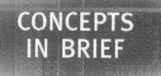

- When two parties to a transaction have different amounts of information, we call this asymmetric information. Asymmetric information before a transaction can result in adverse selection. Adverse selection causes borrowers who are the worst credit risks to be the ones most likely to seek loans.

- Asymmetric information after a transaction can cause moral hazard. Lenders often face the hazard that borrowers will choose riskier actions after borrowers have taken out loans.
- The separation of ownership and control in today's large corporations can give rise to the principal-agent problem, whereby the agents (managers) may have interests that differ from those of the principals (shareholders).
- Several methods exist for solving the principal-agent and moral hazard problems. They include requiring lenders to post collateral and devising incentive-compatible contracts in which borrowers have a large amount of their own assets at risk.

NETNOMICS

The Economic Effects of On-Line Trading

The biggest appeal of on-line trading for many investors is the low cost per trade—often one-half to one-tenth the cost of dealing with a human being at a full-service stock brokerage. Quite apart the potential for putting money into the pocket of investors, the advent of on-line trading helps make the stock and bond markets more efficient in two ways.

First, on every trade that takes place, fewer resources are used when an investor chooses to make the trade on-line rather than otherwise. But note that one can't merely subtract the difference between the conventional broker's fee and the on-line fee and conclude that the difference is all savings. After all, on-line traders typically have to spend some added amount of their own time and computer resources to make those on-line trades. Suppose, for example, that on a trade of 1,000 shares of stock, the conventional fee would be $250 and the on-line fee is $50. If the investor devotes, say, an additional $35 of her time on research and computer time in making the on-line trade, the net resource savings on the trade are $165 (= $250 − $50 − $35). When added up over thousands of trades that on-line traders across the country are making each day, these savings for the economy can be significant.

The lower costs of on-line trading also improve the efficiency of the securities markets by making more trades possible. When trading costs are high, some people refrain from buying stocks or bonds they believe have upside potential, while others refrain from selling stocks or bonds they feel are headed downward. With lower costs due to on-line trading, both types of investors will be able to do more of what they want to do, thereby making both better off.

Interestingly, the fact that costs per trade are lower on-line has the potential to *raise* the total amount that investors are spending on stock and bond trades! How is this possible? Well, the lower costs per trade encourage more trades, and the total amount spent on trading is the product of price (the fee per trade) times quantity (the number of trades). If the number of trades increases enough—which it will, if the demand for trading services is elastic—the net effect of the lower cost per trade will be more money spent on trading. But note that even if traders end up spending more on trading, this does not wipe out their gains from using on-line services: Indeed, they will continue to use those services only if they accrue net benefits from doing so. What it does mean is that the simple arithmetic of on-line trading doesn't always add up to the correct economics of on-line trading.

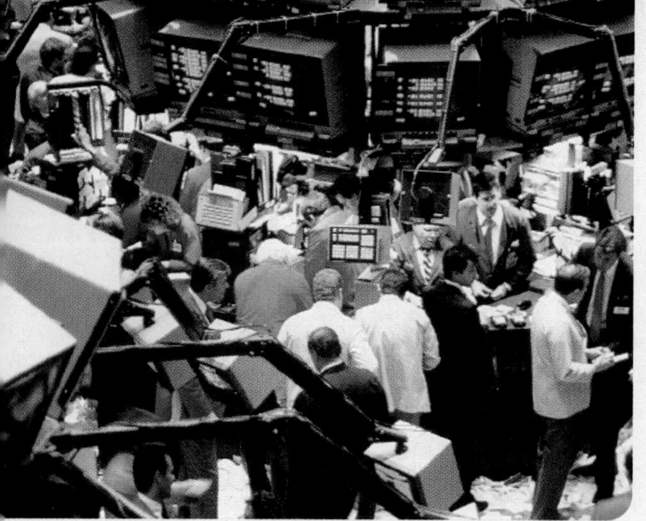

ISSUES & APPLICATIONS

The Spread of Corporate Stock Ownership

Shortly after World War II ended, only one out of 25 Americans owned corporate stock. By 1981, one out of 16 Americans owned stock. At the beginning of the 1990s, the number was one out of four, and by the year 2000, almost one of every two Americans owned stock. Why has this growth in stock ownership taken place, and what does it mean—for the economy and for politics?

No single factor can account for the growing popularity of stock ownership over the past 50 years, although several factors have clearly played a role. The low incidence of stock ownership after World War II was due in part to memories of the Great Depression, heralded by a spectacular drop in stock prices in 1929. As memories of hard times faded, however, more Americans became willing to trust in the stock market.

Concepts Applied

- On-line Stock Trading
- Capital Gains
- Taxation and Regulatory Policies
- Recession

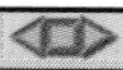

The advent of the Individual Retirement Account (IRA) more than 20 years ago also gave stock ownership a boost. Because the taxes on profits from successful stock trades could be deferred if the stocks were in IRA accounts, stock ownership became much more attractive. The strong economy and booming stock market of the 1980s and 1990s also spurred interest in stock ownership as more and more people realized that unlike objects bound by gravity, stock prices that went up did not have to go down. And when low-cost stock trading over the Internet became possible, interest in stocks became a passion. By the end of the twentieth century, Americans were holding some $12 trillion worth of corporate stocks—more than $40,000 for each person in the country.

How Growing Stock Ownership Matters

Of course, as stock holding in America became more widespread, the consequences of changes in the value of those stocks became broader too. During much of the 1980s and 1990s, rising stock prices helped fuel consumer spending, leading to record-breaking economic expansions. But there can be a downside as well. For example, when stock prices plunged 20 percent in late 1987, it sparked a slowdown in consumer spending. And when stocks dropped sharply again in 1997, consumer spending faltered in several sectors of the economy until stock prices bounced back. Some economists think that with the huge amount of wealth now in the form of corporate stocks, a sudden and sustained 20 percent drop in stock prices might be enough to trigger a recession.

It is on the political front, however, that the implications of America's interest in the stock market can be the most surprising. Once upon a time, stock holding in America was confined to the wealthy and the elderly. This set up a natural sort of "us versus them" rivalry when it came to tax and regulatory policies affecting the bottom line of American corporations. Low-income individuals and young people tended to favor higher corporate and capital gains taxes and heavier regulatory intervention by the government. (Capital gains taxes are levied on the positive difference between the sale and purchase price of an asset, such as corporate stock.) In contrast, the wealthy and the over-40 crowd were more likely to push for policies that enhanced corporate profits and let investors keep more of their gains from higher stock prices. All of this is changing in the new era of stock ownership.

The Role of Internet Trading

More than half of all families with incomes between $25,000 and $50,000 own stock, and although stock ownership is less prevalent among families with incomes below $25,000, stock ownership is increasing faster in this low-income segment than in any other. Moreover, Internet-savvy young people are becoming a growing force in the on-line trading of stocks—and are therefore well aware of which government policies are likely to earn them profits or yield losses. The result is a changing dynamic in American politics.

For example, among individuals with more than $5,000 in stocks or bonds, one poll found nearly two-thirds support lower capital gains taxes, compared to 46 percent among noninvestors. Moreover, support for capital gains tax cuts rises with stock ownership. Perhaps this helps explain the turnaround on this issue in Washington. In the 1980s, Democrats attacked Republicans as being elitists for proposing cuts in the capital gains tax. In the late 1990s, a Democratic president cheerfully signed legislation that cut the rate sharply—and left much more of the profits from the rising stock market in the hands of voters.

The spread of stock ownership is affecting other political areas as well. For example, the growing investor class is expressing increasing support for expanded IRAs (especially the Roth IRA, which allows tax-free withdrawals) and the initiation of personal Social Security accounts under the control of the beneficiary rather than a government bureaucrat. There is even evidence that today's knowledgeable investors are starting to pay attention to the effects of new government regulations on their personal bottom line. And the fact that the investor class is growing will boost support for market-oriented economic policies. The challenge for our political leaders is to turn this support into sensible economic policies.

FOR CRITICAL ANALYSIS

1. Could a drop in the value of U.S. stocks cause a recession in other countries?
2. How does a reduction in the capital gains tax affect the incentives to own corporate stocks and to buy and sell them on a regular basis?

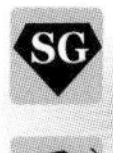

SUMMARY DISCUSSION OF LEARNING OBJECTIVES

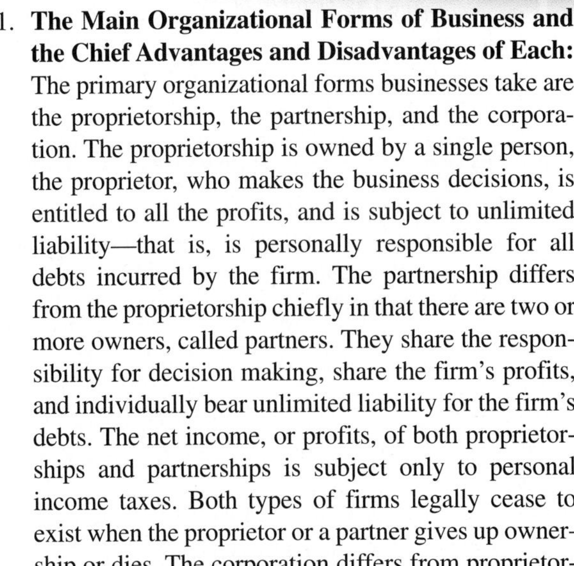

1. **The Main Organizational Forms of Business and the Chief Advantages and Disadvantages of Each:** The primary organizational forms businesses take are the proprietorship, the partnership, and the corporation. The proprietorship is owned by a single person, the proprietor, who makes the business decisions, is entitled to all the profits, and is subject to unlimited liability—that is, is personally responsible for all debts incurred by the firm. The partnership differs from the proprietorship chiefly in that there are two or more owners, called partners. They share the responsibility for decision making, share the firm's profits, and individually bear unlimited liability for the firm's debts. The net income, or profits, of both proprietorships and partnerships is subject only to personal income taxes. Both types of firms legally cease to exist when the proprietor or a partner gives up ownership or dies. The corporation differs from proprietorships and partnerships in three important dimensions. Owners of corporations enjoy limited liability; that is, their responsibility for the debts of the corporation is limited to the value of their ownership shares. In addition, the income from corporations is subject to double taxation—corporate taxation when income is earned by the corporation and personal taxation when after-tax profits are paid as dividends to the owners. Finally, corporations do not legally cease to exist due to a change of ownership or the death of an owner.
2. **The Three Main Sources of Corporate Funds:** The main sources of financial capital for corporations are stocks, bonds, and reinvestment of profits. Stocks are ownership shares, promising a share of profits, sold to investors. Common stocks also embody voting rights regarding the major decisions of the firm; preferred stocks typically have no voting rights but enjoy priority status in the

payment of dividends. Bonds are notes of indebtedness, issued in return for the loan of money. They typically promise to pay interest in the form of annual coupon payments, plus repayment of the original principal amount upon maturity. Bondholders are generally promised payment before any payment of dividends to shareholders, and for this reason bonds are less risky than stocks. Reinvestment involves the purchase of assets by the firm, using retained profits or depreciation reserves it has set aside for this purpose. No new stocks or bonds are issued in the course of reinvestment, although its value is fully reflected in the price of existing shares of stock.

3. **The Differences Between Stocks and Bonds:** Stocks represent ownership in a corporation. They are called equity capital. Bonds represent the debt of a corporation. They are part of the debt capital of a corporation. Bond owners normally receive a fixed interest payment on a regular basis, whereas owners of stock are not normally guaranteed any dividends. If a corporation goes out of business, bondholders have first priority on whatever value still exists in the entity. Owners of stock get whatever is left over. Finally, if the corporation is very successful, owners of stock can reap the increases in the market value of their shares of stock. In contrast, the market value of corporate bonds is not so closely tied to the profits of a corporation but is rather influenced by how interest rates are changing in the economy in general.
4. **The Economic Impact of On-Line Trading of Stocks and Bonds:** On-line trading helps make stock and bond markets more efficient in two ways. First, fewer resources are used when an investor trades on-line rather than through a broker. To calculate the cost savings, one has to add the value of one's time and personal computer costs to the on-line fees and compare that total to what a conventional broker would charge. Added up over thousands of trades that on-line traders make each day, the net savings for the economy can be significant. Second, the lower costs of on-line trading improve the efficiency of the stock market by making more trades possible. When trading costs are high, some people refrain from buying or selling stocks or bonds. Thanks to the lower costs of on-line trading, investors will be able to do more of what they want to do. The fact that costs per trade are lower on-line has the potential to *increase* the total amount that investors are spending on stock and bond trades because lower costs per trade encourage more trades.
5. **The Global Nature of Capital Markets:** Trading in U.S. government securities is one of the fastest-growing 24-hour markets in the world, thanks to sophisticated communications and computer technology. The deregulation of financial markets in foreign countries now permits much more of such trading. Also, since 1984, the United States has allowed foreign investors to buy U.S. government securities tax-free. Moreover, the rapid growth of on-line securities trading has the potential to turn the world's financial markets into one unified market that responds instantly to events, whenever and wherever they occur.
6. **The Problems of Corporate Control:** When two parties to a transaction have different amounts of information, we call this asymmetric information. Asymmetric information before a transaction can result in adverse selection. Adverse selection causes borrowers who are the worst credit risks to be the ones most likely to seek loans. Asymmetric information after a transaction can cause moral hazard. Lenders often face the hazard that borrowers will choose riskier actions after having been granted loans. The separation of ownership and control in today's large corporation has led to the principal-agent problem, whereby the agents (managers) may have interests that differ from those of the principals (shareholders). Several methods exist for solving the principal-agent and moral hazard problems, including requiring lenders to post collateral and devising incentive-compatible contracts in which borrowers have a large amount of their own assets at risk.

Key Terms and Concepts

Bond (509)	Dividends (508)	Inside information (510)
Collateral (518)	Financial capital (506)	Limited liability (508)
Corporation (508)	Incentive-compatible contract (518)	Partnership (507)

Problems

Answers to the odd-numbered problems appear at the back of the book.

21-1. Classify the following items as either financial capital or physical capital.

a. A drill press owned by a manufacturing company

b. $100,000 set aside in an account to purchase a drill press

c. Funds raised through a bond offer to expand plant and equipment

d. A warehouse owned by a shipping company

21-2. Write a brief explanation of the difference between a sole proprietorship, a partnership, and a corporation. In addition, list one advantage and one disadvantage of a sole proprietorship, a partnership, and a corporation.

21-3. Explain the difference between the dividends of a corporation and the profits of a sole proprietorship or partnership, particularly in their tax treatment.

21-4. Outline the differences between common stock and preferred stock.

21-5. The owner of WebCity is trying to decide whether to remain a proprietorship or to incorporate. Suppose that the corporate tax rate on profits is 20 percent and the personal income tax rate is 30 percent. For simplicity, assume that all corporate profits (after corporate taxes are paid) are distributed as dividends in the year they are earned and that such dividends are subject to the personal income tax.

a. If the owner of WebCity expects to earn $100,000 in before-tax profits this year, regardless of whether the firm is a proprietorship or a corporation, which method of organization should be chosen?

b. What is the dollar value of the after-tax advantage of that form of organization?

c. Suppose that the corporate form of organization has cost advantages that will raise before-tax profits by $50,000. Should the owner of WebCity incorporate?

d. By how much will after-tax profits change due to incorporation?

e. Suppose that tax policy is changed to exempt from personal taxation the first $40,000 per year in dividends. Would this change in policy affect the decision made in part (a)?

f. How can you explain the fact that even though corporate profits are subject to double taxation, most business in America is conducted by corporations rather than by proprietorships or partnerships?

21-6. Suppose that you are trying to decide whether to spend $1,000 on stocks issued by WildWeb or on bonds issued by the same company. There is a 50 percent chance that the value of the stock will rise to $2,200 at the end of the year and a 50 percent chance that the stock will be worthless at the end of the year. The bonds promise an interest rate of 20 percent per year, and it is certain that the bonds and interest will be repaid at the end of the year.

a. Assuming that your time horizon is exactly one year, will you choose the stocks or the bonds?

b. By how much is your expected end-of-year wealth reduced if you make the wrong choice?

c. Suppose the odds of success improve for WildWeb: Now there is a 60 percent chance that the value of the stock will be $2,200 at year's end and only a 40 percent chance that it will be worthless. Should you now choose the stocks or the bonds?

d. By how much did your expected end-of-year wealth rise as a result of the improved outlook for WildWeb?

21-7. Lucinda is a financial consultant whose time is worth $120 per hour. Ralph is an accountant whose time is worth $40 per hour. FSB, a full-service brokerage, offers to make stock trades for its clients on the following basis: For each trade there is a fee of $25, plus 10 cents per share for each share traded. WebTrader offers to make trades for a flat rate of $50 per trade, regardless of how many shares are traded. Because of the design of the WebTrader Web site, it takes people 30 minutes more to execute a trade with WebTrader than to execute with FSB.

a. If Lucinda and Ralph are each separately considering a trade involving 100 shares, with whom will each person execute the trade?

b. If Lucinda and Ralph are each separately considering a trade involving 500 shares, with whom will each person execute the trade?

c. If Lucinda and Ralph are each separately considering a trade involving 1,000 shares, with whom will each person execute the trade?

d. In general, will larger or smaller trades be executed with WebTrader or with FSB? Explain your answer.

e. In general, how will the value of a person's time affect the choice of using WebTrader or FSB? Explain.

21-8. After graduating from college with an economics major, Sally Smith started her own consulting firm. After her first year of operation, Sally is contemplating whether to remain a sole proprietorship or to incorporate. Based on her first year's experience, Sally expects to generate $250,000 in pretax profits for the upcoming year. If she remains a sole proprietorship, her profits will be subject to a personal income tax rate of 35 percent. If she incorporates, the corporation faces a 25 percent corporate tax rate. All profits of the corporation will be paid as dividends to Sally as personal income.

a. How do after-tax profits differ under the two types of organizational structure?

b. Based on income considerations alone, which organizational structure should Sally choose?

21-9. Classify each event as an example of asymmetric information, moral hazard, or adverse selection.

a. The Wired Corporation is contemplating starting a string of Internet cafés. Market research shows this to be a very risky venture that will either ensure the success of the company or drive it into bankruptcy. The finance department therefore suggests offering bonds at a rate higher than the market average.

b. Based on your limited knowledge of Internet cafés, you believe that this is a "sure thing" and therefore buy the bonds issued by the Wired Corporation.

c. Instead of setting up a string of Internet cafés as it had promised, the Wired Corporation buys a bankrupt fast-food chain and takes the chance that it can turn the chain around, resell it, and make more profit, albeit at a higher risk.

21-10. Explain the basic differences between a share of stock and a bond.

21-11. Suppose that one of your classmates informs you that he has developed a method of forecasting stock market returns based on past trends. With a monetary investment by you, the two of you could profit handsomely from this forecasting method. How should you respond to your classmate?

Economics on the Net

How the New York Stock Exchange Operates This application gives you the chance to learn about how the New York Stock Exchange functions.

Title: The New York Stock Exchange: How the NYSE Operates

Navigation: Click here to visit the New York Stock Exchange. In the left margin, click Education. Along the top, select the tab named Educational Publications. Then, click on You and the Investment World. Next, click on Chapter 3: How the NYSE Operates.

Application Read the chapter, and answer the following questions.

1. According to the article, the price of a seat on the NYSE can sell for more than $1 million. Why do you suppose that someone would be willing to pay this much for a seat? (Hint: Think about the potential ways that someone could generate earnings from holding an NYSE seat.)
2. List the key functions of a stock exchange specialist. Why is the "Point-of-Sale Display Book" likely to be particularly useful for a specialist?

For Group Study and Analysis Divide the class into groups, and have each group examine and discuss the description of how NYSE trades are executed. Ask each group to compose a listing of the various points at which Internet trading may be a more efficient way to execute a trade, as compared with trading via a traditional brokerage firm. Then go through these as a class, and discuss the following issue: In the New York Stock Exchange, which people cannot be replaced by new information technologies?

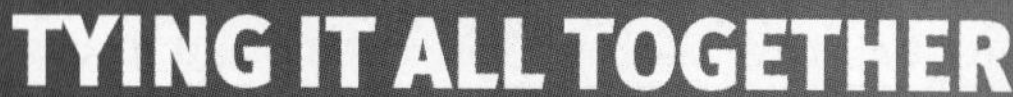

TYING IT ALL TOGETHER

Part 5 Case Problem

Case Background

Top executives for Southern Cola, a privately owned manufacturer and distributor of soft drinks marketed under the names of various grocery store chains throughout the Southwest and Southeast, have decided that the company will enter the vending business in these same U.S. regions. Their next decision is what type of vending machines to purchase. They must balance their desire to purchase high-tech vending machines with the constraints they will face in financing this major investment.

Management Issues in the Emerging High-Tech Vending Business Southern Cola's executives can choose among several lines of vending machines, ranging from the standard, no-frills coin- and bill-operated model to a top-of-the-line, Internet-connected model. One increasingly common feature is to include a card slot that can read credit cards and debit cards. Another new and relatively high-tech feature, which has been available since Coca-Cola's first experiments in 1999, is a device that automatically increases the soft-drink prices in hot weather. This feature requires only a temperature sensor and a computer chip, both of which are now relatively inexpensive "old technologies."

If Southern Cola chooses machines with the latter option, the company can also upgrade to vending machines with a higher-quality microprocessor that enables the machines to perform several other functions. One is keeping track of the time of day and adjusting prices upward during periods of the day when people are most likely to be in buildings or near kiosks where the machines are located.

Another option, which also requires access to a fiber-optic cable or other telecommunications connection, is to automatically keep tabs on the machine's inventories of various soft drinks. In real time, therefore, the machine's microprocessor could inform Southern Cola's central office when the machine is running low on popular soft drinks. Then the company can dispatch employees for just-in-time inventory restocking of the machines, which would keep employees from making unnecessary trips to well-stocked vending machines—thereby reducing the company's employee expenses. Furthermore, the company's central office could readily compile the streams of data obtained from its vending machines to help its marketing force determine which drinks are selling best in which locations. This could help not only in short-term marketing efforts but also in longer-term planning for the introduction of new products in the future.

Real-time inventory management could also allow for pricing adjustments. If one brand is clearly more popular than another, the microprocessor could be programmed to charge a slightly higher price for the more popular brand. In addition, if some brands are temporarily out of stock, Southern Cola could program the vending machine to automatically raise the prices of remaining items somewhat.

Vending is a brand-new business for Southern Cola, however. To finance its entry into this business, the executives realize that they will have to convince the owners of the company to "take it public" via an initial public offering (IPO).

The executives realize that they face an interlocking set of decisions. They must determine if high-tech vending machines are a necessary part of their long-term strategy for succeeding in this new business. If so, a successful IPO would go a long way toward making the new venture a success. A merely adequate IPO, however, might force the company to face the prospect of either scaling back the scope of its market entry or taking on additional debt to finance the grand leapfrogging effort that its executives wish to achieve.

Points to Analyze

1. Which of the vending machine features that Southern Cola's executives are considering would adjust prices to take into account changes in the position of the demand curve at each of the company's vending machines?
2. What vending machine features would adjust soft-drink prices in light of variations in the price elasticity of demand at each vending machine?
3. What are the advantages and disadvantages of making Southern Cola a publicly owned company?
4. Why do the company's executives believe that developing a business plan that demonstrates a significant potential for revenue enhancements and cost efficiencies is crucial to the success of the IPO?

Caving the Internet

1. **Click here to go to Coca-Cola's home page.**
   a. **Click on "Our Company" and then click on "Citizenship." Click on "Environment." Why do you suppose that Coca-Cola is so interested in convincing visitors to its site that it is an environment-friendly corporation? Do you think that this discussion is aimed at consumers, investors, or both? Why?**
   b. **Click here to go to the homepage of PepsiCo, the maker and distributor of Pepsi-Cola and related soft-drink products. In what ways does this homepage differ from the homepage of Coca-Cola? Do you see any similarities between the objectives of the two companies' Web sites? Differences?**
2. **Click here to go to the homepage of Mars Electronics International (MEI). Select a region and language. Then click on "Register Later."**
   a. **Click on "Product Applications," then click on "Soft Drink," and read the description of this business. How many types of vending machines does this company market? Why do you think there are so many models to choose from?**

Part 6

Market Structure, Resource Allocation, and Regulation

CHAPTER

22

THE FIRM: COST AND OUTPUT DETERMINATION

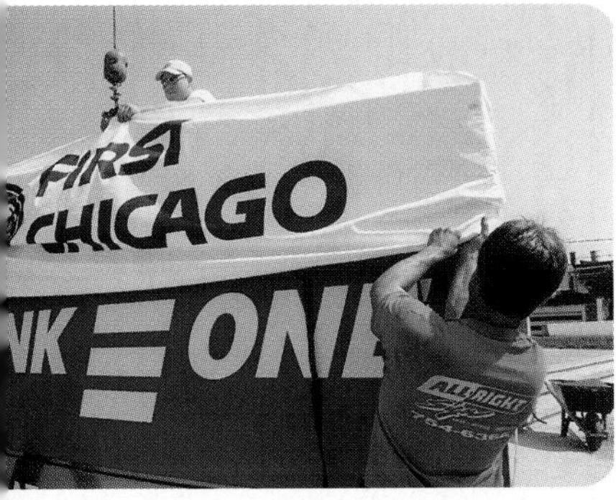

This bank was originally called First Chicago but was acquired by Bank One. There have been over 4,000 bank mergers in the past 10 years. Why do banks want to get bigger by merger?

Since 1989, nearly 4,000 mergers have occurred among U.S. commercial banks—financial firms that issue checking accounts and use the funds they raise from this activity to earn interest returns from loans and holdings of government securities. More than two-thirds of the nation's banking resources have been involved in these mergers. Bank consolidation has also produced some very large banking firms, at least relative to historical standards for the United States. Presumably, bank owners and managers have had good reasons to conclude that bigger is better. The most common rationale that bank owners and managers offer is that large banks are more cost-efficient than small banks. Before you can evaluate this contention, however, you must understand the nature of cost curves that individual businesses face.

LEARNING OBJECTIVES

After reading this chapter, you should be able to:

1. Distinguish between accounting profits and economic profits
2. Discuss the difference between the short run and the long run from the perspective of a firm
3. Understand why the marginal physical product of labor eventually declines as more units of labor are employed
4. Explain the short-run cost curves a typical firm faces
5. Describe the long-run cost curves a typical firm faces
6. Identify situations of economies and diseconomies of scale and define a firm's minimum efficient scale

Chapter Outline

- The Firm
- Short Run Versus Long Run
- The Relationship Between Output and Inputs
- Diminishing Marginal Returns
- Short-Run Costs to the Firm
- The Relationship Between Diminishing Marginal Returns and Cost Curves
- Long-Run Cost Curves
- Why the Long-Run Average Cost Curve Is U-Shaped
- Minimum Efficient Scale

Did You Know That... there are more than 25 steps in the process of manufacturing a simple lead pencil? In the production of an automobile, there are literally thousands. At each step, the manufacturer can have the job done by workers or machines or some combination of the two. The manufacturer must also figure out how much to produce each month. Should a new machine be bought that can replace 10 workers? Should more workers be hired, or should the existing workers be paid overtime? If the price of aluminum is rising, should the company try to make do with plastic? What you will learn about in this chapter is how producers can select the best combination of inputs for any given output that is desired.

Before we look at the firm's costs, we need to define a firm.

THE FIRM

We define a business, or **firm,** as follows:

> A firm is an organization that brings together factors of production—labor, land, physical capital, human capital, and entrepreneurial skill—to produce a product or service that it hopes can be sold at a profit.

A typical firm will have an organizational structure consisting of an entrepreneur, managers, and workers. The entrepreneur is the person who takes the risks, mainly of losing his or her personal wealth. In compensation, the entrepreneur will get any profits that are made. Recall from Chapter 2 that entrepreneurs take the initiative in combining land, labor, and capital to produce a good or a service. Entrepreneurs are the ones who innovate in the form of new production and new products. The entrepreneur also decides whom to hire to manage the firm. Some economists maintain that the true quality of an entrepreneur becomes evident with his or her selection of managers. Managers, in turn, decide who should be hired and fired and how the business generally should be set up. The workers ultimately use the other inputs to produce the products or services that are being sold by the firm. Workers and managers are paid contractual wages. They receive a specified amount of income for a specified time period. Entrepreneurs are not paid contractual wages. They receive no reward specified in advance. The entrepreneurs make profits if there are any, for profits accrue to those who are willing to take risks. (Because the entrepreneur gets only what is left over after all expenses are paid, he or she is often referred to as a *residual claimant.* The entrepreneur lays claim to the residual—whatever is left.)

Firm 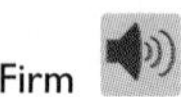
A business organization that employs resources to produce goods or services for profit. A firm normally owns and operates at least one plant in order to produce.

Profit and Costs

Most people think of profit as the difference between the amount of revenues a business takes in and the amount it spends for wages, materials, and so on. In a bookkeeping sense, the following formula could be used:

$$\text{Accounting profits} = \text{total revenues} - \text{explicit costs}$$

where **explicit costs** are expenses that the business managers must take account of because they must actually be paid out by the firm. This definition of profit is known as **accounting profit.** It is appropriate when used by accountants to determine a firm's taxable income. Economists are more interested in how firm managers react not just to changes in explicit costs but also to changes in **implicit costs,** defined as expenses that business managers do not have to pay out of pocket but are costs to the firm nonetheless because they

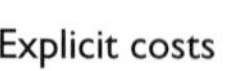
Explicit costs 
Costs that business managers must take account of because they must be paid; examples are wages, taxes, and rent.

Accounting profit 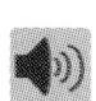
Total revenues minus total explicit costs.

represent an opportunity cost. These are noncash costs—they do not involve any direct cash outlay by the firm and must therefore be measured by the alternative cost principle. That is to say, they are measured by what the resources (land, capital) currently used in producing a particular good or service could earn in other uses. Economists use the full opportunity cost of all resources (including both explicit and implicit costs) as the figure to subtract from revenues to obtain a definition of profit. Another definition of implicit cost is therefore the opportunity cost of using factors that a producer does not buy or hire but already owns.

Implicit costs 
Expenses that managers do not have to pay out of pocket and hence do not normally explicitly calculate, such as the opportunity cost of factors of production that are owned; examples are owner-provided capital and owner-provided labor.

Opportunity Cost of Capital

Firms enter or remain in an industry if they earn, at minimum, a **normal rate of return.** People will not invest their wealth in a business unless they obtain a positive normal (competitive) rate of return—that is, unless their invested wealth pays off. Any business wishing to attract capital must expect to pay at least the same rate of return on that capital as all other businesses (of similar risk) are willing to pay. Put another way, when a firm requires the use of a resource in producing a particular product, it must bid against alternative users of that resource. Thus the firm must offer a price that is at least as much as other potential users are offering to pay. For example, if individuals can invest their wealth in almost any publishing firm and get a rate of return of 10 percent per year, each firm in the publishing industry must *expect* to pay 10 percent as the normal rate of return to present and future investors. This 10 percent is a *cost to the firm,* the **opportunity cost of capital.** The opportunity cost of capital is the amount of income, or yield, that could have been earned by investing in the next-best alternative. Capital will not stay in firms or industries in which the expected rate of return falls below its opportunity cost, that is, what could be earned elsewhere. If a firm owns some capital equipment, it can either use it or lease it and earn a return. If the firm uses the equipment for production, part of the cost of using that equipment is the forgone revenue that the firm could have earned had it leased out that equipment.

Normal rate of return 
The amount that must be paid to an investor to induce investment in a business; also known as the *opportunity cost of capital.*

Opportunity cost of capital 
The normal rate of return, or the available return on the next-best alternative investment. Economists consider this a cost of production, and it is included in our cost examples.

Opportunity Cost of Owner-Provided Labor and Capital

Single-owner proprietorships often grossly exaggerate their profit rates because they understate the opportunity cost of the labor that the proprietor provides to the business. Here we are referring to the opportunity cost of labor. For example, you may know people who run a small grocery store. These people will sit down at the end of the year and figure out what their "profits" are. They will add up all their sales and subtract what they had to pay to other workers, what they had to pay to their suppliers, what they had to pay in taxes, and so on. The end result they will call "profit." They normally will not, however, have figured into their costs the salary that they could have made if they had worked for somebody else in a similar type of job. By working for themselves, they become residual claimants—they receive what is left after all explicit costs have been accounted for. However, part of the costs should include the salary the owner-operator could have received working for someone else.

Consider a simple example of a skilled auto mechanic working 14 hours a day at his own service station, six days a week. Compare this situation to how much he could earn as a trucking company mechanic 84 hours a week. This self-employed auto mechanic might have an opportunity cost of about $20 an hour. For his 84-hour week in his own service station, he is forfeiting $1,680. Unless his service station shows accounting profits of more than that per week, he is losing money in an economic sense.

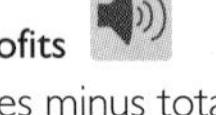
Click here to obtain the most recent estimates of U.S. firms' annual revenues and payroll expenses.

Another way of looking at the opportunity cost of running a business is that opportunity cost consists of all explicit and implicit costs. Accountants only take account of explicit costs. Therefore, accounting profit ends up being the residual after only explicit costs are subtracted from total revenues.

This same analysis can apply to owner-provided capital, such as land or buildings. The fact that the owner owns the building or the land with which he or she operates a business does not mean that it is "free." Rather, use of the building and land still has an opportunity cost—the value of the next-best alternative use for those assets.

Accounting Profits Versus Economic Profits

Economic profits
Total revenues minus total opportunity costs of all inputs used, or the total of all implicit and explicit costs.

The term *profits* in economics means the income that entrepreneurs earn, over and above all costs including their own opportunity cost of time, plus the opportunity cost of the capital they have invested in their business. Profits can be regarded as total revenues minus total costs—which is how accountants think of them—but we must now include *all* costs. Our definition of **economic profits** will be the following:

$$\text{Economic profits} = \text{total revenues} - \text{total opportunity cost of all inputs used}$$

or

$$\text{Economic profits} = \text{total revenues} - (\text{explicit} + \text{implicit costs})$$

Remember that implicit costs include a normal rate of return on invested capital. We show this relationship in Figure 22-1.

The Goal of the Firm: Profit Maximization 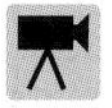

When we examined the theory of consumer demand, utility (or satisfaction) maximization by the individual provided the basis for the analysis. In the theory of the firm and production, *profit maximization* is the underlying hypothesis of our predictive theory. The goal of

FIGURE 22-1
Simplified View of Economic and Accounting Profit
We see on the right column that accounting profit is the difference between total revenues and total explicit accounting costs. Conversely, we see on the left column that economic profit is equal to total revenues minus economic costs. Economic costs equal explicit accounting costs plus all implicit costs, including a normal rate of return on invested capital.

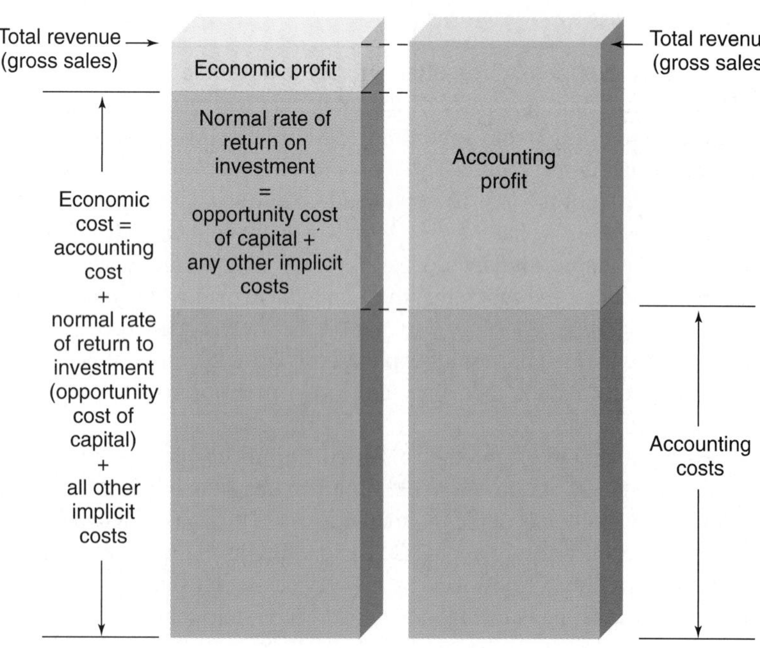

the firm is to maximize economic profits, and the firm is expected to try to make the positive difference between total revenues and total costs as large as it can.

Our justification for assuming profit maximization by firms is similar to our belief in utility maximization by individuals. To obtain labor, capital, and other resources required to produce commodities, firms must first obtain financing from investors. In general, investors are indifferent about the details of how a firm uses the money they provide. They are most interested in the earnings on this money and the risk of obtaining lower returns or losing the money they have invested. Firms that can provide relatively higher risk-corrected returns will therefore have an advantage in obtaining the financing needed to continue or expand production. Over time we would expect a policy of profit maximization to become the dominant mode of behavior for firms that survive.

FAQ

Haven't the profit rates of American corporations been growing?

No, after accounting for year-to-year variations arising from cyclical factors, pretax U.S. corporate profit rates have generally declined since the 1970s. Between 1950 and the mid-1970s, pretax corporate profits averaged about 11 percent of GDP. Over the period since the mid-1970s, pretax profits have averaged slightly less than 8 percent of GDP. The rate of *after*-tax profits relative to GDP has remained relatively stable, within a range of about 4 to 6 percent.

CONCEPTS IN BRIEF

- Accounting profits differ from economic profits. Economic profits are defined as total revenues minus total costs, where costs include the full opportunity cost of all of the factors of production plus all other implicit costs.
- Single-owner proprietorships often fail to consider the opportunity cost of the labor services provided by the owner.
- The full opportunity cost of capital invested in a business is generally not included as a cost when accounting profits are calculated. Thus accounting profits often overstate economic profits.
- We assume throughout these chapters that the goal of the firm is to maximize economic profits.

SHORT RUN VERSUS LONG RUN

In Chapter 20, we discussed short-run and long-run price elasticities of supply and demand. For consumers, the long run meant the time period during which all adjustments to a change in price could be made, and anything shorter than that was considered the short run. For suppliers, the long run was the time in which all adjustments could be made, and anything shorter than that was the short run.

Now that we are discussing firms only, we will maintain a similar distinction between the short and the long run, but we will be more specific. In the theory of the firm, the **short run** is defined as any time period that is so short that there is at least one input, such as current **plant size,** that the firm cannot alter.* In other words, during the short run, a firm makes do with whatever big machines and factory size it already has, no matter how much more it wants to produce because of increased demand for its product. We consider the plant and heavy equipment, the size or amount of which cannot be varied in the short run,

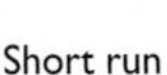

Short run
The time period when at least one input, such as plant size, cannot be changed.

Plant size
The physical size of the factories that a firm owns and operates to produce its output. Plant size can be defined by square footage, maximum physical capacity, and other physical measures.

*There can be many short runs but only one long run. For ease of analysis, in this section we simplify the case to one short run and talk about short-run costs.

as fixed resources. In agriculture and in some other businesses, land may be a fixed resource.

There are, of course, variable resources that the firm can alter when it wants to change its rate of production. These are called *variable inputs* or *variable factors of production.* Typically, the variable inputs of a firm are its labor and its purchases of raw materials. In the short run, in response to changes in demand, the firm can, by definition, change only the amounts of its variable inputs.

Long run
The time period in which all factors of production can be varied.

The **long run** can now be considered the period of time in which *all* inputs can be varied. Specifically, in the long run, the firm can alter its plant size. How long is the long run? That depends on each individual industry. For Wendy's or McDonald's, the long run may be four or five months, because that is the time it takes to add new franchises. For a steel company, the long run may be several years, because that's how long it takes to plan and build a new plant. An electric utility might need over a decade to build a new plant, as another example.

Short run and *long run* in our discussion are in fact management planning terms that apply to decisions made by managers. The firm can operate only in the short run in the sense that decisions must be made in the present. The same analysis applies to your own behavior. You may have many long-run plans about graduate school, vacations, and the like, but you always operate in the short run—you make decisions every day about what you do every day.

THE RELATIONSHIP BETWEEN OUTPUT AND INPUTS

A firm takes numerous inputs, combines them using a technological production process, and ends up with an output. There are, of course, a great many factors of production, or inputs. We classify production inputs into two broad categories (ignoring land)—labor and capital. The relationship between output and these two inputs is as follows:

$$\text{Output per time period} = \text{some function of capital and labor inputs}$$

In simple math, the production relationship can be written $Q = f(K, L)$, where Q = output per time period, K = capital, and L = labor.

Production
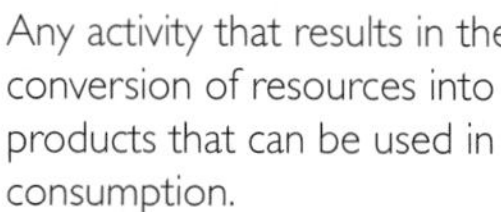
Any activity that results in the conversion of resources into products that can be used in consumption.

We have used the word *production* but have not defined it. **Production** is any process by which resources are transformed into goods or services. Production includes not only making things but also transporting them, retailing, repackaging them, and so on. Notice that if we know that production occurs, we do not necessarily know the value of the output. The production relationship tells nothing about the worth or value of the inputs or the output.

INTERNATIONAL EXAMPLE

Europeans Use More Capital

Since 1970, the 15 nations of the European Union (EU) have increased their total annual output of goods and services relatively steadily. But over this same time period, the EU has dramatically increased the amount of capital relative to the amount of labor it uses in its production processes. Business managers in the EU have substituted capital for labor much more than in the United States because the cost of labor (wages corrected for inflation) has increased by almost 60 percent in the EU but by only 15 percent in the United States.

For Critical Analysis

How does a firm decide when to buy more machines?

The Production Function: A Numerical Example

The relationship between maximum physical output and the quantity of capital and labor used in the production process is sometimes called a **production function.** The production function is a technological relationship between inputs and output. Firms that are inefficient or wasteful in their use of capital and labor will obtain less output than the production function in theory will show. No firm can obtain more output than the production function shows, however. The production function specifies the maximum possible output that can be produced with a given amount of inputs. It also specifies the minimum amount of inputs necessary to produce a given level of output. The production function depends on the technology available to the firm. It follows that an improvement in technology that allows the firm to produce more output with the same amount of inputs (or the same output with fewer inputs) results in a new production function.

Production function 
The relationship between inputs and maximum physical output. A production function is a technological, not an economic, relationship.

Look at panel (a) of Figure 22-2 on page 538. It shows a production function relating total output in column 2 to the quantity of labor measured in workers per week in column 1. When there are zero workers per week of input, there is no output. When there are 5 workers per week of input (given the capital stock), there is a total output of 50 bushels per week. (Ignore for the moment the rest of that panel.) Panel (b) of Figure 22-2 shows this particular hypothetical production function graphically. Note again that it relates to the short run and that it is for an individual firm.

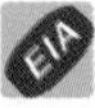

The Theory of Firm Production
Gain further understanding of the production function for a firm.

Panel (b) shows a total physical product curve, or the maximum amount of physical output that is possible when we add successive equal-sized units of labor while holding all other inputs constant. The graph of the production function in panel (b) is not a straight line. In fact, it peaks at 7 workers per week and starts to go down. To understand why it starts to go down with an individual firm in the short run, we have to analyze in detail the **law of diminishing (marginal) returns.**

Law of diminishing (marginal) returns 
The observation that after some point, successive equal-sized increases in a variable factor of production, such as labor, added to fixed factors of production, will result in smaller increases in output.

But before that, let's examine the meaning of columns 3 and 4 of panel (a) of Figure 22-2—that is, average and marginal physical product.

Average and Physical Marginal Product

The definition of **average physical product** is straightforward: It is the total product divided by the number of worker weeks. You can see in column 3 of panel (a) of Figure 22-2 that the average physical product of labor first rises and then steadily falls after two workers are hired.

Average physical product 
Total product divided by the variable input.

Remember that *marginal* means "additional." Hence the **marginal physical product** of labor is the change in total product that occurs when a worker joins an existing production process. (The term *physical* here emphasizes the fact that we are measuring in terms of physical units of production, not in dollar terms.) It is also the *change* in total product that occurs when that worker quits or is laid off an existing production process. The marginal physical product of labor therefore refers to the *change in output caused by a one-unit change in the labor input.* (Marginal physical product is also referred to as *marginal product* and *marginal return.*)

Marginal physical product 
The physical output that is due to the addition of one more unit of a variable factor of production; the change in total product occurring when a variable input is increased and all other inputs are held constant; also called *marginal product* or *marginal return.*

DIMINISHING MARGINAL RETURNS

The concept of diminishing marginal returns—also known as diminishing marginal product—applies to many situations. If you put a seat belt across your lap, a certain amount of safety is obtained. If you add another seat belt over your shoulder, some additional safety

FIGURE 22-2

Diminishing Returns, the Production Function, and Marginal Product: A Hypothetical Case

Marginal product is the addition to the total product that results when one additional worker is hired. Thus the marginal product of the fourth worker is eight bushels of wheat. With four workers, 44 bushels are produced, but with three workers, only 36 are produced; the difference is 8. In panel (b), we plot the numbers from columns 1 and 2 of panel (a). In panel (c), we plot the numbers from columns 1 and 4 of panel (a). When we go from 0 to 1, marginal product is 10. When we go from one worker to two workers, marginal product increases to 16. After two workers, marginal product declines, but it is still positive. Total product (output) reaches its peak at seven workers, so after seven workers marginal product is negative. When we move from seven to eight workers, marginal product becomes −1 bushel.

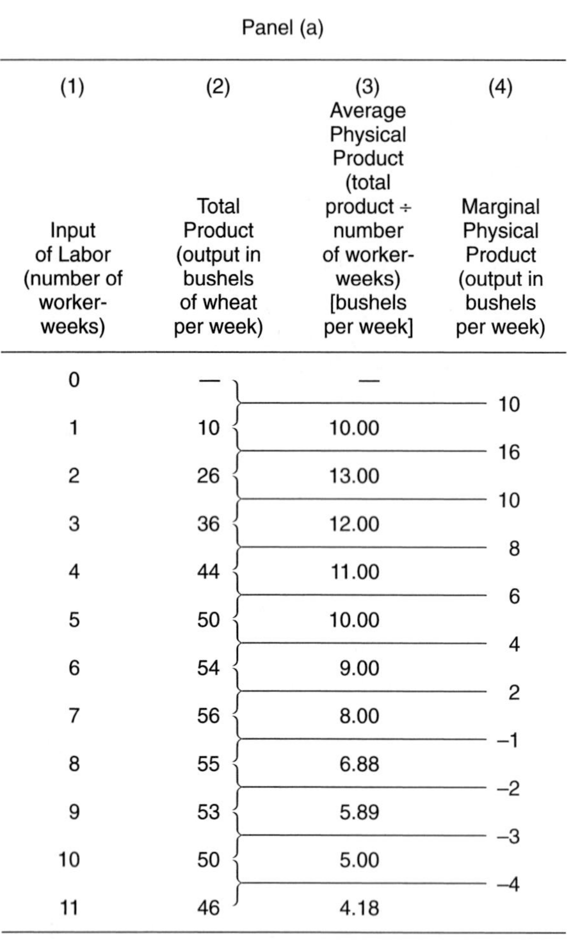

Panel (a)

(1) Input of Labor (number of worker-weeks)	(2) Total Product (output in bushels of wheat per week)	(3) Average Physical Product (total product ÷ number of worker-weeks) [bushels per week]	(4) Marginal Physical Product (output in bushels per week)
0	—	—	
			10
1	10	10.00	
			16
2	26	13.00	
			10
3	36	12.00	
			8
4	44	11.00	
			6
5	50	10.00	
			4
6	54	9.00	
			2
7	56	8.00	
			–1
8	55	6.88	
			–2
9	53	5.89	
			–3
10	50	5.00	
			–4
11	46	4.18	

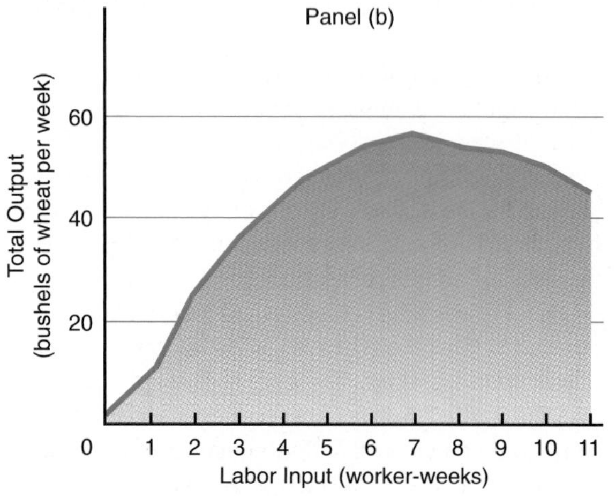

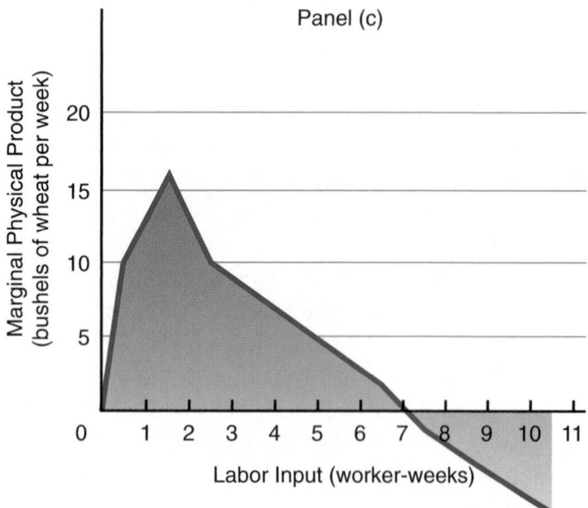

is obtained, but less than when the first belt was secured. When you add a third seat belt over the other shoulder, the amount of *additional* safety obtained is even smaller.

The same analysis holds for firms in their use of productive inputs. When the returns from hiring more workers are diminishing, it does not necessarily mean that more workers won't be hired. In fact, workers will be hired until the returns, in terms of the *value* of the *extra* output produced, are equal to the additional wages that have to be paid for those workers to produce the extra output. Before we get into that decision-making process, let's demonstrate that diminishing returns can be represented graphically and can be used in our analysis of the firm.

Measuring Diminishing Returns

How do we measure diminishing returns? First, we limit the analysis to only one variable factor of production (or input)—let's say the factor is labor. Every other factor of production, such as machines, must be held constant. Only in this way can we calculate the marginal returns from using more workers and know when we reach the point of diminishing marginal returns.

Click here to consider an additional numerical illustration of a production function and diminishing returns.

The marginal productivity of labor may increase rapidly at the very beginning. A firm starts with no workers, only machines. The firm then hires one worker, who finds it difficult to get the work started. But when the firm hires more workers, each is able to *specialize,* and the marginal product of those additional workers may actually be greater than the marginal product of the previous few workers. Beyond some point, however, diminishing returns must set in—*not* because new workers are less qualified but because each worker has, on average, fewer machines with which to work (remember, all other inputs are fixed). In fact, eventually the firm will become so crowded that workers will start to get in each other's way. At that point, marginal physical product becomes negative, and total production declines.

Using these ideas, we can define the law of diminishing returns as follows:

> As successive equal increases in a variable factor of production are added to fixed factors of production, there will be a point beyond which the extra, or marginal, product that can be attributed to each additional unit of the variable factor of production will decline.

Note that the law of diminishing returns is a statement about the *physical* relationships between inputs and outputs that we have observed in many firms. If the law of diminishing returns were not a fairly accurate statement about the world, what would stop firms from hiring additional workers forever?

An Example of the Law of Diminishing Returns

Agriculture provides an example of the law of diminishing returns. With a fixed amount of land, fertilizer, and tractors, the addition of more farm workers eventually yields decreasing increases in output. After a while, when all the tractors are being used, additional farm workers will have to start farming manually. They obviously won't be as productive as the first farm workers who manned the tractors. The marginal physical product of an additional farm worker, given a specified amount of capital, must eventually be less than that for the previous workers.

A hypothetical set of numbers illustrating the law of diminishing marginal returns is presented in panel (a) of Figure 22-2. The numbers are presented graphically in panel (c). Marginal productivity (returns from adding more workers) first increases, then decreases, and finally becomes negative.

When one worker is hired, total output goes from 0 to 10. Thus marginal physical product is 10 bushels of wheat per week. When the second worker is hired, total product goes from 10 to 26 bushels of wheat per week. Marginal physical product therefore increases to 16 bushels of wheat per week. When a third worker is hired, total product again increases, from 26 to 36 bushels of wheat per week. This represents a marginal physical product of only 10 bushels of wheat per week. Therefore, the point of diminishing marginal returns occurs after two workers are hired.

Notice that after 7 workers per week, marginal physical product becomes negative. That means that the hiring of an eighth worker would create a situation that reduces total product. Sometimes this is called the *point of saturation,* indicating that given the amount of fixed inputs, there is no further positive use for more of the variable input. We have entered the region of negative marginal returns.

EXAMPLE

Microsoft Confronts the Law of Diminishing Marginal Returns

One of the great success stories of the computer age has been Microsoft's Windows, which for some time has been the dominant operating system for personal computers. Many businesses and households have also come to rely on another Microsoft desktop software package called Office, a "suite" of programs, including Word, Excel, PowerPoint, and Access. In 1999, Microsoft released Office 2000, which incorporated Internet-friendly features. The scheduled 2002 release of Office 2003 promises speech-recognition programs that may make certain keyboard and mouse functions redundant.

In spite of these features, Microsoft has had to work harder at promoting each new version of the software package. The reason is that many users of Office increasingly find that its programs are so crammed with features that they cannot begin to exhaust the possibilities. According to some estimates, even enterprising users with lots of time on their hands are unlikely to use more than a quarter of the features of the Word 2000 word processing program. Consequently, a large number of computer users are concluding that upgrading to bigger, more sophisticated versions of the Office suite does little to enhance their productivity.

Because so many users of Office are confronting diminishing marginal returns from adding further to the already extensive software code stored on their hard drives, Microsoft is working hard on the suite's new speech-recognition features. Presumably, the company is hoping that if nothing else, people will appreciate having their computers do what they tell them to do.

For Critical Analysis

Under what circumstances could adding computer software yield a *negative* marginal product, at least within a period following installation of the software?

CONCEPTS IN BRIEF

- The technological relationship between output and input is called the production function. It relates output per time period to the several inputs, such as capital and labor.
- After some rate of output, the firm generally experiences diminishing marginal returns.
- The law of diminishing returns states that if all factors of production are held constant except one, equal increments in that one variable factor will eventually yield decreasing increments in output.

SHORT-RUN COSTS TO THE FIRM

You will see that costs are the extension of the production ideas just presented. Let's consider the costs the firm faces in the short run. To make this example simple, assume that there are only two factors of production, capital and labor. Our definition of the short run will be the time during which capital is fixed but labor is variable.

In the short run, a firm incurs certain types of costs. We label all costs incurred **total costs.** Then we break total costs down into total fixed costs and total variable costs, which we will explain shortly. Therefore,

Total costs 

The sum of total fixed costs and total variable costs.

Total costs (TC) = total fixed costs (TFC) + total variable costs (TVC)

Remember that these total costs include both explicit and implicit costs, including the normal rate of return on investment.

After we have looked at the elements of total costs, we will find out how to compute average and marginal costs.

Total Fixed Costs

Let's look at an ongoing business such as Dell Computer. The decision makers in that corporate giant can look around and see big machines, thousands of parts, huge buildings, and a multitude of other components of plant and equipment that have already been bought and are in place. Dell has to take account of the technological obsolescence of this equipment, no matter how many computers it produces. The payments on the loans taken out to buy the equipment will all be exactly the same. The opportunity costs of any land that Dell owns will all be exactly the same. These costs are more or less the same for Dell no matter how many computers it produces.

We also have to point out that the opportunity cost (or normal rate of return) of capital must be included along with other costs. Remember that we are dealing in the short run, during which capital is fixed. If investors in Dell have already put $100 million into a new factory addition, the opportunity cost of that capital invested is now, in essence, a *fixed cost.* Why? Because in the short run, nothing can be done about that cost; the investment has already been made. This leads us to a very straightforward definition of fixed costs: All costs that do not vary—that is, all costs that do not depend on the rate of production—are called **fixed costs.**

Fixed costs 

Costs that do not vary with output. Fixed costs include such things as rent on a building. These costs are fixed for a certain period of time; in the long run, they are variable.

Let's now take as an example the fixed costs incurred by an assembler of pocket calculators. This firm's total fixed costs will equal the cost of the rent on its equipment and the insurance it has to pay. We see in panel (a) of Figure 22-3 on page 542 that total fixed costs per day are $10. In panel (b), these total fixed costs are represented by the horizontal line at $10 per day. They are invariant to changes in the output of calculators per day—no matter how many are produced, fixed costs will remain at $10 per day.

Total Variable Costs

Total **variable costs** are costs whose magnitude varies with the rate of production. One obvious variable cost is wages. The more the firm produces, the more labor it has to hire; therefore, the more wages it has to pay. Another variable cost is parts. In the assembly of calculators, for example, microchips must be bought. The more calculators that are made, the more chips must be bought. Part of the rate of depreciation (the rate of wear and tear) on machines that are used in the assembly process can also be considered a variable cost if depreciation depends partly on how long and how intensively the machines are used. Total variable costs are given in column 3 in panel (a) of Figure 22-3. These are translated into the total variable cost curve in panel (b). Notice that the total variable cost curve lies below the total cost curve by the vertical distance of $10. This vertical distance represents, of course, total fixed costs.

Variable costs 

Costs that vary with the rate of production. They include wages paid to workers and purchases of materials.

FIGURE 22-3

Cost of Production: An Example

In panel (a), the derivation of columns 4 through 9 are given in parentheses in each column heading. For example, column 6, average variable costs, is derived by dividing column 3, total variable costs, by column 1, total output per day. Note that marginal cost (MC) in panel (c) intersects average variable costs (AVC) at the latter's minimum point. Also, MC intersects average total costs (ATC) at that latter's minimum point. It is a little more difficult to see that MC equals AVC and ATC at their respective minimum points in panel (a) because we are using discrete one-unit changes. You can see, though, that the marginal cost of going from 4 units per day to 5 units per day is $2 and increases to $3 when we move to 6 units per day. Somewhere in the middle it equals AVC of $2.60, which is in fact the minimum average variable cost. The same analysis holds for ATC, which hits minimum at 7 units per day at $4.28 per unit. MC goes from $4 to $5 and just equals ATC somewhere in between.

Panel (a)

(1) Total Output (*Q*/day)	(2) Total Fixed Costs (TFC)	(3) Total Variable Costs (TVC)	(4) Total Costs (TC) (4) = (2) + (3)	(5) Average Fixed Costs (AFC) (5) = (2) ÷ (1)	(6) Average Variable Costs (AVC) (6) = (3) ÷ (1)	(7) Average Total Costs (ATC) (7) = (4) ÷ (1)	(8) Total Costs (TC) (4)	(9) Marginal Cost (MC) (9) = change in (8) / change in (1)
0	$10	$ 0	$10	—	—	—	$10	
								$5
1	10	5	15	$10.00	$5.00	$15.00	15	
								3
2	10	8	18	5.00	4.00	9.00	18	
								2
3	10	10	20	3.33	3.33	6.67	20	
								1
4	10	11	21	2.50	2.75	5.25	21	
								2
5	10	13	23	2.00	2.60	4.60	23	
								3
6	10	16	26	1.67	2.67	4.33	26	
								4
7	10	20	30	1.43	2.86	4.28	30	
								5
8	10	25	35	1.25	3.13	4.38	35	
								6
9	10	31	41	1.11	3.44	4.56	41	
								7
10	10	38	48	1.00	3.80	4.80	48	
								8
11	10	46	56	.91	4.18	5.09	56	

Panel (b)

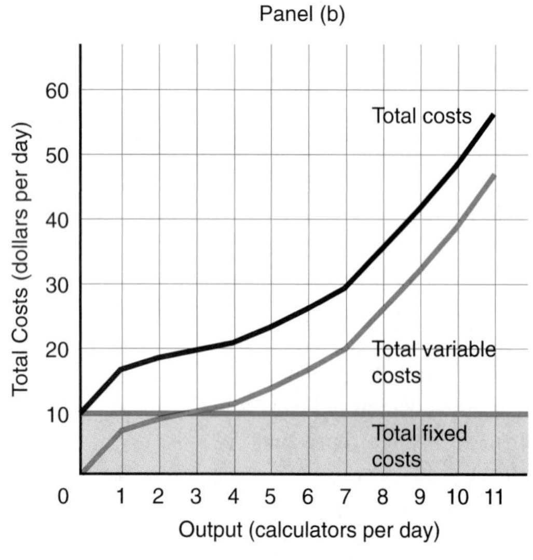

Panel (c)

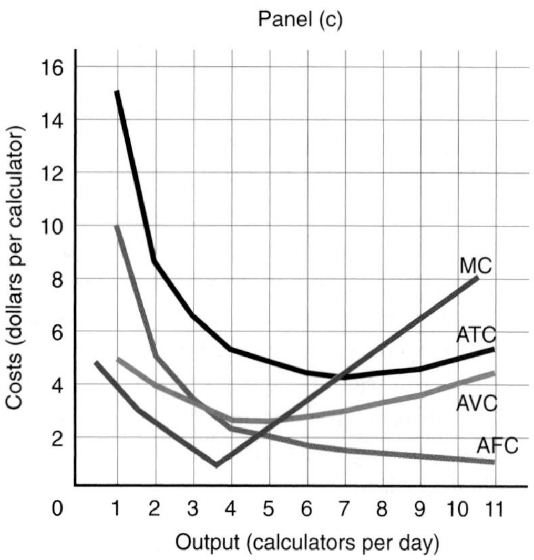

Short-Run Average Cost Curves

In panel (b) of Figure 22-3, we see total costs, total variable costs, and total fixed costs. Now we want to look at average cost. The average cost concept is one in which we are measuring cost per unit of output. It is a matter of simple arithmetic to figure the averages of these three cost concepts. We can define them as follows:

$$\text{Average total costs (ATC)} = \frac{\text{total costs (TC)}}{\text{output } (Q)}$$

$$\text{Average variable costs (AVC)} = \frac{\text{total variable costs (TVC)}}{\text{output } (Q)}$$

$$\text{Average fixed costs (AFC)} = \frac{\text{total fixed costs (TFC)}}{\text{output } (Q)}$$

The arithmetic is done in columns 5, 6, and 7 in panel (a) of Figure 22-3. The numerical results are translated into a graphical format in panel (c). Because total costs (TC) equal variable costs (TVC) plus fixed costs (TFC), the difference between average total costs (ATC) and average variable costs (AVC) will always be identical to average fixed costs (AFC). That means that average total costs and average variable costs move together as output expands.

Now let's see what we can observe about the three average cost curves in Figure 22-3.

Average Fixed Costs (AFC). **Average fixed costs** continue to fall throughout the output range. In fact, if we were to continue panel (c) (see diagram) farther to the right, we would find that average fixed costs would get closer and closer to the horizontal axis. That is because total fixed costs remain constant. As we divide this fixed number by a larger and larger number of units of output, the resulting AFC has to become smaller and smaller. In business, this is called "spreading the overhead."

Average fixed costs 
Total fixed costs divided by the number of units produced.

Average Variable Costs (AVC). We assume a particular form of the curve for **average variable costs.** The form that it takes is U-shaped: First it falls; then it starts to rise. It is possible for the AVC curve to take other shapes in the long run.

Average variable costs 
Total variable costs divided by the number of units produced.

Average Total Costs (ATC). This curve has a shape similar to that of the AVC curve. However, it falls even more dramatically in the beginning and rises more slowly after it has reached a minimum point. It falls and then rises because **average total costs** are the summation of the AFC curve and the AVC curve. Thus when AFC and AVC are both falling, ATC must fall too. At some point, however, AVC starts to increase while AFC continues to fall. Once the increase in the AVC curve outweighs the decrease in the AFC curve, the ATC curve will start to increase and will develop its familiar U shape.

Average total costs 
Total costs divided by the number of units produced; sometimes called *average per-unit total costs.*

Marginal Cost

We have stated repeatedly that the basis of decisions is always on the margin—movement in economics is always determined at the margin. This dictum also holds true within the firm. Firms, according to the analysis we use to predict their behavior, are very interested in their **marginal costs.** Because the term *marginal* means "additional" or "incremental" (or "decremental," too) here, marginal costs refer to costs that result from a one-unit

Marginal costs 
The change in total costs due to a one-unit change in production rate.

change in the production rate. For example, if the production of 10 calculators per day costs a firm \$48 and the production of 11 calculators costs it \$56 per day, the marginal cost of producing 11 rather than 10 calculators per day is \$8.

Marginal costs can be measured by using the formula

$$\text{Marginal cost} = \frac{\text{change in total cost}}{\text{change in output}}$$

We show the marginal costs of calculator production per day in column 9 of panel (a) in Figure 22-3, calculated according to the formula just given. In our example, we have changed output by one unit every time, so we can ignore variations in the denominator in that particular formula.

This marginal cost schedule is shown graphically in panel (c) of Figure 22-3. Just like average variable costs and average total costs, marginal costs first fall and then rise. The U shape of the marginal cost curve is a result of increasing and then diminishing marginal returns. At lower levels of output, the marginal cost curve declines. The reasoning is that as marginal physical product increases with each addition of output, the marginal cost of this last unit of output must fall. Conversely, when diminishing marginal returns set in, marginal physical product decreases (and eventually becomes negative); it follows that the marginal cost must rise when the marginal product begins its decline. These relationships are clearly reflected in the geometry of panels (b) and (c) of Figure 22-3.

In summary:

As long as marginal physical product rises, marginal cost will fall, and when marginal physical product starts to fall (after reaching the point of diminishing marginal returns), marginal cost will begin to rise.

POLICY EXAMPLE

Can "Three Strikes" Laws Reduce Crime?

Crime and violence have been the top concern of Americans for at least a decade. At both the federal and the state level, politicians have responded with a variety of policies aimed at reducing crime. One popular new law has been labeled "three strikes and you're out." A defendant with a prior conviction for two serious or violent offenses faces mandatory life imprisonment for a third offense.

Such legislation has dramatically affected the marginal cost of violence and murder to potential criminal defendants who have already been convicted of two felonies. Here is what one career criminal, Frank Schweickert, said in a *New York Times* interview: "Before, if I was doing a robbery and getting chased by cops, I'd lay my gun down. . . . But now you are talking about a life sentence. Why isn't it worth doing whatever it takes to get away? If that meant shooting a cop, if that meant shooting a store clerk, if that meant shooting someone innocent in my way, well, they'd have gotten shot. Because what is the worst thing that could happen to me: life imprisonment? If I'm getting a murder sentence anyway, I might as well do whatever it takes to maybe get away." In other words, the "three strikes" legislation has reduced to zero the marginal cost of murder (in non-capital-punishment states) committed while engaging in a criminal activity after two prior felony convictions.

For Critical Analysis

Do criminals subject to the new legislation have to understand the concept of marginal cost in order for our theory to predict well? Explain.

The Relationship Between Average and Marginal Costs

Let us now examine the relationship between average costs and marginal costs. There is always a definite relationship between averages and marginals. Consider the example of 10 football players with an average weight of 200 pounds. An eleventh player is added. His weight is 250 pounds. That represents the marginal weight. What happens now to the average weight of the team? It must increase. Thus when the marginal player weighs more than the average, the average must increase. Likewise, if the marginal player weighs less than 200 pounds, the average weight will decrease.

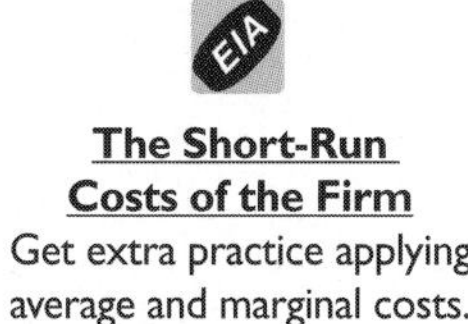

The Short-Run Costs of the Firm
Get extra practice applying average and marginal costs.

There is a similar relationship between average variable costs and marginal costs. When marginal costs are less than average costs, the latter must fall. Conversely, when marginal costs are greater than average costs, the latter must rise. When you think about it, the relationship makes sense. The only way for average variable costs to fall is for the extra cost of the marginal unit produced to be less than the average variable cost of all the preceding units. For example, if the average variable cost for two units of production is $4.00 a unit, the only way for the average variable cost of three units to be less than that of two units is for the variable costs attributable to the last unit—the marginal cost—to be less than the average of the past units. In this particular case, if average variable cost falls to $3.33 a unit, total variable cost for the three units would be three times $3.33, or almost exactly $10.00. Total variable cost for two units is two times $4.00, or $8.00. The marginal cost is therefore $10.00 minus $8.00, or $2.00, which is less than the average variable cost of $3.33.

A similar type of computation can be carried out for rising average variable costs. The only way for average variable costs to rise is for the average variable cost of additional units to be more than that for units already produced. But the incremental cost is the marginal cost. In this particular case, the marginal costs have to be higher than the average variable costs.

There is also a relationship between marginal costs and average total costs. Remember that average total cost is equal to total cost divided by the number of units produced. Remember also that marginal cost does not include any fixed costs. Fixed costs are, by definition, fixed and cannot influence marginal costs. Our example can therefore be repeated substituting *average total cost* for *average variable cost.*

These rising and falling relationships can be seen in Figure 22-3, where MC intersects AVC and ATC at their respective minimum points.

Minimum Cost Points

At what rate of output of calculators per day does our representative firm experience the minimum average total costs? Column 7 in panel (a) of Figure 22-3 shows that the minimum average total cost is $4.28, which occurs at an output rate of seven calculators per day. We can also find this minimum cost by finding the point in panel (c) of Figure 22-3 at which the marginal cost curve intersects the average total cost curve. This should not be surprising. When marginal cost is below average total cost, average total cost falls. When marginal cost is above average total cost, average total cost rises. At the point where average total cost is neither falling nor rising, marginal cost must then be equal to average total cost. When we represent this graphically, the marginal cost curve will intersect the average total cost curve at the latter's minimum.

The same analysis applies to the intersection of the marginal cost curve and the average variable cost curve. When are average variable costs at a minimum? According to panel (a) of Figure 22-3, average variable costs are at a minimum of $2.60 at an output rate of five calculators per day. This is where the marginal cost curve intersects the average variable cost curve in panel (c) of Figure 22-3.

CONCEPTS IN BRIEF

- Total costs equal total fixed costs plus total variable costs.
- Fixed costs are those that do not vary with the rate of production; variable costs are those that do vary with the rate of production.
- Average total costs equal total costs divided by output (ATC=TC/Q).
- Average variable costs equal total variable costs divided by output (AVC=TVC/Q).
- Average fixed costs equal total fixed costs divided by output (AFC=TFC/Q).
- Marginal cost equals the change in total cost divided by the change in output (MC=ΔTC/ΔQ, where Δ means "change in").
- The marginal cost curve intersects the minimum point of the average total cost curve and the minimum point of the average variable cost curve.

THE RELATIONSHIP BETWEEN DIMINISHING MARGINAL RETURNS AND COST CURVES

There is a unique relationship between output and the shape of the various cost curves we have drawn. Let's consider specifically the relationship between marginal cost and the example of diminishing marginal physical returns in panel (a) of Figure 22-4. It turns out that if wage rates are constant, the shape of the marginal cost curve in panel (d) of Figure 22-4 is both a reflection of and a consequence of the law of diminishing returns. Let's assume that each unit of labor can be purchased at a constant price. Further assume that labor is the only variable input. We see that as more workers are hired, marginal physical product first rises and then falls after the point at which diminishing returns are encountered. Thus the marginal cost of each extra unit of output will first fall as long as marginal physical product is rising, and then it will rise as long as marginal physical product is falling. Recall that marginal cost is defined as

$$\text{MC} = \frac{\text{change in total cost}}{\text{change in output}}$$

Because the price of labor is assumed to be constant, the change in total cost depends solely on the constant price of labor, *W*. The change in output is simply the marginal physical product (MPP) of the one-unit increase in labor. Therefore, we see that

$$\text{Marginal cost} = \frac{W}{\text{MPP}}$$

This means that initially, when there are increasing returns, marginal cost falls (we are dividing *W* by increasingly larger numbers), and later, when diminishing returns set in and marginal physical product is falling, marginal cost must increase (we are dividing *W* by smaller numbers). As marginal physical product increases, marginal cost decreases, and as marginal physical product decreases, marginal cost must increase. Thus when marginal physical product reaches its maximum, marginal cost necessarily reaches its minimum. To illustrate this, let's return to Figure 22-2 and consider specifically panel (a). Assume that a worker is paid $100 a week. When we go from zero labor input to one unit, output increases by 10 bushels of wheat. Each of those 10 bushels of wheat has a marginal cost of $10. Now the second unit of labor is hired, and it too costs $100 per week. Output increases by 16. Thus the marginal cost is $100 ÷ 16 = $6.25. We continue the experiment. We see that the next unit of labor yields only 10 additional bushels of wheat, so marginal cost starts to rise again back to $10. The following unit of labor increases marginal physical product by only 8, so marginal cost becomes $100 ÷ 8 = $12.50.

Panel (a)

(1) Labor Input	(2) Total Product (number of pairs sold)	(3) Average Physical Product (pairs per salesperson) (3) = (2) ÷ (1)	(4) Marginal Physical Product	(5) Average Variable Cost (5) = *W* ($100) ÷ (3)	(6) Marginal Cost (6) = *W* ($100) ÷ (4)
0	0	—	—	—	—
1	50	50	50	$2.00	$2.00
2	110	55	60	1.82	1.67
3	180	60	70	1.67	1.43
4	240	60	60	1.67	1.67
5	290	58	50	1.72	2.00
6	330	55	40	1.82	2.50
7	360	51	30	1.96	3.33

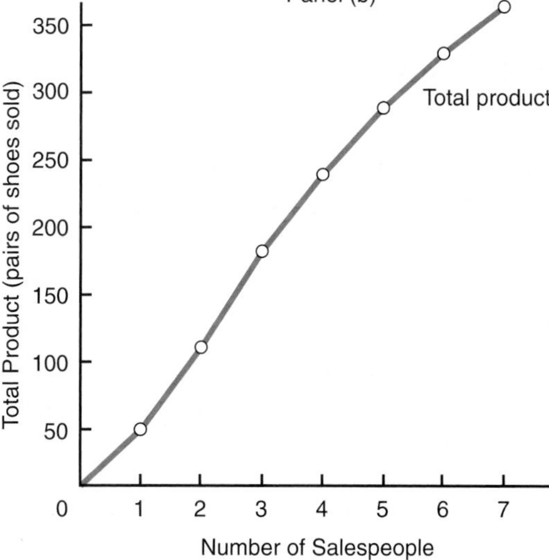

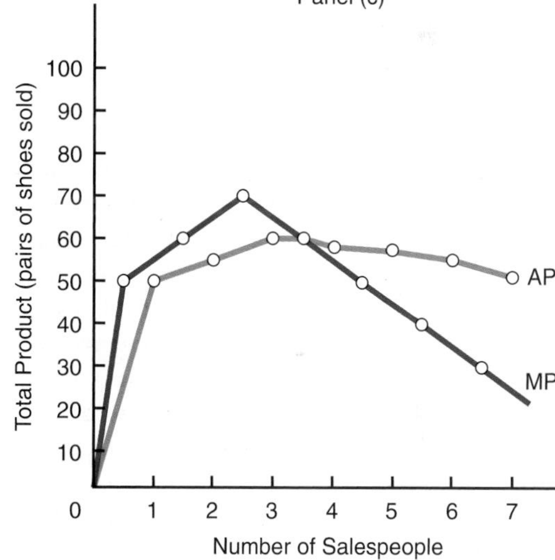

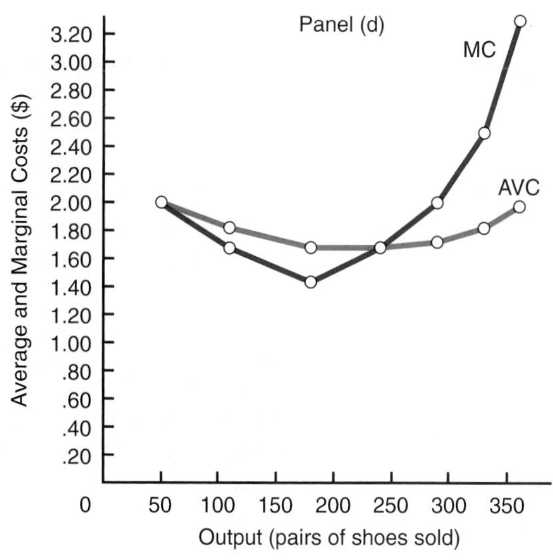

FIGURE 22-4

The Relationship Between Physical Output and Costs

As the number of salespeople increases, the total number of pairs of shoes sold rises, as shown in panels (a) and (b). In panel (c), marginal physical product (MPP) first rises and then falls. Average physical product (APP) follows. The mirror image of panel (c) is shown in panel (d), in which MC and AVC first fall and then rise.

All of the foregoing can be restated in relatively straightforward terms:

> Firms' short-run cost curves are a reflection of the law of diminishing marginal returns. Given any constant price of the variable input, marginal costs decline as long as the marginal product of the variable resource is rising. At the point at which diminishing marginal returns begin, marginal costs begin to rise as the marginal product of the variable input begins to decline.

The result is a marginal cost curve that slopes down, hits a minimum, and then slopes up. The average total cost curve and average variable cost curve are of course affected. They will have their familiar U shape in the short run. Again, to see this, recall that

$$\text{AVC} = \frac{\text{total variable costs}}{\text{total output}}$$

As we move from zero labor input to one unit in panel (a) of Figure 22-2, output increases from zero to 10 bushels. The total variable costs are the price per worker, *W* ($100), times the number of workers (1). Because the average product of one worker (column 3) is 10, we can write the total product, 10, as the average product, 10, times the number of workers, 1. Thus we see that

$$\text{AVC} = \frac{\$100 \times 1}{10 \times 1} = \frac{\$100}{10} = \frac{W}{\text{AP}}$$

From column 3 in panel (a) of Figure 22-2 we see that the average product increases, reaches a maximum, and then declines. Because AVC = *W*/AP, average variable cost decreases as average product increases and increases as average product decreases. AVC reaches its minimum when average product reaches its maximum. Furthermore, because ATC = AVC+AFC, the average total cost curve inherits the relationship between the average variable cost and diminishing returns.

To illustrate, consider a shoe store that employs salespeople to sell shoes. Panel (a) of Figure 22-4 presents in column 2 the total number of pairs of shoes sold as the number of salespeople increases. Notice that the total product first increases at an increasing rate and later increases at a decreasing rate. This is reflected in column 4, which shows that the marginal physical product increases at first and then falls. The average physical product too first rises and then falls. The marginal and average physical products are graphed in panel (c) of Figure 22-4. Our immediate interest here is the average variable and marginal costs. Because we can define average variable cost as $100/AP (assuming that the wage paid is constant at $100), as the average product rises from 50 to 55 to 60 pairs of shoes sold, the average variable cost falls from $2.00 to $1.82 to $1.67. Conversely, as average product falls from 60 to 50, average variable cost rises from $1.67 to $2.00. Likewise, because marginal cost can also be defined as *W*/MPP, we see that as marginal physical product rises from 50 to 70, marginal cost falls from $2.00 to $1.43. As marginal physical product falls to 30, marginal cost rises to $3.33. These relationships are also expressed in panels (b), (c), and (d) of Figure 22-4.

LONG-RUN COST CURVES

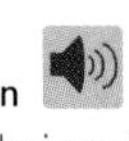
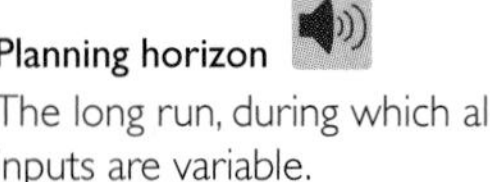
Planning horizon
The long run, during which all inputs are variable.

The long run is defined as a time period during which full adjustment can be made to any change in the economic environment. Thus in the long run, *all* factors of production are variable. Long-run curves are sometimes called *planning curves,* and the long run is sometimes called the **planning horizon.** We start out our analysis of long-run cost curves by

FIGURE 22-5

Preferable Plant Size and the Long-Run Average Cost Curve

If the anticipated permanent rate of output per unit time period is Q_1, the optimal plant to build would be the one corresponding to SAC_1 in panel (a) because average costs are lower. However, if the permanent rate of output increases to Q_2, it will be more profitable to have a plant size corresponding to SAC_2. Unit costs fall to C_3.

If we draw all the possible short-run average cost curves that correspond to different plant sizes and then draw the envelope (a curve tangent to each member of a set of curves) to these various curves, SAC_1–SAC_8, we obtain the long-run average cost curve, or the planning curve, as shown in panel (b).

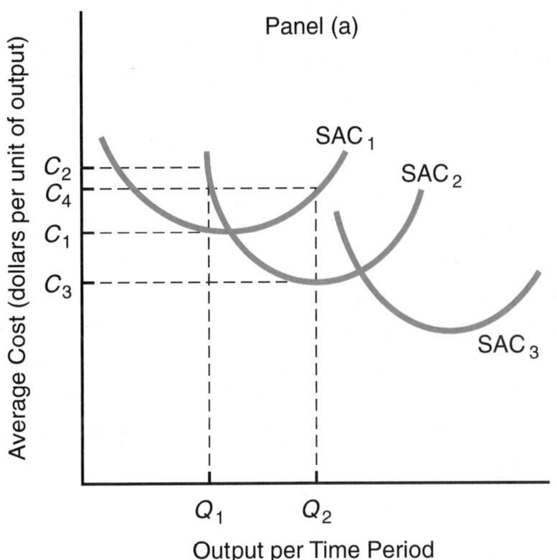

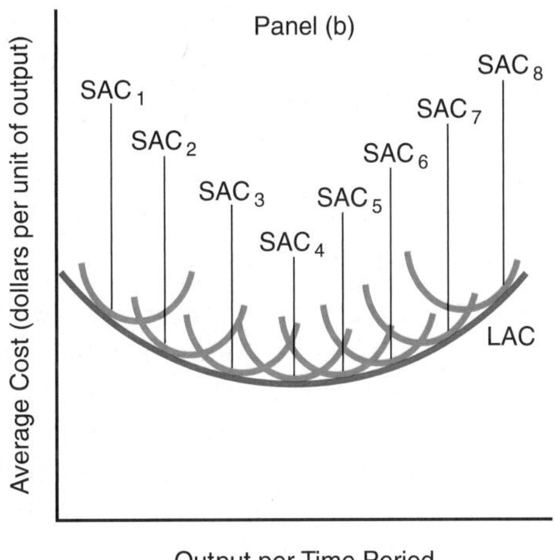

considering a single firm contemplating the construction of a single plant. The firm has three alternative plant sizes from which to choose on the planning horizon. Each particular plant size generates its own short-run average total cost curve. Now that we are talking about the difference between long-run and short-run cost curves, we will label all short-run curves with an *S* and long-run curves with an *L;* short-run average (total) costs will be labeled SAC; and long-run average cost curves will be labeled LAC.

Panel (a) of Figure 22-5 shows three short-run average cost curves for three successively larger plants. Which is the optimal size to build? That depends on the anticipated normal, sustained (permanent) rate of output per time period. Assume for a moment that the anticipated normal, sustained rate is Q_1. If a plant of size 1 is built, the average costs will be C_1. If a plant of size 2 is built, we see on SAC_2 that the average costs will be C_2, which is greater than C_1. Thus if the anticipated rate of output is Q_1, the appropriate plant size is the one from which SAC_1 was derived.

However, if the anticipated permanent rate of output per time period goes from Q_1 to Q_2 and a plant of size 1 had been decided on, average costs would be C_4. If a plant of size 2 had been decided on, average costs would be C_3, which is clearly less than C_4.

In choosing the appropriate plant size for a single-plant firm during the planning horizon, the firm will pick the size whose short-run average cost curve generates an average cost that is lowest for the expected rate of output.

Long-Run Average Cost Curve

If we now assume that the entrepreneur faces an infinite number of choices of plant sizes in the long run, we can conceive of an infinite number of SAC curves similar to the three in panel (a) of Figure 22-5. We are not able, of course, to draw an infinite number; we have drawn quite a few, however, in panel (b) of Figure 22-5. We then draw the "envelope" to all these various short-run average cost curves. The resulting envelope is the **long-run average cost curve.** This long-run average cost curve is sometimes called the **planning curve,** for it represents the various average costs attainable at the planning stage of the firm's decision making. It represents the locus (path) of points giving the least unit cost of producing any given rate of output. Note that the LAC curve is *not* tangent to each individual SAC curve at the latter's minimum points. This is true only at the minimum point of the LAC curve. Then and only then are minimum long-run average costs equal to minimum short-run average costs.

Long-run average cost curve
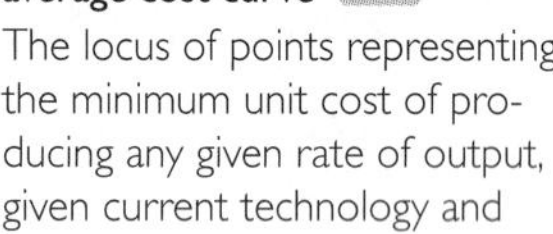
The locus of points representing the minimum unit cost of producing any given rate of output, given current technology and resource prices.

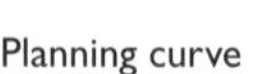
Planning curve
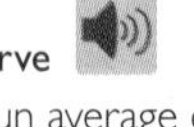
The long-run average cost curve.

WHY THE LONG-RUN AVERAGE COST CURVE IS U-SHAPED

Notice that the long-run average cost curve, LAC, in panel (b) of Figure 22-5 is U-shaped, similar to the U shape of the short-run average cost curve developed earlier in this chapter. The reason behind the U shape of the two curves is not the same, however. The short-run average cost curve is U-shaped because of the law of diminishing marginal returns. But the law cannot apply to the long run, because in the long run, all factors of production are variable; there is no point of diminishing marginal returns because there is no fixed factor of production.

Economies of scale
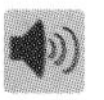
Decreases in long-run average costs resulting from increases in output.

Constant returns to scale
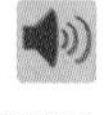
No change in long-run average costs when output increases.

Diseconomies of scale

Increases in long-run average costs that occur as output increases.

Why, then, do we see the U shape in the long-run average cost curve? The reasoning has to do with economies of scale, constant returns to scale, and diseconomies of scale. When the firm is experiencing **economies of scale,** the long-run average cost curve slopes downward—an increase in scale and production leads to a fall in unit costs. When the firm is experiencing **constant returns to scale,** the long-run average cost curve is at its minimum point, such that an increase in scale and production does not change unit costs. When the firm is experiencing **diseconomies of scale,** the long-run average cost curve slopes upward—an increase in scale and production increases unit costs. These three sections of the long-run average cost curves are broken up into panels (a), (b), and (c) in Figure 22-6.

Reasons for Economies of Scale 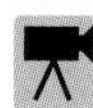

We shall examine three of the many reasons why a firm might be expected to experience economies of scale: specialization, the dimensional factor, and improved productive equipment.

Specialization. As a firm's scale of operation increases, the opportunities for specialization in the use of resource inputs also increase. This is sometimes called *increased division of tasks* or *operations.* Gains from such division of labor or increased specialization are well known. When we consider managerial staffs, we also find that larger enterprises may be able to put together more highly specialized staffs.

Dimensional Factor. Large-scale firms often require proportionately less input per unit of output simply because certain inputs do not have to be physically doubled in order to double

FIGURE 22-6

Economies of Scale, Constant Returns to Scale, and Diseconomies of Scale Shown with the Long-Run Average Cost Curve

Long-run average cost curves will fall when there are economies of scale, as shown in panel (a). They will be constant (flat) when the firm is experiencing constant returns to scale, as shown in panel (b). They will rise when the firm is experiencing diseconomies of scale, as shown in panel (c).

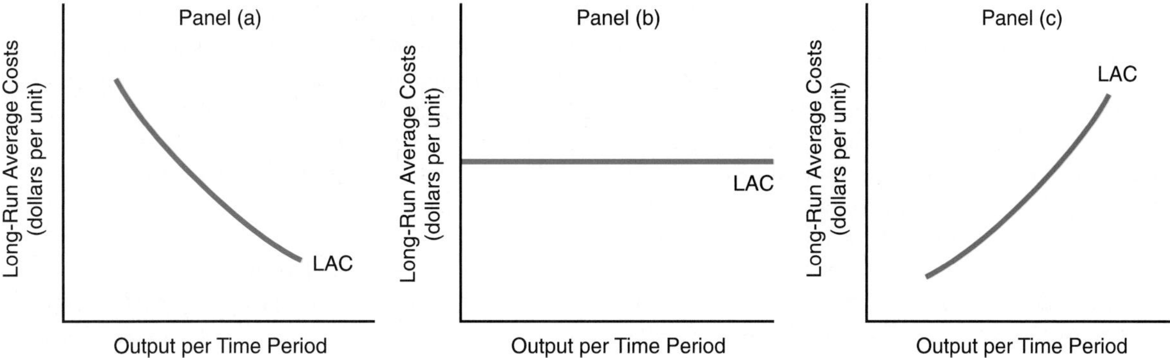

the output. Consider the cost of storage of oil. The cost of storage is basically related to the cost of steel that goes into building the storage container; however, the amount of steel required goes up less than in proportion to the volume (storage capacity) of the container (because the volume of a container increases more than proportionately with its surface area).

Improved Productive Equipment. The larger the scale of the enterprise, the more the firm is able to take advantage of larger-volume (output capacity) types of machinery. Small-scale operations may not be able profitably to use large-volume machines that can be more efficient per unit of output. Also, smaller firms often cannot use technologically more advanced machinery because they are unable to spread out the high cost of such sophisticated equipment over a large output.

For any of these reasons, the firm may experience economies of scale, which means that equal percentage increases in output result in a decrease in average cost. Thus output can double, but total costs will less than double; hence average cost falls. Note that the factors listed for causing economies of scale are all *internal* to the firm; they do not depend on what other firms are doing or what is happening in the economy.

EXAMPLE

Measuring the Value of Ideas

When contemplating the appropriate scale for production, it is relatively straightforward for a business to evaluate the amount of machines and buildings available for the production of the goods or services it produces. Another fundamental internal factor that a firm must take into account is assessing the scale of its operations, however, is its internal base of knowledge and ideas. Today more than ever, the physical aspects of a business's plants and equipment are supplemented and even overshadowed by more intangible factors, such as patents, computer software, research and development programs, and the expertise—the ideas—of managers and employees.

A reflection of problems in measuring these intangible factors is the fact that since the 1970s, the median ratio of the stock market values of public U.S. companies relative to their book values (values as measured by accountants) has more than doubled. The gap between market values and book values has increased particularly among companies for which intangible factors such as ideas are most crucial—software developers and manufacturers, Internet marketers, and the like.

To improve their ability to measure ideas and other intangible factors of production, some companies have begun to develop "intellectual capital reports" that take into account the educational attainments of staff, the age profile of employees, and investments in research and development. These companies hope to be able to use these reports alongside traditional measures of capital resources when determining the current scale of their enterprises. For instance, after taking into account the value of ideas and knowledge, Baruch Lev of New York University estimates that Merck, a pharmaceutical company, has "knowledge capital" worth about $50 billion and that DuPont, a manufacturer of chemicals and plastics, has knowledge capital in excess of $25 billion.

In the past, companies have regarded the wages they pay their employees solely as short-run costs. Nevertheless, every time an employee leaves a company, the company loses a bit of the intangible knowledge capital locked up in that employee's mind. Recognition of this fact has induced more companies to consider the information contained in intellectual capital reports so that they can better gauge the long-run implications of their staffing decisions.

For Critical Analysis

What problems are companies likely to encounter when they attempt to measure the value of knowledge and ideas?

Why a Firm Might Experience Diseconomies of Scale

One of the basic reasons that a firm can expect to run into diseconomies of scale is that there are limits to the efficient functioning of management. Moreover, as more workers are hired, a more than proportionate increase in managers and staff people may be needed, and this could cause increased costs per unit. This is so because larger levels of output imply successively larger *plant* size, which in turn implies successively larger *firm* size. Thus, as the level of output increases, more people must be hired, and the firm gets bigger. As this happens, however, the support, supervisory, and administrative staff and the general paperwork of the firm all increase. As the layers of supervision grow, the costs of information and communication grow more than proportionately; hence the average unit cost will start to increase.

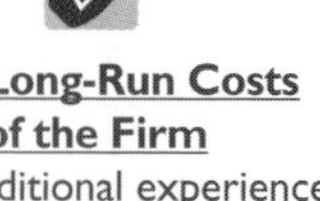

The Long-Run Costs of the Firm
Gain additional experience with the concepts of long-run costs and scale economies.

Some observers of corporate giants claim that many of them have been experiencing some diseconomies of scale. Witness the problems that General Motors and IBM had in the early 1990s. Some analysts say that the financial problems they encountered were at least partly a function of their size relative to their smaller, more flexible competitors, who could make decisions more quickly and then take advantage of changing market conditions more rapidly. This was particularly true for IBM. Initially, the company adapted very slowly to the fact that the large mainframe computer business was declining as micro- and mini-computers became more and more powerful. Finally, by the end of the 1990s, IBM had adjusted to a more appropriate scale.

MINIMUM EFFICIENT SCALE

Economists and statisticians have obtained actual data on the relationship between changes in all inputs and changes in average cost. It turns out that for many industries, the long-run average cost curve does not resemble that shown in panel (b) of Figure 22-5. Rather, it

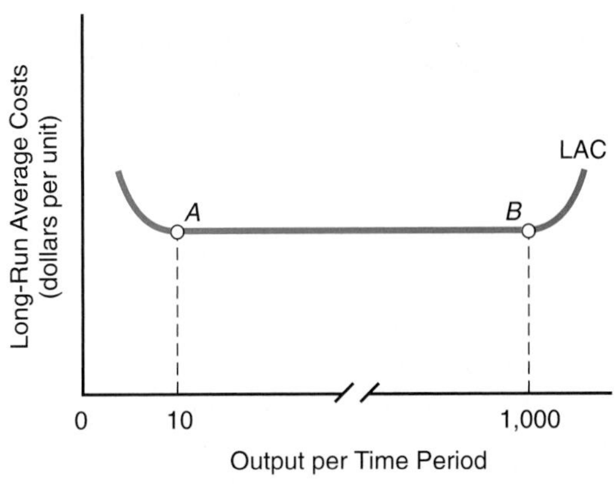

FIGURE 22-7

Minimum Efficient Scale

This long-run average cost curve reaches a minimum point at *A*. After that point, long-run average costs remain horizontal, or constant, and then rise at some later rate of output. Point *A* is called the minimum efficient scale for the firm because that is the point at which it reaches minimum costs. It is the lowest rate of output at which the average long-run costs are minimized.

more closely resembles Figure 22-7. What you can observe there is a small portion of declining long-run average costs (economies of scale) and then a wide range of outputs over which the firm experiences relatively constant economies of scale. At the output rate when economies of scale end and constant economies of scale start, the **minimum efficient scale (MES)** for the firm is encountered. It occurs at point *A*. (The point is, of course, approximate. The more smoothly the curve declines into its flat portion, the more approximate will be our estimate of the MES.) The minimum efficient scale will always be the lowest rate of output at which long-run average costs are minimized. In any industry with a long-run average cost curve similar to the one in Figure 22-7, larger firms will have no cost-saving advantage over smaller firms as long as the smaller firms have at least obtained the minimum efficient scale at point *A*.

Minimum efficient scale (MES) 
The lowest rate of output per unit time at which long-run average costs for a particular firm are at a minimum.

Among its uses, the minimum efficient scale gives us a rough measure of the degree of competition in an industry. If the MES is small relative to industry demand, the degree of competition in that industry is likely to be high because there is room for many efficiently sized plants. Conversely, when the MES is large relative to industry demand, the degree of competition is likely to be small because there is room for a relatively small number of efficiently sized plants or firms. Looked at another way, if it takes a very large scale of plant to obtain minimum long-run average cost, the output of just a few of these very large firms can fully satisfy total market demand. This means that there isn't room for a large number of smaller plants if maximum efficiency is to be obtained in the industry.

CONCEPTS IN BRIEF

- The long run is often called the planning horizon. The long-run average cost curve is the planning curve. It is found by drawing a line tangent to one point on a series of short-run average cost curves, each corresponding to a different plant size.
- The firm can experience economies of scale, diseconomies of scale, and constant returns to scale, all according to whether the long-run average cost curve slopes downward, slopes upward, or is horizontal (flat). Economies of scale refer to what happens to average cost when all factors of production are increased.
- We observe economies of scale for a number of reasons, among which are specialization, improved productive equipment, and the dimensional factor, because large-scale firms require proportionately less input per unit of output. The firm may experience diseconomies of scale primarily because of limits to the efficient functioning of management.
- The minimum efficient scale occurs at the lowest rate of output at which long-run average costs are minimized.

NETNOMICS

Classified Ads That Fido Can't Chew Up

The typical American consumer makes 80 percent of all purchases within 20 miles of home. A traditional "local purchase" is the hometown newspaper. After all, that is where one can find local movie and concert listings, classified ads, and news. Never mind that getting a newspaper printed and delivered is a complicated task involving lots of paper and ink, subscription clerks, and home delivery personnel. Where else can you go to find out what is going on in your neighborhood?

Microsoft Corporation came up with a possible answer. It is called Sidewalk. In mid-1997, Microsoft set up Sidewalk Web sites for three cities: Boston, New York, and Seattle. The company geared these sites toward local residents rather than tourists, offering listings of concerts, movies, and restaurants, information about planned civic events, and so on. Today, you can find a Sidewalk Web site for Birmingham, Alabama; Flint, Michigan; Winston-Salem, North Carolina; and about 100 other cities.

Why was Microsoft interested in providing people with hometown information? The reason was that the company wanted a share of the revenues earned by local newspapers and other local media—an estimated $70 billion is spent on such advertisements. Sidewalk sells space on its site to local advertisers, just as newspapers sell portions of their pages for print ads.

Why was Microsoft convinced that Sidewalk could compete? In its view, it has a big cost advantage over newspapers. Instead of running the presses each day and churning out a lot of paper that people throw out or recycle the next day, Sidewalk employees simply change the data for Sidewalk Web sites electronically. It is as if your local newspaper could get by with just a staff of reporters armed with word processors but no presses, paper, or delivery people. A potential result may be a big efficiency advantage in the form of much lower average variable costs for providing the same basic services that local newspapers have traditionally provided.

Some media experts believe that local newspapers will lose at least $2 billion in local ad revenues to on-line services such as Sidewalk over the next few years. And if heightened competition from Internet services also pushes down the market price of ads, local papers stand to lose even more.

ISSUES & APPLICATIONS

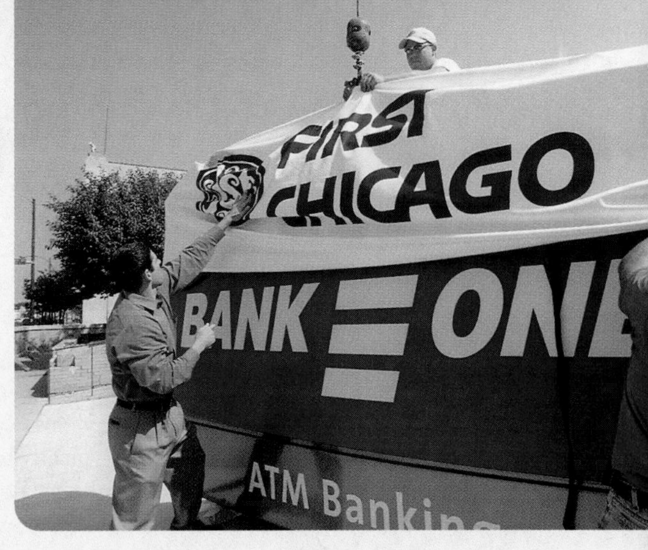

Are Bigger Banks Necessarily More Efficient?

Since the late 1980s, U.S. commercial banking has experienced a wave of mergers (combinations of existing banks) and acquisitions (purchases of banks by other banks). As you can see in Table 22-1, thousands of banks have been involved in mergers and acquisitions since 1989. Hundreds of millions of dollars in bank assets—loans, securities, and cash—are being consolidated within a smaller number of banks. The average bank is getting bigger. Most banking experts anticipate that this trend will persist for several more years.

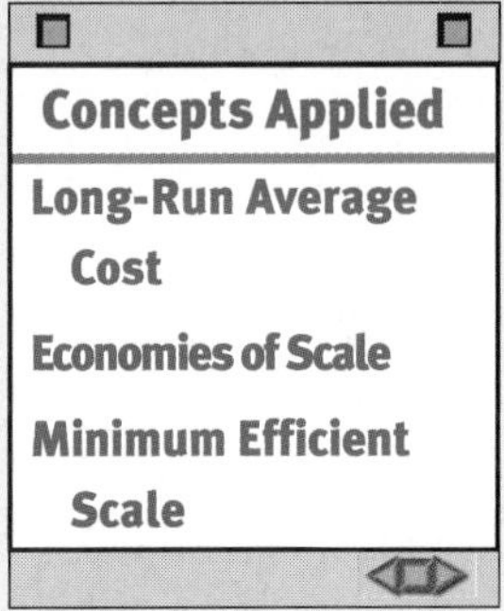

Concepts Applied
Long-Run Average Cost
Economies of Scale
Minimum Efficient Scale

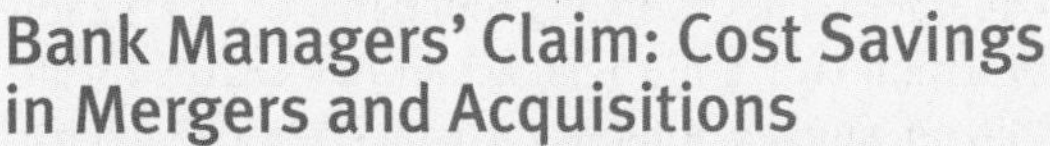

Bank Managers' Claim: Cost Savings in Mergers and Acquisitions

Combining banks into a single financial services company is a time-consuming and expensive task. Nevertheless, bank managers promote mergers and acquisitions as a means of achieving reductions in the long-run costs of operating new, enlarged institutions. Combining banks, they argue, permits banks to pool more loans under the management of fewer lending officers, to apply computer technologies to managing financial risks for a bigger set of assets, and to handle check clearing for more customers using equipment housed within a single bank.

According to this rationale, therefore, merged banks can reduce labor expenses by shedding employees and can slash other operating expenses by using fewer computers and

Year	New Bank Startups Less Bank Failures	Reduction Due to Mergers and Acquisitions	Total Number of U.S. Banks at Year End
1990	25	−393	12,329
1991	26	−446	11,909
1992	−32	−428	11,449
1993	−25	−480	10,944
1994	34	−547	10,431
1995	99	−609	9,921
1996	142	−553	9,510
1997	213	−599	9,124
1998	195	−563	8,756
1999	241	−417	8,580
2000	212	−404	8,388
Total Change, 1990–2000	1,130	−5,439	−4,309

Source: Federal Deposit Insurance Corporation *Historical Banking Statistics*, 2000.
*Author's estimates based on first-quarter data.

TABLE 22-1
Bank Mergers and the Declining Number of U.S. Banks
About 1,130 more new banks have opened than those that have failed since 1990. Nevertheless, an estimated 5,439 ceased to exist because of mergers. On net, therefore, the total number of U.S. commercial banks has declined by more than one-third since 1989.

other capital goods. In short, by expanding to a larger size, consolidated banks can lower their long-run average cost. They can take advantage of economies of scale.

Does the Reality of Bank Mergers and Acquisitions Support the Claim?

Nevertheless, many economists have had trouble finding evidence of economies of scale in banking. Banking output is notoriously hard to measure, but no matter what output gauge economists have used—total assets, total deposits, index measures of banking services—studies have typically found that the minimum efficient scale in banking is no greater than about $50 million. To explain the existence of multibillion-dollar behemoths such as Citibank or Bank of America, economists often relied on the idea that there might be "economies of scope" in banking: Banks might achieve lower long-run average costs by pooling all kinds of financial services in a single big company.

Studies of bank mergers that occurred during the late 1980s and early 1990s seemed to provide a more cynical rationale for bank mergers. They typically found that one of the few unambiguous effects of a merger or acquisition was a big increase in the salaries of the managers who survived staffing cuts. Although studies of these early mergers and acquisitions found glimmers of evidence of cost savings, the efficiency gains were generally insignificant. Managers seemed to benefit the most.

More recent studies, however, have given new life to bank managers' claims that bigger banks really are more efficient. Consolidations that have taken place since the mid-1990s appear to have reduced long-run average costs for merged banks by as much as 20 percent. In addition, some banks created by earlier consolidations have found ways to reduce their costs, albeit more slowly than originally promised.

Why are consolidated banks more cost-efficient now than in earlier years? One possible reason is that recent regulatory changes allowing banks to expand the scope of their activities—notably, permitting them to sell insurance and mutual funds—have helped them realize cost savings from greater size. Another is that bigger banks may have a cost advantage in operating on-line banking services and using other financial services technologies that were not available when the banking consolidation wave began. If new technologies are responsible for the reduction in costs, then the managers of banks that merged earlier were either quite prophetic, or, more likely, just plain lucky.

FOR CRITICAL ANALYSIS

1. If big banks are more efficient, why are there thousands of small banks in the United States?
2. Why would difficulties in measuring a bank's output make determining its minimum efficient scale more complicated?

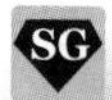

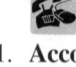

SUMMARY DISCUSSION OF LEARNING OBJECTIVES

1. **Accounting Profits Versus Economic Profits:** A firm's accounting profits equal its total revenues minus its total explicit costs, which are expenses directly paid out by the firm. Economic profits equal accounting profits minus implicit costs, which are expenses that managers do not have pay out of pocket, such as the opportunity cost of factors of production dedicated to the firm's production process. Owners of a firm seek to maximize the firm's economic profits to ensure that they earn at least a normal rate of return, meaning that the firm's total revenues at least cover explicit costs and implicit opportunity costs.
2. **The Short Run Versus the Long Run from a Firm's Perspective:** The short run for a firm is a period during which at least one input, such as plant size, cannot be altered. Inputs that cannot be changed in the short run are fixed inputs, whereas factors of production that may be adjusted in the short run are variable inputs. The long run is a period in which a firm may vary all factors of production.
3. **The Law of Diminishing Marginal Returns:** The production function is the relationship between inputs and the maximum physical output, or total product, that a firm can produce. Typically, a firm's marginal physi-

cal product—the physical output resulting from the addition of one more unit of a variable factor of production—increases with the first few units of the variable factor of production that it employs. Eventually, however, as the firm adds more and more units of the variable input, the marginal physical product begins to decline. This is the law of diminishing returns.

4. **A Firm's Short-Run Cost Curves:** The expenses for a firm's fixed inputs are its fixed costs, and the expenses for its variable inputs are variable costs. The total costs of a firm are the sum of its fixed costs and variable costs. Dividing fixed costs by various possible output levels traces out the firm's average fixed cost curve, which slopes downward because dividing fixed costs by a larger total product yields a lower average fixed cost. Average variable cost equals total variable cost divided by total product, and average total cost equals total cost divided by total product; doing these computations at various possible output levels yields U-shaped curves. Finally, marginal cost is the change in total cost resulting from a one-unit change in production. A firm's marginal cost curve typically declines as the firm produces the first few units of output, but at the point of diminishing marginal returns, the marginal cost curve begins to slope upward. The marginal cost curve also intersects the minimum points of the average variable cost curve and average total cost curve.
5. **A Firm's Long-Run Cost Curves:** Over a firm's long-run, or planning, horizon, it can choose all factors of production, including plant size. Thus it can choose a long-run scale of production along a long-run average cost curve. The long-run average cost curve, which for most firms is U-shaped, is traced out by the short-run average cost curves corresponding to various plant sizes.
6. **Economies and Diseconomies of Scale and a Firm's Minimum Efficient Scale:** Along the downward-sloping range of a firm's long-run average cost curve, the firm experiences economies of scale, meaning that its long-run production costs decline as it increases its plant size and thereby raises its output scale. By contrast, along the upward-sloping portion of the long-run average cost curve, the firm encounters diseconomies of scale, so that its long-run costs of production rises as it increases its output scale. The minimum point of the long-run average cost curve occurs at the firm's minimum efficient scale, which is the lowest rate of output at which the firm can achieve minimum long-run average cost.

Key Terms and Concepts

Accounting profit (532)
Average fixed costs (543)
Average physical product (537)
Average total costs (543)
Average variable costs (543)
Constant returns to scale (550)
Diseconomies of scale (550)
Economic profits (534)
Economies of scale (550)
Explicit costs (532)
Firm (532)
Fixed costs (541)
Implicit costs (532)
Law of diminishing (marginal) returns (537)
Long run (536)
Long-run average cost curve (550)
Marginal costs (543)
Marginal physical product (537)
Minimum efficient scale (MES) (553)
Normal rate of return (533)
Opportunity cost of capital (533)
Planning curve (550)
Planning horizon (548)
Plant size (535)
Production (536)
Production function (537)
Short run (535)
Total costs (541)
Variable costs (541)

Problems

Answers to the odd-numbered problems appear at the back of the book.

22-1. After graduation, you face a choice. One option is to work for a multinational consulting firm and earn a starting salary (benefits included) of $40,000. The other option is to use $5,000 in savings to start your own consulting firm. You could have earned an interest return of 5 percent on your savings. You choose to start your own consulting firm. At the end of the first year, you add up all of your expenses and revenues. Your total includes $12,000 in rent, $1,000 in office supplies, $20,000 for office staff, and $4,000 in telephone expenses. What are your total explicit costs and total implicit costs?

22-2. Suppose, as in Problem 22-1, that you choose to start your own consulting firm upon graduation. At the end of the first year, your total revenues are $77,250. Based on the information in Problem 22-1, what is your accounting profit and what is your economic profit?

22-3. The academic calendar for a university is August 15 through May 15. A professor commits to a contract that binds her to a teaching position at this university for this period. Based on this information, explain the short run and long run that the professor faces.

22-4. The short-run production function for a manufacturer of DVD drives is as follows:

Input of Labor (workers per week)	Total Output of DVD Drives
0	0
1	25
2	60
3	85
4	105
5	115
6	120

Based on this information, calculate the average physical product at each quantity of labor.

22-5. Using the information provided in Problem 22-4, calculate the marginal physical product labor at each quantity of labor.

22-6. For the manufacturer of DVD drives in Problems 22-4 and 22-5, at what point do diminishing marginal returns set in?

22-7. At the end of the year, a firm produced 10,000 laptop computers. Its total costs were $5 million, and its fixed costs were $2 million. What are the average variable costs of this firm?

22-8. The cost structure of a manufacturer of cable modems is described in the following table. The firm's fixed costs equal $30 per day.

Output (cable modems per day)	Total Cost of Output ($ thousands)
0	10
25	60
50	95
75	150
100	220
125	325
150	465

Calculate the average variable cost, average fixed cost, and average total cost at each output level.

22-9. Calculate the marginal cost that the manufacturer of cable modems in Problem 22-8 faces at each daily output rate, including the first cable modem it produces. At what production rate do diminishing marginal returns set in?

22-10. A watch manufacturer finds that at 1,000 units of output, its marginal costs are below average total costs. If it produces an additional watch, will its average total costs rise, fall, or stay the same?

22-11. A manufacturing firm with a single plant is contemplating changing its plant size. It must choose from among seven alternative plant sizes. In the table below, plant size A is the smallest it might build, and size G is the largest. Currently, the firm's plant size is B.

Plant Size	Average Total Cost ($)
A (smallest)	5,000
B	4,000
C	3,500
D	3,100
E	3,000
F	3,250
G (largest)	4,100

a. Is this firm currently experiencing economies of scale or diseconomies of scale?

b. What is the firm's minimum efficient scale?

Economics on the Net

Industry-Level Corporate Profits In this chapter, you learned how to measure profits. This Internet application provides you with an opportunity to take a look at the rates of profitability of various industries in the United States.

Title: Corporate Profits by Industry

Navigation: Click here to view the Bureau of Economic Analysis page about Corporate Profits. Select Table 11, Corporate Profits by Industry.

Application Consider the categories under Durable Goods.

1. Is the BEA reporting economic profits or accounting profits?
2. Which industry generates the greatest amount of profit in the United States? Which industry generates the least amount of profit in the United States?
3. Which industry experienced the greatest growth in profits over the past year? Which industry experienced the greatest decline in profit over the past year?

For Group Discussion and Analysis Which industries generated the greatest increase in their rate of return on investment over the past year? Discuss why you believe these industries do so well. Which industries generated the greatest decline in their rate of return on investment over the past year? Discuss why you believe these industries do so poorly. (Hint: Think of some companies that serve as examples for these industries.)

CHAPTER

23

PERFECT COMPETITION

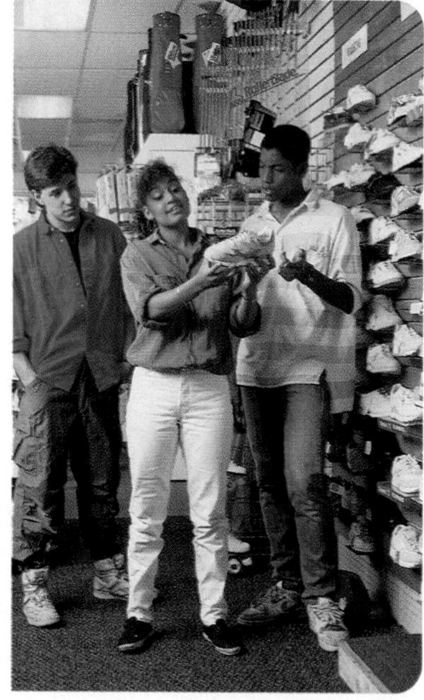

Today, there are more brands and styles of sports footwear than ever before. Does this mean that the American marketplace is more competitive today than in the past? If so, should the profits of large corporations be falling or rising?

Few Americans today would say that competition does not exist in the United States. After all, since the early 1990s, a multitude of new firms, ranging from corner bakeries to Internet booksellers to software developers, have jumped into the marketplace. But has all this activity really produced a more competitive American economy? In the world of perfect competition, which you will read about in this chapter, consumers can choose among virtually identical baked goods, books, and software produced by a host of suppliers. Within each industry, therefore, there is widespread substitutability among goods or services produced by rival firms. Is the American marketplace truly more competitive today than in years past? To answer this question, you need to learn about the model of perfect competition and its assumptions.

LEARNING OBJECTIVES

After reading this chapter, you should be able to:

1. Identify the characteristics of a perfectly competitive market structure
2. Discuss the process by which a perfectly competitive firm decides how much output to produce
3. Understand how the short-run supply curve for a perfectly competitive firm is determined
4. Explain how the equilibirum price is determined in perfectly competitive market
5. Describe what factors induce firms to enter or exit a perfectly competitive industry
6. Distinguish among constant-, increasing-, and decreasing-cost industries based on the shape of the long-run industry supply curve

Did You Know That... in the United States, there are tens of thousands of copy shops? There are also several thousand desktop publishing companies offering their services. The number of companies wanting to sell only Web site development is much smaller but growing. The number of companies offering to write software applications is somewhere in between, but that is only in the United States. Today, because of the cheapness and rapidity of modern telecommunications, much of the software code that goes in today's computer applications programs produced by American companies is written in India and elsewhere.

Competition is the word that applies to all of these situations. As used in common speech, *competition* simply means "rivalry." In perfectly competitive situations, individual buyers and sellers cannot affect the market price—it is determined by the market forces of demand and supply. In this chapter, we examine what has become known as perfect competition.

Chapter Outline 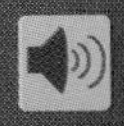

CHARACTERISTICS OF A PERFECTLY COMPETITIVE MARKET STRUCTURE

We are interested in studying how a firm acting within a perfectly competitive market structure makes decisions about how much to produce. In a situation of **perfect competition,** each firm is such a small part that it cannot affect the price of the product in question. That means that each **perfectly competitive firm** in the industry is a **price taker**—the firm takes price as a given, something determined *outside* the individual firm.

This definition of a competitive firm is obviously idealized, for in one sense the individual firm *has* to set prices. How can we ever have a situation in which firms regard prices as set by forces outside their control? The answer is that even though every firm sets its own prices, a firm in a perfectly competitive situation will find that it will eventually have no customers at all if it sets its price above the competitive price. The best example is in agriculture. Although the individual farmer can set any price for a bushel of wheat, if that price doesn't coincide with the market price of a bushel of similar-quality wheat, no one will purchase the wheat at a higher price; nor would the farmer be inclined to reduce revenues by selling below the market price.

Let's examine the reasons why a firm in a perfectly competitive industry ends up being a price taker.

1. *There must be a large number of buyers and sellers.* When this is the case, the quantity demanded by an individual buyer or the quantity supplied by the seller is negligible relative to the market quantity. No one buyer or one seller has any influence on price.
2. *The product sold by the firms in the industry must be homogeneous.* The product sold by each firm in the industry must be a perfect substitute for the product sold by each other firm. Buyers must be able to choose from a large number of sellers of a product that the buyers believe to be the same.
3. *Any firm can enter or leave the industry without serious impediments.* Firms in a competitive industry cannot be hampered in their ability to get resources or relocate resources. They move labor and capital in pursuit of profit-making opportunities to whatever business venture gives them their highest expected rate of return on their investment.
4. *Both buyers and sellers have equal access to information.* Consumers have to be able to find out about lower prices charged by competing firms. Firms have to be able to

Perfect competition 
A market structure in which the decisions of individual buyers and sellers have no effect on market price.

Perfectly competitive firm 
A firm that is such a small part of the total industry that it cannot affect the price of the product it sells.

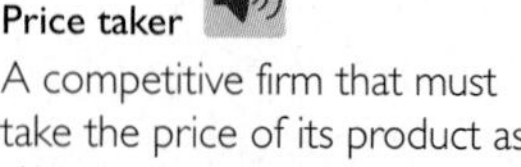

Price taker
A competitive firm that must take the price of its product as given because the firm cannot influence its price.

find out about cost-saving innovations in order to lower production costs and prices, and they have to be able to learn about profitable opportunities in other industries.

INTERNATIONAL EXAMPLE

A Common Pricing Denominator in Europe

Perfect competition is more likely to thrive in an environment in which buyers and sellers have more nearly complete and equal access to information. Historically, a factor hindering the development of European-wide competitive markets has been that a consumer in a country such as Portugal who was contemplating whether to buy substitute goods manufactured by a German, Italian, or Belgian firm had to compare prices quoted in German marks, Italian lire, and Belgian francs.

Making accurate price comparisons of this sort required that every consumer stay abreast of the latest currency conversion rates, making it harder for consumers to shop around for the best buys. This contributed to great variability in the prices of the same goods from nation to nation within Europe. Figure 23-1 shows average price variations for several products for nine European nations: Austria, Belgium, France, Germany, Ireland, Italy, the Netherlands, Portugal, and Spain. Across these countries, the average price of a Big Mac varied by more than 10 percent. The typical fee for a bank account varied by well over 50 percent from one country to the next.

Beginning in 2002, European price differentials should start to narrow, thanks to a coordinated policy decision on the part of the governments of these nine European nations, plus Finland and Luxembourg. At the beginning of that year, the euro, a unit of account created in 1999, will replace national currencies. When

FIGURE 23-1
Variability in the Domestic Prices of Selected Products in Nine European Nations
In advance of the adoption of the euro as a single currency, the prices of products sold in European nations varied from just under 5 percent for the Volkswagen Golf to more than 50 percent for financial products such as insurance and bank accounts.

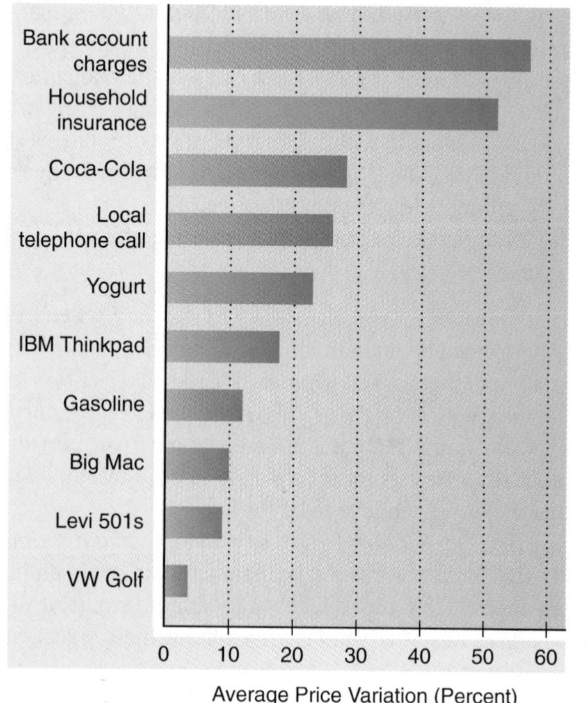

all prices are quoted in euros, the nearly 300 million consumers residing in these 11 countries will have an easier time spotting the best buys. This change should go long way toward promoting more competitive markets in Europe.

For Critical Analysis

Are regional price differences likely to disappear completely following full adoption of the euro as a hand-to-hand currency? (Hint: Are there regional dollar price differences for the same goods in the United States?)

THE DEMAND CURVE OF THE PERFECT COMPETITOR

When we discussed substitutes in Chapter 20, we pointed out that the more substitutes there were and the more similar they were to the commodity in question, the greater was the price elasticity of demand. Here we assume for the perfectly competitive firm that it is producing a homogeneous commodity that has perfect substitutes. That means that if the individual firm raises its price one penny, it will lose all of its business. This, then, is how we characterize the demand schedule for a perfectly competitive firm: It is the going market price as determined by the forces of market supply and market demand—that is, where the market demand curve intersects the market supply curve. The demand curve for the product of an individual firm in a perfectly competitive industry is perfectly elastic at the going market price. Remember that with a perfectly elastic demand curve, any increase in price leads to zero quantity demanded.

We show the market demand and supply curves in panel (a) of Figure 23-2. Their intersection occurs at the price of $5. The commodity in question is computer minidisks. Assume for the purposes of this exposition that all minidisks are perfect substitutes for all others. At the going market price of $5 apiece, a hypothetical individual demand curve for a minidisk producer who sells a very, very small part of total industry production is shown in panel (b). At the market price, this firm can sell all the output it wants. At the market price of $5 each, which is where the demand curve for the individual producer lies, consumer demand for the minidisks of that one producer is perfectly elastic. This can be seen by noting that if the firm raises its price, consumers, who are assumed to know that this supplier is charging more than other producers, will buy elsewhere, and the producer in

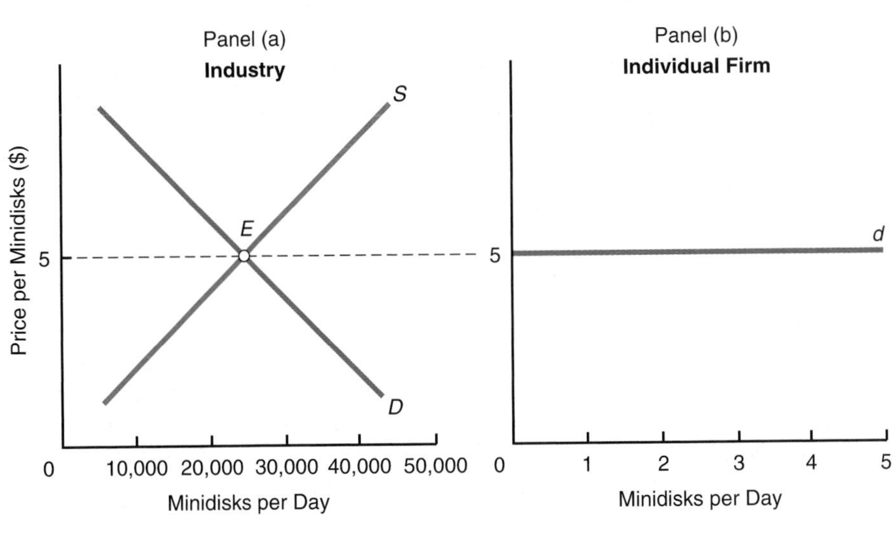

FIGURE 23-2

The Demand Curve for a Minidisk Producer

At $5—where market demand, *D*, and market supply, *S*, intersect—the individual firm faces a perfectly elastic demand curve, *d*. If it raises its price even one penny, it will sell no minidisks at all. Notice the difference in the quantities of minidisks represented on the horizontal axis of panels (a) and (b).

question will have no sales at all. Thus the demand curve for that producer is perfectly elastic. We label the individual producer's demand curve *d,* whereas the *market* demand curve is always labeled *D.*

HOW MUCH SHOULD THE PERFECT COMPETITOR PRODUCE?

As we have shown, a perfect competitor has to accept the price of the product as a given. If the firm raises its price, it sells nothing; if it lowers its price, it earns lower revenues per unit sold than it otherwise could. The firm has one decision left: How much should it produce? We will apply our model of the firm to this question to come up with an answer. We'll use the *profit-maximization model,* which assumes that firms attempt to maximize their total profits—the positive difference between total revenues and total costs. This also means that firms seek to minimize any losses that arise in times when total revenues may be less than total costs.

Total Revenues

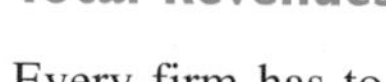

Total revenues The price per unit times the total quantity sold.

Every firm has to consider its *total revenues,* or TR. **Total revenues** are defined as the quantity sold multiplied by the price. (They are the same as total receipts from the sale of output.) The perfect competitor must take the price as a given.

Look at Figure 23-3. Much of the information in panel (a) comes from panel (a) of Figure 22-3, but we have added some essential columns for our analysis. Column 3 is the market price, *P,* of $5 per minidisk. Column 4 shows the total revenues, or TR, as equal to the market price, *P,* times the total output per day, or *Q*. Thus TR = *PQ*.

For the perfect competitor, price is also equal to average revenue (AR) because

$$\text{AR} = \frac{\text{TR}}{Q} = \frac{PQ}{Q} = P$$

where *Q* stands for quantity. If we assume that all units sell for the same price, it becomes apparent that another name for the demand curve is the *average revenue curve* (this is true regardless of the type of market structure under consideration).

We are assuming that the market supply and demand schedules intersect at a price of $5 and that this price holds for all the firm's production. We are also assuming that because our minidisk maker is a small part of the market, it can sell all that it produces at that price. Thus panel (b) of Figure 23-3 shows the total revenue curve as a straight green line. For every unit of sales, total revenue is increased by $5.

Comparing Total Costs with Total Revenues

Total costs are given in column 2 of panel (a) of Figure 23-3 and plotted in panel (b). Remember, the firm's costs always include a normal rate of return on investment. So whenever we refer to total costs, we are talking not about accounting costs but about economic costs. When the total cost curve is above the total revenue curve, the firm is experiencing losses. When it is below the total revenue curve, the firm is making profits.

By comparing total costs with total revenues, we can figure out the number of minidisks the individual competitive firm should produce per day. Our analysis rests on the assumption that the firm will attempt to maximize total profits. In panel (a) of Figure 23-3, we see that total profits reach a maximum at a production rate of either seven or eight mindisks per

Panel (a)

(1) Total Output and Sales per Day (*Q*)	(2) Total Costs (TC)	(3) Market Price (*P*)	(4) Total Revenue (TR) (4) = (3) x (1)	(5) Total Profit (TR – TC) (5) = (4) – (2)	(6) Average Total Cost (ATC) (6) = (2) ÷ (1)	(7) Average Variable Cost (AVC)	(8) Marginal Cost (MC) (8) = Change in (2) / Change in (1)	(9) Marginal Revenue (MR) (9) = Change in (4) / Change in (1)
0	$10	$5	$ 0	–$10	—	—	$5	$5
1	15	5	5	– 10	$15.00	$5.00	3	5
2	18	5	10	– 8	9.00	4.00	2	5
3	20	5	15	– 5	6.67	3.33	1	5
4	21	5	20	– 1	5.25	2.75	2	5
5	23	5	25	2	4.60	2.60	3	5
6	26	5	30	4	4.33	2.67	4	5
7	30	5	35	**5**	4.28	2.86	5	5
8	35	5	40	**5**	4.38	3.12	6	5
9	41	5	45	4	4.56	3.44	7	5
10	48	5	50	2	4.80	3.80	8	5
11	56	5	55	– 1	5.09	4.18		

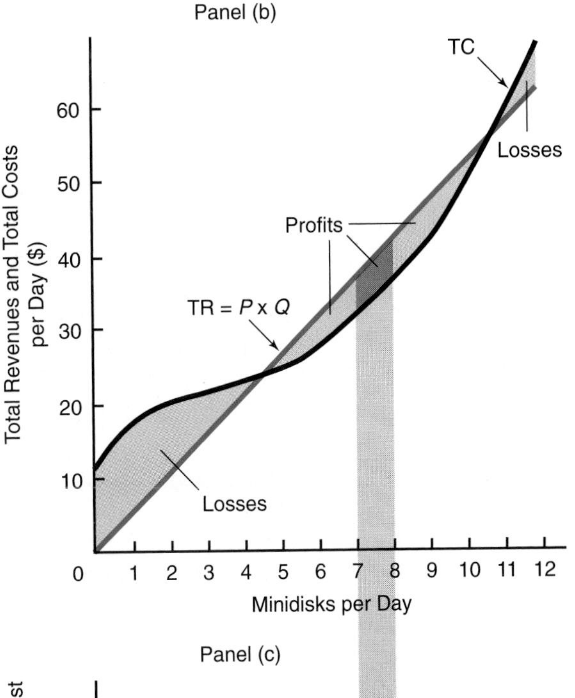

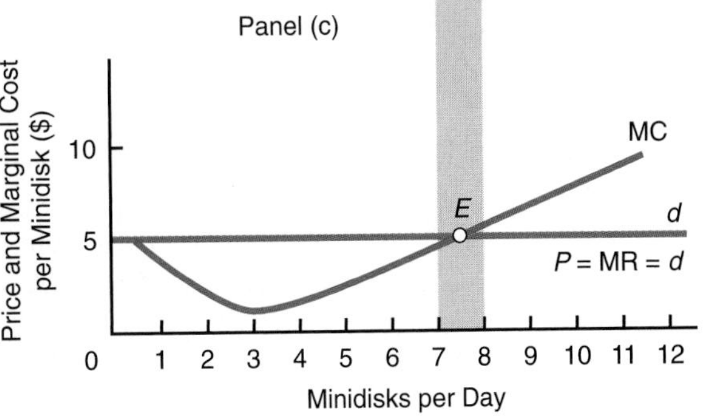

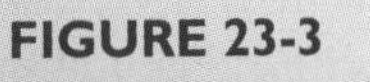

FIGURE 23-3

Profit Maximization

Profit maximization occurs where marginal revenue equals marginal cost. Panel (a) indicates that this point occurs at a rate of sales of between seven and eight minidisks per day. In panel (b), we find maximum profits where total revenues exceed total costs by the largest amount. This occurs at a rate of production and sales per day of seven or eight minidisks. In panel (c), the marginal cost curve, MC, intersects the marginal revenue curve at a rate of output and sales of somewhere between seven and eight minidisks per day.

day. We can see this graphically in panel (b) of the figure. The firm will maximize profits where the total revenue curve exceeds the total curve by the greatest amount. That occurs at a rate of output and sales of either seven or eight minidisks per day; this rate is called the **profit-maximizing rate of production.** (If output were continuously divisible or we were dealing with extremely large numbers of minidisks, we would get a unique profit-maximizing output.)

Profit-maximizing rate of production

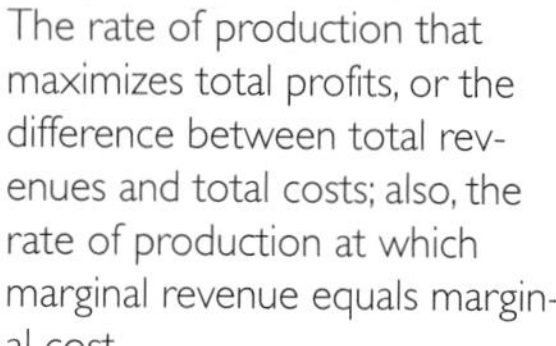

The rate of production that maximizes total profits, or the difference between total revenues and total costs; also, the rate of production at which marginal revenue equals marginal cost.

We can also find this profit-maximizing rate of production for the individual competitive firm by looking at marginal revenues and marginal costs.

USING MARGINAL ANALYSIS TO DETERMINE THE PROFIT-MAXIMIZING RATE OF PRODUCTION

It is possible—indeed, preferred—to use marginal analysis to determine the profit-maximizing rate of production. We end up with the same results derived in a different manner, one that focuses more on where decisions are really made—on the margin. Managers examine changes in costs and relate them to changes in revenues. In fact, we almost always compare changes in cost with changes in benefits, where change is occurring at the margin, whether it be with respect to how much more or less to produce, how many more workers to hire or fire, or how much more to study or not study.

Marginal revenue 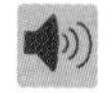

The change in total revenues resulting from a change in output (and sale) of one unit of the product in question.

Marginal revenue represents the change in total revenues attributable to changing production by one unit of the product in question. Hence a more formal definition of marginal revenue is

$$\text{Marginal revenue} = \frac{\text{change in total revenues}}{\text{change in output}}$$

In a perfectly competitive market, the marginal revenue curve is exactly equivalent to the price line or the individual firm's demand curve. Each time the firm produces and sells one more unit, total revenues rise by an amount equal to the (constant) market price of the good. Thus in Figure 23-2 on page 563, the demand curve, *d,* for the individual producer is at a price of $5—the price line is coincident with the demand curve. But so is the marginal revenue curve, for marginal revenue in this case also equals $5.

The marginal revenue curve for our competitive minidisk producer is shown as a line at $5 in panel (c) of Figure 23-3. Notice again that the marginal revenue curve is equal to the price line, which is equal to the individual firm's demand, or average revenue, curve, *d.*

When Are Profits Maximized?

Now we add the marginal cost curve, MC, taken from column 8 in panel (a) of Figure 23-3. As shown in panel (c) of that figure, the marginal cost curve first falls and then starts to rise because of the law of diminishing returns, eventually intersecting the marginal revenue curve and then rising above it. Notice that the numbers for both the marginal cost schedule, column 8 in panel (a), and the marginal revenue schedule, column 9 in panel (a), are printed *between* the rows on which the quantities appear. This indicates that we are looking at a *change* between one rate of output and the next.

In panel (c), the marginal cost curve intersects the marginal revenue curve somewhere between seven and eight minidisks per day. The firm has an incentive to produce and sell until the amount of the additional revenue received from selling one more mindisk just equals the additional costs incurred for producing and selling that minidisk. This is how the firm maximizes profit. Whenever marginal cost is less than marginal revenue, the firm will always make more profit by increasing production.

Now consider the possibility of producing at an output rate of 10 minidisks per day. The marginal cost curve at that output rate is higher than the marginal revenue (or *d*) curve. The firm would be spending more to produce that additional output than it would be receiving in revenues; it would be foolish to continue producing at this rate.

But how much should it produce? It should produce at point *E*, where the marginal cost curve intersects the marginal revenue curve from below.* The firm should continue production until the cost of increasing output by one more unit is just equal to the revenues obtainable from that extra unit. This is a fundamental rule in economics:

Profit maximization normally occurs at the rate of output at which marginal revenue equals marginal cost.

For a perfectly competitive firm, this is at the intersection of the demand schedule, *d*, and the marginal cost curve, MC. When MR exceeds MC, each additional unit of output adds more to total revenues than to total costs, causing losses to decrease or profits to increase. When MC is greater than MR, each unit produced adds more to total cost than to total revenues, causing profits to decrease or losses to increase. Therefore, profit maximization occurs when MC equals MR. In our particular example, our profit-maximizing, perfectly competitive minidisk producer will produce at a rate of either seven or eight minidisks a day. (If we were dealing with a very large rate of output, we would come up with an exact profit-maximizing rate.)

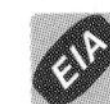

Output and Price Determination Under Perfect Competition
Get more practice thinking through how perfectly competitive firms determine how much to produce.

CONCEPTS IN BRIEF

- Four fundamental characteristics of the market in perfect competition are (1) a large number of buyers and sellers, (2) a homogeneous product, (3) unrestrained exit from and entry into the industry by other firms, and (4) good information in the hands of both buyers and sellers.
- A perfectly competitive firm is a price taker. It has no control over price and consequently has to take price as a given, but it can sell all that it wants at the going market price.
- The demand curve for a perfect competitor is a line at the going market price. The demand curve is also the perfect competitor's marginal revenue curve because marginal revenue is defined as the change in total revenue due to a one-unit change in output.
- Profit is maximized at the rate of output where the positive difference between total revenues and total costs is the greatest. This is the same level of output at which marginal revenue equals marginal cost. The perfectly competitive firm produces at an output rate at which marginal cost equals the price per unit of output, because $MR \equiv P$.

SHORT-RUN PROFITS

To find what our competitive individual minidisk producer is making in terms of profits in the short run, we have to add the average total cost curve to panel (c) of Figure 23-3. We take the information from column 6 in panel (a) and add it to panel (c) to get Figure 23-4 on page 568. Again the profit-maximizing rate of output is between seven and eight mini-

*The marginal cost curve, MC, also cuts the marginal revenue curve, *d*, from above at an output rate of less than 1 in this example. This intersection should be ignored because it is irrelevant to the firm's decisions.

FIGURE 23-4

Measuring Total Profits

Profits are represented by the shaded area. The height of the profit rectangle is given by the difference between average total costs and price ($5), where price is also equal to average revenue. This is found by the vertical difference between the ATC curve and the price, or average revenue, line *d,* at the profit-maximizing rate of output of between seven and eight minidisks per day.

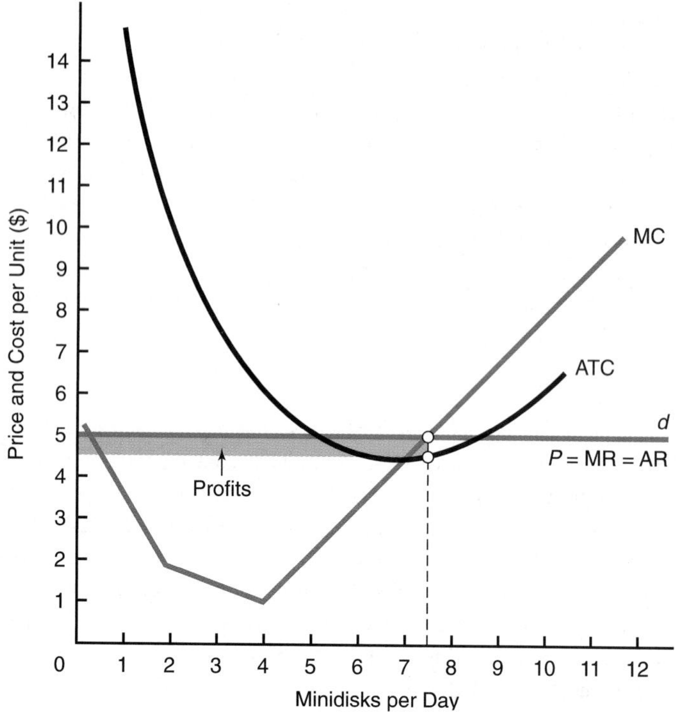

disks per day. If we have production and sales of seven minidisks per day, total revenues will be $35 a day. Total costs will be $30 a day, leaving a profit of $5 a day. If the rate of output in sales is eight minidisks per day, total revenues will be $40 and total costs will be $35, again leaving a profit of $5 a day. In Figure 23-4, the lower boundary of the rectangle labeled "Profits" is determined by the intersection of the profit-maximizing quantity line represented by vertical dashes and the average total cost curve. Why? Because the ATC curve gives us the cost per unit, whereas the price ($5), represented by *d,* gives us the revenue per unit, or average revenue. The difference is profit per unit. So the height of the rectangular box representing profits equals profit per unit, and the length equals the amount of units produced. When we multiply these two quantities, we get total profits. Note, as pointed out earlier, that we are talking about *economic profits* because a normal rate of return on investment is included in the average total cost curve, ATC.

It is certainly possible, also, for the competitive firm to make short-run losses. We give an example in Figure 23-5, where we show the firm's demand curve shifting from d_1 to d_2. The going market price has fallen from $5 to $3 per minidisk because of changes in market supply or demand conditions (or both). The firm will do the best it can by producing where marginal revenue equals marginal cost. We see in Figure 23-5 that the marginal revenue (d_2) curve is intersected (from below) by the marginal cost curve at an output rate of about $5\frac{1}{2}$ minidisks per day. The firm is clearly not making profits because average total costs at that output rate are greater than the price of $3 per minidisk. The losses are shown in the shaded area. By producing where marginal revenue equals marginal cost, however, the firm is minimizing its losses; that is, losses would be greater at any other output.

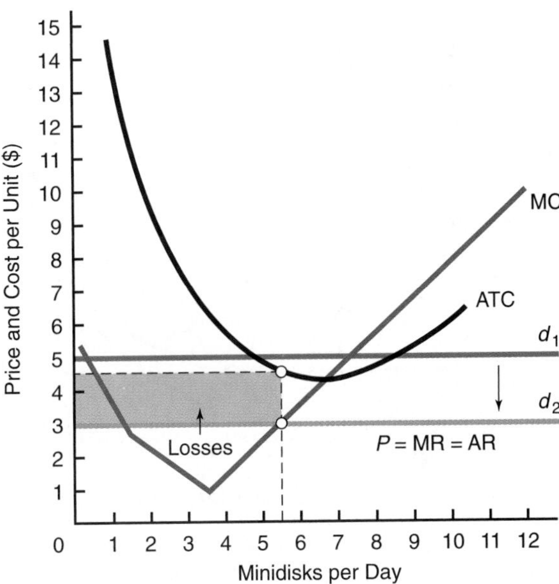

FIGURE 23-5
Minimization of Short-Run Losses
In cases in which average total costs exceed the average revenue, or price (and price is greater than or equal to average variable cost), profit maximization is equivalent to loss minimization. This again occurs where marginal cost equals marginal revenue. Losses are shown in the shaded area.

THE SHORT-RUN SHUTDOWN PRICE 

In Figure 23-5, the firm is sustaining economic losses. Will it go out of business? In the long run it will, but in the short run the firm will not necessarily go out of business. As long as the loss from staying in business is less than the loss from shutting down, the firm will continue to produce. A firm *goes out of business* when the owners sell its assets to someone else. A firm temporarily *shuts down* when it stops producing, but it still is in business.

Now how can we tell when the firm is sustaining economic losses in the short run and it is still worthwhile not to shut down? The firm must compare the cost of producing (while incurring losses) with the cost of closing down. The cost of staying in production in the short run is given by the total *variable* cost. Looking at the problem on a per-unit basis, as long as average variable cost (AVC) is covered by average revenues (price), the firm is better off continuing to produce. If average variable costs are exceeded even a little bit by the price of the product, staying in production produces some revenues in excess of variable costs that can be applied toward covering fixed costs.

A simple example will demonstrate this situation. The price of a product is \$8, and average total costs equal \$9 at an output of 100. In this example, average total costs are broken up into average variable costs of \$7 and average fixed costs of \$2. Total revenues, then, equal \$8 × 100, or \$800, and total costs equal \$9 × 100, or \$900. Total losses therefore equal \$100. However, this does not mean that the firm will shut down. After all, if it does shut down, it still has fixed costs to pay. And in this case, because average fixed costs equal \$2 at an output of 100, the fixed costs are \$200. Thus the firm has losses of \$100 if it continues to produce, but it has losses of \$200 (the fixed costs) if it shuts down. The logic is fairly straightforward:

> As long as the price per unit sold exceeds the average *variable* cost per unit produced, the firm will be covering at least part of the opportunity cost of the investment in the business—that is, part of its fixed costs.

FIGURE 23-6

Short-Run Shutdown and Break-Even Prices

We can find the short-run break-even price and the short-run shutdown price by comparing price with average total costs and average variable costs. If the demand curve is d_1, profit maximization occurs at output E_1, where MC equals marginal revenue (the d curve). Because the ATC curve includes all relevant opportunity costs, point E_1 is the break-even point, and zero economic profits are being made. The firm is earning a normal rate of return. If the demand curve falls to d_2, profit maximization (loss minimization) occurs at the intersection of MC and MR (the d_2 curve), or E_2. Below this price, it does not pay for the firm to continue in operation because its average variable costs are not covered by the price of the product.

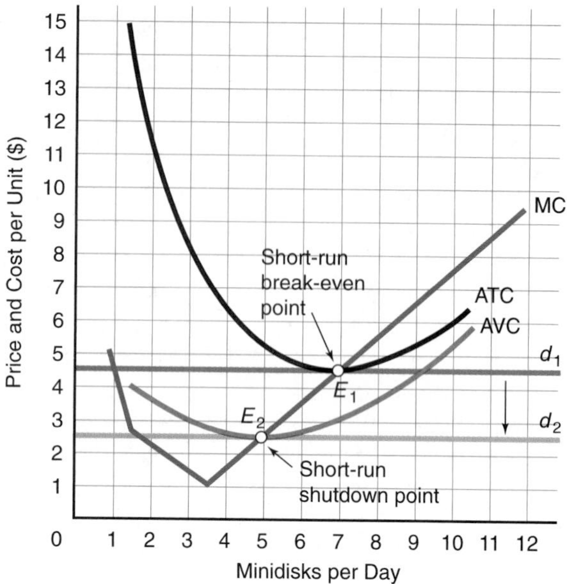

Calculating the Short-Run Break-Even Price

Look at demand curve d_1 in Figure 23-6. It just touches the minimum point of the average total cost curve, which, as you will remember, is exactly where the marginal cost curve intersects the average total cost curve. At that price, which is about $4.30, the firm will be making exactly zero short-run economic profits. That price is called the **short-run break-even price,** and point E_1 therefore occurs at the short-run break-even price for a competitive firm. It is the point at which marginal revenue, marginal cost, and average total cost are all equal (that is, at which P = MC and P = ATC). The break-even price is the one that yields zero short-run economic profits or losses.

Short-run break-even price 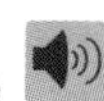
The price at which a firm's total revenues equal its total costs. At the break-even price, the firm is just making a normal rate of return on its capital investment. (It is covering its explicit and implicit costs.)

Calculating the Short-Run Shutdown Price

To calculate the firm's shutdown price, we must introduce the average variable cost (AVC) to our graph. In Figure 23-6, we have plotted the AVC values from column 7 in panel (a) of Figure 23-3. For the moment, consider two possible demand curves, d_1 and d_2, which are also the firm's respective marginal revenue curves. Therefore, if demand is d_1, the firm will produce at E_1, where that curve intersects the marginal cost curve. If demand falls to d_2, the firm will produce at E_2. The special feature of the hypothetical demand curve, d_2, is that it just touches the average variable cost curve at the latter's minimum point, which is also where the marginal cost curve intersects it. This price is the **short-run shutdown price.** Why? Below this price, the firm would be paying out more in variable costs than it is receiving in revenues from the sale of its product. Each unit it sold would add to its losses. Clearly, the way to avoid incurring these additional losses, if price falls below the shutdown point, is in fact to shut down operations.

Short-run shutdown price 
The price that just covers average variable costs. It occurs just below the intersection of the marginal cost curve and the average variable cost curve.

The intersection of the price line, the marginal cost curve, and the average variable cost curve is labeled E_2. The resulting short-run shutdown price is valid only for the short run because, of course, in the long run the firm will not stay in business at a yield less than a normal rate of return and hence at least zero economic profits.

THE MEANING OF ZERO ECONOMIC PROFITS 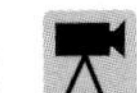

The fact that we labeled point E_1 in Figure 23-6 the break-even point may have disturbed you. At point E_1, price is just equal to average total cost. If this is the case, why would a firm continue to produce if it were making no profits whatsoever? If we again make the distinction between accounting profits and economic profits, then at that price the firm has zero economic profits but positive accounting profits. Recall that accounting profits are total revenues minus total explicit costs. What is ignored in such accounting is the reward offered to investors—the opportunity cost of capital—plus all other implicit costs.

Click here for an analysis of whether the drug market fits the model of perfect competition.

In economic analysis, the average total cost curve includes the full opportunity cost of capital. Indeed, the average total cost curve includes the opportunity cost of *all* factors of production used in the production process. At the short-run break-even price, economic profits are, by definition, zero. Accounting profits at that price are not, however, equal to zero; they are positive. Consider an example. A baseball bat manufacturer sells bats at some price. The owners of the firm have supplied all the funds in the business. They have borrowed no money from anyone else, and they explicitly pay the full opportunity cost to all factors of production, including any managerial labor that they themselves contribute to the business. Their salaries show up as a cost in the books and are equal to what they could have earned in the next-best alternative occupation. At the end of the year, the owners find that after they subtract all explicit costs from total revenues, they have earned $100,000. Let's say that their investment was $1 million. Thus the rate of return on that investment is 10 percent per year. We will assume that this turns out to be equal to the rate of return that, on average, all other baseball bat manufacturers make in the industry.

This $100,000, or 10 percent rate of return, is actually, then, a competitive, or normal, rate of return on invested capital in that industry or in other industries with similar risks. If the owners had made only $50,000, or 5 percent on their investment, they would have been able to make higher profits by leaving the industry. The 10 percent rate of return is the opportunity cost of capital. Accountants show it as a profit; economists call it a cost. We include that cost in the average total cost curve, similar to the one shown in Figure 23-6. At the short-run break-even price, average total cost, including this opportunity cost of capital, will just equal that price. The firm will be making zero economic profits but a 10 percent *accounting* rate of return.

Now we are ready to derive the firm's supply curve.

The Perfect Competitor's Short-Run Supply Curve

What does the supply curve for the individual firm look like? Actually, we have been looking at it all along. We know that when the price of minidisks is $5, the firm will supply seven or eight of them per day. If the price falls to $3, the firm will supply five or six minidisks per day. And if the price falls below $3, the firm will shut down in the short run. Hence in Figure 23-7, the firm's supply curve is the marginal cost curve above the short-run shutdown point. This is shown as the solid part of the marginal cost curve. ***The definition, then, of the individual firm's short-run supply curve in a competitive industry is its marginal cost curve equal to and above the point of intersection with the average variable cost curve.***

The Short-Run Industry Supply Curve

In Chapter 3, we indicated that the market supply curve was the summation of individual supply curves. At the beginning of this chapter, we drew a market supply curve in Figure 23-2. Now we want to derive more precisely a market, or industry, supply curve to reflect individual

FIGURE 23-7

The Individual Firm's Short-Run Supply Curve

The individual firm's short-run supply curve is the portion of its marginal cost curve above the minimum point on the average variable cost curve.

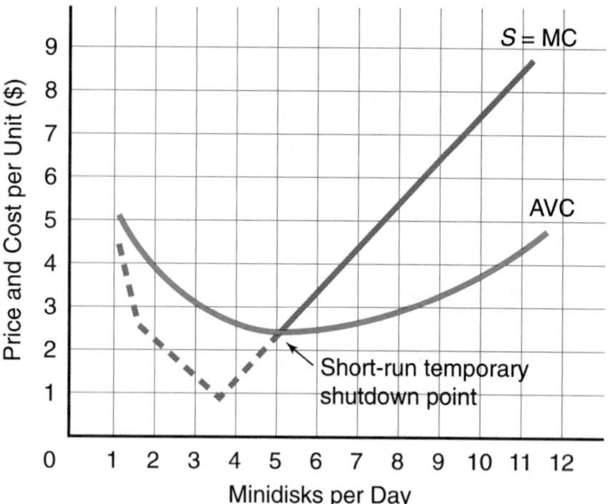

producer behavior in that industry. First we must ask, What is an industry? It is merely a collection of firms producing a particular product. Therefore, we have a way to figure out the total supply curve of any industry: We add the quantities that each firm will supply at every possible price. In other words, we sum the individual supply curves of all the competitive firms *horizontally.* The individual supply curves, as we just saw, are simply the marginal cost curves of each firm.

Consider doing this for a hypothetical world in which there are only two minidisk producers in the industry, firm A and firm B. These two firms' marginal cost curves are given in panels (a) and (b) of Figure 23-8. The marginal cost curves for the two separate firms are presented as MC_A in panel (a) and MC_B in panel (b). Those two marginal cost curves are

FIGURE 23-8

Deriving the Industry Supply Curve

Marginal cost curves above average minimum variable cost are presented in panels (a) and (b) for firms A and B. We horizontally sum the two quantities supplied, q_{A1} and q_{B1}, at price P_1. This gives us point *F* in panel (c). We do the same thing for the quantities at price P_2. This gives us point *G*. When we connect those points, we have the industry supply curve, *S,* which is the horizontal summation [represented by the Greek letter sigma (Σ)] of the firms' marginal cost curves above their respective average minimum costs.

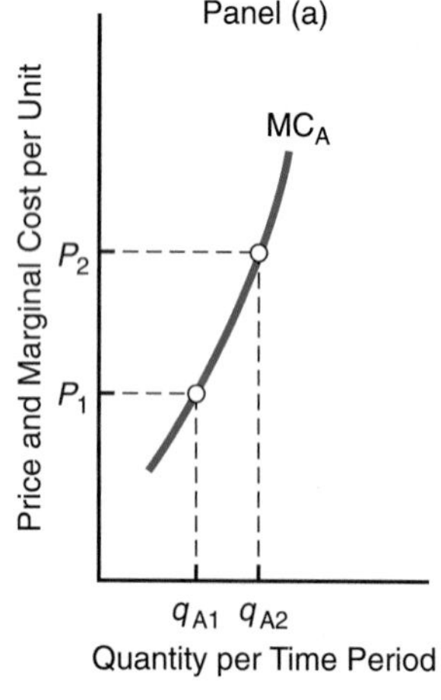

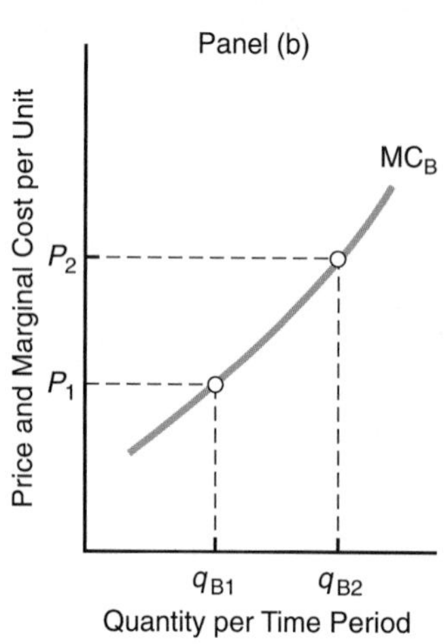

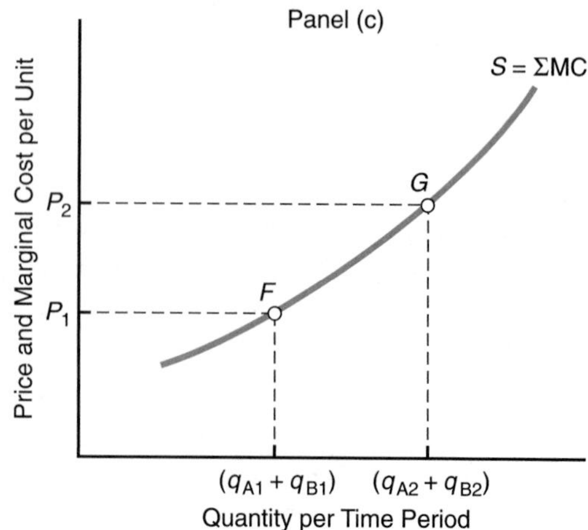

drawn only for prices above the minimum average variable cost for each respective firm. Hence we are not including any of the marginal cost curves below minimum average variable cost. In panel (a), for firm A, at price P_1, the quantity supplied would be q_{A1}. At price P_2, the quantity supplied would be q_{A2}. In panel (b), we see the two different quantities that would be supplied by firm B corresponding to those two prices. Now for price P_1 we add horizontally the quantity of q_{A1} and q_{B1}. This gives us one point, *F*, for our short-run **industry supply curve,** *S*. We obtain the other point, *G*, by doing the same horizontal adding of quantities at P_2. When we connect points *F* and *G*, we obtain industry supply curve *S*, which is also marked ΣMC, indicating that it is the horizontal summation of the marginal cost curves (above the respective minimum average variable cost of each firm).* Because the law of diminishing returns makes marginal cost curves rise, the short-run supply curve of a perfectly competitive industry must be upward-sloping.

Industry supply curve 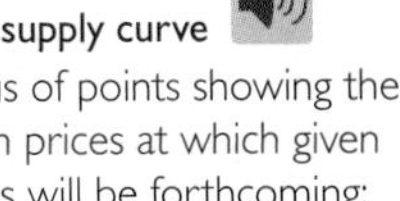
The locus of points showing the minimum prices at which given quantities will be forthcoming; also called the *market supply curve*.

Factors That Influence the Industry Supply Curve

As you have just seen, the industry supply curve is the horizontal summation of all of the individual firms' marginal cost curves above their respective minimum average variable cost points. This means that anything that affects the marginal cost curves of the firm will influence the industry supply curve. Therefore, the individual factors that will influence the supply schedule in a competitive industry can be summarized as the factors that cause the variable costs of production to change. These are factors that affect the individual marginal cost curves, such as changes in the individual firm's productivity, in factor costs (wages paid to labor, prices of raw materials, etc.), in taxes, and in anything else that would influence the individual firm's marginal cost curve.

All of these are *ceteris paribus* conditions of supply. Because they affect the position of the marginal cost curve for the individual firm, they affect the position of the industry supply curve. A change in any of these will shift the market supply curve.

CONCEPTS IN BRIEF

- Short-run average profits or average losses are determined by comparing average total costs with price (average revenue) at the profit-maximizing rate of output. In the short run, the perfectly competitive firm can make economic profits or economic losses.
- The competitive firm's short-run break-even output occurs at the minimum point on its average total cost curve, which is where the marginal cost curve intersects the average total cost curve.
- The competitive firm's short-run shutdown output is at the minimum point on its average variable cost curve, which is also where the marginal cost curve intersects the average variable cost curve. Shutdown will occur if price falls below average variable cost.
- The firm will continue production at a price that exceeds average variable costs even though the full opportunity cost of capital is not being met; at least some revenues are going toward paying fixed costs.
- At the short-run break-even price, the firm is making zero economic profits, which means that it is just making a normal rate of return in that industry.
- The firm's short-run supply curve is the portion of its marginal cost curve equal to or above minimum average variable costs. The industry short-run supply curve is a horizontal summation of the individual firms' marginal cost curves above their respective minimum average variable costs.

*The capital Greek sigma, Σ, is the symbol for summation.

FIGURE 23-9

Industry Demand and Supply Curves and the Individual Firm Demand Curve

The industry demand curve is represented by D in panel (a). The short-run industry supply curve is S and equal to ΣMC. The intersection of the demand and supply curves at E determines the equilibrium or market clearing price at P_e. The individual firm demand curve in panel (b) is set at the market clearing price determined in panel (a). If the producer has a marginal cost curve MC, this producer's individual profit-maximizing output level is at q_e. For AC_1, economic profits are zero; for AC_2, profits are negative; and for AC_3, profits are positive.

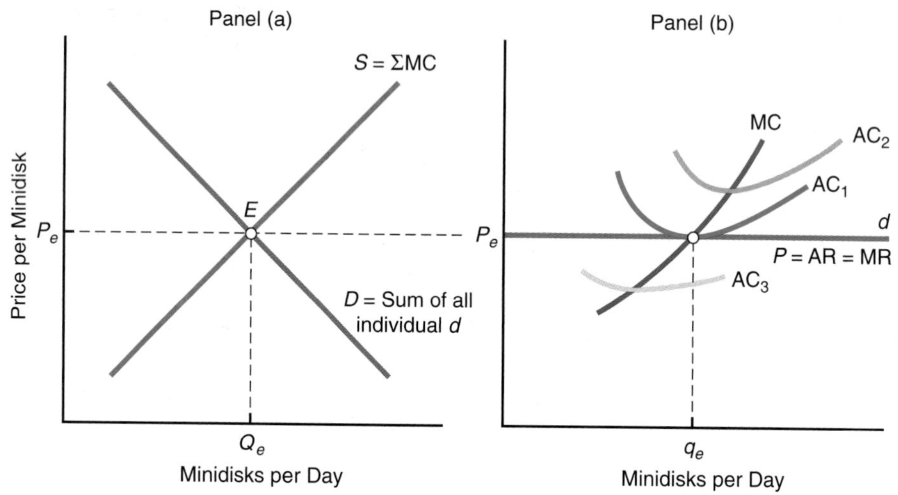

COMPETITIVE PRICE DETERMINATION

How is the market, or "going," price established in a competitive market? This price is established by the interaction of all the suppliers (firms) and all the demanders. The market demand schedule, *D,* in panel (a) of Figure 23-9 represents the demand schedule for the entire industry, and the supply schedule, *S,* represents the supply schedule for the entire industry. Price P_e is established by the forces of supply and demand at the intersection of *D* and the short-run industry supply curve, *S.* Even though each individual firm has no control or effect on the price of its product in a competitive industry, the interaction of *all* the producers and buyers determines the price at which the product will be sold. We say that the price P_e and the quantity Q_e in panel (a) of Figure 23-9 constitute the competitive solution to the pricing-quantity problem in that particular industry. It is the equilibrium where quantity demanded equals quantity supplied, and both suppliers and demanders are maximizing. The resulting individual firm demand curve, *d,* is shown in panel (b) of Figure 23-9 at the price P_e.

In a purely competitive industry, the individual producer takes price as a given and chooses the output level that maximizes profits. (This is also the equilibrium level of output from the producer's standpoint.) We see in panel (b) of Figure 23-9 that this is at q_e. If the producer's average costs are given by AC_1, q_e is also the short-run break-even output (see Figure 23-6); if its average costs are given by AC_2, at q_e, AC exceeds price (average revenue), and the firm is incurring losses. Alternatively, if average costs are given by AC_3, the firm will be making economic profits at q_e. In the former case, we would expect, over time, that firms will cease production (exit the industry), causing supply to shift inward, whereas in the latter case, we would expect new firms to enter the industry to take advantage of the economic profits, thereby causing supply to shift outward. We now turn to these long-run considerations.

EXAMPLE

Even Harvard Can't Charge an Above-Market Price

How things have changed since 1991. In that year, the U.S. Department of Justice filed suit against Ivy League universities. It claimed that they had conspired in their financial aid decisions, thereby forestalling the competitive determination of tuition rates for their students. Recently, however, Princeton University began to offer full scholarships to academically qualified students with family incomes below $40,000, and it increased its aid offers for students from middle-income families. Not long afterward, Yale also announced more financial aid for middle-income students, as did Brown and Cornell. Then Stanford and MIT (outside the Ivy League, but close competitors nonetheless) established similar aid plans.

Finally, the nation's oldest and most distinguished university, Harvard, sent a letter to each newly admitted student. In part, it said, "We expect that some of our students will have particularly attractive offers from the institutions with new aid programs, and those students should not assume that we will not respond." Translation: We'll meet the market price. Even Harvard is a perfect competitor in the market for top-notch higher education.

For Critical Analysis

According to the perfect competition model, all sellers charge the market price. But if sellers conspire to fix prices, they also charge the same price. How might one discern if sellers are charging competitive or noncompetitive prices for their products?

THE LONG-RUN INDUSTRY SITUATION: EXIT AND ENTRY

In the long run in a competitive situation, firms will be making zero economic profits. In the long run, we surmise that perfectly competitive firms will tend to have average total cost curves that just touch the price (marginal revenue) curve, or individual demand curve *d*. How does this occur? It is through an adjustment process that depends on economic profits and losses.

Exit and Entry of Firms

Go back and look at Figures 23-4 (p. 568) and 23-5 (p. 569). The existence of either profits or losses is a signal to owners of capital both within and outside the industry. If the industry is characterized by firms showing economic profits as represented in Figure 23-4, this will signal owners of capital elsewhere in the economy that they, too, should enter this industry. If, by contrast, there are firms in the industry like the ones suffering economic losses represented in Figure 23-5, this signals resource owners outside the industry to stay out. It also signals resource owners within the industry not to reinvest and if possible to leave the industry. It is in this sense that we say that profits direct resources to their highest-valued use. In the long run, capital will flow into industries in which profitability is highest and will flow out of industries in which profitability is lowest.

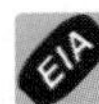

Long-Run Adjustments
Gain more experience thinking about long-run equilibrium under perfect competition.

The price system therefore allocates capital according to the relative expected rates of return on alternative investments. Entry restrictions will thereby hinder economic efficiency, and thus welfare, by not allowing resources to flow to their highest-valued use. Similarly, exit restrictions (such as laws that require firms to give advance notice of closings) will act to trap resources (temporarily) in sectors in which their value is below that in alternative uses. Such laws will also inhibit the ability of firms to respond to changes in the domestic and international marketplace.

Not every industry presents an immediate source of opportunity for every firm. In a brief period of time, it may be impossible for a firm that produces tractors to switch to the production of computers, even if there are very large profits to be made. Over the long run, however, we would expect to see such a change, whether or not the tractor producers want to change over to another product. In a market economy, investors supply firms in the more profitable industry with more investment funds, which they take from firms in less profitable industries. (Also, profits give existing firms internal investment funds for expansion.) Consequently, resources useful in the production of more profitable goods, such as labor, will be bid away from lower-valued opportunities. Investors and other suppliers of resources respond to market **signals** about their highest-valued opportunities.

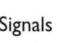

Signals
Compact ways of conveying to economic decision makers information needed to make decisions. A true signal not only conveys information but also provides the incentive to react appropriately. Economic profits and economic losses are such signals.

Market adjustment to changes in demand will occur regardless of the wishes of the managers of firms in less profitable markets. They can either attempt to adjust their product line to respond to the new demands, be replaced by managers who are more responsive to new conditions, or see their firms go bankrupt as they find themselves unable to replace worn-out plant and equipment.

In addition, when we say that in a competitive long-run equilibrium situation firms will be making zero economic profits, we must realize that at a particular point in time it would be pure coincidence for a firm to be making *exactly* zero economic profits. Real-world information is not as precise as the curves we use to simplify our analysis. Things change all the time in a dynamic world, and firms, even in a very competitive situation, may for many reasons not be making exactly zero economic profits. We say that there is a *tendency* toward that equilibrium position, but firms are adjusting all the time to changes in their cost curves and in their individual demand curves.

EXAMPLE

Who Really Shops at Club Warehouses?

One of the most pervasive competitive innovations in retailing in the United States has been the club warehouse phenomenon. These now ubiquitous retail outlets were first developed by San Diego's Sol Price. He started the Price Club chain in 1976. Since then, entry into the club warehouse business has been aggressive. It is dominated today by Wal-Mart-owned Sam's Club and Costco, the successor to the original Price Club. Smaller club warehouse chains, such as B.J.'s (a subsidiary of Waban, Inc.), dominate regional markets.

One interesting aspect of club warehouses involves who shops there and their reasons for doing so. One might assume at first glance that poorer American families would patronize club warehouses more heavily because of the their lower prices. The reality is just the opposite—the average family shopping at a club warehouse has above-average income. What accounts for that? A club warehouse stocks only a few branded goods in each product category. In essence, the club warehouse has done each customer's comparison shopping and obtained the best terms from the vendors. Individuals who have a relatively higher opportunity cost of time (usually those who make higher incomes) find this a value-added service.

For Critical Analysis

Why do you think the club warehouse market is dominated by a few large firms?

Long-Run Industry Supply Curves

In panel (a) of Figure 23-9 on page 574, we drew the summation of all of the portions of the individual firms' marginal cost curve above each firm's respective minimum average variable costs as the upward-sloping supply curve of the entire industry. We should be aware, however, that a relatively steep upward-sloping supply curve may be appropriate only in the short run. After all, one of the prerequisites of a competitive industry is free entry.

Remember that our definition of the long run is a period of time in which all adjustments can be made. The **long-run industry supply curve** is a supply curve showing the relationship between quantities supplied by the entire industry at different prices after firms have been allowed to either enter or leave the industry, depending on whether there have been positive or negative economic profits. Also, the long-run industry supply curve is drawn under the assumption that entry and exit have been completed. Thus along the long-run industry supply curve, firms in the industry earn zero economic profits.

Long-run industry supply curve 
A market supply curve showing the relationship between prices and quantities forthcoming after firms have been allowed the time to enter into or exit from an industry, depending on whether there have been positive or negative economic profits.

The long-run industry supply curve can take one of three shapes, depending on whether input costs stay constant, increase, or decrease as the number of firms in the industry changes. In Chapter 22, we assumed that input prices remained constant to the firm regardless of the firm's rate of output. When we look at the entire industry, when all firms are expanding and new firms are entering, they may simultaneously bid up input prices.

Constant-Cost Industries. In principle, there are industries that use such a small percentage of the total supply of inputs required for industrywide production that firms can enter the industry without bidding up input prices. In such a situation, we are dealing with a **constant-cost industry.** Its long-run industry supply curve is therefore horizontal and is represented by S_L in panel (a) of Figure 23-10.

Constant-cost industry 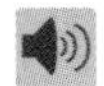
An industry whose total output can be increased without an increase in long-run per-unit costs; an industry whose long-run supply curve is horizontal.

We can work through the case in which constant costs prevail. We start out in panel (a) with demand curve D_1 and supply curve S_1. The equilibrium price is P_1. Market demand shifts rightward to D_2. In the short run, the equilibrium price rises to P_2. This generates positive economic profits for existing firms in the industry. Such economic profits induce capital to flow into the industry. The existing firms expand or new firms enter (or both). The short-run supply curve shifts outward to S_2. The new intersection with the new demand

FIGURE 23-10
Constant-Cost, Increasing-Cost, and Decreasing-Cost Industries
In panel (a), we show a situation in which the demand curve shifts from D_1 to D_2. Price increases from P_1 to P_2; however, in time the short-run supply curve shifts outward because positive profits are being earned, and the equilibrium shifts from E_2 to E_3. The market clearing price is again P_1. If we connect points such as E_1 and E_3, we come up with the long-run supply curve S_L. This is a constant-cost industry. In panel (b), costs are increasing for the industry, and therefore the long-run supply curve slopes upward and long-run prices rise from P_1 to P_2. In panel (c), costs are decreasing for the industry as it expands, and therefore the long-run supply curve slopes downward such that long-run prices decline from P_1 to P_2.

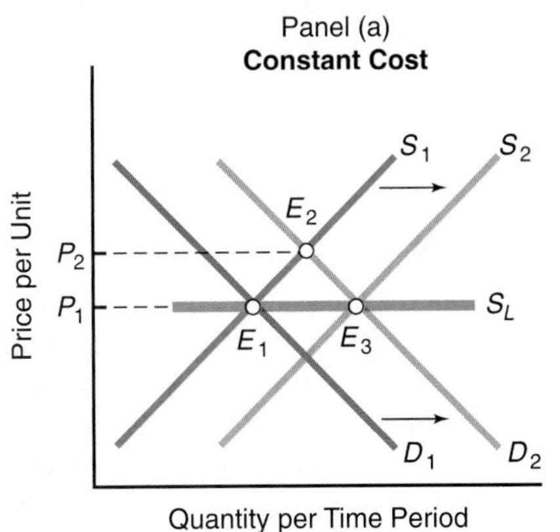

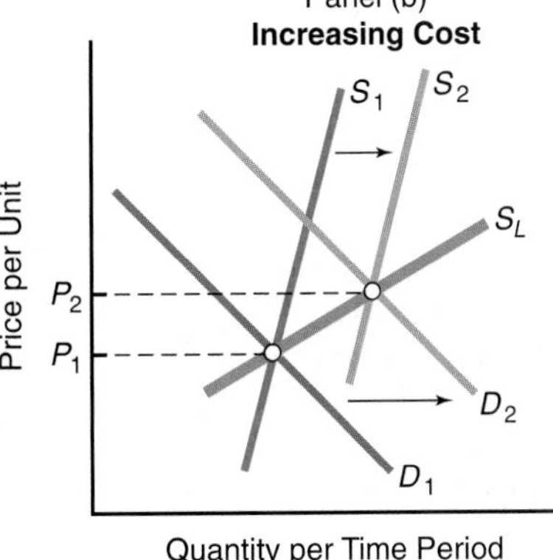

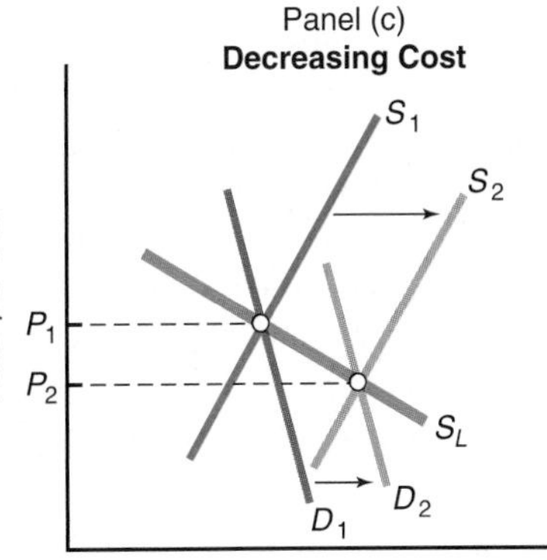

curve is at E_3. The new equilibrium price is again P_1. The long-run supply curve is obtained by connecting the intersections of the corresponding pairs of demand and supply curves, E_1 and E_3. Labeled S_L, it is horizontal; its slope is zero. In a constant-cost industry, long-run supply is perfectly elastic. Any shift in demand is eventually met by an equal shift in supply so that the long-run price is constant at P_1.

Retail trade is often given as an example of such an industry because output can be expanded or contracted without affecting input prices. Banking is another example.

Increasing-cost industry An industry in which an increase in industry output is accompanied by an increase in long-run per-unit costs, such that the long-run industry supply curve slopes upward.

Increasing-Cost Industries. In an **increasing-cost industry,** expansion by existing firms and the addition of new firms cause the price of inputs specialized within that industry to be bid up. As costs of production rise, the ATC curve and the firms' MC curves shift upward, causing short-run supply curves (each firm's marginal cost curve) to shift upward. The result is a long-run industry supply curve that slopes upward, as represented by S_L in panel (b) of Figure 23-10. Examples are residential construction and coal mining—both use specialized inputs that cannot be obtained in ever-increasing quantities without causing their prices to rise.

Decreasing-cost industry An industry in which an increase in output leads to a reduction in long-run per-unit costs, such that the long-run industry supply curve slopes downward.

Decreasing-Cost Industries. An expansion in the number of firms in an industry can lead to a reduction in input costs and a downward shift in the ATC and MC curves. When this occurs, the long-run industry supply curve will slope downward. An example is given in panel (c) of Figure 23-10. This is a **decreasing-cost industry.**

LONG-RUN EQUILIBRIUM

In the long run, the firm can change the scale of its plant, adjusting its plant size in such a way that it has no further incentive to change. It will do so until profits are maximized. Figure 23-11 shows the long-run equilibrium of the perfectly competitive firm. Given a price of P and a marginal cost curve, MC, the firm produces at output Q_e. Because profits must be zero in the long run, the firm's short-run average costs (SAC) must equal P at Q_e, which occurs at minimum SAC. In addition, because we are in long-run equilibrium, any economies of scale must be exhausted so that we are on the minimum point of the long-run average cost curve (LAC). In other words, the long-run equilibrium position is where "everything is equal," which is at point E in Figure 23-11. There, *price* equals *marginal revenue* equals *marginal cost* equals *average cost* (minimum, short-run, and long-run).

Perfect Competition and Minimum Average Total Cost

Look again at Figure 23-11. In long-run equilibrium, the perfectly competitive firm finds itself producing at output rate Q_e. At that rate of output, the price is just equal to the minimum long-run average cost as well as the minimum short-run average cost. In this sense, perfect competition results in the production of goods and services using the least costly combination of resources. This is an important attribute of a perfectly competitive long-run equilibrium, particularly when we wish to compare the

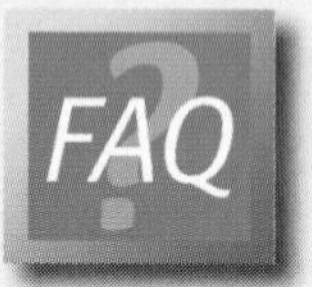

In the long run, don't national boundaries limit the extent to which firms can compete?

National borders can restrain competition only to the extent that governments are successful in erecting enforceable barriers to foreign competition. Emerging information technologies are doing an end run around many of these barriers. Anyone can shop on the Internet, as long as there are relatively few restraints on their ability to receive goods from delivery services. Even in markets for traditional goods such as agricultural products, artificial restraints on trade have ultimately given way to the forces of competition. Today, U.S. consumers buy fruit grown in South America, and African consumers purchase grains harvested in the American Midwest. Furthermore, agricultural businesses around the world enter and exit in response to price changes that occur in a global marketplace.

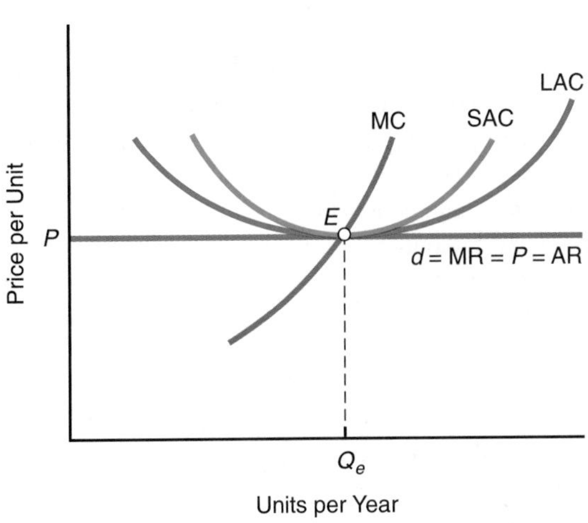

FIGURE 23-11

Long-Run Firm Competitive Equilibrium

In the long run, the firm operates where price, marginal revenue, marginal cost, short-run minimum average cost, and long-run minimum average cost are all equal. This occurs at point *E*.

market structure of perfect competition with other market structures that are less than perfectly competitive. We will examine these other market structures in later chapters.

COMPETITIVE PRICING: MARGINAL COST PRICING

In a perfectly competitive industry, each firm produces where its marginal cost curve intersects its marginal revenue curve from below. Thus perfectly competitive firms always sell their goods at a price that just equals marginal cost. This represents an optimal pricing situation because the price that consumers pay reflects the opportunity cost to society of producing the good. Recall that marginal cost is the amount that a firm must spend to purchase the additional resources needed to expand output by one unit. Given competitive markets, the amount paid for a resource will be the same in all of its alternative uses. Thus MC reflects relative resource input use; that is, if the MC of good 1 is twice the MC of good 2, one more unit of good 1 requires twice the resource input of one more unit of good 2. Because price equals marginal cost under perfect competition, the consumer, in determining allocation of income on purchases on the basis of relative prices, is actually allocating income on the basis of relative resource input use.

Click here to find out how the Congressional Budget Office tries to judge whether banks engage in marginal cost pricing with automated teller machines.

Marginal Cost Pricing

The competitive firm produces up to the point at which the market price just equals the marginal cost. Herein lies the element of the optimal nature of a competitive solution. It is called **marginal cost pricing.** The competitive firm sells its product at a price that just equals the cost to society—the opportunity cost—for that is what the marginal cost curve represents. (But note here that it is the self-interest of firm owners that causes price to equal the additional cost to society.) In other words, the marginal benefit to consumers, given by the price that they are willing to pay for the last unit of the good purchased, just equals the marginal cost to society of producing the last unit. [If the marginal benefit exceeds the marginal cost ($P >$ MC), too little is being produced in that people value additional units more than the cost to society of producing them; if $P <$ MC, the opposite is true.]

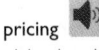

Marginal cost pricing 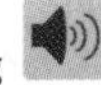
A system of pricing in which the price charged is equal to the opportunity cost to society of producing one more unit of the good or service in question. The opportunity cost is the marginal cost to society.

When an individual pays a price equal to the marginal cost of production, the cost to the user of that product is equal to the sacrifice or cost to society of producing that quantity of that good as opposed to more of some other good. (We are assuming that all marginal social costs are accounted for.) The competitive solution, then, is called *efficient,* in the economic sense of the word. Economic efficiency means that it is impossible to increase the output of any good without lowering the *value* of the total output produced in the economy. No juggling of resources, such as labor and capital, will result in an output that is higher in total value than the value of all of the goods and services already being produced. In an efficient situation, it is impossible to make one person better off without making someone else worse off. All resources are used in the most advantageous way possible, and society therefore enjoys an efficient allocation of productive resources. All goods and services are sold at their opportunity cost, and marginal cost pricing prevails throughout.

Market failure 
A situation in which an unrestrained market operation leads to either too few or too many resources going to a specific economic activity.

Lemons problem 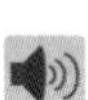
The situation in which consumers, who do not know details about the quality of a product, are willing to pay no more than the price of a low-quality product, even if a higher-quality product at a higher price exists.

Market Failure

Although perfect competition does offer many desirable results, situations arise when perfectly competitive markets cannot efficiently allocate resources. Either too many or too few resources are used in the production of a good or service. These situations are instances of **market failure.** Externalities and public goods are examples. For reasons discussed in later chapters, perfectly competitive markets cannot efficiently allocate resources in these situations, and alternative allocation mechanisms are called for. In some cases, alternative market structures, or government intervention, *may* improve the economic outcome.

● The competitive price is determined by the intersection of the market demand curve and the market supply curve; the market supply curve is equal to the horizontal summation of

POLICY EXAMPLE

Can the Government Cure Market Failure Due to Asymmetric Information, or Are Lemons Here to Stay?

One kind of market failure may occur when assumption 4 (p. 561) with respect to perfect competition is violated. Specifically, if information is not the same for buyers and sellers, markets may be dominated by low-quality products. This is a situation of asymmetric information. It has been called the **lemons problem** because cars, particularly used cars, that turn out to be "bad deals" are called lemons. The potential buyer of a used car has relatively little information about the true quality of the car—its motor, transmission, brakes, and so on. The only way the buyer can find out is to purchase the car and use it for a time. In contrast, the seller usually has much greater information about the quality of the car, for the seller has been using it for some time. The owner of the used car knows whether or not it is a lemon. In situations like this, with asymmetric information between buyer and seller, buyers tend to want to pay only a price that reflects the lower quality of the typical used car in the market, not a price that reflects the higher value of a truly good used car.

From the car seller's point of view, given that the price of used cars will tend to reflect average qualities, all of the owners of known lemons will want to put their cars up for sale. The owners of high-quality used cars will be more reluctant to do so. The logical result of this adverse selection is a disproportionate number of lemons on the used car market and consequently relatively fewer sales than would exist if information were symmetric.

So lemons will be overpriced and great-running used cars will be underpriced. Is there room for government policy to improve this market? Because the government has no better information than used-car buyers, it cannot provide any improved information. What the government has done, though, is require mileage certificates on all used cars and the disclosure of major defects and work that has been performed on them. What the market has done is use brand names both for cars and for firms that sell used cars. Used-car retailers also offer extended warranties.

For Critical Analysis

If used-car dealers depend on repeat customers, is the lemons problem reduced or eliminated?

CONCEPTS IN BRIEF

the portions of the individual marginal cost curves above their respective minimum average variable costs.

- In the long run, competitive firms make zero economic profits because of entry and exit of firms into and out of the industry whenever there are industrywide economic profits or economic losses.
- A constant-cost industry will have a horizontal long-run supply curve. An increasing-cost industry will have a upward-sloping long-run supply curve. A decreasing-cost industry will have a downward-sloping long-run supply curve.
- In the long run, a competitive firm produces where price, marginal revenue, marginal cost, short-run minimum average cost, and long-run minimum average cost are all equal.
- Competitive pricing is essentially marginal cost pricing, and therefore the competitive solution is called efficient because marginal cost represents the social opportunity cost of producing one more unit of the good; when consumers face a price equal to the full opportunity cost of the product they are buying, their purchasing decisions will lead to an efficient use of available resources.

NETNOMICS

Emerging Competitive Market for International Communications Services

Ask your parents about the "bad old days" of telecommunications, during which the typical American house contained a single telephone. Families had no choice but to lease that telephone from a single licensed company, and they were stuck with that company's rates on local calls. For long-distance service, the "choice" was either to pay the rates established by a single company or not to make long-distance calls at all. Of course, deregulation changed all that. Today, many families have four or more wired telephones and at least one cellular phone. They can choose among long-distance phone services, and a growing number of people can even choose which local phone company will get their business.

The international telephone business has been slower to experience heightened competition. Various restraints on competition among national phone companies have led to profit margins on international phone calls in excess of 60 percent. As a result, national phone companies earn more than $25 billion in annual global revenues from international calls.

This state of affairs may not last much longer, however. It is now possible to use the Internet to send not only e-mail but also relatively inexpensive fax, verbal, and video transmissions. The technology has existed for several years, but until recently, Internet-based calls have suffered from lags and inferior voice quality compared to traditional phone calls. But now that the technology of Internet-based communications promises to improve over the next few years, a number of Internet-based companies are likely to begin offering communications services, directly competing with traditional phone companies. This heralds a more competitive market in international communications services.

Such a development could pose particular problems for the world's biggest provider of international calling services, AT&T. U.S. callers tend to spend more time on the phone during international calls, which helps explain why AT&T earns about a third of world revenues from international calls. But U.S. residents also spend more time on-line than others around the world. Consequently, they may be the quickest to defect to AT&T's emerging Internet rivals. Some experts on the international telecommunications industry estimate that e-mail and Internet communications technologies have already siphoned away as much as $350 million in revenues that AT&T once earned from international phone calls. AT&T and other traditional providers of international telephone services are now considering whether they should get into the Internet telephony business.

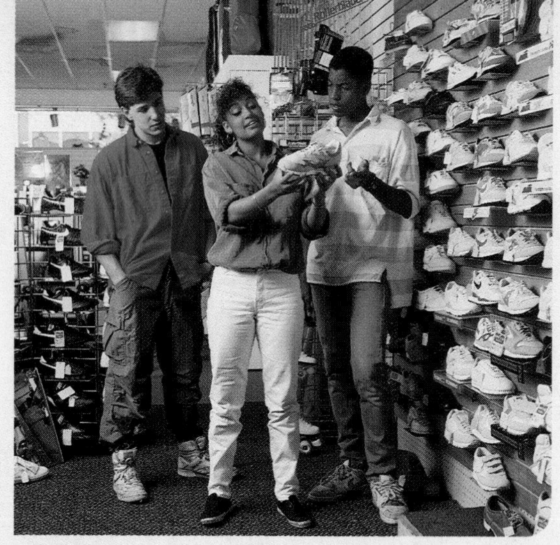

ISSUES & APPLICATIONS

Has the U.S. Economy Become More Competitive?

It is commonplace to read, see, and hear media accounts of "how much more competitive" the U.S. economy has become. Consumers report enjoying a greater range of substitution when they shop for goods and services. Businesspeople complain about the "pricing pressures" they face in today's marketplace. According to General Electric CEO John Welch, "There's no pricing power at all" in U.S. markets; that is, firms are price takers. Perception is one thing, but reality is another. Is the overall U.S. economy really more competitive than it used to be?

Concepts Applied

Perfect Competition

Competitive Price Determination

Groundwork for Greater Competition: Deregulation in the 1970s and 1980s

There is good reason to think that many American industries ought to be more competitive than they once were. Table 23-1 lists key regulatory changes enacted in the 1970s and 1980s. As you can see, common descriptors for regulatory initiatives adopted for various

TABLE 23-1
Significant Deregulation Since the 1970s

Industry	Major Initiatives
Airlines	CAB Liberalization of Entry and Discount Fare Experiments (mid 1970s)
	Airline Deregulation Act (1978)
Trucking	ICC Liberalization of Truck Rates (late 1970s)
	Motor Carrier Reform Act (1980)
Railroads	ICC Liberalization of Rail Rates and Contracting (late 1970s)
	Staggers Rail Act (1980)
Telecommunications	Federal Communications Commission (FCC) Court Decisions (late 1960s–mid 1970s)
	Execunet Decision (1977)
	AT&T Settlement (1982)
Cable television	FCC Rulemakings and other Regulatory Proceedings (late 1970s)
	Cable Television Deregulation Act (1984)
Brokerage	Securities Acts Amendments (1975)
Banking	Depository Institution Deregulation and Monetary Control Act (1980)
	Garn–St. Germain Depository Institutions Act (1982)
Petroleum	Decontrol of crude oil and refined petroleum products (executive orders beginning in 1979)
Natural gas	Natural Gas Policy Act (1978)

major industries for were "liberalization" and "deregulation." The U.S. government clearly sought to lay the groundwork for more competition a generation ago.

Some Evidence: Trying to Measure Overall Competition

If the American economy has truly become more competitive, firm profits should be closer to normal levels, indicating heightened rivalry among firms. With more scope for consumers to substitute among competing products, firms should be unable to set prices in excess of average production costs. One way to evaluate whether the entire U.S. economy is more competitive might be to examine each and every American industry in search of evidence that these predictions are better satisfied today than before. If this were true for most industries, we might feel comfortable saying that competition really has increased in the United States.

Another approach, however, is to take a "big picture" perspective. Economists have sought to do this by examining aggregate profit data for all U.S. firms. This is the approach taken by John Duca of the Federal Reserve Bank of Dallas and David VanHoose of the University of Alabama. They use data on aggregate U.S. business profits since the early 1950s to develop year-to-year estimates of the extent to which companies have been able to "mark up" their prices over and above their average costs of production. Naturally, the

FIGURE 23-12

Aggregate Competition in the United States

Aggregate year-to-year markups of prices over average production costs implied by data on the total profits of American companies yield an index measure of U.S. competition. This competition index has trended upward.

Source: John Duca and David VanHoose, "Has Greater Competition Restrained Inflation?" *Southern Economic Journal,* January 2000.

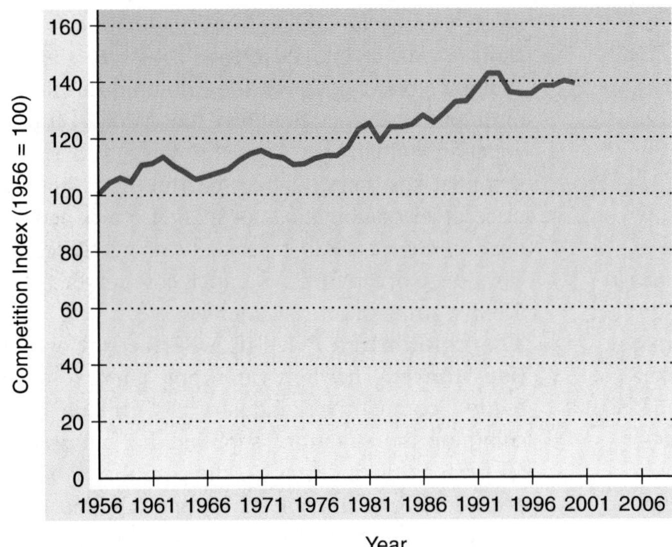

perfect competition model indicates that a greater range of substitution among goods that firms produce should restrain the size of price markups over average cost. Consequently, Duca and VanHoose's estimates of aggregate year-to-year price markups implied by total profit data essentially yield an aggregate measure of how substitutable the products of American firms have been over time. In short, they yield an index measure of "overall competition" in the U.S. economy.

Annual estimates of this index measure are plotted in Figure 23-12. Although there is some year-to-year variability in this aggregate competition index, it exhibits a definite upward trend. This is particularly notable since the 1970s, when widespread deregulation of a number U.S. industries began to reduce many barriers to entry and exit. The index has continued to increase as the information technology revolution has further enhanced the ability of consumers to shop for the best price among the products of rival firms. Aggregate profit data, therefore, indicate that the U.S. economy is indeed more competitive than it used to be.

FOR CRITICAL ANALYSIS

1. Based on the evidence in Figure 23-12, was the average U.S. company more or less likely to earn above-zero economic profits in the 1960s, compared with today?
2. Does a higher degree of overall U.S. competition today necessarily mean that every U.S. industry conforms more closely with the perfect competition model relative to earlier years?

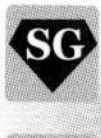

SUMMARY DISCUSSION OF LEARNING OBJECTIVES

1. **The Characteristics of a Perfectly Competitive Market Structure:** There are four fundamental characteristics of a perfectly competitive industry: (1) there are a large number of buyers and sellers, (2) firms in the industry produce and sell a homogeneous product, (3) there are insignificant barriers to industry entry or exit, and (4) information is equally accessible to both buyers and sellers. These characteristics imply that each firm in a perfectly competitive industry is a price taker, meaning that the firm takes the market price as given and outside its control.
2. **How a Perfectly Competitive Firm Decides How Much to Produce:** Because a perfectly competitive firm sells the amount that it wishes at the market price, the additional revenue it earns from selling an additional unit of output is the market price. Thus the firm's marginal revenue curve is horizontal at the market price, and this marginal revenue curve is the firm's own perfectly elastic demand curve. The firm maximizes economic profits when marginal cost equals marginal revenue, as long as the market price is not below the short-run shutdown price, where the marginal cost curve crosses the average variable cost curve.
3. **The Short-Run Supply Curve of a Perfectly Competitive Firm:** If the market price is below the short-run shutdown price, the firm's total revenues fail to cover its variable costs. Then the firm would be better off halting production and incurring only its fixed costs, thereby minimizing its economic loss in the short run. If the market price is above the short-run shutdown price, however, the firm produces the rate of output where marginal revenue, the market price, equals marginal cost. Thus the range of the firm's marginal cost curve above the short-run shutdown price gives combinations of market prices and production choices of the perfectly competitive firm. This range of the firm's marginal cost curve is therefore the firm's short-run supply curve.
4. **The Equilibrium Price in a Perfectly Competitive Market:** The short-run supply curve for a perfectly competitive industry is obtained by summing the quantities supplied at each price by all firms in the industry. At the equilibrium market price, the total amount of output supplied by all firms is equal to the total amount of output demanded by all buyers.

5. **Incentives to Enter or Exit a Perfectly Competitive Industry:** In the short run, a perfectly firm will continue to produce output as long as the market price exceeds the short-run shutdown price. This is so even if the market price is below the short-run break-even point where the marginal cost curve crosses the firm's average total cost curve. Even though the firm earns an economic loss, it minimizes the amount of the loss by continuing to produce in the short run. In the long run, however, an economic loss is a signal that the firm is not engaged in the highest-value activity available to its owners, and continued economic losses in the long run will induce the firm to exit the industry. Conversely, persistent economic profits induce new firms to enter a perfectly competitive industry. In long-run equilibrium, the market price is equal to the minimum average total cost of production for the firms in the industry, because at this point firms earn zero economic profits.
6. **The Long-Run Industry Supply Curve and Constant-, Increasing-, and Decreasing-Cost Industries:** The long-run industry supply curve in a perfectly competitive industry shows the relationship between prices and quantities after firms have the opportunity to enter or leave the industry in response to economic profits or losses. In a constant-cost industry, total output can increase without a rise in long-run per-unit production costs, so the long-run industry supply curve is horizontal. In an increasing-cost industry, however, per-unit costs increase with a rise in industry output, so that the long-run industry supply curve slopes upward. By contrast, per-unit costs decline as industry output increases, and the long-run industry supply curve slopes downward.

Key Terms and Concepts

Constant-cost industry (577)
Decreasing-cost industry (578)
Increasing-cost industry (578)
Industry supply curve (573)
Lemons problem (580)
Long-run industry supply curve (577)
Marginal cost pricing (579)
Marginal revenue (566)
Market failure (580)
Perfect competition (561)
Perfectly competitive firm (561)
Price taker (562)
Profit-maximizing rate of production (566)
Short-run break-even price (570)
Short-run shutdown price (570)
Signals (576)
Total revenues (564)

Problems

Answers to the odd-numbered problems appear at the back of the book.

23-1. Explain why each of the following examples is not a competitive industry.

a. Even though one firm produces a large portion of the industry's total output, there are many firms in the industry, and their products are indistinguishable. Firms can easily exit and enter the industry.

b. There are many buyers and sellers in the industry. Consumers have equal information about the prices of firms' products, which differ slightly in quality from firm to firm.

c. There are many taxicabs that compete in a city. The city's government requires all taxicabs to provide identical service. Taxicabs are virtually identical, and all drivers must wear a designated uniform. The government also controls the number of taxicab companies that can operate within the city's boundaries.

23-2. Illustrate the following situation in the market for video rentals, which is perfectly competitive: The supply curve slopes upward, the demand curve slopes downward, and the equilibrium rental price equals \$3.50. Next, illustrate the demand curve that a single independent video rental store faces. Finally, illustrate how an increase in the market demand for video rentals affects the market price and the demand curve faced by the individual rental store.

23-3. The campus barber faces stiff competition from the large number of shops that surround the campus area. For all practical purposes, therefore, this is a competitive market. He charges $6 for a haircut and cuts hair for 15 people a day. His shop is open five days a week. Calculate his weekly total revenue, average revenue, and marginal revenue.

23-4. The following table represents the hourly output and cost structure for a local pizza shop. The market is perfectly competitive, and the market price of a pizza in the area is $10. Total costs include all implicit opportunity costs.

Total Output and Sales of Pizzas	Total Cost ($)
0	5
1	9
2	11
3	12
4	14
5	18
6	24
7	32
8	42
9	54
10	68

a. Calculate the total revenue and total economic profit for this pizza shop at each rate of output.

b. Assuming that the pizza shop always produces and sells at least one pizza per hour, does this appear to be a situation of short-run or long-run equilibrium?

23-5. Using the information provided in Problem 23-4, calculate the pizza shop's marginal cost and marginal revenue at each rate of output. Based on marginal analysis, what is the profit-maximizing rate of output for the pizza shop?

23-6. Based on the information in Problems 23-4 and 23-5 and your answers to them, draw a diagram depicting the short-run marginal revenue and marginal cost curves for this pizza shop, and illustrate the determination of its profit-maximizing output rate.

23-7. Consider the information provided in Problem 23-4. Suppose the market price drops to only $5 per pizza. In the short run, should this pizza shop continue to make pizzas, or will it maximize its economic profits (that is, minimize its economic loss) by shutting down?

23-8. Suppose that a firm in a competitive industry finds that at its current output rate, marginal revenue exceeds the minimum average total cost of producing any feasible rate of output. Furthermore, the firm is producing an output rate for which marginal cost at that output rate is less than the average total cost of that rate of output. Is the firm maximizing its economic profits? Why or why not?

23-9. A perfectly competitive industry is initially in a short-run equilibrium in which all firms are earning zero economic profits but in which firms are operating below their minimum efficient scale. Explain the long-run adjustments that will take place for the industry to attain long-run equilibrium with firms operating at their minimum efficient scale.

23-10. A perfectly competitive industry is initially in a long-run equilibrium at which the market price of its output is $40 per unit and total industry output is 500,000 units. Then there is a decline in demand for the product that the industry produces. Some firms exit in response to declining profits, and eventually the industry reattains a long-run equilibrium at a market price of $35 per unit and total industry output of 450,000 units.

a. Draw the long-run supply curve for this industry.

b. Is this a decreasing-, constant-, or increasing-cost industry?

Economics on the Net

The Cost Structure of the Movie Theater Business A key idea in this chapter is that competition among firms in an industry can influence the long-run cost structure within the industry. Here you get a chance to apply this concept to a multinational company that owns movie theaters.

Title: AMC International

Navigation: Click here to visit American Multi-Cinema's homepage.

Application Answer the following questions.

1. Click on Investor Relations. What is the average number of screens in an AMC theater? How many theaters does it own and manage?

2. Click on AMC International and select Locations. Select the theater in Toyohashi City, Japan. This is the largest megaplex theater in Japan. How many screens does the megaplex have?

3. Based on the average number of screens at an AMC theater and the number of screens at the new Japanese facility, what can you conclude about the cost structure of this industry? Illustrate the long-run average cost curve for this industry.

For Group Discussion and Analysis Is the Japanese facility the largest multiplex? What do you think constrains the size of a multiplex in Japan? Given the location of AMC's headquarters, how does that affect the cost structure of the firm? Is it easier for AMC to have fewer facilities that are larger in size?

CHAPTER

24

MONOPOLY

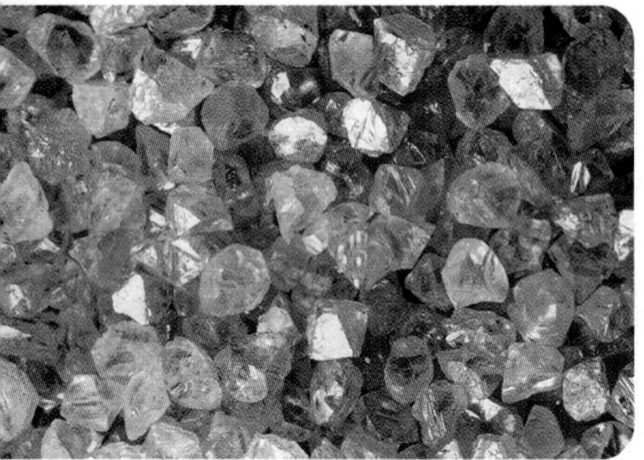

An extremely high percentage of all jewelry-quality diamonds are marketed through the De Beers company's selling organization. Has this monopoly guaranteed De Beers perpetually high diamond prices?

"Diamonds are forever." For decades, the expression has applied not just to diamonds but also to South Africa's De Beers diamond cartel. In any given year, its marketing arm, the London-based Central Selling Organization (CSO), sells about 70 percent of the world's rough-cut diamonds. The CSO's annual revenues range from $3 billion to $5 billion, approximately 10 percent of which is typically profit. Each year, however, the company withholds from the marketplace a stockpile of $4 billion to $5 billion in uncut diamonds. Why would the CSO choose to forgo additional revenues that it could earn if it were to sell these additional diamonds? To understand the CSO's motivation, you need to know about the theory of monopoly.

LEARNING OBJECTIVES

After reading this chapter, you should be able to:

1. **Identify situations that can give rise to monopoly**
2. **Describe the demand and marginal revenue conditions a monopolist faces**
3. **Discuss how a monopolist determines how much output to produce and what price to charge**
4. **Evaluate the profits earned by a monopolist**
5. **Understand price discrimination**
6. **Explain the social cost of monopolies**

Did You Know That... from the Great Depression of the 1930s until 1996, New York City kept the number of taxicab licenses (called "medallions") fixed at 11,787? The owner of a medallion can use or lease the medallion by the day or the week, and the owner can require a taxi driver to supply a car and provide insurance. In 1996, bidders for 53 new medallions paid an average of $177,000 for the right to sell taxi services. Today, the medallions are valued at more than $300,000. Why has there been such a big price increase? The reason is that there are so few taxis relative to the population in New York City. The absolute limit on the number of sellers of taxi services permits those sellers to extract the maximum amount of profit possible.

In some instances, there is only one seller of a good or service. Single sellers of goods and services exist all around you. The company that sells food in your school cafeteria has most probably been granted the exclusive right to do so by your college or university. The ski resort that offers you food at the top of the mountain does not allow anyone else to open a restaurant next to it. When you run a business that is the only one of its type in a particular location, you can usually charge a higher price per constant-quality unit than when there is intense competition. In this chapter, you will read more about situations in which competition is restricted. We call these situations *monopoly.*

Chapter Outline

DEFINITION OF A MONOPOLIST

The word *monopoly* probably brings to mind notions of a business that gouges the consumer, sells faulty products, and gets unconscionably rich in the process. But if we are to succeed in analyzing and predicting the behavior of noncompetitive firms, we will have to be more objective in our definition. Although most monopolies in the United States are relatively large, our definition will be equally applicable to small businesses: A **monopolist** is the *single supplier* of a good or service for which there is no close substitute.

Monopolist 
A single supplier that comprises its entire industry for a good or service for which there is no close substitute.

In a monopoly market structure, the firm (the monopolist) and the industry are one and the same. Occasionally there may be a problem in identifying an industry and therefore determining if a monopoly exists. For example, should we think of aluminum and steel as separate industries, or should we define the industry in terms of basic metals? Our answer depends on the extent to which aluminum and steel can be substituted in the production of a wide range of products.

As we shall see in this chapter, a seller prefers to have a monopoly than to face competitors. In general, we think of monopoly prices as being higher than prices under perfect competition and of monopoly profits as being higher than profits under perfect competition (which are, in the long run, merely equivalent to a normal rate of return). How does a firm obtain a monopoly in an industry? Basically, there must be *barriers to entry* that enable firms to receive monopoly profits in the long run. Barriers to entry are restrictions on who can start a business or who can stay in a business.

BARRIERS TO ENTRY 

For any amount of monopoly power to continue to exist in the long run, the market must be closed to entry in some way. Either legal means or certain aspects of the industry's technical or cost structure may prevent entry. We will discuss several of the barriers to entry that have allowed firms to reap monopoly profits in the long run (even if they are not pure monopolists in the technical sense).

Ownership of Resources Without Close Substitutes

Preventing a newcomer from entering an industry is often difficult. Indeed, some economists contend that no monopoly acting without government support has been able to prevent entry into the industry unless that monopoly has had the control of some essential natural resource. Consider the possibility of one firm's owning the entire supply of a raw material input that is essential to the production of a particular commodity. The exclusive ownership of such a vital resource serves as a barrier to entry until an alternative source of the raw material input is found or an alternative technology not requiring the raw material in question is developed. A good example of control over a vital input is the Aluminum Company of America (Alcoa), a firm that prior to World War II controlled the world's bauxite, the essential raw material in the production of aluminum. Such a situation is rare, though, and is ordinarily temporary.

Problems in Raising Adequate Capital

Certain industries require a large initial capital investment. The firms already in the industry can, according to some economists, obtain monopoly profits in the long run because no competitors can raise the large amount of capital needed to enter the industry. This is called the "imperfect" capital market argument employed to explain long-run, relatively high rates of return in certain industries. These industries are generally ones in which large fixed costs must be incurred merely to start production. Their fixed costs are generally for expensive machines necessary to the production process.

EXAMPLE

"Intel Inside"

Many observers of today's high-stakes high-technology world argue that the world's largest manufacturer of microprocessors, Intel, is a monopoly. They point out that to compete effectively with Intel, a potential adversary would have to invest billions of dollars. Intel provides the critical microprocessor chip that goes into the majority of the world's personal computers. Each new generation of microprocessor quickly becomes the industry standard for all IBM-compatible personal computers. Apple computers for years used a Motorola-made chip. In an attempt to fight back against Intel, Apple, Motorola, and IBM formed an alliance that did develop the Power PC microprocessor. So far, though, it has not made serious inroads into Intel's market. A few companies have attempted to clone Intel's chips, but they have not been very successful for both legal and technical reasons.

For Critical Analysis

Intel spends billions of dollars developing each new generation of microprocessor. Would it spend more or less if it had a smaller share of the microprocessor market?

Economies of Scale

Sometimes it is not profitable for more than one firm to exist in an industry. This is so if one firm would have to produce such a large quantity in order to realize lower unit costs that there would not be sufficient demand to warrant a second producer of the same product. Such a situation may arise because of a phenomenon we discussed in Chapter 22, economies of scale. When economies of scale exist, total costs increase less than proportionately to the increase in output. That is, proportional increases in output yield proportionately smaller increases in total costs, and per-unit costs drop. The advantage in

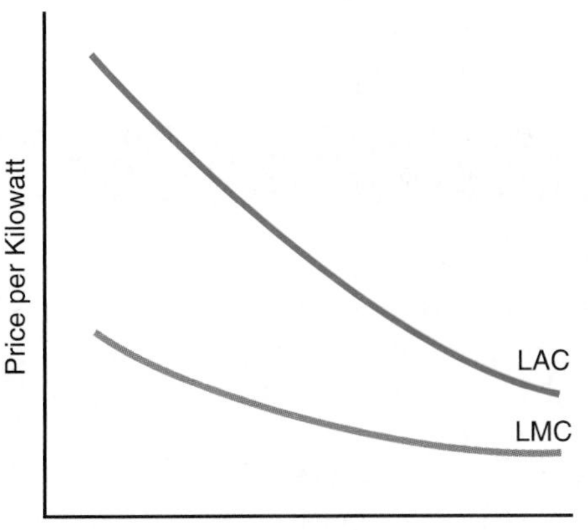

FIGURE 24-1

The Cost Curves That Might Lead to a Natural Monopoly: The Case of Electricity

Whenever long-run average costs are falling, so, too, will be long-run marginal costs. Also, long-run marginal costs (LMC) will always be below long-run average costs (LAC). A natural monopoly might arise in such a situation. The first firm to establish the low-unit-cost capacity would be able to take advantage of the lower average total cost curve. This firm would drive out all rivals by charging a lower price than the others could sustain at their higher average costs.

economies of scale lies in the fact that larger firms (with larger output) have lower costs that enable them to charge lower prices, and that drives smaller firms out of business.

When economies of scale occur over a wide range of outputs, a **natural monopoly** may develop. The natural monopoly is the firm that first takes advantage of persistent declining long-run average costs as scale increases. The natural monopolist is able to underprice its competitors and eventually force all of them out of the market.

Natural monopoly 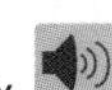
A monopoly that arises from the peculiar production characteristics in an industry. It usually arises when there are large economies of scale relative to the industry's demand such that one firm can produce at a lower average cost than can be achieved by multiple firms.

In Figure 24-1, we have drawn a downward-sloping long-run average cost curve (LAC). Recall that when average costs are falling, marginal costs are less than average costs. We can apply the same analysis in the long run. When the long-run average cost curve (LAC) is falling, the long-run marginal cost curve (LMC) will be below the LAC.

In our example, long-run average costs are falling over such a large range of production rates that we would expect only one firm to survive in such an industry. That firm would be the natural monopolist. It would be the first one to take advantage of the decreasing average costs; that is, it would construct the large-scale facilities first. As its average costs fell, it would lower prices and get an increasingly larger share of the market. Once that firm had driven all other firms out of the industry, it would set its price to maximize profits.

Legal or Governmental Restrictions

Governments and legislatures can also erect barriers to entry. These include licenses, franchises, patents, tariffs, and specific regulations that tend to limit entry.

Licenses, Franchises, and Certificates of Convenience. In many industries, it is illegal to enter without a government license, or a "certificate of convenience and public necessity." For example, in some states you still cannot form an electrical utility to compete with the electrical utility already operating in your area. You would first have to obtain a certificate of convenience and public necessity from the appropriate authority, which is usually the state's public utility commission. Yet public utility commissions in these states rarely, if ever, issue a certificate to a group of investors who want to compete directly in the same geographic area with an existing electrical utility; hence entry into the industry in a particular geographic area is prohibited, and long-run monopoly profits could conceivably be earned by the electrical utility already serving the area.

To enter interstate (and also many intrastate) markets for pipelines, television and radio broadcasting, and transmission of natural gas, to cite a few such industries, it is often necessary to obtain similar permits. Because these franchises or licenses are restricted, long-run monopoly profits might be earned by the firms already in the industry.

INTERNATIONAL EXAMPLE

Will Mexico Ever Hang Up on Its Telephone Monopoly?

Suppose that two businesspeople are competing to close a deal with a firm based in London. One is from the United States, and the other is from Mexico. Each person makes five four-minute calls. The American will typically pay $5 or $6 for the calls. The Mexican will pay $25 to $30. The reason for this big price disparity is simple: There are numerous competing long-distance providers in the United States, but there is one national phone company in Mexico.

Under the terms of a 1995 Mexican telecommunications law, this company, Telmex, is a regulated monopoly. A government agency is charged with regulating the company's rate of return. Telmex is the second-largest corporation in Mexico, and it is the largest company listed on the Mexican Stock Exchange. In recent years, the Mexican government has aimed for high and stable Mexican stock prices. Instead of taking the interests of consumers into account, the Mexican government has encouraged Telmex to maximize its profits to keep the prices of its shares high in the stock market.

As the monopoly model suggests, the result has been hefty telephone rates for consumers. In one year alone, Telmex raised the prices of local phone services throughout Mexico by 67 percent. Many Mexican residents have responded by forgoing phone service altogether. On average, there are only 10 telephones per 100 residents in Mexico.

For Critical Analysis

How would telephone rates and usage change if the Mexican government allowed other firms to compete with Telemex?

Patents. A patent is issued to an inventor to provide protection from having the invention copied or stolen for a period of 20 years. Suppose that engineers working for Ford Motor Company discover a way to build an engine that requires half the parts of a regular engine and weighs only half as much. If Ford is successful in obtaining a patent on this discovery, it can (in principle) prevent others from copying it. The patent holder has a monopoly. It is the patent holder's responsibility to defend the patent, however. That means that Ford—like other patent owners—must expend resources to prevent others from imitating its invention. If in fact the costs of enforcing a particular patent are greater than the benefits, the patent may not bestow any monopoly profits on its owner. The policing costs would be just too high.

Click here to learn more about patents and trademarks;
Click here to learn all about copyrights.

EXAMPLE

Patents as Intellectual Property

A patent may bestow on its owner a monopoly for a given time period. So, too, may copyrights. Trademarks don't actually bestow monopoly power, but they do in certain cases have extreme value. Coca-Cola can exploit its trademark by licensing it for clothes and paraphernalia. So, too, can Harley-Davidson. Both of those companies have done so. Copyrights, trademarks, patents, and the like are all part of what is known as intellectual property. Songs, music, computer programs, and designs are all intellectual property. Indeed, some economists believe that the world value of intellectual property now exceeds the value of physical property, such as real estate, buildings, and equipment. Not surprisingly, in the corporate world, when a business buys another business, the acquiring company's lawyers have to worry a great deal about the acquired company's intellectual property portfolio. What intellectual property rights in terms of patents, trademarks, and copyrights does the soon-to-be-acquired company actually own?

For Critical Analysis

Why doesn't the ownership of a well-known trademark bestow true monopoly power on its owner?

Tariffs. **Tariffs** are special taxes that are imposed on certain imported goods. Tariffs have the effect of making imports relatively more expensive than their domestic counterparts, so that consumers switch to the relatively cheaper domestically made products. If the tariffs are high enough, domestic producers gain monopoly advantage as the sole suppliers. Many countries have tried this protectionist strategy by using high tariffs to shut out foreign competitors.

Tariffs 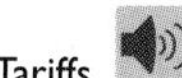

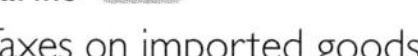
Taxes on imported goods.

Regulations. During much of the twentieth century, government regulation of the American economy has increased, especially along the dimensions of safety and quality. For example, pharmaceutical quality-control regulations enforced by the Food and Drug Administration may require that each pharmaceutical company install a $2 million computerized testing machine that requires elaborate monitoring and maintenance. Presumably, this large fixed cost can be spread over a larger number of units of output by larger firms than by smaller firms, thereby putting the smaller firms at a competitive disadvantage. It will also deter entry to the extent that the scale of operation of a potential entrant must be sufficiently large to cover the average fixed costs of the required equipment. We examine regulation in more detail in Chapter 26.

Cartels

"Being the only game in town" is preferable because such a monopoly position normally allows the monopolist to charge higher prices and make greater profits. Not surprisingly, manufacturers and sellers have often attempted to form an organization (which often is international) that acts as one. This is called a **cartel.** Cartels are an attempt by their members to earn higher than competitive profits. They set common prices and output quotas for their members. The key to the success of a cartel is keeping one member from competing against other members by expanding production and thereby lowering price. Apparently, one of the most successful international cartels ever was the Organization of Petroleum Exporting Countries (OPEC), an association of the world's largest oil-producing countries, including Saudi Arabia, which at times has accounted for a significant percentage of the world's crude oil output. OPEC effectively organized a significant cutback on the production of crude oil in the wake of the so-called Yom Kippur War in the Middle East in 1973. Within one year, the spot price of crude oil jumped from $2.12 to $7.61 per barrel on the world market. By the early 1980s, the price had risen to over $30.

Cartel 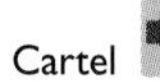

An association of producers in an industry that agree to set common prices and output quotas to prevent competition.

Most cartels have not had as much success.

INTERNATIONAL EXAMPLE

"We're Just Trying to Keep the Market Stable"

The stated goal of most international cartels is keeping markets "stable." In reality, cartel members are seeking higher prices (and profits) for their product. But to achieve their aims, the producing countries have to be willing to withhold some of their production from the world market.

Nowhere are international cartels as prevalent as in the market for commodities. The International Coffee Organization lasted 30 years until the United States pulled out; it was succeeded by the Association of Coffee Producing Countries. Cocoa has the International Cocoa Organization. There is even an ostrich cartel called the Little Karoo Agricultural Cooperative.

The U.S. government has at times sanctioned the equivalent of a cartel. A meeting in Washington, D.C., involving executives from a dozen global aluminum producers and government officials representing the United States, the European Union, and four other nations ultimately resulted in an agreement by all those attending to reduce aluminum production. All such reductions were voluntary except by Russia. In exchange for cutting primary aluminum production by 500,000 tons over a two-year period, Russia received the promise of $250 million of U.S. taxpayers' money for equity investments. U.S. government officials claim that "the markets are still open" nonetheless.

For Critical Analysis

The price of gasoline today (corrected for inflation) is less than what it was in 1984. What does that tell you about the long-run effectiveness of global cartels?

CONCEPTS IN BRIEF

- A monopolist is defined as a single seller of a product or a good for which there is no good close substitute.
- To maintain a monopoly, there must be barriers to entry. Barriers to entry include ownership of resources without close substitutes; large capital requirements in order to enter the industry; economies of scale; legally required licenses, franchises, and certificates of convenience; patents; tariffs; and safety and quality regulations.

THE DEMAND CURVE A MONOPOLIST FACES

A *pure monopolist* is the sole supplier of *one* product, good, or service. A pure monopolist faces a demand curve that is the demand curve for the entire market for that good.

The monopolist faces the industry demand curve because the monopolist is the entire industry.

Because the monopolist faces the industry demand curve, which is by definition downward-sloping, its decision-making process with respect to how much to produce is not the same as for a perfect competitor. When a monopolist changes output, it does not automatically receive the same price per unit that it did before the change.

Profits to Be Made from Increasing Production

How do firms benefit from changing production rates? What happens to price in each case? Let's first review the situation among perfect competitors.

Marginal Revenue for the Perfect Competitor. Recall that a competitive firm has a perfectly elastic demand curve. That is because the competitive firm is such a small part of the market that it cannot influence the price of its product. It is a *price taker.* If the forces of supply and demand establish that the price per constant-quality pair of shoes is $50, the individual firm can sell all the pairs of shoes it wants to produce at $50 per pair. The average revenue is $50, the price is $50, and the marginal revenue is also $50.

Let us again define marginal revenue:

Marginal revenue equals the change in total revenue due to a one-unit change in the quantity produced and sold.

In the case of a competitive industry, each time a single firm changes production by one unit, total revenue changes by the going price, and price is always the same. Marginal revenue never changes; it always equals price, or average revenue. Average revenue was defined as total revenue divided by quantity demanded, or

$$\text{Average revenue} = \frac{\text{TR}}{Q} = \frac{PQ}{Q} = P$$

Hence marginal revenue, average revenue, and price are all the same for the price-taking firm.

Marginal Revenue for the Monopolist. What about a monopoly firm? Because a monopoly is the entire industry, the monopoly firm's demand curve is the market demand curve. The market demand curve slopes downward, just like the other demand curves that we have seen. Therefore, to sell more of a particular product, given the industry demand curve, the monopoly firm must lower the price. Thus the monopoly firm moves *down* the demand curve. If all buyers are to be charged the same price, the monopoly must lower the price on all units sold in order to sell more. It cannot just lower the price on the *last* unit sold in any given time period in order to sell a larger quantity.

Put yourself in the shoes of a monopoly ferryboat owner. You have a government-bestowed franchise, and no one can compete with you. Your ferryboat goes between two islands. If you are charging \$1 per crossing, a certain quantity of your services will be demanded. Let's say that you are ferrying 100 people a day each way at that price. If you decide that you would like to ferry more individuals, you must lower your price to all individuals—you must move *down* the existing demand curve for ferrying services. To calculate the marginal revenue of your change in price, you must first calculate the total revenues you received at \$1 per passenger per crossing and then calculate the total revenues you would receive at, say, 90 cents per passenger per crossing.

It is sometimes useful to compare monopoly markets with perfectly competitive markets. The only way the monopolist can increase its total revenues is by getting consumers to spend more of their incomes on the monopolist's product and less on all other products combined. Thus the monopolist is constrained by the entire market demand curve for its product. We see this in Figure 24-2, which compares the demand curves of the perfect competitor and the monopolist.

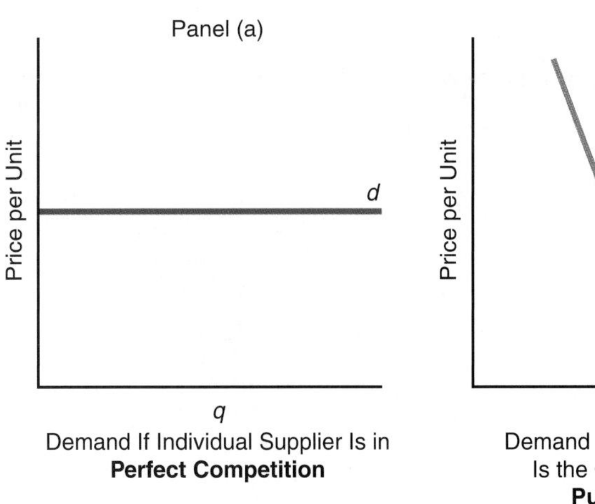

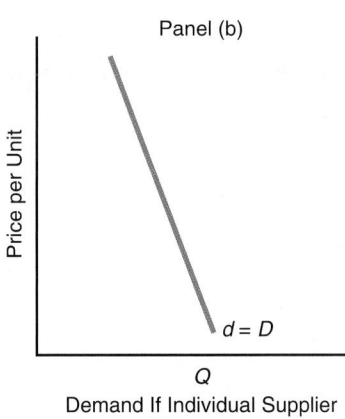

FIGURE 24-2
Demand Curves for the Perfect Competitor and the Monopolist
The perfect competitor in panel (a) faces a perfectly elastic demand curve, *d*. The monopolist in panel (b) faces the entire industry demand curve, which slopes downward.

Here we see the fundamental difference between the monopolist and the competitor. The competitor doesn't have to worry about lowering price to sell more. In a purely competitive situation, the competitive firm accounts for such a small part of the market that it can sell its entire output, whatever that may be, at the same price. The monopolist cannot. The more the monopolist wants to sell, the lower the price it has to charge on the last unit (and on *all* units put on the market for sale). Obviously, the extra revenues the monopolist receives from selling one more unit are going to be smaller than the extra revenues received from selling the next-to-last unit. The monopolist has to lower the price on the last unit to sell it because it is facing a downward-sloping demand curve and the only way to move down the demand curve is to lower the price on all units.

The Monopolist's Marginal Revenue: Less than Price

An essential point is that for the monopolist, marginal revenue is always less than price. To understand why, look at Figure 24-3, which shows a unit increase in output sold due to a reduction in the price of a commodity from P_1 to P_2. After all, the only way that the firm can sell more output, given a downward-sloping demand curve, is for the price to fall. Price P_2 is the price received for the last unit. Thus price P_2 times the last unit sold represents revenues received from the last unit sold. That is equal to the vertical column (area A). Area A is one unit wide by P_2 high.

But price times the last unit sold is *not* the addition to *total* revenues received from selling that last unit. Why? Because price had to be reduced on all previous units sold (Q) in order to sell the larger quantity $Q + 1$. The reduction in price is represented by the vertical distance from P_1 to P_2 on the vertical axis. We must therefore subtract area B from area A to come up with the *change* in total revenues due to a one-unit increase in sales. Clearly, the change in total revenues—that is, marginal revenue—must be less than price because marginal revenue is always the difference between areas A and B in Figure 24-3. For example, if the initial price is \$8 and quantity demanded is 3, to increase quantity to 4 units, it is necessary to decrease price to \$7, not just for the fourth unit, but on all three previous units as well. Thus at a price of \$7, marginal revenue is \$7 − \$3 = \$4 because there is a \$1 per unit price reduction on three previous units. Hence marginal revenue, \$4, is less than price, \$7.

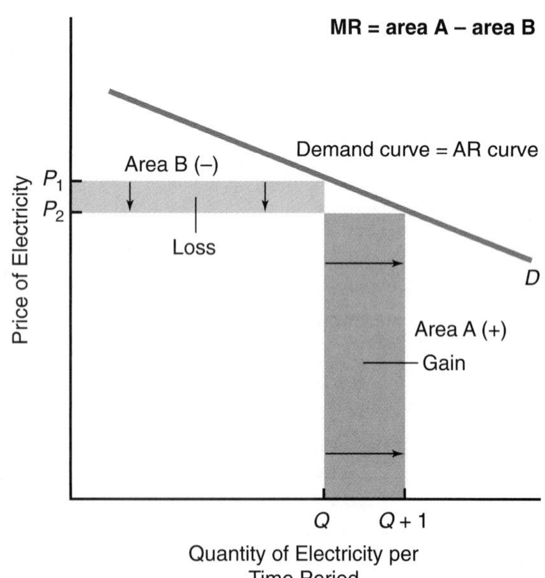

FIGURE 24-3

Marginal Revenue: Always Less than Price

The price received for the last unit sold is equal to P_2. The revenues received from selling this last unit are equal to P_2 times one unit, or the area of the vertical column. However, if a single price is being charged for all units, total revenues do not go up by the amount of the area represented by that column. The price had to be reduced on all the previous Q units that were being sold at price P_1. Thus we must subtract area B—the rectangle between P_1 and P_2 from the origin to Q—from area A in order to derive marginal revenue. Marginal revenue is therefore always less than price.

ELASTICITY AND MONOPOLY 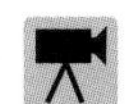

The monopolist faces a downward-sloping demand curve (its average revenue curve). That means that it cannot charge just *any* price with no changes in quantity (a common misconception) because, depending on the price charged, a different quantity will be demanded.

Earlier we defined a monopolist as the single seller of a well-defined good or service with no *close* substitute. This does not mean, however, that the demand curve for a monopoly is vertical or exhibits zero price elasticity of demand. (Indeed, as we shall see, the profit-maximizing monopolist will never operate in a price range in which demand is inelastic.) After all, consumers have limited incomes and alternative wants. The downward slope of a monopolist's demand curve occurs because individuals compare the marginal satisfaction they will receive to the cost of the commodity to be purchased. Take the example of telephone service. Even if miraculously there were absolutely no substitute whatsoever for telephone service, the market demand curve would still slope downward. At lower prices, people will add more phones and separate lines for different family members.

Furthermore, the demand curve for telephone service slopes downward because there are at least several *imperfect* substitutes, such as letters, e-mails, in-person conversations, and Internet telephony. Thus even though we defined a monopolist as a single seller of a commodity with no *close* substitute, we can talk about the range of *imperfect* substitutes. The more such imperfect substitutes there are, and the better these substitutes are, the more elastic will be the monopolist's demand curve, all other things held constant.

CONCEPTS IN BRIEF

- The monopolist estimates its marginal revenue curve, where marginal revenue is defined as the change in total revenues due to a one-unit change in quantity sold.
- For the perfect competitor, price equals marginal revenue equals average revenue. For the monopolist, price is always greater than marginal revenue. For the monopolist, marginal revenue is always less than price because price must be reduced on all units to sell more.
- The price elasticity of demand for the monopolist depends on the number and similarity of substitutes. The more numerous and more similar the substitutes, the greater the price elasticity of demand of the monopolist's demand curve.

COSTS AND MONOPOLY PROFIT MAXIMIZATION

To find out the rate of output at which the perfect competitor would maximize profits, we had to add cost data. We will do the same thing now for the monopolist. We assume that profit maximization is the goal of the pure monopolist, just as for the perfect competitor. The perfect competitor, however, has only to decide on the profit-maximizing rate of output because price is given. The competitor is a price taker. For the pure monopolist, we must seek a profit-maximizing *price-output combination* because the monopolist is a **price searcher.** We can determine this profit-maximizing price-output combination with either of two equivalent approaches—by looking at total revenues and total costs or by looking at marginal revenues and marginal costs. We shall examine both approaches.

Price searcher 
A firm that must determine the price-output combination that maximizes profit because it faces a downward-sloping demand curve.

The Total Revenues–Total Costs Approach

We show hypothetical demand (rate of output and price per unit), revenues, costs, and other data in panel (a) of Figure 24-4. In column 3, we see total revenues for our hypothetical monopolist, and in column 4, we see total costs. We can transfer these two columns to

FIGURE 24-4

Monopoly Costs, Revenues, and Profits

In panel (a), we give hypothetical demand (rate of output and price per unit), revenues, costs, and other relevant data. As shown in panel (b), the monopolist maximizes profits where the positive difference between TR and TC is greatest. This is at an output rate of between 9 and 10. Put another way, profit maximization occurs where marginal revenue equals marginal cost, as shown in panel (c). This is at the same output rate of between 9 and 10. (The MC curve must cut the MR curve from below.)

Panel (a)

(1) Output (units)	(2) Price per Unit	(3) Total Revenues (TR) (3) = (2) x (1)	(4) Total Costs (TC)	(5) Total Profit (5) = (3) – (4)	(6) Marginal Cost (MC)	(7) Marginal Revenue (MR)
0	$8.00	$ .00	$10.00	–$10.00		
					$4.00	$7.80
1	7.80	7.80	14.00	– 6.20		
					3.50	7.40
2	7.60	15.20	17.50	– 2.30		
					3.25	7.00
3	7.40	22.20	20.75	1.45		
					3.05	6.60
4	7.20	28.80	23.80	5.00		
					2.90	6.20
5	7.00	35.00	26.70	8.30		
					2.80	5.80
6	6.80	40.80	29.50	11.30		
					2.75	5.40
7	6.60	46.20	32.25	13.95		
					2.85	5.00
8	6.40	51.20	35.10	16.10		
					3.20	4.60
9	6.20	55.80	38.30	17.50		
					4.00	4.20
10	6.00	60.00	42.30	17.70		
					6.00	3.80
11	5.80	63.80	48.30	15.50		
					9.00	3.40
12	5.60	67.20	57.30	9.90		

Panel (b)

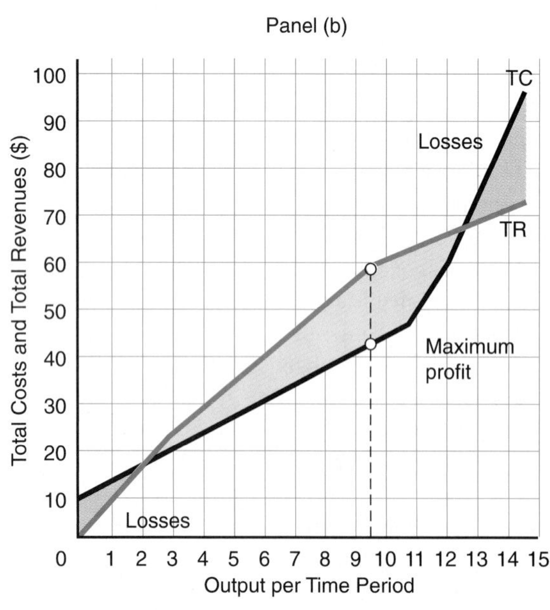

Panel (c)

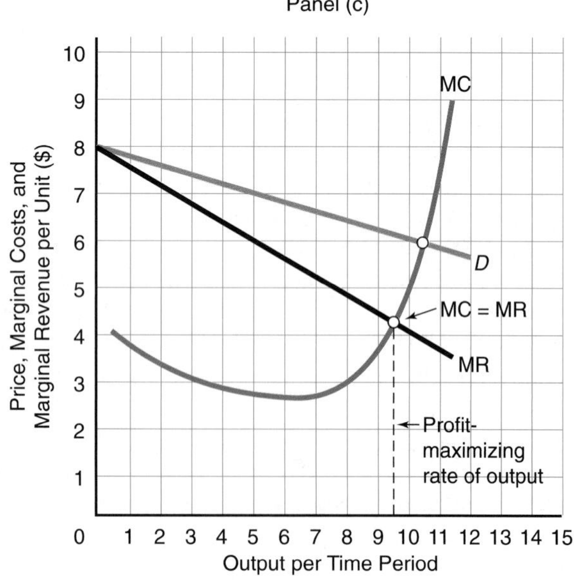

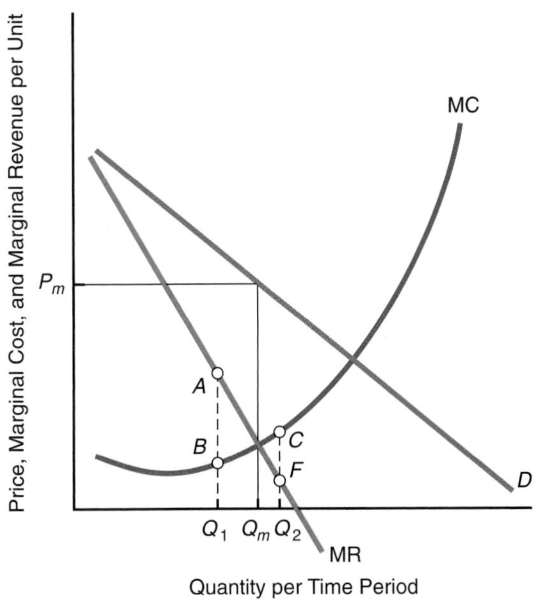

FIGURE 24-5
Maximizing Profits
The profit-maximizing production rate is Q_m, and the profit-maximizing price is P_m. The monopolist would be unwise to produce at the rate Q_1 because here marginal revenue would be Q_1A and marginal costs would be Q_1B. Marginal revenue exceeds marginal cost. The firm will keep producing until the point Q_m, where marginal revenue just equals marginal cost. It would be foolish to produce at the rate Q_2, for here marginal cost exceeds marginal revenue. It behooves the monopolist to cut production back to Q_m.

panel (b). The only difference between the total revenue and total cost diagram in panel (b) and the one we showed for a perfect competitor in Chapter 23 is that the total revenue line is no longer straight. Rather, it curves. For any given demand curve, in order to sell more, the monopolist must lower the price. Thus, the basic difference between a monopolist and a perfect competitor has to do with the demand curve for the two types of firms. Monopoly market power is derived from facing a downward-sloping demand curve.

Click here to see how effective OPEC has been in trying to act as an oil market monopolist.

Profit maximization involves maximizing the positive difference between total revenues and total costs. This occurs at an output rate of between 9 and 10 units.

The Marginal Revenue–Marginal Cost Approach

Profit maximization will also occur where marginal revenue equals marginal cost. This is as true for a monopolist as it is for a perfect competitor (but the monopolist will charge a higher price). When we transfer marginal cost and marginal revenue information from columns 6 and 7 in panel (a) of Figure 24-4 to panel (c), we see that marginal revenue equals marginal cost at an output rate of between 9 and 10 units. Profit maximization occurs at the same output as in panel (b).

Why Produce Where Marginal Revenue Equals Marginal Cost? If the monopolist goes past the point where marginal revenue equals marginal cost, marginal cost will exceed marginal revenue. That is, the incremental cost of producing any more units will exceed the incremental revenue. It just would not be worthwhile, as was true also in perfect competition. But if the monopolist produces

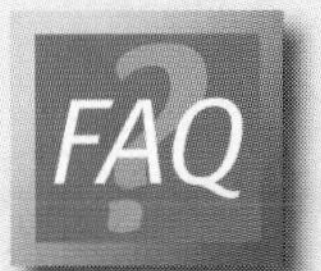

Is the Organization of Petroleum Exporting Countries (OPEC) an effective oil monopoly?

Not any more. In the 1970s, OPEC succeeded in restraining world oil production and driving up prices for several years. Today, however, there are so many oil producers that it is hard to induce them all to withhold oil from the market. For instance, in the summer of 1998, OPEC's biggest producers, Saudi Arabia, Mexico, and Venezuela, agreed to cut back on output in an effort to stem a big decline in oil prices. This simply opened up sales opportunities for smaller producers, however. Within four months, Venezuelan companies had broken the terms of the OPEC agreement.

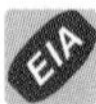

Monopoly Output and Price Determination
Gain further understanding of how a monopolist sets its output rate and product price.

less than that, it is also not making maximum profits. Look at output rate Q_1 in Figure 24-5. Here the monopolist's marginal revenue is at *A*, but marginal cost is at *B*. Marginal revenue exceeds marginal cost on the last unit sold; the profit for that *particular* unit, Q_1, is equal to the vertical difference between *A* and *B*, or the difference between marginal revenue and marginal cost. The monopolist would be foolish to stop at output rate Q_1 because if output is expanded, marginal revenue will still exceed marginal cost, and therefore total profits will rise. In fact, the profit-maximizing monopolist will continue to expand output and sales until marginal revenue equals marginal cost, which is at output rate Q_m. The monopolist won't produce at rate Q_2 because here, as we see, marginal costs are *C* and marginal revenues are *F*. The difference between *C* and *F* represents the *reduction* in total profits from producing that additional unit. Total profits will rise as the monopolist reduces its rate of output back toward Q_m.

POLICY EXAMPLE

Limiting Limos in Las Vegas

Las Vegas, Nevada, is one of the leading convention centers on the planet. It welcomes 25 million visitors per year. When they reach the city's airport, these visitors typically hire taxicabs and limousines. The city has not allowed a single new taxi in over 25 years, so enterprising limo operators began to offer their services.

In 1997, however, the Nevada legislature passed a law creating the state Transportation Services Authority. Its main source of funds is money it raises from application fees and fines it assesses on violators of limitations on limousine services. The law requires an applicant for a limo license to prove that a new limo in the market will "not unreasonably and adversely affect other carriers." A recent applicant submitted more than 1,000 pages of documentation and incurred $15,000 in application fees and expenses. His application was rejected. So was an application by a quadriplegic who wanted to provide specialized limo services to wheelchair-bound people. The rationale for both rejections was that additional limos would cut into the profits currently earned by existing operators. Keeping those profits up requires restricting the quantity of limo services available for use by visitors.

For Critical Analysis

Some cities, such as Denver and Indianapolis, have opened their markets for taxi and limo services to increased competition. How do you predict that the quantity and prices of these transportation services changed in these cities?

What Price to Charge for Output?

How does the monopolist set prices? We know the quantity is set at the point at which marginal revenue equals marginal cost. The monopolist then finds out how much can be charged—how much the market will bear—for that particular quantity, Q_m, in Figure 24-5. We know that the demand curve is defined as showing the *maximum* price for which a given quantity can be sold. That means that our monopolist knows that to sell Q_m, it can charge only P_m because that is the price at which that specific quantity, Q_m, is demanded. This price is found by drawing a vertical line from the quantity, Q_m, to the market demand curve. Where that line hits the market demand curve, the price is determined. We find that price by drawing a horizontal line from the demand curve over to the price axis; that gives us the profit-maximizing price, P_m.

In our detailed numerical example, at a profit-maximizing rate of output of a little less than 10 in Figure 24-4, the firm can charge a maximum price of about $6 and still sell all the goods produced, all at the same price.

The basic procedure for finding the profit-maximizing short-run price-quantity combination for the monopolist is first to determine the profit-maximizing rate of output, by either the total revenue-total cost method or the marginal revenue-marginal cost method, and then to determine by use of the demand curve, *D*, the maximum price that can be charged to sell that output.

Don't get the impression that just because we are able to draw an exact demand curve in Figure 24-4 and Figure 24-5, real-world monopolists have such perfect information. The process of price searching by a less than perfect competitor is just that—a process. A monopolist can only estimate the actual demand curve and therefore can only make an educated guess when it sets its profit-maximizing price. This is not a problem for the perfect competitor because price is given already by the intersection of market demand and market supply. The monopolist, in contrast, reaches the profit-maximizing output-price combination by trial and error.

CALCULATING MONOPOLY PROFIT

We have talked about the monopolist's profit, but we have yet to indicate how much profit the monopolist makes. We have actually shown total profits in column 5 of panel (a) in Figure 24-4. We can also find total profits by adding an average total cost curve to panel (c) of that figure. We do that in Figure 24-6. When we add the average total cost curve, we find that the profit that a monopolist makes is equal to the shaded area [or total revenues minus total costs (ATC × *Q*)]. Given the demand curve and a uniform pricing system (i.e., all units sold at the same price), there is no way for a monopolist to make greater profits than those shown by the shaded area. The monopolist is maximizing profits where marginal cost equals marginal revenue. If the monopolist produces less than that, it will be forfeiting some profits. If the monopolist produces more than that, it will be forfeiting some profits.

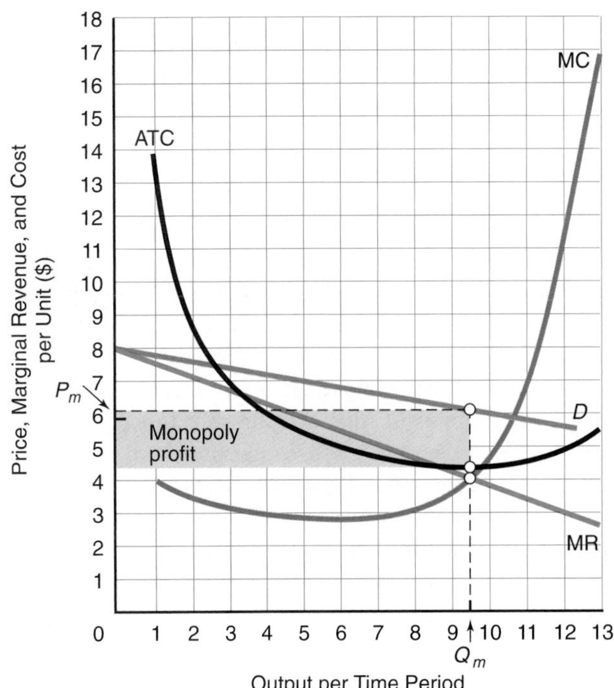

FIGURE 24-6
Monopoly Profit
We find monopoly profit by subtracting total costs from total revenues at an output rate of almost 10, labeled Q_m, which is the profit-maximizing rate of output for the monopolist. The profit-maximizing price is therefore about $6 and is labeled P_m. Monopoly profit is given by the shaded area, which is equal to total revenues (P × *Q*) minus total costs (ATC × *Q*). This diagram is similar to panel (c) of Figure 24-4, with the short-run average total cost curve (ATC) added.

FIGURE 24-7

Monopolies: Not Always Profitable

Some monopolists face the situation shown here. The average total cost curve, ATC, is everywhere above the average revenue, or demand, curve, D. In the short run, the monopolist will produce where MC = MR at point E. Output Q_m will be sold at price P_m, but average total cost per unit is C_1. Losses are the shaded rectangle. Eventually, the monopolist will go out of business.

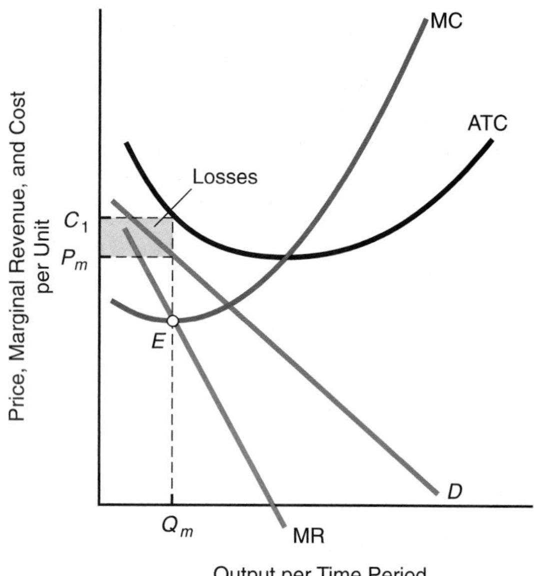

The same is true of a perfect competitor. The competitor produces where marginal revenues equal marginal costs because it produces at the point where the marginal cost curve intersects the perfectly elastic firm demand curve. The perfectly elastic firm demand curve represents the marginal revenue curve for the pure competitor, for the same average revenues are obtained on all the units sold. Perfect competitors maximize profits at MR = MC, as do pure monopolists. But the perfect competitor makes no true economic profits in the long run; rather, all it makes is a normal, competitive rate of return.

In Chapter 23, we talked about companies experiencing short-run economic profits because they had, for example, invented something new. Competition, though, gradually eroded those higher than normal profits. The fact that a firm experiences higher than normal profits today does not mean that it has a monopoly forever. Try as companies may, keeping competitors away is never easy.

No Guarantee of Profits

The term *monopoly* conjures up the notion of a greedy firm ripping off the public and making exorbitant profits. However, the mere existence of a monopoly does not guarantee high profits. Numerous monopolies have gone bankrupt. Figure 24-7 shows the monopolist's demand curve as D and the resultant marginal revenue curve as MR. It does not matter at what rate of output this particular monopolist operates; total costs cannot be covered. Look at the position of the average total cost curve. It lies everywhere above D (the average revenue curve). Thus there is no price-output combination that will allow the monopolist even to cover costs, much less earn profits. This monopolist will, in the short run, suffer economic losses as shown by the shaded area. The graph in Figure 24-7 depicts a situation for millions of typical monopolies that exist; they are called inventions. The owner of a patented invention or discovery has a pure legal monopoly, but the demand and cost curves may be such that production is not profitable. Every year at inventors' conventions, one can see many inventions that have never been put into production because they were deemed "uneconomic" by potential producers and users.

CONCEPTS IN BRIEF

- The basic difference between a monopolist and a perfect competitor is that a monopolist faces a downward-sloping demand curve, and therefore marginal revenue is less than price.
- The monopolist must choose the profit-maximizing price-output combination—the output at which marginal revenue equals marginal cost and the highest price possible as given by the demand curve for that particular output rate.
- Monopoly short-run profits are found by looking at average total costs compared to price per unit. This difference multiplied by quantity sold at that price determines monopoly profit.
- A monopolist does not necessarily earn a profit. If the average total cost curve lies entirely above the demand curve for a monopoly, production will not be profitable.

ON MAKING HIGHER PROFITS: PRICE DISCRIMINATION 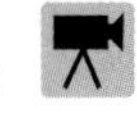

In a perfectly competitive market, each buyer is charged the same price for every unit of the particular commodity (corrected for differential transportation charges). Because the product is homogeneous and we also assume full knowledge on the part of the buyers, a difference in price cannot exist. Any seller of the product who tried to charge a price higher than the going market price would find that no one would purchase it from that seller.

In this chapter we have assumed until now that the monopolist charged all consumers the same price for all units. A monopolist, however, may be able to charge different people different prices or different unit prices for successive units sought by a given buyer. When there is no cost difference, either one or a combination of these strategies is called **price discrimination.** A firm will engage in price discrimination whenever feasible to increase profits. A price-discriminating firm is able to charge some customers more than other customers.

Price discrimination 
Selling a given product at more than one price, with the price difference being unrelated to differences in cost.

It must be made clear at the outset that charging different prices to different people or for different units that reflect differences in the cost of service to those particular people does not amount to price discrimination. This is **price differentiation:** differences in price that reflect differences in marginal cost.

Price differentiation 
Establishing different prices for similar products to reflect differences in marginal cost in providing those commodities to different groups of buyers.

We can also say that a uniform price does not necessarily indicate an absence of price discrimination. Charging all customers the same price when production costs vary by customer is actually a case of price discrimination.

Necessary Conditions for Price Discrimination

Four conditions are necessary for price discrimination to exist:

1. The firm must face a downward-sloping demand curve.
2. The firm must be able to separate markets at a reasonable cost.
3. The buyers in the various markets must have different price elasticities of demand.
4. The firm must be able to prevent resale of the product or service.

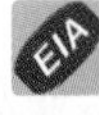

Monopolistic Price Discrimination
See how a monopolist can segment a market for its product to allow it to engage in price discrimination.

For example, charging students a lower price than nonstudents for a movie can be done relatively easily. The cost of checking student IDs is apparently not significant. Also, it is fairly easy to make sure that students do not resell their tickets to nonstudents.

EXAMPLE

Cheaper Airfares for Some, Exorbitant Fares for Others

First-class airfares are often stunningly higher than coach class—far higher than any additional marginal cost warrants. This is a good example of price discrimination. And even in coach class, there may be fare differences of 800 percent. All coach passengers are packed in like sardines, so why the difference in price among them? The answer is again price discrimination, but this time it is based on how badly a person wants to fly. If you are a businessperson who is called to a meeting for the next day, you want to fly very badly. The fact that your company will not allow you to fly first class will not save you from having to pay, say, $2,000 to fly round-trip from Cincinnati to Los Angeles, particularly if you do not stay over on a Saturday. The Saturday stay-over requirement for low fares neatly differentiates individuals who must travel from those who have the time to stay over—people on business trips versus people on leisure trips. If you have a relatively high price elasticity of demand, you will also want to take advantage of low fares that require 7 days', 14 days', or longer advance purchase. The more price-sensitive you are, the more you will pay attention to such cheap-fare requirements, and the lower will be the fare you are likely to pay.

Airlines, with sophisticated computer programs performing what is known as yield management, are also able to change prices constantly. Such programs allow them to project relatively precisely how many last-minute business travelers are going to pay full fare to get on a flight. Computerized yield management works so well because of a mathematical formula that Bell Laboratories patented in 1988. It allows rapid calculations on fare problems with thousands of variables. The airlines compare historical databases on ridership with what is happening in terms of bookings right now. A typical flight will be divided into seven fare "buckets" that may have a differential of as much as 800 percent. The yield management computers constantly adjust the number of seats available in each bucket. When advance bookings are few, more seats are added to the low-fare buckets. When advance bookings are above normal, more seats are added to the highest-fare buckets. The result is lower fares for many and much higher fares for a few. In essence, the airlines are attempting to hit every "price point" on the demand curve for airline travel, as is shown in Figure 24-8.

For Critical Analysis

Assuming that the Bell Laboratories mathematical formula had been available 25 years ago, why couldn't airlines have used it then?

FIGURE 24-8

Toward Perfect Price Discrimination

What the airlines attempt to do by dividing any particular round-trip fare into "buckets" is to price-discriminate as finely as possible. Here we show the airlines setting seven different prices for the same round trip. Those who pay price P_7 are the ones who are the last to ask for a reservation. Those who pay price P_1 are the ones who planned furthest in advance or happened to hit it lucky when seats were added to the low-fare bucket.

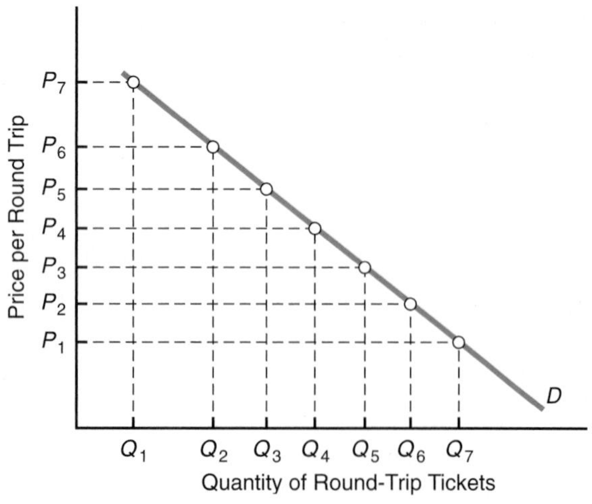

THE SOCIAL COST OF MONOPOLIES

Let's run a little experiment. We will start with a purely competitive industry with numerous firms, each one unable to affect the price of its product. The supply curve of the industry is equal to the horizontal sum of the marginal cost curves of the individual producers above their respective minimum average variable costs. In panel (a) of Figure 24-9, we show the market demand curve and the market supply curve in a perfectly competitive situation. The competitive price in equilibrium is equal to P_e, and the equilibrium quantity at that price is equal to Q_e. Each individual competitor faces a demand curve (not shown) that is coincident with the price line P_e. No individual supplier faces the market demand curve, *D*.

Now let's assume that a monopolist comes in and buys up every single competitor in the industry. In so doing, we'll assume that the monopolist does not affect any of the marginal cost curves or demand. We can therefore redraw *D* and *S* in panel (b) of Figure 24-9, exactly the same as in panel (a).

How does this monopolist decide how much to charge and how much to produce? If the monopolist is profit-maximizing, it is going to look at the marginal revenue curve and produce at the output where marginal revenue equals marginal cost. But what is the marginal cost curve in panel (b) of Figure 24-9? It is merely *S*, because we said that *S* was equal to

FIGURE 24-9

The Effects of Monopolizing an Industry

In panel (a), we show a competitive situation in which equilibrium is established at the intersection of *D* and *S* at point *E*. The equilibrium price would be P_e, and the equilibrium quantity would be Q_e. Each individual competitive producer faces a demand curve that is a horizontal line at the market clearing price, P_e. What happens if the industry is suddenly monopolized? We assume that the costs stay the same; the only thing that changes is that the monopolist now faces the entire downward-sloping demand curve. In panel (b), we draw the marginal revenue curve. Marginal cost is *S* because that is the horizontal summation of all the individual marginal cost curves. The monopolist therefore produces at Q_m and charges price P_m. This price P_m in panel (b) is higher than P_e in panel (a), and Q_m is less than Q_e. We see, then, that a monopolist charges a higher price and produces less than an industry in a competitive situation.

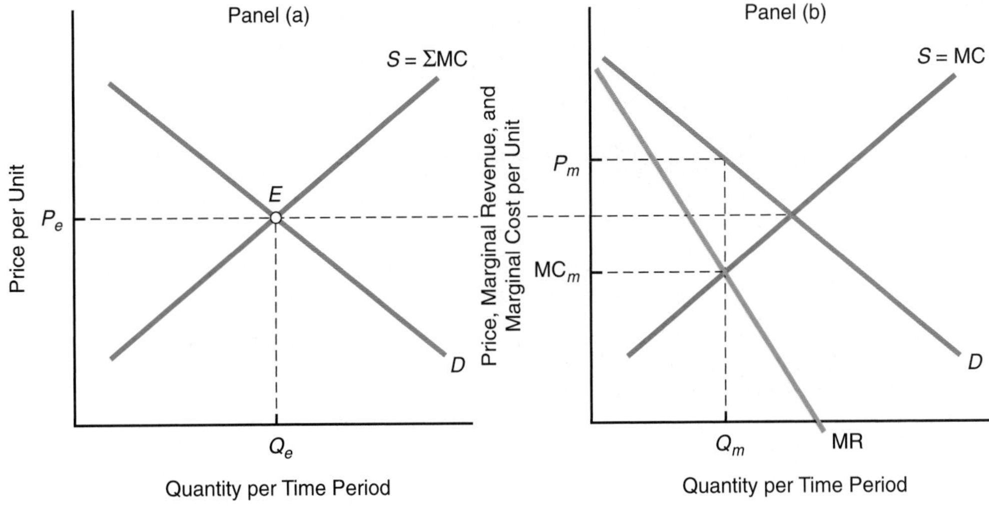

the horizontal summation of the portions of the individual marginal cost curves above each firm's respective minimum average variable cost. The monopolist therefore produces quantity Q_m and sells it at price P_m. Notice that Q_m is less than Q_e and that P_m is greater than P_e. A monopolist therefore produces a smaller quantity and sells it at a higher price. This is the reason usually given when economists criticize monopolists. Monopolists raise the price and restrict production, compared to a competitive situation. For a monopolist's product, consumers are forced to pay a price that exceeds the marginal cost of production. Resources are misallocated in such a situation—too few resources are being used in the monopolist's industry, and too many are used elsewhere.

Notice from Figure 24-9 that by setting MR = MC, the monopolist produces at a rate of output where $P > \text{MC}$ (compare P_m to MC_m). The marginal cost of a commodity (MC) represents what society had to give up in order to obtain the last unit produced. Price, by contrast, represents what buyers are willing to pay to acquire that last unit. Thus the price of a good represents society's valuation of the last unit produced. The monopoly outcome of $P > \text{MC}$ means that the value to society of the last unit produced is greater than its cost (MC); hence not enough of the good is being produced. As we have pointed out before, these differences between monopoly and competition arise not because of differences in costs but rather because of differences in the demand curves the individual firms face. The monopolist has monopoly power because it faces a downward-sloping demand curve. The individual perfect competitor faces a perfectly elastic demand curve.

Before we leave the topic of the cost to society of monopolies, we must repeat that our analysis is based on a heroic assumption. That assumption is that the monopolization of the perfectly competitive industry does not change the cost structure. If monopolization results in higher marginal cost, the cost to society is even greater. Conversely, if monopolization results in cost savings, the cost, if any, to society is less than we infer from our analysis. Indeed, we could have presented a hypothetical example in which monopolization led to such a dramatic reduction in average cost that society actually benefited. Such a situation is a possibility in industries in which economies of scale exist for a very great range of outputs.

CONCEPTS IN BRIEF

- Four conditions are necessary for price discrimination: (1) The firm must face a downward-sloping demand curve, (2) the firm must be able to distinguish markets, (3) buyers in different markets must have different price elasticities of demand, and (4) resale of the product or service must be preventable.
- A monopolist can make higher profits if it can price-discriminate. Price discrimination requires that two or more identifiable classes of buyers exist whose price elasticities of demand for the product or service are different and that these two classes of buyers can be distinguished at little cost.
- Price differentiation should not be confused with price discrimination. The former occurs when differences in price reflect differences in marginal cost.
- Monopoly results in a lower quantity being sold, because the price is higher than it would be in an ideal perfectly competitive industry in which the cost curves were essentially the same as the monopolist's.

NETNOMICS

Arrest That Software! It's Practicing Law Without a License!

Not long ago, a U.S. district court judge in Texas ruled that Internet downloads and computer shop purchases of Quicken Family Lawyer, a software program, are illegal activities in that state. Why? The program was too good. It went beyond allowing users to print out prepackaged versions of wills and other legal documents. It permitted users to *customize* legal documents by asking questions such as how many children they had or where they lived—in other words, soliciting the kind of information for which people lavishly pay lawyers to incorporate into customized wills.

Arguments in favor of making the software available to Texas consumers fell on deaf ears. The judge ruled that the software enabled the "unauthorized practice of law," and only lawyers, he decided, can customize legal documents. In other words, lawyers have the legal right to be free of competition from computer software.

Critics of the decision questioned the state's capability to enforce the decision. They wondered if Texas police will search people for minidisks at the Oklahoma border or if all Internet traffic will have to be routed through state offices. A more basic question was whether it is legal, under the judge's ruling, to purchase a legal textbook. After all, a textbook can teach a person to do everything the software program does, thereby permitting anyone to compete with lawyers and reduce their market power.

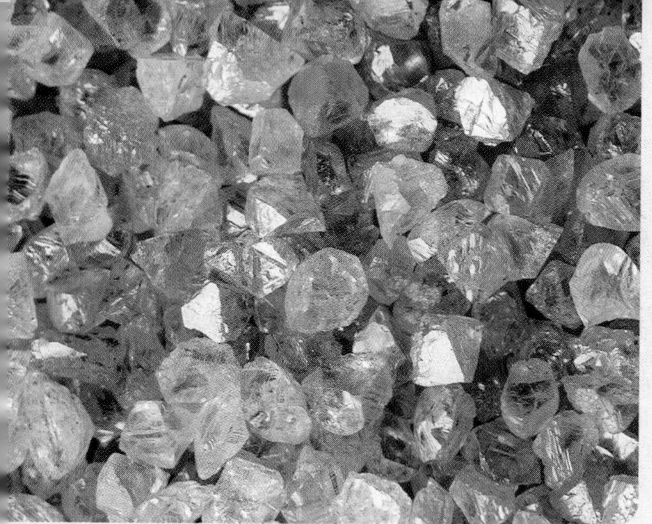

Issues & Applications

Trying to Open a Crack in the Diamond Cartel

The De Beers diamond cartel is so named because the De Beers diamond-mining company of South Africa coordinates its actions. At the center of the cartel's operations is the De Beers marketing subsidiary, the Central Selling Organization (CSO). By restricting diamond sales each year, the CSO aims to maximize profits earned by De Beers and other members of a global cartel of diamond producers.

Concepts Applied

- Market Power
- Monopoly
- Entry
- Competition

Tough Times in the Diamond Cartel

A key to the cartel's profit-maximizing effort has been a coordinated attempt to restrict world diamond sales. To ensure that only a carefully regulated quantity of diamonds makes its way into the marketplace, the CSO regularly purchases diamonds from companies that are not part of the cartel. Between 1986 and 1998, the result was a 50 percent increase in diamond prices.

Since 1998, however, things have not gone so smoothly for the cartel. On the one hand, there was a 5 percent drop in the world demand for diamonds. On the other hand, Russian producers, squeezed by a weakening national economy, violated their contract with the CSO and began selling large volumes of low-quality, so-called near-gem diamonds. When the CSO retaliated by sharply reducing the price it would pay to buy low-quality diamonds, British and Australian companies that also sold near-gem diamonds responded by breaking with the CSO's restraints on diamond sales. Both of these events combined to push down diamond prices by as much as 20 percent. Overall, De Beers's 1998 revenues from diamond sales dropped by more than one-fourth, the second-biggest one-year drop in the company's sales since the end of the Great Depression.

Segmenting the Diamond Market

The De Beers cartel has not given up on keeping its market power, however. Because it produces so many of the world's high-quality diamonds, De Beers has sought to distinguish its diamonds from those produced by others. The demand for these "true-gem" diamonds tends to be less elastic, and that permits De Beers to earn more profits if it can maintain a higher price. To emphasize the higher quality of the diamonds it produces—and hence reinforce the demand for "true gems"—De Beers has begun etching serial numbers on the diamonds it sells. These numbers, plus a De Beers logo also etched into the gems, are invisible to the human eye but can be viewed with special instruments. In the meantime, the CSO continues to restrict the supply of high-quality gems to the world's market. Its stockpile of unsold diamonds has continued to grow.

Simultaneously, the CSO let the world price of low-quality diamonds drop so low that Russian producers found themselves losing money. In the end, most Russian diamond firms rejoined the De Beers cartel and stopped "leaking" low-quality gems into the market. Nevertheless, some experts predict that open competition in diamonds will emerge eventually—at least in the low-quality market. In the market for high-quality diamonds, however, the De Beers cartel still has a firm grip on production and pricing. Indeed, De Beers has been trying to bolster the CSO's market share by seeking joint ventures with other miners of high-quality gems. A key feature of these ventures, of course, is an agreement by the parties to sell only a fraction of the diamonds that are mined.

FOR CRITICAL ANALYSIS

1. Why is withholding a large stockpile of diamonds from the marketplace in the interests of De Beers?
2. Why can other individual mining companies gain, at least in the short term, from violating CSO contracts to restrict their production and sales of diamonds?

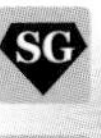

SUMMARY DISCUSSION OF LEARNING OBJECTIVES

1. **Why Monopoly Can Occur:** Monopoly, a situation in which a single firm produces and sells a good or service, can occur when there are significant barriers to market entry by other firms. Examples of barriers to entry include (1) ownership of important resources for which there are no close substitutes, (2) problems in raising adequate capital to begin production, (3) economies of scale for even large ranges of output, or natural monopoly conditions, (4) legal or governmental restrictions, and (5) associations of productions called cartels that work together to stifle competition.
2. **Demand and Marginal Revenue Conditions a Monopolist Faces:** Because a monopolist constitutes the entire industry, it faces the entire market demand curve. When it reduces the price of its product, it is able to sell more units at the new price, which pushes up its revenues, but it also sells other units at this lower price, which pushes its revenues down somewhat. For this reason, the monopolist's marginal revenue at any given quantity of production is less than the price at which it sells that quantity of output. Hence the monopolist's marginal revenue curve slopes downward and lies below the demand curve it faces.
3. **How a Monopolist Determines How Much Output to Produce and What Price to Charge:** A monopolist is a price searcher, meaning that it seeks to charge the price consistent with the production level that maximizes its economic profits. It maximizes its profits by producing to the point at which marginal revenue equals marginal cost. The monopolist then charges the maximum price for this amount of output, which is the price that consumers are willing to pay for that quantity of output.
4. **A Monopolist's Profits:** The amount of profit earned by a monopolist is equal to the difference between the price it charges and its average production cost times the amount of output it produces and sells. At the profit-maximizing output rate, the monopolist's price is at the point on the demand curve corresponding to this output rate, and its average total cost of producing this output rate is at the corresponding point on the monopolist's average total cost curve. Typically, a monopolist earns positive economic profits, but situations can arise in which average total cost exceeds the profit-maximizing price. In this case, the maximum profit is negative, and the monopolist earns an economic loss.
5. **Price Discrimination:** If a monopolist engages in price discrimination, it sells its product at more than one price, with the price difference being unrelated to differences in production costs. To be able to engage successfully in price discrimination, a monopolist must be able to identify and separate buyers with different price elasticities of demand. This allows the monopolist to sell some of its output at higher prices to consumers with less elastic demand. Even then, however, the monopolist must be able to prevent resale of its product by those with less elastic demand who can buy it at a lower price.
6. **Social Cost of Monopolies:** Because a monopoly is a price searcher, it is able to charge the highest price that people are willing to pay for the amount of output it produces. This price exceeds the marginal cost of producing the output. In addition, if the monopolist's marginal cost curve corresponds to the sum of the marginal cost curves for a number of firms that would exist if the industry were perfectly competitive instead, then the monopolist produces and sells less output than perfectly competitive firms would have produced and sold. Consequently, a monopolist sells output at a higher price and produces less output than would be produced under perfect competition.

Key Terms and Concepts

Cartel (593)

Monopolist (589)

Natural monopoly (591)

Price differentiation (603)

Price discrimination (603)

Price searcher (597)

Tariffs (593)

Problems

Answers to the odd-numbered problems appear at the back of the book.

24-1. An international coffee cartel exists to smooth market supply and price fluctuations over the growing seasons. Since the 1960s, the number of coffee-exporting countries has grown dramatically. Explain the likely effect of this trend on the prospects for maintaining a successful coffee cartel.

24-2. Discuss the difference in the price elasticity of demand for an individual firm in a perfectly competitive industry as compared with a monopolist. Explain, in economic terms, why the price elasticities are different.

24-3. The following table depicts the daily output, price, and costs of the only dry cleaner located near the campus of a small college town in a remote location. The dry cleaner is effectively a monopolist.

Output (suits cleaned)	Price per Suit ($)	Total Costs ($)
0	8.00	3.00
1	7.50	6.00
2	7.00	8.50
3	6.50	10.50
4	6.00	11.50
5	5.50	13.50
6	5.00	16.00
7	4.50	19.00
8	4.00	24.00

a. Calculate the dry cleaner's total revenue and total profit at each output level.

b. What is the profit-maximizing level of output?

24-4. Given the information in Problem 24-3, calculate the dry cleaner's marginal revenue and marginal cost at each output level. Based on marginal analysis, what is the profit-maximizing level of output?

24-5. A manager of a monopoly firm notices that the firm is producing output at a rate at which average total cost is falling but is not at its minimum feasible point. The manager argues that surely the firm must not be maximizing its economic profits. Is this argument correct? Explain.

24-6. Referring to the accompanying diagram, answer the following questions.

a. What is monopolist's profit-maximizing rate of output?

b. At the profit-maximizing output rate, what are the monopolist's average total cost and average revenue?

c. At the profit-maximizing output rate, what are the monopolist's total cost and total revenue?

d. What is the maximum profit?

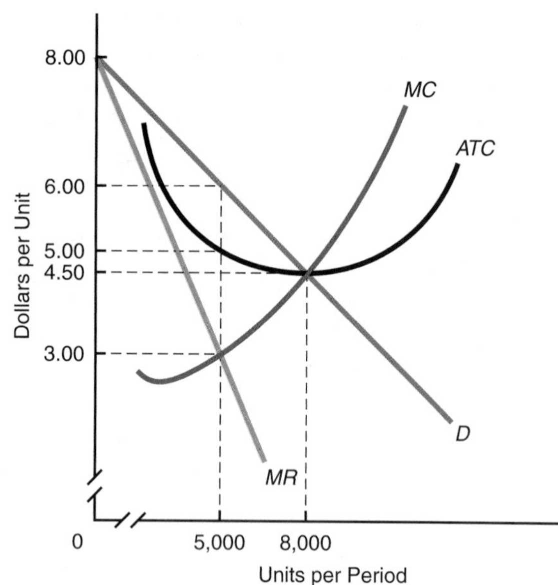

24-7. Using the diagram for Problem 24-6, suppose that the marginal cost and average total cost curves also illustrate the horizontal summation of the individual firms in a competitive industry in the long run. Based on this, what would the market price and equilibrium output be if the market were competitive? Explain the economic cost to society of allowing a monopoly to exist in this industry.

24-8. For each of the following examples, explain how and why a firm with monopoly power would attempt to price-discriminate.

a. Providing air travel for business people and tourists

b. A fastfood restaurant that serves business people and retired people

c. A theater that shows the same movie to large families and to individuals and couples

24-9. A monopolist finds that it is currently producing output at a rate at which the total revenue it earns varies directly with the price it charges. Is the monopolist maximizing its economic profits? Why or why not?

24-10. A new competitor enters the industry and competes with a second firm, which up to this point had been a monopolist. The second firm finds that although demand is not perfectly elastic, it is now relatively more elastic. What will happen to the marginal revenue curve and to the profit-maximizing price that the monopolist charges?

24-11. Because of an increase in the price of resources that are inputs in its production process, a monopolist finds that its marginal cost curve has shifted upward. What is likely to happen to the monopolist's price, output rate, and economic profits?

Economics on the Net

Patents, Trademarks, and Intellectual Property Governments often grant legal protections against efforts to copy new products. This Internet application gives you the opportunity to explore one company's view on the advantages of alternative forms of protection.

Title: Intellectual Property

Navigation: Click here to visit the GlaxoSmithKline Web site. Select Investor Relations, then Financial Reports. View the GlaxoWellcome Annual Report 1999. Scroll down to Intellectual Property (Page 18.)

Application Read the statement on intellectual property and the accompanying table.

1. What does intellectual property include? What are the differences between patents, trademarks, and registered designs and copyrights?
2. What are GlaxoWellcome's objectives regarding intellectual property? What seems to be more important, patents or trademarks? In what areas of medical research does GlaxoWellcome excel?

For Group Discussion and Analysis In 1969, GlaxoWellcome developed Ventolin, a treatment for asthma symptoms. Though the patent and trademark have long expired, the company still retains over a third of the market in this treatment. Explain, in economic terms, the source of GlaxoWellcome's strength in this area. Discuss whether patents and trademarks are beneficial for the development and discovery of new treatments.

CHAPTER

25

MONOPOLISTIC COMPETITION, OLIGOPOLY, AND STRATEGIC BEHAVIOR

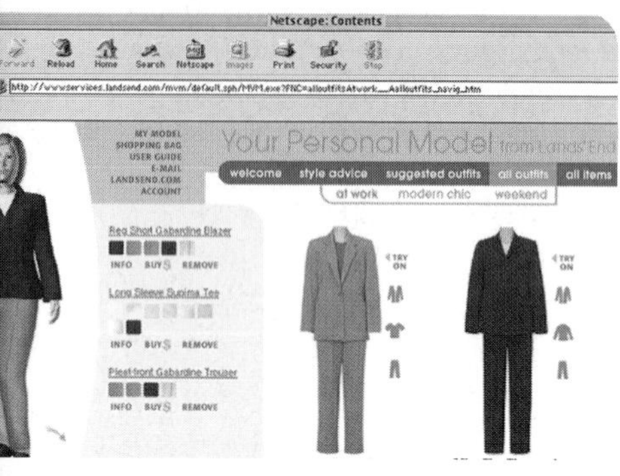

Here is a Web page from the Lands' End site, where Internet shoppers can "try on" different styles and combinations of clothes. Will on-line customization of clothing affect traditional retailers?

If you shop at the Web site of direct retailer Lands' End, you can create a "3-D, personalized shopping model" with your exact measurements. Do you want to see how a blue, nine-button blouse will look with plaid pants? Just click and drag the clothes together for a look. The company's Web site has other features, including a personalized e-mail service alerting customers to sales on the latest in their favorite fashions. By making its Web site interesting and useful, Lands' End seeks to differentiate its brand name from those of its many rivals. The company wants to grab customers away from other apparel sellers, and it wants to keep those customers. To understand the actions of firms that sell similar but differentiated goods, you must learn about monopolistic competition, one subject of this chapter.

LEARNING OBJECTIVES

After reading this chapter, you should be able to:

1. Discuss the key characteristics of a monopolistically competitive industry
2. Contrast the output and pricing decisions of monopolistically competitive firms with those of perfectly competitive firms
3. Outline the fundamental characteristics of oligopoly
4. Understand how to apply game theory to evaluate the pricing strategies of oligopolistic firms
5. Explain the kinked demand theory of oligopolistic price rigidity
6. Describe theories of how firms may deter market entry by potential rivals

Did You Know That... 80 percent of initial customer contacts for General Motors' Saturn division now originate on the Internet? GM's first Saturn Web site offered lots of car specifications and dealer referrals, but few people visited the site. Then the company added more useful features, such as an auto lease pricing calculator, an interactive design shop for experimenting with the looks of alternative car options, and on-line order forms for Saturns. GM vigorously promoted these on-line features in a television commercial showing a college student buying a Saturn over the Internet. Within weeks, the number of Web surfers visiting the Saturn site tripled to as many as 7,000 per day.

In their quest to let people know of their existence and products, American businesses will leave no stone unturned—and no corner of cyberspace unexplored. Companies pull out all the stops to inform people about what they sell, where people can buy it, and at what price.

Advertising did not show up in our analysis of perfect competition. Nevertheless, it plays a large role in industries that cannot be described as perfectly competitive but cannot be described as pure monopolies either. A combination of consumers' preferences for variety and competition among producers has led to similar but *differentiated* products in the marketplace. This situation has been described as *monopolistic competition,* the subject of the first part of this chapter. In the second part of the chapter, we look at firms that are neither perfect competitors nor pure monopolists that do not have to worry about actual competitors. And clearly, perfect competitors cannot make any strategic decisions, for they must take the market price as given. We call firms that have the ability to make strategic decisions *oligopolies,* which we will define more formally later in this chapter.

Chapter Outline 

MONOPOLISTIC COMPETITION 

In the 1920s and 1930s, economists became increasingly aware that there were many industries for which both the perfectly competitive model and the pure monopoly model did not apply and did not seem to yield very accurate predictions. Theoretical and empirical research was instituted to develop some sort of middle ground. Two separately developed models of **monopolistic competition** resulted. At Harvard, Edward Chamberlin published *Theory of Monopolistic Competition* in 1933. The same year, Britain's Joan Robinson published *The Economics of Imperfect Competition.* In this chapter, we will outline the theory as presented by Chamberlin.

Monopolistic competition 
A market situation in which a large number of firms produce similar but not identical products. Entry into the industry is relatively easy.

Chamberlin defined monopolistic competition as a market structure in which there is a relatively large number of producers offering similar but differentiated products. Monopolistic competition therefore has the following features:

1. Significant numbers of sellers in a highly competitive market
2. Differentiated products
3. Sales promotion and advertising
4. Easy entry of new firms in the long run

Even a cursory look at the American economy leads to the conclusion that monopolistic competition is an important form of market structure in the United States. Indeed, that is true of all developed economies.

Number of Firms

In a perfectly competitive situation, there is an extremely large number of firms; in pure monopoly, there is only one. In monopolistic competition, there is a large number of firms, but not as many as in perfect competition. This fact has several important implications for a monopolistically competitive industry.

1. *Small share of market.* With so many firms, each firm has a relatively small share of the total market.
2. *Lack of collusion.* With so many firms, it is very difficult for all of them to get together to collude—to cooperate in setting a pure monopoly price (and output). Price rigging in a monopolistically competitive industry is virtually impossible. Also, barriers to entry are minor, and the flow of new firms into the industry makes collusive agreements less likely. The large number of firms makes the monitoring and detection of cheating very costly and extremely difficult. This difficulty is compounded by differentiated products and high rates of innovation; collusive agreements are easier for a homogeneous product than for heterogeneous ones.
3. *Independence.* Because there are so many firms, each one acts independently of the others. No firm attempts to take into account the reaction of all of its rival firms—that would be impossible with so many rivals. Rivals' reactions to output and price changes are largely ignored.

Product Differentiation

Product differentiation 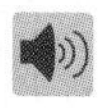
The distinguishing of products by brand name, color, and other minor attributes. Product differentiation occurs in other than perfectly competitive markets in which products are, in theory, homogeneous, such as wheat or corn.

Perhaps the most important feature of the monopolistically competitive market is **product differentiation.** We can say that each individual manufacturer of a product has an absolute monopoly over its own product, which is slightly differentiated from other similar products. This means that the firm has some control over the price it charges. Unlike the perfectly competitive firm, it faces a downward-sloping demand curve.

Consider the abundance of brand names for toothpaste, soap, gasoline, vitamins, shampoo, and most other consumer goods and a great many services. We are not obliged to buy just one type of television set, just one type of jeans, or just one type of footwear. There are usually a number of similar but differentiated products from which to choose. One reason is that the greater a firm's success at product differentiation, the greater the firm's pricing options.

Each separate differentiated product has numerous similar substitutes. This clearly has an impact on the price elasticity of demand for the individual firm. Recall that one determinant of price elasticity of demand is the availability of substitutes: The greater the number and closeness of substitutes available, other things being equal, the greater the price elasticity of demand. If the consumer has a vast array of alternatives that are just about as good as the product under study, a relatively small increase in the price of that product will lead many consumers to switch to one of the many close substitutes. Thus the ability of a firm to raise the price above the price of *close* substitutes is very small. The result of this is that even though the demand curve slopes downward, it does so only slightly. In other words, it is relatively elastic (over that price range) compared to a monopolist's demand curve. In the extreme case, with perfect competition, the substitutes are perfect because we are dealing with only one particular undifferentiated product. In that case, the individual firm has a perfectly elastic demand curve.

Ease of Entry

For any current monopolistic competitor, potential competition is always lurking in the background. The easier—that is, the less costly—entry is, the more a current monopolistic competitor must worry about losing business.

A good example of a monopolistic competitive industry is the computer software industry. Many small firms provide different programs for many applications. The fixed capital costs required to enter this industry are small; all you need are skilled programmers. In addition, there are few legal restrictions. The firms in this industry also engage in extensive advertising in over 150 computer publications.

Sales Promotion and Advertising

Monopolistic competition differs from perfect competition in that no individual firm in a perfectly competitive market will advertise. A perfectly competitive firm, by definition, can sell all that it wants to sell at the going market price anyway. Why, then, would it spend even one penny on advertising? Furthermore, by definition, the perfect competitor is selling a product that is identical to the product that all other firms in the industry are selling. Any advertisement that induces consumers to buy more of that product will, in effect, be helping all the competitors, too. A perfect competitor therefore cannot be expected to incur any advertising costs (except for all firms in an industry collectively agreeing to advertise to urge the public to buy more beef or drink more milk).

But because the monopolistic competitor has at least *some* monopoly power, advertising may result in increased profits. Advertising is used to increase demand and to differentiate one's product. How much advertising should be undertaken? It should be carried to the point at which the additional revenue from one more dollar of advertising just equals that one dollar of marginal cost.

Advertising as Signaling Behavior. Recall from Chapter 23 that signals are compact gestures or actions that convey information. For example, high profits in an industry are signals that resources should flow to that industry. Individual companies can explicitly engage in signaling behavior. They do so by establishing brand names or trademarks, and then promoting them heavily. This is a signal to prospective consumers that this is a company that plans to stay in business. Before the modern age of advertising, banks in America faced a problem of signaling their soundness. They chose to make the bank building large, imposing, and constructed out of marble and granite. Stone communicated permanence. The effect was to give the bank's customers confidence that they were not doing business with a fly-by-night operation.

When Dell Computer advertises its brand name heavily, it incurs substantial costs. The only way it can recoup those costs is by selling lots of Dell computers over a long period of time. Thus heavy advertising of its brand name is a signal to personal computer buyers that Dell is interested in each customer's repeat business.

But what about advertising that does not seem to convey any information, not even about price? What good is an advertisement for, say, Wal-Mart that simply states, "We give you value that you can count on"?

EXAMPLE

Can Advertising Lead to Efficiency?

Advertising budgets by major retailers may just seem like an added expense, not a step on the road to economic efficiency. According to research by economists Kyle Bagwell of Northwestern University and Garey Ramey of the University of California at San Diego, just the opposite is true. When retailers advertise heavily, they increase the number of shoppers that come to their store. Such increased traffic allows retailers to offer a wider selection of goods, to invest in cost-reduction technology (such as computerized inventory and satellite communications), and to exploit manufacturers' quantity discounts. Such cost reductions can help explain the success of Wal-Mart, Circuit City, and Home Depot. Consequently, Bagwell and Ramey conclude that advertising can help promote efficiency even if it provides no "hard" information. Advertising signals to consumers where they can find big-company, low-priced, high-variety stores.

For Critical Analysis

Which is true, then: "We are bigger because we are better" or "We are better because we are bigger"?

CONCEPTS IN BRIEF

- Monopolistic competition is a market structure that lies between pure monopoly and perfect competition.
- A monopolistically competitive market structure has (1) a large number of sellers, (2) differentiated products, (3) advertising, and (4) easy entry of firms in the long run.
- Because of the large number of firms, each has a small share of the market, making collusion difficult; the firms are independent.

PRICE AND OUTPUT FOR THE MONOPOLISTIC COMPETITOR

Now that we are aware of the assumptions underlying the monopolistic competition model, we can analyze the price and output behavior of each firm in a monopolistically competitive industry. We assume in the analysis that follows that the desired product type and quality have been chosen. We further assume that the budget and the type of promotional activity have already been chosen and do not change.

The Individual Firm's Demand and Cost Curves

Because the individual firm is not a perfect competitor, its demand curve slopes downward, as is shown in all three panels of Figure 25-1. Hence it faces a marginal revenue curve that is also downward-sloping and below the demand curve. To find the profit-maximizing rate of output and the profit-maximizing price, we go to the output where the marginal cost curve intersects the marginal revenue curve from below. That gives us the profit-maximizing output rate. Then we draw a vertical line up to the demand curve. That gives us the price that can be charged to sell exactly that quantity produced. This is what we have done in Figure 25-1. In each panel, a marginal cost curve intersects the marginal revenue curve at *E*. The profit-maximizing rate of output is q_e, and the profit-maximizing price is *P*.

Short-Run Equilibrium

In the short run, it is possible for a monopolistic competitor to make economic profits—profits over and above the normal rate of return or beyond what is necessary to keep that firm in that industry. We show such a situation in panel (a) of Figure 25-1. The average total cost curve is drawn in below the demand curve, *d*, at the profit-maximizing rate of output, q_e. Economic profits are shown by the shaded rectangle in that panel.

Losses in the short run are clearly also possible. They are presented in panel (b) of Figure 25-1. Here the average total cost curve lies everywhere above the individual firm's demand curve, *d*. The losses are marked as the shaded rectangle.

FIGURE 25-1

Short-Run and Long-Run Equilibrium with Monopolistic Competition

In panel (a), the typical monopolistic competitor is shown making economic profits. If that were the situation, there would be entry into the industry, forcing the demand curve for the individual monopolistic competitor leftward. Eventually, firms would find themselves in the situation depicted in panel (c), where zero economic profits are being made. In panel (b), the typical firm is in a monopolistically competitive industry making economic losses. If that were the case, firms would leave the industry. Each remaining firm's demand curve would shift outward to the right. Eventually, the typical firm would find itself in the situation depicted in panel (c).

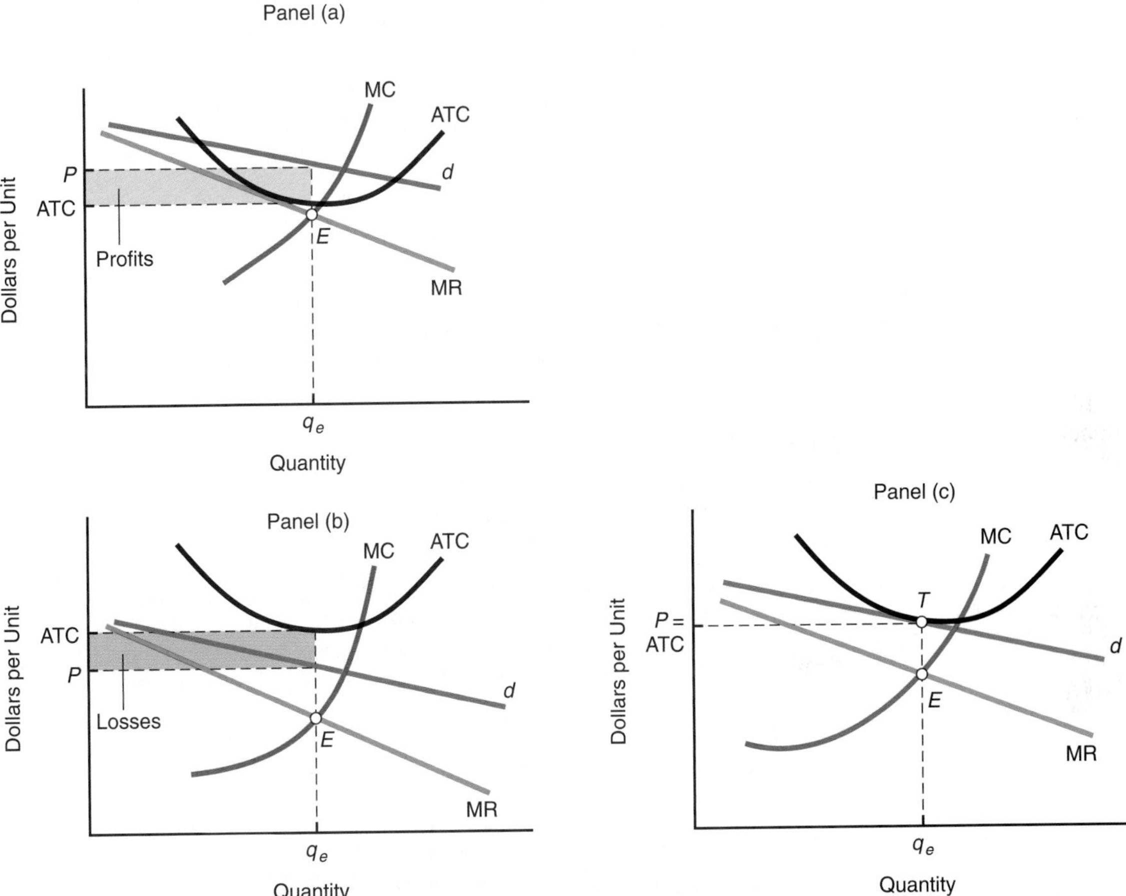

Just as with any market structure or any firm, in the short run it is possible to observe either economic profits or economic losses. (In the long run such is not the case with monopolistic competition, however.) In either case, the price does not equal marginal cost but rather is above it. Therefore, there is some misallocation of resources, a topic that we will discuss later in this chapter.

The Long Run: Zero Economic Profits

The long run is where the similarity between perfect competition and monopolistic competition becomes more obvious. In the long run, because so many firms produce substitutes for the product in question, any economic profits will disappear with competition. They

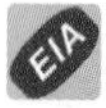

Monopolistic Competition
Further study monopolistic competition.

will be reduced to zero either through entry by new firms seeing a chance to make a higher rate of return than elsewhere or by changes in product quality and advertising outlays by existing firms in the industry. (Profitable products will be imitated by other firms.) As for economic losses in the short run, they will disappear in the long run because the firms that suffer them will leave the industry. They will go into another business where the expected rate of return is at least normal. Panels (a) and (b) of Figure 25-1 therefore represent only short-run situations for a monopolistically competitive firm. In the long run, the individual firm's demand curve *d* will just touch the average total cost curve at the particular price that is profit-maximizing for that particular firm. This is shown in panel (c) of Figure 25-1.

A word of warning: This is an idealized, long-run equilibrium situation for each firm in the industry. It does not mean that even in the long run we will observe every single firm in a monopolistically competitive industry making *exactly* zero economic profits or *just* a normal rate of return. We live in a dynamic world. All we are saying is that if this model is correct, the rate of return will *tend toward* normal—economic profits will *tend toward* zero.

COMPARING PERFECT COMPETITION WITH MONOPOLISTIC COMPETITION

If both the monopolistic competitor and the perfect competitor make zero economic profits in the long run, how are they different? The answer lies in the fact that the demand curve for the individual perfect competitor is perfectly elastic. Such is not the case for the individual

FIGURE 25-2

Comparison of the Perfect Competitor with the Monopolistic Competitor

In panel (a), the perfectly competitive firm has zero economic profits in the long run. The price is set equal to marginal cost, and the price is P_1. The firm's demand curve is just tangent to the minimum point on its average total cost curve, which means that the firm is operating at an optimum rate of production. With the monopolistically competitive firm in panel (b), there are also zero economic profits in the long run. The price is greater than marginal cost; the monopolistically competitive firm does not find itself at the minimum point on its average total cost curve. It is operating at a rate of output to the left of the minimum point on the ATC curve.

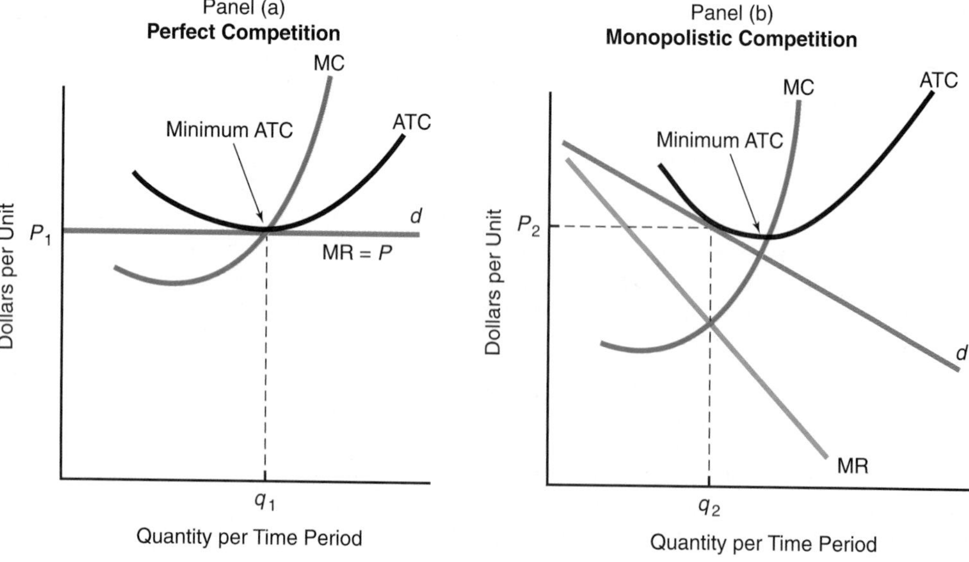

monopolistic competitor; its demand curve is less than perfectly elastic. This firm has some control over price. Price elasticity of demand is not infinite.

We see the two situations in Figure 25-2. Both panels show average total costs just touching the respective demand curves at the particular price at which the firm is selling the product. Notice, however, that the perfect competitor's average total costs are at a minimum. This is not the case with the monopolistic competitor. The equilibrium rate of output is to the left of the minimum point on the average total cost curve where price is greater than marginal cost. The monopolistic competitor cannot expand output to the point of minimum costs without lowering price, and then marginal cost would exceed marginal revenue. A monopolistic competitor at profit maximization charges a price that exceeds marginal cost. In this respect it is similar to the monopolist.

It has consequently been argued that monopolistic competition involves waste because minimum average total costs are not achieved and price exceeds marginal cost. There are too many firms, each with excess capacity, producing too little output. According to critics of monopolistic competition, society's resources are being wasted.

Chamberlin had an answer to this criticism. He contended that the difference between the average cost of production for a monopolistically competitive firm in an open market and the minimum average total cost represented what he called the cost of producing "differentness." Chamberlin did not consider this difference in cost between perfect competition and monopolistic competition a waste. In fact, he argued that it is rational for consumers to have a taste for differentiation; consumers willingly accept the resultant increased production costs in return for choice and variety of output.

CONCEPTS IN BRIEF

- In the short run, it is possible for monopolistically competitive firms to make economic profits or economic losses.
- In the long run, monopolistically competitive firms will make zero economic profits—that is, they will make a normal rate of return.
- Because the monopolistic competitor faces a downward-sloping demand curve, it does not produce at the minimum point on its average total cost curve. Hence we say that a monopolistic competitor has higher average total costs per unit than a perfect competitor would have.
- Chamberlin argued that the difference between the average cost of production for a monopolistically competitive firm and the minimum average total cost at which a competitive firm would produce is the cost of producing "differentness."

OLIGOPOLY

There is another market structure that we have yet to discuss, and it is an important one indeed. It involves a situation in which a few large firms dominate an entire industry. They are not competitive in the sense that we have used the term; they are not even monopolistically competitive. And because there are several of them, a pure monopoly does not exist. We call such a situation an **oligopoly,** which consists of a small number of interdependent sellers. Each firm in the industry knows that other firms will react to its changes in prices, quantities, and qualities. An oligopoly market structure can exist for either a homogeneous or a differentiated product.

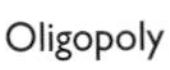

Oligopoly
A market situation in which there are very few sellers. Each seller knows that the other sellers will react to its changes in prices and quantities.

Characteristics of Oligopoly

Oligopoly is characterized by the small number of interdependent firms that constitute the entire market.

Small Number of Firms. How many is "a small number of firms"? More than two but less than 100? The question is not easy to answer. Basically, though, oligopoly exists when a handful of firms dominate the industry enough to set prices. The top few firms in the industry account for an overwhelming percentage of total industry output.

Oligopolies usually involve three to five big companies that produce the bulk of industry output. Between World War II and the 1970s, three firms—General Motors, Chrysler, and Ford—sold nearly all the output of the U.S. automobile industry. Among manufacturers of chewing gum and coin-operated amusement games, four large firms sell essentially the entire output of each industry.

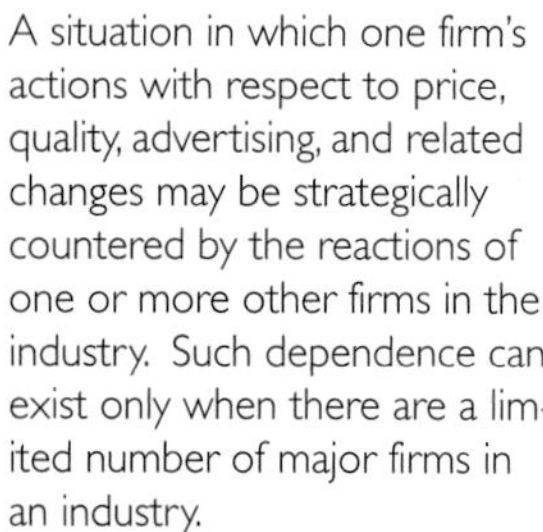

Strategic dependence
A situation in which one firm's actions with respect to price, quality, advertising, and related changes may be strategically countered by the reactions of one or more other firms in the industry. Such dependence can exist only when there are a limited number of major firms in an industry.

Interdependence. All markets and all firms are, in a sense, interdependent. But only when a few large firms dominate an industry does the question of **strategic dependence** of one on the others' actions arise. The firms must recognize that they are interdependent. Any action on the part of one firm with respect to output, price, quality, or product differentiation will cause a reaction on the part of other firms. A model of such mutual interdependence is difficult to build, but examples of such behavior are not hard to find in the real world. Oligopolists in the cigarette industry, for example, are constantly reacting to each other.

Recall that in the model of perfect competition, each firm ignores the behavior of other firms because each firm is able to sell all that it wants at the going market price. At the other extreme, the pure monopolist does not have to worry about the reaction of current rivals because there are none. In an oligopolistic market structure, the managers of firms are like generals in a war: *They must attempt to predict the reaction of rival firms.* It is a strategic game.

Why Oligopoly Occurs

Why are some industries dominated by a few large firms? What causes an industry that might otherwise be competitive to tend toward oligopoly? We can provide some partial answers here.

Economies of Scale. Perhaps the strongest reason that has been offered for the existence of oligopoly is economies of scale. Recall that economies of scale are defined as a situation in which a doubling of output results in less than a doubling of total costs. When economies of scale exist, the firm's average total cost curve will slope downward as the firm produces more and more output. Average total cost can be reduced by continuing to expand the scale of operation. Smaller firms in such a situation will have a tendency to be inefficient. Their average total costs will be greater than those incurred by a large firm. Little by little, they will go out of business or be absorbed into the larger firm.

Barriers to Entry. It is possible that certain barriers to entry have prevented more competition in oligopolistic industries. They include legal barriers, such as patents, and control and ownership over critical supplies. Indeed, we can find periods in the past when firms maintained market power because they were able not only to erect a barrier to entry but also to keep it in place year after year. In principle, the chemical, electronics, and aluminum industries have been at one time or another either monopolistic or oligopolistic because of the ownership of patents and the control of strategic inputs by specific firms.

Oligopoly by Merger. Another reason that oligopolistic market structures may sometimes develop is that firms merge. A merger is the joining of two or more firms under single ownership or control. The merged firm naturally becomes larger, enjoys greater economies of scale as output increases, and may ultimately have a greater ability to influence the market price for the industry's output.

There are two types of mergers, horizontal and vertical. A **horizontal merger** involves firms selling a similar product. If two shoe manufacturing firms merge, that is a horizontal merger. If a group of firms, all producing steel, merge into one, that is also a horizontal merger. A **vertical merger** occurs when one firm merges with either a firm from which it purchases an input or a firm to which it sells its output. Vertical mergers occur, for example, when a coal-using electrical utility purchases a coal-mining firm or when a shoe manufacturer purchases retail shoe outlets. (Obviously, vertical mergers cannot create oligopoly as we have defined it.)

We have been talking about oligopoly in a theoretical manner until now. It is time to look at the actual picture of oligopolies in the United States.

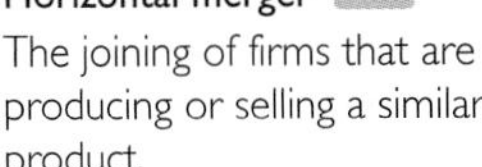

Horizontal merger
The joining of firms that are producing or selling a similar product.

Vertical merger
The joining of a firm with another to which it sells an output or from which it buys an input.

Click here to simulate the effects of an industry merger.

Measuring Industry Concentration

As we have stated, oligopoly is a situation in which a few interdependent firms produce a large part of total output in an industry. This has been called *industry concentration.* Before we show the concentration statistics in the United States, let's determine how industry concentration can be measured.

Concentration Ratio. The most popular way to compute industry concentration is to determine the percentage of total sales or production accounted for by the top four or top eight firms in an industry. This gives the four-or eight-firm **concentration ratio.** An example of an industry with 25 firms is given in Table 25-1. We can see in that table that the four largest firms account for almost 90 percent of total output in the hypothetical industry. That is an example of an oligopoly.

Concentration ratio
The percentage of all sales contributed by the leading four or leading eight firms in an industry; sometimes called the *industry concentration ratio.*

TABLE 25-1
Computing the Four-Firm Concentration Ratio

Firm	Annual Sales ($ millions)		
1	150		
2	100	= 400	Total number of firms in industry = 25
3	80		
4	70		
5 through 25	50		
Total	450		

Four-firm concentration ratio $= \frac{400}{450} = 88.9\%$

TABLE 25-2
Four-Firm Domestic Concentration Ratios for Selected U.S. Industries

Industry	Share of Value of Total Domestic Shipments Accounted for by the Top Four Firms (%)
Tobacco products	93
Breakfast cereals	85
Domestic motor vehicles	84
Soft drinks	69
Primary aluminum	59
Household vacuum cleaners	59
Electronic computers	45
Printing and publishing	23

Source: U.S. Bureau of the Census.

U.S. Concentration Ratios. Table 25-2 shows the four-firm *domestic* concentration ratios for various industries. Is there any way that we can show or determine which industries to classify as oligopolistic? There is no definite answer. If we arbitrarily picked a four-firm concentration ratio of 75 percent, we could indicate that tobacco products, breakfast cereals, and domestic motor vehicles were oligopolistic. But we would always be dealing with an arbitrary definition.

Oligopoly, Efficiency, and Resource Allocation

Reaction function
(For Page 623)
The manner in which one oligopolist reacts to a change in price, output, or quality made by another oligopolist in the industry.

Although oligopoly is not the dominant form of market structure in the United States, oligopolistic industries do exist. To the extent that oligopolists have *market power*—an ability to *individually* affect the *market* price for the industry's output—they lead to resource misallocations, just as monopolies do. Oligopolists charge prices that exceed marginal cost. But what about oligopolies that occur because of economies of scale? One could argue that consumers end up paying lower prices than if the industry were composed of numerous smaller firms.

All in all, there is no definite evidence of serious resource misallocation in the United States because of oligopolies. In any event, the more U.S. firms face competition from the rest of the world, the less any current oligopoly will be able to exercise market power.

CONCEPTS IN BRIEF

- An oligopoly is a market situation in which there are a small number of interdependent sellers.
- Oligopoly may result from (1) economies of scale, (2) barriers to entry, and (3) mergers.
- Horizontal mergers involve the joining of firms selling a similar product.
- Vertical mergers involve the merging of one firm either with the supplier of an input or the purchaser of its output.
- Industry concentration can be measured by the percentage of total sales accounted for by the top four or top eight firms.

Game theory 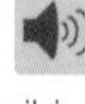
A way of describing the various possible outcomes in any situation involving two or more interacting individuals when those individuals are aware of the interactive nature of their situation and plan accordingly. The plans made by these individuals are known as *game strategies*.

STRATEGIC BEHAVIOR AND GAME THEORY

At this point, we should be able to show oligopoly price and output determination in the way we showed it for perfect competition, pure monopoly, and monopolistic competition, but we cannot. Whenever there are relatively few firms competing in an industry, each can and does react to the price, quantity, quality, and product innovations that the others undertake. In other words, each oligopolist has a **reaction function.** Oligopolistic competitors are interdependent. Consequently, the decision makers in such firms must employ strategies. And we must be able to model their strategic behavior if we wish to predict how prices and outputs are determined in oligopolistic market structures. In general, we can think of reactions of other firms to one firm's actions as part of a *game* that is played by all firms in the industry. Not surprisingly, economists have developed **game theory** models to describe firms' rational interactions. Game theory is the analytical framework in which two or more individuals, companies, or nations compete for certain payoffs that depend on the strategy that the others employ. Poker is such a game situation because it involves a strategy of reacting to the actions of others.

Some Basic Notions About Game Theory

Games can be either cooperative or noncooperative. If firms get together to collude or form a cartel, that is considered a **cooperative game.** Whenever it is too costly for firms to negotiate such collusive agreements and to enforce them, they are in a **noncooperative game** situation. Most strategic behavior in the marketplace would be described as a noncooperative game.

Games can be classified by whether the payoffs are negative, zero, or positive. A **zero-sum game** is one in which one player's losses are offset by another player's gains; at any time, sum totals are zero. If two retailers have an absolutely fixed total number of customers, the customers that one retailer wins over are exactly equal to the customers that the other retailer loses. A **negative-sum game** is one in which players as a group lose at the end of the game (although one perhaps by more than the other, and it's possible for one or more players to win). A **positive-sum game** is one in which players as a group end up better off. Some economists describe all voluntary exchanges as positive-sum games. After an exchange, both the buyer and the seller are better off than they were prior to the exchange.

Strategies in Noncooperative Games. Players, such as decision makers in oligopolistic firms, have to devise a **strategy,** which is defined as a rule used to make a choice. The goal of the decision maker is to devise a strategy that is more successful than alternative strategies. Whenever a firm's decision makers can come up with certain strategies that are generally successful no matter what actions competitors take, these are called **dominant strategies.** The dominant strategy always yields the unique best action for the decision maker no matter what action the other "players" undertake. Relatively few business decision makers over a long period of time have successfully devised dominant strategies. We know this by observation: Few firms in oligopolistic industries have maintained relatively high profits consistently over time.

Cooperative game 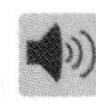
A game in which the players explicity cooperate to make themselves better off. As applied to firms, it involves companies colluding in order to make higher than competitive rates of return.

Noncooperative game 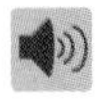
A game in which the players neither negotiate nor cooperate in any way. As applied to firms in an industry, this is the common situation in which there are relatively few firms and each has some ability to change price.

Zero-sum game 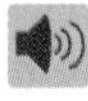
A game in which any gains within the group are exactly offset by equal losses by the end of the game.

Negative-sum game 
A game in which players as a group lose at the end of the game.

Positive-sum game 
A game in which players as a group are better off at the end of the game.

Strategy 
Any rule that is used to make a choice, such as "Always pick heads"; any potential choice that can be made by players in a game.

Dominant strategies 
Strategies that always yield the highest benefit. Regardless of what other players do, a dominant strategy will yield the most benefit for the player using it.

EXAMPLE

The Prisoners' Dilemma

One real-world example of game theory occurs when two people involved in a bank robbery are caught. What should they do when questioned by police? The result has been called the **prisoners' dilemma.** The two suspects, Sam and Carol, are interrogated separately (they cannot communicate with each other) and are given various alternatives. The interrogator indicates to Sam and Carol the following:

1. If both confess to the bank robbery, they will both go to jail for five years.
2. If neither confesses, they will each be given a sentence of two years on a lesser charge.
3. If one prisoner turns state's evidence and confesses, that prisoner goes free and the other one, who did not confess, will serve 10 years on bank robbery charges.

You can see the prisoners' alternatives in the **payoff matrix** in Figure 25-3. The two possibilities for each prisoner are "confess" and "don't confess." There are four possibilities:

1. Both confess.
2. Neither confesses.
3. Sam confesses (turns state's evidence) but Carol doesn't.
4. Carol confesses (turns state's evidence) but Sam doesn't.

In Figure 25-3, all of Sam's possible outcomes are shown on the upper half of each rectangle, and all of Carol's possible outcomes are shown on the lower half.

By looking at the payoff matrix, you can see that if Carol confesses, Sam's best strategy is to confess also—he'll get only 5 years instead of 10. Conversely, if Sam confesses, Carol's best strategy is also to confess—she'll get 5 years instead of 10. Now let's say that Sam is being interrogated and Carol doesn't confess. Sam's best strategy is still to confess, because then he goes free instead of serving two years. Conversely, if Carol is being interrogated, her best strategy is still to confess even if Sam hasn't. She'll go free instead of serving 10 years. To confess is a dominant strategy for Sam. To confess is also a dominant strategy for Carol. The situation is exactly symmetrical. So this is the prisoners' dilemma. The prisoners know that both of them will be better off if neither confesses. Yet it is in each individual prisoner's interest to confess, even though the *collective* outcome of each prisoner's pursuing his or her own interest is inferior for both.

For Critical Analysis

Can you apply the prisoners' dilemma to the firms in a two-firm industry that agree to share market sales equally? (Hint: Think about the payoff to cheating on the market-sharing agreement.)

FIGURE 25-3

The Prisoners' Dilemma Payoff Matrix

Regardless of what the other prisoner does, each person is better off if he or she confesses. So confessing is the dominant strategy and each ends up behind bars for five years.

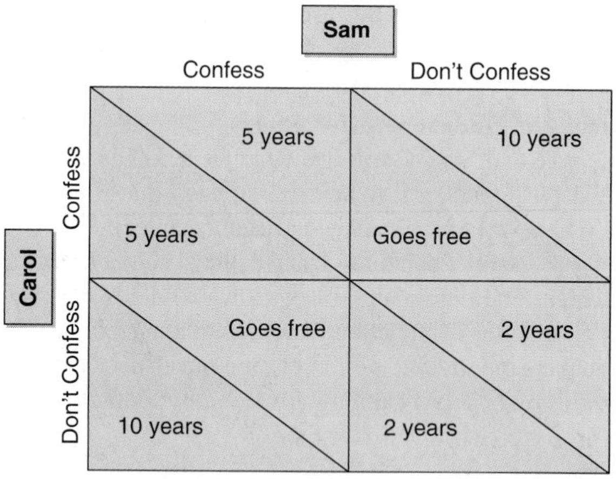

Carol \ Sam	Confess	Don't Confess
Confess	Sam: 5 years / Carol: 5 years	Sam: 10 years / Carol: Goes free
Don't Confess	Sam: Goes free / Carol: 10 years	Sam: 2 years / Carol: 2 years

Prisoners' dilemma

A famous strategic game in which two prisoners have a choice between confessing and not confessing to a crime. If neither confesses, they serve a minimum sentence. If both confess, they serve a maximum sentence. If one confesses and the other doesn't, the one who confesses goes free. The dominant strategy is always to confess.

Payoff matrix

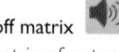

A matrix of outcomes, or consequences, of the strategies available to the players in a game.

Applying Game Theory to Pricing Strategies

We can apply game strategy to two firms—oligopolists—that have to decide on their pricing strategy. Each can choose either a high or a low price. Their payoff matrix is shown in Figure 25-4. If they each choose high prices, they can each make \$6 million, but if they each choose low prices, they will only make \$4 million each. If one sets a high price and the other a low one, the low-priced firm will make \$8 million, but the high-priced firm will only make \$2 million. As in the prisoners' dilemma, in the absence of collusion, they will end up choosing low prices.

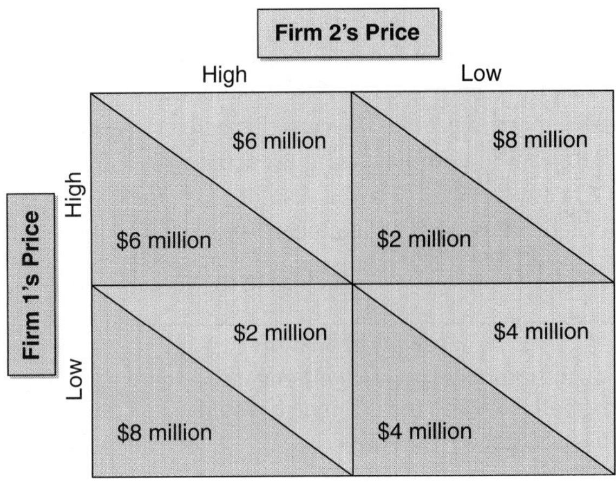

FIGURE 25-4
Game Theory and Pricing Strategies
This payoff matrix shows that if both oligopolists choose a high price, each makes $6 million. If they both choose a low price, each makes $4 million. If one chooses a low price and the other doesn't, the low-priced firm will make $8 million. Unless they collude, however, they will end up at the low-priced solution.

Opportunistic Behavior 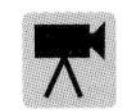

In the prisoners' dilemma, it was clear that cooperative behavior—both parties standing firm without admitting to anything—leads to the best outcome for both players. But each prisoner (player) stands to gain by cheating. Such action is called **opportunistic behavior.** Our daily economic activities involve the equivalent of the prisoners' dilemma all the time. We could engage in opportunistic behavior. You could write a check for a purchase knowing that it is going to bounce because you have just closed that bank account. When you agree to perform a specific task for pay, you could perform your work in a substandard way. When you go to buy an item, the seller might be able to cheat you by selling you a defective item.

Opportunistic behavior
Actions that ignore the possible long-run benefits of cooperation and focus solely on short-run gains.

In short, if all of us—sellers and buyers—engaged in opportunistic behavior all of the time, we would always end up in the upper left-hand box of the prisoners' dilemma payoff matrix in Figure 25-3. We would constantly be acting in a world of noncooperative behavior. That is not the world in which most of us live, however. Why not? Because most of us engage in *repeat transactions.* Manufacturers would like us to keep purchasing their products. Sellers would like us to keep coming back to their stores. As a seller of labor services, each of us would like to keep our jobs, get promotions, or be hired away by another firm at a higher wage rate. We engage in a **tit-for-tat strategic behavior.** In tit-for-tat strategy, manufacturers and sellers continue to guarantee their merchandise, in spite of cheating by a small percentage of consumers.

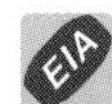

Strategic Behavior
Practice applying game theory.

Tit-for-tat strategic behavior
In game theory, cooperation that continues so long as the other players continue to cooperate.

INTERNATIONAL EXAMPLE

Strategically Relating Loan Subsidies to Nuclear Weapons

Companies are not the only entities that can engage in opportunistic behavior. Nations can do so, too, particularly in their interactions with international agencies such as the International Monetary Fund (IMF). The IMF routinely offers loans to developing countries and to nations that suffer foreign exchange crises. Typically, the IMF grants loans only after receiving promises of "economic self-discipline." The IMF might require, for instance, that a nation reduce its inflation rate, cut its fiscal deficit, improve its legal system, and so on. That is the tack the IMF took when it loaned Pakistan $1.6 billion in the latter part of the 1990s. In 1999, the IMF discovered that in 1998 and 1999 the Pakistani government fudged its budget deficit figures to hide

$2 billion in government spending. Much of this spending was directed toward Pakistan's military budget, including development of nuclear weapons.

From July 1999 to the spring of 2000, the IMF withheld loan installments from the Pakistani government. Soon the government of Pakistan found itself facing default on its debt. The country's military government was already struggling to deal with declines in national saving, investment, exports, and output, and the nation only had sufficient foreign exchange reserves to cover six weeks of imports. Faced with a weakening economy, Pakistan's military leaders began to hint that they might forgo more nuclear tests if Western governments, which fund the IMF, encouraged the international agency to back a debt-rescheduling plan for Pakistan. The IMF gave Pakistan a reprieve until 2001, which gave its leaders some breathing room to get the government's budget in order.

Pakistani government officials acted opportunistically toward the IMF. They did so because they knew they could get away with it, at least for a while.

For Critical Analysis

Why might a foreign government engage in more opportunistic behavior with the IMF than it would with a private lending institution?

PRICE RIGIDITY AND THE KINKED DEMAND CURVE

Let's hypothesize that the decision makers in an oligopolistic firm assume that rivals will react in the following way: They will match all price decreases (in order not to be undersold) but not price increases (because they want to capture more business). There is no collusion. The implications of this reaction function are rigid prices and a kinked demand curve.

Nature of the Kinked Demand Curve

In Figure 25-5, we draw a kinked demand curve, which is implicit in the assumption that oligopolists match price decreases but not price increases. We start off at a given price of P_0 and assume that the quantity demanded at the price for this individual oligopolist is q_0. The starting price of P_0 is usually the stable market price. If the oligopolist assumes that rivals will not react, it faces demand curve d_1d_1 with marginal revenue curve MR_1. Conversely, if it assumes that rivals will react, it faces demand curve d_2d_2 with marginal revenue curve MR_2. More than likely, the oligopoly firm will assume that if it lowers price, rivals will react by matching that reduction to avoid losing their respective shares of the market. The oligopolist that initially lowers its price will not greatly increase its quantity demanded. So when it lowers its price, it believes that it will face demand curve d_2d_2. But if it increases price above P_0, rivals will probably not follow suit. Thus a higher price than P_0 will cause quantity demanded to decrease rapidly. The demand schedule to the left of and above point E will be relatively elastic, as represented by d_1d_1. At prices above P_0, the relevant demand curve is d_1d_1, whereas below price P_0, the relevant demand curve will be d_2d_2. Consequently, at point E there will be a *kink* in the resulting demand curve. This is shown in panel (b) of Figure 25-5, where the demand curve is labeled d_1d_2. The resulting marginal revenue curve is labeled MR_1MR_2. It has a discontinuous portion, or gap, represented by the boldfaced dashed vertical lines in both panels.

Price Rigidity

The kinked demand curve analysis may help explain why price changes might be infrequent in an oligopolistic industry without collusion. Each oligopolist can see only harm in a price change: If price is increased, the oligopolist will lose many of its customers to rivals

FIGURE 25-5

The Kinked Demand Curve

If the oligopolist firm assumes that rivals will not match price changes, it faces demand curve d_1d_1 and marginal revenue curve MR_1. If it assumes that rivals will match price changes, it faces demand curve d_2d_2 and marginal revenue curve MR_2. If the oligopolist believes that rivals will not react to price increases but will react to price decreases, at prices above P_0 it faces demand curve d_1d_1 and at prices below P_0 it faces the other demand curve, d_2d_2. The overall demand curve will therefore have a kink, as is seen in panel (b) at price P_0. The marginal revenue curve will have a vertical break, as shown by the dashed line in panel (b).

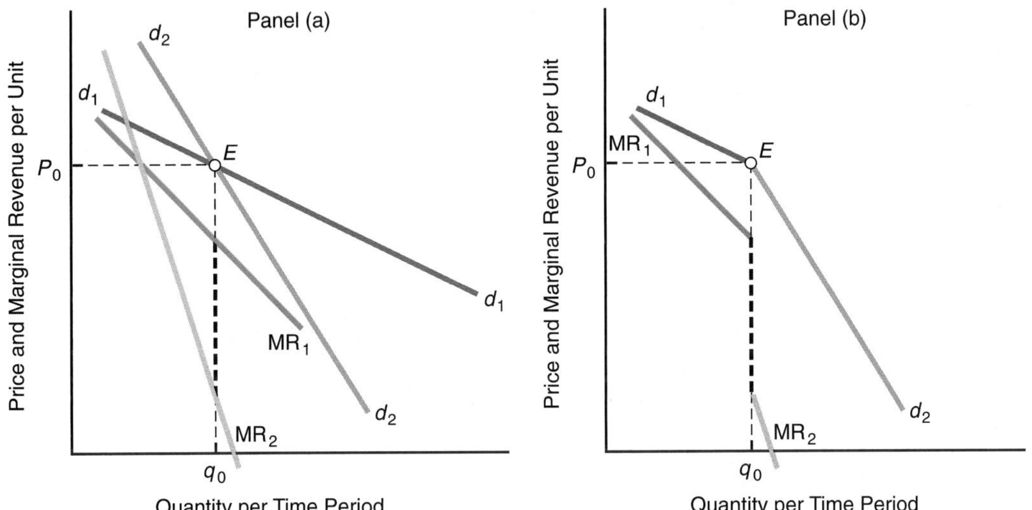

who do not raise their prices. That is to say, the oligopolist moves up from point E along demand curve d_1 in panel (b) of Figure 25-5. However, if an oligopolist lowers its price, given that rivals will lower their prices too, its sales will not increase very much. Moving down from point E in panel (b) of Figure 25-5, we see that the demand curve is relatively inelastic. If the elasticity is less than 1, total revenues will fall rather than rise with the lowering of price. Given that the production of a larger output will increase total costs, the oligopolist's profits will fall. The lowering of price by the oligopolist might start a *price war* in which its rival firms will charge an even lower price.

The theoretical reason for price inflexibility under the kinked demand curve model has to do with the discontinuous portion of the marginal revenue curve shown in panel (b) of Figure 25-5, which we reproduce in Figure 25-6. Assume that marginal cost is represented by MC. The profit-maximizing rate of output is q_0, which can be sold at a price of P_0. Now assume that the marginal cost curve rises to MC′. What will happen to the profit-maximizing rate of output? Nothing. Both quantity and price will remain the same for this oligopolist.

Remember that the profit-maximizing rate of output is where marginal revenue equals marginal cost. The shift in the marginal cost curve to MC′ does not change the profit-maximizing rate of output in Figure 25-6 because MC′ still cuts the marginal revenue curve in the latter's discontinuous portion. Thus the equality between marginal revenue and marginal cost still holds at output rate q_0 even when the marginal cost curve shifts upward. What will happen when marginal costs fall to MC″? Nothing. This oligopolist will continue to produce at a rate of output q_0 and charge a price of P_0. Whenever the marginal cost curve cuts the discontinuous portion of the marginal revenue curve, fluctuations (within limits) in marginal cost will not affect output or price because the profit-maximizing condition MR = MC will hold. The result

FIGURE 25-6

Changes in Cost May Not Alter the Profit-Maximizing Price and Output

As long as the marginal cost curve intersects the marginal revenue curve in the latter's discontinuous portion, the profit-maximizing price P_0 (and output q_0) will remain unchanged even with changes in MC. (However, the firm's rate of profit will change.)

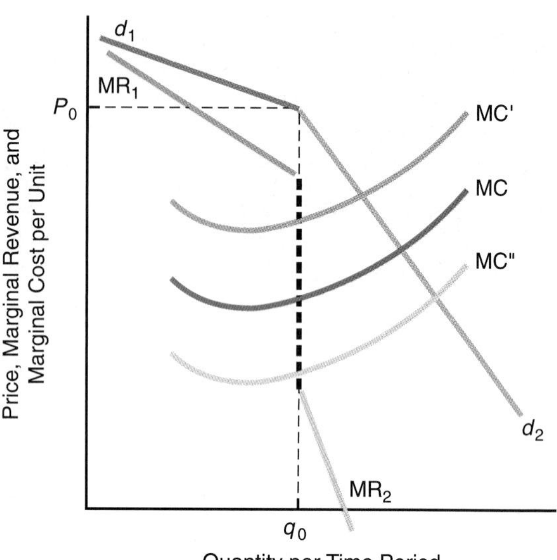

is that even when firms in an oligopolistic industry such as this experience increases or decreases in costs, their prices do not change as long as MC cuts MR in the discontinuous portion. Hence prices are seen to be rigid in oligopolistic industries if oligopolists react the way we assume they do in this model.

Criticisms of the Kinked Demand Curve

One of the criticisms directed against the kinked demand curve is that we have no idea how the existing price, P_0, came to be. If every oligopolistic firm faced a kinked demand curve, it would not pay for it to change prices. The problem is that the kinked demand curve does not show us how demand and supply originally determine the going price of an oligopolist's product.

As far as the evidence goes, it is not encouraging. Oligopoly prices do not appear to be as rigid, particularly in the upward direction, as the kinked demand curve theory implies. During the 1970s and early 1980s, when prices in the economy were rising overall, oligopolistic producers increased their prices frequently. Evidence of price changes during the Great Depression showed that oligopolies changed prices much more frequently than monopolies.

EXAMPLE

Do Pet Products Have Nine Lives?

H. J. Heinz's Pet Products Company knows all about the kinked demand curve. It makes 9-Lives cat food. To meet increased competition (at lower prices) from Nestlé, Quaker, Grand Metropolitan, and Mars, Heinz dropped prices by over 22 percent on the wholesale price of a case of 9-Lives. Finally, it had "had enough." It decided to buck the trend by *raising* prices. The result? A disaster, because none of Heinz's four major competitors increased their prices. Heinz's market share dropped from 23 percent to 15 percent almost overnight.

For Critical Analysis

What does Heinz's experience with 9-Lives perhaps suggest about the price elasticity of demand for its product?

CONCEPTS IN BRIEF

- Each oligopolist has a reaction function because oligopolistic competitors are interdependent. They must therefore engage in strategic behavior. One way to model this behavior is to use game theory.
- Games can be either cooperative or noncooperative. A cartel is cooperative. When a cartel breaks down and its members start cheating, the industry becomes a noncooperative game. In a zero-sum game, one player's losses are exactly offset by another player's gains. In a negative-sum game, all players collectively lose, perhaps one more than the others. In a positive-sum game, the players as a group end up better off.
- Decision makers in oligopolistic firms must devise a strategy. A dominant strategy is one that is generally successful no matter what actions competitors take.
- The kinked demand curve oligopoly model predicts that major shifts in marginal cost will cause any change in industry price.

STRATEGIC BEHAVIOR WITH IMPLICIT COLLUSION: A MODEL OF PRICE LEADERSHIP

What if oligopolists do not actually collude to raise prices and share markets but do so implicitly? There are no formal cartel arrangements and no formal meetings. Nonetheless, there is *tacit collusion.* One example of this is the model of **price leadership.**

Price leadership 
A practice in many oligopolistic industries in which the largest firm publishes its price list ahead of its competitors, who then match those announced prices. Also called *parallel pricing.*

In this model, the basic assumption is that the dominant firm, usually the biggest, sets the price and allows other firms to sell all they can at that price. The dominant firm then sells the rest. The dominant firm always makes the first move in a price leadership model. By definition, price leadership requires that one firm be the leader. Because of laws against collusion, firms in an industry cannot communicate this directly. That is why it is often natural for the largest firm to become the price leader. In the automobile industry during the period of General Motors' dominance (until the 1980s), that company was traditionally the price leader. At various times in the breakfast food industry, Kellogg was the price leader. Some observers have argued that Harvard University was once the price leader among Ivy League schools. In the banking industry, various dominant banks have been price leaders in announcing changes in the prime rate, the interest rate charged on loans offered to the best credit risks. One day a large New York–based bank, such as Chase Manhattan, would announce an increase or decrease in its prime rate. Five or six hours later, all other banks would announce the same change in their prime rate.

Price Wars

Price leadership may not always work. If the price leader ends up much better off than the firms that follow, the followers may in fact not set prices according to those set by the dominant firm. The result may be a **price war.** The dominant firm lowers its prices a little bit, but the other firms lower theirs even more. Price wars have occurred in many industries. Supermarkets within a given locale often engage in price wars, especially during holiday periods. One may offer turkeys at so much per pound on Wednesday; competing stores cut their price on turkeys on Thursday, so the first store cuts its price even more on Friday. We see price wars virtually every year in the airline industry.

Price war 
A pricing campaign designed to capture additional market share by repeatedly cutting prices.

EXAMPLE

Cigarette Price Wars

Price wars occur commonly between long-distance telephone companies, between airlines, and between the makers of cigarettes, soft drinks, computer disc drives, diapers, frozen dinners, and personal computer hardware and software. They do not always lead to the desired result for the company that started the price war. Consider the case of Philip Morris, which cut the price of Marlboro cigarettes by 40 cents a pack to about $1.80. Its main competitor, RJR Nabisco, matched the price cut for Camels. Philip Morris claimed victory because Marlboro's market share increased from 22.1 percent to 27.3 percent. But the domestic operating profits for both companies plummeted in the process; so, too, did the trading value of their stocks. According to business consultants Mike Marn and Robert Garda of McKinsey & Company, the reason is that most companies are unable to offset lower prices with higher volume because variable costs do not start falling until sales increase by about 20 percent. When Philip Morris cut its prices by 18 percent, unit sales increased by only 12.5 percent and profits fell by 25 percent.

For Critical Analysis

How do price wars fit into the tit-for-tat strategic behavior of game theory?

DETERRING ENTRY INTO AN INDUSTRY

Some economists believe that all decision making by existing firms in a stable industry involves some type of game playing. An important part of game playing does not have to do with how existing competitors might react to a decision by others. Rather, it has to do with how *potential* competitors might react. Strategic decision making requires that existing firms in an industry come up with strategies to deter entrance into that industry. One important way is, of course, to get a local, state, or federal government to restrict entry. Adopting certain pricing and investment strategies may also deter entry.

Increasing Entry Costs

Entry deterrence strategy
Any strategy undertaken by firms in an industry, either individually or together, with the intent or effect of raising the cost of entry into the industry by a new firm.

One **entry deterrence strategy** is to raise the cost of entry by a new firm. The threat of a price war is one technique. To sustain a long price war, existing firms might invest in excess capacity so that they can expand output if necessary. When existing firms invest in excess capacity, they are signaling potential competitors that they will engage in a price war.

Another way that existing domestic firms can raise the entry cost of foreign firms is by getting the U.S. government to pass stringent environmental or health and safety standards. These typically raise costs more for foreign producers, often in developing countries, than for domestic producers.

EXAMPLE

Should Hair Braiders Be Licensed?

Many service industries have raised entry costs by getting legislation passed that requires extensive training and licensing before someone can enter the industry. Physicians and lawyers are good examples. Less well known are the high entry costs imposed on individuals who wish to give therapeutic massages or trim and style hair. For example, in California, a license to style hair requires the expenditure of about $6,000 for 1,600 hours of cosmetology classes. Hairstylists in California spend about $600 million a year on classes and test administration fees.

Enter hair braiders, who are hairstylists for the African-American community. Individuals entering this business long assumed that because they use no chemicals, they would not be required to take extensive classes in the use of chemicals. But the California Barbering and Cosmetology Board has recently ruled otherwise. Given that there are about 10,000 hair braiders in America, this issue affects more than California. Currently, there are several lawsuits challenging the licensing requirement for hair braiders. Hair braiders offer a lower-cost alternative to regular beauty salons, and the latter are fighting to prevent this new competition.

For Critical Analysis

Besides currently licensed hairstylists, who else might favor required cosmetology licensing for hair braiders?

Limit-Pricing Strategies

Sometimes existing firms will make it clear to potential competitors that the existing firms would not change their output rate if new firms were to enter the industry. Instead, the existing firms would simply lower the market price (moving down their demand curves) enough to sell the same quantity as they currently do. This new price would be below the level at which an entering firm could earn a normal profit, and that prospect effectively discourages entry. This is called the **limit-pricing model.**

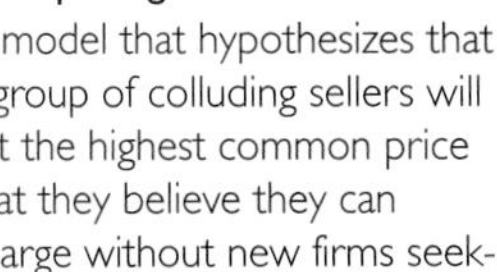

Limit-pricing model
A model that hypothesizes that a group of colluding sellers will set the highest common price that they believe they can charge without new firms seeking to enter that industry in search of relatively high profits.

EXAMPLE

Giving Away Services on the Web: Thwarting an Emerging Rival, Limit Pricing, or Both?

eBay, the Internet auctioneer, earns revenues by assessing commissions based on sales prices. It is a popular site for selling anything from concert tickets to computers to antiques. It is so popular, in fact, that some businesses began to run ads on eBay's Web site because they knew so many people were visiting it. That is how eBay got into the Web advertisement business.

This development alarmed Yahoo! and other Internet search engines because it constituted a threat to a core part of their business. People who use Yahoo!, for example, are exposed to the ads on its site, ads that generate significant revenues for Yahoo!. Yahoo! felt it had to make a strategic response. So it began to offer free auction services. Although Yahoo! leaves it to buyers and sellers to finalize agreements, its service performs the basic auctioneer function of matching the two. Launching this free service allowed Yahoo! to establish an initial presence in the market for on-line auctions. At the same time, however, it established a limit price of zero for other firms that might contemplate becoming auctioneers as a means of horning in on its bread-and-butter on-line advertising business.

In spite of Yahoo!'s action and competition from other Internet sellers such as Onsale.com and Amazon.com, eBay remains the most popular auction site on the Internet. Most observers agree that its popularity is the key to its success, because when sellers list items in auctions, they want to be certain that there will be lots of potential buyers. In addition, eBay continues to provide a wider range of auctioneering services.

For Critical Analysis

How can eBay continue to charge auction commissions while Yahoo! offers its auction services at no charge?

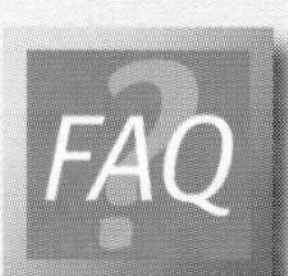

Doesn't a company like Amazon.com have to be really big before it can sell books on the Net at discounted prices?

No, as demonstrated by Lyle Bowlin of the University of Northern Iowa. He is a book lover who decided to contact the same wholesalers from whom Amazon buys the books that it markets. Bowlin learned that to get essentially the same volume discounts that Amazon gets, he had to buy only five copies of each book he ordered. He calculated that if he maintained a Web site, his daughter did his accounting, and his wife handled the shipping, he could beat Amazon's prices. Soon he had gotten into the Internet bookselling business himself, with customers in half the U.S. states and Canada.

Raising Customers' Switching Costs

If an existing firm can make it more costly for customers to switch from its product or service to a competitor's, the existing firm can deter entry. There are a host of ways in which existing firms can raise customers' switching costs. Makers of computer equipment have in the past produced operating systems and software that would not run on competitors' computers. Any customer wanting to change from one computer system to another faced a high switching cost.

CONCEPTS IN BRIEF

- One type of strategic behavior involving implicit collusion is price leadership. The dominant firm is assumed to set the price and then allows other firms to sell all that they want to sell at that price. Whatever is left over is sold by the dominant firm. The dominant firm always makes the first move in a price leadership model. If the nondominant firms decide to compete, they may start a price war.
- One strategic decision may be to attempt to raise the cost of entry of new firms into an industry. The threat of a price war is one technique. Another is to lobby the federal government to pass stringent environmental or health and safety standards in an attempt to keep out foreign competition.
- If existing firms limit prices to a level above competitive prices before entry but are willing to reduce it, this is called a limit-pricing model.
- Another way to raise the cost to new firms is to make it more costly for customers to switch from one product or service to a competitor's.

COMPARING MARKET STRUCTURES

Now that we have looked at perfect competition, pure monopoly, monopolistic competition, and oligopoly, we are in a position to compare the attributes of these four different market structures. We do this in summary form in Table 25-3, in which we compare the number of sellers, their ability to set price, and whether product differentiation exists, and we give some examples of each of the four market structures.

TABLE 25-3
Comparing Market Structures

Market Structure	Number of Sellers	Unrestricted Entry and Exit	Ability to Set Price	Long-Run Economic Profits Possible	Product Differentiation	Nonprice Competition	Examples
Perfect competition	Numerous	Yes	None	No	None	None	Agriculture, coal
Monopolistic competition	Many	Yes	Some	No	Considerable	Yes	Toothpaste, toilet paper, soap, retail trade
Oligopoly	Few	Partial	Some	Yes	Frequent	Yes	Cigarettes, steel
Pure monopoly	One	No (for entry)	Considerable	Yes	None (product is unique)	Yes	Some electric companies, some local telephone companies

NETNOMICS

Will Shopbots Make Internet Sellers More Competitive, or Will They Make the Kinked Demand Curve More Relevant?

Shopbots are software programs that consumers can use to search the Net for the best prices. Most observers have argued that they will be a boon for consumers. Enthusiasts contend that by enabling consumers to flock to Web sites that post the lowest prices, shopbots encourage firms to keep their prices at the marginal cost of production. Any Internet seller that tries to raise its price above this level would lose customers rapidly, they argue.

Hal Varian, an economist at the University of California at Berkeley, thinks that the story isn't quite so simple. He points out that there is nothing to stop Internet sellers from using shopbot programs, too. Indeed, some firms are already programming shopbots to keep tabs on the Web sites of rival sellers, permitting them to respond almost instantaneously to price cuts by competitors. If all rivals in the marketplace follow the same strategy—and know that they do—then the price rigidity predicted by the kinked demand curve can arise. Price can then exceed marginal and average cost, and Internet-based oligopolists will be able to earn economic profits.

Varian argues that which outcome eventually prevails depends on whether consumers or producers move faster in spotting and responding to price differences. In his view, there is good reason to think that consumers will be at a disadvantage in this regard. They will unleash their shopbots only when they happen to be shopping for a specific item. But producers will keep their shopbots busy checking out rivals' prices. A number of Internet sellers, for instance, engage in real-time monitoring of the Web sites of their competitors and automatically match any price cut.

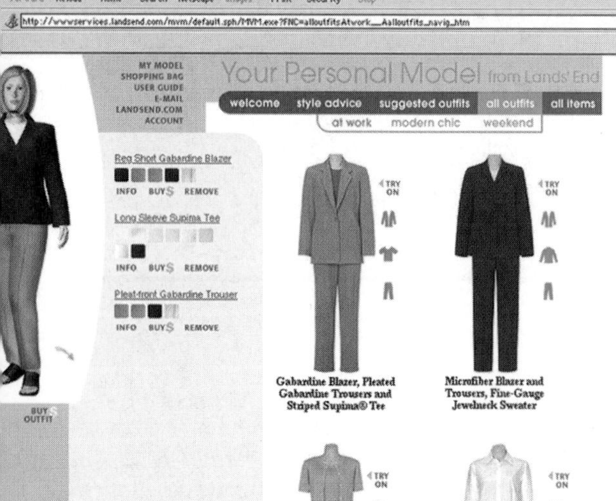

ISSUES & APPLICATIONS

Product Differentiation on the Web

"To do it well is worth millions." This is one marketing specialist's evaluation of the gain from making a big splash on the Internet. As the older mass media of print, radio, and television have become more fragmented, building brands via these advertising vehicles is difficult. For companies whose product lines "grew up" with television, solving the puzzle of marketing on the Net may be the key to continued success or ultimate failure amid an array of competing brand names.

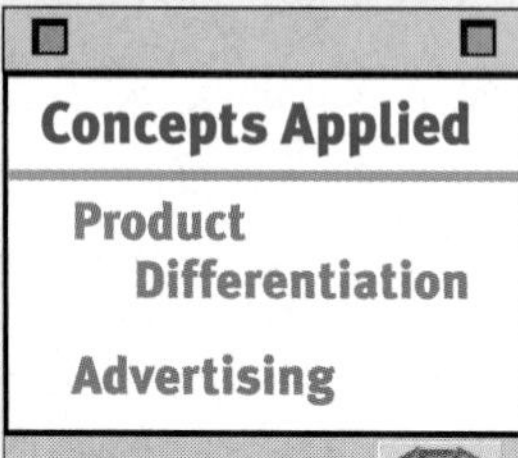

Learning from Current and Past Successes

Some Internet-based companies have scored huge successes. Notable examples are America Online and Yahoo!, which within a few years catapulted into the top echelons of American business. For these companies, forging a recognized brand name has been crucial. Because their actual and potential customers evaluate their products by viewing images in small spaces on flat computer screens, these firms have spent fortunes—and gained even greater fortunes in return—finding ways to make themselves into household names.

One lesson from these successes is that in cyberspace, anybody with sufficient resources to purchase space on a server and build some brand recognition is a potentially threatening rival. Both old companies trying to develop an Internet presence and new Internet start-ups have found that one route to success is to emulate successful firms on the Net. It is no accident, for instance, that the Web site of Barnes & Noble, a traditional bookseller, and Books.com, the Net-based rival Barnes & Noble gobbled up, looked so much like the Amazon.com site. The people at Amazon.com discovered a successful way to sell books on the Net, and its rivals copied that proven strategy.

Another lesson learned by companies hoping to market their brands on the Net is that just posting a Web site full of colorful banners does not necessarily attract customers. Cyberspace can be a lonely place when there are only a few routes to a Web site. Taking out ad space on search engines is one way to attract attention to a company's Web site. Another, however, is to use the old-fashioned communications media. Amazon.com, for instance, advertises heavily in print and on television.

The Key to Internet Selling: Give People Something to Do

Some old approaches have not panned out, however. For instance, Bell Atlantic Corporation tried running a weekly soap opera on its Web site. It couldn't find much evidence that anyone tuned in, and within weeks the soap opera was history.

What Bell Atlantic and other companies have discovered is that potential customers watch television to be passively entertained, but they surf the Internet to *do* something. This is why Lands' End provides on-line birthday reminder services, Macy's offers personal shopping assistance via e-mail, and Toys 'Я' Us provides a Web gift registry for kids with upcoming birthdays. The importance of activity-based selling on the Internet may be bad news for makers of packaged and bottled goods. Consider the example of Coca-Cola, which developed a Cherrycoke.com Web site as an entertainment gateway to interesting Web sites. The company discovered that the average visitor to the site spent no more than 90 seconds there before surfing away. For sellers of soda pop, finding something useful for Web surfers to do while they learn about a brand may prove to be a real challenge.

FOR CRITICAL ANALYSIS

1. McDonald's has a Web site with financial data, kids' games, and maps displaying locations of its stores. In what ways is this a potentially successful way to market hamburgers?
2. How might a breakfast cereal manufacturer effectively promote its brands on the Internet?

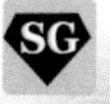

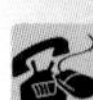

SUMMARY DISCUSSION OF LEARNING OBJECTIVES

1. **The Key Characteristics of a Monopolistically Competitive Industry:** A monopolistically competitive industry consists of a large number of firms that sell differentiated products that are close substitutes. Firms can easily enter or exit a monopolistically competitive industry. Because monopolistically competitive firms can increase their profits if they can successfully distinguish their products from those of their rivals, they have an incentive to engage in sales promotions and advertising.
2. **Contrasting the Output and Pricing Decisions of Monopolistically Competitive Firms with Those of Perfectly Competitive Firms:** In the short run, a monopolistically competitive firm produces output to the point where marginal revenue equals marginal cost. The price it charges for this output, which is the maximum price that people are willing to pay as determined by the demand for its product, can exceed both marginal cost and average total cost in the short run, and the resulting economic profits can induce new firms to enter the industry. As they do, existing firms in the industry experience declines in the demand for their products and reduce their prices to the point at which price equals average total cost. In the long run, therefore, monopolistically competitive firms, like perfectly competitive firms, earn zero economic profits. In contrast to perfectly competitive firms, however, price still exceeds marginal cost in the long-run equilibrium for monopolistically competitive firms.
3. **The Fundamental Characteristics of Oligopoly:** Economies of scale, certain barriers to entry, and horizontal mergers among firms that sell similar products can result in a few firms' producing the bulk of an industry's total output, which is a situation of oligopoly. To measure the extent to which a few firms account for an industry's production and sales, economists calculate concentration ratios, which are the percentages of total sales or total production by the top handful of firms in an industry. Strategic dependence is an important characteristic of oligopoly. One firm's decisions concerning price, product quality, or advertising can bring about responses by other firms. Thus one firm's choices can affect the prices charged by other firms in the industry.
4. **Applying Game Theory to Evaluate the Pricing Strategies of Oligopolistic Firms:** Game theory is the analytical framework that economists apply to evaluate how two or more individuals, companies, or nations compete for payoffs that depend on the strategies that others employ. When firms get together to collude or form a cartel, they participate in cooperative games, but when they cannot work together, they engage in noncooperative games. One important type of game often applied to oligopoly situations is the prisoners' dilemma, in which inability to cooperate in determining prices of their products can cause firms to choose lower prices than they otherwise would prefer.
5. **The Kinked Demand Theory of Oligopolistic Price Rigidity:** If an oligopolistic firm believes that no other firms selling similar products will raise their prices in response to an increase in the price of its product, it perceives the demand curve for its product to be relatively elastic at prices above the price it currently charges. At the same time, if the firm believes that all other firms would respond to a cut in the price of its product by reducing the prices of their products, it views the demand for its product as relatively inelastic at prices below the current price. Hence in this situation, the firm perceives the demand for its product to be kinked, which means that its marginal revenue curve has a break at the current price. Changes in the firm's marginal cost will therefore not necessarily induce the firm to change its production and pricing decisions, so price rigidity may result.
6. **How Firms May Deter Market Entry by Potential Rivals:** To strategically deter market entry by potential competitors, firms in an industry may seek to raise the entry costs that such potential rivals would face. For example, existing firms may invest in excess productive capacity to signal that they could outlast other firms in sustained price wars, or they might engage in lobbying efforts to forestall competition from potential foreign entrants into domestic markets. Existing firms may also engage in limit pricing, signaling to potential entrants that the entry of new rivals would cause them to reduce prices so low that entering the market is no longer economically attractive. Existing firms may also develop ways to make it difficult for current customers to switch to products produced by new entrants.

Key Terms and Concepts

Concentration ratio (621)
Cooperative game (623)
Dominant strategies (623)
Entry deterrence strategy (630)
Game theory (622)
Horizontal merger (621)
Limit-pricing model (631)
Monopolistic competition (613)
Negative-sum game (623)
Noncooperative game (623)
Oligopoly (619)
Opportunistic behavior (625)
Payoff matrix (624)
Positive-sum game (623)
Price leadership (629)
Price war (629)
Prisoners' dilemma (625)
Product differentiation (614)
Reaction function (623)
Strategic dependence (620)
Strategy (623)
Tit-for-tat strategic behavior (625)
Vertical merger (621)
Zero-sum game (623)

Problems

Answers to the odd-numbered problems appear at the back of the book.

25-1. Explain why the following are examples of monopolistic competition.

a. There are a number of fast-food restaurants in town, and they compete fiercely. Some restaurants cook their hamburgers over open flames. Others fry their hamburgers. In addition, some serve broiled fish sandwiches, while others serve fried fish sandwiches. A few serve ice-cream cones for dessert, while others offer frozen ice-cream pies.

b. There is a vast number of colleges and universities across the country. Each competes for top students. All offer similar courses and programs, but some have better programs in business, while others have stronger programs in the arts and humanities. Still others are academically stronger in the sciences.

25-2. A father goes to the pharmacy late at night for cold medicine for a sick child. There are many liquid cold medicines, each of which has almost exactly the same ingredients. Yet medicines with brand names that the man recognizes from television commercials sell for more than the generic versions. Explain, in economic terms, this perplexing situation to the father.

25-3. The following table depicts the prices and total costs a local used bookstore faces. The bookstore competes with a number of similar stores, but it capitalizes on its location and the word-of-mouth reputation of the coffee it serves to its customers.

Output	Price per Book ($)	Total Costs ($)
0	6.00	2.00
1	5.75	5.00
2	5.50	7.50
3	5.25	9.50
4	5.00	10.50
5	4.75	12.50
6	4.50	15.00
7	4.00	18.00

Calculate the store's total revenue, total profit, marginal revenue, and marginal cost. Based on marginal analysis, what is the profit-maximizing level of output for this business?

25-4. Calculate average total costs for the bookstore in Problem 25-3. Illustrate the store's short-run situation by plotting demand, marginal revenue, average total costs, and marginal costs. What is its total profit?

25-5. Suppose that after long-run adjustments take place in the used book market, the business in Problem 25-3 ends up producing 4 units of output. What are the market price and economic profits of this monopolistic competitor in the long run?

25-6. The soft drink market is dominated by a very small number of firms that produce a wide spectrum of drinks and spend vast amounts on advertising. There is very little variation in the prices charged by the leading companies. What is likely to happen if the number one company runs a major new ad campaign and reduces its prices by 5 percent?

25-7. Characterize the followwing examples as a positive-sum game, zero-sum game, or negative-sum game.

a. You play a card game in your dorm room with three other students. Each player brings $5 to the game.

b. Two nations exchange goods in a mutually beneficial transaction.

c. A thousand people buy $1 lottery tickets with a single payoff of $800.

25-8. Last weekend, Bob attended the university football game. At the opening kickoff, the crowd stood up. Bob, therefore, had to stand up as well in order to see the game. For the crowd, not the football team, explain the outcomes of a cooperative game and a noncooperative game. Explain what Bob's "tit-for-tat strategic behavior" would be.

25-9. One of the three shops on campus that sell university logo clothing has found that if it sells a sweatshirt for $30 or more, the other two shops keep their prices constant and the store loses money. If, however, the shop reduces its price below $30, the other stores react by lowering their prices. What kind of market structure does this store face? If the store's marginal costs fluctuate up and down very slightly, how should the store adjust its prices?

25-10. At the beginning of each semester, the university cafeteria posts the prices of its sandwiches. Business students note that as soon as the university posts these prices, the area delis adjust their prices accordingly. The business students argue that this is price collusion and that the university should be held liable. Are the students correct?

Economics on the Net

Current Concentration Ratios in U.S. Manufacturing Industries As you learned in this chapter, economists typically use concentration ratios to evaluate whether industries are oligopolies. In this application, you will make your own determination using the most recent data available.

Title: Concentration Ratios in Manufacturing

Navigation: Click here to start at the U.S. Census Department's homepage. Click on the letter C in the subject area on the left-hand side of the page. Scroll down to and click on Concentration Ratios. Click on Concentration Ratios in Manufacturing.

Application

1. Find the four-firm concentration ratios for the following industries: milk (2026), women's dresses (2335), greeting cards (2771), plumbing fixtures (3261).
2. Which industries are characterized by a high level of competition? Which industries are characterized by a low level of competition? Which industries qualify as oligopolies?
3. Name some of the firms that operate in the industries that qualify as oligopolies.

For Group Discussion and Analysis Discuss whether the four-industry concentration ratio is a good measure of competition. Consider some of the firms you named in item 3. Do you consider these firms to be "competitive" in their pricing and output decisions? Consider the four-firm concentration ratio for ready-mix concrete (3273). Do you think that on a local basis, this industry is competitive? Why or why not?

CHAPTER

26

REGULATION AND ANTITRUST POLICY IN A WORLD OF MULTINATIONAL FIRMS

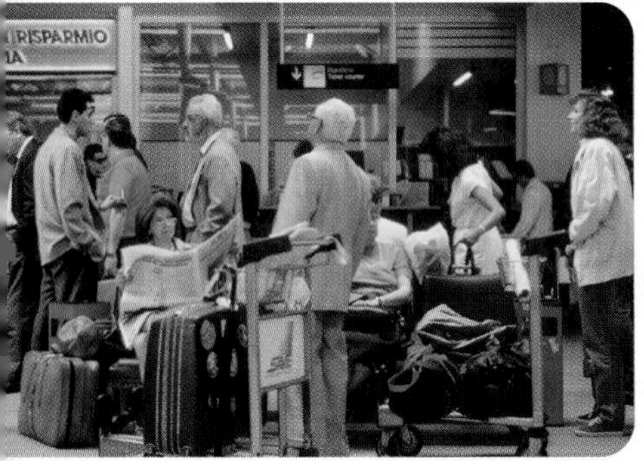

This crowd waiting to be checked in is typical at most airports today. Might such increasing numbers of air travelers be related to the deregulation of airfares? How?

The U.S. government has long regulated the airline industry. A key feature of airline regulation is enforcement of safety rules under the auspices of the Federal Aviation Administration. Today, there are no more than 20 to 30 accidents by any aircraft for every 100,000 hours of flight by all U.S. planes.

Passenger safety is not the only motivation for government regulation of airlines. Traditionally, the federal government has also done everything from regulating flight schedules to defining permissible in-flight passenger services. In the late 1970s, the government took a more hands-off approach to such regulation. Recently, however, the Justice Department and the Transportation Department have begun to study whether to regulate airline pricing. Would this be a sensible area for government regulatory involvement? Before you answer this question, you need to know about regulation and antitrust policy.

LEARNING OBJECTIVES

After reading this chapter, you should be able to:

1. **Recognize practical difficulties that arise when regulating the prices charged by natural monopolies**
2. **Explain the main rationales for government regulation of business**
3. **Identify alternative theories aimed at explaining the behavior of regulators**
4. **Describe short-run and long-run economic effects of deregulation**
5. **Understand the foundations of antitrust laws and regulations**
6. **Discuss basic issues that arise in efforts to enforce antitrust laws**

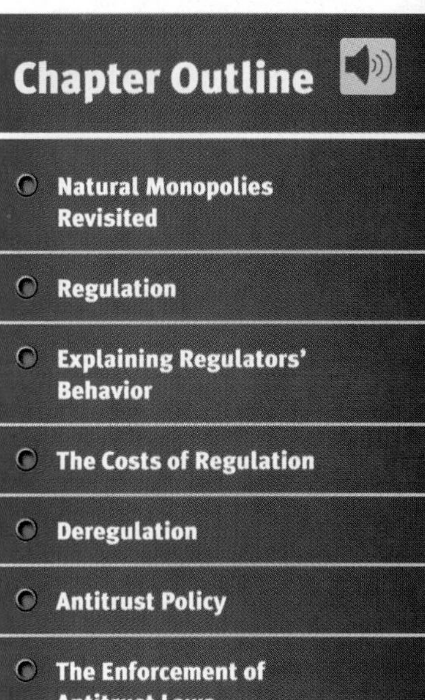

Chapter Outline
Natural Monopolies Revisited
Regulation
Explaining Regulators' Behavior
The Costs of Regulation
Deregulation
Antitrust Policy
The Enforcement of Antitrust Laws

Did You Know That... each year about 75,000 pages of new or modified federal regulations are published? These regulations, found in the *Federal Register,* cover virtually every aspect of the way business can be conducted, products can be built, and services can be offered. In addition, every state and municipality publishes regulations relating to worker safety, restaurant cleanliness, and the number of lights needed in each room in a day-care center. There is no question about it, American business activities are highly regulated. Consequently, how regulators should act to increase economic efficiency and how they actually act are important topics for understanding our economy today. In addition to regulation, the government has one additional weapon to use in its attempts to prevent restraints of trade. It is called antitrust law, and it is the subject of the later part of this chapter.

Let's look first at how government might best regulate a single firm that has obtained a monopoly because of constantly falling long-run average costs, a situation known as a natural monopoly.

NATURAL MONOPOLIES REVISITED

You will recall from our discussion of natural monopolies in Chapter 24 that whenever a single firm has the ability to produce all of the industry's output at a lower per-unit cost than other firms attempting to produce less than total industry output, a natural monopoly arises. Natural gas and electric utilities are examples. Long-run average costs for those firms typically fall as output increases. In a natural monopoly, economies of large-scale production dominate, leading to a single-firm industry.

The Pricing and Output Decision of the Natural Monopolist

A monopolist (like any other firm) will set the output rate where marginal revenue is equal to marginal cost. We draw the market demand curve, *D,* and the revenue curve, MR, in panel (a) of Figure 26-1 on page 640. The intersection of the marginal revenue curve and the marginal cost curve is at point *A*. The monopolist would therefore produce quantity Q_m and charge a price of P_m.

What do we know about a monopolist's solution to the price-quantity question? When compared to a competitive situation, we know that consumers end up paying a higher price for the product, and consequently they purchase less of it than they would purchase under competition. The monopoly solution is economically inefficient from society's point of view; the price charged for the product is higher than the opportunity cost to society, and consequently there is a misallocation of resources. That is, the price does not equal the true marginal cost of producing the good because the true marginal cost is at the intersection *A,* not at price P_m.

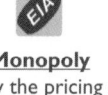

Monopoly
Review the pricing and output choices that a monopolist makes.

Regulating the Natural Monopolist

Assume that the government wants the natural monopolist to produce at an output at which price equals marginal cost, so that the value of the satisfaction that individuals receive from the marginal unit purchased is just equal to the marginal cost to society. Where is that solution in panel (b) of Figure 26-1? It is at the intersection of the marginal cost curve and the demand curve, point *B*. Recall how we derived the competitive industry supply curve. We

FIGURE 26-1

Profit Maximization and Regulation Through Marginal Cost Pricing

The profit-maximizing natural monopolist here would produce at the point in panel (a) where marginal costs equal marginal revenue—that is, at point *A*, which gives the quantity of production Q_m. The price charged would be P_m. If a regulatory commission attempted to regulate natural monopolies so that price equaled long-run marginal cost, the commission would make the monopolist set production at the point where the marginal cost curve intersects the demand schedule. This is shown in panel (b). The quantity produced would be Q_1, and the price would be P_1. However, average costs at Q_1 are equal to AC_1. Losses would ensue, equal to the shaded area. It would be self-defeating for a regulatory commission to force a natural monopolist to produce at an output rate at which MC = *P* without subsidizing some of its costs because losses would eventually drive the natural monopolist out of business.

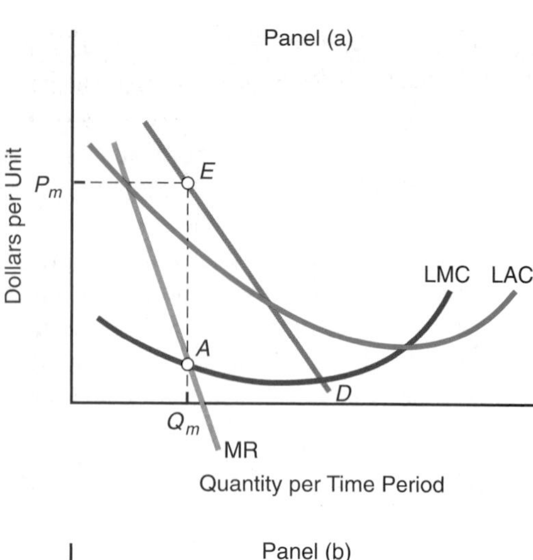

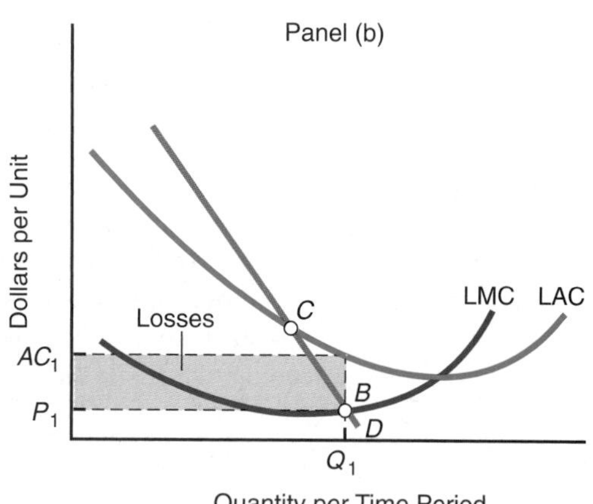

looked at all of the upward-sloping portions of actual and potential firms' marginal cost curves above their respective average variable costs. We then summed all of these portions of the firms' supply curves; that gave us the industry supply curve. We assume that a regulatory commission forces the natural monopolist to engage in marginal cost pricing and hence to produce at quantity Q_1 and to sell the product at price P_1. How large will the monopolist's profits be? Profits, of course, are the *positive* difference between total revenues and total costs. In this case, total revenues equal P_1 times Q_1, and total costs equal average costs times the number of units produced. At Q_1, average cost is equal to AC_1. Average costs are higher than the price that the regulatory commission forces our natural monopolist to charge. Profits turn out to be losses and are equal to the shaded area in panel (b) of Figure 26-1. Thus regulation that forces a natural monopolist to produce and price as if it were in a competitive situation would also force that monopolist into negative profits, or losses. Obviously, the monopolist would rather go out of business than be subject to such regulation.

As a practical matter, then, regulators can't force a natural monopolist to engage in marginal cost pricing. Consequently, regulation of natural monopolies has often taken the form of allowing the regulated natural monopolist to set price where LAC intersects the demand curve *D* at point *C* in panel (b) of Figure 26-1. This is called *average cost pricing.* Average cost includes what the regulators deem a "fair" rate of return on investment.

POLICY EXAMPLE

Power Surges at Electric Utilities: Shocking?

When we discussed natural monopolies, we used a few examples. Panel (a) of Figure 26-1 seems to apply to electric utilities. Technology is changing in that situation, however. Efficient high-voltage transmission lines now exist. This means that the market for electricity generation can transcend local and even national boundaries. This led governments to remove most restrictions on the sale of electric power, thereby permitting competition in the electric utility market. The Department of Energy forecast that by 2010, greater competition in electricity generation could cause the average retail price of electricity to fall to three-fourths of its 1997 level.

Shortly after deregulation began, however, a Midwest heatwave induced two energy-trading companies to default on contracts to deliver electric power to Chicago-based Commonwealth Edison Company. It then had to pay up to $5,000 per megawatt-hour to buy electricity on the spot market—more than 100 times the price that had prevailed during preceding weeks. Commonwealth Edison cut power to manufacturers, and the utility sent out emergency notices prevailing on households to conserve electricity. A number of congressional representatives immediately called for rolling back recent legislation authorizing the new competition in electricity generation.

An interesting thing happened, however. The incident helped convince an independent power producer to invest in a $100 million gas turbine power-generating plant near Chicago. That is, higher electricity prices induced market entry. This reduced the likelihood of a similar problem arising in Chicago in the future. Just as the competition model predicts, price boosts induce new firms to enter the market, which ultimately helps push market prices down toward competitive levels.

For Critical Analysis

Is there really any true natural monopoly left in the world?

CONCEPTS IN BRIEF

- A natural monopoly arises when one firm can produce all of an industry's output at a lower per-unit cost than other firms.
- The first firm to take advantage of the declining long-run average cost curve can undercut the prices of all other sellers, forcing them out of business, thereby obtaining a natural monopoly.
- A natural monopolist allowed to maximize profit will set quantity where marginal revenue equals long-run marginal cost. Price is determined from the demand curve at that quantity.
- A natural monopolist that is forced to set price equal to long-run marginal cost will sustain losses.

REGULATION

The U.S. government began regulating social and economic activity early in the nation's history, but the amount of government regulation has increased in the twentieth century. There are three types of government regulation: regulation of natural monopolies; regulation of inherently competitive industries; and regulation for public welfare across all industries, or so-called social regulation. For example, various state commissions regulate the rates and quality of service of electric power companies, which are considered natural monopolies. Trucking and interstate moving companies are inherently competitive industries but have nonetheless been made subject to government regulation in the past. And federal and state governments impose occupational, health, and safety rules on a wide variety of employers.

Objectives of Economic Regulation

Economic regulation is typically intended to control the prices that regulated enterprises are allowed to charge. Various public utility commissions throughout the United States regulate the rates (prices) of electrical utility companies and some telephone operating companies. This has usually been called rate regulation. The goal of rate regulation has, in principle, been the prevention of both monopoly profits and predatory competition.

Cost-of-service regulation Regulation based on allowing prices to reflect only the actual cost of production and no monopoly profits.

Rate-of-return regulation Regulation that seeks to keep the rate of return in the industry at a competitive level by not allowing excessive prices to be charged.

Two traditional methods of rate regulation have involved cost-of-service regulation and rate-of-return regulation. A regulatory commission using **cost-of-service regulation** allows the regulated companies to charge only prices that reflect the actual average cost of providing the services to the customer. In a somewhat similar vein, regulatory commissions using the **rate-of-return regulation** method allow regulated companies to set prices that ensure a normal, or competitive, rate of return on the investment in the business. We implicitly analyzed these two types of regulation when discussing panel (b) of Figure 26-1. If the long-run average cost curve in that figure includes a competitive rate of return on investment, regulating the price at AC_1 is an example of rate-of-return regulation.

A major problem with regulating monopolies concerns the quality of the service or product involved. Consider the many facets of telephone service: getting a dial tone, hearing other voices clearly, getting the operator to answer quickly, having out-of-order telephone lines repaired rapidly, putting through a long-distance call quickly and efficiently—the list goes on and on. But regulation of a telephone company usually dealt with the prices charged for telephone service. Of course, regulators were concerned with the quality of service, but how could that be measured? Indeed, it cannot be measured very easily. Therefore, it is extremely difficult for any type of regulation to be successful in regulating the *price per constant-quality unit.* Certainly, it is possible to regulate the price per unit, but we don't really know that the quality remains unchanged when the price is not allowed to rise "enough." Thus if regulation doesn't allow prices to rise, quality of service may be lowered, thereby raising the price per constant-quality unit.

Social Regulation

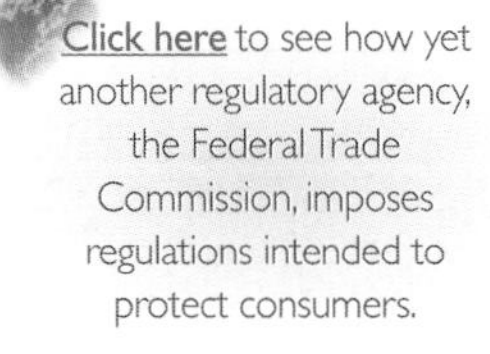
Click here to see how yet another regulatory agency, the Federal Trade Commission, imposes regulations intended to protect consumers.

As mentioned, social regulation reflects concern for public welfare across all industries. In other words, regulation is focused on the impact of production on the environment and society, the working conditions under which goods and services are produced, and sometimes the physical attributes of goods. The aim is a better quality of life for all through a less polluted environment, better working conditions, and safer and better products. For example, the Food and Drug Administration (FDA) attempts to protect against impure and unsafe foods, drugs, cosmetics, and other potentially hazardous products; the Consumer Product Safety Commission (CPSC) specifies minimum standards for consumer products in an attempt to reduce "unreasonable" risks of injury; the Environmental Protection Agency (EPA) watches over the amount of pollutants released into the environment; the Occupational Safety and Health Administration (OSHA) attempts to protect workers against work-related injuries and illnesses; and the Equal Employment Opportunity Commission (EEOC) seeks to provide fair access to jobs.

Table 26-1 lists some major federal regulatory agencies and their areas of concern. Although most people agree with the idea behind such social regulation, many disagree on whether we have too much regulation—whether it costs us more than the benefits we receive. Some contend that the costs that firms incur in abiding by regulations run into the hundreds of billions of dollars per year. The result is higher production costs, which are then passed on

TABLE 26-1
Some Federal Regulatory Agencies

Agency	Jurisdiction	Date Formed	Major Regulatory Functions
Federal Communications Commission (FCC)	Product markets	1934	Regulates broadcasting, telephone, and other communication services.
Federal Trade Commission (FTC)	Product markets	1914	Responsible for preventing businesses from engaging in unfair trade practices and in monopolistic actions, as well as protecting consumer rights.
Equal Employment Opportunity Commission (EEOC)	Labor markets	1964	Investigates complaints of discrimination based on race, religion, sex, or age in hiring, promotion, firing, wages, testing, and all other conditions of employment.
Securities and Exchange Commission (SEC)	Financial markets	1934	Regulates all public securities markets to promote full disclosure.
Environmental Protection Agency (EPA)	Environment	1970	Develops and enforces environmental standards for air, water, toxic waste, and noise.
Occupational Safety and Health Administration (OSHA)	Health and safety	1970	Regulates workplace safety and health conditions.

to consumers. Also, the resources invested in complying with regulatory measures could be invested in other uses. Furthermore, extensive regulation may have an anticompetitive effect because it may represent a relatively greater burden for smaller firms than for larger ones.

But the *potential* benefits of more social regulation are many. For example, the water we drink in some cities is known to be contaminated with cancer-causing chemicals; air pollution from emissions and toxic wastes from production processes cause many illnesses. Some contaminated areas have been cleaned up, but many other problem areas remain.

The benefits of social regulation may not be easy to measure and may accrue to society for a long time. Furthermore, it is difficult to put a dollar value on safer working conditions and a cleaner environment. In any case, the debate goes on. However, it should be pointed out that the controversy is generally not about whether we should have social regulation but about when and how it is being done and whether we take *all* of the costs and benefits into account. For example, is regulation best carried out by federal, state, or local authorities? Is a specific regulation economically justified through a complete cost-benefit analysis?

INTERNATIONAL POLICY EXAMPLE

Conflicting Social Regulations in a World of Multinational Firms

The Data Protection Directive recently took effect in all nations of the European Union. This law governs how firms collect and export personal data about European citizens. Under the rule, any company doing business within the European Union must obtain consumers' permission to collect information about them, disclose how they will use the information, and reveal why it is being collected.

European backers of the law argue that it protects consumers against Big Brother–style corporate intrusion. For U.S. multinational firms, however, the law is a headache. The European requirements run counter to standard business practice in the United States, where it is relatively common to gather information about customers and corporate rivals without their knowledge. Some American business leaders have argued that because information on U.S. firms and consumers is so readily available, the directive gives European firms an unfair advantage in compiling information about competitors and potential business partners in the United States. Indeed, the law will severely limit the ability of U.S. firms to do the same in Europe. In this regard, the directive effectively acts as a protectionist mechanism to hinder U.S. and other foreign companies from competing in Europe.

The law is particularly burdensome for multinational financial firms. Major U.S. banks have had to set up separate systems for American and European customers. In addition, U.S. bankers and government officials worry that criminals will use the directive as a way to learn about investigations of their activities. The directive requires all firms to give customers unlimited access to the information held on them, including files opened as part of investigations into money laundering. Such investigative records are closed in the United States. Some law enforcement officials are already forecasting that money laundering will soon become a big business in Europe.

For Critical Analysis

Critics of the gathering and sale of information about consumers argue that many firms do it to earn higher profits. Why are companies willing to buy this information from other firms?

Creative Response and Feedback Effects: Results of Regulation 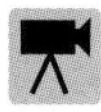

Creative response
Behavior on the part of a firm that allows it to comply with the letter of the law but violate the spirit, significantly lessening the law's effects.

Regulated firms commonly try to avoid the effects of regulation whenever they can. In other words, the firms engage in **creative response,** which is a response to a regulation that conforms to the letter of the law but undermines its spirit. Take state laws requiring male-female pay-equity: The wages of women must be on a par with those paid to males who are performing the same tasks. Employers that pay the same wages to both males and females are clearly not in violation of the law. Yet wages are only one component of total employee compensation. Another component is fringe benefits, such as on-the-job training. Because on-the-job training is difficult to observe from outside the firm, employers could offer less on-the-job training to women and still not be in technical violation of pay-equity laws. This unobservable difference would mean that males were able to acquire skills that could raise their future income even though current wages among males and females were equal, in compliance with the law.

Individuals have a type of creative response that has been labeled a *feedback effect.* Regulation may alter individuals' behavior after the regulation has been put into effect. If regulation requires fluoridated water, then parents know that their children's teeth have significant protection against tooth decay. Consequently, the feedback effect on parents' behavior is that they may be less concerned about how many sweets their children eat.

EXAMPLE

The Effectiveness of Auto Safety Regulation

A good example of the feedback effect has to do with automotive safety regulation. Since the 1960s, the federal government has required automobile manufacturers to make cars increasingly safer. Some of the earlier requirements involved nonprotruding door handles, collapsible steering columns, and shatterproof glass. More recent requirements involve I-beams in the doors, better seat belts, and airbags. The desired result was fewer injuries and deaths for drivers involved in accidents. According to economist Sam Peltzman, however, due to the feedback effect, drivers have gradually started driving more recklessly. Automobiles with more safety features have been involved in a disproportionate number of accidents.

For Critical Analysis

The feedback effect has also been called the law of unintended consequences. Why?

EXPLAINING REGULATORS' BEHAVIOR

Regulation has usually been defended by contending that government regulatory agencies are needed to correct market imperfections. We are dealing with a nonmarket situation because regulators are paid by the government and their decisions are not determined or constrained by the market. A number of theories have been put forward to describe the behavior of regulators. These theories can help us understand how regulation has often harmed consumers through higher prices and less choice and benefited producers through higher profits and fewer competitive forces. Two of the best-known theories of regulatory behavior are the *capture hypothesis* and the *share-the-gains, share-the-pains theory.*

The Capture Hypothesis

It has been observed that with the passage of time, regulators often end up adopting the views of the regulated. According to the **capture hypothesis,*** no matter what the reason for a regulatory agency's having been set up, it will eventually be captured by the special interests of the industry that is being regulated. Consider the reasons.

Capture hypothesis 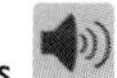
A theory of regulatory behavior that predicts that the regulators will eventually be captured by the special interests of the industry being regulated.

Who knows best about the industry that is being regulated? The people already in the industry. Who, then, will be asked to regulate the industry? Again, people who have been in the industry. And people who used to be in the industry have allegiances and friendships with others in the industry.

Also consider that whenever regulatory hearings are held, the affected consumer groups will have much less information about the industry than the people already in the industry, the producers. Furthermore, the cost to any one consumer to show up at a regulatory hearing to express concern about a change in the rate structure will certainly exceed any perceived benefit that that consumer could obtain from going to the rate-making hearing.

Because they have little incentive to do so, consumers and taxpayers will not be well organized, nor will they be greatly concerned with regulatory actions. But the special interests of the industry are going to be well organized and well defined. Political entrepreneurs within the regulatory agency see little payoff in supporting the views of consumers and taxpayers anyway. After all, few consumers understand the benefits deriving from regulatory agency actions. Moreover, how much could a consumer directly benefit someone who works in an agency? Regulators have the most incentive to support the position of a well-organized special-interest group within the industry that is being regulated.

---

*See George Stigler, *The Citizen and the State: Essays on Regulation* (Chicago: University of Chicago Press, 1975).

"Share the Gains, Share the Pains"

Share-the-gains, share-the-pains theory 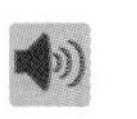
A theory of regulatory behavior in which the regulators must take account of the demands of three groups: legislators, who established and who oversee the regulatory agency; members of the regulated industry; and consumers of the regulated industry's products or services.

A somewhat different view of regulators' behavior is given in the **share-the-gains, share-the-pains theory.*** This theory looks at the specific aims of the regulators. It posits that a regulator simply wants to continue in the job. To do so, the regulator must obtain the approval of both the legislators who established and oversee the regulatory agency and the industry that is being regulated. A third group that must be taken into account is, of course, the customers of the industry.

Under the capture hypothesis, only the special interests of the industry being regulated had to be taken into account by the regulators. The share-the-gains, share-the-pains model contends that such a position is too risky because customers who are really hurt by improper regulation will complain to legislators, who might fire the regulators. Thus each regulator has to attach some weight to these three separate groups. What happens if there is an abrupt increase in fuel costs for electrical utilities? The capture theory would predict that regulators would relatively quickly allow for a rate increase in order to maintain the profits of the industry. The share-the-gains, share-the-pains theory, however, would predict that there will be an adjustment in rates, but not as quickly or as completely as the capture theory would predict. The regulatory agency is not completely captured by the industry; it has to take account of legislators and consumers.

POLICY EXAMPLE

"The Toys Are Safe, But Would You Please Halt Production Anyway?"

A couple of years ago, the Consumer Product Safety Commission (CPSC) did what it does every year around Christmastime: It released a list of toys that can scratch, cut, trap, or choke a child. The CPSC also did something new. It released a study evaluating whether a certain plastic (diisononyl phthalate) used in squeezable children's toys could cause kidney and liver damage, including cancer. The study concluded that "few, if any, children are at risk from liver or other organ toxicity . . . from these products. This is because the amount they might ingest does not reach a level that would be harmful." At the same time the CPSC released these conclusions, however, it told parents of infants to throw away toys containing the plastic. The CPSC also suggested to toy manufacturers and retailers that they should "voluntarily remove" toys containing the plastic from the marketplace. Of course, the companies did. After all, the CPSC's warning to parents and request of manufacturers and retailers could be used in court by a lawyer representing any child who had ever chewed a rattle containing the plastic and then happened to come down with a liver or kidney disease. The risk of future litigation was simply too high for the toymakers and sellers. For the CPSC, however, all turned out well. It had satisfied consumer activists, and at the same time it hadn't issued any mandates for companies to stop selling the squeeze toys.

For Critical Analysis

Does the CPSC appear to have applied cost-benefit analysis in releasing its conflicting statements concerning the use of diisononyl phthalate in squeezable toys?

THE COSTS OF REGULATION

There is no truly accurate way to measure the costs of regulation. Panel (a) of Figure 26-2 shows regulatory spending in 1998 dollars. Except in the years 1981–1985, regulatory spending by federal agencies has increased. This is consistent with what has happened to the number of pages in the *Federal Register,* which publishes all the new federal regulatory

*See Sam Peltzman, "Towards a More General Theory of Regulation," *Journal of Law and Economics,* 19 (1976), pp. 211–240.

FIGURE 26-2

Regulation on the Rise

In panel (a), federal government regulatory spending is shown to exceed $16 billion per year today. State and local spending is not shown. In panel (b), the number of pages in the *Federal Register* per year has been rising since about 1990.

Sources: Institute for University Studies; *Federal Register,* various issues.

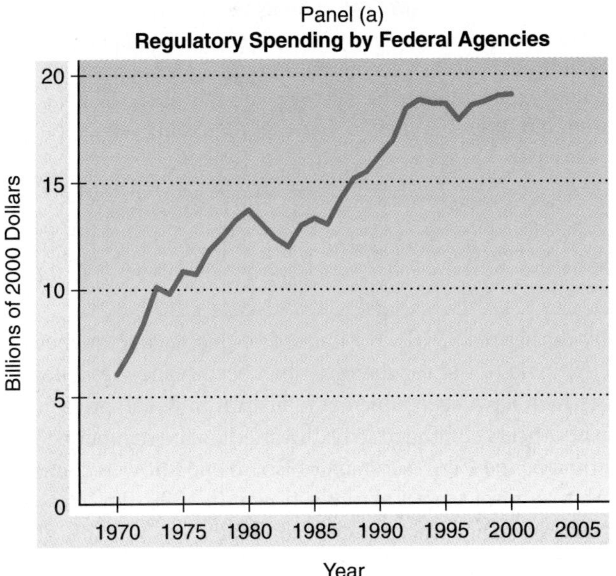

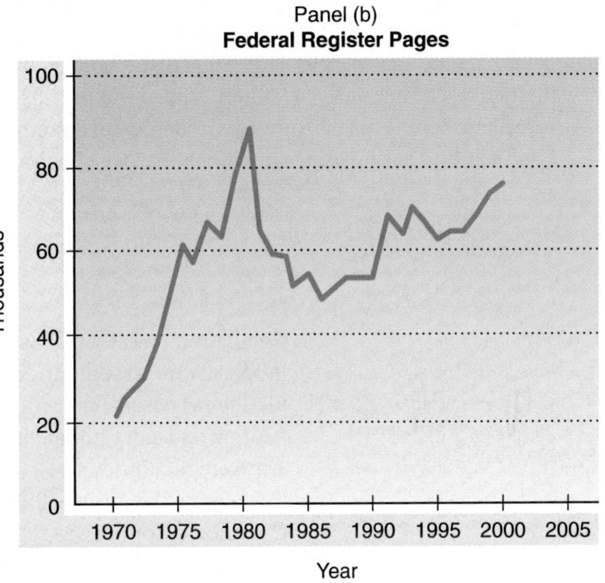

rules; you can see that in panel (b). But actual direct costs to taxpayers are only a small part of the overall cost of regulation. Pharmaceutical-manufacturing safety standards raise the price of drugs. Automobile safety standards raise the price of cars. Environmental controls on manufacturing raise the price of manufactured goods. All of these increased prices add to the cost of regulation. According to economist Thomas Hopkins at the Rochester Institute of Technology, the economic cost of environmental and safety regulation exceeds $200 billion a year. When he adds the cost of all other kinds of regulations, he comes up with a grand total of over $700 billion a year, or about 8 percent of each year's total income in this country. Not surprisingly, the increasing cost of regulation on occasion has brought about cries for deregulation.

POLICY EXAMPLE

Dueling Regulators: What's a Bank to Do?

Recently, the Securities and Exchange Commission (SEC) announced a major enforcement action against a bank known as one of the most conservatively managed in the country, SunTrust Bank of Florida. SunTrust, the SEC claimed, had intentionally manipulated year-to-year changes in its "loan loss reserves," which are anticipated liabilities of the bank resulting from future defaults by a bank's borrowers. According to the SEC, SunTrust had overstated its likely loan losses during a long stretch of good economic times when borrower defaults were unlikely to occur. A possible aim of adding "too much" to loan loss reserves, the SEC concluded, was to intentionally understate the bank's net income, thereby deceiving its shareholders, to whom it distributed dividends that were based on its reported earnings.

The problem was that the bank was following a long-standing practice favored by the Federal Reserve, the Comptroller of the Currency, and the Federal Deposit Insurance Corporation, which are charged with regulating banks to limit failures. Traditionally, these banking regulators have encouraged banks to add to their loan loss reserves in good times so that they will be better prepared when bad times hit and squeeze bank balance sheets. Suddenly SunTrust—and, shortly thereafter, a number of other banks—found itself forced to defend itself from SEC charges of earnings falsification for engaging in actions that were helping generate high ratings from banking regulators. This regulatory squeeze kept the bank's accounting and legal staffs tied up in knots for months, at least until the SEC and banking regulators reached "tentative agreement" on the issue.

For Critical Analysis

Time devoted to dealing with the SEC's complaint was time that SunTrust's accountants could have spent developing expense-reducing systems for the bank. In what way did the SEC action impose regulatory costs on SunTrust?

DEREGULATION

Deregulation
The elimination or phasing out of regulations on economic activity.

Regulation increased substantially during the 1970s. By the end of that decade, numerous proposals for **deregulation**—the removal of old regulations—had been made. Most deregulation proposals and actions since then have been aimed at industries in which price competition and entry competition by new firms continued to be thwarted by the regulators. The Air Deregulation Act of 1978 eliminated the Civil Aeronautics Board and allowed competition among the airlines themselves to control fares and routes flown. In 1980, the Interstate Commerce Commission's power over interstate trucking rates and routes was virtually eliminated, and the same occurred for buses in 1982. Savings account interest rates were deregulated in 1980. Railroad pricing was made more flexible during the same year.

Even prior to this spate of deregulatory acts by Congress, the Federal Communications Commission (FCC) had started in 1972 to deregulate the television broadcast industry. The result has been an increased number of channels, more direct satellite broadcasting, and more cable television transmissions. (Further deregulation occurred in 1996.) In 1975, the Securities and Exchange Commission (SEC) deregulated brokerage fees charged by brokers on the New York Stock Exchange.

Short-Run Versus Long-Run Effects of Deregulation

The short-run effects of deregulation are not the same as the long-run effects. In the short run, a regulated industry that becomes deregulated may experience numerous temporary adjustments. One is the inevitable shakeout of higher-cost producers with the concomitant removal of excess monopoly profits. Another is the sometimes dramatic displacement of workers who have labored long and hard in the formerly regulated industry. The level of service for some consumers may fall; for example, after the deregulation of the telephone industry, some aspects of telephone service decreased in quality. When airlines were deregulated, service to some small cities was eliminated or became more expensive. The power of unions in the formerly regulated industry may decrease. And bankruptcies may cause disruptions, particularly in the local economy where the headquarters of the formerly regulated firm are located.

Proponents of deregulation, or at least of less regulation, contend that there are long-run, permanent benefits. These include lower prices that are closer to marginal cost. Furthermore, fewer monopoly profits are made in the deregulated industry. Such proponents argue that deregulation has had positive *net* benefits.

Deregulation and Contestable Markets 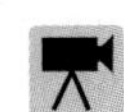

A major argument in favor of deregulation is that when government-imposed barriers to entry are removed, competition will cause firms to enter markets that previously had only a few firms due to those entry barriers. Potential competitors will become actual competitors, and prices will fall toward a competitive level. This argument has been bolstered by a model of efficient firm behavior that predicts competitive prices in spite of a lack of a large number of firms. This model is called the **theory of contestable markets.** Under the theory of contestable markets, most of the outcomes predicted by the theory of perfect competition will occur in certain industries with relatively few firms. Specifically, where the theory of contestable markets is applicable, the few firms may still produce the output at which price equals marginal cost in both the short run and the long run. These firms will receive zero economic profits in the long run.

Theory of contestable markets 
A hypothesis concerning pricing behavior that holds that even though there are only a few firms in an industry, they are forced to price their products more or less competitively because of the ease of entry by outsiders. The key aspect of a contestable market is relatively costless entry into and exit from the industry.

Unconstrained and Relatively Costless Entry and Exit. For a market to be perfectly contestable, firms must be able to enter and leave the industry easily. Freedom of entry and exit implies an absence of nonprice constraints and of serious fixed costs associated with a potential competitor's decision to enter a contestable market. Such an absence of important fixed costs results if the firm need buy no specific durable inputs in order to enter, if it uses up all such inputs it does purchase, or if all of its specific durable inputs are salable upon exit without any losses beyond those normally incurred from depreciation. The important issue is whether or not a potential entrant can easily get his or her investment out at any time in the future.

The mathematical model of perfect contestability is complex, but the underlying logic is straightforward. As long as conditions for free entry prevail, any excess profits, or any inefficiencies on the part of incumbent firms, will serve as an inducement for potential entrants to enter. By entering, new firms can temporarily profit at no risk to themselves from the less than competitive situation in the industry. Once competitive conditions are again restored, these firms will leave the industry just as quickly.

Benefits of Contestable Markets. Contestable markets have several desirable characteristics. One has to do with profits. Profits that exceed the opportunity cost of capital will not exist in the long run because of freedom of entry, just as in a perfectly competitive industry. The elimination of "excess" profits can occur even with only a couple of firms in an industry. The threat of entry will cause them to expand output to eliminate excess profit.

Also, firms that have cost curves that are higher than those of the most efficient firms will find that they cannot compete. These firms will be replaced by entrants whose cost curves are consistent with the most efficient technology. In other words, in contestable markets, there will be no cost inefficiencies in the long run.

Rethinking Regulation Using Cost-Benefit Analysis

Rather than considering deregulation as the only solution to "too much" regulation, some economists argue that regulation should simply be put to a cost-benefit test. Specifically, the cost of existing and proposed regulations should be compared to the benefits. Unless it can be demonstrated that regulations generate net positive benefits (benefits greater than costs), such regulations should not be in effect.

CONCEPTS IN BRIEF

- It is difficult to regulate the price per constant-quality unit because it is difficult to measure all dimensions of quality.
- The capture hypothesis holds that regulatory agencies will eventually be captured by special interests of the industry. This is because consumers are a diffuse group who individually are not affected greatly by regulation, whereas industry groups are well focused and know that large amounts of potential profits are at stake and depend on the outcome of regulatory proceedings.
- In the share-the-gains, share-the-pains theory of regulation, regulators must take account of the interests of three groups: the industry, legislators, and consumers.
- The 1970s and 1980s were periods of deregulation during which formerly regulated industries became much more competitive. The short-run effects of deregulation in some industries were numerous bankruptcies and disrupted service. The long-run results in many deregulated industries included better service, more variety, and lower costs. One argument in favor of deregulation involves the theory of contestable markets—if entry and exit are relatively costless, the number of firms in an industry is irrelevant in terms of determining whether consumers pay competitive prices.

ANTITRUST POLICY

It is the expressed aim of our government to foster competition in the economy. To this end, numerous attempts have been made to legislate against business practices that seemingly destroy the competitive nature of the system. This is the general idea behind antitrust legislation: If the courts can prevent collusion among sellers of a product, monopoly prices will not result; there will be no restriction of output if the members of an industry are not allowed to join together in restraint of trade. Remember that the competitive solution to the price-quantity problem is one in which the price of the item produced is equal to its marginal social opportunity cost. Also, no *economic* profits are made in the long run.

The Sherman Antitrust Act of 1890

Click here to for more details on the history of antitrust regulation.

The Sherman Antitrust Act was passed in 1890. It was the first attempt by the federal government to control the growth of monopoly in the United States. The most important provisions of that act are as follows:

Section 1: Every contract, combination in the form of trust or otherwise, or conspiracy, in restraint of trade or commerce among the several states, or with foreign nations, is hereby declared to be illegal.

Section 2: Every person who shall monopolize, or attempt to monopolize, or combine or conspire with any other person or persons to monopolize any part of the trade or commerce . . . shall be guilty of a misdemeanor.*

Notice how vague this act really is. No definition is given for the terms *restraint of trade* or *monopolization*. Despite this vagueness, however, the act was used to prosecute the infamous Standard Oil trust of New Jersey. Standard Oil of New Jersey was charged with violations of Sections 1 and 2 of the Sherman Antitrust Act. This was in 1906, when Standard Oil controlled over 80 percent of the nation's oil-refining capacity. Among other things, Standard Oil was accused of both predatory price cutting to drive rivals out of business and obtaining preferential price treatment from the railroads for transporting Standard Oil products, thus allowing Standard to sell at lower prices.

*This is now a felony.

Standard Oil was convicted in a district court. The company then appealed to the Supreme Court, which ruled that Standard's control of and power over the oil market created "a *prima facie* presumption of intent and purpose to maintain dominancy . . . not as a result from normal methods of industrial development, but by means of combination." Here the word *combination* meant taking over other businesses and obtaining preferential price treatment from railroads. The Supreme Court forced Standard Oil of New Jersey to break up into many smaller companies.

POLICY EXAMPLE

Microsoft: Gentle Giant or Big Bad Wolf?

A few years back, Netscape was the dominant seller of Web browser software. Its product was called Navigator. Microsoft developed similar features for its Internet Explorer browser. For a while, the two systems competed side by side. But when Microsoft decided to include a new version of Internet Explorer as part of its Windows software, Netscape raised a ruckus—and understandably so: 80 percent of the world's personal computers use the Windows operating system. If Microsoft started "bundling" browser software with Windows, few PC users would need Navigator, and that would quickly drive Netscape out of business. In May 1998, the U.S. Department of Justice took Netscape's side, arguing that "Microsoft possesses (and for several years has possessed) monopoly power in the market for personal computer operating systems." By bundling Internet Explorer within Windows, Justice alleged, "Microsoft is unlawfully taking advantage of its Windows monopoly to protect and extend that monopoly." A federal judge's findings of fact in November 1999 generally supported the Justice Department's interpretation, and thereafter Justice pressed its case for a legal remedy that will entail splitting Microsoft into two different companies.

Monopolies charge prices that are higher than they would be if competition prevailed. Nevertheless, in the software markets, prices have been falling, and the prices of Microsoft's products have not been immune to this downward drift. When someone pointed this out to a Justice Department official, he stated that Justice had to look to the future. In other words, the Justice Department believed that it could predict what will happen in the computer industry, and that was why it was trying to prevent Microsoft from bundling Internet Explorer with Windows.

Of course, none of us can be sure our future predictions will be borne out by events. In fact, in the midst of the Microsoft antitrust action, everyone, including the Justice Department, was taken by surprise when America Online acquired Netscape. Then in 2000 America Online aquired Time Warner in a deal valued at nearly $200 billion, creating a corporate giant rivaling Microsoft. Indeed, some economists began to wonder if Microsoft would be able to compete with America Online's new multimedia empire. Nevertheless, the antitrust action against Microsoft continued.

For Critical Analysis

Why do you suppose that the Justice Department did not drop its antitrust action against Microsoft after America Online purchased Netscape and Time Warner?

The Clayton Act of 1914

Click here to learn more about antitrust policy.

The Sherman Act was so vague that in 1914 a new law was passed to sharpen its antitrust provisions. This law was called the Clayton Act. It prohibited or limited a number of very specific business practices, which again were said to be "unreasonable" attempts at restraining trade or commerce. Section 2 of that act made it illegal to "discriminate in price between different purchasers" except in cases in which the differences are due to actual differences in selling or transportation costs. Section 3 stated that producers cannot sell goods "on the condition, agreement or understanding that the . . . purchaser thereof shall not use or deal in the goods . . . of a competitor or competitors of the seller." And Section 7 provided that corporations cannot hold stock in another company if the effect "may be to substantially lessen competition."

The Federal Trade Commission Act of 1914 and Its 1938 Amendment

The Federal Trade Commission Act was designed to stipulate acceptable competitive behavior. In particular, it was supposed to prevent cutthroat pricing—so-called excessively aggressive competition which would tend to eliminate too many competitors. One of the basic features of the act was the creation of the Federal Trade Commission (FTC), charged with the power to investigate unfair competitive practices. The FTC can do this on its own or at the request of firms that feel they have been wronged. It can issue cease and desist orders where "unfair methods of competition in commerce" are discovered. In 1938, the Wheeler-Lea Act amended the 1914 act. The amendment expressly prohibits "unfair or deceptive acts or practices in commerce." Pursuant to that act, the FTC engages in what it sees as a battle against false or misleading advertising, as well as the misrepresentation of goods and services for sale in the marketplace.

The Robinson-Patman Act of 1936

In 1936, Section 2 of the Clayton Act was amended by the Robinson-Patman Act. The Robinson-Patman Act was aimed at preventing producers from driving out smaller competitors by means of selected discriminatory price cuts. The act has often been referred to as the "Chain Store Act" because it was meant to protect *independent* retailers and wholesalers from "unfair discrimination" by chain stores.

The act was the natural outgrowth of increasing competition that independents faced when chain stores and mass distributors started to develop after World War I. The essential provisions of the act are as follows:

1. It was made illegal to pay brokerage fees unless an independent broker was employed.
2. It was made illegal to offer concessions, such as discounts, free advertising, or promotional allowances, to one buyer of a firm's product if the firm did not offer the same concessions to all buyers of that product.
3. Other forms of discrimination, such as quantity discounts, were also made illegal whenever they "substantially" lessened competition.
4. It was made illegal to charge lower prices in one location than in another or to sell at "unreasonably low prices" if such marketing techniques were designed to "destroy competition or eliminate a competitor."

Exemptions from Antitrust Laws

Numerous laws exempt the following industries and business practices from antitrust legislation:

1. Labor unions
2. Public utilities—electric, gas, and telephone companies
3. Professional baseball
4. Cooperative activities among American exporters
5. Hospitals
6. Public transit and water systems

7. Suppliers of military equipment
8. Joint publishing arrangement in a single city by two or more newspapers

THE ENFORCEMENT OF ANTITRUST LAWS

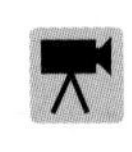

Most antitrust enforcement today is based on the Sherman Act. The Supreme Court has defined the offense of **monopolization** as involving the following elements: "(1) the possession of monopoly power in the relevant market and (2) the willful acquisition or maintenance of that power, as distinguished from growth or development as a consequence of a superior product, business acumen, or historical accident."

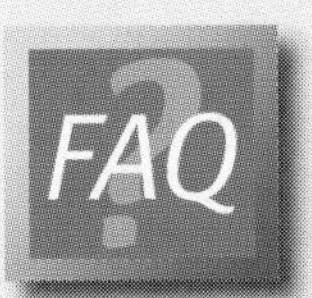

Doesn't an antitrust exemption for major league baseball benefit team owners at the expense of all professional baseball players?

Yes and no. Certainly, the antitrust exemption makes it easier for team owners to work together to restrict the ability of players to negotiate the best possible contract with the team of their choice. Nevertheless, if Congress did away with the antitrust exemption, it might also make it illegal for major league players to have union representation. This might have the effect of pushing down the average salaries of players who are not stars. In addition, without antitrust protection, teams would be unable to bind minor league players to a major league team under the "reserve clause" of major league baseball. This would remove a key incentive for major league teams to support minor league teams, thereby depressing the salaries of minor league players.

Monopoly Power and the Relevant Market

The Sherman Act does not define monopoly. Monopoly clearly is not a single entity. Also, monopoly is not a function of size alone. For example, a "mom and pop" grocery store located in an isolated desert town is a monopolist in at least one sense.

Monopolization 
The possession of monopoly power in the relevant market and the willful acquisition or maintenance of that power, as distinguished from growth or development as a consequence of a superior product, business acumen, or historical accident.

It is difficult to define and measure market power precisely. As a workable proxy, courts often look to the firm's percentage share of the "relevant market." This is the so-called **market share test.** A firm is generally considered to have monopoly power if its share of the relevant market is 70 percent or more. This is not an absolute dictum, however. It is only a loose rule of thumb; in some cases, a smaller share may be held to constitute monopoly power.

Market share test 
The percentage of a market that a particular firm supplies, used as the primary measure of monopoly power.

The relevant market consists of two elements: a relevant product market and a relevant geographic market. What should the relevant product market include? It must include all products produced by different firms that have identical attributes, such as sugar. Yet products that are not identical may sometimes be substituted for one another. Coffee may be substituted for tea, for example. In defining the relevant product market, the key issue is the degree of interchangeability between products. If one product is a sufficient substitute for another, the two products are considered to be part of the same product market.

The second component of the relevant market is the geographic boundaries of the market. For products that are sold nationwide, the geographic boundaries of the market encompass the entire United States. If a producer and its competitors sell in only a limited area (one in which customers have no access to other sources of the product), the geographic market is limited to that area. A national firm may thus compete in several distinct areas and have monopoly power in one area but not in another.

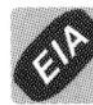

Concentration Ratios
See how to calculate market shares.

Cross-Border Mergers and the Relevant Market

An emerging challenge to the application of antitrust laws is cross-border mergers. How should antitrust authorities define the "relevant market" when Daimler-Benz of Germany desires to merge with Chrysler Corporation or when Deutsche Bank, also of Germany, wishes to purchase one of the nation's largest banks, Banker's Trust? U.S. authorities

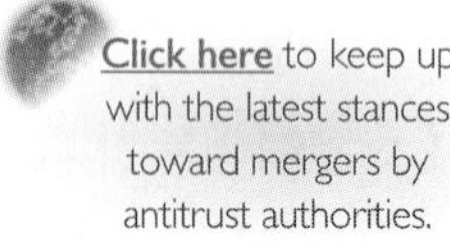
Click here to keep up with the latest stances toward mergers by antitrust authorities.

approved both of these mergers. Their conclusion was that the automotive and banking markets have become global in scope, thereby justifying these cross-border combinations. It remains to be seen whether U.S. antitrust authorities will be so open-minded if the cross-national merger wave continues in these industries or spreads to others in future years. Undoubtedly, internal pressures will emerge to restrain merger activity intended to make home industries more competitive internationally.

Consider the recent experience of the Canadian banking industry. For all its massive geographic size, Canada's population is slightly smaller than California's. The nation has four dominant Toronto-based banking institutions—the Royal Bank of Canada, the Bank of Montreal, the Toronto-Dominion Bank, and the Canadian Imperial Bank of Commerce—which serve as depositories for two-thirds of all funds in Canadian banks. In 1998, the four institutions proposed merging into two, with Royal Bank of Canada set to merge with the Bank of Montreal and the Toronto-Dominion Bank poised to merge with the Canadian Imperial Bank of Commerce. The four institutions wanted to consolidate to assist in fending off competition from big U.S. banks. They also wanted to embark on an effort to compete more successfully in the United States, thereby diversifying their operations geographically. Canadian authorities disallowed both merger requests, however, ruling that the "relevant banking market" was Canada alone. For the banks that had proposed to merge, however, this was a serious blow to their long-range plans regarding their ability to compete effectively in the *international* banking markets that *they* felt were most relevant.

CONCEPTS IN BRIEF

- The first national antitrust law was the Sherman Antitrust Act, passed in 1890, which made illegal every contract and combination in the form of a trust in restraint of trade.
- The Clayton Act made price discrimination and interlocking directorates illegal.
- The Federal Trade Commission Act of 1914 established the Federal Trade Commission. The Wheeler-Lea Act of 1938 amended the 1914 act to prohibit "unfair or deceptive acts or practices in commerce."
- The Robinson-Patman Act of 1936 was aimed at preventing large producers from driving out small competitors by means of selective discriminatory price cuts.

NETNOMICS

Is the Internet Destined to Be Regulated?

According to J. Bradford De Long of the University of California at Berkeley and law professor A. Michael Froomkin of the University of Miami, some of the very characteristics that have driven the rapid adoption of information technology could prove to be its undoing. Recall from Chapter 5 that only one person at a time can consume a *private good.* For instance, when a computer repairperson is working on someone else's hard drive, that individual cannot work at the same time to repair your DVD drive. On the Internet, however, the situation is not quite as clear-cut. If one person is using a Web site, a thousand can. If a thousand are, ten thousand might as well. Indeed, in the network economy, if more people are consuming a good, it becomes more valuable. A dozen people trying to share the same phone booth have a problem, but tens of millions who have access to e-mail may have a distinct advantage over those who don't, because this makes it easier for each one to communicate with the others. Among economists who specialize in Internet economics, the expression "network externalities" is commonly used to describe this situation.

According to De Long and Froomkin, network externalities may yield significant economies of scale that pave the way for domination of portions of cyberspace by individual Internet firms. They suggest that in coming years, this could induce many consumers to clamor for regulating these companies' activities. In addition, De Long and Froomkin note that because digital data are so easy to copy, getting users to pay could become increasingly difficult. As a result, the *excludability principle* discussed in Chapter 5 may not always apply. Sellers may have difficulty inducing consumers to pay for all that they use on their Web sites, so sellers themselves may also perceive advantages in government intervention.

Thus De Long and Froomkin envision a future ablaze with disagreements about whether Internet commerce should be subjected to the same kinds of governmental interventions that traditional firms have experienced. If they are correct, the virtual world of the Web could end up looking a lot like the nonvirtual reality we inhabited before the advent of the Internet.

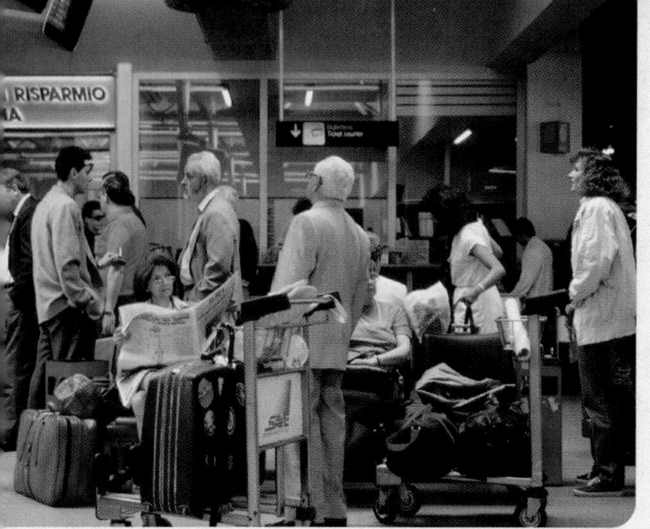

ISSUES & APPLICATIONS

Putting Government Behind the Airline Ticket Counter: Should Airlines Be Forced to Raise Their Fares?

If you have ever shopped around for an airline ticket, you may have been surprised to learn that a round-trip flight from, say, Nashville, Tennessee, to the Raleigh-Durham airport in neighboring North Carolina might cost $600 on one airline but only $200 on another. The second fare looks, comparatively, like a great deal for consumers. To the Department of Justice and the Department of Transportation, however, it is a possible indication of "predatory pricing," a common epithet applied to discriminatory price cuts that are illegal under the Robinson-Patman Act.

Concepts Applied

- Regulation
- Capture Hypothesis
- Share-the-Gain, Share-the-Pain Theory

Fair or Foul?

Some government officials contend that big airlines have entrenched themselves at "fortress hubs"—for instance, the United hub in Denver, the Delta hub in Atlanta, and the Northwest hub in Minneapolis—where their planes often account for more than three-fourths of all flights. Using these hubs, government critics argue, the big carriers can undercut any rival that dares to enter "their" airports.

What is their alleged weapon? According to some officials, it is rock-bottom fares that please consumers for a time but remain in effect only long enough to prevent rivals from establishing a market niche.

Mixed Weather for Airline Markets

There are a number of contrary signals about airline competition. Since 1978, when Congress lifted many economic restrictions on airlines, average airfares have dropped by 40 percent in real terms. The number of flights has risen by 50 percent, and annual passenger boardings have jumped from 275 million to about 600 million. Air travel used to be the domain of businesspeople and the well-off. Now it has become accessible to many ordinary people. Firms in service industries where market power is prevalent tend to charge higher prices and restrict sales of their services. There is little evidence this has been happening in the airline industry.

In addition, the government has since 1969 reserved a number of landings and takeoffs at Chicago's O'Hare airport, Washington's Reagan National Airport, and New York's La Guardia and Kennedy airports. These landing and takeoff "slots," as they are known, are by government edict the "property" of a handful of carriers. There were only two minor expansions in the numbers of government-awarded slots at these airports since 1969. Not until 1998 did the government grant slot exemptions at O'Hare and La Guardia for previously excluded minor carriers trying to break into those markets. Thus the government itself has made it difficult to establish a market niche at four of the nation's busiest airports.

So far there is no sign of any consideration of reducing the competition-stifling regulation of landing slots at major airports. In the meantime, however, the Justice Department has launched an antitrust investigation of possible predatory pricing by major airlines, and the Transportation Department has proposed rules establishing steep fines for airlines that set their fares "too low." Essentially, the government seems intent on establishing price floors in the airline industry. What remains to be seen is how this action would benefit consumers.

FOR CRITICAL ANALYSIS

1. Why do you suppose that the government restricts landing and takeoff slots at big airports?
2. If the government were to establish a "floor airfare" that is above the equilibrium fare that would prevail in a free market, what can you predict would be the likely result?

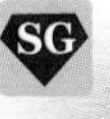

SUMMARY DISCUSSION OF LEARNING OBJECTIVES

1. **Practical Difficulties in Regulating the Prices Charged by Natural Monopolies:** To try to ensure that a monopolist charges a price consistent with the marginal cost to it and to society of producing the good or service that it produces, a government regulator might contemplate requiring the firm to set price equal to marginal cost. This is the point where the demand curve the monopolist faces crosses its marginal cost curve. A problem arises, however, in the case of a natural monopoly, for which the long-run average total cost curve and the long-run marginal cost curve slope downward as a firm's output rate increases. In this situation, long-run marginal cost is typically less than long-run average total cost, so requiring marginal cost pricing forces the natural monopoly to earn an economic loss. As a practical matter, therefore, regulators normally aim for a natural monopoly to charge a price equal to average total cost so that the firm earns zero economic profits.
2. **Rationales for Government Regulation of Business:** There are three types of government regulation of business: regulation of natural monopolies, regulation of inherently competitive industries, and social regulation aimed at ensuring public welfare. Regulation of natural monopolies often takes the form of cost-of-service regulation that seeks to achieve average-cost pricing and rate-of-return regulation aimed at attaining a competitive, zero-profit rate of return. Regulation of otherwise competitive industries is typically designed to address perceived market failures. Social regulations, however, encompass a broad set of objectives concerning such issues as the quality of products, product safety, and conditions under which employees work.
3. **Alternative Theories of Regulator Behavior:** The capture theory of regulator behavior predicts that because people with expertise about a regulated industry are most likely to be selected to regulate the industry, these regulators eventually find themselves supporting the positions of the firms that they regulate. An alternative view, called the share-the-gains, share-the pains theory, predicts that a regulator takes into account the preferences of legislators and consumers as well as the regulated firms themselves. Thus a regulator tries to satisfy all constituencies, at least in part.
4. **Short- and Long-Run Economic Effects of Deregulation:** A number of industries have been deregulated since the late 1970s. The short-run effects of deregulation are typically a number of temporary adjustments, such as failures of high-cost producers, some cutbacks in products or services to some consumers, and the loss of jobs by some workers in the industry. As these adjustments are completed, profits fall toward competitive levels, and prices drop closer to marginal cost. The key issue in assessing deregulation is whether these long-term benefits for society outweigh the short-term adjustment costs.
5. **Foundations of Antitrust:** There are four key antitrust laws. The Sherman Act of 1890 forbids attempts to monopolize an industry. The Clayton Act of 1914 clarified antitrust law by prohibiting specific types of business practices that Congress determined were aimed at restraining trade. In addition, the Federal Trade Commission Act of 1914, as amended in 1938, seeks to prohibit deceptive business practices and to prevent "cutthroat pricing," which Congress felt could unfairly eliminate too many competitors. Finally, the Robinson-Patman Act of 1936 outlawed price cuts that Congress determined to be discriminatory and predatory.
6. **Issues in Enforcing Antitrust Laws:** Because antitrust laws are relatively vague, enforcement of the laws is based on Supreme Court interpretations of their meaning. The Supreme Court has defined monopolization as possessing monopoly pricing power in the "relevant market" or engaging in willful efforts to obtain such power. Authoities charged with enforcing antitrust laws typically use a market share test in which they examine the percentage of market production or sales by the firm under investigation. A key issue in applying the market share test is defining the relevant market. Recent increases in international competition have complicated efforts to do this.

Key Terms and Concepts

Capture hypothesis (645)
Cost-of-service regulation (642)
Creative response (644)
Deregulation (648)
Market share test (653)
Monopolization (653)
Rate-of-return regulation (642)
Share-the-gains, share-the-pains theory (646)
Theory of contestable markets (649)

Problems

Answers to the odd-numbered problems appear at the back of the book.

26-1. Local cable companies are usually granted monopoly rights to service a particular territory of a metropolitan area. The companies typically pay special taxes and license fees to local municipalities. Why might a municipality give monopoly rights to a cable company?

26-2. "A local cable company, the sole provider of cable television service, is regulated by the municipal government. The owner of the company claims that she is opposed to regulation by government but asserts that regulation is necessary because local residents would not want a large number of different cables spanning the skies of the city. Why do you think the owner is defending regulation by the city?

26-3. The following table depicts the cost and demand structure a natural monopoly faces.

Quantity	Price($)	Long-Run Total Cost ($)
0	100	0
1	95	90
2	90	175
3	85	255
4	80	330
5	75	405
6	70	485

If this firm were allowed to operate as a monopolist, what would be the quantity produced and price charged by the firm? What is the amount of monopoly profit?

26-4. If regulators required the firm in Problem 26-3 to practice marginal cost pricing, what quantity would it produce, and what price would it charge? What is the firm's profit under this regulatory framework?

26-5. If regulators required the firm in Problem 26-3 to practice average cost pricing, what quantity would it produce, and what price would it charge? What is the firm's profit under this regulatory framework?

26-6. Discuss the major strength and weakness of the two traditional approaches to economic regulation.

26-7. Contrast the major objectives of economic regulation and social regulation.

26-8. Research into genetically modified crops has led to significant productivity gains for countries such as the United States that employ these techniques. Countries such as the European Union member nations, however, have imposed controls on the import of these products, citing concern for public health. Is the European Union's regulation of genetically modified crops social regulation or economic regulation?

26-9. Using the example in Problem 26-8, do you think this is most likely an example of the capture hypothesis or the share-the-gains, share-the-pains theory? Why?

26-10. In spite of a number of available sites to establish a business, few regulations, and minimum zoning problems, there is only one fast-food restaurant bordering campus. Given the significant potential for entry by other competitors, will this monopoly necessarily maximize its potential monopoly profits?

Economics on the Net

Guidelines for U.S. Antitrust Merger Enforcement How does the U.S. government apply anitrust laws to mergers? This application gives you the opportunity to learn about the standards applied by the Antitrust Division of the U.S. Department of Justice when it evaluates a proposed merger.

Title: U.S. Department of Justice Antitrust Merger Enforcement Guidelines

Navigation: Click here to start at the homepage of the Antitrust Division of the U.S. Department of Justice. Click on Public Documents and then on Merger Enforcement.

Application

1. Click on Horizontal Merger Guidelines. In section 1, click on Overview, and read this section. What factors do U.S. antitrust authorities consider when evaluating the potential for a horizontal merger to "enhance market power"—that is, to place the combination in a monopoly situation?
2. Back up to the page titled Merger Enforcement Guidelines, and click on Non-Horizontal Merger Guidelines. Read the guidelines. In what situations will the antitrust authorities most likely question a nonhorizontal merger?

For Group Study and Analysis Have three groups of students from the class examine sections 1, 2, and 3 of the Horizontal Merger Guidelines discussed in item 1. After each group reports on the all the factors that the antitrust authorities consider when evaluating a horizontal merger, discuss why it is that large teams of lawyers and many economic consultants are typically involved when the Antitrust Division of the Department of Justice alleges that a proposed merger would be "anticompetitive."

TYING IT ALL TOGETHER

Part 6 Case Problem

Case Background

Readme.com is a new company created by two book lovers who wish to emulate the success of Amazon.com and other Internet-based booksellers. These entrepreneurs, who have raised considerable funds from investors, believe that they have developed systems for processing book orders and shipping that are superior than those used by other booksellers on the Web. The problem they face, however, is that they must find a way to establish a presence in an already crowded bookselling market in cyberspace.

Lessons from the Battle Between Amazon.com and Barnes & Noble
Amazon.com first cracked the bookselling market by opening up shop on the Internet in 1995. Between December 1995 and late 1997, the average number of daily visits to Amazon.com's Web site increased from 2,000 to 1 million. It transformed its online catalog into a virtual index of book titles and detailed information about those titles, including outside reviews and even reviews by its own customers. The company also attracted customers by advertising in traditional print publications. It also developed an "associates program" that allowed other Internet sellers to display hot links to Amazon.com and offer books of interest to their customers, and Amazon.com paid other companies referral fees for revenues generated by such orders.

The day in 1997 that Barnes & Noble launched its Web-based bookselling system, Amazon.com expanded its list of discounted books and nearly doubled the fees it paid to Internet sellers in its associates program. Amazon.com also continued to advertise heavily in traditional media, and it built a new warehouse near the East Coast to speed deliveries in the eastern part of the nation.

Assessing the Market for Books on the Web The owners and managers of Readme.com wish to evaluate how Amazon.com, Barnes & Noble, and other firms already in the Internet-bookselling market may respond to the entry of their firm. They are wrestling with the following questions:

1. Will other Internet booksellers respond to the market entry of Readme.com with noticeable price cuts on a wide range of books?
2. If so, will these price cuts be so steep that if Readme.com fails to match them, it will not be able to cover its costs?
3. If Readme.com is able to establish a market presence and capture enough customers to keep its investors on board, will its low-cost operating system for selling books permit it to earn a normal rate of return in the long run?
4. Will the bookselling market eventually become dominated by a few large firms, including Amazon.com and Barnes & Noble, or will it remain a highly splintered market with a large number of sellers? Over the longer term, what scale size should Readme.com seek to attain?

Points to Analyze

1. In what ways does the bookselling market exhibit characteristics of perfect competition?
2. In what ways does the market have features of imperfect competition?
3. Is there any specific theory of imperfect competition that appears to be a potential "fit" for the bookselling market?
4. Based on the foregoing information, does it appear to you that Readme.com should be concerned about the possible use of limit-pricing strategies by Amazon.com, Barnes & Noble, and other major booksellers? Why or why not?
5. Do there appear to be economies of scale in bookselling? Are diseconomies of scale likely to arise for booksellers when they operate at sufficiently high sales levels? Why or why not?

Casing the Internet

1. **Click on each link to visit the Web sites of both Amazon.com and Barnes & Noble. Now, answer the following questions.**
   a. **What are the similarities between the two Web sites? Are there notable differences?**
   b. **In what ways are the products that these two companies market over the Internet homogeneous? In what respects do the companies market differentiated products?**
2. **Chapter 4 discussed the role that middlemen—market intermediaries between buyers and sellers—play in reducing transaction costs for buyers and sellers. Click here to go to the Web site of Anaconda! Partners. This is a company that markets programs that assist companies in linking their Web sites to those of other firms.**
   a. **Review the basic set of available Anaconda! products. In what sense does it appear that Anaconda! Partners is a market middleman?**
   b. **Why would an Internet seller want to link its Web site to the sites of other companies? That is, how might a client of Anaconda! Partners gain from "creating useful informational or affiliate websites that can earn [it] money," as claimed in the heading above the product descriptions?**
   c. **In your view, are Web links among firms likely to make the markets for products sold by firms over the Internet more or less competitive? Support your position.**

Part 7

Productive Factors, Poverty, Health Care, and the Environment

CHAPTER

27

LABOR DEMAND AND SUPPLY

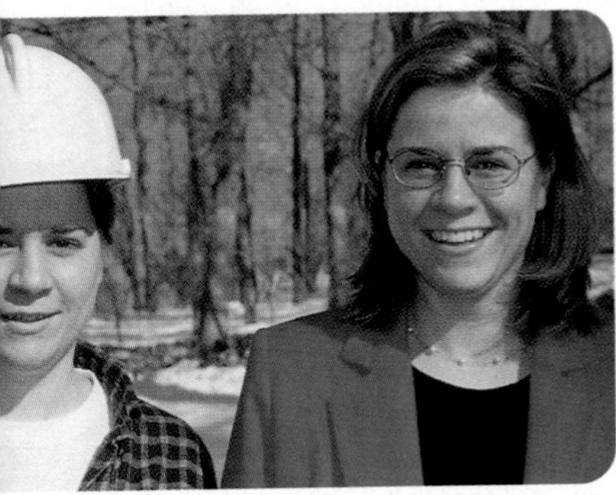

These identical twins pursued different educational paths. Typically, a twin who goes to college will earn 67 percent more in monthly wages than one who joins the work force immediately upon graduating from high school.

Medical researchers, psychologists, and other scientists often conduct studies of identical twins. This allows them to hold constant heredity, early home life, and other factors. Economists have also learned a lot from identical twins. A study by Orley Ashenfelter and Alan Krueger of Princeton University tracked the earning patterns of more than 250 pairs of identical twins. These researchers found that each additional year of schooling increased wages by nearly 16 percent. A twin who attended four years of college earned monthly wages averaging 67 percent higher than those of the sibling with no college. To understand why additional and specialized training can have such dramatic effects on the wages that people earn, you need to understand the basic model of labor demand and supply.

LEARNING OBJECTIVES

After reading this chapter, you should be able to:

1. **Understand why a firm's marginal revenue product curve is its labor demand curve**
2. **Explain in what sense the demand for labor is a "derived" demand**
3. **Identify the key factors influencing the elasticity of demand for inputs**
4. **Describe how equilibrium wage rates are determined for perfectly competitive firms**
5. **Discuss alternative theories of wage determination**
6. **Contrast the demand for labor and wage determination by a product market monopolist with outcomes that would arise under perfect competition**

Chapter Outline

Did You Know That... the top 350 executives in America's biggest corporations are compensated, on the average, $2.5 million each, or about 60 times more than the median family income of a little over $40,000? Recently, the head of the Walt Disney Company, Michael Eisner, was paid more than $100 million in one year. You, in contrast, as a typical college student will probably make between $25,000 and $50,000 a year, or approximately one two-thousandth of Eisner's annual salary. To comprehend why firms pay different employees such vastly different salaries, you must understand how the laws of demand and supply apply to labor.

A firm's demand for inputs can be studied in much the same manner as we studied the demand for output in different market situations. Again, various market situations will be examined. Our analysis will always end with the same commonsense conclusion: A firm will hire employees up to the point beyond which it isn't profitable to hire any more. It will hire employees to the point at which the marginal benefit of hiring a worker will just equal the marginal cost. Basically, in every profit-maximizing situation, it is most profitable to carry out an activity up to the point at which the marginal benefit equals the marginal cost. Remembering that guideline will help you in analyzing decision making at the firm level. We will start our analysis under the assumption that the market for input factors is perfectly competitive. We will further assume that the output market is perfectly competitive. This provides a benchmark against which to compare other situations in which labor markets or product markets are not perfectly competitive.

COMPETITION IN THE PRODUCT MARKET

Let's take as our example a compact disk (CD) manufacturing firm that is in competition with many companies selling the same kind of product. Assume that the laborers hired by our CD manufacturing firm do not need any special skills. This firm sells its product in a perfectly competitive market. A CD manufacturer also buys labor (its variable input) in a perfectly competitive market. A firm that hires labor under perfectly competitive conditions hires only a minuscule proportion of all the workers who are potentially available to the firm. By "potentially available" we mean all the workers in a given geographic area who possess the skills demanded by our perfect competitor. In such a market, it is always possible for the individual firm to pick up extra workers without having to offer a higher wage. Thus the supply of labor to the firm is perfectly elastic at the going wage rate established by the forces of supply and demand in the entire labor market. The firm is a price taker in the labor market.

MARGINAL PHYSICAL PRODUCT

Marginal physical product (MPP) of labor 
The change in output resulting from the addition of one more worker. The MPP of the worker equals the change in total output accounted for by hiring the worker, holding all other factors of production constant.

Look at panel (a) of Figure 27-1. In column 1, we show the number of workers per week that the firm can hire. In column 2, we show total physical product (TPP) per week, the total *physical* production that different quantities of the labor input (in combination with a fixed amount of other inputs) will generate in a week's time. In column 3, we show the additional output gained when a CD manufacturing company adds workers to its existing manufacturing facility. This column, the **marginal physical product (MPP) of labor,** represents the extra (additional) output attributed to employing additional units of the variable input factor. If this firm employs seven workers rather than six, the MPP is 118. The law of diminishing marginal returns predicts that additional units of a variable factor will, after some point, cause the MPP to decline, other things being held constant.

FIGURE 27-1

Marginal Revenue Product

In panel (a), column 4 shows marginal revenue product (MRP), which is the amount of additional revenue the firm receives for the sale of that additional output. Marginal revenue product is simply the amount of money the additional worker brings in—the combination of that worker's contribution to production and the revenue that that production will bring to the firm. For this perfectly competitive firm, marginal revenue is equal to the price of the product, or $6 per unit. At a weekly wage of $498, the profit-maximizing employer will pay for only 12 workers because then the marginal revenue product is just equal to the wage rate or weekly salary.

Panel (a)

(1) Labor Input (workers per week)	(2) Total Physical Product (TPP) CDs per Week	(3) Marginal Physical Product (MPP) CDs per Week	(4) Marginal Revenue (MR = P = $6 net) x MPP = Marginal Revenue Product (MRP) ($ per additional worker)	(5) Wage Rate ($ per week) = Marginal Factor Cost (MFC) = Change in Total Costs / Change in Labor
6	882			
		118	$708	$498
7	1,000			
		111	666	498
8	1,111			
		104	624	498
9	1,215			
		97	582	498
10	1,312			
		90	540	498
11	1,402			
		83	498	498
12	1,485			
		76	456	498
13	1,561			

In panel (b), we find the number of workers the firm will want to hire by observing the wage rate that is established by the forces of supply and demand in the entire labor market. We show that this employer is hiring labor in a perfectly competitive labor market and therefore faces a perfectly elastic supply curve represented by *s* at $498 per week. As in all other situations, we basically have a supply and demand model; in this example, the demand curve is represented by MRP, and the supply curve is *s*. Equilibrium occurs at their intersection.

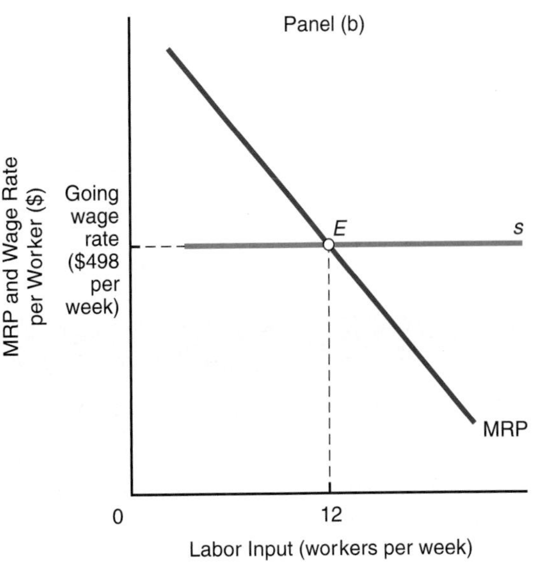

Why the Decline in MPP?

We are assuming all other nonlabor factors of production are held constant. So if our CD manufacturing firm wants to add one more worker to its production line, it has to crowd all the existing workers a little closer together because it does not increase its capital stock (the production equipment). Therefore, as we add more workers, each one has a smaller and smaller fraction of the available capital stock with which to work. If one worker uses one machine, adding another worker usually won't double the output because the machine can run only so fast and for so many hours per day. In other words, MPP declines because of the law of diminishing marginal returns.

Marginal Revenue Product

We now need to translate into a dollar value the physical product that results from hiring an additional worker. This is done by multiplying the marginal physical product by the marginal revenue of the firm. Because our CD firm is selling its product in a perfectly competitive market, marginal revenue is equal to the price of the product. If employing seven workers rather than six yields an MPP of 118 and the marginal revenue is $6 per CD, the **marginal revenue product (MRP)** is $708 (118 × $6). The MRP is shown in column 4 of panel (a) of Figure 27-1. *The marginal revenue product represents the incremental worker's contribution to the firm's total revenues.*

Marginal revenue product (MRP)
The marginal physical product (MPP) times marginal revenue. The MRP gives the additional revenue obtained from a one-unit change in labor input.

When a firm operates in a competitive product market, the marginal physical product times the product price is also sometimes referred to as the *value of marginal product (VMP).* Because price and marginal revenue are the same for a perfectly competitive firm, the VMP is also the MRP for such a firm.

In column 5 of panel (a) of Figure 27-1, we show the wage rate, or *marginal factor cost,* of each worker. The marginal cost of workers is the extra cost incurred in employing an additional unit of that factor of production. We call that cost the **marginal factor cost (MFC).** Otherwise stated,

Marginal factor cost (MFC) 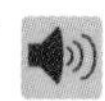
The cost of using an additional unit of an input. For example, if a firm can hire all the workers it wants at the going wage rate, the marginal factor cost of labor is the wage rate.

$$\text{Marginal factor cost} \equiv \frac{\text{change in total cost}}{\text{change in amount of resource used}}$$

Because each worker is paid the same competitively determined wage of $498 per week, the MFC is the same for all workers. And because the firm is buying labor in a perfectly competitive labor market, the wage rate of $498 per week really represents the supply curve of labor to the firm. That curve is perfectly elastic because the firm can purchase all labor at the same wage rate, considering that it is a minuscule part of the entire labor-purchasing market. (Recall the definition of perfect competition.) We show this perfectly elastic supply curve as *s* in panel (b) of Figure 27-1.

EXAMPLE

Does Attractiveness Lead to Higher Marginal Revenue Product?

Economist Daniel Hamermesh of the University of Texas, Austin, and Jeff Biddle of Michigan State University discovered that "plain-looking" people earn 5 to 10 percent less than people of "average" looks, who in turn earn 5 percent less than those who are considered "good-looking." Surprisingly, their research showed that the "looks effect" on wages was greater for men than for women. This wage differential related to appearance is not, contrary to popular belief, evident only in modeling, acting, or working directly with the public. Looks seem to account for higher earnings in jobs such as bricklaying, factory work, and telemarketing.

According to Hamermesh and Biddle, part of the wage differential may be created by the fact that attractiveness leads to higher marginal revenue product. More attractive individuals may have higher self-esteem, which in turn causes them to be more productive on the job.

For Critical Analysis

What are some of the other possible reasons that more attractive people tend to earn more?

General Rule for Hiring

Virtually every optimizing rule in economics involves comparing marginal benefits with marginal cost. The general rule, therefore, for the hiring decision of a firm is this:

> The firm hires workers up to the point at which the additional cost associated with hiring the last worker is equal to the additional revenue generated by that worker.

In a perfectly competitive market, this is the point at which the wage rate just equals the marginal revenue product. If the firm hired more workers, the additional wages would not be covered by additional increases in total revenue. If the firm hired fewer workers, it would be forfeiting the contributions that those workers could make to total profits.

Therefore, referring to columns 4 and 5 in panel (a) of Figure 27-1, we see that this firm would certainly employ at least seven workers because the MRP is $708 while the MFC is only $498. The firm would continue to employ workers up to the point at which MFC = MRP because as workers are added, they contribute more to revenue than to cost.

The MRP Curve: Demand for Labor

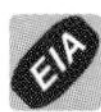

The Marginal Revenue Product of Labor

Gain more experience working with the marginal revenue product (MRP) curve.

We can also use panel (b) of Figure 27-1 to find how many workers our firm should hire. First, we draw a straight line across from the going wage rate, which is determined by demand and supply in the labor market. The straight line is labeled *s* to indicate that it is the supply curve of labor for the *individual* firm purchasing labor in a perfectly competitive labor market. That firm can purchase all the labor it wants of equal quality at $498 per worker. This perfectly elastic supply curve, *s*, intersects the marginal revenue product curve at 12 workers per week. At the intersection, *E*, the wage rate is equal to the marginal revenue product. Equilibrium for the firm is obtained when the firm's demand curve for labor, which turns out to be its MRP curve, intersects the firm's supply curve for labor, shown as *s*. The firm in our example would not hire the thirteenth worker, who will add only $456 to revenue but $498 to cost. If the price of labor should fall to, say, $456 per worker per week, it would become profitable for the firm to hire an additional worker; there is an increase in the quantity of labor demanded as the wage decreases.

DERIVED DEMAND

We have identified an individual firm's demand for labor curve, which shows the quantity of labor that the firm will wish to hire at each wage rate, as its MRP curve. Under conditions of perfect competition in both product and labor markets, MRP is determined by multiplying MPP times the product's price. This suggests that the demand for labor is a **derived demand.** That is to say that our CD firm does not want to purchase the services of labor just for the services themselves. Factors of production are rented or purchased not because they give any intrinsic satisfaction to the firms' owners but because they can be used to manufacture output that is expected to be sold for profit.

Derived Demand 

Input factor demand derived from demand for the final product being produced.

FIGURE 27-2

Demand for Labor, a Derived Demand

The demand for labor is derived from the demand for the final product being produced. Therefore, the marginal revenue product curve will shift whenever the price of the product changes. If we start with the marginal revenue product curve MRP at the going wage rate of $498 per week, 12 workers will be hired. If the price of CDs goes down, the marginal product curve will shift to MRP_1, and the number of workers hired will fall to 10. If the price of CDs goes up, the marginal revenue product curve will shift to MRP_2, and the number of workers hired will increase to 15.

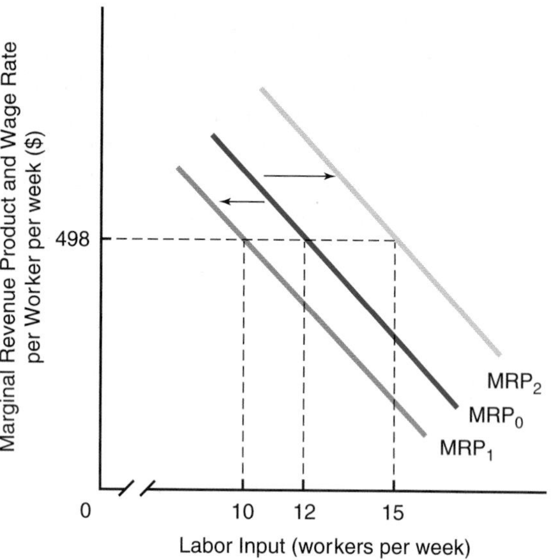

We know that an increase in the market demand for a given product raises the product's price (all other things held constant), which in turn increases the marginal revenue product, or demand for the resource. Figure 27-2 illustrates the effective role played by changes in product demand in a perfectly competitive product market. The MRP curve shifts whenever there is a change in the price of the final product that the workers are producing. Suppose, for example, that the market price of CDs declines. In that case, the MRP curve will shift downward to the left from MRP_0 to MRP_1. We know that MRP $\equiv$ MPP $\times$ MR. If marginal revenue (here the output price) falls, so does the demand for labor. At the same going wage rate, the firm will hire fewer workers. This is because at various levels of labor use, the marginal revenue product of labor is now lower. At the initial equilibrium, therefore, the price of labor (here the MFC) becomes greater than MRP. Thus the firm would reduce the number of workers hired. Conversely, if the marginal revenue (output price) rises, the demand for labor will also rise, and the firm will want to hire more workers at each and every possible wage rate.

We just pointed out that MRP $\equiv$ MPP $\times$ MR. Clearly, then, a change in marginal productivity, or in the marginal physical product of labor, will shift the MRP curve. If the marginal productivity of labor decreases, the MRP curve, or demand curve, for labor will shift inward to the left. Again, this is because at every quantity of labor used, the MRP will be lower. A lower quantity of labor will be demanded at every possible wage rate.

EXAMPLE

"If a Regular Job Doesn't Work Out, Perhaps *Saturday Night Live* Is an Option"

At many firms, the most productive employees are those who can think fast on their feet. Put yourself in the position of an employee of the Chicago-based advertising firm APL/Columbian Advertising. After you pitch carefully prepared proposals to a big client, the client cuts you off and says he hates them. Drawing on comic improvisation techniques that were included in your company's basic employee-training program, you and your colleagues quickly rethink the entire marketing plan and keep your client.

A number of firms, such as the investment company PricewaterhouseCoopers and the advertising company Ogilvy and Mather, send their employees for special training at Second City, the comedy company whose alumni include comic actors Bill Murray and John Belushi, or at Improv Olympic, the rival firm that launched the career of Mike Myers, another standup comedian and actor. Second City is getting so much interest from companies that want to turn wallflowers into rapid-fire communicators that it now has training centers in Chicago, New York, and Toronto and plans to open new centers in Los Angeles and Cleveland. Classes at Second City begin with exercises such as variations on the children's running game called Duck Duck Goose and impromptu skits in which students must carry on conversations using only gibberish. Then students proceed into development of off-the-cuff skits. To the businesses that send their employees to these classes, the idea behind training in stand-up comedy is to prepare their workers to do the kind of speedy thinking that they will have to do each day on the job. This, the companies hope, will raise their employees' productivity.

For Critical Analysis

If companies are correct that comedic training makes their employees more productive, and if more marketing students get such training, what will happen to the demand for these students' skills, other things being equal?

THE MARKET DEMAND FOR LABOR

The downward-sloping portion of each individual firm's marginal revenue product curve is also its demand curve for the one variable factor of production—in our example, labor. When we go to the entire market for a particular type of labor in a particular industry, we find that quantity of labor demanded will vary as the wage rate changes. Given that the market demand curve for labor is made up of the individual firm's downward-sloping demand curves for labor, we can safely infer that the market demand curve for labor will look like *D* in panel (b) of Figure 27-3: It will slope downward. That market demand curve for labor in the CD industry shows the quantities of labor demanded by all of the firms in the industry at various wage rates.

FIGURE 27-3

Derivation of the Market Demand Curve for Labor

The market demand curve for labor is not simply the horizontal summation of each individual firm's demand curve for labor. If wage rates fall from \$20 to \$10, all 200 firms will increase employment and therefore output, causing the price of the product to fall. This causes the marginal revenue product curve of each firm to shift inward, as from d_0 to d_1 in panel (a). The resulting market demand curve, *D*, in panel (b) is therefore less elastic around prices from \$10 to \$20 than it would be if output price remained constant.

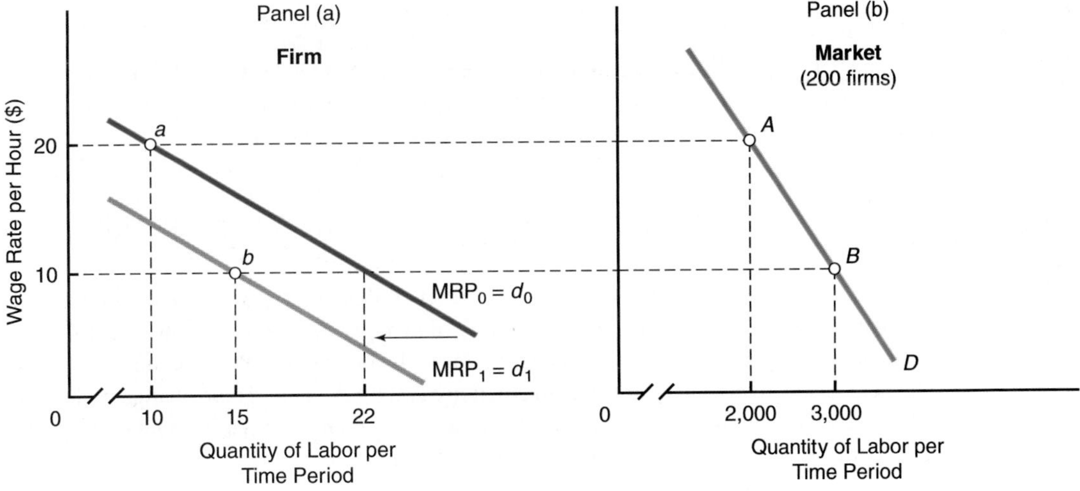

It is important to note that the market demand curve for labor is not a simple horizontal summation of the labor demand curves of all individual firms. Remember that the demand for labor is a derived demand. Even if we hold labor productivity constant, the demand for labor still depends on both the wage rate and the price of the final output. Assume that we start at a wage rate of $20 per hour and employment level 10 in panel (a) of Figure 27-3. If we sum all such employment levels—point *a* in panel (a)—across 200 firms, we get a market quantity demanded of 2,000—point *A* in panel (b)—at the wage rate of $20. A decrease in the wage rate to $10 per hour induces individual firms' employment level to increase toward a quantity demanded of 22. As all 200 firms simultaneously increase employment, however, there is a shift in the product supply curve such that output increases. Hence the price of the product must fall. The fall in the output price in turn causes a downward shift of each firm's MRP curve (d_0) to MRP_1 (d_1) in panel (a). Thus each firm's employment of labor increases to 15 rather than to 22 at the wage rate of $10 per hour. A summation of all such 200 employment levels gives us 3,000—point *B*—in panel (b).

INTERNATIONAL POLICY EXAMPLE

Labor Demand Curves Slope Downward—Except in France

In France, the unemployment rate has exceeded 10 percent for several years now. In an effort to do something about the problem, the French government cut the legal workweek from 39 hours to 35 hours for both hourly and salaried workers. Only senior executives are exempted from the restriction. To enforce the law, the government has issued thousands of citations charging companies with working their employees too many hours. Legal penalties, levied on the chief executive officers of offending companies, include fines up to $1 million and jail terms up to two years.

This has induced some French corporations to install electronic time clocks in hallways. Workers swipe ID cards to record arrival and departure times and coffee and lunch breaks. To allow for some flexibility in the policy, the government permits workers to build up hourly "work credits" in weeks when they exceed the 35-hour threshold. The maximum allowable credit is 15 hours. Managers are required to contact workers who overstep that limit and assist them in drawing up a plan to reduce the backlog. Workaholics who exceed the 15-hour limit by wide margins receive special counseling services to help them figure out how to reduce their time on the job.

This policy has an interesting implication. Lower-paid workers at companies are often blue-collar workers and salaried white-collar clerical staff. The law restricts the hours that these people can work for their relatively lower wages. But the highest-paid senior managers of a company can burn the midnight oil and work as many hours as they wish every week. Thus in France there is now a positive relationship between the wage rate and the quantity of hours that a firm employs workers. In this sense, the law has effectively produced an upward-sloping labor demand curve.

For Critical Analysis

What effect is the French workweek regulation likely to have on the ability of French companies to compete in the face of ever-tougher global competition?

DETERMINANTS OF DEMAND ELASTICITY FOR INPUTS 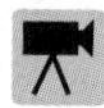

Just as we were able to discuss the price elasticity of demand for different commodities in Chapter 20, we can discuss the price elasticity of demand for inputs. The price elasticity of demand for labor is defined in a manner similar to the price elasticity of demand for goods: the percentage change in quantity demanded divided by the percentage change in the price of labor. When the numerical value of this ratio is less than 1, demand is inelastic; when it is 1, demand is unit-elastic; and when it is greater than 1, demand is elastic.

There are four principal determinants of the price elasticity of demand for an input. The price elasticity of demand for a variable input will be greater:

1. The greater the price elasticity of demand for the final product
2. The easier it is for a particular variable input to be substituted for by other inputs
3. The larger the proportion of total costs accounted for by a particular variable input
4. The longer the time period being considered

Consider some examples. An individual radish farmer faces an extremely elastic demand for radishes, given the existence of many competing radish growers. If the farmer's laborers tried to obtain a significant wage increase, the farmer couldn't pass on the resultant higher costs to radish buyers. So any wage increase to the individual radish farmer would lead to a large reduction in the quantity of labor demanded.

Clearly, the easier it is for a producer to switch to using another factor of production, the more responsive that producer will be to an increase in an input's price. If plastic and aluminum can easily be substituted in the production of, say, car bumpers, then a price rise in aluminum will cause automakers to reduce greatly their quantity of aluminum demanded.

When a particular input's costs account for a very large share of total costs, any increase in that input's price will affect total costs relatively more. If labor costs are 80 percent of total costs, a company will cut back on employment more aggressively than if labor costs were only 8 percent of total costs, for any given wage increase.

Finally, over longer periods, firms have more time to figure out ways to economize on the use of inputs whose prices have gone up. Furthermore, over time, technological change will allow for easier substitution in favor of relatively cheaper inputs and against inputs whose prices went up. At first, a pay raise obtained by a strong telephone company union may not result in many layoffs, but over time, the telephone company will use new technology to replace many of the now more expensive workers.

CONCEPTS IN BRIEF

- The change in total output due to a one-unit change in one variable input, holding all other inputs constant, is called the marginal physical product (MPP). When we multiply marginal physical product times marginal revenue, we obtain the marginal revenue product (MRP).
- A firm will hire workers up to the point at which the additional cost of hiring one more worker is equal to the additional revenues generated. For the individual firm, therefore, its MRP of labor curve is also its demand for labor curve.
- The demand for labor is a derived demand, derived from the demand for final output. Therefore, if the price of final output changes, this will cause a shift in the MRP curve (which is also the firm's demand for labor curve).
- Input price elasticity of demand depends on final product elasticity, the ease of other input substitution, the relative importance of the input's cost in total costs, and the time allowed for adjustment.

WAGE DETERMINATION

Having developed the demand curve for labor (and all other variable inputs) in a particular industry, let's turn to the labor supply curve. By adding supply to the analysis, we can come up with the equilibrium wage rate that workers earn in an industry. We can think in terms of a supply curve for labor that slopes upward in a particular industry. At higher wage rates, more workers will want to enter that particular industry. The individual firm, however, does

FIGURE 27-4

The Equilibrium Wage Rate and the CD Industry

The industry demand curve for labor is *D*. We put in a hypothetical upward-sloping labor supply curve for the CD industry, *S*. The intersection is at point *E*, giving an equilibrium wage rate of $498 per week and an equilibrium quantity of labor demanded of Q_1. At a wage above $498 per week, there will be an excess quantity of workers supplied. At a wage below $498 per week, there will be an excess quantity of workers demanded.

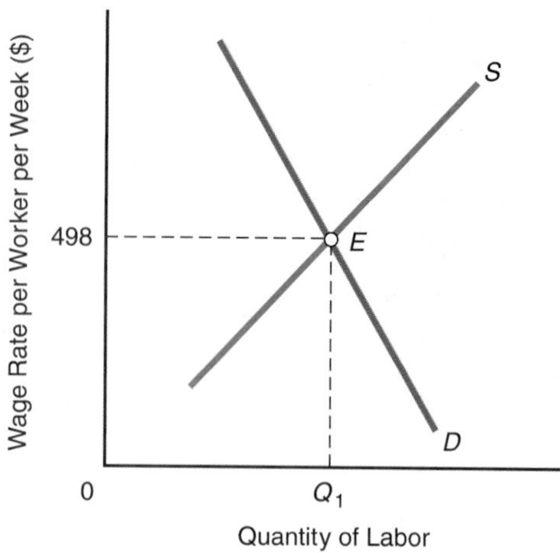

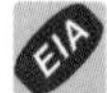

The Equilibrium Wage Rate

Practice thinking through the interaction between labor demand and labor supply.

not face the entire *market* supply curve. Rather, in a perfectly competitive case, the individual firm is such a small part of the market that it can hire all the workers that it wants at the going wage rate. We say, therefore, that the industry faces an upward-sloping supply curve but that the individual *firm* faces a perfectly elastic supply curve for labor.

The demand curve for labor in the CD industry is *D* in Figure 27-4, and the supply curve of labor is *S*. The equilibrium wage rate of $498 a week is established at the intersection of the two curves. The quantity of workers both supplied and demanded at that rate is Q_1. If for some reason the wage rate fell to $400 a week, in our hypothetical example, there would be an excess number of workers demanded at that wage rate. Conversely, if the wage rate rose to $600 a week, there would be an excess quantity of workers supplied at that wage rate. In either case, competition would quickly force the wage back to the equilibrium level.

We have just found the equilibrium wage rate for the entire CD industry. The individual firm must take that equilibrium wage rate as given in the competitive model used here because the individual firm is a very small part of the total demand for labor. Thus each firm purchasing labor in a perfectly competitive market can purchase all of the input it wants at the going market price.

EXAMPLE

Labor Supply Curves for Individuals Eventually Bend Backward

Figure 27-4 depicts an upward-sloping market labor supply curve, which is consistent with evidence that the total quantity of labor supplied by all workers increases with a rise in the market wage. Imagine, however, that you find a job with a company that emerges from initial obscurity to become a market leader. As its fortunes improve, your effective hourly wage rises and rises and then rises some more. It may be stretching your imagination, but mightn't you reach a point where you would prefer to spend more of your time in leisure activities instead of working? That is, isn't there some wage rate high enough to induce you to work *fewer* hours instead of more hours?

In case you can't imagine yourself in this kind of situation, think about this real-life example. Microsoft's wage payments to its employees have included stock in the company. Current estimates are that people who have been with Microsoft since 1994 have earned options on company stock valued at more than $3 million per person. Old-timers who have been with the company since it first went public in 1986 have benefited from a share price rise of more than 700 percent. Some who have held stock in the company all that time are estimated to hold shares valued in excess of $100 million each. All told, about a third of Microsoft's permanent employees are millionaires.

Some are having trouble getting motivated to keep putting in long hours at work. The senior vice-president who supervised Windows 95 and played a key role in developing Internet Explorer switched to part-time status. Another vice-president recently took a year's leave to spend his time sharpening his bowling skills. For most of us, higher wages induce us to substitute *away* from leisure to more time on the job. For people like these Microsoft employees, however, wages are sufficiently high that an *income effect* predominates. Their wages are so high that they prefer to work *less*.

For Critical Analysis

In most occupations, wages are not sufficiently high for workers to become millionaires (at least not very quickly). Does this observation help explain why market labor supply curves slope upward?

ALTERNATIVE THEORIES OF WAGE DETERMINATION

The relatively straightforward analysis of the supply and demand of labor just presented may not fully explain the equilibrium level of wages under certain circumstances. There are two important alternative theories of wage determination that may apply to at least some parts of the economy: efficiency wages and insiders versus outsiders. We analyze those two theories now.

Efficiency Wages

Let's say that in the CD industry, employers can hire as many workers as they want at the equilibrium weekly wage rate of $498. Associated with that weekly wage rate is a specified amount of employment in each firm. Within each firm, though, there is turnover. Some workers quit to go on to other jobs. Turnover costs are significant. Workers have to be trained. What if a firm, even though it could hire workers at $498 a week, offered employment at $600 a week? Several things might occur. First, current employees would have less desire to look elsewhere to find better jobs. There would be less turnover. Second, those workers who applied for openings might be of higher quality, being attracted by the higher wage rate. Third, workers on the job might actually become more productive because they do not want to lose their jobs. They know that alternative competitive wages are $498 a week.

The higher-than-competitive wage rates offered by such a firm have been designated **efficiency wages.** The underlying assumption is that firms operate more efficiently if they pay their workers a higher wage rate. Doing so, goes the efficiency wage argument, gives workers an incentive to be more productive, thereby making firms more cost-efficient.

Efficiency wages 
Wages set above competitive levels to increase labor productivity and profits by enhancing the efficiency of the firm through lower turnover, ease of attracting higher-quality workers, and better efforts by workers.

Insiders Versus Outsiders

A related view of the labor market involves the notion of insiders within a firm. The insiders are those current employees who have the "inside track" and can maintain their positions because the firm would have to incur costs to replace them. These employee insiders are therefore able to exercise some control over the terms under which new employees (outsiders) are hired by the firm. They keep other potential workers out by not allowing them to offer themselves for work at a lower real wage rate than that being earned by the insiders. As pointed out earlier, the costs of hiring and firing workers are significant.

Insider-outsider theory 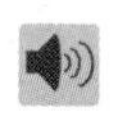
A theory of labor markets in which workers who are already employed have an influence on wage bargaining in such a way that outsiders who are willing to work for lower real wages cannot get a job.

Indeed, the cost of firing one worker may sometimes be relatively high: termination wages, retraining payments, and litigation if the worker believes termination was unjustified. All such costs might contribute to the development of insider-dominated labor markets. They contain significant barriers to entry by outsiders.

So the **insider-outsider theory** predicts that wages may remain higher than the standard supply and demand model would predict even though outsiders are willing to work at lower real wages.

EXAMPLE

What Corporations Have in Common with Street Gangs: A Quest for the Boss's Job

Although efficiency wage theory and the insider-outsider theory may explain wages that are somewhat above a competitive level, they have a harder time explaining really big differences in wages within a firm's management structure. CEOs tend to make many times more than vice-presidents do. Senior vice-presidents, in turn, earn double what a regular vice-president is paid.

According to one theory, which Edward Lazear of Stanford University and Sherwin Rosen of the University of Chicago call the *tournament theory*, corporations create these big salary differentials not in an attempt to reward recipients but rather to create a structure of powerful incentives to get people in the organization to work harder. Pay is based on *relative* performance, relative to one's peers within the management organization. The pay of the vice-president is not what motivates that vice-president; it is the pay of the CEO, to whose job the vice-president aspires. Thus vice-presidents and others under them are involved in a series of tournaments. At each level, the winner moves up to the next higher level. All aspire to the highest level, that of the CEO.

Steven Levitt of the University of Chicago and Sudhir Venkatesh of the Harvard Society of Fellows found a similar pattern of earnings among members of an inner-city gang that deals in crack cocaine. The typical street-corner crack vendor, at the lowest rung on the ladder within the gang, earns as little as $200 per month, well below what could be earned in a minimum-wage job. "Warriors" who fight during periods of intergang warfare earn about $2,000 per month. A sizable 20 percent of the gang's revenue is split among a small number of leaders, with the head of the gang earning $100,000 per year.

For Critical Analysis

If luck plays an unusually large role in an underling's rise to the top of a corporation or a gang, will the pay differential between CEOs or gang chiefs and the next highest group have to be relatively larger or smaller compared with a situation in which luck is not important?

FAQ: *Doesn't the average American stay employed with a company for a relatively long time?*

Not unless you consider about $3\frac{1}{2}$ years a long time. This is the average time that a typical U.S. worker now stays with a company before switching jobs. Just a few years ago, the average worker stuck with the same job closer to four years. That employment with a single firm is so relatively brief casts some doubt on the insider-outsider theory's relevance for most U.S. labor markets. In the United States, the theory probably works best for unionized industries and government agencies—and at least some colleges, where tenured professors often appear to be the ultimate "insiders."

SHIFTS IN THE MARKET DEMAND FOR AND SUPPLY OF LABOR

Just as we discussed shifts in the supply curve and the demand curve for various products in Chapter 3, we can discuss the effects of shifts in supply and demand in labor markets.

Reasons for Labor Demand Curve Shifts

Many factors can cause the demand curve for labor to shift. We have already discussed a number of them. Clearly, because the demand for labor or any other variable input is a derived demand, the labor demand curve will shift if there is a shift in the demand for the final product. There are two other important determinants of the position of the demand curve for labor: changes in labor's productivity and changes in the price of related factors of production (substitutes and complements).

Labor Markets

Practice thinking through factors that shift the market demand for and supply of labor.

Changes in Demand for Final Product. The demand for labor or any other variable input is derived from the demand for the final product. The marginal revenue product is equal to marginal physical product times marginal revenue. Therefore, any change in the price of the final product will change MRP. This happened when we derived the market demand for labor. The general rule of thumb is as follows:

> A change in the demand for the final product that labor (or any other variable input) is producing will shift the market demand curve for labor in the same direction.

Changes in Labor Productivity. The second part of the MRP equation is MPP, which relates to labor productivity. We can surmise, then, that, other things being equal,

> A change in labor productivity will shift the market labor demand curve in the same direction.

Labor productivity can increase because labor has more capital or land to work with, because of technological improvements, or because labor's quality has improved. Such considerations explain why the real standard of living of workers in the United States is higher than in most countries. American workers generally work with a larger capital stock, have more natural resources, are in better physical condition, and are better trained than workers in many countries. Hence the demand for labor in America is, other things held constant, greater. Conversely, labor is relatively more scarce in the United States than it is in many other countries. One result of relatively greater demand and relatively smaller supply is a relatively higher wage rate.

Change in the Price of Related Factors. Labor is not the only resource used. Some resources are substitutes and some are complements. If we hold output constant, we have the following general rule:

> A change in the price of a substitute input will cause the demand for labor to change in the same direction. This is typically called the *substitution effect.*

Note, however, that if the cost of production falls sufficiently, the firm will find it more profitable to produce and sell a larger output. If this so-called *output effect* is great enough, it will override the substitution effect just mentioned, and the firm will end up employing not only more of the relatively cheaper variable input but also more labor. This is exactly what happened for many years in the American automobile industry. Auto companies employed more machinery (capital), but employment continued to increase in spite of rising wage rates. The reason: Technological improvement caused the marginal physical productivity of labor to rise faster than its wage rate.

With respect to complements, we are referring to inputs that must be used jointly. Assume now that capital and labor are complementary. In general, we predict the following:

> A change in the price of a complementary input will cause the demand for labor to change in the opposite direction.

If the cost of machines goes up but they must be used with labor, fewer machines will be purchased and therefore fewer workers will be used.

Determinants of the Supply of Labor

There are a number of reasons why labor supply curves will shift in a particular industry. For example, if wage rates for factory workers in the CD industry remain constant while wages for factory workers in the computer industry go up dramatically, the supply curve of factory workers in the CD industry will shift inward to the left as these workers shift to the computer industry.

Changes in working conditions in an industry can also affect its labor supply curve. If employers in the CD industry discover a new production technique that makes working conditions much more pleasant, the supply curve of labor to the CD industry will shift outward to the right.

Job flexibility also determines the position of the labor supply curve. For example, in an industry in which workers are allowed more flexibility, such as the ability to work at home via computer, the workers are likely to work more hours. That is to say, their supply curve will shift outward to the right. Some industries in which firms offer *job sharing,* particularly to people raising families, have found that the supply curve of labor has shifted outward to the right.

CONCEPTS IN BRIEF

- The individual competitive firm faces a perfectly elastic supply curve—it can buy all the labor it wants at the going market wage rate. The industry supply curve of labor slopes upward.
- By plotting an industrywide supply curve for labor and an industrywide demand curve for labor on the same coordinate system, we obtain the equilibrium wage rate in an industry.
- Efficiency wage theory predicts that wages paid above market wages may lead to high productivity because of lower turnover rates and better work effort by existing workers.
- The labor demand curve can shift because (1) the demand for the final product shifts, (2) labor productivity changes, or (3) the price of a related (substitute or complementary) factor of production changes.

MONOPOLY IN THE PRODUCT MARKET

So far we've considered only a perfectly competitive situation, both in selling the final product and in buying factors of production. We will continue our assumption that the firm purchases its factors of production in a perfectly competitive factor market. Now, however, we will assume that the firm sells its product in an *imperfectly* competitive output market. In other words, we are considering the output market structures of monopoly, oligopoly, and monopolistic competition. In all such cases, the firm, be it a monopolist, an oligopolist, or a monopolistic competitor, faces a downward-sloping demand curve for its product. Throughout the rest of this chapter, we will simply refer to a monopoly output situation for ease of analysis. The analysis holds for all industry structures that are less than perfectly competitive. In any event, the fact that our firm now faces a downward-sloping demand curve for its product means that if it wants to sell more of its product (at a uniform price), it has to lower the price, *not just on the last unit, but on all preceding units.* The *marginal revenue* received from selling an additional unit is continuously falling (and is less than price) as the firm attempts to sell more and more. This is certainly different from our earlier discussions in this chapter in which the firm could sell all it wanted at a constant price. Why? Because the firm we discussed until now was a perfect competitor.

Constructing the Monopolist's Input Demand Curve

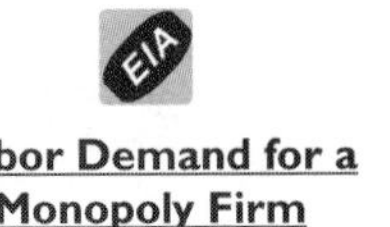

Labor Demand for a Monopoly Firm

Practice working with a monopolist's demand for labor.

In reconstructing our demand schedule for an input, we must account for the facts that (1) the marginal *physical* product falls because of the law of diminishing returns as more workers are added and (2) the price (and marginal revenue) received for the product sold also falls as more is produced and sold. That is, for the monopolist, we have to account for both the diminishing marginal physical product and the diminishing marginal revenue. Marginal revenue is always less than price for the monopolist. The marginal revenue curve is always below the downward-sloping demand curve.

Marginal revenue for the perfect competitor is equal to the price of the product because all units can be sold at the going market price. In our CD example, we assumed that the perfect competitor could sell all it wanted at $6 per compact disc. A one-unit change in sales always led to a $6 change in total revenues. Hence marginal revenue was always equal to $6 for that perfect competitor.

The monopolist, however, cannot simply calculate marginal revenue by looking at the price of the product. To sell the additional output from an additional unit of input, the monopolist has to cut prices on all previous units of output. As output is increasing, then, marginal revenue is falling. The underlying concept is, of course, the same for both the perfect competitor and the monopolist. We are asking exactly the same question in both cases: When an additional worker is hired, what is the benefit? In either case, the benefit is obviously the change in total revenues due to the one-unit change in the variable input, labor. In our discussion of the perfect competitor, we were able simply to look at the marginal physical product and multiply it by the *constant* per-unit price of the product because the price of the product never changed (for the perfect competitor, P = MR).

A single monopolist ends up hiring fewer workers than all of the competitive firms added together. To see this, we must consider the marginal revenue product for the monopolist which varies with each one-unit change in the monopolist's labor input. This is what we do in panel (a) of Figure 27-5 on page 680, where column 5, headed "Marginal Revenue Product," gives the monopolistic firm a quantitative notion of how additional workers and additional production generates additional revenues. The marginal revenue product curve for this monopolist has been plotted in panel (b) of the figure. To emphasize the lower elasticity of the monopolist's MRP curve, MRP_m, the sum of the MRP curves is for a perfectly competitive industry in Figure 27-1, labeled $\Sigma\text{MRP}_c = D$, the labor demand curve under perfect competition, has been plotted on the same graph.

Why does MRP_m represent the monopolist's input demand curve? As always, our profit-maximizing monopolist will continue to hire labor as long as additional profits result. Profits are made as long as the additional cost of more workers is outweighed by

FIGURE 27-5 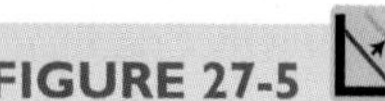

A Monopolist's Marginal Revenue Product

The monopolist hires just enough workers to make marginal revenue product equal to the going wage rate. If the going wage rate is $498 per week, as shown by the labor supply curve, *s*, the monopolist would want to hire approximately 10 workers per week. That is the profit-maximizing amount of labor. The MRP curve for the perfect competitor from Figure 27-1 is also plotted (MRP_c). The monopolist's MRP curve will always be less elastic than it would be if marginal revenue were constant.

Panel (a)

(1) Labor Input (workers per week)	(2) Marginal Physical Product (MPP) CDs per week	(3) Price of Product (*P*)	(4) Marginal Revenue (*MR*)	(5) Marginal Revenue Product (MRP_m) = (2) x (4)
8	110	$8.00	$6.00	$660.00
9	104	7.80	5.60	582.40
10	96	7.60	5.20	499.20
11	88	7.40	4.80	422.40
12	77	7.20	4.40	338.80
13	65	7.00	4.00	260.00

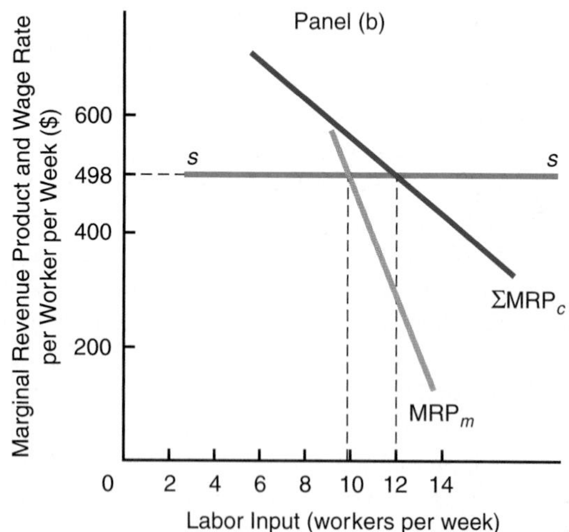

the additional revenues made from selling the output of those workers. When the wage rate equals these additional revenues, the monopolist stops hiring. That is, it stops hiring when the wage rate is equal to the marginal revenue product because additional workers would add more to cost than to revenue.

Why the Monopolist Hires Fewer Workers

Because we have used the same numbers as in Figure 27-1, we can see that the monopolist hires fewer worker-weeks than firms in a perfect competitive market would. That is to say, if we could magically change the CD industry in our example from one in which there is perfect competition in the output market to one in which there is monopoly in the output market, the amount of employment would fall. Why? Because the monopolist must take account of the declining product price that must be charged in order to sell a larger number of CDs. Remember that every firm hires up to the point at which marginal benefit equals marginal cost. The marginal benefit to the monopolist of hiring an additional worker is not simply the additional output times the price of the product. Rather, the monopolist faces a reduction in the price charged on all units sold in order to be able to sell more. So the monopolist ends up hiring fewer workers than all of the perfect competitors taken together, assuming that all other factors remain the same for the two hypothetical examples. But this should not come as a surprise. In considering product markets, by implication we saw that a monopolized CD industry would produce less output than a competitive one. Therefore, the monopolized CD industry would want fewer workers.

OTHER FACTORS OF PRODUCTION

The analysis in this chapter has been given in terms of the demand for the variable input labor. The same analysis holds for any other variable factor input. We could have talked about the demand for fertilizer or the demand for the services of tractors by a farmer instead of the demand for labor and reached the same conclusions. The entrepreneur will hire or buy any variable input up to the point at which its price equals the marginal revenue product.

A further question remains: How much of each variable factor should the firm use when all the variable factors are combined to produce the product? We can answer this question by looking at either the profit-maximizing side of the question or the cost-minimizing side.*

Profit Maximization Revisited

If a firm wants to maximize profits, how much of each factor should be hired (or bought)? As we just saw, the firm will never hire a factor of production unless the marginal benefit from hiring that factor is at least equal to the marginal cost. What is the marginal benefit? As we have pointed out several times, the marginal benefit is the change in total revenues due to a one-unit change in use of the variable input. What is the marginal cost? In the case of a firm buying in a competitive market, it is the price of the variable factor—the wage rate if we are referring to labor.

The profit-maximizing combination of resources for the firm will be where, in a perfectly competitive situation,

$$\begin{aligned} \text{MRP of labor} &= \text{price of labor (wage rate)} \\ \text{MRP of land} &= \text{price of land (rental rate per unit)} \\ \text{MRP of capital} &= \text{price of capital (cost per unit of service)} \end{aligned}$$

*Many economic problems involving maximization of profit or other economic variables have *duals,* or precise restatements, in terms of *minimization* rather than maximization. The problem "How do we maximize our output, given fixed resources?" for example, is the dual of the problem "How do we minimize our cost, given fixed output?" Noneconomists sometimes confuse their discussions of economic issues by mistakenly believing that a problem and its dual are two problems rather than one. Asking, for example, "How can we maximize our profits while minimizing our costs?" makes about as much sense as asking, "How can we cross the street while getting to the other side?"

The marginal revenue product of each of a firm's resources must be exactly equal to its price. If the MRP of labor were \$20 and its price were only \$15, the firm would be underemploying labor.

Cost Minimization

From the cost minimization point of view, how can the firm minimize its total costs for a given output? Assume that you are an entrepreneur attempting to minimize costs. Consider a hypothetical situation in which if you spend \$1 more on labor, you would get 20 more units of output, but if you spend \$1 more on machines, you would get only 10 more units of output. What would you want to do in such a situation? Most likely you would wish to hire more workers or sell off some of your machines, for you are not getting as much output per last dollar spent on machines as you are per last dollar spent on labor. You would want to employ factors of production so that the marginal products per last dollar spent on each are equal. Thus the least-cost, or cost minimization, rule will be as follows:

> To minimize total costs for a particular rate of production, the firm will hire factors of production up to the point at which the marginal physical product per last dollar spent on each factor of production is equalized.

That is,

$$\frac{\text{MPP of labor}}{\text{Price of labor (wage rate)}} = \frac{\text{MPP of capital}}{\text{price of capital (cost per unit of service)}} = \frac{\text{MPP of land}}{\text{price of land (rental rate per unit)}}$$

All we are saying here is that the profit-maximizing firm will always use *all* resources in such combinations that cost will be minimized for any given output rate. This is commonly called the *least-cost combination of resources*. There is an exact relationship between the profit-maximizing combination of resources and the least-cost combination of resources. In other words, either rule can be used to yield the same cost-minimizing rate of use of each variable resource.*

INTERNATIONAL EXAMPLE

Why Are European Businesses Using More Robots and Fewer Workers than U.S. Businesses?

What a strange world we live in, you might say. European countries are experiencing the highest levels of unemployment since the Great Depression. Typical unemployment rates exceed 10 percent throughout the European Union; they are over 10 percent in France and Italy and well over 13 percent in Spain. Compare this with the below 5 percent unemployment rate in the United States, and you can tell that Europe is in trouble. One would expect, therefore, that European firms could easily replace capital with labor and that there would be general pressure toward lower wages. The opposite has occurred. For example, in Germany, department stores use robots in shoe storerooms to seek out the shoes that a salesperson wants. In Denmark, milk warehouses have gone robotic. All in all, the market for automated systems in Europe has grown by more than 10 percent a year, a much greater rate than in the United States. The reason is that businesses in Europe have concluded that it is cheaper to use robots than people. In Germany, an industrial robot costs about \$10 an hour to operate. An

---

*This can be proved as follows: Profit maximization requires that the price of every input must equal that input's marginal revenue product (the general case). Let i be the input. Then $P_i = \text{MRP}_i$. But MRP_i is defined as marginal revenue times marginal physical product of the input. Therefore, for every input i, $P_i = \text{MR} \times \text{MPP}_i$. If we divide both sides by MPP_i, we get $P_i/\text{MPP}_i = \text{MR}$. If we take the reciprocal, we obtain $\text{MPP}_i/P_i = 1/\text{MR}$, which must be true for each and every input. That is another way of stating our cost minimization rule.

industrial worker may cost as much as $37 an hour. And while compensation to workers has continued to rise in Germany and elsewhere since the early 1990s, the operating costs of robots have fallen.

There are many reasons why wages remain so high in spite of massive unemployment in Europe. First of all, minimum wages there may be as much as 50 percent higher than in the United States. And social security contributions that employers have to pay for each worker often equal or even exceed the wages that the worker takes home. In addition, a firm must pay significant severance penalties if it fires a worker. Finally, many workers will not take low-paying jobs in some European countries because they are actually better off receiving unemployment and welfare benefits.

For Critical Analysis

Why have robots not taken over many jobs in the United States?

CONCEPTS IN BRIEF

- When a firm sells its output in a monopoly market, marginal revenue is less than price.
- Just as the MRP is the perfectly competitive firm's input demand curve, the MRP is also the monopolist's demand curve.
- For a less than perfectly competitive firm, the profit-maximizing combination of factors will occur when each factor is used up to the point at which its MRP is equal to its unit price.
- To minimize total costs for a given output, the profit-maximizing firm will hire each factor of production up to the point at which the marginal physical product per last dollar spent on each factor is equal to the marginal physical product per last dollar spent on each of the other factors of production.

NETNOMICS

Banking on the Web as an Employee Communication Tool

According to Pitney Bowes, Inc., each day the average American worker sends and receives 201 messages. An increasing number of these messages are e-mail transmissions. To help its 150,000 employees in 100 countries keep all their interoffice memos and other miscellaneous messages organized, Citibank provides Citiweb. This is a company Web site managed by a dozen full-time employees. About half of the company's employees reach Citiweb using the Internet, and the remainder access it through Citibank's proprietary network.

The site provides bank employees with special e-mail facilities. Citiweb also includes a search engine, automated distribution lists, employee forms and job postings, newsletters from business units within the bank, information about savings plans and benefits, a company events calendar, and internal and external news feeds. In addition, the site has special Citibank billboards, chat rooms, and software tools. Although employees can use Citweb to do on-line personal shopping for items such as flowers and health and beauty aids, they also use it to process corporate purchases of computers and other office equipment.

Citibank reports that the site has raised employee productivity by eliminating the need to maintain distribution lists, print newsletters, or send information in the mail. In addition, Citiweb offers Internet-based training programs that employees can use to develop additional skills. Furthermore, Citibank encourages its employees to use the site to help test new on-line banking services, which helps the bank's software developers identify program bugs before the bank offers the services to the general public.

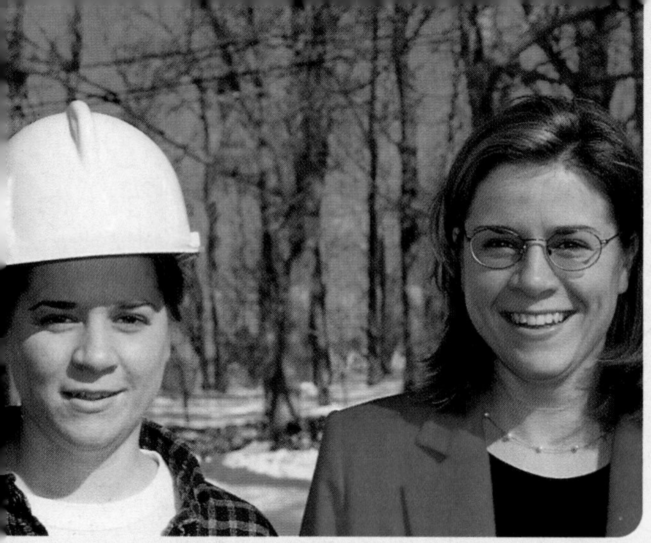

ISSUES & APPLICATIONS

Taking This Course (and Others, of Course) Should Pay Off, at Least in the Near Term

Concepts Applied

- Demand for Labor
- Value of Marginal Product
- Derived Demand
- Substitute Inputs

Often students start to doubt whether they have done the right thing by going on for technical certification or a college degree after high school. If you are one of those students going through some natural soul-searching, stop! There are currently big payoffs to education beyond high school. Whether these sizable relative gains will persist in future years cannot be predicted with certainty, but right now postsecondary education has definite rewards.

An Education-Oriented Labor Market

Take a look at Table 27-1 and at Figure 27-6. Table 27-1 provides estimates going back to 1940 of the breakdown of U.S. employment for high school dropouts, high school graduates, people with some college, and college graduates. As you can see, in 1940, high school dropouts accounted for just over two-thirds of employed workers in the United States. In 1998, they comprised less than 10 percent of the employed workforce. People with any training beyond high school accounted for a share of less than 13 percent of total employment in 1940, but today that share exceeds 57 percent. Today, some college education greatly improves the odds of being employed.

Figure 27-6 shows a ratio-scale plot of the wages of a typical college graduate relative to the wages of a typical high school graduate. The wages of college graduates relative to high school graduates have remained substantially higher, reaching historical levels in recent years. The "higher education wage premium" earned by people who study beyond high school is real and sizeable.

Will the Education Advantage Last?

It is tempting to conclude that people with less education will forever be left behind. This is not necessarily true, however, as reference to Figure 27-6 indicates. Between the 1940s and the 1980s, college graduates' wages relative to those of high school graduates cycled

TABLE 27-1
Full-Time-Equivalent Employment Share, by Education Level

Year	High School Dropouts (%)	High School Graduates(%)	Some College (%)	College Graduates (%)
1940	67.9	19.2	6.5	6.4
1950	58.6	24.4	9.2	7.8
1960	49.5	27.7	12.2	10.6
1970	35.9	34.7	15.6	13.8
1980	20.7	36.1	22.8	20.4
1990	11.4	33.0	30.2	24.4
1998	9.4	33.2	28.3	29.1

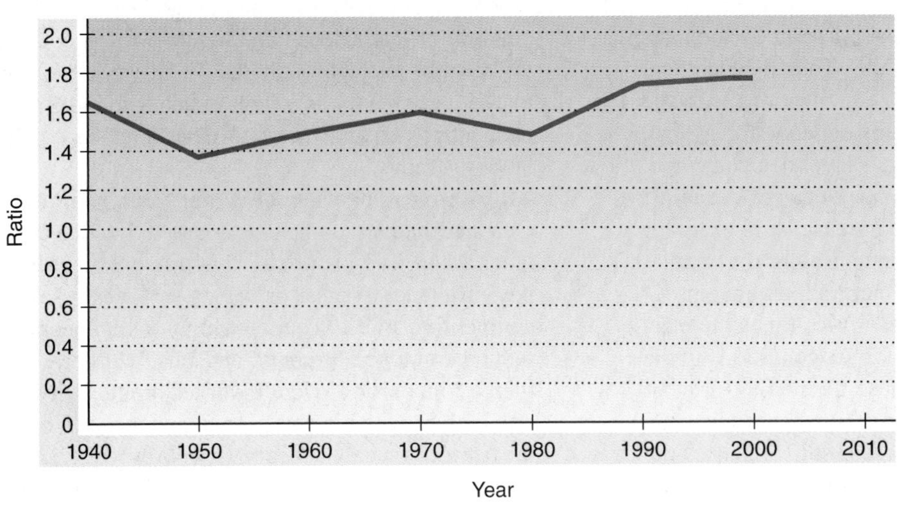

FIGURE 27-6
Wages of College Graduates Relative to Wages of High School Graduates

The ratio of college graduates' average wages to the average wages of high school graduates declined after World War II before rising over the next two decades and then falling off slightly between 1970 and 1980. Since 1980, however, this ratio has risen noticeably.

Source: Lawrence Katz, "Technological Change, Computerization, and the Wage Structure," paper presented at the U.S. Department of Commerce conference "Understanding the Digital Economy," Washington, D.C., May 1999.

up and down. There is nothing to guarantee that a similar downward movement may not take place again.

Indeed, recent software developments may eventually make a difference. One in particular is called electronic performance support systems (EPSS). This software automates many job-related mental tasks and provides quick instructions to help users make the human judgments that are still required for many jobs. For instance, many banks now provide their customer support staff with EPSS software that guides them when they receive calls complaining about features of their credit card accounts. Once the bank's customer service representative enters the caller's account number into a computer, the EPSS software immediately reviews the caller's customer records and evaluates whether the account holder has been profitable for the bank. If so, a green light flashes to cue the bank's customer service representative to satisfy the customer, and directions appear on the screen for, say, upgrading the customer's credit card. If a red light flashes, the bank's employee knows to be unsympathetic. This requires no special skills for the employee beyond an ability to talk with callers. In addition, little training is required to do the job, because the program does most of the work.

Thus EPSS software, a form of capital good, may begin to help replace college-educated employees with others who have less education. Ultimately, the higher education wage premium accruing to college graduates may begin to decline.

FOR CRITICAL ANALYSIS

1. If EPSS software becomes a common feature at most American companies, how do you think the employment distribution in Table 27-1 will change over the next decade or two?
2. What are some pitfalls in trying to forecast how the higher education wage premium may vary in future years?

SG

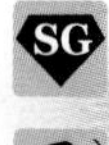

SUMMARY DISCUSSION OF LEARNING OBJECTIVES

1. **Why a Firm's Marginal Revenue Product Curve Is Its Labor Demand Curve:** The marginal revenue product of labor equals marginal revenue times the marginal physical product of labor. Because of the law of diminishing marginal utility, the marginal revenue product curve slopes downward. To maximize profits, a firm hires labor to the point where the marginal factor cost of labor—the addition to total input costs resulting from employing an additional unit of labor. For firms that hire labor in competitive labor markets, the market wage rate is the marginal factor cost of labor, so profit maximization requires hiring

labor to the point where the wage rate equals marginal revenue product, which is a point on the marginal revenue product schedule. Thus the marginal revenue product curve gives combinations of wage rates and desired employment of labor for a firm, which means that it is the firm's labor demand curve.

2. **The Demand for Labor as a Derived Demand:** For firms that are perfect competitors in their product markets, marginal revenue equals the market price of their output, so the marginal revenue product of labor equals the product price times the marginal physical product of labor. As conditions in the product market vary and cause the market price at which firms sell their output to change, their marginal revenue product curves shift. Hence the demand for labor by perfectly competitive firms is derived from the demand for the final products these firms produce.
3. **Key Factors Affecting the Elasticity of Demand for Inputs:** The price elasticity of the demand for an input, such as labor, is equal to the percentage change in the quantity of the input demanded divided by the percentage change in the price of the input, such as the wage rate. The price elasticity of demand for a particular input is relatively high when any one of the following is true: (i) the price elasticity of demand for the final product is relatively high; (ii) it is relatively easy to substitute other inputs in the production process; (iii) the proportion of total costs accounted for by the input is relatively large; or (iv) the firm has a longer time period to adjust to the change in the input's price.
4. **How Equilibrium Wage Rates at Perfectly Competitive Firms Are Determined:** For perfectly competitive firms, the market labor demand curve is the sum of the individual labor demand curves for all firms, which in turn are the firms' marginal revenue product curves. At the equilibrium wage rate, the quantity of labor demanded by all firms is equal to the quantity of labor supplied by all workers in the marketplace. At this wage rate, each firm looks to its own labor demand curve to determine how much labor to employ.
5. **Alternative Theories of Wage Determination:** One alternative to the basic derived-demand-for-labor theory is an approach that proposes that firms pay efficiency wages, or wages sufficiently above competitive levels to attract high-quality workers, reduce employee turnover, and raise worker effort, thereby increasing overall worker productivity and reducing production costs. Another approach, called the insider-outsider theory, proposes that current employees are insiders who are able to influence conditions under which prospective employers are hired, which can make the costs of hiring new workers higher, thereby pushing wages above competitive levels.
6. **Contrasting the Demand for Labor and Wage Determination Under Monopoly with Outcomes Under Perfect Competition:** If a firm that is a monopolist in its product market competes with firms of other industries for labor in a competitive labor market, it takes the market wage rate as given. Its labor demand curve, however, lies to the left of the labor demand curve for the industry that would have arisen if the industry included a number of perfectly competitive firms. The reason is that marginal revenue is less than price for a monopolist, so the marginal revenue product of the monopolist is lower than under competition. Thus at the competitively determined wage rate, a monopolized industry employs fewer workers than the industry otherwise would if it were perfectly competitive.

Key Terms and Concepts

Derived demand (669)
Efficiency wages (675)
Insider-outsider theory (676)
Marginal factor cost (MFC) (668)
Marginal physical product (MPP) of labor (666)
Marginal revenue product (MRP) (668)

Problems

Answers to the odd-numbered problems appear at the back of the book.

27-1. The following table depicts the output of a firm that manufactures computer printers. The printers sell for $100 each.

Labor Input (workers per week)	Total Physical Output (printers per week)
10	200
11	218
12	234
13	248
14	260
15	270
16	278

Calculate the marginal physical product and marginal revenue product for this firm.

27-2. Suppose that the firm in Problem 27-1 has chosen to hire 15 workers. What is the maximum wage the firm would be willing to pay?

27-3. The weekly wages paid by computer printer manufacturers in a perfectly competitive market is $1,200. Using the information provided in the table that accompanies Problem 27-1, how many workers will the profit-maximizing employer hire?

27-4. Suppose that there is an increase in the demand for personal computer systems. Explain the likely effects on marginal revenue product, marginal factor cost, and the number of workers hired by the firm in Problem 27-1.

27-5. Explain what happens to the elasticity of demand for labor in a given industry after each of the following events.

a. A new manufacturing technique makes capital easier to substitute for labor.

b. There is an increase in the number of substitutes for the final product that labor produces.

c. After a drop in the prices of capital inputs, labor accounts for a larger portion of a firm's factor costs.

27-6. Explain how the following events would affect the demand for labor.

a. A new education program administered by the company increases the efficiency of labor.

b. The firm completes a new plant with a larger workspace and new machinery.

27-7. The following table depicts the product market and labor market a portable stereo manufacturer faces.

Labor Input (workers per day)	Total Physical Product	Product Price ($)
10	100	50
11	109	49
12	116	48
13	121	47
14	124	46
15	125	45

Given the information in the table, calculate the firm's marginal physical product, total revenue, and marginal revenue product.

27-8. The firm in Problem 27-7 competes in a perfectly competitive labor market, and the market wage it faces is $100. How many workers will the profit-maximizing employer hire?

27-9. The current market wage rate is $10, the rental rate of land is $1,000, and the rental rate of capital is $500. Production managers at a firm find that under their current allocation of factors of production, the marginal revenue product of labor is 100, the marginal revenue product of land is $10,000, and the marginal revenue product of capital is $4,000. Is the firm maximizing profit? Why or why not?

27-10. The current wage rate is $10, and the rental rate of capital is $500. Production managers at a firm find that the marginal physical product of labor is 200 and the marginal physical product of capital is 20,000. Is the firm maximizing profits for the given cost outlay? Why or why not?

Economics on the Net

How the Minimum Wage Affects the Poor Federal, state, and local minimum-wage laws can affect employment levels around the United States. This Internet application helps you think through the full effects of these laws on many of the poorest individuals that the laws are intended to benefit.

Title: Will Increasing the Minimum Wage Help the Poor?

Navigation: Click here to start at Federal Reserve Bank of Cleveland's home page. Click on Publications. Scroll down, and click on Economic Commentary. Select 1999. Select the article titled "Will Increasing the Minimum Wage Help the Poor?"

Application In this chapter, you read about the market determination of wage rate. Read the article titled "Will Increasing the Minimum Wage Help the Poor?" Then answer the following questions.

1. What type of market control is a minimum wage? What is the primary rationale for increasing the minimum wage rate?

2. Based on the article, will an increase in the minimum wage help the poor? Do you agree? Why or why not?

For Group Discussion and Analysis: Identify the positive economic analysis and the normative issues in this article. What is the consensus view of the economists surveyed on the effect of a minimum wage increase? What alternatives to an increase in the minimum wage can the group propose?

CHAPTER 28

UNIONS AND LABOR MARKET MONOPOLY POWER

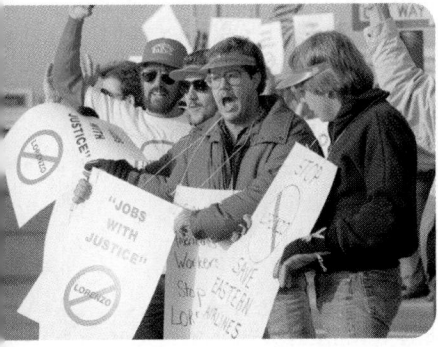

These union demonstrators are part of a dwindling fraction of the labor force. In the private sector of the U.S. economy, only about one worker in 10 belongs to a union. Why has union membership declined?

In the early 1960s, one out of every four American workers was a union member. Today, only about one in 10 belongs to a union. Union strike activity also has waned. Why were there so many union members four decades ago? Why has union membership declined since? Has there been a corresponding decline in the importance of unionized industries in the U.S. economy? Is there any likelihood that the American labor movement that spawned unions could revive in the future? Before you can answer these questions, you need to know about monopoly power in the market for labor.

LEARNING OBJECTIVES

After reading this chapter, you should be able to:

1. Outline the essential history of the American labor union movement
2. Discuss the current status of labor unions in the United States
3. Describe the basic economic goals and strategies of labor unions
4. Evaluate the potential effects of labor unions on wages and productivity
5. Explain how a monopsonist determines how much labor to employ and what wage rate to pay
6. Compare wage and employment decisions by a monopsonistic firm with the choices made by firms in industries with alternative market structures

Chapter Outline

- The American Labor Movement
- Unions and Collective Bargaining Contracts
- Union Goals
- Have Unions Raised Wages?
- Can Unions Increase Productivity?
- The Benefits of Labor Unions
- Monopsony: A Buyer's Monopoly

Did You Know That... in 1971, some 2.5 million workers were involved in strikes, but in the past few years, fewer than 250,000 have been involved? More than 12 times the number of workdays were lost to strikes in the 1950s than are lost to them today. The labor landscape has been changing in the United States. That does not mean that concerted activity on the part of groups of workers is insignificant in our economy, though. Some workers are able to earn more than they would in a competitive labor market because they have obtained a type of monopoly power. These are members of effective **labor unions,** workers' organizations that seek to secure economic improvements for their members. In forming unions, a certain monopoly element enters into the supply of labor equation. That is because we can no longer talk about a perfectly competitive labor supply situation when active and effective unions bargain as a single entity with management. The entire supply of a particular group of workers is controlled by a single source. Later in the chapter, we will examine the converse—a single employer who is the sole user of a particular group of workers.

THE AMERICAN LABOR MOVEMENT

Labor unions 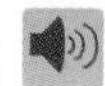
Worker organizations that seek to secure economic improvements for their members; they also seek to improve the safety, health, and other benefits (such as job security) of their members.

Craft unions 
Labor unions composed of workers who engage in a particular trade or skill, such as baking, carpentry, or plumbing.

The American labor movement started with local **craft unions.** These were groups of workers in individual trades, such as shoemaking, printing, or baking. Initially, in the United States, laborers struggled for the right to band together to bargain as a unit. In the years between the Civil War and the Great Depression (1861–1930s), the Knights of Labor, an organized group of both skilled and unskilled workers, demanded an eight-hour workday, equal pay for women and men, and the replacement of free enterprise with the socialist system. In 1886, a dissident group from the Knights of Labor formed the American Federation of Labor (AFL) under the leadership of Samuel Gompers. Until World War I, the government supported business's opposition to unions by offering the use of police personnel to break strikes. During World War I, the image of the unions improved and membership increased to more than 5 million. But after the war, the government decided to stop protecting labor's right to organize. Membership began to fall.

Then came the Great Depression. Franklin Roosevelt's National Industrial Recovery Act of 1933 gave labor the federal right to bargain collectively, but that act was declared unconstitutional. The 1935 National Labor Relations Act (NLRA), otherwise known as the Wagner Act, took its place. The NLRA guaranteed workers the right to start unions, to engage in **collective bargaining** (bargaining between management and representatives of all union members), and to be members in any union that was started.

INTERNATIONAL EXAMPLE

European Merchant Guilds: The Original Craft Unions

The origin of today's modern craft unions is found in a type of association that flourished in continental Europe and England during the Middle Ages. Around the eleventh century, merchants started traveling from market to market in a caravan to protect themselves from bandits. The members of the caravan elected a leader whose rules they pledged to obey. The name of such a caravan was *Gilde* in the Germanic countries of Europe. When the members of the caravan returned home, they frequently stayed in close association. They soon found it beneficial to seek exclusive rights to a particular trade from a feudal lord or, later, from the city government itself. Soon merchant guilds obtained a monopoly over an industry and its related commerce in a city. A guild supervised the crafts and the wholesale and retail selling of commodities manufactured in that city. Nonmember merchants were not allowed to sell goods at retail and were subject to many restrictions from which members of the guild were exempt.

For Critical Analysis

Analyze the medieval guild in terms of the insider-outsider theory presented in Chapter 27.

Industrial Unions

In 1938, the Congress of Industrial Organizations (CIO) was formed by John L. Lewis, the president of the United Mine Workers. Prior to the formation of the CIO, most labor organizations were craft unions. The CIO was composed of **industrial unions** with membership from an entire industry such as steel or automobiles. In 1955, the CIO and the AFL merged. Organized labor's failure to grow at a continuing rapid rate caused leadership in both associations to seek the merger.

Three important industrial unions declared in 1995 that they, too, planned eventually to merge. Sometime soon the United Auto Workers, the United Steelworkers of America, and the International Association of Machinists will have formed a single industrial union with nearly 2 million members.

Collective bargaining 
Bargaining between the management of a company or of a group of companies and the management of a union or a group of unions for the purpose of setting a mutually agreeable contract on wages, fringe benefits, and working conditions for all employees in all the unions involved.

Industrial unions 
Labor unions that consist of workers from a particular industry, such as automobile manufacturing or steel manufacturing.

Congressional Control over Labor Unions

Since the Great Depression, Congress has occasionally altered the relationship between labor and management through significant legislation. One of the most important pieces of legislation was the Taft-Hartley Act of 1947 (the Labor Management Relations Act). Among other things, it allows individual states to pass their own **right-to-work laws.** A right-to-work law makes it illegal for union membership to be a requirement for continued employment in any establishment.

More specifically, the Taft-Hartley Act makes a **closed shop** illegal; a closed shop requires union membership before employment can be obtained. A **union shop,** however, is legal; a union shop does not require membership as a prerequisite for employment, but it can, and usually does, require that workers join the union after a specified amount of time on the job. (Even a union shop is illegal in states with right-to-work laws.)

Jurisdictional disputes, sympathy strikes, and secondary boycotts are also made illegal by the Taft-Hartley Act as well. A **jurisdictional dispute** involves two or more unions fighting (and striking) over which should have control in a particular jurisdiction. For example, should a carpenter working for a steel manufacturer be part of the steelworkers' union or the carpenters' union? A **sympathy strike** occurs when one union strikes in sympathy with another union's cause or strike. For example, if the retail clerks' union in an area is striking grocery stores, Teamsters may refuse to deliver products to those stores in sympathy with the retail clerks' demands for higher wages or better working conditions. A **secondary boycott** is the boycotting of a company that deals with a struck company. For example, if union workers strike a baking company, the boycotting of grocery stores that continue to sell that company's products is a secondary boycott. The secondary boycott brings pressure on third parties to force them to stop dealing with an employer who is being struck.

In general, the Taft-Hartley Act outlawed unfair labor practices of unions, such as make-work rules and forcing unwilling workers to join a particular union. Perhaps the most famous aspect of the Taft-Hartley Act is its provision that the president can obtain a court

Right-to-work laws 
Laws that make it illegal to require union membership as a condition of continuing employment in a particular firm.

Closed shop 
A business enterprise in which employees must belong to the union before they can be hired and must remain in the union after they are hired.

Union shop 
A business enterprise that allows the hiring of nonunion members, conditional on their joining the union by some specified date after employment begins.

Jurisdictional dispute 
A dispute involving two or more unions over which should have control of a particular jurisdiction, such as a particular craft or skill or a particular firm or industry.

Sympathy strike 
A strike by a union in sympathy with another union's strike or cause.

Secondary boycott
(From page 691)
A boycott of companies or products sold by companies that are dealing with a company being struck.

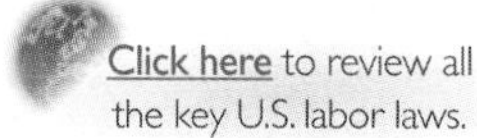
Click here to review all the key U.S. labor laws.

injunction that will stop a strike for an 80-day cooling-off period if the strike is expected to imperil the nation's safety or health.

The Current Status of Labor Unions

You can see from Figure 28-1 that organized labor's heyday occurred from the 1940s through the 1970s. Since then, union membership has fallen almost every year. Currently, it is hovering around 15 percent of the civilian labor force. If you remove labor unions in the public sector—federal, state, and local government workers—private-sector union membership in the United States is only about 11 percent of the civilian labor force.

Part of the explanation for the decline in union membership has to do with the shift away from manufacturing. Unions were always strongest in blue-collar jobs. In 1948, workers in goods-producing industries, transportation, and utilities constituted 51.2 percent of private nonagricultural employment. Today, that number is only 25 percent. Manufacturing jobs account for only 16 percent of all employment. In addition, persistent illegal immigration has weakened the power of unions. Much of the unskilled and typically nonunionized work in the United States is done by foreign-born workers, some of whom are undocumented. They are unlikely targets for union organizers.

The deregulation of certain industries has also led to a decline in unionism. More intense competition in formally regulated industries, such as the airlines, has led to a movement toward nonunionized labor. Undoubtedly, increased global competetion has also played a role. Finally, increased labor force participation by women has led to a decline in

FIGURE 28-1

Decline in Union Membership

Numerically, union membership in the United States has increased dramatically since the 1930s, but as a percentage of the labor force, union membership peaked around 1960 and has been falling ever since. Most recently, the absolute number of union members has also diminished.

Sources: L. Davis et al., *American Economic Growth* (New York: HarperCollins, 1972), p. 220; U.S. Department of Labor, Bureau of Labor Statistics.

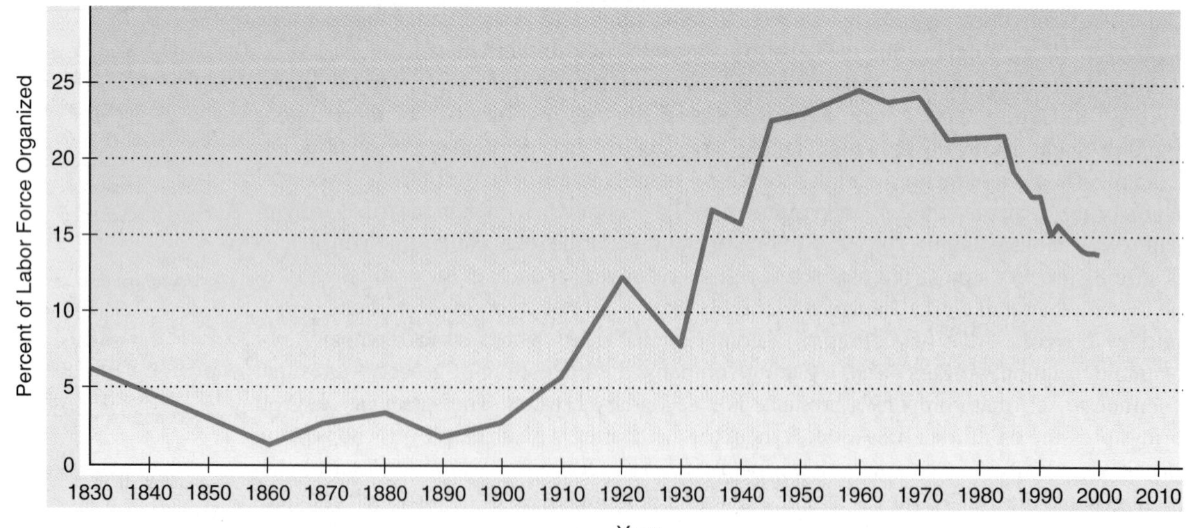

union importance. Women have traditionally been less inclined to join unions than their male counterparts.

INTERNATIONAL EXAMPLE

Europe's Management-Labor Councils

Unionization rates are much higher in the European Union (EU) than in the United States, averaging 48 percent. Perhaps more important, most EU countries have institutionalized the concept of *management-labor councils.* In Germany, legislation dating back to the early 1950s created such councils, requiring that management and labor reach decisions jointly and unanimously. German management-labor councils use up a significant amount of management time. At H. C. Asmussen, a small German distilling company with 300 workers, there are five work councils, some of which meet weekly.

On a pan-European basis, an EU directive has forced 1,500 of the European Union's largest companies to set up Europe-wide worker-management consultative committees. In the United States, no such legislation exists, although there is a management desire to create more "quality circles" (to improve quality and to reduce costs) that involve workers and management. These are often used as a threat to unions or even a substitute for them. In fact, some American unions have succeeded in getting the federal government, through the National Labor Relations Board, to disband such quality circles.

For Critical Analysis

Why do you think American unions might be against quality circles involving management and workers?

CONCEPTS IN BRIEF

- The American Federation of Labor (AFL), composed of craft unions, was formed in 1886 under the leadership of Samuel Gompers. Membership increased until after World War I, at which time the government temporarily stopped protecting labor's right to organize.
- During the Great Depression, legislation was passed that allowed for collective bargaining. The National Labor Relations Act of 1935 guaranteed workers the right to start unions. The Congress of Industrial Organizations (CIO), composed of industrial unions, was formed during the Great Depression.

UNIONS AND COLLECTIVE BARGAINING CONTRACTS

Unions can be regarded as setters of minimum wages. Through collective bargaining, unions establish minimum wages below which no individual worker can offer his or her services. Each year, collective bargaining contracts covering wages as well as working conditions and fringe benefits for about 8 million workers are negotiated. Union negotiators act as agents for all members of the bargaining unit. They bargain with management about the provisions of a labor contract. Once union representatives believe that they have an acceptable collective contract, they will submit it to a vote of the union members. If approved by the members, the contract sets wage rates, maximum workdays, working conditions, fringe benefits, and other matters, usually for the next two or three years. Typically, collective bargaining contracts between management and the union apply also to nonunion members who are employed by the firm or the industry.

Strike: The Ultimate Bargaining Tool

Whenever union-management negotiations break down, union negotiators may turn to their ultimate bargaining tool, the threat or the reality of a strike. The first recorded strike in U.S. history occurred shortly after the Revolutionary War, when Philadelphia printers walked out in 1786 over a demand for a weekly minimum wage of $6. Strikes make headlines, but in less than 4 percent of all labor-management disputes does a strike occur before the contract is signed. In the other 96 percent of cases, contracts are signed without much public fanfare.

The purpose of a strike is to impose costs on recalcitrant management to force its acceptance of the union's proposed contract terms. Strikes disrupt production and interfere with a company's or an industry's ability to sell goods and services. The strike works both ways, though, because workers draw no wages while on strike (though they may be partly compensated out of union strike funds). Striking union workers may also be eligible to draw state unemployment benefits.

The impact of a strike is closely related to the ability of striking unions to prevent nonstriking (and perhaps nonunion) employees from continuing to work for the targeted company or industry. Therefore, steps are usually taken to prevent others from working for the employer. **Strikebreakers** can effectively destroy whatever bargaining power rests behind a strike. Numerous methods have been used to prevent strikebreakers from breaking strikes. Violence has been known to erupt, almost always in connection with attempts to prevent strikebreaking.

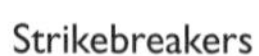

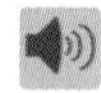

Temporary or permanent workers hired by a company to replace union members who are striking.

EXAMPLE

Taking On the Teamsters: The "Big" UPS Strike

As unionization rates have fallen, so have the number of labor strikes. As you can see in Figure 28-2, the highest number of strikes took place in 1953 and peaked again in the late 1960s and the mid-1970s. Strike activity has declined sharply since then.

Major strikes used to have significant disruptive effects on the overall economy, but that is rarely the case today. The last strike to bring at least part of the economy to a halt was the 1997 Teamsters strike against United Parcel Service (UPS). For several weeks, mail-order companies, college book publishers, and hundreds of thousands of other firms scrambled to replace UPS shipments with alternatives. Federal Express and Airborne Express in particular gained handsomely from the Teamsters strike against UPS.

FIGURE 28-2

The Declining Number of Labor Strikes

Since about 1974, the number of labor walkouts each year has declined steadily. The power of unions seems to be on the wane.

Source: U.S. Bureau of Labor Statistics.

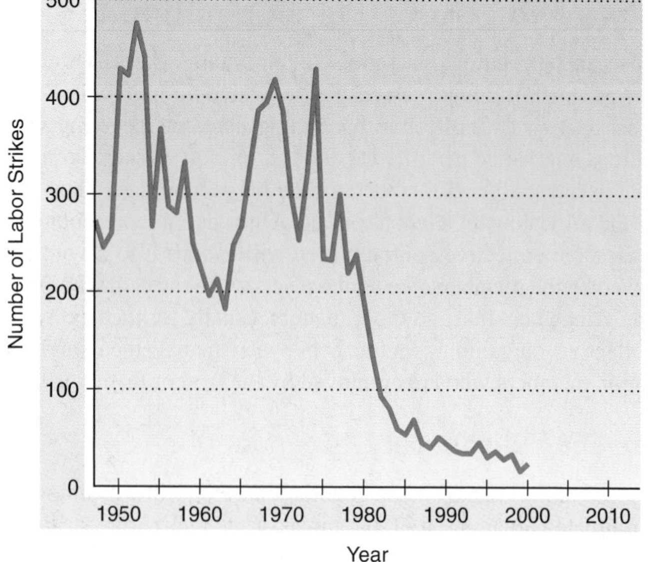

Many media pundits concluded that the strike yielded a big victory for the Teamsters and for organized labor as a whole. The Economic Policy Foundation, however, calculated that the typical UPS worker lost about $1,850 in income as a result of the strike. It calculated that relative to the final prestrike contract offer by UPS, a typical worker would require five years to come out ahead on net after the strike. Furthermore, after the strike the average part-time worker at UPS actually earned slightly *less* relative to what he or she would have earned under the company's prestrike offer. Finally, the higher costs that the new contract imposed on UPS pushed up shipping costs for manufacturing industries that are more heavily unionized, thereby raising prices of manufactured goods and reducing the quantity demanded by consumers. This tends to push down manufacturing wages. So in a sense the Teamsters' gain at UPS translated into a loss for union members in other industries.

For Critical Analysis

In what way may the Teamsters' "victory" have *helped* organized labor?

UNION GOALS 

We have already pointed out that one of the goals of unions is to set minimum wages. In many situations, any wage rate set higher than a competitive market clearing wage rate will reduce total employment in that market. This can be seen in Figure 28-3. We have a competitive market for labor. The market demand curve is D, and the market supply curve is S. The market clearing wage rate will be W_e; the equilibrium quantity of labor will be Q_e. If the union establishes by collective bargaining a minimum wage rate that exceeds W_e, an excess quantity of labor will be supplied (assuming no change in the labor demand schedule). If the minimum wage established by union collective bargaining is W_U, the quantity supplied would be Q_S; the quantity demanded would be Q_D. The difference is the excess quantity supplied, or surplus. Hence the following point becomes clear:

> One of the major roles of a union that establishes a wage rate above the market clearing wage rate is to ration available jobs among the excess number of workers who wish to work in unionized industries.

Note also that the surplus of labor is equivalent to a shortage of jobs at wage rates above equilibrium.

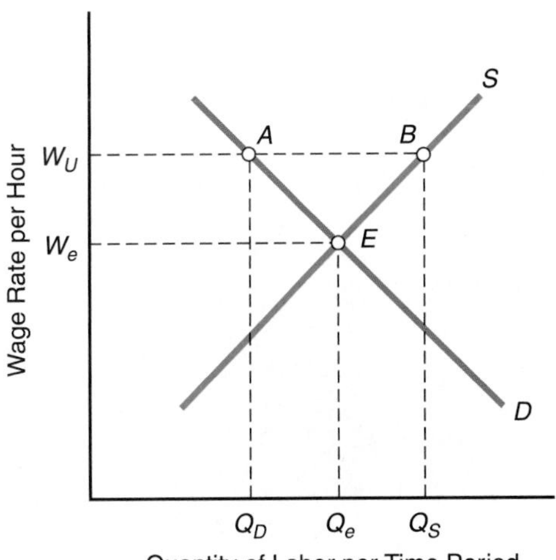

FIGURE 28-3

Unions Must Ration Jobs

If the union succeeds in obtaining wage rate W_U, the quantity of labor demanded will be Q_D, but the quantity of labor supplied will be Q_S. The union must ration a limited number of jobs to a greater number of workers; the surplus of labor is equivalent to a shortage of jobs at that wage rate.

The union may use a system of seniority, a lengthening of the apprenticeship period to discourage potential members from joining, and other such rationing methods. This has the effect of shifting the supply of labor curve to the left in order to support the higher wage, W_U.

There is a trade-off here that any union's leadership must face: Higher wages inevitably mean a reduction in total employment—a smaller number of positions. (Moreover, at higher wages, more workers will seek to enter the industry, thereby adding to the surplus that occurs because of the union contract.) Facing higher wages, management may replace part of the workforce with machinery.

Union Strategies

Goals of Unions
Further review union goals and strategies.

If we view unions as monopoly sellers of a service, we can identify three different wage and employment strategies that they use: ensuring employment for all members of the union, maximizing aggregate income workers, and maximizing wage rates for some workers.

Employing All Members in the Union. Assume that the union has Q_1 workers. If it faces a labor demand curve such as D in Figure 28-4, the only way it can "sell" all of those workers' services is to accept a wage rate of W_1. This is similar to any other demand curve. The demand curve tells the maximum price that can be charged to sell any particular quantity of a good or service. Here the service happens to be labor.

Maximizing Member Income. If the union is interested in maximizing the gross income of its members, it will normally want a smaller membership than Q_1—namely, Q_2 workers, all employed and paid a wage rate of W_2. The aggregate income to all members of the union is represented by the wages of only the ones who work. Total income earned by union members is maximized where the price elasticity of demand is numerically equal to 1. That occurs where marginal revenue equals zero. In Figure 28-4, marginal revenue equals zero at a quantity of labor Q_2. So we know that if the union obtains a wage rate equal to W_2, and therefore Q_2 workers are demanded, the total income to the union membership will be maximized. In other words, $Q_2 \times W_2$ (the shaded area) will be greater than any other combination of wage rates and quantities of union workers demanded. It is, for example, greater than $Q_1 \times W_1$. Note that in this situation, if the union started out with Q_1 members, there

FIGURE 28-4
What Do Unions Maximize?
Assume that the union wants to employ all its Q_1 members. It will attempt to get wage rate W_1. If the union wants to maximize total wage receipts (income), it will do so at wage rate W_2, where the elasticity of the demand for labor is equal to 1. (The shaded area represents the maximum total income that the union would earn at W_2.) If the union wants to maximize the wage rate for a given number of workers, say, Q_3, it will set the wage rate at W_3.

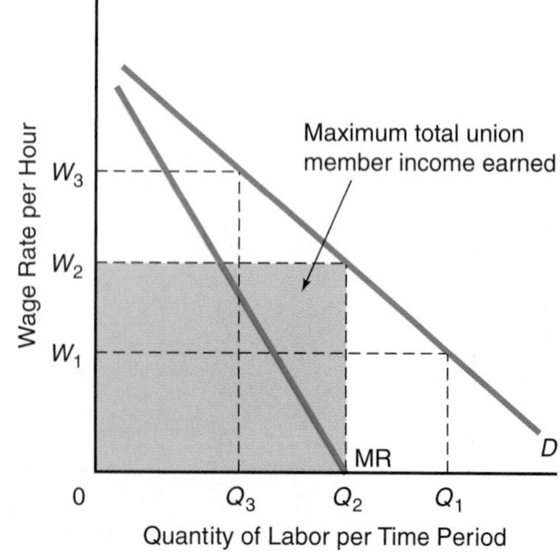

would be $Q_1 - Q_2$ members out of *union* work at the wage rate W_2. (Those out of union work either remain unemployed or go to other industries, which has a depressing effect on wages in nonunion industries due to the increase in supply of nonunion workers there.)

Maximizing Wage Rates for Certain Workers. Assume that the union wants to maximize the wage rates for some of its workers—perhaps those with the most seniority. If it wanted to keep a quantity of Q_3 workers employed, it would seek to obtain a wage rate of W_3. This would require deciding which workers should be unemployed and which workers should work and for how long each week or each year they should be employed.

Limiting Entry over Time

One way to raise wage rates without specifically setting wages is for unions to limit the size of their membership to the size of their employed workforce when the union was first organized. No workers are put out of work at the time the union is formed. Over time, as the demand for labor in the industry increases, there is no net increase in union membership, so larger wage increases are obtained than would otherwise be the case. We see this in Figure 28-5. Union members freeze entry into their union, thereby obtaining a wage rate of $16 per hour instead of allowing a wage rate of $15 per hour with no restriction on labor supply.

Altering the Demand for Union Labor

Another way in which unions can increase wages is to shift the demand curve for labor outward to the right. This approach compares favorably with the supply restriction approach because it increases both wage rates and employment level. The demand for union labor can be increased by increasing worker productivity, increasing the demand for union-made goods, and decreasing the demand for non-union-made goods.

Increasing Worker Productivity. Supporters of unions have argued that unions provide a good system of industrial jurisprudence. The presence of unions may induce workers to feel that they are working in fair and just circumstances. If so, they work harder, increasing

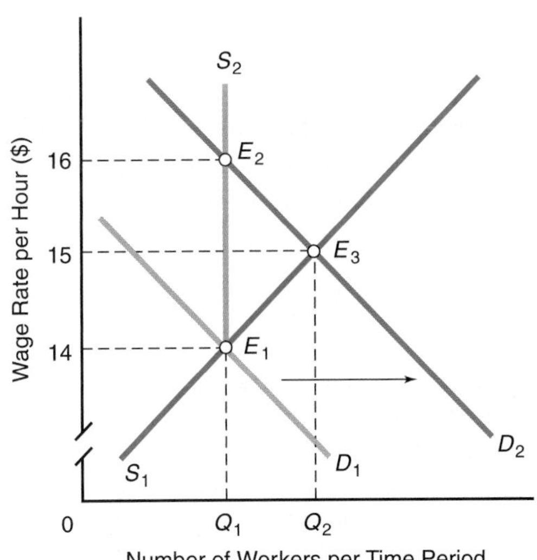

FIGURE 28-5 

Restricting Supply over Time

When the union was formed, it didn't affect wage rates or employment, which remained at $14 and Q_1 (the equilibrium wage rate and quantity). However, as demand increased—that is, as the demand schedule shifted outward to D_2 from D_1—the union restricted membership to its original level of Q_1. The new supply curve is S_1S_2, which intersects D_2 at E_2, or at a wage rate of $16. Without the union, equilibrium would be at E_3 with a wage rate of $15 and employment of Q_2.

labor productivity. Productivity is also increased when unions resolve differences and reduce conflicts between workers and management, thereby providing a smoother administrative environment.

Increasing Demand for Union-Made Goods. Because the demand for labor is a derived demand, a rise in the demand for products produced by union labor will increase the demand for union labor itself. One way in which unions attempt to increase the demand for union-labor-produced products is by advertising "Look for the union label."

Decreasing the Demand for Non-Union-Made Goods. When the demand for goods that are competing with (or are substitutes for) union-made goods is reduced, consumers shift to union-made goods, increasing the demand. A good example is when various unions campaign against imports; restrictions on imported cars are supported by the United Auto Workers as strongly as the Textile Workers Unions support restrictions on imported textile goods. The result is greater demand for goods "made in the USA," which in turn presumably increases the demand for American union (and nonunion) labor.

HAVE UNIONS RAISED WAGES?

We have seen that unions are able to raise the wages of their members if they are successful at limiting the supply of labor in a particular industry. They are also able to raise wages above what wages would otherwise be to the extent that they can shift the demand for union labor outward to the right. This can be done using the methods we have just discussed, including collective bargaining agreements that require specified workers for any given job—for example, by requiring a pilot, a copilot, and an engineer in the cockpit of a jet airplane even if an engineer is not needed on short flights. Economists have done extensive research to determine the actual increase in union wages relative to nonunion wages. They have found that in certain industries, such as construction, and in certain occupations, such as commercial airline pilot, the union wage differential can be 50 percent or more. That is to say, unions have been able in some industries and occupations to raise wage rates 50 percent or more above what they would be in the absence of unions.

In addition, the union wage differential appears to increase during recessions. This is because unions often, through collective bargaining, have longer-term contracts than nonunion workers so that they do not have to renegotiate wage rates, even when overall demand in the economy falls.

On average, unions appear to be able to raise the wage rates of their members relative to nonunion members by 10 to 20 percent. Note, though, that when unions increase wages beyond what productivity increases would permit, some union members will be laid off. A redistribution of income from low- to high-seniority union workers is not equivalent to higher wages for *all* union members.

CAN UNIONS INCREASE PRODUCTIVITY?

Featherbedding 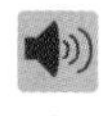
Any practice that forces employers to use more labor than they would otherwise or to use existing labor in an inefficient manner.

A traditional view of union behavior is that unions decrease productivity by artificially shifting the demand curve for union labor outward through excessive staffing and make-work requirements. For example, some economists have traditionally felt that unions tend to bargain for excessive use of workers, as when requiring an engineer on all flights. This is referred to as **featherbedding.** Many painters' unions, for example, resisted the use of paint sprayers and required that their members use only brushes. They even specified the maximum width of the brush. Moreover, whenever a union strikes, productivity drops, and this reduction in productivity in one sector of the economy can spill over into other sectors.

This traditional view against unions has been countered by a view that unions can actually increase productivity. Some labor economists contend that unions act as a collective voice for their members. In the absence of a collective voice, any dissatisfied worker either simply remains at a job and works in a disgruntled manner or quits. But unions, as a collective voice, can listen to worker grievances on an individual basis and then apply pressure on the employer to change working conditions and other things. The individual worker does not run the risk of being singled out by the employer and harassed. Also, the individual worker doesn't have to spend time trying to convince the employer that some change in the working arrangement should be made. Given that unions provide this collective voice, worker turnover in unionized industries should be less, and this should contribute to productivity. Indeed, there is strong evidence that worker turnover is reduced when unions are present. Of course, this evidence may also be consistent with the fact that wage rates are so attractive to union members that they will not quit unless working conditions become truly intolerable.

THE BENEFITS OF LABOR UNIONS 

It should by now be clear that there are two opposing views about unions. One portrays them as monopolies whose main effect is to raise the wage rate of high-seniority members at the expense of low-seniority members. The other contends that they can increase labor productivity through a variety of means. Harvard economists Richard B. Freeman and James L. Medoff argue that the truth is somewhere in between. They came up with the following conclusions:

1. Unionism probably raises social efficiency, thereby contradicting the traditional monopoly interpretation of what unions do. Even though unionism reduces employment in the unionized sector, it does permit labor to develop and implement workplace practices that are more valuable to workers. In some settings, unionism is associated with increased productivity.
2. Unions appear to reduce wage inequality.
3. Unions seem to reduce profits.
4. Internally, unions provide a political voice for all workers, and unions have been effective in promoting general social legislation.
5. Unions tend to increase the stability of the workforce by providing services, such as arbitration proceedings and grievance procedures.

Freeman and Medoff take a positive view of unionism. But their critics point out that they may have overlooked the fact that many of the benefits that unions provide do not require that unions engage in restrictive labor practices, such as the closed shop. Unions could still do positive things for workers without restricting the labor market.

CONCEPTS IN BRIEF

- When unions raise wage rates above market clearing prices, they face the problem of rationing a restricted number of jobs to a more than willing supply of workers.
- Unions may pursue any one of three goals: (1) to employ all members in the union, (2) to maximize total income of the union's workers, or (3) to maximize wages for certain, usually high-seniority, workers.

- Unions can increase the wage rate of members by engaging in practices that shift the union labor supply curve inward or shift the demand curve for union labor outward (or both).
- Some economists believe that unions can increase productivity by acting as a collective voice for their members, thereby freeing members from the task of convincing their employers that some change in working arrangements should be made. Unions may reduce turnover, thus improving productivity.

MONOPSONY: A BUYER'S MONOPOLY 

Let's assume that a firm is a perfect competitor in the product market. The firm cannot alter the price of the product it sells, and it faces a perfectly elastic demand curve for its product. We also assume that the firm is the only buyer of a particular input. Although this situation may not occur often, it is useful to consider. Let's think in terms of a factory town, like those dominated by textile mills or in the mining industry. One company not only hires the workers but also owns the businesses in the community, owns the apartments that workers live in, and hires the clerks, waiters, and all other personnel. This buyer of labor is called a **monopsonist,** the single buyer.

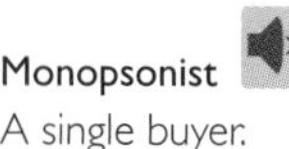

Monopsonist
A single buyer.

What does an upward-sloping supply curve mean to a monopsonist in terms of the costs of hiring extra workers? It means that if the monopsonist wants to hire more workers, it has to offer higher wages. Our monopsonist firm cannot hire all the labor it wants at the going wage rate. If it wants to hire more workers, it has to raise wage rates, including the wage of all its current workers (assuming a non-wage-discriminating monopsonist). It therefore has to take account of these increased costs when deciding how many more workers to hire.

EXAMPLE

Monopsony in College Sports

How many times have you read stories about colleges and universities violating National Collegiate Athletic Association (NCAA) rules? If you keep up with the sports press, these stories about alleged violations occur every year. About 600 four-year colleges and universities belong to the NCAA, which controls more than 20 sports. In effect, the NCAA operates an intercollegiate cartel that is dominated by universities that operate big-time athletic programs. It operates as a cartel with monopsony (and monopoly) power in four ways:

1. It regulates the number of student athletes that universities can recruit.
2. It often fixes the prices that the university charges for tickets to important intercollegiate sporting events.
3. It sets the prices (wages) and the conditions under which the universities can recruit these student athletes.
4. It enforces its regulations and rules with sanctions and penalties.

The NCAA rules and regulations expressly prohibit bidding for college athletes in an overt manner. Rather, the NCAA requires that all athletes be paid only for tuition, fees, room, board, and books. Moreover, the NCAA limits the number of athletic scholarships that can be given by a particular university. These rules are ostensibly to prevent the richest universities from "hiring" the best student athletes.

Not surprisingly, from the very beginning of the NCAA, individual universities and colleges have attempted to cheat on the rules in order to attract better athletes. The original agreement among the colleges was to pay no wages. Almost immediately after this agreement was put into effect, colleges switched to offering athletic scholarships, jobs, free room and board, travel expenses, and other enticements. It was not unusual for athletes to be paid $10 an hour to rake leaves when the going wage rate for such work was only $5 an hour. Finally, the NCAA had to agree to permit wages up to a certain amount per year.

If all universities had to offer exactly the same money wages and fringe benefits, the academically less distinguished colleges in metropolitan areas (with a large potential number of ticket-buying fans) would have the most inducement to violate the NCAA agreements (to compensate for the lower market value of their degrees). They would figure out all sorts of techniques to get the best student athletes. Indeed, such schools have in fact cheated more than other universities and colleges, and their violations have been detected and punished with a greater relative frequency than those of other colleges and universities.

For Critical Analysis

College and university administrators argue that the NCAA rules are necessary to "keep business out of higher education." How can one argue that college athletics is related to academics?

Marginal Factor Cost

The monopsonist faces an upward-sloping supply curve of the input in question because as the only buyer, it faces the entire market supply curve. Each time the monopsonist buyer of labor, for example, wishes to hire more workers, it must raise wage rates. Thus the marginal cost of another unit of labor is rising. In fact, the marginal cost of increasing its workforce will always be greater than the wage rate. This is because in the situation in which the monopsonist pays the same wage rate to everyone in order to obtain another unit of labor, the higher wage rate has to be offered not only to the last worker but also to all its other workers. We call the additional cost to the monopsonist of hiring one more worker the marginal factor cost (MFC).

The marginal factor cost for the last worker is therefore his or her wages plus the increase in the wages of all other existing workers. As we pointed out in Chapter 27, marginal factor cost is equal to the change in total variable cost due to a one-unit change in the one variable factor of production—in this case, labor. In Chapter 27, marginal factor cost was simply the competitive wage rate because the employer could hire all workers at the same wage rate.

Derivation of a Marginal Factor Cost Curve

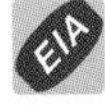

Monopsony
Gain further understanding of marginal factor cost for a monopsonist.

Panel (a) of Figure 28-6 on page 702 shows the quantity of labor purchased, the wage rate per hour, the total cost of the quantity of labor supplied per hour, and the marginal factor cost per hour for the additional labor bought.

We translate the columns from panel (a) to the graph in panel (b) of the figure. We show the supply curve as *S*, which is taken from columns 1 and 2. (Note that this is the same as the *average* factor cost curve; hence you can view Figure 28-6 as showing the relationship between average factor cost and marginal factor cost.) The marginal factor cost curve (MFC) is taken from columns 1 and 4. The MFC curve must be above the supply curve whenever the supply curve is upward-sloping. If the supply curve is upward-sloping, the firm must pay a higher wage rate in order to attract a larger amount of labor. This higher wage rate must be paid to all workers; thus the increase in total costs due to an increase in the labor input will exceed the wage rate. Note that in a perfectly competitive input market, the supply curve is perfectly elastic and the marginal factor cost curve is identical to the supply curve.

FIGURE 28-6

Derivation of a Marginal Factor Cost Curve

The supply curve, *S,* in panel (b) is taken from columns 1 and 2 of panel (a). The marginal factor cost curve (MFC) is taken from columns 1 and 4. It is the increase in the total wage bill resulting from a one-unit increase in labor input.

Panel (a)

(1) Quantity of Labor Supplied to Management	(2) Required Hourly Wage Rate	(3) Total Wage Bill (3) = (1) x (2)	(4) Marginal Factor Cost (MFC) = $\frac{\text{Change in (3)}}{\text{Change in (1)}}$
0	—	—	
			$1.00
1	$1.00	$1.00	
			3.00
2	2.00	4.00	
			3.20
3	2.40	7.20	
			4.00
4	2.80	11.20	
			6.80
5	3.60	18.00	
			7.20
6	4.20	25.20	

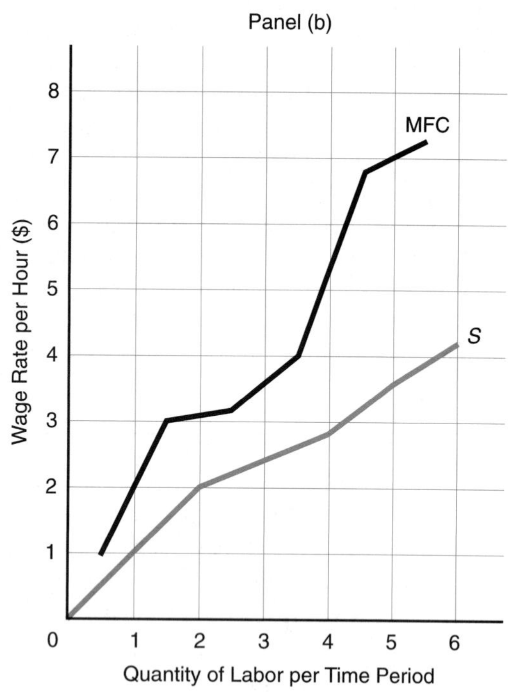

Employment and Wages Under Monopsony

To determine the number of workers that a monopsonist desires to hire, we compare the marginal benefit to the marginal cost of each hiring decision. The marginal cost is the marginal factor cost curve, and the marginal benefit is the marginal revenue product curve. In Figure 28-7, we assume competition in the output market and monopsony in the input market. A monopsonist finds its profit-maximizing quantity of labor demanded at *E,* where the marginal revenue product is just equal to the marginal factor cost.

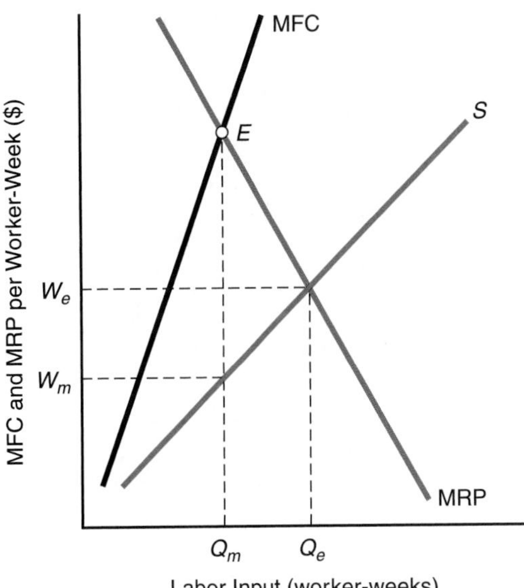

FIGURE 28-7

Marginal Factor Cost Curve for a Monopsonist

The monopsonist firm looks at a marginal cost curve, MFC, that slopes upward and is above its labor supply curve, *S*. The marginal benefit of hiring additional workers is given by the firm's MRP curve. The intersection of MFC with MRP, at point *E*, determines the number of workers hired. The firm hires Q_m workers but has to pay them only W_m in order to attract them. Compare this with the competitive solution, in which the wage rate would have to be W_e and the quantity of labor would be Q_e.

How much is the firm going to pay these workers? In a nonmonopsonistic situation it would face a given wage rate in the labor market, but because it is a monopsonist, it faces the entire supply curve, *S*.

A monopsonist faces an *upward-sloping* supply curve for labor. Firms do not usually face the market supply curve; most firms can hire all the workers they want at the going wage rate and thus usually face a perfectly elastic supply curve for each factor of production. The market supply curve, however, slopes upward.

The monopsonist therefore sets the wage rate so that it will get exactly the quantity, Q_m, supplied to it by its "captive" labor force. We find that wage rate is W_m. There is no reason to pay the workers any more than W_m because at that wage rate, the firm can get exactly the quantity it wants. The actual quantity used is established at the intersection of the marginal factor cost curve and the marginal revenue product curve for labor—that is, at the point at which the marginal revenue from expanding employment just equals the marginal cost of doing so.

Notice that the profit-maximizing wage rate paid to workers (W_m) is lower than the marginal revenue product. That is to say that workers are paid a wage that is less than their contribution to the monopsonist's revenues. This is sometimes referred to as **monopsonistic exploitation** of labor. The monopsonist is able to do this because each individual worker has little power in bargaining for a higher wage. The organization of workers into a union, though, creates a monopoly supplier of labor, which gives the union some power to bargain for higher wages.

Monopsonistic exploitation 
Exploitation due to monopsony power. It leads to a price for the variable input that is less than its marginal revenue product. Monopsonistic exploitation is the difference between marginal revenue product and the wage rate.

What happens when a monopsonist meets a monopolist? This is the situation called **bilateral monopoly,** defined as a market structure in which a single buyer faces a single seller. An example is a state education employer facing a single teachers' union in the labor market. Another example is a professional players' union facing an organized group of team owners. Such bilateral monopoly situations have indeed occurred in professional baseball and football. To analyze bilateral monopoly, we would have to look at the interaction of both sides, buyer and seller. The price outcome turns out to be indeterminate.

Bilateral monopoly 
A market structure consisting of a monopolist and a monopsonist.

We have studied the pricing of labor in various situations, including perfect competition in both the output and input markets and monopoly in both the output and input markets. Figure 28-8 on page 704 shows four possible situations graphically.

FIGURE 28-8

Summary of Pricing and Employment Under Various Market Conditions

In panel (a), the firm operates in perfect competition in both input and output markets. It purchases labor up to the point where the going rate W_e is equal to MRP_c. It hires quantity Q_e of labor. In panel (b), the firm is a perfect competitor in the input market but has a monopoly in the output market. It purchases labor up to the point where W_e is equal to MRP_m. It hires a smaller quantity of labor, Q_m, than in panel (a). In panel (c), the firm is a monopsonist in the input market and a perfect competitor in the output market. It hires labor up to the point where MFC = MRP_c. It will hire quantity Q_1 and pay wage rate W_c. Panel (d) shows a situation in which the firm is both a monopolist in the market for its output and a monopsonist in its labor market. It hires the quantity of labor Q_2 at which MFC = MRP_m and pays the wage rate W_m.

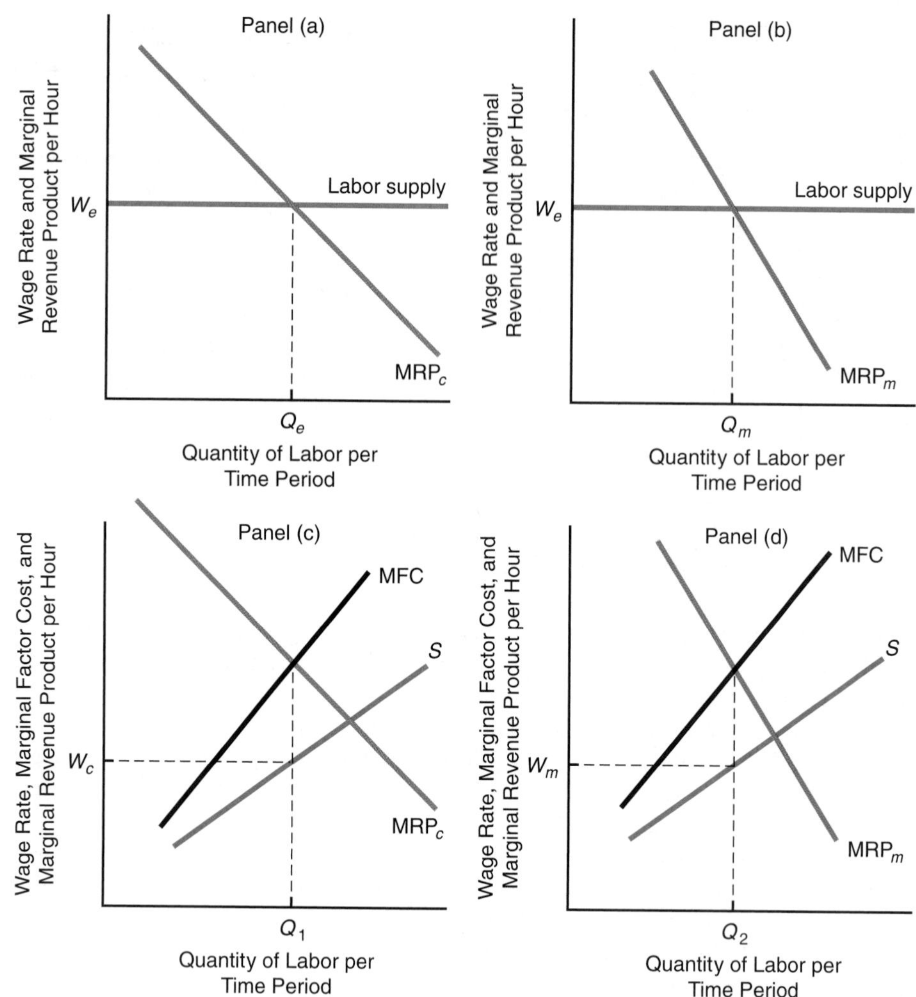

FAQ

Isn't the gender pay gap evidence of employer exploitation of women?

The fact that the average weekly wages of females continue to equal only about three-fourths of average male wages does not necessarily imply that employers exploit female workers. Although wage discrimination against women by some employers undoubtedly occurs, other factors contribute to the gender wage gap. One is that women tend to interrupt their careers to have children and continue in many households to bear the brunt of home responsibilities. Another is that even though there are growing ranks of highly trained female college graduates, the elimination of traditional welfare programs has increased the workforce participation of poorly educated women who have few marketable skills. Francine Blau and Lawrence Kahn of Cornell University have found that after accounting for education, experience, and occupations, women now earn wages no more than 12 percent less than men. Thus the gender wage gap may be somewhat overstated by direct wage comparisons.

EXAMPLE

Will Internet Job-Hunting Services Finally Make Monopsony an Irrelevant Economic Concept?

The classic example of monopsony is the "company town"—a small community in which a single firm is the dominant employer. In extreme examples, companies have owned and managed all housing, stores, and health care facilities in such towns. In these unusual situations, the companies had both monopoly and monopsony power.

Of course, the age of the automobile and commuting brought an end to most company towns. It did not necessarily bring a complete end to monopsony power for some businesses, however. For instance, imagine being a licensed practical nurse in a remote area with relatively few doctors and a single hospital largely managed by those same doctors. Avoiding some monopsonistic exploitation could prove difficult, and it might be hard for you to obtain information about alternative job openings for nurses, say, in home health care or in nursing care facilities within commuting distance of your home.

Today, however, the opportunities for a nurse in this situation are likely to brighten considerably if she logs on to her Internet service provider and types in "www." followed by "careermosaic.com," "careerpath.com," or "nationjob.com." These and other Web sites post job listings sent by company recruiters and help wanted ads from all over. Some sites have facilities for job hunters to post their résumés, and others even collect data from job seekers and then e-mail them potential matches given their talents and locational preferences. Increasingly, the Internet is blurring the distinctions among "local," "regional," and "national" labor markets, making it harder for any firm to exercise much monopsony power.

For Critical Analysis

If a local hospital faces little or no competition from other hospitals, is it possible for it to exploit its nursing employees even if it has no monopsony power?

CONCEPTS IN BRIEF

- A monopsonist is a single buyer. The monopsonist faces an upward-sloping supply curve of labor.
- Because the monopsonist faces an upward-sloping supply curve of labor, the marginal factor cost of increasing the labor input by one unit is greater than the wage rate. Thus the marginal factor cost curve always lies above the supply curve.
- A monopsonist will hire workers up to the point at which marginal factor cost equals marginal revenue product. Then the monopsonist will find what minimal wage is necessary to attract that number of workers. This is taken from the supply curve.

NETNOMICS

Working at Home: A Return to Sweatshops or a New Kind of Liberation?

By the 1890s, many American city-dwellers, adults and children alike, worked in what became known as "sweatshops." These were factories set up in large rooms in urban buildings. Women who worked for textile firms sometimes brought sewing work back to their tenement apartments and had their children assist them. In this way, some homes became extensions of the sweatshops. Today, some labor leaders are expressing concern about the potential for homes to become sweatshops of a different sort, largely as a result of widespread access to the Internet. Already, about 9 million U.S. workers are classified as "telecommuters." These are workers who work out of their homes, interacting with their employers via Internet links, e-mail and fax transmissions, and telephone communications. In addition, a growing number of people and their families now operate on-line businesses out of their homes.

One concern of labor leaders is that some telecommuters or home business operators may begin to pass a portion of their work along to their spouses and children, thereby violating child labor laws. More broadly, however, they fear that companies may increasingly *promote* telecommuting as a way to move work out of traditional plants, shops, and offices that unions have been able to organize. This, they believe, could make it easier for employers to exploit their workers. Certainly, a movement toward more telecommuting will not make it easier for unions to grow.

It is true that companies themselves are beginning to promote telecommuting. Many are cutting back on space. Increasingly, workers share offices and phones with two or three other people. In addition, companies are swayed by studies showing that many people are actually more productive at home, where there are fewer distractions.

Nevertheless, there are many factors pushing more people toward *choosing* to work at home. For one thing, it is easier for a father to make an afternoon transition to "quality time" with his child—say, finding time to take her to softball practice or gymnastics—if he is already at home, where he can e-mail a memo to his boss before departing with his daughter for the diamond or the gym. Likewise, it is easier for a mother to pick her son up at preschool on time each afternoon if she can download sales data from her company's Web site to analyze at home instead of having to stay late at the office to get the work done. Indeed, for some people, the biggest danger associated with using the Internet and e-mail to get their work done may be their computer's location under the same roof as their refrigerator. The waistlines of compulsive snackers may not benefit from the work-at-home revolution made possible by the Internet.

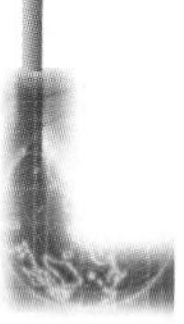

ISSUES & APPLICATIONS

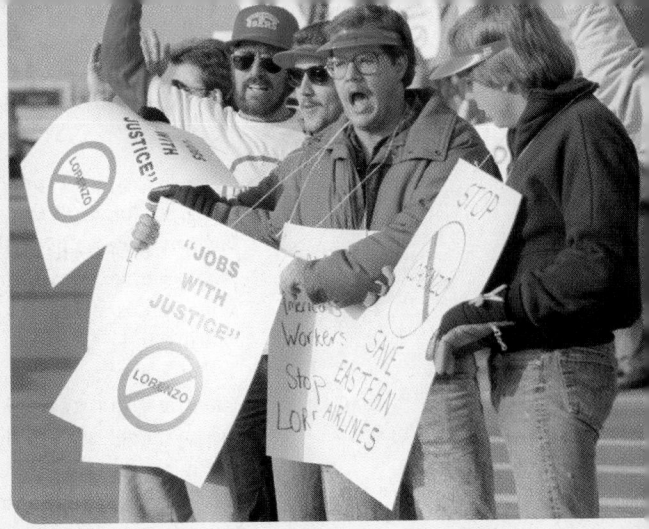

Is Profit Sharing Making Unions Obsolete?

Many economists have contended that the best wage-setting arrangement entails automatic adjustments of wages to firm profitability. Some proponents of profit sharing argue that it can help stabilize employment, because effective wage reductions would accompany profit declines, thereby reducing firms' wage costs and consequent layoffs. Some also contend that increased profit sharing could actually raise overall employment by effectively reducing the net cost of employing each additional unit of labor.

Concepts Applied

- Labor Unions
- Union Membership
- Employee-business Relations

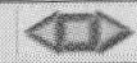

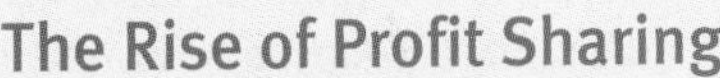

The Rise of Profit Sharing

Panel (a) of Figure 28-9 displays estimates of the proportion of workers employed under contracts with profit-sharing clauses in the nine countries with the largest numbers of workers covered by such contracts. France leads the list, with over a fourth of its workers covered by profit-sharing schemes, which is well above Japan's 15 percent profit-sharing coverage rate. Somewhat contradictory to proponents' arguments, France is infamous for strikes and other manifestations of labor disgruntlement. Labor produc-

FIGURE 28-9

Profit-Sharing Arrangements

Panel (a) indicates the proportion of workers covered by contracts containing profit-sharing arrangements in countries where profit sharing is most prevalent. Panel (b) shows that in the United States, profit sharing has been on the rise in the form of deferred profit-sharing pension plans.

Sources: Organization for Economic Cooperation and Development; John Duca, "The New Labor Paradigm: More Market-Responsive Rules of Work and Pay," Federal Reserve Bank of Dallas *Southwest Economy,* May-June 1998; author's estimates.

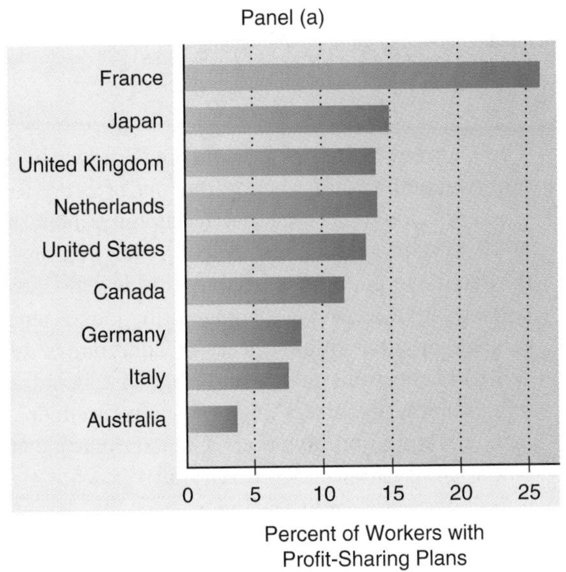

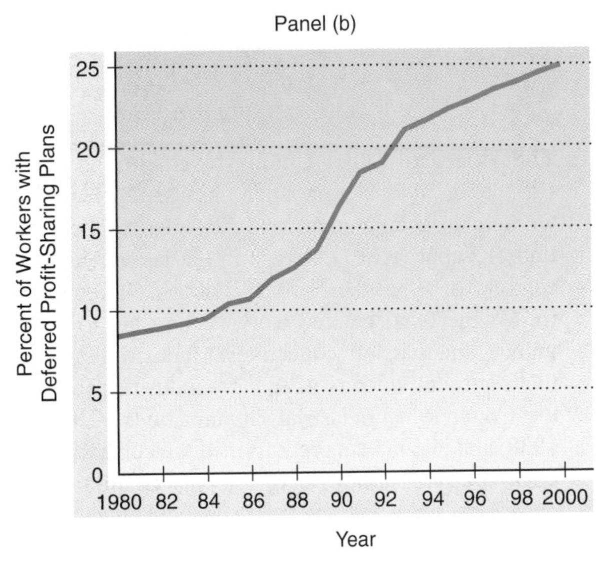

tivity growth in France also lags behind many other countries, and it suffers from a double-digit unemployment rate. Is France a "special case"? The answer is yes. French laws *require* firms with over 50 employees to offer government-designed profit-sharing plans. Hence government edict determines the structure of French profit-sharing plans. This makes it less likely that French workers and firms benefit as much from profit sharing.

Nevertheless, governmental policies also influence the degree of profit sharing in other countries. For example, in Britain, profit-based bonuses are tax-free up to a threshold income level, and in the United States, over 10 percent of workers covered under profit-sharing plans are employed by businesses that receive special tax credits for offering the programs. The Japanese government also gives favored tax treatment to certain profit-sharing schemes. Thus profit sharing is at present not a fully market-determined process. It remains to be seen how widespread profit-sharing arrangements may become in the absence of governmental stimulus.

Panel (b) of Figure 28-9 shows that the proportion of U.S. workers covered by deferred profit-sharing pension plans has risen steadily since 1980. Today, an estimated one in four workers is covered by deferred profit-sharing pension plans. Some of these workers and others also participate in employee stock ownership plans, or ESOPs. Workers in ESOPs receive shares of their companies' stocks as a form of payment. Because firms' rates of profitability influence increases in share prices and stock dividends, this is another way that firms can share profits with workers.

Does a Profit Inducement Lower the Incentive to Unionize?

If you look back at Figure 28-1 on page 692, you will note that the proportion of U.S. workers in unions began its most recent sustained decline during the 1980s. As panel (b) of Figure 28-9 indicates, this is also when profit sharing became more common. Undoubtedly, increased competition in the U.S. marketplace has influenced both patterns.

FOR CRITICAL ANALYSIS

1. If a worker's effective wage falls because of a decline in an employer's profitability, does this give the worker a greater incentive to go on strike or to increase his or her productivity?
2. Is profit sharing necessarily incompatible with unionization?

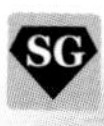

SUMMARY DISCUSSION OF LEARNING OBJECTIVES

1. **The American Labor Union Movement:** The first U.S. labor unions were craft unions, representing workers in specific trades, and the American Federation of Labor (AFL) emerged in the late nineteenth century. In 1935, the National Labor Relations Act (or Wagner Act) granted workers the right to form unions and bargain collectively. Industrial unions that represent workers of specific industries formed the Congress of Industrial Organizations (CIO) in 1938, and in 1955 a merger formed the current AFL-CIO. The Taft-Hartley Act of 1947 placed limitations on unions' rights to organize, strike, and boycott.

2. **The Current Status of U.S. Labor Unions:** In the mid-twentieth century, nearly one out of every four workers belonged to a union. Today only about one in 10 workers is a union member. A key reason for the decline in union membership rates is undoubtedly the relative decline in manufacturing jobs as a percentage of total employment. In addition, in less skilled occupations that would otherwise be attractive to union organizers, many workers are undocumented, foreign-born workers. Greater domestic and global competition has probably also had a part in bringing about a decline in unions.

3. **Basic Goals and Strategies of Labor Unions:** A key goal of most unions is to achieve higher wages. Often this entails bargaining for wages above competitive levels, which produces surplus labor. Thus a major task of many unions is to ration available jobs among the excess number of individuals who desire to work at the wages established by collective bargaining agreements. One strategy that unions often use to address this trade-off between wages and the number of jobs is to maximize the total income of members. If the focus of union objectives is the well-being of current members only, the union may bargain for limits on entry of new workers and seek to maximize the wages only of current union members. Another way for unions to try to push up wages is to try to increase worker productivity and lobby consumers to increase their demands for union-produced goods and reduce their demands for goods produced by nonunionized industries.
4. **Effects of Labor Unions on Wages and Productivity:** Economists have found that wages of unionized workers are typically higher than those of workers who are not union members. This is especially true during recessions, when the wages of nonunionized workers decline while those of unionized workers covered by collective bargaining agreements remain unchanged. On average, union wages are 10 to 20 percent higher than wages of nonunionized workers. It is less clear how unions affect worker productivity. On the one hand, some collective bargaining rules specifying how jobs are performed appear to reduce productivity. On the other hand, unionization reduces job turnover, which may enhance productivity.
5. **How a Monopsonist Determines How Much Labor to Employ and What Wage Rate to Pay:** A monopsony is the only firm that buys a particular input, such as labor. For a monopsonist in a labor market, paying a higher wage to attract an additional unit of labor increases its total factor costs for all other labor employed. For this reason, the marginal factor cost of labor is always higher than the wage rate, so the marginal factor cost schedule lies above the labor supply schedule. The labor market monopsonist employs labor to the point where the marginal factor cost of labor equals the marginal revenue product of labor. It then pays the workers it hires the wage at which they are willing to work, as determined by the labor supply curve that lies below the marginal factor cost curve. As a result, the monopsonist pays workers a wage that is less than their marginal revenue product, thereby engaging in monopsonistic exploitation of labor.
6. **Comparing a Monopsonist's Wage and Employment Decisions with Choices by Firms in Industries with Other Market Structures:** Firms that are perfect competitors or monopolies in their product markets but hire workers in perfectly competitive labor markets take the wage rate as market-determined, meaning that their individual actions are unable to influence the market wage rate. A product market monopolist tends to employ fewer workers than would be employed if the monopolist's industry were perfectly competitive, but the product market monopolist nonetheless cannot affect the market wage rate. By contrast, a monopsonist is the only employer of labor, so it searches for the wage rate that maximizes its profit. This wage rate is less than the marginal revenue product of labor, so monopsonistic exploitation results. In a situation in which a firm is both a product market monopolist and a labor market monopsonist, the firm's demand for labor is also lower than it would be if the firm's product market were competitive, and hence the firm hires fewer workers as well.

Key Terms and Concepts

Problems

Answers to the odd-numbered problems appear at the back of the book.

28-1. Discuss three aspects of collective bargaining that society might deem desirable.

28-2. Give three reasons why a government might seek to limit the power of a union.

28-3. What effect do strikebreakers have on the collective bargaining power of a union or other collective bargaining arrangement?

28-4. Suppose that the objective of a union is to maximize the total dues paid to the union by its membership. Explain the union strategy, in terms of the wage level and employment level, under the following two scenarios.

a. Union dues are a percentage of total earnings of the union membership.
b. Union dues are paid as a flat amount per union member employed.

28-5. Explain why, in economic terms, the total income of union membership is maximized when marginal revenue is zero.

28-6. Explain the impact of each of the following events on the market for union labor.

a. Union-produced commercials convince consumers to buy domestically manufactured clothing instead of imported clothing.
b. The union sponsors periodic training programs that instruct union laborers about the most efficient use of machinery and tools.

28-7. In the short run, a tool manufacturer has a fixed amount of capital. Labor is a variable input. The cost and output structure that the firm faces is depicted in the following table:

Labor Supplied	Total Physical Product	Required Hourly Wage Rate ($)
10	100	5
11	109	6
12	116	7
13	121	8
14	124	9
15	125	10

Derive, at each level of labor supplied, the firm's total wage bill and marginal factor cost.

28-8. Suppose that for the firm in Problem 28-7, the goods market is perfectly competitive. The market price of the product the firm produces is $4 at each quantity supplied by the firm. What is the amount of labor that this profit-maximizing firm will hire, and what wage rate will it pay?

28-9. A firm finds that the price of its product changes with the rate of output. In addition, the wage it pays its workers varies with the amount of labor it employs. The price and wage structure that the firm faces is depicted in the following table.

Labor Supplied	Total Physical Product	Required Hourly Wage Rate ($)	Product Price ($)
10	100	5	3.11
11	109	6	3.00
12	116	7	2.95
13	121	8	2.92
14	124	9	2.90
15	125	10	2.89

This firm maximizes profits. How many units of labor will it hire? What wage will it pay?

28-10. What is the amount of monopsonistic exploitation that takes place at the firm examined in Problem 28-9?

Economics on the Net

Evaluating Union Goals As discussed in this chapter, unions can pursue any of a number of goals. The AFL-CIO's homepage provides links to the Web sites of several unions, and reviewing these sites can help you determine the objectives these unions have selected.

Title: American Federation of Labor–Congress of Industrial Organizations

Navigation: Click here to visit the AFL-CIO's homepage.

Application Perform the indicated operations, and answer the following questions:

1. Click on About the AFL-CIO. Then click on AFL-CIO's Mission. Does the AFL-CIO claim to represent the interests of all workers or just workers in specific firms or industries? Can you discern what broad wage and employment strategy the AFL-CIO pursues?

2. Click on Partners and Links. Explore two or three of these Web sites. Do these unions appear to represent the interests of all workers or just workers in specific firms or industries? What general wage and employment strategies do these unions appear to pursue?

For Group Study and Analysis Divide up all the unions affiliated with the AFL-CIO among groups, and have each group explore the Web sites listed under Partners and Links at the AFL-CIO Web site. Have each group report on the wage and employment strategies that appear to prevail for the unions it examined.

CHAPTER

29

RENT, INTEREST, AND PROFITS

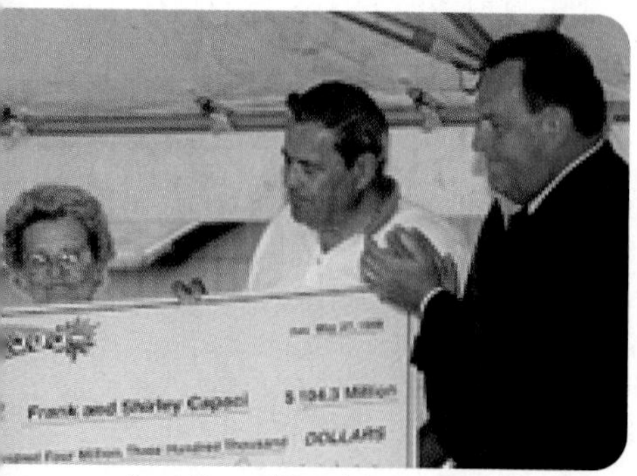

State lotteries advertise their "jackpots" regularly. Most winnings, though, are paid out over 20 years. Is it correct to add up the yearly payments and call the total the jackpot?

A few years ago, a retired electrician from Streamwood, Illinois, purchased $5 in Wisconsin lottery tickets that entered him in a Powerball lottery jointly operated by 20 states. The states sold a total of 138 million Powerball tickets, and the electrician beat odds of 80 million to one to win a single-ticketholder jackpot. Even though he could have received a total of $195 million paid in equal installments over 25 years, the retiree opted for immediate receipt of a lump-sum payment of $104 million. Why did this man choose $104 million immediately instead of $195 million to be received over the course of 25 years? To understand the answer to this question, you must learn about interest rates and the present value of future sums, which are key topics of this chapter.

LEARNING OBJECTIVES

After reading this chapter, you should be able to:

1. Understand the concept of economic rent
2. Evaluate the role of economic rent in the allocation of resources
3. Explain how market interest rates are determined
4. Discuss how the interest rate performs a key role in allocating resources
5. Calculate the present discounted value of a payment to be received at a future date
6. Describe the fundamental role of economic profits

Did You Know That... in America, presumably one of the most industrialized countries in the world, compensation for labor services makes up over 70 percent of national income every year? But what about the other 30 percent? It consists of compensation to the owners of the other factors of production that you read about in Part 1: land, capital, and entrepreneurship. Somebody who owns real estate downtown may earn monthly commercial rents that are higher for one square foot than you might pay to rent a whole apartment. Land is a factor of production, and it has a market clearing price. Businesses also have to use capital. Compensation for that capital is interest, and it, too, has a market clearing level. Finally, some of you may have entrepreneurial ability that you offer to the marketplace. Your compensation is called profit. In this chapter, you will also learn about the sources and functions of profit.

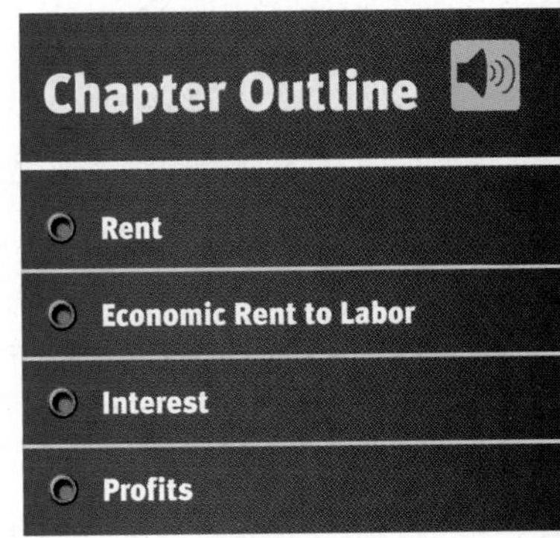

RENT

When you hear the term *rent,* you are accustomed to having it mean the payment made to property owners for the use of land or dwellings. The term *rent* has a different meaning in economics. **Economic rent** is payment to the owner of a resource in excess of its opportunity cost—the payment that would be necessary to call forth production of that amount of the resource.

Economic rent 
A payment for the use of any resource over and above its opportunity cost.

Economists originally used the term *rent* to designate payment for the use of land. What was thought to be important about land was that its supply is completely inelastic. Hence the supply curve for land is a vertical line; no matter what the prevailing market price for land, the quantity supplied will remain the same.

Determining Land Rent

The concept of economic rent is associated with the British economist David Ricardo (1772–1823). He looked at two plots of land on which grain was growing, one of which happened to be more fertile than the other. The owners of these two plots sold the grain that came from their land, but the one who owned the more fertile land grew more grain and therefore made more profits. According to Ricardo, the owner of the fertile land was receiving economic rents that were due not to the landowner's hard work or ingenuity but rather to an accident of nature. Ricardo asked his readers to imagine another scenario, that of walking up a hill that starts out flat with no rocks and then becomes steeper and rockier. The value of the land falls as one walks up the hill. If a different person owns the top of the hill than the bottom, the highland owner will receive very little in payment from, say, a farmer who wants to cultivate land for wheat production.

Here is how Ricardo analyzed economic rent for land. He first simplified his model by assuming that all land is equally productive. Then Ricardo assumed that the quantity of land in a country is *fixed.* Graphically, then, in terms of supply and demand, we draw the supply curve of land vertically (zero price elasticity). In Figure 29-1 on the next page, the supply curve of land is represented by S. If the demand curve is D_1, it intersects the supply curve, S, at price P_1. The entire amount of revenues obtained, $P_1 \times Q_1$, is labeled "Economic rent." If the demand for land increased to D_2, the equilibrium price would rise to P_2. Additions to economic rent are labeled "More economic rent." Notice that the quantity of land remains insensitive to the change in price. Another way of stating this is that the supply curve is perfectly inelastic.

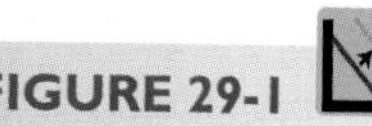

FIGURE 29-1

Economic Rent

If indeed the supply curve of land were completely price inelastic in the long run, it would be depicted by *S*. At the quantity in existence, Q_1, any and all revenues are economic rent. If demand is D_1, the price will be P_1; if demand is D_2, price will rise to P_2. Economic rent would be $P_1 \times Q_1$ and $P_2 \times Q_1$, respectively.

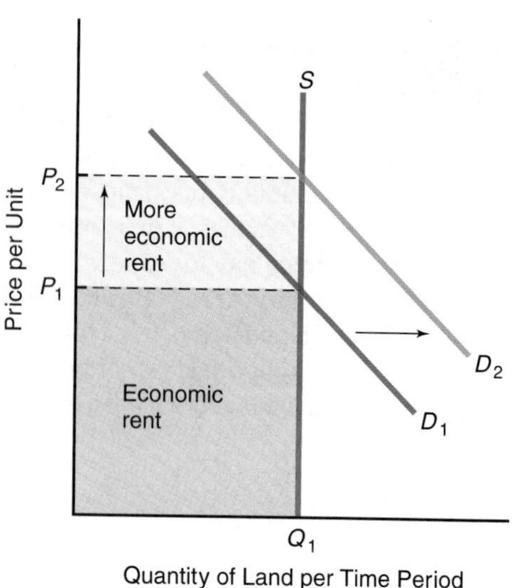

ECONOMIC RENT TO LABOR

Land and natural resources are not the only factors of production to which the analysis of economic rent can be applied. In fact, the analysis is probably more often applicable to labor. Here is a list of people who provide different labor services, some of whom probably receive large amounts of economic rent:

Professional sports superstars
Rock stars
Movie stars
World-class models
Successful inventors and innovators
World-famous opera stars

Just apply the definition of economic rent to the phenomenal earnings that these people make. They would undoubtedly work for much, much less than they earn. Therefore, much of their earnings constitutes economic rent (but not all, as we shall see). Economic rent occurs because specific resources cannot be replicated exactly. No one can duplicate today's most highly paid entertainment figures, and therefore they receive economic rent.

Economic Rent and the Allocation of Resources 

If an extremely highly paid movie star would make the same number of movies at half his or her current annual earnings, does that mean that 50 percent of his or her income is unnecessary? To answer the question, consider first why the superstar gets such a high income. The answer can be found in Figure 29-1. Substitute *entertainment activities of the superstars* for the word *land.* The high "price" received by the superstar is due to the demand for his or her services. If Leonardo Di Caprio announces that he will work for a measly $1 million a movie and do two movies a year, how is he going to know which production company values his services the most highly? Di Caprio and other movie stars let the market decide where their resources should be used. In this sense, we can say the following:

Economic rent allocates resources to their highest-valued use.

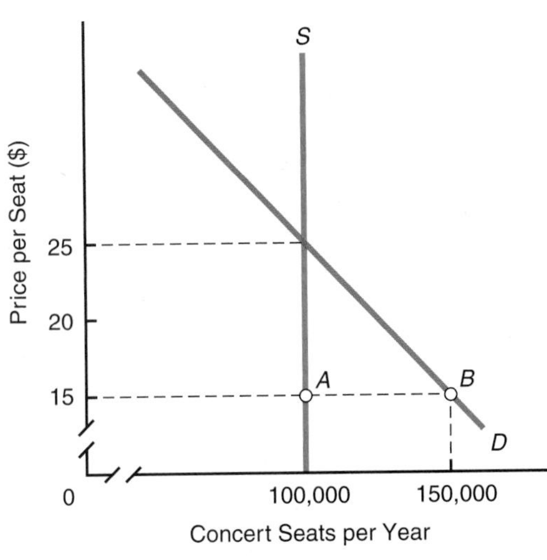

FIGURE 29-2

The Allocative Function of Rent

If the performer agrees to give five concerts a year "at any price" and there are 20,000 seats in each concert hall, the supply curve of concerts, *S*, is vertical at 100,000 seats per year. The demand curve is given by *D*. The performer wants a price of only $15 to be charged. At that price, the quantity of seats demanded per year is 150,000. The excess quantity demanded is equal to the horizontal distance between points *A* and *B*, or 50,000 seats per year.

Otherwise stated, economic rent directs resources to the people who can most efficiently use them.

A common counterexample involves rock stars who claim that promoters try to overprice their tickets. Consequently, the artists agree to perform, say, five concerts with all tickets being sold at the same price, $15. Assume that a star performs these concerts in halls with 20,000 seats. A total of 100,000 individuals per year will be able to see this particular performer. This is represented by point *A* in Figure 29-2. By assumption, this performer is still receiving some economic rent because we are assuming that the supply curve of concerts is vertical at 100,000 seats per year. At a price per ticket of $15, however, the annual quantity of seats demanded will be 150,000, represented by point *B*. The difference between points *A* and *B* is the excess quantity of tickets demanded at the below-market-clearing price of $15 a seat. The *additional* economic rent that could be earned by this performer by charging the clearing price of $25 per seat in this graph would serve as the rationing device that would make the quantity demanded equal to the quantity supplied.

In such situations, part of the economic rent that could have been earned is dissipated—it is captured, for example, by radio station owners in the form of promotional gains when they are allowed to give away a certain number of tickets on the air (even if they have to pay $15 per ticket) because the tickets are worth $25. Ticket holders who resell tickets at higher prices ("scalpers") also capture part of the rent. Conceivably, at 100,000 seats per year, this performer could charge the market clearing price of $25 per ticket and give away to charity the portion of the economic rent ($10 per ticket) that would be dissipated. In such a manner, the performer could make sure that the recipients of the rent are worthy in his or her own esteem.

EXAMPLE

Do Entertainment Superstars Make Super Economic Rents?

Superstars certainly do well financially. Table 29-1 on the next page shows the earnings of selected individuals in the entertainment industry as estimated by *Forbes* magazine. Earnings are totaled for a two-year period. How much of these earnings can be called economic rent? The question is not easy to answer, because an entertainment newcomer would almost certainly work for much less than he or she earns, thereby making high

TABLE 29-1
Superstar Earnings

Name	Occupation	Earnings (two years, millions of dollars)
Jerry Seinfeld	Actor, comedian	267
Larry David	Producer	242
Steven Spielberg	Director, producer, studio owner	175
Oprah Winfrey	Talk show host	125
James Cameron	Director, producer	115
Tim Allen	Actor, comedian	77
Michael Crichton	Writer, producer	65
Harrison Ford	Actor	58
Rolling Stones	Rock group	57
Master P	Rapper, actor	57

Source: Forbes, 2000.

economic rents. The same cannot necessarily be said for entertainers who have been raking in millions for years. They probably have very high accumulated wealth and also a more jaded outlook about their work. It is therefore not clear how much they would work if they were not offered those huge sums of money.

For Critical Analysis

Even if some superstar entertainers would work for less, what forces cause them to make so much income anyway?

Taxing Away Economic Rent

Some people have argued in favor of imposing high taxes on economic rent. For example, drug companies that have developed *successful* patented drugs make large amounts of economic rent during the life of the patent. That is to say, the marginal cost of production is much less than the price charged. If the government taxed this economic rent completely, those successful drugs already on the market would in fact stay on the market. But there would be long-run consequences. Drug companies would invest fewer resources in discovering new successful drugs. So economic rent is typically a *short-run* phenomenon. In the long run, it constitutes a source of reward for risk taking in society. This is true not only in the drug business but also in entertainment and professional sports.

CONCEPTS IN BRIEF

- Economic rent is defined as payment for a factor of production that is completely inelastic in supply. It is payment for a resource over and above what is necessary to keep that resource in existence at its current level in the long run.
- Economic rent serves an allocative function by guiding available supply to the most efficient use.

Interest 
The payment for current rather than future command over resources; the cost of obtaining credit. Also, the return paid to owners of capital.

INTEREST

The term **interest** is used to mean two different things: (1) the price paid by debtors to creditors for the use of loanable funds and (2) the market return earned by (nonfinancial) capital as a factor of production. Owners of capital, whether directly or indirectly, obtain interest income. Often businesses go to credit markets to obtain so-called money capital in order to invest in physical capital from which they hope to make a satisfactory return. In other words, in our complicated society, the production of capital goods often occurs because of the existence of credit markets in which borrowing and lending take place. For the moment, we will look only at the credit market.

Interest and Credit

When you obtain credit, you actually obtain money to have command over resources today. We can say, then, that interest is the payment for current rather than future command over resources. Thus interest is the payment for obtaining credit. If you borrow $100 from me, you have command over $100 worth of goods and services today. I no longer have that command. You promise to pay me back $100 plus interest at some future date. The interest that you pay is usually expressed as a percentage of the total loan, calculated on an annual basis. If at the end of one year you pay me back $110, the annual interest is $10 ÷ $100, or 10 percent. When you go out into the marketplace to obtain credit, you will find that the interest rate charged differs greatly. A loan to buy a house (a mortgage) may cost you 7 to 10 percent annual interest. An installment loan to buy an automobile may cost you 9 to 14 percent annual interest. The federal government, when it wishes to obtain credit (issue U.S. Treasury securities), may have to pay only 3 to 8 percent annual interest. Variations in the rate of annual interest that must be paid for credit depend on the following factors.

1. *Length of loan.* In some (but not all) cases, the longer the loan will be outstanding, other things being equal, the greater will be the interest rate charged.
2. *Risk.* The greater the risk of nonrepayment of the loan, other things being equal, the greater the interest rate charged. Risk is assessed on the basis of the creditworthiness of the borrower and whether the borrower provides collateral for the loan. Collateral consists of any asset that will automatically become the property of the lender should the borrower fail to comply with the loan agreement.
3. *Handling charges.* It takes resources to set up a loan. Papers have to be filled out and filed, credit references have to be checked, collateral has to be examined, and so on. The larger the amount of the loan, the smaller the handling (or administrative) charges as a percentage of the total loan. Therefore, we would predict that, other things being equal, the larger the loan, the lower the interest rate.

What Determines Interest Rates?

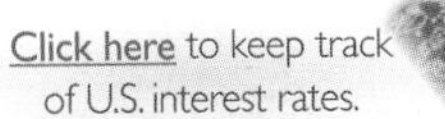

Click here to keep track of U.S. interest rates.

The overall level of interest rates can be described as the price paid for loanable funds. As with all commodities, price is determined by the interaction of supply and demand. Let's first look at the supply of loanable funds and then at the demand for them.

The Supply of Loanable Funds. The supply of loanable funds (credit available) depends on individuals' willingness to save.* When you save, you exchange rights to current consumption for rights to future consumption. The more current consumption you give up, the more valuable is a marginal unit of present consumption in comparison with future consumption.

*Actually, the supply of loanable funds also depends on business and government saving and on the behavior of the monetary authorities and the banking system. For simplicity of discussion, we ignore these components here.

Recall from our discussion of diminishing marginal utility that the more of something you have, the less you value an additional unit. Conversely, the less of something you have, the more you value an additional unit. Thus when you give up current consumption of a good—that is, have less of it—you value an additional unit more. The more you save today, the more utility you attach to your last unit of today's consumption. So to be induced to save more—to consume less—you have to be offered a bigger and bigger reward to match the marginal utility of current consumption you will give up by saving. Because of this, if society wants to induce people to save more, it must offer a higher rate of interest. Hence we expect that the supply curve of loanable funds will slope upward. At higher rates of interest, savers will be willing to offer more current consumption to borrowers, other things being constant.* When the income of individuals increases or when there is a change in individual preferences toward more saving, the supply curve of loanable funds will shift outward to the right, and vice versa.

The Demand for Loanable Funds. There are three major sources of the demand for loanable funds:

1. Households that want loanable funds for the purchase of services and nondurable goods, as well as consumer durables such as automobiles and homes
2. Businesses that want loanable funds to make investments
3. Governments that want loanable funds, usually to cover deficits—the excess of government spending over tax revenues

We will ignore the government's demand for loanable funds and consider only consumers and businesses.

Loans are taken out both by consumers and by businesses. It is useful for us to separate the motives underlying the demand for loans by these two groups of individuals. We will therefore treat consumption loans and investment loans separately. In the discussion that follows, we will assume that there is no inflation—that is, that there is no persistent increase in the overall level of prices.

Consumer Demand for Loanable Funds In general, consumers demand loanable funds because they tend to prefer earlier consumption to later consumption. That is to say, people subjectively value goods obtained immediately more than the same goods of the same quality obtained later on. Consider that sometimes an individual household's present income falls below the average income level expected over a lifetime. Individuals may go to the credit market to borrow whenever they perceive a temporary dip in their current income—assuming that they expect their income to go back to normal later on. Furthermore, by borrowing, they can spread out purchases more evenly during their lifetimes. In so doing, they're able to increase their lifetime total utility.

Consumers' demand for loanable funds will be inversely related to the cost of borrowing—the rate of interest. Why? For the same reason that all demand curves slope downward: A higher rate of interest means a higher cost of borrowing, and a higher cost of borrowing must be

*A complete discussion would include the income effect: At higher interest rates, households receive a higher yield on savings, permitting them to save less to achieve any given target.

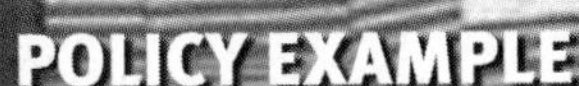

Should Payday Lenders Be Regulated?

Payday lenders are companies that typically offer an individual a small amount of cash, from $100 to $300, in exchange for a personal check. The lender holds on to the check until the individual receives his or her next paycheck and then cashes the check. Payday lending is a booming business. Since 1995, the number of payday lenders in Indiana has increased from 11 to more than 60, and payday loans in that state rose from $13 million to $98 million. Check Into Cash opened its first payday store in 1993 and now has a chain of 432 stores in 16 states, including more than 30 in Illinois.

Payday lenders provide their services for a fee that typically ranges from 15 to 25 percent of the face value of the check. That is, they charge interest on loans that they effectively make to individuals who use their services. When the interest rates on these loans are converted to an annual percentage interest rate, the numbers can be shocking. For instance, a *Chicago Sun-Times* survey of Illinois payday loan lenders found the average annual interest rate charged by the lenders to be 569 percent.

The Consumer Federation of America calls payday lending "legal loan-sharking" and argues that payday lenders prey on the poor while making exorbitant profits. It calls for regulating the interest rates charged by payday lenders. But the key reason that payday lenders charge high rates is that the risk of bad checks is very high. There is also a big benefit to consumers: The ability to borrow $500 reduces the likelihood that someone who is poor will suffer a "spell of hardship," such as not having enough money for food. Thus for someone who cannot obtain a speedy loan any other way, the only thing worse than borrowing $200 at an annual interest rate exceeding 500 percent might be not being able borrow $200 at all.

For Critical Analysis

Payday lenders like to compare payday loans to taxicab transportation, which may be cost-effective for short distances but not for long-distance travel. Does this analogy seem reasonable to you?

weighed against alternative uses of limited income. At higher costs of borrowing, consumers will forgo some current consumption.

Business Demand for Loanable Funds Businesses demand loanable funds to make investments that they believe will increase productivity or profit. Whenever a business believes that by making an investment, it can increase revenues (net of other costs) by more than the cost of capital, it will make the investment. Businesses compare the interest rate they must pay in the loanable funds market with the rate of return they think they can earn by investing. This comparison helps them decide whether to invest.

In any event, we hypothesize that the demand curve for loanable funds by firms for investment purposes will be negatively sloped. At higher interest rates, fewer investment projects will make economic sense to businesses because the cost of capital (loanable funds) will exceed the net revenues derivable from the capital investment. Conversely, at lower rates of interest, more investment projects will be undertaken because the cost of capital will be less than the expected rate of return on the capital investment.

The Equilibrium Rate of Interest

When we add together the demand for loanable funds by households and businesses (and government in more complex models), we obtain a demand curve for loanable funds, as given in Figure 29-3 (p. 720). The supply curve is *S*. The equilibrium rate of interest is i_e.

FIGURE 29-3 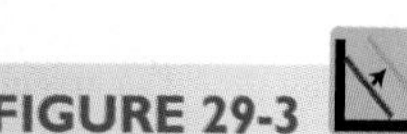

The Supply of and Demand for Loanable Funds

We draw *D* as the demand curve for all loanable funds by households and businesses (and governments). It slopes downward. *S* is the supply curve of credit, or loanable funds. It slopes upward. The intersection of *S* and *D* gives the equilibrium rate of interest at i_e.

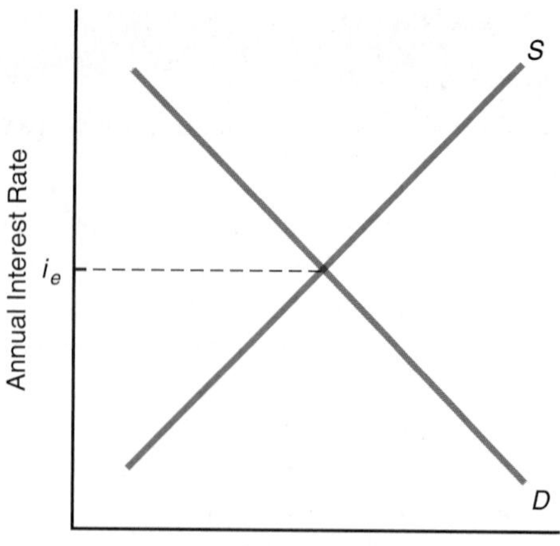

INTERNATIONAL EXAMPLE

Combating Japanese Loan Sharks with "Instant Cash Loans"

Japan has a reputation for trying to keep foreign competition away from its shores. In 1978, however, Japan's Ministry of Finance invited U.S. finance companies to open up shop in the country. Its hope was that American financiers would have the wherewithal to compete with one of Japan's most notorious industries, loan-shark operations, many of which had links to organized crime.

A number of U.S. finance companies, including Household International, Inc., Beneficial Corporation, and Associates First Capital, gave it a try. Initially, it was tough to convince Japanese residents to borrow yen from U.S. companies. Two factors ultimately worked in these companies' favor, however. One was that Japanese banks were so protected from competition in lending to corporations that they did not even try to compete for many individual and small-business customers in the 1980s. Another was that when Japan's banks had problems during the recession that hit East Asia in the late 1990s, even customers who had previously been bank borrowers had trouble getting loans. Many of these former bank customers began to turn to the U.S. finance companies.

Today, finance companies offer credit in the form of "instant cash loans," many of which borrowers can access using electronic dispensers that shoot out currency, typically in the form of 10,000-yen bills (about $100 each). The total volume of finance company credit outstanding in Japan now exceeds $60 billion. Associates First Capital alone has been increasing its lending in Japan at a rate in excess of 20 percent per year, and it now has 600 branches across the country. Associates and other U.S. finance companies typically charge 30 percent interest for loans. The companies pay a rate of 6 percent to raise funds to lend.

For Critical Analysis

There is a lot of competition among U.S. finance companies to extend instant cash loans in Japan. What factors might explain the high interest rate on these loans?

Real Versus Nominal Interest Rates

Nominal rate of interest The market rate of interest expressed in today's dollars.

We have been assuming that there is no inflation. In a world of inflation—a persistent rise in an average of all prices—the **nominal rate of interest** will be higher than it would be in a world with no inflation. Basically, nominal, or market, rates of interest rise to take account of the anticipated rate of inflation. If, for example, there is no inflation and no inflation is expected, the nominal rate of interest might be 5 percent for home mortgages. If the rate of inflation goes to 10 percent a year and stays there, everybody will anticipate that inflation rate. The nominal rate of interest will rise to about 15 percent to take account of the anticipated rate of inflation. If the interest rate did not rise to 15 percent, the principal plus interest earned at 5 percent would be worth less in the future because inflation would have eroded its purchasing power. We can therefore say that the nominal, or market, rate of interest is approximately equal to the real rate of interest plus the anticipated rate of inflation, or

$$i_n = i_r + \text{anticipated rate of inflation}$$

where i_n equals the nominal rate of interest and i_r equals the real rate of interest. In short, you can expect to see high nominal rates of interest in periods of high inflation rates. The **real rate of interest** may not necessarily be high, though. We must first correct the nominal rate of interest for the anticipated rate of inflation before determining whether the real interest rate is in fact higher than normal.

Real rate of interest 
The nominal rate of interest minus the anticipated rate of inflation.

FAQ

Aren't high nominal interest rates always an indication that real interest rates are high?

No, in many instances real interest rates are relatively low in countries with high nominal rates of interest. The reason for double- and triple-digit interest rates in some countries—such as interest rates exceeding 100 percent in Russia in the early 1990s and above 40 percent in Brazil more recently—has often been that people anticipated high rates of inflation. Real interest rates in double digits are very rare.

The Allocative Role of Interest

In Chapter 4, we talked about the price system and the role that prices play in the allocation of resources. Interest is a price that allocates loanable funds (credit) to consumers and to businesses. Within the business sector, interest allocates loanable funds to different firms and therefore to different investment projects. Investment, or capital, projects with rates of return higher than the market rate of interest in the credit market will be undertaken, given an unrestricted market for loanable funds. For example, if the expected rate of return on the purchase of a new factory in some industry is 15 percent and loanable funds can be acquired for 11 percent, the investment project may proceed. If, however, that same project had an expected rate of return of only 9 percent, it would not be undertaken. In sum, the interest rate allocates loanable funds to industries whose investments yield the highest returns—where resources will be the most productive.

It is important to realize that the interest rate performs the function of allocating money capital (loanable funds) and that this ultimately allocates real physical capital to various firms for investment projects.

Interest Rates and Present Value 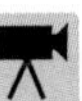

Click here for additional review of present value.

Businesses make investments in which they often incur large costs today but don't make any profits until some time in the future. Somehow they have to be able to compare their investment cost today with a stream of future profits. How can they relate present cost to future benefits?

Interest rates are used to link the present with the future. After all, if you have to pay $110 at the end of the year when you borrow $100, that 10 percent interest rate gives you a measure of the premium on the earlier availability of goods and services. If you want to have things today, you have to pay the 10 percent interest rate in order to have current purchasing power.

The question could be put this way: What is the present value (the value today) of $110 that you could receive one year from now? That depends on the market rate of interest, or the rate of interest that you could earn in some appropriate savings institution, such as in a

Present value 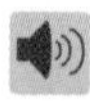
The value of a future amount expressed in today's dollars; the most that someone would pay today to receive a certain sum at some point in the future.

savings account. To make the arithmetic simple, let's assume that the rate of interest is 10 percent. Now you can figure out the **present value** of \$110 to be received one year from now. You figure it out by asking the question, How much money must I put aside today at the market interest rate of 10 percent to receive \$110 one year from now? Mathematically, we represent this equation as

$$(1 + .1)PV_1 = \$110$$

where PV_1 is the sum that you must set aside now.

Let's solve this simple equation to obtain PV_1:

$$PV_1 = \frac{\$110}{1.1} = \$100$$

That is to say, \$100 will accumulate to \$110 at the end of one year with a market rate of interest of 10 percent. Thus the present value of \$110 one year from now, using a rate of interest of 10 percent, is \$100. The formula for present value of any sums to be received one year from now thus becomes

$$PV_1 = \frac{FV_1}{1 + i}$$

Click here to calculate present value on the Internet.

where

PV_1 = present value of a sum one year hence

FV_1 = future sum of money paid or received one year hence

i = market rate of interest

Present Values for More Distant Periods. The present-value formula for figuring out today's worth of dollars to be received at a future date can now easily be seen. How much would have to be put in the same savings account today to have \$110 two years from now if the account pays a rate of 10 percent per year compounded annually?

After one year, the sum that would have to be set aside, which we will call PV_2, would have grown to $PV_2 \times 1.1$. This amount during the second year would increase to $PV_2 \times 1.1 \times 1.1$, or $PV_2 \times (1.1)^2$. To find the PV_2 that would grow to \$110 over two years, let

$$PV_2 \times (1.1)^2 = \$110$$

and solve for PV_2:

$$PV_2 = \frac{\$110}{(1.1)^2} = \$90.91$$

Thus the present value of \$110 to be paid or received two years hence, discounted at an interest rate of 10 percent per year compounded annually, is equal to \$90.91. In other words, \$90.91 put into a savings account yielding 10 percent per year compounded interest would accumulate to \$110 in two years.

Discounting 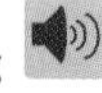
The method by which the present value of a future sum or a future stream of sums is obtained.

The General Formula for Discounting. The general formula for **discounting** becomes

$$PV_t = \frac{FV_t}{(1 + i)^t}$$

TABLE 29-2
Present Value of a Future Dollar
This table shows how much a dollar received at the end of a certain number of years in the future is worth today. For example, at 5 percent a year, a dollar to be received 20 years in the future is worth 37.7 cents; if received in 50 years, it isn't even worth a dime today. To find out how much $10,000 would be worth a certain number of years from now, just multiply the figures in the table by 10,000. For example, $10,000 received at the end of 10 years discounted at a 5 percent rate of interest would have a present value of $6,140.

	Compounded Annual Interest Rate				
Year	3%	5%	8%	10%	20%
1	.971	.952	.926	.909	.833
2	.943	.907	.857	.826	.694
3	.915	.864	.794	.751	.578
4	.889	.823	.735	.683	.482
5	.863	.784	.681	.620	.402
6	.838	.746	.630	.564	.335
7	.813	.711	.583	.513	.279
8	.789	.677	.540	.466	.233
9	.766	.645	.500	.424	.194
10	.744	.614	.463	.385	.162
15	.642	.481	.315	.239	.0649
20	.554	.377	.215	.148	.0261
25	.478	.295	.146	.0923	.0105
30	.412	.231	.0994	.0573	.00421
40	.307	.142	.0460	.0221	.000680
50	.228	.087	.0213	.00852	.000109

where t refers to the number of periods in the future the money is to be paid or received.

Table 29-2 gives the present value of $1 to be received in future years at various interest rates. The interest rate used to derive the present value is called the **rate of discount.**

Rate of discount 
The rate of interest used to discount future sums back to present value.

POLICY EXAMPLE

Should the "Pre-Death" Business Be Regulated?

Many Americans with terminal illnesses have life insurance policies that they would like to sell in order to use the proceeds while they are alive. To satisfy this demand, viatical ("provisions for a journey") companies make a present value calculation to determine how much they will pay to the person who is going to die. A terminally ill person with a life insurance policy may have an expected life of, say, four years. If the life insurance policy is sold to a viatical business, the latter must estimate the present value of receiving the payoff from the life insurance policy in four years. The company also has to determine an appropriate discount rate. The viatical business, which started around 1988, has enjoyed a rate of return of around 20 percent a year. Cries in favor of state regulation of the business are now heard virtually everywhere. After all, dying people may be too willing to sell their life insurance policies at a low price because they do not have enough information. Already, state insurance commissioners have agreed that terminally ill patients with six months to live should be paid at least 80 percent of the face value of their policies.

For Critical Analysis

What alternatives do terminally ill life insurance policy holders have? (Hint: How could they use the policy as collateral?)

CONCEPTS IN BRIEF

- Interest is the price paid for the use of capital. It is also the cost of obtaining credit. In the credit market, the rate of interest paid depends on the length of the loan, the risk, and the handling charges, among other things.
- The interest rate is determined by the intersection of the supply curve of credit, or loanable funds, and the demand curve for credit, or loanable funds. The major sources for the demand for loanable funds are households, businesses, and governments.
- Nominal, or market, interest rates include a factor to take account of the anticipated rate of inflation. Therefore, during periods of high anticipated inflation, nominal interest rates will be relatively high.
- Payments received or costs incurred in the future are worth less than those received or incurred today. The present value of any future sum is lower the further it occurs in the future and the greater the discount rate used.

PROFITS

In Chapter 2, we identified entrepreneurship, or entrepreneurial talent, as a factor of production. Profit is the reward that this factor earns. You may recall that entrepreneurship involves engaging in the risk of starting new businesses. In a sense, then, nothing can be produced without an input of entrepreneurial skills.

Until now, we have been able to talk about the demand for and supply of labor, land, and capital. We can't talk as easily about the demand for and supply of entrepreneurship. For one thing, we have no way to quantify entrepreneurship. What measure should we use? We do know that entrepreneurship exists. We cannot, however, easily present a supply and demand analysis to show the market clearing price per unit of entrepreneurship. We must use a different approach, focusing on the reward for entrepreneurship—profit. First we will determine what profit is *not.* Then we will examine the sources of true, or economic, profit. Finally, we will look at the functions of profits in a market system.

Distinguishing Between Economic Profit and Business, or Accounting, Profit

In our discussion of rent, we had to make a distinction between the common notions of rent and the economist's concept of economic rent. We must do the same thing when we refer to profit. We always have to distinguish between **economic profit** and **accounting profit.** The accountant calculates profit for a business as the difference between total explicit revenues and total explicit costs. Consider an extreme example. You are given a large farm as part of your inheritance. All of the land, fertilizer, seed, machinery, and tools has been fully paid for by your deceased relative. You take over the farm and work on it diligently with half a dozen workers. At the end of the year, you sell the output for $1 million. Your accountant then subtracts your actual ("explicit") expenses, mainly the wages you paid.

Economic profit 
The difference between total revenues and the opportunity cost of all factors of production.

Accounting profit 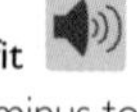
Total revenues minus total explicit costs.

The difference is called profit, but it is not economic profit. Why? Because no accounting was taken of the *implicit* costs of using the land, seed, tools, and machinery. The only explicit cost considered was the workers' wages. But as long as the land could be rented out, the seed could be sold, and the tools and machinery could be leased, there was an opportunity cost to using them. To derive the economic profit that you might have earned last year from the farm, you must subtract from total revenues the full opportunity cost of all factors of production used (which will include both implicit and explicit costs).

In summary, then, accounting profit is used mainly to define taxable income and, as such, may include some returns to both the owner's labor and capital. Economic profit, by contrast, represents a return over and above the opportunity cost of all resources (including a normal return on, or payment for, the owner's entrepreneurial abilities).

When viewed in this light, it is possible for economic profit to be negative, even if accounting profit is positive. Turning to our farming example again, what if the opportunity cost of using all of the resources turned out to be \$1.1 million? The economic profit would have been a *negative* \$100,000. You would have suffered economic losses.

In sum, the businessperson's accounting definition and the economist's economic definition of profit usually do not coincide. Economic profit is a residual. It is whatever remains after all economic, or opportunity, costs have been taken into account.

Explanations of Economic Profit

Alternative sources of profit are numerous. Let us examine a few of them: restrictions on entry, innovation, and reward for bearing uninsurable risks.

Restrictions on Entry. We pointed out in Chapter 24 that monopoly profits—a special form of economic profits—are possible when there are barriers to entry, and these profits are often called monopoly rents by economists. Entry restrictions exist in many industries, including taxicabs, cable television franchises, and prescription drugs and eyeglasses. Basically, monopoly profits are built into the value of the business that owns the particular right to have the monopoly.

Innovation. A number of economists have maintained that economic profits are created by innovation, which is defined as the creation of a new organizational strategy, a new marketing strategy, or a new product. This source of economic profit was popularized by Harvard economics professor Joseph Schumpeter (1883–1950). The innovator creates new economic profit opportunities through innovation. The successful innovator obtains a temporary monopoly position, garnering temporary economic profits. When other firms catch up, those temporary economic profits disappear.

Reward for Bearing Uninsurable Risks

There are risks in life, including those involved in any business venture. Many of these risks can be insured, however. You can insure against the risk of losing your house to fire, flood, hurricane, or earthquake. You can do the same if you own a business. You can insure against the risk of theft also. Insurance companies are willing to sell you such insurance because they can predict relatively accurately what percentage of a class of insured assets will suffer losses each year. They charge each insured person or business enough to pay for those fully anticipated losses and to make a normal rate of return.

But there are risks that cannot be insured. If you and a group of your friends get together and pool your resources to start a new business, no amount of statistical calculations can accurately predict whether your business will still be running a year from now or 10 years from now. Consequently, you can't, when you start your business, buy insurance against losing money, bad management, miscalculations about the size of the market, aggressive competition by big corporations, and the like. Entrepreneurs therefore incur uninsurable risks. According to a theory of profits advanced by economist Frank H. Knight (1885–1973), this is the origin of economic profit.

The Function of Economic Profit

In a market economy, the expectation of profits induces firms to discover new products, new production techniques, and new marketing techniques—literally all the new ways to make higher profits. Profits in this sense spur innovation and investment.

Profits also cause resources to move from lower-valued to higher-valued uses. Prices and sales are dictated by the consumer. If the demand curve is close to the origin, there will be few sales and few profits, if any. The lack of profits therefore means that there is insufficient demand to cover the opportunity cost of production. In the quest for higher profits, businesses will take resources out of areas in which lower than normal rates of return are being made and put them into areas in which there is an expectation of higher profits. The profit reward is an inducement for an industry to expand when demand and supply conditions warrant it. Conversely, the existence of economic losses indicates that resources in the particular industry are not valued as highly as they might be elsewhere. These resources therefore move out of that industry, or at least no further resources are invested in it. Therefore, resources follow the businessperson's quest for higher profits. Profits allocate resources, just as wages and interest do.

CONCEPTS IN BRIEF

- Profit is the reward for entrepreneurial talent, a factor of production.
- It is necessary to distinguish between accounting profit and economic profit. Accounting profit is measured by the difference between total revenues and all explicit costs. Economic profit is measured by the difference between total revenues and the total of all opportunity costs of all factors of production.
- Theories of why profits exist include restriction on entry, innovation, and payment to entrepreneurs for taking uninsurable risks.
- The function of profits in a market economy is to allocate scarce resources. Resources will flow to wherever profits are highest.

ISSUES & APPLICATIONS

Accepting Millions of Dollars in Lottery Winnings Is Harder than You Might Imagine

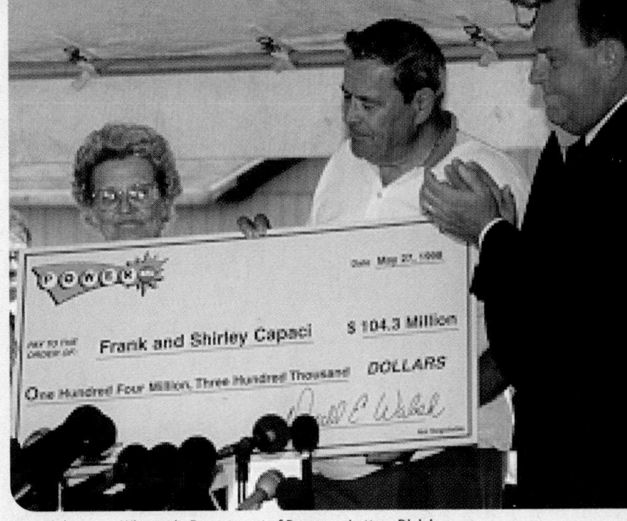

Copyright 2000–Wisconsin Department of Revenue–Lottery Division

When 67-year-old Frank Capaci won the 1998 Wisconsin Powerball jackpot, he opted for a lump-sum payment of $104 million instead of $195 million paid in annual installments of $7.8 million over 25 years. Was this his best choice? One argument for taking a lump-sum amount was his age. But his 63-year-old wife probably had a longer life expectancy. In addition, they might have had children and grandchildren about whom they cared deeply. Assuming that he cared about his loved ones, wouldn't Capaci want them to be guaranteed receipt of $7.8 million per year even after his death?

Concepts Applied

- Present Value
- Interest Rates

Determining the Value of Lottery Payments

Put yourself in Frank Capaci's place. The Powerball lottery administrators notified him that he could either receive $104 million instantly or $7.8 million every year for 25 years. What Capaci had to do was compare the present value of $7.8 million per year for a total of 25 years with an immediate $104 million lump sum.

Look back at Table 29-2 on page 723. How could Capaci calculate the present value of 25 years' worth of lottery payments? The answer is that he could use the present-value figures in Table 29-2 to convert each year's $7.8 million payment into present-value terms. For instance, at an interest rate of 5 percent, the present value of $7.8 million received a year later would be .952 times $7.8 million, or $7,425,600. The present value of $7.8 million two years later would be .907 times $7.8 million, or $7,074,600. Using the 5 percent column of Table 29-2 in this way (after filling in years 11–14, 16–19, and 21–24 in the table), he could calculate 25 years' worth of present values of annual payments of $7.8 million. Then he could sum these to come up with a grand total present value of the payments to compare with the $104 million lump sum he was offered.

A Retired Electrician Who Understood Interest and Present Value

The same calculations can be performed at each interest rate in Table 29-2. Table 29-3 gives the resulting present-value sums (rounded to the nearest hundred thousand dollars) for the 25 years of annual payments. As you can see, the present value of these payments was $115.4 million at an interest rate of 5 percent. At an interest rate of 8 percent, however, the present value of the payments was only $90.3 million.

TABLE 29-3
Present Values of Lottery Payments at Different Interest Rates

	Interest Rate				
	3%	5%	8%	10%	20%
Present Value ($ million)	139.9	115.4	90.3	77.9	46.3

Thus, if Frank Capaci cared about his loved ones as much as he did himself, he knew that one key issue was what he expected market interest returns to be over the next 25 years. At the time he won the lottery, most bonds were offering annual returns ranging from 7 to 8 percent. Much higher average (though riskier) annual returns were available in the stock market. Thus if Frank Capaci saved his lump-sum payment by holding a mix of bonds and stocks, he could feel reasonably certain that he and his loved ones would be better off than if he accepted 25 years' worth of payments instead. (Capaci did not indicate an intention to spend all the money quickly. He said that he planned to buy a Harley-Davidson motorcycle.)

FOR CRITICAL ANALYSIS

1. Why was the present value of the annual lottery payments higher at lower interest rates?
2. Initial press accounts said that Capaci won a $195 million jackpot. Were they accurate?

Of Course, There Are Always Complications

Other factors surely influenced Frank Capaci's decision. For instance, if he decided to leave all his wealth to his wife, then there would be no inheritance taxes on that sum. Annual payments would be subject to inheritance taxes.

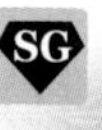

SUMMARY DISCUSSION OF LEARNING OBJECTIVES

1. **The Concept of Economic Rent:** Owners of a resource in fixed supply, meaning that the resource supply curve is perfectly inelastic, are paid economic rent. Originally, this term was used to refer to payment for the use of land or any other natural resource that is considered to be in fixed supply. More generally, however, economic rent is a payment for use of any resource that exceeds the opportunity cost of the resource.
2. **Economic Rent and Resource Allocation:** Owners of any productive factors with inelastic supply earn economic rent because competition among potential users of those factors bids up the prices of these factors. Hence people who provide labor services that are difficult for others to provide, such as sports superstars, movie stars, and the like, typically receive earnings well in excess of the earnings that would otherwise have been sufficient to induce them to provide their services. Nevertheless, the economic rents that they earn reflect the maximum market valuation of their value, so economic rent allocates resources to their highest-valued use.
3. **How Market Interest Rates Are Determined:** Interest is a payment for the ability to use resources today instead of in the future. The equilibrium rate of interest is determined by the intersection of the demand for loanable funds (the demand for credit) with the supply of loanable funds (the supply of credit). Other factors that influence interest rates are the length of the term of a loan, the loan's risk, and handling charges. The nominal interest rate includes a factor that takes into account the anticipated inflation rate. Therefore, during periods of high anticipated inflation, current market (nominal) interest rates are high.
4. **The Key Role the Interest Rate Performs in Allocating Resources:** The rate of interest is a price that induces lenders to allocate loanable funds to consumers and to businesses. Comparing the market interest rate with the rate of return on prospective capital investment projects enables owners of loanable funds to determine the highest-valued uses of the funds. Thus the interest rate allocates loanable funds to industries whose investments yield the highest returns, thereby ensuring that available resources will be put to their most productive uses.
5. **Calculating the Present Discounted Value of a Payment to Be Received at a Future Date:** The present value of a future payment is the value of the future amount expressed in today's dollars, and it is equal to the most that someone would pay today to receive that amount in the future. The method by which the present value of a future sum is calculated is called *discounting*. This method implies that the

present value of a sum to be received a year from now is equal to the future amount divided by 1 plus the appropriate rate of interest, which is called the *rate of discount.*

6. **The Fundamental Role of Economic Profits:** A positive economic profit of a firm is a return over and above the opportunity cost of all resources, including a payment for the entrepreneurial abilities of the firms' owners. Hence economic profit reflects implicit opportunity costs of directing entrepreneurial resources to one line of business instead of a different line of business. A firm earning positive accounting profit, in which total revenues exceed explicit, out-of-pocket expenses, can still earn negative economic profits. This occurs if the accounting profit fails to cover the opportunity cost of entrepreneurship allocated to that business. In response to a negative economic profit in one business, an owner has an incentive to redirect resources to a different business, thereby allocating them to their highest-valued use.

Key Terms and Concepts

Accounting profit (724)	Economic rent (713)	Present value (722)
Discounting (722)	Interest (716)	Rate of discount (723)
Economic profit (724)	Nominal rate of interest (720)	Real rate of interest (721)

Problems

Answers to odd-numbered problems appear at the back of the book.

29-1. Which of the following would you expect to have a high level of economic rent, and which would you expect to have a low level of economic rent? Explain why for each.

a. Bob has a highly specialized medical skill that is in great demand.

b. Sally has never attended school. She is 25 years old and is an internationally known supermodel.

c. Tim is a high school teacher and sells insurance part time.

29-2. Though he has retired from hockey, Wayne Gretzky still earns a sizable annual income from endorsements. Explain why, in economic terms, his level of economic rent is still so high.

29-3. Michael Jordan once retired from basketball to play baseball. As a result, his annual dollar income dropped from the millions to the thousands. Eventually Jordan quit baseball and returned to basketball. What can be said about the role of economic rents in his situation?

29-4. A British pharmaceutical company spent several years and considerable funds on the development of a treatment for HIV patients. Now, with the protection afforded by patent rights, the company has the potential to reap enormous gains. The government, in response, has threatened to tax away any rents the company may earn. Is this an advisable policy? Why or why not?

29-5. Explain how the following events would likely affect the relevant interest rate.

a. A major bond-rating agency has improved the risk rating of a developing nation.

b. To regulate and protect the public, the government has passed legislation that requires a considerable increase in the reporting paperwork when a bank makes a loan.

c. At the time of graduation, you elect to pay off your student loan in five years instead of 10.

29-6. Explain how each of the following would affect the rate of interest.

a. Because of expected higher future prices of durable goods, consumers borrow money to buy these items today.

b. Pessimistic views on business prospects lead businesses to postpone capital expenditures.

29-7. Suppose that the government enacts a binding ceiling on interest rates. What is the impact of this legislation on the market for loanable funds and on the economy in general?

29-8. Suppose that the rate of interest in Japan is only 2 percent, while the comparable rate in the United States is 4 percent. Japan's rate of inflation is .5 percent, while the U.S. inflation rate is 3 percent. Which economy has the higher real interest rate?

29-9. You expect to receive a payment of $104 one year from now. Your discount rate is 4 percent. What is the present value of the payment to be received? Suppose that the discount rate is 5 percent. What is the present value of the payment to be received?

29-10. An individual leaves a college faculty, where she was earning $40,000 a year, to begin a new venture. She invests her savings of $10,000, which were earning 10 percent annually. She then spends $20,000 on office equipment, hires two students at $30,000 a year each, rents office space for $12,000, and has other variable expenses of $40,000. At the end of the year, her revenues were $200,000. What are her accounting profit and her economic profit for the year?

Economics on the Net

Interest Rates in Mexico As discussed in this chapter, there are many different types of interest rates in the United States. Indeed, any nation has a number of different market interest rates. In this application, you will contemplate various interest rates in Mexico.

Title: The Bank of Mexico

Navigation: Click here to begin at the Bank of Mexico's homepage. Select "Economic and Financial Indicators," then "Financial Markets and Interest Rates". Scroll down to "Information Structures" and then click on the daily "Money Market Representative Interest Rates".

Application Record the most recent 28-day TIIE rate, bank funding rate, and government funding rate.

Next, click here to visit the Federal Reserve Web site. Select the most recent release, and find the U.S. prime lending rate.

1. On the Bank of Mexico's site, back up to the main "Economic and Financial Indicators" page. Click on "Prices" and select to view the monthly Main Price Index. Record the percent change in the Consumer Price Index for the most recent month with respect to the same month of the previous year. What was the annual rate of inflation for Mexico over the past year? Using the three one-month rates you collected, which are quoted in annual terms, calculate the real rate of each.

For Group Discussion and Analysis Based on the data you collected, why do you think the U.S. prime lending rate is lower than the TIIE rate? Does this necessarily mean that U.S. prime customers are less risky than the Mexican government? (Hint: Discuss the how anticipated changes in exchange rates likely affect the amount of interest charged.)

CHAPTER 30

INCOME, POVERTY, AND HEALTH CARE

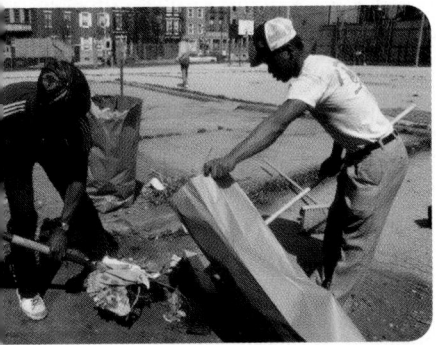

These workers are cleaning up in the South Shore neighborhood of Chicago, where many residents are officially listed as earning below the poverty line. Yet during the 1990s, consumer spending increased more in South Shore than in any other part of Chicago. Can you explain this anomaly?

A few years ago, a Chicago group called Social Compact sought to evaluate the opportunities for regenerating neighborhoods on the south side of the city. It focused on a largely African-American neighborhood called South Shore, where U.S. government data indicated that 27 percent of residents were mired in poverty. To the group's surprise, it found that spending in parts of the South Shore economy was actually booming. Over the previous 10-year period, South Shore residents had increased their use of electricity by double the average rate of growth of the rest of Chicago. Supermarket sales in the area placed the stores among the top Chicago outlets. Insurers reported that sales of homeowners' insurance policies were increasing twice as fast as elsewhere in the city. What is the right way to measure "poverty"? This is one of the questions you will contemplate as you read this chapter.

LEARNING OBJECTIVES

After reading this chapter, you should be able to:

1. **Describe how to use a Lorenz curve to represent a nation's income distribution**
2. **Identify the key determinants of income differences across individuals**
3. **Discuss theories of desired income distribution**
4. **Distinguish among alternative approaches to measuring and addressing poverty**
5. **Recognize the major reasons for rising health care costs**
6. **Describe alternative approaches to paying for health care**

Chapter Outline

- Income
- Determinants of Income Differences
- Theories of Desired Income Distribution
- Poverty and Attempts to Eliminate It
- Health Care

Did You Know That... 20 percent of the world's people consume 86 percent of its goods and services? This highest-income portion of the population also uses more than half the world's annual energy output and devours close to half its meat and fish. Even as a billion of the world's poorest individuals struggle to meet their basic dietary requirements, Americans spend $8 billion a year on cosmetics, and Europeans spend $50 billion a year on cigarettes. Why is it that some people can earn more income and spend more than others? Why is the **distribution of income** the way it is? Economists have devised various theories to explain income distribution. We will present some of these theories in this chapter. We will also present some of the more obvious institutional reasons why income is not distributed equally in the United States and examine what might be done about health care problems.

INCOME

Distribution of income 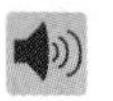
The way income is allocated among the population.

Income provides each of us with the means of consuming and saving. Income can be derived from a payment for labor services or a payment for ownership of one of the other factors of production besides labor—land, physical capital, and entrepreneurship. In addition, individuals obtain spendable income from gifts and government transfers. (Some individuals also obtain income by stealing, but we will not treat this matter here.) Right now, let us examine how money income is distributed across classes of income earners within the United States.

Lorenz curve 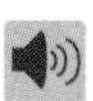
A geometric representation of the distribution of income. A Lorenz curve that is perfectly straight represents complete income equality. The more bowed a Lorenz curve, the more unequally income is distributed.

Measuring Income Distribution: The Lorenz Curve

We can represent the distribution of money income graphically with what is known as the **Lorenz curve,** named after a U.S.-born statistician, Max Otto Lorenz, who proposed it in 1905. The Lorenz curve shows what portion of total money income is accounted for by different proportions of the nation's households. Look at Figure 30-1. On the horizontal axis, we measure the *cumulative* percentage of households, lowest-income households first. Starting at the left corner, there are zero households; at the right corner, we have 100 percent

FIGURE 30-1 
The Lorenz Curve
The horizontal axis measures the cumulative percentage of households, with lowest-income households first, from 0 to 100 percent. The vertical axis measures the cumulative percentage of money income from 0 to 100. A straight line at a 45-degree angle cuts the box in half and represents a line of complete income equality, along which 25 percent of the families get 25 percent of the money income, 50 percent get 50 percent, and so on. The Lorenz curve, showing actual money income distribution, is not a straight line but rather a curved line as shown. The difference between complete money income equality and the Lorenz curve is the inequality gap.

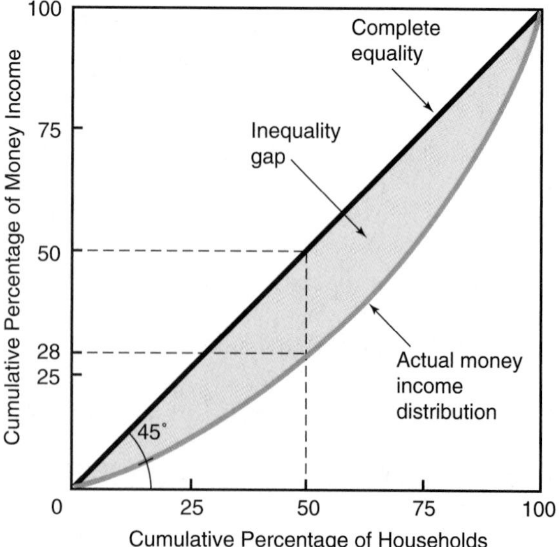

of households; and in the middle, we have 50 percent of households. The vertical axis represents the cumulative percentage of money income. The 45-degree line represents complete equality: 50 percent of the households obtain 50 percent of total income, 60 percent of the households obtain 60 percent of total income, and so on. Of course, in no real-world situation is there such complete equality of income; no actual Lorenz curve would be a straight line. Rather, it would be some curved line, like the one labeled "Actual money income distribution" in Figure 30-1. For example, the bottom 50 percent of households in the United States receive about 28 percent of total money income.

In Figure 30-2, we again show the actual money income distribution Lorenz curve, and we also compare it to the distribution of money income in 1929. Since that year, the Lorenz curve has become less bowed; that is, it has moved closer to the line of complete equality.

Criticisms of the Lorenz Curve. In recent years, economists have placed less and less emphasis on the shape of the Lorenz curve as an indication of the degree of income inequality in a country. There are five basic reasons why the Lorenz curve has been criticized:

1. The Lorenz curve is typically presented in terms of the distribution of *money* income only. It does not include **income in kind,** such as government-provided food stamps, education, or housing aid, and goods or services produced and consumed in the home or on the farm.
2. The Lorenz curve does not account for differences in the size of households or the number of wage earners they contain.
3. It does not account for age differences. Even if all families in the United States had exactly the same *lifetime* incomes, chances are that young families would have lower incomes, middle-aged families would have relatively high incomes, and retired families would have low incomes. Because the Lorenz curve is drawn at a moment in time, it could never tell us anything about the inequality of *lifetime* income.
4. The Lorenz curve ordinarily reflects money income *before* taxes.
5. It does not measure unreported income from the underground economy, a substantial source of income for some individuals.

Income in kind 

Income received in the form of goods and services, such as housing or medical care; to be contrasted with money income, which is simply income in dollars, or general purchasing power, that can be used to buy *any* goods and services.

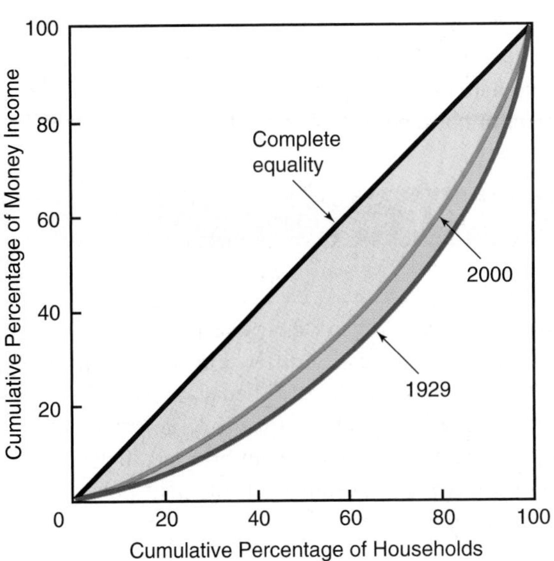

FIGURE 30-2

Lorenz Curves of Income Distribution, 1929 and 2000

Since 1929, the Lorenz curve has moved slightly inward toward the straight line of perfect income equality.

Source: U.S. Department of Commerce.

TABLE 30-1
Percentage Share of Money Income for Households Before Direct Taxes

Income Group	1998	1975	1960	1947
Lowest fifth	3.6	4.4	4.8	5.1
Second fifth	9.0	10.5	12.2	11.8
Third fifth	15.0	17.1	17.8	16.7
Fourth fifth	23.2	24.8	24.0	23.2
Highest fifth	49.2	43.2	41.3	43.3

Source: U.S. Bureau of the Census.
Note: Figures may not sum to 100 percent due to rounding.

Income Distribution in the United States

Click here to view the most recent data on U.S. income distribution. Click on the most recent year next to "Money Income in the United States."

We could talk about the percentage of income earners within specific income classes—those earning between $20,001 and $30,000 per year, those earning between $30,001 and $40,000 per year, and so on. The problem with this type of analysis is that we live in a growing economy. Income, with some exceptions, is going up all the time. If we wish to make comparisons of the relative share of total income going to different income classes, we cannot look at specific amounts of money income. Instead, we talk about a distribution of income over five groups. Then we can talk about how much the bottom fifth (or quintile) makes compared with the top fifth, and so on. In Table 30-1, we see the percentage share of income for households before direct taxes. The table groups households according to whether they are in the lowest 20 percent of the income distribution, the second lowest 20 percent, and so on. We see that in 1998, the lowest 20 percent had a combined money income of 3.6 percent of the total money income of the entire population. This is a little less than the lowest 20 percent had at the end of World War II. Accordingly, the conclusion has been drawn that there have been only slight changes in the distribution of money income. Indeed, considering that the definition of money income used by the U.S. Bureau of the Census includes only wage and salary income, income from self-employment, interest and dividends, and such government transfer payments as Social Security and unemployment compensation, we have to agree that the distribution of money income has not changed. *Money* income, however, understates *total* income for individuals who receive in-kind transfers from the government in the form of food stamps, public housing, education, and so on. In particular, since World War II, the share of total income—money income plus in-kind benefits—going to the bottom 20 percent of households has probably more than doubled.

INTERNATIONAL EXAMPLE

Relative Income Inequality Throughout the Richest Countries

The United States wins again—it has, according to the World Bank, the greatest amount of income inequality of any of the major industrialized countries. Look at Figure 30-3. There you see the ratio of income of the richest 20 percent of households to the poorest 20 percent of households. Should something be done about such income inequality?

Public attitudes toward the government's role in reducing income inequality differ dramatically in the United States and elsewhere. Whereas fewer than 30 percent of Americans believe that government should reduce income differentials, between 60 and 80 percent of Britons, Germans, Italians, and Austrians believe it is the government's job.

FIGURE 30-3
Relative Income Inequality in the World
The United States has greater income inequality than other developed countries.
Source: World Bank.

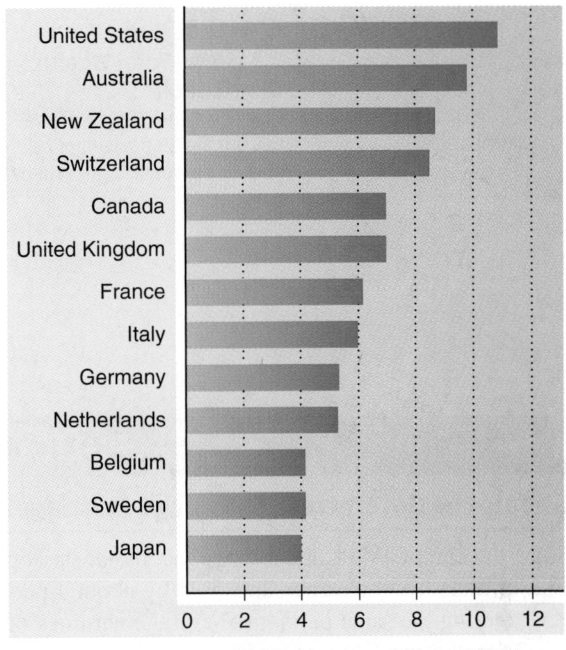

For Critical Analysis

Does it matter whether the same families stay in the lowest fifth of income earners over time? Otherwise stated, do we need to know anything about mobility across income groups?

The Distribution of Wealth

We have been referring to the distribution of income in the United States. We must realize that income—a flow—can be viewed as a return on wealth (both human and nonhuman)—a stock. A discussion of the distribution of income in the United States is not the same thing as a discussion of the distribution of wealth. A complete concept of wealth would include tangible objects, such as buildings, machinery, land, cars, and houses—nonhuman wealth—as well as people who have skills, knowledge, initiative, talents, and so on—human wealth. The total of human and nonhuman wealth in the United States makes up our nation's capital stock. (Note that the terms *wealth* and *capital* are often used only with reference to nonhuman wealth.) The capital stock consists of anything that can generate utility to individuals in the future. A fresh ripe tomato is not part of our capital stock. It has to be eaten before it turns rotten, and once it has been eaten, it can no longer generate satisfaction.

Figure 30-4 (p. 736) shows that the richest 10 percent of U.S. households hold about two-thirds of all wealth. The problem with those data, gathered by the Federal Reserve System, is that they do not include many important assets. The first of these is workers' claims on private pension plans, which equal at least $4 trillion according to economist Lawrence B. Lindsey. If you add the value of these pensions, household wealth increases by almost a quarter, meaning that the majority of U.S. households belong to middle-income households (popularly known as the *middle class*). Also omitted is future Social Security liabilities, estimated at about $13 trillion. Again, most of this is "owned" by the middle class.

FIGURE 30-4
Measured Total Wealth Distribution
The top 10 percent of households have 69 percent of all *measured* wealth.
Source: Board of Governors of the Federal Reserve.

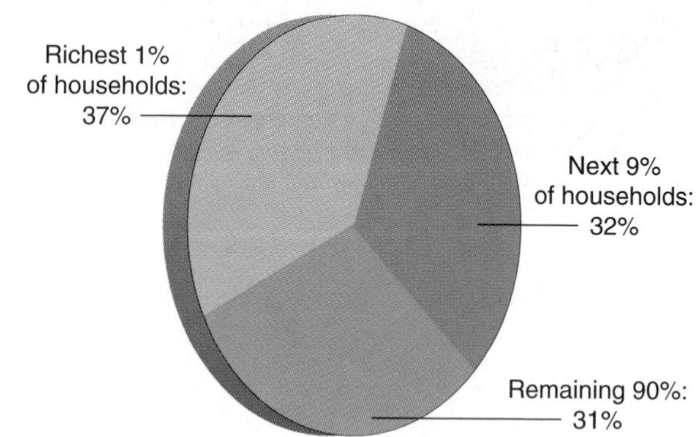

POLICY EXAMPLE

Should the Government Encourage Marriage?

Since the end of 1970s, the average income of the top fifth of male income earners has risen by about 4 percent. During the same period, the average earnings of men in the bottom fifth fell by 44 percent. A key reason for this disparity is that poor men today are less likely to be married. In 1979, almost three out of every five of the men among the poorest 20 percent of income earners were married. Today, however, only about two out of five are married.

The reason this drop in marriage rates among lowest-income men makes such a big difference is that the incomes of women have risen. Today, about 65 percent of women with poor husbands work, up only slightly from 61 percent in 1979. The wages of these women have increased by about two-thirds, however. If the poorest males were marrying at the same rate as before, fewer lower-income households would have suffered big drops in their average earnings. Marriage has only added to the gains experienced by the households of the highest-income men. In 1979, just over half of the women with the highest-income husbands worked. Today, three-fourths of these women work, and their average wages have risen by more than 70 percent. This has further enriched the households of the highest-income males.

Based on these data, some economists argue that the government should develop policies that encourage higher marriage rates among the poorest individuals. At a minimum, they recommend eliminating policies that discourage marriage, such as taxing married couples at higher rates than single individuals at the same income levels.

For Critical Analysis

Some poor men are probably less likely to be married because their sharp income drop has hurt their marriage prospects. What, if anything, can or should the government do about this?

CONCEPTS IN BRIEF

- The Lorenz curve graphically represents the distribution of income. If it is a straight line, there is complete equality of income. The more it is bowed, the more inequality of income exists.
- The distribution of wealth is not the same as the distribution of income. Wealth includes assets such as houses, stocks, and bonds. Although the apparent distribution of wealth seems to be more concentrated at the top, the data used are not very accurate, and most summary statistics fail to take account of workers' claims on private and public pensions, which are substantial.

DETERMINANTS OF INCOME DIFFERENCES 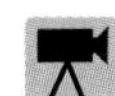

We know that there are income differences—that is not in dispute. A more important question is why these differences in income occur, for if we know why income differences occur, perhaps we can change public policy, particularly with respect to helping people in the lowest income classes climb the income ladder. What is more, if we know the reasons for income differences, we can ascertain whether any of these determinants have changed over time. We will look at four income difference determinants: age, marginal productivity, inheritance, and discrimination.

Age

Age turns out to be a determinant of income because with age comes, usually, more education, more training, and more experience. It is not surprising that within every class of income earners, there seem to be regular cycles of earning behavior. Most individuals earn more when they are middle-aged than when they are younger or older. We call this the **age-earnings cycle.**

Age-earnings cycle 
The regular earnings profile of an individual throughout his or her lifetime. The age-earnings cycle usually starts with a low income, builds gradually to a peak at around age 50, and then gradually curves down until it approaches zero at retirement.

The Age-Earnings Cycle. Every occupation has its own age-earnings cycle, and every individual will probably experience some variation from the average. Nonetheless, we can characterize the typical age-earnings cycle graphically in Figure 30-5. Here we see that at age 18, earnings from wages are relatively low. Earnings gradually rises until they peak at about age 50. Then they fall until retirement, when they become zero (that is, currently earned wages become zero, although retirement payments may then commence). The reason for such a regular cycle in earnings is fairly straightforward.

When individuals start working at a young age, they typically have no work-related experience. Their ability to produce is less than that of more seasoned workers—that is, their productivity is lower. As they become older, they obtain more training and accumulate more experience. Their productivity rises, and they are therefore paid more. They also generally start to work longer hours. As the age of 50 approaches, the productivity of individual workers usually peaks. So, too, do the number of hours per week that are worked. After this peak in the age-earnings cycle, the detrimental effects of aging—decreases in stamina, strength, reaction time, and the like—usually outweigh any increases in training

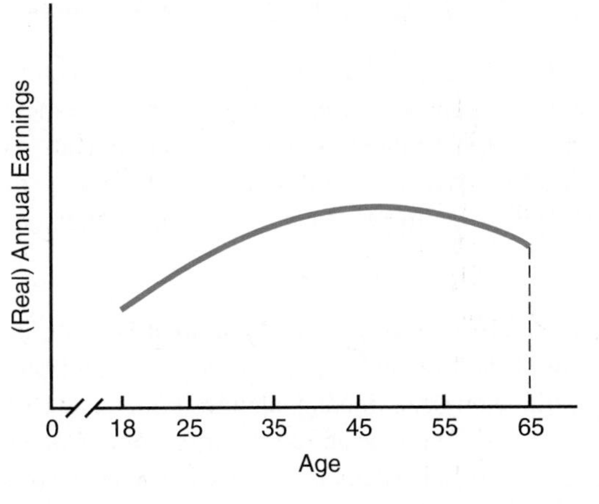

FIGURE 30-5 

Typical Age-Earnings Profile

Within every class of income earners there is usually a typical age-earnings profile. Earnings from wages are lowest when starting work at age 18, reach their peak at around age 50, and then taper off until retirement around age 65, when they become zero for most people. The rise in earnings up to age 50 is usually due to increased experience, longer working hours, and better training and schooling. (We abstract from economywide productivity changes that would shift the entire curve upward.)

or experience. Also, hours worked usually start to fall for older people. Finally, as a person reaches retirement, both productivity and hours worked diminish rather drastically.

Note that general increases in overall productivity for the entire workforce will result in an upward shift in the typical age-earnings profile given in Figure 30-5. Thus even at the end of the age-earnings cycle, when just about to retire, the worker would not receive a really low wage compared with the starting wage 45 years earlier. The wage would be higher due to factors that contribute to rising real wages for everyone, regardless of the stage in the age-earnings cycle.

Now we have some idea why specific individuals earn different incomes at different times in their lives, but we have yet to explain why different people are paid different amounts of money for their labor. One way to explain this is to recall the marginal productivity theory developed in Chapter 27.

Marginal Productivity

When trying to determine how many workers a firm would hire, we had to construct a marginal revenue product curve. We found that as more workers were hired, the marginal revenue product fell due to diminishing marginal returns. If the forces of demand and supply established a certain wage rate, workers would be hired until their marginal physical product times marginal revenue (which equals the marketing price under perfect competition) was equal to the going wage rate. Then the hiring would stop. This analysis suggests what workers can expect to be paid in the labor market: They can each expect to be paid their marginal revenue product (assuming that there are low-cost information flows and that the labor and product markets are competitive).

In a competitive situation, with mobility of labor resources (at least on the margin), workers who are being paid less than their marginal revenue product will be bid away to better employment opportunities. Either they will seek better employment themselves, or other employers will offer them a higher wage rate. This process will continue until each worker is being paid his or her marginal revenue product.

You may balk at the suggestion that people are paid their marginal revenue product because you may personally know individuals whose MRP is more or less than what they are being paid. Such a situation may, in fact, exist because we do not live in a world of perfect information or in a world with perfectly competitive input and output markets. Employers cannot always find the most productive employees available. It takes resources to research the past records of potential employees, their training, their education, and their abilities. Nonetheless, competition creates a tendency toward equality of wages and MRP.

Determinants of Marginal Productivity. If we accept marginal revenue product theory, we have a way to find out how people can earn higher incomes. If they can increase their marginal physical product, they can expect to be paid more. Some of the determinants of marginal physical product are talent, education, experience, and training. Most of these are means by which marginal physical product can be increased. Let's examine them in greater detail.

Talent This factor is the easiest to explain but difficult to acquire if you don't have it. Innate abilities and attributes can be very strong, if not overwhelming, determinants of a person's potential productivity. Strength, coordination, and mental alertness are facets of nonacquired human capital and thus have some bearing on the ability to earn income. Someone who is extremely tall has a better chance of being a basketball player than someone who is short. A person born with a superior talent for abstract thinking has a better chance of earning a relatively high income as a mathematician or a physicist than someone who is not born with that knack.

Experience Additional experience at particular tasks is another way to increase productivity. Experience can be linked to the well-known *learning curve* that applies when the same task is done over and over. The worker repeating a task becomes more efficient: The worker can do the same task in less time or in the same amount of time but better. Take an example of a person going to work on an automobile assembly line. At first she is able to fasten only three bolts every two minutes. Then the worker becomes more adept and can fasten four bolts in the same time plus insert a rubber guard on the bumper. After a few more weeks, another task can be added. Experience allows this individual to improve her productivity. The more effectively people learn to do something, the quicker they can do it and the more efficient they are. Hence we would expect experience to lead to higher productivity. And we would expect people with more experience to be paid more than those with less experience. More experience, however, does not guarantee a higher wage rate. The *demand* for a person's services must also exist. Spending a long time to become a first-rate archer in modern society would probably add very little to a person's income. Experience has value only if the output is demanded by society.

Training Training is similar to experience but is more formal. Much of a person's increased productivity is due to on-the-job training. Many companies have training programs for new workers. On-the-job training is perhaps responsible for as much of an increase in productivity as is formal education beyond grade school.

EXAMPLE

Economists, Aging, and Productivity

Do the actions of professional economists fit the model that predicts a decrease in productivity after some peak at around age 50? Yes, according to University of Texas economist Daniel Hamermesh. One measure of productivity of economics professors is the number of articles they publish in professional journals. Whereas the over-50 economists constitute 30 percent of the profession, they contribute a mere 6 percent of the articles published in leading economics journals. Whereas 56 percent of economists between ages 36 and 50 submit articles on a regular basis, only 14 percent of economists over 50 do so.

For Critical Analysis

Why should we predict that an economist closer to retirement will submit fewer professional journal articles for publication than a younger economist?

Investment in Human Capital. Investment in human capital is just like investment in any other thing. If you invest in yourself by going to college, rather than going to work after high school and earning more current income, you will presumably be rewarded in the future with a higher income or a more interesting job (or both). This is exactly the motivation that underlies the decision of many college-bound students to obtain a formal higher education. Undoubtedly there would be students going to school even if the rate of return on formal education were zero or negative. But we do expect that the higher the rate of return on investing in ourselves, the more such investment there will be. U.S. Labor Department data demonstrate conclusively that, on average, high school graduates make more than grade school graduates and that college graduates make more than high school graduates. The estimated annual income of a full-time worker with four years of college in the early 2000s was about $65,000. That person's high school counterpart was estimated to earn only $32,000, which gives a "college premium" of about 57 percent. Generally, the rate of return on investment in human capital is on a par with the rate of return on investment in other areas.

To figure out the rate of return on an investment in a college education, we first have to figure out the marginal costs of going to school. The main cost is not what you have to pay for books, fees, and tuition but rather the income you forgo. *The main cost of education is the income forgone—the opportunity cost of not working.* In addition, the direct expenses of college must be paid for. Not all students forgo all income during their college years. Many work part time. Taking account of those who work part time and those who are supported by state tuition grants and other scholarships, the average rate of return on going to college ranges between 12 and 18 percent. This is not a bad rate. Of course, this type of computation does leave out all the consumption benefits you get from attending college. Also omitted from the calculations is the change in personality after going to college. You undoubtedly come out a different person. Most people who go through college feel that they have improved themselves both culturally and intellectually in addition to having increased their potential marginal revenue product so that they can make more income. How do we measure the benefit from expanding our horizons and our desire to experience different things in life? This is not easy to measure, and such nonmoney benefits from investing in human capital are not included in normal calculations.

Inheritance

It is not unusual to inherit cash, jewelry, stocks, bonds, homes, or other real estate. Yet only about 10 percent of income inequality in the United States can be traced to differences in wealth that was inherited. If for some reason the government confiscated all property that had been inherited, there would be only a modest change in the distribution of income in the United States. In any event, at both federal and state levels of taxation, substantial inheritance taxes are levied on the estates of relatively wealthy deceased Americans (although there are some legally valid ways to avoid certain estate taxes).

Discrimination

Economic discrimination occurs whenever workers with the same marginal revenue product receive unequal pay due to some noneconomic factor such as their race, sex, or age. Alternatively, it occurs when there is unequal access to labor markets. It is possible—and indeed quite obvious—that discrimination affects the distribution of income. Certain groups in our society are not paid wages at rates comparable to those received by other groups, even when we correct for productivity. Differences in income remain between whites and nonwhites and between men and women. For example, the median income of black families is about 60 percent that of white families. The median wage rate of women is about 70 percent that of men. Some people argue that all of these differences are due to discrimination against nonwhites and against women. We cannot simply accept *any* differences in income as due to discrimination, though. What we need to do is discover why differences in income between groups exist and then determine if factors other than discrimination in the labor market can explain them. The unexplained part of income differences can rightfully be considered the result of discrimination.

Access to Education. African Americans and other minorities have faced discrimination in the acquisition of human capital. The amount and quality of schooling offered black Americans has generally been inferior to that offered whites. Even if minorities attend school as long as whites, their scholastic achievement can be lower because they are typically allotted fewer school resources than their white counterparts. Nonwhite urban individuals are more likely to live in lower-income areas, which have fewer resources to allocate to education due to the lower tax base. One study showed that nonwhite urban males receive between 23 and 27 percent less income than white urban males because of lower-quality education. This would mean that even if employment discrimination were substantially reduced, we would still expect to see a difference between white and nonwhite income because of the low quality of schooling received by the nonwhites and the resulting lower level of productivity. We say, therefore, that among other things, African Americans and certain other minority groups, such as Hispanics, suffer from too small an investment in human capital. Even when this difference in human capital is taken into account, however, there still appears to be an income differential that cannot be explained. The unexplained income differential between whites and blacks is often attributed to discrimination in the labor market. Because no better explanation is offered, we will stick with the notion that discrimination in the labor market does indeed exist.

EXAMPLE

Removing Racial Barriers: The Colorful but Color-Blind Internet

When a white customer asks an African-American salesman if a different salesperson can assist her, the salesman may suspect that his race may have cost him a sale. Likewise, when a white banker turns down an African-American loan applicant, there is always the chance that race made a difference. To explain why race or other factors might affect people's economic choices, economists have developed the *cultural affinity hypothesis.* It indicates that lenders find it less costly to evaluate applicants who share their own backgrounds. This hypothesis could also help explain why applicants for loans might prefer to apply at banks that are owned and managed by people who share their characteristics or why customers might prefer to do business with certain salespersons rather than others.

Documenting or explaining differential interactions on the basis of different characteristics does nothing for people who feel that their racial, ethnic, or gender status causes them to lose out on earnings. For many African-American entrepreneurs, the Internet is increasingly providing a means to avoid such lost opportunities. For instance, Autonetwork.com is a booming Web site that offers auto broker services and leasing information, but there is no reason for anyone looking for a good deal on an auto lease to know—or care—that the site is owned by an African-American man who earns more than $200,000 per year in advertising revenue alone from operating the site. Likewise, all a college student who wants to do better in biology class cares about is whether Cyberstudy101.com can help him, without regard to the fact that this successful on-line business was the brainchild of an African-American woman.

For Critical Analysis

Some on-line businesses advertise that they are owned by people of a particular race, ethnicity, or gender and offer products aimed at people who share that characteristic. Could the cultural affinity hypothesis help explain this phenomenon?

The Doctrine of Comparable Worth. Discrimination against women can occur because of barriers to entry in higher-paying occupations and because of discrimination in the acquisition of human capital, just as has occurred for African Americans. Consider the distribution of highest-paying and lowest-paying occupations. The lowest-paying jobs are

Comparable-worth doctrine 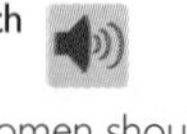
The belief that women should receive the same wages as men if the levels of skill and responsibility in their jobs are equivalent.

dominated by females, both white and nonwhite. For example, the proportion of women in secretarial, clerical, janitorial, and food service jobs ranges from 70 percent (food service) to 97 percent (secretarial). Proponents of the **comparable-worth doctrine** feel that female secretaries, janitors, and food service workers should be making salaries comparable to those of male truck drivers or construction workers, assuming that the levels of skill and responsibility in these jobs are comparable. These advocates also believe that a comparable-worth policy would benefit the economy overall. They contend that adjusting the wages of workers in female-dominated jobs upward would create a move toward more efficient and less discriminatory labor markets.

THEORIES OF DESIRED INCOME DISTRIBUTION

We have talked about the factors affecting the distribution of income, but we have not yet mentioned the normative issue of how income *ought* to be distributed. This, of course, requires a value judgment. We are talking about the problem of economic justice. We can never completely resolve this problem because there are always going to be conflicting values. It is impossible to give all people what each thinks is just. Nonetheless, two particular normative standards for the distribution of income have been popular with economists. These are income distribution based on productivity and income distribution based on equality.

Productivity

The *productivity standard* for the distribution of income can be stated simply as "To each according to what he or she produces." This is also called the *contributive standard* because it is based on the principle of rewarding according to the contribution to society's total output. It is also sometimes referred to as the *merit standard* and is one of the oldest concepts of justice. People are rewarded according to merit, and merit is judged by one's ability to produce what is considered useful by society.

However, just as any standard is a value judgment, so is the productivity standard. It is rooted in the capitalist ethic and has been attacked vigorously by some economists and philosophers, including Karl Marx, who felt that people should be rewarded according to need and not according to productivity.

We measure a person's productive contribution in a capitalist system by the market value of that person's output. We have already referred to this as the marginal revenue product theory of wage determination.

Do not immediately jump to the conclusion that in a world of income distribution determined by productivity, society will necessarily allow the aged, the infirm, and the disabled to die of starvation because they are unproductive. In the United States today, the productivity standard is mixed with a standard based on people's "needs" so that the aged, the disabled, the involuntarily unemployed, the very young, and other unproductive (in the market sense of the word) members of the economy are provided for through private and public transfers.

Equality

The *egalitarian principle* of income distribution is simply "To each exactly the same." Everyone would have exactly the same amount of income. This criterion of income distribution has been debated as far back as biblical times. This system of income distribution has been considered equitable, meaning that presumably everybody is dealt with fairly and equally. There are problems, however, with an income distribution that is completely equal.

Some jobs are more unpleasant or more dangerous than others. Should the people undertaking these jobs be paid exactly the same as everyone else? Indeed, under an equal distribution of income, what incentive would there be for individuals to take risky, hazardous, or unpleasant jobs at all? What about overtime? Who would be willing to work overtime without additional pay? There is another problem: If everyone earned the same income, what incentive would there be for individuals to invest in their own human capital—a costly and time-consuming process?

Just consider the incentive structure within a corporation. Recall from Chapter 27 that much of the pay differential between, say, the CEO and all of the vice-presidents is meant to create competition among the vice-presidents for the CEO's job. The result is higher productivity. If all incomes were the same, much of this competition would disappear, and productivity would fall.

There is some evidence that differences in income lead to higher rates of economic growth. Future generations are therefore made better off. Elimination of income differences may reduce the rate of economic growth and cause future generations to be poorer than they otherwise might have been.

CONCEPTS IN BRIEF

- Most people follow an age-earnings cycle in which they earn relatively small incomes when they first start working, increase their incomes until about age 50, and then slowly experience a decrease in their real incomes as they approach retirement.
- If we accept the marginal revenue product theory of wages, workers can expect to be paid their marginal revenue product. However, full adjustment is never obtained, so some workers may be paid more or less than their MRP.
- Marginal physical productivity depends on talent, education, experience, and training.
- Going to school and receiving on-the-job training can be considered an investment in human capital. The main cost of education is the opportunity cost of not working.
- Discrimination is most easily observed in various groups' access to high-paying jobs and to quality education. Minorities and women are disproportionately underrepresented in high-paying jobs. Also, minorities sometimes do not receive access to higher education of the same quality offered to majority-group members.
- Proponents of the comparable-worth doctrine contend that disparate jobs can be compared by examining efforts, skill, and educational training and that wages should therefore be paid on the basis of this comparable worth.
- Two normative standards for income distribution are income distribution based on productivity and income distribution based on equality.

POVERTY AND ATTEMPTS TO ELIMINATE IT

Throughout the history of the world, mass poverty has been accepted as inevitable. However, this nation and others, particularly in the Western world, have sustained enough economic growth in the past several hundred years so that *mass* poverty can no longer be said to be a problem for these fortunate countries. As a matter of fact, the residual of poverty in the United States strikes us as bizarre, an anomaly. How can there still be so much poverty in a nation of such abundance? Having talked about the determinants of the distribution of income, we now have at least some ideas of why some people are destined to remain low-income earners throughout their lives.

FIGURE 30-6

Official Number of Poor in the United States

The number of individuals classified as poor fell steadily from 1959 through 1969. From 1970 to 1981, the number stayed about the same. It then increased during the 1981–1982 recession, dropped off for a while, rose in the early 1990s, and then fell.

Source: U.S. Department of Labor.

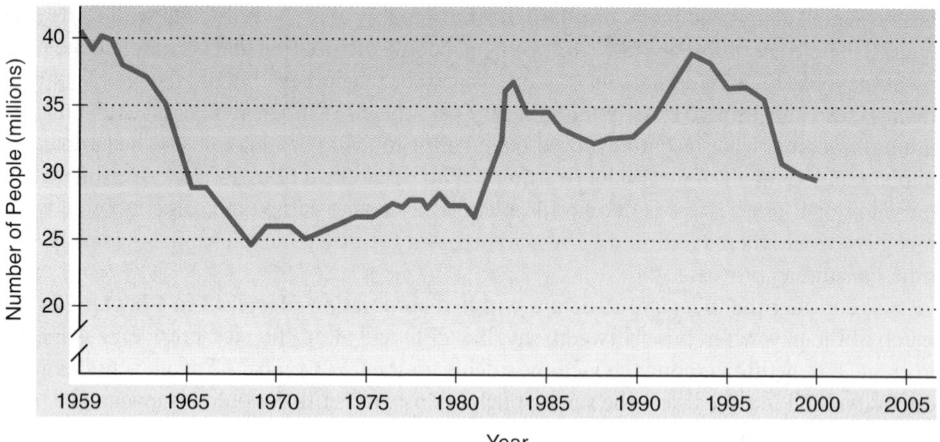

There are methods of transferring income from the relatively well-to-do to the relatively poor, and as a nation we have been using them for a long time. Today, we have a vast array of welfare programs set up for the purpose of redistributing income. However, we know that these programs have not been entirely successful. Are there alternatives to our current welfare system? Is there a better method of helping the poor? Before we answer these questions, let's look at the concept of poverty in more detail and at the characteristics of the poor. Figure 30-6 shows that those classified as poor fell steadily from 1959 to 1969, then leveled off until the recession of 1981–1982. The number started to rise dramatically, fell back during the late 1980s, rose again after the recession in the early 1990s, and has been falling slowly since then.

INTERNATIONAL EXAMPLE

Poverty Rates in the European Union

For years, politicians throughout much of the European Union have proclaimed their unwillingness to adopt the more laissez-faire, "let the chips fall where they may" economic model that prevails in the United States. They are convinced that the result is too much poverty. But they were shocked to discover in an article published in the newspaper *Le Monde* in 1997 that the poverty rate for the European Union was more than 17 percent—fully 57 million people out of a population of 330 million. Whereas the poverty rate in the United States has hovered between 13 and 15 percent of the population since the 1970s, the rate in Europe has increased over the same period from 10 percent to the current 17 percent. One-third of the officially poor in the European Union work, one-third are retired, and one-third are unemployed.

For Critical Analysis

What problems might there be in comparing poverty rates across nations?

Defining Poverty 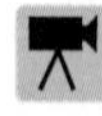

The threshold income level, which is used to determine who falls into the poverty category, was originally based on the cost of a nutritionally adequate food plan designed by the U.S. Department of Agriculture for emergency or temporary use. The threshold was determined by multiplying the food plan cost by 3 on the assumption that food expenses comprise approximately one-third of a poor family's income. Annual revisions of the threshold level were based only on price changes in the food budget. In 1969, a federal interagency committee looked at the calculations of the threshold and decided to set new standards, with adjustments made on the basis of changes in the Consumer Price Index. For example, in 2000, the official poverty level for an urban family of four was around $17,000. It goes up each year to reflect whatever inflation has occurred.

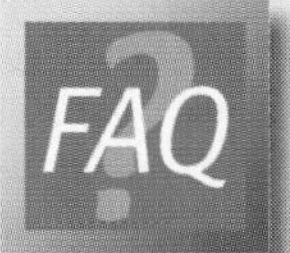

Don't nations with higher average incomes also have higher average life expectancies?

On net, the answer is yes. In Africa, one of the lowest-income regions of the world, more than three-fourths of deaths were of people under the age of 50. In Europe, by contrast, only 15 percent of people die before reaching 50. Nevertheless, higher-income nations also experience a greater incidence of so-called "diseases of affluence"—heart disease, strokes, and cancer—that are associated with high-fat, low-exercise lifestyles. Deaths from circulatory diseases and cancer have increased steadily as the world's population has become relatively more affluent, even as deaths from infectious and parasitic diseases have fallen off. As a result, worldwide deaths from diseases of affluence now exceed deaths from infectious and parasitic diseases by several million per year.

Absolute Poverty

Because the low-income threshold is an absolute measure, we know that if it never changes in real terms, we will reduce poverty even if we do nothing. How can that be? The reasoning is straightforward. Real incomes in the United States have been growing at a compounded annual rate of almost 2 percent per capita for at least the past century and at about 2.5 percent since World War II. If we define the poverty line at a specific real level, more and more individuals will make incomes that exceed that poverty line. Thus in absolute terms, we will eliminate poverty (assuming continued per capita growth and no change in income distribution).

Click here to learn about the World Bank's programs intended to combat global poverty.

Relative Poverty

Be careful with this analysis, however. Poverty can also be defined in relative terms; that is, it is defined in terms of the income levels of individuals or families relative to the rest of the population. As long as the distribution of income is not perfectly equal, there will always be some people who make less income than others, even if their relatively low income is high by historical standards. Thus in a relative sense, the problem of poverty will always exist, although it can be reduced. In any given year, for example, the absolute poverty level *officially* decided on by the U.S. government is far above the average income in many countries in the world.

Transfer Payments as Income

The official poverty level is based on pretax income, including cash but not in-kind subsidies—food stamps, housing vouchers, and the like. If we correct poverty levels for such benefits, the percentage of the population that is below the poverty line drops dramatically. Some economists argue that the way the official poverty level is calculated makes no sense in a nation that redistributed over $850 billion in cash and noncash transfers in 2000.

Furthermore, some of the nation's official poor partake in the informal, or underground, sectors of the economy without reporting their income from these sources. And some of the officially defined poor obtain benefits from owning their own home (40 percent of all poor households do own their own homes). Look at Figure 30-7 (p. 746) for two different views of what has happened to the relative position of this nation's poor. The graph shows the ratio of the top fifth of the nation's households to the bottom fifth of the nation's households. If

FIGURE 30-7

Relative Poverty: Comparing Household Incomes and Household Spending

This graph shows, on the vertical axis, the ratio of the top 20 percent of income-earning households to the bottom 20 percent. If measured household income is used, there appears to be increasing income inequality, particularly during the early to mid-1980s. If we look at household *spending*, though, inequality appears to remain constant.

Sources: U.S. Bureau of Labor Statistics; U.S. Bureau of the Census.

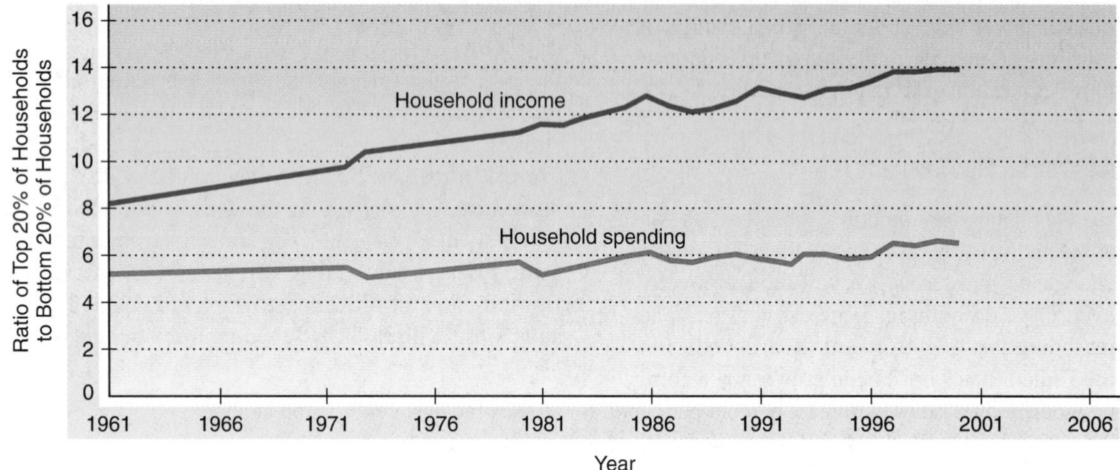

we look only at measured income, it appears that the poor are getting relatively poorer compared to the rich (the top line). If we compare household spending (consumption), a different picture emerges. The nation's poorest households are in fact holding their own.

Attacks on Poverty: Major Income Maintenance Programs

There are a variety of income maintenance programs designed to help the poor. We examine a few of them here.

Social Security. For the retired, the unemployed, and the disabled, social insurance programs provide income payments in prescribed situations. The best known is Social Security, which includes what has been called old-age, survivors', and disability insurance (OASDI). As discussed in Chapter 6, this is essentially a program of compulsory saving financed from compulsory payroll taxes levied on both employers and employees. Workers pay for Social Security while working and receive the benefits after retirement. The benefit payments are usually made to people who have reached retirement age. When the insured worker dies, benefits accrue to the survivors, including widows and children. Special benefits provide for disabled workers. Over 90 percent of all employed persons in the United States are covered by OASDI. Social Security was originally proposed as a social insurance program that workers paid for themselves and under which they received benefits that varied with the size of past contributions. Today, it is simply an intergenerational income transfer that is only vaguely related to past earnings. It transfers income from Americans who work—the young through the middle-aged—to those who do not work—older retired persons.

In 2000, more than 52 million people were receiving OASDI checks averaging about $742 a month. Benefit payments from OASDI redistribute income to some degree. However, benefit payments are not based on recipient need. Participants' contributions give them the right to benefits even if they would be financially secure without them. Social Security is not really an insurance program because people are not guaranteed that the benefits they receive will be in line with the contributions they have made. It is not a personal savings account. The benefits are legislated by Congress. In the future, Congress may not be as sympathetic toward older people as it is today. It could (and probably will have to) legislate for lower real levels of benefits instead of higher ones.

Supplemental Security Income (SSI) and Temporary Assistance to Needy Families (TANF). Many people who are poor but do not qualify for Social Security benefits are assisted through other programs. The federally financed and administered Supplemental Security Income (SSI) program was instituted in 1974. The purpose of SSI is to establish a nationwide minimum income for the aged, the blind, and the disabled. SSI has become one of the fastest-growing transfer programs in America. Whereas in 1974 less than $8 billion was spent, the prediction for 2001 is $35.4 billion. Americans currently eligible for SSI include children and individuals claiming mental disabilities, including drug addicts and alcoholics.

Temporary Assistance to Needy Families (TANF) is a state-administered program, financed in part by federal grants. The program provides aid to families in need. TANF replaced Aid to Families with Dependant Children (AFDC). TANF is intended to be temporary. Projected expenditures for TANF are $21.4 billion in 2001.

Food Stamps. Food stamps are government-issued coupons that can be used to purchase food. The food stamp program was started in 1964, seemingly, in retrospect, mainly to shore up the nation's agricultural sector by increasing demand for food through retail channels. In 1964, some 367,000 Americans were receiving food stamps. In 2000, the estimate is over 28 million recipients. The annual cost has jumped from $860,000 to more than $30 billion. In 2000, almost one in every nine citizens (including children) was using food stamps. The food stamp program has become a major part of the welfare system in the United States. The program has also become a method of promoting better nutrition among the poor.

The Earned Income Tax Credit Program (EITC). In 1975, the EITC was created to provide rebates of Social Security taxes to low-income workers. Over one-fifth of all tax returns claim an earned-income tax credit. In some states, such as Mississippi, as well as the District of Columbia, nearly half of all families are eligible for EITC. The program works as follows: Households with a reported income of less than $25,300 (exclusive of welfare payments) receive EITC benefits up to $2,528. There is a catch, though. Those with earnings between $8,425 and $11,000 get a flat $2,528. But families earning between $11,000 and $25,300 get penalized 17.68 cents for every dollar they earn above $11,000. This constitutes a punitive tax. Thus the EITC discourages work by a low- or moderate-income earner more than it rewards work. In particular, it discourages low-income earners from taking on a second job. The General Accounting Office estimates that hours worked by working wives in EITC-beneficiary households have consequently decreased by 10 percent. The average EITC recipient works 1,300 hours compared to a normal work year of 2,000 hours.

No Apparent Reduction in Poverty Rates

In spite of the numerous programs in existence and the hundreds of billions of dollars transferred to the poor, the officially defined rate of poverty in the United States has shown no long-run tendency to decline. From 1945 until the early 1970s, the percentage of Americans in poverty fell steadily every year. It reached a low of around 11 percent in 1973, shot back up beyond 15 percent in 1983, fell steadily to 13.1 percent in 1990, and has stayed about that ever since. Why this has happened is a real puzzlement. Since the War on Poverty was launched under President Lyndon B. Johnson in 1965, nearly $4 trillion has been transferred to the poor, and yet more Americans are poor today than ever before. This fact created the political will to pass the Welfare Reform Act of 1996, putting limits on people's use of welfare. The goal is now to get people off welfare and onto "workfare."

CONCEPTS IN BRIEF

- If poverty is defined in absolute terms, economic growth eventually decreases the number of officially defined poor. If poverty is defined relatively, however, we will never eliminate it.
- Major attacks on poverty have been social insurance programs in the form of Social Security, Supplemental Security Income, Aid to Families with Dependent Children, the earned-income tax credit, and food stamps.
- Although the relative lot of the poor measured by household income seems to have worsened, household spending by the bottom 20 percent of households compared to the top 20 percentile has shown little change since the 1960s.

HEALTH CARE

It may seem strange to be reading about health care in a chapter on the distribution of income and poverty. Yet health care is in fact intimately related to those two topics. For example, sometimes people become poor because they do not have adequate health insurance (or have none at all), fall ill, and deplete all of their wealth on care. Moreover, sometimes individuals remain in certain jobs simply because their employer's health care package seems so good that they are afraid to change jobs and risk not being covered by health care insurance in the process. Finally, as you will see, much of the cause of the increased health care spending in America can be attributed to a change in the incentives that Americans face.

America's Health Care Situation

Spending for health care is estimated to account for 14 percent of the total annual income created in the U.S. economy. You can see from Figure 30-8 that in 1965, about 6 percent of annual income was spent on health care, but that percentage has been increasing ever since. Per capita spending on health care is greater in the United States than anywhere else in the world today. On a per capita basis, we spend more than twice as much as citizens of Luxembourg, Austria, Australia, Japan, and Denmark. We spend almost three times as much on a per capita basis as citizens of Spain and Ireland.

Why Have Health Care Costs Risen So Much? There are numerous explanations for why health care costs have risen so much. At least one has to do with changing demographics: The U.S. population is getting older.

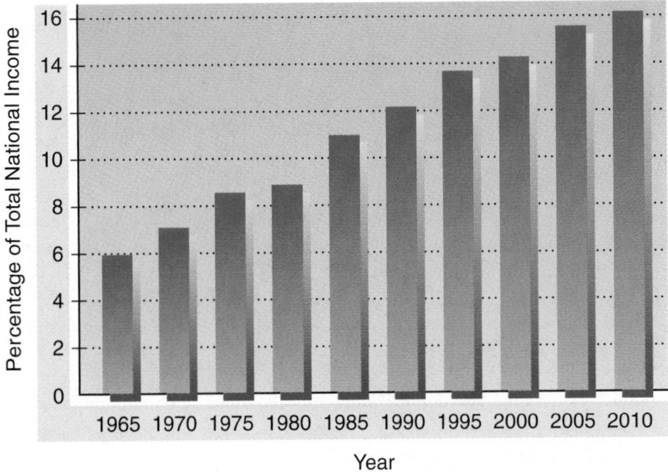

FIGURE 30-8

Percentage of Total National Income Spent on Health Care in the United States

The portion of total national income spent on health care has risen steadily since 1965.

Sources: U.S. Department of Commerce; U.S. Department of Health and Human Services; Deloitte and Touche LLP; VHA, Inc.

The Age–Health Care Expenditure Equation The top 5 percent of health care users incur over 50 percent of all health costs. The bottom 70 percent of health care users account for only 10 percent of health care expenditures. Not surprisingly, the elderly make up most of the top users of health care services. Nursing home expenditures are made primarily by people older than 70. The use of hospitals is also dominated by the aged.

The U.S. population is aging steadily. More than 12 percent of the current 275 million Americans are over 65. It is estimated that by the year 2035, senior citizens will comprise about 22 percent of our population. This aging population stimulates the demand for health care. The elderly consume more than four times the per capita health care services than the rest of the population uses. In short, whatever the demand for health care services is today, it is likely to be considerably higher in the future as the U.S. population ages.

New Technologies Another reason that health care costs have risen so dramatically is high technology. A CT (computerized tomography) scanner costs around $1 million. An MRI (magnetic resonance imaging) scanner can cost over $2 million. A PET (positron emission tomography) scanner costs around $4 million. All of these machines became increasingly available in the 1980s, 1990s, and 2000s and are desired throughout the country. Typical fees for procedures using them range from $300 to $500 for a CT scan to as high as $2,000 for a PET scan. The development of new technologies that help physicians and hospitals prolong human life is an ongoing process in an ever-advancing industry. New procedures at even higher prices can be expected in the future.

Third-Party Financing Currently, government spending on health care constitutes over 40 percent of total health care spending (of which the *federal* government pays about 70 percent). Private insurance accounts for a little over 35 percent of payments for health care. The remainder—less than 20 percent—is paid directly by individuals. Figure 30-9 on the next page shows the change in the payment scheme for medical care in the United States since 1930. Medicare and Medicaid are the main sources of hospital and other medical benefits to 35 million Americans, most of whom are over 65. Medicaid—the joint state-federal program—provides long-term health care, particularly for people living in nursing homes. Medicare, Medicaid, and private insurance companies are considered **third parties** in the medical care equation. Caregivers and patients are the two primary parties. When third parties step in to pay for medical care, the quantity demanded for those services increases. For example, when

Third parties 
Parties who are not directly involved in a given activity or transaction. For example, in the relationship between caregivers and patients, fees may be paid by third parties (insurance companies, government).

FIGURE 30-9

Third Party Versus Out-of-Pocket Health Care Payments

Out-of-pocket payments for health care services have been falling steadily since the 1930s. In contrast, third-party payments for health care have risen to the point that they account for over 80 percent of all such outlays today.

Sources: Health Care Financing Administration; U.S. Department of Health and Human Services.

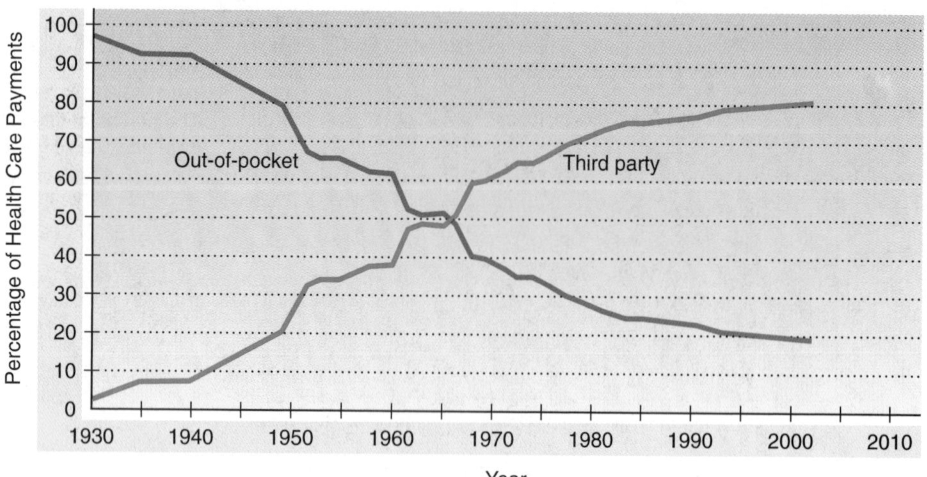

Medicare and Medicaid went into effect in the 1960s, the volume of federal government–reimbursed medical services increased by more than 65 percent.

The availability of third-party payments for costly medical care has generated increases in the availability of hospital beds. Between 1974 and 2000, the number of hospital beds increased by over 50 percent. Present occupancy rates are only around 65 percent.

Price, Quantity Demanded, and the Question of Moral Hazard. While some people may think that the demand for health care is insensitive to price changes, theory clearly indicates otherwise. Look at Figure 30-10. There you see a hypothetical demand curve for health care services. To the extent that third parties—whether government or private insurance—pay for health care, the out-of-pocket cost, or net price, to the individual will drop. In an extreme example, all medical expenses are paid for by third parties so that the price is zero in Figure 30-10 and the quantity demanded is many times what it would be at a higher price.

One of the issues here has to do with the problem of moral hazard. Consider two individuals with two different health insurance policies. The first policy pays for all medical expenses, but in the second the individual has to pay the first $1,000 a year (this amount is known as the *deductible*). Will the behavior of the two individuals be different? Generally, the answer is yes. The individual with no deductible may be more likely to seek treatment for health problems after they develop rather than try to avoid them and will generally expect medical attention on a more regular basis. In contrast, the individual who faces the

FIGURE 30-10

The Demand for Health Care Services

At price P_1, the quantity of health care services demanded per year would hypothetically be Q_1. If the price falls to zero (third-party payment with zero deductible), the quantity demanded expands to Q_2.

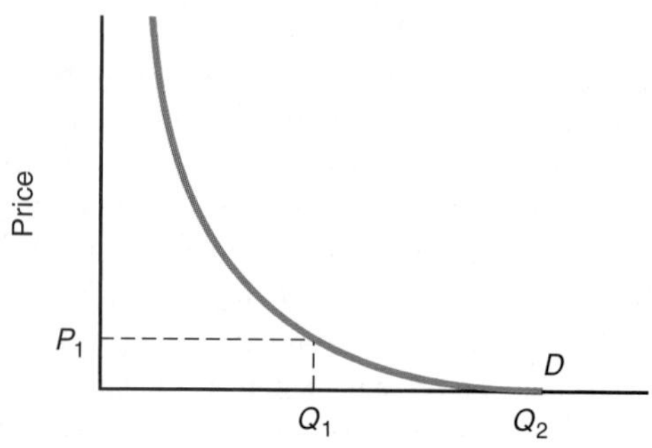

first $1,000 of medical expenses each year will tend to engage in more wellness activities and will be less inclined to seek medical care for minor problems. The moral hazard here is that the individual with the zero deductible for medical care expenses may engage in a lifestyle that is less healthful than will the individual with the $1,000 deductible.

Moral Hazard as It Affects Physicians and Hospitals. The issue of moral hazard also has a direct effect on the behavior of physicians and hospital administrators. Due to third-party payments, patients rarely have to worry about the expense of operations and other medical procedures. As a consequence, both physicians and hospitals order more procedures. Physicians are typically reimbursed on the basis of medical procedures; thus they have no financial interest in trying to keep hospital costs down. Indeed, many have an incentive to raise costs.

Such actions are most evident with terminally ill patients. A physician may order a CT scan and other costly procedures for a terminally ill patient. The physician knows that Medicare or some other type of insurance will pay. Then the physician can charge a fee for analyzing the CT scan. Fully 30 percent of Medicare expenditures are for Americans who are in the last six months of their lives.

Rising Medicare expenditures are one of the most serious problems facing the federal government today. The number of beneficiaries has increased from 19.1 million in 1966 (first year of operation) to an estimated 40 million in 2000. Figure 30-11 shows that federal spending on Medicare has been growing at over 10 percent a year, adjusted for inflation.

Is National Health Insurance the Answer?

Proponents of a national health care system believe that the current system relies too heavily on private insurers. They argue in favor of a Canadian-style system. In Canada, the government sets the fees that are paid to each doctor for seeing a patient and prohibits private practice. The Canadian government also imposes a cap on the incomes that any doctor can receive in a given year. The Canadian federal government provides a specified amount of funding to hospitals, leaving it to them to decide how to allocate the funds. If we were to follow the

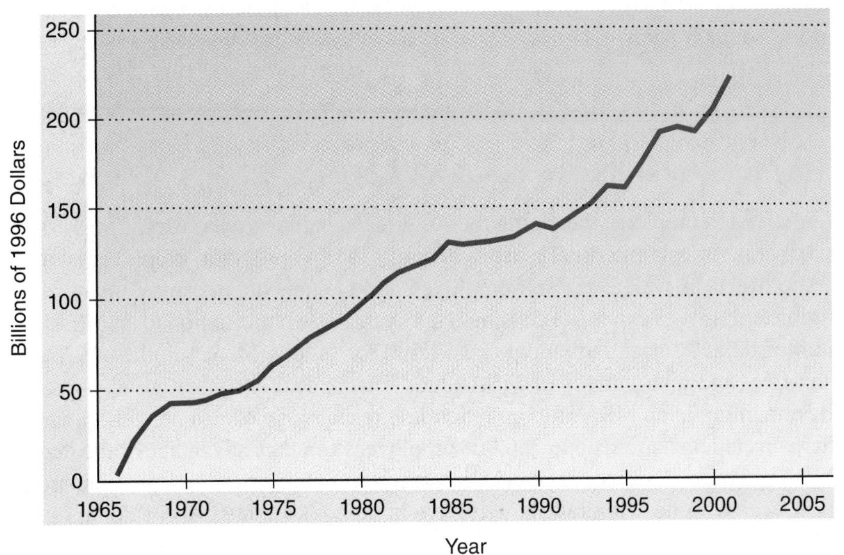

FIGURE 30-11
Federal Medicare Spending
Federal spending on Medicare has increased about 10 percent a year, after adjusting for inflation, since its inception in 1966. (All figures expressed in constant 1996 dollars.)
Sources: Economic Report of the President; U.S. Bureau of Labor Statistics.

Canadian model, the average American would receive fewer health services than at present. Hospital stays would be longer, but there would be fewer tests and procedures.

Alternatives to a national health care policy involve some type of national health insurance, perhaps offered only to people who qualify on the basis of low annual income. A number of politicians have offered variations on such a program. The over 40 million Americans who have no health insurance at some time during each year would certainly benefit. The share of annual national income that goes to health care expenditures would rise, however. Also, federal government spending might increase by another $30 billion to $50 billion (or more) per year to pay for the program.

INTERNATIONAL EXAMPLE

While Americans Complain About Health Care Expenses, Canadians Wait in Line

In Chapter 4, you learned about several ways to ration goods and services. Although government programs and some private programs engage in nonprice rationing in the United States, the primary rationing device continues to be the price mechanism. A disadvantage of this approach is that some people may not wish to pay market prices for the best-quality care. A large number of U.S. residents do not have health insurance at some time each year.

In Canada, the government provides a "single-payer" national health system under which all citizens are promised "free care." In recent years, proponents of a national U.S. health care system have held up the Canadian system as a model for the United States to emulate. Within the past few years, dramatic events highlighted the pitfalls of the Canadian system. For instance, a pregnant woman died of a brain hemorrhage when her doctors could not locate a neurosurgical facility that had room for her. After months of postponed appointments, a woman suffering from stomach pains died of cancer that might have been treatable if detected earlier. Other patients with suspected cancers had to sign waiting lists *to get on to* true waiting lists for magnetic resonance imaging (MRI) devices.

Offering free health care encourages patients to seek as much care as they can get. Of course, a government that promises care must incur costs to provide it. These costs have put a severe strain on Canadian federal and provincial governments. To cope with rising costs, Canadian officials have closed hospitals and limited the hours that physicians can treat patients. They have depended on *rationing by queues*. For people who can get treatment in Canada, the quality of care is very good. The problem is that people typically have to wait in line to get it—and some die waiting.

For Critical Analysis

What identifiable groups stand to gain from allowing market prices to ration health care? Do any specific groups gain from health care rationing by queues?

Countering the Moral Hazard Problem: A Medical Savings Account

Medical savings account (MSA)
A tax-exempt health care account into which individuals would pay on a regular basis and out of which medical care expenses could be paid.

As an alternative to completely changing the American health care industry, Congress has legislated the experimental **medical savings account (MSA)** program. Employers with 50 or fewer employees, as well as the self-employed and the uninsured, can set up a tax-free MSA. Eligible employees can make an annual tax-deductible contribution to an MSA up to a maximum of $2,250 for an individual and $4,500 for family. Money in the MSA accumulates tax-free, and distributions of MSA funds for medical expenses are also exempt. Any funds remaining in an MSA after an individual reaches age 65 can be withdrawn tax-free. Under current legislation, up to 750,000 employees can take advantage of the demonstration MSA program. The benefits can be impressive. A single person depositing around $1,500 each year with no withdrawals will have hundreds of thousands of dollars in the account after 40 years.

Combating Moral Hazard. A major benefit of an MSA is that the moral hazard problem is reduced. Individuals ultimately pay for their own minor medical expenses. They do not have the incentive to seek medical care as frequently for minor problems. In addition, they have an incentive to engage in wellness activities. Finally, for those using an MSA, the physician-patient relationship remains intact, for third parties (insurance companies or the government) do not intervene in paying or monitoring medical expenses. Patients with MSAs will not allow physicians to routinely order expensive tests for every minor ache or pain because they get to keep any money saved in the MSA.

Critics' Responses. Some critics argue that because individuals get to keep whatever they don't spend from their MSAs, they will forgo necessary visits to medical care facilities and may develop more serious medical problems as a consequence. Other critics argue that MSAs will sabotage managed care plans. Under managed care plans, deductibles are either reduced or eliminated completely. In exchange, managed health care plan participants are extremely limited in physician choice. Just the opposite would occur with MSAs—high deductibles and unlimited choice of physicians.

CONCEPTS IN BRIEF

- Health care costs have risen because (1) our population has been getting older and the elderly use more health care services, (2) new technologies and medicine cost more, and (3) third-party financing—private and government-sponsored health insurance—reduces the incentive for individuals to reduce their spending on health care services.
- National health insurance has been proposed as an answer to our current problems, but it does little to alter the reasons why health care costs continue to rise.
- An alternative to a national health care program might be medical savings accounts, which allow individuals to set aside money that is tax exempt, to be used only for medical care. Whatever is left over becomes a type of retirement account.

NETNOMICS

Cyberdocs Versus Cyberquacks

It is estimated that more than 30 million people per year log on to the Internet to look for information or assistance with a medical or personal problem. Doctors, psychologists, and health care firms have noticed. Since 1997, at least $250 million in venture capital has been invested in Net-related health care sites. The nation's largest health maintenance organization, Kaiser Permanente, now has a Web site that allows its 9.2 million members to register for office visits, send e-mail questions to nurses and pharmacists, learn about the results of lab tests, and refill prescriptions. Former U.S. Surgeon General C. Everett Koop operates a consumer health site called drkoop.com, and the Mayo Clinic's Health Oasis Web site receives hundreds of thousands of visitors each month. Anyone today can access Web sites offering a wide array of medical research and news, as well as links to databases that explain diseases and drugs in laymen's terms. Some offer on-line chats with physicians and nurses, personal medical pages with customized data, and risk assessment services that rate a person's health based on lifestyle and medical information. A growing number of sites sell health-related products ranging from vitamins to health insurance.

Some medical experts hope that the Web will ultimately link physicians, patients, and insurers much like human nerve cells link to form the body's nervous system. Creating a

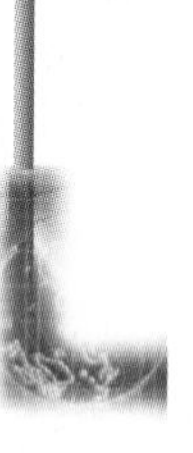

Net-based "electronic nervous system" for the health care industry, they argue, could help avoid wasting funds on unnecessary and duplicated medical treatments, thereby saving about a third of the more than $1 trillion that Americans spend on health care.

Nevertheless, there are hazards to Net-based health advice and care. Recall the lemons problem discussed in Chapter 23: If consumers do not know the details about the quality of a product, they may be willing to pay no more than the price of a low-quality product, even if a higher-quality product is available at a higher price. There are now at least 15,000 health-related Web sites, and undoubtedly some charge consumers for bad or misleading information. A few cyberspace health practitioners undoubtedly market low-priced "home remedies" that do little, if anything, to cure real diseases. To combat this problem, the non-profit Health on the Net Foundation certifies and monitors health-related Web sites. The U.S. Department of Health and Human Services has even set up a Web site, www.healthfinder.gov, which is aimed at helping consumers distinguish legitimate sites from those that practice cyberquackery.

ISSUES & APPLICATIONS

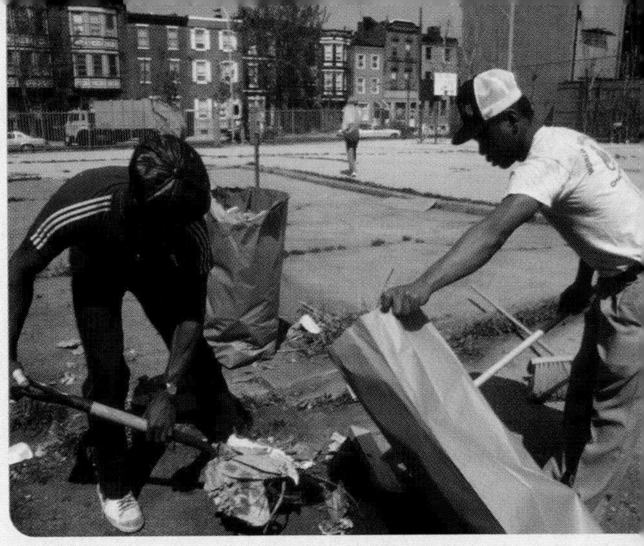

Why Is Measuring Poverty So Hard?

When officers of financial firms in Chicago formed Social Compact and launched their study of opportunities for bringing about economic renewal in official poverty-stricken portions of the city, they were surprised to see how well African-American South Side was doing. In addition, figures that Social Compact compiled in its study of low-income Chicago neighborhoods led to a particularly startling conclusion: People in some of the neighborhoods appeared to be spending more than official income data showed that they were earning.

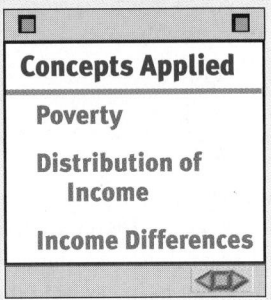

Concepts Applied

- Poverty
- Distribution of Income
- Income Differences

Problems in Relying on Incomes to Measure Poverty

Many economists are not surprised that spending has increased in poor neighborhoods. Studies of the earnings and spending of Americans who, according to government figures, earn between $10,000 and $20,000 per year find that overall they spend 40 percent more than their reported incomes. People who report earning less than $10,000 per year spend more than 150 percent more than their reported incomes.

What explains these discrepancies? One possible explanation, of course, is measurement errors. Perhaps people aren't really spending that much more than they report earnings. Nevertheless, study after study indicates the same pattern. A second, and more likely, explanation is that many low-income people report less income than they actually earn. Again, there may be reporting errors. Nevertheless, a plausible inference is that a lot of low-income people want to avoid paying taxes on the little income they do earn. So they do not report all their income.

Consumption as a Measure of Poverty

As you learned in this chapter, the government officially defines poverty on the basis of income levels. A number of economists have questioned this method for years, because incomes are not particularly useful measures of well-being. A person's reported income typically does not include earnings from informal work, and it does not take into account the value of health and education subsidies received from the government. This has led some economists to propose defining poverty in terms of *consumption* levels.

To do this, economists such as Dale Jorgenson of Harvard University and Robert Triest of the Federal Reserve Bank of Boston have used the federal government's Survey of Consumer Expenditures to fill in blanks and pick up details missed by income surveys. For instance, data from consumption surveys reveal when a low-income household can get by relatively well because it lives in a comfortable house inherited from parents. In addition, they indicate general improvements in standard of living, such as increased ownership of washing machines and automatic dishwashers. Of course, some consumption patterns have ambiguous implications. For example, if people consume less beef, is it because they are worse off and cannot afford to buy as much, or is it because they are better off and want to switch to a more healthful diet?

An Old Problem Rears Its Ugly Head

One of the biggest problems with consumption-based measures of poverty, however, has to do with tracking changes in the cost of living over time. Economists have found that there are significant measurement problems in determining changes in consumer prices. It turns out that depending on how economists measure price changes over time, they reach different conclusions about whether the poverty problem is worsening or improving. It seems that no matter where economists turn in their quest to define poverty, measurement problems abound.

FOR CRITICAL ANALYSIS

1. Why might similar households with identical incomes consume different amounts?
2. How might economists define an official "poverty" level of consumption?

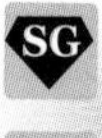

SUMMARY DISCUSSION OF LEARNING OBJECTIVES

1. **Using a Lorenz Curve to Represent a Nation's Income Distribution:** A Lorenz curve is a diagram that illustrates the distribution of income geometrically by measuring the percentage of households in relation to the cumulative percentage of income earnings. A perfectly straight Lorenz curve depicts perfect income equality, because at each percentage of households measured along a straight-line Lorenz curve, those households earn exactly the same percentage of income. The more bowed a Lorenz curve, the more unequally income is distributed.
2. **Key Determinants of Income Differences Across Individuals:** Because of the age-earnings cycle, in which people typically begin working at relatively low incomes when young, age is an important factor influencing income differences. So are marginal productivity differences, which arise from differences in talents, experience, and training due to different human capital investments. Discrimination likely plays a role as well, and economists attribute some of the unexplained portions of income differences across people to factors that relate to discrimination.
3. **Theories of Desired Income Distribution:** Economists agree that determining how income ought to be distributed is a normative issue influenced by alternative notions of economic justice. Nevertheless, two theories of desired income distribution receive considerable attention. One is the productivity standard (also called the contributive or merit standard), according to which each person receives income according to the value of what the person produces. The other is the egalitarian principle of income distribution, which proposes that each person should receive exactly the same income.
4. **Alternative Approaches to Measuring and Addressing Poverty:** One approach to defining poverty is to define an absolute poverty standard, such as a specific and unchanging income level. If an absolute measure of poverty is used and the economy experiences persistent real growth, poverty eventually will disappear. Another approach defines poverty in terms of income levels relative to the rest of the population. Under this definition, poverty exists as long as the distribution of incomes is unequal. Official poverty measures are often based on pretax income and fail to take transfer payments into account. Currently, the U.S. government seeks to address poverty via income maintenance programs such as Social Security, Supplemental Security Income, Temporary Assistance to Needy Families, food stamps, and the Earned Income Tax Credit program.
5. **Major Reasons for Rising Health Care Costs:** Spending on health care as a percentage of total U.S. spending has increased during recent decades. One reason is that the U.S. population is aging, and older people typically experience more health problems. Another contributing factor is the adoption of higher-priced technologies for diagnosing and treating health problems. In addition, third-party financing of health care expenditures by private and government insurance programs gives covered individuals an incentive to purchase more health care than they would if they paid all expenses out of pocket. Moral hazard problems can also arise, because consumers

may be more likely to seek treatment for insured health problems after they develop instead of trying to avoid them, and doctors and hospitals may order more procedures than they otherwise would require.

6. **Alternative Approaches to Paying for Health Care:** An alternative approach to funding health care would be to rely less on private insurers and more on governmental funding of care for all citizens. Under such a system, the government typically sets fees and establishes limits on access to care. Another approach would be to establish a national health insurance program that is income-based, in which only lower-income people would qualify for government assistance in meeting their health care expenses. Another option is provide incentives for people to save some of their income in medical savings accounts, from which they can draw funds to pay for health care expenses in the future.

Key Terms and Concepts

Age-earnings cycle (737)
Comparable-worth doctrine (742)
Distribution of income (732)
Income in kind (733)
Lorenz curve (732)
Medical savings account (MSA) (752)
Third parties (749)

Problems

Answers to the odd-numbered problems appear at the back of the book.

30-1. Consider the accompanying graph, which depicts Lorenz curves for countries X, Y, and Z.

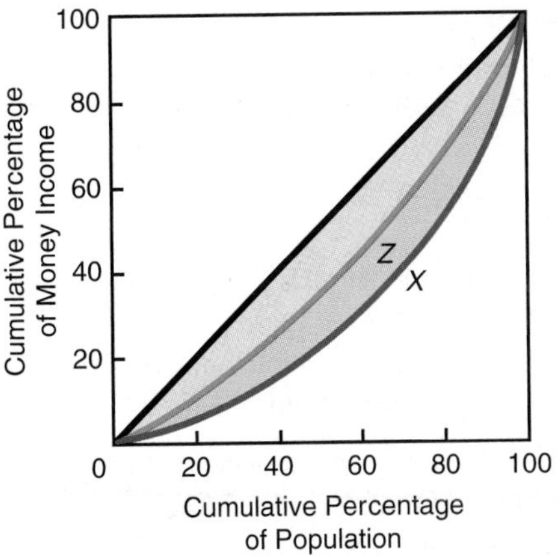

a. Which country has the least income inequality?
b. Which country has the most income inequality?
c. Countries Y and Z are identical in all but one respect: population distribution. The share of the population made up of children below working age is much higher in country Z. Recently, however, birthrates have declined in country Z and risen in country Y. Assuming that the countries remain identical in all other respects, would you expect that in 20 years the Lorenz curves for the two countries will be closer together or farther apart?

30-2. Consider the following income distribution estimates from the 1990s. Use graph paper or a hand-drawn diagram to draw rough Lorenz curves for each country. Which has the most nearly equal distribution, based on your diagram?

Country	Poorest 40%	Next 30%	Next 20%	Richest 10%
Bolivia	13	21	26	40
Chile	13	20	26	41
Uruguay	22	26	26	26

30-3. Estimates indicate that during the 1990s, the poorest 40 percent of the population earned about 15 percent of total income in Argentina. In Brazil, the poorest 40 percent earned about 10 percent of total income. The next-highest 30 percent of income earners in Argentina received roughly 25 percent of total income. By contrast, in Brazil, the next-highest 30 percent of income earners received approximately 20 percent of total income. Can you determine, without drawing a diagram (though you can if you wish), which country's Lorenz curve was bowed out farther to the right?

30-4. A retired 72-year-old man currently draws Social Security and a small pension from his previous employment. He is in very good health and would like to take on a new challenge, and he decides to go back to work. He determines that under the rules of Social Security and his pension plan, if he were to work full time, he would face a marginal tax rate of 110 percent for the last hour he works each week. What does this mean?

30-5. In what ways might policies aimed at achieving complete income equality across all households be incompatible with economic efficiency?

30-6. Some economists have argued that if the government wishes to subsidize health care, it should instead provide predetermined sums of money (based on the type of health care problems experienced) directly to patients, who then would be free to choose their health care providers. Whether or not you agree, can you provide an economic rationale for this approach to governmental health care funding?

30-7. Suppose that a government agency guarantees to pay all of an individual's future health care expenses after the end of this year, so that the effective price of health care for the individual will be zero from that date onward. In what ways might this well-intended policy induce the individual to consume "excessive" health care services in future years?

30-8. Suppose that a group of doctors establishes a joint practice in a remote area. This group provides the only health care available to people in the local community, and its objective is to maximize total economic profits for the group's members. Draw a diagram illustrating how the price and quantity of health care will be determined in this community.

30-9. A government agency determines that the entire community discussed in Problem 30-8 qualifies for a special program in which the government will pay for a number of health care services that most residents previously had not consumed. Many residents immediately make appointments with the community physicians' group. Given the information in Problem 30-8, what is the likely effect on the profit-maximizing price and the equilibrium quantity of health care services provided by the physicians' group in this community?

30-10. A government agency notifies the physicians' group in Problem 30-8 that to continue providing services in the community, the group must document its activities. The resulting paperwork expenses raise the cost of each unit of health care services that the group provides. What is the likely effect on the profit-maximizing price and the equilibrium quantity of health care services provided by the physicians' group in this community?

Economics on the Net

Measuring Poverty Many economists believe that there are problems with the current official measure of poverty. In this application, you will learn about some of these problems and will be able to examine an alternative poverty measure that one group of economists has proposed.

Title: Joint Center for Poverty Research (JCPR)

Navigation: Click here to visit the JCPR's homepage. Click on Publications. Select the complete listing of policy briefs. Click on the Policy Brief titled "Measuring Poverty—A New Approach."

Application Read the article; then answer the following questions.

1. How is the current official poverty income level calculated? What is the main problem with this way of calculating the threshold income for classifying impoverished households?
2. What is the alternative conceptual measure of poverty that the authors propose? How does it differ from the current measure?

For Group Study and Analysis Discuss the two measures of poverty discussed in the article. What people would no longer be classified as living in poverty under the proposed measure of poverty? What people would join the ranks of those classified as among the impoverished in America? How might adopting the new measure of poverty affect efforts to address the U.S. poverty problem?

CHAPTER

31

ENVIRONMENTAL ECONOMICS

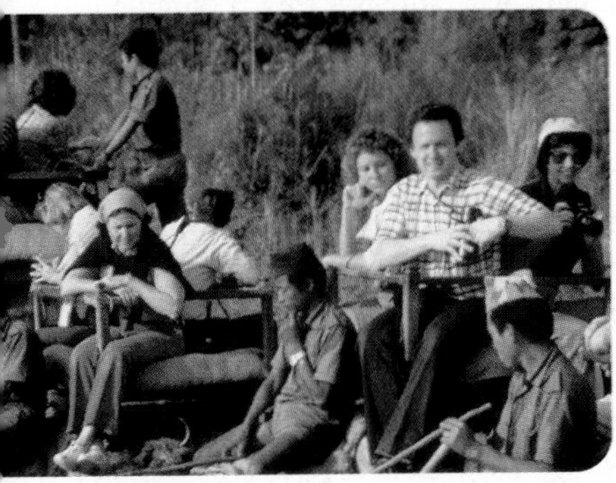

These tourists are on a Nepalese tiger safari. They are willing to pay large sums of money to observe tigers in the wild. Can you use this fact to devise a policy to preserve Asian tigers?

It is estimated that at the beginning of the twentieth century, there were more than 100,000 tigers that roamed Asia. Today there are at most 7,300. Furthermore, despite concerted international efforts—bans on hunting, government-operated tiger reserves, and restraints on trade in tiger body parts—over more than three decades, the number of tigers continues to dwindle. Can economists contribute to continuing efforts to save the tiger? To understand what economics can add to wildlife conservation efforts, as well as to broader efforts to prevent environmental degradation, you must first learn about environmental economics. You will be looking at the costs and benefits of every action, including those already undertaken and those proposed to solve any problem of global dimension.

LEARNING OBJECTIVES

After reading this chapter, you should be able to:

1. **Distinguish between private costs and social costs**
2. **Understand market externalities and possible ways to correct externalities**
3. **Describe how economists can conceptually determine the optimal quantity of pollution**
4. **Explain the roles of private and common property rights in alternative approaches to addressing the problem of pollution**
5. **Discuss how the assignment of property rights may influence the fates of endangered species**
6. **Contrast the benefits and costs of recycling scarce resources**

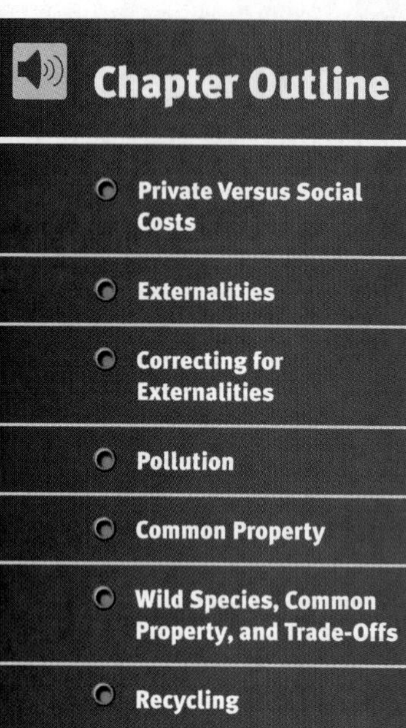

Did You Know That... within three months after the Pilgrims landed at Plymouth Rock, half of them had died from malnutrition and illness because of the harsh conditions they encountered? Some of the surviving Pilgrims gave up and returned with the *Mayflower* when it sailed back across the Atlantic. The remaining Pilgrims struggled with famine. After three years of enduring conditions bordering on starvation, and after some Pilgrims became so desperate that they took to stealing from the others, the colonists began to reconsider a key method they had adopted in an effort to promote their new society. This was the practice of "farming in common," which entailed pooling what they produced and then rationing this "common property" in equal allotments. Following much thought and discussion, the colonists decided instead to parcel the *land* equally among families, who could then either consume or trade all fruits of their labors. This change in the Pilgrims' incentive structure worked wonders. Soon they had such bountiful harvests that they decided to have a day of thanksgiving—the forerunner of the modern American Thanksgiving holiday.

How to design incentives for people to use common property in ways that is in the interest of society as a whole is an important economic problem. Certainly, it is in the interest of today's societies and of future generations to find a mix of incentives that induce human beings to protect our most important form of common property, our environment. It should not surprise you that the economic way of thinking about the environment has to do with costs.

For example, are you willing to give up driving your car in order to have a cleaner environment? Or would you pay $4 for a gallon of gas to help clean up the environment? In a phrase, how much of your current standard of living are you willing to give up to help the environment? The economic way of looking at ecological issues is often viewed as anti-ecological. But this is not so. Economists want to help citizens and policymakers opt for informed policies that have the maximum possible *net* benefits (benefits minus costs). As you will see, every decision in favor of "the environment" involves a trade-off.

PRIVATE VERSUS SOCIAL COSTS

Human actions often give rise to unwanted side effects—the destruction of our environment is one. Human actions generate pollutants that go into the air and the water. The question that is often asked is, Why can individuals and businesses continue to create pollution without necessarily paying directly for the negative consequences?

Until now, we've been dealing with situations in which the costs of an individual's actions are borne directly by the individual. When a business has to pay wages to workers, it knows exactly what its labor costs are. When it has to buy materials or build a plant, it knows quite well what these will cost. An individual who has to pay for car repairs or a theater ticket knows exactly what the cost will be. These costs are what we term *private costs*. **Private costs** are borne solely by the individuals who incur them. They are *internal* in the sense that the firm or household must explicitly take account of them.

Private costs 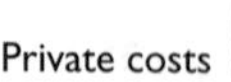
Costs borne solely by the individuals who incur them. Also called *internal costs*.

What about a situation in which a business dumps the waste products from its production process into a nearby river or in which an individual litters a public park or beach? Obviously, a cost is involved in these actions. When the firm pollutes the water, people downstream suffer the consequences. They may not want to swim in or drink the polluted water. They may also be unable to catch as many fish as before because of the pollution. In the case of littering, the people who come along after our litterer has cluttered the park or the beach are the ones who bear the costs. The cost of these actions is borne by people other than those who commit the actions. The creator of the cost is not the sole bearer. The costs are not internalized by the individual or firm; they are external. When we add *external* costs to *internal,* or private, costs, we get **social costs.** Pollution problems—indeed, all problems pertaining to the environment—may be viewed as situations in which social costs exceed private costs. Because some economic participants don't pay the full social costs of their actions but rather only the smaller private costs, their actions are socially "unacceptable." In such situations in which there is a divergence between social and private costs, we therefore see "too much" steel production, automobile driving, and beach littering, to pick only a few of the many possible examples.

Social costs 
The full costs borne by society whenever a resource use occurs. Social costs can be measured by adding private, or internal, costs to external costs.

The Costs of Polluted Air

Why is the air in cities so polluted from automobile exhaust fumes? When automobile drivers step into their cars, they bear only the private costs of driving. That is, they must pay for the gas, maintenance, depreciation, and insurance on their automobiles. But they cause an additional cost, that of air pollution, which they are not forced to take account of when they make the decision to drive. Air pollution is a cost because it causes harm to individuals—burning eyes, respiratory ailments, and dirtier clothes, cars, and buildings. The air pollution created by automobile exhaust is a cost that individual operators of automobiles do not yet bear directly. The social cost of driving includes all the private costs plus at least the cost of air pollution, which society bears. Decisions made only on the basis of private costs lead to too much automobile driving or, alternatively, to too little money spent on the reduction of automobile pollution for a given amount of driving. Clean air is a scarce resource used by automobile drivers free of charge. They will use more of it than they would if they had to pay the full social costs.

EXTERNALITIES

When a private cost differs from a social cost, we say that there is an **externality** because individual decision makers are not paying (internalizing) all the costs. (We briefly covered this topic in Chapter 5.) Some of these costs remain external to the decision-making process. Remember that the full cost of using a scarce resource is borne one way or another by all who live in the society. That is, society must pay the full opportunity cost of any activity that uses scarce resources. The individual decision maker is the firm or the customer, and external costs and benefits will not enter into that individual's or firm's decision-making processes.

Externality 
A situation in which a private cost (or benefit) diverges from a social cost (or benefit); a situation in which the costs (or benefits) of an action are not fully borne (or gained) by the two parties engaged in exchange or by an individual engaging in a scarce-resource-using activity.

We might want to view the problem as it is presented in Figure 31-1 on the next page. Here we have the market demand curve, D, for the product X and the supply curve, S_1, for product X. The supply curve, S_1, includes only internal, or private, costs. The intersection of the demand and supply curves as drawn will be at price P_1 and quantity Q_1 (at E_1). We now assume that the production of good X involves externalities that the private firms did not take into account. Those externalities could be air pollution, water pollution, scenery destruction, or anything of that nature.

We know that the social costs of producing product X exceed the private costs. We show this by drawing curve S_2. It is above the original supply curve S_1 because it includes the full social costs of producing the product. If firms could be made to bear these costs, the price would be P_2 and the quantity Q_2 (at E_2). The inclusion of external costs in the decision-making process leads to a higher-priced product and a decline in quantity produced. Thus we see that when social costs are not being fully borne by the creators of those costs, the quantity produced is "excessive," because the price is too low.

FIGURE 31-1

Reckoning with Full Social Costs

The supply curve, S_1, is equal to the horizontal summation (Σ) of the individual marginal cost curves above the respective minimum average variable costs of all the firms producing good X. These individual marginal cost curves include only internal, or private, costs. If the external costs were included and added to the private costs, we would have social costs. The supply curve would shift upward to S_2. In the uncorrected situation, the equilibrium price would be P_1 and the equilibrium quantity would be Q_1. In the corrected situation, the equilibrium price would rise to P_2 and the equilibrium quantity would fall to Q_2.

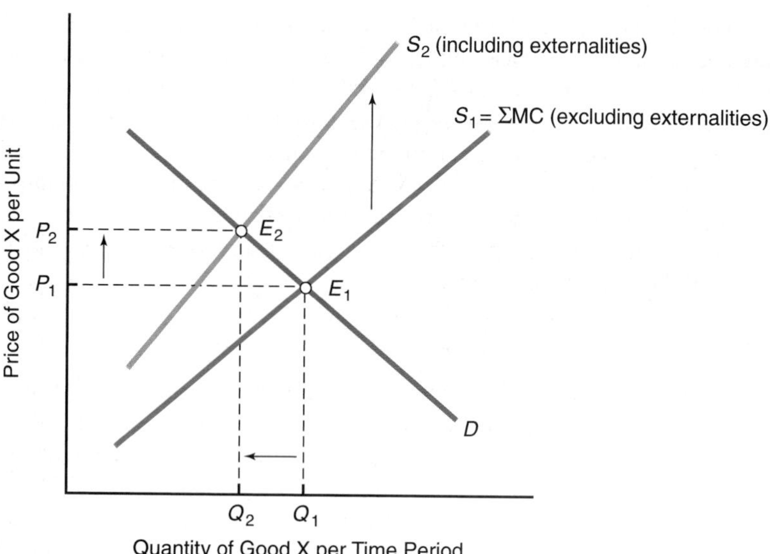

CORRECTING FOR EXTERNALITIES

We can see here a method for reducing pollution and environmental degradation. Somehow the signals in the economy must be changed so that decision makers will take into account *all* the costs of their actions. In the case of automobile pollution, we might want to devise some method by which motorists are taxed according to the amount of pollution they cause. In the case of a firm, we might want to devise a system whereby businesses are taxed according to the amount of pollution for which they are responsible. In this manner, they would have an incentive to install pollution abatement equipment.

The Polluters' Choice

Facing an additional private cost for polluting, firms will be induced to (1) install pollution abatement equipment or otherwise change production techniques so as to reduce the amount of pollution, (2) reduce pollution-causing activity, or (3) simply pay the price to pollute. The relative costs and benefits of each option for each polluter will determine which one or combination will be chosen. Allowing the choice is the efficient way to decide who pollutes and who doesn't. In principle, each polluter faces the full social cost of its actions and makes a production decision accordingly.

Is a Uniform Tax Appropriate?

It may not be appropriate to levy a *uniform* tax according to physical quantities of pollution. After all, we're talking about external costs. Such costs are not necessarily the same everywhere in the United States for the same action.

Essentially, we must establish the amount of the *economic damages* rather than the amount of the physical pollution. A polluting electrical plant in New York City will cause much more damage than the same plant in remote Montana. There are already innumerable demands on the air in New York City, so the pollution from smokestacks will not be cleansed away naturally. Millions of people will breathe the polluted air and thereby incur the costs of sore throats, sickness, emphysema, and even early death. Buildings will become dirtier faster because of the pollution, as will cars and clothes. A given quantity of pollution will cause more harm in concentrated urban environments than it will in less dense rural environments. If we were to establish some form of taxation to align private costs with social costs and to force people to internalize externalities, we would somehow have to come up with a measure of *economic* costs instead of *physical* quantities. But the tax, in any event, would fall on the private sector and modify private-sector economic agents' behavior. Therefore, because the economic cost for the same physical quantity of pollution would be different in different locations according to population density, the natural formation of mountains and rivers, and so forth, so-called optimal taxes on pollution would vary from location to location. (Nonetheless, a uniform tax might make sense when administrative costs, particularly the cost of ascertaining the actual economic costs, are relatively high.)

POLICY EXAMPLE

Should Car Antitheft Devices Be Subsidized?

Externalities exist for many activities. Consider the theft of automobiles. About 1.5 million cars are stolen in the United States every year. If you own an expensive car, you run a risk of having it stolen when you park on the street. Enter an antitheft device called Lojack, first used in 1986. A tiny transmitter is hidden in each Lojack-equipped car. When a car is stolen, in any of 20 major cities, the police can turn on the transmitter. About 95 percent of Lojack-equipped stolen cars are recovered and sustain less damage than other recovered stolen cars. Researchers Ian Ayres and S. D. Levitt of the National Bureau of Economic Research estimate that positive externalities are worth 15 times more than the benefit received by the Lojack-equipped car owner—when there are lots of Lojacks in the area, thieves leave the area, meaning that they don't steal non-Lojack-equipped cars either. One auto theft is eliminated annually for every three Lojacks installed in central cities.

For Critical Analysis

Who might want to subsidize Lojacks?

CONCEPTS IN BRIEF

- Private costs are costs that are borne directly by consumers and producers when they engage in any resource-using activity.
- Social costs are private costs plus any other costs that are external to the decision maker. For example, the social costs of driving include all the private costs plus any pollution and congestion caused.
- When private costs differ from social costs, externalities exist because individual decision makers are not internalizing all the costs that society is bearing.
- When social costs exceed private costs, we say that there are externalities.

POLLUTION

The term *pollution* is used quite loosely and can refer to a variety of by-products of any activity. Industrial pollution involves mainly air and water but can also include noise and such concepts as aesthetic pollution, as when a landscape is altered in a negative way. For the most part, we will be analyzing the most common forms, air and water pollution.

When asked how much pollution there should be in the economy, many people will respond, "None." But if we ask those same people how much starvation or deprivation of consumer products should exist in the economy, many will again say, "None." Growing and distributing food or producing consumer products creates pollution, however. In effect, therefore, there is no correct answer to how much pollution should be in an economy because when we ask how much pollution there *should* be, we are entering the realm of normative economics. We are asking people to express values. There is no way to disprove somebody's value system scientifically. One way we can approach a discussion of the "correct" amount of pollution would be to set up the same type of marginal analysis we used in our discussion of a firm's employment and output decisions. That is to say, we should pursue measures to reduce pollution only up to the point at which the marginal benefit from further reduction equals the marginal cost of further reduction.

Click here to see a review of possible economic effects of alternative pollution reduction scenarios.

Look at Figure 31-2. On the horizontal axis, we show the degree of cleanliness of the air. A vertical line is drawn at 100 percent cleanliness—the air cannot become any cleaner. Consider the benefits of obtaining a greater degree of air cleanliness. These benefits are represented by the marginal benefit curve, which slopes downward because of the law of diminishing marginal utility.

When the air is very dirty, the marginal benefit from air that is a little cleaner appears to be relatively high, as shown on the vertical axis. As the air becomes cleaner and cleaner, however, the marginal benefit of a little bit more air cleanliness falls.

Consider the marginal cost of pollution abatement—that is, the marginal cost of obtaining cleaner air. In the 1960s, automobiles had no pollution abatement devices. Eliminating only 20 percent of the pollutants emitted by internal-combustion engines entailed a relatively small cost per unit of pollution removed. The cost of eliminating the next 20 percent rose, though. Finally, as we now get to the upper limits of removal of pollutants from the emissions of internal-combustion engines, we find that the elimination of one more percentage point of the amount of pollutants becomes astronomically expensive. To go from 97 percent cleanliness to 98 percent cleanliness involves a marginal cost that is many times greater than going from 10 percent cleanliness to 11 percent cleanliness.

It is realistic, therefore, to draw the marginal cost of pollution abatement as an upward-sloping curve, as shown in Figure 31-2. (The marginal cost curve slopes up because of the law of diminishing returns.)

FIGURE 31-2

The Optimal Quantity of Air Pollution

As we attempt to get a greater degree of air cleanliness, the marginal cost rises until even the slightest attempt at increasing air cleanliness leads to a very high marginal cost, as can be seen at the upper right of the graph. Conversely, the marginal benefit curve slopes downward: The more pure air we have, the less we value an additional unit of pure air. Marginal cost and marginal benefit intersect at point *E*. The optimal degree of air cleanliness is something less than 100 percent at Q_0. The price that we should pay for the last unit of air cleanup is no greater than P_0, for that is where marginal cost equals marginal benefit.

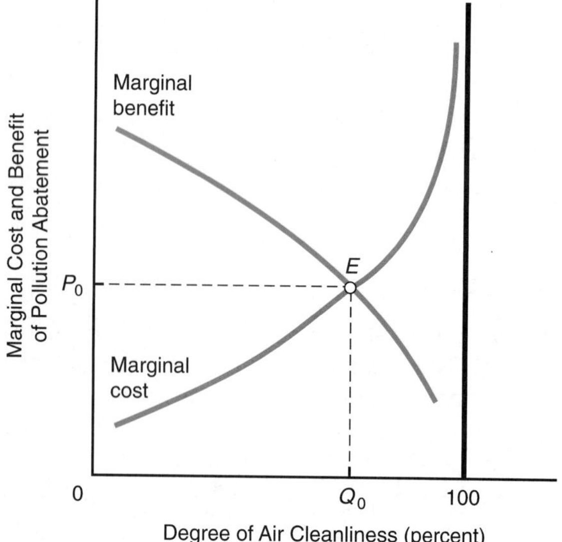

The Optimal Quantity of Pollution

The **optimal quantity of pollution** is defined as the level of pollution at which the marginal benefit equals the marginal cost of obtaining clean air. This occurs at the intersection of the marginal benefit curve and the marginal cost curve in Figure 31-2, at point *E*, which is analytically exactly the same as for every other economic activity. If we increased pollution control by one more unit greater than Q_0, the marginal cost of that small increase in the degree of air cleanliness would be greater than the marginal benefit to society.

Optimal quantity of pollution 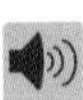
The level of pollution for which the marginal benefit of one additional unit of clean air just equals the marginal cost of that additional unit of clean air.

As is usually the case in economic analysis, the optimal quantity of just about anything occurs when marginal cost equals marginal benefit. That is, the optimal quantity of pollution occurs at the point at which the marginal cost of reducing (or abating) pollution is just equal to the marginal benefit of doing so. The marginal cost of pollution abatement rises as more and more abatement is achieved (as the environment becomes cleaner and cleaner, the *extra* cost of cleansing rises). The state of technology is such that early units of pollution abatement are easily achieved (at low cost), but attaining higher and higher levels of environmental quality becomes progressively more difficult (as the extra cost rises to prohibitive levels). At the same time, the marginal benefits of a cleaner and cleaner environment fall; the marginal benefit of pollution abatement declines as the concept of a cleaner and cleaner environment moves from human life-support requirements to recreation to beauty to a perfectly pure environment. The point at which the increasing marginal cost of pollution abatement equals the decreasing marginal benefit of pollution abatement defines the (theoretical) optimal quantity of pollution.

Click here to learn about a market-oriented government program for reducing pollution.

Recognizing that the optimal quantity of pollution is not zero becomes easier when we realize that it takes scarce resources to reduce pollution. It follows that a trade-off exists between producing a cleaner environment and producing other goods and services. In that sense, nature's ability to cleanse itself is a resource that can be analyzed like any other resource, and a cleaner environment must take its place with other societal wants.

INTERNATIONAL POLICY EXAMPLE

Will Anyone Be Able to Tell If Abiding by the Kyoto Protocol Affects Global Temperatures?

In December 1997, the United States government tentatively agreed at a United Nations meeting held in Kyoto, Japan, to reduce nationwide emissions of greenhouse gases by 7 percent below 1990 levels. This goal would be achieved by reducing the combustion of fossil fuels sufficiently to diminish emission levels in 2010 to 41 percent below where they would end up at current rates of emission growth. Although any estimates of the overall economic effects of the agreement are fraught with uncertainties, economists estimated that abiding by the agreement could reduce U.S. GDP growth by as much as 2.3 percentage points per year.

Scientists using a climate model developed at the National Center for Atmospheric Research also had trouble coming up with very precise estimates of the likely effect of the proposed emissions reduction on global temperatures. Their best estimate was that such a reduction in emissions might reduce planetary warming by 0.19 degree Celsius (0.32 degree Fahrenheit) over a 50-year period—a barely discernible reduction in the earth's potential warming trend. Another problem is that the networks of surface thermometers that scientists use to monitor the earth's overall average temperature are unable to differentiate such a small temperature change from normal year-to-year variations. Even accounting for improved temperature-measuring capabilities 50 years in the future, measuring the ultimate environmental impact of implementing the Kyoto Protocol on Greenhouse Emissions might prove impossible. Consequently, determining the marginal social benefit of emissions reductions, at least from a global-warming standpoint, may be impracticable.

For Critical Analysis

If the effects of greenhouse emission abatement on global temperatures are too hard to measure, how else might the marginal benefit of emission abatement be determined?

FAQ

Aren't carbon emissions polluting the atmosphere?

Not all of them. The earth's oceans absorb a third of all emissions of carbon emitted by autos, trucks, and other motorized vehicles. Recent studies indicate that as much as another fourth of all carbon emissions may be absorbed by the "North American carbon sink," consisting of the continent's forests and plants. This is more than the carbon output of the United States and Canada resulting from the burning of fossil fuels. Thus it is actually conceivable that North America may be contributing to a net reduction in the world's carbon levels. This further complicates measuring the marginal benefit of emission abatement limitations intended to slow global warming.

CONCEPTS IN BRIEF

- The marginal cost of cleaning up the environment rises as we get closer to 100 percent cleanliness. Indeed, it rises at an increasing rate.
- The marginal benefit of environmental cleanliness falls as we have more of it.
- The optimal quantity of pollution is the quantity at which the marginal cost of cleanup equals the marginal benefit of cleanup.
- Pollution abatement is a trade-off. We trade off goods and services for cleaner air and water, and vice versa.

COMMON PROPERTY

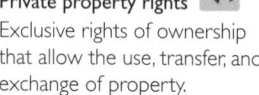

Private property rights
Exclusive rights of ownership that allow the use, transfer, and exchange of property.

Common property 
Property that is owned by everyone and therefore by no one. Air and water are examples of common property resources.

In most cases, you do not have **private property rights**—exclusive ownership rights—to the air surrounding you, nor does anyone else. Air is a **common property**—nonexclusive—resource. Therein lies the crux of the problem. When no one owns a particular resource, no one has any incentive (conscience aside) to consider misuse of that resource. If one person decides not to pollute the air, there normally will be no significant effect on the total level of pollution. If one person decides not to pollute the ocean, there will still be approximately the same amount of ocean pollution—provided, of course, that the individual was previously responsible for only a small part of the total amount of ocean pollution.

Basically, pollution occurs where we have poorly defined private property rights, as in air and common bodies of water. We do not, for example, have a visual pollution problem in people's attics. That is their own property, which they choose to keep as clean as they want, given their preferences for cleanliness as weighed against the costs of keeping the attic neat and tidy.

Where private property rights exist, individuals have legal recourse to any damages sustained through the misuse of their property. When private property rights are well defined, the use of property—that is, the use of resources—will generally involve contracting between the owners of those resources. If you own land, you might contract with another person who wants to use your land for raising cows. The contract would most likely be written in the form of a lease agreement.

INTERNATIONAL POLICY EXAMPLE

Dead Dogs in the Hills of Italy

Each September, about 110 miles north of Rome, a truffle hunt breaks out across 1,000 square miles of public land. Some 1,833 licensed "hunters" try their luck at finding truffles (a rare and hence expensive edible fungus), which grow wild on the buried roots of various trees. Truffle hunters use trained dogs to sniff out the hidden treasure. Each year, some of those dogs do not survive the truffle-hunting season. They are poisoned by bits of meat laced with strychnine—placed there by other truffle hunters seeking to reduce competition. In a recent year, more than 50 dogs died this way. The number of dogs poisoned turns out to be directly related to the market price of white Italian truffles. Several years ago, owing to a dry summer, the truffle crop dropped in half, the market price skyrocketed—and the number of dogs poisoned doubled from the previous year. Clearly, if the public land on which the truffles grow were not common property, the situation would be different.

For Critical Analysis

Assume that you owned all of the land in which Italian truffles grew. What system would you use for harvesting each year's crop?

Voluntary Agreements and Transaction Costs

Is it possible for externalities to be internalized via voluntary agreement? Take a simple example. You live in a house with a nice view of a lake. The family living below you plants a tree. The tree grows so tall that it eventually starts to cut off your view. In most cities, no one has property rights to views; therefore, you cannot usually go to court to obtain relief. You do have the option of contracting with your neighbor, however.

Voluntary Agreements: Contracting. You have the option of paying your neighbors (contracting) to cut back the tree. You could start out with an offer of a small amount and keep going up until your neighbors agree or until you reach your limit. Your limit will equal the value you place on having an unobstructed view of the lake. Your neighbors will be willing if the payment is at least equal to the reduction in their intrinsic property value due to a stunted tree. Your offering the payment makes your neighbors aware of the social cost of their actions. The social cost here is equal to the care of the tree plus the cost suffered by you from an impeded view of the lake.

In essence, then, your offer of money income to your neighbors indicates to them that there is an opportunity cost to their actions. If they don't comply, they forfeit the money that you are offering them. The point here is that *opportunity cost always exists, whoever has property rights.* Therefore, we would expect under some circumstances that voluntary contracting will occur to internalize externalities.* The question is, When will voluntary agreements occur?

Transaction Costs. One major condition for the outcome just outlined is that the **transaction costs**—all costs associated with making and enforcing agreements—must be low relative to the expected benefits of reaching an agreement. (We already looked at this

Transaction costs 
All costs associated with making, reaching, and enforcing agreements.

*This analysis is known as the *Coase theorem,* named after its originator, Nobel laureate Ronald Coase, who demonstrated that negative or positive externalities do not necessarily require government intervention in situations in which property rights are defined and enforceable and transaction costs are relatively low.

topic briefly in Chapter 4.) If we expand our example to a much larger one such as air pollution, the transaction costs of numerous homeowners trying to reach agreements with the individuals and companies that create the pollution are relatively high. Consequently, we don't expect voluntary contracting to be an effective way to internalize the externality of air pollution.

Changing Property Rights

In considering the problem of property rights, we can approach it by assuming that initially in a society, many property rights to resources are not defined. But this situation does not cause a problem so long as no one cares to use the resources for which there are no property rights or so long as enough of these resources are available that people can have as much as they want at a zero price. Only when and if a use is found for a resource or the supply of a resource is inadequate at a zero price does a problem develop. The problem requires that something be done about deciding property rights. If not, the resource will be wasted and possibly even destroyed. Property rights can be assigned to individuals who will then assert control; or they may be assigned to government, which can maintain and preserve the resource, charge for its use, or implement some other rationing device. What we have seen with common property such as air and water is that governments have indeed attempted to take over the control of those resources so that they cannot be wasted or destroyed.

Another way of viewing the pollution problem is to argue that property rights are "sacred" and that there are property rights in every resource that exists. We can then say that each individual does not have the right to act on anything that is not his or her property. Hence no individual has the right to pollute because that amounts to using property that the individual does not specifically own.

Clearly, we must fill the gap between private costs and social costs in situations in which property rights are not well defined or assigned. There are three ways to fill this gap: taxation, subsidization, and regulation. Government is involved in all three. Unfortunately, government does not have perfect information and may not pick the appropriate tax, subsidy, or type of regulation. We also have to consider cases in which taxes are hard to enforce or subsidies are difficult to give out to "worthy" recipients. In such cases, outright prohibition of the polluting activity may be the optimal solution to a particular pollution problem. For example, if it is difficult to monitor the level of a particular type of pollution that even in small quantities can cause severe environmental damage, outright prohibition of activities that cause such pollution may be the only alternative.

Are There Alternatives to Pollution-Causing Resource Use?

Some people cannot understand why, if pollution is bad, we still use pollution-causing resources such as coal and oil to generate electricity. Why don't we forgo the use of such polluting resources and opt for one that apparently is pollution free, such as solar energy? The plain fact is that the cost of generating solar power in most circumstances is much higher than generating that same power through conventional means. We do not yet have the technology that allows us the luxury of driving solar-powered cars. Moreover, with current technology, the solar panels necessary to generate the electricity for the average town would cover massive sections of the countryside, and the manufacturing of those solar panels would itself generate pollution.

WILD SPECIES, COMMON PROPERTY, AND TRADE-OFFS

One of the most distressing common property problems concerns endangered species, usually in the wild. No one is too concerned about not having enough dogs, cats, cattle, sheep, and horses. The reason is that virtually all of those species are private property. Spotted owls, bighorn mountain sheep, condors, and the like are typically common property. No one has a vested interest in making sure that they perpetuate in good health.

Click here to contemplate the issue of endangered species.

The federal government passed the Endangered Species Act in an attempt to prevent species from dying out. Initially, few individuals were affected by the rulings of the Interior Department regarding which species were listed as endangered. Eventually, however, as more and more species were put on the endangered list, a trade-off became apparent. Nationwide, the trade-off was brought to the public's attention when the spotted owl was declared an endangered species in the Pacific Northwest. Ultimately, thousands of logging jobs were lost when the courts upheld the ban on logging in the areas presumed to be the spotted owl's natural habitat. Then another small bird, the marbled murrelet, was found in an ancient forest, causing the Pacific Lumber Company to cut back its logging practices. In 1995, the U.S. Supreme Court ruled that the federal government did have the right to regulate activities on private land in order to save endangered species.

The issues are not straightforward. Today, the earth has only 0.02 percent of all of the species that have ever lived, and nearly all the 99.08 percent of extinct species became extinct *before* humans appeared. Every year, 1,000 to 3,000 new species are discovered and classified. Estimates of how many species are actually dying out vary from a high of 50,000 a year (based on an assumption that undiscovered insect species are dying off before being discovered) to a low of one every four years.

INTERNATIONAL POLICY EXAMPLE

Preventing Overfishing by Trading Quotas

Under the European Union's Common Fisheries Policy, countries are allocated quotas for the amounts of different kinds of fish that their fishermen can catch in various areas of the sea. In most European nations, governments control the allocation of fishing rights under these quotas. When a fisherman retires or dies, his quota goes into a pool to be reallocated. In the United Kingdom, however, fishermen can buy, sell, or lease their quotas. It turns out that this has had beneficial side effects for fish conservation.

The reason is that because many fishermen would like to catch more fish than their quotas permit them to catch, there is always a temptation to exceed quota limits. If a British fisherman thinks that he is more efficient at hauling in fish than another fisherman, he can buy or lease the other fisherman's quota. If he is right, he earns higher profits than he would by overfishing and trying to sell his excess catch (which the fishermen call "black fish") illegally in the black market.

Indeed, many British fishermen might be pleased if the European Union were to cut quotas in a further effort to repopulate stocks of fish. Their current incomes would fall, but the market value of their quotas would rise. The values of quotas are already relatively high. When a tragic accident recently led to the sinking of a fishing boat off the coast of Scotland, the deceased owner's quotas for herring, mackerel, and other fish sold for about $10 million.

For Critical Analysis

How does the existence of a market for quotas help keep the stocks of fish off the shores of Europe from dwindling?

CONCEPTS IN BRIEF

- A common property resource is one that no one owns—or, otherwise stated, that everyone owns.
- Common property exists when property rights are indefinite or nonexistent.
- When no property rights exist, pollution occurs because no one individual or firm has a sufficient economic incentive to care for the common property in question, be it air, water, or scenery.
- Private costs will not equal social costs when common property is at issue unless only a few individuals are involved and they are able to contract among themselves.

RECYCLING 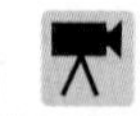

Recycling 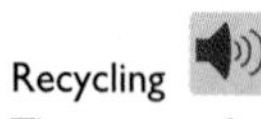
The reuse of raw materials derived from manufactured products.

As part of the overall ecology movement, there has been a major push to save scarce resources via recycling. **Recycling** involves reusing paper products, plastics, glass, and metals rather than putting them into solid waste dumps. Many cities have instituted mandatory recycling programs.

The benefits of recycling are straightforward. Fewer *natural* resources are used. But some economists argue that recycling does not necessarily save *total* resources. For example, recycling paper products may not necessarily save trees, according to A. Clark Wiseman, an economist for Resources for the Future in Washington, D.C. He argues that an increase in paper recycling will eventually lead to a reduction in the demand for virgin paper and thus for trees. Because most trees are planted specifically to produce paper, a reduction in the demand for trees will mean that certain land now used to grow trees will be put to other uses. The end result may be smaller rather than larger forests, a result that is probably not desired in the long run.

Recycling's Invisible Costs

The recycling of paper can also pollute. Used paper has ink on it that has to be removed during the recycling process. According to the National Wildlife Federation, the product of 100 tons of deinked (bleached) fiber generates 40 tons of sludge. This sludge has to be disposed of, usually in a landfill. A lot of recycled paper companies, however, are beginning to produce unbleached paper. In general, recycling does create waste that has to be disposed of.

There is another issue involved in the use of resources: Recycling requires human effort. The labor resources involved in recycling are often many times more costly than the potential savings in scarce resources not used. That means that net resource use, counting all resources, may sometimes be greater with recycling than without it.

Landfills

One of the arguments in favor of recycling is to avoid a solid waste "crisis." Some people believe that we are running out of solid waste dump sites in the United States. This is perhaps true in and near major cities, and indeed the most populated areas of the country might ultimately benefit from recycling programs. In the rest of the United States, however, the data do not seem to indicate that we are running out of solid waste landfill sites. Throughout the United States, the disposal price per ton of city garbage has actually fallen. Prices vary, of course, for the 200 million tons of trash disposed of each year. In San Jose, California, it costs $50 a ton to dump, whereas in Morris County, New Jersey, it costs $131 a ton.

Currently, municipal governments can do three things with solid waste: burn it, bury it, or recycle it. The amount of solid waste dumped in landfills is dropping, even as total trash output rises. Consider, though, that the total garbage output of the United States for the entire twenty-first century could be put in a square landfill 35 miles on a side that is 100 yards deep. Recycling to reduce solid waste disposal may end up costing society more resources simply because putting such waste into a landfill may be a less costly alternative.

INTERNATIONAL POLICY EXAMPLE

Can Citizens Recycle Too Much? The Case of Germany

Recycling is popular throughout the European Union, but the Germans have raised it to an art form—a very expensive art form. Germany has a law requiring that manufacturers or retailers take back their packaging or ensure that 80 percent of it is collected rather than thrown away. What is collected must be recycled or reused. The law covers about 40 percent of the country's garbage. The problem is that German consumers responded more enthusiastically than anticipated. The administrative costs of the program run by the company in charge of recycling Germany's trash, Duales System Deutschland, have ballooned to more than $2 billion, and these funds are raised through licensing fees paid by manufacturers and retailers, who pass some of these additional costs on to consumers in the form of higher prices. Public dissatisfaction has encouraged competition to emerge. The Lahn-Dill district in the German state of Hessen recently implemented a new waste-processing program that can handle nearly as many recyclables at about half the expense. One of Lahn-Dill's biggest cost-saving features is a simple rule common in the United States: requiring citizens themselves to sort through their garbage and place recyclables in a separate container.

For Critical Analysis

How is it possible that German citizens might have recycled "too much" of their trash?

Should We Save Scarce Resources?

Periodically, the call for recycling focuses on the necessity of saving scarce resources because "we are running out." There is little evidence to back up this claim because virtually every natural resource has fallen in price (corrected for inflation) over the past century. In 1980, the late Julian Simon made a $1,000 bet with well-known environmentalist Paul Erlich. Simon bet $200 per resource that any five natural resources that Erlich picked would decline in price (corrected for inflation) by the end of the 1980s. Simon won. (When Simon asked Erlich to renew the bet for $20,000 for the 1990s, Erlich declined.) During the 1980s and 1990s, the price of virtually every natural resource fell (corrected for inflation), and so did the price of every agricultural commodity. The same was true for every forest product. Though few people remember the dire predictions of the 1970s, many noneconomists throughout the world argued at that time that the world's oil reserves were vanishing. If this were true, the pretax, inflation-corrected price of gasoline would not be the same today as it was in the 1950s (which it is).

In spite of predictions in the early 1980s by World Watch Institute president Lester Brown, real food prices did not rise. Indeed, the real price of food fell by more than 30 percent for the major agricultural commodities during the 1980s and even more during the 1990s. A casual knowledge of supply and demand tells you that because the demand for food did not decrease, supply must have increased faster than demand.

With respect to the forests, at least in the United States and Western Europe, there are more forests today than there were 100 years ago. In this country, the major problems of deforestation seem to be on land owned by the United States Forest Service for which private timber companies are paid almost $1 billion a year in subsidies to cut down trees.

EXAMPLE

Earning Profits from Conserving Natural Wonders

In Virginia's Shenandoah Valley, 230 miles southwest of Washington, D.C., stands a 215-foot-tall rock arch called Natural Bridge. A tributary of the James River flows beneath. A 347-foot cavern lies inside a park surrounding Natural Bridge. The 1,600-acre park receives about 300,000 visitors per year. This park has been in private hands since 1774, when Thomas Jefferson paid King George III 20 shillings for it. Today, the park belongs to Natural Bridge of Virginia, Inc., a private company controlled by a Washington, D.C., real estate developer who purchased it in 1988 for $6.6 million. The reason he paid so much is that the park earns a tidy annual profit, estimated at about $5 million. A park visitor pays $8 to see the bridge and another $7 for a tour of a cave and a wax museum. A visitor also can buy souvenirs at park shops, purchase food at one or more of its three on-site restaurants, and pay to stay in one of the park's 180 guest rooms. To attract these profit-generating visitors, the company pays close attention to details. It pays botanists to plant and care for native plants, and it stocks the river with rainbow trout. The park is kept free of graffiti; the last known person to carve his initials into Natural Bridge was a young surveyor by the name of George Washington.

Some economists have argued that lands currently owned by the government and administered by state and national park services might receive better long-term care if they were privately owned and administered instead. Natural Bridge is one example of a part of the environment that the profit motive is helping to preserve.

For Critical Analysis

Why does the profit motive encourage environmental conservation efforts at a private park?

CONCEPTS IN BRIEF

- Recycling involves reusing paper, glass, and other materials rather than putting them into solid waste dumps. Recycling does have a cost both in the resources used for recycling and in the pollution created during recycling, such as the sludge from deinking paper for reuse.
- Landfills are an alternative to recycling. Expansion of these solid waste disposal sites is outpacing demand increases.
- Resources may not be getting scarcer. The inflation-corrected price of most resources has been falling for decades.

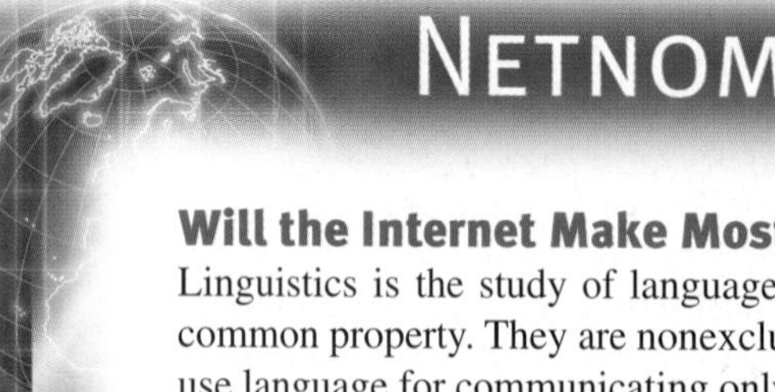

NETNOMICS

Will the Internet Make Most Languages Obsolete?

Linguistics is the study of languages and their structure. By their nature, languages are common property. They are nonexclusive resources. In some instances, of course, we may use language for communicating only with ourselves, such as when we take notes for later reference. For the most part, however, we use language to communicate with others.

Today, the Internet is emerging as one of the world's key communications media. Roughly 80 percent of all information stored on the world's computers is in English. The same proportion of Internet transmissions—e-mail messages, file transfers, and the like—are in English. This has added to existing incentives for non-English speakers around the globe to learn English. Berlitz International, the world's largest language school, reports that 70 percent of the 5 million language lessons it gives each year are for English. Many experts today argue that English is now such an intrinsic part of the global communications revolution that its dominance is unassailable. This has led some to worry about loss of national identities as English "replaces" other languages. A former French president went so far as to call the Internet "a major risk for humanity."

In fact, there are good economic reasons to believe that global use of the Internet could actually *improve* the odds that many languages will survive the onslaught from English. Because they rely on one-way transmissions, broadcast media such as television and radio force languages to compete. For instance, the time that a European transmission of a *Star Wars* movie dubbed in Danish takes on a given bandwidth could instead be devoted to transmission of the original English version, which more people could understand, thereby increasing the chances that advertisers will reach more customers. In cyberspace, however, transmissions in various languages do not compete directly. Promoters of a Danish rock festival can post Internet advertisements for the festival in English, but they can also post them in Danish, as well as German Norwegian, Swedish, and any other language whose speakers might be interested.

Ultimately, the languages that survive will do so because of gains in specialization. People will continue to use their native language when they want to communicate with others who share that tongue, whether across a shared fence, in local newspapers, or via Internet chat rooms. They will use other languages, such as English today, primarily for formal communications with others around the globe. In the process, the "professional" version of English itself could begin to diverge from traditional English. Someday, English speakers may even have to know two languages: the English they read and speak at home and the "techie English" they use in their Web-based communications.

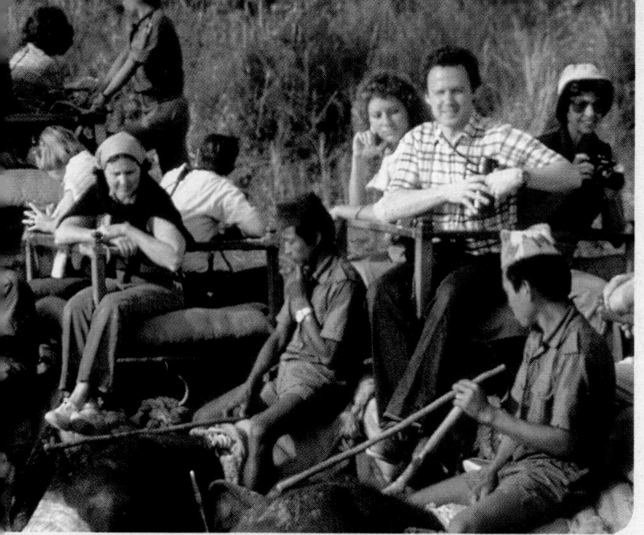

ISSUES & APPLICATIONS

What Mix of Economic Incentives Will Save the Tiger?

The tiger's worldwide population has declined by almost 93 percent during the past 100 years. Trying to understand why this has occurred, and determining how to stop it from continuing, requires thinking about economic incentives.

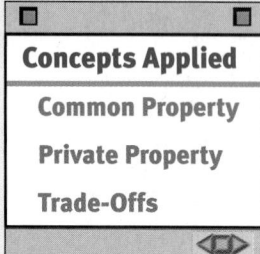

The Private Incentives All Point Toward Tiger Extinction

If you have ever viewed tigers at a zoo, you probably noticed that the zoo's operators designed the exhibit so that both space and iron bars separated you from the tigers. There is a reason for this. Tigers are natural predators. They are very good at killing other animals, including humans. In their natural habitats in nations such as India, Indonesia, and Nepal, wild tigers frequently attack and kill both livestock and the animals' owners. This gives people who live near tigers powerful incentives to kill the giant felines, either in acts of self-defense or as "preemptive strikes." Furthermore, several highly prized traditional East Asian medicines use powder from the bones of tigers as a prime ingredient. As a result, tiger bones command high prices on the black market, providing yet another incentive to destroy these creatures. In the private marketplace, private benefits derive mainly from tiger deaths, not tiger population enhancement.

Are There Market Solutions for Repopulating Tigers?

Nearly anyone who has seen a tiger, however, would agree that they are beautiful animals. Society, therefore, might determine that the species is a form of common property that should be preserved. The issue is how best to change human incentives. So far bans on hunting and set-asides of public lands have not succeeded.

There are at least four possible changes that might promote tiger repopulation. All entail giving people incentives.

1. *Private property rights:* South Africa already has adopted a private property law to protect the rhinoceros. Conservationists who own private reserves naturally wish to keep the animals on their reserves alive. They are also often more successful than governments, who face competing demands for public moneys, at raising funds specifically aimed at supporting and caring for animals on their lands.
2. *Promoting trourism:* In 1995, Nepal's government gave a local group land management rights in a tiger habitat adjoining a national park. Local residents build nature trails for elephant-back safaris and a viewing tower with hotel accommodations for overnight guests. Income generated from tiger-based tourism helps fund education and health care for local residents—giving them strong incentives to protect the tigers on their reserve.

3. *Limited hunting:* Selling rights to hunt endangered animals to people who have always dreamed of big game hunting may seem counterproductive—after all, the hunters kill the animals, don't they? Nevertheless, South Africa has turned this into a trade-off that ultimately helps white rhinos. Fees paid by white rhino hunters, amounting to hundreds of thousands of dollars a year, are used to help preserve the species as a whole. The same approach could work for tigers.
4. *Legalized farming:* Unlike some animals, tigers breed readily in captivity. Farmers could breed tigers for eventual sale of their bones. This would drive down the price of tiger bones, greatly reducing the incentive for illegal poaching.

FOR CRITICAL ANALYSIS

1. Which people would stand to lose the most from legalized tiger farming?
2. Which of these proposals might help protect endangered aquatic species?

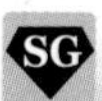

SUMMARY DISCUSSION OF LEARNING OBJECTIVES

1. **Private Costs Versus Social Costs:** Private, or internal, costs are borne solely by individuals who use resources. Social costs are the full costs that society bears whenever resources are used. Pollution problems and other problems related to the environment arise when individuals take into account only private costs instead of the broader social costs arising from their use of resources.
2. **Market Externalities and Ways to Correct Them:** A market externality is a situation in which a private cost (or benefit) differs from the social cost (or benefit) associated with a market transaction between two parties or from use of a scarce resource. Correcting an externality arising from differences between private and social costs, such as pollution, requires forcing individuals to take all the social costs of their actions into account. This might be accomplished by taxing those who create externalities, such as polluters.
3. **Determining the Optimal Amount of Pollution:** The marginal benefit of pollution abatement, or the additional benefit to society from reducing pollution, declines as the quality of the environment improves. At the same time, however, the marginal cost of pollution abatement, or the additional cost to society from reducing pollution, increases as more and more resources are devoted to bringing about an improved environment. The optimal quantity of pollution is the amount of pollution for which the marginal benefit of pollution abatement just equals the marginal cost of pollution abatement. Beyond this level of pollution, the additional cost of cleaning the environment exceeds the additional benefit.
4. **Private and Common Property Rights and the Pollution Problem:** Private property rights are exclusive individual rights of ownership that permit the use and exchange of a resource. Common property is owned by everyone and therefore by no single individual. A pollution problem often arises because air and many water resources are common property, and private property rights relating to them are not well defined. Therefore, no one has an individual incentive to take the long-run pernicious effects of excessive pollution into account. This is a common rationale for using taxes, subsidies, or regulations to address the pollution problem.
5. **Endangered Species and the Assignment of Property Rights:** Many members of such species as dogs, pigs, and horses are the private property of human beings. Thus people have economic incentives—satisfaction derived from pet ownership, the desire for pork as a food product, a preference for animal-borne transport—to protect members of these species. By contrast, most members of species such as spotted owls, condors, or tigers are common property, so no specific individuals have incentives to keep these species in good health. One way to address the endangered species problem is government involvement via taxes, subsidies, or regulations. Another is to find a way to assign private property rights to at least some members of species that are endangered.
6. **Benefits and Costs of Recycling:** Recycling entails reusing paper, glass, and other materials instead of putting them in solid waste dumps. Recycling has a clear benefit of limiting the use of natural resources. It also entails costs, however. One cost might be lost benefits of forests, because a key incentive for perpetuating forests is the future production of paper and other wood-based products. Recycling also requires the use of labor, and the costs of these human resources can exceed the potential savings in scarce resources not used because of recycling.

Key Terms and Concepts

Common property (766)
Externality (761)
Optimal quantity of pollution (765)
Private costs (760)
Private property rights (766)
Recycling (770)
Social costs (761)
Transaction costs (767)

Problems

Answers to the odd-numbered problems appear at the back of the book.

31-1. The market price of insecticide is initially $10 per unit. To address a negative externality in this market, the government decides to charge producers of insecticide for the privilege of polluting during the production process. A fee that fully takes into account the social costs of pollution is determined, and once it is put into effect, the market supply curve for insecticide shifts upward by $4 per unit. The market price of insecticide also increases, to $12 per unit. What is the fee that the government is charging insecticide manufacturers?

31-2. A tract of land is found to contain a plant from which drug companies can extract a newly discovered cancer-fighting medicine. This variety of plant does not grow anywhere else in the world. Initially, the many owners of lots within this tract, who had not planned to use the land for anything other than its current use as a scenic locale for small vacation homes, announced that they would put all their holdings up for sale to drug companies. Because the land is also home to an endangered lizard species, however, a government agency decides to limit the number of acres in this tract that drug companies can purchase and use for their drug-producing operations. The government declares that the remaining portion of the land must be left in its current state. What will happen to the market price of the acreage that is available for extraction of cancer-fighting medicine? What will happen to the market price of the land that the government declares to be usable only for existing vacation homes?

31-3. When a government charges firms for the privilege of polluting, a typical result is a rise in the market price of the good or service produced by those firms. Consequently, consumers of the good or service usually have to pay a higher price to obtain it. Why might this be socially desirable?

31-4. Most wild Asian tigers are the common property of the humans and governments that control the lands they inhabit. Why does this pose a significant problem for maintaining the wild tiger population in the future?

31-5. In several African countries where the rhinoceros was once a prevalent species, the animal is now nearly extinct. In most of these nations, rhinoceros horns are used as traditional ingredients in certain medicines. Why might making rhinoceros farming legal do more to promote preservation of the species than imposing stiff penalties on people who are caught engaging in rhinoceros hunting?

31-6. Why is it possible for recycling of paper or plastics to use up more resources than the activity saves?

31-7. Examine the following marginal costs and marginal benefits associated with water cleanliness in a given locale.

Quantity of Clean Water (%)	Marginal Cost ($)	Marginal Benefit ($)
0	3,000	200,000
20	15,000	120,000
40	50,000	90,000
60	85,000	85,000
80	100,000	40,000
100	Infinite	0

a. What is the optimal degree of water cleanliness?

b. What is the optimal degree of water pollution?

c. Suppose that a company creates a food additive that offsets most of the harmful effects of drinking polluted water. As a result, the marginal benefit of water cleanliness declines by $40,000 at each degree of water cleanliness at or less than 80 percent. What is the optimal degree of water cleanliness after this change?

31-8. Examine the following marginal costs and marginal benefits associated with air cleanliness in a given locale:

Quantity of Clean Air (%)	Marginal Cost ($)	Marginal Benefit ($)
0	50,000	600,000
20	150,000	360,000
40	200,000	200,000
60	300,000	150,000
80	400,000	120,000
100	Infinite	0

a. What is the optimal degree of air cleanliness?
b. What is the optimal degree of air pollution?
c. Suppose that a state provides subsidies for a company to build plants that contribute to air pollution. Cleaning up this pollution causes the marginal cost of air cleanliness to rise by$210,000 at each degree of water cleanliness. What is the optimal degree of air cleanliness after this change?

31-9. The following table displays hypothetical annual total costs and total benefits of conserving wild tigers at several possible worldwide tiger population levels.

Population of Wild Tigers	Total Cost ($ million)	Total Benefit ($ million)
0	0	40
2,000	5	90
4,000	15	130
6,000	30	160
8,000	55	185
10,000	90	205
12,000	140	215

a. Calculate the marginal costs and benefits.
b. Given the data, what is the socially optimal world population of wild tigers?
c. Suppose that tiger farming is legalized and that this has the effect of reducing the marginal cost of tiger conservation by $15 million for each 2,000-tiger population increment in the table. What is the new socially optimal population of wild tigers?

Economics on the Net

Economic Analysis at the Environmental Protection Agency In this chapter, you learned how to use economic analysis to think about environmental problems. Does the U.S. government use economic analysis? This application helps you learn the extent to which the government uses economics in its environmental policymaking.

Title: The Environmental Protection Agency: Environmental Economics Research at the EPA

Navigation: Click here to visit the EPA's homepage. Click on Browse EPA Topics, then Economics, and finally on Economy and the Environment. Select Other Information, then Environmental Economics in Plain English. Click on Regulatory Economic Analysis at the EPA and view the table of contents. Read the Introduction.

Application Read this section of the article; then answer the following questions:

1. According to the article, what are the key objectives of the EPA? What role does cost-benefit analysis appear to play in the EPA's efforts? Does the EPA appear to take other issues into account in its policymaking?

2. Back up to Table of Contents, and in Section 1: Introduction, click on Statutory Authorities for Economic Analysis. In what ways does this discussion help clarify your answers in item 1?

For Group Study and Analysis Have a class discussion of the following question: Should the EPA apply economic analysis in all aspects of its policymaking? If not, why not? If so, in what manner should economic analysis be applied?

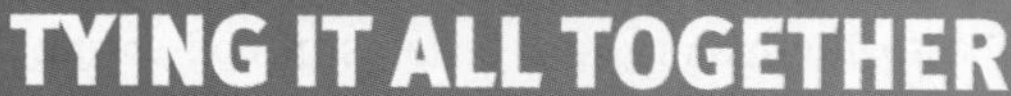

TYING IT ALL TOGETHER

Part 7 Case Problem

Case Background

Modular Systems, Inc. (MSI), manufacturers and sells four products for personal computers: modems, diskette drives, CD-ROM drives, and DVD drives. Until now its workforce has not been unionized. Recently, however, professional union organizers from two unions have held meetings with a large portion of MSI's employees.

The Derived Demands for Labor at a Firm That Sells Multiple Products MSI has separate plants for each of the four products it produces, and its workforce is divided among these four facilities. Workers rarely move from one plant to another. The markets for modems and diskette drives contain large numbers of buyers and sellers, and MSI competes for labor with a number of other manufacturers of modems and diskette drives.

MSI is the only producer and seller of a new external, wireless-connection CD-ROM drive. It competes with many other manufacturers of CD-ROM drives for workers, however. MSI is also the only producer and seller of a new external, wireless-connection DVD drive. The employees that have developed and now manufacture this product have highly specialized skills, and they have found that many potential employers regard them as overspecialized. Consequently, those who have interviewed for jobs with other DVD drive manufacturers have not received job offers. For these workers, MSI is their only good match for jobs, at least in the near term. Recently, some workers in the company's DVD drive facility staged a work slowdown to express their displeasure with what they perceive to be low pay for their highly specialized skills in developing MSI's new DVD drive product offering. They are particularly unhappy that they earn lower wages than workers in MSI's other three facilities. They are also disgruntled about recent company layoffs of a few workers who have had trouble finding jobs in any industry because of the region's faltering economic climate.

MSI is located in a union shop state. In contrast to the experience of much of the rest of the country, the state's economy has faltered in recent months, which has reduced the overall demand for labor on the part of most other employers in the state.

One complication arose when the two union organizers conducted their visits with MSI's employees in successive weeks. The second visitor disputed the first organizer's claim that her union is the "better fit" for MSI's workers and hence should have the first opportunity to conduct a unionization vote.

Determining the Appropriate Company Response MSI's owners and managers were shocked by the recent work slowdown in the DVD drive facility. They decide that the company should contemplate the following options:

1. No response whatsoever
2. Attempting to convince employees that wages are stagnant because of the recent weakening in economic conditions within the state

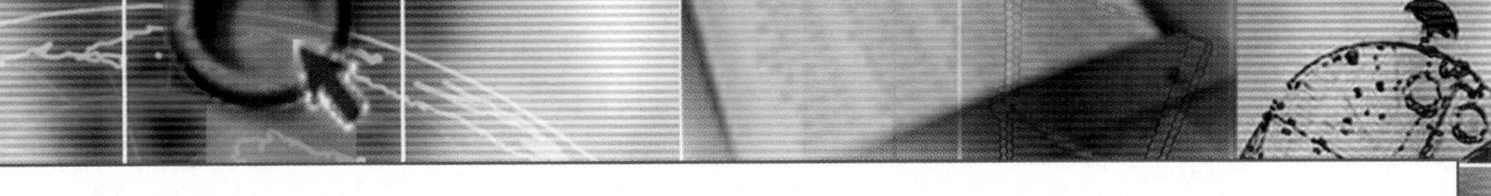

3. Separate meetings of senior management with the workers in each plant to allow the workers to air their grievances and to discuss steps the company might take to address them
4. Turning each facility into a separate company owned by an umbrella corporation, in the hope that workers in at least two of the current facilities would vote not to unionize the new companies
5. Moving its operations to a right-to-work state
6. Making a dramatic change in how the company compensates its workers, including one or all of the following: (a) improving worker health benefits; (b) offering company-subsidized child care at each of its manufacturing facilities; (c) offering employee stock ownership plans, bonus plans, and other forms of company profit sharing

Points to Analyze

1. In which of the markets for its products is MSI more likely to be a perfectly competitive firm? In which is it more likely to be a monopolist?
2. In which of its facilities is it more likely that MSI employees supply their time and skills in perfectly competitive labor markets? In monopsonistic labor markets?
3. Could MSI's management make a case that weak economic conditions help explain relatively low wages? Could the workers contend that this argument is contrived?
4. Workers are equally productive, and the per-unit price of each of the company's products happens to be the same. List each facility according to which is likely to employ the largest number of workers and which is likely to employ the fewest number.
5. What are the advantages and disadvantages of moving MSI's production facilities to a right-to-work state?
6. Which of the options for changing the company's compensation of its workers is most likely to help address the concerns of the DVD-drive workers? Why?

Casing the Internet

1. **Click here to go to the AFL-CIO's homepage. Click on "Partners and Links." Explore several of these Web sites; then answer the following questions.**
   a. **Does it appear that these unions are engaged in actively recruiting new members?**
   b. **Do you see any potential jurisdictional disputes that could arise as a result of efforts by these various unions to increase their memberships?**
2. **Click here to go to the homepage of the National Right to Work Legal Defense Foundation, Inc.**
   a. **Click on "About the Foundation," and then click on "Right to Work Frequently Asked Questions." Read this page. Do you see any regional concentration among the states that have right-to-work laws?**
   b. **In states without right-to-work laws, how much flexibility do workers have to avoid paying union dues and associated fees?**

Part 8
Global Economics

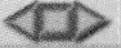

CHAPTER

32

COMPARATIVE ADVANTAGE AND THE OPEN ECONOMY

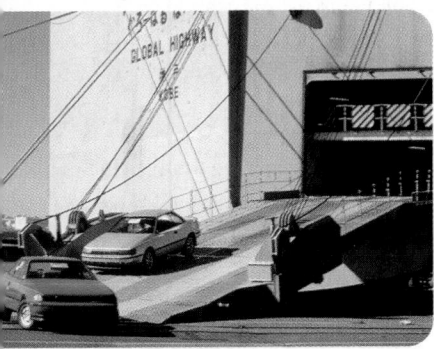

These cars built in Japan are being unloaded in Baltimore. Who would lose and who would gain if imports of Japanese cars were outlawed?

An American businessman visiting an emerging economy came upon a team of about 100 workers using shovels to move earth next to a stream. His guide told him that several days earlier, a local government agency had assigned the people to build a dam. Later, the businessman told a local official about a U.S. company that was offering discounts on earth-moving machines. "With such a machine," the businessman boasted, "one worker could build that dam in a single afternoon." The official replied, "Of course. But think of all the unemployment that importing such a machine would create." The businessman then said, "Oh, I thought you were building a dam. If it's jobs you want to create, take away the workers' shovels and give them spoons!"

In this chapter, you will learn that U.S. exports to other nations do not necessarily cause workers in those nations to lose their jobs or earn lower pay. Nor do American imports of goods from other nations necessitate *net* job losses or pay cuts in the United States. Nevertheless, workers in certain industries often unite with owners and managers to oppose free trade. In this chapter, you will learn the elements of international trade, as well as the arguments for and against free trade.

LEARNING OBJECTIVES

After reading this chapter, you should be able to:

1. Discuss the worldwide importance of international trade
2. Explain why nations can gain from specializing in production and engaging in international trade
3. Distinguish between comparative advantage and absolute advantage
4. Understand common arguments against free trade
5. Describe ways that nations restrict foreign trade
6. Identify key international agreements and organizations that adjudicate trade disputes among nations

Chapter Outline

- The Worldwide Importance of International Trade
- Why We Trade: Comparative Advantage and Mutual Gains from Exchange
- The Relationship Between Imports and Exports
- International Competitiveness
- Arguments Against Free Trade
- Ways to Restrict Foreign Trade

Did You Know That... most U.S. imports come from a few developed countries? In fact, about two-thirds of imported goods and services are produced in nations that economists classify as high-wage countries. Only 10 percent of U.S. imports come from countries classified as low-wage nations. The remainder of U.S. imports are produced in middle-income countries located mainly in Latin America and Southeast Asia.

The workers residing in nations from which Americans import most of their goods earn relatively high wages. Recent studies indicate that manufacturing wages paid to workers who live and work in twenty-five nations that engage in the most trade with the United States have have risen steadily. In 1975, manufacturing workers in these top U.S. trading partners earned 65 percent of the U.S. compensation level. Today, the wages of these workers have reached 95 percent of the U.S. compensation level.

Without international trade, many people who work to produce goods for sale to other nations would have to find other employment. Some might even have trouble finding work. Nevertheless, other people in these countries would undoubtedly stand to gain from restricting international trade. Learning about international trade will help you understand why this is so.

THE WORLDWIDE IMPORTANCE OF INTERNATIONAL TRADE

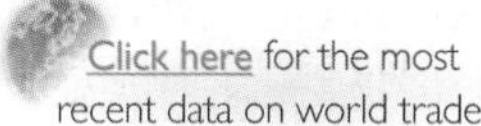
Click here for the most recent data on world trade.

Look at panel (a) of Figure 32-1. Since the end of World War II, world output of goods and services (world gross domestic product, or GDP) has increased almost every year until the present, when it is almost six times what it was. Look at the top line in panel (a). World trade has increased to more than 13 times what it was in 1950.

The United States figured prominently in this expansion of world trade. In panel (b) of Figure 32-1, you see imports and exports expressed as a percentage of total annual yearly income (GDP). Whereas imports added up to barely 4 percent of annual national income in 1950, today they account for over 12 percent. International trade has definitely become more important to the economy of the United States. Trade may become even more important in the United States as other countries start to loosen their trade restrictions.

INTERNATIONAL EXAMPLE

The Importance of International Trade in Various Countries

Whereas both imports and exports in the United States each account for more than 10 percent of total annual national income, in some countries the figure is much greater (see Table 32-1). Consider that Luxembourg must import practically everything!

Another way to understand the worldwide importance of international trade is to look at trade flows on the world map in Figure 32-2 on page 786. You can see that the United States trades more with Europe than with other parts of the world.

For Critical Analysis

How can Luxembourg have a strong economy if it imports so many goods and services?

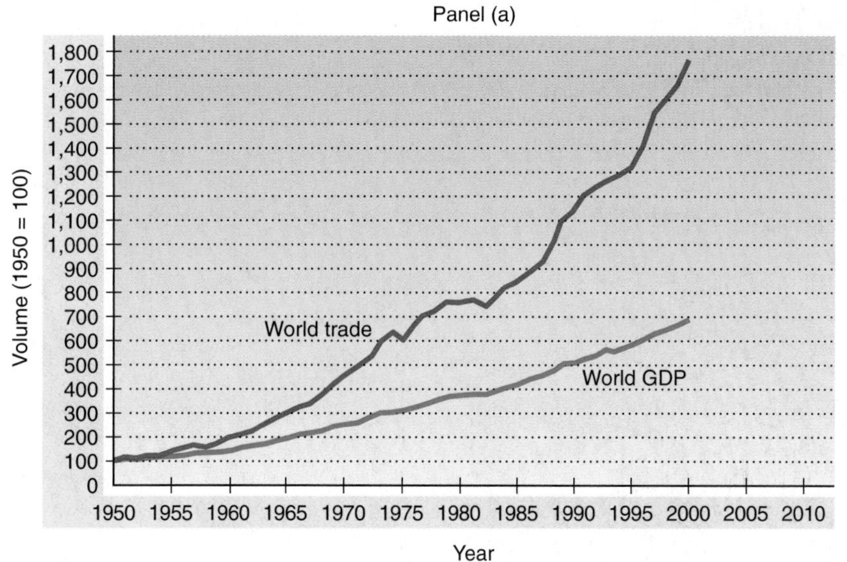

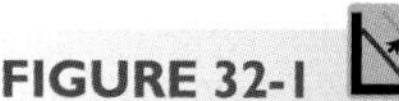

FIGURE 32-1

The Growth of World Trade

In panel (a), you can see the growth in world trade in relative terms because we use an index of 100 to represent real world trade in 1950. By the early 2000s, that index had increased to over 1,700. At the same time, the index of world GDP (annual world income) had gone up to only around 700. World trade is clearly on the rise: Both imports and exports, expressed as a percentage of annual national income (GDP) in panel (b), have been rising.

Sources: Steven Husted and Michael Melvin, *International Economics,* 3d ed. (New York: HarperCollins, 1995), p. 11, used with permission; World Trade Organization; Federal Reserve System; U.S. Department of Commerce.

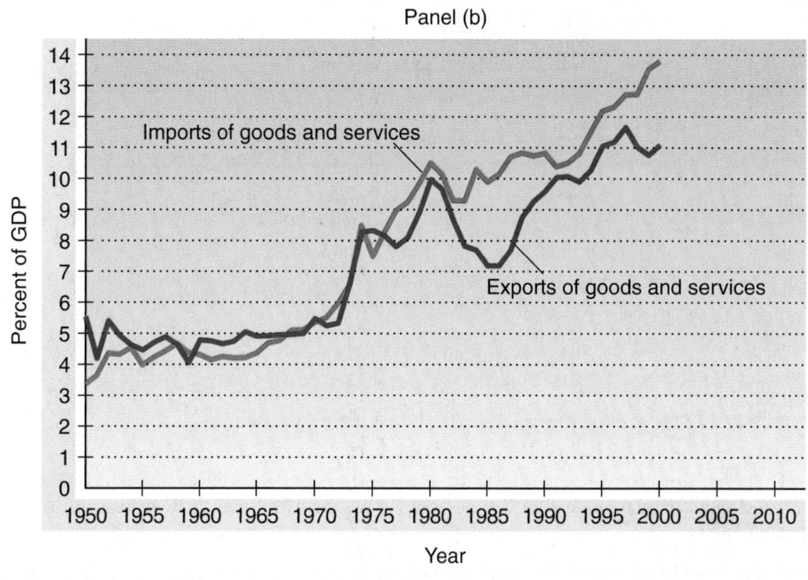

TABLE 32-1

Importance of Imports in Selected Countries

Residents of some nations spend much of their incomes on imported goods and services.

Country	Imports as a Percentage of Annual National Income
Luxembourg	95.0
Netherlands	58.0
Norway	30.0
Canada	23.5
Germany	23.0
United Kingdom	21.0
China	19.0
France	18.4
Japan	6.8

Source: International Monetary Fund.

FIGURE 32-2
World Trade Flows
International merchandise trade amounts to over $3 trillion worldwide. The percentage figures show the proportion of trade flowing in the various directions.
Source: World Trade Organization (data are for 2000).

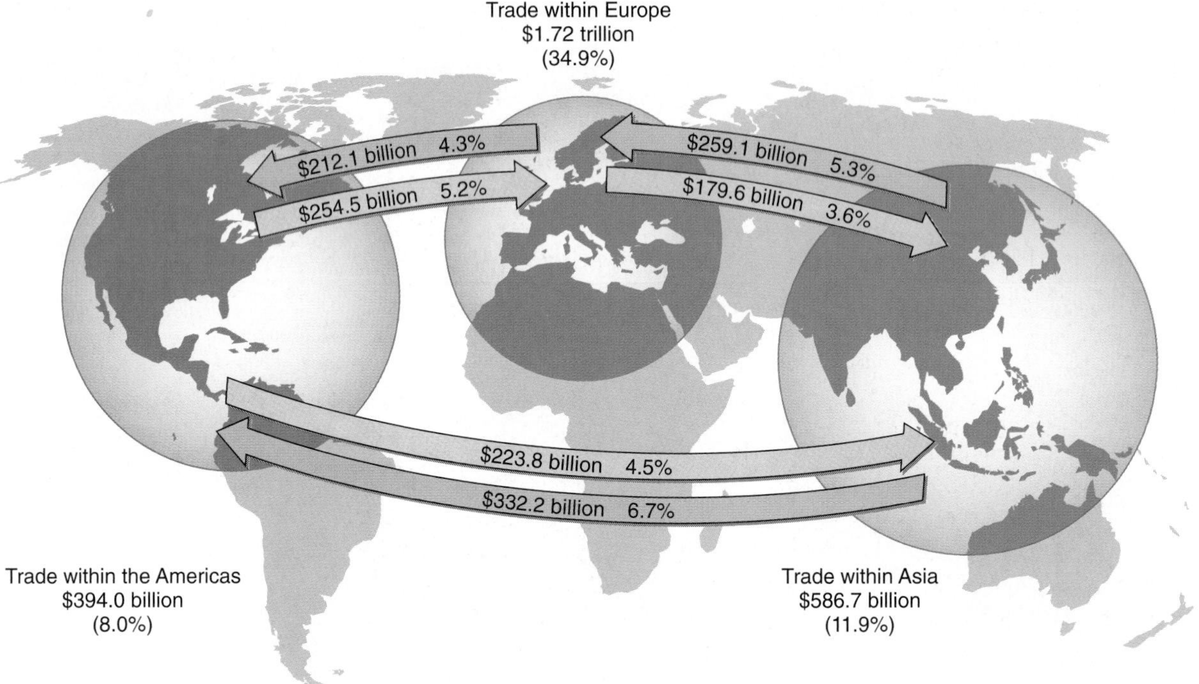

WHY WE TRADE: COMPARATIVE ADVANTAGE ANDMUTUAL GAINS FROM EXCHANGE

You have already been introduced to the concept of specialization and mutual gains from trade in Chapter 2. These concepts are worth repeating because they are essential to understanding why the world is better off because of more international trade. The best way to understand the gains from trade among nations is first to understand the output gains from specialization between individuals.

The Output Gains from Specialization 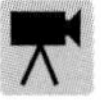

Suppose that a creative advertising specialist can come up with two pages of ad copy (written words) an hour or generate one computerized art rendering per hour. At the same time, a computer artist can write one page of ad copy per hour or complete one computerized art rendering per hour. Here the ad specialist can come up with more pages of ad copy per hour than the computer specialist and seemingly is just as good as the computer specialist at doing computerized art renderings. Is there any reason for the creative specialist and the computer specialist to "trade"? The answer is yes, because such trading will lead to higher output.

Consider the scenario of no trading. Assume that during each eight-hour day, the ad specialist and the computer whiz devote half of their day to writing ad copy and half to computerized art rendering. The ad specialist would create eight pages of ad copy (4 hours × 2) and four computerized art renderings (4 × 1). During that same period, the computer specialist would create four pages of ad copy (4 × 1) and four computerized art renderings (4 × 1). Each day, the combined output for the ad specialist and the computer specialist would be 12 pages of ad copy and eight computerized art renderings with no decline in art renderings.

Click here for data on U.S. trade with all other nations of the world.

If the ad specialist specialized only in writing ad copy and the computer whiz specialized only in creating computerized art renderings, their combined output would rise to 16 pages of ad copy (8 × 2) and eight computerized art renderings (8 × 1). Overall, production would increase by four pages of ad copy per day.

The creative advertising employee has a comparative advantage in writing ad copy, and the computer specialist has a comparative advantage in doing computerized art renderings. **Comparative advantage** derives from the ability to produce something at a lower opportunity cost than other producers, as we pointed out in Chapter 2.

Comparative advantage 
The ability to produce a good or service at a lower opportunity cost than other producers.

Specialization Among Nations

To demonstrate the concept of comparative advantage for nations, let's take the example of France and the United States. In Table 32-2, we show the comparative costs of production of wine and beer in terms of worker-days. This is a simple two-country, two-commodity world in which we assume that labor is the only factor of production. As you can see from the table, in the United States, it takes one worker-day to produce 1 liter of wine, and the same is true for 1 liter of beer. In France, it takes one worker-day to produce 1 liter of wine but two worker-days for 1 liter of beer. In this sense, Americans appear to be just as good at producing wine as the French and actually have an **absolute advantage** in producing beer.

Absolute advantage 
The ability to produce more output from given inputs of resources than other producers can.

Trade will still take place, however, which may seem paradoxical. How can trade take place if we can seemingly produce both goods at least as cheaply as the French can? Why don't we just produce both ourselves? To understand why, let's assume first that there is no trade and no specialization and that the workforce in each country consists of 200 workers. These 200 workers are, by assumption, divided equally in the production of wine and beer. We see in Table 32-3 on the next page that 100 liters of wine and 100 liters of beer are produced per day in the United States. In France, 100 liters of wine and 50 liters of beer are produced per day. The total daily world production in our two-country world is 200 liters of wine and150 liters of beer.

Now the countries specialize. What can France produce more cheaply? Look at the comparative costs of production expressed in worker-days in Table 32-2. What is the cost of producing 1 liter more of wine? One worker-day. What is the cost of producing 1 liter more of beer? Two worker-days. We can say, then, that in terms of the value of beer given up, in France the opportunity cost of producing wine is lower than in the United States. France will specialize in the activity that has the lower opportunity cost. In other words, France will specialize in its comparative advantage, which is the production of wine.

TABLE 32-2
Comparative Costs of Production

Product	United States (worker-days)	France (worker-days)
Wine (1 liter)	1	1
Beer (1 liter)	1	2

TABLE 32-3
Daily World Output Before Specialization
It is assumed that 200 workers are available in each country.

	United States		France		
Product	Workers	Output (liters)	Workers	Output (liters)	World Output (liters)
Wine	100	100	100	100	200
Beer	100	100	100	50	150

According to Table 32-4, after specialization, the United States produces 200 liters of beer and France produces 200 liters of wine. Notice that the total world production per day has gone up from 200 liters of wine and 150 liters of beer to 200 liters of wine and 200 liters of beer per day. This was done without any increased use of resources. The gain, 50 "free" liters of beer, results from a more efficient allocation of resources worldwide. World output is greater when countries specialize in producing the goods in which they have a comparative advantage and then engage in foreign trade. Another way of looking at this is to consider the choice between two ways of producing a good. Obviously, each country would choose the less costly production process. One way of "producing" a good is to import it, so if in fact the imported good is cheaper than the domestically produced good, we will "produce" it by importing it. Not everybody, of course, is better off when free trade occurs. In our example, U.S. wine makers and French beer makers are worse off because those two *domestic* industries have disappeared.

TABLE 32-4
Daily World Output After Specialization
It is assumed that 200 workers are available in each country.

	United States		France		
Product	Workers	Output (liters)	Workers	Output (liters)	World Output (liters)
Wine	—	—	200	200	200
Beer	200	200	—	—	200

Some people are worried that the United States (or any country, for that matter) might someday "run out of exports" because of overaggressive foreign competition. The analysis of comparative advantage tells us the contrary. No matter how much other countries compete for our business, the United States (or any other country) will always have a comparative advantage in something that it can export. In 10 or 20 years, that something may not be what we export today, but it will be exportable nonetheless because we will have a comparative advantage in producing it.

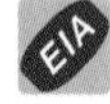

Why Do People Trade?
Practice applying the concepts of comparative and absolute advantage.

Other Benefits from International Trade: The Transmission of Ideas

Beyond the fact that comparative advantage results in an overall increase in the output of goods produced and consumed, there is another benefit to international trade. International trade bestows benefits on countries through the international transmission of ideas. According to economic historians, international trade has been the principal means by which new goods, services, and processes have spread around the world. For example, coffee was initially grown in Arabia near the Red Sea. Around A.D. 675, it began to be roasted and consumed as a beverage. Eventually, it was exported to other parts of the world, and the Dutch started cultivating it in their colonies during the seventeenth century and the French in the eighteenth century. The lowly potato is native to the Peruvian Andes. In the sixteenth century, it was brought to Europe by Spanish explorers. Thereafter, its cultivation and consumption spread rapidly. It became part of the American agricultural scene in the early eighteenth century.

All of the *intellectual property* that has been introduced throughout the world is a result of international trade. This includes new music, such as rock and roll in the 1950s and hip-hop and grunge in the 1990s. It includes the software applications that are common for computer users everywhere.

New processes have been transmitted through international trade. One of those involves the Japanese manufacturing innovation that emphasized redesigning the system rather than running the existing system in the best possible way. Inventories were reduced to just-in-time levels by reengineering machine setup methods. Just-in-time inventory control is now common in American factories.

INTERNATIONAL EXAMPLE

International Trade and the Alphabet

Even the alphabetic system of writing that appears to be the source of most alphabets in the world today was spread through international trade. According to some scholars, the Phoenicians, who lived on the long, narrow strip of Mediterranean coast north of Israel from the ninth century B.C. to around 300 B.C., created the first true alphabet. Presumably, they developed the alphabet to keep international trading records on their ships rather than having to take along highly trained scribes.

For Critical Analysis

Before alphabets were used, how might have people communicated in written form?

THE RELATIONSHIP BETWEEN IMPORTS AND EXPORTS

The basic proposition in understanding all of international trade is this:

In the long run, imports are paid for by exports.*

The reason that imports are ultimately paid for by exports is that foreigners want something in exchange for the goods that are shipped to the United States. For the most part, they want goods made in the United States. From this truism comes a remarkable corollary:

Any restriction of imports ultimately reduces exports.

Click here to view the most recent trade statistics for the United States.

This is a shocking revelation to many people who want to restrict foreign competition to protect domestic jobs. Although it is possible to protect certain U.S. jobs by restricting foreign competition, it is impossible to make *everyone* better off by imposing import restrictions. Why? Because ultimately such restrictions lead to a reduction in employment in the export industries of the nation.

*We have to modify this rule by adding that in the short run, imports can also be paid for by the sale (or export) of real and financial assets, such as land, stocks, and bonds, or through an extension of credit from other countries.

INTERNATIONAL EXAMPLE

The Importation of Priests into Spain

Imports affect not only goods but also services and the movement of labor. In Spain, some 3,000 priests retire each year, but barely 250 young men are ordained to replace them. Over 70 percent of the priests in Spain are now over the age of 50. The Spanish church estimates that by 2005, the number of priests will have fallen to half the 20,441 who were active in Spain in 1990. The Spanish church has had to seek young seminarians from Latin America under what it calls Operation Moses. It is currently subsidizing the travel and training of an increasing number of young Latin Americans to take over where native Spaniards have been before.

For Critical Analysis

How might the Catholic church in Spain induce more native Spaniards to become priests?

INTERNATIONAL COMPETITIVENESS

"The United States is falling behind." "We need to stay competitive internationally." These and similar statements are often heard in government circles when the subject of international trade comes up. There are two problems with this issue. The first has to do with a simple definition. What does "global competitiveness" really mean? When one company competes against another, it is in competition. Is the United States like one big corporation, in competition with other countries? Certainly not. The standard of living in each country is almost solely a function of how well the economy functions *within that country,* not relative to other countries.

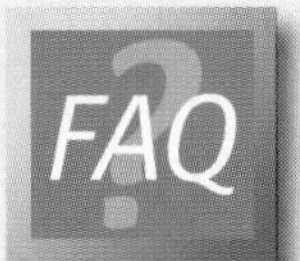

Don't productivity improvements in other countries erode the competitive position of the United States?

International trade is not a zero-sum game: If China becomes more productive, this does not mean that the United States is now less productive. A more productive China will certainly have more products to market to American consumers. It will also have higher-quality products to sell at lower prices than before, which benefits consumers in the United States who buy Chinese goods. Furthermore, China's national income will rise as a result of its productivity improvement. Consequently, it will become a bigger potential market for U.S. exports. Thus other nations can experience economic success without in any way reducing the ability of U.S. firms to produce efficiently and compete with foreign producers.

Another problem arises with respect to the real world. According to the Institute for Management Development in Lausanne, Switzerland, the United States continues to lead the pack in overall productive efficiency, ahead of Japan, Germany, and the rest of the European Union. According to the report, America's top-class ranking is due to the sustained U.S. economic recovery following its 1990–1991 recession, widespread entrepreneurship, and a decade of economic restructuring. Other factors include America's sophisticated financial system and large investments in scientific research.

CONCEPTS IN BRIEF

- Countries can be better off materially if they specialize in producing goods for which they have a comparative advantage.
- It is important to distinguish between absolute and comparative advantage; the former refers to the ability to produce a unit of output with fewer physical units of input; the latter refers to producing output that has the lowest opportunity cost for a nation.
- Different nations will always have different comparative advantages because of differing opportunity costs due to different resource mixes.

ARGUMENTS AGAINST FREE TRADE 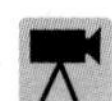

Numerous arguments are raised against free trade. They mainly point out the costs of trade; they do not consider the benefits or the possible alternatives for reducing the costs of free trade while still reaping benefits.

The Infant Industry Argument

A nation may feel that if a particular industry were allowed to develop domestically, it could eventually become efficient enough to compete effectively in the world market. Therefore, if some restrictions were placed on imports, domestic producers would be given the time needed to develop their efficiency to the point where they would be able to compete in the domestic market without any restrictions on imports. In graphic terminology, we would expect that if the protected industry truly does experience improvements in production techniques or technological breakthroughs toward greater efficiency in the future, the supply curve will shift outward to the right so that the domestic industry can produce larger quantities of each and every price. National policymakers often conclude that this **infant industry argument** has some merit in the short run. They have used it to protect a number of industries in their infancy around the world.

Infant industry argument The contention that tariffs should be imposed to protect from import competition an industry that is trying to get started. Presumably, after the industry becomes technologically efficient, the tariff can be lifted.

Such a policy can be abused, however. Often the protective import-restricting arrangements remain even after the infant has matured. If other countries can still produce more cheaply, the people who benefit from this type of situation are obviously the stockholders (and specialized factors of production that will earn economic rents) in the industry that is still being protected from world competition. The people who lose out are the consumers, who must pay a price higher than the world price for the product in question. In any event, it is very difficult to know beforehand which industries will eventually survive. In other words, we cannot predict very well the specific infant industries that policymakers might deem worthy of protection. Note that when we speculate about which industries "should" be protected, we are in the realm of *normative economics.* We are making a value judgment, a subjective statement of what *ought to be.*

EXAMPLE

An Infant Industry Blossoms Due to Protection from Foreign Imports: Marijuana

Marijuana was made illegal in the United States in the 1930s, but just as for many other outlawed drugs, a market for it remained. Until about 25 years ago, virtually all the marijuana consumed in the United States was imported. Today, earnings from the burgeoning and increasingly high-tech "pot" industry are estimated at $35 billion a year, making it the nation's biggest cash crop (compared to corn at $15 billion). Starting with President Richard Nixon in the 1970s, the federal government has ended up protecting the domestic marijuana industry from imports by declaring a war on drugs. Given virtually no foreign competition, the American marijuana industry expanded and invested millions in developing both more productive and more potent seeds as well as more efficient growing technologies. Domestic marijuana growers now dominate the high end of a market in which consumers pay $300 to $500 an ounce for a reengineered home-grown product. New growing technologies allow domestic producers, using high-intensity sodium lights, carbon dioxide, and advances in genetics, to produce a kilogram of the potent sinsemilla variety every two months in a space no bigger than a phone booth.

For Critical Analysis

What has spurred domestic producers to develop highly productive indoor growing methods?

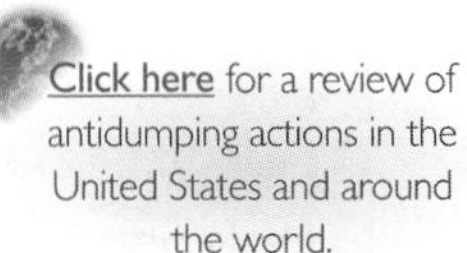

Click here for a review of antidumping actions in the United States and around the world.

Countering Foreign Subsidies and Dumping

Another strong argument against unrestricted foreign trade has to do with countering other nations' subsidies to their own producers. When a foreign government subsidizes its producers, our producers claim that they cannot compete fairly with these subsidized foreigners. To the extent that such subsidies fluctuate, it can be argued that unrestricted free trade will seriously disrupt domestic producers. They will not know when foreign governments are going to subsidize their producers and when they are not. Our competing industries will be expanding and contracting too frequently.

Dumping 
Selling a good or a service abroad below the price charged in the home market or at a price below its cost of production.

The phenomenon called *dumping* is also used as an argument against unrestricted trade. **Dumping** is said to occur when a producer sells its products abroad below the price that is charged in the home market or at a price below its cost of production. When a foreign producer is accused of dumping, further investigation usually reveals that the foreign nation is in the throes of a recession. The foreign producer does not want to slow down its production at home. Because it anticipates an end to the recession and doesn't want to hold large inventories, it dumps its products abroad at prices below home prices. U.S. competitors may also allege that it sells its output at prices below its costs in an effort to cover at least part of its variable costs of production. Dumping does disrupt international trade. It also creates instability in domestic production and therefore may impair commercial well-being at home.

INTERNATIONAL POLICY EXAMPLE

Who's Dumping on Whom?

Claims of dumping are handled on a case-by-case basis under international rules. Only a few firms in an industry have to lodge a claim to justify a dumping investigation. Under international law, antidumping rules permit governments to impose *duties*—special taxes on imported goods—on the products sold by firms of offending nations. Take a look at Figure 32-3. As you can see, in the early 1990s, developed nations filed an

FIGURE 32-3
Claims to the World Trade Organization for Antidumping Relief
In recent years, developing nations have filed at least as many claims seeking antidumping relief as the number filed by developed nations.
Source: World Trade Organization.

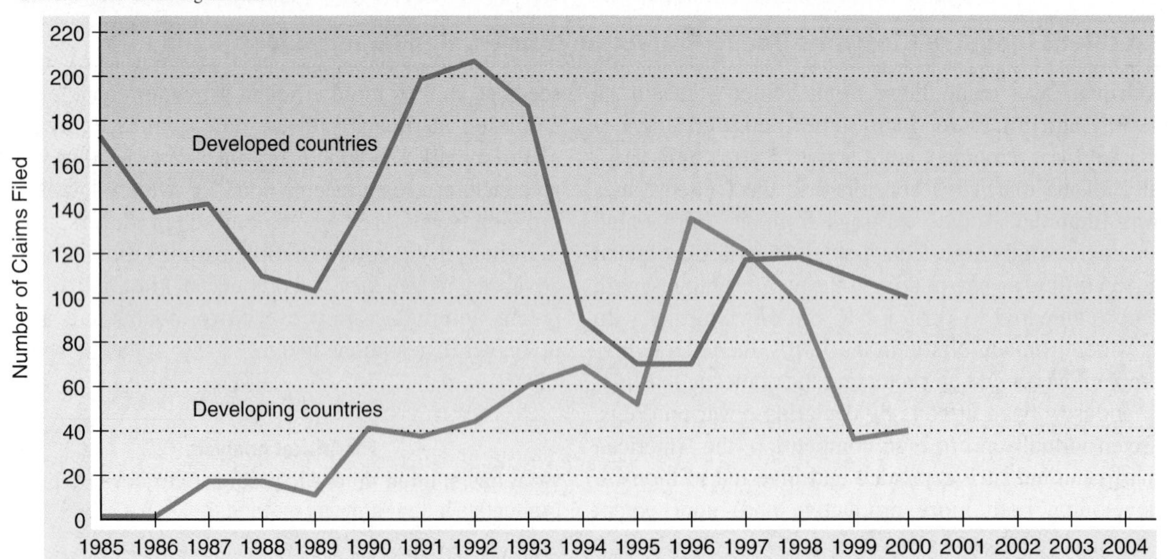

increasing number of claims seeking antidumping relief. The biggest filer of dumping claims during this period was the United States, which launched cases mainly against companies based in South America and Asia. The United States began to cut back on dumping claims beginning in the mid-1990s. Nevertheless, dumping claims by emerging economies—notably Argentina, Brazil, Mexico, and South Africa—rose precipitously. Whom did these emerging economies accuse of dumping? Firms in the United States, of course.

For Critical Analysis

Why did dumping claims by emerging nations fall as their economies expanded after the early 1990s?

Protecting American Jobs

Perhaps the argument used most often against free trade is that unrestrained competition from other countries will eliminate American jobs because other countries have lower-cost labor than we do. (Less restrictive environmental standards in other countries might also lower their private costs relative to ours.) This is a compelling argument, particularly for politicians from areas that might be threatened by foreign competition. For example, a representative from an area with shoe factories would certainly be upset about the possibility of constituents' losing their jobs because of competition from lower-priced shoe manufacturers in Brazil and Italy. But of course this argument against free trade is equally applicable to trade between the states.

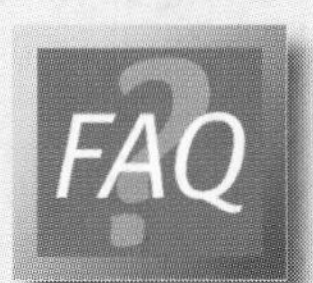

In the long run, aren't workers who have to leave their jobs because of foreign competition the biggest losers from free trade?

Some economists would argue that this is the opposite of the truth. Americans who leave their jobs rather than take wage cuts to match lower labor costs of new foreign competitors are presumably the ones who cared the least about their jobs in the first place. From this perspective, the biggest losers in the U.S. workplace are the Americans who value their jobs highly enough to keep them and absorb the full effects of the wage cuts. Because these workers presumably lack skills that they need to switch to jobs in industries with a comparative advantage over foreign producers, they are more likely to be "stuck" in low-paying jobs.

Economists David Gould, G. L. Woodbridge, and Roy Ruffin examined the data on the relationship between increases in imports and the rate of unemployment. Their conclusion was that there is no causal link between the two. Indeed, in half the cases they studied, when imports increased, unemployment fell.

Another issue has to do with the cost of protecting American jobs by restricting international trade. The Institute for International Economics examined just the restrictions on foreign textiles and apparel goods. U.S. consumers pay $9 billion a year more to protect jobs in those industries. That comes out to $50,000 a year for each job saved in an industry in which the average job pays only $20,000 a year. Similar studies have yielded similar results: Restrictions on the imports of Japanese cars have cost $160,000 *per year* for every job saved in the auto industry. Every job preserved in the glass industry has cost $200,000 each and every year. Every job preserved in the U.S. steel industry has cost an astounding $750,000 per year.

Click here to learn about the domestic costs of trade restrictions.

Emerging Arguments Against Free Trade

In recent years, two new antitrade arguments have been advanced. One of these focuses on environmental concerns. For instance, many environmentalists have raised concerns that genetic engineering of plants and animals could lead to accidental production of new diseases. These worries have induced the European Union to restrain trade in such products.

Another argument against free trade arises from national defense concerns. Major espionage successes by China in the late 1990s led some U.S. strategic experts to propose sweeping restrictions on exports of new technology.

Free trade proponents counter that at best these are arguments for the judicial regulation of trade. They continue to argue that by and large, broad trade restrictions mainly harm the interests of the nations that impose them.

CONCEPTS IN BRIEF

- The infant industry argument against free trade contends that new industries should be protected against world competition so that they can become technologically efficient in the long run.
- Unrestricted foreign trade may allow foreign governments to subsidize exports or foreign producers to engage in dumping—selling products in other countries below their cost of production. To the extent that foreign export subsidies and dumping create more instability in domestic production, they may impair our well-being.

WAYS TO RESTRICT FOREIGN TRADE

There are many ways in which international trade can be stopped or at least stifled. These include quotas and taxes (the latter are usually called *tariffs* when applied to internationally traded items). Let's talk first about quotas.

Quotas

Quota system A government-imposed restriction on the quantity of a specific good that another country is allowed to sell in the United States. In other words, quotas are restrictions on imports. These restrictions are usually applied to one or several specific countries.

Under the **quota system,** individual countries or groups of foreign producers are restricted to a certain amount of trade. An import quota specifies the maximum amount of a commodity that may be imported during a specified period of time. For example, the government might not allow more than 50 million barrels of foreign crude oil to enter the United States in a particular year.

Consider the example of quotas on textiles. Figure 32-4 presents the demand and the supply curves for imported textiles. In an unrestricted import market, the equilibrium quantity imported is 900 million yards at a price of $1 per yard (expressed in constant-quality units). When an import quota is imposed, the supply curve is no longer *S*. Rather, the supply

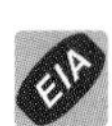

Trade Restrictions and Their Effects
See how trade restrictions work.

FIGURE 32-4
The Effect of Quotas on Textile Imports
Without restrictions, 900 million yards of textiles would be imported each year into the United States at the world price of $1.00 per yard. If the federal government imposes a quota of only 800 million yards, the effective supply curve becomes vertical at that quantity. It intersects the demand curve at a new equilibrium price of $1.50 per yard.

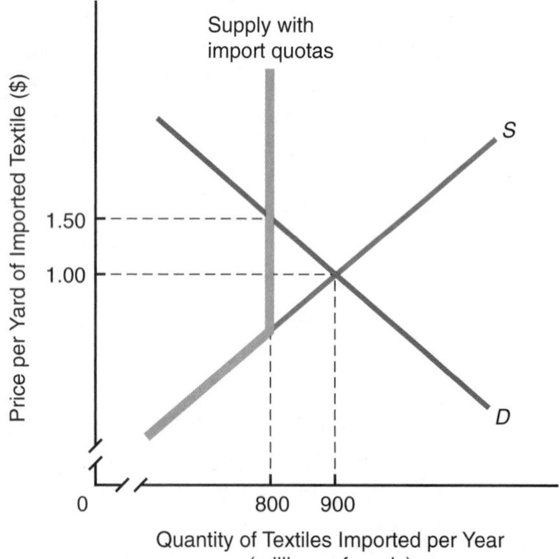

curve becomes vertical at some amount less than the equilibrium quantity—here, 800 million yards per year. The price to the American consumer increases from $1.00 to $1.50. Thus the output restriction induced by the textile quota also has the effect of influencing the price that domestic suppliers can charge for their goods. This benefits domestic textile producers by raising their revenues and therefore their profits.

INTERNATIONAL POLICY EXAMPLE

The U.S. Textile Industry: A Quota Agency of Its Very Own

Recently, American textile companies decided that they did not want so much foreign competition. Under normal circumstances, an industry might have to band together with others to lobby Congress for new laws imposing tariffs or quotas. Since the 1970s, however, the U.S. textile industry has had a special arrangement known as CITA—the Committee for the Implementation of Textile Agreements. CITA is comprised of appointees from the U.S. departments of Commerce, Labor, State, and Treasury, along with the chief textile negotiator of the Office of the President.

CITA holds no open meetings. Yet in a recent four-year period, CITA reduced or threatened to reduce quotas on specific types of textile imports. For instance, it placed limits on men's underwear from the Dominican Republic, cotton nightwear from Jamaica, and wool coats from Honduras. The annual benefit of CITA quotas for U.S. textile firms has been estimated to be as high as $12 billion in additional profits. In 2005, the United States is committed to international treaties that will phase out most textile quotas. Until then, however, CITA's quotas will be the law of the land.

For Critical Analysis

How are CITA quotas on textile imports likely to affect the prices that American consumers pay for underwear, nightwear, and coats?

Voluntary Quotas. Quotas do not have to be explicit and defined by law. They can be "voluntary." Such a quota is called a **voluntary restraint agreement (VRA).** In the early 1980s, the United States asked Japan voluntarily to restrain its exports to the United States. The Japanese government did so, limiting itself to exporting 2.8 million Japanese automobiles. Today, there are VRAs on machine tools and textiles.

Voluntary restraint agreement (VRA) 
An official agreement with another country that "voluntarily" restricts the quantity of its exports to the United States.

The opposite of a VRA is a **voluntary import expansion (VIE).** Under a VIE, a foreign government agrees to have its companies import more foreign goods from another country. The United States almost started a major international trade war with Japan in 1995 over just such an issue. The U.S. government wanted Japanese automobile manufacturers voluntarily to increase their imports of U.S.-made automobile parts. Ultimately, Japanese companies did make a token increase in the imports of U.S. auto parts.

Voluntary import expansion (VIE) 
An official agreement with another country in which it agrees to import more from the United States.

Tariffs

We can analyze tariffs by using standard supply and demand diagrams. Let's use as our commodity laptop computers, some of which are made in Japan and some of which are made domestically. In panel (a) of Figure 32-5 on the next page, you see the demand and supply of Japanese laptops. The equilibrium price is $1,000 per constant-quality unit, and the equilibrium quantity is 10 million per year. In panel (b), you see the same equilibrium price of $1,000, and the *domestic* equilibrium quantity is 5 million units per year.

Click here to take a look at the U.S. State Department's reports on economic policy and trade practices.

Now a tariff of $500 is imposed on all imported Japanese laptops. The supply curve shifts upward by $500 to S_2. For purchasers of Japanese laptops, the price increases to $1,250. The quantity demanded falls to 8 million per year. In panel (b), you see that at the

FIGURE 32-5

The Effect of a Tariff on Japanese-Made Laptop Computers

Without a tariff, the United States buys 10 million Japanese laptops per year at an average price of \$1,000, as shown in panel (a). American producers sell 5 million domestically made laptops, also at \$1,000 each, as shown in panel (b). A \$500-per-laptop tariff will shift the Japanese import supply curve to S_2 in panel (a), so that the new equilibrium is at E_2, with price \$1,250 and quantity sold reduced to 8 million per year. The demand curve for American-made laptops (for which there is no tariff) shifts to D_2 in panel (b). Domestic sales increase to 6.5 million per year.

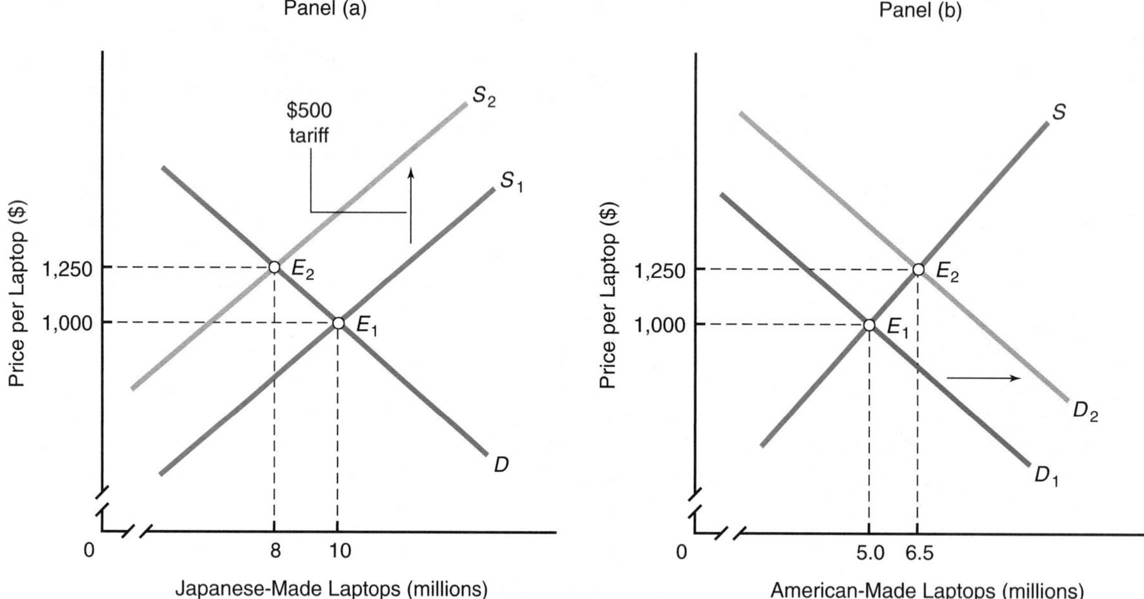

higher price of imported Japanese laptops, the demand curve for American-made laptops shifts outward to the right to D_2. The equilibrium price increases to \$1,250, but the equilibrium quantity increases to 6.5 million units per year. So the tariff benefits domestic laptop producers because it increases the demand for their products due to the higher price of a close substitute, Japanese laptops. This causes a redistribution of income from American consumers of laptops to American producers of laptops.

Tariffs in the United States. In Figure 32-6, we see that tariffs on all imported goods have varied widely. The highest rates in the twentieth century occurred with the passage of the Smoot-Hawley Tariff in 1930.

POLICY EXAMPLE

Did the Smoot-Hawley Tariff Worsen the Great Depression?

By 1930, the unemployment rate had almost doubled in a year. Congress and President Hoover wanted to do something that would help stimulate U.S. production and reduce unemployment. The result was the Smoot-Hawley Tariff, which set tariff schedules for over 20,000 products, raising duties on imports by an average of 52 percent. This attempt to improve the domestic economy at the expense of foreign economies backfired. Each trading partner of the United States in turn imposed its own high tariffs, including the United Kingdom, the Netherlands, France, and Switzerland. The result was a massive reduction in international trade by an incredible 64 percent in three years. Some believe that the ensuing world Great Depression was partially caused by such tariffs.

For Critical Analysis

The Smoot-Hawley Tariff has been labeled a "beggar thy neighbor" policy. Explain why.

Current Tariff Laws. The Trade Expansion Act of 1962 gave the president the authority to reduce tariffs by up to 50 percent. Subsequently, tariffs were reduced by about 35 percent. In 1974, the Trade Reform Act allowed the president to reduce tariffs further. In 1984, the Trade and Tariff Act resulted in the lowest tariff rates ever. All such trade agreement obligations of the United States were carried out under the auspices of the **General Agreement on Tariffs and Trade (GATT),** which was signed in 1947. Member nations of GATT account for more

General Agreement on Tariffs and Trade (GATT) 
An international agreement established in 1947 to further world trade by reducing barriers and tariffs.

FIGURE 32-6
Tariff Rates in the United States Since 1820
Tariff rates in the United States have bounced around like a football; indeed, in Congress, tariffs are a political football. Import-competing industries prefer high tariffs. In the twentieth century, the highest tariff we had was the Smoot-Hawley Tariff of 1930, which was almost as high as the "tariff of abominations" in 1828.
Source: U.S. Department of Commerce.

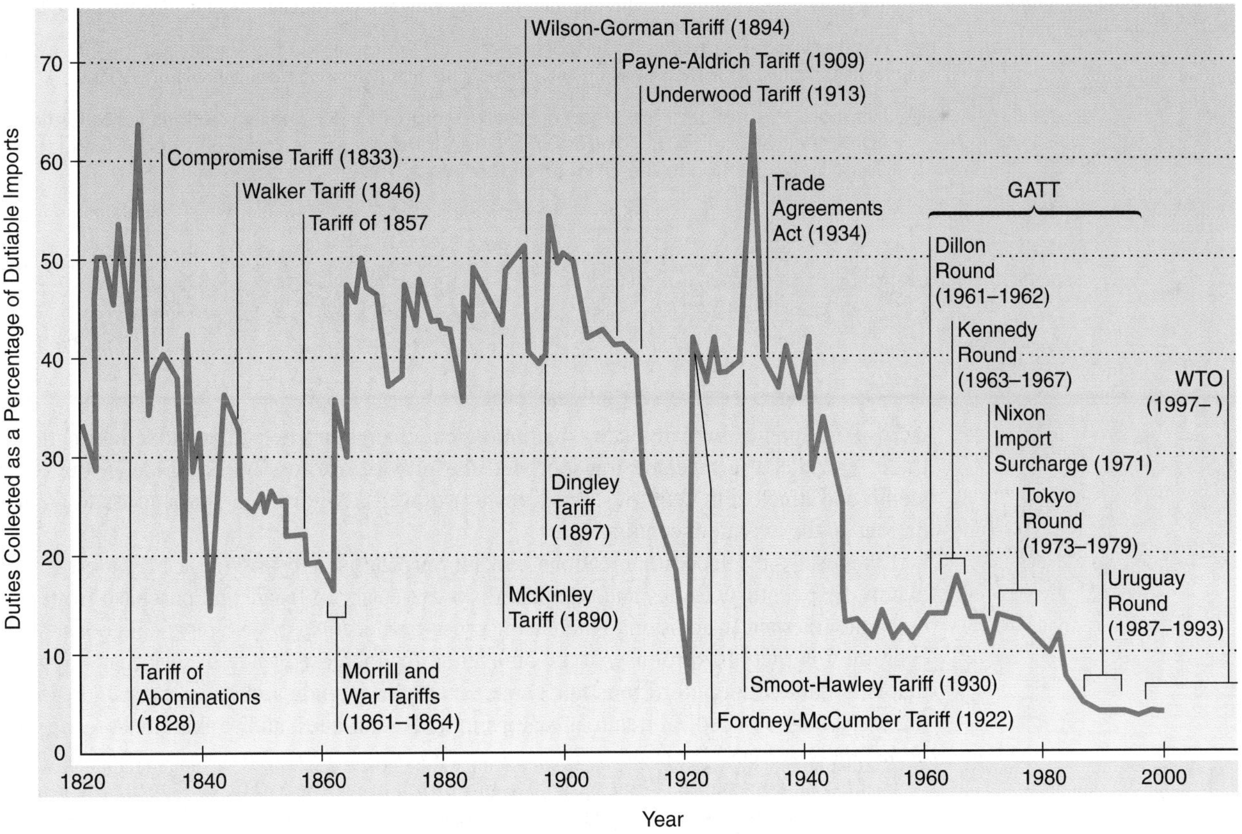

than 85 percent of world trade. As you can see in Figure 32-6 on page 797, there have been a number of rounds of negotiations to reduce tariffs since the early 1960s. The latest round was called the Uruguay Round because that is where the meetings were held.

The World Trade Organization (WTO)

World Trade Organization (WTO) 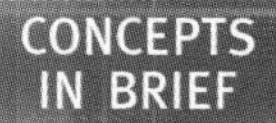
The successor organization to GATT, it handles all trade disputes among its 135 member nations.

The Uruguay Round of the General Agreement on Tariffs and Trade (GATT) was ratified by 117 nations at the end of 1993. A year later, in a special session of Congress, the entire treaty was ratified. On January 1, 1995, the new **World Trade Organization (WTO)** replaced GATT. As of 2000, the WTO had 135 member nations, plus 32 observer governments, all but two of which have applied for membership. WTO decisions have concerned such topics as the European Union's "banana wars," in which the EU's policies were determined to favor unfairly many former European colonies in Africa, the Caribbean, and the Pacific at the expense of banana-exporting countries in Latin America. Now those former colonies no longer have a privileged position in European markets.

On a larger scale, the WTO fostered the most important and far-reaching global trade agreement ever covering financial institutions, including banks, insurers, and investment companies. The more than 100 signatories to this new treaty have legally committed themselves to giving foreigners more freedom to own and operate companies in virtually all segments of the financial services industry.

CONCEPTS IN BRIEF

- One means of restricting foreign trade is a quota system. Beneficiaries of quotas are the importers who get the quota rights and the domestic producers of the restricted good.
- Another means of restricting imports is a tariff, which is a tax on imports only. An import tariff benefits import-competing industries and harms consumers by raising prices.
- The main international institution created to improve trade among nations is the General Agreement on Tariffs and Trade (GATT). The latest round of trade talks under GATT, the Uruguay Round, led to the creation of the World Trade Organization.

NETNOMICS

WTO: "Wired Trade Organization"?

Across the span of human history, technological change has helped advance international trade. Speedier transoceanic transport fed the growth of cross-border trade in the eighteenth and nineteenth centuries. Air transport played a key role in spurring trade among nations in the twentieth century.

Likewise, the telecommunications revolution promises to provide a big boost in the twenty-first century. Books and compact disks are easier to locate and purchase from afar using the Internet. In addition to increasing cross-border trade in such physical goods, however, the Internet also promises to be an avenue for increased trade in services. Anything that is tradable in digital form is fair game. Examples include architectural designs, information about new medical treatments and surgical techniques, and banking, insurance, and brokerage services.

Electronic commerce is emerging as a big problem for the WTO. WTO rules work differently for tariffs versus quotas. In most nations, goods are subjected to tariffs. By contrast, many nations have chosen to apply quotas to services by placing restrictions on access to national markets.

The Internet and digital technology are blurring the distinctions between traded goods and traded services, however. Under current interpretation, a recording by a top rap artist that crosses a national border while resident on a CD is a good subject to tariffs. Is the same recording sent over the Internet in digital form a service under WTO rules? Or is it no different from a CD and thus subject to the WTO's tariff guidelines? Likewise, if an architectural firm ships detailed drawings to a customer in another country, the drawings are treated as goods, and tariffs apply. But what if the firm sends the drawings to its client in the form of an e-mail attachment?

These examples illustrate how WTO rules concerning how to define goods and services might exert significant effects on the choice between physical and digital methods of trade. National authorities are already having trouble keeping track of the proliferation of Internet-based service offerings. If quotas on cross-border Internet services are difficult for national authorities to enforce, people will have a strong incentive to shift even more trade to the Internet.

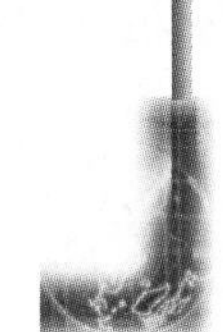

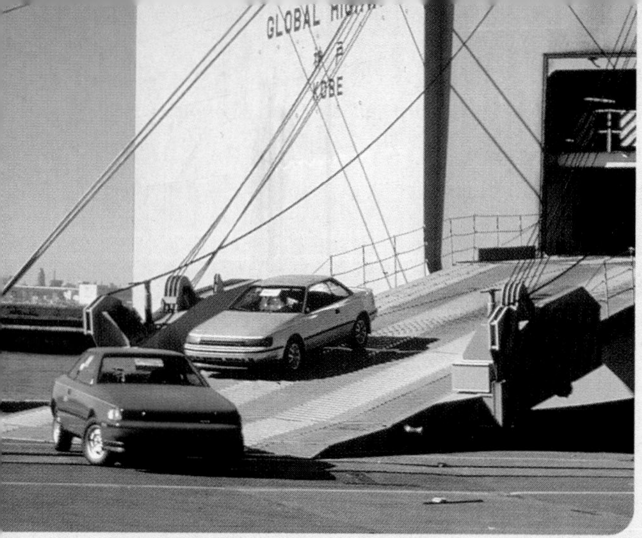

Issues & Applications

Does Importing Goods Hurt Low-Wage Workers at Home?

Once the U.S. economy got past the 1990–1991 recession, it entered a lengthy period of simultaneous low inflation and low unemployment. For many Americans, the 1990s were a time of higher real wages, increased fringe benefits, and soaring stock values.

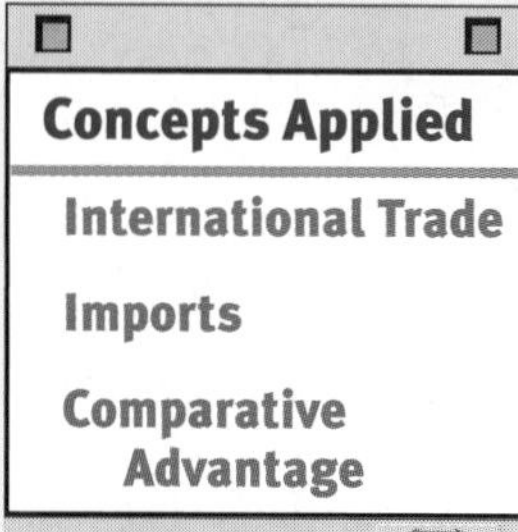

Rising Earnings Inquality

Not all Americans shared in these gains, however. Since the 1970s, the real pay of male workers among the 10 percent at the top of the U.S. income distribution has risen by over 10 percent, but the real compensation received by the 10 percent at the bottom has not increased by much. Female workers in the bottom 10 percent of the U.S. income distribution have done a little better than their male counterparts: Their earnings have risen by just under 5 percent. Women in the top 10 percent have made considerable strides, however. These high-income women have seen their earnings increase by nearly 30 percent.

Some politicians and union leaders blamed this growing U.S. earnings inequality on international trade. In the early 1970s, they point out, only one-sixth of U.S. imports of manufactured goods came from emerging economies. Today, the proportion is about one-third. There must be a simple line of causation, they claim. Extrapolating from these data, they conclude that to keep from losing his job to foreign workers, the pay of an "average Joe" is falling. The "average Jane," they contend, has barely been holding her own in the face of this same competition from abroad.

FIGURE 32-7
U.S. Manufacturing Wages and Trade with Developing Countries
In recent decades, wages earned by workers in manufacturing in nations that trade with the United States have increased relative to the wages of U.S. manufacturing workers. Some observers argue that the implied relative decline in U.S. manufacturing wages is due in part to increased trade with developing countries.

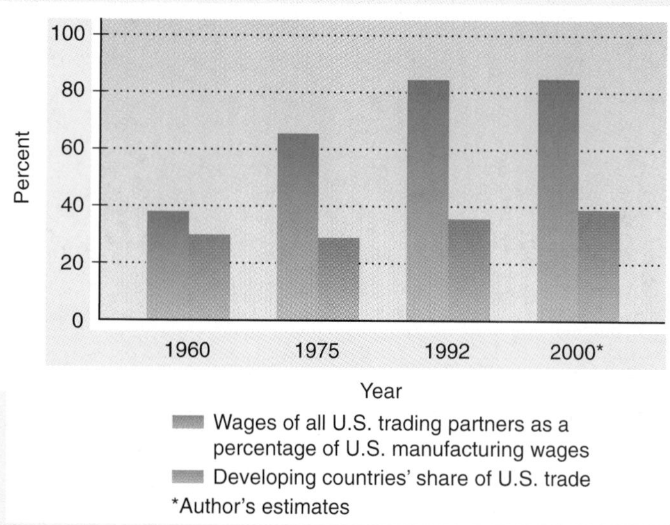

Is Free Trade the Culprit?

Take a look at Figure 32-7. It shows that American consumers have slightly increased the share of products they buy from developing countries. It also shows that the wages of all U.S. trading partners, including emerging economies, have increased relative to the wages of American manufacturing workers. One interpretation of these data is that the politicians and union leaders are correct: By purchasing more goods from emerging nations, American consumers end up reducing the wages of American workers relative to low-wage workers in those countries. Thus, goes the argument, Americans are losing out from freer trade, and the United States should put up barriers against imports from emerging nations.

As you have learned in this chapter, however, the story is not nearly this simple. The whole point of free trade is that it induces nations to specialize in producing goods for which they have a comparative advantage. Thus when trade barriers are removed—as many of them were in the United States during the 1970s and 1980s—resources naturally shift into industries in nations with a comparative advantage. They shift away from industries that lack a comparative advantage. Although this change undoubtedly works in favor of the U.S. economy as a whole, in the short run it can also work to the disadvantage of people with fewer marketable skills. One result can be a relative decline in the real earnings of lower-paid workers, at least in the near term.

FOR CRITICAL ANALYSIS

1. Do the data in Figure 32-7 necessarily indicate that U.S. manufacturing wages are declining? (Hint: A ratio can rise even if both the numerator and denominator increase, if the numerator increases faster.)
2. If American industries are losing out to foreign competition, what are some policy alternatives to dealing with the plight faced by lower-wage U.S. workers, aside from telling all American consumers that they cannot buy products from emerging nations?

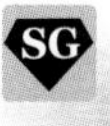
 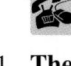

SUMMARY DISCUSSION OF LEARNING OBJECTIVES

1. **The Worldwide Importance of International Trade:** Total trade among nations has been growing faster than total world GDP. The growth of U.S. exports and imports relative to U.S. GDP parallels this global trend. Exports and imports now equal more than 10 percent of total national production. In some countries, trade accounts for much higher shares of total economic activity.
2. **Why Nations Can Gain from Specializing in Production and Engaging in Trade:** A country has a comparative advantage in producing a good if it can produce that good at a lower opportunity cost, in terms of forgone production of a second good, than another nation. If the other nation has a comparative advantage in producing the second good, both nations can gain by specializing in producing the goods in which they have a comparative advantage and engaging in international trade. Together they can then produce and consume more than they would have produced and consumed in the absence of specialization and trade.
3. **Comparative Advantage Versus Absolute Advantage:** Whereas a nation has a comparative advantage in producing a good when it can produce the good at lower opportunity cost relative to the opportunity cost of producing the good in another nation, a nation has an absolute advantage when it can produce more output with a given set of inputs than can be produced in the other country. Nevertheless, trade can still take place if both nations have a comparative advantage in producing goods that they can agree to exchange. The reason is that it can still benefit the nation with an absolute advantage to specialize in production.
4. **Arguments Against Free Trade:** One argument against free trade is that temporary import restrictions might permit an "infant industry" to develop to the point where it could compete without such

restrictions. Another argument concerns dumping, in which foreign companies allegedly sell some of their output in domestic markets at prices below the prices in the companies' home markets or even below the companies' costs of production. In addition, some environmentalists contend that nations should restrain foreign trade to prevent exposing their countries to environmental hazards to plants, animals, or even humans. Finally, some contend that countries should limit exports of technologies that could pose a threat to their national defense.

5. **Ways That Nations Restrict Foreign Trade:** One way to restrain trade is to impose a quota, or a limit on imports of a good. This action restricts the supply of the good in the domestic market, thereby pushing up the equilibrium price of the good. Another way to reduce trade is to place a tariff on imported goods. This reduces the supply of foreign-made goods and increases the demand for domestically produced goods, which brings about a rise in the price of the good.
6. **Key International Agreements and Organizations That Adjudicate Trade Disputes:** From 1947 to 1995, nations agreed to abide by the General Agreement on Trades and Tariffs (GATT), which laid an international legal foundation for relaxing quotas and reducing tariffs. Since 1995, the World Trade Organization (WTO) has adjudicated trade disputes that arise between or among nations.

Key Terms and Concepts

Absolute advantage (787)
Comparative advantage (787)
Dumping (792)
General Agreement on Tariffs and Trade (GATT) (797)
Infant industry argument (791)
Quota system (794)
Voluntary import expansion (VIE) (795)
Voluntary restraint agreement (VRA) (795)
World Trade Organization (WTO) (798)

Problems

Answers to the odd-numbered problems appear at the back of the book.

32-1. The following hypothetical example depicts the number of calculators and books that Norway and Sweden can produce with one unit of labor.

Country	Calculators	Books
Norway	2	1
Sweden	4	1

If each country has 100 workers and the country splits its labor force evenly between the two industries, how much of each good can the nations produce individually and jointly? Which nation has an absolute advantage in calculators, and which nation has an absolute advantage in books?

32-2. Suppose that the two nations in Problem 32-1 do not trade.

a. What would be the price of books in terms of calculators for each nation?

b. What is the opportunity cost of producing one calculator in each nation?

c. What is the opportunity cost of producing one book in each nation?

32-3. Consider the nations in Problem 32-1 when answering the following questions.

a. Which has a comparative advantage in calculators and which in books?

b. What is total or joint output if the two nations specialize in the good for which they have a comparative advantage?

32-4. Illustrate the production possibilities frontiers for the two nations in Problem 32-1 in a graph with books depicted on the vertical axis and calculators on the horizontal axis. What is the significance of the differing slopes of the PPFs for these two nations?

32-5. Suppose that the two nations in Problem 32-1 trade with each other at a rate where one book exchanges for three calculators. Using this rate of exchange, explain, in economic terms, whether their exchange is a zero-sum game, a positive-sum game, or a negative-sum game. (Hint: Review Chapter 25 if necessary to answer this question.)

32-6. The marginal physical product of a worker in an advanced nation (MPP_A) is 100 and the wage (W_A) is \$25. The marginal physical product of a worker in a developing nation (MPP_D) is 15 and the wage (W_D) is \$5. As a cost-minimizing business manager in the developing nation, would you be enticed to move your business to the developing nation to take advantage of the lower wage?

32-7. You are a policymaker of a major exporting nation. Your main export good has a price elasticity of demand of −.50. Is there any economic reason why you would voluntarily agree to export restraints?

32-8. The following table depicts the bicycle industry before and after a nation has imposed quota restraints.

	Before Quota	After Quota
Quantity imported	1,000,000	900,000
Price paid	\$50	\$60

Draw a diagram illustrating conditions in the imported bicycle market before and after the quota, and answer the following questions.

a. What are the total expenditures of consumers before and after the quota?

b. What is the price elasticity of demand for bicycles?

c. Who benefits from the imposition of the quota?

32-9. The following diagrams illustrate the markets for imported Korean-made and U.S. manufactured televisions before and after a tariff is imposed on imported TVs.

a. What was the amount of the tariff?

b. What was the total revenue of Korean television exports before the tariff? After the tariff?

c. What is the tariff revenue earned by the U.S. government?

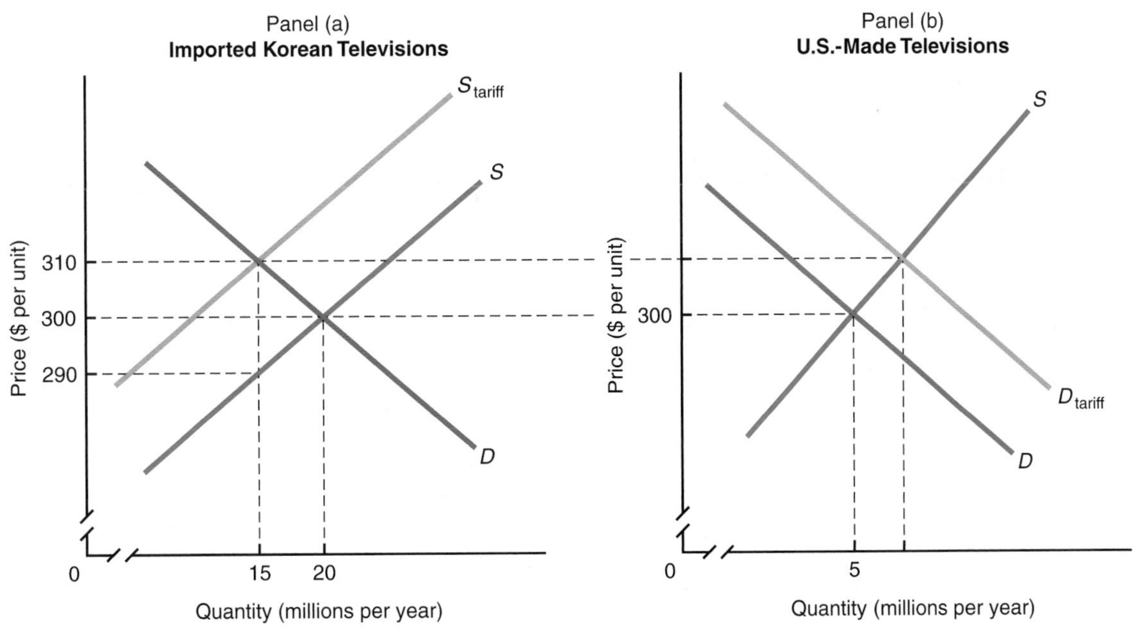

32-10. Base your answers to the following questions on the graph accompanying Problem 32-9.

a. What was the revenue of U.S. television manufacturers before the tariff was imposed?

b. What is their total revenue after the tariff?

c. Who has gained from the tariff and who has it made worse off?

Economics on the Net

How the World Trade Organization Settles Trade Disputes A key function of the WTO is to adjudicate trade disagreements that arise among nations. This application helps you learn about the process that the WTO follows when considering international trade disputes.

Title: The World Trade Organization: Settling Trade Disputes

Navigation: Click here to begin at the WTO's homepage. Select the A-Z List of Topics. Then click on Disputes, and click on How Does the WTO Settle Disputes?

Application Read the first article. Then answer the following questions.

1. As the article discusses, settling trade disputes often takes at least a year. What aspects of the WTO's dispute settlement process take the longest time?
2. Does the WTO actually "punish" a country it finds has broken international trading agreements? If not, who does impose sanctions?

For Group Study and Analysis Read the Beyond the Agreements section, which lists areas that the WTO is currently exploring for future action. Have a class discussion of the pros and cons of WTO involvement in each of these areas. Which are most important for promoting world trade? Which are least important?

CHAPTER 33

EXCHANGE RATES AND THE BALANCE OF PAYMENTS

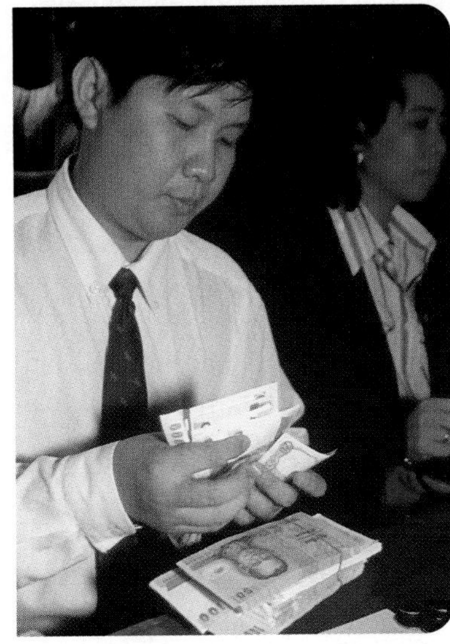

During the Asian currency crisis, the Thai government launched a campaign to keep the national currency, the baht, from falling in value. The government asked Thais to turn in their foreign currencies in exchange for baht. Why?

In 1997, an international payments crisis swept Southeast Asia. Investors from around the world began selling off their holdings of bonds and stocks denominated in the Thai baht, Indonesian rupiah, and Malaysian ringgit. The prime minister of Malaysia, Mahathir Mohamad, said that the crisis was caused by currency speculators—individuals and firms that seek to profit solely from the activity of buying currencies at low values and selling them at higher values. During the summer of 1997, a number of currency speculators earned sizable profits by conjecturing that Southeast Asian nations, including Malaysia, could not maintain the value of their currencies. According to Mahathir, these were ill-gotten gains. Speculative currency trading, Mahathir contended, "is unnecessary, unproductive, and immoral." Are currency speculators really unproductive individuals engaged in an unnecessary and immoral business? To evaluate this question, you must first learn more about international payments and exchange rates.

LEARNING OBJECTIVES

After reading this chapter, you should be able to:

1. Distinguish between the balance of trade and the balance of payments
2. Identify the key accounts within the balance of payments
3. Outline how exchange rates are determined in the markets for foreign exchange
4. Discuss factors that can induce changes in equilibrium exchange rates
5. Understand how policymakers can go about attempting to fix exchange rates
6. Explain alternative approaches to limiting exchange rate variability

Chapter Outline

- The Balance of Payments and International Capital Movements
- Determining Foreign Exchange Rates
- The Gold Standard and the International Monetary Fund
- Fixed Versus Floating Exchange Rates

Did You Know That... every day, around the clock, over $1 trillion in foreign currencies is traded? Along with that trading come news headlines, such as "The dollar weakened today," "The dollar is clearly overvalued," "The dollar is under attack," and "Members of the Group of Seven acted to prevent the dollar from rising." If you are confused by such newspaper headlines, join the crowd. Surprisingly, though, if you regard the dollar, the pound, the euro, the yen, and the baht as assets that are subject to the laws of supply and demand, the world of international finance can be quickly demystified. Perhaps the first step is to examine the meaning of the terms used with respect to U.S. international financial transactions during any one-year period.

THE BALANCE OF PAYMENTS AND INTERNATIONAL CAPITAL MOVEMENTS

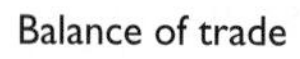

Balance of trade
The difference between exports and imports of goods.

Balance of payments
A system of accounts that measures transactions of goods, services, income, and financial assets between domestic households, businesses, and governments and residents of the rest of the world during a specific time period.

Governments typically keep track of each year's economic activities by calculating the gross domestic product—the total of expenditures on all newly produced final domestic goods and services—and its components. In the world of international trade also, a summary information system has been developed. It relates to the balance of trade and the balance of payments. The **balance of trade** refers specifically to exports and imports of goods as discussed in Chapter 32. When international trade is in balance, the value of exports equals the value of imports. When the value of imports exceeds the value of imports, we are running a deficit in the balance of trade. When the value of exports exceeds the value of imports, we are running a surplus.

The **balance of payments** is a more general concept that expresses the total of all economic transactions between a nation and the rest of the world, usually for a period of one year. Each country's balance of payments summarizes information about that country's exports, imports, earnings by domestic residents on assets located abroad, earnings on domestic assets owned by foreign residents, international capital movements, and official transactions by central banks and governments. In essence, then, the balance of payments is a record of all the transactions between households, firms, and the government of one country and the rest of the world. Any transaction that leads to a *payment* by a country's residents (or government) is a deficit item, identified by a negative sign (−) when we examine the actual numbers that might be in Table 33-1. Any transaction that leads to a *receipt* by a country's residents (or government) is a surplus item and is identified by a plus sign (+) when actual numbers are considered. Table 33-1 gives a listing of the surplus and deficit items on international accounts.

Accounting Identities

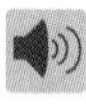

Accounting identities
Values that are equivalent by definition.

Accounting identities—definitions of equivalent values—exist for financial institutions and other businesses. We begin with simple accounting identities that must hold for families and then go on to describe international accounting identities.

If a family unit is spending more than its current income, such a situation necessarily implies that the family unit must be doing one of the following:

1. Reducing its money holdings, or selling stocks, bonds, or other assets
2. Borrowing
3. Receiving gifts from friends or relatives

TABLE 33-1
Surplus (+) and Deficit (−) Items on the International Accounts

Surplus Items (+)	Deficit Items (−)
Exports of merchandise	Imports of merchandise
Private and governmental gifts from foreigners	Private and governmental gifts to foreigners
Foreign use of domestically owned transportation	Use of foreign-owned transportation
Foreign tourists' expenditures in this country	Tourism expenditures abroad
Foreign military spending in this country	Military spending abroad
Interest and dividend receipts from foreign entities	Interest and dividends paid to foreigners
Sales of domestic assets to foreigners	Purchases of foreign assets
Funds deposited in this country by foreigners	Funds placed in foreign depository institutions
Sales of gold to foreigners	Purchases of gold from foreigners
Sales of domestic currency to foreigners	Purchases of foreign currency

4. Receiving public transfers from a government, which obtained the funds by taxing others (a transfer is a payment, in money or in goods or services, made without receiving goods or services in return)

We can use this information to derive an identity: If a family unit is currently spending more than it is earning, it must draw on previously acquired wealth, borrow, or receive either private or public aid. Similarly, an identity exists for a family unit that is currently spending less than it is earning: It must be increasing its money holdings or be lending and acquiring other financial assets, or it must pay taxes or bestow gifts on others. When we consider businesses and governments, each unit in each group faces its own identities or constraints. Ultimately, net lending by households must equal net borrowing by businesses and governments.

Disequilibrium. Even though our individual family unit's accounts must balance, in the sense that the identity discussed previously must hold, sometimes the item that brings about the balance cannot continue indefinitely. *If family expenditures exceed family income and this situation is financed by borrowing, the household may be considered to be in disequilibrium because such a situation cannot continue indefinitely.* If such a deficit is financed by drawing on previously accumulated assets, the family may also be in disequilibrium because it cannot continue indefinitely to draw on its wealth; eventually, it will become impossible for that family to continue such a lifestyle. (Of course, if the family members are retired, they may well be in equilibrium by drawing on previously acquired assets to finance current deficits; this example illustrates that it is necessary to understand circumstances fully before pronouncing an economic unit in disequilibrium.)

Equilibrium. Individual households, businesses, and governments, as well as the entire group of households, businesses, and governments, must eventually reach equilibrium. Certain economic adjustment mechanisms have evolved to ensure equilibrium. Deficit households must eventually increase their income or decrease their expenditures. They will find that they have to pay higher interest rates if they wish to borrow to finance their deficits. Eventually, their credit sources will dry up, and they will be forced into equilibrium. Businesses, on occasion, must lower costs or prices—or go bankrupt—to reach equilibrium.

TABLE 33-2
U.S. Balance of Payments Account, 2000 (in billions of dollars)

Current Account		
(1) Exports of goods	+711.6	
(2) Imports of goods	−1,135.3	
(3) Balance of trade		−423.7
(4) Exports of services	+311.2	
(5) Imports of services	−213.4	
(6) Balance of services		+97.8
(7) Balance on goods and services [(3) + (6)]		−325.9
(8) Net unilateral transfers	−34.2	
(9) Balance on current account		−360.1
Capital Account		
(10) U.S. private capital going abroad	−642.2	
(11) Foreign private capital coming into the United States	+987.1*	
(12) Balance on capital account [(10) + (11)]		+344.9
(13) Balance on current account plus balance on capital account [(9) + (12)]		−15.2
Official Reserve Transactions Account		
(14) Official transactions balance		+15.2
(15) Total (balance)		.00

Sources: U.S. Department of Commerce, Bureau of Economic Analysis; U.S. Department of the Treasury.
*Includes a $26 billion statistical discrepancy, probably unaccounted capital inflows, many of which relate to the illegal drug trade.

An Accounting Identity Among Nations. When nations trade or interact, certain identities or constraints must also hold. Nations buy goods from people in other nations; they also lend to and present gifts to people in other nations. If a nation interacts with others, an accounting identity ensures a balance (but not an equilibrium, as will soon become clear). Let's look at the three categories of balance of payments transactions: current account transactions, capital account transactions, and official reserve account transactions.

Current Account Transactions

During any designated period, all payments and gifts that are related to the purchase or sale of both goods and services constitute the current account in international trade. The four major types of current account transactions are the exchange of merchandise, the exchange of services, unilateral transfers, and net investment income.

Merchandise Trade Exports and Imports. The largest portion of any nation's balance of payments current account is typically the importing and exporting of merchandise goods. During 2000, for example, as can be seen in lines 1 and 2 of Table 33-2, the United States exported $711.6 billion of merchandise and imported $1,135.3 billion. The balance of merchandise trade is defined as the difference between the value of merchandise exports and the value of merchandise imports. For 2000, the United States had a balance of merchandise trade deficit because the value of its merchandise imports exceeded the value of its merchandise exports. This deficit amounted to $423.7 billion (line 3).

Service Exports and Imports. The balance of (merchandise) trade has to do with tangible items—you can feel them, touch them, and see them. Service exports and imports have to do with invisible or intangible items that are bought and sold, such as shipping, insurance, tourist expenditures, and banking services. Also, income earned by foreigners on U.S. investments and income earned by U.S. residents on foreign investments are part of service imports and exports. As can be seen in lines 4 and 5 of Table 33-2, in 2000, service exports were $311.2 billion and service imports were $213.4 billion. Thus the balance of services was about $97.8 billion in 2000 (line 6). Exports constitute receipts or inflows into the United States and are positive; imports constitute payments abroad or outflows of money and are negative.

When we combine the balance of merchandise trade with the balance of services, we obtain a balance of goods and services equal to −$325.9 billion in 2000 (line 7).

Unilateral Transfers. U.S. residents give gifts to relatives and others abroad, the federal government grants gifts to foreign nations, foreigners give gifts to U.S. residents, and some foreign governments have granted money to the U.S. government. In the current account, we see that net unilateral transfers—the total amount of gifts given by U.S. residents minus the total amount received by U.S. residents from abroad—came to −$34.2 billion in 2000 (line 8). The fact that there is a minus sign before the number for unilateral transfers means that U.S. residents gave more to foreigners than foreigners gave to U.S. residents.

Balancing the Current Account. The balance on current account tracks the value of a country's exports of goods and services (including military receipts plus income on investments abroad) and transfer payments (private and government) relative to the value of that country's imports of goods and services and transfer payments (private and government). In 2000, it was −$360.1 billion.

If the sum of net exports of goods and services plus unilateral transfers plus net investment income exceeds zero, a current account surplus is said to exist; if this sum is negative, a current account deficit is said to exist. A current account deficit means that we are importing more than we are exporting. Such a deficit must be paid for by the export of money or money equivalent, which means a capital account surplus.

Click here for latest U.S. balance-of-payments figures.

Capital Account Transactions

In world markets, it is possible to buy and sell not only goods and services but also real and financial assets. This is what the capital accounts are concerned with in international transactions. Capital account transactions occur because of foreign investments—either by foreign residents investing in the United States or by U.S. residents investing in other countries. The purchase of shares of stock on the London stock market by a U.S. resident causes an outflow of funds from the United States to Britain. The building of a Japanese automobile factory in the United States causes an inflow of funds from Japan to the United States. Any time foreign residents buy U.S. government securities, that is an inflow of funds from other countries to the United States. Any time U.S. residents buy foreign government securities, there is an outflow of funds from the United States to other countries. Loans to and from foreign residents cause outflows and inflows.

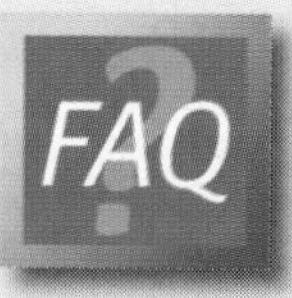

The United States has large trade deficits. Does this mean we have a weak economy?

It is true that the current account in the United States has been in deficit continuously since the early 1980s, but this was also true during the 1880s. So it is not a new phenomenon. (Note also that we were a creditor nation from 1914 to 1985.) Figure 33-1 shows that whenever the United States is in deficit in its current account, it is in surplus in its capital account. The United States does not have a trade deficit because its economy is weak and it cannot compete in world markets. Rather, the United States is a good place to invest capital because we have strong prospects for growth. As long as foreign residents wish to invest more in the United States than U.S. residents wish to invest abroad, there will *always* be a current account deficit. The U.S. is better off, not worse off, because of it.

Line 10 of Table 33-2 indicates that in 2000, the value of private and government capital going out of the United States was −$642.2 billion, and line 11 shows that the value of private and government capital coming into the United States (including a statistical discrepancy) was $987.1 billion. U.S. capital going abroad constitutes payments or outflows and is therefore negative. Foreign capital coming into the United States constitutes receipts or inflows and is therefore positive. Thus there was a positive net capital movement of $344.9 billion into the United States (line 12). This is also called the balance on capital account.

There is a relationship between the current account and the capital account, assuming no interventions by the finance ministries or central banks of nations.

In the absence of interventions by finance ministries or central banks, the current account and the capital account must sum to zero. Stated differently, the current account deficit must equal the capital account surplus when governments or central banks do not engage in foreign exchange interventions. In this situation, any nation experiencing a current account deficit, such as the United States, must also be running a capital account surplus.

Official Reserve Account Transactions

The third type of balance of payments transaction concerns official reserve assets, which consist of the following:

1. Foreign currencies
2. Gold
3. **Special drawing rights (SDRs),** which are reserve assets that the International Monetary Fund created to be used by countries to settle international payment obligations
4. The reserve position in the International Monetary Fund
5. Financial assets held by an official agency, such as the U.S. Treasury Department

Special drawing rights (SDRs) 
Reserve assets created by the International Monetary Fund for countries to use in settling international payment obligations.

To consider how official reserve account transactions occur, look again at Table 33-2. The surplus in the U.S. capital account was $344.9 billion. But the deficit in the U.S. current account was −$360.1 billion, so the United States had a net deficit on the combined accounts (line 13) of −$15.2 billion. In other words, the United States obtained less in foreign money in all its international transactions than it used. How is this deficiency made up? By our central bank drawing down its existing balances of foreign moneys, shown by the +$15.2 billion in official transactions shown on line 14 in Table 33-2. There is a plus sign on line 14 because this represents an *inflow* of foreign exchange into our international transactions.

The balance (line 15) in Table 33-2 is zero, as it must be with double-entry bookkeeping. The U.S. balance of payments deficit is measured by the official transactions figure on line 14.

FIGURE 33-1

The Relationship Between the Current Account and the Capital Account

To some extent, the capital account is the mirror image of the current account. We can see this in the years since 1970. When the current account was in surplus, the capital account was in deficit. When the current account was in deficit, the capital account was in surplus. Indeed, virtually the only time foreigners can invest in America is when the current account is in deficit.

Sources: International Monetary Fund; *Economic Indicators.*

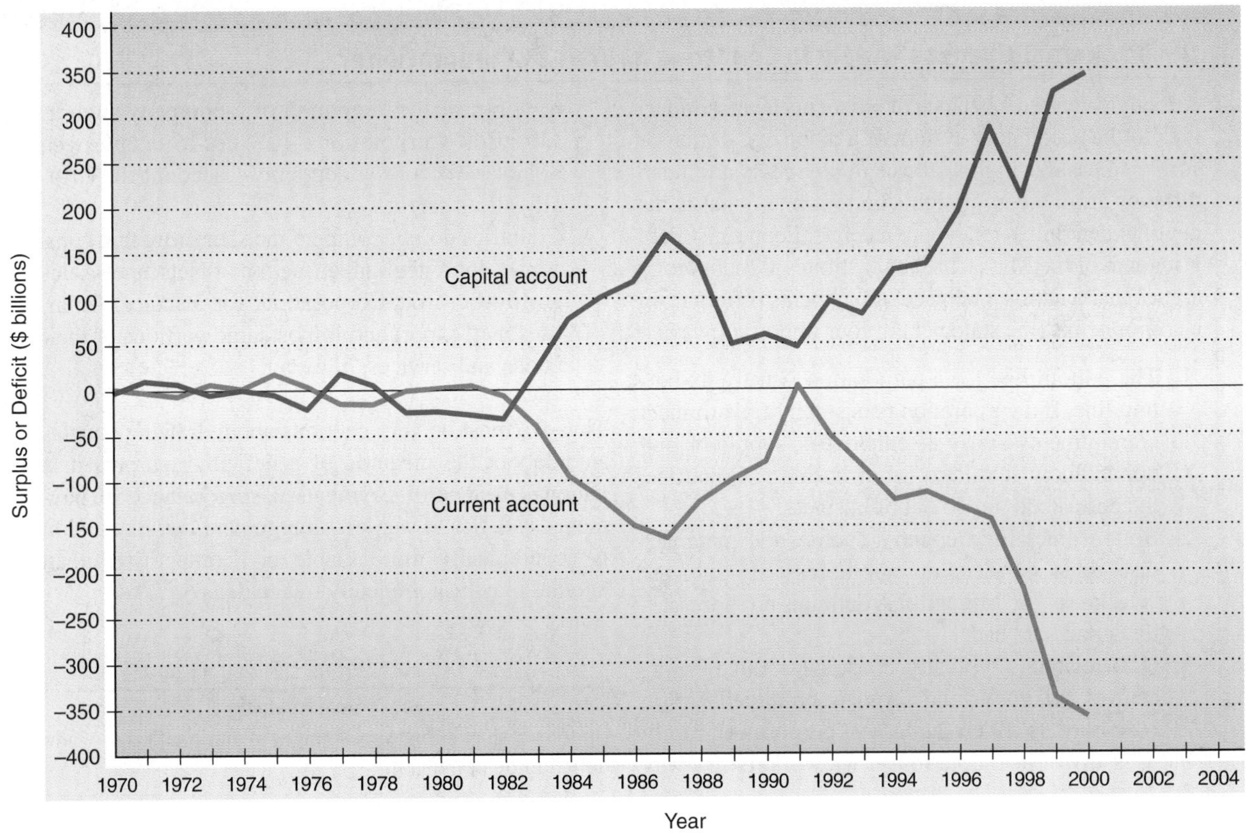

What Affects the Balance of Payments?

A major factor affecting any nation's balance of payments is its rate of inflation relative to that of its trading partners. Assume that the rates of inflation in the United States and in Japan are equal. Now suppose that all of a sudden, the U.S. inflation rate increases. The Japanese will find that U.S. products are becoming more expensive, and U.S. firms will export fewer of them to Japan. At the current exchange rate, U.S. residents will find Japanese products relatively cheaper, and they will import more. The converse will occur if the U.S. inflation rate suddenly falls relative to that of Japan. All other things held constant, whenever the U.S. rate of inflation exceeds that of its trading partners, we expect to see a larger deficit in the U.S. balance of trade and payments. Conversely, when the U.S. rate of inflation is less than that of its trading partners, other things being constant, we expect to see a smaller deficit in the U.S. balance of trade and payments.

Another important factor that sometimes influences a nation's balance of payments is its relative political stability. Political instability causes *capital flight.* Owners of capital in countries anticipating or experiencing political instability will often move assets to countries that are politically stable, such as the United States. Hence the U.S. capital account balance, and so its balance of payments, is likely to increase whenever political instability looms in other nations in the world.

POLICY EXAMPLE

Does "Competitiveness" Apply to Countries as Well as Corporations?

Although a nation's balance of payments bears similarities to the accounting system of a company, deficit or surplus measures in the balance of payments are much different from a corporation's bottom line—that is, its net of expenditures relative to receipts. Economist Paul Krugman of the Massachusetts Institute of Technology argues that a nation's balance of payments differs from a corporate income statement in four important ways:

1. The bottom line for a corporation is truly its bottom line. If a corporation persistently fails to meet commitments to pay its employees, suppliers, and bondholders, it will go out of business. Countries, in contrast, do not go out of business.
2. Bottom lines for a country, such as the merchandise trade balance, do not necessarily indicate "weakness" or "strength." A deficit is not necessarily "good" or "bad."
3. U.S. residents typically consume about 90 percent of the goods and services produced within U.S. borders. Even the largest corporation rarely sells any of its output to its own workers. By way of contrast, the "exports" of a company such as Microsoft Corporation—its sales to people who do not work for the company—account for virtually all its sales.
4. Countries do not compete the same way that companies do. A negligible fraction of Netscape's sales go to Microsoft Corporation, for instance. Countries may export and import large portions of their goods and services, however.

Thus we must be very cautious about drawing conclusions about the meaning of a deficit or surplus in a nation's balance of payments. Using balance of payments statistics to support an argument that one nation is economically more viable or "competitive" than another may be completely misguided.

For Critical Analysis

Under what circumstances might a nation find a trade deficit to be beneficial?

CONCEPTS IN BRIEF

- The balance of payments reflects the value of all transactions in international trade, including goods, services, financial assets, and gifts.
- The merchandise trade balance gives us the difference between exports and imports of tangible items. Merchandise trade transactions are represented by exports and imports of tangible items.
- Included in the current account along with merchandise trade are service exports and imports relating to commerce in intangible items, such as shipping, insurance, and tourist expenditures. The current account also includes income earned by foreign residents on U.S. investments and income earned by U.S. residents on foreign investments.
- Unilateral transfers involve international private gifts and federal government grants or gifts to foreign nations.
- When we add the balance of merchandise trade and the balance of services and take account of net unilateral transfers and net investment income, we come up with the balance on the current account, a summary statistic.

- There are also capital account transactions that relate to the buying and selling of financial and real assets. Foreign capital is always entering the United States, and U.S. capital is always flowing abroad. The difference is called the balance on capital account.
- Another type of balance of payments transaction concerns the official reserve assets of individual countries, or what is often simply called official transactions. By standard accounting convention, official transactions are exactly equal to a nation's balance of payments but opposite in sign.
- A nation's balance of payments can be affected by its relative rate of inflation and by its political stability relative to other nations.

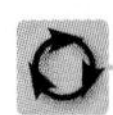

DETERMINING FOREIGN EXCHANGE RATES

When you buy foreign products, such as a Japanese-made laptop computer, you have dollars with which to pay the Japanese manufacturer. The Japanese manufacturer, however, cannot pay workers in dollars. The workers are Japanese, they live in Japan, and they must have yen to buy goods and services in that country. There must therefore be some way of exchanging dollars for yen that the computer manufacturer will accept. That exchange occurs in a **foreign exchange market,** which in this case specializes in exchanging yen and dollars. (When you obtain foreign currencies at a bank or an airport currency exchange, you are participating in the foreign exchange market.)

Foreign exchange market
A market in which households, firms, and governments buy and sell national currencies.

Exchange rate
The price of one nation's currency in terms of the currency of another country.

The particular **exchange rate** between yen and dollars that prevails—the dollar price of the yen—depends on the current demand for and supply of yen and dollars. In a sense, then, our analysis of the exchange rate between dollars and yen will be familiar, for we have used supply and demand throughout this book. If it costs you 1 cent to buy 1 yen, that is the foreign exchange rate determined by the current demand for and supply of yen in the foreign exchange market. The Japanese person going to the foreign exchange market would need 100 yen to buy 1 dollar.

We will continue our example in which the only two countries in the world are Japan and the United States. Now let's consider what determines the demand for and supply of foreign currency in the foreign exchange market.

Demand for and Supply of Foreign Currency

You wish to purchase a Japanese-made laptop computer direct from the manufacturer. To do so, you must have Japanese yen. You go to the foreign exchange market (or your U.S. bank). Your desire to buy the Japanese laptop computer therefore causes you to offer (supply) dollars to the foreign exchange market. Your demand for Japanese yen is equivalent to your supply of U.S. dollars to the foreign exchange market.

> Every U.S. transaction involving the importation of foreign goods constitutes a supply of dollars and a demand for some foreign currency, and the opposite is true for export transactions.

In this case, the import transaction constitutes a demand for Japanese yen.

In our example, we will assume that only two goods are being traded, Japanese laptop computers and U.S. microprocessors. The U.S. demand for Japanese laptop computers creates a supply of dollars and demand for yen in the foreign exchange market. Similarly, the Japanese demand for U.S. microprocessors creates a supply of yen and a demand for dollars in the foreign exchange market. Under a system of **flexible exchange rates,** the supply of and demand for dollars and yen in the foreign exchange market will determine the

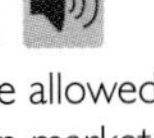

Flexible exchange rates
Exchange rates that are allowed to fluctuate in the open market in response to changes in supply and demand. Sometimes called *floating exchange rates.*

equilibrium foreign exchange rate. The equilibrium exchange rate will tell us how many yen a dollar can be exchanged for—that is, the dollar price of yen—or how many dollars (or fractions of a dollar) a yen can be exchange for—the yen price of dollars.

The Equilibrium Foreign Exchange Rate

To determine the equilibrium foreign exchange rate, we have to find out what determines the demand for and supply of foreign exchange. We will ignore for the moment any speculative aspect of buying foreign exchange. That is, we assume that there are no individuals who wish to buy yen simply because they think that their price will go up in the future.

Click here for recent data on the exchange value of the U.S. dollar relative to the major currencies of the world.

The idea of an exchange rate is no different from the idea of paying a certain price for something you want to buy. If you like coffee, you know you have to pay about 75 cents a cup. If the price went up to $2.50, you would probably buy fewer cups. If the price went down to 5 cents, you might buy more. In other words, the demand curve for cups of coffee, expressed in terms of dollars, slopes downward following the law of demand. The demand curve for yen slopes downward also, and we will see why.

Let's think more closely about the demand schedule for yen. Let's say that it costs you 1 cent to purchase 1 yen; that is the exchange rate between dollars and yen. If tomorrow you had to pay $1\frac{1}{4}$ cents ($.0125) for the same yen, the exchange rate would have changed. Looking at such an increase with respect to the yen, we would say that there has been an **appreciation** in the value of the yen in the foreign exchange market. But another way to view this increase in the value of the yen is to say that there has been a **depreciation** in the value of the dollar in the foreign exchange market. The dollar used to buy 100 yen; tomorrow, the dollar will be able to buy only 80 yen at a price of $1\frac{1}{4}$ cents per yen. If the dollar price of yen rises, you will probably demand fewer yen. Why? The answer lies in looking at the reason you and others demand yen in the first place.

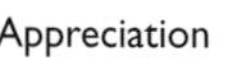

Appreciation

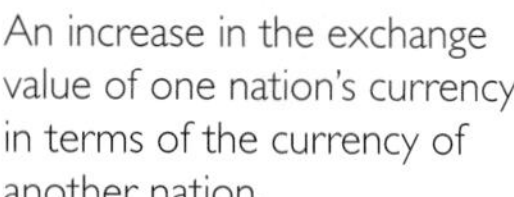

An increase in the exchange value of one nation's currency in terms of the currency of another nation.

Depreciation

A decrease in the exchange value of one nation's currency in terms of the currency of another nation.

Appreciation and Depreciation of Japanese Yen. Recall that in our example, you and others demand yen to buy Japanese laptop computers. The demand curve for Japanese laptop computers, we will assume, follows the law of demand and therefore slopes downward. If it costs more U.S. dollars to buy the same quantity of Japanese laptop computers, presumably you and other U.S. residents will not buy the same quantity; your quantity demanded will be less. We say that your demand for Japanese yen is *derived from* your demand for Japanese laptop computers. In panel (a) of Figure 33-2, we present the hypothetical demand schedule for Japanese laptop computers by a representative set of U.S. consumers during a typical week. In panel (b), we show graphically the U.S. demand curve for Japanese yen in terms of U.S. dollars taken from panel (a).

An Example of Derived Demand. Let us assume that the price of a Japanese laptop computer in Japan is 100,000 yen. Given that price, we can find the number of yen required to purchase up to 500 Japanese laptop computers. That information is given in panel (c) of Figure 33-2. If one laptop computer requires 100,000 yen, 500 laptop computers require 50 million yen. Now we have enough information to determine the derived demand curve for Japanese yen. If 1 yen costs 1 cent, a laptop computer would cost $1,000 (100,000 yen per computer × 1 cent per yen = $1,000 per computer). At $1,000 per computer, the representative group of U.S. consumers would, we see from panel (a) of Figure 33-2, demand 500 laptop computers.

From panel (c), we see that 50 million yen would be demanded to buy the 500 laptop computers. We show this quantity demanded in panel (d). In panel (e), we draw the derived demand curve for yen. Now consider what happens if the price of yen goes up to $1\frac{1}{4}$ cents

Panel (a)
Demand Schedule for Japanese Laptop Computers in the United States per Week

Price per Unit	Quantity Demanded
$1,500	100
1,250	300
1,000	500
750	700

Panel (b)
American Demand Curve for Japanese Laptop Computers

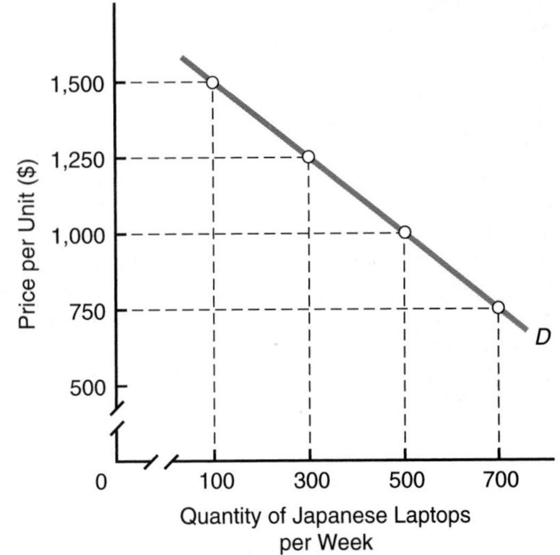

Panel (c)
Yen Required to Purchase Quantity Demanded (at P = 100,000 yen per computer)

Quantity Demanded	Yen Required (millions)
100	10
300	30
500	50
700	70

Panel (d)
Derived Demand Schedule for Yen in the United States with Which to Pay for Imports of Laptops

Dollar Price of One Yen	Dollar Price of Computers	Quantity of Computers Demanded	Quantity of Yen Demanded per Week (millions)
$ .0150	$1,500	100	10
.0125	1,250	300	30
.0100	1,000	500	50
.0075	750	700	70

Panel (e)
American Derived Demand for Yen

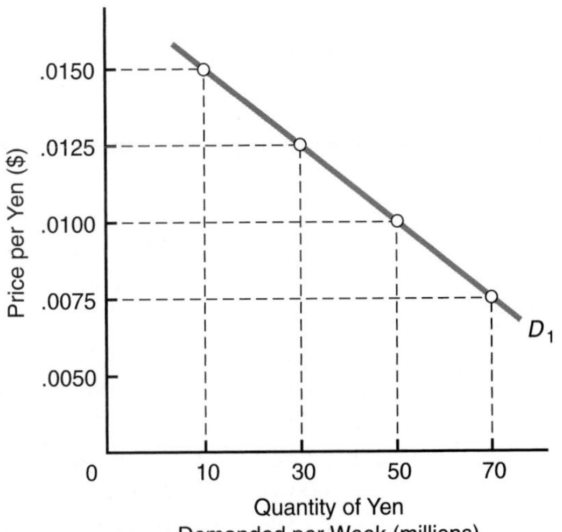

FIGURE 33-2
Deriving the Demand for Yen
In panel (a), we show the demand schedule for Japanese laptop computers in the United States, expressed in terms of dollars per computer. In panel (b), we show the demand curve, *D*, which slopes downward. In panel (c), we show the number of yens required to purchase up to 700 laptop computers. If the price per laptop computer in Japan is 100,000 yen, we can now find the quantity of yen needed to pay for the various quantities demanded. In panel (d), we see the derived demand for yen in the United States in order to purchase the various quantities of computers given in panel (a). The resultant demand curve, D_1, is shown in panel (e). This is the American derived demand for yen.

FIGURE 33-3

The Supply of Japanese Yen

If the market price of a U.S.-produced microprocessor is $200, then at an exchange rate of $.0100 per yen (1 cent per yen), the price of the microprocessor to a Japanese consumer is 20,000 yen. If the exchange rate rises to $.0125 per yen, the Japanese price of the microprocessor falls to 16,000 yen. This induces an increase in the quantity of microprocessors demanded by Japanese consumers and consequently an increase in the quantity of yen supplied in exchange for dollars in the foreign exchange market. By contrast, if the exchange rate falls to $.0075 per yen, the Japanese price of the microprocessor rises to 26,667 yen. This causes a decrease in the quantity of microprocessors demanded by Japanese consumers. As a result, there is a decline in the quantity of yen supplied in exchange for dollars in the foreign exchange market.

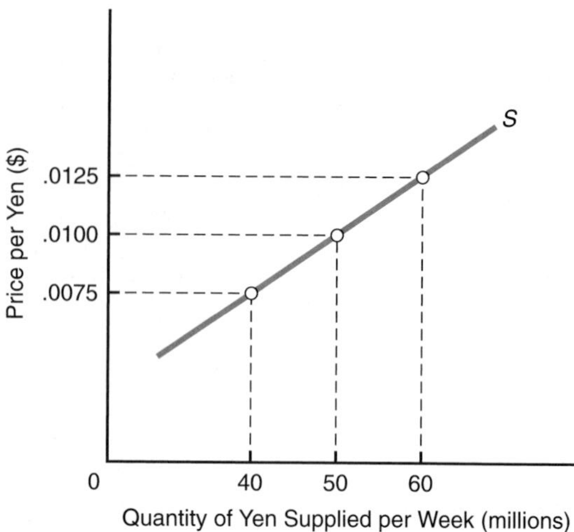

($.0125). A Japanese laptop computer priced at 100,000 yen in Japan would now cost $1,250. From panel (a), we see that at $1,250 per computer, 300 laptop computers will be imported from Japan into the United States by our representative group of U.S. consumers. From panel (c), we see that 300 computers would require 30 million yen to be purchased; thus in panels (d) and (e), we see that at a price of $1\frac{1}{4}$ cents per yen, the quantity demanded will be 30 million yen.

We continue similar calculations all the way up to a price of $1\frac{1}{2}$ cents ($.0150) per yen. At that price, a Japanese laptop computer costing 100,000 yen in Japan would cost $1,500, and our representative U.S. consumers would import only 100 laptop computers.

Downward-Sloping Derived Demand. As can be expected, as the price of yen rises, the quantity demanded will fall. The only difference here from the standard demand analysis developed in Chapter 3 and used throughout this text is that the demand for yen is derived from the demand for a final product—Japanese laptop computers in our example.

Supply of Japanese Yen. Assume that Japanese laptop manufacturers buy U.S. microprocessors. The supply of Japanese yen is a derived supply in that it is derived from the Japanese demand for U.S. microprocessors. We could go through an example similar to the one for laptop computers to come up with a supply schedule of Japanese yen in Japan. It slopes upward. Obviously, the Japanese want dollars to purchase U.S. goods. Japanese residents will be willing to supply more yen when the dollar price of yen goes up, because they can then buy more U.S. goods with the same quantity of yen. That is, the yen would be worth more in exchange for U.S. goods than when the dollar price for yen was lower.

An Example. Let's take an example. Suppose a U.S.-produced microprocessor costs $200. If the exchange rate is 1 cent per one yen, a Japanese resident will have to come up with 20,000 yen (= $200 at $.0100 per yen) to buy one microprocessor. If, however, the exchange rate goes up to $1\frac{1}{4}$ cents for yen, a Japanese resident must come up with only 16,000 yen (= $200 at $.0125 per yen) to buy a U.S. microprocessor. At a lower price (in yen) of U.S. microprocessors, the Japanese will demand a larger quantity. In other words, as the price of Japanese yen goes up in terms of dollars, the quantity of U.S. microprocessors demanded will go up, and hence the quantity of Japanese yen supplied will go up.

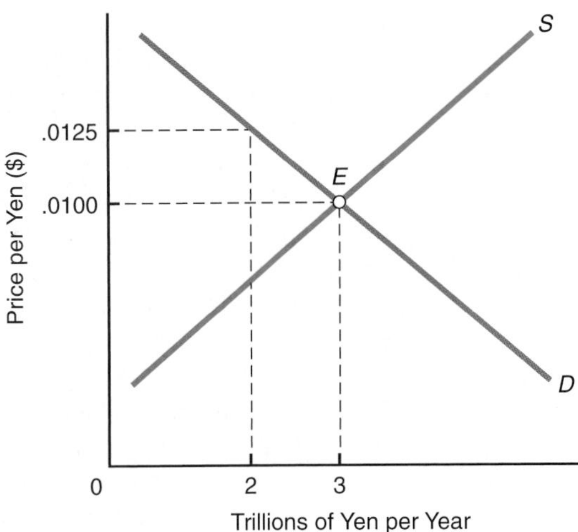

FIGURE 33-4

Total Demand for and Supply of Japanese Yen

The market supply curve for Japanese yen results from the total demand for U.S. microprocessors. The demand curve, *D,* slopes downward like most demand curves, and the supply curve *S,* slopes upward. The foreign exchange price, or the U.S. dollar price of yen, is given on the vertical axis. The number of yen is represented on the horizontal axis. If the foreign exchange rate is $.0125—that is, if it takes $1\frac{1}{4}$ cents to buy 1 yen—Americans will demand 2 trillion yen. The equilibrium exchange rate is at the intersection of *D* and *S.* The equilibrium exchange rate is $.0100 (1 cent). At this point, 3 trillion yen are both demanded and supplied each year.

Therefore, the supply schedule of yen, which is derived from the Japanese demand for U.S. goods, will slope upward.*

We could easily work through a detailed numerical example to show that the supply curve of Japanese yen slopes upward. Rather than do that, we will simply draw it as upward-sloping in Figure 33-3 on the previous page. In our hypothetical example, assuming that there are only representative groups of laptop computer consumers in the United States and microprocessor consumers in Japan, the equilibrium exchange rate will be set at 1 cent per yen, or 100 yen to 1 dollar.

Total Demand for and Supply of Japanese Yen. Let us now look at the total demand for and supply of Japanese yen. We take all demanders of Japanese laptop computer and U.S. microprocessors and put their demands for and supplies of yen together into one diagram. Thus we are showing the total demand for and total supply of Japanese yen. The horizontal axis in Figure 33-4 represents a quantity of foreign exchange—the number of yen per year. The vertical axis represents the exchange rate—the price of foreign currency (yen) expressed in dollars (per yen). The foreign currency price of $.0125 per yen means it will cost you $1\frac{1}{4}$ cents to buy 1 yen. At the foreign currency price of $.0100 per yen, you know that it will cost you 1 cent to buy 1 yen. The equilibrium is again established at 1 cent for 1 yen.

This equilibrium is not established because U.S. residents like to buy yen or because the Japanese like to buy dollars. Rather, the equilibrium exchange rate depends on how many microprocessors the Japanese want and how many Japanese laptop computers U.S. residents want (given their respective incomes, their tastes, and the relative price of laptop computers and microprocessors).†

*Actually, the supply schedule of foreign currency will be upward-sloping if we assume that the demand for U.S. imported microprocessors on the part of the Japanese is price elastic. If the demand schedule for microprocessors is inelastic, the supply schedule will be negatively sloped. In the case of unit elasticity of demand, the supply schedule for yen will be a vertical line. Throughout the rest of this chapter, we will assume that demand is price elastic. Remember that the price elasticity of demand tells us whether or not total expenditures by microprocessor purchasers in Japan will rise or fall when the Japanese yen drops in value. In the long run, it is quite realistic to think that the price elasticity of demand for imports is numerically greater than 1 anyway.

†Remember that we are dealing with a two-country world in which we are considering only the exchange of U.S. microprocessors and Japanese laptop computers. In the real world, more than just goods and services are exchanged among countries. Some U.S. residents buy Japanese financial assets; some Japanese residents buy U.S. financial assets. We are ignoring such transactions for the moment.

A Shift in Demand. Assume that a successful advertising campaign by U.S. computer importers has caused U.S. demand for Japanese laptop computers to rise. U.S. residents demand more laptop computers at all prices. Their demand curve for Japanese laptop computers has shifted outward to the right.

The increased demand for Japanese laptop computers can be translated into an increased demand for yen. All U.S. residents clamoring for laptop computers will supply more dollars to the foreign exchange market while demanding more Japanese yen to pay for the computers. Figure 33-5 presents a new demand schedule, D_2, for Japanese yen; this demand schedule is to the right of the original demand schedule. If the Japanese do not change their desire for U.S. microprocessors, the supply schedule for Japanese yen will remain stable.

A new equilibrium will be established at a higher exchange rate. In our particular example, the new equilibrium is established at an exchange rate of $.0120 per yen. It now takes 1.2 cents to buy 1 Japanese yen, whereas formerly it took 1 cent. This will be translated into an increase in the price of Japanese laptop computers to U.S. residents and as a decrease in the price of U.S. microprocessors to the Japanese. For example, a Japanese laptop computer priced at 100,000 yen that sold for $1,000 in the United States will now be priced at $1,200. Conversely, a U.S. microprocessor priced at $50 that previously sold for 5,000 yen in Japan will now sell for 4,167 yen.

A Shift in Supply. We just assumed that the U.S. demand for Japanese laptop computers had shifted due to a successful ad compaign. Because the demand for Japanese yen is a derived demand by U.S. residents for laptop computers, this is translated into a shift in the demand curve for yen. As an alternative exercise, we might assume that the supply curve of Japanese yen shifts outward to the right. Such a supply shift could occur for many reasons, one of which is a relative rise in the Japanese price level. For example, if the price of all Japanese-manufactured computer components went up 100 percent in yen, U.S. microprocessors would become relatively cheaper. That would mean that Japanese residents would want to buy more U.S. microprocessors. But remember that when they want to buy more U.S. microprocessors, they supply more yen to the foreign exchange market.

Thus we see in Figure 33-6 that the supply curve of Japanese yen moves from S to S_1. In the absence of restrictions—that is, in a system of flexible exchange rates—the new

FIGURE 33-5

A Shift in the Demand Schedule

The demand schedule for Japanese laptop computers shifts to the right, causing the derived demand schedule for yen to shift to the right also. We have shown this as a shift from D_1 to D_2. We have assumed that the Japanese supply schedule for yen has remained stable—that is, Japanese demand for American microprocessors has remained constant. The old equilibrium foreign exchange rate was $.0100 (1 cent). The new equilibrium exchange rate will be E_2; it will now cost $.0120 (1.2 cents) to buy 1 yen. The higher price of yen will be translated into a higher U.S. dollar price for Japanese laptop computers and a lower Japanese yen price for American microprocessors.

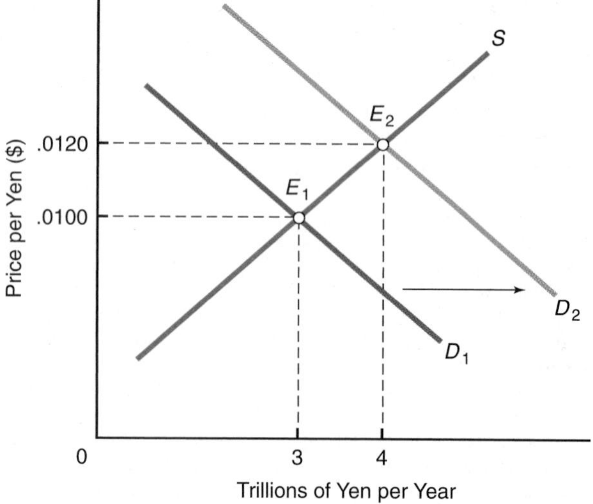

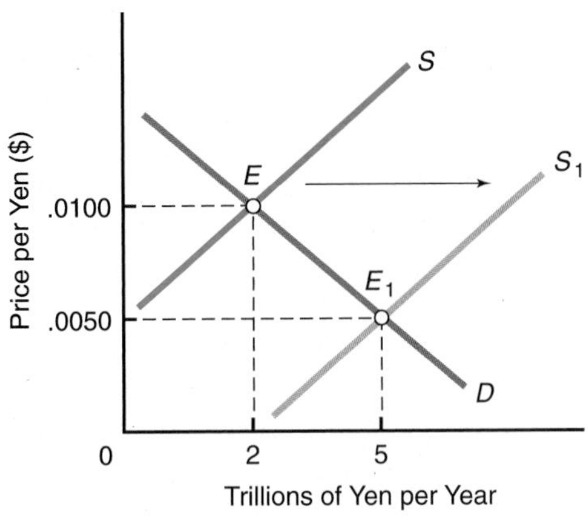

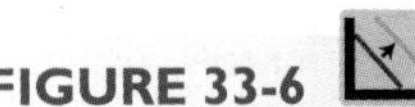

FIGURE 33-6

A Shift in the Supply of Japanese Yen

There has been a shift in the supply curve for Japanese yen. The new equilibrium will occur at E_1, meaning that \$.0050 ($\frac{1}{2}$ cent), rather than \$.0100 (1 cent), will now buy 1 yen. After the exchange rate adjustment, the amount of yen demanded and supplied will increase to 5 trillion per year.

equilibrium exchange rate will be 1 yen equals \$.0050, or $\frac{1}{2}$ cent equals 1 yen. The quantity of yen demanded and supplied will increase from 2 trillion per year to 5 trillion per year. We say, then, that in a flexible international exchange rate system, shifts in the demand for and supply of foreign currencies will cause changes in the equilibrium foreign exchange rates. Those rates will remain in effect until supply or demand shifts.

Market Determinants of Exchange Rates 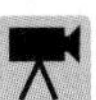

The foreign exchange market is affected by many other variables in addition to changes in relative price levels, including the following:

1. *Changes in real interest rates.* If the United States interest rate, corrected for people's expectations of inflation, abruptly increases relative to the rest of the world, international investors elsewhere will increase their demand for dollar-denominated assets, thereby increasing the demand for dollars in foreign exchange markets. An increased demand for dollars in foreign exchange markets, other things held constant, will cause the dollar to appreciate and other currencies to depreciate.
2. *Changes in productivity.* Whenever one country's productivity increases relative to another's, the former country will become more price competitive in world markets. At lower prices, the quantity of its exports demanded will increase. Thus there will be an increase in the demand for its currency.
3. *Changes in consumer preferences.* If Germany's citizens suddenly develop a taste for U.S.-made automobiles, this will increase the derived demand for U.S. dollars in foreign exchange markets.
4. *Perceptions of economic stability.* As already mentioned, if the United States looks economically and politically more stable relative to other countries, more foreign residents will want to put their savings into U.S. assets than in their own domestic assets. This will increase the demand for dollars.

CONCEPTS IN BRIEF

- The foreign exchange rate is the rate at which one country's currency can be exchanged for another's.
- The demand for foreign exchange is a derived demand; it is derived from the demand for foreign goods and services (and financial assets). The supply of foreign exchange is derived from foreign residents' demands for domestic goods and services.

- The demand curve of foreign exchange slopes downward, and the supply curve of foreign exchange slopes upward. The equilibrium foreign exchange role occurs at the intersection of the demand and supply curves for a currency.
- A shift in the demand for foreign goods will result in a shift in the demand for foreign exchange, thereby changing the equilibrium foreign exchange rate. A shift in the supply of foreign currency will also cause a change in the equilibrium exchange rate.

THE GOLD STANDARD AND THE INTERNATIONAL MONETARY FUND

The current system of more or less freely floating exchange rates is a recent development. We have had, in the past, periods of a gold standard, fixed exchange rates under the International Monetary Fund, and variants of these two.

The Gold Standard

Until the 1930s, many nations were on a gold standard. The value of their domestic currency was tied directly to gold. Nations operating under this gold standard agreed to redeem their currencies for a fixed amount of gold at the request of any holder of that currency. Although gold was not necessarily the means of exchange for world trade, it was the unit to which all currencies under the gold standard were pegged. And because all currencies in the system were linked to gold, exchange rates between those currencies were fixed. Indeed, the gold standard has been offered as the prototype of a fixed exchange rate system. The heyday of the gold standard was from about 1870 to 1914.

There was (and always is) a relationship between the balance of payments and changes in domestic money supplies throughout the world. Under a gold standard, the international financial market reached equilibrium through the effect of gold flows on each country's money supply. When a nation suffered a deficit in its balance of payments, more gold would flow out than in. Because the domestic money supply was based on gold, an outflow of gold to foreign residents caused an automatic reduction in the domestic money supply. This caused several things to happen. Interest rates rose, thereby attracting foreign capital and reducing any deficit in the balance of payments. At the same time, the reduction in the money supply was equivalent to a restrictive monetary policy, which caused national output and prices to fall. Imports were discouraged and exports were encouraged, thereby again improving the balance of payments.

Two problems plagued the gold standard. One was that by varying the value of its currency in response to changes in the quantity of gold, a nation gave up control of its domestic monetary policy. Another was that the world's commerce was at the mercy of gold discoveries. Throughout history, each time new veins of gold were found, desired expenditures on goods and services increased. If production of goods and services failed to increase, however, prices of goods and services increased, so inflation resulted.

International Monetary Fund (IMF)

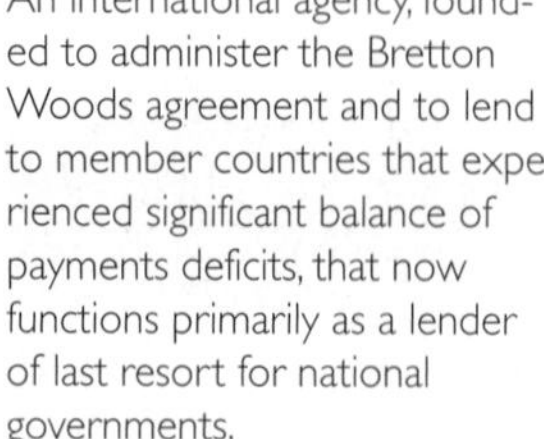

An international agency, founded to administer the Bretton Woods agreement and to lend to member countries that experienced significant balance of payments deficits, that now functions primarily as a lender of last resort for national governments.

Bretton Woods and the International Monetary Fund

In 1944, as World War II was ending, representatives from the world's capitalist countries met in Bretton Woods, New Hampshire, to create a new international payment system to replace the gold standard, which had collapsed during the 1930s. The Bretton Woods Agreement Act was signed on July 31, 1945, by President Harry Truman. It created a new permanent institution, the **International Monetary Fund (IMF),** to administer the agreement and to lend to member countries that were experiencing significant balance of payments deficits. The arrangements thus provided are now called the old IMF system or the Bretton Woods system.

Member governments were obligated to intervene to maintain the value of their currencies in foreign exchange markets within 1 percent of the declared **par value**—the officially determined value. The United States, which owned most of the world's gold stock, was similarly obligated to maintain gold prices within a 1 percent margin of the official rate of $35 an ounce. Except for a transitional arrangement permitting a onetime adjustment of up to 10 percent in par value, members could alter exchange rates thereafter only with the approval of the IMF.

Par value 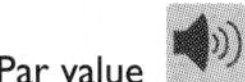
The officially determined value of a currency.

On August 15, 1971, President Richard Nixon suspended the convertibility of the dollar into gold. On December 18, 1971, the United States officially devalued the dollar—that is, lowered its official value—relative to the currencies of 14 major industrial nations. Finally, on March 16, 1973, the finance ministers of the European Economic Community (now the European Union) announced that they would let their currencies float against the dollar, something Japan had already begun doing with its yen. Since 1973, the United States and most other trading countries have had either freely floating exchange rates or managed ("dirty") floating exchange rates, in which their governments or central banks intervene from time to time to try to influence market exchange rates.

FIXED VERSUS FLOATING EXCHANGE RATES

The United States went off the Bretton Woods system of fixed exchange rates in 1973. As Figure 33-7 indicates, many other nations of the world have been less willing to permit the values of their currencies to vary in the foreign exchange markets.

Fixing the Exchange Rate

How did nations fix their exchange rates in years past? How do many countries accomplish this today? Figure 33-8 on the next page shows the market for baht, the currency of Thailand. At the initial equilibrium point E_1, U.S. residents had to give up $0.40 to obtain 1 baht. Suppose now that there is an increase in the supply of baht for dollars, perhaps because Thai residents wish to buy more U.S. goods. Other things being equal, the result would be a movement to point E_2 in Figure 33-8. The dollar value of the baht would fall to $0.30.

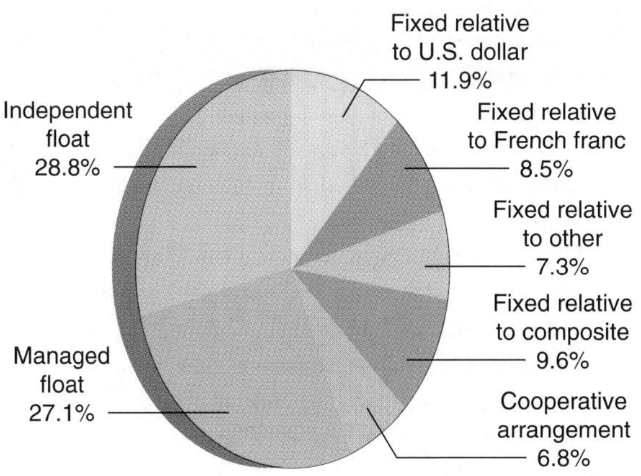

FIGURE 33-7

Current Foreign Exchange Rate Arrangements

Currently, 56 percent of the member nations of the International Monetary Fund have an independent float or managed float exchange rate arrangement. Among countries with a fixed exchange rate, nearly one in three uses a fixed U.S. dollar exchange rate. Fixing the exchange rate relative to a composite or basket of currencies is the next most common arrangement.

Source: International Monetary Fund.

FIGURE 33-8

A Fixed Exchange Rate

This figure illustrates how the Bank of Thailand could fix the dollar-baht exchange rate in the face of an increase in the supply of baht caused by a rise in the demand for U.S. goods by Thai residents. In the absence of any action by the Bank of Thailand, the result would be a movement from point E_1 to point E_2. The dollar value of the baht would fall from \$0.40 to \$0.30. The Bank of Thailand can prevent this exchange rate change by purchasing baht with dollars in the foreign exchange market, thereby raising the demand for baht. At the new equilibrium point E_3, the baht's value remains at \$0.40.

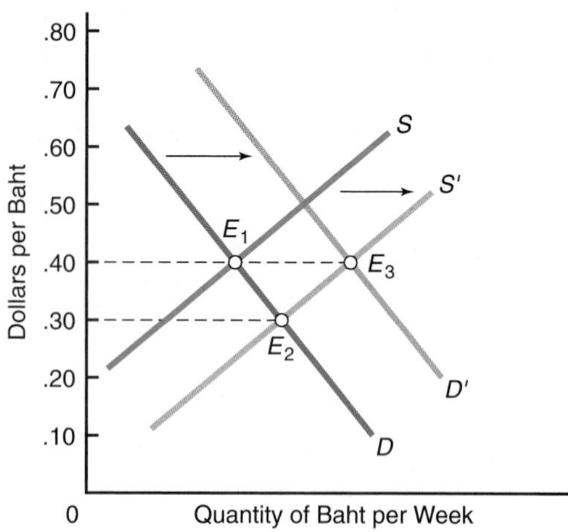

To prevent a baht depreciation from occurring, however, the Bank of Thailand, the central bank, could increase the demand for baht in the foreign exchange market by purchasing baht with dollars. The Bank of Thailand can do this using dollars that it had on hand as part of its *foreign exchange reserves.* All central banks hold reserves of foreign currencies. Because the U.S. dollar is a key international currency, the Bank of Thailand and other central banks typically hold billions of dollars in reserve so that they can, if they wish, make transactions such as the one in this example. Note that a sufficiently large purchase of baht could, as shown in Figure 33-8, cause the demand curve to shift rightward to achieve the new equilibrium point E_3, at which the baht's value remains at \$0.40. Provided that it has enough dollar reserves on hand, the Bank of Thailand could maintain—effectively fix—the exchange rate in the face of the sudden fall in the demand for baht.

This is the manner in which the Bank of Thailand fixed the dollar-baht exchange rate until 1997. This basic approach—varying the amount of the national currency demanded at any given exchange rate in foreign exchange markets when necessary—is also the way that *any* central bank seeks to keep its nation's currency value unchanged in light of changing market forces.

Central banks can keep exchange rates fixed as long as they have enough foreign exchange reserves available to deal with potentially long-lasting changes in the demand for or supply of their nation's currency.

INTERNATIONAL POLICY EXAMPLE

Can Foreign Exchange Rates Be Fixed Forever?

Trying to keep the exchange rate fixed in the face of foreign exchange market volatility can be a difficult policy to pursue. Consider Thailand's experience. At the beginning of 1997, the Bank of Thailand was holding \$40 billion in foreign exchange reserves. Within 10 months, those reserves had fallen to \$3 billion. Whatever the Bank of Thailand promised about not devaluing, it no longer had credibility. Not surprisingly, the baht's value relative to the dollar fell by more than 25 percent in July 1997 alone.

The Thai experience was repeated on a larger scale throughout Southeast Asia in 1997 and 1998 as efforts by the central banks of Indonesia, Malaysia, South Korea, and Vietnam to fix exchange rates ultimately collapsed, leading to sizable devaluations. Even the previously stalwart exchange rate arrangements of

Singapore, Taiwan, and Hong Kong became increasingly less credible. These nations learned an old lesson: Trying to protect residents from foreign exchange risks works only as long as foreign exchange market traders believe that central banks have the financial wherewithal to keep exchange rates unchanged. Otherwise, a fixed exchange rate policy can ultimately prove unsustainable.

For Critical Analysis

Why do you think governments attempt to maintain the foreign exchange value of their domestic currencies?

Pros and Cons of a Fixed Exchange Rate 

Why might a nation such as Thailand wish to keep the value of its currency from fluctuating? One reason is that changes in the exchange rate can affect the market values of assets that are denominated in foreign currencies. This can increase the financial risks that a nation's residents face, thereby forcing them to incur costs to avoid these risks.

Foreign Exchange Risk. The possibility that variations in the market value of assets can take place as a result of changes in the value of a nation's currency is called the **foreign exchange risk** that residents of a country face because their nation's currency value can vary. For instance, if companies in Thailand had many loans denominated in dollars but earned nearly all their revenues in baht from sales within Thailand, a decline in the dollar value of the baht would mean that Thai companies would have to allocate a larger portion of their earnings to make the same *dollar* loan payments as before. Thus a fall in the baht's value would increase the operating costs of these companies, thereby reducing their profitability and raising the likelihood of eventual bankruptcy.

Foreign exchange risk 
The possibility that changes in the value of a nation's currency will result in variations in market values of assets.

Limiting foreign exchange risk is a classic rationale for adopting a fixed exchange rate. Nevertheless, a country's residents are not defenseless against foreign exchange risk. They can **hedge** against such risk, meaning that they can adopt strategies intended to offset the risk arising from exchange rate variations. For example, a company in Thailand that has significant euro earnings from sales in Germany but sizable loans from U.S. investors could arrange to convert its euro earnings into dollars via special types of foreign exchange contracts called *currency swaps.* The Thai company could thereby avoid holdings of baht and shield itself—*hedge*—against variations in the baht's value.

Hedge 
A financial strategy that reduces the chance of suffering losses arising from foreign exchange risk.

The Exchange Rate as a Shock Absorber. If fixing the exchange rate limits foreign exchange risk, why do so many nations allow the exchange rates to float? The answer must be that there are potential drawbacks associated with fixing exchange rates. One is that exchange rate variations can actually perform a valuable service for a nation's economy. Consider a situation in which residents of a nation speak only their own nation's language, which is so difficult that hardly anyone else in the world takes the trouble to learn it. As a result, the country's residents are very *immobile:* They cannot trade their labor skills outside of their own nation's borders.

Now think about what happens if this nation chooses to fix its exchange rate. Imagine a situation in which other countries begin to sell products that are close substitutes for the products its people specialize in producing, causing a sizable drop in worldwide demand for the nation's goods. Over a short-run period in which prices and wages cannot adjust, the result will be a sharp decline in production of goods and services, a fall-off in national income, and higher unemployment. Contrast this situation with one in which the exchange rate floats. In this case, a sizable decline in outside demand for the nation's products will cause it to experience a trade deficit, which will lead to a significant drop in the demand for the nation's currency. As a result, the nation's currency will experience a sizable depreciation, making the goods that the nation offers to sell abroad much less expensive in other countries. People abroad who continue to consume the nation's products will increase their purchases, and the nation's exports will increase. Its production will begin to recover somewhat, as will its residents' incomes. Unemployment will begin to fall

This example illustrates how exchange rate variations can be beneficial, especially if a nation's residents are relatively immobile. It can be much more difficult, for example, for a Polish resident who has never studied Portuguese to make a move to Lisbon, even if she is highly qualified for available jobs there. If many residents of Poland face similar linguistic or cultural barriers, Poland could be better off with a floating exchange rate even if its residents must incur significant costs hedging against foreign exchange risk as a result.

Splitting the Difference: Dirty Floats and Target Zones

In recent years, national policymakers have tried to soften the choice of either adopting a fixed exchange rate or allowing exchange rates full flexibility in the foreign exchange markets by "splitting the difference" between the two extremes.

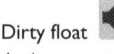

Dirty float
Active management of a floating exchange rate on the part of a country's government, often in cooperation with other nations.

A Dirty Float. One way to split the difference is to let exchange rates float most of the time but "manage" exchange rate movements part of the time. U.S. policymakers have occasionally engaged in what is called a **dirty float,** the management of flexible exchange rates. The management of flexible exchange rates has usually come about through international policy cooperation. For example, the Group of Five (G-5) nations—France, Germany, Japan, the United Kingdom, and the United States—and the Group of Seven (G-7) nations—the G-5 nations plus Italy and Canada—have for some time shared information on their economic policy objectives and procedures. They do this through regular meetings between economic policy secretaries, ministers, and staff members. One of their principal objectives has been to "smooth out" foreign exchange rates.

Is it possible for these groups to "manage" foreign exchange rates? Some economists do not think so. For example, economists Michael Bordo and Anna Schwartz studied the foreign exchange intervention actions coordinated by the Federal Reserve and the U.S. Treasury during the second half of the 1980s. Besides showing that such interventions were sporadic and variable, Bordo and Schwartz came to an even more compelling conclusion: Exchange rate interventions were trivial relative to the total trading of foreign exchange on a daily basis. For example, in April 1989, total foreign exchange trading amounted to \$129 billion per day, yet the American central bank purchased only \$100 million in deutsche marks and yen during that entire month (and did so on a single day). For all of 1989, Fed purchases of marks and yen were only \$17.7 billion, or the equivalent of less than 13 percent of the amount of an average day's trading in April of that year. Their conclusion is that neither the U.S. central bank nor the central banks of the other G-7 nations can influence exchange rates in the long run.

Crawling peg
An exchange rate arrangement in which a country pegs the value of its currency to the exchange value of another nation's currency but allows the par value to change at regular intervals.

Crawling Pegs. Another approach to splitting the difference between fixed and floating exchange rates is called a **crawling peg.** This is an automatically adjusting target for the value of a nation's currency. For instance, a central bank might announce that it wants the value of its currency relative to the U.S. dollar to decline at an annual rate of 5 percent, a rate of depreciation that it feels is consistent with long-run market forces. The central bank would then try to buy or sell foreign exchange reserves in sufficient quantities to be sure that the currency depreciation takes place gradually, thereby reducing the foreign exchange risk faced by the nation's residents.

In this way, a crawling peg functions like a floating exchange rate in the sense that the exchange rate can change over time. But it is like a fixed exchange rate in the sense that the central bank always tries to keep the exchange rate close to a target value. In this way, a crawling peg has elements of both kinds of exchange rate systems.

Target Zones. A third way to try to split the difference between fixed and floating exchange rates is to adopt an exchange rate **target zone.** Under this policy, a central bank announces that there are specific upper and lower *bands,* or limits, for permissible values for the exchange rate. Within those limits, which define the exchange rate target zone, the central bank permits the exchange rate to move flexibly. The central bank commits itself, however, to intervene in the foreign exchange markets to ensure that its nation's currency value will not rise above the upper band or fall below the lower band. For instance, if the exchange rate approaches the upper band, the central bank must sell foreign exchange reserves in sufficient quantities to prevent additional depreciation of its nation's currency. If the exchange rate approaches the lower band, the central bank must purchase sufficient amounts of foreign exchange reserves to halt any further currency appreciation.

Target zone 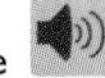
A range of permitted exchange rate variations between upper and lower exchange rate bands that a central bank defends by selling or buying foreign exchange reserves.

Starting in 1999, officials from the European Union attempted to get the United States, Japan, and several other countries' governments to agree to target zones for the exchange rate between the newly created euro and the dollar, yen, and some other currencies. Officials in the United States were not in favor. So far no target zones have been created, and the euro has floated freely—mostly downward.

CONCEPTS IN BRIEF

- The International Monetary Fund was developed after World War II as an institution to maintain fixed exchange rates in the world. Since 1973, however, fixed exchange rates have disappeared in most major trading countries. For these nations, exchange rates are largely determined by the forces of demand and supply in foreign exchange markets.
- Many other nations, however, have tried to fix their exchange rates, with varying degrees of success. Although fixing the exchange rate helps protect a nation's residents from foreign exchange risk, this policy makes less mobile residents susceptible to greater volatility in income and employment. It can also expose the central bank to sporadic currency crises arising from unpredictable changes in world capital flows.
- Countries have experimented with exchange rate systems between the extremes of fixed and floating exchange rates. Under a dirty float, a central bank permits the value of its nation's currency to float in foreign exchange markets but intervenes from time to time to influence the exchange rate. Under a crawling peg, a central bank tries to push its nation's currency value in a desired direction. Pursuing a target zone policy, a central bank aims to keep the exchange rate between upper and lower bands, intervening only when the exchange rate approaches either limit.

NETNOMICS

Making Foreign Exchange Markets More Efficient

The buying and selling of foreign exchange can involve considerable transaction costs. This is particularly true for companies that do not engage in large orders. The Internet has allowed for increased efficiency in this market, at least measured by real-time access and lower implicit commission rates for such transactions.

Back in 1993, a company called E-FOREX was founded to take advantage of Internet technology to develop a new marketplace for foreign exchange. In October 1995, E-FOREX completed its first Internet-based foreign exchange trade. Initially, E-FOREX was conceived as an on-line brokerage company, similar to E*Trade for stocks. Starting in 1996, though, E-FOREX began to license its Internet platforms to other financial institutions. Banks, brokers, and asset managers, for companies, pension plans, and governments, are using E-FOREX to trade today.

Consider a client that wishes to convert U.S. dollars to pay a 13 million yen invoice from its Japanese parts supplier. Even though a foreign exchange trading company would charge only a $50 commission on such a trade, it would also impose a large "spread" between the buying and selling price of yen. E-FOREX charges no commission but makes its profit on a small spread. In this transaction, the savings would be over $500 to the client. Throughout a year's worth of transactions, these savings might become considerable.

With large quantities of dollars, yen, euros, baht, and other currencies being traded over the Internet, security is a major issue. E-FOREX incorporates the latest 128-bit encryption technology and uses digital certificates from Versign as well as firewalls, which prevent outsiders from entering the secure system.

To avoid disaster, if one computer system fails, E-FOREX, similar to other Internet-based brokerage companies, operates two or more systems for routers and database servers. In addition, a remote backup data center supports those systems redundantly. In the event of a service interruption at any facility, no data are lost.

Finally, E-FOREX provides so-called 100 percent double-blind dealing. The party who takes the other side of a client's trade does not know who the client is, and vice versa. This increases foreign exchange efficiency because no clients can guess at the direction of trades and skew rates to earn trading profits in excess of a normal profit.

ISSUES & APPLICATIONS

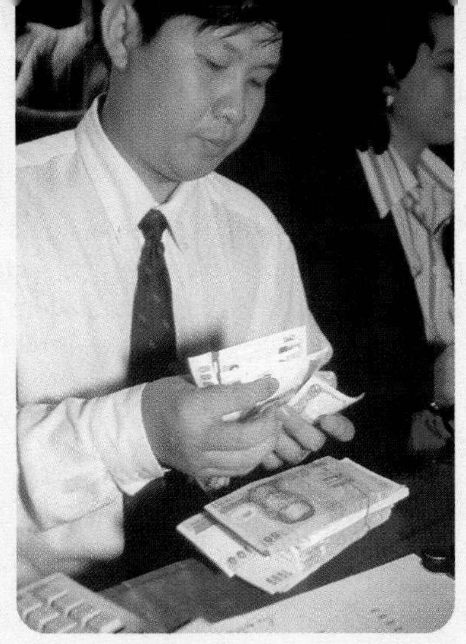

Are Currency Speculators Unproductive?

When the exchange value of the pound sterling plummeted more than 30 years ago, British politicians blamed the fall on "gnomes of Zurich"—currency speculators based in Switzerland. More recently, when Mahathir Mohamad, the Malaysian prime minister, decried currency speculators as "immoral," he particularly had in mind a speculator named George Soros, the chief executive of Quantum Fund, a firm that sought to earn speculative trading profits for its clients.

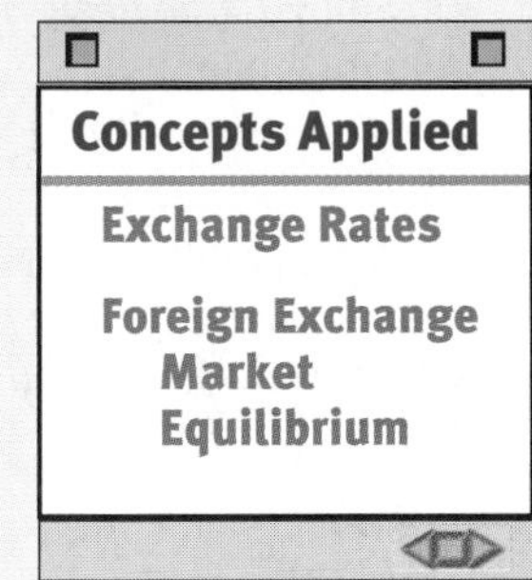

Speculative Attacks

In Mahathir's view, Quantum Fund reaped millions of dollars in trading profits at the expense of Malaysia when Soros correctly speculated that Malaysia could not maintain a fixed exchange rate for the Malaysian ringgit relative to the U.S. dollar. Quantum Fund and other individuals and firms conducted large numbers of currency trades with an aim to profit from a decline in the ringgit's value, thereby engaging in what economists call a *speculative attack* on the Malaysian currency.

Perhaps not surprisingly, Mahathir has argued that speculative currency trading is "excessive." He points to the trend highlighted in Figure 33-9: The growth of total foreign exchange trading has far outpaced the growth of total world trade in goods and services. Much of the growth in foreign exchange trading arises from increased purchases and sales of currencies by speculators. Much of this trading, Mahathir concludes, is "unnecessary" and "unproductive."

Some economists and policymakers agree with this assessment. They worry that foreign exchange markets may experience excessive volatility because of the activities of currency

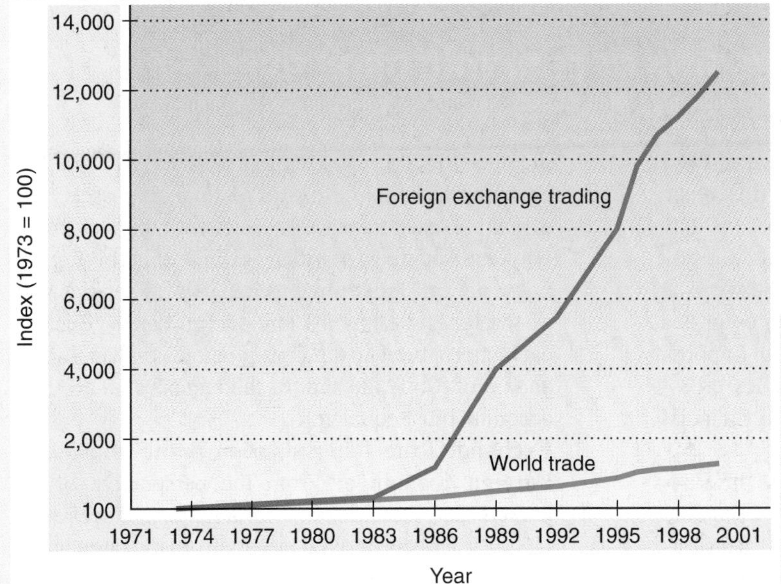

FIGURE 33-9
Foreign Exchange Trading and World Trade Since 1973
This figure displays index measures (1973 = 100) of the dollar volumes of total world trade and foreign exchange trading. At least a portion of the much faster growth of foreign exchange trading undoubtedly reflects an increase in speculative currency trading.
Sources: Bank for International Settlements; World Trade Organization.

speculators. To address this concern, Nobel laureate James Tobin has proposed taxing foreign exchange transactions to reduce the incentive to engage in currency speculation. In 1999, a United Nations study proposed imposing this "Tobin tax" and transferring the proceeds to the less developed nations of the world.

The Economic Role of Currency Speculators

There are, however, reasons to argue that the activities of currency speculators have social value. Firms such as Quantum Fund devote considerable time to studying the economic and political factors that play a fundamental role in determining exchange rates. This helps the firms seek out economic imbalances that are ultimately likely to force exchange rates to move into line with these fundamental factors at some point in the future. For currency speculators, such imbalances—such as, in the case of Malaysia in 1997, a fixed exchange rate that conflicts with the nation's economic policies—offer profitable opportunities. It is arguable that these imbalances could eventually pose serious economic problems in nations that experience them. By forcing countries to deal with imbalances sooner rather than later, speculative attacks may help prevent national policymakers from following misguided policies.

Speculative currency trading also plays an important economic role by making foreign exchange markets more liquid. Suppose that currency speculation were inhibited, for instance, by high taxes on foreign exchange transactions or by regulations requiring anyone who buys a foreign-currency-denominated asset to keep it for a specified period, regardless of changes in economic conditions. In such a situation, there might not be a strong incentive to hold the currency at all. This could make it hard for someone who wants to engage in the cross-border exchange of a real good or service to find willing buyers or sellers of currency required to finance the transaction. Thus the activities of currency speculators may contribute to the liquidity of foreign exchange markets and thereby contribute to the growth of world trade in goods and services. Stopping currency speculation could hinder or even reverse global growth of international trade.

FOR CRITICAL ANALYSIS

1. Why might it be desirable for a country's government to alter policies that are contributing to national economic imbalances sooner rather than later?
2. If defenders of currency speculators are correct, does Figure 33-9 indicate that foreign exchange markets have become more or less liquid in recent years?

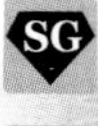

SUMMARY DISCUSSION OF LEARNING OBJECTIVES

1. **The Balance of Trade Versus the Balance of Payments:** The balance of trade is the difference between exports of goods and imports of goods during a given period. The balance of payments is a system of accounts for all transactions between a nation's residents and the residents of other countries of the world. In addition to exports and imports, therefore, the balance of payments includes cross-border exchanges of services, income, and financial assets within a given time interval.
2. **The Key Accounts Within the Balance of Payments:** There are three important accounts within the balance of payments. The current account measures net exchanges of goods and services, transfers, and income flows across a nation's borders. The capital account measures net flows of financial assets. The official reserve transactions account tabulates cross-border exchanges of financial assets involving the home nation's governments and central bank as well as foreign governments and central banks. Because each international exchange generates both an inflow and an outflow, the sum of the balances on all three accounts must equal zero.
3. **Exchange Rate Determination in the Market for Foreign Exchange:** From the perspective of the United States, the demand for a nation's currency by U.S. residents is derived largely from the demand for imports from that nation. Likewise, the supply of a

nation's currency is derived mainly from the supply of U.S. exports to that country. The equilibrium exchange rate is the rate of exchange between the dollar and the other nation's currency at which the quantity of the currency demanded is equal to the quantity supplied.

4. **Factors That Can Induce Changes in Equilibrium Exchange Rates:** The equilibrium exchange rate changes in response to changes in the demand for or supply of another nation's currency. Changes in desired flows of exports or imports, real interest rates, productivity in one nation relative to productivity in another nation, tastes and preferences of consumers, and perceptions of economic stability are key factors that can affect the positions of the demand and supply curves in foreign exchange markets. Thus changes in these factors can induce variations in equilibrium exchange rates.
5. **How Policymakers Can Attempt to Keep Exchange Rates Fixed:** If the current price of another nation's currency in terms of the home currency starts to fall below the level where the home country wants it to remain, the home country's central bank can use reserves of the other nation's currency to purchase the home currency in foreign exchange markets. This raises the demand for the home currency and thereby pushes up the currency's value in terms of the other nation's currency. In this way, the home country can keep the exchange rate fixed at a desired value, as long as it has sufficient reserves of the other currency to use for this purpose.
6. **Alternative Approaches to Limiting Exchange Rate Variability:** Today, many nations permit their exchange rates to vary in foreign exchange markets. Others pursue policies that limit the variability of exchange rates. Some engage in a dirty float, in which they manage exchange rates, often in cooperation with other nations. Some establish crawling pegs, in which the target value of the exchange rate is adjusted automatically over time. And some establish target zones, with upper and lower limits on the extent to which exchange rates are allowed to vary.

Key Terms and Concepts

Accounting identities (806)
Appreciation (814)
Balance of payments (806)
Balance of trade (806)
Crawling peg (824)
Depreciation (814)
Dirty float (824)
Exchange rate (813)
Flexible exchange rates (813)
Foreign exchange market (813)
Foreign exchange risk (823)
Hedge (823)
International Monetary Fund (IMF) (820)
Par value (821)
Special drawing rights (SDRs) (810)
Target zone (825)

Problems

Answers to the odd-numbered problems appear at the back of the book.

33-1. Over the course of a year, a nation tracked its foreign transactions and arrived at the following amounts:

Merchandise exports	500
Service Exports	75
Net unilateral exports	10
Domestic assets abroad (capital outflows)	−200
Foreign assets at home (capital inflows)	300
Changes in official reserves	−35
Merchandise imports	600
Service imports	50

What is this nation's balance of trade, current account balance, and capital account balance?

33-2. Whenever the United States reaches record levels on its current account deficit, Congress flirts with the idea of restricting imported goods. Would trade restrictions like those studied in Chapter 32 be an appropriate response?

33-3. Explain how the following events would affect the market for the Mexican peso.

a. Improvements in Mexican production technology yield superior guitars, and many musicians desire these guitars.

b. Perceptions of political instability surrounding regular elections in Mexico make international investors nervous about future business prospects in Mexico.

33-4. On Wednesday, the exchange rate between the euro and the U.S. dollar was $1.07 per euro. On Thursday, it was $1.05. Did the euro appreciate or depreciate against the dollar? By how much?

33-5. On Wednesday, the exchange rate between the euro and the U.S. dollar was $1.07 per euro and the exchange rate between the Canadian dollar and the U.S. dollar was U.S. $.68 per Canadian dollar. What is the exchange rate between the Canadian dollar and the euro?

33-6. Suppose that signs of an improvement in the Japanese economy lead international investors to resume lending to the Japanese government and businesses. Policymakers, however, are worried about how this will influence the yen. How would this event affect the market for the yen? How should the central bank, the Bank of Japan, respond to this event if it wants to maintain the value of the yen?

33-7. Briefly explain the differences between a flexible exchange rate system, a fixed exchange rate system, a dirty float, and a target zone.

33-8. Explain how each of the following would affect Canada's balance of payments.

a. Canada's rate of inflation falls below that of the United States, its main trading partner.

b. The possibility of Quebec's separating from the federation frightens international investors.

33-9. Suppose that under a gold standard, the U.S. dollar is pegged to gold at a rate of $35 per ounce and the pound sterling is pegged to gold at a rate of £17.50 per ounce. Explain how the gold standard constitutes an exchange rate arrangement. What is the exchange rate between the U.S. dollar and the pound sterling?

33-10. Suppose that under the Bretton Woods System, the dollar is pegged to gold at a rate of $35 per ounce and the pound sterling is pegged to the dollar at a rate of $2 = £1. If the dollar is devalued against gold and the pegged rate is changed to $40 per ounce, what does this imply for the exchange value of the pound?

Economics on the Net

Daily Exchange Rates It is an easy matter to keep up with changes in exchange rates every day using the Web site of the Federal Reserve Bank of New York. In this application, you will learn how hard it is to predict exchange rate movements, and you will get some practice thinking about what factors can cause exchange rates to change.

Title: The Federal Reserve Bank of New York: Foreign Exchange 12 Noon Rates

Navigation: Click here to visit the Federal Reserve Bank of New York's homepage. Select Statistics. Click on Foreign Exchange 12 Noon Rates.

Application

1. For each currency listed, how many dollars does it take to purchase a unit of the currency in the spot foreign exchange market?
2. For each day during a given week (or month), choose a currency from those listed and keep track of its value relative to the dollar. Based on your tabulations, try to predict the value of the currency at the end of the week *following* your data collections. Use any information you may have, or just do your best without any additional information. How far off did your prediction turn out to be?

For Group Study and Analysis Each day, you can also click on a report titled "Foreign Exchange 10 a.m. Rates," which shows exchange rates for a subset of countries listed in the noon report. Assign each country in the 10 A.M. report to a group. Ask the group to determine whether the currency's value appreciated or depreciated relative to the dollar between 10 A.M. and noon. In addition, ask each group to discuss what kinds of demand or supply shifts could have caused the change that occurred during this interval.

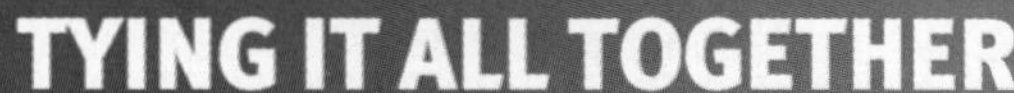

TYING IT ALL TOGETHER

Part 8 Case Problem

Case Background

The president of a small, less developed Latin American nation has big problems. The annual inflation rate is running above 100 percent, the value of the country's currency is dropping like a rock, and foreign savers are rushing to sell off their shares in investment within the country. The president has appointed a working group of economists to study alternative approaches to achieving the president's goal of fixing the nation's exchange rate relative to the U.S. dollar.

A Currency Board Versus Dollarization It does not take long for the working group to narrow down the choices. One means of establishing a truly fixed rate of exchange for a nation's currency is by establishing a currency board. This is an institution that issues currency fully backed by reserves of a foreign currency. That is, the currency board pledges to redeem its domestic currency for a foreign "hard currency," such as the U.S. dollar, at a fixed rate of exchange. With full backing of outstanding currency, the government board can fulfill this pledge.

Establishing a currency board would preclude a couple of activities associated with central banking. Most obviously, this nation could no longer conduct an independent monetary policy if it cannot vary the quantity of its currency that is in circulation. In the event of unexpected outflows of funds—such as the one the country has recently experienced—there would be pressure for the nation's currency to depreciate. To prevent this from occurring, the currency board would simply sell some of its foreign reserves. The second central-banking activity that a currency board often cannot undertake is lending to liquidity-constrained banks and other financial institutions to thwart a bank run or similar financial crisis. Some nations, such as Argentina, have preserved this central-banking role for their currency boards by permitting the currency board to hold some domestic securities. In the event of a liquidity crunch, the currency board can lend financial institutions funds from that available pool of domestic assets.

In addition, there can be an explicit cost of operating a currency board. Financial instruments of developing nations often yield higher returns than those of a developed country such as the United States. Because a currency board would hold dollar-denominated reserves instead of domestic securities, the government of this Latin American country would have to forgo some interest earnings that it normally could use to help fund public expenditures.

An even more dramatic way to achieve a permanently fixed exchange rate is dollarization, which entails the abandonment of the nation's own currency in favor of making the U.S. dollar the country's only legal currency. In this event, there really would be no exchange rate, of course; the currency circulating in the Latin American nation would be the U.S. currency. But the rate of exchange of home currency for U.S. currency would be, as the president wishes, one for one, so in this sense dollarization is the most extreme form of a fixed exchange rate.

In a fully dollarized economy, the nation's monetary policymaker's job would simply be to facilitate the replacement of worn-out dollars. To get to the point of complete dollarization, the nation would obtain the dollars by issuing dollar-denominated debts, and the interest it would have to pay on these debts would be an explicit cost of dollarization. As with a currency board, this forgone interest income could be used to help fund public expenditures. Another cost would be the expense of transporting new dollars and coins from the United States when setting up the system and when old U.S. currency eventually wears out and has to be replaced.

Points to Analyze

1. What is the fundamental difference between a fixed-exchange-rate policy as implemented by a central bank as compared with a fixed exchange rate policy as pursued by a currency board? Why might foreign savers perceive that the latter is less risky than the former?
2. Is there any point in retaining a central bank if there is a currency board? If the economy is dollarized?
3. Why might adopting a currency board or dollarization help stabilize cross-border flows of funds and international trade in goods and services?
4. Why are foreign savers likely to believe that dollarization is a more credible commitment to stable terms of international exchange than a currency board would be?
5. Suppose that the nation decides to dollarize its economy. Who in this country would pay for this change? (Hint: Who pays for the public expenditures that in the past have been partly funded with government revenues from interest on domestic security holdings?)
6. Is an irrevocably fixed exchange rate more desirable than a floating exchange rate? Why?

Casing the Internet

1. **Click here to learn more about how currency boards have functioned. Click on "Introduction." Read the article, and then answer the following questions:**
   a. **What are the key features of an "orthodox" currency board?**
   b. **In what ways have Argentina and Bulgaria's currency board arrangements differed from those of an orthodox currency board?**
   c. **The article lists a number of countries that have used currency board arrangements in the past and present. Make a list of nations that have had either good or poor experience with currency boards. What factors appear to influence how well a currency board works?**
2. **Click here to go to the Web site of the Hong Kong Monetary Authority. Answer the following questions:**
   a. **Click on "THE HKMA," and after you read the page, at the top click on "Advisory Committee". Read about the Exchange Fund Advisory Committee. In the context of our case description of a currency board, what exactly is the Hong Kong "Exchange Fund"?**
   b. **Back up to the homepage, and under "Monetary Stability" click on "Currency Board System". Why does the Hong Kong Monetary Authority refer to its system as "Linked Exchange Rate System"?**

Answers to Odd-Numbered Problems

CHAPTER 1

1-1. This issue involves choice and therefore can be approached using the economic way of thinking. In the case of health care, an individual typically has an unlimited desire for good health. The individual has a limited budget and limited time, however. She must allocate her budget across other desirable goods, such as housing and food, and must allocate their time across waiting in the doctor's office, work, leisure, and sleep. Hence choices must be made in light of limited resources.

1-3. Sally is displaying rational behavior if all of these activities are in her self-interest. For example, Sally likely derives intrinsic value from volunteer and extracurricular activities and may believe that these activities, along with good grades, improve her prospects of finding a job after she completes her studies. Hence these activities are in her self-interest even though they take away some study time.

1-5. Suppose that you desire to earn an A (90 percent) in economics and merely to pass (60 percent) in French. If your model indicates that you earn 15 percentage points on each exam for every hour you spend studying, you would spend 6 hours ($6 \times 15 = 90$) studying economics and 4 hours ($4 \times 15 = 60$) studying French.

1-7. Positive economic analysis deals with the outcome of economics models, whereas normative analysis includes social values in the choice as well.

1-9. a. An increase in the supply of laptop computers, perhaps because of the entry of new computer manufacturers into the market, pushes their price back down.
b. Another factor, such as higher hotel taxes at popular vacation destinations, makes vacation travel more expensive.
c. Some other factor, such as a fall in wages that workers earn, discourages people from working additional hours.

APPENDIX A

A-1. a. Independent: price; dependent: quantity
b. Independent: work-study hours; dependent: credit hours
c. Independent: hours of study; dependent: economics grade

A-3. a. Above *x* axis; left of *y* axis
b. Below *x* axis; right of *y* axis
c. Above *x* axis; on *y* axis

A-5.

y	*x*
−20	−4
−10	−2
0	0
10	2
20	4

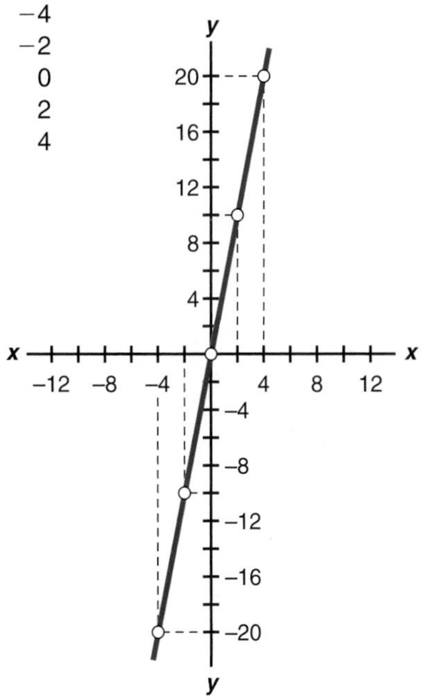

A-7. 5

A-9. a. Positive
b. Positive
c. Negative

CHAPTER 2

2-1. Each additional 10 points earned in economics costs 10 additional points in biology, so this PPC illustrates *constant* opportunity costs.

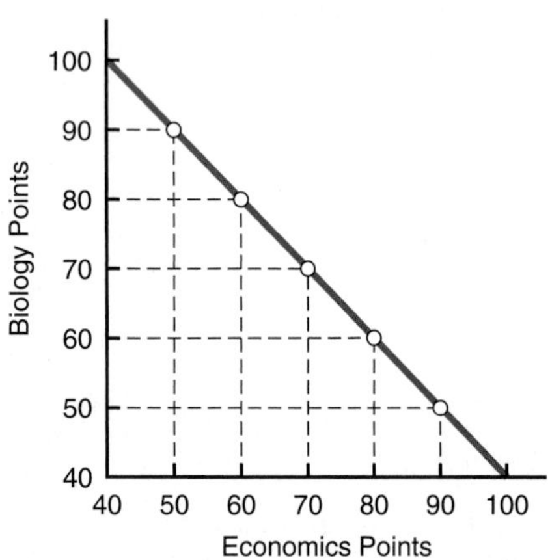

2-3. The \$4,500 paid for tuition, room and board, and books consists of explicit costs, not opportunity costs. The \$3,000 in lost wages is a forgone opportunity, as is the 3 percent interest that could have been earned on the \$4,500. Hence the total opportunity cost is equal to \$3,000 + (\$4,500 × 0.03) = \$3,000 + \$135 = \$3,135.

2-5.

a.

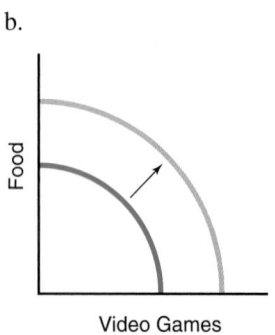

Food

Video Games

b.

Food

Video Games

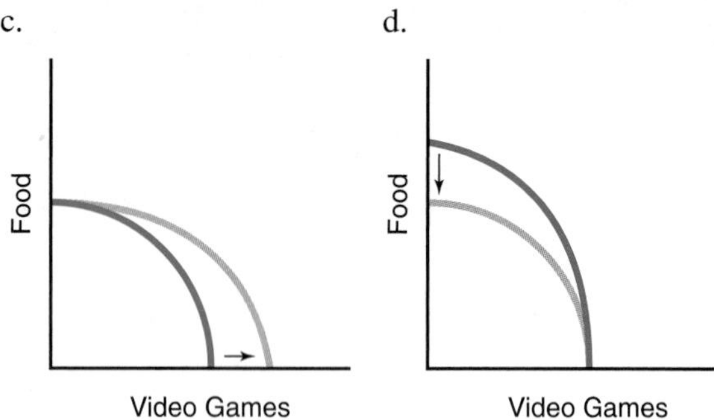

2-7. Because it takes you less time to do laundry, you have an absolute advantage in laundry. Neither you nor your roommate has an absolute advantage in meal preparation. You require two hours to fold a basket of laundry, so your opportunity cost of folding a basket of laundry is two meals. Your roommate's opportunity cost of folding a basket of laundry is three meals. Hence you have a comparative advantage in laundry, and your roommate has a comparative advantage in meal preparation.

2-9. If countries produce the goods for which they have a comparative advantage and trade for those for which they are at a comparative disadvantage, the distribution of resources is more efficient in each nation, yielding gains for both. Artificially restraining trade that would otherwise yield such gains thereby imposes social losses on the residents of both nations.

2-11. a. If the two nations have the same production possibilities, they face the same opportunity costs of producing consumption goods and capital goods. Thus at present neither has a comparative advantage in producing either good.
b. Because country B produces more capital goods today, it will be able to produce more of both goods in the future. Consequently, country B's PPC will shift outward by a greater amount next year.
c. Country B now has a comparative advantage in producing capital goods, and country A now has a comparative advantage in producing consumer goods.

CHAPTER 3

3-1. The equilibrium price is $11 per CD, and the equilibrium quantity is 80 million CDs. At a price of $10 per CD, the quantity of CDs demanded is 90 million, and the quantity of CDs supplied is 60 million. Hence there is a shortage of 30 million CDs at a price of $10 per CD.

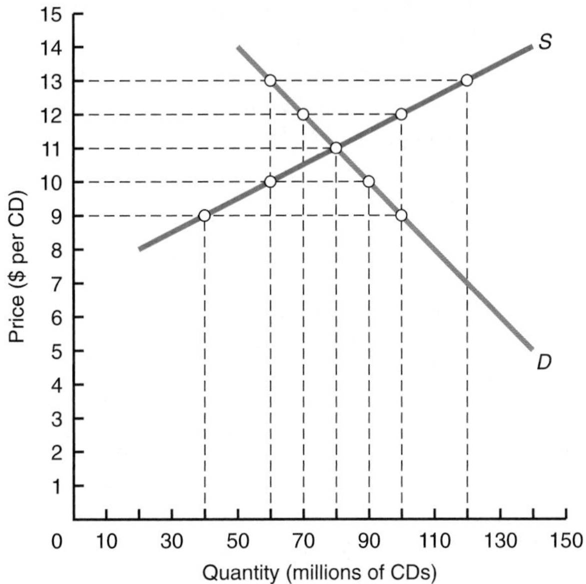

3-3. a. This fall in the price of an input used to produce rock music CDs causes the supply of these CDs to increase. The results are a decline in the market price of rock music CDs and an increase in the equilibrium quantity of rock music CDs.

b. Because CD players and CDs are complements in consumption, a decrease in the price of CD players causes the demand for rock music CDs to increase. This results in an increase in the market price of rock music CDs and an increase in the equilibrium quantity of these CDs.

c. Because cassette tapes and CDs are substitutes in consumption, an increase in the price of cassette tapes increases the demand for rock music CDs. This causes an increase in the market price of rock music CDs and an increase in the equilibrium quantity of rock music CDs.

d. As long as a CD is a normal good, an increase in the income of the typical rock music CD consumer results in an increase in the demand for rock music CDs, which causes the market price of rock music CDs to rise and the equilibrium quantity of these CDs to increase.

e. This shift in preferences would cause a decrease in the demand for rock music CDs, so the market price of these CDs would decline, and the equilibrium quantity of rock music CDs would decrease.

3-5. The imposition of this tax would decrease the supply of Roquefort cheese, which would cause the supply curve to shift leftward. The market price would increase, and equilibrium quantity would fall.

3-7. a. Because memory chips are an input in the production of laptop computers, a decrease in the price of memory chips causes an increase in the supply of laptop computers. The market supply curve shifts to the right, causing the market price to fall and the equilibrium quantity to increase.

b. A decrease in the price of memory chips used in desktop personal computers causes the supply of desktop computers to increase, thereby bringing about a decline in the market price of desktop computers, which are substitutes for laptop computers. This causes a decrease in the demand for laptop computers. The market demand curve shifts leftward, which causes declines in the market price and equilibrium quantity of laptop computers.

c. An increase in the number of manufactures of laptop computers causes an increase in the supply of laptop computers. The market supply curve shifts rightward. The market price of laptop computers declines, and the equilibrium quantity of laptop computers increases.

d. Because computer peripherals are complements, decreases in their prices induce an increase in the demand for laptop computers. Thus the market demand curve shifts to the right, and the market price and equilibrium quantity of laptop computers increase.

3-9. a. The demand for tickets declines, and there will be a surplus of tickets.

b. The demand for tickets rises, and there will be a shortage of tickets.

c. The demand for tickets increases, and there will be a shortage of tickets.

d. The demand for tickets falls, and there will be a surplus of tickets.

CHAPTER 4

4-1. To the band, its producer, and consumers, the market price of the CD provides an indication of the popularity of the band's music; for instance, if the market price rises relative to other CDs, this signals that the band should continue to record its music for sale.

4-3. The market rental rate is $500 per apartment, and 2,000 apartments are rented at this price. At a ceiling price of $450 per month, students wishing to live off campus wish to rent 2,500 apartments, but apartment owners are willing to supply only 1,800 apartments. Thus there is a shortage of 700 apartments at the ceiling price.

4-5. At the above-market price of sugar in the U.S. sugar market, U.S. businesses that use sugar as an input in their products (such as chocolate manufacturers) face higher costs, which shifts the market supply curve leftward. This pushes up the market price of chocolate products and reduces the equilibrium quantity. U.S. sugar producers also sell surplus sugar in foreign sugar markets, which causes the supply curve to shift rightward in foreign markets. This reduces the market price of foreign sugar and raises the equilibrium quantity in the international market.

U.S. Chocolate Market

S' S P_2 P_1 Price D Q_2 Q_1 Quantity

Foreign Sugar Market

S S' P_1 P_2 Price D Q_1 Q_2 Quantity

4-7. The market price is $400, and the equilibrium quantity of seats is 1,600. If airlines cannot sell tickets to more than 1,200 passengers, passengers are willing to pay $600 per seat, but airlines are willing to sell each ticket for $200.

4-9. Before the price support program, total revenue for farmers was $5 million. After the program, total revenue is $10 million. The cost of the program for taxpayers is $5 million.

CHAPTER 5

5-1. a. As shown in the figure, if the social costs associated with groundwater contamination were reflected in the costs incurred by pesticide manufacturers, the supply schedule would be *S*' instead of *S*, and the market price would be higher. The equilibrium quantity of pesticides produced would be lower.

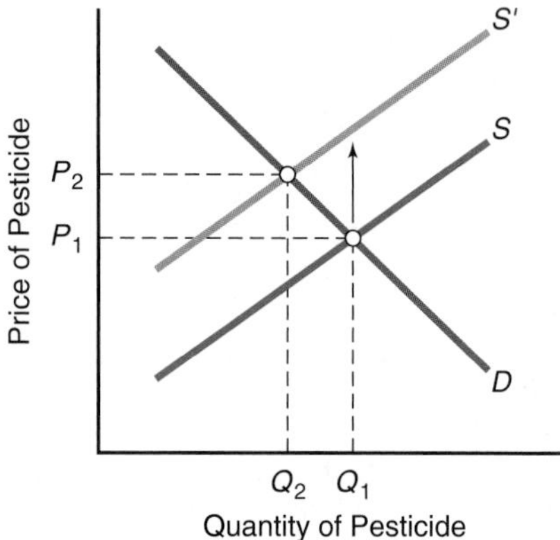

b. The government could tax the production and sale of pesticides, thereby shifting the supply curve upward and to the left.

5-3 a. As shown in the figure, if the social benefits associated with bus ridership were taken into account, the demand schedule would be *D*' instead of *D*, and the market price would be higher. The equilibrium quantity of bus rides would be higher.

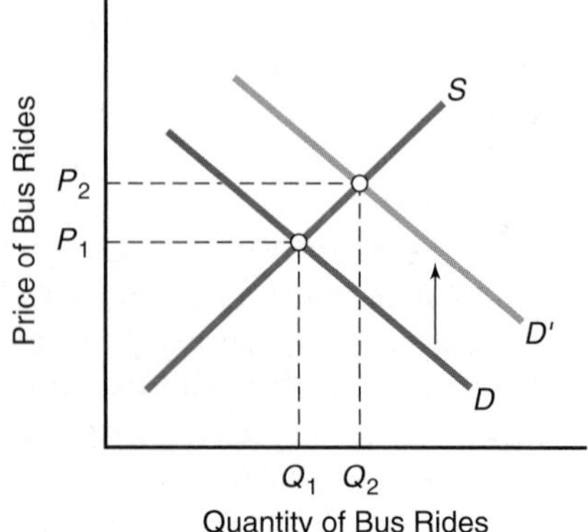

b. The government could pay commuters a subsidy to ride the bus, thereby shifting the demand curve upward and to the right. This would increase the market price and equilibrium number of bus rides.

5-5. The problem is that although most people around the lighthouse will benefit from its presence, there is no incentive for people to contribute voluntarily if they believe that others ultimately will pay for it. That is, the city is likely to face a free-rider problem in its efforts to raise its share of the funds required for the lighthouse.

5-7. Because the marginal tax rate increases as workers' earnings decline, this tax system is regressive.

5-9. Seeking to increase budget allocations in future years and to make workers' jobs more interesting is similar to the goals of firms in private markets. Achieving these goals via majority rule and regulatory coercion, however, are aspects that are specific to the public sector.

CHAPTER 6

6-1. 50 percent

6-3. No more than $9 per hour

6-5. a. Equilibrium price = $500; society's total expense = $40 million
b. 100,000 tests
c. Producers' per-unit cost = $700; society's total expense = $70 million
d. Government's per-unit subsidy = $600; total subsidy = $60 million

CHAPTER 7

7-1. By the time you would begin employment with employer B, the purchasing power of the salary you would earn from that job would have dropped by 5 percent. Thus a year from now, the purchasing power of the $25,000 salary will have dropped to $25,000/1.05 = $23,809.52. Furthermore, additional inflation during the following year will continue to erode the salary's purchasing power. In contrast, you anticipate that the purchasing power of the job offer from employer A will remain unchanged at $24,000. Because you are indifferent between the jobs in other respects, you should accept job A.

7-3. a. 3 percent
b. 5 percent
c. 6 percent
d. 8 percent

7-5. a. 5 percent
b. One month
c. Two months
d. 10 percent

7-7. 105.0

7-9. a. The homeowner gains; the savings bank loses.
b. The tenants gain; the landlord loses.
c. The auto buyer gains; the bank loses.
d. The employer gains; the pensioner loses.

CHAPTER 8

8-1. a. GDP = $14.6 trillion; NDP = $13.3 trillion; NI = $12.5 trillion.
b. GDP in 2006 will equal $13.5 trillion.
c. If the value of depreciation were to exceed gross private domestic investment in 2006, the nation's capital stock would decline. Because capital is a productive resource, the nation's future productivity likely would decline, and this decline would worsen if the situation were to continue beyond 2006.

8-3. a. Gross domestic income = $14.6 trillion; GDP = $14.6 trillion.
b. Gross private domestic investment = $2 trillion.
c. Personal income = $12 trillion; personal disposable income = $10.3 trillion.

8-5. a. Measured GDP declines.
b. Measured GDP increases.
c. Measured GDP does not change (the firearms are not newly produced).

8-7. a. Nominal GDP for 1997 is $2,300; for 2002, $2,832.
b. Real GDP for 1997 is $2,300; for 2002, $2,229.

8-9. The market transactions included in GDP would be the $15 million paid to construction companies and the $5 million paid to salvage companies, for a total of $20 million included in real GDP. Any lost market value of existing homes not reclaimed would be a wealth loss not captured in GDP, because it is a loss in the value of a *stock* of resources. In addition, the $3 million in time that some devote to the reconstruction of their homes would be nonmarket transactions not included in GDP. Also not included would be the reduction in the general state of happiness-which is not valued in the marketplace-for everyone affected by the hurricane.

CHAPTER 9

9-1. a. *B*
b. *C*

9-3. 1.77 times higher after 20 years; 3.16 times higher after 40 years

9-5. Five years

9-7. 4 percent

CHAPTER 10

10-1. Unemployment would consist of only frictional and structural unemployment.

10-3. $2 trillion

10-5. There are three effects of a rise in the price level. First, there is a real-balance effect, because the rise in the price level reduces real money balances, inducing people to cut back on their spending. In addition, there is an interest rate effect as a higher price level pushes up interest rates, thereby reducing the attractiveness of purchasing autos, houses, and business assets. Finally, there is an open economy effect as home residents respond to the higher price level by reducing purchases of domestically produced goods in favor of foreign-produced goods, while foreign residents cut back on their purchases of home-produced goods. All three effects entail a reduction in purchases of goods and services, so the aggregate demand curve slopes downward.

10-7. a. At the price level P_2 above the equilibrium price level P_1, the total quantity of real output that people plan to consume is less than the total quantity that is consistent with firms' production plans. One reason is that at the higher-than-equilibrium price level, real money balances are lower, which reduces real wealth and induces lower planned consumption. Another is that interest rates are higher at the higher-than-equilibrium price level, which generates a cutback in consumption spending. Finally, at the higher-than equilibrium price level P_2, people tend to cut back on purchasing domestic goods in favor of foreign-produced goods, and foreign residents reduce purchases of domestic goods. As unsold inventories of output accumulate, the price level drops toward the equilibrium price level P_1, which ultimately causes planned consumption to rise toward equality with total production.
b. At the price level P_3 below the equilibrium price level P_1, the total quantity of real output that people plan to consume exceeds the total quantity that is consistent with firms' production plans. One reason is that at the lower-than-equilibrium price level, real money balances are higher, which raises real wealth and induces higher planned consumption. Another is that interest rates are lower at the higher-than-equilibrium price level, which generates an increase in consumption spending. Finally, at the lower-than equilibrium price level P_2, people tend to raise their purchases of domestic goods and cut back on buying foreign-produced goods, and foreign residents increase purchases of domestic goods. As inventories of output are depleted, the price level begins to rise toward the equilibrium price level P_1, which ultimately causes planned consumption to fall toward equality with total production.

10-9. Unexpected inflation transfers resources. For example, unanticipated inflation harms creditors but benefits debtors. Unpredictable nonstationarity of the price level results in such transfers.

CHAPTER 11

11-1. a. Because saving increases at any given interest rate, the desired saving curve shifts rightward. This causes the equilibrium interest rate to decline.

b. There is no effect on current output, however, because in the classical model the vertical long-run aggregate supply curve always applies.

c. A change in the saving rate does not directly affect the demand for labor or the supply of labor in the classical model, so equilibrium employment does not change.

d. The decrease in the equilibrium interest rate generates a rightward and downward movement along the demand curve for investment. Consequently, desired investment declines.

e. The fall in current investment implies lower capital accumulation. Other things being equal, this will imply lower future production.

11-3. Because there is full information and speedy adjustment of wages and prices in the classical model, the aggregate demand curve shifts leftward along the vertical long-run aggregate supply curve. The equilibrium price level decreases, but there is no change in equilibrium national output.

11-5. a. A decline in nominal wages is one factor. A decrease in the cost of any other important input, such as energy, is another.

b. A technological improvement is one factor. Greater capital accumulation or increased labor force participation are others.

11-7. At this point, the actual unemployment rate is below the natural rate of unemployment. The reason is that the economy is producing a level of output per year that exceeds its long-run capability, which entails employing workers that in normal times would be frictionally or structurally unemployed.

11-9. This will make it relatively more expensive for businesses to purchase inputs from abroad, thereby pushing up their operating costs. Thus the short-run aggregate supply curve will shift leftward. Although it also makes home-produced products cheaper to foreign residents and foreign-produced products more expensive for home residents, the amount of trade is said to be low, so aggregate demand does not shift rightward by much. On net, therefore, the equilibrium price level is likely to fall, and the equilibrium level of real output is likely to decline.

CHAPTER 12

12.1 a, b.

Disposable Income	Saving	Consumption	APS	APC
$ 200	$−40	$240	−0.20	1.20
400	0	400	0.00	1.00
600	40	560	0.07	0.93
800	80	720	0.10	0.90
1,000	120	880	0.12	0.88
1,200	160	1,040	0.13	0.87

c. MPS = 40/200 = 0.20; MPC = 120/200 = 0.8.

12-3. a. Yes, because the rate of return on the investment exceeds the market interest rate

b. No, because the rate of return on the investment is now less than the market interest rate

12-5. a.

Real Income	Consumption	Saving	Investment
$ 2,000	$ 2,000	$ 0	$ 1,200
4,000	3,600	400	1,200
6,000	5,200	800	1,200
8,000	6,800	1,200	1,200
10,000	8,400	1,600	1,200
12,000	10,000	2,000	1,200

MPC = 1,600/2000 = 0.8; MPS = 400/2,000 = 0.2.

b, c.

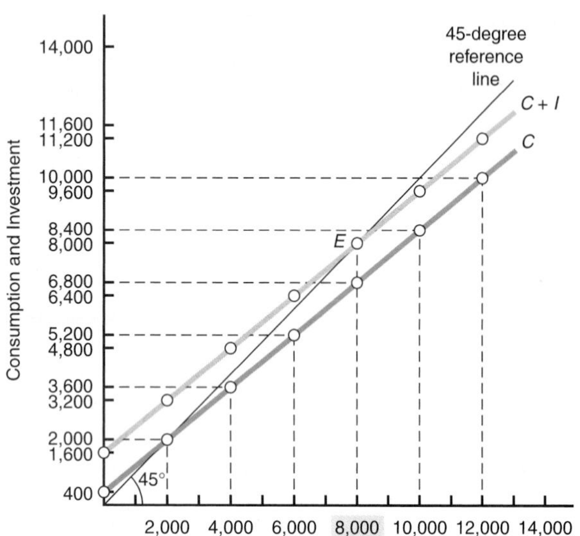

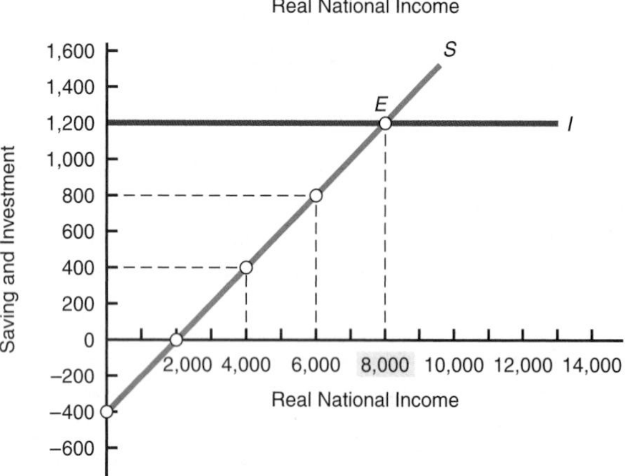

Equilibrium real national income on both graphs equals $8,000.

d. 5

e. 0.15

f. If autonomous consumption were to rise by $100, equilibrium real national income would increase by $100 × 5, or $500.

CHAPTER 13

13-1. a. A key factor that could help explain why the actual multiplier effect may turned out to be lower is the crowding-out effect. Some government spending may have directly crowded out private expenditures on a dollar-for-dollar basis. In addition, indirect crowding out may have occurred. Because the government did not change taxes, it probably sold bonds to finance its increased expenditures, and this action likely pushed up interest rates, thereby discouraging private investment. Furthermore, the increase in government spending likely pushed up aggregate demand, which may have caused a short-run increase in the price level. This may in turn have induced foreign residents to reduce their expenditures on U.S. goods. It could also have reduced real money holdings sufficiently to discourage consumers from spending as much as before. On net, therefore, real GDP rose in the short run but not by the full multiple amount.

b. In the long run, as the increased spending raised aggregate demand, wages and other input prices likely increased in proportion to the resulting increase in the price level. Thus in the long run, the aggregate supply schedule was vertical, and the increase in government spending induced only a rise in the price level.

13-3. Because of the recognition time lag entailed in gathering information about the economy, policymakers may be slow to respond to a downturn in real national income. Congressional approval of policy actions to address the downturn may be delayed, causing an action time lag. Finally, there is an effect time lag, because policy actions take time to exert their full effects on the economy. If these lags are sufficiently long, it is possible that by the time a policy to address a downturn has begun to have its effects, real national income might already be rising. If so, the policy action might push real GDP up faster than intended, thereby making real national income less stable.

13-5. b, d

13-7. One possibility would be a government spending decrease of just the right amount to shift the aggregate demand curve leftward to a new equilibrium point on the long-run aggregate supply curve. Another would be a tax increase designed to achieve the same outcome.

13-9. A cut in the tax rate should induce a rise in consumption and consequently a multiple increase in equilibrium real income. In addition, however, a tax rate reduction reduces the automatic stabilizer properties of the tax system, so equilibrium real income would be less stable in the face of changes in autonomous spending.

APPENDIX C

C-1. a. The marginal propensity to consume is equal to $1 - \text{MPS}$, or $\frac{6}{7}$.
b. Investment or government spending must increase by $50 billion.
c. The government would have to cut taxes by $58.33 billion.

C-3. a. The aggregate expenditure curve shifts upward by $1 billion; equilibrium real income increases by $5 billion.
b. The aggregate expenditures curve shifts downward by the MPC times the tax increase, or $0.8 \times \$1$ billion = 0.8 billion; equilibrium real income falls by $4 billion.
c. The aggregate expenditures curve shifts upward by $(1 - \text{MPC}) \times \$1$ billion = 0.8 billion. Equilibrium real income rises by $1 billion.
d. No change; no change.

CHAPTER 14

14-1. Medium of exchange; store of value; standard of deferred payment

14-3. Store of value; standard of deferred payment

14-5. a. Both
b. Neither
c. M2
d. M2
e. M2

14-7. This is an example of adverse selection, in which a prospective borrower had information not possessed by potential lenders.

14-9. It provides banking services such as check clearing for other banks and for the U.S. Treasury, just as a private bank provides such services for its customers. Unlike a private bank, however, the Federal Reserve serves as a lender of last resort, a regulator, and a policymaker.

CHAPTER 15

15-1. $13.5 million

15-3. Yes, the bank holds $50 million in excess reserves.

15-5. $850,000

15-7. 25 percent (or 0.25)

15-9. The money supply declines by $5 billion.

CHAPTER 16

16-1. The bank's total costs from issuing smart cards are $400,000, and its expected revenues will $500,000, so the bank will anticipate profiting and should issue the smart cards.

16-3. Yes. Unless many people carry and use smart cards, retailers will be less likely to accept them, which reduces any given individual's incentive to carry one.

16-5. If FinCEN discovers half of $100 million in laundered funds each year, or $50 million, it can bring in half that amount, or $25 million, in taxes and penalties. If it spends $20 million each year investigating laundering activities and bringing perpetrators to justice, on net it earns $5 million for the government. Ignoring any other factors, this would give FinCEN a rationale for conducting these activities.

16-7. The money supply implications are the same no matter which mechanism people use to make payments.

16-9. The maximum potential value of the money multiplier would remain unchanged at 1 divided by the required reserve ratio. If new on-line banking institutions hold excess reserves in the same proportion to checkable deposits that they issue online and if their customers hold the same relative quantities of currency or digital cash that regular bank customers hold, the actual money multiplier also would be the same.

CHAPTER 17

17-1. a. $10,000
b. Its price falls to $5,000.

17-3. a. One possible policy action would be an open market sale of securities, which would reduce the money supply and shift the aggregate demand curve leftward.
b. In principle, the Fed's action would reduce inflation more quickly.

17-5. Because a contractionary monetary policy causes interest rates to increase, financial capital begins to flow into the United States. This causes the demand for dollars to rise, which pushes up the value of the dollar and makes U.S. exports more expensive to foreign residents. They cut back on their purchases of U.S. products, which tends to reduce U.S. real national income.

17-7. The price level doubles.

17-9. 10

APPENDIX D

D-1. By its purchase of $1 billion in bonds, the Fed increased excess reserves by $1 billion. This ultimately caused a $3 billion increase in the money supply after full multiple expansion. The 1 percent drop in the interest rate, from 10 to 9 percent, caused investment to rise by $25 billion, from $200 billion to $225 billion. An investment multiplier of 3 indicates that equilibrium national income rose by $75 billion to $2,075 trillion.

CHAPTER 18

18-1. a. The actual unemployment rate would decline.
b. Natural unemployment rate estimates would also be lower.
c. The logic of the short- and long-run Phillips curves would not be altered. The government might wish to make this change if it feels that members of the military do "hold jobs" and should therefore be counted as employed persons in the U.S. economy.

18-3. The "long run" is an interval sufficiently long that input prices fully adjust and people have full information. Adoption of more sophisticated computer and communications technology provides people with more immediate access to information, which can reduce this interval.

18-5. No, because then the new classical theory indicates that workers and firms will speedily adjust nominal wages and other input prices when the price level changes in response to Fed policy actions. As a result, real GDP will not change, so the actual unemployment rate will remain unaltered.

18-7. The explanation would be that aggregate demand has increased at a faster pace than the rise in aggregate supply caused by economic growth. On net, therefore, the price level has risen during the past few years.

18-9. If there is widespread price stickiness, the short-run aggregate supply curve would be horizontal (see Chapter 11), and real GDP would respond strongly to a policy action that affects aggregate demand. By contrast, if prices are highly flexible, the short-run aggregate supply curve slopes upward, and real GDP is less responsive to the change in aggregate demand.

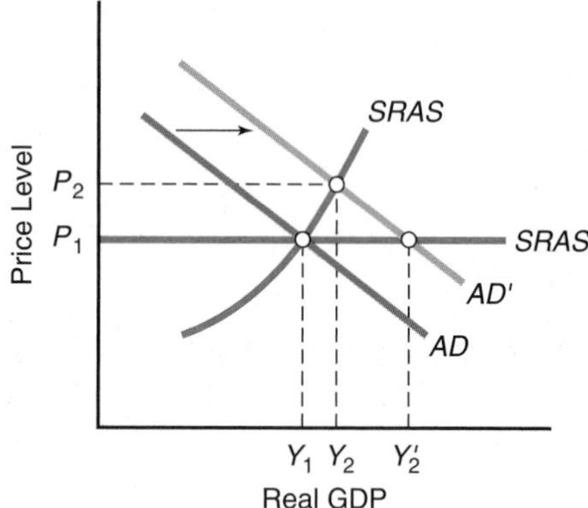

APPENDIX E

E-1. The indifference curve is convex to the origin because of a diminishing marginal rate of substitution. That is, as an individual consumes more and more of an item, the less they are willing to forgo of the other item. The diminishing marginal rate of substitution is due to a diminishing marginal utility.

E-3. Sue's marginal rate of substitution is calculated as follows:

Combination of Bottled Water and Soft Drinks	Bottled Water per Month	Soft Drinks Per Month	MRS
A	5	11	
B	10	7	5:4
C	15	4	5:3
D	20	2	5:2
E	25	1	5:1

The diminishing marginal rate of substitution of soft drinks for water shows Sue's diminishing marginal utility of bottled water. She is willing to forgo fewer and fewer soft drinks to get an additional five bottles of water.

E-5. Given that water is on the horizontal axis and soft drinks on the vertical axis, the slope of Sue's budget constraint is the price of water divided by the price of soft drinks, $P_W/P_S = \frac{1}{2}$. The only combination of bottled water and soft drink that is on Sue's indifference curve and budget constraint is at point *C*, where total expenditures on water and soft drink total $23.

E-7. Given that water is on the horizontal axis and soft drinks on the vertical axis, the slope of Sue's budget constraint is the price of water divided by the price of soft drinks, $P_W/P_S = 1$. The only combination of bottled water and soft drink that is on Sue's indifference curve and budget constraint is at point *C*, where total expenditures on water and soft drink total $23.

E-9. Yes, Sue's revealed preferences indicate that her demand for soft drinks obeys the law of demand. As the price of soft drinks declines from $2 to $1, her quantity demanded rises from 4 to 8.

CHAPTER 19

19-1. The campus pizzeria indicates by its pricing policy that it recognizes the principle of diminishing marginal utility. Because the marginal utility of the second pizza is typically lower than the first, the customer is likely to value the second less and is therefore less willing to pay full price for it.

19-3. The total utility of the third, fourth, and fifth cheeseburger is 48, 56, and 60, respectively. The marginal utility of the first and second cheeseburger is 20 and 16, respectively. The total utility of the first, second, and third bag of french fries is 8, 14, and 18, respectively. The marginal utility of the fourth and fifth bag of french fries is 2 and 0, respectively.

19-5. When total utility is rising, the only thing we can say for certain about marginal utility is that it is positive.

19-7. The student should compare the marginal utility per tuition dollar spent at the two universities. Assuming that a "unit" of college is a degree, the student should divide the notional value of an education at each university by the total tuition it would take to earn a degree at each institution. The university with the higher marginal utility per tuition dollar is the one the student should attend.

19-9. The new utility-maximizing combination is four cheeseburgers and two orders of french fries. The substitution effect is shown by the increase in the relatively less expensive good, cheeseburgers, relative to french fries. The income effect is illustrated by greater total consumption.

CHAPTER 20

20-1. $\frac{(200 - 150)/(350/2)}{(9 - 10)/(19/2)} = 2.7$

20-3. $\frac{(100 - 200)/(300/2)}{(2 - 1)/(3/2)} = 1.0$

20-5. a. Nearly perfectly elastic
b. Nearly perfectly inelastic
c. Nearly perfectly inelastic
d. Nearly perfectly inelastic

20-7. Within the first range, demand is elastic. As price falls, therefore, total revenue rises, and the total revenue curve is increasing. Within the second range, demand is at first elastic and then inelastic. When price falls, therefore, total revenue and the total revenue curve are initially rising. Eventually total revenue and the total revenue curve reach the maximum point, which corresponds to the point of unit elasticity. Beyond this point, total revenue declines.

20-9. Goods X and Y are substitutes; goods X and Z are complements; therefore, goods Y and Z are substitutes.

20-11. Income elasticity of demand is measured as the percentage change in demand divided by the percentage change in income. A negative income elasticity of demand indicates that as income rises, demand falls. This type of good is defined in Chapter 3 as an inferior good. A positive income elasticity of demand therefore indicates that the good is a normal good, as defined in Chapter 3. Hence we can conclude that a hot dog is an inferior good and that lobster is a normal good.

CHAPTER 21

21-1. a. Physical capital
b. Financial capital
c. Financial capital
d. Physical capital

21-3. The dividends of a corporation result from the corporation's profits, which are subject to corporate income taxation. The dividends are then paid out to shareholders, who must pay taxes on them as personal income. The profits of a partnership or proprietorship are subject only to individual income tax.

21-5. a. The owner of WebCity faces both tax rates if the firm is a corporation, but if it is a proprietorship, the owner faces only the 30 percent personal income tax rate.
b. If WebCity is a corporation, the $100,000 in corporate earnings is taxed at a 20 percent rate, so after-tax dividends are $80,000, and these are taxed at the personal income tax rate of 30 percent, leaving $56,000 in after-tax income for the owner. Hence the firm should be organized as a proprietorship so that the after-tax earnings are $70,000.
c. In this case, incorporation raises earnings to $150,000, which are taxed at a rate of 20 percent, yielding after-tax dividends of $120,000 that are taxed at the personal rate of 30 percent. This leaves an after-tax income for the owner of $84,000, which is higher than the after-tax earnings of $70,000 if WebCity is a proprietorship that earns lower pretax income taxed at the personal rate.
d. After-tax profits rise from $56,000 to $84,000, or by $28,000.
e. This policy change would only increase the incentive to incorporate.
f. A corporate structure provides limited liability for owners, which can be a major advantage. Furthermore, owners may believe that the corporate structure will yield higher pretax earnings.

21-7. a. For both, trading 100 shares with FSB entails paying the $25 flat fee plus the volume fee of $10, or $35. Including the opportunity cost of 30 minutes, Lucinda's cost of trading with WebTrader instead is $65 higher, and Ralph's is $35 higher. Both should execute their trades with FSB.
b. For both, trading 500 shares with FSB entails paying the $25 flat fee plus the volume fee of $50, or $75. Including the opportunity cost of 30 minutes, Lucinda's cost of trading with WebTrader instead is $35 higher, but Ralph's is $5 lower. Lucinda should execute her trade with FSB, but Ralph should do so with WebTrader.
c. For both, trading 1,000 shares with FSB entails paying the $25 flat fee plus the volume fee of $100, or $125. Including the opportunity cost of 30 minutes, Lucinda's cost of trading with WebTrader instead is $15 lower, and Ralph's is $55 lower. Both should execute their trades with WebTrader.
d. In general, larger trades will be executed with WebTrader, because FSB's total fees rise with the number of share trades that the broker executes, but the total cost of having WebTrader execute trades does not.
e. A person with a higher opportunity cost of time is more likely to have FSB execute trades.

21-9. a. Adverse selection
b. Asymmetric information
c. Moral hazard

21-11. You should point out to your classmate that stock prices tend to follow a random walk. That is, yesterday's price is the best guide to today's price, and there are no predictable trends that can be used to "beat" the market.

CHAPTER 22

22-1. Explicit costs are $12,000 in rent, $1,000 in office supplies, $20,000 for office staff, and $4,000 in telephone expenses, for a total of $37,000. Implicit costs are the forgone $40,000 salary and the 5 percent interest on the $5,000 savings ($250), for a total of $40,250.

22-3. The short run is a time period in which the academic cannot enter the job market and find employment elsewhere. This is the nine-month period from August 15 through May 15. The academic can find employment elsewhere after the contract has been fulfilled, so the short run is nine months and the long run is greater than nine months.

22-5.

Input of Labor (workers per month)	Total Output of DVD Drives	Marginal Physical Product
0	0	—
100	25	0.25
200	60	0.35
300	85	0.25
400	105	0.20
500	115	0.10
600	120	0.05

22-7. Variable costs are equal to total costs, $5 million, less fixed costs, $2 million. Variable costs are therefore equal to $3 million. Average variable costs are equal to total variable costs divided by the number of units produced. Average variable costs therefore equal $3 million divided by 10,000, or $300.

22-9. Increasing marginal cost occurs as the firm moves from producing 50 cable modems to 75 cable modems.

Output (cable modems per month)	Total Cost of Output ($ thousands)	Marginal Costs ($ thousands)
0	10	—
25	60	2.0
50	95	1.4
75	150	2.2
100	220	2.8
125	325	4.2
150	465	5.6

22-11. a. Diseconomies of scale
b. Plant size E

CHAPTER 23

23-1. a. The single dominant firm can affect price. Therefore, this is not a competitive industry.
b. The output of each firm is not homogeneous, so this is not a competitive industry.
c. Firms cannot easily enter the industry, so this is not a competitive industry.

23-3. During the course of a week, the barber cuts hair for $15 \times 5 = 75$ people. His total revenue for a week is $75 \times \$6 = \$450$. Because this is a competitive market, marginal revenue equals market price, $6.

23-5. The profit-maximizing rate of output is where marginal cost equals marginal revenue, which occurs at 8 pizzas.

Total Output and Sales of Pizzas	Total Cost ($)	Marginal Cost ($)	Marginal Revenue ($)
0	5	0	10
1	9	4	10
2	11	2	10
3	12	1	10
4	14	2	10
5	18	4	10
6	24	6	10
7	32	8	10
8	42	10	10
9	54	12	10
10	68	14	10

23-7. Even though the price of pizzas, and hence marginal revenue, falls to only $5, this covers average variable cost. Thus the shop should stay open.

23-9. Because firms experience diseconomies of scale, they will increase their output at the current market price level. This causes the market supply schedule to shift rightward. The market price declines, and some firms begin to earn negative economic profits and leave the industry. This causes the supply schedule to shift back to the left and the market price to rise somewhat. In the final long-run equilibrium, the market price is equal to the minimum long-run average cost, and each surviving firm produces output at the minimum point of its long-run average cost curve.

CHAPTER 24

24-1. Because the objective of each cartel member is to maximize economic profits, there is an incentive for an individual member to cheat. Preventing members from cheating becomes harder and harder as the number of members grows. Hence the large number of coffee growers that exists today makes it unlikely that the cartel will be effective in the long run.

24-3. a. The total revenue and total profits of the dry cleaner are as follows.

Output (suits cleaned)	Price per Suit ($)	Total Costs ($)	Total Revenue ($)	Total Profit ($)
0	8.00	3.00	0	−3.00
1	7.50	6.00	7.50	1.50
2	7.00	8.50	14.00	5.50
3	6.50	10.50	19.50	9.00
4	6.00	11.50	24.00	12.50
5	5.50	13.50	27.50	14.00
6	5.00	16.00	30.00	14.00
7	4.50	19.00	31.50	12.50
8	4.00	24.00	32.00	8.00

b. The profit-maximizing rate of output is 5 or 6 units.

24-5. This statement is not true. Profit maximization occurs at the output rate where marginal revenue and marginal cost are equal. This rate of output may well occur before the point of minimum average total cost.

24-7. In a perfectly competitive market, price is $4.50 and quantity is 8,000. Because the monopolist produces less and charges a higher price than under perfect competition, price exceeds marginal cost at the profit-maximizing level of output. The difference between the price and marginal cost is the per-unit cost to society of a monopolized industry.

24-9. If price varies positively with total revenue, the monopolist is operating on the inelastic portion of the demand curve. This corresponds to the range where marginal revenue is negative. The monopolist cannot therefore be at the point where its profits are maximized. In other words, the monopolist is not producing where marginal cost equals marginal revenue.

24-11. Because marginal cost have risen, the monopolist will be operating at a lower rate of output and charging a higher price.

CHAPTER 25

25-1. a. There are many rival fast food restaurants that sell heterogeneous products. Both features of this industry are consistent with the theory of monopolistic competition.

b. There is a large number of colleges and universities, but each specializes in different academic areas and hence produces heterogeneous products, as in the theory of monopolistic competition.

25-3.

Output	Price ($)	Total Costs ($)	Total Revenue ($)	Marginal Cost ($)	Marginal Revenue ($)
0	6.00	2.00	0	—	—
1	5.75	5.00	5.75	3.00	5.75
2	5.50	7.50	11.00	2.50	5.25
3	5.25	9.50	15.75	2.00	4.75
4	5.00	10.50	20.00	1.00	4.25
5	4.75	12.50	23.75	2.00	3.75
6	4.50	15.00	27.00	2.50	3.25
7	4.00	18.00	28.00	3.00	1.00

25-5. The market price is $5.00 per unit, and the firm's economic profits equal $9.50.

25-7. a. Zero-sum game
b. Positive-sum game
c. Negative-sum game

25-9. This is an oligopoly structure that is consistent with the kinked demand curve. If the store's marginal cost curve shifts only slightly, it probably will not choose to vary its prices.

CHAPTER 26

26-1. If cable service is an industry that enjoys diminishing long-run average total costs, the city may wish to have a single, large firm that produces at a lower long-run average cost and to regulate the firm's activity.

26-3. If the firm were allowed to operate as a monopolist, it would produce at the level where marginal cost equals marginal revenue, which occurs at 2 units. Price is $90 at this level of output, so monopoly profit is $180 − $175 = $5.

26-5. Average cost pricing occurs where long-run average total cost equals demand, which is at 3 units. Price is $85, so profit is zero at this level.

26-7. Economic regulation seeks to keep prices low. Social regulation seeks to improve the working conditions of the firm and minimize adverse spillovers of production.

26-9. If European regulation is designed to protect domestic farm interests, it is an example of the capture hypothesis. If there are legitimate health concerns, it is an example of share-the-pains, share-the-gains hypothesis.

CHAPTER 27

27-1.

Labor Input (workers per week)	Total Physical Output (printers per week)	Marginal Physical Product ($)	Marginal Revenue Product ($)
10	200	—	—
11	218	18	1,800
12	234	16	1,600
13	248	14	1,400
14	260	12	1,200
15	270	10	1,000
16	278	8	800

27-3. The profit-maximizing employer will hire 14 workers, as this is the level where marginal revenue product equals marginal factor cost.

27-5. a. The greater the substitutability of capital, the more elastic the demand for labor.
b. Because the demand for labor is a derived demand, the greater the elasticity of demand for the final product, the greater the elasticity of demand for labor.
c. The larger the portion of factor costs accounted for by labor, the larger the price elasticity of demand for labor.

27-7.

Labor Input (workers per day)	Total Physical	Product Price ($)	Marginal Physical Product	Total Revenue ($)	Marginal Revenue Product ($)
10	100	50	—	5,000	—
11	109	49	9	5,341	341
12	116	48	7	5,568	227
13	121	47	5	5,687	119
14	124	46	3	5,704	17
15	125	45	1	5,625	−79

27-9. To maximize profits, a firm should hire inputs up to the point where marginal revenue product per dollar spent is equalized across all factors. This is not true in this example, so the firm is not maximizing profits. The firm should reduce the number of capital units it uses and increase its use of labor and land.

CHAPTER 28

28-1. Individual workers can air grievances to the collective voice, who then takes the issue to the employer. The individual does not run the risk of being singled out by an employer. The individual employee does not waste work time trying to convince employers that changes are needed in the workplace.

28-3. Because strikebreakers can replace union employees, they diminish the collective bargaining power of a union.

28-5. When marginal revenue is zero, the price elasticity of demand is equal to unity. At this point, total revenue is neither rising nor falling. Hence it is at a maximum point.

28-7.

Labor Supplied	Total Physical Product	Required Hourly Wage Rate ($)	Total Wage Bill ($)	Marginal Factor Cost ($)
10	100	5	50	—
11	109	6	66	16
12	116	7	84	18
13	121	8	104	20
14	124	9	126	22
15	125	10	150	24

28-9.

Labor Supplied	Total Physical Product	Required Hourly Wage Rate ($)	Product Price ($)	Total Revenue ($)	Marginal Revenue Product ($)
10	100	5	3.11	311	—
11	109	6	3.00	327	16.00
12	116	7	2.95	342.20	15.20
13	121	8	2.92	353.32	11.12
14	124	9	2.90	359.60	6.28
15	125	10	2.89	361.25	1.65

At 11 units of labor, the marginal revenue product is $16. This is equal to the marginal factor cost at this level of employment, as seen in the answer to Problem 28-7. The firm will therefore hire 11 units of labor and pay a wage of $6 an hour.

CHAPTER 29

29-1. a. Bob earns a high economic rent. With a specialized skill that is in great demand, his income is likely to be high and his opportunity cost relatively low.

b. Sally earns a high economic rent. As a supermodel, her income is likely to be high and, without any education, her opportunity cost relatively low.

c. If Tim were to leave teaching, not a relatively high-paying occupation, he could sell insurance full time. Hence his opportunity cost is high relative to his income, and his economic rent is low.

29-3. The economic rents that Michael Jordan would enjoy as a basketball player relative to those he enjoyed as a baseball player surely played a large role in his decision to return to basketball. Hence they help direct his talent (resources) into their most efficient use.

29-5. a. The debt issued by this country will not appear as risky to individuals, and they would therefore not require as high an interest rate. The interest rate will decline.

b. Increases in reporting requirements increase the cost of issuing a loan. The lender will increase rates to compensate for this. The interest rate will rise.

c. By shortening the length of the loan, the interest rate will decline.

29-7. The binding ceiling generates a shortage of loanable funds. Overall there is a decrease in loanable funds activity and a decrease in capital improvement projects.

29-9. The present value is $PV_1 = \$104/1.04 = \$100$. With a 5 percent discount rate, the present value is $\$104/1.05 = \$99.05$.

CHAPTER 30

30-1. a. X

b. Z

c. Closer

30-3. Brazil's

30-5. To achieve complete equality of incomes, such policies would remove individual gains from maximizing the economic value of resources and minimizing production costs. Enacting policies aimed at complete income equality could therefore significantly reduce overall efficiency in an economy.

30-7. First, a moral hazard problem will exist, because government action would reduce the individual's incentive to continue a healthy lifestyle, thereby increasing the likelihood of greater health problems that will require future treatment. Second, an individual who currently has health problems will have an incentive to substitute future care that will be available at a zero price for current care that the individual must purchase at a positive price. Finally, in future years the patient will no longer have an incentive to contain health care expenses, nor will health care providers have an incentive to minimize their costs.

30-9. The profit-maximizing price and the equilibrium quantity of health care services will increase.

CHAPTER 31

31-1. \$4 per unit

31-3. At the previous, lower market price, consumers failed to pay a price that reflected the social costs, including those relating to pollution, of resources that the firms use to produce the good or service.

31-5. Penalizing rhino hunting discourages most people from engaging in the activity, which reduces the supply of rhino horns and drives up their market price. This in turn makes illegal poaching a more lucrative activity, which can lead to an increase in illegal hunting of the few remaining rhinos. If raising rhinos as stock animals were legalized, more rhino horns would be produced-via an increase in the number of rhinos on farms-and the market price of rhino horns would decline. This would reduce the incentive for poaching wild rhinos.

31-7. a. 60 percent

b. 40 percent

c. 40 percent

31-9. a.

Population of Wild Tigers	Marginal Cost	Marginal Benefit
0	—	—
2,000	5	50
4,000	10	40
6,000	15	30
8,000	25	25
10,000	35	20
12,000	50	10

b. 8,000 tigers
c. 6,000 tigers

CHAPTER 32

32-1. Norway can produce 100 calculators and 50 books, while Sweden can produce 200 calculators and 50 books. Their total output, therefore, is 300 calculators and 100 books. Sweden has an absolute advantage in calculators. Neither country has an absolute advantage in books.

32-3. a. Norway has a comparative advantage in the production of books and Sweden has a comparative advantage in the production of calculators.
b. If they specialize, total production is 400 calculators and 100 books.

32-5. Without trade, Norway would have to forgo 1/2 book to obtain 1 calculator. With trade, however, Norway can obtain 1 calculator for 1/3 book. Without trade, Sweden would have to forgo 4 calculators to obtain 1 book. With trade, however, Sweden can obtain 1 book for 3 calculators. By trading, both nations can obtain the good at a price that is less than the opportunity cost of producing it. They are both better off with trade, so this is a positive-sum game.

32-7. A price elasticity of demand less than unity indicates inelastic demand, and therefore price and total revenue move in the same direction. If the nation restricts its exports, the price of the product rises and so does total revenue, even though the nation is selling fewer units.

32-9. a. Because the supply curve shifts by the amount of the tariff, the diagram indicates that the tariff is $20 per television.
b. Total revenue was $6 billion before the tariff and $4.35 billion after the tariff.
c. The tariff revenue earned by the U.S. government is $20 × 15 million, or $300 million.

CHAPTER 33

33-1. The trade balance is a deficit of 100, the current account balance is a deficit of 65, and the capital account balance is a surplus of 100.

33-3. a. The increase in demand for Mexican-made guitars increases the demand for the Mexican peso, and the peso appreciates.
b. International investors will move their capital out of Mexico. The increase in the supply of the peso in the foreign exchange market will cause the peso to depreciate.

33-5. The Canadian dollar–euro rate is found by dividing the U.S. dollar–euro rate by the U.S. dollar–Canadian dollar rate. Thus the Canadian dollar–euro rate = 1.07/0.68 = 1.57.

33-7. A flexible exchange rate system allows the exchange value of a currency to be determined freely in the foreign exchange market with no intervention by the government. A fixed exchange rate pegs the value of the currency, and the authorities responsible for the value of the currency intervene in foreign exchange markets to maintain this value. A dirty float involves occasional intervention by the exchange authorities. A target zone allows the exchange value to fluctuate, but only within a given range of values.

33-9. When the U.S. dollar is pegged to gold at a rate of $35 and the pound sterling at a rate of $17.50, an implicit value between the dollar and the pound is established. The exchange value is $35/£17.50 = $2 per pound.

Glossary

Absolute advantage The ability to produce more units of a good or service using a given quantity of labor or resource inputs. Equivalently, the ability to produce the same quantity of a good or service using fewer units of labor or resource inputs. *Can also be viewed as* the ability to produce more output from given inputs of resources than other producers can.

Accounting identities Values that are equivalent by definition.

Accounting profit Total revenues minus total explicit costs.

Action time lag The time between recognizing an economic problem and implementing policy to solve it. The action time lag is quite long for fiscal policy, which requires congressional approval.

Active (discretionary) policymaking All actions on the part of monetary and fiscal policymakers that are undertaken in response to or in anticipation of some change in the overall economy.

Adverse selection The likelihood that individuals who seek to borrow money may use the funds that they receive for unworthy, high-risk projects.

Age-earnings cycle The regular earnings profile of an individual throughout his or her lifetime. The age-earnings cycle usually starts with a low income, builds gradually to a peak at around age 50, and then gradually curves down until it approaches zero at retirement.

Aggregate demand The total of all planned expenditures for the entire economy.

Aggregate demand curve A curve showing planned purchase rates for all final goods and services in the economy at various price levels, all other things held constant.

Aggregate demand shock Any shock that causes the aggregate demand curve to shift inward or outward.

Aggregates Total amounts or quantities; aggregate demand, for example, is total planned expenditures throughout a nation.

Aggregate supply The total of all planned production for the economy.

Aggregate supply shock Any shock that causes the aggregate supply curve to shift inward or outward.

Anticipated inflation The inflation rate that we believe will occur; when it does, we are in a situation of fully anticipated inflation.

Antitrust legislation Laws that restrict the formation of monopolies and regulate certain anticompetitive business practices.

Appreciation An increase in the exchange value of one nation's currency in terms of the currency of another nation.

Asset demand Holding money as a store of value instead of other assets such as certificates of deposit, corporate bonds, and stocks.

Assets Amounts owned; all items to which a business or household holds legal claim.

Asymmetric information Possession of information by one party in a financial transaction but not by the other party.

Automated clearinghouse (ACH) A computer-based clearing and settlement facility that replaces check transactions by interchanging credits and debits electronically.

Automated teller machine (ATM) network A system of linked depository institution computer terminals that are activated by magnetically encoded bank cards.

Automatic, or **built-in, stabilizers** Special provisions of certain federal programs that cause changes in desired aggregate expenditures without the action of Congress and the president. Examples are the federal tax system and unemployment compensation.

Autonomous consumption The part of consumption that is independent of (does not depend on) the level of disposable income. Changes in autonomous consumption shift the consumption function.

Average fixed costs Total fixed costs divided by the number of units produced.

Average physical product Total product divided by the variable input.

Average propensity to consume (APC) Consumption divided by disposable income; for any given level of income, the proportion of total disposable income that is consumed.

Average propensity to save (APS) Saving divided by disposable income; for any given level of income, the proportion of total disposable income that is saved.

Average tax rate The total tax payment divided by total income. It is the proportion of total income paid in taxes.

Average total costs Total costs divided by the number of units produced; sometimes called average per-unit total costs.

Average variable costs Total variable costs divided by the number of units produced.

Balance of payments A system of accounts that measures transactions of goods, services, income, and financial assets between domestic households, businesses, and governments and residents of the rest of the world during a specific time period.

Balance of trade The difference between exports and imports of goods.

Balance sheet A statement of the assets and liabilities of any business entity, including financial institutions and the Federal Reserve System. Assets are what is owned; liabilities are what is owed.

Bank runs Attempts by many of a bank's depositors to convert checkable and time deposits into currency out of fear for the bank's solvency.

Barter The direct exchange of goods and services for other goods and services without the use of money.

Base year The year that is chosen as the point of reference for comparison of prices in other years.

Bilateral monopoly A market structure consisting of a monopolist and a monopsonist.

Black market A market in which goods are traded at prices above their legal maximum prices or in which illegal goods are sold.

Bond A legal claim against a firm, usually entitling the owner of the bond to receive a fixed annual coupon payment, plus a lump-sum payment at the bond's maturity date. Bonds are issued in return for funds lent to the firm.

Budget constraint All of the possible combinations of goods that can be purchased (at fixed prices) with a specific budget.

Business fluctuations The ups and downs in overall business activity, as evidenced by changes in national income, employment, and the price level.

Capital consumption allowance Another name for depreciation, the amount that businesses would have to save in order to take care of the deterioration of machines and other equipment.

Capital controls Legal restrictions on the ability of a nation's residents to hold and trade assets denominated in foreign currencies.

Capital gain The positive difference between the purchase price and the sale price of an asset. If a share of stock is bought for $5 and then sold for $15, the capital gain is $10.

Capital goods Producer durables; nonconsumable goods that firms use to make other goods.

Capital loss The negative difference between the purchase price and the sale price of an asset.

Capture hypothesis A theory of regulatory behavior that predicts that the regulators will eventually be captured by the special interests of the industry being regulated.

Cartel An association of producers in an industry that agree to set common prices and output quotas to prevent competition.

Central bank A banker's bank, usually an official institution that also serves as a country's treasury's bank. Central banks normally regulate commercial banks.

Certificate authority A group charged with supervising the terms governing how buyers and sellers can legitimately make digital cash transfers.

Certificate of deposit (CD) A time deposit with a fixed maturity date offered by banks and other financial institutions.

***Ceteris paribus* [KAY-ter-us PEAR-uh-bus] assumption** The assumption that nothing changes except the factor or factors being studied.

Checkable deposits Any deposits in a thrift institution or a commercial bank on which a check may be written.

Clearing House Interbank Payment System (CHIPS) A large-value wire transfer system linking about 100 banks that permits them to transmit large sums of money related primarily to foreign exchange and Eurodollar transactions.

Closed shop A business enterprise in which employees must belong to the union before they can be hired and must remain in the union after they are hired.

Collateral An asset pledged to guarantee the repayment of a loan.

Collective bargaining Bargaining between the management of a company or of a group of companies and the management of a union or a group of unions for the purpose of setting a mutually agreeable contract on wages, fringe benefits, and working conditions for all employees in all the unions involved.

Collective decision making How voters, politicians, and other interested parties act and how these actions influence nonmarket decisions.

Common property Property that is owned by everyone and therefore by no one. Air and water are examples of common property resources.

Comparable-worth doctrine The belief that women should receive the same wages as men if the levels of skill and responsibility in their jobs are equivalent.

Comparative advantage The ability to produce a good or service at a lower opportunity cost compared to other producers.

Complements Two goods are complements if both are used together for consumption or enjoyment—for example, coffee and cream. The more you buy of one, the more you buy of the other. For complements, a change in the price of one causes an opposite shift in the demand for the other.

Concentration ratio The percentage of all sales contributed by the leading four or leading eight firms in an industry; sometimes called the *industry concentration ratio*.

Constant dollars Dollars expressed in terms of real purchasing power using a particular year as the base or standard of comparison, in contrast to current dollars.

Constant returns to scale No change in long-run average costs when output increases.

Constant-cost industry An industry whose total output can be increased without an increase in long-run per-unit costs; an industry whose long-run supply curve is horizontal.

Consumer optimum A choice of a set of goods and services that maximizes the level of satisfaction for each consumer, subject to limited income.

Consumer Price Index (CPI) A statistical measure of a weighted average of prices of a specified set of goods and services purchased by wage earners in urban areas.

Consumption Spending on new goods and services out of a household's current income. Whatever is not consumed is saved. Consumption includes such things as buying food and going to a concert. *Can also be viewed as* the use of goods and services for personal satisfaction.

Consumption function The relationship between amount consumed and disposable income. A consumption function tells us how much people plan to consume at various levels of disposable income.

Consumption goods Goods bought by households to use up, such as food, clothing, and movies.

Contraction A business fluctuation during which the pace of national economic activity is slowing down.

Cooperative game A game in which the players explicity cooperate to make themselves better off. As applied to firms, it involves companies colluding in order to make higher than competitive rates of return.

Corporation A legal entity that may conduct business in its own name just as an individual does; the owners of a corporation, called shareholders, own shares of the firm's profits and enjoy the protection of limited liability.

Cost-of-living adjustments (COLAs) Clauses in contracts that allow for increases in specified nominal values to take account of changes in the cost of living.

Cost-of-service regulation Regulation based on allowing prices to reflect only the actual cost of production and no monopoly profits.

Cost-push inflation Inflation caused by a continually decreasing short-run aggregate supply curve.

Craft unions Labor unions composed of workers who engage in a particular trade or skill, such as baking, carpentry, or plumbing.

Crawling peg An exchange rate arrangement in which a country pegs the value of its currency to the exchange value of another nation's currency but allows the par value to change at regular intervals.

Creative response Behavior on the part of a firm that allows it to comply with the letter of the law but violate the spirit, significantly lessening the law's effects.

Credit risk The risk of loss that might occur if one party to an exchange fails to honor the terms under which the exchange was to take place.

Cross price elasticity of demand (E_{xy}) The percentage change in the demand for one good (holding its price constant) divided by the percentage change in the price of a related good.

Crowding-out effect The tendency of expansionary fiscal policy to cause a decrease in planned investment or planned consumption in the private sector; this decrease normally results from the rise in interest rates.

Crude quantity theory of money and prices The belief that changes in the money supply lead to proportional changes in the price level.

Cyclical unemployment Unemployment resulting from business recessions that occur when aggregate (total) demand is insufficient to create full employment.

Debit card A plastic card that allows the bearer to transfer funds to a merchant's account, provided that the bearer authorizes the transfer by providing personal identification.

Decreasing-cost industry An industry in which an increase in output leads to a reduction in long-run per-unit costs, such that the long-run industry supply curve slopes downward.

Deflation The situation in which the average of all prices of goods and services in an economy is falling.

Demand A schedule of how much of a good or service people will purchase at any price during a specified time period, other things being constant.

Demand curve A graphical representation of the demand schedule; a negatively sloped line showing the inverse relationship between the price and the quantity demanded (other things being equal).

Demand-pull inflation Inflation caused by increases in aggregate demand not matched by increases in aggregate supply.

Demerit good A good that has been deemed socially undesirable through the political process. Heroin is an example.

Dependent variable A variable whose value changes according to changes in the value of one or more independent variables.

Depository institutions Financial institutions that accept deposits from savers and lend those deposits out at interest.

Depreciation Reduction in the value of capital goods over a one-year period due to physical wear and tear and also to obsolescence; also called *capital consumption allowance*. *Can also be viewed as* a decrease in the exchange value of one nation's currency in terms of the currency of another nation.

Depression An extremely severe recession.

Deregulation The elimination or phasing out of regulations on economic activity.

Derived demand Input factor demand derived from demand for the final product being produced.

Development economics The study of factors that contribute to the economic development of a country.

Digital cash Funds contained on computer software, in the form of secure programs stored on microchips and other computer devices.

Diminishing marginal utility The principle that as more of any good or service is consumed, its extra benefit declines. Otherwise stated, increases in total utility from the consumption of a good or service become smaller and smaller as more is consumed during a given time period.

Direct expenditure offsets Actions on the part of the private sector in spending income that offset government fiscal policy actions. Any increase in government spending in an area that competes with the private sector will have some direct expenditure offset.

Direct relationship A relationship between two variables that is positive, meaning that an increase in one variable is associated with an increase in the other and a decrease in one variable is associated with a decrease in the other.

Dirty float Active management of a floating exchange rate on the part of a country's government, often in cooperation with other nations.

Discounting The method by which the present value of a future sum or a future stream of sums is obtained.

Discount rate The interest rate that the Federal Reserve charges for reserves that it lends to depository institutions. It is sometimes referred to as the rediscount rate or, in Canada and England, as the bank rate.

Discouraged workers Individuals who have stopped looking for a job because they are convinced that they will not find a suitable one.

Diseconomies of scale Increases in long-run average costs that occur as output increases.

Disposable personal income (DPI) Personal income after personal income taxes have been paid.

Dissaving Negative saving; a situation in which spending exceeds income. Dissaving can occur when a household is able to borrow or use up existing assets.

Distribution of income The way income is allocated among the population.

Dividends Portion of a corporation's profits paid to its owners (shareholders).

Division of labor The segregation of a resource into different specific tasks; for example, one automobile worker puts on bumpers, another doors, and so on.

Dominant strategies Strategies that always yield the highest benefit. Regardless of what other players do, a dominant strategy will yield the most benefit for the player using it.

Dumping Selling a good or a service abroad below the price charged in the home market or at a price below its cost of production.

Durable consumer goods Consumer goods that have a life span of more than three years.

Economic goods Goods that are scarce, for which the quantity demanded exceeds the quantity supplied at a zero price.

Economic growth Increases in per capita real GDP measured by its rate of change per year.

Economic profits Total revenues minus total opportunity costs of all inputs used, or the total of all implicit and explicit costs. *Can also be viewed as* the difference between total revenues and the opportunity cost of all factors of production.

Economic rent A payment for the use of any resource over and above its opportunity cost.

Economics The study of how people allocate their limited resources to satisfy their unlimited wants.

Economies of scale Decreases in long-run average costs resulting from increases in output.

Effect time lag The time that elapses between the onset of policy and the results of that policy.

Efficiency wage theory The hypothesis that the productivity of workers depends on the level of the real wage rate.

Efficiency The case in which a given level of inputs is used to produce the maximum output possible. Alternatively, the situation in which a given output is produced at minimum cost.

Efficiency wages Wages set above competitive levels to increase labor productivity and profits by enhancing the efficiency of the firm through lower turnover, ease of attracting higher-quality workers, and better efforts by workers.

Effluent fee A charge to a polluter that gives the right to discharge into the air or water a certain amount of pollution. Also called a *pollution tax*.

Elastic demand A demand relationship in which a given percentage change in price will result in a larger percentage change in quantity demanded. Total expenditures and price changes are inversely related in the elastic region of the demand curve.

Empirical Relying on real-world data in evaluating the usefulness of a model.

Endowments The various resources in an economy, including both physical resources and such human resources as ingenuity and management skills.

Entrepreneurship The factor of production involving human resources that perform the functions of raising capital, organizing, managing, assembling other factors of production, and making basic business policy decisions. The entrepreneur is a risk taker.

Entry deterrence strategy Any strategy undertaken by firms in an industry, either individually or together, with the intent or effect of raising the cost of entry into the industry by a new firm.

Equation of exchange The formula indicating that the number of monetary units times the number of times each unit is spent on final goods and services is identical to the price level times output (or nominal national income).

Equilibrium The situation when quantity supplied equals quantity demanded at a particular price.

Eurodollar deposits Deposits denominated in U.S. dollars but held in banks outside the United States, often in overseas branches of U.S. banks.

Excess reserves The difference between legal reserves and required reserves.

Exchange rate The price of one nation's currency in terms of the currency of another country.

Exclusion principle The principle that no one can be excluded from the benefits of a public good, even if that person hasn't paid for it.

Expansion A business fluctuation in which overall business activity is rising at a more rapid rate than previously or at a more rapid rate than the overall historical trend for the nation.

Expenditure approach A way of computing national income by adding up the dollar value at current market prices of all final goods and services.

Explicit costs Costs that business managers must take account of because they must be paid; examples are wages, taxes, and rent.

Externality A consequence of an economic activity that spills over to affect third parties. Pollution is an externality. *Can also be viewed as* a situation in which a private cost (or benefit) diverges from a social cost (or benefit); a situation in which the costs (or benefits) of an action are not fully borne (or gained) by the two parties engaged in exchange or by an individual engaging in a scarce-resource-using activity.

Featherbedding Any practice that forces employers to use more labor than they would otherwise or to use existing labor in an inefficient manner.

The Fed The Federal Reserve System; the central bank of the United States.

Federal Deposit Insurance Corporation (FDIC) A government agency that insures the deposits held in banks and most other depository institutions; all U.S. banks are insured this way.

Federal funds market A private market (made up mostly of banks) in which banks can borrow reserves from other banks that want to lend them. Federal funds are usually lent for overnight use.

Federal funds rate The interest rate that depository institutions pay to borrow reserves in the interbank federal funds market.

Fedwire A large-value wire transfer system operated by the Federal Reserve that is open to all depository institutions that legally must maintain required reserves with the Fed.

Fiduciary monetary system A system in which currency is issued by the government and its value is based uniquely on the public's faith that the currency represents command over goods and services.

Final goods and services Goods and services that are at their final stage of production and will not be transformed into yet other goods or services. For example, wheat is not ordinarily considered a final good because it is usually used to make a final good, bread.

Financial capital Money used to purchase capital goods such as buildings and equipment.

Financial intermediaries Institutions that transfer funds between ultimate lenders (savers) and ultimate borrowers.

Financial intermediation The process by which financial institutions accept savings from businesses, households, and governments and lend the savings to other businesses, households, and governments.

Financial trading system A mechanism linking buyers and sellers of stocks and bonds.

Firm A business organization that employs resources to produce goods or services for profit. A firm normally owns and operates at least one plant in order to produce.

Fiscal policy The discretionary changing of government expenditures or taxes to achieve national economic goals, such as high employment with price stability.

Fixed costs Costs that do not vary with output. Fixed costs include such things as rent on a building. These costs are fixed for a certain period of time; in the long run, they are variable.

Fixed investment Purchases by businesses of newly produced producer durables, or capital goods, such as production machinery and office equipment.

Flexible exchange rates Exchange rates that are allowed to fluctuate in the open market in response to changes in supply and demand. Sometimes called *floating exchange rates.*

Flow A quantity measured per unit of time; something that occurs over time, such as the income you make per week or per year or the number of individuals who are fired every month.

Foreign exchange market A market in which households, firms, and governments buy and sell national currencies.

Foreign exchange rate The price of one currency in terms of another.

Foreign exchange risk The possibility that changes in the value of a nation's currency will result in variations in market values of assets.

45-degree reference line The line along which planned real expenditures equal real national income per year.

Fractional reserve banking A system in which depository institutions hold reserves that are less than the amount of total deposits.

Free-rider problem A problem that arises when individuals presume that others will pay for public goods so that, individually, they can escape paying for their portion without causing a reduction in production.

Frictional unemployment Unemployment due to the fact that workers must search for appropriate job offers. This takes time, and so they remain temporarily unemployed.

Full employment An arbitrary level of unemployment that corresponds to "normal" friction in the labor market. In 1986, a 6.5 percent rate of unemployment was considered full employment. Today, it is assumed to be 5 percent or possibly even less.

Game theory A way of describing the various possible outcomes in any situation involving two or more interacting individuals when those individuals are aware of the interactive nature of their situation and plan accordingly. The plans made by these individuals are known as *game strategies*.

GDP deflator A price index measuring the changes in prices of all new goods and services produced in the economy.

General Agreement on Tariffs and Trade (GATT) An international agreement established in 1947 to further world trade by reducing barriers and tariffs.

Goods All things from which individuals derive satisfaction or happiness.

Government, or **political, goods** Goods (and services) provided by the public sector; they can be either private or public goods.

Gross domestic income (GDI) The sum of all income—wages, interest, rent, and profits—paid to the four factors of production.

Gross domestic product (GDP) The total market value of all final goods and services produced by factors of production located within a nation's borders.

Gross private domestic investment The creation of capital goods, such as factories and machines, that can yield production and hence consumption in the future. Also included in this definition are changes in business inventories and repairs made to machines or buildings.

Gross public debt All federal government debt irrespective of who owns it.

Hedge A financial strategy that reduces the chance of suffering losses arising from foreign exchange risk.

Horizontal merger The joining of firms that are producing or selling a similar product.

Human capital The accumulated training and education of workers.

Implicit costs Expenses that managers do not have to pay out of pocket and hence do not normally explicitly calculate, such as the opportunity cost of factors of production that are owned; examples are owner-provided capital and owner-provided labor.

Import quota A physical supply restriction on imports of a particular good, such as sugar. Foreign exporters are unable to sell in the United States more than the quantity specified in the import quota.

Incentive-compatible contract A loan contract under which a significant amount of the borrower's assets are at risk, providing an incentive for the borrower to look after the lender's interests.

Incentives Rewards for engaging in a particular activity.

Incentive structure The system of rewards and punishments individuals face with respect to their own actions.

Income approach A way of measuring national income by adding up all components of national income, including wages, interest, rent, and profits.

Income elasticity of demand (E_i) The percentage change in demand for any good, holding its price constant, divided by the percentage change in income; the responsiveness of demand to changes in income, holding the good's relative price constant.

Income in kind Income received in the form of goods and services, such as housing or medical care; to be contrasted with money income, which is simply income in dollars, or general purchasing power, that can be used to buy *any* goods and services.

Income velocity of money The number of times per year a dollar is spent on final goods and services; equal to GDP divided by the money supply.

Income-consumption curve The set of optimum consumption points that would occur if income were increased, relative prices remaining constant.

Increasing-cost industry An industry in which an increase in industry output is accompanied by an increase in long-run per-unit costs, such that the long-run industry supply curve slopes upward.

Independent variable A variable whose value is determined independently of, or outside, the equation under study.

Indifference curve A curve composed of a set of consumption alternatives, each of which yields the same total amount of satisfaction.

Indirect business taxes All business taxes except the tax on corporate profits. Indirect business taxes include sales and business property taxes.

Industrial unions Labor unions that consist of workers from a particular industry, such as automobile manufacturing or steel manufacturing.

Industry supply curve The locus of points showing the minimum prices at which given quantities will be forthcoming; also called the *market supply curve*.

Inefficient point Any point below the production possibilities curve at which resources are being used inefficiently.

Inelastic demand A demand relationship in which a given percentage change in price will result in a less than proportionate percentage change in the quantity demanded. Total expenditures and price are directly related in the inelastic region of the demand curve.

Infant industry argument The contention that tariffs should be imposed to protect from import competition an industry that is trying to get started. Presumably, after the industry becomes technologically efficient, the tariff can be lifted.

Inferior goods Goods for which demand falls as income rises.

Inflation The situation in which the average of all prices of goods and services in an economy is rising.

Inflation-adjusted return A rate of return that is measured in terms of real goods and services, that is, after the effects of inflation have been factored out.

Inflationary gap The gap that exists whenever the equilibrium level of real national income per year is greater than the full-employment level as shown by the position of the long-run aggregate supply curve.

Innovation Transforming an invention into something that is useful to humans.

Inside information Information that is not available to the general public about what is happening in a corporation.

Insider-outsider theory A theory of labor markets in which workers who are already employed have an influence on wage bargaining in such a way that outsiders who are willing to work for lower real wages cannot get a job.

Interest The payment for current rather than future command over resources; the cost of obtaining credit. Also, the return paid to owners of capital.

Interest rate effect One of the reasons that the aggregate demand curve slopes downward is that higher price levels increase the interest rate, which in turn causes businesses and consumers to reduce desired spending due to the higher price of borrowing.

Intermediate goods Goods used up entirely in the production of final goods.

International financial diversification Financing investment projects in more than one country.

International Monetary Fund (IMF) An international agency, founded to administer the Bretton Woods agreement and to lend to member countries that experienced significant balance of payments deficits, that now functions primarily as a lender of last resort for national governments.

Inventory investment Changes in the stocks of finished goods and goods in process, as well as changes in the raw materials that businesses keep on hand. Whenever inventories are decreasing, inventory investment is negative; whenever they are increasing, inventory investment is positive.

Inverse relationship A relationship between two variables that is negative, meaning that an increase in one variable is associated with a decrease in the other and a decrease in one variable is associated with an increase in the other.

Investment Any use of today's resources to expand tomorrow's production or consumption. *Can also be viewed as* the spending by businesses on things such as machines and buildings, which can be used to produce goods and services in the future. The investment part of total output is the portion that will be used in the process of producing goods in the future.

Job leaver An individual in the labor force who quits voluntarily.

Job loser An individual in the labor force whose employment was involuntarily terminated.

Jurisdictional dispute A dispute involving two or more unions over which should have control of a particular jurisdiction, such as a particular craft or skill or a particular firm or industry.

Keynesian short-run aggregate supply curve The horizontal portion of the aggregate supply curve in which there is unemployment and unused capacity in the economy.

Labor Productive contributions of humans who work, involving both mental and physical activities.

Labor force Individuals aged 16 years or older who either have jobs or are looking and available for jobs; the number of employed plus the number of unemployed.

Labor force participation rate The percentage of noninstitutionalized working-age individuals who are employed or seeking employment.

Labor productivity Total real domestic output (real GDP) divided by the number of workers (output per worker).

Labor unions Worker organizations that seek to secure economic improvements for their members; they also seek to improve the safety, health, and other benefits (such as job security) of their members.

Land The natural resources that are available from nature. Land as a resource includes location, original fertility and mineral deposits, topography, climate, water, and vegetation.

Large-value wire transfer system A payment system that permits the electronic transmission of large dollar sums.

Law of demand The observation that there is a negative, or inverse, relationship between the price of any good or service and the quantity demanded, holding other factors constant.

Law of diminishing (marginal) returns The observation that after some point, successive equal-sized increases in a variable factor of production, such as labor, added to fixed factors of production, will result in smaller increases in output.

Law of increasing relative cost The observation that the opportunity cost of additional units of a good generally increases as society attempts to produce more of that good. This accounts for the bowed-out shape of the production possibilities curve.

Law of supply The observation that the higher the price of a good, the more of that good sellers will make available over a specified time period, other things being equal.

Leading indicators Factors that economists find to exhibit changes before changes in business activity.

Legal reserves Reserves that depository institutions are allowed by law to claim as reserves—for example, deposits held at Federal Reserve district banks and vault cash.

Lemons problem The situation in which consumers, who do not know details about the quality of a product, are willing to pay no more than the price of a low-quality product, even if a higher-quality product at a higher price exists.

Liabilities Amounts owed; the legal claims against a business or household by nonowners.

Limited liability A legal concept whereby the responsibility, or liability, of the owners of a corporation is limited to the value of the shares in the firm that they own.

Limit-pricing model A model that hypothesizes that a group of colluding sellers will set the highest common price that they believe they can charge without new firms seeking to enter that industry in search of relatively high profits.

Liquidity The degree to which an asset can be acquired or disposed of without much danger of any intervening loss in *nominal* value and with small transaction costs. Money is the most liquid asset.

Liquidity approach A method of measuring the money supply by looking at money as a temporary store of value.

Liquidity risk The risk of loss that may occur if a payment is not received when due.

Long run The time period in which all factors of production can be varied.

Long-run aggregate supply curve A vertical line representing real output of goods and services after full adjustment has occurred. *Can also be viewed as* representing the real output of the economy under conditions of full employment—the full-employment level of real GDP.

Long-run average cost curve The locus of points representing the minimum unit cost of producing any given rate of output, given current technology and resource prices.

Long-run industry supply curve A market supply curve showing the relationship between prices and quantities forthcoming after firms have been allowed the time to enter into or exit from an industry, depending on whether there have been positive or negative economic profits.

Lorenz curve A geometric representation of the distribution of income. A Lorenz curve that is perfectly straight represents complete income equality. The more bowed a Lorenz curve, the more unequally income is distributed.

Lump-sum tax A tax that does not depend on income or the circumstances of the taxpayer. An example is a $1,000 tax that every family must pay, irrespective of its economic situation.

M1 The money supply, taken as the total value of currency plus checkable deposits plus traveler's checks not issued by banks.

M2 M1 plus (1) savings and small-denomination time deposits at all depository institutions, (2) overnight repurchase agreements at commercial banks, (3) overnight Eurodollars held by U.S. residents other than banks at Caribbean branches of member banks, (4) balances in retail money market mutual funds, and (5) money market deposit accounts (MMDAs).

Macroeconomics The study of the behavior of the economy as a whole, including such economywide phenomena as changes in unemployment, the general price level, and national income.

Majority rule A collective decision-making system in which group decisions are made on the basis of more than 50 percent of the vote. In other words, whatever more than half of the electorate votes for, the entire electorate has to accept.

Marginal cost pricing A system of pricing in which the price charged is equal to the opportunity cost to society of producing one more unit of the good or service in question. The opportunity cost is the marginal cost to society.

Marginal costs The change in total costs due to a one-unit change in production rate.

Marginal factor cost (MFC) The cost of using an additional unit of an input. For example, if a firm can hire all the workers it wants at the going wage rate, the marginal factor cost of labor is the wage rate.

Marginal physical product The physical output that is due to the addition of one more unit of a variable factor of production; the change in total product occurring when a variable input is increased and all other inputs are held constant; also called *marginal product* or *marginal return*.

Marginal physical product (MPP) of labor The change in output resulting from the addition of one more worker. The MPP of the worker equals the change in total output accounted for by hiring the worker, holding all other factors of production constant.

Marginal propensity to consume (MPC) The ratio of the change in consumption to the change in disposable income. A marginal propensity to consume of 0.8 tells us that an additional $100 in take-home pay will lead to an additional $80 consumed.

Marginal propensity to save (MPS) The ratio of the change in saving to the change in disposable income. A marginal propensity to save of 0.2 indicates that out of an additional $100 in take-home pay, $20 will be saved. Whatever is not saved is consumed. The marginal propensity to save plus the marginal propensity to consume must always equal 1, by definition.

Marginal revenue The change in total revenues resulting from a change in output (and sale) of one unit of the product in question.

Marginal revenue product (MRP) The marginal physical product (MPP) times marginal revenue. The MRP gives the additional revenue obtained from a one-unit change in labor input.

Marginal tax rate The change in the tax payment divided by the change in income, or the percentage of additional dollars that must be paid in taxes. The marginal tax rate is applied to the highest tax bracket of taxable income reached.

Marginal utility The change in total utility due to a one-unit change in the quantity of a good or service consumed.

Market All of the arrangements that individuals have for exchanging with one another. Thus we can speak of the labor market, the automobile market, and the credit market.

Market clearing, or **equilibrium, price** The price that clears the market, at which quantity demanded equals quantity supplied; the price where the demand curve intersects the supply curve.

Market demand The demand of all consumers in the marketplace for a particular good or service. The summing at each price of the quantity demanded by each individual.

Market failure A situation in which an unrestrained market operation leads to either too few or too many resources going to a specific economic activity.

Market share test The percentage of a market that a particular firm supplies, used as the primary measure of monopoly power.

Median age The age that divides the older half of the population from the younger half.

Medical savings account (MSA) A tax-exempt health care account into which individuals would pay on a regular basis and out of which medical care expenses could be paid.

Medium of exchange Any asset that sellers will accept as payment.

Merit good A good that has been deemed socially desirable through the political process. Museums are an example.

Microeconomics The study of decision making undertaken by individuals (or households) and by firms.

Minimum efficient scale (MES) The lowest rate of output per unit time at which long-run average costs for a particular firm are at a minimum.

Minimum wage A wage floor, legislated by government, setting the lowest hourly rate that firms may legally pay workers.

Models, or **theories** Simplified representations of the real world used as the basis for predictions or explanations.

Monetarists Macroeconomists who believe that inflation is always caused by excessive monetary growth and that changes in the money supply affect aggregate demand both directly and indirectly.

Monetary rule A monetary policy that incorporates a rule specifying the annual rate of growth of some monetary aggregate.

Money Any medium that is universally accepted in an economy both by sellers of goods and services as payment for those goods and services and by creditors as payment for debts.

Money illusion Reacting to changes in money prices rather than relative prices. If a worker whose wages double when the price level also doubles thinks he or she is better off, the worker is suffering from money illusion.

Money market deposit accounts (MMDAs) Accounts issued by banks yielding a market rate of interest with a minimum balance requirement and a limit on transactions. They have no minimum maturity.

Money market mutual funds Funds of investment companies that obtain funds from the public that are held in common and used to acquire short-maturity credit instruments, such as certificates of deposit and securities sold by the U.S. government.

Money multiplier The reciprocal of the required reserve ratio, assuming no leakages into currency and no excess reserves. It is equal to 1 divided by the required reserve ratio.

Money price The price that we observe today, expressed in today's dollars. Also called the *absolute* or *nominal price*.

Money supply The amount of money in circulation.

Monopolist A single supplier that comprises its entire industry for a good or service for which there is no close substitute.

Monopolistic competition A market situation in which a large number of firms produce similar but not identical products. Entry into the industry is relatively easy.

Monopolization The possession of monopoly power in the relevant market and the willful acquisition or maintenance of that power, as distinguished from growth or development as a consequence of a superior product, business acumen, or historical accident.

Monopoly A firm that has great control over the price of a good. In the extreme case, a monopoly is the only seller of a good or service.

Monopsonist A single buyer.

Monopsonistic exploitation Exploitation due to monopsony power. It leads to a price for the variable input that is less than its marginal revenue product. Monopsonistic exploitation is the difference between marginal revenue product and the wage rate.

Moral hazard The possibility that a borrower might engage in riskier behavior after a loan has been obtained.

Multiplier The ratio of the change in the equilibrium level of real national income to the change in autonomous expenditures; the number by which a change in autonomous investment or autonomous consumption, for example, is multiplied to get the change in the equilibrium level of real national income.

National income (NI) The total of all factor payments to resource owners. It can be obtained by subtracting indirect business taxes from NDP.

National income accounting A measurement system used to estimate national income and its components; one approach to measuring an economy's aggregate performance.

Natural monopoly A monopoly that arises from the peculiar production characteristics in an industry. It usually arises when there are large economies of scale relative to the industry's demand such that one firm can produce at a lower average cost than can be achieved by multiple firms.

Natural rate of unemployment The rate of unemployment that is estimated to prevail in long-run macroeconomic equilibrium, when all workers and employers have fully adjusted to any changes in the economy.

Near moneys Assets that are almost money. They have a high degree of liquidity; they can be easily converted into money without loss in value. Time deposits and short-term U.S. government securities are examples.

Negative-sum game A game in which players as a group lose at the end of the game.

Net domestic product (NDP) GDP minus depreciation.

Net investment Gross private domestic investment minus an estimate of the wear and tear on the existing capital stock. Net investment therefore measures the change in capital stock over a one-year period.

Net public debt Gross public debt minus all government interagency borrowing.

Net worth The difference between assets and liabilities.

New classical model A modern version of the classical model in which wages and prices are flexible, there is pure competition in all markets, and the rational expectations hypothesis is assumed to be working.

New entrant An individual who has never held a full-time job lasting two weeks or longer but is now seeking employment.

New growth theory A theory of economic growth that examines the factors that determine why technology, research, innovation, and the like are undertaken and how they interact.

New Keynesian economics A macroeconomic approach that emphasizes that the prices of some goods and services adjust sluggishly in response to changing market conditions. Thus an unexpected decrease in the price level results in some firms with higher-than-desired prices. A consequence is a reduction in sales for those firms.

Nominal rate of interest The market rate of interest expressed in today's dollars.

Nominal values The values of variables such as GDP and investment expressed in current dollars, also called money values; measurement in terms of the actual market prices at which goods are sold.

Nonaccelerating inflation rate of unemployment (NAIRU) The rate of unemployment below which the rate of inflation tends to rise and above which the rate of inflation tends to fall.

Noncooperative game A game in which the players neither negotiate nor cooperate in any way. As applied to firms in an industry, this is the common situation in which there are relatively few firms and each has some ability to change price.

Nondurable consumer goods Consumer goods that are used up within three years.

Nonincome expense items The total of indirect business taxes and depreciation.

Nonprice rationing devices All methods used to ration scarce goods that are price-controlled. Whenever the price system is not allowed to work, nonprice rationing devices will evolve to ration the affected goods and services.

Normal goods Goods for which demand rises as income rises. Most goods are considered normal.

Normal rate of return The amount that must be paid to an investor to induce investment in a business; also known as the *opportunity cost of capital.*

Normative economics Analysis involving value judgments about economic policies; relates to whether things are good or bad. A statement of what ought to be.

Number line A line that can be divided into segments of equal length, each associated with a number.

Oligopoly A market situation in which there are very few sellers. Each seller knows that the other sellers will react to its changes in prices and quantities.

Open economy effect One of the reasons that the aggregate demand curve slopes downward is that higher price levels result in foreigners' desiring to buy fewer American-made goods while Americans now desire more foreign-made goods, thereby reducing net exports. This is equivalent to a reduction in the amount of real goods and services purchased in the United States.

Open market operations The purchase and sale of existing U.S. government securities (such as bonds) in the open private market by the Federal Reserve System.

Opportunistic behavior Actions that ignore the possible long-run benefits of cooperation and focus solely on short-run gains.

Opportunity cost The highest-valued, next-best alternative that must be sacrificed to obtain something or to satisfy a want.

Opportunity cost of capital The normal rate of return, or the available return on the next-best alternative investment. Economists consider this a cost of production, and it is included in our cost examples.

Optimal quantity of pollution The level of pollution for which the marginal benefit of one additional unit of clean air just equals the marginal cost of that additional unit of clean air.

Origin The intersection of the *y* axis and the *x* axis in a graph.

Par value The officially determined value of a currency.

Partnership A business owned by two or more joint owners, or partners, who share the responsibilities and the profits of the firm and are individually liable for all of the debts of the partnership.

Passive (nondiscretionary) policymaking Policymaking that is carried out in response to a rule. It is therefore not in response to an actual or potential change in overall economic activity.

Patent A government protection that gives an inventor the exclusive right to make, use, or sell an invention for a limited period of time (currently, 20 years).

Payment intermediary An institution that facilitates the transfer of funds between buyer and seller during the course of any purchase of goods, services, or financial assets.

Payment system An institutional structure by which consumers, businesses, governments, and financial institutions exchange payments.

Payoff matrix A matrix of outcomes, or consequences, of the strategies available to the players in a game.

Perfect competition A market structure in which the decisions of individual buyers and sellers have no effect on market price.

Perfectly competitive firm A firm that is such a small part of the total industry that it cannot affect the price of the product it sells.

Perfectly elastic demand A demand that has the characteristic that even the slightest increase in price will lead to zero quantity demanded.

Perfectly elastic supply A supply characterized by a reduction in quantity supplied to zero when there is the slightest decrease in price.

Perfectly inelastic demand A demand that exhibits zero responsiveness to price changes; no matter what the price is, the quantity demanded remains the same.

Perfectly inelastic supply A supply for which quantity supplied remains constant, no matter what happens to price.

Personal income (PI) The amount of income that households actually receive before they pay personal income taxes.

Phillips curve A curve showing the relationship between unemployment and changes in wages or prices. It was long thought to reflect a trade-off between unemployment and inflation.

Physical capital All manufactured resources, including buildings, equipment, machines, and improvements to land that is used for production.

Planning curve The long-run average cost curve.

Planning horizon The long run, during which all inputs are variable.

Plant size The physical size of the factories that a firm owns and operates to produce its output. Plant size can be defined by square footage, maximum physical capacity, and other physical measures.

Point-of-sale (POS) network System in which consumer payments for retail purchases are made by means of direct deductions from their deposit accounts at depository institutions.

Policy irrelevance proposition The new classical and rational expectations conclusion that policy actions have no real effects in the short run if the policy actions are anticipated and none in the long run even if the policy actions are unanticipated.

Positive economics Analysis that is strictly limited to making either purely descriptive statements or scientific predictions; for example, "If A, then B." A statement of what is.

Positive-sum game A game in which players as a group are better off at the end of the game.

Precautionary demand Holding money to meet unplanned expenditures and emergencies.

Present value The value of a future amount expressed in today's dollars; the most that someone would pay today to receive a certain sum at some point in the future.

Price ceiling A legal maximum price that may be charged for a particular good or service.

Price controls Government-mandated minimum or maximum prices that may be charged for goods and services.

Price differentiation Establishing different prices for similar products to reflect differences in marginal cost in providing those commodities to different groups of buyers.

Price discrimination Selling a given product at more than one price, with the price difference being unrelated to differences in cost.

Price elasticity of demand (E_p) The responsiveness of the quantity demanded of a commodity to changes in its price; defined as the percentage change in quantity demanded divided by the percentage change in price.

Price elasticity of supply (E_s) The responsiveness of the quantity supplied of a commodity to a change in its price; the percentage change in quantity supplied divided by the percentage change in price.

Price floor A legal minimum price below which a good or service may not be sold. Legal minimum wages are an example.

Price index The cost of today's market basket of goods expressed as a percentage of the cost of the same market basket during a base year.

Price leadership A practice in many oligopolistic industries in which the largest firm publishes its price list ahead of its competitors, who then match those announced prices. Also called *parallel pricing*.

Price searcher A firm that must determine the price-output combination that maximizes profit because it faces a downward-sloping demand curve.

Price system An economic system in which relative prices are constantly changing to reflect changes in supply and demand for different commodities. The prices of those commodities are signals to everyone within the system as to what is relatively scarce and what is relatively abundant.

Price taker A competitive firm that must take the price of its product as given because the firm cannot influence its price.

Price war A pricing campaign designed to capture additional market share by repeatedly cutting prices.

Price-consumption curve The set of consumer optimum combinations of two goods that the consumer would choose as the price of one good changes, while money income and the price of the other good remain constant.

Principal-agent problem The conflict of interest that occurs when agents—managers of firms—pursue their own objectives to the detriment of the goals of the firms' principals, or owners.

Principle of rival consumption The recognition that individuals are rivals in consuming private goods because one person's consumption reduces the amount available for others to consume.

Principle of substitution The principle that consumers and producers shift away from goods and resources that become priced relatively higher in favor of goods and resources that are now priced relatively lower.

Prisoners' dilemma A famous strategic game in which two prisoners have a choice between confessing and not confessing to a crime. If neither confesses, they serve a minimum sentence. If both confess, they serve a maximum sentence. If one confesses and the other doesn't, the one who confesses goes free. The dominant strategy is always to confess.

Private costs Costs borne solely by the individuals who incur them. Also called *internal costs*.

Private goods Goods that can be consumed by only one individual at a time. Private goods are subject to the principle of rival consumption.

Private property rights Exclusive rights of ownership that allow the use, transfer, and exchange of property.

Producer durables, or **capital goods** Durable goods having an expected service life of more than three years that are used by businesses to produce other goods and services.

Producer Price Index (PPI) A statistical measure of a weighted average of prices of commodities that firms produce and sell.

Product differentiation The distinguishing of products by brand name, color, and other minor attributes. Product differentiation occurs in other than perfectly competitive markets in which products are, in theory, homogeneous, such as wheat or corn.

Production Any activity that results in the conversion of resources into products that can be used in consumption.

Production function The relationship between inputs and maximum physical output. A production function is a technological, not an economic, relationship.

Production possibilities curve (PPC) A curve representing all possible combinations of total output that could be produced assuming (1) a fixed amount of productive resources of a given quality and (2) the efficient use of those resources.

Profit-maximizing rate of production The rate of production that maximizes total profits, or the difference between total revenues and total costs; also, the rate of production at which marginal revenue equals marginal cost.

Progressive taxation A tax system in which as income increases, a higher percentage of the additional income is taxed. The marginal tax rate exceeds the average tax rate as income rises.

Property rights The rights of an owner to use and to exchange property.

Proportional rule A decision-making system in which actions are based on the proportion of the "votes" cast and are in proportion to them. In a market system, if 10 percent of the "dollar votes" are cast for blue cars, 10 percent of the output will be blue cars.

Proportional taxation A tax system in which regardless of an individual's income, the tax bill comprises exactly the same proportion. Also called a *flat-rate tax*.

Proprietorship A business owned by one individual who makes the business decisions, receives all the profits, and is legally responsible for all the debts of the firm.

Public goods Goods to which the principle of rival consumption does not apply; they can be jointly consumed by many individuals simultaneously at no additional cost and with no reduction in quality or quantity.

Purchasing power The value of money for buying goods and services. If your money income stays the same but the price of one good that you are buying goes up, your effective purchasing power falls, and vice versa.

Purchasing power parity Adjustment in exchange rate conversions that takes into account differences in the true cost of living across countries.

Quota system A government-imposed restriction on the quantity of a specific good that another country is allowed to sell in the United States. In other words, quotas are restrictions on imports. These restrictions are usually applied to one or several specific countries.

Random walk theory The theory that there are no predictable trends in securities prices that can be used to "get rich quick."

Rate of discount The rate of interest used to discount future sums back to present value.

Rate of return An economic system in which relative prices are constantly changing to reflect changes in supply and demand for different commodities. The prices of those commodities are signals to everyone within the system as to what is relatively scarce and what is relatively abundant.

Rate-of-return regulation Regulation that seeks to keep the rate of return in the industry at a competitive level by not allowing excessive prices to be charged.

Rational expectations hypothesis A theory stating that people combine the effects of past policy changes on important economic variables with their own judgment about the future effects of current and future policy changes.

Rationality assumption The assumption that people do not intentionally make decisions that would leave them worse off.

Reaction function The manner in which one oligopolist reacts to a change in price, output, or quality made by another oligopolist in the industry.

Real-balance effect The change in expenditures resulting from the real value of money balances when the price level changes, all other things held constant. Also called the wealth effect.

Real business cycle theory An extension and modification of the theories of the new classical economists of the 1970s and 1980s, in which money is neutral and only real, supply-side factors matter in influencing labor employment and real output.

Real-income effect The change in people's purchasing power that occurs when, other things being constant, the price of one good that they purchase changes. When that price goes up, real income, or purchasing power, falls, and when that price goes down, real income increases.

Real rate of interest The nominal rate of interest minus the anticipated rate of inflation.

Real values Measurement of economic values after adjustments have been made for changes in the average of prices between years.

Recession A period of time during which the rate of growth of business activity is consistently less than its long-term trend or is negative.

Recessionary gap The gap that exists whenever the equilibrium level of real national income per year is less than the full-employment level as shown by the position of the long-run aggregate supply curve.

Recognition time lag The time required to gather information about the current state of the economy.

Recycling The reuse of raw materials derived from manufactured products.

Reentrant An individual who used to work full time but left the labor force and has now reentered it looking for a job.

Regressive taxation A tax system in which as more dollars are earned, the percentage of tax paid on them falls. The marginal tax rate is less than the average tax rate as income rises.

Reinvestment Profits (or depreciation reserves) used to purchase new capital equipment.

Relative price The price of one commodity divided by the price of another commodity; the number of units of one commodity that must be sacrificed to purchase one unit of another commodity.

Rent control The placement of price ceilings on rents in particular cities.

Repricing, or **menu, cost of inflation** The cost associated with recalculating prices and printing new price lists when there is inflation.

Repurchase agreement (REPO, or **RP)** An agreement made by a bank to sell Treasury or federal agency securities to its customers, coupled with an agreement to repurchase them at a price that includes accumulated interest.

Required reserve ratio The percentage of total deposits that the Fed requires depository institutions to hold in the form of vault cash or deposits with the Fed.

Required reserves The value of reserves that a depository institution must hold in the form of vault cash or deposits with the Fed.

Reserves In the U.S. Federal Reserve System, deposits held by Federal Reserve district banks for depository institutions, plus depository institutions' vault cash.

Resources Things used to produce other things to satisfy people's wants.

Retained earnings Earnings that a corporation saves, or retains, for investment in other productive activities; earnings that are not distributed to stockholders.

Ricardian equivalence theorem The proposition that an increase in the government budget deficit has no effect on aggregate demand.

Right-to-work laws Laws that make it illegal to require union membership as a condition of continuing employment in a particular firm.

Saving The act of not consuming all of one's current income. Whatever is not consumed out of spendable income is, by definition, saved. *Saving* is an action measured over time (a flow), whereas *savings* are a stock, an accumulation resulting from the act of saving in the past.

Savings deposits Interest-earning funds that can be withdrawn at any time without payment of a penalty.

Say's law A dictum of economist J. B. Say that supply creates its own demand; producing goods and services generates the means and the willingness to purchase other goods and services.

Scarcity A situation in which the ingredients for producing the things that people desire are insufficient to satisfy all wants.

Seasonal unemployment Unemployment resulting from the seasonal pattern of work in specific industries. It is usually due to seasonal fluctuations in demand or to changing weather conditions, rendering work difficult, if not impossible, as in the agriculture, construction, and tourist industries.

Secondary boycott A boycott of companies or products sold by companies that are dealing with a company being struck.

Secular deflation A persistent decline in prices resulting from economic growth in the presence of stable aggregate demand.

Securities Stocks and bonds.

Separation of ownership and control The situation that exists in corporations in which the owners (shareholders) are not the people who control the operation of the corporation (managers). The goals of these two groups are often different.

Services Mental or physical labor or help purchased by consumers. Examples are the assistance of doctors, lawyers, dentists, repair personnel, housecleaners, educators, retailers, and wholesalers; things purchased or used by consumers that do not have physical characteristics.

Share of stock A legal claim to a share of a corporation's future profits; if it is *common stock*, it incorporates certain voting rights regarding major policy decisions of the corporation; if it is *preferred stock*, its owners are accorded preferential treatment in the payment of dividends.

Share-the-gains, share-the-pains theory A theory of regulatory behavior in which the regulators must take account of the demands of three groups: legislators, who established and who oversee the regulatory agency; members of the regulated industry; and consumers of the regulated industry's products or services.

Short run The time period when at least one input, such as plant size, cannot be changed.

Short-run aggregate supply curve The relationship between aggregate supply and the price level in the short run, all other things held constant. If prices adjust gradually in the short run, the curve is positively sloped.

Short-run break-even price The price at which a firm's total revenues equal its total costs. At the break-even price, the firm is just making a normal rate of return on its capital investment. (It is covering its explicit and implicit costs.)

Short-run shutdown price The price that just covers average variable costs. It occurs just below the intersection of the marginal cost curve and the average variable cost curve.

Shortage A situation in which quantity demanded is greater than quantity supplied at a price below the market clearing price.

Signals Compact ways of conveying to economic decision makers information needed to make decisions. A true signal not only conveys information but also provides the incentive to react appropriately. Economic profits and economic losses are such signals.

Slope The change in the *y*-value divided by the corresponding change in the *x* value of a curve; the "incline" of the curve.

Small menu cost theory A hypothesis that it is costly for firms to change prices in response to demand changes because of the cost of renegotiating contracts, printing price lists, and so on.

Smart card A card containing a microprocessor that permits storage of funds via security programming, can communicate with other computers, and does not require on-line authorization for funds transfers.

Social costs The full costs borne by society whenever a resource use occurs. Social costs can be measured by adding private, or internal, costs to external costs.

Social Security contributions The mandatory taxes paid out of workers' wages and salaries. Although half are supposedly paid by employers, in fact the net wages of employees are lower by the full amount.

Special drawing rights (SDRs) Reserve assets created by the International Monetary Fund for countries to use in settling international payment obligations.

Specialization The division of productive activities among persons and regions so that no one individual or one area is totally self-sufficient. An individual may specialize, for example, in law or medicine. A nation may specialize in the production of coffee, computers, or cameras.

Standard of deferred payment A property of an asset that makes it desirable for use as a means of settling debts maturing in the future; an essential property of money.

Stock The quantity of something, measured at a given point in time—for example, an inventory of goods or a bank account. Stocks are defined independently of time, although they are assessed at a point in time.

Store of value The ability to hold value over time; a necessary property of money.

Stored-value card A card bearing magnetic stripes that hold magnetically encoded data, providing access to stored funds.

Strategic dependence A situation in which one firm's actions with respect to price, quality, advertising, and related changes may be strategically countered by the reactions of one or more other firms in the industry. Such dependence can exist only when there are a limited number of major firms in an industry.

Strategy Any rule that is used to make a choice, such as "Always pick heads"; any potential choice that can be made by players in a game.

Strikebreakers Temporary or permanent workers hired by a company to replace union members who are striking.

Structural unemployment Unemployment resulting from a poor match of workers' abilities and skills with current requirements of employers.

Subsidy A negative tax; a payment to a producer from the government, usually in the form of a cash grant.

Substitutes Two goods are substitutes when either one can be used for consumption to satisfy a similar want—for example, coffee and tea. The more you buy of one, the less you buy of the other. For substitutes, the change in the price of one causes a shift in demand for the other in the same direction as the price change.

Substitution effect The tendency of people to substitute cheaper commodities for more expensive commodities.

Supply A schedule showing the relationship between price and quantity supplied for a specified period of time, other things being equal.

Supply curve The graphical representation of the supply schedule; a line (curve) showing the supply schedule, which generally slopes upward (has a positive slope), other things being equal.

Supply-side economics The notion that creating incentives for individuals and firms to increase productivity will cause the aggregate supply curve to shift outward.

Surplus A situation in which quantity supplied is greater than quantity demanded at a price above the market clearing price.

Sweep account A depository institution account that entails regular shifts of funds from transaction deposits that are subject to reserve requirements to savings deposits that are exempt from reserve requirements.

Sympathy strike A strike by a union in sympathy with another union's strike or cause.

Systemic risk The risk that some payment intermediaries may not be able to meet the terms of their credit agreements because of failures by other institutions to settle other transactions.

Target zone A range of permitted exchange rate variations between upper and lower exchange rate bands that a central bank defends by selling or buying foreign exchange reserves.

Tariffs Taxes on imported goods.

Tax bracket A specified interval of income to which a specific and unique marginal tax rate is applied.

Tax incidence The distribution of tax burdens among various groups in society.

Technology Society's pool of applied knowledge concerning how goods and services can be produced.

Terms of exchange The terms under which trading takes place. Usually the terms of exchange are equal to the price at which a good is traded.

Theory of contestable markets A hypothesis concerning pricing behavior that holds that even though there are only a few firms in an industry, they are forced to price their products more or less competitively because of the ease of entry by outsiders. The key aspect of a contestable market is relatively costless entry into and exit from the industry.

Theory of public choice The study of collective decision making.

Third parties Parties who are not directly involved in a given activity or transaction. For example, in the relationship between caregivers and patients, fees may be paid by third parties (insurance companies, government).

Thrift institutions Financial institutions that receive most of their funds from the savings of the public; they include mutual savings banks, savings and loan associations, and credit unions.

Time deposit A deposit in a financial institution that requires notice of intent to withdraw or must be left for an agreed period. Withdrawal of funds prior to the end of the agreed period may result in a penalty.

Tit-for-tat strategic behavior In game theory, cooperation that continues so long as the other players continue to cooperate.

Total costs The sum of total fixed costs and total variable costs.

Total income The yearly amount earned by the nation's resources (factors of production). Total income therefore includes wages, rent, interest payments, and profits that are received, respectively, by workers, landowners, capital owners, and entrepreneurs.

Total revenues The price per unit times the total quantity sold.

Transaction costs All of the costs associated with exchanging, including the informational costs of finding out price and quality, service record, and durability of a product, plus the cost of contracting and enforcing that contract.

Transactions accounts Checking account balances in commercial banks and other types of financial institutions, such as credit unions and mutual savings banks; any accounts in financial institutions on which you can easily write checks without many restrictions.

Transactions approach A method of measuring the money supply by looking at money as a medium of exchange.

Transactions demand Holding money as a medium of exchange to make payments. The level varies directly with nominal national income.

Transfer payments Money payments made by governments to individuals for which in return no services or goods are concurrently rendered. Examples are welfare, Social Security, and unemployment insurance benefits.

Transfers in kind Payments that are in the form of actual goods and services, such as food stamps, subsidized public housing, and medical care, and for which in return no goods or services are rendered concurrently.

Traveler's checks Financial instruments purchased from a bank or a nonbanking organization and signed during purchase that can be used as cash upon a second signature by the purchaser.

Unanticipated inflation Inflation at a rate that comes as a surprise, either higher or lower than the rate anticipated.

Unemployment The total number of adults (aged 16 years or older) who are willing and able to work and who are actively looking for work but have not found a job.

Union shop A business enterprise that allows the hiring of nonunion members, conditional on their joining the union by some specified date after employment begins.

Unit elasticity of demand A demand relationship in which the quantity demanded changes exactly in proportion to the change in price. Total expenditures are invariant to price changes in the unit-elastic region of the demand curve.

Unit of accounting A measure by which prices are expressed; the common denominator of the price system; a central property of money.

Universal banking Environment in which banks face few or no restrictions on their power to offer a full range of financial services and to own shares of stock in corporations.

Unlimited liability A legal concept whereby the personal assets of the owner of a firm can be seized to pay off the firm's debts.

Util A representative unit by which utility is measured.

Utility The want-satisfying power of a good or service.

Utility analysis The analysis of consumer decision making based on utility maximization.

Value added The dollar value of an industry's sales minus the value of intermediate goods (for example, raw materials and parts) used in production.

Variable costs Costs that vary with the rate of production. They include wages paid to workers and purchases of materials.

Vertical merger The joining of a firm with another to which it sells an output or from which it buys an input.

Voluntary exchange An act of trading, done on a voluntary basis, in which both parties to the trade are subjectively better off after the exchange.

Voluntary import expansion (VIE) An official agreement with another country in which it agrees to import more from the United States.

Voluntary restraint agreement (VRA) An official agreement with another country that "voluntarily" restricts the quantity of its exports to the United States.

Wants What people would buy if their incomes were unlimited.

Wealth The stock of assets owned by a person, household, firm, or nation. For a household, wealth can consist of a house, cars, personal belongings, stocks, bonds, bank accounts, and cash.

World index fund A portfolio of bonds issued in various nations whose yields generally move in offsetting directions, thereby reducing the overall risk of losses.

World Trade Organization (WTO) The successor organization to GATT, it handles all trade disputes among its 135 member nations.

***x* axis** The horizontal axis in a graph.

***y* axis** The vertical axis in a graph.

Zero-sum game A game in which any gains within the group are exactly offset by equal losses by the end of the game.

Index

Note: Page numbers followed by n indicate footnotes.